THE COMPLETE DIRECTORY FOR

Pediatric Disorders

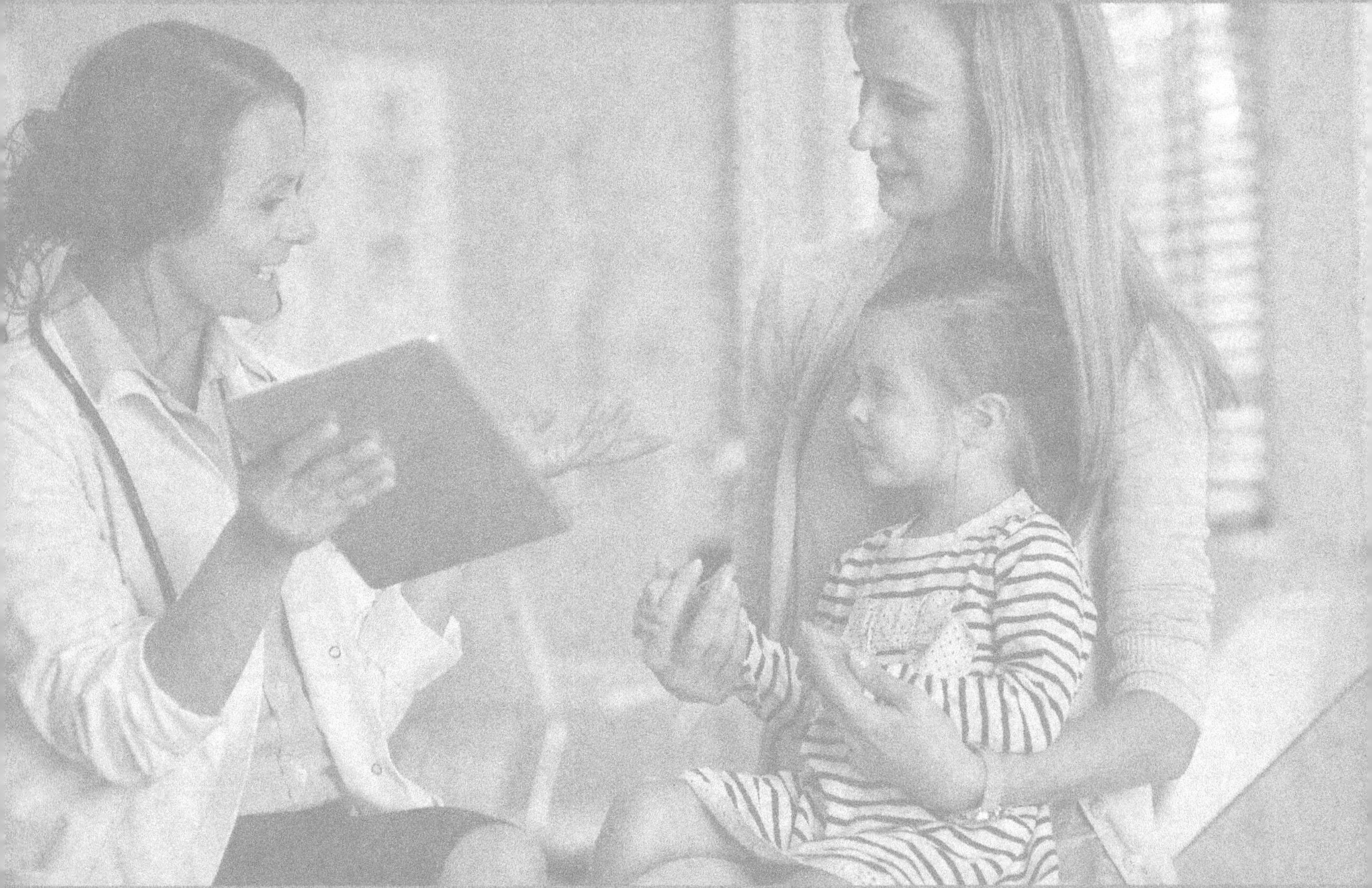

THE COMPLETE DIRECTORY FOR

Pediatric Disorders

2017/18
NINTH
EDITION

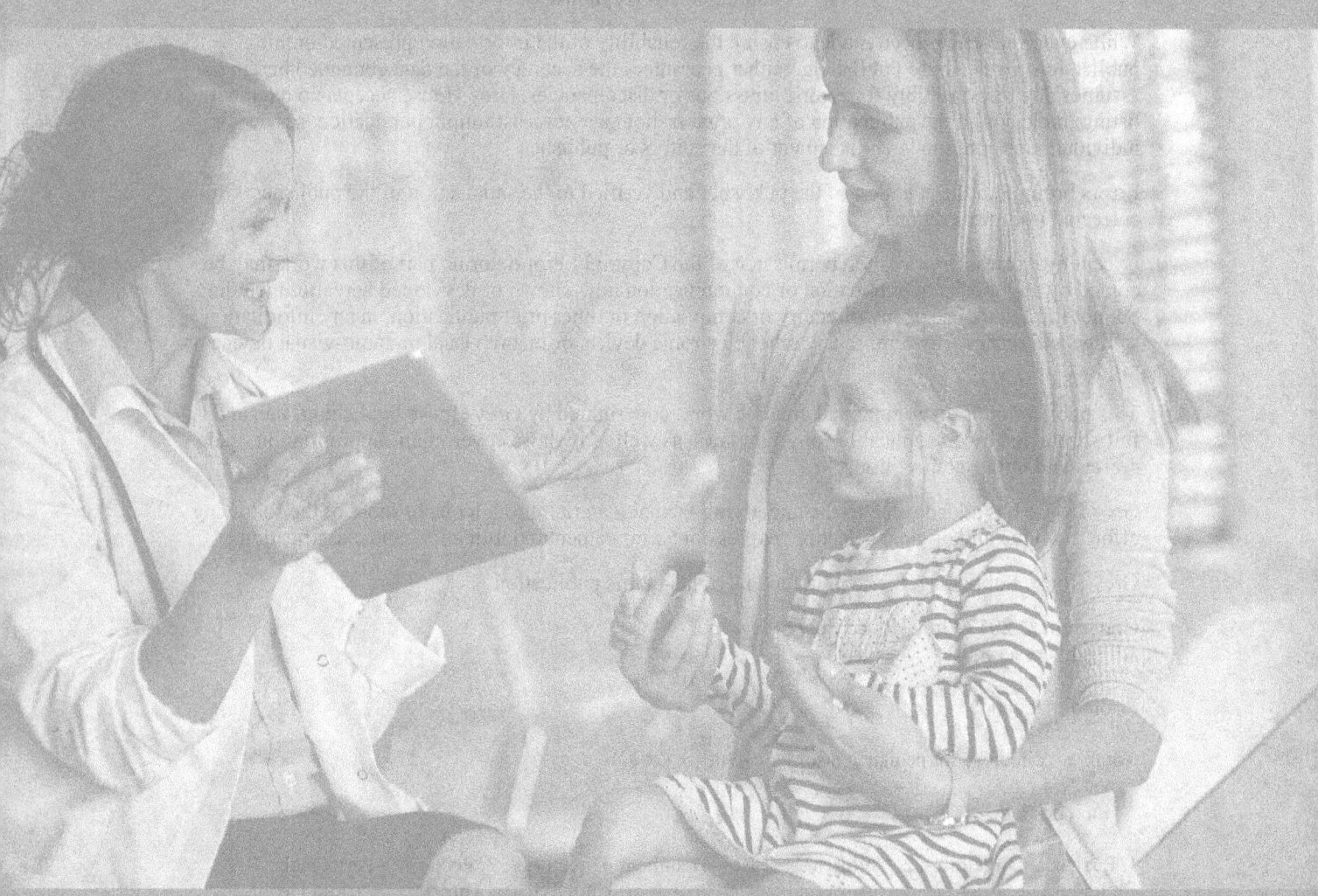

A SEDGWICK PRESS BOOK

GREY HOUSE PUBLISHING

PUBLISHER: Leslie Mackenzie
EDITORIAL DIRECTOR: Laura Mars

PRODUCTION MANAGER & COMPOSITION: Kristen Hayes
MARKETING DIRECTOR: Jessica Moody

A Sedgewick Press Book
Grey House Publishing, Inc.
4919 Route 22
Amenia, NY 12501
518.789.8700
FAX 845.373.6390
www.greyhouse.com
e-mail: books@greyhouse.com

Complete directory for pediatric disorders – 9th ed. (2017)-
    v.; 27.5 cm.
    Includes index.

1. Pediatric–Directories. 2. Children–Diseases–Treatment–Directories. 3. Pediatrics–Periodicals. 4. Children–Diseases–Treatments–Periodicals. 5. Pediatrics–United States–Directory. 6. Child Health Services–United States–Directory. 7. Information Services–United States–Directory. 8. Self-Help Groups–United States–Directory. I. Grey House Publishing, Inc. II. Title: Directory for pediatric disorders.

RJ61.C728
618.92

ISBN: 978-1-68217-360-2
ISSN: 1537-7180

Table of Contents

Introduction xi
Glossaries xiii
Guidelines for Additional Resources xix
Disorders by Biologic System xxv
Modest Increase in Kids' Physical Activity Could Avert Billions in Medical
   and Other Costs xxxiii

Section I: Pediatric Disorders
   Achondroplasia 1
   Acute Gastrointestinal Infections 4
   Acute Lymphoblastic Leukemia 9
   Acute Myeloid Leukemia 16
   Albinism 22
   Alopecia Areata 26
   Alpha-1-Antitrypsin Deficiency 28
   Anencephaly 30
   Aniridia 32
   Ankylosing Spondylitis 34
   Anorectal Malformations 36
   Aortic Stenosis 39
   Apnea of Prematurity 41
   Arnold-Chiari Malformation 43
   Arrhythmias 45
   Arthrogryposis Multiplex Congenita 48
   Asperger Syndrome 50
   Asthma 56
   Ataxia 67
   Atrial Septal Defects 76
   Attention Deficit Hyperactivity Disorder 78
   Autistic Disorder 89
   Bell's Palsy 117
   Biliary Atresia 119
   Bipolar Disorder 121
   Brain Tumors 126
   Bronchopulmonary Dysplasia 144
   Burn Injuries 146
   Celiac Disease 149
   Cerebral Palsy 153
   Charcot-Marie-Tooth Disease 171
   Childhood Dermatomyositis 174
   Childhood Schizophrenia 179
   Chorea 186
   Cleft Lip and Cleft Palate 188
   Clubfoot 192
   Coarctation of the Aorta 194
   Colic 196
   Conduct Disorder 198

Table of Contents

Congenital Adrenal Hyperplasia 203
Congenital Cataracts 205
Congenital Diaphragmatic Hernia 217
Congenital Dysplasia of the Hip 219
Congenital Glaucoma 221
Conjunctivitis 233
Cornelia de Lange Syndrome 235
Craniosynostosis 237
Crohn's Disease 240
Cryptorchidism 249
Cushing's Syndrome 251
Cystic Fibrosis 253
Cytomegalovirus 264
Dental Conditions 266
Depression 272
Diabetes Mellitus 282
DiGeorge Syndrome 289
Down Syndrome 292
Dyslexia 307
Dystonia 311
Eating Disorders 315
Ectodermal Dysplasias 330
Eczema 333
Ehlers-Danlos Syndrome 337
Encephalocele 339
Encopresis 342
Epidermolysis Bullosa 344
Erb's Palsy 346
Erythema Infectiosum 348
Esophageal Atresia 350
Ewing's Sarcoma 352
Familial Dysautonomia 355
Fetal Alcohol Syndrome 357
Fetal Retinoid Syndrome 360
Fragile X Syndrome 362
Galactosemia 365
Gaucher's Disease 367
Growth Hormone Deficiency 369
Guillain-Barre Syndrome 375
HIV Infection 377
Head Injuries 385
Hearing Impairment/Deafness 399
Hemangiomas and Lymphangiomas 447
Hemolytic Disease of the Newborn 450
Hemophilia 452
Hepatitis 469
Hereditary Fructose Intolerance 473
Herpes Simplex 475
Hirschsprung Disease 477

Histiocytosis 480
Hodgkin's Disease. 482
Homocystinuria 485
Hydrocephalus 487
Hypertrophic Cardiomyopathy 494
Hypoplastic Left Heart Syndrome. 496
Hypothyroidism 500
Ichthyosis. 503
Intraventricular Hemorrhage 506
Juvenile Rheumatoid Arthritis. 507
Kawasaki Disease 511
Keloids. 513
Kernicterus. 515
Klinefelter Syndrome. 517
Klippel-Feil Syndrome 519
Lazy Eye 521
Lead Poisoning 525
Learning Disability/Reading Dyslexia 527
Legg-Calve-Perthes Disease 533
Leukodystrophies. 535
Lissencephaly 537
Lyme Disease. 540
Macrocephaly 543
Maple Syrup Urine Disease. 545
Marfan Syndrome 547
McCune-Albright Syndrome 549
Meningitis 551
Mental Retardation 553
Microcephaly 559
Microdontia 561
Migraine Headaches 562
Milk Protein Allergy/Lactose Intolerance 567
Mucolipidoses 569
Mucopolysaccharidoses. 571
Muscular Dystrophies 573
Narcolepsy. 580
Neonatal Herpes Simplex 587
Neonatal Jaundice 589
Nephrotic Syndrome 591
Neurofibromatosis 593
Neuroblastoma. 599
Neutropenia 602
Nightmares. 604
Night Terrors 607
Nocturnal Enuresis 610
Non-Hodgkin's Lymphoma. 612
Noonan Syndrome 616
Nystagmus 618
Obesity. 629

Table of Contents

Obsessive-Compulsive Disorder 635
Omphalocele 641
Oppositional Defiant Disorder 643
Osteogenesis Imperfecta 645
Otitis Media 650
Passive-Aggressive Behavior 652
Patent Ductus Arteriosus 655
Pemphigus 657
Phenylketonuria (PKU) 660
Phobias 662
Photosensitivity 668
Physical & Sexual Abuse 671
PICA 678
Pinworm (Enterobius Vermicularis) 680
Pityriasis Rosea 681
Pneumonia 683
Polydactyly 685
Porphyria 687
Post-Traumatic Stress Disorder 689
Prader-Willi Syndrome 693
Precocious Puberty 700
Prematurity 702
Preventable Childhood Infections 705
Protein C Deficiency 713
Psoriasis 715
Ptosis 720
Pulmonary Hypertension 722
Pulmonary Valve Stenosis 724
Pyloric Stenosis 726
Refraction Disturbances 728
Respiratory Distress Syndrome of the Newborn 739
Respiratory Syncytial Virus Infection 741
Retinitis Pigmentosa 743
Retinoblastoma 745
Retinopathy of Prematurity 749
Rhinitis 751
Sarcoidosis 755
Scleroderma 761
Scoliosis 766
Seizures 772
Sickle Cell Disease 784
Sleep Apnea 789
Sleepwalking 792
Social Anxiety Disorder 794
Speech Impairment 798
Spina Bifida 804
Spinal Muscular Atrophies 814
Strabismus 817
Stuttering 819

Subacute Sclerosing Panencephalitis (SSPE) 822
Sudden Infant Death Syndrome. 824
Syncope 835
Syndactyly 837
Systemic Lupus Erythematosus. 839
Tay-Sachs Disease. 843
Telangiectasia 848
Tetralogy of Fallot. 852
Thalassemias 855
Thrombocytopenias 861
Thumbsucking 863
Tics 865
Tourette Syndrome 868
Toxoplasmosis. 880
Transposition of the Great Arteries 882
Trisomy 18 Syndrome 884
Trisomy 13 Syndrome 886
Tuberculosis. 888
Tuberous Sclerosis. 891
Turner Syndrome. 894
Ulcerative Colitis. 900
Urticaria. 904
Ventricular Septal Defects. 906
Violence by Children & Teenagers 907
Williams Syndrome. 917
Wilms Tumor. 919
Wilson Disease 922

Section II: General Resources
Government Agencies 925
National Associations and Support Groups. 928
State Agencies & Support Groups. 948
Libraries & Resource Centers 980
Research Centers 990
Conferences 991
Audio/Video 993
Web Sites. 994
Book Publishers. 999
Magazines 999
Journals 999
Newsletters 999
Pamphlets. 1000
Camps 1002
Grant a Wish Foundations 1012

Section III: The Human Body
Cardiovascular System 1015
Cells. 1017
Dermatologic System. 1021
Digestive System. 1023

Table of Contents

Endocrine System 1026
Growth and Development 1029
Hematologic System 1032
Immune System 1034
Musculoskeletal System 1036
Nervous System 1037
Reproductive System 1041
Respiratory System 1043
Sensory Organs 1045
Urologic System 1047

Section IV: Indexes
Entry Index 1049
Geographic Index 1091
Disorder & Related Term Index 1109

Introduction

This ninth edition of *The Complete Directory for Pediatric Disorders* provides current, understandable medical information, resources and support services for 213 pediatric disorders. A repeat winner of the National Health Information Awards "Honoring the Nation's Best Consumer Health Information Programs and Materials," this reference work provides vital information for afflicted children and their support network, including family, friends, and medical professionals.

Praise for previous editions:

> *"The strength of this source is in the information referral portion for each entry: the wide range of resources and organizations presented that can assist with additional information and support."*
>
> —ARBA

> *"...thousands of resources are provided covering a diverse range of services... All entries offer resource descriptions, as well as full contact information. Three indexes assist readers in locating specific information..."*
>
> —Against the Grain

> *"...It will be particularly useful for libraries serving parents of young children and youth, and for medical professionals working in the pediatrics field...the information is comprehensive and current."*
>
> —Choice

The disorders and issues covered in this directory have been determined to be most prevalent in the pediatric population, ages 0-18. They include both physical and mental conditions, and range from cancer to nightmares.

The front matter for *The Complete Directory for Pediatric Disorders* includes:
- NEW article: "Modest Increase in Kids' Physical Activity Could Avert Billions in Medical and Other Costs"
- Two glossaries. The first is a guide to medical terminology that provides important navigational tips and more than 200 commonly used medical prefixes, roots and suffixes to help readers decipher terms they may encounter in the disorder descriptions or in other resources they are using. The second glossary includes medical acronyms, especially as they relate to vaccines.
- Guidelines for Obtaining Additional Information and Research. These guidelines assist parents and caregivers who are interested in obtaining more information on such diverse topics as physicians who specialize in certain pediatric disorders, accredited hospitals, approved drugs or medical devices for certain pediatric conditions, or current clinical trials that are investigating possible new therapies for particular diseases.
- A valuable list of Disorders by Biologic System.

This reference work includes 8,843 listings. Each listing has updated contact data – address, phone, fax, web site, e-mail – and helpful descriptions. You will find 6,344 fax numbers, 6,035 e-mail addresses, 7,910 web sites and 14,625 key executives.

This Directory is a one-stop resource, enabling professionals and the families they serve to obtain immediate, important information from one comprehensive source. It is organized in the following six sections:

Section I – Disorders

This section includes 213 major disorder chapters that comprise more than 266 specific disorders, diseases, or conditions. They are arranged in alphabetical order, from Achondroplasia to Wilson Disease. Each chapter begins with an extensive description, written in understandable language. The descriptions in this eighth edition have been reviewed by medical professionals to include the most up-to-date methods of diagnoses and treatment. Each description includes: Disorder name and synonyms; Primary symptoms; Physical findings; Related Disorders; Cause: Body system affected; Standard treatment.

Following each description are *disorder-specific resources*, including Associations, Federal and State Agencies, Support Groups, Libraries, Resource Centers, Research Centers, Web sites, Media Resources and Camps. The more prevalent a disorder is, the more resources there are available.

The Complete Directory for Pediatric Disorders also includes care centers, medical organizations, and advocacy groups that offer extended information on a great variety of conditions. These combined resources offer the most comprehensive coverage available of the most prevalent pediatric disorders being diagnosed in pediatrician's offices around the country.

Section II – General Resources

This section includes 1,014 resources, including Government Agencies, National Associations, State Agencies, Support Groups, Newsletters, Books, Magazines, Camps and Wish Foundations. These may not be limited to a specific disorder, but offer information and support for categories of disorders.

Users will find resources on not only physical pediatric disorders, but also on mental and emotional conditions that affect our younger population. There are also resources that deal with multi-disorder conditions.

Section III – The Human Body

This educational element is comprised of 14 detailed descriptions of body systems or medical categories. This section is designed to provide a comprehensive overview of the human body, enabling the user to broaden his or her understanding of how a particular disorder affects a specific body system(s) and further, how it may relate to the body as a whole. It includes twelve specific body systems, from Cardiovascular to Urologic, plus two additional chapters: Human Cells and Child Growth & Development.

Section IV – Indexes

The Complete Directory for Pediatric Disorders contains three indexes to help readers access the information from several places:

- **Entry Index** is an alphabetical listing of all entry names.
- **Geographic Index** groups listings by state.
- **Disorder & Related Term Index** is an alphabetical list of pediatric disorders, condition names, synonyms, and related disorders.

The Complete Directory for Pediatric Disorders is available for subscription online at http://gold.greyhouse.com, for even faster, easier access to this vast array of information. With a subscription, users can search by disorder, keyword, geographic area, bodily system, and much more. Visit the site or call (800) 562-2139 to set up a free trial of the Online Database.

Glossary
A Concise Guide to Medical Terminology

This Guide is designed to help the reader decipher some unfamiliar terms used in the disorder descriptions. It is helpful to divide medical terms into their basic elements: prefix, root, and suffix. Following these examples are 249 commonly used medical prefixes, roots, and suffixes - over a dozen more than last edition.

Example 1: The medical term *microcephaly* is a combination of "micr(o)," meaning small, and "cephal(o)," which means head. Therefore, microcephaly denotes an abnormally small head. In contrast, "macr(o)" means large. Thus, *macrocephaly* indicates an unusually large head.

Example 2: The word *polydactyly* includes "poly," meaning much or many, and "dactyl," which refers to fingers or toes. Thus, the medical term *polydactyly* means the presence of extra fingers or toes. Accordingly, because "brachy" means short, the word *brachydactyly* indicates abnormally short fingers or toes.

Example 3: The term *myositis* is a combination of "my(o)," which denotes muscle, and "itis," meaning inflammation. Therefore, *myositis* means muscle inflammation. When "cardi(o)," meaning heart, is added, forming the term *myocarditis,* the meaning becomes inflammation of heart muscle.

Medical Prefixes, Roots, and Suffixes

A	absence of, without	cent.	one hundred
Ab	away from	centr(o)	center
Acou	hear	cephal(o)	head
aden(o)	gland	cerebr(o)	brain
-algia	pain	cervic	neck
all(o)	other, different	chole.	bile
andr(o)	man	chondr(o)	cartilage
angi(o)	vessel	circum	around
ankyl(o)	bent, crooked	-coele	body/organ cavity
ante	before	contra	against, counter
anti	against, counter	cost(o)	rib
arteri(o)	artery	crani(o)	skull
arthr(o)	joint	cry(o)	cold
audio	hearing, sound	crypt(o)	conceal, hide
auri	ear	cyan	blue
aut(o)	self	cyst(o)	bladder
bacteri(o)	bacteria	cyt(o)	cell
bio	life	de	away from, down
blast(o)	bud, early embryonic budding	dent(o)	tooth
-blast	formative cell, germinal layer	dermat(o)	skin
blephar(o)	eyelid	di	two
brachi(o)	arm	dia	apart, through
brachy	short	digit	finger or toe
brady	slow	dipl(o)	double
bronch(o)	bronchi	dors(o)	back
bucc(o)	cheek	dys	abnormal, bad
carcin(o)	cancer	ect(o)	outside, out of place
cardi(o)	heart	-emia	blood
-cele	hernia, protrusion, tumor	en	in, on

end(o)	inside, within	lien(o)	spleen
enter(o)	intestine	lingu(o)	tongue
epi	above, upon	lip(o)	fat
erythr(o)	red	lith(o)	stone
eso	inside, within	lymph(o)	water
esthesi(o)	feel, perceive	macr(o)	large
eu	normal, well	mal	abnormal, bad
ex	away from, outside	malac(o)	soft
extra	beyond, in addition, outside of	mamm(o)	breast
flav(o)	yellow	mast(o)	breast
galact(o)	milk	medi	middle
gastr(o)	stomach	mega	great, large
gen(o)	gene or reproduction	megal(o)	great, large
gloss(o)	tongue	melan(o)	black
glyc(o)	sweet	mening(o)	membrane
gnath(o)	jaw	mes(o)	middle
gram	draw, record, write	meta	after, beyond
graph(o)	record, write	metr(o)	uterus
gynec(o)	woman	micr(o)	small
hemat(o)	blood	mill(i)	one thousand
hemi	half	mon(o)	only, single, sole
hepat(o)	liver	morph(o)	form, shape, structure
hex	six	myel(o)	marrow
hidr(o)	sweat	my(o)	muscle
hist(o)	tissue	myx(o)	mucus
hom(o)	common, same	narc(o)	stupor
hydr(o)	water	nas(o)	nose
hyper	above, beyond, excessive	necr(o)	corpse, death
hypn(o)	sleep	neo	new
hyp(o)	below, deficient, low	nephr(o)	kidney
hyster(o)	uterus	neur(o)	nerve
iatr(o)	physician	noci	pain
idi(o)	distinct, separate	noso	disease
ili(o)	intestines	ocul(o)	eye
inter	among, between	odont(o)	tooth
intra	inside, within	-odyn(o)	distress, pain
ischi(o)	hip	olig(o)	deficient, few, little
-itis	inflammation	-oma neoplasm	tumor
kary(o)	nucleus	omphal(o)	navel
kilo	one thousand	onc(o)	mass, tumor
kinet(o)	move	onych(o)	nail
labio	lips	oo	egg
lact(o)	milk	ophthalm(o)	eye
lapar(o)	flank, loin	orchi(o)	testicle
laryng(o)	larynx	oro	mouth
latero	side	-osis	process, disease from
leuc(o)	white	osse(o)	bone
leuk(o)	white	oste(o)	bone

ot(o)	ear	rheo	flow
ovari(o)	ovary	rhin(o)	nose
oxy	sharp	sangui	blood
pachy	thick	sarc(o)	flesh
pan	whole, all	scler(o)	hard
para	beside, beyond, resembling	-scope	instrument for examining
path(o)	disease	semi	half
ped(o)	child	sial(o)	saliva
pen	around	somat(o)	body
penia	abnormal reduction, deficiency	somn(i)	sleep
pent(a)	five	spasm(o)	spasm
per	through	spermat(o)	seed
phag(o)	consume, eat	splen(o)	spleen
pharmaco	drug, medicine	spondyl(o)	vertebra
pharyng(o)	throat	spor(o)	spore
phleb(o)	vein	steat(o)	fat
phon(o)	sound	sten(o)	compressed, narrow
phot(o)	light	stomat(o)	mouth, opening
physi(o)	natural, physical	sub	below, near, under
pil(o)	hair	super	above, beyond, excessive
-plasia	development, formation	syn	together, with
platy	broad, flat	tachy	fast, rapid
pleur(o)	rib, side	tel(o)	end
-pnea	breathing	tetra	four
pneumat(o)	air, breathing	therm(o)	heat
pneum(o)	air, breath, lung	thorac(o)	chest
pod(o)	foot	thromb(o)	clot
poly	many, much	-tome	instrument for cutting
post	after, behind	tox(o)	poison
pre	before, in front of	trans	through, across
pro	before, in front of	traumat(o)	wound
proct(o)	rectum	tri	three
pseud(o)	false	trich(o)	hair
psych(o)	mind	troph(o)	food, nourishment
pulmon(o)	lung	-uria	urine
pyel(o)	pelvis	vas(o)	vessel
pyr(o)	fire, heat	vertebr(o)	vertebrae
quadri	four	vesic(o)	bladder or blister
rachi(o)	spine	xanth(o)	yellow
radio	radiation	xen(o)	foreign, different
re	again, back	xer(o)	dry
ren(o)	kidneys	zyg(o)	junction, union
retr(o)	backward, behind		

GLOSSARY OF ACRONYMS

Note: Compound acronyms denote vaccine combinations.
'DTPHibHepIPV', for example, denotes DTP, Hib, HepB and IPV vaccines combined.

AMC	advanced market commitment
aP	acellular pertussis vaccine
BCG	bacille Calmette-Guérin (vaccine against tuberculosis)
CBAW	childbearing-aged women; refers to ages 15-45 unless otherwise noted
Dip	diphtheria toxoid vaccine
DT	diphtheria toxoid
DTaP	diphtheria and tetanus toxoid with acellular pertussis vaccine
DTP	diphtheria and tetanus toxoid with pertussis vaccine
DTP1	first dose of diphtheria and tetanus toxoid with pertussis vaccine
DTP3	third dose of diphtheria and tetanus toxoid with pertussis vaccine
DTwP	diphtheria and tetanus toxoid with whole-cell pertussis vaccine
EPI	Expanded Programme on Immunization
GAVI	Global Alliance for Vaccines and Immunisation
GNI	gross national income (US)
H1N1	monovalent vaccine against the 2009 influenza A (H1N1) virus
HepA	hepatitis A vaccine
HepB	hepatitis B vaccine
HepB3	third dose of hepatitis B vaccine
HFRS	hemorrhagic fever with renal syndrome (hantavirus) vaccine
Hib	Haemophilus infl uenzae type b vaccine
Hib3	third dose of Haemophilus influenzae type b vaccine
HPV	human papilloma virus vaccine
IPV	inactivated polio vaccine
JE	Japanese encephalitis
MCV	measles-containing vaccine
MCV2	second dose of measles-containing vaccine
MenA	meningococcal A vaccine; this monovalent vaccine protects against meningitis serogroup A

MenAC	meningococcal AC vaccine; this bivalent vaccine protects against meningitis serogroups A and C
MenACW	meningococcal ACWY vaccine; this quadrivalent vaccine protects against meningitis serogroups A, C and W-135
MenACWY	meningococcal ACWY vaccine; this quadrivalent vaccine protects against meningitis serogroups A, C, Y and W-135
MenBC	meningococcal BC vaccine; this bivalent vaccine protects against meningitis serogroups B and C
MenC	meningococcal C vaccine; this monovalent vaccine protects against meningitis serogroup C
MenC_conj	meningococcal C conjugate vaccine
MM	measles and mumps vaccine
MMR	measles-mumps-rubella vaccine
MMRV	measles-mumps-rubella-varicella vaccine
MR	measles and rubella vaccine
OPV	oral polio vaccine
PAB	protected at birth against tetanus
Pneumo_conj	pneumococcal conjugate vaccine
Pneumo_ps	pneumococcal polisaccharide vaccine
Pol3	third dose of poliomyelitis vaccine
PPP	purchasing power parity
Pw	whole-cell pertussis vaccine
TBE	tick-borne encephalitis vaccine
TBD	to be determined
Td	tetanus toxoid with reduced amount of diphtheria toxoid
Tdap	tetanus toxoid vaccine (full dose) with acellular pertussis vaccine (reduced dose)
TT	tetanus toxoid

Source: http://www.unicef.org and www.who.int

Guidelines for Obtaining Additional Information and Resources

Many parents and caregivers are interested in obtaining information regarding *physicians* who specialize in certain pediatric disorders, accredited *hospitals, approved drugs or medical devices* for certain pediatric conditions, or current *clinical trials* that are investigating possible new therapies for particular diseases. In addition, some individuals may wish to have access to medical journal articles and other medical literature that may be available on their child's disorder, disease, or condition. Following are several tips that may be shared with parents and caregivers in their efforts to obtain such information and resources.

Disease-Specific Resources: Many of the disease-specific resources in this *Directory* maintain listings of physicians who are experts in a particular pediatric disorder. They may also offer information on accredited hospitals with appropriate specialty departments. In addition, many may provide information on standard therapies for certain pediatric conditions and ongoing clinical trials that are investigating possible new therapies. Some of these organizations, such as certain national voluntary health associations (NVHAs) or support groups, function as patient registries, working closely with expert physicians, researchers, and university medical centers specializing in specific pediatric disorders.

Online "Physician Finder" Services: Several professional medical associations provide searchable databases on the Internet as a public service for individuals who wish to obtain information on physicians.

Example: The *American Medical Association (AMA) Physician Select* database provides information on licensed physicians in the United States, including credential data that has been verified by medical schools, residency training programs, certifying and licensing boards, and accrediting agencies. AMA Physician Select enables online visitors to search for physicians by name, medical specialty, or geographic location. This online service is located at http://www.webapps.ama-assn.org/doctorfinder.

Example: The *American Board of Medical Specialties (ABMS) Public Education Program* offers an online physician locator and information service. This service, which lists all physicians certified by ABMS Member Boards, allows online visitors to verify board certification status, specialty, and location of physicians who are certified by one or more of the ABMS Member Boards. The ABMS also provides the *Certified/Doctor Locator Service,* which lists physicians certified by ABMS Member Boards who have subscribed to the service. Such listings include board certification(s), address, telephone number, and hospital affiliation(s). These online services may be accessed at www.abms.org.

Example: The U.S. federal government has an online service known as *healthfinder®* that serves as a Web portal or directory for those who are interested in locating current, high quality health information and resources on the Internet. The site is located at www.healthfinder.gov.

Hospital Accreditation: Individuals who are interested in learning about a particular medical facility's accreditation status may consider contacting the *Joint Commission,* which is the the United States' leading health care quality evaluator and accredits approximately 15,000 health care facilities, organizations, and programs. Accreditation is recognized as a *"Gold Seal of Approval"* indicating that the hospital meets certain standards of performance and is committed to meeting state-of-the-art performance expectations. The Joint Commission offers an online service known as *Quality Check* that enables online visitors to obtain information about an organization's accreditation, such as how it was rated during its most recent quality report. This service is located at www.qualitycheck.org. Callers may also receive information concerning a hospital's accreditation status by calling the Joint Commission, at (630) 792-5800 or visiting www.jointcommission.org.

Hospital Public Information Lines and Web Sites: Many hospitals are creating and strongly promoting special public information lines. Such help lines are often publicized within local or regional newspapers and in the introductory sections of local phone books. In addition, many hospitals are creating Web sites that: offer information on their services and programs; link to sites offered by different departments or facilities; discuss ongoing research; provide searchable physician directories; publish newsletters, various reports, press releases, and other materials; and offer a variety of additional information. These Web sites may be located by visiting various search engines and using the name of the facility as a search term. (For more information, see *Search Engines* below.)

Academic Hospitals: If children have been diagnosed with a chronic, difficult-to-treat, or relatively uncommon disorder or if they remain undiagnosed after visits to several primary care or specialist pediatricians, parents or other caregivers may wish to consider taking their children to a major academic medical center. Generally, such teaching hospitals use state-of-the-art testing techniques, have comprehensive evaluation centers, and follow multidisciplinary approaches to diagnosis and treatment. In addition, such centers are often affiliated with medical schools where clinical research is conducted.

Food and Drug Administration: Individuals who are interested in learning more about approved drug therapies or medical devices for certain pediatric disorders may wish to contact the *U. S. Food and Drug Administration (FDA)*. The FDA is the U.S. agency that enforces federal regulations to prevent the sale and distribution of dangerous or impure substances, such as unsafe foods, impure cosmetics, or unsafe or ineffective drugs or medical devices. For example, according to the FDA Modernization Act of 1997, one of the agency's primary objectives is "to promote the public health by promptly and efficiently reviewing clinical research and taking appropriate action on the marketing of regulated products in a timely manner." The agency is a branch of the U.S. Department of Health and Human Services. The FDA's Web site provides: FAQs (Frequently Asked Questions) areas; Consumer Drug Information Sheets; information on new and generic drug approvals, medical device product approvals, and drug labeling changes; health advisories; and access to MedWatch, the FDA's *Safety Information and Adverse Event Reporting Program*. MedWatch enables consumers and health care professionals to report adverse reactions to approved medical products directly to the FDA and/or the manufacturers. The primary purpose of MedWatch is to ensure the rapid identification of potential health hazards associated with approved medical products and the prompt communication of safety information to the health care and medical communities. The FDA's Web site is located at www.fda.gov/medwatch. The agency's address follows:

FDA
10903 New Hampshire Ave.
Silver Spring, MD 20993-0002
Toll-free: (888) INFO-FDA or (888) 463-6332

Clinical Research: A clinical protocol is a scientific study that evaluates the safety or effectiveness (efficacy) of a particular drug therapy or medical device in humans. Clinical studies enable researchers and physicians to determine new and more effective ways to prevent, diagnose, manage, and treat disease. Medications and treatments that are found to be safe and effective during laboratory and animal testing must then prove safe and effective in humans before they are approved for use by the general public. Participation in clinical studies may only occur if individuals volunteer and are fully informed and understanding of both the potential benefits and risks of such participation ("informed consent"). Participants may voluntarily leave a clinical study at any time.
Research on new drugs, which are known as *investigational new drug applications* or *INDS,* is conducted in three phases:

Phase I Study - The main objective of a Phase I study is to establish the *safety* of the investigational new drug. Such studies:
• may take several months

• typically involve a relatively small number of participants who are healthy volunteers

• are designed to evaluate the INDs biologic activities in the human body (e.g., absorption, metabolism, etc.) and its potential side effects as drug dosages are raised

Phase II Study - The purpose of a Phase II study is to establish the *safety and efficacy* of the investigational new drug in treating a specific disease. Such studies:

• may take from several months to a few years

• may include a relatively small number or up to several hundred patients

• usually involve randomized, double-blind trials. During such studies, one group of participants receives the drug (experimental group) and the other group is given a harmless, unmedicated substance (placebo) or a standard, well-established therapy (control group). The information concerning which patients are included in which group is hidden from both the patients and the researchers.

Phase III Study - The purpose of a Phase III study is to evaluate the overall *safety, efficacy, possible adverse effects, and benefits* of the investigational new drug in a large number of patients and to compare such therapy with the use of well-established treatments or with an untreated disease course. Such studies:

• may last for several years

• may involve hundreds or thousands of patients

• may include research teams from multiple national or international clinical centers

• typically involve randomized, double-blind trials

If an investigational new drug application successfully completes Phase III studies, the drug's sponsor may request FDA approval for marketing to the public, which is known as a *New Drug Approval* (NDA). In some cases, additional clinical research may be conducted:

Phase IV Study – The purpose of a Phase IV study may be to:
• monitor the drug's long-term efficacy

• compare the drug with other medications that have been available for longer periods

As mentioned above, disease-specific organizations and registries, support groups, and online services may serve as essential sources of information concerning clinical studies for a particular disease. There are also several additional, more general resources that promote and provide information on clinical trials:

Example: The *Warren Grant Magnuson Clinical Center,* which is part of the National Institutes of Health (NIH), is a federally funded biomedical research hospital. The Clinical Center was designed to support studies conducted by the NIH. Only individuals with conditions or disorders under NIH investigation are admitted for treatment, and all patients must be referred by their physicians. The Clinical Center's Web site includes a clinical research database that enables online visitors to search for current research studies by certain predefined parameters, such as primary disease category, or specific diagnosis, symptom, sign, or other keywords. The Clinical Center's Web site is located at www.cc.nih.gov and its Protocol Database may be accessed at http://clinicalstudies.info.nih.gov. The Clinical Center's address follows:

Department of Health and Human Services
Public Health Service
National Institutes of Health (NIH)
Warren G. Magnuson Clinical Center
Patient Recruitment and Referral Center
9000 Rockville Pike
Bethesda, MD 20892
Toll-free: (800) 411-1222

E-mail: prpl@mail.cc.nih.gov

Example: *CenterWatch, Inc.* provides a *Clinical Trials Listing Service*™ on its Web site for patients and research professionals. The site provides listings of over 7 ,000 national and international clinical trials that are searchable by geographic region and therapeutic area. Interested individuals may also sign up for CenterWatch's confidential *Patient Notification Service,* which provides notification via e-mail of future clinical trial postings in a certain therapeutic area. CenterWatch's Clinical Trials Service also provides: a listing of NIH-funded clinical research programs that are currently being conducted at the NIH's Warren Grant Magnuson Clinical Center; a general explanation of clinical trials, profiles of clinical research centers; listings of medications recently approved by the FDA; and linkage to health-related sites for patients and patient advocates. The Clinical Trials Listing Service™ is located at www.centerwatch.com. CenterWatch's address follows:

CenterWatch, Inc.
100 North Washington St., Ste. 301
Boston, MA 02114
Phone: (617) 948-5100
Fax: (617) 948-5101
Toll-Free: 866-219-3440
E-Mail: customerservice@centerwatch.com

Example: The *National Cancer Institute (NCI)* offers an online service known as *CancerNet*™ that provides information for patients and family members, health professionals, and researchers. The site offers: information on current clinical trials; summaries on cancer prevention, screening, treatment, and supportive care; cancer fact sheets; and linkage to the *Physician Data Query* or *PDQ® Cancer Information Service,* the NCI's cancer database. PDQ contains a registry of open and closed cancer clinical trials as well as directories of organizations, physicians, and genetic counselors who provide cancer care. CancerNet™ also provides access to *cancerTrials,* a clinical trials information center, and *CANCERLIT®,* a bibliographic database. CancerNet™ is located at http://cancer.gov. The NCI also offers a Cancer Information Service (CIS) for callers Monday through Friday from 9 a.m. to 4:30 p.m., Eastern Standard Time. The CIS may be reached at (800) 422-6237. Individuals with hearing impairment who have TTY equipment may call (800) 332-8615.

Example: *OncoLink* is an online resource on the Internet that is affiliated with the University of Pennsylvania Medical Center and the University of Pennsylvania Cancer Center. The site provides: information on cancer clinical trials; symptom management; personal experiences and psychosocial support; cancer causes, prevention, and screening; FAQs (frequently asked questions); financial issues for cancer patients; and additional topics. The site is located at www.oncolink.upenn.edu.

Search Engines. If individuals are interested in locating a particular organization's Web site but do not have its address or wish to determine what online services may be available in a certain subject area, Internet search engines are an essential resource. Search engines enable online visitors to conduct general or targeted searches for information within their areas of interest and appropriate to their needs. In addition to searching for and providing direct linkage to certain Web sites, many search engines enable users to search for e-mail discussion groups (listservs), UseNet newsgroups, FAQs (frequently asked questions), or other tools. Following is a sample listing of some of the search engines available on the Web:

Altavista: www.altavista.com
Dogpile: www.dogpile.com
Excite: www.excite.com
HotBot: www.hotbot.com
Lycos: www.lycos.com
Metacrawler: www.metacrawler.com
Snap.com: www.snap.com

Yahoo: www.yahoo.com

General Medical and Professional Association Sites: Some individuals may be interested in visiting medical sites that offer general information on disease and health issues. In addition, many professional medical associations and societies have Web sites that provide access to patient and professional information, press releases, journals, clinical updates, and other areas that may be helpful to those interested in pediatric disorder topics. Following is a brief listing of such sites:

American Academy of Family Physicians: www.aafp.org
American Academy of Pediatrics: www.aap.org
American Medical Association: www.ama-assn.org
MyOptumHealth: www.myoptumhealth.com
Johns Hopkins Health Information: www.hopkinshospital.org/health_info
Mayo Clinic Health Information: www.mayoclinic.com
Medical Matrix: www.medmatrix.org/reg/login.asp
Medscape: www.medscape.com
US Pharmacopeia (information on medications): www.usp.org

Medical Journal Articles. Individuals who are interested in accessing abstracts summarizing medical journal articles may visit the National Library of Medicine's (NLM's) *PubMed.* The PubMed search service provides free access to the approximately 17 million medical journal citations within NLM's *MEDLINE.* MEDLINE is essentially the online version of *Index Medicus,* a monthly subject/author guide to articles in thousands of medical journals. Online visitors to PubMed may conduct searches for medical journal citations and abstracts by journal title and date, author, and topic. In addition to providing access to selected journal abstracts, PubMed offers links to participating online journals and enables registered users to order full-text articles for a fee. (If individuals are interested in accessing other medical journal sites, such online journals may often be located by using various search engines.) PubMed may be accessed at www.pubmed.gov. In addition, several general medical sites provide access to PubMed and enable users to order full-text journal articles for a fee.

Online Mendelian Inheritance in Man (OMIM). Individuals who wish to access comprehensive and timely medical information on genetic disorders may be interested in visiting OMIM™ or *Online Mendelian Inheritance in Man,* a database of genetic disorders and human genes. This searchable database, which is written and edited by Dr. Victor A. McKusick and colleagues at Johns Hopkins University and other locations, was developed for the Web by the National Center for Biotechnology Information (NCBI). OMIM™ contains entries on genetic diseases, clinical synopses, links to relevant MEDLINE citations, and more. OMIM™ is located at www.ncbi.nlm.nih.gov/omim/.

Disorders by Biologic System Affected

Cardiovascular Disorders; see also *Cardiovascular System*, page 1015.
Aortic Stenosis
Arrhythmias
Atrial Septal Defects
Coarctation of the Aorta
Hypertrophic Cardiomyopathy
Hypoplastic Left Heart Syndrome (HLHS)
Kawasaki Disease
Marfan Syndrome
Noonan's Syndrome
Patent Ductus Arteriosus
Pulmonary Hypertension
Pulmonary Valve Stenosis
Syncope
Tetralogy of Fallot
Transposition of the Great Arteries
Ventricular Septal Defects
Williams Syndrome

Connective Tissue Disorders; see also *Cells*, page 1017.
Childhood Dermatomyositis
Ehlers-Danlos Syndrome
Sarcoidosis
Scleroderma

Dental Disorders; see also *Digestive System*, page 1023.
Dental Conditions
Ectodermal Dysplasia
Microdontia

Dermatologic Disorders; see also *Dermatologic System*, page 1021.
Albinism
Alopecia Areata
Burn Injuries
Childhood Dermatomyositis
Cleft Life and Cleft Palate
Ectodermal Dysplasia
Eczema
Epidermolysis Bullosa
Hemangiomas and Lymphangiomas
Icthyosis
Keloids
Neurofibromatosis
Pemphigus
Photosensitivity
Pityriasis Rosea
Tuberous Sclerosis
Psoriasis

Telangiectasia
Urticaria

Developmental, Behavioral and Psychiatric Disorders; see also *Growth and Development*, page 1029.
Asperger Syndrome
Attention Deficit Hyperactivity Disorder
Autistic Disorder
Bipolar Disorder
Childhood Schizophrenia
Conduct Disorder
Depression
Eating Disorders
Encopresis
Lead Poisoning
Learning Disability, Reading Disability Dyslexia
Mental Retardation
Migraine Headaches
Nightmares
Night Terrors
Nocturnal Enuresis
Obesity
Obsessive-Compulsive Disorder
Oppositional Defiant Behavior
Passive-Aggressive Behavior
Phobias
Physical and Sexual Abuse
PICA
Post-Traumatic Stress Disorder
Sleepwalking
Stuttering
Thumbsucking
Violence by Children & Teenagers

Endocrinologic Disorders; see also *Endocrine System*, page 1026.
Congenital Adrenal Hyperplasia
Cushing's Syndrome
Diabetes Mellitus
Growth Hormone Deficiency
Hypothyroidism
McCune-Albright Syndrome
Obesity
Prader-Willi Syndrome
Precocious Puberty

Gastrointestinal Disorders; see also *Digestive System*, page 1023.
Acute Gastrointestinal Infections
Alpha-1-Antitrypsin Deficiency
Anorectal Malformations
Biliary Atresia

Celiac Disease
Colic
Congenital Diaphragmatic Hernia
Crohn's Disease
Encopresis
Esophageal Atresia
Galactosemia
Hepatitis
Hirschsprung Disease
Milk Protein Allergy and Lactose Intolerance
Omphalocele
Pyloric Stenosis
Ulcerative Colitis
Wilson's Disease

Genetic/Chromosomal/Syndrome/Metabolic Disorders; see also *Growth and Development*, page 1029.
Achondroplasia
Albinism
Alpha-1-Antitrypsin Deficiency
Asperger Syndrome
Congenital Cataracts
Cornelia de Lange Syndrome
DiGeorge Syndrome
Down Syndrome
Familial Dysautonomia
Fetal Alcohol Syndrome
Fragile X Syndrome
Galactosemia
Gaucher's Disease
Hereditary Fructose Intolerance
Homocystinuria
Klinefelter Syndrome
Klipple-Feil Syndrome
Leukodystrophies
Maple Syrup Urine Disease
Marfan Syndrome
McCune-Albright Syndrome
Mucolipidoses
Mucopolysaccharidoses
Noonan's Syndrome
Osteogenesis Imperfecta
Phenylketonuria
Polydactyly
Prader-Willi Syndrome
Tay-Sachs Disease
Trisomy 18 Syndrome
Trisomy 13 Syndrome
Turner Syndrome
Williams Syndrome

Hematologic and Oncologic Disorders; see also *Hematologic System*, page 1032.

Acute Lymphoblastic Leukemia
Acute Myeloid Leukemia
Ewing's Sarcoma
Hemolytic Disease of the Newborn
Hemophilia
Histiocytosis
Hodgkins Disease
Neuroblastoma
Neutropenia
Non-Hodgkins Lymphoma
Porphyria
Protein C Deficiency
Retinoblastoma
Sickle Cell Disease
Thalasemias
Thrombocytopenias
Wilm's Tumor

Immunologic and Rheumatologic Disorders; see also *Immune System*, page 1034.

Alopecia Areata
DiGeorge Syndrome
HIV Infection
Juvenile Rheumatoid Arthritis
Kawasaki Disease
Subacute Sclerosing Panencephalitis (SSPE)
Systemic Lupus Erythematosus

Infectious Diseases; see also *Immune System*, page 1034.

Acute Gastrointestinal Infections
Conjunctivitis
Cytomegalovirus
Erythema Infectiosum
HIV Infection
Hepatitis
Herpes Simplex
Lyme Disease
Meningitis
Neonatal Herpes Simplex
Otitis Media
Pinworm
Pityriasis Rosea
Pneumonia
Preventable Childhood Infections
Respiratory Syncytial Virus
Toxoplasmosis
Tuberculosis

Neonatal and Infant Disorders; see also *Growth and Development*, page 1029.
Apnea of Prematurity
Bronchopulmonary Dysplasia
Colic
Congenital Dysplasia of the Hip
Hemolytic Disease of the Newborn
Interventricular Hemorrhage
Kernicterus
Neonatal Herpes Simplex
Neonatal Jaundice
Omphalocele
Prematurity
Respiratory Distress Syndrome of the Newborn
Retinopathy of Prematurity
Sudden Infant Death Syndrome

Neurologic Disorders; see also *Nervous System*, page 1037.
Anencephaly
Arnold-Chiari Malformation
Asperger Syndrome
Ataxia
Autistic Disorder
Brain Tumors
Bell's Palsy
Cerebral Palsy
Chorea
Dyslexia
Dystonia
Encephalocele
Erb's Palsy
Familial Dysautonomia
Guillain-Barre Syndrome
Head Injuries
Hearing Impairment/Deafness
Hydrocephalus
Interventricular Hemorrhage
Lead Poisoning
Leukodystrophies
Lissencephaly
Macrocephaly
Meningitis
Mental Retardation
Microcephaly
Muscular Dystrophies
Narcolepsy
Nystagmus
Ptosis
Seizures
Speech Impairment
Spina Bifida

Spinal Muscular Atrophies
Strabismus
Stuttering
Subacute Sclerosing Panencephalitis (SSPE)
Tics
Tourette Syndrome
Tuberous Sclerosis

Ophthalmologic Disorders; see also *Sensory Organs*, page 1045.
Aniridia
Congenital Cataracts
Congenital Glaucoma
Conjunctivitis
Lazy Eye
Nystagmus
Ptosis
Refraction Disturbances
Retinitis Pigmentosa
Retinoblastoma
Retinopathy of Prematurity
Strabismus

Orthopedic and Muscle Disorders; see also *Musculoskeletal System*, page 1036.
Achondroplasia
Ankylosing Spondylitis
Arthorogryposis Multiplex Congenita
Cerebral Palsy
Charcot-Marie-Tooth Disease
Childhood Dermatomyositis
Cleft Lip and Cleft Palate
Clubfoot
Congenital Dysplasia of the Hip
Craniosynostosis
Dystonia
Ewing's Sarcoma
Legg-Calve-Perthes Disease
Marfan Syndrome
Muscular Dystrophies
Neurofibromatosis
Osteogenesis Imperfecta
Polydactyly
Scoliosis
Spina Bifida
Spinal Muscular Atrophies
Strabismus
Syndactyly

Renal and Urologic Disorders; see also *Urologic System*, page 1047.
Cryptorchidism
Nephrotic Syndrome
Nocturnal Enuresis

Respiratory Disorders; see also *Respiratory System*, page 1043.
Alpha-1-Antitrypsin Deficiency
Apnea of Prematurity
Asthma
Bronchopulmonary Dysplasia
Congenital Diaphragmatic Hernia
Cystic Fibrosis
Pneumonia
Pulmonary Hypertension
Respiratory Distress Syndrome of the Newborn
Respiratory Syncytial Virus Infection
Rhinitis
Sleep Apnea
Tuberculosis

Modest Increases in Kids' Physical Activity Could Avert Billions in Medical and Other Costs

Johns Hopkins Bloomberg School of Public Health

Even getting in just a little more can reduce obesity and related illnesses in adulthood.

Increasing the percentage of elementary school children in the United States who participate in 25 minutes of physical activity three times a week from 32 percent to 50 percent would avoid $21.9 billion in medical costs and lost wages over the course of their lifetimes, new Johns Hopkins Bloomberg School of Public Health research suggests.

The findings, published May 1 in the journal Health Affairs, suggest that just a small increase in the frequency of exercise among children ages 8 through 11 would also result in 340,000 fewer obese and overweight youth, a reduction of more than 4 percent. If all current 8– through 11–year–olds in the United States exercised 25 minutes a day, three times a week, the researchers suggest that $62.3 billion in medical costs and lost wages over the course of their lifetimes could be avoided and 1.2 million fewer youths would be overweight or obese.

These numbers represent cost savings for one cohort of 8–to–11 year olds, so every year that children in this age group reach those levels of physical activity, over $60 billion more would be saved.

"Physical activity not only makes kids feel better and helps them develop healthy habits, it's also good for the nation's bottom line," says study leader Bruce Y. Lee, MD, MBA, executive director of the Global Obesity Prevention Center at the Bloomberg School. "Our findings show that encouraging exercise and investing in physical activity such as school recess and youth sports leagues when kids are young pays big dividends as they grow up."

For the study, Lee and his colleagues, including team members from the Bloomberg School and the Pittsburgh Supercomputing Center at Carnegie Mellon University, developed a computational simulation model utilizing their VPOP (Virtual Population for Obesity Prevention) software platform to represent the current population of U.S. children and to show how changes in levels of physical activity could affect them throughout their lifetime and the resulting economic impact. The model relied on data from the 2005 and 2013 National Health and Nutrition Examination Survey (NHANES) and on information from the National Center for Health Statistics. The medical costs and the lost wages were calculated in the second model, which looked at the lifetime effects of physical activity.

The researchers also looked at various levels of healthy physical activity, starting with the current average of 32 percent of children 8 to 11 who exercise for 25 minutes a day, three days a week, up to 100 percent doing so. That is a guideline developed by the Sports and Fitness Industry Association. The researchers found that maintaining the current level of physical activity would result in 8.1 million of these youths being overweight or obese by 2020, which would cost $2.8 trillion in additional medical costs and lost wages over their lifetimes. An overweight person's lifetime medical costs average $62,331 and lost wages average $93,075. For an obese person, these amounts are even greater.

"Even modest increases in physical activity could yield billions of dollars in savings," Lee says.

The costs averted are likely an underestimate, he says, as there are other benefits of physical activity that don't impact weight, such as improving bone density, improving mood and building muscle.

Lee says that the spending averted by healthy levels of physical activity would more than make up for costs of programs designed to increase activity levels.

"As the prevalence of childhood obesity grows, so will the value of increasing physical activity," he says. "We need to be adding physical education programs and not cutting them. We need to encourage kids to be active, to reduce screen time and get them running around again. It's important for their physical health."

Reprinted with permission from MDLinx/A division of M3.

DESCRIPTION

2   ACHONDROPLASIA
Synonyms: Chondrodystrophy, Fetal Rickets
Involves the following Biologic System(s):
Genetic/Chromosomal/Syndrome/Metabolic Disorders, Orthopedic and Muscle Disorders

Achondroplasia is a disorder of the skeletal system that occurs in about one of every 20,000 newborn infants. It belongs to a group of disorders known as chondrodystrophies. These disorders involve a disturbance in the cartilage at the ends of the body's long bones (arms and legs). In Achondroplasia, this disturbance interferes with the conversion of cartilage into bone in the regions known as epiphyses, where these bones normally grow in length. This occurs in infancy and childhood, preventing the bones from growing normally and resulting in shortened limbs and a short stature. Achondroplasia does not affect intelligence.

Achondroplasia is caused by a defect in a single, specific gene that permits the body to make a protein known as fibroblast growth factor-3 (FGF3). Normally, FGF3 limits bone growth, and a decline in the production of this protein is what permits growth during childhood and adolescence. The genetic defect in Achondroplasia, however, causes the body to continue to produce FGF3, leading to an excess of this protein that sharply limits growth. Genetically, Achondroplasia is called an autosomal dominant disorder, because the defective FGF3 gene needs to be inherited from only one parent for Achondroplasia to be present.

Symptoms and characteristic findings include a disproportionately large head with a protruding and prominent forehead (frontal bossing); a flattened nasal bridge; an underdeveloped upper jaw and prominent lower jaw (prognothism); a well-developed but shortened trunk; and short, bowed arms and legs. The upper portions of the arms and legs are proportionately shorter than the lower parts of these limbs, and the elbows may have a limited range of motion. Usually, the fingers and toes are also short, with a V-shaped gap between the third and fourth fingers, and the hands are relatively wide. As children with Achondroplasia grow, their pelvis tilts forward, resulting in a pronounced spinal curvature known as lumbar lordosis, that causes prominence of the abdomen and buttocks. Other effects of Achondroplasia can include decreased muscle tone and muscle weakness.

Diagnosis of Acondroplasia is made from physical examination and findings on X-ray images of the skeleton. Identification of this condition early in life facilitates family and medical planning for treatment and care.

Complications associated with Achondroplasia may include dental problems such as malocclusion, in which the upper and lower teeth do not meet in the proper alignment, and chronic and severe middle ear infections (otitis media) that can result in a loss of conductive hearing. Potentially life-threatening complications include temporary cessations of breathing during sleep, known as sleep apnea, caused by obstruction of the airways by the craniofacial abnormalities in Achondroplasia, and/or from compression of the spinal cord at the point where the cord passes from the spine into the skull. Additionally, this may obstruct the normal flow of cerebrospinal fluid (CSF) between the brain and spinal cord, resulting in hydrocephalus, a condition in which the cerebrospinal fluid collects in and around the brain, with potentially life-threatening effects.

Treatment with human growth hormone (HGH) is often used to improve growth and height in persons with Achondroplasia, and the availability of recombinant human growth hormone, or somatotropin, has revolutionized the treatment of short stature. Surgical lengthening of the limbs can produce improvement in some patients. Other treatment is directed at preventing or correcting complications of the condition. Monitoring head growth during infancy to insure normal growth limits is effective for detecting hydrocephalus. Physiotherapy, dental treatment and orthopedic appliances such as braces can correct or prevent a number of the complications caused by Achondroplasia. Appropriate counseling can provide emotional and psychological support to persons with the condition and their family members.

Government Agencies

3   NIH/National Institute of Arthritis and Musculoskeletal and Skin Diseases
1 AMS Circle
Bethesda, MD 20892
301-495-4484
877-226-4267
Fax: 301-718-6366
TTY: 301-565-2966
niamsinfo@mail.nih.gov
www.niams.nih.gov

The mission of the NIAMS, a part of the NIH, is to support research into the causes, treatment and prevention of arthritis and musculosketal and skin diseases, the training of basic and clinical scientists to carry out this research, and the dissemination of information on research progress in these diseases.
Stephen I Katz MD PhD, Director
Robert H Carter MD, Deputy Director
Gahan Breithaupt, Assoc Dir. Management & Operations

4   NIH/National Institute of Environmental Health Sciences (NIEHS)
111 T.W. Alexander Drive
RTP, NC 27709
919-541-3345
Fax: 301-480-2978
webcenter@niehs.nih.gov.
www.niehs.nih.gov

NIEHS reduces the burden of human illness and dysfunction from environmental causes by defining how environmental exposures, genetics and age interact to affect an individual's health.
Linda S Birnbaum, PhD, Director
Richard Woychik, PhD, Deputy Director
Chris Long, Executive Officer

5   NIH/National Institute on Drug Abuse (NIDA)
6001 Executive Boulevard/Ste 5274
Bethesda, MD 20892
301-443-1124
Fax: 301-443-7397
information@nida.nih.gov
www.drugabuse.gov

NIDA leads the nation in bringing the power of science to bear on drug abuse and addiction through support and conduct of research across all disciplines and rapid and effective dissemination of results of that research to improve drug abuse and addiction prevention and treatment.
Nora D. Volkow MD, Director
Wilson Compton, MD, MPE, Deputy Director
Joellen Austin, MP, Associate Director for Management

National Associations & Support Groups

6 **American Academy of Pediatrics**
141 Northwest Point Boulevard
Elk Grove Village, IL 60007
847-434-4000
800-433-9016
Fax: 847-434-8000
www.aap.org

The American Academy of Pediatrics and its member pediatricians are committed to the attainment of optimal physical, mental and social health and well-being for all infants, children, adolescents, and young adults.

Fernando Stein, MD, FAAP, President
Colleen A Kraft, MD, FAAP, President-Elect
Karen Remley, MD, CEO/Executive Vice President

7 **Human Growth Foundation**
997 Glen Cove Avenue, Suite 5
Glen Head, NY 11545
516-671-4041
800-451-6434
Fax: 516-671-4055
hgf1@hgfound.org
www.hgfound.org

A voluntary, nonprofit organization whose mission is to help children and adults with disorders of growth and growth hormones through research, education, support and advocacy. The foundation is dedicated to helping medical science to better understand the process of growth. It is composed of concerned parents and friends of children and adults with growth problems; and interested health professionals.

Pisit Pitukcheewanont MD, President/Executive Committee Board
Patricia D Costa, Executive Director
Emily Germain Lee, MD, Vice President/Executive Committee

8 **Little People of America**
250 El Camino Real, Suite 218
Tustin, CA 92780
714-368-3689
888-572-2001
Fax: 714-368-3367
info@lpaonline.org
www.lpaonline.org

A nonprofit organization that provides support and information to people of short stature and their families.

Gary Arnold, President
April Brazier, Senior Vice President
Jon North, Programs Director

9 **MAGIC Foundation: Major Aspects of Growth in Children**
4200 Cantera Drive, #106
Warrenville, IL 60555
630-836-8200
800-362-4423
Fax: 630-836-8181
ContactUs@magicfoundation.org
www.magicfoundation.org

A national nonprofit organization providing support and education regarding growth disorders in children and related adult disorders. Provides educational information, networking, a national conference, a kids' program and an extensive medical library.

10,000 members

Dianne Kremidas, Executive Director
Mary Andrews, CEO
Teresa Tucker, Patient Advocacy

Libraries & Resource Centers

10 **NIH/National Library of Medicine (NLM)**
8600 Rockville Pike
Bethesda, MD 20894
301-594-5983
888-346-3656
Fax: 301-402-1384
TDD: 800-735-2258
custserv@nlm.nih.gov
www.nlm.nih.gov

NLM collects, organizes and makes available biomedical science information to scientists, health professionals and the public. The library's databases, including PubMed/Medline and MedlinePlus, are used extensively around the world. NLM conducts and supports research in biometric communications; creates information resources for molecular biology, biotechnology, toxicology, and environmental health; and provides grant support for training, medical library resources, and biomedical informatics.

Patricia Flatley Brennan, Director
Betsy Humphreys, Deputy Director
Paul Kiehl, Deputy Executive Officer

Conferences

11 **Adult Endocrine Disorders/GHD Educational Convention**
Magic Foundation
4200 Cantera Drive, #106
Warrenville, IL 60555
630-836-8200
800-362-4423
Fax: 630-836-8181
contactus@magicfoundation.org
www.magicfoundation.org

An educational program for adults who are affected with Growth Hormone Deficiency and/or other endocrine disorders.

June

Dianne Kremidas, Executive Director
Rich Buckley, Chairman
Mary Andrews, Chief Executive Officer

12 **LPA National Conference**
Little People of America
250 El Camino Real, Suite 218
Tustin, CA 92780
714-368-3689
888-572-2001
Fax: 714-368-3367
info@lpaonline.org
www.lpaonline.org

July

Leah Smith, Public Relations Director
Gary Arnold, President
April Brazier, Senior Vice President

Web Sites

13 **Achondroplasia UK**
52 Vernham Grove
Odd down, Bath, Avon, BA2 2
admin@achondroplasia.co.uk
www.achondroplasia.co.uk

Offers information on health supervision for children of all ages, divided into the following growth stages: newborn; infancy; early childhood; late childhood; and adolescence to early adulthood.

14 **Human Growth Foundation**
997 Glen Cove Ave., Suite 5
Glen Head, NY 11545
800-451-6434
Fax: 516-671-4055
hgf1@hgfound.org
www.hgfound.org

The Human Growth Foundation is a voluntary, non-profit organization whose mission is to help children and adults with disorders of growth and growth horomone through research, education, support, and advocacy.

Pisit Pitukcheewanont, MD, President
Patricia D. Costa, Executive Director
Emily Y. Germain-Lee, MD, Vice President

15 **Little People of America**
250 El Camino Real, Suite 218
Tustin, CA 92780
714-368-3689
888-LPA-2001
Fax: 714-368-3367
info@lpaonline.org
www.lpaonline.org

Offers resources pertaining to dwarfism and Little People of America, medical data, instructions on how to join an e-mail discussion group, and links to numerous other dwarfism-related sites.

Gary Arnold, President
April Brazier, Executive Director
Jon North, Programs Director

16   MAGIC Foundation: Major Aspects of Growth in Children
4200 Cantera Drive, #106
Warrenville, IL 60555   630-836-8200
                                               800-362-4423
                                          Fax: 630-836-8181
                             ContactUs@magicfoundation.org
                                www.magicfoundation.org

Provides educational information regarding growth disorders.

Dianne Kremidas, Executive Director
Mary Andrews, Chief Executive Officer
Teresa Tucker, Patient Advocacy

17   Medical College of Wisconsin
8701 Watertown Plank Road
Milwaukee, WI 53226   414-955-8296
                                               www.mcw.edu

A private, academic institution dedicated to leadership and excellence in education, research, patient care, and service.

John R. Raymond, Sr., MD, President/ CEO
Joseph E. Kerschner, MD, Dean/ EVP
Ravi Misra, PhD, Dean/ Professor of Biochemistry

18   Online Mendelian Inheritance in Man
National Library of Medicine, Building 38A
Bethesda, MD 20894   888-346-3656
                                            info@ncbi.nlm.nih.gov
                                            www.ncbi.nlm.nih.gov

This database is a catalog of human genes and genetic disorders.

Christine E. Seidman, M.D., Chair
David J. Lipman, M.D., Executive Secretary

19   Restricted Growth Association
www.rgaonline.org.uk

Provides medical advice, welfare and counseling services with the support of Regional Coordinators, and offers contact with others and the sharing of helpful information through an information magazine, advisory booklets, meetings, social events and conventions.

Pamphlets

20   Achondroplasia
Human Growth Foundation
977 Glen Cove Avenue, Suite 5
Glen Head, NY 11545   516-671-4041
                                               800-451-6434

Signs, causes, and prevention of achondroplasia.

DESCRIPTION

21   ACUTE GASTROINTESTINAL INFECTIONS
Covers these related disorders: Acute infectious diarrhea, Gastroenteritis
Involves the following Biologic System(s):
Gastrointestinal Disorders, Infectious Disorders

Acute gastrointestinal infections are conditions of the gastrointestinal tract caused by various microorganisms such as certain bacteria, viruses, and parasites (more common outside the U.S.) and are usually characterized by diarrhea and vomiting. Such microorganisms may be transmitted through fecal-oral contamination or contamination of food or water. Bacterial gastrointestinal infection may result from the release of toxins by bacteria or by bacterial growth inside or outside the walls of the intestines. Viral infection by gastroenteritis viruses, especially the rotavirus, is a major source of diarrhea-causing infection in the U.S. Although infectious gastroenteritis often resolves on its own, some patients experience acute or prolonged symptoms that may require treatment, as well as identification of the causative agent.

Symptoms and findings associated with infectious gastroenteritis depend upon the cause of the infection and the age and general health of the patient. The most common manifestation of infection is watery or bloody diarrhea that usually appears suddenly and lasts from a few days to two weeks or longer. Other symptoms may include nausea, vomiting, loss of appetite, and abdominal cramping or distress. Infants and those with compromised immune systems are at risk for potentially severe illness. Diarrhea and vomiting in infants younger than six months, and severe episodes in any child, may result in a potentially life-threatening and excessive fluid loss (dehydration) as well as the loss of essential substances, known as electrolytes, in the fluid portion of the blood (e.g., sodium, potassium, and calcium). Symptoms associated with dehydration may include fever, thirst, less-than-average urinary output, dry mouth, and poor feeding. In addition, severely dehydrated infants and children may become weak, listless, or sleepy and their eyes may have a sunken, dry appearance. Bacteria associated with gastroenteritis sometimes cause infection outside the gastrointestinal tract and may involve the urinary tract, eyes, vaginal areas in females, as well as inflammation of the membranes surrounding the brain and spinal cord (meningitis), the liver (hepatitis), the lungs (pneumonia), the bone and bone marrow (osteomyelitis), and other tissues. In addition, certain food-borne or water-borne infections caused by bacterial or other toxins may produce severe, sudden, and potentially life-threatening symptoms including neurologic involvement such as numbness and paralysis.

Acute infectious diarrhea symptoms are similar to those associated with infectious gastroenteritis. In addition, a temporary inability to properly digest milk may result from damage to the mucosal lining of the small intestine.

Prevention of some types of infectious gastroenteritis may include vaccination against certain infectious diseases when traveling to countries in which these illnesses are widespread. In addition, care in handling and preparing foods may help to alleviate certain types of food-borne illness. Treatment for both infectious gastroenteritis and acute infectious diarrhea is first directed toward the replacement of body fluids and electrolytes through oral preparations or, in the case of more severe dehydration, intravenously. Once dehydration is corrected, breast-feeding, or feeding with lactose-free formula, gradually followed by regular formula, may resume. If indicated, identification of the cause may then be established through evaluation of family history including recent travels, foods eaten, other similar family illness as well as physical examination and testing of stool specimens. Although some cases of acute infectious diarrhea will resolve spontaneously, other treatment may be directed at the underlying cause. Bacterial infections may be treated with appropriate antibiotics. Prevention of this potentially severe condition may often be accomplished by attention to good hygienics such as frequent hand washing, etc. Other treatment is symptomatic and supportive.

Government Agencies

22   NIH/National Institute of Allergy and Infectious Diseases
5601 Fishers Lane, MSC 9806
Bethesda, MD 20892
301-496-5717
866-284-4107
Fax: 301-402-3573
TDD: 800-877-8339
ocpostoffice@niaid.nih.gov
www.niaid.nih.gov

Conducts and supports basic and applied research to better understand, treat, and ultimately prevent infectious, immunologic, and allergic diseases.

Anthony S Fauci MD, Director

National Associations & Support Groups

23   American Academy of Pediatrics
141 Northwest Point Boulevard
Elk Grove Village, IL 60007
847-434-4000
800-433-9016
Fax: 847-434-8000
www.aap.org

The American Academy of Pediatrics and its member pediatricians are committed to the attainment of optimal physical, mental and social health and well-being for all infants, children, adolescents, and young adults.

Fernando Stein, MD, FAAP, President
Karen Remley, MD, CEO/Executive VP

24   American College of Gastroenterology
6400 Goldsboro Road, Suite 200
Bethesda, MD 20817
301-263-9000
info@acg.gi.org
www.gi.org

The American College of Gastroenterology was founded in 1932 to advance the scientific study and medical practice of diseases of the GI tract.

13,000 members

Carol A. Burke, MD, FACG, President

25   American Gastroenterological Association
4930 Del Ray Avenue
Bethesda, MD 20814
301-654-2055
Fax: 301-654-5920
member@gastro.org
www.gastro.org

Society of physicians, surgeons, scientists and other individuals within the healthcare community interested in the functions and disorders of the digestive system.

Timothy C. Wang, MD, President
Tom Serena, Executive VP

26 **Digestive Disease National Coalition**
507 Capitol Court NE, Suite 200
Washington, DC 20002   202-544-7497
                                        Fax: 202-546-7105
                                        hpayne@hmcw.org
                                        www.ddnc.org

Advocacy organization comprised of over 30 voluntary and professional societies concerned with the many diseases of the digestive tract and liver.

Lynn Seim, Chairperson
Ralph McKibbin, President
Cathy Griffith, Vice Chairperson

27 **International Foundation for Functional Gastrointestinal Disorders**
PO Box 170864
Milwaukee, WI 53217   414-964-1799
                                        Fax: 414-964-7176
                                        iffgd@iffgd.org
                                        www.iffgd.org

The organization offers responses to those commonly asked questions for families and individuals whose lives have been touched by gastrointestinal disorders.

Nancy J. Norton, President & Director
William Norton, Co-Founder
Eleanor Cautley, Vice President

28 **North American Society for Pediatric Gastroenterology/Hepatology/Nutrition**
714 N Bethlehem Pike, Suite 300
Ambler, PA 19002   215-641-9800
                                        Fax: 215-641-1995
                                        naspghan@naspghan.org
                                        www.naspghan.org

Strives to improve the care of infants, children and adolescents with digestive disorders by promoting advances in clinical care of children with chronic abdominal pain, diarrhea, constipation, vomiting, bleeding from the GI tract, inflammatory bowel disease, liver diseases, diseases of the pancreas, poor weight gain and nutritional problems.

Margaret K Stallings, Executive Director
Kim Rose, Associate Director
Donna Murphy, Membership

29 **Oley Foundation**
43 New Scotland Avenue, MC-28
Albany, NY 12208   518-262-5079
                                        800-776-6539
                                        Fax: 518-262-5528
                                        info@oley.org
                                        www.oley.org

Helping people whose daily survival depends on home intravenous or tube-fed nutrition.

Joan Bishop, Executive Director
Roslyn Dahl, Director, Communications
Lisa Crosby Metzger, Director, Community Engagement

30 **World Health Organization**
Avenue Appia 20
CH-1211 Geneva 27,
Switzerland   www.who.int

WHO is the directing and coordinating authority for health within the United Nations system.

Dr Margaret Chan, Director General
Dr.Anarfi Asamoa-Baah, Deputy Director-General
Bruce Aylward, Assistant Director General

Libraries & Resource Centers

31 **National Digestive Diseases Information Clearinghouse**
9000 Rockville Pike
Bethesda, MD 20892   301-496-3583
                                        800-860-8747
                                        Fax: 301-907-8906
                                        healthinfo@niddk.nih.gov
                                        www.niddk.nih.gov

The National Institute of Diabetes and Digestive and Kidney Diseases conducts and supports research on many of the most serious diseases affecting public health. The Institute supports much of the clinical research on the diseases of internal medicine and related subspecialty fields as well as many basic science disciplines.

Dr. Griffin P. Rodgers, Director
Dr. Gregory G. Germino, Deputy Director
Camille M. Hoover, M.S.W., Executive Officer

Conferences

32 **IFFGD Professional Symposia**
Int'l Foundation for Functional Gastrointestinal
PO Box 170864
Milwaukee, WI 53217   414-964-1799
                                        888-964-2001
                                        Fax: 414-964-7176
                                        iffgd@iffgd.org
                                        www.iffgd.org

Aimed at promoting education and awareness among professionals from multiple disciplines who treat gastrointestinal disorders and incontinence.

April

Nancy J Norton, President/Director/Co-Founder
William Norton, Vice President/Director/Co-Founder
Eleanor Cautley, Vice President/Director

33 **NASPGHAN Annual Meeting and Postgraduate Course**
NASPGHAN
714 N. Bethlehem Pike, Ste 300
Ambler, PA 19002   215-641-9800
                                        Fax: 215-641-1995
                                        naspghan@naspghan.org
                                        www.naspghan.org

November

Margaret K Stallings, Executive Director
Kim Rose, Associate Director
Donna Murphy, Membership

34 **Oley Foundation Annual Conference**
Oley Foundation
43 New Scotland Ave, MC-28, Albany Medical Center
Albany, NY 12208   518-262-5079
                                        800-776-6539
                                        Fax: 518-262-5528
                                        info@oley.org
                                        www.oley.org

Helping people whose daily survival depends on home intravenous or tube-fed nutrition.

July

Joan Bishop, Executive Director
Roslyn Dahl, Communications Director

Computer Software

35 **Digestive Diseases Self-Education Program (DDSEP 5.0)**
American Gastroenterological Association
4930 Del Ray Avenue
Bethesda, MD 20814   301-654-2055
                                        Fax: 301-654-5920
                                        member@gastro.org
                                        www.gastro.org

Provides an in-depth review of core topics in gastroenterology and hepatology. gastroenterologists use this software to assess and update their knowledge and earn CME credit.

Eugene Chang, MD, Editor
John F Kuemmerle, MD, Associate Editor

Web Sites

36   American Gastroenterological Association
4930 Del Ray Avenue
Bethesda, MD 20814
301-654-2055
Fax: 301-654-5920
member@gastro.org
www.gastro.org

Information regarding prevention, treatment and cure of digestive diseases.

Timothy C. Wang, MD, President
Tom Serena, Executive VP

37   Baby Center
163 Freelon Street
San Francisco, CA 94107
www.babycenter.com

The Academy is committed to the attainment of optimal physical, mental and social health for all infants, children, adolescents, and young adults. To this end, the members of the Academy dedicate their efforts and resources.

Colleen Hancock, SVP/ Global COO
Linda J. Murray, SVP/ Global Editor-in-Chief
Clarence Wilhelm, Chief Information Officer

38   Health Research Project (HaRP)
www.harpnet.org

harp@kmsgh.org
www.harpnet.org

A program by USAID, the project strives to improve the health status of infants, children, mothers and families through the development and research of new tools, technologies, policies and approaches.

39   Hepatitis A
NIDDK Health Information Center
Bethesda, MD 20892
800-860-8747
TTY: 866-569-1162
healthinfo@niddk.nih.gov
www.niddk.nih.gov

Explains the prevention, causes, symptoms, modes of transmission, and treatment of Hepatitis A.

Dr. Griffin P. Rodgers, Director
Dr. Gregory G. Germino, Deputy Director

40   Hepatitis B
NIDDK Health Information Center
Bethesda, MD 20892
800-860-8747
TTY: 866-569-1162
healthinfo@niddk.nih.gov
www.niddk.nih.gov

Explains the prevention, causes, symptoms, modes of transmission, and treatment of Hepatitis B.

Dr. Griffin P. Rodgers, Director
Dr. Gregory G. Germino, Deputy Director

41   Hepatitis C
NIDDK Health Information Center
Bethesda, MD 20892
800-860-8747
TTY: 866-569-1162
healthinfo@niddk.nih.gov
www.niddk.nih.gov

Explains the prevention, causes, symptoms, modes of transmission, and treatment of Hepatitis C.

Dr. Griffin P. Rodgers, Director
Dr. Gregory G. Germino, Deputy Director

42   National Digestive Diseases Information Clearinghouse
9000 Rockville Pike
Bethesda, MD 20892
301-496-3583
www.digestive.niddk.nih.gov

Information regarding digestive and kidney diseases.

Griffin P. Rodgers, M.D., M.A.C.P., Director
Kevin Abbott, Program Director
Kristin Abraham, Program Director

Book Publishers

43   Digestive Diseases Dictionary
NIDDK Health Information Center
Bethesda, MD 20892
800-860-8747
TTY: 866-569-1162
healthinfo@niddk.nih.gov
catalog.niddk.nih.gov/catalog/

Defines words that are often used when talking or writing about digestive diseases.

Dr. Griffin P. Rodgers, Director
Dr. Gregory G. Germino, Deputy Director
Camille M. Hoover, Executive Officer

Journals

44   American Journal of Gastroenterology
American College of Gastroenterology
6400 Goldsboro Rd, Ste 200
Bethesda, MD 20817
301-263-9000
gi.org

Publishes scientific papers relevant to the practice of clinical gastroenterology, Features outstanding original research, review articles and consensus papers related to new drugs and therapeutic modalities.

Stephen B. Hanauer, MD, FACG, President
Carol A. Burke, MD, FACG, Vice President
Sunanda V. Kane, MD, MSPH, FACG, Secretary

45   Journal of Pediatric Gastroenterology and Nutrition
Lippincott Williams & Wilkins
Two Commerce Square, 2001 Market Street
Philadelphia, PA 19103
215-521-8300
Fax: 215-521-8902
www.wolterskluwerhealth.com

Provides a forum for original papers and reviews dealing with nutrition in normal and abnormal functions of the alimentary tract and its associated organs including the salivary glands, pancreas, gallbladder, and liver. Particular emphasis is on development and its relation to infant and childhood nutrition.

Bob Becker, President/ CEO
Susan Yules, Chief Financial Officer
Cathy Wolfe, President/ CEO, Medical Research

Newsletters

46   NASPGHAN News
714 N. Bethlehem Pike, Ste 300
Ambler, PA 19002
215-641-9800
Fax: 215-641-1995
naspghan@naspghan.org
www.naspgn.org

Publication of the North American Society for Pediatric Gastroenterolgy, Hepatology and Nutrition, which strives to improve the care of infants, children and adolescents with digestive disorders by promoting advances in clinical care of children with chronic abdominal pain, diarrhea, constipation, vomiting, bleeding from the GI tract, inflammatory bowel disease, liver diseases, diseases of the pancreas, poor weight gain and nutritional problems.

Margaret K Stallings, Executive Director
Kim Rose, Associate Director
Donna Murphy, Membership

Pamphlets

47   Bleeding in the Digestive Tract
NIDDK Publications Catalog
1 Information Way
Bethesda, MD 20892   800-860-8747
                                                  TTY: 866-569-1162
                                         healthinfo@niddk.nih.gov
                                              catalog.niddk.nih.gov

Includes information on the causes of bleeding in the digestive tract and how the bleeding is recognized, diagnosed, and treated.

6 pages Spanish

Griffin P. Rodgers, M.D., Director

48   Cyclic Vomiting Syndrome
NDDIC
2 Information Way
Bethesda, MD 20892   301-654-3810
                                                        800-891-5389
                                                  Fax: 703-738-4929
                                                  TTY: 866-569-1162
                                           nddic@info.niddk.nih.gov
                                                  www.niddk.nih.gov

Describes the four phases of cyclic vomiting syndrome and the current treatment options available. Outlines the complications associated with the disorder and provides additional resources.

4 pages

Griffin P. Rodgers, M.D., M.A.C.P, Director
Kevin Abbott, Program Director
Kristin Abraham, Program Director

49   Diagnostic Tests
NDDIC
2 Information Way
Bethesda, MD 20892   301-654-3810
                                                        800-891-5389
                                                  Fax: 703-738-4929
                                                  TTY: 866-569-1162
                                           nddic@info.niddk.nih.gov
                                                  www.niddk.nih.gov

Contains patient education fact sheets on seven diagnostic tests for gastrointestinal disorders (Colonoscopy, Sigmoidoscopy, Upper Endoscopy, Lower GI Series, ERCP, Liver Biopsy). Designed to be photocopy masters for health professionals to copy and distribute to patients.

Griffin P. Rodgers, M.D., M.A.C.P, Director
Kevin Abbott, Program Director
Kristin Abraham, Program Director

50   Diarrhea
NDDIC
2 Information Way
Bethesda, MD 20892   301-654-3810
                                                        800-891-5389
                                                  Fax: 703-738-4929
                                                  TTY: 866-569-1162
                                           nddic@info.niddk.nih.gov
                                                  www.niddk.nih.gov

Includes general information on diarrhea and what can cause it. Also provides information about diagnosis, treatment, and prevention.

6 pages

Griffin P. Rodgers, M.D., M.A.C.P, Director
Kevin Abbott, Program Director
Kristin Abraham, Program Director

51   Diverticular Disease
NIDDK Health Information Center
1 Information Way
Bethesda, MD 20892   800-860-8747
                                                  TTY: 866-569-1162
                                         healthinfo@niddk.nih.gov
                                              catalog.niddk.nih.gov

Provides clear definitions of diverticulosis and diverticulitis, along with information on symptoms, causes, complications, and treatments.

6 pages

Griffin P. Rodgers, M.D., Director

52   Facts & Fallacies About Digestive Diseases
NDDIC
2 Information Way
Bethesda, MD 20892   301-654-3810
                                                        800-891-5389
                                                  Fax: 703-738-4929
                                                  TTY: 866-569-1162
                                           nddic@info.niddk.nih.gov
                                                  www.niddk.nih.gov

Provides information about common digestive disorders, including ulcers, inflammatory bowel disease, and constipation, in true/false format.

4 pages

Griffin P. Rodgers, M.D., M.A.C.P, Director
Kevin Abbott, Program Director
Kristin Abraham, Program Director

53   Gallstones
NDDIC
2 Information Way
Bethesda, MD 20892   301-654-3810
                                                        800-891-5389
                                                  Fax: 703-738-4929
                                                  TTY: 866-569-1162
                                           nddic@info.niddk.nih.gov
                                                  www.niddk.nih.gov

Provides general information on gallstones, including what causes them, who is at risk, and how they are diagnosed and treated.

6 pages

Griffin P. Rodgers, M.D., M.A.C.P, Director
Kevin Abbott, Program Director
Kristin Abraham, Program Director

54   Gas in the Digestive Tract
NDDIC
2 Information Way
Bethesda, MD 20892   301-654-3810
                                                        800-891-5389
                                                  Fax: 703-738-4929
                                                  TTY: 866-569-1162
                                           nddic@info.niddk.nih.gov
                                                  www.niddk.nih.gov

Describes what causes gas, discusses the symptoms and the problems they cause, and provides information on treatment.

8 pages

Griffin P. Rodgers, M.D., M.A.C.P, Director
Kevin Abbott, Program Director
Kristin Abraham, Program Director

55   Gastroesophageal Reflux Disease in Children
NDDIC
2 Information Way
Bethesda, MD 20892   301-654-3810
                                                        800-891-5389
                                                  Fax: 703-738-4929
                                                  TTY: 866-569-1162
                                           nddic@info.niddk.nih.gov
                                                  www.niddk.nih.gov

Describes gastroesophageal reflux (GER) in children and adolescents, including information about the causes, symptoms, and diagnosis of this condition, as well as its treatment.

4 pages

Griffin P. Rodgers, M.D., M.A.C.P, Director
Kevin Abbott, Program Director
Kristin Abraham, Program Director

56 Heart Burn, Hiatal Hernia, and Gastroesophageal Reflux Disease
NDDIC
2 Information Way
Bethesda, MD 20892

301-654-3810
800-891-5389
Fax: 703-738-4929
TTY: 866-569-1162
nddic@info.niddk.nih.gov
www.niddk.nih.gov

Defines gastroesophageal reflux disease (GERD) and describes the role of hiatal hernia. Provides general information on heartburn, as well as treatments for GERD, including surgery.

6 pages

Griffin P. Rodgers, M.D., M.A.C.P, Director
Kevin Abbott, Program Director
Kristin Abraham, Program Director

57 Hemochromatosis
NDDIC
2 Information Way
Bethesda, MD 20892

301-654-3810
800-891-5389
Fax: 703-738-4929
TTY: 866-569-1162
nddic@info.niddk.nih.gov
www.niddk.nih.gov

Provides information about the causes, risk factors, symptoms, diagnosis, treatment, diagnostic tests for, and current research about hemochromatosis. Includes a list of additional resources.

6 pages

Griffin P. Rodgers, M.D., M.A.C.P, Director
Kevin Abbott, Program Director
Kristin Abraham, Program Director

58 Irritable Bowel Syndrome
NDDIC
2 Information Way
Bethesda, MD 20892

301-654-3810
800-891-5389
Fax: 703-738-4929
TTY: 866-569-1162
nddic@info.niddk.nih.gov
www.niddk.nih.gov

Describes causes, symptoms, tests to rule out more serious intestinal diseases, and lifestyle and medical approaches to syptom management.

4 pages

Griffin P. Rodgers, M.D., M.A.C.P, Director
Kevin Abbott, Program Director
Kristin Abraham, Program Director

59 Ulcerative Colitis
NDDIC
2 Information Way
Bethesda, MD 20892

301-654-3810
800-891-5389
Fax: 703-738-4929
TTY: 866-569-1162
nddic@info.niddk.nih.gov
www.niddk.nih.gov

Outlines the symptoms, diagnostic procedures, and risks and benefits of several drugs and kinds of surgery to treat this disease.

6 pages

Griffin P. Rodgers, M.D., M.A.C.P, Director
Kevin Abbott, Program Director
Kristin Abraham, Program Director

60 Your Digestive System & How it Works
NDDIC
2 Information Way
Bethesda, MD 20892

301-654-3810
800-891-5389
Fax: 703-738-4929
TTY: 866-569-1162
nddic@info.niddk.nih.gov
www.niddk.nih.gov

Providees general information about the organs of the digestive system, the digestive process, and the absorption of nutrients. Includes a list of additional readings.

6 pages

Griffin P. Rodgers, M.D., M.A.C.P, Director
Kevin Abbott, Program Director
Kristin Abraham, Program Director

DESCRIPTION

61   ACUTE LYMPHOBLASTIC LEUKEMIA

Synonyms: Acute lymphocytic leukemia, ALL

Involves the following Biologic System(s):

Hematologic and Oncologic Disorders

Acute lymphoblastic leukemia (ALL) is a malignant disease characterized by excessive production of immature white blood cells known as lymphoblasts. ALL is the most common type of leukemia in children, having a slightly greater incidence, or rate of occurrence, in boys than in girls. Although ALL may develop during adolescence or occasionally in adulthood, it occurs most commonly in children between 3 and 7 years of age. The outcome in childhood ALL is related to a multitude of factors, including age, numbers of lymphoblasts and other blood cells found in the blood and bone marrow, and various genetic factors.

The lymphoblasts involved in ALL are produced in the bone marrow, and normally go on to develop into the white blood cells called lymphocytes, which are primarily responsible for fighting infection. In ALL, these lymphoblasts go through an uncontrolled proliferation that results in their accumulation in huge numbers in the bone marrow, impairing its ability to produce the other types of blood cells that originate in the marrow. The lymphoblasts responsible for ALL also proliferate in organs other than the marrow, particularly the liver, spleen, and lymph nodes.

The lymphoblasts affected by ALL evolve into either of two types of mature lymphocytes. One of these types are T-lymphocytes, which migrate from the bone marrow to the thymus gland in the neck, where they complete their maturation. The second type of lymphocytes, called B-lymphocytes mature entirely within the bone marrow. Because of this difference, ALL itself is divided into two categories — T-cell and B-cell. The technique used for differentiating the two kinds of ALL is known as "immunophenotyping." B-cell ALL is more common than T-cell, which tends to occur more often in boys, after the age of 10 years. Treatment of the two types of ALL may also differ, depending upon age, results of clinical and laboratory tests, and other factors.

All forms of ALL originate from abnormalities in the genetic structure of the cells that give rise to lymphoblasts. These abnormalities include changes in the structure of specific genes, breaks in the chainlike strands of genes known as chromosomes, with the broken parts joining other parts of the same chromosome or to other chromosomes where they do not belong, and other kinds of damage to the chromosomes or genes.

The chromosomal or genetic abnormalities in ALL are responsible for both the uncontrolled proliferation of lymphocytes and a cessation in the development of these cells, preventing them from maturing normally into lymphocytes.

Factors that may increase the risk for developing childhood ALL include Trisomy 21, the chromosomal abnormality responsible for Down syndrome; certain genetic disorders, such as Fanconi's anemia; presence of the aberrant chromosome known as the Philadelphia chromosome, created by the breakage of a specific chromosome and entry of its broken part into another; exposure to radiation, some drugs used for chemotherapy, and certain chemicals such as benzene.

Many of the symptoms and effects of ALL in children and young adults are related to their uncontrolled proliferation of leukemic cells in the marrow or other organs. Overpopulation of the marrow by the diseased lymphoblasts in ALL may impede the formation of red blood cells, which also develop in the marrow; of the cells known as platelets, which are essential to blood clotting; and of the cells known as granulocytes, that normally team up with lymphocytes to fight off infection. The resulting symptoms typically include pallor, loss of appetite (anorexia), weight loss, and a generalized feeling of ill health (malaise); fatigue and weakness, from decreased numbers of the circulating red blood cells that carry oxygen to the body's tissues (anemia);bleeding from the gums or nose, easy bruising, and the development of small red or purple spots on the skin (petechiae) from decreased levels of the blood platelets responsible forblood clotting; and infection and fever from decreased numbers of mature white blood cells and granulocytes. Other symptoms of ALL may include headache and bone or joint pain. In many cases, effects of ALL include swollen lymph glands and an enlarged spleen (splenomegaly).

The diagnosis of ALL is established by the presence of lymphoblasts in a bone marrow sample obtained through biopsy. Treatment of ALL is directed toward destroying leukemic cells through the use of specific drugs, known as chemotherapy, which is sometimes given together with treatment delivered by high-energy radiation, such as that of X-rays. Treatment of ALL typically involves several stages, or "phases," and may cover a period of many months. The first stage of treatment, known as the "induction phase," is directed at maximum destruction of leukemic cells in the blood and bone marrow. This is commonly followed by what is known as "remission," in which the activity and effects of ALL are markedly reduced. The second phase of treatment, known as the "consolidation phase," is begun during remission and designed to eradicate any residual leukemic cells that may remain anywhere in the body and become reactivated, causing a recurrence or relapse of ALL. The third phase of therapy is known as "maintenance" or "continuation" therapy. The eradication of leukemic cells that have entered the brain, the membranes surrounding the brain and spinal cord (meninges), or the cerebrospinal fluid that surrounds these organs may require direct injection of a chemotherapeutic agent into the cerebrospinal fluid (intrathecal injection). Alternatively, X-ray or other irradiation may be focused on the brain or spinal cord to eliminate residual leukemic cells (intrathecal radiation). In some cases, immature blood cells are taken from the bone marrow of a donor and given to children with ALL to replace cells destroyed by chemotherapy or radiation therapy, with the goal of allowing these immature cells to grow to maturity and restore the patient's production of red and white blood cells and platelets.

Supportive measures in the treatment of ALL may include blood transfusions to alleviate anemia and bleeding irregularities, as well as the administration of antibiotics to treat infections resulting from the white cell abnormalities associated with both ALL and its treatment. Relapse of ALL after successful initial remission therapy usually results from lymphoblasts that have remained in the bone marrow and brain, and may require one or more additional courses of chemotherapy.

Government Agencies

62   NIH/National Cancer Institute
BG 9609 / 9609 Medical Center Drive
Bethesda, MD 20892
800-422-6237
www.cancer.gov

The National Cancer Institute coordinates the National Cancer Program, which conducts and supports research, training, health information dissemination, and other programs with respect to the cause, diagnosis, prevention, and treatment of cancer, rehabilitation from cancer, and the continuing care of cancer patients and the families of cancer patients.

Douglas R. Lowy, MD, Acting Director
James Doroshow, MD, Deputy Director
Henry P. Ciolino, PhD, Acting Director, Cancer Centers

63   NIH/National Heart, Lung and Blood Institute
National Institute of Health
31 Center Dr MSC 2486, Bldg 31, Room 5A52
Bethesda, MD 20892
301-592-8573
Fax: 240-629-3246
TTY: 240-629-3255
NHLBIinfo@nhlbi.nih.gov
www.nhlbi.nih.gov

Primary responsibility of this organization is the scientific investigation of heart, blood vessel, lung and blood disorders. Oversees research, demonstration, prevention, education, control and training activities in these fields and emphasizes the prevention and control of heart diseases.

Gary H Gibbons, MD, Director
Nakela Cook, MD, Chief of Staff

National Associations & Support Groups

64   American Academy of Pediatrics
141 Northwest Point Boulevard
Elk Grove Village, IL 60007
847-434-4000
800-433-9016
Fax: 847-434-8000
www.aap.org

The American Academy of Pediatrics and its member pediatricians are committed to the attainment of optimal physical, mental and social health and well-being for all infants, children, adolescents, and young adults.

Fernando Stein, MD, FAAP, President
Karen Remley, MD, CEO/Executive VP

**65   American Childhood Cancer Organization (fo rmerly
Candlelighters Childhood Cancer)**
PO Box 498
Kensington, MD 20895
301-962-3520
855-858-2226
Fax: 310-962-3521
staff@acco.org
www.acco.org

The American Childhood Cancer Organization (ACCO) was founded in 1970 by a group of parents whose children had been diagnosed with cancer. Today, ACCO is one of the largest grassroots, national organizations dedicated to improving the lives of children and adolescents with cancer and their families.

Ruth I. Hoffman, MPH, Executive Director
Jessica DiBenedetto, Program Coordinator
Christy Perry, Director, Marketing/Communications

66   Association of Child Life Professionals
1820 N Fort Myer Drive, Ste 520
Arlington, VA 22209
501-483-4500
800-252-4515
Fax: 501-483-4482
aclpadmin@childlife.org
www.childlife.org

Professionals who strive to reduce the impact of stressful or traumatic life events and situations which affect the development, health and well being of infants, children, youth and families. They embrace the value of play as a healing modality while working to enhance the normal growth and development of children through assessment, intervention, prevention, advocacy and education. The council offers publications, annual conferences, professional certification and more.

Jennifer Lipsey, Interim CEO
Yvonne Kassimatis, Marketing & Communications
Ramona Spencer, Manager, Conferences & Events

67   B.A.S.E. Camp Children's Cancer Foundation
650 North Wymore Rd, #103
Winter Park, FL 32789
407-673-5060
Fax: 407-673-5095
info@basecamp.org
www.basecamp.org

Provides a year round base of support for children and families facing the challenge of living with cancer, hemophilia and other blood related illnesses.

Terri Jones, President
Cindy Whitaker, Parent & Program Coordinator
Rachel Perez, Office Administrator

68   Believe In Tomorrow - National Children's Foundation
6601 Frederick Road, PO Box 21243
Baltimore, MD 21228
410-744-1032
Fax: 410-744-1984
info@believeintomorrow.org
www.believeintomorrow.org

Provides exceptional hospital and retreat housing services to critically ill children and their families.

Brian Morrison, Founder & CEO
Richard E. McCready, Chairman
David Reymann, Vice Chairman

69   CancerCare
275 7th Avenue
New York, NY 10001
212-712-8400
800-813-4673
Fax: 212-712-8495
info@cancercare.org
www.cancercare.org

Dedicated to providing emotional support, information, and practical help to people with cancer and their loved ones. CancerCare is the oldest, largest, nonprofit agency devoted to offering professional services.

Patricia J Goldsmith, CEO
John Rutigliano, Chief Operating Officer
Ahuva Morris, Children's Program Coordinator

70   Childhood Cancer Canada Foundation
21 St. Clair Avenue East, Suite 801
Toronto, Ontario,
Canada
416-489-6440
800-363-1062
Fax: 416-489-9812
info@childhoodcancer.ca
www.childhoodcancer.ca

Founded in 1987, Childhood Cancer Canada (CCC) is the country's leading Foundation dedicated entirely to the fight against childhood cancer. Through their unique partnership will all of Canada's 17 childhood cancer hospitals and treatment centres, CCC can ensure that children with cancer are exposed to kinder and gentler treatments that will not only cure them but leave them with an improved quality of life into adulthood.

Glenn Fraser, Chair
Megan Davidson, President & CEO
Alan Zimmermann, VP, Operations

71   Children's Cancer & Blood Foundation
333 E 38th Street, Suite 830
New York, NY 10016
212-297-4336
Fax: 212-297-4340
info@childrenscbf.org
www.childrenscbf.org

The foundation's major emphasis is on blood diseases affecting children: leukemia, thalassemia, hemophilia, sickle cell anemia, platelet disorders, retinoblastoma and cancer.

Drew Phillips, President
Greg Karakashian, Operations Associate

72   Children's Leukemia Association
National Leukemia Research Association
585 Stewart Avenue, Suite 18
Garden City, NY 11530

516-222-1944
Fax: 516-222-0457
info@childrensleukemia.org
www.childrensleukemia.org

A not-for-profit organization dedicated to raising funds to support research efforts towards finding the causes and cure for Leukemia.

Anthony Pasqua, President
Henry Green, Esq., Vice President
William Regina, Secretary/Treasurer

73   Dreams Come True Emery Clinic-Peds
1365 Clfton Road NE
Atlanta, GA 30322

404-778-5000
800-223-6679
patient.relations@emoryhealthcare.org
www.emoryhealthcare.org

Serves any child with cancer or chronic blood disease treated at Emory University Homo/Onc Clinic. Dreams submitted by children.

S. Wright Caughman, MD, Chairman
John T. Fox, President/CEO
Robert J. Bachman, CEO

74   Hair Club for Kids: Hair Club for Men
270 Farmington Avenue, Suite 232 (Second Floor)
Farmington, CT 06032

860-674-0202
888-888-8986
Fax: 860-676-0805
www.hairclub.com/hairclub-for-kids.php

Since 1992, Hair Club has offered free hair restoration services to children who suffer from diseases that lead to hair loss or alopecia. Hair Club for Kids is a non-profit program funded entirely by Hair Club that's available at no charge to children ages 6-17.

Sy Sperling, Founder
Steven Barth, President
Lydia Cassarino, Manager

75   Just In Time
PO Box 27693
Philadelphia, PA 19118

215-247-8777
Fax: 215-247-0956
tome@softhats.com
www.softhats.com

All cotton headwear for girls and women who have experienced hair loss.

Verlay Platt, President

76   Leukemia & Lymphoma Society
3 International Drive, Ste 200
Rye Brook, NY 10573

914-949-5213
Fax: 914-949-6691
infocenter@lls.org
www.lls.org

Largest voluntary health organization dedicated to funding blood cancer research, education and patient services.

Louis J. DeGennaro, PhD, President & CEO
Andrew Coccari, Chief Product Officer
Danielle Gee, Chief of Staff

77   National Bone Marrow Transplant Link
20411 W 12 Mile Road, Suite 108
Southfield, MI 48076

248-358-1886
800-546-5268
Fax: 248-358-1889
info@nbmtlink.org
www.nbmtlink.org

The mission of the National Bone Marrow Transplant Link is to help patients, caregivers, and families cope with the social and emotional challenges of bone marrow/stem cell transplant from diagnosis through survivorship by providing vital information and personalized support services.

Myra Jacobs, Founding Director
Barbara Saltz, Program & Administrative Assistant
Cindy Goldman, Patient & Caregiver Support Coordin

78   National Childhood Cancer Foundation
4600 East West Highway, Suite 600
Bethesda, MD 20814

301-718-0042
800-458-6223
Fax: 301-718-0047
info@curesearch.org
www.curesearch.org

CureSearch for Children's Cancer is a national non-profit foundation that accelerates the cure for children's cancer by driving innovation, eliminating research barriers and solving the field's most challenging problems.They fight every day to make treatment possible and a cure probable for the 36 children diagnosed with cancer daily.

Stuart Siegal MD, Chair of the Board
Timothy Harmon, Vice Chair
Mary Payne, Treasurer

79   National Coalition for Cancer Survivorship
1010 Wayne Road, Suite 770
Silver Spring, MD 20910

301-650-9127
888-650-9127
Fax: 301-565-9670
info@canceradvocacy.org
www.canceradvocacy.org

NCCS advocates for quality cancer care for all people touched by cancer and provides tools that empower people to advocate for themselves. Founded by and for cancer survivors, NCCS created the widely accepted definition of survivorship and defines someone as a cancer survivor from the time of diagnosis and for the balance of life.

Michael L Kappel, Chair
Samira K Beckwith, Vice Chair
Barbara Hoffman J.D, Secretary

State Agencies & Support Groups

Alaska

80   Leukemia & Lymphoma Society - Washington/ Alaska Chapter
Leukemia & Lymphoma Society
5601 6th Avenue, Ste 182
Seattle, WA 98108

206-628-0777
anne.gillingham@lls.org
www.lls.org/washingtonalaska

Dedicated to finding cures for leukemia and related cancers and to improving the quality of life for patients and their families.

Anne Gillingham, Executive Director
Courtney Hale, Operations Director
Victoria Wenick, Senior Campaign Director

North Carolina

81   Leukemia & Lymphoma Society - North Carolina Chapter
Leukemia & Lymphoma Society
401 Harrison Oaks Blvd, Ste 200
Cary, NC 27513

919-367-4100
800-888-9934
Fax: 704-998-5010
emily.blust@lls.org
www.lls.org/north-carolina

The mission of The Leukemia & Lymphoma Society (LLS) is to Cure leukemia, lymphoma, Hodgkin's disease and myeloma, and improve the quality of life of patients and their families.LLS is the world's largest voluntary health agency dedicated to blood cancer. LLS funds lifesaving blood cancer research around the world and provides free information and support services.

Emily Blust, Executive Director

Ohio

82 Leukemia & Lymphoma Society - Central Ohio Chapter
2215 Citygate Drive, Suite A
Columbus, OH 43219
614-476-7194
800-686-CURE
Fax: 614-476-7189
breana.shawver@lls.org
www.lls.org/central-ohio

Dedicated to finding cures for leukemia and related cancers and to improving the quality of life for patients and their families.

Breana Shawver, Executive Director
Dan Swisher, Operations Manager

83 Leukemia & Lymphoma Society - Northern Ohio Chapter
5700 Brecksville Road 3rd Floor
Independence, OH 44131
216-264-5680
800-589-5721
Fax: 440-617-2879
lindsay.silverstein@lls.org
www.lls.org/northern-ohio

Dedicated to finding cures for leukemia and related cancers and to improving the quality of life for patients and their families.

Lindsay Silverstein, Executive Director
Deborah Kending, Patient Services Manager

84 Leukemia & Lymphoma Society - Tri-State Southern Ohio Chapter
4370 Glendale Milford Road
Cincinnati, OH 45242
513-698-2828
Fax: 513-351-5386
tom.carleton@lls.org
www.lls.org/tri-state-southern-ohio

Dedicated to finding cures for leukemia and related cancers and to improving the quality of life for patients and their families. This chapter serves a 22-county geographic area that includes Adams, Brown, Butler, Clermont, Clinton, Darke, Gallia, Greene, Hamilton, Highland, Jackson, Lawrence, Meigs, Miami, Montgomery, Pike, Preble, Scioto and Warren counties in Ohio and Boone, Campbell and Kenton counties in Kentucky.

Tom Carleton, Executive Director
Cris Peterson, Dayton Area Director

Oklahoma

85 Leukemia & Lymphoma Society - Oklahoma Chapter
Leukemia & Lymphoma Society
500 N Broadway, Suite 250
Oklahoma City, OK 73102
405-943-8888
888-828-4572
Fax: 405-945-8355
jeannine.laughlin@lls.org
www.lls.org/oklahoma

Our Mission: Cure leukemia, lymphoma, Hodgkin's disease and myeloma, and improve the quality of life for patients and their families.

Jeannine Laughlin, Business Developmnt Mgr In Training

Oregon

86 Leukemia & Lymphoma Society - Oregon Chapter
9320 SW Barbur Boulevard Suite 350
Portland, OR 97219
503-245-9866
800-466-6572
Fax: 503-245-9865
stephanie.carlson@lls.org
www.lls.org

Dedicated to finding cures for leukemia and related cancers and to improving the quality of life for patients and their families.

Stephanie Carlson, Executive Director

Pennsylvania

87 Leukemia & Lymphoma Society - Western Pennsylvania/West Virginia Chapter
333 E. Carson Street, Ste, 441
Pittsburgh, PA 15219
412-263-2873
800-726-2873
Fax: 412-395-2888
christina.massari@lls.org
www.lls.org

Dedicated to finding cures for leukemia and related cancers and to improving the quality of life for patients and their families.

Tina Massari-Thompson, Executive Director
Jeanne Caliguiri, Director of Development
Robert Stout, Operations Director

Tennessee

88 Leukemia & Lymphoma Society, Tennessee Chapter
404 BNA Drive, Suite 102
Nashville, TN 37217
615-331-2980
800-332-2980
Fax: 615-331-2941
jeff.parsley@lls.org
www.lls.org/tennessee

To better serve the needs of Tennesseans - offers contribution-funded community services, family support groups, free educational materials and financial assistance for those affected by leukemia, Hodgkin's disease, myeloma and the lymphomas.

Jeff Parsley, Executive Director

Texas

89 Leukemia & Lymphoma Society - North Texas Chapter
8111 LBJ Freeway, Suite 425
Dallas, TX 75251
972-996-5900
800-800-6702
Fax: 972-239-0892
carol.withers@lls.org
www.lls.org

Dedicated to finding cures for leukemia and related cancers and to improving the quality of life for patients and their families.

Patricia Thomson, Executive Director
Stacey Russell, Deputy Executive Director
Kacy Lowe, Senior Director

90 Leukemia & Lymphoma Society - South Central Texas - San Antonio Chapter
1218 Arion Parkway, Ste 102
San Antonio, TX 78216
210-998-5400
800-683-2458
clarissa.flores@lls.org
www.lls.org/south-central-texas

Dedicated to finding cures for leukemia and related cancers and to improving the quality of life for patients and their families.

Clarissa Flores, Executive Director
Alana Seger, Area Director
Linda Juarez, Director, Operations

91 Leukemia & Lymphoma Society - Texas Gulf Coast Chapter
5433 Westheimer Suite 300
Houston, TX 77056
713-840-0483
Fax: 281-683-9504
billiesue.parris@lls.org
www.lls.org/texas-gulf-coast

Dedicated to finding cures for leukemia and related cancers and to improving the quality of life for patients and their families.

Billie Sue Parris, Executive Director
Charley Tauer, Development Director

Virginia

92 **Leukemia & Lymphoma Society - National Capital Area Chapter**
Leukemia & Lymphoma Society
3601 Eisenhower Avenue, Ste 450
Alexandria, VA 22304
703-399-2900
Fax: 703-960-0920
beth.gorman@lls.org
www.lls.org/national-capital-area

Serves the greater Washington DC metropolitan area, including Northern Virginia, Prince George's and Montgomery counties.

Beth Gorman, Executive Director
Jaclyn Toll, Deputy Executive Director
Mary Angelo, Sr Campaign Director, Special Event

Washington

93 **Leukemia & Lymphoma Society - Washington/ Alaska Chapter**
Leukemia & Lymphoma Society
5601 6th Avenue, Ste 182
Seattle, WA 98108
206-628-0777
anne.gillingham@lls.org
www.lls.org/washingtonalaska

Dedicated to finding cures for leukemia and related cancers and to improving the quality of life for patients and their families.

Anne Gillingham, Executive Director
Courtney Hale, Operations Director
Victoria Wenick, Senior Campaign Director

Wisconsin

94 **Leukemia & Lymphoma Society - Wisconsin Chapter**
4125 North 124th Street, No A
Brookfield, WI 53005
262-790-4701
800-261-7399
Fax: 262-790-4706
liz.klug@lls.org
www.lls.org/wisconsin

To serve Wisconsites touched by leukemia, lymphoma, Hodgkin's disease and myeloma.

Liz Klug, Executive Director
Karen Ropel, Deputy Executive Director
Naomi Gould, Director, Light The Night

Libraries & Resource Centers

95 **Children's National Health System**
George Washington University
111 Michigan Avenue NW
Washington, DC 20010
202-476-5000
888-884-2327
tbear@childrensnational.org
www.childrensnational.org

Children's National serves as the regional referral center for pediatric emergency, cancer, trauma, cardiac and critical care as well as neonatology, orthopaedic surgery, neurology, and neurosurgery.

Kurt Newman, MD, President and CEO
Vittorio Gallo, PhD, Chief Research Officer
Mark Batshaw, Executive VP & CAO

Research Centers

96 **International Bone Marrow Transplant Registry**
Medical College of Wisconsin
9200 W Wisconsin Avenue Suite C5500
Milwaukee, WI 53226
414-805-0700
Fax: 414-805-0714
contactus@cibmtr.org
www.cibmtr.org/pages/index.aspx

CIBMTR collaborates with the global scientific community to advance hematopoietic cell transplantation and cellular therapy research worldwide.

Jeffery Chell MD, Executive Leader
Mary Horowitz MD, Executive Leader
J. Douglas Rizzo MD, MS, Executive Leader

Conferences

97 **ACLP Annual Conference**
Association of Child Life Professionals
1820 N Fort Myer Drive, Ste 520
Arlington, VA 22209
501-483-4500
800-252-4515
Fax: 501-483-4482
aclpadmin@childlife.org
www.childlife.org

The premier educational experience for child life professionals. The largest gathering of child life specialists of the year, offers ample opportunities for both formal and informal networking with peers.

1,000 May

Jennifer Lipsey, Interim CEO
Ramona Spencer, Manager, Conferences & Events

Audio Video

98 **Coping with Childhood Cancer**
Films for the Humanities and Sciences
132 West 31st Street
New York, NY 10001
800-257-5126
Fax: 609-275-0266
custserv@films.com
www.ffh.films.com

Coping with chronic and perhaps fatal disease and gaining control over their lives is something that childhood cancer victims must learn. This program presents open and honest interviews with five family members of childhood cancer patients. The stress on the family is intense; ofteh, the brothers and sisters of children with cancer or any chronic life-threatening illness are most severely affected emotionally.

28 minutes
ISBN: 1-421320-42-7

99 **My Hair's Falling Out...Am I Still Pretty?**
Necessary Pictures
7 W 20th Street, Suite 2F
New York, NY 10011
212-675-1809
800-221-3170

Moving film about two children with cancer who are hospital roommates. Using dance, animation and music, the video explores the feelings of the patients, families, and friends while it sensitively informs and educates the viewers about the emotional and physical aspects of childhood cancer. The child with leukemia grows up to become a doctor, while her roommate with a tumor dies. For school-age children and their families. Purchase is $25 for families and $79 for professionals.

22 minutes
ISBN: 0-965083-20-9

Web Sites

100 ALL Kids
www.all-kids.org/

ALL Kids is an Internet mailing list providing support for families and caregivers of children with Acute Lymphoblastic Leukemia.

101 CancerCare
275 Seventh Avenue
New York, NY 10001

212-712-8400
800-813-4673
Fax: 212-712-8495
info@cancercare.org
www.cancercare.org

CancerCare is a national nonprofit, 501(c)(3) organization that provides free, professional support services to anyone affected by cancer: people with cancer, caregivers, children, loved ones, and the bereaved. CancerCare programs - including counseling and support groups, education, financial assistance and practical help - are provided by professional oncology social workers and are completely free of charge.

Patricia J Goldsmith, CEO
John Rutigliano, Chief Operating Officer
Ahuva Morris, Children's Program Coordinator

102 Children's Cancer Web
www.cancerindex.org/ccw

An independent nonprofit site, established to provide a directory of childhood cancer resources.

103 Leukemia & Lymphoma Society
3 International Drive, Ste 200
Rye Brook, NY 10573

914-949-5213
Fax: 914-949-6691
www.lls.org

Is the largest voluntary health organization dedicated to funding blood cancer research, education and patient services. The mission is to cure leukemia, lymphoma, Hodgkin's disease and myeloma, and to improve the quality of life of patients and their families.

Louis J. DeGennaro, Ph.D., President/ CEO
Andrew Coccari, Chief Product Officer
Danielle Gee, Chief of Staff

Book Publishers

104 Blood & Circulatory Disorders Sourcebook 4th Edition
Omnigraphics
615 Griswold, Ste 901
Detroit, MI 48226

800-234-1340
contact@omnigraphics.com
www.omnigraphics.com

Basic consumer health information on blood and its components, anemias, leukemias, bleeding disorders, and circulatory system disorders, including aplastic anemia, thrombophilia, RH disease and hemophilia.

600 pages
ISBN: 0-780817-46-9

105 Childhood Leukemia: A Guide for Families, Friends & Caregivers
O'Reilly & Associates
1005 Gravenstein Highway North
Sebastopol, CA 95472

707-827-7019
800-889-8969
Fax: 707-824-8268
orders@oreilly.com
www.oreilly.com

Features a wealth of tools to help parents become strong advocates for their child, detailed and precise medical information, and day-to-day practical advice to help cope with procedures, hospitalization, family and friends, schools, social, emotional and financial issues.

528 pages Softcover
ISBN: 0-596500-15-7

Tim O'Reilly, Founder/CEO

106 Draw Me a Picture
Cancervive
11636 Chayote Street
Los Angeles, CA 90049

310-203-9232
800-486-2873
Fax: 310-471-4618
cancervivr@aol.com
www.cancervive.org

A fun coloring book for children with cancer (ages three to six). Marty Bunny talks about how it was when he was in the hospital for cancer and invites readers to draw about their experiences.

107 Having Leukemia Isn't So Bad, of Course, It Wouldn't Be My First Choice
Sargasso Enterprises
18 Ginn Road
Winchester, MA 01890

781-729-9037
Fax: 781-729-2726
cak@krumme.com

Personal story of Catherine Krumme, diagnosed with leukemia at age four, relapsed at age seven, finished treatment at age ten. Catherine graduated from college in 1998 and went on to graduate school. The book is a supportive resource for families with cancer, for their friends, and for teachers working with children with health issues.

149 pages Softcover
ISBN: 0-963555-44-8

Ann Combs

108 Kathy's Hats: A Story of Hope
Albert Whitman and Company
250 South Northwest Highway, Suite 320
Park Ridge, IL 60068

847-232-2800
800-255-7675
Fax: 847-581-0039
mail@albertwhitman.com
www.albertwhitman.com

A charming book for ages five to ten about chemotherapy and the loss of Kathy's hair.

32 pages Hardcover
ISBN: 0-807541-16-8

Trudy Krisher, Author

109 Let's Talk About Going to the Hospital
Rosen Publishing Group's PowerKids Press
29 E 21st Street
New York, NY 10010

212-777-3017
800-237-9932
Fax: 888-436-4643
rosenpub@tribeca.ios.com
www.rosenpublishing.com

If a child has to check into the hospital, chances are he or she is already upset about being ill. Knowing how a hospital functions and what the procedures are, such as when family members can visit, will help in what is already a stressful situation. Grades K-5.

24 pages
ISBN: 0-823950-36-0

110 Pediatric Cancer Sourcebook
Omnigraphics
PO Box 31-1640
Detroit, PA 48231

800-234-1340
Fax: 800-875-1340
info@omnigraphics.com
omnigraphics.com

Basic consumer health information about leukemias, brain tumors, sarcomas, lymphomas and other cancers in infants, children and adolescents.

587 pages
ISBN: 0-780802-45-4

111 Surviving Childhood Cancer: A Guide for Families
New Harbinger Publications
5674 Shattuck Avenue
Oakland, CA 94609
510-652-0215
800-748-6273
Fax: 800-652-1613
customerservice@newharbinger.com
newharbinger.com

Cancer in a child is an overwhelming experience for a family. This book explains common medical procedures and offers readers practical advice about how to cope with emotions and stress during this time.

1998 215 pages
ISBN: 1-572241-02-0

Magazines

112 Coping with Cancer Magazine
PO Box 682268
Franklin, TN 37068
615-790-2400
Fax: 615-614-3986
info@copingmag.com
www.copingmag.com

A bimonthly publication devoted to people whose lives have been touched by cancer.

Paula Chadwell, Vice President

Pamphlets

113 Resource Center for the American Alliance of Cancer - Pain Initiatives
Wisconsin Cancer Pain Initiative
1300 University Avenue, Room 4720
Madison, WI 53706
608-262-0978
Fax: 608-265-4014
trc@mailplus.wisc.edu
www.aacpi.org

A booklet that helps parents determine if their child is in pain and provides methods to manage the pain. Single copy free. Also available, a Handbook of Cancer Pain Management, 5th edition.

12 pages Paperback

Camps

114 Arizona Camp Sunrise & Sidekicks
PO Box 27872
Tempe, AZ 85285
480-382-8564
melissa@azcampsunrise.org
www.azcampsunrise.org

The camp is dedicated to provide an exciting, medically safe camp program for children whose families have been affected by cancer.

Melissa Lee, Camp Director

115 Big Sky Kids Cancer Camp
6901 Goldenstein Lane
Bozeman, MT 59715
406-586-1781
Fax: 406-586-5794
bigskykids@eaglemount.org
www.eaglemount.org

Provides a positive environment and give children, teens, and their parents emotional support, a sense of normalcy, and a network of friends who share similar experiences.

Mary Peterson, Executive Director
Chad Biggerstaff, Big Sky Program Director
Kara Erickson, Director

116 Camp Catch-A-Rainbow
American Cancer Society
1755 Abbey Rd
East Lansing, MI 48823
517-332-3300
kwilson@ymcastorercamps.org
www.cancer.org

Open to any child, ages 7 thru 15, who has, or has had, cancer.

Katie Wilson, Coordinator

117 Camp Fantastic
Special Love
117 Youth Development Court
Winchester, VA 22602
504-667-3774
888-930-2707
Fax: 540-667-8144
www.specialove.org

Nonprofit organization that provides enriching programs for children with cancer, including Camp Fantastic.

Dave Smith, CEO
Angela Ashman, Program Director

118 Camp Sunshine Dreams
PO Box 28232
Fresno, CA 93729
contact@campsunshinedreams.com
www.campsunshinedreams.com

Summer camp for children with cancer.

Anthony Aiello, Board Member

119 Des Moines YMCA Camp
1192 166th Drive
Boone, IA 50036
515-432-7558
Fax: 515-432-5414
ycamp@dmymca.org
www.y-camp.org

For boys and girls with cancer, diabetes, asthma, cystic fibrosis, hearing impaired and other disabilities.

David Sherry, Executive Director
Alex Kretzinger, Program Director

120 Okizu Foundation Camps
16 Digital Drive, Suite 130
Novato, CA 94949
415-382-9083
Fax: 415-382-8384
info@okizu.org
www.okizu.org

This foundation runs family camp programs for children who have cancer and their families, and for children who have or had a parent with cancer.

Lori Sparrow, Executive Director
Heather Ferrier, Camp Director of Operations

DESCRIPTION

121   ACUTE MYELOID LEUKEMIA
Synonyms: Acute granulocytic leukemia, Acute myeloblastic leukemia, Acute myelocytic leukemia, Acute myelogenous leukemia, Acute myelomonocytic leukemia, AML
Involves the following Biologic System(s):
Hematologic and Oncologic Disorders

Acute myeloid leukemia (AML) is a malignant disease, or cancer, characterized by excessive production in the bone marrow of the white blood cells called myelocytes, sometimes also known as granulocytes, which are vital in helping the body to combat and prevent infection. Although AML is primarily a disease of adulthood (median age at onset is 60 years), it is responsible for about 20% of all childhood leukemias.

The symptoms and characteristic findings associated with AML result from the accumulation of myelocytes in the bone marrow, eventually impairing the ability of the marrow to produce mature blood cells. In addition, myelocytes are released into the general blood circulation and carried to other organs, where they continue to grow at a rapid rate.

Children and young adults with AML exhibit fatigue, fever, lethargy, headache and bone or joint pain. In older adults, AML tends to have a slow, progressive onset, with lethargy, loss of appetite, and shortness of breath. Other findings may include enlargement of the liver and spleen (hepatosplenomegaly) and swollen lymph glands. Some children with AML may have swollen gums, as well as swelling of the salivary glands, which are located in front of the ears. Other effects of AML can include small leukemic cell tumors (chloromas) that develop under the skin or on the membranes surrounding the brain and spinal cord, and are followed by inflammation of these membranes (meningitis). Most children with AML develop irregularities in the blood, such as an abnormal deficiency in the numbers of circulating red blood cells (anemia) and platelets (thrombocytopenia), although the white blood cell count may range from low to high. Because AML directly affects cells that enable the body to fight off infection, one of its most serious effects is an increased susceptibility to severe, frequent infections.

AML results from mutations in the genes of myeloblasts or myelocytes, or from damage to these genes or chromosomes. This damage distorts the functions of the affected genes in such a way as to cause uncontrolled cell division and a subsequent rapid increase in the numbers of leukemic blood cells. Factors that may increase the risk for developing AML include genetic disorders such as trisomy 21 (the chromosome abnormality responsible for Down syndrome), Bloom syndrome (caused by a gene mutation and marked by small red lesions and sensitivity to light), Fanconi anemia (caused by any of several gene mutations), and certain other inherited disorders. Chemotherapy or radiation for earlier malignancies, as well as exposure to benzene or cigarette smoke, can also increase the risk of developing AML.

The diagnosis of AML is confirmed from a bone marrow sample obtained through biopsy. Treatment of AML is directed initially toward destroying leukemic cells through the use of drugs (chemotherapy) in an initial, induction phase intended to destroy leukemic cells and induce remission. This is followed with a second phase of chemotherapy to destroy any remaining leukemic cells, and by a further, "remission" phase of therapy to ensure lasting destruction of such cells. The chemotherapy used against AML may be given intravenously by infusion into the blood, or by infusion into the spinal canal. In some cases, radiation is directed at the brain and spinal cord to destroy leukemic cells. Chemotherapy or radiation directed at the brain and spinal cord is known as "intrathecal therapy." In some cases, bone marrow from a suitable donor is given to patients with AML to "reconstitute" or restore their capacity to produce normal myelocytes, and better enable them to defend themselves against infection and other effects of the disease.

Because the potent drugs used in chemotherapy also suppress white blood cell production, thus increasing susceptibility to infection, antibiotic therapy is often given to prevent infection. In some patients, transfusions of red blood cells and platelets are given to ease anemia and bleeding irregularities. Greater than 70% of adults younger than 60 achieve complete remission with treatment for AML. For some patients, a bone marrow or cord blood transplant may offer the best chance for a long-term remission.

Government Agencies

122   NIH/National Cancer Institute
BG 9609 / 9609 Medical Center Drive
Bethesda, MD 20892   800-422-6237
                                                    www.cancer.gov

The National Cancer Institute coordinates the National Cancer Program, which conducts and supports research, training, health information dissemination, and other programs with respect to the cause, diagnosis, prevention, and treatment of cancer, rehabilitation from cancer, and the continuing care of cancer patients and the families of cancer patients.
Douglas R. Lowy, MD, Acting Director
James Doroshow, MD, Deputy Director
Henry P. Ciolino, PhD, Acting Director, Cancer Centers

123   NIH/National Heart, Lung and Blood Institute
National Institute of Health
31 Center Dr MSC 2486, Bldg 31, Room 5A52
Bethesda, MD 20892   301-592-8573
                                              Fax: 240-629-3246
                                              TTY: 240-629-3255
                                         nhlbiinfo@nhlbi.nih.gov
                                                 www.nhlbi.nih.gov

The National Heart, Lung, and Blood Institute (NHLBI) provides global leadership for a research, training, and education program to promote the prevention and treatment of heart, lung, and blood diseases and enhance the health of all individuals so that they can live longer and more fulfilling lives.
Gary H Gibbons, MD, Director
Nakela Cook, MD, Chief of Staff

National Associations & Support Groups

124   American Academy of Pediatrics
141 Northwest Point Boulevard
Elk Grove Village, IL 60007   847-434-4000
                                                    800-433-9016
                                              Fax: 847-434-8000
                                                    www.aap.org

The American Academy of Pediatrics and its member pediatricians are committed to the attainment of optimal physical, mental and social health and well-being for all infants, children, adolescents, and young adults.

Fernando Stein, MD, FAAP, President
Karen Remley, MD, CEO/Executive VP

125   American Childhood Cancer Organization (fo rmerly Candlelighters Childhood Cancer)
PO Box 498
Kensington, MD 20895

301-962-3520
855-858-2226
Fax: 310-962-3521
staff@acco.org
www.acco.org

The American Childhood Cancer Organization (ACCO) was founded in 1970 by a group of parents whose children had been diagnosed with cancer. Today, ACCO is one of the largest grass-roots, national organizations dedicated to improving the lives of children and adolescents with cancer and their families.

Ruth I. Hoffman, MPH, Executive Director
Jessica DiBenedetto, Program Coordinator
Christy Perry, Director, Marketing/Communications

126   Association of Child Life Professionals
1820 N Fort Myer Drive, Ste 520
Arlington, MD 22209

501-483-4500
800-252-4515
Fax: 501-483-4482
aclpadmin@childlife.org
www.childlife.org

Professionals who strive to reduce the impact of stressful or trau-matic life events and situations which affect the development, health and well being of infants, children, youth and families. They embrace the value of play as a healing modality while work-ing to enhance the normal growth and development of children through assessment, intervention, prevention, advocacy and edu-cation. The council offers publications, annual conferences, professional certification and more.

Jennifer Lipsey, Interim CEO
Yvonne Kassimatis, Marketing & Communications
Ramona Spencer, Manager, Conferences & Events

127   B.A.S.E. Camp Children's Cancer Foundation
650 North Wymore Rd, #103
Winter Park, FL 32789

407-673-5060
Fax: 407-673-5095
info@basecamp.org
www.basecamp.org

Provides a year round base of support for children and families facing the challenge of living with cancer, hemophilia and other blood related illnesses.

Terri Jones, President
Cindy Whitaker, Program Coordinator
Rachel Perez, Office Administrator

128   Believe In Tomorrow Children's Foundation
6601 Frederick Road
Baltimore, MD 21228

410-744-1032
Fax: 410-744-1984
info@believeintomorrow.org
www.believeintomorrow.org

Provides housing services and a variety of special services and programs (such as beach and mountain retreats or attending Ori-oles games) to any child up to 18 years of age who is being treated for cancer. Services are provided free of charge and are available on an ongoing basis throughout treatment.

Brian Morrison, Founder and CEO
Richard E McCready, Chairman
David Reymann, Vice Chairman

129   CancerCare
275 7th Avenue
New York, NY 10001

212-712-8400
800-813-4673
Fax: 212-712-8495
info@cancercare.org
www.cancercare.org

CancerCare provides free, professional support services to indi-viduals, families, caregivers and the bereaved to help them cope with and manage the emotional and practical challenges of cancer.

Patricia J Goldsmith, CEO
John Rutigliano, Chief Operating Officer
Ahuva Morris, Children's Program Coordinator

130   Children's Cancer & Blood Foundation
333 E 38th Street, Suite 830
New York, NY 10016

212-297-4336
Fax: 212-297-4340
info@childrenscbf.org
www.childrenscbf.org

The foundation's major emphasis is on blood diseases affecting children: leukemia, thalassemia, hemophilia, sickle cell anemia, platelet disorders, retinoblastoma and cancer.

Drew Phillips, President
Greg Karakashian, Operations Associate

131   Children's Leukemia Association
National Leukemia Research Association
585 Stewart Avenue, Suite 18
Garden City, NY 11530

516-222-1944
Fax: 516-222-0457
info@childrensleukemia.org
www.childrensleukemia.org

A not-for-profit organization dedicated to raising funds to sup-port research efforts towards finding the causes and cure for leukemia.

Anthony Pasqua, President
Henry Green, Esq., Vice President
William Regina, Secretary/Treasurer

132   Dreams Come True Emery Clinic-Peds
1365 Clfton Road NE
Atlanta, GA 30322

404-778-5000
800-753-6679
www.emoryhealthcare.org

Serves any child with cancer or chronic blood disease treated at Emory University Homo/Onc Clinic. Dreams submitted by chil-dren.

John T. Fox, President/ CEO
Anne Adams, JD, Chief Compliance Officer
William A. Bornstein, MD, PhD, Chief Quality Officer

133   Hair Club for Kids: Hair Club for Men
270 Farmington Avenue, Suite 232 (Second Floor)
Farmington, CT 06032

860-674-0202
800-269-7384
Fax: 860-676-0805
www.hairclub.com/hairclub-for-kids.php

Since 1992, Hair Club has offered free hair restoration services to children who suffer from diseases that lead to hair loss or alope-cia. Hair Club for Kids is a non-profit program funded entirely by Hair Club that's available at no charge to children ages 6-17.

Sy Sperling, Founder
Steven Barth, President
Lydia Cassarino, Manager

134   ICARE
PO Box 341657
Bethesda, MD 20814

301-652-3461
800-422-7361
contact@icare.org
www.icare.org

The International Care Alliance for Research and Education (ICARE) is a nonprofit organization which provides high-quality, focused, user-friendly, cancer information to each patient as well as their physician on an on-going, and person to person basis.

David Hankins, Executive Director

135   Just In Time
PO Box 27693
Philadelphia, PA 19118

215-247-8777
Fax: 215-247-0956
tome@softhats.com
www.softhats.com

All cotton headwear for girls and women who have experienced hair loss.

Verlay Platt, President

136 Leukemia & Lymphoma Society
3 International Drive, Ste 200
Rye Brook, NY 10573
914-949-5213
Fax: 914-949-6691
infocenter@lls.org
www.lls.org

Largest voluntary health organization dedicated to funding blood cancer research, education and patient services.

Louis J. DeGennaro, PhD, President & CEO
Andrew Coccari, Chief Product Officer
Danielle Gee, Chief of Staff

137 National Bone Marrow Transplant Link
20441 W 12 Mile Road, Suite 108
Southfield, MI 48076
248-358-1886
800-546-5268
info@nbmtlink.org
www.nbmtlink.org

Publications designed to help you understand and deal with the logistics of bone marrow transplantation, finances and medical insurance, information about the National Bone Marrow Transplant Link and its peer support program, and a celebration of BMT survivor stories.

Myra Jacobs, Founding Director
Denise Lillvis, Executive Director
Cindy Goldman, Patient & Caregiver Support Coordin

138 National Coalition for Cancer Survivorship
1010 Wayne Road, Suite 770
Silver Spring, MD 20910
301-650-9127
888-650-9127
Fax: 301-565-9670
info@canceradvocacy.org
www.canceradvocacy.org

NCCS advocates for quality cancer care for all people touched by cancer and provides tools that empower people to advocate for themselves. Founded by and for cancer survivors, NCCS created the widely accepted definition of survivorship and defines someone as a cancer survivor from the time of diagnosis and for the balance of life.

Michael L Kappel, Chair
Samira K Beckwith, Vice Chair
Barbara Hoffman J.D, Secretary

State Agencies & Support Groups

New York

139 Leukemia & Lymphoma Society - Westchester/ Connecticut/Hudson Valley Chapter
3 Landmark Square, Suite 330
Stamford, CT 06901
203-388-9160
deborah.barker@lls.org
www.lls.org

Cure leukemia, lymphoma, Hodgkin's disease and myeloma and improve the quality of life of patients and their families.

Deborah Barker, Executive Director
Brandy Sinisi, Operations Manager

140 Leukemia & Lymphoma Society - Western & Central New York Chapter
4043 Maple Road, Suite 105
Amherst, NY 14226
716-834-2578
800-955-4572
nancy.hails@lls.org
www.lls.org/western-central-new-york

Dedicated to finding cures for leukemia and related cancers and to improving the quality of life for patients and their families.

Nancy Hails, Executive Director
Luann Burgio, Deputy Executive Director
Sue Michalak, Operations Manager

North Carolina

141 Leukemia & Lymphoma Society - North Carolina Chapter
Leukemia & Lymphoma Society
401 Harrison Oaks Blvd, Ste 200
Cary, NC 27513
919-367-4100
800-888-9934
emily.blust@lls.org
www.lls.org/north-carolina

Dedicated to finding cures for leukemia and related cancers and to improving the quality of life for patients and their families.

Emily Blust, Executive Director

Ohio

142 Leukemia & Lymphoma Society - Central Ohio Chapter
2215 Citygate Drive, Suite A
Columbus, OH 43219
614-476-7194
800-686-CURE
Fax: 614-476-7189
breana.shawver@lls.org
www.lls.org/central-ohio

Dedicated to finding cures for leukemia and related cancers and to improving the quality of life for patients and their families.

Breana Shawver, Executive Director
Dan Swisher, Operations Manager

143 Leukemia & Lymphoma Society - Northern Ohio Chapter
5700 Brecksville Road 3rd Floor
Independence, OH 44131
216-264-5680
800-589-5721
Fax: 440-617-2879
lindsay.silverstein@lls.org
www.lls.org/northern-ohio

Dedicated to finding cures for leukemia and related cancers and to improving the quality of life for patients and their families.

Lindsay Silverstein, Executive Director
Deborah Kending, Patient Services Manager

144 Leukemia & Lymphoma Society - Tri-State Southern Ohio Chapter
4370 Glendale Milford Road
Cincinnati, OH 45242
513-698-2828
Fax: 513-351-5386
tom.carleton@lls.org
www.lls.org/tri-state-southern-ohio

Dedicated to finding cures for leukemia and related cancers and to improving the quality of life for patients and their families. This chapter serves a 22-county geographic area that includes Adams, Brown, Butler, Clermont, Clinton, Darke, Gallia, Greene, Hamilton, Highland, Jackson, Lawrence, Meigs, Miami, Montgomery, Pike, Preble, Scioto and Warren counties in Ohio and Boone, Campbell and Kenton counties in Kentucky.

Tom Carleton, Executive Director
Cris Peterson, Dayton Area Director
Roseann Hayes, Campaign Director, Special Events

Oklahoma

145 Leukemia & Lymphoma Society - Oklahoma Chapter
Leukemia & Lymphoma Society
500 N Broadway, Suite 250
Oklahoma City, OK 73102
405-943-8888
888-828-4572
Fax: 405-945-8355
jeannine.laughlin@lls.org
www.lls.org/oklahoma

Our Mission: Cure leukemia, lymphoma, Hodgkin's disease and myeloma, and improve the quality of life for patients and their families.

Jeannine Laughlin, Business Developmnt Mgr In Training

Oregon

146 Leukemia & Lymphoma Society - Oregon Chapter
9320 SW Barbur Boulevard Suite 350
Portland, OR 97219   503-245-9866
                                    800-466-6572
                               Fax: 503-245-9865
                          stephanie.carlson@lls.org
                                     www.lls.org

Dedicated to finding cures for leukemia and related cancers and
to improving the quality of life for patients and their families.

Stephanie Carlson, Executive Director

Pennsylvania

**147 Leukemia & Lymphoma Society - Western Pennsylvania/West
Virginia Chapter**
333 E. Carson Street, Ste. 441
Pittsburgh, PA 15219   412-263-2873
                                    800-726-2873
                               Fax: 412-395-2888
                          christina.massari@lls.org
                                     www.lls.org

Dedicated to finding cures for leukemia and related cancers and
to improving the quality of life for patients and their families.

Tina Massari, Executive Director
Jeanne Caliguiri, Director of Development
Robert Stout, Operations Director

Tennessee

148 Leukemia & Lymphoma Society, Tennessee Chapter
404 BNA Drive, Suite 102
Nashville, TN 37217   615-331-2980
                                    800-332-2980
                               Fax: 615-331-2941
                            jeff.parsley@lls.org
                             www.lls.org/tennessee

To better serve the needs of Tennesseans - offers contribution-funded community services, family support groups, free educational materials and financial assistance for those affected by
leukemia, Hodgkin's disease, myeloma and the lymphomas.

Jeff Parsley, Executive Director

Texas

149 Leukemia & Lymphoma Society - North Texas Chapter
8111 LBJ Freeway, Suite 425
Dallas, TX 75251   972-996-5900
                                    800-800-6702
                               Fax: 972-239-0892
                            carol.withers@lls.org
                                     www.lls.org

Dedicated to finding cures for leukemia and related cancers and
to improving the quality of life for patients and their families.

Patricia Thomson, Executive Director
Stacey Russell, Deputy Executive Director
Kacy Lowe, Senior Director

**150 Leukemia & Lymphoma Society - South Central Texas - San
Antonio Chapter**
1218 Arion Parkway, Ste 102
San Antonio, TX 78216   210-998-5400
                                    800-683-2458
                           clarissa.flores@lls.org
                        www.lls.org/south-central-texas

Dedicated to finding cures for leukemia and related cancers and
to improving the quality of life for patients and their families.

Clarissa Flores, Executive Director
Alana Seger, Area Director
Linda Juarez, Director, Operations

151 Leukemia & Lymphoma Society - Texas Gulf Coast Chapter
5433 Westheimer Suite 300
Houston, TX 77056   713-840-0483
                               Fax: 281-683-9504
                          billiesue.parris@lls.org
                           www.lls.org/texas-gulf-coast

Dedicated to finding cures for leukemia and related cancers and
to improving the quality of life for patients and their families.

Billie Sue Parris, Executive Director
Charley Tauer, Development Director

Virginia

**152 Leukemia & Lymphoma Society - National Capital Area
Chapter**
3601 Eisenhower Avenue, Ste 450
Alexandria, VA 22304   703-399-2900
                               Fax: 703-960-0920
                             beth.gorman@lls.org
                        www.lls.org/national-capital-area

Serves the greater Washington DC metropolitan area, including
Northern Virginia, Prince George's and Montgomery counties.

Beth Gorman, Executive Director
Jaclyn Toll, Deputy Executive Director
Mary Angelo, Sr Campaign Dir, Special Events

Wisconsin

153 Leukemia & Lymphoma Society - Wisconsin Chapter
200 S. Executive Drive Suite 203
Brookfield, WI 53005   262-790-4701
                                    800-261-7399
                               Fax: 262-790-4706
                               liz.klug@lls.org
                             www.lls.org/wisconsin

To serve Wisconsites touched by leukemia, lymphoma, Hodgkin's disease and myeloma.

Liz Klug, Executive Director
Karen Ropel, Deputy Executive Director
Naomi Gould, Director, Light The Night

Libraries & Resource Centers

154 Children's National Health System
George Washington University
111 Michigan Avenue NW
Washington, DC 20010   202-476-5000
                                    888-884-2327
                        tbear@childrensnational.org
                         www.childrensnational.org

Children's National serves as the regional referral center for pediatric emergency, cancer, trauma, cardiac and critical care as
well as neonatology, orthopaedic surgery, neurology, and
neurosurgery.

Kurt Newman, MD, President/CEO
Vittorio Gallo, PhD, Chief Research Officer
Mark Batshaw, Executive VP & CAO

Audio Video

155 Coping with Childhood Cancer
Films for the Humanities and Sciences
132 West 31st Street
New York, NY 10001   800-257-5126
                               Fax: 609-275-0266
                             custserv@films.com
                               www.ffh.films.com

Coping with chronic and perhaps fatal disease and gaining control over their lives is something that childhood cancer victims must learn. This program presents open and honest interviews with five family members of childhood cancer patients. The stress on the family is intense; ofteh, the brothers and sisters of children with cancer or any chronic life-threatening illness are most severely affected emotionally.

28 minutes
ISBN: 1-421320-42-7

Web Sites

156   CancerCare
275 Seventh Avenue
New York, NY 10001
800-813-4673
info@cancercare.org
www.cancercare.org

CancerCare is a national nonprofit, 501(c)(3) organization that provides free, professional support services to anyone affected by cancer: people with cancer, caregivers, children, loved ones, and the bereaved. CancerCare programs - including counseling and support groups, education, financial assistance and practical help - are provided by professional oncology social workers and are completely free of charge.

Patricia J Goldsmith, CEO
John Rutigliano, Chief Operating Officer
Ahuva Morris, Children's Program Coordinator

157   Children's Cancer Web
www.cancerindex.org/ccw

An independent nonprofit site, established to provide a directory of childhood cancer resources.

158   Leukemia & Lymphoma Society
3 International Drive, Ste 200
Rye Brook, NY 10573
914-949-5213
Fax: 914-949-6691
www.lls.org

Is the largest voluntary health organization dedicated to funding blood cancer research, education and patient services. The mission is to cure leukemia, lymphoma, Hodgkin's disease and myeloma, and to improve the quality of life of patients and their families.

Louis J. DeGennaro, Ph.D., President/ CEO
Andrew Coccari, Chief Product Officer
Danielle Gee, Chief of Staff

159   Mediconsult
www.mediconsult.com

We are committed to provide excellent and professional services to our business partners. Through a team approach we will develop, provide and continuously improve our knowledge and competency. We work towards the betterment of healthcare delivery systems for the community.

Book Publishers

160   Blood & Circulatory Disorders Sourcebook 4th Edition
Omnigraphics
615 Griswold, Ste 901
Detroit, MI 48226
800-234-1340
Fax: 800-875-1340
contact@omnigraphics.com
www.omnigraphics.com

Basic consumer health information on blood and its components, anemias, leukemias, bleeding disorders, and circulatory system disorders, including aplastic anemia, thrombophilia, RH disease and hemophilia.

600 pages
ISBN: 0-780817-46-9

161   Let's Talk About Going to the Hospital
Rosen Publishing Group's PowerKids Press
29 E 21st Street
New York, NY 10010
212-777-3017
800-237-9932
Fax: 888-436-4643
rosenpub@tribeca.ios.com
www.rosenpublishing.com

If a child has to check into the hospital, chances are he or she is already upset about being ill. Knowing how a hospital functions and what the procedures are, such as when family members can visit, will help in what is already a stressful situation. Grades K-5.

24 pages
ISBN: 0-823950-36-0

162   Let's Talk About when Kids Have Cancer
Rosen Publishing Group's PowerKids Press
29 E 21st Street
New York, NY 10010
212-777-3017
800-237-9932
Fax: 888-436-4643
customerservice@rosenpub.com
www.rosenpublishing.com

In a straightforward yet comforting way, this book explains what cancer is, what kinds of treatments surround the disease and how to cope if a child has cancer.

24 pages
ISBN: 0-823951-95-2

163   Pediatric Cancer Sourcebook
Omnigraphics
PO Box 31-1640
Detroit, PA 48231
800-234-1340
Fax: 800-875-1340
info@omnigraphics.com
omnigraphics.com

Basic consumer health information about leukemias, brain tumors, sarcomas, lymphomas and other cancers in infants, children and adolescents.

587 pages
ISBN: 0-780802-45-4

164   Surviving Childhood Cancer: A Guide for Families
New Harbinger Publications
5674 Shattuck Avenue
Oakland, CA 94609
510-652-0215
800-748-6273
Fax: 800-652-1613
customerservice@newharbinger.com
newharbinger.com

Cancer in a child is an overwhelming experience for a family. This book explains common medical procedures and offers readers practical advice about how to cope with emotions and stress during this time.

1998 215 pages
ISBN: 1-572241-02-0

Pamphlets

165   Acute Lymphocytic Leukemia
Leukemia & Lymphoma Society
3 International Drive, Ste 200
Rye Brook, NY 10573
914-949-5213
Fax: 914-949-6691
www.lls.org

Information about acute lymphocytic leukemia for patients and their families and a glossary of terms to help readers understand technical terms.

16 pages

Louis J. DeGennaro, Ph.D., President/ CEO
Rosemarie Loffredo, CAO/ CFO
Mark Roithmayr, Chief Development Officer

Camps

166   Arizona Camp Sunrise & Sidekicks
PO Box 27872
Tempe, AZ 85285   480-382-8564
                                         928-478-4564
                                melissa@azcampsunrise.org
                                  www.azcampsunrise.org

The camp is dedicated to provide an exciting, medically safe
camp program for children whose families have been affected by
cancer.

Melissa Lee, Camp Director

167   Camp Catch-A-Rainbow
American Cancer Society
1205 E Saginaw Street
Lansing, MI 48906   517-371-2920
                                         800-227-2345
                              kwilson@ymcastorercamps.org
                                www.cancer.org/camprainbow

Open to any child, age 7 thru 15, who has, or has had, cancer.

Katie Wilson, Coordinator

168   Camp Fantastic
Special Love
117 Youth Development Court
Winchester, VA 22602   703-667-3774
                                         888-930-2707
                                       www.specialove.org

Nonprofit organization that provides enriching programs for children with cancer, including Camp Fantastic.

Dave Smith, CEO
Angela Ashman, Program Director

169   Camp Sunshine Dreams
PO Box 28232
Fresno, CA 93729   contact@campsunshinedreams.com
                          www.campsunshinedreams.com

Summer camp for children with cancer.

Anthony Aiello, Board Member

170   Des Moines YMCA Camp
1192 166th Drive
Boone, IA 50036   515-432-7558
                                    Fax: 515-432-5414
                                     ycamp@dmymca.org
                                       www.y-camp.org

For boys and girls with cancer, diabetes, asthma, cystic fibrosis,
hearing impaired and other disabilities.

David Sherry, Executive Director
Mike Havlik, Program Director
Alex Kretzinger, Program Director- Summer Camp

171   Okizu Foundation Camps
16 Digital Drive, Suite 130
Novato, CA 94949   415-382-9083
                                    Fax: 415-382-8384
                                        info@okizu.org
                                         www.okizu.org

This foundation runs family camp programs for children who
have cancer and their families, and for children who have or had a
parent with cancer.

Lori Sparrow, Executive Director
Heather Ferrier, Camp Director of Operations

DESCRIPTION

172 ALBINISM

Covers these related disorders: Tyrosinase negative albinism, Oculocutaneous albinism, Waardenburg syndrome

Involves the following Biologic System(s):
Dermatologic Disorders,
Genetic/Chromosomal/Syndrome/Metabolic Disorders

Albinism refers to a condition that is present at birth (congenital) and results from an inability of the body to produce and distribute the pigment melanin, which normally gives the skin, hair, and eyes their coloration. Albinism occurs in all races and in about one in 20,000 individuals worldwide.

Although there are several types of albinism, and all are caused by genetic defects, two major forms of the condition - tyrosinase-negative, and tyrosinase-positive - have been identified.

Tyrosinase-negative, or type I, albinism is the most severe form of generalized oculocutaneous albinism, or OCA. It results from a genetic defect that reduces or eliminates the activity of tyrosinase, an enzyme essential to the proper metabolism of melanin. Because of the absence of this enzyme, type I is characterized by a complete lack of melanin in the hair, skin, and eyes, resulting in pink or white skin, white hair, and eyes that may appear pink or bluish-gray. Other eye-related or optical irregularities also occur in type I, such as involuntary, flickering-type movements of the eyes (nystagmus), nearsightedness (myopia), and sensitivity or intolerance to bright light (photophobia). OCA type 1 is an autosomal recessive condition, meaning that it develops only when both parents carry the gene responsible for OCA type 1. A variant form of OCA type 1, in which some pigmentation develops in the skin, hair, and eyes with age, occurs in Amish communities in the United States. The optical irregularities in this variant form of OCA type 1 are usually less severe than in the more common form of the condition.

Tyrosinase-positive, or type II OCA is more common and less severe than type I. Rather than being caused by an absence of the enzyme tyrosinase, this type of albinism is thought to result from an inborn error in the transport of the substance known as tyrosinea which the body normally transforms into melanin. Newborns with OCA type II may have little to no melanin at birth, but it may accumulate in their skin, hair, and eyes as these children grow, producing some darkening of skin color during the course of childhood. Moreover, ocular abnormalities present at birth may ease over the course of childhood. Like OCA type I, OCA type II is caused by a genetic defect and is inherited as an autosomal recessive trait. Several variant forms of tyrosinase-positive albinism may be present as a part of several syndromes that affect other organs or systems of the body in addition to its pigmentation. Among these syndromes are Hermansky-Pudlak syndrome, Chediak-Higashi syndrome, and Cross-McKusick-Breen syndrome.

Types of albinism other than OCA types I and II may include ocular albinism that chiefly affects the pigmentation of the eyes and is characterized by photophobia; nystagmus; and decreased visual acuity. The hair and eyes of such persons may be of lighter than average color, but not excessively so. In what are known as Nettleship-Falls type ocular albinism and Forsius-Eriksson syndrome, ocular albinism may be inherited as a trait, or characteristic, that is associated with or "linked to" the X chromosome, which is inherited from an individual's mother. Ocular albinism may also be inherited as an autosomal dominant trait, in which it results from only a single copy of a defective gene, inherited from either a mother or a father.

Besides these various types of albinism, some individuals may have partial albinism, sometimes called piebaldism, which is characterized by patchy, unpigmented areas of hair or skin. In some individuals this type of albinism may be manifested only by a lock of white hair near the forehead. Piebaldism is inherited as an autosomal dominant trait, and may be part of the condition known as Waardenburg syndrome, which is also characterized by hearing impairment.

Because people with albinism have an increased risk of developing skin cancer from exposure to the sun, protection of their skin is highly important. This may be accomplished with suitable clothing and the use of an appropriate sunscreen of SPF 15 or greater. The deficit in pigmentation of the eyes in albinism may require the use of tinted or dark glasses to reduce light sensitivity. Children with albinism should have early evaluation and treatment for any visual irregularities caused by the condition, to minimize any difficulties at school. Other treatment is symptomatic and supportive.

Government Agencies

173 NIH/ Eunice Kennedy Shriver National Institute of Child Health & Human Development
31 Center Drive, Building 31
Bethesda, MD 20892
301-496-5113
800-370-2943
Fax: 866-760-5947
TTY: 888-320-6942
nichdpress@mail.nih.gov
www.nichd.nih.gov

Established in 1962 by congress, today the institute conducts and supports laboratory research, clinical trials, and epidemiological studies that explore health processes; examines the impact of disabilities, diseases, and variations on the lives of individuals; and sponsors training programs for scientists, health care providers, and researchers to ensure that NICHD research can continue.

Diana W. Bianchi, Director
Paul Williams, Director, Communications

National Associations & Support Groups

174 American Academy of Pediatrics
141 Northwest Point Boulevard
Elk Grove Village, IL 60007
847-434-4000
800-433-9016
Fax: 847-434-8000
www.aap.org

The American Academy of Pediatrics and its member pediatricians are committed to the attainment of optimal physical, mental and social health and well-being for all infants, children, adolescents, and young adults.

Fernando Stein, MD, FAAP, President
Karen Remley, MD, CEO/Executive VP

175   American Council of the Blind
1703 Beauregard Street, Ste 420
Alexandria, VA 22311   202-467-5081
                                         800-424-8666
                                         Fax: 703-465-5085
                                         info@acb.org
                                         www.acb.org

The council strives to improve the well being of all blind and visually impaired people by serving as a representative national organization of blind people, elevating the social, ecomonic and
cultural levels of blind people, improving educational and rehabilitation facilities and opportunities and cooperating with the
public and private institutions and organizations concerned with
blind services.

Eric Bridges, Executive Director
Anthony Stephens, Director, Advocacy/Govt'l Affairs
Nancy Marks-Becker, Chief Accountant

176   American Foundation for the Blind
2 Penn Plaza, Suite 1102
New York, NY 10121   212-502-7600
                                         800-232-5463
                                         Fax: 888-545-8331
                                         afbinfo@afb.net
                                         www.afb.org

The American Foundation of the Blind, has been eliminating barriers the prevent people who are blind or visually impaired from
reaching their potential. AFB is dedicated to addressing the most
critical issues of facing this growing population: independent living, literacy, employment, and technology.

Kirk Adams, President & CEO
Adrianna Montague-Devaud, Chief Communications/Mkting Officer

177   American School Counselor Association
1101 King Street, Suite 310
Alexandria, VA 22314   703-683-2722
                                         800-306-4722
                                         Fax: 703-997-7572
                                         asca@schoolcounselor.org
                                         www.schoolcounselor.org

The mission of ASCA is to represent professional school counselors and to promote professionalism and ethical practices.

Richard Wong, Executive Director
Jeff Broderson, Information Technology Admin.
Kathleen M Rakestraw, Director of Communications

178   Genetic Alliance
4301 Connecticut Avenue NW, Suite 404
Washington, DC 20008   202-966-5557
                                         800-336-4363
                                         Fax: 202-966-8553
                                         info@geneticalliance.org
                                         www.geneticalliance.org

World's leading nonprofit health advocacy organization committed to transforming health through genetics and promoting an environment of openness centered on the health of individuals,
families, and communities.

Sharon Terry, President/CEO
Tetyana Murza, Managing Director
Natasha Bonhomme, VP, Strategic Development

179   Hermansky-Pudlak Syndrome Network
One South Road
Oyster Bay, NY 11771   516-922-3440
                                         800-789-9477
                                         Fax: 516-922-0640
                                         info@hpsnetwork.org
                                         www.hpsnetwork.org

A volunteer, support group for people and families dealing with
Hermansky-Pudlak Syndrome (HPS) and related disorders such as
Chediak Higashi Syndrome.

Donna Jean Appell, Founder & President
Heather Kirkwood, VP, Director of Outreach
Richard Appell, Treasurer

180   Natalie's Way Foundation
16 Lyle Court
Staten Island, NY 10306   718-351-0806
                                         admin@natalieswayfoundation.com
                                         www.ourwebpage.org

Conducts fundraising for research into albinism and children's
eye disorders.

Robert Stasi, President
Annette Stasi, VP

181   National Mental Health Consumers' Self-Help Clearinghouse
1211 Chestnut Street, Suite 1207
Philadelphia, PA 19107   215-751-1810
                                         800-553-4539
                                         Fax: 215-636-6312
                                         info@mhselfhelp.org
                                         www.mhselfhelp.org

The Clearinghouse works to foster peer empowerment through
our website, up-to-date news and information announcements, a
directory of peer-driven services, electronic and printed publications, training packages, and individual and onsite consultation

Joseph Rogers, Executive Director & Founder
Susan Rogers, Director of Special Projects
Britani Nestel, Program Specialist

182   National Organization for Albinism and Hypopigmentation
PO Box 959
East Hampstead, NH 03826   603-887-2310
                                         800-473-2310
                                         Fax: 800-648-2310
                                         webmaster@albinism.org
                                         www.albinism.org

NOAH is a volunteer organization for persons and families involved with the condition of albinism. It does not diagnose, treat,
or provide genetic counseling. It is involved in self-help, while
trying to promote research and education.

Mike McGowan, Executive Director & Founder
Sheila Adamo, Chair
Donna Appell, Vice Chair

183   Positive Exposure
Rick Guidotti
43 E 20th Street, 6th Floor
New York, NY 10003   212-420-1931
                                         Fax: 212-228-0592
                                         rick@positiveexposure.org
                                         www.rickguidotti.com

Utilizes photography and video interviews to investigate the social and psychological experiences of people with albinism of all
ages and ethnocultural heritages. This innovative program challenges the stigma associated with difference, attacks public fears
about difference and celebrates the richness of genetic variation.

Rick Guidotti, Founder and Director
Liz Matejka Grossman, Executive Director
Cecilia Burbridge, Administrative Assistant

184   Society for Pediatric Dermatology
8365 Keystone Crossing, Suite 107
Indianapolis, IN 46240   317-202-0224
                                         Fax: 317-205-9481
                                         info@pedsderm.net
                                         www.pedsderm.net

The objective of the Society is to promote, develop and advance
education, research and care of skin disease in all pediatric age
groups.

Kent Lindeman, Executive Director
Karen Wiss, President
Andrea Zaenglen, President-Elect

185   Vision of Children Foundation
4310 Genesee Ave, Suite 101
San Diego, CA 92117   858-560-5181
                                         Fax: 858-560-1926
                                         frontoffice@visionsource-drsneag.com
                                         www.visionsource-drsneag.com

Provides information, promotes research and assists the families of blind and visually impaired children, including those with ocular albinism, in locating organizations and service providers who can give support.

Gary Sneag, Manager
Vivian L Hardage, Chairman & Co-Founder
Stephanie Durso, Executive Director

Conferences

186 Annual World Symposium on Ocular Albinism
11975 El Camino Real, Suite 104
San Diego, CA 92130
858-314-7917
Fax: 858-314-7920
info@visionofchildren.org
www.visionofchildren.org

The Vision of Children Foundation's team of doctors, scientists and researchers will collaborate on their research efforts in Ocular Albinism.

March

Samuel A Hardage, Chairman & Co-Founder
Vivian L Hardage, Co-Founder
Debora B Farber, Chief Scientific Advisor

187 Genetic Alliance Annual Conference
Genetic Alliance
4301 Connecticut Avenue NW, Suite 404
Washington, DC 20008
202-966-5557
800-336-4363
Fax: 202-966-8553
info@geneticalliance.org
www.geneticalliance.org

Consistently inspirational and enables partnership among all stakeholders: advocates and community leaders, health and industry professionals, policymakers, and academicians.

July

Sharon Terry, President/CEO
Tetyana Murza, Managing Director
Natasha Bonhomme, VP, Strategic Development

188 Hermansky-Pudlak Syndrome Network Annual Family Conference
One South Road
Oyster Bay, NY 11771
516-922-3440
800-789-9477
Fax: 516-922-4022
appell@worldnet.att.net
www.medhelp.org/web/hpsn.htm

A volunteer, nonprofit, self-help support group for persons and families dealing with the syndrome. Assists in networking families and doctors, maintains a bibliography of materials and promotes research.

Donna Jean Appell, Founder & President

189 NFB National Convention
American Foundation for the Blind
2 Penn Plaza, Suite 1102
New York, NY 10121
212-502-7600
800-232-5463
Fax: 212-502-7777
afbinfo@afb.net
www.afb.org

The largest disability conference of its kind.

3000

Carl R Augusto, President/CEO
Paul Schroeder, Vice President
Rick Bozeman, CFO

190 National Organization for Albinism and Hypopigmentation Bi-Annual Conference
PO Box 959
East Hampstead, NH 03826
603-887-2310
800-473-2310
Fax: 800-648-2310
webmaster@albinism.org
www.albinism.org

NOAH holds a national conference every other year (even years).

191 Society for Pediatric Dermatology Annual Meeting
8365 Keystone Crossing, Suite 107
Indianapolis, IN 46240
317-202-0224
Fax: 317-205-9481
info@pedsderm.net
www.pedsderm.net

Kent Lindeman, Executive Director

Audio Video

192 Assistive Media
400 Maynard Street, Suite 404
Ann Arbor, MI 48104
734-332-0369
info@assistivemedia.org
www.assistivemedia.org/

The mission of Assistive Media is to heighten the educational, cultural, and quality-of-living standard for people with disabilites and help achieve independence and become better integrated within the mainstream of society and community life in general. Assistve Media accomplishes this by providing free-of-charge, copyright-approved, high caliber audio literary works to the world-wide disability community via the internet effectively, inexpensively, and efficiently.

David Henry Erdody, Founder

Web Sites

193 International Albinism Center
www.cbc.umn.edu/iac/
IAC is a team of dedicated research professionals interested in understanding the basis of albinism in humans. We are a munlti-disciplinary group of researchers that include interests in clinical genetics, molecular biology, ophthalmology, dermatology, and biochemistry, all with a central theme of understnading the cause and effect of albinism and other forms of pigment loss in humans.

Journals

194 Pediatric Dermatology Journal
Society for Pediatric Dermatology
8365 Keystone Crossing, Suite 107
Indianapolis, IN 46240
317-202-0224
Fax: 317-205-9481
info@pedsderm.net
www.pedsderm.net

6 issues/yr

Kent Lindeman, Executive Director

Newsletters

195 Hermansky-Pudlak Syndrome Network Newsletter
One South Road
Oyster Bay, NY 11771
516-922-3440
800-789-9477
Fax: 516-624-0640
info@hpsnetwork.org
www.hpsnetwork.org

A volunteer, nonprofit, self-help support group for persons and families dealing with the syndrome. Assists in networking families and doctors, maintains a bibliography of materials and promotes research.

Donna Jean Appell, R.N., Founder/President
Heather Kirkwood, VP/ Director of Outreach
Richard Appell, Treasurer

Camps

196 Camp Discovery
American Academy of Dermatology
930 E Woodfield Road
Schaumburg, IL 60173

847-240-1280
866-503-7546
Fax: 847-240-1859
jmueller@aad.org
www.campdiscovery.org

A camp for young people with chronic skin conditions. There is no fee and transportation is provided. Three locations: Camp Horizon in Millville, PA, Camp Knutson in Crosslake, MN, and Camp Dermadillo in Burton, TX.

David M Pariser, MD, President
Janine Mueller, Program Coordinator

DESCRIPTION

197   ALOPECIA AREATA

Synonyms: Alopecia circumscripta, Androgenetic alopecia, Pelade

Involves the following Biologic System(s):

Dermatologic Disorders, Immunologic and Rheumatologic Disorders

Alopecia is partial or complete loss of hair (baldness) and may result from genetic factors, aging or local or systemic disease. Alopecia areata is characterized by the sudden, localized loss of patches of scalp hair and other areas of hair growth, such as the eyelashes and eyebrows. These patches are usually well-defined, round or oval in shape, and most often appear on the scalp or beard area. On rare occasions, progression of hair loss may result in the total loss of scalp hair in a condition called alopecia totalis. If the disease progresses to include the total loss of both scalp and body hair, the condition is called alopecia universalis. Another uncommon form of alopecia areata called ophiasis involves the loss of hair in a continuous band around the head. If hair loss associated with alopecia areata is not widespread, the condition is usually reversible, with most patients exhibiting new hair growth within a few months to a year; however, recurrences are quite common. Children who develop this condition at a very young age, patients who experience recurring episodes, and those who have extensive involvement are less likely to experience spontaneous remission. Although this disease occurs most commonly in the adult population, approximately 20 percent of those affected develop the disorder between birth and 20 years of age. This type of hair loss is different than male pattern baldness, an inherited condition.

Although the skin in the area of hair loss may appear unremarkable, microscopic examination may reveal the presence of inflammation. In addition, some individual hairs that appear at the margins of the bald, patchy areas may be easily removed and, upon microscopic examination, reveal a lightly-pigmented, tapered hair shaft that ends in a hair root that is reduced in size (exclamation hairs). Symptoms or characteristic findings sometimes associated with alopecia areata include the development of irregularities such as nail pitting and ridging, allergic or hypersensitivity reactions, and opacities of the lenses of the eye (cataracts). Alopecia areata may also be associated with certain autoimmune diseases such as Addison disease, Hashimoto thyroiditis, vitiligo, and others. In addition, approximately seven percent of children with Trisomy 21 exhibit the symptoms associated with alopecia areata.

The exact cause of alopecia areata is not known; however, approximately 25 percent of those affected are believed to inherit the disease through autosomal dominant transmission. Other suggested causes include autoimmune responses or emotional factors related to stress. Because alopecia areata so often resolves spontaneously, treatment for this disease in young children may simply include ongoing observation. A variety of treatments can be tried. Steroid injections and cream to the scalp have been used for many years. Other medications include minoxidil, irritants (anthralin or topical coal tar), and topical immunotherapy (cyclosporine), each of which are sometimes used in different combinations. The use of hairpieces and other cosmetic considerations may be beneficial to the emotional well-being of children, especially adolescents, with alopecia areata.

National Associations & Support Groups

198   American Academy of Dermatology
PO Box 4014
Schaumburg, IL 60168

866-503-7546
Fax: 847-240-1859
MRC@aad.org
www.aad.org

The AAD is the largest, and most representative dermatology group in the United States.

Dirk M. Elston, President
Lisa A. Garner MD, Vice President
Brett M Coldiron MD, President-Elect

199   American Academy of Pediatrics
141 Northwest Point Boulevard
Elk Grove Village, IL 60007

847-434-4000
800-433-9016
Fax: 847-434-8000
www.aap.org

The American Academy of Pediatrics and its member pediatricians are committed to the attainment of optimal physical, mental and social health and well-being for all infants, children, adolescents, and young adults.

Fernando Stein, MD, FAAP, President
Karen Remley, MD, CEO/Executive VP

200   American Autoimmune Related Diseases Association, Inc.
22100 Gratiot Avenue
Eastpointe, MI 48021

586-776-3900
800-598-4668
Fax: 586-776-3903
aarda@aarda.org
www.aarda.org

The American Autoimmune Related Diseases Association is dedicated to the eradication of autoimmune diseases and the alleviation of suffering and the socioeconomic impact of autoimmunity through fostering and facilitating collaboration in the areas of education, public awareness, research, and patient services in an effective, ethical and efficient manner.

Virginia T. Ladd, President/Executive Director
Patricia Barber, Assistant Director
Deb Patrick, Events Specialist

201   American Hair Loss Association
23679 Calabasas Road #682
Calabasas, CA 91301

inquire@americanhairloss.org
www.americanhairloss.org

The American Hair Loss Association is committed to educating and improving the lives of all those affected by hair loss. It is their goal to create public awareness of this devastating disease of the spirit, and to legitimize hair loss of all forms in the eyes of our medical community, the media and society as a whole.

202   Children's Alopecia Project
PO Box 6036
Wyomissing, PA 19610

610-468-1011
info@childrensalopeciaproject.org
www.childrensalopeciaproject.org

The mission is to help any child in need who is living with hair loss due to all forms of Alopecia.

Betsy Woytovich, Executive Director
Wayne Gehris, President
Christine Cieplinski, Vice President

203   National Alopecia Areata Foundation
14 Mitchell Boulevard
San Rafael, CA 94903

415-472-3780
Fax: 415-472-5343
info@naaf.org
www.naaf.org

NAAF supports research to find a cure or acceptable treatment for alopecia areata, supports those with the disease, and educates the public about alopecia areata. NAAF is widely regarded as the largest, most influential and most representative foundation associated with alopecia areata.

Maureen McGettigan, Chair
Bob Flint, Chief Financial Officer
Hoy Lanning, Secretary

204   Society for Pediatric Dermatology
8365 Keystone Crossing, Suite 107
Indianapolis, IN 46240

317-202-0224
Fax: 317-205-9481
info@pedsderm.net
www.pedsderm.net

The objective of the Society is to promote, develop and advance education, research and care of skin disease in all pediatric age groups.

Kent Lindeman, Executive Director
Karen Wiss, President
Andrea Zaenglen, President-Elect

Conferences

205   National Alopecia Areata Foundation Annual Conference
National Alopecia Areata Foundation
14 Mitchell Boulevard
San Rafael, CA 94903

415-472-3780
Fax: 415-472-5343
info@naaf.org
www.naaf.org

A four day conference for people of all ages who have alopecia areata or care about someone who has alopecia areata. Provides the attendee with the latest medical and research updates, to better understand and manage alopecia areata, and also provides them with a wealth of support.

June

Vicki Kalabokes, President/CEO
Jeanne Rappoport, VP Administration/Meetings

Web Sites

206   Children's Alopecia Project
www.childrensalopeciaproject.org

The mission is to help any child in need who is living with hair loss due to all forms of Alopecia.

Jeff Woytovich, Founder/Director
Betsy Woytovich, Co-Founder
Christine Cieplinski, President

Journals

207   Pediatric Dermatology Journal
Society for Pediatric Dermatology
8365 Keystone Crossing, Suite 107
Indianapolis, IN 46240

317-202-0224
Fax: 317-205-9481
info@pedsderm.net
www.pedsderm.net

6 issues/yr
Kent Lindeman, Executive Director

Newsletters

208   Infocus Newsletter
American Autoimmune Related Diseases Associaion
22100 Gratiot Avenue
Eastpointe, MI 48021

586-776-3900
Fax: 586-776-3903
www.aarda.org

The national newsletter of AARDA.

The Rev. Herbert G. Ford, D. Min., Chairman of the Board
Stanley M. Finger, Ph.D., Vice Chairperson
Virginia T. Ladd, President/ Executive Director

209   National Alopecia Areata Foundation Newsletter
National Alopecia Areata Foundation
65 Mitchell Boulevard, Suite 200-B
San Rafael, CA 94903

415-472-3780
Fax: 415-480-1800
info@naaf.org
www.naaf.org

NAAF publishes their award winning newsletter four times a year. It is a great resource and is written especially for the alopecia areata community.

Vicki Kalabokes, President/CEO
Jeanne Rappoport, Chief Administrative Officer
Maureen Smith, Chief Development Strategist

DESCRIPTION

210 ALPHA-1-ANTITRYPSIN DEFICIENCY
Involves the following Biologic System(s):
Gastrointestinal Disorders,
Genetic/Chromosomal/Syndrome/Metabolic Disorders, Respiratory
Disorders

Alpha-1-antitrypsin (AAT) deficiency is a hereditary metabolic disorder characterized by deficiency of alpha-1-antitrypsin, an enzyme that is produced by the liver and inhibits the actions of other enzymes that break down certain proteins. Deficiency of alpha-1-antitrypsin may result in emphysema, a progressive destructive change in the lungs. In addition, some patients may experience liver disease that is thought to result from abnormal retention of the alpha-1-antitrypsin enzyme in liver cells. Alpha-1-antitrypsin deficiency is caused by certain changes (mutations) of a gene known as Pi (protease inhibitor). Alpha-1-antitrypsin deficiency is typically inherited as an autosomal recessive trait due to inheritance of two deficiency-causing genes (homozygosity).

The specific symptoms associated with alpha-1-antitrypsin deficiency as well as the age of onset vary from patient to patient. Shortly after birth, a small percentage of affected children may develop suppression or cessation of the flow of bile (neonatal cholestasis). Bile, a liquid secreted by the liver, carries waste products away from the liver and assists in the digestion of fats in the small intestine. During the first week of life, affected infants may have yellowish discoloration of the skin, whites of the eyes, and mucous membranes (jaundice); abnormal enlargement of the liver (hepatomegaly); and the presence of unabsorbed fat in the feces. Jaundice often spontaneously resolves within two to four months after birth. Affected infants and children may appear to have no further associated symptoms (asymptomatic), may have chronic liver disease, or, in the most severe cases, may experience scarring of the liver and gradual impairment of liver function (cirrhosis). Older children may develop chronic liver disease or cirrhosis and associated high blood pressure within veins from the spleen and intestines to the liver (portal hypertension). In some patients with portal hypertension, there may be a diversion of portal circulation to veins in the walls of the stomach and esophagus, causing abnormal widening of such blood vessels (esophageal varices). Without treatment, some patients with liver disease may experience potentially life-threatening complications.

In general, AAT deficiency leads to emphysema, progressive degeneration of and destructive changes in the air sacs (alveoli) of the lungs in the fourth decade of life in smokers and a decade later in nonsmokers. (emphysema).

In children with alpha-1-antitrypsin deficiency, the treatment of associated liver disease is primarily symptomatic and supportive. AAT deficiency is the main cause of liver transplantation in children. Preventing or slowing the progression of lung disease is the major goal of AAT deficiency management. No treatment for emphysema has a greater effect on survival than quitting smoking. Other options include prompt, aggressive treatment of respiratory infections and provision of oxygen therapy. Medications are available to improve lung function. In addition, patients should avoid exposure to tobacco smoke, aerosol sprays, and other lung irritants. Alpha-1-antitrypsin enzyme replacement therapy (e.g., prolastin therapy) is also available. Two surgical approaches may help selected patients with AAT deficiency - volume-reduction surgery and lung transplantation.

National Associations & Support Groups

211 AlphaNet, Inc.
2937 SW 27 Avenue, Suite 305
Coconut Grove, FL 33133
305-442-1776
800-577-2638
Fax: 305-442-1803
info@alphanet.org
www.alphanet.org

Founded to improve the lives of individuals affected by Alpha-1 Antitrypsin Deficiency.AlphaNet provides a wide range of specialized programs and services designed to meet the specific needs of the Alphas it serves.

Robert Barrett, CEO
Robert A. Sandhaus, Medical Director
Janis Berend, Clinical Specialist

212 American Academy of Pediatrics
141 Northwest Point Boulevard
Elk Grove Village, IL 60007
847-434-4000
800-433-9016
Fax: 847-434-8000
www.aap.org

The American Academy of Pediatrics and its member pediatricians are committed to the attainment of optimal physical, mental and social health and well-being for all infants, children, adolescents, and young adults.

Fernando Stein, MD, FAAP, President
Karen Remley, MD, CEO/Executive VP

213 American Liver Foundation
39 Broadway, Suite 2700
New York, NY 10006
212-668-1000
800-465-4837
Fax: 212-483-8179
info@liverfoundation.org
www.liverfoundation.org

The American Liver Foundation is the nation's leading nonprofit organization promoting liver health and disease prevention. ALF provides research, education and advocacy for those affected by liver-related diseases, including hepatitis.

Thomas F Nealon III, Chairman of the Board of Directors
Daniel E Weil, Treasurer and Member of the Executi
Carlo Frappolli, Secretary and Member of the Transit

214 American Lung Association
55 W. Wacker Drive, Suite 1150
Chicago, IL 60601
312-801-7628
800-548-8252
info@lung.org
www.lung.org

The American Lung Association is the leading organization working to save lives by improving lung health and preventing lung disease through Education, Advocacy and Research. With the generous support of the public, we are Fighting for Air.

Harold P. Wimmer, National President & CEO
Susan Rappaport, National VP, Research/Scientific
Sue Swan, Chief Development Officer

215 Children's Liver Association for Support Services
PO Box 15061
Monaca, PA 15061
724-888-2568
info@classkids.org
www.classkids.org

CLASS is an all volunteer, nonprofit organization dedicated to serving the emotional, educational and financial needs of families coping with childhood liver disease and transplantation. Our goal is to be both a service to families and a valuable resource for the medical community.

Diane Sumner, Co-Founder
Mark Sumner, Co-Founder
Aimee Seningen, MD, Treasurer

216 Genetic Alliance
4301 Connecticut Avenue NW, Suite 404
Washington, DC 20008
202-966-5557
800-336-4363
Fax: 202-966-8553
info@geneticalliance.org
www.geneticalliance.org

World's leading nonprofit health advocacy organization committed to transforming health through genetics and promoting an environment of openness centered on the health of individuals, families, and communities.

Sharon Terry, President/CEO
Tetyana Murza, Managing Director
Natasha Bonhomme, VP, Strategic Development

217 March of Dimes Foundation
1275 Mamaroneck Avenue
White Plains, NY 10605
914-997-4488
888-663-4637
Fax: 914-997-4763
answers@marchofdimes.com
www.marchofdimes.com

March of Dimes help moms have full-term pregnancies and research the problems that threaten the health of babies. The March of Dimes also acts globally: sharing best practices in perinatal health and helping improve birth outcomes where the needs are the most urgent.

Stacey D. Stewart, President

Conferences

218 Genetic Alliance Annual Conference
Genetic Alliance
4301 Connecticut Avenue NW, Suite 404
Washington, DC 20008
202-966-5557
800-336-4363
Fax: 202-966-8553
info@geneticalliance.org
www.geneticalliance.org

Consistently inspirational and enables partnership among all stakeholders: advocates and community leaders, health and industry professionals, policymakers, and academicians.

July

Sharon Terry, President/CEO
Tetyana Murza, Managing Director
Natasha Bonhomme, VP, Strategic Development

Web Sites

219 Children's Liver Association for Support Services
www.classkids.org

CLASS is an all volunteer, nonprofit organization dedicated to serving the emotional, educational and financial needs of families coping with childhood liver disease and transplantation. Our goal is to be both a service to families and a valuable resource for the medical community.

220 Online Mendelian Inheritance in Man
National Library of Medicine, Building 38A
Bethesda, MD 20894
888-346-3656
info@ncbi.nlm.nih.gov
www.ncbi.nlm.nih.gov

This database is a catalog of human genes and genetic disorders.

Christine E. Seidman, M.D., Chair
David J. Lipman, M.D., Executive Secretary

Book Publishers

221 Let's Talk About Going to the Hospital
Rosen Publishing Group's PowerKids Press
29 E 21st Street
New York, NY 10010
212-777-3017
800-237-9932
Fax: 888-436-4643
rosenpub@tribeca.ios.com
www.powerkidspress.com

If a child has to check into the hospital, chances are he or she is already upset about being ill. Knowing how a hospital functions and what the procedures are, such as when family members can visit, will help in what is already a stressful situation. Grades K-5.

24 pages
ISBN: 0-823950-36-0

DESCRIPTION

222 ANENCEPHALY

Involves the following Biologic System(s):

Neurologic Disorders

Anencephaly is an abnormality that is present at birth (congenital) and belongs to a group of birth defects known as neural tube defects. This condition is characterized by the absence of a major portion of the brain, skull, and scalp. Approximately one of 1,000 infants is born with anencephaly.

During the early stages of pregnancy, a specialized layer of tissue extends along the back portion of the developing embryo. As the embryo grows, this tissue, known as the neural plate, forms a groove that is bordered by folds. This groove eventually deepens and closes to form the neural tube. Later in development, the neural tube gives rise to tissue that later forms the brain and spinal cord. The neural tube is surrounded and protected by the bones of the back (vertebrae). Failure in this sequence of developmental events results in a neural tube defect.

Anencephaly represents a type of neural tube defect that is incompatible with life. Infants with this disorder are born without a forebrain, the largest part of the brain consisting mainly of the cerebral hemispheres which are responsible for higher level cognition, i.e., thinking. The remaining brain tissue is often exposed - not covered by bone or skin. Infants born with anencephaly are usually blind, deaf, unconscious, and unable to feel pain. Additional physical findings associated with this abnormality include folded ears, incomplete closure of the palate (cleft palate), and congenital heart defects. The cause of anencephaly is unknown, although it is thought to occur as the result of genetic or environmental factors, alone or in combination. Neural tube defects do not follow direct patterns of heredity. However, the theory of a genetic predisposition to anencephaly is supported by the fact that the risk of additional children being born with this defect rises with each pregnancy.

Supplementation with high-dose folic acid, initiated before and given during pregnancy, reduces the risk of neural tube defects to 1%.

Government Agencies

223 NIH/ Eunice Kennedy Shriver National Insti tute of Child Health & Human Development
31 Center Drive, Building 31
Bethesda, MD 20892

301-496-5113
800-370-2943
Fax: 866-760-5947
TTY: 888-320-6942
nichdpress@mail.nih.gov
www.nichd.nih.gov

Established in 1962 by congress, today the institute conducts and supports laboratory research, clinical trials, and epidemiological studies that explore health processes; examines the impact of disabilities, diseases, and variations on the lives of individuals; and sponsors training programs for scientists, health care providers, and researchers to ensure that NICHD research can continue.

Diana W. Bianchi, Director
Paul Williams, Director, Communications

National Associations & Support Groups

224 American Academy of Pediatrics
141 Northwest Point Boulevard
Elk Grove Village, IL 60007

847-434-4000
800-433-9016
Fax: 847-434-8000
www.aap.org

The American Academy of Pediatrics and its member pediatricians are committed to the attainment of optimal physical, mental and social health and well-being for all infants, children, adolescents, and young adults.

Fernando Stein, MD, FAAP, President
Karen Remley, MD, CEO/Executive VP

225 Anencephaly Support Foundation
20311 Sienna Pines Ct.
Spring, TX 77379

281-364-9222
888-206-7526
www.anencephaly.net

A nonprofit religious foundation dedicated to serving parents, families and educational communities. Offered are information, personal stories and medical articles regarding the neural tube defect of anencephaly, support and encouragement to parents who have chosen to carry an anencephalic pregnancy to term, and information regarding possible causations, prevention theories, and support group referrals.

226 Birth Defect Research for Children
976 Lake Baldwin Lane, Suite 104
Orlando, FL 10023

407-895-0802
Fax: 407-895-0824
staff@birthdefects.org
www.birthdefects.org

Birth Defect Research for Children is a non-profit organization that provides parents and expectant parents with information about birth defects and support services for their children.

Betty Mekdeci, Executive Director

227 Genetic Alliance
4301 Connecticut Avenue NW, Suite 404
Washington, DC 20008

202-966-5557
800-336-4363
Fax: 202-966-8553
info@geneticalliance.org
www.geneticalliance.org

World's leading nonprofit health advocacy organization committed to transforming health through genetics and promoting an environment of openness centered on the health of individuals, families, and communities.

Sharon Terry, President/CEO
Tetyana Murza, Managing Director
Natasha Bonhomme, VP, Strategic Development

228 March of Dimes Foundation
1275 Mamaroneck Avenue
White Plains, NY 10605

914-997-4488
888-663-4637
Fax: 914-997-4763
answers@marchofdimes.com
www.marchofdimes.com

March of Dimes help moms have full-term pregnancies and research the problems that threaten the health of babies.The March of Dimes also acts globally: sharing best practices in perinatal health and helping improve birth outcomes where the needs are the most urgent.

Stacey D. Stewart, President

229 National Dissemination Center for Children with Disabilities
1825 Connecticut Avenue NW , Suite 700
Washington, DC 10026

202-884-8200
800-695-0285
Fax: 202-884-8441
nichcy@fhi360.org
www.nichcy.org

A national information and referral center for families, educators and other professionals on: disabilities in children and youth; programs and services; IDEA, the nation's special education law; and research-based information on effective practices.

Suzanne Ripley, Executive Director

Conferences

230 Genetic Alliance Annual Conference
Genetic Alliance
4301 Connecticut Avenue NW, Suite 404
Washington, DC 20008

202-966-5557
800-336-4363
Fax: 202-966-8553
info@geneticalliance.org
www.geneticalliance.org

Consistently inspirational and enables partnership among all stakeholders: advocates and community leaders, health and industry professionals, policymakers, and academicians.

July

Sharon Terry, President/CEO
Tetyana Murza, Managing Director
Natasha Bonhomme, VP, Strategic Development

Web Sites

231 Online Mendelian Inheritance in Man
National Library of Medicine, Building 38A
Bethesda, MD 20894

888-346-3656
info@ncbi.nlm.nih.gov
www.ncbi.nlm.nih.gov

This database is a catalog of human genes and genetic disorders.

Christine E. Seidman, M.D., Chair
David J. Lipman, M.D., Executive Secretary

232 Rare Genetic Diseases in Children (NYU)
www.med.nyu.edu/rgdc/homenow.htm

We target issues arising from rare genetic diseases affecting children. And to assist in the endeavor to bring knowledge and hope to those for whom there is, at present, so little.

DESCRIPTION

233 ANIRIDIA

Synonym: Hypoplasia of iris

Involves the following Biologic System(s):

Ophthalmologic Disorders

Aniridia is a birth defect characterized by absence of all or a portion of the colored area of the eye (iris). Both eyes are typically affected (bilateral aniridia). The term aniridia may be a misnomer, since an undeveloped (vestigial) portion of the iris is usually present (i.e., apparent upon slit-lamp examination or gonioscopy). The iris is an involuntary circular muscle that is visible through the transparent, front portion of the eye (cornea). When certain fibers in the iris contract, the hole in the center of the iris (pupil) either widens or constricts, allowing in additional or less light.

In some infants with aniridia, the corneas of the eyes are also abnormally small. In addition, many affected infants and children experience loss of transparency of the lenses of the eyes (cataracts) or displacement of the lenses, which are located behind the pupils. Aniridia is often associated with underdevelopment (hypoplasia) of the macula, the central portion of the retina that distinguishes detail in the central field of vision.

Additional eye abnormalities often associated with aniridia include rapid, involuntary movements of the eyes (nystagmus); reduced fields of vision; abnormally increased sensitivity to light (photophobia); and progressively increased fluid pressure within the eyes (glaucoma). In most cases, glaucoma is not apparent during the first month of life (neonatal period).

Depending upon the range and severity of associated eye abnormalities, children with aniridia may have varying levels of visual impairment. However, in most cases, affected children may have visual acuity of approximately 20/200 or even further reductions in vision. The clearness or sharpness of vision (i.e., visual acuity) is typically measured on a scale comparing a patient's vision at 20 feet with that of an unaffected individual with full visual acuity. Thus, a person with 20/200 vision sees at 20 feet what someone with full visual acuity sees at 200 feet.

Aniridia may be an isolated condition or may occur in association with certain syndromes, such as WAGR syndrome, a rare disorder characterized by kidney tumors (Wilms tumor), aniridia, genitourinary anomalies (abnormalities of the reproductive and urinary tracts), due to spontaneous genetic changes (mutations), and retardation. WAGR is inherited as an autosomal dominant trait; in very rare cases, aniridia is inherited as an autosomal recessive trait (e.g., aniridia-cerebellar ataxia-mental deficiency). Medical care for aniridia is directed toward prevention of glaucoma and control of intraocular pressure (fluid pressure inside the eye. Other measures focus on specific problems, such as nystagamus, sensitivity to light (photophobia) and supportive measures, such as removal of cataracts. Visual aids, such as artificial pupil contact lenses, may also be used.

Government Agencies

234 NIH/National Eye Institute
31 Center Drive MSC 2510
Bethesda, MD 20892
301-496-5248
2020@nei.nih.gov
www.nei.nih.gov

Conducts and supports research that helps prevent and treat eye diseases and other disorders of vision. This research leads to sight-saving treatments, reduces visual impairment and blindness, and improves the quality of life for people of all ages. NEI-supported research has advanced our knowledge of how the eye functions in health and disease.

Paul A Sieving M.D., Ph.D., Director

National Associations & Support Groups

235 American Academy of Pediatrics
141 Northwest Point Boulevard
Elk Grove Village, IL 60007
847-434-4000
800-433-9016
Fax: 847-434-8000
www.aap.org

The American Academy of Pediatrics and its member pediatricians are committed to the attainment of optimal physical, mental and social health and well-being for all infants, children, adolescents, and young adults.

Fernando Stein, MD, FAAP, President
Karen Remley, MD, CEO/Executive VP

236 Genetic Alliance
4301 Connecticut Avenue NW, Suite 404
Washington, DC 20008
202-966-5557
800-336-4363
Fax: 202-966-8553
info@geneticalliance.org
www.geneticalliance.org

World's leading nonprofit health advocacy organization committed to transforming health through genetics and promoting an environment of openness centered on the health of individuals, families, and communities.

Sharon Terry, President/CEO
Tetyana Murza, Managing Director
Natasha Bonhomme, VP, Strategic Development

237 Lighthouse Guild
15 West 65th Street
New York, NY 10023
212-769-6200
800-284-4422
info@lighthouseguild.org
www.lighthouseguild.org

Since 1905, Lighthouse International has led the charge in the fight against vision loss through prevention, treatment and empowerment. In 2013, it merged with Jewish Guild Healthcare to form a leading non profit vision and healthcare organization.

Alan R. Morse, President/CEO
Mark G. Ackermann, Executive VP/COO
Maura J. Sweeney, Senior VP, Programs & Services

238 March of Dimes Foundation
1275 Mamaroneck Avenue
White Plains, NY 10605
914-997-4488
888-663-4637
Fax: 914-997-4763
answers@marchofdimes.com
www.marchofdimes.com

March of Dimes help moms have full-term pregnancies and research the problems that threaten the health of babies.The March of Dimes also acts globally: sharing best practices in perinatal health and helping improve birth outcomes where the needs are the most urgent.

Stacey D. Stewart, President

239 National Eye Research Foundation
910 Skokie Boulevard, Suite 207A
Northbrook, IL 10031   847-564-4652
                                        800-621-2258
                                        Fax: 847-564-0807
                                        info@nerf.org
                                        www.nerf.org

Devoted to the enhancement of care and study of eye related diseases.

Conferences

240 Genetic Alliance Annual Conference
Genetic Alliance
4301 Connecticut Avenue NW, Suite 404
Washington, DC 20008   202-966-5557
                                        800-336-4363
                                        Fax: 202-966-8553
                                        info@geneticalliance.org
                                        www.geneticalliance.org

Consistently inspirational and enables partnership among all
stakeholders: advocates and community leaders, health and industry professionals, policymakers, and academicians.

July

Sharon Terry, President/CEO
Tetyana Murza, Managing Director
Natasha Bonhomme, VP, Strategic Development

Web Sites

241 Aniridia Network
22 Cornish House, Adelaide Lane
Sheffield, S3 8B   077-2 8-7 94
                                        info@aniridia.org.uk
                                        aniridia.org.uk

We are an international support group which aims to bring people
with aniridia closer together as well as providing practical support and information.

242 Aniridia Web Site
22 Cornish House, Adelaide Lane
Sheffield, S3 8B   077-2 8-7 94
                                        info@aniridia.org.uk
                                        aniridia.org.uk

The Aniridia Network is an international nonprofit organization
dedicated to supporting people with aniridia and their families,
increasing awareness of aniridia and improving the quality of information about aniridia around the world.

243 National Association for Visually Handicapped
111 E 59th St
New York, NY 10022   800-284-4422
                                        info@lighthouseguild.org
                                        www.lighthouseguild.org

Provides information on large print books, textbooks and educational tools.

244 Online Mendelian Inheritance in Man
National Library of Medicine, Building 38A
Bethesda, MD 20894   888-346-3656
                                        info@ncbi.nlm.nih.gov
                                        www.ncbi.nlm.nih.gov

This database is a catalog of human genes and genetic disorders.

Christine E. Seidman, M.D., Chair
David J. Lipman, M.D., Executive Secretary

Book Publishers

245 Children with Visual Impairments: A Parents' Guide
Peytral Publications
PO Box 1162
Minnetonka, MN 55345   952-949-8707
                                        877-739-8725
                                        Fax: 952-906-9777
                                        help@peytral.com
                                        www.peytral.com

Covers visual impairments ranging from low vision to total blindness. Offers authoritative information and empathy, parental insight on diagnosis and treatment, orientation and mobility,
literacy, legal issues and more. Valuable to parents, educators and
support staff.

395 pages

M Cay Holbrook PhD, Editor

246 Let's Talk About Going to the Hospital
Rosen Publishing Group's PowerKids Press
29 E 21st Street
New York, NY 10010   212-777-3017
                                        800-237-9932
                                        Fax: 888-436-4643
                                        rosenpub@tribeca.ios.com
                                        www.rosenpublishing.com

If a child has to check into the hospital, chances are he or she is
already upset about being ill. Knowing how a hospital functions
and what the procedures are, such as when family members can
visit, will help in what is already a stressful situation. Grades
K-5.

24 pages
ISBN: 0-823950-36-0

DESCRIPTION

247 ANKYLOSING SPONDYLITIS

Synonyms: AS, Marie-Strumpell spondylitis

Involves the following Biologic System(s):

Orthopedic and Muscle Disorders

Ankylosing spondylitis (AS) is a chronic, progressive, inflammatory disease that affects joints of the spine and results in pain, stiffness, and possible loss of spinal mobility. In most patients, the joints between the spine and the hipbones (sacroiliac joints) are affected. In addition, joints in the spinal column of the lower back (lumbosacral spine) and the neck (cervical spine) may be involved to varying degrees. Although the disease usually becomes apparent during young adulthood or middle age, it may also begin during childhood. Males are more commonly affected than females.

In most cases, children initially present with periodic inflammation and discomfort in the joints of the arms and legs (transient peripheral arthritis), particularly the large joints of the legs. Many also experience arthritis in the shoulders, the lower jaw bone (i.e., temporomandibular joints), and the feet. Such inflammation results in swelling, pain, abnormal warmth (erythema), and possible limited movement of affected joints. In children with AS, involvement of the sacroiliac joints may be apparent at the disorder's onset or may develop over several months or years. The different regions of the spine may then be progressively affected, usually beginning in the spinal column of the lower back (lumbar spine) and eventually involving the upper back (thoracic spine) and the cervical spine. Children with the disease experience periodic pain and stiffness that may be alleviated by movement. Many have hip, thigh, and lower back pain that is more severe at night and experience stiffness of affected areas in the mornings. In addition, some children have involvement of the joints that connect the ribs to the spine (costovertebral joints). The resulting inflammation, pain, and stiffness may limit expansion of the chest when taking deep breaths. Disease progression may spontaneously cease at any stage; however, in some cases, all regions of the spine may gradually be affected, potentially resulting in severely impaired spinal mobility.

Other symptoms associated with ankylosing spondylitis include fatigue, low-grade fever, lack of appetite (anorexia), low levels ofred blood cells (anemia), growth retardation, and repeated inflammation of the colored region of the eye (iritis) and its muscle (iridocyclitis). Inflammation of the aorta, the largest artery of the body (aoritis), is a finding that is often seen in adults with ankylosing spondylitis, but is rarely seen in affected children.

Research has shown that approximately 95 percent of affected individuals have a specific human leukocyte antigen or HLA. Antigens are proteins that stimulate the body to produce certain antibodies in response to invading microorganisms or foreign tissues. Most individuals with ankylosing spondylitis have a specific genetically determined HLA known as HLA-B27. The possible role of HLA-B27 in predisposing an individual to the disorder has not been determined. Anklosing spondylitis is thought to be an autosomal dominant disorder. In some cases, individuals with a defective gene for AS may not experience symptoms and findings associated with the

disorder (reduced penetrance). AS is thought to have a higher penetrance among males.

Although HLA-B27 is present in most individuals with ankylosing spondylitis, it is not considered diagnostic for the disorder. AS is typically diagnosed based upon a complete patient and family history, characteristic physical findings, and specialized x-ray techniques. Treatment of children is primarily directed toward relieving pain and ensuring proper posture to help preserve spinal mobility. Certain medications may be prescribed to help alleviate or manage pain (e.g., indomethacin or other nonsteroidal antiinflammatory medications [NSAIDs]). Special exercises may be recommended to help strengthen back muscles and maintain proper posture. In addition, certain lifestyle changes may be suggested, including avoiding thick pillows and using a firm mattress. Additional treatment is usually symptomatic and supportive.

Government Agencies

248 NIH/National Institute of Arthritis and Musculoskeletal and Skin Diseases
1 AMS Circle
Bethesda, MD 20892
                                              301-495-4484
                                              877-226-4267
                                    Fax: 301-718-6366
                                    TTY: 301-565-2966
                                    TDD: 301-565-2966
                              niamsinfo@mail.nih.gov
                                    www.niams.nih.gov

The mission of the National Institute of Arthritis and Musculoskeletal and Skin Diseases is to support research into the causes, treatment, and prevention of arthritis and musculoskeletal and skin diseases; the training of basic and clinical scientists to carry out this research; and the dissemination of information on research progress in these diseases

Stephen I Katz MD PhD, Director
Robert H Carter MD, Deputy Director
Gahan Breithaupt, Assoc Dir. Management & Operations

National Associations & Support Groups

249 American Academy of Pediatrics
141 Northwest Point Boulevard
Elk Grove Village, IL 60007
                                              847-434-4000
                                              800-433-9016
                                    Fax: 847-434-8000
                                              www.aap.org

The American Academy of Pediatrics and its member pediatricians are committed to the attainment of optimal physical, mental and social health and well-being for all infants, children, adolescents, and young adults.

Fernando Stein, MD, FAAP, President
Karen Remley, MD, CEO/Executive VP

250 American Autoimmune Related Diseases Association
22100 Gratiot Avenue
Eastpointe, MI 48021
                                              586-776-3900
                                              800-598-4668
                                    Fax: 586-776-3903
                                    aarda@aarda.org
                                        www.aarda.org

The American Autoimmune Related Diseases Association is dedicated to the eradication of autoimmune diseases and the alleviation of suffering and the socioeconomic impact of autoimmunity through fostering and facilitating collaboration in the areas of education, public awareness, research, and patient services in an effective, ethical and efficient manner.

Virginia T. Ladd, President/Executive Director
Patricia Barber, Assistant Director
Deb Patrick, Events Specialist

251 American Juvenile Arthritis Organization
1330 W. Peachtree Street.; Suite 100
Atlanta, GA 10034
404-237-8771
800-933-7023
Fax: 404-237-8153
TTY: 404-965-7904
info.ga@arthritis.org
www.arthritis.org

The Arthritis Foundation is committed to raising awareness and reducing the unacceptable impact of arthritis, a disease which must be taken as seriously as other chronic diseases because of its devastatng consequences.

Daniel T. McGowan, Chair
Rowland W. (Bing) Chang, Vice Chair
Patricia Novak Nelson, Vice Chair

252 Arthritis Foundation
1330 W. Peachtree Street.; Suite 100
Atlanta, GA 10035
404-872-7100
800-568-4045
Fax: 404-872-0457
TTY: 404-965-7904
info.ga@arthritis.org
www.arthritis.org

The Arthritis Foundation is committed to raising awareness and reducing the unacceptable impact of arthritis, a disease which must be taken as seriously as other chronic diseases because of its devastatng consequences.

Daniel T. McGowan, Chair
Rowland W. (Bing) Chang, Vice Chair
Patricia Novak Nelson, Vice Chair

253 March of Dimes Foundation
1275 Mamaroneck Avenue
White Plains, NY 10605
914-997-4488
888-663-4637
Fax: 914-997-4763
answers@marchofdimes.com
www.marchofdimes.com

March of Dimes help moms have full-term pregnancies and research the problems that threaten the health of babies. The March of Dimes also acts globally: sharing best practices in perinatal health and helping improve birth outcomes where the needs are the most urgent.

Stacey D. Stewart, President

254 Spondylitis Association of America
PO Box 5872
Sherman Oaks, CA 10037
818-981-1616
800-777-8189
Fax: 818-892-1611
info@spondylitis.org
www.spondylitis.org

Founded in 1983 SAA was the first and remains the largest resource in the United States for people seeking information on AS and related diseases.

Craig Gimbel DDS, Chair
Charlotte K Howard, Vice Chair
Leslie Kautz CFA, Treasurer

Web Sites

255 American Autoimmune Related Diseases Association
22100 Gratiot Ave.
Eastpointe, MI 48021
586-776-3900
800-598-4668
Fax: 586-776-3903
www.aarda.org

Dedicated to the eradiction of autoimmune diseases and the alleviation of suffering and the socio-economic impact of autoimmunity through fostering and facilitating collaboration in the areas of education, public awareness, research and patient services in an effective, ethical and efficient manner.

Virginia T. Ladd, President/ Executive Director
Patricia Barber, Asst. Director

256 Online Mendelian Inheritance in Man
National Library of Medicine, Building 38A
Bethesda, MD 20894
888-346-3656
info@ncbi.nlm.nih.gov
www.ncbi.nlm.nih.gov

This database is a catalog of human genes and genetic disorders.

Christine E. Seidman, M.D., Chair
David J. Lipman, M.D., Executive Secretary

Pamphlets

257 Ankylosing Spondylitis
Arthritis Foundation
1330 W. Peachtree Street, Suite 100
Atlanta, GA 30309
404-872-7100
800-568-4045
Fax: 404-872-0457
www.arthritis.org

An informative pamphlet published by the Arthritis Foundation.

Ann M. Palmer, President/ CEO
Meagan Fulmer, Chief Development Officer
Wayne Guthrie, SPHR, SVP, Staff Operations

DESCRIPTION

258   ANORECTAL MALFORMATIONS

Covers these related disorders: Anal atresia, Anal fistula, Anal stenosis, Ectopic anus, Imperforate anus

Involves the following Biologic System(s):

Gastrointestinal Disorders

Anorectal malformations are a group of birth defects affecting the rectum, the anus, or both. The rectum is the final straight portion of the large intestine that terminates at an external opening known as the anus. Anorectal malformations are birth defects in which the anus and rectum do not develop normally and vary in severity. For example, the anal opening may be in its normal location but may be unusually small or narrow (e.g., anal stenosis or imperforate anus). Some anorectal malformations may not be apparent upon physical examination (e.g., imperforate anus or anal atresia). In infants with imperforate anus, the anal opening is partially or completely closed due to the presence of a thin membrane (i.e., cloacal membrane). In anal atresia, the rectum may end blindly due to absence (atresia) of the anal canal. In addition, in many affected infants, an abnormal channel (fistula) may be present between the rectum and certain other unusual locations. Anorectal malformations affect approximately one in 4,000 newborns.

Most newborns with anorectal malformations experience lower intestinal obstruction within 24 hours after birth due to incomplete passage of meconium, the thick, darkish green material that accumulates in the fetal intestines and forms a newborn's first stool. Newborns normally pass meconium during the first 24 to 48 hours after birth. Affected infants may also have incomplete or infrequent bowel movements or experience difficulty passing stools (constipation) within days or weeks after birth. Associated findings may include rectal bleeding; periodic episodes of diarrhea following constipation and associated abrasions of the skin (e.g., of the perineum and the buttocks); and abnormal enlargement of a segment of the large intestine (megacolon). In affected males with a channel between the rectum and the urinary tract, there can be passage of gas (pneumaturia) and meconium in the urine.

When newborns are diagnosed with anorectal malformations, physicians may consider surgical measures to prevent intestinal or urinary obstruction. Therapies for affected newborns or infants depend upon the nature and location of the anorectal malformation and, in some cases, other associated birth defects that may be present. Treatment measures, which may be conducted during the newborn period or later during infancy, may include surgical correction of anorectal malformations (e.g., anoplasty) and widening (dilatation) of the anal opening or other supportive measures; a colostomy is often needed.

Anorectal malformations are thought to result from abnormalities in the development of the embryonic structures that form the rectum and portions of the urinary tract. In cases in which anorectal malformations occur as isolated findings, such malformations are thought to result from abnormal changes (mutations) of one or several different genes, possibly in association with certain environmental factors (multifactorial). However, familial cases have also been reported that appear to have autosomal dominant, autosomal re-

cessive, X-linked, or multifactorial inheritance. In approximately 50 percent of affected infants, anorectal malformations occur in association with other birth defects or underlying malformation syndromes, such as VACTERL association, a rare disorder that may be characterized by (V)ertebral abnormalities, (A)nal atresia, (C)ardiac defects, (T)racheo(E)sophageal fistula, (R)enal malformations, and (L)imb defects. Therefore, it is essential that newborns diagnosed with anorectal malformations are thoroughly examined and carefully monitored to ensure the detection and appropriate treatment of associated abnormalities.

National Associations & Support Groups

259   American Academy of Pediatrics
141 Northwest Point Boulevard
Elk Grove Village, IL 60007   847-434-4000
                                               800-433-9016
                                               Fax: 847-434-8000
                                               www.aap.org

The American Academy of Pediatrics and its member pediatricians are committed to the attainment of optimal physical, mental and social health and well-being for all infants, children, adolescents, and young adults.

Fernando Stein, MD, FAAP, President
Karen Remley, MD, CEO/Executive VP

260   American College of Gastroenterology
6400 Goldsboro Road, Suite 200
Bethesda, MD 20817   301-263-9000
                                               info@acg.gi.org
                                               www.gi.org

The American College of Gastroenterology was founded in 1932 to advance the scientific study and medical practice of diseases of the GI tract.

13,000 members

Carol A. Burke, MD, FACG, President

261   Digestive Disease National Coalition
507 Capitol Court NE, Suite 200
Washington, DC 20002   202-544-7497
                                               Fax: 202-546-7105
                                               hpayne@hmcw.org
                                               www.ddnc.org

Advocacy organization comprised of over 30 voluntary and professional societies concerned with the many diseases of the digestive tract and liver.

Lynn Seim, Chairperson
Ralph McKibbin, President
Cathy Griffith, Vice Chairperson

262   International Foundation for Functional Gastrointestinal Disorders
PO Box 170864
Milwaukee, WI 53217   414-964-1799
                                               Fax: 414-964-7176
                                               iffgd@iffgd.org
                                               www.iffgd.org

Founded in 1991 by Nancy Norton and William Norton, IFFGD has been working with patients (both adults and children), families, physicians, practitioners, investigators, employers, regulators, and others to broaden understanding about gastrointestinal disorders and support or encourage research.

Nancy J. Norton, President & Director
William Norton, Co-Founder
Eleanor Cautley, Vice President

263   Intestinal Disease Foundation
1 E Station Square Drive
Pittsburgh, PA 10042   412-261-5888
                                               877-587-9606
                                               Fax: 412-471-2722
                                               info@intestinalfoundation.org
                                               www.intestinalfoundation.org

Nonprofit organization whose mission is to improve the quality of life of adults and children affected by chronic digestive illness through information, guidance and support. IDF offers a quarterly newsletter, Intestinal Fortitude, educational seminars, volunteer phone network, and Pittsburgh area support groups.

264 March of Dimes Foundation
1275 Mamaroneck Avenue
White Plains, NY 10605   914-997-4488
                                     888-663-4637
                                Fax: 914-997-4763
                            answers@marchofdimes.com
                            www.marchofdimes.com

March of Dimes help moms have full-term pregnancies and research the problems that threaten the health of babies. The March of Dimes also acts globally: sharing best practices in perinatal health and helping improve birth outcomes where the needs are the most urgent.

Stacey D. Stewart, President

265 National Dissemination Center for Children with Disabilities
1825 Connecticut Avenue NW , Suite 700
Washington, DC 10044   202-884-8200
                                     800-695-0285
                                Fax: 202-884-8441
                                nichcy@fhi360.org
                                www.nichcy.org

A national information and referral center that provides information on disabilities and disability-related issues for families, educators and other professionals.

Suzanne Ripley, Executive Director

266 North American Society for Pediatric Gastroenterology/Hepatology/Nutrition
714 N Bethlehem Pike, Suite 300
Ambler, PA 19002   215-641-9800
                                Fax: 215-641-1995
                            naspghan@naspghan.org
                            www.naspghan.org

Strives to improve the care of infants, children and adolescents with digestive disorders by promoting advances in clinical care of children with chronic abdominal pain, diarrhea, constipation, vomiting, bleeding from the GI tract, inflammatory bowel disease, liver diseases, diseases of the pancreas, poor weight gain and nutritional problems.

Margaret K Stallings, Executive Director
Kim Rose, Associate Director
Donna Murphy, Membership

267 Oley Foundation
43 New Scotland Avenue, MC-28, Albany Medical Ctr
Albany, NY 12208   518-262-5079
                                     800-776-6539
                                Fax: 518-262-5528
                                info@oley.org
                                www.oley.org

Helping people whose daily survival depends on home intravenous or tube-fed nutrition.

Joan Bishop, Executive Director
Roslyn Dahl, Director, Communications & Develop
Lisa Crosby Metzger, Director, Community Engagement

268 Pull-Thru Network
1705 Wintergreen Parkway
Normal, IL 10045   309-262-0786
                            pullthrunetwork@gmail.com
                            www.pullthrunetwork.org

Pull-thru Network (PTN) was founded in 1988 and has grown to be one of the largest organizations in the world dedicated to the needs of those born with an anorectal malformation or colon disease and any of the associated diagnoses.

Bonnie McElroy, President
Alberto Pena, Director
Charles Paidas, Chief of Pediatric Surgery

Libraries & Resource Centers

269 National Digestive Diseases Information Clearinghouse
9000 Rockville Pike
Bethesda, MD 20892   301-496-3583
                                     800-860-8747
                                Fax: 301-907-8906
                            healthinfo@niddk.nih.gov
                            www.niddk.nih.gov

The National Institute of Diabetes and Digestive and Kidney Diseases conducts and supports research on many of the most serious diseases affecting public health. The Institute supports much of the clinical research on the diseases of internal medicine and related subspecialty fields as well as many basic science disciplines.

Dr. Griffin P. Rodgers, Director
Dr. Gregory G. Germino, Deputy Director
Camille M. Hoover, M.S.W., Executive Officer

Conferences

270 IFFGD Professional Symposia
Int'l Foundation for Functional Gastrointestinal
PO Box 170864
Milwaukee, WI 53217   414-964-1799
                                     888-964-2001
                                Fax: 414-964-7176
                                iffgd@iffgd.org
                                www.iffgd.org

Founded in 1991 by Nancy Norton and William Norton to help patients (both adults and children), families, physicians, practitioners, investigators, employers, regulators, and others broaden understanding about gastrointestinal disorders and support and encourage research.

April

Nancy J Norton, Founder
William Norton, Co-Founder
Eleanor Cautley, Vice President

271 NASPGHAN Annual Meeting and Postgraduate Course
NASPGHAN
714 N. Bethlehem Pike, Ste 300
Ambler, PA 19002   215-641-9800
                                Fax: 215-641-1995
                            naspghan@naspghan.org
                            www.naspghan.org

November

Margaret K Stallings, Executive Director
Kim Rose, Associate Director
Donna Murphy, Membership

272 Oley Foundation Annual Conference
Oley Foundation
43 New Scotland Ave, MC-28, Albany Medical Center
Albany, NY 12208   518-262-5079
                                     800-776-6539
                                Fax: 518-262-5528
                                info@oley.org
                                www.oley.org

Helping people whose daily survival depends on home intravenous or tube-fed nutrition.

July

Joan Bishop, Executive Director

273 PTN National Conference
Pull-Thru Network
1705 Wintergreen Parkway
Normal, IL 61761   205-978-2930
                            pullthrunetwork@gmail.com
                            www.pullthrunetwork.org

July

Bonnie McElroy, President

Web Sites

274 Baby Center
163 Freelon Street
San Francisco, CA 94107   www.babycenter.com

The Academy is committed to the attainment of optimal physical, mental and social health for all infants, children, adolescents, and young adults. To this end, the members of the Academy dedicate their efforts and resources.

Colleen Hancock, SVP/Global COO
Linda J. Murray, SVP/Global Editor-in-Chief
Clarence Wilhelm, Chief Information Officer

275 Health Research Project (HaRP)
www.harpnet.org

harp@kmsgh.org
www.harpnet.org

A program by USAID, the project strives to improve the health status of infants, children, mothers and families through the development and research of new tools, technologies, policies and approaches.

276 National Digestive Diseases Information Clearinghouse
www.digestive.niddk.nih.gov

Supports clinical research on the diseases of internal medicine and related subspecialty fields as well as many basic science disciplines.

Journals

277 Journal of Pediatric Gastroenterology and Nutrition (NASPGHAN)
Lippincott Williams & Wilkins
Two Commerce Square, 2001 Market Street
Philadelphia, PA 19103   215-521-8300
Fax: 215-521-8902
www.wolterskluwerhealth.com

Publication of the North American Society for Pediatric Gastroenterolgy, Hepatology and Nutrition, which strives to improve the care of infants, children and adolescents with digestive disorders by promoting advances in clinical care of children with chronic abdominal pain, diarrhea, constipation, vomiting, bleeding from the GI tract, inflammatory bowel disease, liver diseases, diseases of the pancreas, poor weight gain and nutritional problems.

Bob Becker, President/ CEO
Susan Yules, Chief Financial Officer
Cathy Wolfe, President/ CEO, Medical Research

Newsletters

278 NASPGHAN News
714 N. Bethlehem Pike, Ste 300
Ambler, PA 19002   215-641-9800
Fax: 215-641-1995
naspghan@naspghan.org
www.naspghan.org

Publication of the North American Society for Pediatric Gastroenterolgy, Hepatology and Nutrition, which strives to improve the care of infants, children and adolescents with digestive disorders by promoting advances in clinical care of children with chronic abdominal pain, diarrhea, constipation, vomiting, bleeding from the GI tract, inflammatory bowel disease, liver diseases, diseases of the pancreas, poor weight gain and nutritional problems.

Margaret K Stallings, Executive Director
Kim Rose, Associate Director
Donna Murphy, Membership

279 PTN News
1705 Wintergreen Parkway
Normal, IL 61761   205-978-2930
pullthrunetwork@gmail.com
www.pullthrunetwork.org

Newsletter of the Pull-thru Network, a chapter of the United Ostomy Association and a nonprofit service organization dedicated to the support of children and adults with anorectal malformations.

Quarterly

Pamphlets

280 Anorectal Malformations- A Parent's Guide
1705 Wintergreen Parkway
Normal, IL 61761   205-978-2930
pullthrunetwork@gmail.com
www.pullthrunetwork.org

Brochure distributed free to physicians, nurses and hospitals by the Pull-thru Network, a chapter of the United Ostomy Association and a nonprofit service organization dedicated to the support of children and adults with anorectal malformations.

Quarterly

DESCRIPTION

281 AORTIC STENOSIS

Synonym: Aortic stenosis

Involves the following Biologic System(s):

Cardiovascular Disorders

Aortic stenosis is a condition characterized by abnormal narrowing (stenosis) of the aortic valve, through which blood flows from the left ventricle of the heart to the aorta, the major artery of the body. Such stenosis may occur alone, as a sole abnormality, or together with other inborn abnormalities within or outside the heart. Narrowing of the aortic valve prevents the left ventricle from pumping its full load of blood into the aorta and therefore throughout the body. Effects of the diminished blood flow resulting from aortic stenosis include a deficient supply of blood-borne oxygen and nutrients to the body's tissues, including the muscle tissue of the ventricle, damaging these tissues. In an attempt to overcome this reduced blood supply by pumping blood more forcefully through a narrowed or stenotic aortic value and into the aorta, the muscular wall of the left ventricle may gradually thicken (hypertrophy). With its continued effort to pump blood through a stenotic aortic value, the left ventricle can eventually become enlarged and weakened, reducing its ability to pump blood and thereby leaving an increasing volume of residual blood and an increased blood pressure within the heart. Congestive heart failure, in which the heart ultimately becomes unable to pump blood, is a potentially life-threatening effect of aortic valve stenosis.

Normally, the aortic valve consists of three leaflets (cusps) that meet along their outer edges and overlap one another to prevent blood that is in the aorta from pushing back into the heart between heartbeats. These valves open when the heart contracts, permitting the left ventricle to pump blood out of itself and into the aorta. Most cases of aortic stenosis result from abnormalities in the leaflets or cusps of the valve. One such abnormality is an aortic valve that has only a single leaflet rather than the usual three leaflets. Such a monocuspid valve can occur either as an inherited, genetic effect or as the result of fusion of the valve's leaflets with one another. The inborn or congenital abnormality known as a bicuspid aortic valve is characterized by a valve that has only two cusps or leaflets instead of the usual three, and while many such valves work reasonably well, they are more often narrower than the normal aortic valve. Aortic stenosis can also result from genetic or inherited narrowing of the aortic valve, degenerative diseases, and inflammatory diseases that affect the heart, such as rheumatic fever.

Aortic valve stenosis is identified in as many as 15% of patients before the age of 1 year. Among other persons, the condition presents during childhood, adolescence, or adulthood. Congestive heart failure can be a major effect of aortic valve stenosis in newborns. In older children, a heart murmur is often the first indication of such stenosis. Fatigue soon after beginning a physical activity, dizziness, and chest pain may be other indications of aortic valve stenosis in older children.

Symptoms of aortic valve stenosis depend upon the severity of the abnormality. Valve obstruction that occurs in early infancy may be characterized by a weak pulse, a low output of urine difficulty in breathing, enlargement of the heart (cardiomegaly), congestive heart failure, and abnormal accumulation of fluid in the lungs (pulmonary edema). Severe aortic valve stenosis may be life-threatening to infants and older children. Children with less severe aortic stenosis may have no symptoms other than a heart murmur detected during a physical examination, while those with more severe involvement may experience fatigue, dizziness, and chest pain.

Treatment for aortic valve stenosis depends upon the severity of the obstruction. In some cases it is successfully corrected through the procedure known as balloon valvuloplasty, in which a thin, hollow tube (catheter), with a small balloon attached at its tip, is passed into the valve and the balloon is then inflated, increasing the size of the valve opening. The most frequent treatment for aortic satenosis is surgery to repair the valve if possible or to replace it if necessary. During such surgery, a heart bypass machine takes the place of the heart and lungs, oxygenating the patient's blood and pumping it through the body. In the procedure known as valvotomy, the aortic valve is surgically rebuilt so as to allow it to effectively pass blood from the ventricle into the aorta. In the technique known as the Ross procedure, achild's own pulmonary valve, which normally controls the flow of blood from the heart's right ventricle to the lungs, is used to replace a stenotic aortic valve, and is itself then replaced with a surgically implanted pulmonary valve.

Government Agencies

282 NIH/ Eunice Kennedy Shriver National Insti tute of Child Health & Human Development
31 Center Drive, Building 31
Bethesda, MD 20892

301-496-5113
800-370-2943
Fax: 866-760-5947
TTY: 888-320-6942
nichdpress@mail.nih.gov
www.nichd.nih.gov

Established in 1962 by congress, today the institute conducts and supports laboratory research, clinical trials, and epidemiological studies that explore health processes; examines the impact of disabilities, diseases, and variations on the lives of individuals; and sponsors training programs for scientists, health care providers, and researchers to ensure that NICHD research can continue.

Diana W. Bianchi, Director
Paul Williams, Director, Communications

283 NIH/National Heart, Lung and Blood Institu te
National Institute of Health
31 Center Dr MSC 2486, Bldg 31, Room 5A52
Bethesda, MD 20892

301-592-8573
Fax: 240-629-3246
TTY: 240-629-3255
nhlbiinfo@nhlbi.nih.gov
www.nhlbi.nih.gov

The National Heart, Lung, and Blood Institute (NHLBI) provides global leadership for a research, training, and education program to promote the prevention and treatment of heart, lung, and blood diseases and enhance the health of all individuals so that they can live longer and more fulfilling lives.

Gary H Gibbons, MD, Director
Nakela Cook, MD, Chief of Staff

National Associations & Support Groups

284 American Academy of Pediatrics
141 Northwest Point Boulevard
Elk Grove Village, IL 60007

847-434-4000
800-433-9016
Fax: 847-434-8000
www.aap.org

The American Academy of Pediatrics and its member pediatricians are committed to the attainment of optimal physical, mental and social health and well-being for all infants, children, adolescents, and young adults.

Fernando Stein, MD, FAAP, President
Karen Remley, MD, CEO/Executive VP

285 American Heart Association
7272 Greenville Avenue
Dallas, TX 75231   214-373-6300
                                          800-242-8721
                                     Fax: 214-706-1341
                                      inquire@amhrt.org
                                 www.heart.org/HEARTORG/

Our mission is to build healthier lives, free of cardiovascular diseases and stroke. That single purpose drives all we do. The need for our work is beyond question

Nancy Brown, CEO
Dr. Stephen Houser, President
Suzie Upton, Chief Operating Officer

286 Genetic Alliance
4301 Connecticut Avenue NW, Suite 404
Washington, DC 20008   202-966-5557
                                          800-336-4363
                                     Fax: 202-966-8553
                                  info@geneticalliance.org
                                  www.geneticalliance.org

World's leading nonprofit health advocacy organization committed to transforming health through genetics and promoting an environment of openness centered on the health of individuals, families, and communities.

Sharon Terry, President/CEO
Tetyana Murza, Managing Director
Natasha Bonhomme, VP, Strategic Development

287 March of Dimes Foundation
1275 Mamaroneck Avenue
White Plains, NY 10605   914-997-4488
                                          888-663-4637
                                     Fax: 914-997-4763
                                 answers@marchofdimes.com
                                  www.marchofdimes.com

Partnership of volunteers and professionals dedicates to improving the health of babies by preventing birth defects and infant mortality. Over 100 chapters are located across the country and can be located through the National Office.

Stacey D. Stewart, President

Conferences

288 Genetic Alliance Annual Conference
Genetic Alliance
4301 Connecticut Avenue NW, Suite 404
Washington, DC 20008   202-966-5557
                                          800-336-4363
                                     Fax: 202-966-8553
                                  info@geneticalliance.org
                                  www.geneticalliance.org

Consistently inspirational and enables partnership among all stakeholders: advocates and community leaders, health and industry professionals, policymakers, and academicians.

July

Sharon Terry, President/CEO
Tetyana Murza, Managing Director
Natasha Bonhomme, VP, Strategic Development

Web Sites

289 Southern Illinois University School of Medicine
PO Box 19639
Springfield, IL 62794   217-545-8000
                                          800-342-5748
                                     TDD: 217-545-8038
                                   admin@siuhealthcare.org
                                www.siumed.edu/peds/index.htm

Mission is to meet the health care needs of children and their families in Central and Southern Illinois through the provision of high quality, coordinated care of children with acute and chronic heart conditions with inpatient, ambulatory, and community-based programs.

290 Yale University School of Medicine
333 Cedar Street
New Haven, CT 6510   203-432-4771
                                      medicine.yale.edu

Information on congenital heart conditions, including Aortic Stenosis — symptoms, treatments and support.

Peter Salovey, President of the University
Richard Belitsky, M.D., Deputy Dean for Education
Benjamin Polak, B.A., M.A., Ph.D., Provost of the University

Book Publishers

291 Congenital Disorders Sourcebook
Omnigraphics
PO Box 31-1640
Detroit, PA 48231   800-234-1340
                                     Fax: 800-875-1340
                                  info@omnigraphics.com
                                  www.omnigraphics.com

Provides basic consumer health information about the most common types of nonhereditary birth defects and disorders related to prematurity, gestational injuries, congenital infections, and birth complications, including disorders of the heart, brain, gastrointestinal tract, musculoskeletal system, urinary tract, and reproductive system, craniofacial disorders, cerebral palsy, spina bifida, and fetal alcohol syndrome, and detailing the causes, diagnostic tests, and treatments for each.

650 pages
ISBN: 0-780809-45-9

DESCRIPTION

292 APNEA OF PREMATURITY

Synonym: Idiopathic apnea of prematurity

Involves the following Biologic System(s):

Neonatal and Infant Disorders, Respiratory Disorders

Apnea is a condition characterized by a temporary cessation of breathing. Newborns may experience episodes of apnea due to several underlying disorders or conditions, including certain respiratory, neurologic, digestive, cardiovascular, metabolic, or infectious diseases. However, in newborns with apnea of prematurity, apneic episodes occur in the absence of identifiable, underlying disorders (idiopathic). The condition primarily affects premature infants who are born before 34 weeks of pregnancy (gestation). In general, the greater the degree of prematurity, the greater the frequency of the condition.

Apnea of prematurity is thought to occur due to immaturity of the region of the brain that controls breathing (respiratory centers of the medulla), causing failed stimulation of respiratory muscles. Resulting episodes of apnea, which are referred to as central apnea, are characterized by an absence of airflow as well as of chest wall movements. Apnea of prematurity may also be caused by obstruction of the upper airways due to improper coordination of the tongue and upper airway muscles, instability of the throat (pharynx), or other factors. Resulting episodes of apnea, known as obstructive apnea, are characterized by absence of airflow but ongoing chest wall movements. Most infants with apnea of prematurity experience both central and obstructive apnea.

With infant apnea, more appropriately called an apparent life-threatening event, initial episodes of apnea typically occur on the second to the seventh day of life. Such episodes are defined as serious if breathing spontaneously ceases for more than 15 to 20 seconds or if they result in decreased levels of oxygen in the blood and associated bluish discoloration of the skin and mucous membranes (cyanosis) and slowing of the heart rate (bradycardia).

The frequency of apnea episodes typically increases during the cycle of sleep that is associated with rapid eye movements (REMs), dreaming, increased levels of brain activity, and involuntary muscle jerks. During REM sleep, infants are more likely to experience abnormal chest wall movements during breathing, such as relaxation of the chest muscles while inhaling rather than exhaling. Abnormal chest wall movements as well as inhibition of muscle tone (particularly of the throat) during REM sleep contribute to the increased frequency of apneic episodes.

Infants at risk for episodes of apnea should be monitored with devices that detect abnormal changes in chest wall movements, heart rate, and respiratory activity. These devices, known as apnea monitors, sound an alarm when spontaneous breathing temporarily ceases. In infants who experience mild, occasional episodes of apnea, supportive measures may be sufficient, such as gentle skin stimulation and massage. In patients with severe, prolonged, and recurrent apnea episodes, treatment should include close monitoring, immediate measures to assist breathing (e.g., bag and maskentilation) and oxygen therapy to ensure sufficient oxygen supply to body

tissues. Infants with apnea may be monitored at home which can have a significant impact on caregivers. In general, as the child matures, the cause of the ALTE is diagnosed and treated or spontaneously resolves.

Government Agencies

293 NIH/ Eunice Kennedy Shriver National Insti tute of Child Health & Human Development
31 Center Drive, Building 31
Bethesda, MD 20892

301-496-5113
800-370-2943
Fax: 866-760-5947
TTY: 888-320-6942
nichdpress@mail.nih.gov
www.nichd.nih.gov

Established in 1962 by congress, today the institute conducts and supports laboratory research, clinical trials, and epidemiological studies that explore health processes; examines the impact of disabilities, diseases, and variations on the lives of individuals; and sponsors training programs for scientists, health care providers, and researchers to ensure that NICHD research can continue.

Diana W. Bianchi, Director
Paul Williams, Director, Communications

294 NIH/National Institute of Neurological Dis orders and Stroke (NINDS)
PO Box 5801
Bethesda, MD 20824

301-496-5751
800-352-9424
Fax: 301-496-0296
TTY: 301-468-5981
www.ninds.nih.gov

Works to reduce the burden of neurological disease by conducting, fostering, coordinating and guiding research on the causes, prevention, diagnosis and treatment of neurological disorders and stroke, while supporting basic research in related scientific areas.

Walter J. Koroshetz, MD, Director

National Associations & Support Groups

295 American Academy of Pediatrics
141 Northwest Point Boulevard
Elk Grove Village, IL 60007

847-434-4000
800-433-9016
Fax: 847-434-8000
www.aap.org

The American Academy of Pediatrics and its member pediatricians are committed to the attainment of optimal physical, mental and social health and well-being for all infants, children, adolescents, and young adults.

Fernando Stein, MD, FAAP, President
Karen Remley, MD, CEO/Executive VP

296 American Sleep Apnea Association
641 S Street NW, 3rd Floor
Washington, DC 20001

202-293-3650
Fax: 202-293-3656
asaa@sleepapnea.org
www.sleepapnea.org

Dedicated to reducing injury, disability and death from sleep apnea and to enhancing the well-being of those affected by this common disorder. They promote education and awareness. Network of voluntary mutual support groups, research, and continuous improvement of care.

Will Headapohl, Chair (Emeritus)
Justine Amdur, Program Coordinator, AWAKE
Valerie Danielson, Program Coordinator, CPAP

297 National Sleep Foundation
1010 N Glebe Road
Arlington, VA 22201

703-243-1697
Fax: 202-347-3472
nsf@sleepfoundation.org
www.sleepfoundation.org

Works to improve the quality of life for millions of Americans who suffer from sleep disorders, and to prevent the catastrophic accidents that are related to poor or disordered sleep through research, education and the dissemination of information towards the cause of the Narcolepsy Project. Seeks patients to aid new research project targeting the cause of the disorder.

David Cloud, CEO

Web Sites

298 Apnea of Prematurity
395 Hudson Street, 3rd Floor
New York, NY 10014   212-301-6700
                    emedicine.medscape.com/article/974971-overview

Provides information on how to tell if an unborn baby has sleep apnea.

Dharmendra J. Nimavat, MD, FAAP, Author
Ted Rosenkrantz, MD, Chief Editor

Camps

299 VACC Camp
Nicklaus Children's Hospital
3200 SW 60th Court, Suite 203
Miami, FL 33155
                                       305-662-8222
                                  Fax: 786-268-1765
                                  bela.florentin@mch.com
                                  www.vacccamp.com

Free, week-long, overnight camp for ventilation assisted children (children needing a tracheotomy ventilator, C-PAP, BiPAP, or oxygen to support breathing) and their families. Gives families a fun oppourtinity to socialize with peers and enjoy activities not readily accessible to technology dependent children.

Bela Florentin, Camp Coordinator
Rose Ann Farrell, Volunteer Assistants Coordinator
Alyssa Garcia, Operations

DESCRIPTION

300   ARNOLD-CHIARI MALFORMATION

Synonyms: ACM, Arnold-Chiari deformity, Arnold-Chiari syndrome, Chiari malformation

Covers these related disorders: Arnold-Chiari malformation type I, Arnold-Chiari malformation type II

Involves the following Biologic System(s):

Neurologic Disorders

Arnold-Chiari malformation is a developmental abnormality characterized by deformities at the base of the brain that are present at birth (congenital). Such deformities typically include abnormal elongation of a portion of the cerebellum (cerebellar tonsils) and the lowest region of the brain stem (medulla oblongata), resulting in protrusion of these regions through the large opening (foramen magnum) in the base of the skull and into the upper spinal canal (cervical canal). The cerebellum is a region of the brain that plays an essential role in coordinating voluntary movement and maintaining posture and balance. The brain stem, which is the lowest section of the brain and connects it with the spinal cord, helps to relay motor and sensory impulses between other regions of the brain and the spinal cord, and connects with most of the cranial nerves, which conduct impulses involved in such functions as taste, vision, swallowing, and facial expression, as well as movements of the tongue, head, and shoulders. Although the exact cause of Arnold-Chiari malformation is unknown, researchers have suggested that it may result from the interaction of several genes, environmental influences, or both (multifactorial inheritance).

In some affected newborns, Arnold-Chiari malformation occurs in association with myelomeningocele, a developmental abnormality characterized by protrusion (herniation) of a portion of the spinal cord and its protective membranes (meninges) through an abnormalopening in the bone of the spinal column. Arnold-Chiari malformation without a myelomeningocele is termed Arnold-Chiari malformation type I. When it is accompanied by a myelomeningocele, the condition is known as Arnold-Chiari malformation type II. In both types of the condition, the foramen magnum is abnormally large. Additionally, the base of the skull is flattened and may be pushed upward by the upper vertebrae (cervical vertebrae) surrounding the spinal cord.

Infants and children with Arnold-Chiari malformation type II experience progressive hydrocephalus, a condition characterized by the abnormal accumulation of cerebrospinal fluid (CSF) in the brain. This accumulation of CSF, which comes from obstruction of the normal flow of this fluid between the brain and spine, or its impaired absorption results in increased fluid pressure within cavities (ventricles) of the brain. Other findings in Arnold-Chiari malformation type II may include abnormal enlargement of the chambers within the brain that contain its CSF, known as the ventricles, potential enlargement of the head, and other associated symptoms and findings. Some infants with Arnold-Chiari malformation type II may also experience abnormalities due to pressure or damage to lower cranial nerves. Such abnormalities, which vary in range and severity, include uncontrollable twitching (fasciculations) of the tongue, a high-pitched sound upon inhalation (i.e., laryngeal stridor), facial weakness, hearing impairment, lagging of the head (sternomastoid paralysis), or weakness or impaired control of muscles that turn the eyes outward (bilateral abducens palsies). During later childhood, some patients with Arnold-Chiari malformation type II may experience increased stiffness (rigidity), causing restriction of movement (spasticity); abnormalities in walking (abnormal gait); and progressive lack of coordination. During later childhood or adolescence, individuals with this condition may also experience symptoms and findings often associated with Arnold-Chiari malformation type I.

These symptoms may also first occur in adolescence or adulthood rather than in childhood, and often occur without hydrocephalus. Associated symptoms and findings may include recurrent headaches; neck pain; impaired control of voluntary movements (ataxia); or progressive muscle weakness, degeneration (atrophy), spasticity, and potential sensory loss affecting the lower and, in some cases, the upper limbs.

Treatment of Arnold-Chiari malformation depends on the severity of the malformation and associated symptoms and findings. If symptoms are only mild, treatment includes regular monitoring and symptomatic and supportive measures as required, such as the use of medication to relieve pain. However, surgery is the only means of correcting the structural problem in Arnold-Chiari malformation, and is required in more severe cases of this condition. The surgery for Arnold-Chiari malformation is directed at uncrowding the area at the base of the cerebellum where this part of the brain is pushing against the brain stem and spinal cord. This is done by removing a small portion of bone at the base of the skull, and often also by removing a part of the back of the first and occasionally other upper segments of the spinal column (e.g., upper cervical laminectomy).

Government Agencies

301   NIH/ Eunice Kennedy Shriver National Institute of Child Health & Human Development
31 Center Drive, Building 31
Bethesda, MD 20892
301-496-5113
800-370-2943
Fax: 866-760-5947
TTY: 888-320-6942
nichdpress@mail.nih.gov
www.nichd.nih.gov

Established in 1962 by congress, today the institute conducts and supports laboratory research, clinical trials, and epidemiological studies that explore health processes; examines the impact of disabilities, diseases, and variations on the lives of individuals; and sponsors training programs for scientists, health care providers, and researchers to ensure that NICHD research can continue.

Diana W. Bianchi, Director
Paul Williams, Director, Communications

National Associations & Support Groups

302   American Academy of Pediatrics
141 Northwest Point Boulevard
Elk Grove Village, IL 60007
847-434-4000
800-433-9016
Fax: 847-434-8000
www.aap.org

The American Academy of Pediatrics and its member pediatricians are committed to the attainment of optimal physical, mental and social health and well-being for all infants, children, adolescents, and young adults.

Fernando Stein, MD, FAAP, President
Karen Remley, MD, CEO/Executive VP

303 Genetic Alliance
4301 Connecticut Avenue NW, Suite 404
Washington, DC 20008
202-966-5557
800-336-4363
Fax: 202-966-8553
info@geneticalliance.org
www.geneticalliance.org

World's leading nonprofit health advocacy organization committed to transforming health through genetics and promoting an environment of openness centered on the health of individuals, families, and communities.

Sharon Terry, President/CEO
Tetyana Murza, Managing Director
Natasha Bonhomme, VP, Strategic Development

304 March of Dimes Foundation
1275 Mamaroneck Avenue
White Plains, NY 10605
914-997-4488
888-663-4637
Fax: 914-997-4763
answers@marchofdimes.com
www.marchofdimes.com

March of Dimes help moms have full-term pregnancies and research the problems that threaten the health of babies. The March of Dimes also acts globally: sharing best practices in perinatal health and helping improve birth outcomes where the needs are the most urgent.

Stacey D. Stewart, President

305 World Arnold-Chiari Malformation Association
31 Newtown Woods Road
Newtown Square, PA 10059
610-353-4737
chiari-owner@yahoogroups.com
www.pressenter.com/~wacma/

Staffed by volunteers, we are committed to providing support, current information, and understanding to those affected by the Arnold Chiari malformation and syringomyelia. It is also our goal to raise the awareness of, and educate the medical community as to the complex nature of this disease and how it affects the lives of those who have it.

Bernie Meyer, Manager/Moderator
Ann Hood, Manager/Moderator
Sandi Justin, Manager/Moderator

Conferences

306 Genetic Alliance Annual Conference
Genetic Alliance
4301 Connecticut Avenue NW, Suite 404
Washington, DC 20008
202-966-5557
800-336-4363
Fax: 202-966-8553
info@geneticalliance.org
www.geneticalliance.org

Consistently inspirational and enables partnership among all stakeholders: advocates and community leaders, health and industry professionals, policymakers, and academicians.

July

Sharon Terry, President/CEO
Tetyana Murza, Managing Director
Natasha Bonhomme, VP, Strategic Development

Web Sites

307 National Institute of Health NINDS Information Page
PO Box 5801
Bethesda, MD 20824
301-496-5751
800-352-9424
www.ninds.nih.gov

The mission is to reduce the burden of neurological disease — a burden born by every age group, by every segment of society, by people all over the world.

Walter J. Koroshetz, M.D., Acting Director
Alan L. Willard, Ph.D., Acting Deputy Director
Caroline Lewis, Executive Officer

308 Online Mendelian Inheritance in Man
National Library of Medicine, Building 38A
Bethesda, MD 20894
888-346-3656
info@ncbi.nlm.nih.gov
www.ncbi.nlm.nih.gov

This database is a catalog of human genes and genetic disorders.

Christine E. Seidman, M.D., Chair
David J. Lipman, M.D., Executive Secretary

309 Rare Genetic Diseases in Children (NYU)
www.med.nyu.edu/rgdc/homenow.htm

We target issues arising from rare genetic diseases affecting children. And assist in the endeavor to bring knowledge and hope to those for whom there is, at present, so little.

Book Publishers

310 Let's Talk About Going to the Hospital
Rosen Publishing Group's PowerKids Press
29 E 21st Street
New York, NY 10010
212-777-3017
800-237-9932
Fax: 888-436-4643
rosenpub@tribeca.ios.com
www.rosenpublishing.com

If a child has to check into the hospital, chances are he or she is already upset about being ill. Knowing how a hospital functions and what the procedures are, such as when family members can visit, will help in what is already a stressful situation. Grades K-5.

24 pages
ISBN: 0-823950-36-0

DESCRIPTION

311   ARRHYTHMIAS

Covers these related disorders: Supraventricular Tachycardia (SVT), Wolff-Parkinson-White Syndrome (WPW)

Involves the following Biologic System(s):
Cardiovascular Disorders

The term arrhythmia refers to an abnormality in the rhythm of the heartbeat. It may take the form of an abnormally slow or abnormally fast heartbeat or another disturbance in heart rhythm. Any such problem can interfere with the ability of the heart to effectively pump blood to the body's organs and tissues. Many such problems can, however, be treated medically, surgically, or in other ways.

Arrhythmias result from disturbances in the electrical conduction system of the heart, also called the cardiac conduction system. This system consists of pathways, made up of specialized tissues that conduct electrical impulses to the muscle cells of the heart, prompting them to contract and pump blood. Within the cardiac conduction system are also several tissue structures known as nodes, which act as pacemakers, coordinating the sequence of muscle contractions by which the heart pumps blood from each of its four chambers into the next chamber and out into the lungs and body. This coordinated pumping begins in the right atrium or upper right chamber of the heart, which collects blood that re-enters the heart after circulating through the body. The muscle tissue of the right atrium then contracts, pumping this blood downward and into the right ventricle, the chamber of the heart that is located immediately below the right atrium. The right ventricle pumps this blood to the lungs, which supply the blood with oxygen and return it to the left atrium of the heart, which pumps this oxygenated blood downward and into the most muscular of the heart's four chambers, the left ventricle. The left ventricle then pumps the oxygenated blood out of itself and into the body by way of the large main artery known as the aorta.

Most of the arrhythmias caused by aberrations in the cardiac conduction system can be detected with the diagnostic procedure known as electrocardiography. In this procedure, small electrodes that sense the electrical impulses that accompany each heartbeat are pasted to the skin at locations on the chest, arms, and legs. The impulses pass into the electrodes and through wires to an instrument that records, on paper or on a computer screen, the visible tracing known as an electrocardiogram (ECG or EKG), which indicates the intensity, rhythm, and other features of the heartbeat.

Normally, the heart contracts at a rate of 60 to 80 beats per minute when the body is at rest, and this rate increases with exercise to meet the body's increased need for oxygen and blood-borne nutrients. An increased heartbeat rate is known as a tachycardia, while a heartbeat that falls below the normal rate is called a bradycardia. In many instances, both tachycardias and bradycardias are temporary, passing events without serious or dangerous effects. Thus, exercise, excitement, and fever can all cause the typically harmless tachycardia known as sinus tachycardia. The most frequent type of medically important tachycardia in infants and children under the age of 12 is known as supraventricular tachycardia (SVT), sometimes also called paroxysmal supraventricular tachycardia (PSVT) or paroxysmal atrial tachycardia (PAT). As its name indicates, this type of tachycardia comes from a disturbance in the cardiac conduction system that originates at some point above the ventricles. It is characterized by a heart rate of more than 220 beats per minute, but is not typically life-threatening. Infants experiencing an instance of SVT may seem restless, have rapid breathing, or be especially sleepy. SVT requires treatment only if it is frequent or its episodes are long-lasting. Treatment of SVT is based on the specific mechanism responsible for the tachycardia and the age of the patient. A variety of medications (anti-arrhythmia agents) are available for controlling SVT.

More potentially serious than SVT is ventricular tachycardia (VT), caused by an aberration in conduction at some point below the atria of the heart. Although it may occur in the absence of any apparent source, VT is most often the result of damage to or an inborn defect in the conduction system or in another component of the heart. If it occurs in the right ventricle, VT can interfere with pumping of blood to the lungs, and in the left ventricle can interfere with pumping of blood through the entire body. One way in which VT may disrupt the heart's pumping of blood is by triggering the condition known as ventricular fibrillation, in which a weak, flaccid pattern of ventricular contraction replaces the normally forceful, coordinated contractions of these chambers of the heart, preventing them from effectively pumping blood.

A cause of serious disturbances in heart rhythm is the condition known as Wolff-Parkinson-White (WPW) syndrome. This results from an aberration in the cardiac conduction system at some point between the atria and ventricles, and can cause the sudden, complete, and life-threatening cessation of heartbeat known as cardiac arrest. In many cases, WPW syndrome shows no outward signs of its existence, and is first identified only on an electrocardiogram. WPW syndrome often responds to medical treatment with drugs. Destruction or ablation of its source within the cardiac conduction system often corrects WPW syndrome. This technique, known as radiofrequency ablation, involves the passage of an electrical current through a catheter and directly into the source of the syndrome. In other instances surgery is often effective in eliminating WPW syndrome.

Also serious is the condition known as complete heart block, which can occur during childhood and even prenatally. This disorder results from a genetic defect or other damage to the cardiac conduction system that interrupts electrical conduction within the heart, interfering with the pumping of blood from the atria into the ventricles. When this happens, a naturally occurring pacemaker within the ventricles sustains their contraction and pumping of blood, but at a reduced heart rate. If this natural process does not restore an adequate heart rate, heart block may be corrected by implantation of an artificial pacemaker.

Another source of interference with normal heart rhythm is sick sinus syndrome. In this condition, the sinus node, one of the natural pacemakers within the cardiac conduction system, is damaged by illness, injury, or accidentally during heart surgery, triggering intermittent episodes of either tachycardia or of the slowed heartbeat rate known as bradycardia. Symptoms of this condition may include fatigue or faintness. The condition can be treated medically, with drugs, and if necessary by implantation of an artificial pacemaker.

National Associations & Support Groups

312 **American Academy of Pediatrics**
141 Northwest Point Boulevard
Elk Grove Village, IL 60007
847-434-4000
800-433-9016
Fax: 847-434-8000
www.aap.org

The American Academy of Pediatrics and its member pediatricians are committed to the attainment of optimal physical, mental and social health and well-being for all infants, children, adolescents, and young adults.

Fernando Stein, MD, FAAP, President
Karen Remley, MD, CEO/Executive VP

313 **American College of Cardiology**
2400 N Street, NW
Washington, DC 20037
202-375-6000
800-253-4636
Fax: 202-375-7000
resource@acc.org
www.acc.org

The mission of the American College of Cardiology is to advocate for quality cardiovascular care, through education, research promotion, development and application of standards and guidelines, and to influence health care policy.

Shalom Jacobovitz, CEO
Cathleen C. Gates, COO
Brendan Mullen, Executive VP

314 **American Heart Association**
7272 Greenville Avenue
Dallas, TX 75231
214-373-6300
800-242-8721
Fax: 214-706-1341
inquire@amhrt.org
www.heart.org/HEARTORG/

Our mission is to build healthier lives, free of cardiovascular diseases and stroke. That single purpose drives all we do. The need for our work is beyond question

Nancy Brown, CEO
Dr. Stephen Houser, President
Suzie Upton, Chief Operating Officer

315 **Heart Failure Society of America**
6707 Democracy Blvd, Suite 925
Bethesda, MD 20817
301-312-8635
Fax: 888-213-4417
info@hfsa.org
www.hfsa.org

The Heart Failure Society of America, Inc. (HFSA) represents the first organized effort by heart failure experts from the Americas to provide a forum for all those interested in heart function, heart failure, and congestive heart failure (CHF) research and patient care.

Patrick McGary, COO
Jaime Abreu, Executive VP, Educational Programs
Patrice Guzman, Senior Mgr, Programs/Patient Adv.

316 **Rush Children's Heart Center**
1653 W Congress Parkway
Chicago, IL 10064
312-942-5000
888-352-7874
contact_rush@rush.edu
www.rush.edu/rumc/page-1099918801842.html

Rush Children's Hospital, part of at Rush University Medical Center in Chicago, Illinois, provides complete clinical services for the diagnosis and treatment of congenital and acquired heart disease in children and young adults.

Larry J Goodman MD, CEO
Richard M Jaffee, Chairman
Susan Crown, Vice Chair

317 **Sudden Arrhythmia Death Syndromes Foundati on**
4527 South 2300 East, Suite 104
Salt Lake City, UT 84117
801-272-3023
800-786-7723
sads@sads.org
www.sads.org

Our mission is to save the lives and support the families of children and young adults who are genetically predisposed to sudden death due to heart rhythm abnormalities.

Alice Lara, RN, President/CEO
Lynn Johnson, MD, Dairector, Family Support
William Shiflett, MPA, Director, Medical Education/COO

Research Centers

318 **Cardiovascular Research Foundation**
1700 Broadway, 9th Floor
New York, NY 10019
646-434-4500
info@crf.org
www.crf.org

A nonprofit organization with a mission to improve the survival and quality of life for people with cardiovascular disease through research and education.

Gary S Mintz MD, Chief Medical Officer
Eric B Woldenberg Esq, Chairman

Conferences

319 **HFSA Annual Scientific Meeting**
Heart Failure Society of America
2550 University Avenue W
Saint Paul, MN 10062
651-642-1633
Fax: 651-642-1502
info@hfsa.org
www.hfsa.org

The Heart Failure Society of America, Inc. (HFSA) represents the first organized effort by heart failure experts from the Americas to provide a forum for all those interested in heart function, heart failure, and congestive heart failure (CHF) research and patient care.
September

Barry M Massie MD, President

Web Sites

320 **Heart Center Online**
495 East Waterfront Drive Suite 200
Homestead, PA 15120
412-326-0330
www.theheartcenteronline.com

The mission of the Heart Center Online is to be the premier cardiovascular specialized health care site on the Internet, to provide cardiovascular patients, their families and site visitors with tools they need to better understand the complex nature of heart-related conditions, treatments and preventive care, and to provide services and applications that deliver value to cardiovascullar practices.

321 **Rush Children's Heart Center**
www.rush.edu

Provides complete clinical services for the diagnosis and treatment of congenital and acquired heart disease in children and young adults.

322 **Yale University School of Medicine**
333 Cedar Street
New Haven, CT 6510
203-432-4771
medicine.yale.edu

Information on heart conditions, including arrhythmias.

Peter Salovey, President of the University
Richard Belitsky M.D., Deputy Dean for Education
Benjamin Polak, B.A., M.A., Ph.D., Provost of the University

Journals

323 Journal of Cardiac Failure
Cardiac Heart Failure Society of America
6707 Democracy Blvd. Suite 925
Bethesda, MD 20817   301-312-8635
                                     Fax: 888-213-4417
                                          info@hfsa.org
                                          www.hfsa.org

Contains review articles on clinical research, basic human studies, animal studies, and bench research with potential clinical applications to heart failure, pathogenesis, etiology, epidemiology, pathophysiological mechanisms, assessment, prevention and treatment.

6x year

Michele Blair, CEO
JoAnn Lindenfeld, MD, President
Mandeep R. Mehra, MD, Vice President

324 Texas Heart Institute Journal
Texas Heart Institute
6770 Bertner Avenue
Houston, TX 77030   832-355-3792
                                     Fax: 832-355-3714
                                    webmaster@texasheart.org
                                   www.texasheartinstitute.org

The purpose of the Texas Heart Institute Journal is to educate, with emphasis on the dissemination of information to physicians in practice.

Quaterly

Denton A. Cooley, MD, Founder
L. Maximilian Buja, MD, Chief
C. David Collard, MD, Chief

Newsletters

325 Heart Failure Society Newsletter
6707 Democracy Blvd. Suite 925
Bethesda, MD 20817   301-312-8635
                                     Fax: 888-213-4417
                                          info@hfsa.org
                                          www.hfsa.org

Provides information on the society and also on different aspects of heart failure.

Quaterly

Patrick McGary, COO
Anna Leong, Publications Manager

DESCRIPTION

326 ARTHROGRYPOSIS MULTIPLEX CONGENITA
Synonym: AMC
Covers these related disorders: Amyoplasia
Involves the following Biologic System(s):
Orthopedic and Muscle Disorders

Arthrogryposis multiplex congenita (AMC) refers to a group of disorders present at birth (congenital) that are characterized by limited movement or immobility of multiple joints and partial or complete replacement of involved muscle with fibrous or fatty tissue. Affected joints may be permanently flexed or extended in various fixed postures (joint contractures). Approximately 150 syndromes have been identified that are characterized by the presence of congenital multiple contractures. The most common form of arthrogryposis multiplex congenita is known as amyoplasia. This classic form of AMC affects approximately one in 10,000 newborns.

In newborns with amyoplasia, multiple congenital contractures are present that typically affect the upper and lower extremities. In most newborns who are affected, such contractures include abnormal flexion or extension of the elbows; flexion of the wrists toward either the thumb side or pinky side of the hands(radial or ulnar deviation); cupping of the hands; and internal rotation of the shoulders. Many newborns with amyoplasia also have severe deformities of the feet (clubfoot or talipes equinovarus) in which the heels are turned inward and the soles of the feet are flexed (plantar flexion). Additional musculoskeletal deformities are also typically present including abnormal rigidity of the joints between the bones of the thumbs and other fingers (interphalangeal joints); deformities of the palms of the hands; fixed flexion or extension of the knees; and abnormal flexion, extension, rotation, and possible dislocation of the hips. These abnormalities are usually similar from one side of the body to the other (symmetric). Amyoplasia is also characterized by a susceptibility to bone fractures (i.e., perinatal fractures) and progressive abnormal sideways curvature of the spine (scoliosis) that varies in severity and in age at onset. Most newborns with amyoplasia also have distinctive facial abnormalities including short, upturned (anteverted) nostrils; a rounded face; a slightly small jaw (mild micrognathia); and a benign, reddish, purple growth in the midportion of the face (midline frontal hemangioma). Amyoplasia appears to occur randomly for unknown reasons (sporadically), and the underlying causes of amyoplasia and other forms of AMC are not fully understood.

All newborns with multiple congenital joint contractures should receive a thorough neuromuscular evaluation to help detect, confirm, or rule out potential underlying muscular or neurologic abnormalities. The treatment of infants and children with amyoplasia includes symptomatic and supportive measures. The presence of fractures should be ruled out or confirmed (e.g., with x-ray studies) and treated as necessary (e.g., with appropriate immobilization) before physical therapy is begun. Other treatment measures for congenital contractures and associated abnormalities include physical therapy (e.g., passive range of motion exercises) and splinting of extremities to improve the range of motion; the use of casts or other orthopedic appliances; and possible surgical interventions. In addition, orthopedic appliances may be used to help slow the progression of scoliosis. In most patients with severe scoliosis, surgical measures may also be required.

Government Agencies

327 NIH/National Institute of Arthritis and Musculoskeletal and Skin Diseases
1 AMS Circle
Bethesda, MD 20892
301-495-4484
877-226-4267
Fax: 301-718-6366
TTY: 301-565-2966
TDD: 301-565-2966
niamsinfo@mail.nih.gov
www.niams.nih.gov

The mission of the National Institute of Arthritis and Musculoskeletal and Skin Diseases is to support research into the causes, treatment, and prevention of arthritis and musculoskeletal and skin diseases; the training of basic and clinical scientists to carry out this research; and the dissemination of information on research progress in these diseases

Stephen I Katz MD PhD, Director
Robert H Carter MD, Deputy Director
Gahan Breithaupt, Assoc Dir. Management & Operations

National Associations & Support Groups

328 American Academy of Pediatrics
141 Northwest Point Boulevard
Elk Grove Village, IL 60007
847-434-4000
800-433-9016
Fax: 847-434-8000
www.aap.org

The American Academy of Pediatrics and its member pediatricians are committed to the attainment of optimal physical, mental and social health and well-being for all infants, children, adolescents, and young adults.

Fernando Stein, MD, FAAP, President
Karen Remley, MD, CEO/Executive VP

329 Genetic Alliance
4301 Connecticut Avenue NW, Suite 404
Washington, DC 20008
202-966-5557
800-336-4363
Fax: 202-966-8553
info@geneticalliance.org
www.geneticalliance.org

World's leading nonprofit health advocacy organization committed to transforming health through genetics and promoting an environment of openness centered on the health of individuals, families, and communities.

Sharon Terry, President/CEO
Tetyana Murza, Managing Director
Natasha Bonhomme, VP, Strategic Development

330 Human Growth Foundation
997 Glen Cove Avenue, Suite 5
Glen Head, NY 10069
516-671-4041
800-451-6434
Fax: 516-671-4055
hgf1@hgfound.org
www.hgfound.org

A voluntary, nonprofit organization whose mission is to help children and adults with disorders of growth and growth hormones through research, education, support and advocacy. The foundation is dedicated to helping medical science to better understand the process of growth. It is composed of concerned parents and friends of children and adults with growth problems and interested health professionals.

Patricia D Costa, Executive Director
Earl A. Gershenow, Board of Directors
Emily Germain-Lee MD, Vice President

331 MAGIC Foundation: Major Aspects of Growth in Children
4200 Cantera Drive, #106
Warrenville, IL 60555
630-836-8200
800-362-4423
Fax: 630-836-8181
mary@magicfoundation.org
www.magicfoundation.org

A national nonprofit organization providing support and education regarding growth disorders in children and related adult disorders. Provides educational information, networking, a national conference, a kids' program and an extensive medical library.

Dianne Kremidas, Executive Director
Mary Andrews, Chief Executive Officer
Teresa Tucker, Patient Advocacy

332 March of Dimes Foundation
1275 Mamaroneck Avenue
White Plains, NY 10605
914-997-4488
888-663-4637
Fax: 914-997-4763
answers@marchofdimes.com
www.marchofdimes.com

March of Dimes help moms have full-term pregnancies and research the problems that threaten the health of babies. The March of Dimes also acts globally: sharing best practices in perinatal health and helping improve birth outcomes where the needs are the most urgent.

Stacey D. Stewart, President

Conferences

333 Adult Endocrine Disorders/GHD Educational Convention
Magic Foundation
4200 Cantera Drive, #106
Warrenville, IL 60555
630-836-8200
800-362-4423
Fax: 630-836-8181
contactus@magicfoundation.org
www.magicfoundation.org

An educational program for adults who are affected with Growth Hormone Deficiency and/or other endocrine disorders.

June

Rick Buckley, Chairman
Ken Dickard, Vice Chairman
Courtney Lance, Secretary

334 Genetic Alliance Annual Conference
Genetic Alliance
4301 Connecticut Avenue NW, Suite 404
Washington, DC 20008
202-966-5557
800-336-4363
Fax: 202-966-8553
info@geneticalliance.org
www.geneticalliance.org

Consistently inspirational and enables partnership among all stakeholders: advocates and community leaders, health and industry professionals, policymakers, and academicians.

July

Sharon Terry, President/CEO
Tetyana Murza, Managing Director
Natasha Bonhomme, VP, Strategic Development

Web Sites

335 Online Mendelian Inheritance in Man
National Library of Medicine, Building 38A
Bethesda, MD 20894
888-346-3656
info@ncbi.nlm.nih.gov
www.ncbi.nlm.nih.gov

This database is a catalog of human genes and genetic disorders.

Christine E. Seidman, M.D., Chair
David J. Lipman, M.D., Executive Secretary

336 Wheeless' Textbook of Orthopaedics
www.wheelessonline.com

Comprehensive, unparalleled, dynamic online medical textbook that is updated daily.

Clifford R. Wheeless, III, M.D., Author

Book Publishers

337 Let's Talk About Going to the Hospital
Rosen Publishing Group's PowerKids Press
29 E 21st Street
New York, NY 10010
212-777-3017
800-237-9932
Fax: 888-436-4643
rosenpub@tribeca.ios.com
www.rosenpublishing.com

If a child has to check into the hospital, chances are he or she is already upset about being ill. Knowing how a hospital functions and what the procedures are, such as when family members can visit, will help in what is already a stressful situation. Grades K-5.

24 pages
ISBN: 0-823950-36-0

DESCRIPTION

338   ASPERGER SYNDROME
Involves the following Biologic System(s):

Developmental/Behavioral/Psychiatric Disorders, Genetic/Chromosomal/Syndrome/Metabolic Disorders, Neurologic Disorders

Asperger syndrome (AS) is a developmental disorder belonging to the group of neurological conditions known as autism spectrum disorders (ASDs), which are marked by problems in language and communications and confined patterns of thought and behavior. AS usually manifests itself by the age of 3 years, and in some cases may be apparent in infancy through clumsiness and delayed crawling or walking. Children with AS have no difficulty with intelligence or language skills, but may speak in a monotone or in an excessively formal manner or have difficulties with the subtleties of language, such as the slight variations in rhythm and pitch that help to communicate different shades of meaning (prosody). Children with AS also exhibit repetitive or ritualistic behavior; tend to be preoccupied with a single activity or area of personal interest to the exclusion of other activities or interests; have difficulty in their gestures and motor movements, such as those needed for ballplaying or playground activities; and interact poorly with other children of their age group and usually also with adults, manifesting motor symptoms of the syndrome or focusing on their own interests rather than engaging in dialogue. In some cases, AS in children is followed by other psychological problems and symptoms in adolescence and adulthood.

AS occurs in about 2 of every 10,000 children and is more likely to affect boys than girls. Although its precise cause remains unknown, studies suggest that AS stems from aberrations in the structure and function of several regions of the brain, which may come from irregularities in the fetal development and growth of the brain. Recent studies suggest that susceptibility to AS, and the severity with which it affects an individual, may be related to one or more aberrations in a specific group of genes.

The absence of standardized, universally accepted diagnostic criteria for AS has complicated its diagnosis. Currently, several verbal and behavioral procedures are used in diagnostic testing for AS. Because each of these procedures has its own standards, the various procedures can yield different diagnostic results. Moreover, different specialists have different viewpoints about the nature and characteristics of AS, with some considering it a mild form of autism known as high-functioning autism rather than a distinct disorder. In identifying AS, most physicians use a set of criteria based on abnormal eye contact; failure of a child to respond to its name; failure to use gestures to point or indicate an object or item; and a lack of interest in and play with other children of the same age.

The complete examination of a child with suspected AS typically requires a psychologist, psychiatrist, neurologist, and speech therapist, with other professionals called upon as needed. Diagnosis of the syndrome includes testing of intelligence, language and communication skills, motor and other neurologic function, and genetics.

The treatment of AS similarly requires professionals specialized in improving the communications skills, easing the obsessive or repetitive behavioral patterns, and reducing the physical clumsiness of children with the syndrome. This typically involves strengthening the child's interests, actively involving the child in structured activities, and reinforcing socially adaptive behavior through the use of supervised group therapy. Physical and occupational therapy can be used to improve affected childrens' motor skills. Although they usually require these special educational services, children with Asperger syndrome are typically educated in the traditional community setting. If needed, medication can be used to alleviate anxiety and depression in children with AS.

Government Agencies

339   NIH/National Institute of Mental Health
6001 Executive Boulevard, Room 6200, MSC 9663
Bethesda, MD 20892

301-443-4536
866-615-6464
Fax: 301-443-4279
TTY: 301-443-8431
nimhinfo@nih.gov
www.nimh.nih.gov

The mission of NIMH is to transform the understanding and treatment of mental illnesses through basic and clinical research, paving the way for prevention, recovery, and cure.

Joshua Gordon, MD, PhD, Director
Shelli Avenevoli, MD, Deputy Director

340   NIH/National Institute of Neurological Dis orders and Stroke (NINDS)
PO Box 5801
Bethesda, MD 20824

301-496-5751
800-352-9424
Fax: 301-496-0296
TTY: 301-468-5981
www.ninds.nih.gov

The mission of NINDS is to reduce the burden of neurological disease - a burden borne by every age group, by every segment of society, by people all over the world.

Walter J. Koroshetz, MD, Director

341   NIH/National Institute on Deafness and Oth er Communication Disorders (NIDCD)
31 Center Drive, MSC 2320
Bethesda, MD 20892

800-241-1044
TTY: 800-241-1055
nidcdinfo@nidcd.nih.gov
www.nidcd.nih.gov

Conducts and supports biomedical research and research training on normal mechanisms, as well as diseases and disorders of hearing, balance, smell, taste, voice, speech and language.

James F Battey Jr, MD, PhD, Director
Judith A Cooper PhD, Deputy Director
Timothy J Wheeles, Executive Officer

National Associations & Support Groups

342   AASCEND
P.O. Box 591011
San Francisco, CA 94159

info@aascend.org
www.aascend.org

Adults of all ages on the autism spectrum, their families and friends, academics and professionals in the autism field unite as a community in AASCEND.

Greg Yates, Co-chair

343 AHA Association [Asperger Syndrome and Hig h Functioning Autism Association
PO Box 916
Bethpage, NY 11714
888-918-9198
Fax: 888-918-9198
info@ahany.org
www.ahany.org

Serves individuals on the autism spectrum, their families, and the professionals who work with them, providing crucial resources and support as they face challenges, build on their strengths and fulfill their potential.

Pat Schissel, LMSW, President/ Executive Director
Michael A. Buffa, Esq., VP of Board of Directors
Jennifer Feldman, Event Coordinator

344 ASPEN (Asperger Autism SPectrum Education Network)
9 Aspen Circle
Edison, NJ 8820
732-321-0880
aspenorg@aol.com
aspennj.org

ASPEN provides families and individuals whose lives are affected by Autism Spectrum Disorders (Asperger Syndrome, Pervasive Developmental Disorder-NOS, High Functioning Autism), and Nonverbal Learning Disabilities with education, support & advocacy.

Lori Shery, President/Executive Director
Rich Meleo, Vice President
Elizabeth Yamashita, Vice President

345 America's Special Kidz
P.O. Box 2098
Woodland Park, NJ 7424
973-521-0433
Fax: 973-341-7423
joanne@AmericaSpecialKidz.org
americaspecialkidz.org

America's Special Kidz A.S.K understands the importance of healthy families. With a large population of families with special kids-especially single parents-they serve these struggling families.

346 American Academy of Pediatrics
141 Northwest Point Boulevard
Elk Grove Village, IL 60007
847-434-4000
800-433-9016
Fax: 847-434-8000
www.aap.org

The American Academy of Pediatrics and its member pediatricians are committed to the attainment of optimal physical, mental and social health and well-being for all infants, children, adolescents, and young adults.

Fernando Stein, MD, FAAP, President
Karen Remley, MD, CEO/Executive VP

347 American Asperger's Association
1301 Seminole Blvd Suite B-112
Largo, Fl 33770
727-518-7294
Knaus@gmail.com
americanaspergers.forumotion.net

The mission of the American Aspergers Association is to initiate, sponsor, support, and promote activities and projects for the care, treatment and education of children and adults afflicted with Autism and Aspergers Syndrome without regard to faith, creed, race, national origin or ethnic background.

Dr. Ronald Knaus, Medical Director/ Founder

348 American Association for Marriage and Family Therapy
112 South Alfred Street
Alexandria, VA 22314
703-838-9808
Fax: 703-838-9805
www.aamft.org

The American Association for Marriage and Family Therapy (AAMFT) is the professional association for the field of marriage and family therapy.

Marvarene Oliver, EdD, President
Tracy Todd, PhD, Executive Director
Chris Michaels, Chief Operations Officer

349 American School Counselor Association
1101 King Street, Suite 310
Alexandria, VA 22314
703-683-2722
800-306-4722
Fax: 703-997-7572
asca@schoolcounselor.org
www.schoolcounselor.org

The mission of ASCA is to represent professional school counselors and to promote professionalism and ethical practices.

Richard Wong, Executive Director
Jeff Broderson, Information Technology Admin.
Kathleen M Rakestraw, Director of Communications

350 Asperger Autism Spectrum Education Network (ASPEN)
9 Aspen Circle
Edison, NJ 08820
732-321-0880
info@aspennj.org
www.aspennj.org

ASPEN provides families and individuals whose lives are affected by Autism Spectrum Disorders (Asperger Syndrome, Pervasive Developmental Disorder-NOS, High Functioning Autism), and Nonverbal Learning Disabilities.

Lori Shery, President/Executive Director
Rich Meleo, Vice President
Elizabeth Yamashita, Vice President

351 Asperger's Network Support for Well-being Education and Research
12930 30th Ave N
Plymouth, MN 55441
763-227-5059
tnamie@aspergersmn.org
www.aspergersmn.org

ANSWER is a group of advocates for improving awareness, research, education and support of individuals and families impacted by Asperger's Syndrome.

Theresa Namie, Executive Director/ Co-Founder
Kathy Hoffman, Chair
James Namie, Treasurer

352 Asperger/Autism Network
51 Water Street, Suite 206
Watertown, MA 2472
617-393-3824
866-597-AANE
Fax: 617-393-3827
info@aane.org
www.aane.org

The Asperger/Autism Network (AANE) works with individuals, families, and professionals to help people with Asperger Syndrome and similar autism spectrum profiles build meaningful, connected lives.

Jayne Burke, President
Karen Boyd, Vice President
Stephen Burgay, B.A., J.D., Vice President

353 Aspergers Women's Association
www.aspergerwomen.org
AWA serves to educate the public on issues unique to women and girls on the spectrum, as well as their families.

354 Autism Network International
PO Box 35448
Syracuse, NY 13235
315-476-2462
jisincla@syr.edu
www.autismnetworkinternational.org

Supported by individuals who want to make a difference for the sufferers, the foundation provides a variety of support and educational references to inform on the latest changes in the field.

Jim Sinclair, Coordinator
Jame Bordner, List-owner
Sola Shelly, Webmaster

355 **Autism New Jersey**
500 Horizon Drive, Suite 530
Robbinsville, NJ 08691 609-588-8200
800-428-8476
Fax: 609-588-8858
information@autismnj.org
www.autismnj.org

Autism New Jersey is a nonprofit agency committed to ensuring safe and fulfilling lives for individuals with autism, their families, and the professionals who support them. Through awareness, credible information, education, and public policy initiatives, Autism New Jersey leads the way to lifelong individualized services provided with skill and compassion.

Suzanne Buchanan, Executive Director
Elizabeth Neumann, Director, Education/Training
Ellen Schisler, Director, Development/Marketing

356 **Autism Society of America**
4340 East-West Hwy, Suite 350
Bethesda, MD 20814 301-657-0881
800-328-8476
info@autism-society.org
www.autism-society.org

The Autism Society, the nation's leading grassroots autism organization, exists to improve the lives of all affected by autism. We do this by increasing public awareness about the day-to-day issues faced by people on the spectrum, advocating for appropriate services for individuals across the lifespan, and providing the latest information regarding treatment, education, research and advocacy.

Scott Badesch, President & CEO
Matthew Asner, VP Development
Selena Hernandez, Manager, Support Services

357 **Bridges4Kids**
www.bridges4kids.org

info@bridges4kids.org
www.bridges4kids.org

A non-profit organization providing a comprehensive system of information and referral for parents and professionals seeking help for children from birth through transition to adult life.

Deborah K. Canja, CEO
Jackie D. Igafo-Te'o, Webmaster

358 **Center for Autism and Related Disorders**
19019 Ventura Blvd., Suite 300
Tarzana, CA 91356 818-345-2345
855-345-2273
Fax: 818-758-8015
www.centerforautism.com

The Center for Autism and Related Disorders (CARD) uses applied behavior analysis (ABA) in the treatment of autism spectrum disorder.

Doreen Granpeesheh, Founder/ Executive Director

359 **Families of Adults Afflicted with Asperger's Syndrome**
PO Box 514
Centerville, MA 2632 508-790-1930
faaas@faaas.org
faaas.org

Offers support to the family members of adult individuals with Asperger's Syndrome.

Karen E. Rodman, President/ Founder
Jack Kelley, Events Coordinator
Thomas Rodman, Webmaster/ Docmaster

360 **Global and Regional Asperger Syndrome Partnership**
419 Lafayette Street
New York, NY 10003 888-474-7277
info@grasp.org
grasp.org

GRASP works to improve the lives of teens and adults with autism spectrum disorder (ASD). It offers in-school programs to help students with autism learn advocacy skills and improve social skills. Through its website, it educates the public about autism, while also offering free online resources and networking opportunities for individuals with ASD and their families.

361 **NIH/ Eunice Kennedy Shriver National Institute of Child Health & Human Development**
31 Center Drive, Building 31
Bethesda, MD 20892 301-496-5113
800-370-2943
Fax: 866-760-5947
TTY: 888-320-6942
nichdpress@mail.nih.gov
www.nichd.nih.gov

NICHD conducts and supports laboratory research, clinical trials, and epidemiological studies that explore health processes; examines the impact of disabilities, diseases, and variations on the lives of individuals; and sponsors training programs for scientists, health care providers, and researchers to ensure that NICHD research can continue.

Diana W. Bianchi, Director
Paul Williams, Director, Communications

362 **National Alliance on Mental Illness**
3803 N. Fairfax Drive, Suite 100
Arlington, VA 22203 703-524-7600
800-950-6264
Fax: 703-524-9094
info@nami.org
www.nami.org

Grassroots mental health organization dedicated to building better lives for the millions of Americans affected by mental illness. - See more at:
http://www.nami.org/About-NAMI#sthash.IYtjmu5h.dpuf

Jim Payne, J.D., President
David Levy, Chief Financial Officer
Mary Giliberti, J.D., Executive Director

363 **National Association of Special Education Teachers**
1250 Connecticut Avenue, N.W., Suite 200
Washington, DC 20036 800-754-4421
Fax: 800-754-4421
contactus@naset.org
www.naset.org

A membership organization dedicated solely to meeting the needs of special education teachers and those preparing for the field of special education teaching.

Dr. Roger Pierangelo, Co-Executive Director
Dr. George Giuliani, Co-Executive Director

364 **National Autism Association**
One Park Avenue, Suite 1
Portsmouth, RI 02871 401-293-5551
877-622-2884
Fax: 401-293-5342
naa@nationalautism.org
nationalautismassociation.org

NAA is a parent-run advocacy organization and the leading voice on urgent issues related to severe autism, regressive autism, autism safety, autism abuse, and crisis prevention.

Wendy Fournier, President
Kelly Vanicek, Executive Director
Katie Wright, Vice President

365 **National Institute of Environmental Sciences**
P.O. Box 12233, MD K3-16, Research Triangle Park
Research Triangle Park, NC 27709 919-541-1919
Fax: 301-480-2978
webcenter@niehs.nih.gov
www.niehs.nih.gov

The mission of the NIEHS is to discover how the environment affects people in order to promote healthier lives.

Linda S. Birnbaum, Director
Richard Woychik, Ph.D., Deputy Director
Sheila A. Newton, Ph.D., Policy, Planning, and Evaluation

366 National Mental Health Consumers' Self-Help Clearinghouse
1211 Chestnut Street, Suite 1207
Philadelphia, PA 10079
215-751-1810
800-553-4539
Fax: 215-636-6312
info@mhselfhelp.org
www.mhselfhelp.org

The Clearinghouse works to foster peer empowerment through
our website, up-to-date news and information announcements, a
directory of peer-driven services, electronic and printed publications, training packages, and individual and onsite consultation

Joseph Rogers, Executive Director & Founder
Susan Rogers, Director of Special Projects
Britani Nestel, Program Specialist

367 Oasis at MAAP
PO Box 524
Crown Point, IN 10080
219-662-1311
Fax: 219-682-6372
info@aspergersyndrome.org
www.aspergersyndrome.org

MAAP Services is a world wide 501-C-3 non profit organization
providing information, networking, referrals and printed materials
for families, challenged individuals and professionals concerned
with the autism spectrum. Founded in 1984, MAAP Services, adheres to the basic principal that all individuals with autism spectrum challenges have the ability to learn, grow and enjoy a good
quality of life.

Susan Moreno, Founder & President
Lara Blanchard, BCBA

368 US Aspergers Association
5364 Ehrlich Rd. #175
Tampa, FL 33624
813-264-0777
Fax: 813-830-7373
info@usaspergers.org
usaspergersassn.com

A charitable organization that was created to help those children,
adults and their families get the help they need in order to be
properly diagnosed with Asperger's Syndrome.

Philip Bernie, President
Nina Bernie, Vice President

369 US Autism & Asperger Association
P.O. Box 532
Draper, UT 84020
888-9AU-ISM
www.usautism.org

US Autism & Asperger Association (USAAA) is a 501(c)(3) nonprofit organization for autism and Asperger education, support,
and solutions.

Lawrence P. Kaplan, PhD, Chairman/ CEO
Richard Dunie, MPh, MBA, CPA, Secretary/ Treasurer
Phillip C. DeMio, MD, Chief Medical Officer

Conferences

370 ASPEN Annual Fall Conference
Asperger Autism Spectrum Education Network
9 Aspen Circle
Edison, NJ 08820
732-321-0880
info@aspennj.org
www.aspennj.org

Practical strategies for teachers and parents of students with autism spectrum disorders for navigating school, home and life

October

Lori Shery, President/Executive Director
Rich Meleo, Vice President
Ann Hiller, Secretary

371 Autism Society National Conference and Exposition
Autism Society of America
4340 East-West Hwy, Suite 350
Bethesda, MD 20814
301-657-0881
800-328-8476
info@autism-society.org
www.autism-society.org

Addresses the range of issues affecting people with autism including early intervention, education, employment, behavior,
communication, social skills, biomedical interventions and others, across the entire lifespan.

July

Scott Badesch, President/CEO
Matthew Asner, VP Development
Selena Hernandez, Manager, Support Services

372 Autreat
Autism International Network
PO Box 35448
Syracuse, NY 13235
315-476-2462
webmaster@autreat.com
www.autismnetworkinternational.org

A retreat-style conference run by autistic people, for autistic people and friends. Focuses on positive living with autism, not on
causes, cures, or ways to make individuals more normal.

August

Jim Sinclair, Coordinator

Audio Video

373 Asperger's Syndrome: Autism and Obsessive Behavior
Films for the Humanities and Sciences
132 West 31st Street
New York, NY 10001
800-257-5126
Fax: 609-275-0266
custserv@films.com
www.ffh.films.com

This program profiles the symptoms of Asperger's Syndrome and
what sufferers and their families can do to overcome the limitations that it imposes.

28 minutes
ISBN: 1-421387-67-3

374 The Boy Inside
Fanlight Productions
32 Court Street, 21st Floor
Brooklyn, NY 11201
718-488-8900
800-876-1710
Fax: 718-488-8642
info@fanlight.com
www.fanlight.com

The harrowing story of the filmaker's son Adam, a 12-year-old
with Asperger Syndrome, during a tumultuous year in the life of
their family. AS makes Adam's life in seventh grade a minefield,
where he finds himself isollated and bullied. As he struggles to
find a place for himself, his troublees escalate, both at school and
at home. ISBN: DVD: 1-57295-838-3; VHS: 1-57295-449-3

47 minutes DVD or VHS

Web Sites

375 Asperger's Association of New England
51 Water Street, Suite 206
Watertown, MA 2472
617-393-3824
866-597-AANE
Fax: 617-393-3827
info@aane.org
www.aane.org

The immediate goal of austistic.org is to build a global database
of information and resouces by and for persons on the autistic
spectrum.

Jayne Burke, President
Karen Boyd, Vice President
Stephen Burgay, B.A., J.D., Vice President

376 Autism Resources
www.autism-resources.com

Offers information and links regarding the developemental disabilities autism and Asperger's Syndrom.

377 Family Village
www.familyvillage.wisc.edu

A global community that integrates information, resources and communication opportunities on the Internet for persons with cognitive and other disabilities, for their families and for those that provide them services and support.

378 Online Asperger Syndrome Information and Support
P.O. Box 524
Crown Point, IN 46308   219-662-1311
                                         info@aspergersyndrome.org
                                         www.aspergersyndrome.org

Provides parents, professionals and person with the links they need to research anything.

379 University Students with Autism and Asperger's Syndrome Web Site
www.users.dircon.co.uk/~cns/

Helps to develop an understanding of the difficulties people with Asperger Syndrome may face. We also work on a one to one basis with the student and liase with staff and peers. Help is also given in setting up support networks such as mentors and providing effective strategies to aid independent learning.

Book Publishers

380 Asperger Syndrome

A Klin, F Volkmar, S Sparrow, author

Guilford Publications
72 Spring Street
New York, NY 10012   212-431-9800
                                         800-365-7006
                                         Fax: 212-966-6708
                                         info@guilford.com
                                         www.guilford.com

Brings together preeminent scholars and practitioners to offer a definitive statement of what is currently known about Asperger syndrome and to highlight promising leads in research and clinical practice. Sifts through the latest developments in theory and research, discussing key diagnostic and conceptual issues and reviewing what is known about behavioral features and neurobiology. The effects of Asperger syndrome on social development, learning and communication are examined.

Jan 2000 489 pages
ISBN: 1-572305-34-2

381 Asperger Syndrome and Your Child: A Parent's Guide
Autism Society of North Carolina Bookstore
505 Oberlin Road, Suite 230
Raleigh, NC 27605   919-743-0204
                                         800-442-2762
                                         Fax: 919-743-0208
                                         books@autismsociety-nc.org
                                         www.autismbookstore.com

Written primarily for parents, this book provides a clinician's view of Asperger Syndrome.

382 Asperger Syndrome: A Practical Guide for Teachers
ADD WareHouse
300 NW 70th Avenue, Suite 102
Plantation, FL 33317   954-792-8100
                                         800-233-9273
                                         Fax: 954-792-8545
                                         websales@addwarehouse.com
                                         www.addwarehouse.com

A clear and concise guide to effective classroom practice for teachers and support assistants working with children with Asperger Syndrome in school. The authors explain characteristics of children with Asperger Syndrome, discuss methods of assessment and offer practical strategies for effective classroom interventions.

90 pages
ISBN: 1-853464-99-6

383 Asperger Syndrome: Guide for Educators and Parents, Second Edition
Pro-Ed
8700 Shoal Creek Boulevard
Austin, TX 78757   512-451-3246
                                         800-897-3202
                                         Fax: 800-397-7633
                                         info@proedinc.com
                                         www.proedinc.com

A ground-breaking resource on Asperger Syndrome, this text outlines, in lay terms, the characteristics of the syndrome sometimes referred to as higher-functioning autism.

215 pages
ISBN: 0-890798-98-2

384 Asperger's Syndrome: A Guide for Parents and Professionals
ADD WareHouse
300 NW 70th Avenue, Suite 102
Plantation, FL 33317   954-792-8100
                                         800-233-9273
                                         Fax: 954-792-8545
                                         websales@addwarehouse.com
                                         addwarehouse.com

Providing a description and analysis of the unusual characteristics of Asperger's Syndrome, with strategies to reduce those that are most conspicuous or debilitating. This guide brings together the most relevant and useful information on all aspects of the syndrome, from language and social behavior to motor clumsiness.

240 pages
ISBN: 1-853025-77-1

385 Autism and Asperger Syndrome
Autism Society of North Carolina Bookstore
505 Oberlin Road, Suite 230
Raleigh, NC 27605   919-743-0204
                                         800-442-2762
                                         info@autismsociety-nc.org
                                         www.austismsociety-nc.org

Chapters include topics such as the relationship of autism and Asperger Syndrome, living with the syndrome and Asperger Syndrome in adulthood.

247 pages

Beverly Moore, Chairman
Sharon Jeffries-Jones, Vice Chair
Darryl R Marsch, Secretary

386 Can I Tell You About Asperger Syndrome?: A Guide for Friends and Family
Autism Society of North Carolina Bookstore
505 Oberlin Road, Suite 230
Raleigh, NC 27605   919-743-0204
                                         800-442-2762
                                         Fax: 919-743-0208
                                         books@autismsociety-nc.org
                                         www.autismbookstore.com

Written for young people so that they can better understand the challenges faced by a sibling, friend, or classmate who has Asperger Syndrome. For readers ages 7-15.

387 Oasis Guide to Asperger Syndrome
Autism Society of North Carolina Bookstore
505 Oberlin Road, Suite 230
Raleigh, NC 27605   919-743-0204
                                         800-442-2762
                                         Fax: 919-743-0208
                                         books@autismsociety-nc.org
                                         www.autismbookstore.com

Combining the most current information about Asperger Syndrome (AS) diagnosis and treatment with hundreds of practical tips and reosurce listings, this guide is comprehensive in scope.

388 Out-of-Sync Child: Recognizing and Coping with Sensory Processing Disorder
Autism Society of North Carolina Bookstore
505 Oberlin Road, Suite 230
Raleigh, NC 27605
919-743-0204
800-442-2762
Fax: 919-743-0208
books@autismsociety-nc.org
www.autismbookstore.com

The author provides, readers with information on the symptoms and diagnosis of sensory processing disorder (SPD), as well as treatment approach based on early intervention.

389 To Be Me: Understanding What It's Like to Have Asperger's Syndrome
Autism Society of North Carolina Bookstore
505 Oberlin Road, Suite 230
Raleigh, NC 27605
919-743-0204
800-442-2762
Fax: 919-743-0208
books@autismsociety-nc.org
www.autismbookstore.com

Colorfully illustrated book is about a boy named David, who has Asperger Syndrome (AS). Told from David's point of view, the story focuses on his social difficulties, as he struggles to fit in with his classmates at school. For readers ages 9-12.

Pamphlets

390 Asperger Syndrome
NINDS
PO Box 5801
Bethesda, MD 20824
301-496-5751
800-352-9424
www.ninds.nih.gov

Information sheet.
Walter J. Koroshetz, M.D., Acting Director
Alan L. Willard, Ph.D., Acting Deputy Director
Caroline Lewis, Executive Officer

391 Autism Fact Sheet
NINDS
PO Box 5801
Bethesda, MD 20824
301-496-5751
800-352-9424
TTY: 301-468-5981
www.ninds.nih.gov

Also available in Spanish.
Walter J. Koroshetz, M.D., Acting Director
Alan L. Willard, Ph.D., Acting Deputy Director
Caroline Lewis, Executive Officer

Camps

392 Anchor Point Camp
RBM Ministries
PO Box 128
Plainwell, MI 49080
269-342-9879
bobgoodenough@sbcglobal.net
www.rbmministries.org

Accepts mentally and physically handicapped children ages 13 and up.
Bob Goodenough, Executive Director

393 Camp Akeela
1 Thoreau Way
Thetford Center, VT 05075
866-680-4744
Fax: 866-462-2828
info@campakeela.com
www.campakeela.com

A co-ed, overnight camp in Vermont. Within a well-rounded and traditional program we emphasize the social growth of our campers, many of whom have been diagnosed with Asperger's Syndrome or a non verbal learning disability.
Debbie Sasson, Director

394 Camp Northwood
132 State Route 365
Remsen, NY 13438
315-831-3621
Fax: 315-831-5867
northwoodprograms@hotmail.com
www.nwood.com

Specialize in working with non-aggressive children ranging in age from 8-18 classified with Asperger's Syndrome, HFA, Attention Deficits, Language Processing Weaknesses and children with other forms of minimal learning issues.
Gordon Felt, Director

395 Charis Hills
498 Faulkner Road
Sunset, TX 76270
940-964-2145
888-681-2173
Fax: 940-964-2147
info@charishills.org
www.charishills.org

Residential Christian summer camp which helps kids with learning differences build confidence and find success. We welcome kids with ADHD, PDD, Asperger's Syndrome and High Functioning Autism.
Rand Soulhard, President

396 Frontier Travel Camp
2000 NE 197 Terrace
Miami, FL 33179
305-895-1123
866-750-2267
Fax: 305-402-0900
info@frontiertravelcamp.com
www.frontiertravelcamp.com

Established in 1997 as a summer camp alternative for individuals with special needs. We believe that group trips are an ideal way to experience independence, improve social skills, and increase self-esteem in a secure and exciting environment.
Scott Fineman, Director

397 Summer Experience
Vanguard School
PO Box 730
Paoli, PA 19301
610-296-6700; Fax: 610-640-0132
info@vanguardshool-pa.org
www.vanguardschool-pa.org

For students who are experiencing learning difficulties due to neurological impairment, social/emotional disturbance and/or autism/pervasive developmental disorder.
Susan Snyder, Admissions Director
John D Wilson, Education Director

398 Summit Camp
168 Duck Harbor Road
Honesdale, PA 18431
570-253-4381
800-323-9908
Fax: 570-253-2937
info@summitcamp.com
www.summitcamp.com

Provides a summer camp experience for boys and girls, ages 7-17, who have issues of attention. These may include ADD, verbal or non-verbal disabilities, mild social or emotional concerns, and/or Aspergers syndrome.
Eugene Bell, Senior Director

399 Wesley Woods
1001 Fiddlersgreen Rd
Grand Valley, PA 16420
814-430-7802
Fax: 814-436-7669
www.wesleywoods.com

Exceptional children's camp for children with emotional and intellectual handicaps.
Herb West

DESCRIPTION

400   ASTHMA

Synonym: Bronchial asthma

Involves the following Biologic System(s):

Respiratory Disorders

Asthma is a chronic respiratory disorder in which abnormal sensitivity (hyperresponsiveness) to certain stimuli causes inflammation and associated narrowing of the lungs' large and small airways, resulting in shortness of breath and other symptoms. Approximately 14 million adults and 6 million children have asthma. It is the primary cause of chronic illness in children. Up to 10 percent of girls and 15 percent of boys are affected by asthma at some point during childhood. Initial symptoms occur during the first year of life in about 30 percent of patients and before the age of four to five years in approximately 80 to 90 percent.

Episodes may be triggered by exposure to many different stimuli, such as certain foreign substances (allergens) including pollen, mold, house dust, or animal hair. Asthma attacks may also be triggered by respiratory infections or exposure to smoke, certain chemicals or medications, strong odors, cold air, vigorous exercise, or stress. Exposure to such stimuli or precipitating factors may prompt certain cells within the lungs' airways (e.g., mast cells) to release particular substances that may cause spasms of the smooth muscles lining the airways, inflammation and swelling of the airway walls, excessive secretion of mucus, and associated airway narrowing (bronchoconstriction) and obstruction.

Asthma episodes may vary greatly in frequency, severity, and duration. For example, attacks may subside after minutes or have a duration of hours or even days. Some patients may have only occasional, mild episodes of shortness of breath. Others may regularly cough and produce a high-pitched whistling sound while breathing (wheezing) and experience severe asthma episodes upon exposure to certain triggering stimuli. Most children with asthma have only periodic episodes that are mild to moderate in severity. However, a small percentage of children have severe asthma that interferes with regular daily functioning. Interestingly, most patients become relatively free of symptoms within 10 to 20 years after disease onset; however, many may have recurrences at some time during adulthood. Children with severe asthma may experience chronic disease through adulthood.

Asthma episodes may begin suddenly or gradually and are initially characterized by signs of air hunger, such as sighing, yawning, wheezing that may be most apparent while exhaling. Other symptoms include shortness of breath and a hacking, nonproductive cough. As mucus secretions increase, exhaling may become abnormally prolonged; however, this finding may not be obvious in infants and young children. Shortness of breath may become so severe that patients have difficulty walking and become unable to speak other than in a panting manner. These patients may assume a hunched over position in an attempt to make breathing easier. Additional symptoms may include chest tightness, profuse sweating due to exertion and anxiety, nausea, and vomiting. During extremely severe episodes, wheezing may diminish due to lack of airflow in the airways; breathing may become irregular and shallow; and patients may become listless (lethargic), appear confused due to lack of oxygen, and develop abnormal bluish discoloration of the skin and mucous membranes (cyanosis) due to abnormally diminished oxygen levels in the blood. Without immediate treatment, such patients may experience life-threatening complications.

Asthma is classified according to frequency of symptoms and the result of lung (pulmonary) tests. Classification and monitoring assists with the management of asthma and includes minimizing exposure to possible precipitating factors, such as avoiding rapid changes in humidity or temperature and reducing exposure to tobacco smoke, pollen, strong odors, fumes, or other possible irritants. In some cases, specialized tests may help to determine specific triggering stimuli that should be avoided. Asthma medications can be divided into long-term control and quick relief medications. Treatment choices are based on the severity of the patient's underlying asthma and the severity of asthma exacerbations. Treatment should be administered as quickly as possible to open the airways and restore normal breathing and proper oxygen levels in the blood. Drug therapy may include medications that relax and widen the airways (bronchodilators), such as albuterol. Depending upon the specific drugs prescribed or the severity of an episode, such medications may be administered by a metered dose inhaler with a spacer, or by a nebulizer, which produces a mist for inhalation. Inhaled steroids are the most effective anti-inflammatory medications for management of chronic asthma. Intravenous medications may be used in the hospitalized patient. If a patient is unable to be managed at home, or has progression of symptoms requiring intervention more often than every 4 hours, they should seek emergency care. Emergency treatment may include IV corticosteroids, IV bronchodilators, continuous nebulizer treatments and, in the most severe cases, possibly intubation with mechanical ventilation.

Government Agencies

401   NIH/National Heart, Lung and Blood Institute Information Center

NHLBI Information Center
PO Box 30105
Bethesda, MD 20824

301-592-8573
Fax: 301-629-3246
TTY: 240-629-3255
nhlbiinfo@nhlbi.nih.gov
www.nhlbi.nih.gov

The National Heart, Lung, and Blood Institute (NHLBI) provides global leadership for a research, training, and education program to promote the prevention and treatment of heart, lung, and blood diseases and enhance the health of all individuals so that they can live longer and more fulfilling lives.

Gary H Gibbons, MD, Director
Nakela Cook, MD, Chief of Staff

402   NIH/National Institute of Allergy and Disease Council

5601 Fishers Lane, MSC 9806
Bethesda, MD 20892

301-496-5717
Fax: 301-402-3573
ocpostoffice@niaid.nih.gov
www.niaid.nih.gov

The principal advisory board of the NIAID. The council is composed of physicians, scientists and representatives of the public and advises on the conduct and support or research, training and dissemination of health information regarding allergies and infectious diseases.

Anthony S Fauci MD, Director

403 National Advisory Allergic and Infectious Disease Council
5601 Fishers Lane, MSC 9806
Bethesda, MD 20892   301-496-5717
                                                          866-284-4107
                                                       Fax: 301-402-3573
                                                       TDD: 800-877-8339
                                                    ocpostoffice@niaid.nih.gov
                                                         www.niaid.nih.gov

The principal advisory board of the NIAID. The council is composed of physicians, scientists and representatives of the public and advises on the conduct and support or research, training and dissemination of health information regarding allergies and infectious diseases.

Dr. Anthony S. Fauci, M.D., Director

National Associations & Support Groups

404 Air Support America
3435 Wilshire Blvd., Suite #350
Los Angeles, CA 90010   323-937-7859
                                                       Fax: 866-324-8074
                                                         breathmobile.org

The organization provides information, activities, and resources for asthma and allergy patients and their families.

405 Allergy & Asthma Network Mothers of Asthmatics
8201 Greensboro Drive, Suite 300
McLean, VA 22102   800-878-4403
                                                       Fax: 703-288-5271
                                                         info@aanma.org
                                                          www.aanma.org

A nonprofit family health organization dedicated to eliminating suffering and death due to asthma, allergies and related conditions.

Nancy Sander, President/Founder
Marcela Gieminiani, Director of Administration
Sandra Fusco-Walker, Director of Advocacy

406 American Academy of Allergy, Asthma & Immunology
555 East Wells Street, Suite 1100
Milwaukee, WI 10084   414-272-6071
                                                       Fax: 414-272-6070
                                                         info@aaaai.org
                                                          www.aaaai.org

The American Academy of Allergy, Asthma & Immunology is dedicated to the advancement of the knowledge and practice of allergy, asthma and immunology for optimal patient care.

Linda Coz MD, President
James T Li MD, President-Elect
Robert F Lemanske Jr MD, Secretary-Treasurer

407 American Academy of Pediatrics
141 Northwest Point Boulevard
Elk Grove Village, IL 60007   847-434-4000
                                                          800-433-9016
                                                       Fax: 847-434-8000
                                                           www.aap.org

The American Academy of Pediatrics and its member pediatricians are committed to the attainment of optimal physical, mental and social health and well-being for all infants, children, adolescents, and young adults.

Fernando Stein, MD, FAAP, President
Karen Remley, MD, CEO/Executive VP

408 American Association for Respiratory Care
9425 N. MacArthur Blvd. Suite 100
Irving, TX 75063   972-243-2272
                                                         info@aarc.org
                                                          www.aarc.org

The AARC encourages and promotes professional excellence, advances the science and practice of respiratory care, and serves as an advocate for patients and their families, the public, the profession and the respiratory therapist.

409 American Asthma Foundation
Box 0509, UCSF
San Francisco, CA 94143   415-514-0730
                                                       Fax: 415-514-0734
                                                    info@americanasthma.org
                                                  www.americanasthmafoundation.org

They fund innovative research by outstanding investigators from all fields that might impact asthma.

Michael J. Welsh, M.D., Chair
Valerie Dougherty, Program Manager
William E. Seaman, M.D., Research Director

410 American College of Allergy, Asthma and Immunology
85 W Algonquin Road, Suite 550
Arlington Heights, IL 60005   847-427-1200
                                                          800-842-7777
                                                       Fax: 847-427-9656
                                                          mail@acaai.org
                                                          www.acaai.org

The association provides its members with continuing medical education, publications, and representation to managed care organizations, medical organizations, consumer and patient groups, and government and regulatory agencies. The College also develops and disseminates educational information to patients, other physicians, health professionals and health plan administrators.

Rick Slawny, Executive Director
Nancy Ryan, Associate Executive Director
Hollis Heavenrich-Jones, Public Relations Manager

411 American Lung Association
55 W. Wacker Drive, Suite 1150
Chicago, IL 60601   312-801-7628
                                                          800-586-4872
                                                          info@lung.org
                                                           www.lung.org

The American Lung Association fights lung disease in all its forms, with special emphasis on asthma, tobacco control and environmental health. The American Lung Association is funded with contributions from the public, along with gifts and grants from corporations, foundations and government agencies. The association achieves its many successes through the work of thousands of committed volunteers and staff.

Harold P. Wimmer, National President & CEO
Susan Rappaport, National VP, Research/Scientific
Sue Swan, Chief Development Officer

412 American Medical Association
AMA Plaza, 330 North Wabash Ave., Suite 39300
Chicago, IL 60611   800-262-3211
                                                       www.ama-assn.org/ama

AMA is dedicated to ensuring sustainable physician practices that result in better health outcomes for patients.

James L. Madara, MD, CEO/ EVP
Bernard L. Hengesbaugh, Chief Operating Officer
Kenneth J. Sharigian, SVP/ Chief Strategy Officer

413 American School Counselor Association
1101 King Street, Suite 310
Alexandria, VA 22314   703-683-2722
                                                          800-306-4722
                                                       Fax: 703-997-7572
                                                    asca@schoolcounselor.org
                                                      www.schoolcounselor.org

The mission of ASCA is to represent professional school counselors and to promote professionalism and ethical practices.

Richard Wong, Executive Director
Jeff Broderson, Information Technology Admin.
Kathleen M Rakestraw, Director of Communications

414 American Thoracic Society
25 Broadway
New York, NY 10004   212-315-8600
                                                       Fax: 212-315-6498
                                                     ATSInfo@Thoracic.org
                                                         www.thoracic.org

The American Thoracic Society improves global health by advancing research, patient care, and public health in pulmonary disease, critical illness, and sleep disorders. Founded in 1905 to combat TB, the ATS has grown to tackle asthma, COPD, lung cancer, sepsis, acute respiratory distress, and sleep apnea, among other diseases.

Thomas W. Ferkol, MD, President
Atul Malhotra, MD, President-elect
Stephen C. Crane, PhD, MPH, Executive Director

415 Association of Asthma Educators
70 Buckwalter Rd., Ste 900, #330
Royersford, PA 19468   888-988-7747
admin@asthmaeducators.org
www.asthmaeducators.org

The Association of Asthma Educators is the premier inter-professional organization striving for excellence to raise the competency of diverse individuals who educate patients and families living with asthma.

Cindy Cooper, President
Traci Hardin, Vice-President
Michael Shoemaker, Treasurer

416 Asthma and Allergy Foundation of America
8201 Corporate Drive Suite 1000
Landover, MD 10087   800-727-8462
info@aafa.org
www.aafa.org

AAFA is dedicated to improving the quality of life for people with asthma and allergic diseases through education, advocacy and research.

Lynn Hanessian, Chair
Michele Abu Carrick, LICSW, Co-Chair, Governance
Calvin Anderson, Chair, Finance & Treasurer

417 Breathing Association (The)
1520 Old Henderson Road
Columbus, O 43220   614-457-4570
Fax: 614-457-3777
dferraro@breathingassociation.org
www.breathingassociation.org

The Breathing Association serves the community as the leading resource for promoting lung health and preventing lung disease through education, detection, service, and treatment.

Diane L. Habash, Ph.D., RD, LD, Chair
Joanne Spoth, President & CEO
Danni Palmore, Secretary

418 Environmental Protection Agency
1200 Pennsylvania Avenue, N.W.
Washington, DC 20460   202-272-0167
TTY: 202-272-0165
www.epa.gov

EPA promotes scientific understanding of environmental asthma triggers and ways to manage asthma in community settings through research, education and outreach.

Gina McCarthy, Administrator
Stan Meiburg, Acting Deputy Administrator
Gwen Keyes Fleming, Chief of Staff

419 Genetic Alliance
4301 Connecticut Avenue NW, Suite 404
Washington, DC 20008   202-966-5557
800-336-4363
Fax: 202-966-8553
info@geneticalliance.org
www.geneticalliance.org

World's leading nonprofit health advocacy organization committed to transforming health through genetics and promoting an environment of openness centered on the health of individuals, families, and communities.

Sharon Terry, President/CEO
Tetyana Murza, Managing Director
Natasha Bonhomme, VP, Strategic Development

420 Get a Grip on Asthma Programs
2751 Prosperity Avenue, Suite 150
Fairfax, VA 10089   703-641-9595
800-878-4403
Fax: 703-573-7794
info@aanma.org
www.aanma.org

Allergy & Asthma Network Mothers of Asthmatics (AANMA) is the leading nonprofit family health organization dedicated to eliminating suffering and death due to asthma, allergies and related conditions. From diagnosis to control, from diapers to college - AANMA is your one-stop, family-to-family support network.

Nancy Sander, President/Founder
Susan Rogers, Director of Special Projects
Nathan Hulfish, Project & Events Coordinator

421 National Association of School Nurses
1100 Wayne Avenue Suite 925
Silver Spring, MD 20910   240-821-1130
866-627-6767
Fax: 301-585-1791
www.nasn.org

The mission is to advance school nurse practice to keep students healthy, safe and ready to learn.

Donna J. Mazyck, Executive Director
Nichole K. Bobo, Nursing Education Director
Margaret Cellucci, Director of Communications

422 National Asthma Educator Certification Board
4001 E Baseline, Suite 206
Gilbert, AZ 85234   877-408-0072
info@naecb.org
www.naecb.com

The mission of the National Asthma Educator Certification Board is to promote optimal asthma management and quality of life among individuals with asthma, their families and communities, by advancing excellence in asthma education through the certified asthma educator (AE-Cr) process.

John Manning, Chair
Timothy R. Hudd, Vice Chair

423 National Environmental Education Foundation
4301 Connecticut Avenue NW, Suite 160
Washington, DC 20008   202-833-2933
www.neefusa.org

NEEF provides lifelong environmental learning, connecting people to knowledge they use to improve the quality of their lives and the health of the planet.

S. Decker Anstrom, Chairman
Diane Wood, Secretary
Diane W. Wood, President

424 National Institute of Environmental Health Sciences
P.O. Box 12233, MD K3-16, Research Triangle Park
Research Triangle Park, NC 27709   919-541-1919
Fax: 301-480-2978
webcenter@niehs.nih.gov
www.niehs.nih.gov

The mission of the NIEHS is to discover how the environment affects people in order to promote healthier lives.

Linda S. Birnbaum, Director
Richard Woychik, Ph.D., Deputy Director
Sheila A. Newton, Ph.D., Policy, Planning, and Evaluation

425 National Medical Association
8403 Colesville Road, Suite 920
Silver Spring, MD 20910   202-347-1895
Fax: 202-347-0722
www.nmanet.org

The National Medical Association (NMA) is the collective voice of African American physicians and the leading force for parity and justice in medicine and the elimination of disparities in health.

Garfield Clunie, M.D., Chairman of the Board
Lawrence Sanders, President
Martin Hamlette, J.D., M.H.A., Executive Director

426 Respiratory Health Association
1440 W. Washington Blvd.
Chicago, I 60607   312-243-2000
                                          888-880-5864
                                     Fax: 312-243-3954
                                   info@lungchicago.org
                                   www.lungchicago.org

The association addresses asthma, COPD, lung cancer, tobacco control and air quality with a comprehensive approach involving research, education and advocacy activities.

Joel Africk, President/ CEO
Kate McMahon, Senior Director, Programs & Policy
Gina Schwieger, Senior Director, Special Events

427 Support for Asthmatic Youth (SAY) Support Groups
Asthma and Allergy Foundation of America
1080 Glen Cove Avenue
Glen Head, NY 11545   516-621-4348
                                     Fax: 516-625-2976
                                   reneeTheo1@aol.com
                      www.medhelp.org/Support-Groups/4061.htm

A network of educational/support groups for adolescents between the ages of nine and seventeen. All meetings are free and feature guest speakers, informational programs, games and other fun activities.

Renee Theodorakis, MA

428 Support for Asthmatic Youth Pals-Pen Pals
Asthma and Allergy Foundation of America
1080 Glen Cove Avenue
Glen Head, NY 11545   516-621-4348
                                     Fax: 516-625-2976
                                   reneeTheo1@aol.com
                      www.medhelp.org/Support-Groups/4061.htm

A pen pal program that matches adolescents ages 9 to 17 who share similar interests and also happen to have asthma and/or allergies.

Renee Theodorakis, MA, Adolescent Services

State Agencies & Support Groups

Alaska

429 Alaska Chapter of Asthma and Allergy Found ation of America
PO Box 201927
Anchorage, AK 10092   907-349-0637
                                          800-651-4914
                                     Fax: 907-696-4810
                                   aafaalaska@gci.net
                                   www.aafaalaska.com

THE MISSION OF AAFA ALASKA IS TO SERVE PEOPLE AFFECTED BY ASTHMA AND ALLERGIES THROUGH EDUCATION, COMMUNITY RESOURCES, RESEARCH AND SUPPORT

Kathryn Anderson, Board of Directors
Kathleen Bell, Secretary
Mark Glore, CPA, Treasurer

California

430 Northern California Chapter of Asthma and Allergy Foundation of America
5900 Wilshire Boulevard, Suite 710
Los Angeles, CA 90036   323-937-7859
                                          800-624-0044
                                     Fax: 323-937-7815
                               breathingmatters@aafa-ca.org
                                   www.aafa-ca.org

The Foundation was formed to alleviate suffering and loss from asthma and allergy disorders. The Foundation offers a nationwide network of chapters and support groups, and provides education and emotional support for persons with allergies and asthma. Also funds research for improved treatments and ultimately a cure.

Trina Celise, Acting Executive Director

Colorado

431 Parents of Asthmatic/Allergic Children, In c.
1024 S. Lemay Avenue
Fort Collins, CO 80524   970-495-8153
                                     Fax: 970-495-7608
                                        cmc@pvhs.org
                                 www.coloradoallergy.com

Support group for parents and children ages 6 and older, focusing on asthma, and issues such as allergic and non-allergic rhinitis.

Cindy Coopersmith, Coordinator

Maryland

432 Maryland-Greater Washington, DC Chapter As thma and Allergy Foundation of America
1498 Reisterstown Road, Suite 324
Baltimore, MD 10094   410-484-2054
                                          800-727-8462
                                     Fax: 410-484-2043
                                   info@aafa-md.org
                                   www.aafa-md.org

The Maryland-Greater DC Chapter works to help asthma and allergy sufferers successfully manage and control their disease through the support of education, advocacy, referrals and research. Major activities include accredited childcare provider course, school liaison, patient assistance and professional education courses.

Dalton A. Tong, Chairman
Stephanie L. Covington, Board of Directors
Sara Sheckells Hendrickson, Board of Directors

Massachusetts

433 Asthma & Allergy Foundation of America New England Chapter
109 Highland Avenue
Needham, MA 02494   781-444-7778
                                          800-227-8462
                                     Fax: 781-444-7718
                                   aafane@aafane.org
                               www.asthmaandallergies.org

The Foundation was formed to alleviate suffering and loss from asthma and allergy disorders. The Foundation offers a nationwide network of chapters and support groups, and provides education and emotional support for persons with allergies and asthma. Also funds research for improved treatments and ultimately a cure.

Elaine Erenrich Rosenburg, Executive Director

Michigan

434 Michigan Chapter of Allergy and Asthma Foundation of America
2075 Walnut Lake Road
West Bloomfield, MI 10096   248-406-4254
                                          888-444-0333
                                     Fax: 248-757-2102
                                 aafamich@sbcglobal.net
                                   www.aafamich.org

Our mission is to improve the quality of life for individuals affected with asthma and allergic diseases by promoting awareness through education and training.

Kathleen Felice Slonager, Executive Director

Missouri

435 **Allergy and Pulmonary Medicine**
Saint Louis Children's Hospital
One Children's Place
Saint Louis, MO 10097   314-454-6000
                                        Fax: 314-454-2515
                                        www.stlouischildrens.org

Evaluating and treating a child's allergy or pulmonary disorder is only part of the care provided by the professionals at St. Louis Children's Hospital. Many of the difficulties children endure also require extensive treatment at home, therefore, educating parents and caregivers about home care and progress monitoring is a primary concern for the Allergy and Pulmonary Medicine staff. In most cases, the staff works with other team members throughout the hospital.

Stuart C Sweet MD PhD, Secretary

436 **Asthma and Allergy Foundation of America Greater Kansas City Chapter**
400 E Red Bridge Road, Suite 214
Kansas City, MO 10098   816-333-6608
                                        888-542-8252
                                        Fax: 816-333-6684
                                        info@aafakc.org
                                        www.aafakc.org

The Asthma and Allergy Foundation of America, Greater Kansas City Chapter, (AAFA-KC) is committed to enhancing and saving the lives of asthma and allergy sufferers through support, advocacy, education, research and access to treatment.

Mrs Jamie Mayes, Board Chair
Mr Kent Wessely, Vice President
Mr Kevin P Sparks, Treasurer

437 **Asthma and Allergy Foundation of America - Saint Louis Chapter**
1500 South Big Bend, Suite 1S
Saint Louis, MO 10099   314-645-2422
                                        Fax: 314-645-2022
                                        aafa@aafastl.org
                                        www.aafastl.org

The AAFA, St. Louis Chapter (AAFA), a United Way Agency, has been serving the asthmatic and allergic needs of the St. Louis community for over 30 years. AAFA's medical assistance program, Project Concern, provides uninsured and underinsured children with life-saving asthma and allergy medications, equipment, education, and support.

H. James Wedner, M.D, President
Bill Vice President, Vice President
Dave Birkenmeier, Second Vice President

New Jersey

438 **Asthma and Allergy Foundation of America - Southeast Pennsylvania Chapter**
470 Sentry Parkway East, Suite 200
Blue Bell, PA 10100   610-397-1540
                                        800-727-8462
                                        Fax: 856-224-5893
                                        aafasepa@verizon.net
                                        www.aafa.org

Serves southeastern Pennsylvania and portions of New Jersey. Program highlights include the Children at Risk program.

Marijo Washburn, Acting Director

Pennsylvania

439 **SE Pennsylvania Chapter of Asthma and Allergy Foundation of America**
470 Sentry Parkway East, Suite 200
Blue Bell, PA 10101   610-397-1540
                                        800-727-8462
                                        Fax: 856-224-5893
                                        aafasepa@prodigy.net
                                        www.aafa.org

Serves southeastern Pennsylvania and portions of New Jersey. Program highlights include the Children at Risk program.

Debi Maines, Executive Director

Texas

440 **Asthma and Allergy Foundation of America - North Texas Chapter**
3904 Justin Drive
Ft Worth, TX 10102   817-297-3132
                                        888-933-AAFA
                                        Fax: 817-297-6564
                                        info@aafatexas.org
                                        www.aafatexas.org

The mission of the Asthma and Allergy Foundation of America, Texas Chapter (formerly North Texas Chapter), a non-profit organization, is to help asthma and allergy sufferers to successfully manage and control their diseases through education, information, training and referrals.

Jim Rosenthal, President
Laura Steves, Executive Director
William Lumry MD, VP Funding

Libraries & Resource Centers

441 **National Jewish Health**
National Jewish Center for Immunology
1400 Jackson Street
Denver, CO 80206   877-225-5654
                                        800-423-8891
                                        lungline@njhealth.org
                                        www.nationaljewish.org

A free information service answering questions, sending literature and giving advice to patients with immunologic or respiratory illnesses. The Line is an educational service and not a substitute for medical care. Diagnosis or suggested treatment will not be provided for a caller's specific condition. The Line does suggest topics that a patient might want to discuss with his or her doctor.

Micheal Salem, MD, President/CEO
Valerie Hale, Owner
Jerry Gillette, Manager

442 **Physician Referral and Information Line**
American Academy of Allergy, Asthma & Immunology
555 E Wells Street, Suite 1100
Milwaukee, WI 53202   414-272-6071
                                        800-822-2762
                                        Fax: 414-272-6070
                                        info@aaaai.org
                                        www.aaaai.org

Referral line offering information on allergy and asthma, referral to an allergy/immunology specialist.

Kay Whalen, Executive Director
Joy Blackburn, President
Dennis Ledfored, President-Elect

Research Centers

443 Brigham and Women's Hospital, Asthma and Allergic Disease Research Center
75 Francis Street
Boston, MA 10103
617-732-5500
800-294-9999
TTY: 617-732-6458
bwhinfo@partners.org
www.brighamandwomens.org

Brigham and Women's Hospital is world-renowned in virtually every area of adult medicine. As a teaching hospital of Harvard Medical School, our leadership in patient quality and safety, development of state-of-the-art treatments and technologies, and robust research programs have improved the health of people around the world.

Amy Yunes, President
Peter Helms, Vice President
Mary Montuori, Vice President

444 Center for Interdisciplinary Research on Immunologic Diseases
Children's Hospital Medical Center
300 Longwood Avenue
Boston, MA 10104
617-355-6000
800-355-7944
TTY: 617-730-0152
webteam
www.childrenshospital.org

Boston Children's community mission is to Provide the best quality care to our patients and serve as a safety net hospital, Develop and support community programs to make an impact and address the most pressing community health needs-asthma, obesity, mental health and child development and Work with partners to address health and non-health issues that affect the entire community

James Mandell, CEO/Trustee
Sandra Fenwick, President
Margaret Coughlin, Senior Vice President & Chief Admin

445 John Hopkins Arthritis Center
5200 Eastern Avenue, Suite 4100
Baltimore, MD 10105
410-550-0545
Fax: 410-550-2090
jhuarthrities@jhmi.edu
www.hopkins-arthritis.org

The Johns Hopkins Arthritis Center has assembled a team of some of the world's leading experts and specializes in the care of inflammatory arthritis. This includes, most notably, osteoarthritis and rheumatoid arthritis.

Clifton Bingham, III, Director
Susan Bartlett, PhD, Associate Professor of Medicine
Uzma Haque, Assistant Professor of Medicine

446 Johns Hopkins Arthritis Center
5501 Hopkins Bayview Circle
Baltimore, MD 21224
410-550-0545
Fax: 410-550-2090
jhuallergy@jhmi.edu
www.hopkins-arthritis.org

Studies of allergic diseases and individuals with allergic disease, pulmonary diseases and diseases involving inflammation and immunological processes.

Dr. Lawrence Lichtenstein, Director

447 National Jewish Center for Immunology and Respiratory Medicine
1400 Jackson Street
Denver, CO 10107
877-225-5654
800-423-8891
lungline@njhealth.org
www.nationaljewish.org

Since 1899 we have been at the forefront of research and medicine. We integrate the latest scientific research discoveries with coordinated care for lung, heart and immune diseases.

John Cambier PhD, Department Chairman
Rafeul Alam MD PhD, Division Chief

448 National Jewish Medical & Research Center
1400 Jackson Street
Denver, CO 10108
877-225-5654
800-423-8891
lungline@njhealth.org
www.nationaljewish.org

Since 1899 we have been at the forefront of research and medicine. We integrate the latest scientific research discoveries with coordinated care for lung, heart and immune diseases.

Gregory P Downey MD, Executive Vice President
Valerie Hale, Owner

449 Northwestern University Asthma and Allergy Disease Center
420 East Superior Street
Chicago, IL 60611
312-503-8194
Fax: 312-503-0994
medcommunications@northwestern.edu
www.feinberg.northwestern.edu/clinical-services/inde

The school has earned recognition for its research in genetic medicine, nanotechnology, biochemistry, neuroscience, cancer research, and materials sciences. NU partners with the~Argonne National Laboratory, Fermilab, and local universities.

Eric G Neilson, MD, Vice President for Medical Affairs
William L. Lowe, Jr., MD, Vice Dean Academic Affairs
Raymond H. Curry, MD Curry, MD, Vice Dean Education

450 Tulane University Clinical Immunology Section
1430 Tulane Avenue Box SL-57
New Orleans, LA 10110
504-988-5578
800-355-7944
Fax: 504-988-3686
medsch@tulane.edu
www.tulane.edu/som/departments/medicine/medciar/

Tulane Medical Center, an acclaimed teaching, research and medical facility, serving the greater New Orleans area.

Laurianne G Wild, M.D., Director
Mary Brown, MBA, Vice President Health Sciences Syst

451 University of Texas Southwestern Medical Center/Asthma & Allergic Diseases
5323 Harry Hines Boulevard
Dallas, TX 10111
214-648-3111
Fax: 214-648-2102
www.utsouthwestern.edu

Among the nation's best performers in biology and biochemistry basic science research in achieving clinical breakthroughs.

Daniel K. Podolsky, President
J. Gregory Fitz MD, Executive Vice President
Bruce A Meyer MD MBA, Executive Vice President

452 University of Virginia General Clinical Research Center
1215 Lee Street
Charlottesville, VA 10112
434-924-5000
Fax: 434-924-9960
gcrc@virginia.edu
www.healthsystem.virginia.edu

To provide excellence, innovation and superlative quality in the care of patients, the training of health professionals, and the creation and sharing of health knowledge.

David R Jones, Program Director

453 University of Wisconsin Asthma and Allergic Disease Center
600 Highland Avenue
Madison, WI 10113
608-263-6100
877-942-7846
wiasthma@medicine.wisc.edu
www2.medicine.wisc.edu/home/asthma/asthmamain

The University of Wisconsin is known for its strong research environment, and the Department of Medicine has a rich history of academic achievement.

Carl J Getto, Head
Richard Page, Chair

Conferences

454 AAAAI Annual Meeting
American Academy of Allergy, Asthma & Immunology
555 East Wells Street, Suite 1100
Milwaukee, WI 53202
414-272-6071
Fax: 414-272-6070
annualmeeting@aaaai.org
www.aaaai.org

The world's premier gathering of allergy and immunology experts. Attendees include clinicians, academicians, allied health professionals and others interested in allergic and immunologic disease.

March

Dennis K Ledford MD, President

455 ACAAI Annual Meeting
American College Of Allergy, Asthma & Immunology
555 East Wells Street, Suite 1100
Milwaukee, WI 53202
414-272-6071
800-842-7777
Fax: 847-427-1294
mail@acaai.org
www.acaai.org

Offers an array of educational sessions for physicians, allied health professionals, office managers and asthma educators, as well as some fantastic social events.

November

James Slawny, Executive Director
Rick Slawny, Co-Executive Director
Mike Slawny, Director

456 Genetic Alliance Annual Conference
Genetic Alliance
4301 Connecticut Avenue NW, Suite 404
Washington, DC 20008
202-966-5557
800-336-4363
Fax: 202-966-8553
info@geneticalliance.org
www.geneticalliance.org

Consistently inspirational and enables partnership among all stakeholders: advocates and community leaders, health and industry professionals, policymakers, and academicians.

July

Sharon Terry, President/CEO
Tetyana Murza, Managing Director
Natasha Bonhomme, VP, Strategic Development

Audio Video

457 A Regular Kid
American Lung Association
55 W. Wacker Drive, Suite 1150
Chicago, IL 60601
312-801-7630
800-LUN-USA
Fax: 202-452-1805
info@lungusa.org
www.lungusa.org

This film shows how families and children cope with asthma problems. Proven asthma management strategies are presented through the experiences of four children with asthma, ranging in age from toddler to teenager.

Film

Kathryn A. Forbes, CPA, Chair
John F. Emanuel, JD, Vice Chair
Penny J. Siewert, Secretary/Treasurer

458 Allergy & Asthma Issues
American Academy of Allergy, Asthma & Immunology
555 E Wells Street, Suite 1100
Milwaukee, WI 53202
414-272-6071
Fax: 414-272-6070
info@aaaai.org
www.aaaai.org

Patient newsletter covering issues for allergy and asthma patients throughtout the year. Articles discuss and advise on flus, inhalers, allergins, climate change effects on allergins, astham attacks in pregnancy, and much more.Available free online.

Quarterly

Melissa Graham, Media & Member Comm Manager
Megan Brown, Senior Media & Member Comm Manager

459 Allergy Control Begins at Home: House Dust Allergy
Allergy Control Products
1620-D Satellite Blvd
Duluth, GA 30097
800-255-3749
Fax: 800-395-9303
info@allergycontrol.com
www.allergycontrol.com

Shows simple steps to decrease your level of dust mite exposure.

1993 35 minutes

460 Asthma - Understanding and Control
American Academy of Allergy, Asthma & Immunology
555 E Wells Street, Suite 1100
Milwaukee, WI 53202
414-272-6071
Fax: 414-272-6070
info@aaaai.org
www.aaaai.org

This 20 minute public education tool helps patients understand asthma diagnosis, allergic and non-allergic triggers, risk factors, and guidelines for control of the disease. It is a great addition to physician waiting rooms and for patient use at home. This DVD format includes a Spanish version.

Melissa Graham, Media & Member Comm Manager
Megan Brown, Senior Media & Member Comm Manager

461 Baby Breath
Allergy and Asthma Network/Mothers of Asthmatics
8229 Boone Boulevard, Suite 260
Vienna, VA 22182
703-641-9595
800-878-4403
Fax: 703-288-5271
www.aanma.org

Shows babies and toddlers taking a nebulizer treatment.

2003 Video

Tonya Winders, President/ CEO
Beth Gannett, Director of Membership & Marketing
Brenda Silvia-Torma, Project Manager

462 Childhood Asthma
Films for the Humanities and Sciences
132 West 31st Street
New York, NY 10001
800-257-5126
Fax: 609-275-0266
custserv@films.com
www.ffh.films.com

This program deals with the nature of bronchial and allergic asthma and with the diagnosis and treatment of childhood allergies. It explains how asthma attacks can be triggered by allergies, respiratory infections, exervise, and emotional stress; shows by means of animation how the bronchial tubes of asthmatics become inflamed and constricted during an attack; stresses the early diagnosis and treatment of childhood asthma; and explains what treatments are recommended.

28 minutes
ISBN: 1-421339-06-1

463 Managing Childhood Asthma
American Lung Association
50 East Huron Street
Chicago, IL 60611
312-944-6780
800-545-2433
Fax: 312-440-9374
ala@ala.org
www.ala.org

What parents need to know to manage asthma. 22 minutes.

Video

Keith Michael Fiels, Executive Director
Willie Glispie, Senior Administrative Assistant
Lois Ann Gregory-Wood, Secretariat

464   Mastering Asthma
Aquarius Health Care Videos
18 North Main Street
Sherborn, MA 1770   508-650-1616
                                        888-440-2963
                                    Fax: 508-650-1665
                            www.aquariusproductions.com

Mastering Asthma, so it doesn't master you, is an entertaining
and informative video for both parents and children that takes
viewers into the lives of three different families learning about
and living with childhood asthma. Learn what is Asthma and what
causes it. Everything from allergens and triggers to peak flow meters and bronchodialators and more is discussed. Closed
captioned.

ISBN: 1-581402-93-7

465   Pharmacologic Therapy of Pediatric Asthma
American Lung Association
1740 Broadway
New York, NY 10019   212-315-8700

A Learning Resource Program developed by a joint committee of
the American Thoracic Society and the ALA.

Film

466   What School Personnel Should Know About Asthma
American Lung Association
1740 Broadway
New York, NY 10019   212-315-8700

Professionally produced videotape discussing the triggers, symptoms and management of childhood asthma.

Videotape

Web Sites

467   Allergy & Asthma Network Mothers of Asthmatics
www.aanma.org

A national nonprofit network of families whose desire is to overcome not to cope with allergies and asthma.

468   American Academy of Allergy, Asthma and Immunology
555 E Wells Street, Suite 1100
Milwaukee, WI 53202   414-272-6071
                                        info@aaaai.org
                                        www.aaaai.org

The mission of the American Academy of Allergy, Asthma and
Immunology, is the advancement of the knowledge and practice
of allergy, asthma and immunology for optimal patient care: by
discussion at meetings, by fostering the education of students and
the public, by encouraging union and cooperation among those
engaged in the field, and by promoting and stimulating research
and study in allergy, asthma and immunology.

Melissa Graham, Media & Member Comm Manager
Megan Brown, Senior Media & Member Comm Manager

469   American Lung Association
55 W. Wacker Drive, Suite 1150
Chicago, IL 60601   312-801-7628
                                        800-LUN-USA
                                        info@lung.org
                                        www.lung.org

Information regarding lung disease in all its forms, with special
emphasis on asthma, tobacco control and environmental health.

Harold P. Wimmer, National President & CEO
Susan Rappaport, National VP, Research/Scientific
Sue Swan, Chief Development Officer

470   Asthma and Allergy FAQs
www.cs.unc.edu/~kupstas/FAQ.html

The Allergy and Asthma FAQ is an informal gathering of the net
wisdom on allergies and asthma. It includes links to various
(Web and non-Web) sources of information. This started as the
misc.kids Allergy and Asthma FAQ, so a certain amount of this
information is geared towards parents, but there is plenty of information for adults, too.

471   Asthma and Allergy Foundation of America
8201 Corporate Drive, Suite 1000
Landover, MD 20785   800-727-8462
                                        Info@aafa.org
                                        www.aafa.org

Provides information, support and referrals through a national
network of chapters and educational support groups.

Cary Sennett, President/ CEO
Lynda Mitchell, SVP, Community Services
Yolanda Miller, SVP/ COO/ CFO

472   Gazoontite
www.gazoontite.com

We are an employee-owned company of allergy sufferers, dedicated to providing you with the very best allergen control
products.

473   NIH/National Insitute of Allergy and Infectious Diseases
5601 Fishers Lane, MSC 9806
Bethesda, MD 20892   301-496-5717
                                        866-284-4107
                                   Fax: 301-402-3573
                                   TDD: 800-877-8339
                            ocpostoffice@niaid.nih.gov
                                   www.niaid.nih.gov/

The National Institute of Allergy and Infectous Diseases is a
component of the National Institutes of Health. NIAID conducts
and supports research that strives to understand, treat, and ultimately prevent the myriad infectious, immunologic, and allergic
diseases that threaten hundreds of millions of people worldwide.

Dr. Anthony S. Fauci, M.D., Director

474   National Eczema Association for Science and Education
4460 Redwood Highway Suite 16D
San Rafael, CA 94903   415-499-3474
                                        800-818-7546
                              www.nationaleczema.org

Information and education works to improve the health and the
quality of life of persons living with atopic dermatists/eczema,
including those who have the disease as well as their loved ones.

Dinesh Shenoy, CFO
Lisa Choy, Secretary
Julie Block, President & CEO

475   Online Mendelian Inheritance in Man
National Library of Medicine, Building 38A
Bethesda, MD 20894   888-346-3656
                                   info@ncbi.nlm.nih.gov
                                   www.ncbi.nlm.nih.gov

This database is a catalog of human genes and genetic disorders.

Christine E. Seidman, M.D., Chair
David J. Lipman, M.D., Executive Secretary

Book Publishers

476   Asthma
Franklin Watts c/o Grolier
90 Old Sherman Turnpike
Danbury, CT 06816   203-797-3500
                                   Fax: 203-797-3197
                      http://librarypublishing.scholastic.com

This book offers vital information on causes and treatments, plus
advice on how to prevent flare-ups.

128 pages Grades 9 12
ISBN: 0-531113-31-0

477   Asthma Self Help Book
Allergy Control Products
1620-D Satellite Blvd
Duluth, GA 30097   203-438-9580
                                        800-255-3749
                                   Fax: 203-431-8963
                                   TTY: 123-019-99
                            info@allergycontrol.com
                                www.allergycontrol.com

A comprehensive manual on the management of asthma for parents of asthmatic children, adult asthmatics, and for health professionals.

Softcover

478   Best of Superstuff Activity Booklet
American Lung Association
1740 Broadway
New York, NY 10019   212-315-8700

For young children with asthma featuring a series of activities designed to help youngsters cope with asthma.

32 pages Ages 6-8

479   Let's Talk About Going to the Hospital
Rosen Publishing Group's PowerKids Press
29 E 21st Street
New York, NY 10010   212-777-3017
                                       800-237-9932
                                  Fax: 888-436-4643
                      rosenpub@tribeca.ios.com
                      www.rosenpublishing.com

If a child has to check into the hospital, chances are he or she is already upset about being ill. Knowing how a hospital functions and what the procedures are, such as when family members can visit, will help in what is already a stressful situation. Grades K-5.

24 pages
ISBN: 0-823950-36-0

480   Let's Talk About Having Asthma
Rosen Publishing Group's PowerKids Press
29 E 21st Street
New York, NY 10010   212-777-3017
                                       800-237-9932
                                  Fax: 888-436-4643
                      rosenpub@tribeca.ios.com
                      www.rosenpublishing.com

This book talks about the cause and treatments for asthma as well as the precautions sufferers should take. Recommended for grades K-4.

1997 24 pages
ISBN: 0-823950-32-8

481   Living with Asthma
Walker & Company
1385 Broadway 5th Floor
New York, NY 10018   212-419-5300
                                  Fax: 212-727-0984
                      contact@bloomsbury.com
                      www.bloomsbury.com/us/childrens

Dispels the myths surrounding this disease and introduces readers to famous athletes and public figures who deal with it on a daily basis. Explains what asthma is, how to cope with it, what triggers an attack, and what to do if you or somone you are with is having an attack.

2000 112 pages
ISBN: 0-802775-85-3

482   Lung Disorders Sourcebook
Omnigraphics
PO Box 31-1640
Detroit, MI 48231   800-234-1340
                                  Fax: 800-875-1340
                      info@omnigraphics.com
                      omnigraphics.com

Basic consumer health information on lung disorders including tuberculosis, asthma and cystic fibrosis.

2002 678 pages
ISBN: 0-780803-39-6

483   Understanding Asthma
University Press of Mississippi
3825 Ridgewood Road
Jackson, MS 39211   601-432-6205
                                       800-737-7788
                                  Fax: 601-432-6217
                      press@ihl.state.ms.us
                      www.upress.state.ms.us

Noting that understanding and education are key to halting the rise in numbers of asthma cases, Dr. Phil Lieberman has written this book for families and the individual sufferer. Subjects include lungs of an asthmatic, allergies which trigger the disease, and measures used to control asthma. A Choice outstanding book for 2000, and American Journal of Nursing Book of the Year award for 2001.

120 pages Hardcover/Ppbck
ISBN: 1-578061-42-3

484   You Can Control Asthma - Books for the Family & Kids
Asthma and Allergy Foundation of America
8201 Corporate Drive, Suite 1000
Landover, MD 20785   202-466-7643
                                       800-727-8462
                                  Fax: 202-466-8940
                      info@aafa.org
                      www.aafa.org

Here is a set of easy to read workbooks, one for the family and one for children, ages 6-12, to help learn everything one needs to know about asthma. Learn how to keep asthma episodes from starting, what to do when an asthma episode starts, how to use flow meters, spacers, and inhalers through the use of pictures, captions and activities. Kids have their own workbook that helps them to make choices and to feel more in control of their asthma. Workbooks are available in English or Spanish.

45-61 pages

Lynn Hanessian, Chairman
Nancy Kercher, Secretary

Magazines

485   Allergy & Asthma Today
Allergy and Asthma Network/Mothers of Asthmatics
8229 Boone Boulevard, Suite 260
Vienna, VA 22182   703-641-9595
                                       800-878-4403
                                  Fax: 703-288-5271
                      info@aanma.org
                      www.aanma.org

Communicates practical advice and support for the benefit of all people affected by allergies, asthma and related conditions. Seeks to improve health outcomes by providing information in a consumer-friendly format with strategies for implementing behavior changes. Free to AANMA members.

Quarterly

Tonya Winders, President/ CEO
Beth Gannett, Director of Membership & Marketing
Brenda Silvia-Torma, Project Manager

486   Controlling Asthma
American Lung Association
1740 Broadway
New York, NY 10019   212-315-8700

For parents of children with asthma, this newsmagazine tells how parents can help their child deal with the many problems presented by asthma.

16 pages

487   Coping with Allergies and Asthma
PO Box 682268
Franklin, TN 37068   615-790-2400
                                  Fax: 615-614-3986
                      info@copingmag.com
                      www.copingmag.com

A bimonthly publication devoted to people whose lives are affected by difficult breathing conditions.

Paula Chadwell, Vice President

Newsletters

488   **MA Report**
Allergy and Asthma Network Mothers of Asthmatics
8229 Boone Boulevard, Suite 260
Vienna, VA 22182
Fax: 703-288-5271
aanma@aol.com
www.aanma.org

Practical allergy and asthma management information along with the latest allergy and asthma news, recalls, medical updates, product reviews and advocacy initiatives.

8 pages free w/member

Tonya Winders, President/ CEO
Beth Gannett, Director of Membership & Marketing
Brenda Silvia-Torma, Project Manager

Pamphlets

489   **Asthma and Allergy Answers: Patient Education Library**
Asthma and Allergy Foundation of America
8201 Corporate Drive, Suite 1000
Landover, MD 20785
202-466-7643
800-727-8462
Fax: 202-466-8940
Info@aafa.org
www.aafa.org

This resource tool has information on more than forty topics of interest to patients. These reproducible camera ready answers are written in a patient friendly question and answer format. There is space to personalize the handy patient education materials with your practice or facility information. Topics covered are adult onset of asthma and allergies, food allergies, latex allergies, asthma medications, peak flow meters and managing your asthma.

In binder form

Cary Sennett, President/ CEO
Lynda Mitchell, SVP, Community Services
Yolanda Miller, SVP/ COO/ CFO

490   **Childhood Asthma: A Matter of Control**
American Lung Association
1740 Broadway
New York, NY 10019
212-315-8700

A guide for parents of children with asthma, this booklet covers topics such as identifying asthma signs and symptoms as well as controlling the condition.

28 pages

491   **Living with Asthma and Allergies Brochure Series**
Asthma and Allergy Foundation of America
8201 Corporate Drive, Suite 1000
Landover, MD 20785
202-466-7643
800-727-8462
Fax: 202-466-8940
Info@aafa.org
www.aafa.org

This informative series was developed to provide up-to-date, accurate information on common topics. Written in easy to understand language, with helpful illustrations, the brochures covers some of the most commonly asked questions about asthma and allergies. Perfect for individuals, whether newly diagnosed or more experienced, and for distribution to patients. Titles include, Allergy Basics, Seasonal Allergies: Pollens and Molds, Asthma Basics, Exercise and Asthma, and more.

Cary Sennett, President/ CEO
Lynda Mitchell, SVP, Community Services
Yolanda Miller, SVP/ COO/ CFO

492   **Superstuff**
American Lung Association
1740 Broadway
New York, NY 10019
212-315-8700

Kit specifically designed to help the elementary school child with asthma to learn how to manage the condition. The kit contains teaching tools, puzzles, riddles, stories and games.

493   **Teens Talk to Teens About Asthma**
Asthma and Allergy Foundation of America
8201 Corporate Drive, Suite 1000
Landover, MD 20785
202-466-7643
800-727-8462
Fax: 202-466-8940
Info@aafa.org
www.aafa.org

This brochure is a great gift of support to a teen you care about. Includes quotes and thoughts from teens that capture the essenceof what it feels like to live with asthma. Perfect for newly diagnosed teens. Single copies free with two first class stamps on a business-sized, self-addressed envelope.(Order #P-012) Quantities available, please call for prices.

Cary Sennett, President/ CEO
Lynda Mitchell, SVP, Community Services
Yolanda Miller, SVP/ COO/ CFO

494   **There are Solutions for the Student with Asthma**
American Lung Association
1740 Broadway
New York, NY 10017
212-315-8700

Leaflet telling how parents and school personnel can work together to make life easier for children with asthma.

4 pages

495   **Your Child and Asthma**
National Jewish Center for Immunology
1400 Jackson Street
Denver, CO 80206
303-388-4461
877-225-5654
www.nationaljewish.org

A booklet offering information to parents and family about their child with asthma. Offers information on diagnosis, treatments, triggers and family concerns.

Michael Salem, MD, President/ CEO
Richard A. Schierburg, Chair
Robin Chotin, Vice Chairs

Camps

496   **Camp Vacamas**
256 Macopin Road
West Milford, NJ 7480
973-838-0942
Fax: 973-838-7534
info@vacamas.org
www.vacamas.org

Disadvantaged children with asthma or sickle cell anemia, ages 8-16, are offered special programs in canoeing, backpacking, camping, music and leadership training. Sliding scale tuition. Year round programs for groups.

Michael Friedman, Executive Director
Philip Smith, Camp Director

497   **Des Moines YMCA Camp**
1192 166th Drive
Boone, IA 50036
515-432-7558
Fax: 515-432-5414
ycamp@dmymca.org
www.y-camp.org

For boys and girls with cancer, diabetes, asthma, cystic fibrosis, hearing impaired and other disabilities.

David Sherry, Executive Director
Alex Kretzinger, Program Director Camps

498 **VACC Camp**
Nicklaus Children's Hospital
3200 SW 60th Court, Suite 203
Miami, FL 33155

305-662-8222
Fax: 786-268-1765
bela.florentin@mch.com
www.vacccamp.com

Free, week-long, overnight camp for ventilation assisted children (children needing a tracheotomy ventilator, C-PAP, BiPAP, or oxygen to support breathing) and their families. Gives families a fun oppourtinity to socialize with peers and enjoy activities not readily accessible to technology dependent children.

Bela Florentin, Camp Coordinator
Rose Ann Farrell, Volunteer Assistants Coordinator
Alyssa Garcia, Operations

DESCRIPTION

499 ATAXIA

Involves the following Biologic System(s):

Neurologic Disorders

Ataxia is a neuromuscular condition characterized by an impaired ability to coordinate voluntary movements. The condition is caused by abnormalities of or damage to the region of the brain known as the cerebellum, nerve pathways that transmit messages to and from the cerebellum, or certain regions of the spinal cord. The cerebellum plays an essential role in regulating the maintenance of normal postures, sustaining balance, and producing smooth and coordinated movements. The spinal cord conducts sensory and motor impulses to and from the brain. The symptoms associated with ataxia vary, depending upon the specific regions of the brain that are affected; however, symptoms may often include imbalance and an abnormal staggering manner of walking (gait). Ataxia may be the result of certain infection, malformations of the cerebellum of spinal cord that are present at birth (congenital), head injury, brain tumors, exposure to particular medications, or certain genetic disorders. The primary infectious causes of ataxia during childhood include the formation of pus-filled pockets of infection in the cerebellum (cerebellar abscesses); sudden, severe inflammation of the passages within the inner ear (acute labyrinthitis): or acute cerebellar ataxia. Acute labyrinthitis typically occurs due to middle ear infections and may be characterized by vomiting and a sense that one's body or environment is spinning (vertigo). Acute cerebellar ataxia occurs subsequent to certain viral infections, such as chicken pox, and is thought to result from an abnormal immune response causing inflammation of the brain. Acute cerebellar ataxia typically occurs suddenly and may be characterized by impaired control of voluntary movements of the torso (truncal ataxia) and difficulties sitting or standing; involuntary, rapid eye movements (nystagmus); and severe slurring of speech or an inability to speak. Although the condition typically improves within a few weeks, it sometimes is present for up to two months. Most children have a complete recovery; however, some may have residual speech abnormalities and lack of coordination.

Abnormalities present at birth (congenital) that may cause ataxia include absence of the region of the brain between the two sides or hemispheres of the cerebellum (agensis of cerebellar vermis); protrusion of part of the brain through an opening in the skull (encephalocele); or protrusion of certain, malformed regions of the brain through the opening at the base of the skull (foramen magnum) into the upper spinal canal (Arnold-Chiari malformation). Infants and children with such birth defects develop ataxia due to malformation of or damage to certain regions of the cerebellum.

Ataxia may also be an initial symptom associated with certain brain tumors, including tumors affecting the cerebellum or a particular area of the cerebrum where it joins with the cerebellum (i.e., frontal lobe). In addition, brain tumors known as neuroblastomasmay result in progressive ataxia. Neuroblastomas are solid, malignant tumors that may originate in any part of the sympathetic nervous system, which is that part of the nervous system that regulates certain involuntary activities during times of stress, such as raising blood pressure and increasing the heart rate.

In some children, ataxia may result from the administration of certain drugs, such as anticonvulsant medications, particularly phenytoin. In addition, the condition may be caused by exposure to a household pesticide that is commonly used as a rat poison (thallium).

Ataxia may also occur in association with certain inborn errors of metabolism and is a primary feature of many hereditary degenerative disorders of the brain and spinal cord. These degenerative disorders, which may be referred to as hereditay ataxias, include ataxia-telangiectasia and Friedreich's ataxia.

Ataxia-telangiectasia (AT) is a multisystem disorder that is inherited as an autosomal recessive trait. Affected children typically develop ataxia at approximately two years of age, eventually leading to an inability to walk. Friedreich's ataxia is a genetic disorder that is usually inherited as an autosomal recessive trait. The disorder is characterized by degenerative changes of certain regions of the spinal cord and is categorized as a spinocerebellar ataxia. Children with Friedreich's ataxia typically develop ataxia before age 10. The ataxia is slowly progressive and usually affects the legs and feet more severely than the arms and hands. Patients develop unusual high arching and severe muscle weakness of the feet and progressive difficulties walking, typically resulting in the need of a wheelchair. Additional hereditary spinocerebellar ataxia of childhood, such as Roussy-Levy syndrome, cause symptoms and findings similar to those associated with Friedreich's ataxia. Roussy-Levy syndrome often becomes apparent during infancy and is characterized by loss of joint position sensation (sensory ataxia), causing poorly judged, uncoordinated movements. Such ataxia initially affects the legs, causing difficulty walking, and later progresses to affect the hands. Roussy-Levy syndrome is transmitted as an autosomal dominant trait.

Another group of hereditary disorders, known as the olivopontocerebellar atrophics (OPCAs) are associated with ataxia. These disorders are characterized by progressive degeneration of the cerebellum as well as other areas of the brain. Although associated symptoms of most forms of OPCA become apparent during adolescence or adulthood, one form of the disorder is known to occur during infancy (OPCA of neonatal onset). Symptoms may include severely diminished muscle tone; rapidly progressive ataxia; involuntary, rapid eye movements; episodes of abnormally increased electrical activity in the brain (seizures); failure to grow and gain weight at the expected rate (failure to thrive); abnormalities in the structure and function of heart muscle (hypertrophic cardiomyopathy); and other symptoms and findings. Methods used in the management of ataxia may vary and depend upon the condition's underlying cause, the specific form of ataxia present, and other factors. Such measures are typically symptomatic and supportive.

Government Agencies

500 NIH/National Institute of Neurological Dis orders and Stroke (NINDS)
PO Box 5801
Bethesda, MD 20824

301-496-5751
800-352-9424
Fax: 301-496-0296
TTY: 301-468-5981
www.ninds.nih.gov

The mission of NINDS is to reduce the burden of neurological disease - a burden borne by every age group, by every segment of society, by people all over the world.

Walter J. Koroshetz, MD, Director

National Associations & Support Groups

501 American Academy of Pediatrics
141 Northwest Point Boulevard
Elk Grove Village, IL 60007

847-434-4000
800-433-9016
Fax: 847-434-8000
www.aap.org

The American Academy of Pediatrics and its member pediatricians are committed to the attainment of optimal physical, mental and social health and well-being for all infants, children, adolescents, and young adults.

Fernando Stein, MD, FAAP, President
Karen Remley, MD, CEO/Executive VP

502 National Ataxia Foundation
2600 Fernbrook Lane N Suite 119
Minneapolis, MN 10115

763-553-0020
Fax: 763-553-0167
naf@ataxia.org
www.ataxia.org

The National Ataxia Foundation is dedicated to improving the lives of persons affected by ataxia through support, education, and research.

Harry T Orr PhD, Board of Directors
Michael Parent, Executive Director
William P Sweeney, Treasurer

State Agencies & Support Groups

Alabama

503 Birmingham Support Group
National Ataxia Foundation
16 The Oaks Circle
Birmingham, AL 10116

205-987-2883
Fax: 763-553-0167
donnelly613b@aol.com
www.ataxia.org

The primary mission is to encourage and support research into Hereditary Ataxia, a group of neurological disorders which are chronic and progressive conditions affecting coordination.

Fred Donnelly, Contact
Becky Donnelly, Contact

Arizona

504 Arizona Ataxia Support Group
National Ataxia Foundation
7665 E Placita Luna Preciosa
Tucson, AZ 10117

520-885-8326
Fax: 763-553-0167
bbeck15@cox.net
www.ataxia.org/chapters/Tucson/default.aspx

The primary mission is to encourage and support research into Hereditary Ataxia, a group of neurological disorders which are chronic and progressive conditions affecting coordination.

Bart Beck, SG Leader

California

505 Greater North Valley California Support Group
4335 Bourdeaux Drive
Oakley, CA 10118

925-625-0738
www.geocites.com/hotsprings/

The primary mission is to encourage and support research into Hereditary Ataxia, a group of neurological disorders which are chronic and progressive conditions affecting coordination.

Debra Kellerman, Contact

506 Los Angeles Ataxia Support Group
National Ataxia Foundation
339 W Palmer, Apartment A
Glendale, CA 10119

818-246-5758
Fax: 763-553-0167
ccherilynmc@yahoo.com
www.ataxia.org/chapters/losangeles/default.aspx

The primary mission is to encourage and support research into Hereditary Ataxia, a group of neurological disorders which are chronic and progressive conditions affecting coordination.

Sherry McLaughlin, Contact

507 Northern California Support Group
National Ataxia Foundation
1980 Saint George Rd
Danville, CA 10120

925-735-7037
Fax: 763-553-0167
joanneloveland@gmail.com
www.ataxia.org/chapters/northerncalifornia/default.a

The primary mission is to encourage and support research into Hereditary Ataxia, a group of neurological disorders which are chronic and progressive conditions affecting coordination.

Joanne Loveland, Contact

508 Orange County Support Group
National Ataxia Foundation
829 W Gary Ave
Montebello, CA 10121

323-788-7751
Fax: 763-553-0167
danieln27@gmail.com
www.ataxia.org/chapters/orangecounty/default.aspx

The primary mission is to encourage and support research into Hereditary Ataxia, a group of neurological disorders which are chronic and progressive conditions affecting coordination.

Daniel Navar, Leader

509 Pacific Southwest Regional Genetics Group
2151 Berkeley Way
Berkeley, CA 10122

510-540-2696
Fax: 510-540-2966
www.hgen.pitt.edu/counseling/resources/regional04.ht

Coordinates genetic services; promotes communication among genetic professionals and consumers through network newsletter, meetings, and other events; share resources; and promote education and awareness of genetic disorders,

George C Cunningham, Director

510 San Diego Support Group
National Ataxia Foundation
2087 Granite Hills Drive
El Cajon, CA 92019

619-447-3753
Fax: 763-553-0167
sdasg@cox.net
www.ataxia.org

The primary mission is to encourage and support research into Hereditary Ataxia, a group of neurological disorders which are chronic and progressive conditions affecting coordination.

Earl McLaughlin, Contact

511 San Fernando Valley Support Group
19450 Turtle Ridge Lane
Northridge, CA 10124

818-363-5335
www.ataxia.org

The primary mission is to encourage and support research into Hereditary Ataxia, a group of neurological disorders which are chronic and progressive conditions affecting coordination.

Darneal J Myers, Contact

Colorado

512 Colorado Support Group
National Ataxia Foundation
5902 W Maplewood Drive
Littleton, CO 10125   303-794-6351
                                Fax: 763-553-0167
                              tom_sathre@acm.org
                                    www.ataxia.org

The primary mission is to encourage and support research into Hereditary Ataxia, a group of neurological disorders which are chronic and progressive conditions affecting coordination.

Donna Sathre, Leader
Tom Sathre, Leader

513 Mountain States Regional Genetics Services Network
4300 Cherry Creek Drive S
Denver, CO 10126   303-692-2423
                                Fax: 303-782-5576
          www.hgen.pitt.edu/counseling/resources/regional04.ht

Coordinates genetic services; promotes communication among genetic professional and consumers through network newsletters, meetings, and other events; share resources; and promote education and awareness of genetic disorders.

George C Cunningham, Director

Florida

514 Broward County Support Group
10603 NW 49th Place
Coral Springs, FL 10127   954-341-8565
                                Fax: 954-753-6761
                              pathamilto@aol.com
                   community.insidecentralflorida.com/bcfasg/

The primary mission is to encourage and support research into Hereditary Ataxia, a group of neurological disorders which are chronic and progressive conditions affecting coordination.

Patricia B Hamilton, Contact

515 Clearwater, FL Support Group
2363 Mary Lane
Clearwater, FL 10128   727-799-2852
                              joyous7@mciworld.com
                                    www.ataxia.org

The primary mission is to encourage and support research into Hereditary Ataxia, a group of neurological disorders which are chronic and progressive conditions affecting coordination.

Joyce Robbins, Contact

516 NE Florida Support Group
National Ataxia Foundation
8925 Adams Walk Dr
Jacksonville, FL 10129   904-314-2061
                                Fax: 763-553-0167
                              coryhannan@hotmail.com
                                    www.ataxia.org

The primary mission is to encourage and support research into Hereditary Ataxia, a group of neurological disorders which are chronic and progressive conditions affecting coordination.

Cory Hannan, Leader

517 Tampa Support Group
National Ataxia Foundation
306 Caloosa Palm St
Son City Center, FL 10130   charlie@flataxia1.org
                                    www.ataxia.org

The primary mission is to encourage and support research into Hereditary Ataxia, a group of neurological disorders which are chronic and progressive conditions affecting coordination.

Charlie Kirchner, Contact

Georgia

518 Georgia Ataxia Support Group
National Ataxia Foundation
320 Peters Street, Unit 12
Atlanta, GA 10131   404-822-7451
                              rookssgj@yahoo.com
                                    www.ataxia.org

The primary mission is to encourage and support research into Hereditary Ataxia, a group of neurological disorders which are chronic and progressive conditions affecting coordination.

Greg Rooks, Contact

519 Greater Atlanta Area Support Group
National Ataxia Foundation
320 Peters Street, Unit 12
Atlanta, GA 10132   404-822-7451
                   www.geocities.com/atlantaataxia
                              rookssgj@yahoo.com

The primary mission is to encourage and support research into Hereditary Ataxia, a group of neurological disorders which are chronic and progressive conditions affecting coordination.

Greg Rooks, Contact

520 Macon Support Group
116 Summerfield Drive
Macon, GA 10133   912-757-9454
                              rookssgj@yahoo.com
                                    www.ataxia.org

The primary mission is to encourage and support research into Hereditary Ataxia, a group of neurological disorders which are chronic and progressive conditions affecting coordination.

Millard H McWhorter III, MD, Contact

521 Southeast Regional Genetics Group
PO Box 1642
Decatur, GA 10134   404-778-8551
                                Fax: 404-778-8562
                              mlane@sergg.org
                                    www.sergginc.org

SERGG addresses the inequities in genetic service and resources in the region and to expand existing regional capabilities and resources and to develop new regional systems to address these gaps.Another goal is to improve the existing regional communication infrastructure and to facilitate information sharing among providers of genetic services and consumers and to establish collaborative partnerships with other professional organizations.

Hans Andersson, MD, President
Mary Rose Simpson, BS, Secretary/Treasurer

Illinois

522 Chicago, IL Area Ataxia Support Group
National Ataxia Foundation
3400 Wellington Court, #302
Rolling Meadows, IL 10135   847-797-9398
                              caasgz@aol.com
                                    www.ataxia.org

The primary mission is to encourage and support research into Hereditary Ataxia, a group of neurological disorders which are chronic and progressive conditions affecting coordination.

Craig Lisack, Contact

Indiana

523 Central Indiana Support Group
5716 N 225 W
W Lafayette, IN 10136   765-463-3973
                                Fax: 765-463-3972
                              turtle23@mindspring.com
                                    www.ataxia.org

The primary mission is to encourage and support research into Hereditary Ataxia, a group of neurological disorders which are chronic and progressive conditions affecting coordination.

Judy Marten, Contact

524   NE Indiana Support Group
4522 Shenandoah Circle W
Fort Wayne, IN 10137
219-485-0965
Fax: 763-553-0167
naf@ataxia.org
www.ataxia.org

The primary mission is to encourage and support research into Hereditary Ataxia, a group of neurological disorders which are chronic and progressive conditions affecting coordination.

Don & Jenny Roemke, Contact

Louisiana

525   Louisiana Chapter
National Ataxia Foundation
1720 Parker St.
Baton Rouge, LA 10138
985-643-0783
louisiananaf@yahoo.com
www.angelfire.com/la/ataxiachapter/

The primary mission is to encourage and support research into Hereditary Ataxia, a group of neurological disorders which are chronic and progressive conditions affecting coordination.

Elizabeth Tanner, Contact

526   Louisiana Support Group
National Ataxia Foundation
1720 Parker St.
Baton Rouge, LA 10139
985-643-0783
Fax: 763-553-0167
louisiananaf@yahoo.com
www.angelfire.com/la/ataxiachapter/

The primary mission is to encourage and support research into Hereditary Ataxia, a group of neurological disorders which are chronic and progressive conditions affecting coordination.

Elizabeth Tanner, Contact

Maine

527   Maine Support
National Ataxia Foundation
PO Box 113
Bowdoinham, ME 10140
763-553-0020
Fax: 763-553-0167
Kelley3902@myfairpoint.net
www.ataxia.org

The primary mission is to encourage and support research into Hereditary Ataxia, a group of neurological disorders which are chronic and progressive conditions affecting coordination.

Kelly Rollins, Contact

528   New England Regional Genetics Group
PO Box 920288
Needham, MA 10141
781-444-0126
Fax: 781-444-0127
mfgnergg@verizon.net
www.nergg.org

To provide a forum for collaboration among genetic professionals, consumers of genetic services and the Public Health Community in New England by Raising awareness about the impact of genetics on health throughout the lifespan and Promoting and facilitating access to genetic services, education and resources

Lisa Demers MS, CGC, President
Marinell Newton, President Elect
Lisa Brailey MD, Service Provider

Maryland

529   Chesapeake Chapter
National Ataxia Foundation
5938 Rossmore Drive
Bethesda, MD 10142
301-530-4989
Fax: 301-530-2480
carljlauter@erols.com
www.geocities.com/Hotsprings/Oasis/4988/

The primary mission is to encourage and support research into Hereditary Ataxia, a group of neurological disorders which are chronic and progressive conditions affecting coordination.

Carl J Lauter, President

Massachusetts

530   New England Support Group
National Ataxia Foundation
45 Juliette Street
Andover, MA 10143
978-475-8072
Fax: 763-553-0167
naf@ataxia.org
www.ataxia.org

The primary mission is to encourage and support research into Hereditary Ataxia, a group of neurological disorders which are chronic and progressive conditions affecting coordination.

Donna Gorzela, Leader
Richard Gorzela, Leader

Michigan

531   Detroit Michigian Ataxia Support Group
National Ataxia Foundation
20217 Wyoming
Detroit, MI 10144
313-397-7858
Fax: 763-553-0167
tinyt48221@yahoo.com
www.ataxia.org

The primary mission is to encourage and support research into Hereditary Ataxia, a group of neurological disorders which are chronic and progressive conditions affecting coordination.

Tany Tunstull, Leader

Minnesota

532   Minneapolis, MN Support Group
National Ataxia Foundation
2549 32nd Avenue S
Minneapolis, MN 10145
612-724-3784
Fax: 763-553-0167
schultz.lenore@yahoo.com
www.ataxia.org

The primary mission is to encourage and support research into Hereditary Ataxia, a group of neurological disorders which are chronic and progressive conditions affecting coordination.

Lenore Healey Schultz, Contact

Mississippi

533   Mississippi Chapter
National Ataxia Foundation
PO Box 17005
Hattiesburg, MS 10146
763-553-0020
Fax: 763-553-0167
daglio1@bellsouth.net
www.ataxia.org

The primary mission is to encourage and support research into Hereditary Ataxia, a group of neurological disorders which are chronic and progressive conditions affecting coordination.

Camille Daglio, President

Missouri

534 Central Missouri Area Support Group
National Ataxia Foundation
1609 Cocoa Court
Columbia, MO 10147   572-474-7232
                                        Fax: 763-553-0167
                                 rogercooley@localnet.com
                                           www.ataxia.org

The primary mission is to encourage and support research into
Hereditary Ataxia, a group of neurological disorders which are
chronic and progressive conditions affecting coordination.

Roger Colley, Leader

535 Kansas City, Missouri Support Group
National Ataxia Foundation
17700 East 17th Terrace Ct. S #102
Independence, MO 10148   816-257-2428
                                        Fax: 763-553-0167
                               clarkstone9348@sbcglobal.net
                        www.ataxia.org/chapters/kansascity/default.aspx

The primary mission is to encourage and support research into
Hereditary Ataxia, a group of neurological disorders which are
chronic and progressive conditions affecting coordination.

Jim Clark, Contact

536 Springfield Area Support Group
12 Jackson St, Apt 811-B
Jefferson City, MO 10149   drsusie@embarqmail.com
                        www.ataxia.org/chapters/strode/default.aspx

The primary mission is to encourage and support research into
Hereditary Ataxia, a group of neurological disorders which are
chronic and progressive conditions affecting coordination.

Susan Strode, PhD, Contact

New York

537 Genetic Network of the Empire State
Laboratory of Human Genetics
Empire State Plaza
Albany, NY 10150   518-474-7148
                                        Fax: 518-474-8590
                                           www.sergginc.org

Coordinates genetic services; promotes communication among genetic professionals and consumers through network newsletters,
meetings, and other events; share resources; and promote education and awareness of genetic disorders.

Karen Greendale, Coordinator

538 New York City Area Support Group
National Ataxia Foundation
36 West Redoubt Road
Fishkill, NY 10151   845-897-5632
                                    vrabsolutely@aol.com
                        www.ataxia.org/chapters/valerieruggiero/default.aspx

The primary mission is to encourage and support research into
Hereditary Ataxia, a group of neurological disorders which are
chronic and progressive conditions affecting coordination.

Valerie Ruggiero, Contact

539 New York Support Group
National Ataxia Foundation
423 Church Street
North Syracuse, NY 10152   315-683-9486
                                         jtarrants@aol.com
                        www.ataxia.org/chapters/centralnewyork/default.aspx

Primary mission is to encourage and support research into Hereditary Ataxia, a group of neurological disorders which are chronic
and progressive conditions affecting coordination.

Mary Jane Damiano, Contact

540 Tri-State Support Group
National Ataxia Foundation
Northgate 6C
Bronxville, NY 10153   914-720-2179
                                        Fax: 763-553-0167
                                   markmeghan2@gmail.com
                        www.ataxia.org/chapters/tri-state/default.aspx

The primary mission is to encourage and support research into
Hereditary Ataxia, a group of neurological disorders which are
chronic and progressive conditions affecting coordination.

Denise Mitchell, Leader
Mark Mitchell, Contact

Ohio

541 Ohio Support Group
National Ataxia Foundation
7852 Country Court
Mentor, OH 10154   440-255-8284
                                        wurbanski@oh.rr.com
                        www.ataxia.org/chapters/centralohio/default.aspx

The primary mission is to encourage and support research into
Hereditary Ataxia, a group of neurological disorders which are
chronic and progressive conditions affecting coordination.

Cecelia Urbanski, Contact

Oklahoma

542 North Central Oklahoma Support Group
915 Thislewood
Norman, OK 10155   405-447-6085
                                   czechmarkmhd@yahoo.com
                        www.ataxia.org/chapters/Ambassador/default.aspx

The primary mission is to encourage and support research into
Hereditary Ataxia, a group of neurological disorders which are
chronic and progressive conditions affecting coordination.

Mark Dvorak, Contact

Oregon

543 Pacific Northwest Regional Genetics Group
PO Box 574
Portland, OR 10156   503-494-8342
                                        Fax: 503-494-4447
                                           www.sergginc.org

Coordinates genetics services; promotes communication among
genetic professional and consumers through network newsletters,
meetings, and other events; share resources; and promote education and awareness of genetic disorders.

Jonathan Zonana, MD, Director

544 Willamette Valley Ataxia Support Group
Albany General Hospital-National Ataxia Foundation
1046 6th Avenue SW
Albany, OR 10157   541-812-4162
                                        Fax: 541-812-4614
                                     istillwell@samhealth.org
                        www.ataxia.org/chapters/Willamette/default.aspx

The primary mission is to encourage and support research into
Hereditary Ataxia, a group of neurological disorders which are
chronic and progressive conditions affecting coordination.

Ivy Stilwell, Contact

Pennsylvania

545 Central Pennsylvania Area Support Group
3844 West Linden Street
Allentown, PA 18104   610-395-6905
                                         rakshys@ptd.net
                        www.ataxia.org/chapters/rakshys/default.aspx

The primary mission is to encourage and support research into Hereditary Ataxia, a group of neurological disorders which are chronic and progressive conditions affecting coordination.

Christina Rakshys, Contact

546   Mid-Atlantic Regional Human Genetics Network
260 S Broad Street
Philadelphia, PA 10158
215-456-7910
Fax: 215-456-7911
www.sergginc.org

Coordinates genetics services; promotes communication among genetic professional and consumers through network newsletters, meeting, and other events; share resources; and promote education and awareness of genetic disorders.

Deborah Eunpu, MS, President

547   Southeast Pennsylvania Support Group
National Ataxia Foundation
220 Beechwood Road
Norristown, PA 10159
610-272-1502
lizout@aol.com
www.ataxia.org/chapters/sepennsylvania/default.aspx

The primary mission is to encourage and support research into Hereditary Ataxia, a group of neurological disorders which are chronic and progressive conditions affecting coordination.

Liz Nussear, Contact

South Carolina

548   Carolinas Support Group
National Ataxia Foundation
1305 Cely Road
Easley, SC 10160
864-220-3395
cecerussell@hotmal.com
www.ataxia.org/chapters/Carolinas/default.aspx

The primary mission is to encourage and support research into Hereditary Ataxia, a group of neurological disorders which are chronic and progressive conditions affecting coordination.

Cece Russell, Contact

Texas

549   Houston Support Group
National Ataxia Foundation
9405 Hwy 6 South
Houston, TX 10161
281-693-1826
angelahcloud@aol.com
www.ataxia.org/chapters/houston/default.aspx

The primary mission is to encourage and support research into Hereditary Ataxia, a group of neurological disorders which are chronic and progressive conditions affecting coordination.

Angela Cloud, Contact

550   North Texas Support Group
National Ataxia Foundation
7 Wentworth Court
Trophy Club, TX 10162
903-785-7058
cheve11e@sbcglobal.net
www.ataxia.org/chapters/northtexas/default.aspx

The primary mission is to encourage and support research into Hereditary Ataxia, a group of neurological disorders which are chronic and progressive conditions affecting coordination.

David Henry Jr, Contact

Utah

551   Utah Support Group National Ataxia Foundation
University of Utah - Moran Eye Clinic
65 Mario Copecchi Dr.
Salt Lake City, UT 84132
801-587-3020
Lisa.ord@hsc.utah.edu
www.ataxia.org/chapters/Utah/default.aspx

The primary mission is to encourage and support research into Hereditary Ataxia, a group of neurological disorders which are chronic and progressive conditions affecting coordination.

Lisa Ord PhD, Contact

Washington

552   Seattle Area Support Group
National Ataxia Foundation
14104 107th Avenue NE
Kirkland, WA 10164
425-823-6239
ataxiaseattle@comcast.net
www.ataxia.org/chapters/Seattle/default.aspx

The primary mission is to encourage and support research into Hereditary Ataxia, a group of neurological disorders which are chronic and progressive conditions affecting coordination.

Milly Lewendon, Contact

Research Centers

553   Ataxia Telangiectasia Children's Project
5300 W. Hillsboro Blvd. Suite 105
Coconut Creek, FL 10165
954-481-6611
800-543-5728
Fax: 954-725-1153
info@atcp.org
www.atcp.org

Established in the United States in 1993, the A-T Children's Project is a 501c3 nonprofit organization that raises funds to support and coordinate biomedical research projects, scientific conferences and a clinical center aimed at finding life-improving therapies and a cure for ataxia-telangiectasia (A-T). A-T is a rare, genetic disease that attacks children, causing progressive loss of muscle control, cancer, and immune system problems.

Brad Margus, President
Vicki Margus, Founder

554   Ataxia Telangiectasia Medical Research Foundation
16224 Elisa Place
Encino, CA 91436
818-906-2861
Fax: 818-906-2870
atmrf@aol.com
www.ninds.nih.gov/find_people/voluntary_orgs/volorg1

Private nonprofit organization dedicated to finding a cure for ataxia-telangiectasia.

Story C Landis, PhD, Director
Walter J Koroshetz, MD, Deputy Director
Joellen Harper Austin, Associate Director

555   Ataxia Telangiectasia Project
3002 Enfield Road
Austin, TX 10166
512-472-4892
A-TProject@austin.rr.com
www.atproject.org

Nonprofit foundation that supports basic scientific research into treatments for neurological deterioration and cancer in children with ataia-telangiectasia.

Conferences

556   National Ataxia Foundation Annual Membersh ip Meeting
National Ataxia Foundation
2600 Fernbrook Lane, Suite 119
Minneapolis, MN 55447
763-553-0020
Fax: 763-553-0167
naf@ataxia.org
www.ataxia.org

Brings together NAF members and their families to meet and learn from world leading ataxia researchers and neurologists, but also to build new friendships and reunite with old friends.

Mike Parent, Executive Director

Audio Video

557 Diagnostic Approach to the Dysmorphic Patient
Southeastern Resgional Genetics Group, Inc SERGG
PO Box 1642
Decatur, GA 30031   404-778-8551
                                      Fax: 404-778-8562
                                      mlane@sergginc.org
                                      www.sergginc.org

This 2-hour video focuses on learning how to approach, catego-
rize, and conceptualize the patient with multiple congenital anomalies (MCA). Critical terminology is illustrated. Patients are seen
in hospital and clinic settings. Emphasis is placed in prioritizing
clinical features and weighing each feature's value in reaching a
diagnosis. An outline is included with time frames and detailed
explanations of what each statement, definition and
categorization means.

Timothy C. Wood, PhD, President
Mary Rose Simpson, Administrator

558 Pearls of Dysmorphology
Southeastern Resgional Genetics Group, Inc SERGG
PO Box 1642
Decatur, GA 30031   404-778-8551
                                      Fax: 404-778-8562
                                      mlane@sergginc.org
                                      www.sergginc.org

This 1 1/2-hour video which contains 87 individual features considered 'pearls' or 'semi-pearls' relative to their value in reaching
or suspecting a specific diagnosis. Many additional features are
commented on as the formal 'pearls' are presented. There is an
exercise at the end of the tape for helping viewers understand
how dysmorphology pearls can be used to prioritize the diagnostic value of individual features. A handout accompanies this tape,
to help make this exercise fun and educational.

Timothy C. Wood, PhD, President
Mary Rose Simpson, Administrator

559 Syndromes Associated with Multiple Congenital Anomalies
Southeastern Resgional Genetics Group, Inc SERGG
PO Box 1642
Decatur, GA 30031   404-778-8551
                                      Fax: 404-778-8562
                                      mlane@sergginc.org
                                      www.sergginc.org

This 2-hour video includes 30 of the more common malformation
syndromes within the categories of single gene, chromosomal,
teratogens, associations, and sequences. Each disorder is preceded by a Table of Features and each disorder is shown at different ages and often includes some verbal interaction. The vast
majority of the cases are within the hospital or clinic setting.
There is minimal use of slides.

Timothy C. Wood, PhD, President
Mary Rose Simpson, Administrator

560 Together...There Is Hope
National Ataxia Foundation
2600 Fernbrook Lane, Suite 119
Minneapolis, MN 55447   763-553-0020
                                      Fax: 763-553-0167
                                      naf@ataxia.org
                                      www.ataxia.org

A video discussing ataxias genetic patterns of inheritance and the
National Ataxia Foundation and its research efforts.

Charlene Danielson, President
Camille Daglio, Vice-President
William P. Sweeney, Treasurer

Web Sites

561 Gene Clinics
481B Edward H. Ross Drive
Elmwood Park, NJ 7407   888-729-1204
                                      Fax: 201-212-6457
                                      genetests@genetests.org
                                      www.geneclinics.org

By providing current, authoritative information on genetic testing
and its use in diagnosis, management, and genetic counseling,
GeneTests promotes the appropriate use of genetic services in patient care and personal decision making.

Roberta A Pagon, Founder
Amar Kamath, Commercial Director
Deb Eunpu, Program Manager

562 Health Answers
410 Horsham Road
Horsham, PA 19044   215-442-9017
                                      Michael.tague@healthanswers.com
                                      www.healthanswers.com

HealthAnswers offers a breadth of services in medical education,
sales force training, patient support solutions, professional promotion and consumer solutions.

Michael Tague, Managing Director

563 International Network of Ataxia Friends
www.internaf.org
Website mailing list which is maintained by volunteers who have
some form of ataxia.

564 National Ataxia Foundation
2600 Fernbrook Lane, Suite 119
Minneapolis, MN 55447   763-553-0020
                                      Fax: 763-553-0167
                                      naf@ataxia.org
                                      www.ataxia.org

Information regarding support, education, and research for dominant ataxia, recessive ataxia, and sporatic ataxia.

Charlene Danielson, President
Camille Daglio, Vice-President
William P. Sweeney, Treasurer

Book Publishers

565 A Balancing Act: Living with Spinal Cerebellar Ataxia
8600 Rockville Pike
Bethesda, MD 20894   301-594-5983
                                           888-346-3656
                                      Fax: 301-402-1384
                                      TDD: 800-735-2258
                                      custserv@nlm.nih.gov
                                      www.nlm.nih.gov

Describes living with Spinocerebellar Ataxia. Available from
Amazon.com only.
ISBN: 1-889826-00-6

Patricia B Hamilton

566 Directory of National Genetic Voluntary Organizations
Genetic Alliance
4301 Connecticut Avenue NW, Suite 404
Washington, DC 20008   202-966-5557
                                      Fax: 202-966-8553
                                      info@genticalliance.org
                                      www.genticalliance.orgtm

Lists hundreds of organizations and associations dealing with genetic conditions.

Sharon F. Terry, President/CEO
Natasha Bonhomme, Vice President
Lisa Wise, Chief Operating Officer

567 Hereditary Ataxia: A Guidebook for Managing Speech & Swallowing
National Ataxia Foundation
2600 Fernbrook Lane, Suite 119
Minneapolis, MN 55447
763-553-0020
Fax: 763-553-0167
naf@ataxia.org
www.ataxia.org

568 Living with Ataxia
National Ataxia Foundation
2600 Fernbrook Lane, Suite 119
Minneapolis, MN 55447
763-553-0020
Fax: 763-553-0167
naf@ataxia.org
www.ataxia.org

A compassionate resource for people who have or may be at risk of having ataxia, and for their families. This book explains the nature and causes of ataxia, the basic genetics that underlie many kinds of ataxia, discusses medical management of ataxia, provides practical advice for everyday living, points the way to many useful resources and assures that living a good life is an entirely reasonable aspiration, even with ataxia.

112 pages

569 Ten Years to Live
National Ataxia Foundation
2600 Fernbrook Lane, Suite 119
Minneapolis, MN 55447
763-553-0020
Fax: 763-553-0167
naf@ataxia.org
www.ataxia.org

Struggles of the Schut family with hereditary ataxia.
ISBN: 0-962716-63-1

Newsletters

570 A-TMRF Newsletter
A-T Medical Research Foundation
5241 Round Meadow Road
Hidden Hills, CA 91302
818-704-8146
Fax: 818-704-8310

Reports on the two major labs that are supported and funded by us.

571 Alert
Alliance of Genetic Support Groups
4301 Connecticut Ave NW, Suite 404
Washington, DC 20008
202-966-5557
Fax: 202-966-8553
info@geneticalliance.org
www.geneticalliance.org

Functions as a vehicle of communication between the Alliance and its constituency. Provides timely and useful information on genetics research.
Monthly

Sharon Terry, MA, President/ CEO
Natasha Bonhomme, VP, Strategic Development
Ruth Evans, Director of Accounting

572 Generations
National Ataxia Foundation
2600 Fernbrook Lane, Suite 119
Minneapolis, MN 55447
763-553-0020
Fax: 763-553-0167
naf@ataxia.org
www.ataxia.org

Contains reports on the organization and its chapters, offers research, advice and guides to other resources available.

Charlene Danielson, President
Camille Daglio, Vice-President
William P. Sweeney, Treasurer

573 MSRGSN Newsletter
Mountain States Regional Genetics Service Network
4300 Cherry Creek Drive S
Denver, CO 80222
303-692-2423
Fax: 303-782-5576

Joyce Hooker, Coordinator

574 NERG News
New England Regional Genetics Group
PO Box 670
Mount Desert, ME 4660
207-288-2701
Fax: 207-288-2705

575 SERGG Regional News
Southeast Regional Genetics Group
PO Box 1642
Decatur, GA 30031
404-775-8551
Fax: 404-775-8562
mlane@sergginc.org
www.sergginc.org

Provides information on genetics services, public health departments, consumers, and related laboratory services.

Timothy C. Wood, PhD, President
Mary Rose Simpson, Administrator

Pamphlets

576 Alliance Brochure
Alliance of Genetic Support Groups
4301 Connecticut Ave NW, Suite 404
Washington, DC 20008
202-966-5557
Fax: 202-966-8553
info@geneticalliance.org
www.geneticalliance.org

Explains the services and programs offered by the Alliance.

Sharon Terry, MA, President/ CEO
Natasha Bonhomme, VP, Strategic Development
Ruth Evans, Director of Accounting

577 Ataxia Fact Sheet
National Ataxia Foundation
2600 Fernbrook Lane, Suite 119
Minneapolis, MN 55447
763-553-0020
Fax: 763-553-0167
naf@ataxia.org
www.ataxia.org

Describes ataxia as a symptom and its association with other medical problems as well as the hereditary types.

Charlene Danielson, President
Camille Daglio, Vice-President
William P. Sweeney, Treasurer

578 Consumer Indicators of Quality Genetic Services
Alliance of Genetic Support Groups
4301 Connecticut Avenue NW, #404
Washington, DC 20008
202-966-5557
800-336-4363
Fax: 202-966-8553
info@geneticalliance.org
www.geneticalliance.org

Describes the Alliance of Genetic Support Groups Partnership Program, which strives to increase provider awareness of the unique needs and resources of genetic consumers, improve provider access to quality, consumer-oriented support group resources, and develop replacable educational materials for other programs.

Sharon Terry, MA, President/ CEO
Natasha Bonhomme, VP, Strategic Development
Ruth Evans, Director of Accounting

579 Facts About Friedreich's Ataxia
Muscular Dystrophy Association
222 S. Riverside Plaza, Suite 1500
Chicago, IL 60606
520-529-2000
800-572-1717
Fax: 520-529-5300
mda@mdausa.org
mda.org

Explains Friedreich's ataxia in layman's terms and answers commonly asked questions about the disease. Also in Spanish and on-line.

2006

Kristine Welker, Interim President/CEO
Valerie A. Cwik, MD, EVP, Chief Medical & Scientific
Julie Faber, EVP, CFO

580 Friedrich's Ataxia
National Ataxia Foundation
2600 Fernbrook Lane, Suite 119
Minneapolis, MN 55447
763-553-0020
Fax: 763-553-0167
naf@ataxia.org
www.ataxia.org

Describes symptoms, diagnosis, genetics and hints on coping.

Charlene Danielson, President
Camille Daglio, Vice-President
William P. Sweeney, Treasurer

581 Gene Testing for Ataxia
National Ataxia Foundation
2600 Fernbrook Lane, Suite 119
Minneapolis, MN 55447
763-553-0020
Fax: 763-553-0167
naf@ataxia.org
www.ataxia.org

Describes the latest information about who should consider it and where to have it done.

Charlene Danielson, President
Camille Daglio, Vice-President
William P. Sweeney, Treasurer

582 Hereditary Ataxia: The Facts
National Ataxia Foundation
2600 Fernbrook Lane, Suite 119
Minneapolis, MN 55447
612-553-0020
Fax: 612-553-0167
naf@mr.net
www.ataxia.org

Describes recessive and dominant ataxias, information on how hereditary ataxia is transmitted and explanations of the NAF's role in education, service and prevention.

Charlene Danielson, President
Camille Daglio, Vice-President
William P. Sweeney, Treasurer

583 Incorporating Consumers into Regional Genetics Networks
Alliance of Genetic Support Groups
4301 Connecticut Avenue NW, Suite 404
Washington, DC 20008
301-652-5553
Fax: 202-966-8553
alliance@capaccess.org
medhelp.org/www/agsg.htm

584 Informed Consent: Participation in Genetic Research Studies
Alliance of Genetic Support Groups
4301 Connecticut Avenue NW, Suite 404
Washington, DC 20008
202-966-5557
800-336-4363
Fax: 202-966-8553
info@geneticalliance.org
www.geneticalliance.org

This booklet explains the nature of genetic research with its benefits and risks.

Sharon Terry, MA, President/ CEO
Natasha Bonhomme, VP, Strategic Development
Ruth Evans, Director of Accounting

585 Pen-Pal Directory
National Ataxia Foundation
2600 Fernbrook Lane, Suite 119
Minneapolis, MN 55447
763-553-0020
Fax: 763-553-0167
naf@ataxia.org
www.ataxia.org

National, state and international directory of others who are affected by ataxia. Available to NAF Pen-Pal members only.

Charlene Danielson, President
Camille Daglio, Vice-President
William P. Sweeney, Treasurer

DESCRIPTION

586   ATRIAL SEPTAL DEFECTS

Synonyms: ASD, Atrioseptal defects

Involves the following Biologic System(s):

Cardiovascular Disorders

The term atrial septal defect, or ASD, refers to a group of congenital abnormalities characterized by the presence of a hole in the wall (septum) that separates the two upper chambers of the heart (atria). Atrial septal defects are classified according to their location and may occur as a single anomaly or in association with other heart (cardiac) defects. These types of abnormalities occur in approximately 2000 of every 100,000 births.

The upper left chamber of the heart (left atrium) receives blood that is rich with oxygen (oxygenated) from the lungs. The blood then passes into the lower left chamber (left ventricle) from which it is then pumped through the arteries of the body into the general circulation. The right atrium receives blood that has been depleted of oxygen (deoxygenated) that then passes into the right ventricle and is pumped to the lungs where it once again receives oxygen. Atrial septal defects may allow the passage of some oxygenated blood from the upper left side of the heart into the upper right side of the heart where it mixes with blood that is oxygen depleted. In some patients, this results in a reduced oxygen supply to the body and an increase in blood flow to the lungs. Physical findings associated with ASDs may include enlargement of the right atrium, the right ventricle, or both, and characteristic heart sounds. In some patients, symptoms may be completely absent, especially in early childhood. ASDs are often discovered during routine physical examination by the pressure of a systolic heart murmur. Some affected individuals may experience fatigue upon exertion or exercise. Other findings or symptoms may become apparent after the age of 30 years or when an affected woman becomes pregnant. In these patients, symptoms may include fatigue upon exercise (exercise intolerance), valve insufficiencies, and other, more serious problems such as heart failure and or arrhythmias.

The standard method for closure of atrial septal defects has been open-heart surgery. However, a new nonsurgical procedure has been developed and is done in the heart catheterization laboratory, thus avoiding the need for surgery. A patch, usually resembling a small umbrella, is inserted into the damaged area through a catheter. It is then put into place to close the hole.

Government Agencies

587   NIH/ Eunice Kennedy Shriver National Insti tute of Child Health & Human Development
31 Center Drive, Building 31
Bethesda, MD 20892

301-496-5113
800-370-2943
Fax: 866-760-5947
TTY: 888-320-6942
nichdpress@mail.nih.gov
www.nichd.nih.gov

Established in 1962 by congress, today the institute conducts and supports laboratory research, clinical trials, and epidemiological studies that explore health processes; examines the impact of disabilities, diseases, and variations on the lives of individuals; and sponsors training programs for scientists, health care providers, and researchers to ensure that NICHD research can continue.

Diana W. Bianchi, Director
Paul Williams, Director, Communications

588   NIH/National Heart, Lung and Blood Institu te
National Institute of Health
31 Center Dr MSC 2486, Bldg 31, Rm 5A52
Bethesda, MD 20892

301-592-8573
Fax: 240-629-3246
TTY: 240-629-3255
nhlbiinfo@nhlbi.nih.gov
www.nhlbi.nih.gov

The National Heart, Lung, and Blood Institute (NHLBI) provides global leadership for a research, training, and education program to promote the prevention and treatment of heart, lung, and blood diseases and enhance the health of all individuals so that they can live longer and more fulfilling lives.

Gary H Gibbons MD, Director
Nakela Cook MD, Chief of Staff

National Associations & Support Groups

589   American Academy of Pediatrics
141 Northwest Point Boulevard
Elk Grove Village, IL 60007

847-434-4000
800-433-9016
Fax: 847-434-8000
www.aap.org

The American Academy of Pediatrics and its member pediatricians are committed to the attainment of optimal physical, mental and social health and well-being for all infants, children, adolescents, and young adults.

Fernando Stein, MD, FAAP, President
Karen Remley, MD, CEO/Executive VP

590   American Heart Association
7272 Greenville Avenue
Dallas, TX 75231

214-373-6300
800-242-8721
Fax: 214-706-1341
inquire@amhrt.org
www.heart.org/HEARTORG/

Our mission is to build healthier lives, free of cardiovascular diseases and stroke.

Nancy Brown, CEO
Dr. Stephen Houser, President
Suzie Upton, Chief Operating Officer

591   Genetic Alliance
4301 Connecticut Avenue NW, Suite 404
Washington, DC 20008

202-966-5557
800-336-4363
Fax: 202-966-8553
info@geneticalliance.org
www.geneticalliance.org

World's leading nonprofit health advocacy organization committed to transforming health through genetics and promoting an environment of openness centered on the health of individuals, families, and communities.

Sharon Terry, President/CEO
Tetyana Murza, Managing Director
Natasha Bonhomme, VP, Strategic Development

592   March of Dimes Foundation
1275 Mamaroneck Avenue
White Plains, NY 10605

914-997-4488
888-663-4637
Fax: 914-997-4763
answers@marchofdimes.com
www.marchofdimes.com

The March of Dimes helps moms have full-term pregnancies and research the problems that threaten the health of babies.

Stacey D. Stewart, President

Conferences

593 Genetic Alliance Annual Conference
Genetic Alliance
4301 Connecticut Avenue NW, Suite 404
Washington, DC 20008

202-966-5557
800-336-4363
Fax: 202-966-8553
info@geneticalliance.org
www.geneticalliance.org

Consistently inspirational and enables partnership among all stakeholders: advocates and community leaders, health and industry professionals, policymakers, and academicians.

July

Sharon Terry, President/CEO
Tetyana Murza, Managing Director
Natasha Bonhomme, VP, Strategic Development

Web Sites

594 Southern Illinois University School of Medicine
P O Box 19658
Springfield, IL 62794

217-545-8000
www.siumed.edu/peds/index.htm

Mission is to meet the health care needs of children and their families in Central and Southern Illinois through provision of high quality, coordinated care of children with acute and chronic conditions with inpatient, ambulatory, and community-based programs.

595 Yale University School of Medicine
333 Cedar Street
New Haven, CT 6510

203-432-4771
medicine.yale.edu

Offers information on congential heart conditions such as Atrial Septal Defects, including symptoms, causes and treatments.

Peter Salovey, President of the University
Richard Belitsky M.D., Deputy Dean for Education
Benjamin Polak B.A., M.A., Ph.D., Provost of the University

Book Publishers

596 Congenital Disorders Sourcebook 2nd Edition
Omnigraphics
PO Box 31-1640
Detroit, MI 48231

800-234-1340
Fax: 800-875-1340
info@omnigraphics.com
www.omnigraphics.com

Provides basic consumer health information about the most common types of nonhereditary birth defects and disorders related to prematurity, gestational injuries, congenital infections, and birth complications, including disorders of the heart, brain, gastrointestinal tract, musculoskeletal system, urinary tract, and reproductive system craniofacial disorders, cerebral palsy, spina bifida, and fetal alcohol syndrome, and detailing the causes, diagnostic tests, and treatments for each.

650 pages
ISBN: 0-780809-45-9

DESCRIPTION

597   ATTENTION DEFICIT HYPERACTIVITY DISORDER

Synonyms: ADHD, Hyperactive child syndrome, Hyperkinetic syndrome

Involves the following Biologic System(s):

Developmental/Behavioral/Psychiatric Disorders

Attention deficit hyperactivity disorder, or ADHD, is a syndrome of childhood and adolescence characterized by impulsive behavior, motor-related overactivity (hyperactivity), and inattention. The short attention span results in a decreased ability or inability to complete chores, assignments, or other tasks. ADHD is four to six times more prevalent among boys than it is in girls. In approximately 50 percent of cases, this disorder develops before the age of four years, while in others it appears before seven years of age. Over the last decade, it has been increasingly diagnosed in adults. Some behavioral symptoms associated with this disorder may be present at times in children with ADHD or in children with certain other disorders (e.g., conduct disorder, learning disabilities, hearing impairment, etc.). Therefore, specialists often base their diagnosis on the frequent presence of eight or more characteristic findings. Among these are restlessness, difficulty in remaining seated, difficulty in waiting for a turn in group activities, inclination to be easily distracted, impulsively answering questions before they are completed, difficulty following instructions, inability to sustain concentration while performing tasks or playing, shifting to other tasks before completing others, talking excessively, poor ability to play quietly, interrupting or butting in on others, not appearing to listen when others speak, losing things, and frequently taking part in dangerous physical activities.Evaluation of an individual with ADHD involves taking a detailed family and medical history, paying careful attention to such things as activity level, behavior, and temperament during the early years of the life of the affected child. Obtaining this information may be helpful in determining the extent of the disorder and the presence of additional difficulties (e.g., learning disabilities, anxiety disorders, conduct disorders, etc.).

ADHD is currently considered to be a persistent and chronic condition for which no medical cure is available. Although the cause of ADHD is not known, genetic influences may be a factor in the development of this disorder. In addition, children with neurological disorders and other abnormalities related to the central nervous system may be predisposed to the development of ADHD. Treatment of attention deficit hyperactivity disorder may include an ongoing behavioral and psychosocial therapeutic plan that includes the cooperation of school personnel, the child, and the child's parents or caregivers. In addition, psychostimulant drugs or other medications may be prescribed and carefully monitored. Affected children may also benefit from a structured environment at home and in school. Studies show that, in many phases children who receive multifaceted treatment are better able to cope with ADHD through their adolescent years and into adulthood. Other treatment is supportive.

Government Agencies

598   NIH/National Institute of Mental Health
6001 Executive Boulevard, Room 6200, MSC 9663
Bethesda, MD 20892

301-443-4536
866-615-6464
Fax: 301-443-4279
TTY: 301-443-8431
nimhinfo@nih.gov
www.nimh.nih.gov

The mission of NIMH is to transform the understanding and treatment of mental illnesses through basic and clinical research, paving the way for prevention, recovery, and cure.

Joshua Gordon, MD, PhD, Director
Shelli Avenevoli, MD, Deputy Director

599   NIH/National Institute of Neurological Dis orders and Stroke (NINDS)
PO Box 5801
Bethesda, MD 20824

301-496-5751
800-352-9424
Fax: 301-496-0296
TTY: 301-468-5981
www.ninds.nih.gov

The mission of NINDS is to reduce the burden of neurological disease - a burden borne by every age group, by every segment of society, by people all over the world.

Walter J. Koroshetz, MD, Director

National Associations & Support Groups

600   AD-IN: Attention Deficit Information Network
475 Hillside Avenue
Needham, MA 10174

781-455-9895
Fax: 781-444-5466
adin@gis.net
www.addinfonetwork.com

Provides information on training programs and speakers for those who work with individuals with ADD.

601   ADHD Challenge
PO Box 488
West Peabody, MA 01985

978-535-3276
800-233-2322
TDD: 508-535-3276
www.additudemag.com/adhd/article/8643.html

Provision of data and emotional assistance to both sufferers and medical professionals.

602   ARC of the United States
1010 Wayne Avenue, Suite 650
Silver Spring, MD 20910

301-565-3842
Fax: 301-565-5342
info@thearc.org
www.thearc.org

The ARC of the United States advocates for the rights and full participation of all children and adults with intellectual and developmental disabilities. Together with our network of members and affiliated chapters, we improve systems of supports and services; connect families; inspire communities an influence public policy.

Peter V Barns, CEO
Nancy Webster, President
Ronald Brown, Vice President

603   American Academy of Pediatrics
141 Northwest Point Boulevard
Elk Grove Village, IL 60007

847-434-4000
800-433-9016
Fax: 847-434-8000
www.aap.org

The American Academy of Pediatrics and its member pediatricians are committed to the attainment of optimal physical, mental and social health and well-being for all infants, children, adolescents, and young adults.

Fernando Stein, MD, FAAP, President
Karen Remley, MD, CEO/Executive VP

604 Attention Deficit Disorder Association
PO Box 7557
Wilmington, DE 10177

800-939-1019
Fax: 856-439-0525
info@add.org
www.add.org

The Attention Deficit Disorder Association provides information, resources and networking opportunities to help adults with Attention Deficit Hyperactivity Disorder lead better lives.

Evelyn Polk Green, President
Linda Roggli, Vice President
Janet Kramer MD, Treasurer

605 CHADD: Children and Adults with Attention Deficit/Hyperactivity Disorders
8181 Professional Place, Suite 150
Landover, MD 10178

301-306-7070
800-233-4050
Fax: 301-306-7090
www.chadd.org

Children and Adults with Attention-Deficit/Hyperactivity Disorder (CHADD) was founded in 1987 in response to the frustration and sense of isolation experienced by parents and their children with ADHD.

1987

Barbara S Hawkins, President
Michael MacKay, Treasurer

606 Feingold Association of the US
11849 Suncatcher Drive
Fishers, IN 10179

631-369-9340
800-321-3287
Fax: 631-369-2988
help@feingold.org
www.feingold.org

An organization of families and professionals founded in 1976 to provide a dietary management program for both children and adults

Annette Miller, President
Kathleen Bratby, Secretary
Larisa Scarbrough, Vice President

607 Genetic Alliance
4301 Connecticut Avenue NW, Suite 404
Washington, DC 20008

202-966-5557
800-336-4363
Fax: 202-966-8553
info@geneticalliance.org
www.geneticalliance.org

World's leading nonprofit health advocacy organization committed to transforming health through genetics and promoting an environment of openness centered on the health of individuals, families, and communities.

Sharon Terry, President/CEO
Tetyana Murza, Managing Director
Natasha Bonhomme, VP, Strategic Development

608 Learning Disabilities Association of America
4156 Library Road
Pittsburgh, PA 15234

412-341-1515
888-300-6710
Fax: 412-344-0224
info@LDAAmerica.org
www.ldaamerica.org

Helps families of the affected individual through information and referral to professionals in their area. A membership organization with affiliates across the country.

Sheila Buckley, Executive Director

609 March of Dimes Foundation
1275 Mamaroneck Avenue
White Plains, NY 10605

914-997-4488
888-663-4637
Fax: 914-997-4763
answers@marchofdimes.com
www.marchofdimes.com

March of Dimes help moms have full-term pregnancies and research the problems that threaten the health of babies.The March of Dimes also acts globally: sharing best practices in perinatal health and helping improve birth outcomes where the needs are the most urgent.

Stacey D. Stewart, President

610 Mental Health America
500 Montgomery Street, Ste 820
Alexandria, VA 22314

703-684-7722
800-969-6642
Fax: 703-684-5968
TTY: 800-433-5959
info@mentalhealthamerica.net
www.mentalhealthamerica.net

MHA, the leading advocacy organization addressing the full spectrum of mental and substance use conditions and their effects nationwide, works to inform, advocate and enable access to quality behavioral health services for all Americans.

Paul Gionfriddo, President/CEO
Shavonne Carpenter, Sr Assoc., Support & Services
Mallory Pernell, Assoc. Dir, Comments/Marketing

611 National Alliance for the Mentally Ill
3803 N. Fairfax Dr., Suite 100
Arlington, VA 10183

703-525-7600
800-950-6264
Fax: 703-524-9094
TDD: 703-516-7227
info@nami.org
www.nami.org

NAMI is a nonprofit, grassroots, self-help, support and advocacy organization of consumers, families and friends of people with severe mental illness, such as schizophrenia, bipolar disorder, major depressive disorder, obsessive compulsive disorder, anxiety disorders, autism and other severe and persistent mental illnesses that affect the brain.

Keris J„n Myrick, President
Kevin B Sullivan, First Vice President
Jim Payne, Second Vice President

612 National Center for Learning Disabilities
381 Park Avenue S, Suite 1401
New York, NY 10184

212-545-7510
888-575-7373
Fax: 212-545-9665
ncld@ncld.org
www.ncld.org

The National Center for Learning Disabilities improves the lives of all people with learning difficulties and disabilities by empowering parents, enabling young adults, transforming schools, and creating policy and advocacy impact.

Frederic M Poses, CEO
Anne Ford, Chairman Emeritus
Mary Kalikow, Vice Chair

613 National Mental Health Consumers' Self-Help Clearinghouse
1211 Chestnut Street, Suite 1207
Philadelphia, PA 10185

215-751-1810
800-553-4539
Fax: 215-636-6312
info@mhselfhelp.org
www.mhselfhelp.org

The Clearinghouse works to foster peer empowerment through our website, up-to-date news and information announcements, a directory of peer-driven services, electronic and printed publications, training packages, and individual and onsite consultation

Joseph Rogers, Executive Director & Founder
Susan Rogers, Director of Special Projects
Britani Nestel, Program Specialist

614   Option Institute: Son Rise Program
Autism Treatment Center of America
2080 S Undermountain Road
Sheffield, MA 10186   413-229-2100
                                                        800-714-2779
                                                   Fax: 413-229-3202
                                       information@son-rise.org
                                                www.son-rise.org

Describes an effective, loving and respectful method for treating
children with autism. It teaches parents and healing professionals
how to set up a home based program using the child's motivation
to reach their special child.

Barry Neil Kaufman, Co-Founder/Co-Creator
Samahria Lyte Kaufman, Co-Founder/Co-Creator
Bryn Hogan, ATCA Senior Staff

615   The Council For Exceptional Children
2900 Crystal Drive, Suite 1000
Arlington, VA 10187   703-243-0446
                                                        888-232-7733
                                                   Fax: 703-264-9494
                                                   TTY: 866-915-5000
                                               service@cec.sped.org
                                                 www.cec.sped.org

wide mission of the Council for Exceptional Children is to improve educational outcomes for individuals with exceptionalities.

Bruce Ramirez, Executive Director
Veronica Browne-Barnes, Senior Executive Assistant for Gove
Sharon Rodriguez, Senior Executive Assistant for Admi

Conferences

616   Annual International Conference on ADHD
CHADD
8181 Professional Place, Suite 150
Landover, MD 20785   301-306-7070
                                                        800-233-4050
                                                   Fax: 301-306-7090
                                              webmaster@chadd.org
                                                  www.chadd.org

November

Marsha Bokman, Meetings/Events Director

617   Arc's National Convention
ARC
1825 K Street NW, Suite 1200
Washington, DC 20006   202-534-3700
                                                        800-433-5255
                                                   Fax: 202-534-3731
                                                    info@thearc.org
                                                    www.thearc.org

Where members, staff, volunteers, professionals, experts, self advocates and their families gather for a dynamic convention to
meet each other, learn from each other, and tackle the tough issues facing the intellectual and developmental disability (I/DD)
community together.

Nanci Webster, President
Ronald Brown, Vice President
Elise McMillan, Secretary

618   CEC Convention & Expo
Council for Exceptional Children
2900 Crystal Drive Suite 1000
Arlington, VA 22202   703-243-0446
                                                        888-232-7733
                                                   Fax: 703-264-9494
                                                   TTY: 866-915-5000
                                               service@cec.sped.org
                                                 www.cec.sped.org

Offers an unparalleled experience with more than 800 sessions to
help you learn the latest in evidence-based practices; explore innovative technologies, products, and services; and network with
other professionals working with children with exceptionalities
and their families.

April

Bruce Ramirez, Executive Director

619   Genetic Alliance Annual Conference
Genetic Alliance
4301 Connecticut Avenue NW, Suite 404
Washington, DC 20008   202-966-5557
                                                        800-336-4363
                                                   Fax: 202-966-8553
                                              info@geneticalliance.org
                                              www.geneticalliance.org

Consistently inspirational and enables partnership among all
stakeholders: advocates and community leaders, health and industry professionals, policymakers, and academicians.

July

Sharon Terry, President/CEO
Tetyana Murza, Managing Director
Natasha Bonhomme, VP, Strategic Development

620   NAMI Convention
National Alliance on Mental Illness
3803 N Fairfax Drive, Suite 100
Arlington, VA 22203   703-524-7600
                                                        888-999-6264
                                                   Fax: 703-524-9094
                                                   TDD: 703-516-7227
                                                      info@nami.org
                                                      www.nami.org

The NAMI Convention is packed with information, chances to
network, leadership development opportunities, and lots more.

July

Keris Jan Myrick, President
Kevin B Sullivan, Vice President
Clarence Jordan, Secretary

Audio Video

621   ADD From A To Z-Understanding The Diagnosi s &
Treatment of ADD in Children & Adult
Connecticut Association for Children with LD
25 Van Zant Street, Suite 15-5
East Norwalk, CT 6855   203-838-5010
                                                   Fax: 203-866-6108
                                               cacld@optonline.net
                                                    www.cacld.org

Provides a comprehensive overview of this complicated and often
misunderstood subject. Informative, authorative, and entertaining, this video will be useful to anyone who wants a clear understanding of what ADD is and what is not.

107 Minutes

622   ADHD: What Can We Do?
ADD WareHouse
300 NW 70th Avenue, Suite 102
Plantation, FL 33317   954-792-8100
                                                        800-233-9273
                                                   Fax: 954-792-8545
                                         websales@addwarehouse.com
                                              www.addwarehouse.com

Can serve as a companion to ADHD: What Do We Know. This
video focuses on the most effective ways to manage ADHD, both
in the home and in the classroom. Scenes depict the use of behavior management at home and accommodations and interventions
in the classroom which have proven to be effective in the treatment of ADHD. Thirty seven minutes.

1993
ISBN: 0-898629-82-1

623   ADHD: What Do We Know?
Russell A Barkley, author

Guilford Publications
370 Seventh Avenue, Suite 1200
New York, NY 10001   212-431-9800
                                                        800-365-7006
                                                   Fax: 212-966-6708
                                                   info@guilford.com
                                                   www.guilford.com

An introduction for teachers and special education practitioners, school psychologists and parents of ADHD children. Topics outlined in this video include the causes and prevalence of ADHD, ways children with ADHD behave, other conditions that may accompany ADHD and long-term prospects for children with ADHD. DVD'36 minutes, Manual 31 pages.

Oct 2006 31 pages DVD & Manual

624 Concentration Video
Learning disAbilities Resources
PO Box 716
Bryn Mawr, PA 19010
610-525-8336
Fax: 610-525-8337

An instructional video which provides a perspective about attention problems, possible causes and solutions.

Video

625 Educating Inattentive Children
ADD WareHouse
300 NW 70th Avenue, Suite 102
Plantation, FL 33317
954-792-8100
800-233-9273
Fax: 954-792-8545
websales@addwarehouse.com
www.addwarehouse.com

An excellent resources for teachers who encounter inattention and hyperactivity in the classroom. It helps teachers distinguish deliberate misbehavior from the incompetent, nonpurposeful behavior of the inattentive child.

1990 Video

626 How to Help Your Child Succeed in School
Peytral Publications
PO Box 1162
Minnetonka, MN 55345
952-949-8707
877-739-8725
Fax: 952-906-9777
help@peytral.com
www.peytral.com

In this deeply powerful video, Sandra Reif presents the essential information needed by those who work with ADHD and/or Learning Disabilities to help children in school. The focus is on the key for success, a strong partnership in education between home and school.

56 Minutes

Donna Kaufman

627 Medication for ADHD
ADD WareHouse
300 NW 70th Avenue, Suite 102
Plantation, FL 33317
954-792-8100
800-233-9273
Fax: 954-792-8545
websales@addwarehouse.com
www.addwarehouse.com

This comprehensive DVD program addresses the critical questions regarding the use of medicati in the treatment of ADD or ADHD. WGN-TV medical reporter Dina Bair interviews two long-time ADHD experts: psychiatrist Dr Jonathan Bloomberg and clinical psychologist Dr Thomas Phelan.

ISBN: 1-889140-18-X

628 Understanding Attention Deficit Disorder
Connecticut Association for Children with LD
25 Van Zant Street, Suite 15-5
East Norwalk, CT 6855
203-838-5010
Fax: 203-866-6108
cacld@optonline.net
www.cacld.org

A video in an interview format for parents and professionals providing the history, symptoms, methods of diagnosis and three approaches used to ease the effects of attention deficit disorder.

45 minutes

629 Understanding Hyperactivity
Psychiatric Support Services
Houston, TX
281-580-0046

Designed for parents and teachers, a video explaining the symptoms and consequences of attention deficit hyperactivity disorder.

Video

630 Why Can't Michael Pay Attention?
Learning Seed
P.O. Box 617880
Chicago, IL 60661
800-634-4941
Fax: 800-998-0854
info@learningseed.com
www.learningseed.com

After a multi-faceted assessment, six year old, Michael is diagnosed with Attention Deficit Hyperactivity Disorder. Michael's parents learn techniques such as consistent schedules, docking systems, star charts, and self-monitoring to help organize home life. ISBN: DVD 1-55740-973-0; VHS 1-55740-896-3

21 minutes

631 Why Won't My Child Pay Attention?
Wiley Publishing Inc
111 River Street
Hoboken, NJ 07030
317-572-3000
201-748-6000
Fax: 201-748-6088
info@wiley.com
as.wiley.com/WileyCDA/Section/index.html

Practical and reassuring videotape. Noted child psychologist tells parents about two of the most common and complex problems of childhood: inattention and hyperactivity.

1993 Video
ISBN: 0-471303-19-4

Stephen M. Smith, President & CEO
John Kritzmacher, Executive Vice President
Edward J. May, Corporate Secretary

Web Sites

632 Attention Deficit Disorder Association
www.add.org

Provides children, adolescents and adults with ADD information, support groups, publications, videos, and referrals.

Evelyn Polk Green, President
Linda Roggli, Vice President
Celeste A. Jacque, Board of Director

633 Attention Deficit Disorder and Parenting Site
www.LD-ADD.com

Website has been created for parents to help them recognize and manage ADHD/LD in children.

634 Attention Deficit Information Network
www.addinfonetwork.com

Nonprofit volunteer organization. We offer support and information to families of children with ADD and adults with ADD, professionals through a network of AD-IN chapters.

635 CHADD: Children and Adults with Attention Deficit Disorders
4601 Presidents Drive, Suite 300
Lanham, MD 20706
301-306-7070
800-233-4050
Fax: 301-306-7090
help@chadd.org
www.chadd.org

Many children and/or adults have a disorder characterized by deficits in attention span and impulse control, which is frequently accompanied by hyperactivity. C.H.A.D.D. (Children and Adults with Attention Deficit Disorders) provides parents, professionals and adults diagnosed with ADD information, support and educational material dealing with this disorder. C.H.A.D.D. has over 600 chapters across the country and over 28,000 active members.

Michael MacKay, President
April Gower, Chief Operations Officer
Khalilah Long, Director of Membership & Marketing

636 Feingold Association of the US
11849 Suncatcher Drive
Fishers, IN 46037
631-369-9340
help@feingold.org
www.feingold.org

Helps families of children with learning and behavior problems, including attention deficit disorder. Also helps chemically-sensitive and salicylate-sensitive adults. Program is based upon a diet which primarily eliminates certain synthetic food additives.

637 Health Answers
410 Horsham Road
Horsham, PA 19044
215-442-9017
Michael.tague@healthanswers.com
www.healthanswers.com

HealthAnswers offers a breadth of services in medical education, sales force training, patient support solutions, professional promotion and consumer solutions.

Michael Tague, Managing Director

638 Learning Disabilities Association of Ameri ca
www.ldaamerica.org

Helps families of the affected individual through information and referral to professionals in their area. A membership organization with affiliates across the country.

639 National Center for Learning Disabilities
32 Laight Street, Second Floor
New York, NY 10013
212-545-7510
888-575-7373
Fax: 212-545-9665
help@ncld.org
www.ld.org

The mission of the NCLD is to increase opportunities for all individuals with learning disabilities to achieve their potential. NCLD accomplishes this by increasing public awareness and understanding of learning disabilities, conducting educational programs and services that promote research-based knowledge and providing national leadership in shaping public policy.

Frederic M Poses, Chairman
Mary Kalikow, Vice Chairman
William Haney, Secretary

640 Option Institute: Son Rise Program
www.autismtreatmentcenter.org

877-766-7473
www.autismtreatmentcenter.org

Describes an effective, loving and respectful method for treating children with autism. It teaches parents and healing professionals how to set up a home based program using the child's motivation to reach their special child.

Barry Neil Kaufman, Co-Founder
Kate Wilde, Group Facilitator
Samahria Lyte Kaufman, Founder

Book Publishers

641 ADD & Learning Disabilities
Bantam Doubleday Dell Publishing
1745 Broadway, 10th Floor
New York, NY 10019
212-572-6066
Fax: 212-782-9700
webmaster@randomhouse.com
www.randomhouse.com

For parents of children with learning disabilities and attention deficit disorder - and for educational and medical professionals who encounter these children - two experts in the field have devised a handbook to help identify the very best treatments.

256 pages
ISBN: 0-385469-31-4

642 ADD: Helping Your Child
Warner Books
1271 Avenue of the Americas
New York, NY 10020
212-484-2900
Fax: 617-263-2854

1994 224 pages Paperback
ISBN: 0-446670-13-8

643 ADHD Parenting Handbook: Practical Advice for Parents from Parents
Taylor Publishing
1550 W Mockingbird Lane
Dallas, TX 75235
214-637-2800
Fax: 214-819-8141

Provides guidelines, suggestions, and advice to help parents interact with their children who have ADHD.

1994 224 pages Paperback
ISBN: 0-878338-62-4

644 ADHD Survival Guide for Parents and Teachers
Hope Press
PO Box 188
Duarte, CA 91009
818-303-0644
800-321-4039
Fax: 626-358-3520
dcomings@earthlink.net
hopepress.com

Guide for parents and teacher and other caretakers of ADHD children.

ISBN: 1-878267-43-4

645 ADHD in Schools: Assessment and Intervention Strategies
George DuPaul, Gary Stoner, author

Guilford Publications
72 Spring Street
New York, NY 10012
212-431-9800
800-365-7006
Fax: 212-966-6708
info@guilford.com
www.guilford.com

Comprehensive and practical, the book includes several reproducible assessment tools and handouts, and emphasizes a team-based approach to intervention. This is a popular reference providing essential guidance for school-based professionals meeting the challenges of ADHD at any grade level. Available in paperback or hardcover.

Oct 2004 330 pages Paperback
ISBN: 1-593850-89-0

646 ADHD in the Young Child
ADD WareHouse
300 NW 70th Avenue, Suite 102
Plantation, FL 33317
954-792-8100
800-233-9273
Fax: 954-792-8545
websales@addwarehouse.com
www.addwarehouse.com

The authors sensitively and effectively describe what life is like living with a young child with ADHD. With the help of over 75 cartoon illustrations they provide practical solutions to common problems found at home, in school and elsewhere.

2006 202 pages
ISBN: 1-886941-32-7

647 ADHD: Handbook for Diagnosis & Treatment
Guilford Press
72 Spring Street
New York, NY 10012
800-365-7006
Fax: 212-966-6708
info@guilford.com
www.guilford.com

This second edition helps clinicians diagnose and treat Attention Deficit Hyperactivity Disorder. Written by an internationally recognized authority in the field, it covers the history of ADHD, its primary symptoms, associated conditions, developmental course and outcome, and family context. A workbook companion manual is also available.

2005 770 pages
ISBN: 1-593852-10-8

648   All Kinds of Minds
ADD WareHouse
300 NW 70th Avenue, Suite 102
Plantation, FL 33317
954-792-8100
800-233-9273
Fax: 954-792-8545
websales@addwarehouse.com
www.addwarehouse.com

Primary and elementary students with learning disorders can now gain insight into the difficulties they face in school. This book helps all children understand and respect all kinds of minds and can encourage children with learning disorders to maintain their motivation and keep from developing behavior problems stemming from their learning disorders.

1993 283 pages
ISBN: 0-838820-90-5

649   Alphabet Soup: A Recipe for Understanding & Treating ADD
Minerva Books
137 W 14th Street
New York, NY 10011
212-343-6100
Fax: 212-343-6934

1994 50 pages Paperback
ISBN: 0-934695-00-8

650   Attention Deficit Disorder and Learning Disabilities
Random House
1745 Broadway
New York, NY 10019
212-572-6066
webmaster@randomhouse.com
www.randomhouse.com

Realities, myths, and controversial treatments. Section I tries to dispel the myths and discusses proven treatments for ADHD and LD. Section II explains how the scientific community evaluates new treatment methods, and Section III summarizes alternative treatments and discusses scientific evidence pertaining to its usefulness.

256 pages
ISBN: 0-385469-31-4

651   Attention Deficit Disorder: Concise Source of Information for Parents
Temeron Books
6531 111th Street NW
Edmonton, AB T6H 4
Canada
403-283-0900
855-283-0900
Fax: 403-283-6947
contact@brusheducation.ca
www.brusheducation.ca

Help with a frustrating situation that many parents face.

2006 112 pages
ISBN: 1-550590-82-0

Glenn Rollans, Partner
Lauri Seidlitz, Managing Editor

652   Attention Deficit Hyperactivity Disorder: What Every Parent Wants to Know
Paul H Brookes & Company
PO Box 10624
Baltimore, MD 21285
301-337-9580
800-638-3775
Fax: 410-337-8539
custserv@brookspublishing.com
www.brookespublishing.com

The new edition breaks down the complex issues surrounding ADHD today into easy-to-understand, non-technical terms. Now you can quickly get the information you need to help your child with ADHD, without taking the time to wade through heavy research or statistics.

2000 304 pages Paperback
ISBN: 1-557663-98-X

653   Beyond Ritalin: Facts About Medication and Other Strategies for Helping Children
ADD WareHouse
300 NW 70th Avenue, Suite 102
Plantation, FL 33317
954-792-8100
800-233-9273
Fax: 954-792-8545
websales@addwarehouse.com
www.addwarehouse.com

The authors respond to concerns all parents and individuals have about using medication to treat disorders such as ADHD, explain the importance of a treatment program for those with this condition and discuss fads and fallacies in current treatments.

1996 272 pages
ISBN: 0-060977-25-6

654   Distant Drums, Different Drummers: A Guide for Young People with ADHD
ADD WareHouse
300 NW 70th Avenue, Suite 102
Plantation, FL 33317
954-792-8100
800-233-9273
Fax: 954-792-8545
websales@addwarehouse.com
www.addwarehouse.com

This book presents a positive perspective of ADHD - one that stresses the value of individual differences. Written for children and adolescents struggling with ADHD, it offers young readers the opportunity to see themselves in a positive light and motivates them to face challenging problems. Ages 8-14.

1995 39 pages
ISBN: 0-964854-80-5

Barbara Ingersoll, PhD

655   Don't Give Up Kid
ADD WareHouse
300 NW 70th Avenue, Suite 102
Plantation, FL 33317
954-792-8100
800-233-9273
Fax: 954-792-8545
websales@addwarehouse.com
www.addwarehouse.com

Alex, the hero of this book, is one of two million children in the US who have learning disabilities. This book gives children with reading problems and learning disabilities a clear understanding of their difficulties and the necessary courage to learn to live with them. Ages 5-12.

ISBN: 1-884281-10-9

656   Eagle Eyes A Child's View od Attention Deficit Disorder
Connecticut Association for Children with LD
25 Van Zant Street, Suite 15-5
East Norwalk, CT 06855
203-838-5010
Fax: 203-866-6108
cacld@optonline.net
www.cacld.org

Story about a boy with ADHD. A valuable tool for parents and teachers to use with elementary school age children with ADHD, their siblings and classmates to help them understand the strengths as well as weaknesses of this population.

30 pages

657   Eagle Eyes: A Child's View of Attention Deficit Disorder
ADD WareHouse
300 NW 70th Avenue, Suite 102
Plantation, FL 33317
954-792-8100
800-233-9273
Fax: 954-792-8545
websales@addwarehouse.com
www.addwarehouse.com

This book helps readers of all ages understand ADD and gives practical suggestions for organization, social cues and self calming. Expressive illustrations enhance the book and encourage reluctant readers. Ages 5-12.

ISBN: 1-884281-11-7

Jeanne Gehret

658   Eukee the Jumpy, Jumpy Elephant
ADD WareHouse
300 NW 70th Avenue, Suite 102
Plantation, FL 33317

954-792-8100
800-233-9273
Fax: 954-792-8545
websales@addwarehouse.com
www.addwarehouse.com

A story about a bright young elephant who is not like all the other elephants. Eukee moves through the jungle like a tornado, unable to pay attention to the other elephants. He begins to feel sad, but gets help after a visit to the doctor who explains why Eukee is so jumpy and hyperactive. With love, support and help, Eukee learns ways to help himself and gain renewed self-esteem. Ideal for ages 3-8.

1995 22 pages
ISBN: 0-962162-98-1

Cliff Corman, MD
Esther Trevino

659   Getting a Grip on ADD: A Kid's Guide to Understanding & Coping with ADD
Educational Media Corporation
6021 Wish Avenue
Encino, CA 91316

818-708-0962

1994 64 pages Paperback
ISBN: 0-932796-60-3

660   Give Your ADD Teen a Chance: A Guide for Parents of Teenagers with ADD
ADD WareHouse
300 NW 70th Avenue, Suite 102
Plantation, FL 33317

954-792-8100
800-233-9273
Fax: 954-792-8545
websales@addwarehouse.com
www.addwarehouse.com

Parenting teenagers is never easy, especially if your teen suffers from ADD. This book provides parents with expert help by showing them how to determine which issues are caused by 'normal' teenager development and which are caused by ADD.

1996 299 pages
ISBN: 0-891099-77-8

Lynn Weiss, PhD

661   Hyperactive Child, Adolescent, and Adult: ADD Through the Lifespan
Connecticut Association for Children with LD
25 Van Zant Street, Suite 15-5
East Norwalk, CT 06855

203-838-5010
Fax: 203-866-6108
cacld@optonline.net
www.cacld.org

Comprehensive general review. Update on previous research by the author, offering a basic text.

162 pages

662   Hyperactivity: Why Won't My Child Pay Attention?
John Wiley & Sons
1 Wiley Drive
Somerset, NJ 08875

732-469-4400
Fax: 732-302-2300
custserv@wiley.com
www.wiley.com

Deals with children who experience problems paying attention, controlling their emotions and physical actions and acting without forethought. Helps parents and professionals to accept the hyperactive child's behavior and find ways to help the child succeed. Provides and accurate understanding of the current state of science concerning the cause, developmental course, evaluation and outcome of this problem.

224 pages
ISBN: 0-471533-07-6

663   It's So Much Work to Be Your Friend
Active Parenting Publishers
1220 Kennestone Circle, Suite 130
Marietta, GA 30066

770-429-0565
800-825-0060
Fax: 770-429-0334
cservice@activeparenting.com
www.activeparenting.com

Offers practical strategies to help learning disabled children ages six through seventeen navigate the treacherous social waters of their school, home, and community.

448 pages

664   Jumpin' Johnny Get Back to Work! A Child's Guide to ADHD/Hyperactivity
Connecticut Association for Children with LD
25 Van Zant Street, Suite 15-5
East Norwalk, CT 06855

203-838-5010
Fax: 203-866-6108
cacld@optonline.net
www.cacld.org

Written primarily for elementary age youngsters with ADHD to help them understand their disability. Also valuable as an educational tool for parents, siblings, friends, and classmates. Includes two pages on medication.

24 pages

665   Kids With Incredible Potential Parent's Guide
Active Parenting Publishers
1220 Kennestone Circle, Suite 130
Marietta, GA 30066

770-429-0565
800-825-0060
Fax: 770-429-0334
cservice@activeparenting.com
www.activeparenting.com

The guide for parents of ADHD children is designed as an add-on to the Active Parenting Now video and discussion program. Adds an ADHD emphasis that makes the parenting information more immediate and practical for these parents' special needs.

666   Kids with Incredible Potential Leader's Guide
Active Parenting Publishers
1220 Kennestone Circle, Suite 130
Marietta, GA 30066

770-429-0565
800-825-0060
Fax: 770-429-0334
cservice@activeparenting.com
www.activeparenting.com

Allows the facilitator to give parents specialized information that is more immediate and practical to these parents' needs.

667   Learning To Slow Down and Pay Attention
Connecticut Association for Children with LD
25 Van Zant Street, Suite 15-5
East Norwalk, CT 06855

203-838-5010
Fax: 203-866-6108
cacld@optonline.net
www.cacld.org

Written for elementary school age children with ADHD to read with their parents. A checklist helps families decide if attention and concentration are problems. Interventions are given for parents, doctors and teachers. Includes practical strategies for paying better attention, getting more organized and problem solving.

62 pages

668 **Managing Attention Deficit Hyperactivity Disorder in Children**
John Wiley & Sons
1 Wiley Drive
Somerset, NJ 08875 732-469-4400
Fax: 732-302-2300
custserv@wiley.com
www.wiley.com

This book explores symptoms of ADHD, the crossover into adulthood with such a disorder, and the latest and most controversial treatments.

1998 896 pages
ISBN: 0-471121-58-4

669 **Maybe You Know My Kid: A Parent's Guide to Identifying ADHD**
Birch Lane Press
120 Enterprise Avenue S
Secaucus, NJ 07094 212-407-1500
Fax: 212-935-0699

The author writes about her family experiences with their son, David, who has attention deficit disorder. Contains a comprehensive review of important issues plus descriptions of some helpful management techniques.

222 pages

670 **My Brother's a World Class Pain: A Sibling's Guide To ADHD/Hyperactivity**
Connecticut Association for Children with LD
25 Van Zant Street, Suite 15-5
East Norwalk, CT 06855 203-838-5010
Fax: 203-866-6108
cacld@optonline.net
www.cacld.org

A young girl tells what it's like to have a little brother with ADHD. She expresses the frustration, anger, embarrassment and resentment that often develop living with a sibling who has attention deficit. Her parents seek professional help to understand the disability and enlisted in trying to bring about positive changes in the family.

34 pages

671 **Otto Learns About His Medicine A Story About Medication for Hyperative Children**
Connecticut Association for Children with LD
25 Van Zant Street, Suite 15-5
East Norwalk, CT 06855 203-838-5010
Fax: 203-866-6108
cacld@optonline.net
www.cacld.org

A book about Otto, a young, hyperactive car. Otto has difficulty paying attention in school, so his parents take him to a mechanic who prescribes medication that will help him control his behavior.

28 pages

672 **Parenting Children with ADHD: Lessons That Medicine Cannot Teach**
Active Parenting Publishers
1220 Kennestone Circle, Suite 130
Marietta, GA 30066 770-429-0565
800-825-0060
Fax: 770-429-0334
cservice@activeparenting.com
www.activeparenting.com

Gives parents a framework for building a successful parenting program at home. Presents a series of ten lessons that are essential for promoting the success of kids with ADHD.

261 pages

673 **Parents Helping Parents: A Directory of Support Groups for ADD**
CibaGelgy, Pharmaceuticals Division
External Communications
Summit, NJ 07901 908-277-5000
Fax: 973-781-2601
www.add.org

Evelyn Polk Green, President
Linda Roggli, Vice President
Janet Kramer, Treasurer

674 **Parents' Hyperactivity Handbook: Helping the Fidgety Child**
Plenum Press
233 Spring Street
New York, NY 10013 212-620-8000
Fax: 212-463-0742
info@plenum.com

1993 306 pages
ISBN: 0-306444-65-8

675 **Putting On The Brakes - Young People's Guide To Understanding ADHD**
Connecticut Association for Children with LD
25 Van Zant Street, Suite 15-5
East Norwalk, CT 06855 203-838-5010
Fax: 203-866-6108
cacld@optonline.net
www.cacld.org

Written from both a medical and educational perspective. Reviews what it is like to have ADHD. It explains what's going on in the brain, discusses feelings and tries to help children gain some control of their lives.

64 pages

676 **Putting on the Brakes**
Courage To Change
PO Box 486
Wilkes-Barres, PA 18703 800-440-4003
Fax: 800-772-6499
www.couragetochange.com

This book written for kids ages eight to thirteen tells all they need to know about ADHD. Also available is a companion activity book that teaches organizing, setting priorities, problem solving, maintaining control and other life management skills. The activity book is 88 pages and sells for $14.95.

677 **Rethinking Attention Deficit Disorders**
Brookline Books
8 Trumbell Rd, Suite B-001
Northampton, MA 01060 413-584-0184
800-666-2665
Fax: 413-584-6184
brbooks@yahoo.com
www.brooklinebooks.com

Gives the classroom teacher useful information that provides ideas and strategies for working with children suffering from ADD.

ISBN: 1-571290-37-0

678 **Ritalin is Not the Answer**
Jossey-Bass
111 River Street
Hoboken, NJ 07030 201-748-6000
800-956-7739
Fax: 201-748-6088
www.josseybass.com

A healthy, drug-free alternative to Ritalin and an absolute must read for every physician before prescribing it.

224 pages
ISBN: 0-787945-14-5

679 **Self-Control Games & Workbook**
Western Psychological Services
12031 Wilshire Boulevard
Los Angeles, CA 90025 310-478-2061
Fax: 310-478-7838

This game is designed to teach self-control in academic and social situations. Addresses a total of 24 impulsive, inattentive and hyperactive behaviors. The companion workbook reinforces the use of positive self-statements, and problem-solving techniques, instead of expressing anger.

Game

680 Shelley The Hyperactive Turtle
Connecticut Association for Children with LD
25 Van Zant Street, Suite 15-5
East Norwalk, CT 06855
203-838-5010
Fax: 203-866-6108
cacld@optonline.net
www.cacld.org

Delightful picture book for use with very young children. Sensitive text and wonderful colored illustrations help little ones understand ADHD.

20 pages

681 Taking Charge of ADHD: The Complete, Authoritative Guide for Parents
Guilford Press
72 Spring Street
New York, NY 10012
800-365-7006
Fax: 212-966-6708
info@guilford.com
www.guilford.com

Provides a guide to understanding attention-deficit/hyperactivity disorder and relating to the children whose behavior can be frustrating and confusing. Hardcover, paperback, e-book.

2005 321 pages Paperback
ISBN: 1-572305-60-1

682 Teaching the Tiger
Hope Press
PO Box 188
Duarte, CA 91009
800-321-4039
Fax: 626-358-3520
dcomings@earthlink.net
www.hopepress.com

A handbook for individuals involved in the education of students with Attention Deficit Disorder, Tourette Syndrome, or Obsessive Compulsive Disorder.

ISBN: 1-878267-34-5

David E Comings MD, Presenter

683 The 'Putting On The Brakes' Activity Book For Young People With ADHD
Connecticut Association for Children with LD
25 Van Zant Street, Suite 15-5
East Norwalk, CT 06855
203-838-5010
Fax: 203-866-6108
cacld@optonline.net
www.cacld.org

A companion to the book 'Putting On The Brakes: Young People's Guide To Understanfing Attention Deficit Hyperactivity Disorder (ADHD)'. Offers various exercises to help children with ADHD learn to deal with their problems in a positive way. Some activities can be done independently, others need the collaboration of an adult.

88 pages

684 The ADHD Book of Lists
Courage To Change
PO Box 486
Wilkes-Barres, PA 18703
800-440-4003
Fax: 800-772-6499
www.couragetochange.com

Presented in list format and created for parents, school psychologists, and mental health professionals. A reliable source of answers, strategies, tools, interventions, support, and additional resources.

685 The LD Child and the ADHD Child: Ways Parents and Professionals Can Help
John F Blair Publishers
1406 Plaza Drive
Winston-Salem, NC 27103
336-768-1374
800-222-9796
Fax: 336-768-9194
editorial@blairpub.com
www.blairpub.com

The author recommends other options that can be explored to treat LD and ADHD children without drugs.

261 pages Paperback
ISBN: 0-895871-42-4

Carolyn Sakowski, President
Steve Kirk, Editor In Chief

686 You and Your ADD Child
Nelson Publications
1 Gateway Plaza
Port Chester, NY 10573
914-937-8400
Fax: 914-937-8676

1995 252 pages Paperback
ISBN: 0-785278-95-8

Magazines

687 Attention
CHADD
4601 Presidents Drive, Suite 300
Lanham, MD 20706
301-306-7070
800-233-4050
Fax: 301-306-7090
help@chadd.org
www.chadd.org

Available with membership.

Quarterly

Michael MacKay, President
April Gower, Chief Operations Officer
Khalilah Long, Director of Membership & Marketing

Newsletters

688 ADHD Report
Guilford Publications
370 Seventh Avenue, Suite 1200
New York, NY 10001
212-431-9800
800-365-7006
Fax: 212-966-6708
info@guilford.com
www.guilford.com

Presents the most up-to-date information on the evaluation, diagnosis and management of ADHD in children, adolescents and adults. This important newsletter is an invaluable resource for all professionals interested in ADHD. 6 issues per year; content available online.

16 pages Subscription
ISBN: 1-065802-5 -

Russell A. Barkley, PhD, Editor

689 Chadder
CHADD
BOX.8181 Professional Place, Suite 201
Landover, MD 20785
301-306-7070
Fax: 301-306-7090
TTY: 301-429-0641
disabilityresourcejs.weebly.com/adhd.html

Quarterly

690 Pure Facts
Feingold Association of the US
11849 Suncatcher Drive
Fishers, IN 46037
631-369-9340
help@feingold.org
www.feingold.org

Monthly newsletter with articles on nutrition and behavior and lists of approved brand-name foods.

monthly

Deborah Lehner, Executive Director

Pamphlets

691 ADHD
Learning Disabilities Association of America
4156 Library Road
Pittsburgh, PA 15234

412-341-1515
Fax: 412-344-0224
info@LDAAmerica.org
ldaamerica.org

A booklet for parents offering information on Attention Deficit-Hyperactivity Disorders and learning disabilities.

Nancie Payne, President
Ed Schlitt, First Vice President
Beth McGaw, Secretary

692 Attention Deficit Disorders and Hyperactivity
ERIC Clearinghouse on Disabled and Gifted Children
1920 Association Drive
Reston, VA 20191

703-620-3660
Fax: 703-620-2521

Dedicated to improving educational outcomes for individuals with exceptionalities, students with disabilities, and/or the gifted.

693 Attention Deficit-Hyperactivity Disorder: Is it a Learning Disability?
Georgetown University, School of Medicine
3800 Reservoir Road NW, Main Hospital Building, Fi
Washington, DC 20007

202-444-3960
Fax: 202-687-2387
www.medstarhealth.org

Offers information on learning disabilities and related disorders.

Stephen Ray Mitchell, MD, MBA, Dean for Medical Education
Mikey Cassidy, Executive Assistant to the Dean
Diana Kassar, Sr. Associate Dean for Fin & Admin

694 COGREHAB
Life Science Associates
1 Fenimore Road
Bayport, NY 11705

631-472-2111
Fax: 631-472-8146
lifesciassoc@pipeline.com
www.lifesciassoc.home.pipeline.com

Divided into six groups for diagnosis and treatment of attention, memory and perceptual disorders to be used by and under the guidance of a professional.

$95 - $1,950

Frank Manoriota, Vice President

695 Children with ADD: A Shared Responsibility
Council for Exceptional Children
2900 Crystal Drive, Suite 1000
Arlington, VA 22202

703-264-9494
888-232-7733
TTY: 866-915-5000
service@cec.sped.org
www.cec.sped.org

This book represents a consensus of what professionals and parents believe ADD is all about and how children with ADD may best be served. Reviews the evaluation process under IDEA and 504 and presents effective classroom strategies.

35 pages
ISBN: 0-865862-33-8

James P. Heiden, President
Antonis Katsiyannis, President Elect
Sharon Raimondi, Treasurer

696 Coping with Your Inattentive Child
Connecticut Association for Children with LD
25 Van Zant Street, Suite 15-5
East Norwalk, CT 6855

203-838-5010
Fax: 203-866-6108
cacld@optonline.net
www.cacld.org

Lists signs of ADHD and discusses managing the problems of children with ADHD from infancy through elementary school.

13 pages

697 Identification and Treatment of Attention Deficit Disorders
Therapro
225 Arlington Street
Framingham, MA 1701

508-872-9494
800-257-5376
Fax: 508-875-2062

This handbook contains information that is based on research and offers practical suggestions for parents, teachers and other professionals.

698 Out of Darkness
Connecticut Association for Children with LD
25 Van Zant Street, Suite 15-5
East Norwalk, CT 6855

203-838-5010
Fax: 203-866-6108
cacld@optonline.net
www.cacld.org

Article by an adult who discovers at age 30 that he has ADD.

4 pages

699 Parenting Attention Deficit Disordered Teens
Connecticut Association for Children with LD
25 Van Zant Street, Suite 15-5
East Norwalk, CT 6855

203-838-5010
Fax: 203-866-6108
cacld@optonline.net
www.cacld.org

Detailed outline of the various problems of adolescents with ADHD.

14 pages

700 School Based Assessment of Attention Deficit Disorders
National Clearinghouse of Rehabilitation Materials
5202 N Richmond Hill Drive
Stillwater, OK 74078

405-624-7650
800-223-5219
Fax: 405-624-0695
TDD: 405-624-3156
www.nchrtm.okstate,edu

The 1992 OSEP ruling, placing more responsibility on schools for the assessment of students who may have attention deficit disorders, has raised questions concerning the assessment process. This guide was developed to help states formulate new policies. The paper seeks to: present an overview of current thoughts concerning ADD from an educational perspective, contrast traditional assessment strategies with an alternative model, and describe phases of evaluation.

David Brooks, Director
Carolyn Cain

Camps

701 Camp Buckskin
4124 Quebec Ave N, Ste 300
Minneapolis, MN 55427

763-208-4805
Fax: 952-938-6996
info@campbuckskin.com
www.campbuckskin.com

LD and ADD/ADHD youth have often experienced frustration and a lack of success. Buckskin assists these individuals to realize and develop the potentials and abilities which they possess.

Thomas R Bauer, CCD, Camp Director

702   Camp Nuhop
404 Hillcrest Drive
Ashland, OH 44805   419-289-2227
                                          Fax: 419-289-2227
                                          info@campnuhop.org
                                          www.campnuhop.org

A summer residential program for any youngster from 6 to 18
with a learning disability, behavior disorder or Attention Deficit
Disorder. Sixty two campers and 35 staff members live on site in
groups of 7 campers to every 3 counselors. Activities focus on
positive self-concept and behaviors and teach children to learn
how to find their strengths, abilities and talents from a positive,
yet realistic viewpoint.

Jerry Dunlap, Director

703   Dallas Academy
950 Tiffany Way
Dallas, TX 75218   214-324-1481
                                          Fax: 214-327-8537
                                          www.dallas-academy.com

7-week summer session for students who are having difficulty in
regular school classes.

Jim Richardson, Director

704   Developmental Center
6710 86th Avenue N
Pinellas Park, FL 33782   727-541-5716
                                          Fax: 727-544-8186
                                          infopp@centeracademy.com
                                          www.centeracademy.com

Specifically designed for the learning disabled child and other
children with difficulties in concentration, strategy, social skills,
impulsivity, distractibility and study strategies. Programs offered
include: attention training, visual-motor remediation, socialization skills training, relaxation training, horseback riding and
more. The day camp meets weekdays from 9-3 for 3,4 or 5 week
sessions.

Dr. Eric Larson

705   Eagle Hill School - Summer Program
242 Old Petersham Road, PO Box 116
Hardwick, MA 01037   413-477-6000
                                          Fax: 413-477-6837
                                          admission@eaglehillschool.com
                                          www.ehs1.org

For the child, age 9-19, with a specific learning disability or Attention Deficit Disorder, this summer program offers a structured
curriculum designed to build a basic foundation of academic competence. Extracurricular and outdoor activities complement the
educational program.

Erin E Wynne, Dean of Admission

706   Groves Academy
3200 Highway 100 South
Saint Louis Park, MN 55416   952-920-6377
                                          Fax: 952-920-2068
                                          www.grovesacademy.org

A nonprofit day school in Minnesota designed especially for children with learning differences. The Center has a full day academic program from September through June, as well as an 8
week summer program. Groves also offers community services
such as: psychoeducational testing for children and adults, consulting services, workshops on learning disabilities and other special learning needs, and afternoon/evening tutorial services for
children and adults.

John Alexander, Head of School

707   Hill School of Fort Worth
4817 Odessa Avenue
Fort Worth, TX 76133   817-923-9482
                                          Fax: 817-923-4894
                                          admission@hillschool.org
                                          www.hillschool.org

Provides an alternative learning environment for students having
average or above-average intelligence with learning differences.
Hill school is an established leader in North Texas with a 25 year
history of effectively serving LD children. Beginning in 1961 as
a tutorial service, Hill became a formal school in 1973. Our mission is to help those who learn differently develop skills and
strategies to succeed. We do this by developing academic/study
skills, and self-discipline.

Lucille H Helton, Principal
Cathy Allen, Admissions Director
Grey Owens, Principal

708   Lab School of Washington Summer Program
4759 Reservoir Road NW
Washington, DC 20007   202-965-6600
                                          Fax: 202-965-5106
                                          Alexandra.Freeman@labschool.org
                                          www.labschool.org

The Lab School 5-week summer session includes individualized
reading, spelling, writing, study skills, and math programs. A
multisensory approach addresses the needs of bright learning disabled children. Related services such as speech/language therapy
and occupational therapy are integrated into the curriculum. Ele-
mentary/Intermediate; Junior High/High School.

Sally Smith, Founder
Susan Feeley, Admissions Director

709   Maplebrook School
5142 Route 22
Amenia, NY 12501   845-373-8191
                                          Fax: 845-373-7029
                                          jscully@maplebrookschool.org
                                          www.maplebrookschool.org

A coeductional boarding school for students with learning differences and ADD. A New York State registered high school servicing ages 11-18. Post secondary options offered to 18-21.

Donna M Konkolios, Head of School
Jennifer Scully, Director Admissions

710   Round Lake Camp
21 Plymouth Street
Fairfield, NJ 7004   973-575-3333
                                              800-776-5657
                                          Fax: 973-575-4188
                                          rlc@njycamps.org
                                          www.njycamps.org

For ages 7-18, this camp provides individualized academics in
reading, language development and math for children with mild
learning disabilities, Round Lake also offers therapeutic recreation and Jewish cultural values to its participants.

Sheira Director, Asst. Director

711   Tourette Syndrome Camp Organization
6933 N Kedzie, Ste 816
Chicago, IL 60640   773-465-7536
                                          info@tourettecamp.com
                                          www.tourettecamp.com

Dedicated to promoting camping opportunities for children with
Tourette Syndrome and its assocaited disorders, Obsessive Com-
pulsive Disorder (OCD) and Attention Deficit/Hyperactivity
Disorder (ADD/ADHD).

Monica Newman, Camp Director

DESCRIPTION

712 AUTISTIC DISORDER

Synonyms: Infantile autism, Kanner's syndrome

Involves the following Biologic System(s):

Developmental/Behavioral/Psychiatric Disorders, Neurologic Disorders

Autistic disorder, also known as infantile autism, is classified as a developmental disability that results from a disorder of the human central nervous system. It usually becomes apparent by three years of age. It is thought to affect approximately four in 10,000 children and is about three to four times more common in males than females. Autistic disorder is characterized by deficient verbal and nonverbal communication, impaired social interactions, and a restricted range of interests and activities.

Children with autistic disorder may fail to acquire or have poorly developed verbal and nonverbal communication skills. If children do communicate verbally, abnormal speech patterns are typically present, such as repetition of another's words or phrases (echolalia); reversal of the proper use of pronouns, such as use of the term "you" rather than "I" when referring to themselves; and nonsensical rhyming. In addition, affected children may be withdrawn, make little or no eye contact, resist cuddling, lack awareness of others' thoughts or feelings, or fail to seek comfort when distressed. Children also typically engage in solitary play for hours, perform ritualistic behaviors and repeated body movements (e.g., rocking, flicking fingers) and have a strong need for a predictable, consistent environment. Certain behaviors (e.g., rubbing an object or surface) may demonstrate a heightened awareness of particular stimuli, whereas others, such as a lack of reaction to sudden, loud noises, may indicate a lowered sensitivity to other stimuli. In many children with autistic disorder, disruptions of rituals or routines may result in tantrum-like outbursts or rages. In addition, some children may exhibit self-injurious or outwardly aggressive behaviors. Because of impairment of language and socialization skills, it may be difficult to obtain accurate estimates of overall intelligence levels and potential. Although such testing often demonstrates functional retardation, some affected children perform adequately in nonverbal areas, such as spatial and motor skills, and those with speech skills may perform adequately in all test areas.

In most patients, the symptoms and findings associated with autistic disorder continue to affect them throughout life. The Food and Drug Administration (FDA) recently approved the use of an antipsychotic, risperidone, for the treatment of irritability associated with autistic disorder, including symptoms of aggression, deliberate self-injury, temper tantrums, and quickly changing moods. This is the first time the FDA has approved any medication for use in children and adolescents with autism. In addition, the management and treatment of affected children may include integrated, multidisciplinary techniques, such as language therapy, structured play and interpersonal exercises, and other behavioral therapies. Some patients, particularly those with speech development, may lead somewhat independent lives with proper support. However, other individuals with autistic disorder may require special, ongoing care.

The cause of autistic disorder is unknown. However, according to the medical literature, several underlying neurologic, infectious, and other disorders are known to produce or to increase a predisposition toward autistic-like behaviors in children. Genetic abnormalities are also thought to play some role in causing or resulting in susceptibility for the disorder. For example, some researchers theorize that autistic disorder may result from certain brain abnormalities during infancy (e.g., particular biochemical abnormalities, brain injury, etc.), potentially in combination with a genetic predisposition for the condition (multifactorial).

Government Agencies

713 NIH/National Institute of Neurological Disorders and Stroke (NINDS)
PO Box 5801
Bethesda, MD 20824

301-496-5751
800-352-9424
Fax: 301-496-0296
TTY: 301-468-5981
www.ninds.nih.gov

The mission of NINDS is to reduce the burden of neurological disease - a burden borne by every age group, by every segment of society, by people all over the world.

Walter J. Koroshetz, MD, Director

714 NIH/National Institute on Deafness and Other Communication Disorders (NIDCD)
31 Center Drive, MSC 2320
Bethesda, MD 20892

800-241-1044
TTY: 800-241-1055
nidcdinfo@nidcd.nih.gov
www.nidcd.nih.gov

Conducts and supports biomedical research and research training on normal mechanisms, as well as diseases and disorders of hearing, balance, smell, taste, voice, speech and language.

James F Battey Jr, MD, PhD, Director
Judith A Cooper, Deputy Director
Timothy J Wheeles, Executive Officer

National Associations & Support Groups

715 Achieve Beyond
7000 Austin Street, Suite 200
Forest Hills, NY 11375

718-762-7633
Fax: 212-679-7867
info@achievebeyondusa.com
www.achievebeyondusa.com

Achieve Beyond was founded in 1995 to meet the needs of developmentally delayed and disabled children and their families, particularly children with bilingual needs.

Trudy Font Padron, Founder/ Programs Executive Dir
Robert Padron, Executive Director

716 Aging with Autism
704 Marten RD
Princeton, NJ 8540

908-904-9319
contact@agingwithautism.org
www.agingwithautism.org

Aging with Autism is dedicated to enhancing programs and services for individuals with autism and other developmental disabilities as they transition to and through adulthood.

Dr. Cyndy Hayes, Founder/ President
Andria Prather, Administrator

717 American Academy of Pediatrics
141 Northwest Point Boulevard
Elk Grove Village, IL 60007

847-434-4000
800-433-9016
Fax: 847-434-8000
www.aap.org

The American Academy of Pediatrics and its member pediatricians are committed to the attainment of optimal physical, mental and social health and well-being for all infants, children, adolescents, and young adults.

Fernando Stein, MD, FAAP, President
Karen Remley, MD, CEO/Executive VP

718 American Psychological Association
750 First St. NE
Washington, DC 20002
202-336-5500
800-374-2721
TTY: 202-336-6123
www.apa.org

The mission is to advance the creation, communication and application of psychological knowledge to benefit society and improve people's lives.

Norman B. Anderson, PhD, CEO/ EVP
L. Michael Honaker, PhD, Deputy Chief Executive Officer
Ellen G. Garrison, PhD, Senior Policy Advisor

719 American School Counselor Association
1101 King Street, Suite 310
Alexandria, VA 22314
703-683-2722
800-306-4722
Fax: 703-997-7572
asca@schoolcounselor.org
www.schoolcounselor.org

The mission of ASCA is to represent professional school counselors and to promote professionalism and ethical practices.

Richard Wong, Executive Director
Jeff Broderson, Information Technology Admin.
Kathleen M Rakestraw, Director of Communications

720 Asperger/Autism Network
51 Water Street, Suite 206
Watertown, MA 2472
617-393-3824
866-597-AANE
Fax: 617-393-3827
info@aane.org
www.aane.org

The Asperger/Autism Network (AANE) works with individuals, families, and professionals to help people with Asperger Syndrome and similar autism spectrum profiles build meaningful, connected lives.

Jayne Burke, President
Karen Boyd, Vice President
Stephen Burgay, B.A., J.D., Vice President

721 Association for Science in Autism Treatment
PO Box 188
Crosswicks, NJ 08515
781-397-8943
info@asatonline.org

To disseminate accurate information about autism and treatments, and to improve access to effective, science-based treatments for all people with autism.

David Celiberti PhD BCBA, President
Sharon A Reeve PhD BCBA, Vice President

722 Autism Action Network
550 East Chester Street
Long Beach, NY 11561
516-382-0081
Fax: 888-995-6161
jgilmore@autismactionnetwork.org
autismactionnetwork.org

Autism Action Network is a national, non-partisan, grassroots, political action organization formed by parents in support of children and adults with autism, vaccine injuries, and neurodevelopmental and communication disorders.

723 Autism Consortium
10 Shattuck Street
Boston, MA 2115
866-518-0296
Fax: 617-432-6960
autismconsortium@hms.harvard.edu
www.autismconsortium.org

The Autism Consortium catalyzes rapid advances in understanding of autism by fostering collaboration among families, researchers, clinicians, and donors. There mission is to improve the care of children and families affected by autism and other neurological disorders.

Deirdre B. Phillips, Executive Director
Laura K. Farfel, Digital Outreach Coordinator

724 Autism Inclusion Resources
www.autismir.com

info@autismir.com
www.autismir.com

AIR is the creative force behind services and solutions that will enable today's generation of children with autism to participate more fully in the world.

Wendy Ross, MD, FAAP, Founder
Roger Ideishi, JD, OT/L, Collaborator
Angela Jones, PhD, Collaborator

725 Autism National Committee
3 Bedford Green
South Burlington, VT 05403
800-378-0386
sandra.mcclennen@emich.edu
www.autcom.org

Organization dedicated to social justice for all citizens with autism through a shared vision and a commitment to positive approaches.

Anne Bakeman, Treasurer

726 Autism Network International
PO Box 35448
Syracuse, NY 10190
315-476-2462
jisincla@mailbox.syr.edu
www.autismnetworkinternational.org

Supported by individuals who want to make a difference for the sufferers, the foundation provides a variety of support and educational references to inform on the latest changes in the field.

Jim Sinclair, Coordinator
Jame Bordner, List-owner
Sola Shelly, Webmaster

727 Autism Network for Hearing and Visually Impaired Persons
7510 Ocean Front Avenue
Virginia Beach, VA 23451
757-428-9036
Fax: 757-428-0019
www.autism.com

Provides communication, education, research and advocacy for persons with autism combined with a hearing or visual disability, their families, and professionals. Sharing of educational materials, phone help, support groups, referrals and conferences.

Dolores Bartel, Contact
Alan Bartel, Contact

728 Autism Research Foundation
C/O Moss-Rosene Lab, W701
72 East Concord Street, R-1014
Boston, MA 10192
617-414-7012
Fax: 617-414-7207
tarf@ladders.org
www.theautismresearchfoundation.org/

he Autism Research Foundation is a 501(c)3 nonprofit organization dedicated to brain-based research and inclusion programs in the community. Our goal is to fundraise for continuous brain-based research, while providing tangible resources for families and providers managing autism right now.

Margaret Bauman MD, Fouding Director
Thomas Sabin MD, President
Thomas Kemper MD, Vice President

729 Autism Research Institute
4182 Adams Avenue
San Diego, CA 10193
619-281-7165
866-366-3361
Fax: 619-563-6840
media@autismresearchinstitute.com
www.autism.com

ARI advocates for the rights of people with ASD, and operates without funding from special-interest groups. ARI is dedicated to developing a standard of care for individuals with autism spectrum disorders and their families. We rely on the generosity of donors to help us advance autism research and provide needed information and support for families and individuals with autism spectrum disorders.

Stephen Edelson, Executive Director
Jane Johnson, Managing Director
Rebecca McKenney, Office Manager

730   Autism Research Institute Conference
Autism Research Institute
4182 Adams Avenue
San Diego, CA 10194   619-281-7165
                                             866-366-3361
                                          Fax: 619-563-6840
                              www.autism.com/index.php/video

ARI advocates for the rights of people with ASD, and operates without funding from special-interest groups. ARI is dedicated to developing a standard of care for individuals with autism spectrum disorders and their families. We rely on the generosity of donors to help us advance autism research and provide needed information and support for families and individuals with autism spectrum disorders.

Stephen Edelson PhD, Executive Director
Jane Johnson, Managing Director
Rebecca McKenney, Office Manager

731   Autism Science Foundation
28 West 39th Street, Suite #502
New York, NY 10018   212-391-3913
                                          Fax: 212-391-3954
                       contactus@autismsciencefoundation.org
                                 autismsciencefoundation.org

The Autism Science Foundation's mission is to support autism research by providing funding and other assistance to scientists and organizations conducting, facilitating, publicizing and disseminating autism research. The organization also provides information about autism to the general public and serves to increase awareness of autism spectrum disorders and the needs of individuals and families affected by autism.

Alison Singer, Co-Founder/ President
Karen Margulis London, Co-Founder
Gregg E. Ireland, SVP, Capital World Investors

732   Autism Services Center
929 4th Avenue, P.O. Box 507
Huntington, WV 10195   304-525-8014
                                          Fax: 304-525-8026
                              www.autismservicescenter.org

Autism Services Center (ASC) is a nonprofit, licensed behavioral health center that was founded in 1979 by Ruth C. Sullivan, Ph.D. to provide services in Cabell, Wayne, Lincoln and Mason counties in the state of West Virginia. Though specializing in autism, ASC provides comprehensive, community-integrated services to all individuals with intellectual and developmental disabilities.

Mike Grady, CEO
Elaine Harvey, Vice President
Derek Hyman, President & Treasurer of the Greate

733   Autism Society of America
4340 East-West Hwy, Suite 350
Bethesda, MD 20814   301-657-0881
                                             800-328-8476
                                    info@autism-society.org
                                    www.autism-society.org

The Autism Society, the nation's leading grassroots autism organization, exists to improve the lives of all affected by autism.We do this by increasing public awareness about the day-to-day issues faced by people on the spectrum, advocating for appropriate services for individuals across the lifespan, and providing the latest information regarding treatment, education, research and advocacy

Scott Badesch, President & CEO
Matthew Asner, VP Development
Selena Hernandez, Manager, Support Services

734   Autism Solution Center
www.autismsolutioncenter.com

                                       dorrisphilpot@yahoo.com
                                  www.autismsolutioncenter.com

The Autism Solution Center, Inc. (ASC) is a non-profit organization being developed to address an unmet, ongoing need within our communities for autism therapy, support services, research and other assistance.

735   Autism Speaks
1 East 33rd Street 4th Floor
New York, NY 10197   212-252-8584
                                        Fax: 212-252-8676
                           familyservices@autismspeaks.org
                                     www.autismspeaks.org

At Autism Speaks, our goal is to change the future for all who struggle with autism spectrum disorder.We are dedicated to funding global biomedical research into the causes, prevention, treatments, and cure for autism; to raising public awareness about autism and its effects on individuals, families, and society; and to bringing hope to all who deal with the hardships of this disorder.

Liz Feld, President
Peter H Bell, Executive VP
Lisa Goring, Vice President

736   Autism Treatment Center of America
www.autismtreatmentcenter.org

                                             413-229-2100
                                             877-766-7473
                                 www.autismtreatmentcenter.org

Welcome to the Autism Treatment Center of AmericaT, the worldwide teaching center for The Son-Rise Programr , a powerful and effective treatment for children and adults challenged by Autism, Autism Spectrum Disorders, Pervasive Developmental Disorder (PDD) , Asperger's Syndrome, and other developmental difficulties.

737   Autistic Services
4444 Bryant Stratton Way
Williamsville, NY 10198   716-631-5777
                                             888-288-4764
                                        Fax: 716-565-0671
                      tpanzarella@autism-services-inc.org.
                                    www.autisticservices.org

Agency exclusively dedicated to serving the unique lifelong needs of autistic individuals. Also a regional resource for parents, school districts, physicians and other professionals.

Veronica Federiconi, Executive Director

738   Autreat
Autism Network International
PO Box 35448
Syracuse, NY 13235   315-476-2462
                                   jisincla@mailbox.syr.edu
                             www.autismnetworkinternational.org

A retreat-style conference run by autistic people, for autistic people and friends. Focuses on positive living with autism, not on causes, cures, or ways to make individuals more normal.

August

Jim Sinclair, Coordinator
Jame Bordner, List-Owner
Sola Shelly, Webmaster

739   Center for Autism and Related Disorders
19019 Ventura Blvd., Suite 300
Tarzana, CA 91356   818-345-2345
                                             855-345-2273
                                        Fax: 818-758-8015
                                    www.centerforautism.com

The Center for Autism and Related Disorders (CARD) uses applied behavior analysis (ABA) in the treatment of autism spectrum disorder.

Doreen Granpeesheh, Founder/ Executive Director

740 **Community Services for Autistic Adults & Children (CSAAC)**
8615 East Village
Montgomery Village, MD 10201　　　204-912-2220
　　　　　　　　　　　　　　　　Fax: 301-926-9384
　　　　　　　　　　　　　　　　csaac@csaac.org
　　　　　　　　　　　　　　　　www.csaac.org

To enable individuals with autism to achieve their highest potential and contribute as confident individuals to their community

Ian Paregol, Executive Director
Marcee Smith, Ph.D., Assistant Executive Director of Pro

741 **Developmental Delay Resources (DDR)**
5801 Beacon Street
Pittsburgh, PA 10202　　　　　　412-422-3373
　　　　　　　　　　　　　　　　800-497-0944
　　　　　　　　　　　　　　　　Fax: 412-422-1374
　　　　　　　　　　　　　　　　devdelay@mindspring.com
　　　　　　　　　　　　　　　　www.devdelay.org

Dedicated to meeting the needs of those working with children who have developmental delays in sensory, motor, language, social, and emotional areas. Publicizes research into determining identifiable factors that would put a child at risk and maintains a registry, tracking possible trends.

Patricia Lemer, Owner

742 **Facilitated Communication Institute at Syracuse University**
307 Huntington Hall
Syracuse, NY 10203　　　　　　315-443-9379
　　　　　　　　　　　　　　　　Fax: 315-443-2274
　　　　　　　　　　　　　　　　ICIstaff@syr.edu
　　　www.soe.syr.edu/centers_institutes/institute_communi

College offering facilitated learning research into communication with persons who have autism or severe disabilities. Offers books, videos and public awareness information on the research projects.

Timothy Eatman, Director
Kathleen Hinchman, Board of Directors
Nancy Cantor, Chancellor and President

743 **Families for Early Autism Treatment**
PO Box 255722
Sacramento, CA 10204　　　　　916-303-7405
　　　　　　　　　　　　　　　　Fax: 916-303-7405
　　　　　　　　　　　　　　　　feat@feat.org
　　　　　　　　　　　　　　　　www.feat.org

A nonprofit organization of parents and professionals, designed to help families with children who are diagnosed with autism or pervasive developmental disorder. It offers a network of support for families. FEAT has a Lending Library, with information on autism and also offers Support Meetings on the third Wednesday of each month.

Nancy Fellmeth, President
Kathleen Berry, VP
Gordon Hall, Treasurer

744 **Families of Adults Afflicted with Asperger's Syndrome**
PO Box 514
Centerville, MA 2632　　　　　508-790-1930
　　　　　　　　　　　　　　　　faaas@faaas.org
　　　　　　　　　　　　　　　　faaas.org

Offers support to the family members of adult individuals with Asperger's Syndrome.

Karen E. Rodman, President/ Founder
Jack Kelley, Events Coordinator
Thomas Rodman, Webmaster/ Docmaster

745 **Federation of Families for Children's Mental Health**
9605 Medical Center Drive, Suite 280
Rockville, MD 10205　　　　　240-403-1901
　　　　　　　　　　　　　　　　Fax: 240-403-1909
　　　　　　　　　　　　　　　　ffcmh@ffcmh.org
　　　　　　　　　　　　　　　　www.ffcmh.org

The National family run organization is dedicated exclusively to helping children with mental health needs and their families achieve a better quality of life.

Teka Dempson, President
Sherri Luthe, Vice President
Sheila Pires, Treasurer

746 **Generation Rescue**
13636 Ventura Blvd. #259
Sherman Oaks, CA 91423　　　877-98 -UTIS
　　　　　　　　　　　　　　　　www.generationrescue.org

Provides hope, information and immediate treatment assistance to families affected by autism spectrum disorders.

JB Handley, Co-Founder
Lisa Handley, Co-Founder
Jenny McCarthy, President

747 **Genetic Alliance**
4301 Connecticut Avenue NW, Suite 404
Washington, DC 20008　　　　202-966-5557
　　　　　　　　　　　　　　　　800-336-4363
　　　　　　　　　　　　　　　　Fax: 202-966-8553
　　　　　　　　　　　　　　　　info@geneticalliance.org
　　　　　　　　　　　　　　　　www.geneticalliance.org

World's leading nonprofit health advocacy organization committed to transforming health through genetics and promoting an environment of openness centered on the health of individuals, families, and communities.

Sharon Terry, President/CEO
Tetyana Murza, Managing Director
Natasha Bonhomme, VP, Strategic Development

748 **Global and Regional Asperger Syndrome Partnership**
419 Lafayette Street
New York, NY 10003　　　　　888-474-7277
　　　　　　　　　　　　　　　　info@grasp.org
　　　　　　　　　　　　　　　　grasp.org

GRASP works to improve the lives of teens and adults with autism spectrum disorder (ASD). It offers in-school programs to help students with autism learn advocacy skills and improve social skills. Through its website, it educates the public about autism, while also offering free online resources and networking opportunities for individuals with ASD and their families.

749 **Groupworks West**
11140 Washington Blvd.
Culver City, CA 90232　　　　310-287-1640
　　　　　　　　　　　　　　　　Fax: 310-287-0851
　　　　　　　　　　　　　　　　www.groupworkswest.com

GroupWorks West utilizes innovative intervention programs designed to improve the quality of life of children, teens and young adults challenged by developmental, psychiatric, and behavior disorders.

Christopher Mulligan, L.C.S.W., Founder/ Clinical Director

750 **Institute on Communication and Inclusion**
307 Huntington Hall
Syracuse, NY 13244　　　　　315-443-9379
　　　　　　　　　　　　　　　　Fax: 315-443-2274
　　　　　　　　　　　　　　　　icistaff@syr.edu
　　　　　　　　　　　　　　　　www.soe.syr.edu/about/

College offering facilitated learning research into communication with persons who have autism or severe disabilities. Offers books, videos and public awareness information on the research projects.

Douglas Biklen, Ph.D., Director
Christine Ashby, Ph.D., Research Director
Michele Paetow, Lead Trainer

751 **Lovaas Institute**
6167 Bristol Parkway, Suite 130
Culver City, CA 90230　　　　310-410-4450
　　　　　　　　　　　　　　　　Fax: 310-410-4455
　　　　　　　　　　　　　　　　info@lovaas.com
　　　　　　　　　　　　　　　　www.lovaas.com

Committed to providing the highest quality treatment available to children diagnosed with autism or a related disorder.

Scott Wright, President/ CEO:
Simone Stevens, Director of West Coast Ops/ COO
Matthew Sands, Director of East Coast Ops/ CFO

752   March of Dimes Foundation
1275 Mamaroneck Avenue
White Plains, NY 10605   914-997-4488
                                         888-663-4637
                                    Fax: 914-997-4763
                               answers@marchofdimes.com
                               www.marchofdimes.com

March of Dimes help moms have full-term pregnancies and research the problems that threaten the health of babies.The March
of Dimes also acts globally: sharing best practices in perinatal
health and helping improve birth outcomes where the needs are
the most urgent.

Stacey D. Stewart, President

753   Mental Health America
500 Montgomery Street, Ste 820
Alexandria, VA 22314   703-684-7722
                                         800-969-6642
                                    Fax: 703-684-5968
                               info@mentalhealthamerica.net
                               www.mentalhealthamerica.net

MHA, the leading advocacy organization addressing the full spectrum of mental and substance use conditions and their effects nationwide, works to inform, advocate and enable access to quality
behavioral health services for all Americans.

Paul Gionfriddo, President/CEO
Shavonne Carpenter, Sr Assoc., Support & Services
Mallory Pernell, Assoc. Dir, Comments/Marketing

**754   National Association of Residential Providers for Adults with
         Autism**
www.narpaa.org

                                         info@narpaa.org
                                         www.narpaa.org

To assure the availability of residential services and other supports for adults with autism throughout their lives.

Gwen Lee, Treasurer
Mike Storz, Vice President
Barbara Boyett, President

755   National Association of Special Education Teachers
1250 Connecticut Avenue, N.W., Suite 200
Washington, DC 20036   800-754-4421
                                    Fax: 800-754-4421
                               contactus@naset.org
                               www.naset.org

A membership organization dedicated solely to meeting the needs
of special education teachers and those preparing for the field of
special education teaching.

Dr. Roger Pierangelo, Co-Executive Director
Dr. George Giuliani, Co-Executive Director

756   National Autism Association
One Park Avenue, Suite 1
Portsmouth, RI 02871   401-293-5551
                                         877-622-2884
                                    Fax: 401-293-5342
                               naa@nationalautism.org
                               nationalautismassociation.org

NAA is a parent-run advocacy organization and the leading voice
on urgent issues related to severe autism, regressive autism, autism safety, autism abuse, and crisis prevention.

Wendy Fournier, President
Kelly Vanicek, Executive Director
Katie Wright, Vice President

757   National Autism Hotline - Autism Services Center
605 Ninth Street Prichard Bldg PO Box 507
Huntington, WV 25710   304-525-8014
                                    Fax: 304-525-8026
                               info@autismlink.com
                               www.autismlink.com/listing/national_autism_hotline_a

Service agency for individuals with autism and developmental
disabilities, and their families. Assists families and agencies attempting to meet the needs of individuals with autism and other
developmental disabilities. Makes available technical assistance
in designing treatment programs and more. The hotline provides
informational packets to callers re: autism and assists via
telephone when possible.

Cindy Walterman, Director
Rick Bryant, Board Member
Kathy Horvath, Board Member

758   National Dissemination Center for Children with Disabilities
1825 Connecticut Ave NW
Washington, DC 10211   202-884-8200
                                         800-695-0285
                                    Fax: 202-884-8441
                               nichcy@fhi360.org
                               www.nichcy.org

A national information and referral center that provides information on disabilities and disability-related issues for families, educators and other professionals.

Suzanne Ripley, Executive Director

759   National Mental Health Consumers' Self-Help Clearinghouse
1211 Chestnut Street, Suite 1207
Philadelphia, PA 10212   215-751-1810
                                         800-553-4539
                                    Fax: 215-636-6312
                               info@mhselfhelp.org
                               www.mhselfhelp.org

The Clearinghouse works to foster peer empowerment through
our website, up-to-date news and information announcements, a
directory of peer-driven services, electronic and printed publications, training packages, and individual and onsite consultation

Joseph Rogers, Executive Director & Founder
Susan Rogers, Director of Special Projects
Britani Nestel, Program Specialist

760   New England Center for Children
33 Turnpike Road
Southborough, MA 10213   508-481-1015
                                    Fax: 508-485-3421
                               info@necc.org
                               www.necc.org

Serving students between the ages of 3 and 22 diagnosed with autism, learning disabilities, language delays, mental retardation,
behavior disorders and related disabilities; educational curriculum encompasses both the teaching of functional life skills and
traditional academics; communication skills are taught throughout all activities in the school, residence, and community. Tuition
and fees are set by the state. Consulting services also available.

Lisel Macenka, Chair of the Board
James C Burling, Vice Chair of Board
L Vincent Strully Jr, President

761   Oak-Leyden Developmental Services
411 Chicago Avenue
Oak Park, IL 10214   708-524-1050
                                    Fax: 708-524-2469
                               webmaster@oakleyden.org
                               www.oakleyden.org

The mission of Oak-Leyden Developmental Services is to serve
people with developmental disabilities and their families in a
manner which recognizes their dignity, is supportive of their personal choices and promotes their inclusion in the larger
community.

Bob Atkinson, CEO
Nancy Thomas, Director of Human Resources
Mary Taylor, Vice President of Finance

762   Oasis at MAAP
PO Box 524
Crown Point, IN 10215   219-662-1311
                                    Fax: 219-662-0638
                               info@aspergersyndrome.org
                               www.aspergersyndrome.org

MAAP Services is a world wide 501-C-3 non profit organization providing information, networking, referrals and printed materials for families, challenged individuals and professionals concerned with the autism spectrum. Founded in 1984, MAAP Services, adheres to the basic principal that all individuals with autism spectrum challenges have the ability to learn, grow and enjoy a good quality of life.

Susan Moreno, Founder & President
Lara Blanchard, BCBA

763   Option Institute: Son Rise Program
Autism Treatment Center of America
2080 S Undermountain Road
Sheffield, MA 10216
413-229-2100
800-714-2779
Fax: 413-229-3202
information@son-rise.org
www.son-rise.org

Describes an effective, loving and respectful method for treating children with autism. It teaches parents and healing professionals how to set up a home based program using the child's motivation to reach their special child.

Barry Neil Kaufman, Co-Founder/Co-Creator
Samahria Lyte Kaufman, Co-Founder/Co-Creator
Bryn Hogan, ATCA Senior Staff

764   Organization for Autism Research
2000 North 14th Street, Suite 240
Arlington, VA 22201
703-243-9710
www.researchautism.org

The Organization for Autism Research (OAR) was created in December 2001-the product of the shared vision and unique life experiences of OAR's seven founders. Led by these parents and grandparents of children and adults on the autism spectrum, OAR set out to use applied science to answer questions that parents, families, individuals with autism, teachers and caregivers confront daily. No other autism organization has this singular focus.

Peter F. Gerhardt, Ed.D., OAR Scientific Council
Lori Lapin Jones, Vice Chairperson
Michael V. Maloney, Executive Director/ Secretary

765   Raleigh TEACCH Center
University of North Carolina at Chapel Hill
100 Renee Lynne Court
Carrboro, NC 10217
919-966-2174
Fax: 413-229-3202
TEACCH@unc.edu
www.teacch.com

The University of North Carolina TEACCH Autism Program creates and cultivates the development of exemplary community-based services, training programs, and research to enhance the quality of life for individuals with Autism Spectrum Disorder and for their families across the lifespan.

Eric Schopler, Founder & Co-Director

766   Rethink autism
19 West 21st Street, Suite 403
New York, NY 10010
877-988-8871
Fax: 646-257-2926
info@rethinkfirst.com
www.rethinkfirst.com

Offers parents and professionals immediate access to effective and affordable Applied Behavior Analysis-based treatment tools for the growing population affected by autism spectrum disorders.

Daniel A. Etra, Chief Executive Officer
Eran Rosenthal, President/ COO
Jamie Pagliaro, EVP/ Chief Learning Officer

767   Society for Autistic Children
NYS Society for Autistic Children
879 Madison Avenue
Albany, NY 10218
518-459-1418
info@autism-society.org
www.autism-society.org/

The Autism Society, the nation's leading grassroots autism organization, exists to improve the lives of all affected by autism. We do this by increasing public awareness about the day-to-day issues faced by people on the spectrum, advocating for appropriate services for individuals across the lifespan, and providing the latest information regarding treatment, education, research and advocacy.

James Ball, Executive Chair
Ron E Simmons, Vice Chair
Scott Badesch, President & COO

768   Talk About Curing Autism
2222 Martin St., Suite 140
Irvine, CA 92612
949-640-4401
855-726-7810
Fax: 949-640-4424
www.tacanow.org

Talk About Curing Autism (TACA) is a national non-profit 501(c)(3) organization dedicated to educating, empowering and supporting families affected by autism. For families who have just received the autism diagnosis, TACA aims to speed up the cycle time from the autism diagnosis to effective treatments.

Glen Ackerman, President
Lisa Ackerman, Founder/ Secretary
Dan Carney, CFO/ Board Member

769   The Daniel Jordan Fiddle Foundation
www.djfiddlefoundation.org
info@djfiddlefoundation.org
www.djfiddlefoundation.org

The Daniel Jordan Fiddle Foundation is a national organization focused on adults living with Autism Spectrum Disorders (ASD). The mission of the volunteer-run organization is to develop, advocate for and fund our Signature Programs that create innovative blueprints for grassroots organizations and service providers to develop their own programs for the diverse population of adults living with ASD.

Linda J. Walder, Esq., Founder and President
Frederick J. Fiddle, Founder/ Treasurer
James J. Scancarella, VP, Development Co-Chair

770   The Doug Flutie, Jr. Foundation for Autism
PO Box 767
Framingham, MA 1701
508-270-8855
Fax: 508-270-6868
www.flutiefoundation.org

The goal of the Flutie Foundation is to help families affected by autism live life to the fullest.

Douglas Flutie, President/ Co-Founder
Laurie Flutie, Vice President/ Co-Founder
Lisa Borges, Executive Director

771   The Golden Fund for Autism
P.O. BOX 424
Cold Spring Harbor, NY 11724
admin@goldenfundautism.org
www.goldenfundautism.org

The Golden Fund for Autism is a 501(c)(3) tax-exempt organization dedicated to raising funds for children diagnosed with Autism Spectrum Disorders and their families.

Joelle A. Perez, Executive Director

772   The Help Group
13130 Burbank Blvd.
Sherman Oaks, CA 91401
818-781-0360
877-994-3588
Fax: 818-779-5295
www.thehelpgroup.org

Serves children with special needs related to autism spectrum disorder, learning disabilities, ADHD, developmental delays, abuse and emotional problems.

Barbara Firestone, PhD, President/ CEO
Susan Berman, PhD, Chief Operating Officer
Tom Komp, LCSW, Sr. Vice President

773   Train 4 Autism
904 Silver Spur Rd., #373
Rolling Hills Estates, CA 90274   info@train4autism.org
                                          www.train4autism.org

Train 4 Autism is a foundation dedicated to bringing together a community of athletes, physically active, and socially conscious people who are committed to raising awareness and funds for research and treatment for those living with Autism and their families.

Ben Fesagaiga, Founder
Sam Felsenfeld, Director of Technology
Shelly Overton, Director of Chapter Development

774   US Autism & Asperger Association
P.O. Box 532
Draper, UT 84020   888-9AU-ISM
                                          www.usautism.org

US Autism & Asperger Association (USAAA) is a 501(c)(3) non-profit organization for autism and Asperger education, support, and solutions.

Lawrence P. Kaplan, PhD, Chairman/ CEO
Richard Dunie, MPh, MBA, CPA, Secretary/ Treasurer
Phillip C. DeMio, MD, Chief Medical Officer

775   iCanShine
P.O. Box 541
Paoli, PA 19301   610-647-4176
                                          icanshine.org

iCan Shine (formerly, Lose The Training Wheels) is a national charitable nonprofit organization. They collaborate with local organizations and individuals, and refer to as our program 'hosts', to conduct over 100 five-day iCan Bike programs in 32 States and 3 Provinces in Canada serving nearly 3,000 people with disabilities each year.

Lisa Ruby, Founder/ Executive Director
Jeff Sullivan, Co-Founder, Dir of Finance & Admin
Jillian Bonior, Floor Supervisor

New Jersey

776   New Jersey Center for Outreach & Services for the Autism Community (COSAC)
500 Horizon Drive Suite 530
Robbinsville, NJ 08691   609-588-8200
                                          800-428-8476
                                      Fax: 609-588-8858
                                  information@autismnj.org
                                          www.njcosac.org

Autism New Jersey is a nonprofit agency committed to ensuring safe and fulfilling lives for individuals with autism, their families, and the professionals who support them. Through awareness, credible information, education, and public policy initiatives, Autism New Jersey leads the way to lifelong individualized services provided with skill and compassion.

James A. Paone, II, Esq, President
Genare Valiant, Vice President
Mary Jane Weiss, Ph.D., BCBA-D, Vice President

State Agencies & Support Groups

Alabama

777   Autism Society of Alabama
Autism Society of America
4217 Dolly Ridge Rd
Birmingham, AL 10219   205-951-1364
                                          877-428-8476
                                      Fax: 205-951-1366
                                 melanie@autism-alabama.org
                                       www.autism-alabama.org

To improve services for persons with Autism Spectrum Disorders and their families through education and advocacy.

Melanie Jones, Executive Director
Michelle McDaniel, Community & Program Coordinator
Bama Hager, PhD, Program Director

778   Autism Society of North Alabama
Autism Society of America
PO Box 2902
Huntsville, AL 10220   256-773-0549
                                       tntntwhite@msn.com
                                       www.autism-alabama.org

To improve services for persons with Autism Spectrum Disorders and their families through education and advocacy.

Todd Tomerlin, Community/Program Coordinator

Arizona

779   Autism Society of America Greater Phoenix Chapter
PO Box 10543
Phoenix, AZ 10221   480-940-1093
                                 cynthia.macluskie@phxautism.org
                                       www.phxautism.org

The Autism Society of Greater Phoenix provides information, resources, and support to families affected by autism and helps families who have just received the autism diagnosis by providing information on effective treatments.

James B Adams, President
Catina Hoffman, Co-Chair

780   Autism Society of America Southern Arizona Chapter
2600 N Wyatt DR
Tucson, AZ 85712   520-770-1541
                                     Fax: 520-319-5979
                                         info@as-az.org
                                         www.as-az.org

Volunteer organization of parents, professionals, and friends of persons with autism, designed to promote the general welfare of persons with autism.

Jared Perkins, President
Jared Perrine, Treasurer
Lynda Weigel-Firor, Secretary

California

781   Autism Society of America Coachella Valley
Autism Society of America
77564 Country Club Dr.Building B Suite 363
Palm Desert, CA 92211   760-772-1000
                                      coordinator@cvasa.org
                                          www.cvasa.org

The Coachella Valley Autism Society of America (CVASA) exists to provide support for families of individuals with autism in the Coachella Valley and surrounding desert areas.

Thomas Lister-Looker, President
Donna Redman-Bentley, Secretary
Kristen Alvarez, Treasurer

782   Autism Society of America Greater Long Beach/San Gabriel Valley
Autism Society of America
8635 Greenleaf Ave, Unit B
Long Beach, CA 90602   562-943-3335
                                          562-941-1931
                                     Fax: 562-943-3335
                          ca-longbeach@autismsocietyofamerica.org
                               www.greaterlongbeach-asa.org

We provide information and referrals about behavior problems, education and treatment programs, your child's right to a free appropriate public education (FAPE), inclusion, how and where to obtain an evaluation and diagnosis, specialized facilities such as camps or residential programs, federal and state legislation, how to be an advocate for your child and more.

Regina Moreno, President
Penne Fode, Vice President
Roman Castro, Jr, Treasurer

783 Autism Society of America Inland Empire Chapter
Autism Society of America
2276 Griffin Way, Suite 105-194
Corona, CA 10227
909-220-6922
ieautism@att.net
www.ieautism.org

The mission of the Autism Society Inland Empire is to improve
the lives of all affected by an autism spectrum disorder. We do
this by increasing public awareness about the day-to-day issues
faced by people on the spectrum, advocating for appropriate services for individuals across the lifespan, and providing the latest
information regarding treatment, education, research, support and
advocacy.

Beth Burt, President
Lillian Vasquez, Vice President
Philip Hannawi, Treasurer

784 Autism Society of America Los Angeles Chapter
Autism Society of America
21250 Hawthorne Blvd, Ste 500
Los Angeles, CA 90503
562-804-5556
Fax: 562-425-4940
info@autismla.org
www.autismla.org/

To improve the lives of all affected by autism in Los Angeles
County by empowering individuals with autism, their families,
and professionals through advocacy, education, support, and community collaboration.

Andy Kopito, President
Mari-Anne Kehler, VP

785 Autism Society of America North San Diego County Chapter
Autism Society of America
4699 Murphy Canyon Road
San Diego, CA 10230
858-715-0678
Fax: 858-712-1510
info@autismsocietysandiego.org
www.autismsocietysandiego.org/Home.php

Offers chapter meetings, local groups for support and information, family events, and a lending library.

Amy Munera, President
Paul James, Treasurer
Kay Freeman, Administrator

786 Autism Society of America Orange County Chapter
Autism Society of America
582 N. Waverly
Orange, CA 10231
714-282-9005
paulap@mailcity.com
www.asaoc.tripod.com/Index.htm

The Autism Society of Orange County, in unison with the Autism
Society of America, strives to promote lifelong access and opportunities for persons within the autistic spectrum and their families, to be fully included, participating members of their
communities through advocacy, public awareness, education, and
research related to autism.

Paula Peterson, President
Linda Molyneux, Vice President

787 Autism Society of America San Diego Chapter
Autism Society of America
PO Box 420908
San Diego, CA 10232
858-715-0678
Fax: 858-712-1510
info@autismsocietysandiego.org
www.autismsocietysandiego.org/Home.php

Promotes lifelong access and opportunities for persons within the
autism spectrum and their families, to be fully included, participating members of their communities through advocacy, public
awareness, education, and research related to autism.

Shirley Fett, President
Nichole Hope Moore, President Elect
Tina Huston, Treasurer

788 Autism Society of America San Francisco Bay Chapter
Autism Society of America
PO Box 249
San Mateo, CA 94401
650-637-7772
info@sfautismsociety.org
http://sfautismsociety.virtualave.net

Promotes lifelong access and opportunities for persons within the
autism spectrum and their families, to be fully included, participating members of their communities through advocacy, public
awareness, education, and research related to autism.

Connie Boyar, President
Sue Swezey, Secretary
Irma Velasquez, Treasurer

789 Autism Society of America San Gabriel Valley Chapter
Autism Society of America
PO Box 15247
Glendora, CA 10234
626-388-2134
www.greaterlongbeach-asa.org/

We provide information and referrals about behavior problems,
education and treatment programs, your child's right to a free appropriate public education (FAPE), inclusion, how and where to
obtain an evaluation and diagnosis, specialized facilities such as
camps or residential programs, federal and state legislation, how
to be an advocate for your child and more.

Regina Moreno, President
Bronwyn Estephan, Vice President
Joe McNiel, Treasurer

790 Autism Society of America Santa Barbara Chapter
Autism Society of America
PO Box 30364
Santa Barbara, CA 93130
805-560-3762
sdshove@cox.net
www.asasb.org

Promote lifelong access and opportunity for all individuals within
the autism spectrum, and their families, to be fully participating,
included members of their communities. Support, education, advocacy, and an active public awareness from the cornerstones of
ASA Santa Barbara's efforts to carry forth its mission.

Marcia Eichelberger, Co-President
Patti Gaultney, Co-President

791 Autism Society of America Tulare County Chapter
Autism Society of America
3201 West Payson Avenue
Visalia, CA 93291
559-747-2126
lori10677@aol.com
www.autism-society.org

Promote lifelong access and opportunity for all individuals within
the autism spectrum, and their families, to be fully participating,
included members of their community. Support, education, advocacy, and an active public awareness from the cornerstones of
ASA Santa Barbara's efforts to carry forth its mission.

Lori Collins, President

792 Autism Society of California
Autism Society of America
PO Box 1355
Glendora, CA 10236
800-869-7069
ca-california@autismsocietyofamerica.org
www.autismsocietyca.org

The mission of the Autism Society of California is to promote
lifelong access and opportunities for persons within the autism
spectrum and their families, and to be fully included, participating members of their communities through advocacy, public
awareness, education and research related to autism.

Marcia Eichelberger, President
Beth Burt, First Vice President
Sandra Shove, 2nd Vice President

793   Kern Autism Network
Autism Society of America
8200 Stockdale Hwy, M-10#171
Bakersfield, CA 10237   661-588-4235
                                     661-762-7528
                                Fax: 661-588-4235
                            kernautism@gmail.com
                                www.kernautism.org

Autism Society Chapter-Kern Autism Network provides support, awareness, information and education to families, professionals and the public throughout Kern County.

Ramona Puget, parent and advocate
Carl Twisselman, Honorary Lifetime Board Member
Carol Baker-Willey, Parent

Colorado

794   Autism Society of America Larimer County Chapter
3331 Lochwood Dr
Fort Collins, CO 10238   970-377-9640
                            aslc@autismlarimer.org
                                www.autismlarimer.org

The ASLC is a volunteer group of dedicated well-informed parents and professionals working together to increase public awareness about autism and the day-to-day issues faced by individuals with autism, their families and the professionals with whom they interact.

Phyllis Zimmerman, President
Tina Boyer, Vice President
Jennifer Cotton, Treasurer

795   Autism Society of America Pikes Peak Chapter
918 Crown Ridge Drive
Colorado Springs, CO 80904   719-630-7072
                   co-pikespeak@autismsocietyofamerica.org
                                www.asappr.org

Sponsors training opportunities for educators and parents in Southern Colorado to learn best practice strategies that will help students with autism be successful in inclusive classrooms and communities.

Alison Seyler, President

796   Autism Society of America: Colorado Chapter
550 S. Wadsworth Boulevard, Suite 100
Lakewood, CO 10240   720-214-0794
                                Fax: 720-274-2744
                                www.autismcolorado.org

To improve the lives of all affected by Autism.

Kevin Custer, President
John Sheldon, Vice President
Jeffery Nickless, Treasurer

797   Autism Society of American Boulder County Chapter
P.O. Box 270300
Louisville, CO 10241   720-272-8231
                                Fax: 303-604-6656
                            info@autismboulder.org
                                www.autismboulder.org

The Autism Society of Boulder County is an all-volunteer 501(c)(3) non-profit organization that offers all of its services for free to individuals and families affected by autism in Boulder and Broomfield Counties.

Lynn Wysolmierski, President
Allen Richardson, Secretary
Jill Sheldon, Treasurer

Connecticut

798   Autism Society of America Connecticut Chapter
PO Box 1404
Guilford, CT 10242   888-453-4975
                                info@asconn.org
                                www.asconn.org

Worked with parents, educators, state government, and therapeutic and medical professionals to enhance the lives of those touched by Autism Spectrum Disorders. ASCONN serves the entire autism spectrum, across specific diagnosis, needs, challenges, and age ranges.

Sara Reed, Executive Director
Kim Newgass, President
Jonathan Stein, Treasurer

Delaware

799   Autism Society of Delaware
Autism Society of America
924 Old Harmony Road, Suite 201
Newark, DE 10243   302-224-6020
                                     302-472-2639
                                Fax: 302-224-6014
                            delautism@delautism.org
                                www.delautism.org

The Autism Delaware Mission: to create better lives for people with autism and their families in Delaware.

Marcy kempner, President
John Willey II, Vice President
Scott Young, Treasurer

District of Columbia

800   Autism Society of America District of Columbia Chapter
5167 7th Street NE
Washington, DC 10244   202-561-5300
                                     202-561-8634
                        sondrakcunningham@verizon.net
                        www.autism-society.org/chapter130

Provides information and referrals for families affected by autism and related disabilities. Advocate for appropriate services in education, medical and other areas.

Ronald Hampton, President
Rhoda Mcleese Smith, Vice President
Franklin Davis SR, Treasurer

Florida

801   Autism Society of America Broward Chapter
10250 NW 53rd
Sunrise, FL 10245   954-577-4141
                                     954-474-5333
                                www.asabroward.org

ASB's full range of family support, children's programming, public outreach and autism awareness campaigns are available to all interested in the betterment of life for not only individuals and families with autism, but to the community of South Florida as a whole

Hugh J Keough Esq, President
Fabiola Anna Torrez, Vice President
Brent Boucaud, Treasurer

802   Autism Society of America Emerald Coast Chapter
8668 Navarre Parkway Suite # 216
Navarre, FL 10246   850-736-0879
                            myra@ecautismsociety.com
                                www.ecautismsociety.com

Provides information and support.

Myra Fowler, President
Kristen Bowen, Vice-President
Greg Hasty, Treasurer

803   Autism Society of America Florida Chapter
PO Box 450476
Sunrise, FL 10247   954-577-4141
                                     855-529-6807
                                Fax: 954-571-2136
                                ven@autismfl.com
                                www.autismfl.com

The Autism Society of Florida is a statewide organization that supports individuals with autism, their families, and caregivers. It includes individuals with autism and volunteers (including family members, professionals, and other interested persons). The Autism Society of Florida coordinates activities on behalf of people with autism on a statewide basis.

804   Autism Society of America Jacksonville Chapter
1526 University Blvd W #235
Jacksonville, FL 32217   904-399-4490
www.autism-society.org/chapter1003

Mission is to support, inform and empower the families of Jacksonville.

Jeenifer Nunes, President

805   Autism Society of America Manasota Chapter
2380 Wycliff Street, Suite 102
St Paul, MN 10249   651-647-1083
941-780-5237
Fax: 651-642-1230
info@ausm.org
www.ausm.org

Established in 1971, the Autism Society of Minnesota (AuSM) is a self-funded organization committed to education, support and advocacy designed to enhance the lives of those affected by autism from birth through retirement.

Todd Schwartzberg, President
Jean Bender, Vice President
Aaron R Deris, Treasurer

806   Autism Society of America Panhandle Chapter
P.O. Box 30213
Pensacola, FL 32503   850-450-0656
info@autismpensacola.org
www.autismpensacola.org

A nonprofit, tax-exempt association of parents, professionals and other concerned community members dedicated to the education and welfare of children and adults with autism and related disorders of communication and behavior.

Fred Donovan, President
Julian Irby, Vice President
Bonnie Sferes, Treasurer

807   Autism Society of Greater Orlando
Autism Society of America
12720 S. Orange Blossom Trail Suite 8
Orlando, FL 10251   407-855-0235
Fax: 407-855-5129
contact@asgo.org
www.asgo.org

ASGO was founded in 1996 by a group of volunteer parents to better assist families of children and adults with autism in the Central Florida area. The mission or goal of the ASGO is that all individuals within the autism spectrum will be provided a lifetime network of opportunities to become fully accepted, included, and actively participating members of our community, through family support, education, and advocacy, and public awareness.

Donna Lorman, President
Lorienda Crawford, Vice President
Angelica Taylor, Treasurer

Georgia

808   Autism Society of America Greater Georgia Chapter
P.O. Box 3707
Suwanee, GA 10252   770-904-4474
Fax: 678-935-1152
office@asaga.com
www.asaga.com

Chapter of ASA, we offer resource info to individuals and their families and to professionals about autism, add, add and other developmental disabilities

Gailynn Gluth, President
Jason Cavin, 1st Vice President
Jon Basinger, 2nd Vice President

Hawaii

809   Autism Society of Hawaii
Autism Society of America
1600 Kapiolani Blvd. #620
Honolulu, HI 10253   808-282-3676
808-228-0122
autismhi@gmail.com
www.autismhi.org

The Autism Society of Hawaii is a 501(c)(3) organization serving families and individuals touched by autism and autism spectrum disorders.

Dr William Bolman, President
Jessica Wong, Executive Director
John P Dellera, Board Member

Idaho

810   Autism Society of America Treasure Valley Chapter
P.O. Box 44831
Boise, ID 10254   208-336-5676
autism.asatvc@yahoo.com
www.asatvc.org

Top provide advocacy, support and information to individuals with autism, their families, professionals, and communities throughout Treasure Valley Chapter.

Illinois

811   Autism Society of Illinois
Autism Society of America
2200 South Main Street, # 205
Lombard, IL 10255   630-691-1270
888-691-1270
Fax: 630-932-5620
info@autismillinois.org
www.autismillinois.org

Partnering with families and communities living with autism in Illinois by generating awareness and providing education, training, support, and guidance as a compassionate and caring authority.

Mary K Betz, Executive Director
Jean C Thomas, Associate Executive Director
Dave Geslak, Treasurer

Indiana

812   Autism Society of Indiana
Autism Society of America
13295 Illinois Street Suite 213
Carmel, IN 10256   317-695-0252
800-609-8449
info@inautism.org
www.autismsocietyofindiana.org

Since 1998, the Autism Society of America - Indiana (ASI) has worked to raise awareness about autism, to promote early diagnosis and early intervention thereby helping people on the autism spectrum have the fullest and most successful journey possible.

Joshua Carr, Executive Board President
Kylee Hope, Executive Board Vice President
Kelli McKinzie, Executive Board Treasurer

Iowa

813   Autism Society of Iowa
Autism Society of America
4340 East-West Hwy, Suite 350
Bethesda, ML 10257   301-657-0881
800-328-8476
autism50ia@aol.com
www.autism-society.org

The Autism Society, the nation's leading grassroots autism organization, exists to improve the lives of all affected by autism.

Kris Steinmantz, Manager

814   The Link
Autism Society of Iowa
4549 Waterford Drive
West Des Moines, IA 50265   515-327-9075
                                  888-457-7225
                                  autism50ia@aol.com
                                  www.autismia.org

Provides information for parents, professionals and care givers on autism spectrum disorders.

Kris Steinmantz, Manager

Kansas

815   Autism Society of the Heartland
Autism Society of America
PO Box 4455
Olathe, KS 66063   913-706-0042
                                  info@asaheartland.org
                                  www.asaheartland.org

To provide advocacy, support and information to individuals with autism, their families, professionals, and communities throughout state Kansas.

Kathy Bennett, Office Manager

Kentucky

816   Autism Society of America Bluegrass Chapter
Autism Society of America
243 Shady Lane
Lexington, KY 40503   859-299-9000
                                  ky-lexington@autismsocietyofamerica.org
                                  www.asbg.org

A resource and support group for families and professionals in the Central Kentucky area who are involved with autism.

Sara Spragens, President

Louisiana

817   Autism Society of Louisiana
Autism Society of America
PO Box 80162
Baton Rouge, LA 70898   800-955-3760
                                  autismsociety_lastatechapter@yahoo.com
                                  www.lastateautism.org

To provide information and referrals, advocacy and support for individuals with ASD and their families; to help families identify qualified professionals in their communities; to assist families in securing benefits and services provided by law; and, to promote lifelong opportunities for persons with autism spectrum disorder in order to be fully included members of their communities.

Pat Giamanco, President

Maine

818   Autism Society of Maine
Autism Society of America
72 Main Street, Suite B
Winthrop, ME 04364   207-377-9603
                                 800-273-5200
                                 Fax: 207-377-9434
                                 info@asmonline.org
                                 www.asmonline.org

The Autism Society of Maine provides education and resources to support the valued lives of individuals on the autism spectrum and their families.

Janine Collins, President
Laurie Raymond', Vice President
Michael Lamoreau, Treasurer

Maryland

819   Autism Society of America Baltimore Chesapeake Chapter
PO Box 10822
Parkville, MD 21234   410-655-7933
                                  info@baltimoreautismsociety.org
                                  www.bcc-asa.org

Serves families of children and adults with autism spectrum disorders in Baltimore County, Maryland, Baltimore City, and the State of Maryland by providing information, advocacy, and support for families and individuals with autism.

Debbie Page, Co- President
David Savick, Co- President
Kay Holman, Vice President

Massachusetts

820   Autism Society of America Massachusetts Chapter
Autism Society of America
47 Walnut Street
Wellesley Hills, MA 02481   781-237-0272
                                  Fax: 781-237-5020
                                  asamasschapter@hotmail.com
                                  www.massautism.org

Mission is to promote lifelong access and opportunity for all individuals within the autism spectrum and their families to be fully participating, included members of their community.

Barry Neil Kaufman, Co-Founder/Co-Creator
Samahria Lyte Kaufman, Co-Founder/Co-Creator

821   Option Institute: Son Rise Program
Autism Treatment Center of America
2080 S Undermountain Road
Sheffield, MA 01257   413-229-2100
                                  800-714-2779
                                  Fax: 413-229-3202
                                  information@son-rise.org
                                  www.son-rise.org

Since 1983, the Autism Treatment Center of America has provided innovative training programs for parents and professionals caring for children challenged by Autism, Autism Spectrum Disorders, Pervasive Developmental Disorder (PDD) and other developmental difficulties. The Son-Rise Program teaches a specific yet comprehensive system of treatment and education designed to help families and caregivers enable their children to dramatically improve in all areas of learning.

Barry Neil Kaufman, Co-Founder/Co-Creator
Samahria Lyte Kaufman, Co-Founder/Co-Creator
Bryn Hogan, ACTA Senior Staff

Michigan

822   Autism Society of Michigan
Autism Society of America
2178 Commons Parkway
Okemos, MI 48864   517-882-2800
                                  800-223-6722
                                  Fax: 517-862-2816
                                  autism@autism-mi.org
                                  www.autism-mi.org

The Autism Society of Michigan is committed to empowering individuals with autism and their families by offering educational resources and materials, workshops, seminars and other services. ASM advocates that making human connections in a supportive, integrated community is a right of all persons.

Bob Opsommer, President

Minnesota

823 Autism Society of Minnesota
Autism Society of America
2380 Wycliff Street, Suite 102
Saint Paul, MN 55114
651-647-1083
Fax: 651-642-1230
info@ausm.org
www.ausm.org

The Autism Society of Minnesota exists to enhance the lives of individuals with autism spectrum disorders. AuSM seeks to realize its mission through education support, collaboration, and advocacy.

Todd Schwartzberg, President
Jean Bender, Vice President
Aaron R Deris, Treasurer

Mississippi

824 Autism Society of Mississippi
Autism Society of America
5908 Tolar Road
Moss Point, MS 39562   ms-mississippi@autismsocietyofamerica.or
www,autismnow.org/local/autism-society-of-mississipp

Offers information, referrals, and support to parents, professionals and caregivers.

Cathy Pratt, Chairman
Joan Zaro, Executive Director
Lee Grossman, CEO

Missouri

825 Autism Society of America Gateway Chapter
Autism Society of America
7777 Bonhomme Avenue, Suite 1600
St Louis, MO 63105
314-721-0042
Fax: 314-863-7494
pegisues@aol.com

Provides information and support.

Pegi Price, President

Nebraska

826 Autism Society of Nebraska
Autism Society of America
PO Box 83559
Lincoln, NE 68501
402-637-5670
800-580-9279
autismsociety@autismnebraska.org
www.autismnebraska.org

Supports and advocates for individuals with autism and their families through increasing education and awareness, fundraising, and facilitating community involvement for persons with autism spectrum disorders to achieve their potential by becoming a productive, accepted, and integral part of society.

Megan Misegadis, President
Wendy Hamilton, Vice President
Robyn Roberts, Treasurer

Nevada

827 Autism Society of Northern Nevada Chapter
Autism Society of America
3490 Southampton Drive
Reno, NV 89509
775-786-9315
Fax: 775-786-0984
pd1989@yahoo.com
www.nnasa.org

Promote and advocate for the general welfare of persons with autism. To further the education and training of parents and professional personnel for training, educating, and caring for persons with autism.

Dinah Deane, President
Paul Deane, Vice President
Guy McKillip, Web Master

New Hampshire

828 Autism Society of New Hampshire
Autism Society of America
PO Box 68
Concord, NH 03302
603-679-2424
Fax: 301-657-0869
info@nhautism.com
www.autismnow.org/local/autism-society-of-new-hampsh

The Autism Society of New Hampshire is dedicated to individuals with Autism and Pervasive Developmental Disorders.

Stacey Shannon, President

New Jersey

829 New Jersey Center for Outreach & Services for the Autism Community (COSAC)
500 Horizon Drive Suite 530
Robbinsville, NJ 08691
609-588-8200
800-428-8476
Fax: 609-588-8858
information@autismnj.org
www.njcosac.org

Autism New Jersey is a nonprofit agency committed to ensuring safe and fulfilling lives for individuals with autism, their families, and the professionals who support them. Through awareness, credible information, education, and public policy initiatives, Autism New Jersey leads the way to lifelong individualized services provided with skill and compassion.

James A. Paone, II, Esq, President
Genare Valiant, Vice President
Mary Jane Weiss, Ph.D., BCBA-D, Vice President

New Mexico

830 New Mexico Autism Society
Autism Society of America
PO Box 30955
Albuquerque, NM 87190
505-332-0306
www.nmautismsociety.org

Our mission is to promote lifelong access and opportunities for persons within the autism spectrum, and their families, to be fully included participating members of their communities.

Roger Riley,, President
Sarah Baca, Executive Director
Pauline Riley, Treasurer

New York

831 Center for Family Support
333 7th Avenue, #901
New York, NY 10001
212-629-7939
Fax: 212-239-2211
svernikoff@cfsny.org
www.cfsny.org

The Center for Family Support is committed to providing support and assistance to individuals with developmental and related disabilities, and to the family members who care for them.

Steven Vernikoff, Executive Director
Linda Schellenberg, Director, Community Service
Barbara Greenwald, Associate Executive Director

832   New York Autism Network
Autism Society of America
101 State Street
Schenectady, NY 12305   518-355-2191
                                       Fax: 518-355-2191
                                    info@albanyautism.org
                                    www.albanyautism.org

Provide ongoing support to families and professionals, develop
regional networks, provide technical assistance, and conduct conferences related to pervasive developmental disorders.

Gordon Zuckerman, President
Jenny DeBellis, Treasurer
Haley Knox, Secretary

North Carolina

833   Autism Society of North Carolina
Autism Society of America
505 Oberlin Road Suite 230
Raleigh, NC 27605   800-442-2762
                                       Fax: 919-743-0204
                                  info@autismsociety-nc.org
                                  www.autismsociety-nc.org

For over 43 years, the Autism Society of North Carolina (ASNC)
has worked to address areas of need and expand services for the
autism community in North Carolina. ASNC is a statewide organization, supporting North Carolinians affected by autism

Beverly Moore, Chair
Sharon Jeffries-Jones, Vice Chair
Elizabeth Phillippi, Treasurer

Ohio

834   Autism Society of Greater Cincinatti
Autism Society of America
PO Box 58385
Cincinnati, OH 45258   513-561-2300
                                       Fax: 513-561-4748
                                    info@autismcincy.org
                                    www.autismcincy.org

The mission of the Autism Society of Greater Cincinnati is to improve the quality of life for all people with autism spectrum disorders and their families.

Kay Brown, President
Sue Radabaugh, Vice President
James Keller, Treasurer

835   Autism Society of Ohio Tri-County Chapter
Autism Society of America
25 East Boardman Street, Suite 230
Youngstown, OH 44503   330-501-7553
                                       Fax: 614-754-6332
                               mahoningvalley@autismohio.org
                                    www.autismohio.org

To improve the quality of life for all people with autism spectrum
disorders and their families.

Aundrea Cika, Director

Oklahoma

836   Autism Society of Oklahoma
Autism Society of America
PO Box 720103
Norman, OK 73070   405-370-3220
                                       www.asofok.org

Dedicated to the education and welfare of all people with autism
and other pervasive developmental disorders.

Oregon

837   Autism Society of Oregon
Autism Society of America
PO Box 396
Marylhurst, OR 97036   503-636-1676
                                           888-288-4761
                                       Fax: 503-636-1696
                                 www.autismsocietyoregon.org

Promote mutual communication, autism awareness and better service delivery across Oregon.

Tobi Burch, Executive Director
Leigh Ann Chapman, President
Brad Volchok, Treasurer

Pennsylvania

838   Autism Society of America Greater Harrisburg Area Chapter
PO Box 101
Enola, PA 17025   717-732-8400
                                           800-244-2425
                                    www.autismharrisburg.org

To promote opportunities for individuals with autism spectrum
disorders, to participate in the same value life experiences as do
other citizens.

Esther Feirick, President
Kathleen Haigh, Vice President
Diana Fishlock, Treasurer

Rhode Island

839   Autism Society of Rhode Island
Autism Society of America
PO Box 16603
Rumford, RI 02916   401-595-3241
                                        lrego@asa-ri.org
                                        www.asa-ri.org

Provides information and support.

Lisa Rego, President
Claudia Swiader, Vice President

South Carolina

840   Autism Society of South Carolina
Autism Society of America
806 12th Street
West Columbia, SC 29169   803-750-6988
                                           800-438-4790
                                       Fax: 803-750-8121
                                    scas@scautism.org
                                    www.scautism.org

The purpose of the South Carolina Autism Society is to enable all
individuals with autism spectrum disorders to reach their maximum potential.

Susan Kastner, Chair
Alex Holbert, Vice Chair
Mitchell Yell, Treasurer

South Dakota

841   Autism Society of South Dakota Black Hills Chapter
Autism Society of America
3650 Range Road
Rapid City, SD 57702   605-415-3739
                                     info@autismsd.org
                                     www.autismsd.org

We have joined to enable all families and others associated with
an autistic, Asperger's or Pervasive Development Disorder individual to have access to support groups, meetings, additional information and resources.

Tennessee

842   Autism Society of America East Tennessee Chapter
PO Box 30015
Knoxville, TN 37930   865-637-3914
                                       info@asaetc.org
                                       www.asaetc.org

To promote lifelong access and opportunity of all individuals within the autism spectrum, and their families, to be fully participating, included members of their community.

Mike Manfredo, President
Roddey M. Coe, Vice President
Sara Hirtz, Treasurer

Texas

843   Autism Society of America Greater Austin Chapter
Autism Society of America
PO Box 160841
Austin, TX 78716   512-479-4199
                                       austinautismsociety@gmail.com
                                       www.autism-society.org/chapter244

Mission is to promote lifelong access and opportunities for person within the autism spectrum, and their families, to be fully included, participating members of their communities through advocacy, public awareness, education, and research related to Autism.

Ann Hart, President
Sandra Batlouni, Vice President
Tom Ibis, Treasurer

Vermont

844   Autism Society of Vermont
Autism Society of America
PO Box 978
White River Junction, VT 05001   800-559-7398
                                       vt-vermont@autismsocietyofamerica.org
                                       www.asvermont.org

The ASVT is a non-profit corporation serving the needs of Vermont's Autism community.

Cathy Pratt, Chairman
Joan Zaro, Executive Director
Lee Grossman, CEO

Virginia

845   Autism Society of America Northern Virginia Chapter
98 N. Washington Street
Falls Church, VA 22046   703-495-8444
                                       Fax: 703-563-6099
                                       info@asanv.org
                                       www.asanv.org

Provides information and support to individuals with autism and their families in Northern Virginia area.

Scott Campbell, President
Ray Nelson, Vice President
John J Wall, CPA, Treasurer

Washington

846   Autism Society of Washington
Autism Society of America
PO Box 503
Olympia, WA 98507   360-515-8910
                                       888-279-4968
                                       Fax: 253-503-1557
                                       info@autismsocietyofwa.org
                                       www.autismsocietyofwa.org

The mission of the Autism Society of Washington is to promote lifelong access and opportunities for persons within the autism spectrum and their families, and to be fully included, participating members of their communities through advocacy, public awareness, education, and research related to autism.

Jeffrey Foster, President
Teresa McCann, Vice President
Stephen Peters, Treasurer

West Virginia

847   Autism Society of West Virginia
PO Box 7
Huntington, WV 25706   304-748-1331
                                       jfair3@comcast.net
                                       http://autismwv.blogspot.com

ASA-WV is dedicated to increasing public awareness about autism and the day-to-day issues faced by individuals with autism, their families and the professionals with whom they interact. The Society's mission is to provide information and education, support research and advocate for programs and services for the autism population

Christina Lee Fair, President

Wisconsin

848   Autism Society of Wisconsin
Autism Society of America
1477 Kenwood Dr.
Menasha, WI 54952   920-558-4602
                                       888-428-8476
                                       Fax: 920-558-4611
                                       asw@asw4autism.org
                                       www.asw4autism.org

To promote lifelong opportunities for persons within the autism spectrum and their families to be fully included, participating members of their communities through information and referral, advocacy, public awareness, and education and support for local Autism Society of America chapters, professionals and others who support individuals with autism in Wisconsin.

Kristen Cooper, Executive Director
Kelly Brodhagen, Office Manager
Melissa Vande Velden, Events Coordinator/WALN Project Coo

Libraries & Resource Centers

Georgia

849   Emory Autism Resource Center
Emory University
101 Woodruff Circle, Suite 4000
Atlanta, GA 30322   404-727-8382
                                       Fax: 404-727-3969
                                       jsheikh@emory.edu
                                       www.psychiatry.emory.edu/clinical_sites_autism_cente

Offers online bulletin boards which are relevant to autism.

Mark Hyman Rapaport, Chairman

Indiana

850   Indiana Resource Center for Autism
Inst. for the Study of Developmental Disabilities
2853 E 10th Street
Bloomington, IN 47408   812-855-6508
                                       Fax: 812-855-9630
                                       TTY: 812-855-9396
                                       iidc@indiana.edu
                                       www.iidc.indiana.edu/irca

Conducts outreach training and consultation, engage in research, and develops and disseminate information on behalf of individuals across the autism spectrum, including autism, asperger's syndrome, and other pervasive developmental disorders.

Dr. Cathy Pratt, Director

Michigan

851   Burger School for the Autistic
30922 Beechwood Street
Garden City, MI 48135
734-762-8420
Fax: 734-762-8533
www.resa.net/gardencity/burger.htm

Committed to maximizing the potential of each student to gain independence and self-fulfillment.

Mary O'Neill, Manager

Missouri

852   Judevine Center for Autism
1101 Olivette Executive Parkway
Saint Louis, MO 63132
314-432-6200
800-780-6545
Fax: 314-849-2721
contactus@judevine.org
www.judevine.org

Rooted in principles of applied behavior analysis within a social exchange framework, the Judevine Center has provided effective training and treatment to thousands of families locally, nationally and globally.

New Jersey

853   New Jersey Center for Outreach and Service s for the Autism Community (COSAC)
500 Horizon Drive, Suite 530
Robbinsville, NJ 8691
609-588-8200
800-428-8476
Fax: 609-588-8858
information@autismnj.org
www.njcosac.org

Nonprofit agency providing information and advocacy, services, family and professional education and consultation. COSAC encourages responsible basic and applied research that would lead to a lessening of the effects and potential prevention of autism. COSAC is dedicated to ensuring that all people with autism receive appropriate, effective services to maximize their growth potential and to enhance the overall awareness of autism in the general public.

James A Paone, President
Genare Valiant, Vice President
Kathleen Moore, Secretary

New York

854   Institute for Basic Research in Developmental Disabilities
1050 Forest Hill Road
Staten Island, NY 10314
718-494-0600
Fax: 718-698-3803
www.omr.state.ny.us

To conduct basic and clinical research in order to further the prevention and early detection and treatment of mental retardation and developmental disabilities.

W Ted Brown, Manager

855   State University of New York Health Sciences Center
450 Clarkson Avenue, Box 32
Brooklyn, NY 11203
718-270-1000
Fax: 718-778-5397
www.downstate.edu

Child psychiatry research programs.

Richard Kream, Manager

North Carolina

856   Autism Society of North Carolina
505 Oberlin Road, Suite 230
Raleigh, NC 27605
919-743-0204
800-442-2762
Fax: 919-743-0208
books@autismsociety-nc.org
www.autismbookstore.com

Offers a library that carries one of the largest selections of books about autism.

David Lax, Manager

West Virginia

857   Autism Services Center
929 4th Avenue, PO Box 507
Huntington, WV 25710
304-525-8014
Fax: 304-525-8026
www.autismservicescenter.org

Works to improve appropriate and professional training, advocacy, consulting and information for individuals responsible for the welfare and care of autistic individuals and others with developmental disabilities.

Mike Grady, CEO
Derek Hyman, President/Treasurer
Elaine Harvey, Vice President

858   Autism Training Center
Marshall University
1 John Marshall Drive, Suite 316
Huntington, WV 25755
304-696-2332
800-344-5115
Fax: 304-696-2846
wvatc@marshall.edu.
www.marshall.edu/atc/

To provide education, training and treatment programs for West Virginians who have autism, pervasive developmental disorders or Asperger's disorders and have been formally registered with the center.

Barbara Cottrill, Executive Director

Research Centers

859   Autism Research Foundation
BU School of Medicine
72 East Concord Street
Boston, MA 02118
617-414-7012
Fax: 617-414-7207
hello@theautismresearchfoundation.org
www.theautismresearchfoundation.org

A nonprofit, tax-exempt organization dedicated to researching the neurological underpinnings of autism and other related developmental brain disorders. Seeking to rapidly expand and accelerate research into the pervasive developmental disorders. To do this, time and effort goes into investigating the neuropathology of autism in their laboratories, collecting and redistributing brain tissue to promising research groups for use by projects approved by the Tissue Resource Committee.

Margaret Bauman, MD, Founding Director
Thomas Sabin MD, President
Thomas Kemper MD, Vice President

860   Autism Research Institute
4182 Adams Avenue
San Diego, CA 92116
619-281-7165
866-366-3361
Fax: 619-563-6840
media@autismresearchinstitute.com
www.autism.com

ARI advocates for the rights of people with ASD, and operates without funding from special-interest groups. ARI is dedicated to developing a standard of care for individuals with autism spectrum disorders and their families. We rely on the generosity of donors to help us advance autism research and provide needed information and support for families and individuals with autism spectrum disorders.

Stephen Edelson, Executive Director
Jane Johnson, Managing Director
Rebecca McKenney, Office Manager

861 Autism Speaks
1 East 33rd Street 4th Floor
New York, NY 10016   212-252-8584
                                 Fax: 212-252-8676
                      familyservices@autismspeaks.org
                              www.autismspeaks.org

At Autism Speaks, our goal is to change the future for all who struggle with autism spectrum disorder. We are dedicated to funding global biomedical research into the causes, prevention, treatments, and cure for autism; to raising public awareness about autism and its effects on individuals, families, and society; and to bringing hope to all who deal with the hardships of this disorder.

Liz Feld, President
Peter H Bell, Executive VP
Lisa Goring, Vice President

862 Children's Center for Neurodevelopmental Studies
5430 West Glenn Drive
Glendale, AZ 85301   623-915-0345
                                 Fax: 623-937-5425
                               admin@ccnsaz.org
                        www.thechildrenscenteraz.org

The Children's Center is a full service non-profit corporation (501-c3) offering comprehensive educational, therapeutic, and habilitative programs for children and adults

Kent Rideout, Director
Dawna Sterner, Preschool & Education Information
Catherine Orsak, Therapy Information

863 Facilitated Communication Institute at Syracuse University
230 Huntington Hall
Syracuse, NY 13244   315-443-4752
                                 Fax: 315-443-2258
                             scstaff@sued.syr.edu
                           www.soe.syr.edu/about/

Facilitated Communication Institute, the new name, the Institute on Communication and Inclusion, represents a broadened focus developed over the past 20 years, reflecting lines of research, training and public dissemination that focus on school and community inclusion, narratives of disability and ability, and disability rights. Its initiatives stress the important relationship of communication to inclusion.

Robert Bogdan, Distinguished Professor Emeritus
Joan Burstyn, Professor Emerita
John Centra, Professor Emeritus

864 Institute on Communication and Inclusion
203 Huntington Hall
Syracuse, NY 13244   315-443-4752
                                 Fax: 315-443-2258
                                 icistaff@syr.edu
                           www.soe.syr.edu/about/

Facilitated Communication Institute, the new name, the Institute on Communication and Inclusion, represents a broadened focus developed over the past 20 years, reflecting lines of research, training and public dissemination that focus on school and community inclusion, narratives of disability and ability, and disability rights. Its initiatives stress the important relationship of communication to inclusion.

Robert Bogdan, Distinguished Professor Emeritus
Joan Burstyn, Professor Emerita
John Centra, Professor Emeritus

865 State University of New York Health Sciences Center
450 Clarkson Avenue
Brooklyn, NY 11203   718-270-1568
                                 Fax: 718-778-5397
                                 www.downstate.edu

Child psychiatry research programs.

Robert Furchgott, President

866 University of North Carolina at Chapel Hill, Brain Research Center
Matthew Gfeller Center 2207 Stallings-Evans Sports
Chapel Hill, NC 8700   919-962-0409
                                 Fax: 919-962-7060
                                 tbicenter@unc.edu
                www.tbicenter.unc.edu/MAG_Center/Home.html

The Matthew Gfeller Sport-Related Traumatic Brain Injury Research Center demonstrates its commitment to providing the highest level of care for athletes of all ages suffering from sport-related brain injuries, and to assist parents, coaches, and medical professionals in managing these student-athletes.

Kevin M. Guskiewicz, Faculty
Jason P. Mihalik, Faculty
Stephen W. Marshall, Faculty

Conferences

867 Annual TEACCH Conference
University of North Carolina at Chapel Hill
1418 Aversboro Road
Garner, NC 27529   919-662-4625
                                 Fax: 919-662-4634
                          raleighteacch@med.unc.edu
                                 www.teacch.com

May

Eric Schopler, Founder & Co-Director

868 Autism National Committee Conference
Autism National Committee Conference
3 Bedford Green
South Burlington, VT 05403   800-378-0386
                        sandra.mcclennen@emich.edu
                                 www.autcom.org

October

869 Autism Society National Conference & Expo
Austim Society
4340 East-West Way, Suite 350
Bethesda, MD 20814   301-657-0881
                                      800-328-8476
                          info@autism-society.org
                             www.autism-society.org

Addresses the range of issues affecting people with autism including early intervention, education, employment, behavior, communication, social skills, biomedical interventions and others, across the entire lifespan. Bringing together the expertise and experiences of family members, professionals and individuals on the spectrum, attendees are able to learn how to more effectively advocate and obtain supports for the individual with ASD.

July

James Ball, Executive Chair
Ron E Simmons, Vice Chair
Sergio Mariaca, Treasurer

870 FFCMH Annual Conference
Federation of Families for Childrens Mental Health
9605 Medical Center Drive, Suite 280
Rockville, MD 20850   240-403-1901
                                 Fax: 240-403-1909
                                 ffcmh@ffcmh.org
                                 www.ffcmh.org

Address the complex issue of trauma; the impact it has on children and families; the promotion of healing and prevention strategies; knowledge about how to address trauma through resiliency-based interventions, utilizing a familydriven, youth guided approach; and examples of how family organizations and the partners they work with are raising awareness and improving trauma-focused services and supports.

November

Teka Dempson, President
Sherri Luthe, Vice President
Sheila Pires, Treasurer

871 Genetic Alliance Annual Conference
Genetic Alliance
4301 Connecticut Avenue NW, Suite 404
Washington, DC 20008   202-966-5557
                               800-336-4363
                          Fax: 202-966-8553
                          info@geneticalliance.org
                          www.geneticalliance.org

Consistently inspirational and enables partnership among all
stakeholders: advocates and community leaders, health and industry professionals, policymakers, and academicians.

July

Sharon Terry, President/CEO
Tetyana Murza, Managing Director
Natasha Bonhomme, VP, Strategic Development

**872 International Conference On Young Children With Special
Needs & Their Famililies**
Division for Early Childhood
27 Fort Missoula Road, Suite 2
Missoula, MT 59804   406-543-0872
                       Fax: 406-543-0887
                       TTY: 703-264-9446
                       dec@dec-sped.org
                       www.dec-sped.org

Attendees from around the world explore the evidence, present
practical strategies, and engage in discussions that will change
the way one thinks about early childhood special education. Topics include: policy, autism, recommended practices, tiered interventions, challenging behavior, personnel development, research,
assessment, cultural diversity and more.

Bonnie Keilty, President
Juliann Woods, Vice President
Misty Goosen, Secretary

Audio Video

**873 A Sense of Belonging: Including Students with Autism in their
School Community**
Indiana Resource Center for Autism
1905 North Range Rd.
Bloomington, IN 47408   812-855-6508
                          Fax: 812-855-9630
                          TTY: 812-855-9396
                          iidc@indiana.edu
                          www.iidc.indiana.edu

Highlights the efforts of two elementary and one middle school in
Indiana in teaching students with autism in general education settings. Truly involving students in their school community requires teamwork, the adoption of effective instructional practices,
and a school committed to supporting a diverse range of students.

David Mank, Director

874 Autism
Fanflight Productions
32 Court Street, 21st Floor
Brooklyn, NY 11201   718-488-8900
                          800-876-1710
                     Fax: 718-488-8642
                     info@fanlight.com
                     www.fanlight.com

The stories of three families show us what the textbooks and studies cannot — what it's really like to love and care for children
with autism.

28 minutes

Kelli English, Publicity Coordinator

875 Autism Is a World
Syracuse University, Institute on Communication
370 Huntington Hall
Syracuse, NY 13244   315-443-9657
                       Fax: 315-443-2274
                       http://suedweb.syr.edu/thefci

Documentary that takes the viewer on a journey into the mind of
13 year old girl, into her world and her obsessions. Explores
Sue's world world, her writings, and the remarkable friendships
she has created while in college.

Videotape

876 Autism: A Strange, Silent World
Filmakers Library
3212 Duke Street
Alexandria, VA 22314   212-808-4980
                          703-212-8520
                     Fax: 212-808-4983
                     sales@alexanderstreet.com
                     www.academicvideostore.com/filmakers

British educators and medical personnel offer insight into autism's characteristics and treatment approaches through the cam-
eos of three children.

52 Minute

Sue Oscar, Co-President

877 Autism: A World Apart
Fanlight Productions
32 Court Street, 21st Floor
Brooklyn, NY 11201   718-488-8900
                          800-876-1710
                     Fax: 718-488-8642
                     info@fanlight.com
                     www.fanlight.com

In this documentary, three families show us what the textbooks
and studies cannot, what it's like to live with autism day after
day, raise and love children who may be withdrawn and violent
and unable to make personal connections with their families.
ISBN: DVD: 1-57295-950-9; VHS: 1-57295-039-0

29 Minutes DVD or VHS

878 Autism: Being Friends
Indiana Resource Center for Autism
1905 North Range Rd.
Bloomington, IN 47408   812-855-6508
                          800-280-7010
                     Fax: 812-855-9630
                     TTY: 812-855-9396
                     iidc@indiana.edu
                     www.iidc.indiana.edu

This autism awareness videotape was produced specifically for
use with young children. The program portrays the abilities of the
child with autism and describes ways in which peers can help the
child to be a part of the everyday world.

David Mank, Director

879 Autism: The Child Who Couldn't Play
Films for the Humanities and Sciences
132 West 31st Street
New York, NY 10001   800-257-5126
                     Fax: 609-275-0266
                     custserv@films.com
                     www.ffh.films.com

This program is a comprehensive overview of autism, the mysterious disorder that impedes normal child development. It was
once believed that autism was caused by remote, cold parents;
most often the mother was blamed. The program explores the
frontiers of our understanding of autism, which today is recognized as a partly genetic biological disorder.

28 minutes
ISBN: 1-421373-28-7

880 Autism: The Unfolding Mystery
Aquarius Health Care Videos
Lot 2/12 Willmott Ave
Margaret River, WA 6285   508-650-1616
                          888-440-2963
                     Fax: 508-650-1665
                     aquarius33@bigpond.com
                     www.aquariusproductions.com

Explores what it means to be autistic, how you can recognize the
signs of autism in your child, and hear about new tretments and
programs to help children learn to deal with the disorder.

26 Minutes

881 Children and Autism: Time is Brain
Aquarius Health Care Videos
Lot 2/12 Willmott Ave
Margaret River, WA 6285

508-650-1616
888-440-2963
Fax: 508-650-1665
aquarius33@bigpond.com
www.aquariusproductions.com

A mother of an autistic child implores parents who suspect their child may be autisitc not to 'wait and see.' Don't wait, don't be afraid of that diagnosis, diagnosis is a tool, not a stigma. The term 'time is brain' is absolutely accurate for children with autism, because the sooner diagnosed, the sooner they can get excellent care.

27 Minutes
ISBN: 1-581404-44-1

882 Children of the Stars
Fanlight Productions
32 Court Street, 21st Floor
Brooklyn, NY 11201

718-488-8900
800-876-1710
Fax: 718-488-8642
info@fanlight.com
www.fanlight.com

This film explores the harsh reality of raising children with autism in modern day China. It prodives moving insights into the hardships parents face and reminds us painfully of conditions that prevailed in the United States not so very many years ago.

49 Minutes DVD
ISBN: 1-572955-07-4

883 Developing Friendships: Wonderful People to Get to Know
Indiana Resource Center for Autism
1905 North Range Rd.
Bloomington, IN 47408

812-855-6508
Fax: 812-855-9630
TTY: 812-855-9396
iidc@indiana.edu
www.iidc.indiana.edu

Individuals discuss the various social difficulties they experience, such as being bullied, missing subtle social cues, and following and maintaining conversations. Strategies for supporting social interactions are highlighted.

David Mank, Director

884 Developing and Writing IEPs Under the New IDEA
LRP Publications
P.O. Box 24668
West Palm Beach, FL 33416

215-784-0860
800-515-4577
Fax: 215-784-9639
TTY: 215-658-0938
custserve@lrp.com
www.lrp.com

Addresses the new IEP content and IEP team requirements by explaining the new provisions, providing context and background to the changes, and predicting their potential impact on special education programs.

2005 90 minutes

Kenneth F. Kahn, President

885 Educating Students with Autism: Implementa tion of Applied Bahavior Analysis
LRP Publications
P.O. Box 24668
West Palm Beach, FL 33416

215-784-0860
800-515-4577
Fax: 215-784-9639
TTY: 215-658-0938
custserve@lrp.com
www.lrp.com

During this taped audio conference, behavior and autism consultant Dr Susan Catlett discusses the practical aspects of using ABA in your public school programs for students with autism spectrum disorders.

2006 90 Minutes

Kenneth F. Kahn, President

886 Getting Started with Facilitated Communica tion
Syracuse University, Institute On Communication
230 Huntington Hall
Syracuse, NY 13244

315-443-4752
Fax: 315-443-2258
ICIstaff@syr.edu
soe.syr.edu/centers_institutes/institute_communicati

Describes in detail how to help individuals with autism and/or severe communication difficulties to get started with facilitated communication.

Videotape

Christine Ashby, Director
Douglas Biklen, Senior Researcher
Dani Weinstein, Administrative Secretary

887 How I Am (Wie Ich Bin)
Fanlight Productions
32 Court Street, 21st Floor
Brooklyn, NY 11201

718-488-8900
800-876-1710
Fax: 718-488-8642
info@fanlight.com
www.fanlight.com

With the dreams and fears of a teenager, but wisdom beyond his years, Patrick takes us into his emotional world through the words he painstakingly types into his computer.

49 Minutes DVD
ISBN: 1-572955-05-8

888 I Want My Little Boy Back
Autism Treatment Center of America
2080 S Undermountain Road
Sheffield, MA 1257

413-229-2100
877-766-7473
Fax: 413-229-8931
information@son-rise.org
www.autismtreatmentcenter.org

This BBC documentary follows an English family with a child with autism before, during and after their time at the Son Rise Program. It uniquely captures the heart of the Son Rise Program and is extremely useful in understanding our techniques.

1981 379 pages Video
ISBN: 0-449201-08-2

Barry Neil Kaufman, Co-Founder
Kate Wilde, Group Facilitator
Samahria Lyte Kaufman, Founder

889 Sense of Belonging: Including Students with Autism in Their School Community
Indiana Resource Center for Autism
1905 North Range Rd.
Bloomington, IN 47408

812-855-9630
Fax: 812-855-6508
iidc@indiana.edu
www.iidc.indiana.edu

Highlights the efforts of two elementary and one middle school in Indiana in teaching students with autism in general education settings.

20 minutes

David Mank, Director

890 Two Worlds - One Planet
Fanlight Productions
32 Court Street, 21st Floor
Brooklyn, NY 11201

718-488-8900
800-876-1710
Fax: 718-488-8642
info@fanlight.com
www.fanlight.com

This documentary brings Autism syndrome out of the shadows, stressing that young people with developmental disabilities can learn and grow, if their individual needs, styles, and abilities are respected. It takes an upbeat look at students attending a private day school.

62 minutes DVD
ISBN: 1-572954-99-X

891 Understanding Autism
Fanlight Productions
32 Court Street, 21st Floor
Brooklyn, NY 11201   718-488-8900
                                 800-876-1710
                            Fax: 718-488-8642
                            info@fanlight.com
                            www.fanlight.com

Parents of children with autism discuss the nature and symptoms of this lifelong disability, and outline a treatment program based on behavior modification principles. ISBN: DVD: 1-57295-951-7; VHS: 1-572951-11-1

19 minutes DVD or VHS

Kelli English, Publicity Coordinator

892 We've Climbed Mountains: Increasing Our Understanding of Autism Spectrum Disorders
Indiana Resource Center for Autism
1905 North Range Rd.
Bloomington, IN 47408   812-855-6508
                            Fax: 812-855-9630
                            TTY: 812-855-9396
                            iidc@indiana.edu
                            www.iidc.indiana.edu

Provides general information about autism spectrum disorders with the hope of increasing overall awareness, especially about those with high-functioning autism/Asperger's syndrome. Specific topics addressed include sensory challenges, social understanding, and responses to the diagnosis.

David Mank, Director

Web Sites

893 Asperger Autism Spectrum Education Network (ASPEN)
9 Aspen Circle
Edison, NJ 08820   732-321-0880
                            info@aspennj.org
                            www.aspennj.org

Regionally based nonprofit organization headquartered in NJ, with 12 local chapters, providing for families and those individuals affected with Asperger Syndrome, PDD-NOS, High Function Autism, and related disorders.

Lori Shery, President/Executive Director
Rich Meleo, Vice President
Elizabeth Yamashita, Vice President

894 Autism Network International
P.O. Box 35448
Syracuse, NY 13235   webmaster@autreat.com.
                        www.autismnetworkinternational.org

An autistic-run self-help and advocacy organization for autistic people.

895 Autism Network for Dietary Intervention
www.autismndi.com

Providing help and support for families using a gluten and casein free diet in the treatment of autism and related developmental disabilities.

896 Autism Research Institute
4182 Adams Avenue
San Diego, CA 92116   www.autism.com

Provides information based on research to parents and professionals throughout the world.

Stephen Edelson, Executive Director
Jane Johnson, Managing Director
Rebecca McKenney, Office Manager

897 Autism Resources
www.autism-resources.com

Offers information and links regarding the developmental dsabilities of autism and aspergers syndrome.

898 Autism Society of America
4340 East-West Hwy, Suite 350
Bethesda, ML 20814   301-657-0881
                                 800-328-8476
                            info@autism-society.org
                            www.autism-society.org

Information regarding autism.

Scott Badesch, President & CEO
Matthew Asner, VP Development
Selena Hernandez, Manager, Support Services

899 Autism Speaks
1 East 33rd Street, 4th Floor
New York, NY 10016   212-252-8584
                                 888-288-4762
                            Fax: 212-252-8676
                            familyservices@autismspeaks.org
                            www.autismspeaks.org

Information about Autism Research.

Liz Field, President
Lisa Goring, Executive Vice President
Alec M Elbert, Chief Strategy Officer

900 Center for the Study of Autism
www.autism.org

Information about autism to parents and professionals.

901 Community Services for Autistic Adults & Children (CSAAC)
8615 East Village Avenue
Montgomery Village, MD 20886   240-912-2220
                            Fax: 301-926-9384
                            www.csaac.org

Information about autism to parents and professionals.

Ian Paregol, Executive Director
Don Rodrick, Chief Financial Officer
Maree Smith, Assistant Executive Director

902 Families for Early Autism Treatment
P. O. Box 255722
Sacramento, CA 95865   www.feat.org

Information about autism.

903 Institute on Communication and Inclusion
230 Huntington Hall
Syracuse, NY 13244   315-443-4752
                            Fax: 315-443-2258
                            ICIstaff@syr.edu
                  soe.syr.edu/centers_institutes/institute_communicati

College offering facilitated learning research into communication with persons who have autism or severe disabilities. Offers books, videos and public awareness information on the research projects.

Christine Ashby, Director
Douglas Biklen, Senior Researcher
Dani Weinstein, Administrative Secretary

904 Online Mendelian Inheritance in Man
National Library of Medicine, Building 38A
Bethesda, MD 20894   888-346-3656
                            info@ncbi.nlm.nih.gov
                            www.ncbi.nlm.nih.gov

This database is a catalog of human genes and genetic disorders.

Christine E. Seidman, M.D., Chair
David J. Lipman, M.D., Executive Secretary

905 University Students with Autism and Asperger's Syndrome Web Site
www.users.dircon.co.uk/~cns

                                 207-704-7450
                                 77- 56- 774
                            Fax: 207-359-9440
                            judith.kerem@nas.org.uk
                            www.users.dircon.co.uk/~cns

107

Helps to develop and understanding of the difficulties people with Asperger Syndrome may face. We also work on a one to one basis with the student and liase with staff and peers. help is also given in setting up support networks such as mentors and providing effective strategies to aid independent learning.

Book Publishers

906   ABA Program Companion
Autism Society of North Carolina Bookstore
505 Oberlin Road, Suite 230
Raleigh, NC 27605
         919-743-0204
         800-442-2762
         Fax: 919-743-0208
         books@autismsociety-nc.org
         www.autismbookstore.com

A guide developed to help educational teams organize an implement Applied Behavior Analysis (ABA) programs, including home, school, and center-based programs.

907   Activity Schedules for Children with Autism
Autism Society of North Carolina Bookstore
505 Oberlin Road, Suite 230
Raleigh, NC 27605
         919-743-0204
         800-442-2762
         Fax: 919-743-0208
         books@autismsociety-nc.org
         www.autismbookstore.com

Written to help parents and professionals utilize activity schedules to promote independence in children in a variety of settings.

908   Al Capone Does My Shirts: A Novel
Autism Society of North Carolina Bookstore
505 Oberlin Road, Suite 230
Raleigh, NC 27605
         919-743-0204
         800-442-2762
         Fax: 919-743-0208
         books@autismsociety-nc.org
         www.autismbookstore.com

Set in 1935, this colorful novels tells the story of Matthew 'Moose' Flanagan, a 12-year-old boy who moves with his family (including sister with autism) to Alcatraz Island. For readers age 12 and up.

909   Autism Acceptance Book: Being A Friend to Someone With Autism
Autism Society of North Carolina Bookstore
505 Oberlin Road, Suite 230
Raleigh, NC 27605
         919-743-0204
         800-442-2762
         Fax: 919-743-0208
         books@autismsociety-nc.org
         www.autismbookstore.com

Colorfully illustrated activity book was created to help neurotypical children learn about autism spectrum disorder (ASD) and the characteristics that make kids with ASD unique. For readers age 6 and up.

910   Autism Spectrum Disorders: The Complete Guide
Autism Society of North Carolina Bookstore
505 Oberlin Road, Suite 230
Raleigh, NC 27605
         919-743-0204
         800-442-2762
         Fax: 919-743-0208
         books@autismsociety-nc.org
         www.autismbookstore.com

Written to help parents, professionals, and other members of the community learn more about autism spectrum disorder (ASD), and it presents a thorough overview of the disorder, from diagnosis through adulthood.

911   Autism and Learning
David Fulton Publishers
2 Park Square, Milton Park
Abingdon, 0X14 4RN,
United Kingdom
         207-017-7913
         Fax: 207-017-6707
         mail@fultonpublisher.co.uk
         http://catalogue.fultonpublishers.co.uk

This book is about how a cognitive perception on the way in which individuals with autism think and learn may be applied to particular curriculum areas.
1997 180 pages Paperback
ISBN: 1-853464-21-X

912   Autism and the Family: Problems, Prospects and Coping with the Disorder
Charles C Thomas Publishing
2600 S 1st Street
Springfield, IL 62704
         217-789-8980
         800-258-8980
         Fax: 217-789-9130
         books@ccthomas.com
         www.ccthomas.com

Examination of certain issues such as stress, coping and stigma. Contains 33 interviews with parents whose children attended an autistic treatment center. An excellent resource text.
1998 210 pages Softcover
ISBN: 0-398068-43-7

913   Autism as an Executive Director
Oxford University Press
2001 Evans Road
Cary, NC 27513
         919-677-0977
         800-445-9714
         Fax: 919-677-1303
         custserv.us@oup.com
         www.us.oup.com

Provides a new and conroversial perspective from some of the leading researchers in this field.
1998 328 pages
ISBN: 0-198523-49-1

914   Autism: Effective Biomedical Treatments
Autism Society of North Carolina Bookstore
505 Oberlin Road, Suite 230
Raleigh, NC 27605
         919-743-0204
         Fax: 919-743-0208
         books@autismsociety-nc.org
         www.autismbookstore.com

Written for clinicians, professionals, and parents who would like to understand more about specific biomedical treatments for autism spectrum disorder (ASD).

915   Autism: From Tragedy to Triumph
Branden Publishing Company
17 Station Street
Brookline Village, MA 02447
         617-734-2045
         Fax: 617-734-2046
         branden@branden.com
         www.branden.com

A book that deals with the Lovaas method and includes a foreward by Dr. Ivar Lovaas. The book is broken down into two parts — the long road to diagnosis and then treatment.
ISBN: 0-828319-65-0

916   Autism: Mind and Brain
Oxford University Press
2001 Evans Road
Cary, NC 27513
         919-677-0977
         800-445-9714
         Fax: 919-677-1303
         custserv.us@oup.com
         www.us.oup.com

An important work describing the latest advances in autism research.

2004 320 pages
ISBN: 0-198529-24-4

917   Autism: The Facts
Oxford University Press
2001 Evans Road
Cary, NC 27513

919-677-0977
800-445-9714
Fax: 919-677-1303
custserv.us@oup.com
www.us.oup.com

Contains valuable information for families and those afflicted with this condition.

1994 124 pages
ISBN: 0-192623-27-3

918   Beyond the Autism Diagnosis: A Professiona l's Guide to Helping Families
Autism Society of North Carolina Bookstore
505 Oberlin Road, Suite 230
Raleigh, NC 27605

919-743-0204
Fax: 919-743-0208
books@autismsociety-nc.org
www.autismbookstore.com

Helps to change the way professionals communicate with parents of children with autism spectrum disorder (ASD), making the experience more effective and meaningful for all involved.

919   Children With Autism: A Parents Guide
Peytral Publications
P.O. Box 1162
Minnetonka, MN 55345

952-949-8707
877-739-8725
Fax: 952-906-9777
help@peytral.com
www.peytral.com

Informative handbook for parents of children and teens; covers medical, educational, legal, family life, daily care, emotional issues and more.

456 pages

920   Children wIth Starving Brains
Autism Society of North Carolina Bookstore
505 Oberlin Road, Suite 230
Raleigh, NC 27605

919-743-0204
800-442-2762
Fax: 919-743-0208
books@autismsociety-nc.org
www.autismbookstore.com

Written by an experienced physician who is the grandmother of a child with autism spectrum disorder (ASD), this book takes a biomedical approach toward the treatment of ASD.

Eric Schopler, Editor
Gary Mesibov, Co-Editor

921   Children with Autism and Asperger Syndrome A Guide for Practitioners and Carers
John Wiley & Sons
10475 Crosspoint Blvd
Indianapolis, IN 46256

877-762-2974
Fax: 800-597-3299
www.wiley.com

Covers the disorders of autism, understanding the causes and the different approaches of treatment for autistic children.

1999 342 pages
ISBN: 0-471983-28-4

922   Children with Autism: A Developmental Perspective
Harvard University Press
79 Garden Street
Cambridge, MA 02138

401-531-2800
800-405-1619
Fax: 401-531-2801
hup@harvard.edu
www.hup.harvard.edu

Offers a rare close look at the mysterious condition that afflicts approximately 350,000 Americans and millions more.

1997
ISBN: 0-674053-13-3

923   Cowden Preautism Observation Inventory
Jo E. Cowden, author

Charles C Thomas Publisher
2600 S 1st Street
Springfield, IL 62704

217-789-8980
800-258-8980
Fax: 217-789-9130
books@ccthomas.com
www.ccthomas.com

Contains effective intervention activities for sensory motor stimulation and joint attention.

226 pages
ISBN: 0-398086-43-5

Sue F V Rakow, Co-Author
Carol B Carpenter, Co-Author

924   Diagnosis Autism: Now What? 10 Steps to Improve Treatment Outcomes
Autism Society of North Carolina Bookstore
505 Oberlin Road, Suite 230
Raleigh, NC 27605

919-743-0204
800-442-2762
Fax: 919-743-0208
books@autismsociety-nc.org
www.autismbookstore.com

Practical guide was written to help parents of children with autism spectrum disorder (ASD) form successful pediatric partnerships with physicians and other healthcare practitioners involved in their child's diagnosis and treatment.

925   Different Like Me: My Book of Autism Heroe s
Autism Society of North Carolina Bookstore
505 Oberlin Road, Suite 230
Raleigh, NC 27605

919-743-0204
800-442-2762
Fax: 919-743-0208
books@autismsociety-nc.org
www.autismbookstore.com

This beautifully illustrated children's book tells the tales of many famous people throughout history who all had on thing in common: they didn't fit in. It's also possible they may have had autism spectrum disorder (ASD). For readers ages 7-12.

926   Does My Child Have Autism?
Autism Society of North Carolina Bookstore
505 Oberlin Road, Suite 230
Raleigh, NC 27605

919-743-0204
800-442-2762
Fax: 919-743-0208
books@autismsociety-nc.org
www.autismbookstore.com

Written for parents of children age three and younger who have concerns about their child's development.

927   Education and Care for Adolescents and Adults with Autism
Kate Wall, author

Hamill Institute on Disabilities
2455 Teller Road
Thousand Oaks, CA 91320

800-818-7243
Fax: 800-583-2665
info@sagepub.com
www.sagepub.com

Uses case studies and examples that show the reader how to put theory into practice in multi-disciplinary settings, this book clearly explains how changes in policy and provision have affected how young people and adults with autism are cared for and educated. With highlights of up-to-date and accessible information on the nature and affects of ASD, legislation information, family issues, positive intervention programs, and strategies. Hardcover or paperback.

2007 168 pages Paperback
ISBN: 1-412923-82-8

Sara Miller McCune, Founder/Chairman
Blaise R Simqu, President/CEO
Chris Hickok, Senior Vice President/CFO

928   Everybody is Different: A Book for Young People
Autism Society of North Carolina Bookstore
505 Oberlin Road, Suite 230
Raleigh, NC 27605   919-743-0204
                                            800-442-2762
                                       Fax: 919-743-0208
                                 books@autismsociety-nc.org
                                    www.autismbookstore.com

Written for brothers and sisters of young persons with autism
spectrum disorder (ASD). It not only explains the basic
characterisitics of ASD, but also answers the questions often
asked by a sibling of a child with ASD. For readers ages 8-16.

Hardbound

**929   Everyday Solutions: A Practical Guide for Families of
         Children with Autism**
Autism Society of North Carolina Bookstore
505 Oberlin Road, Suite 230
Raleigh, NC 27605   919-743-0204
                                            800-442-2762
                                       Fax: 919-743-0208
                                 books@autismsociety-nc.org
                                    www.autismbookstore.com

Presents 37 everyday situations that may present difficulties for a
child with autism spectrum disorder (ASD), along with recommendations and strategies.

930   Functional Behavior Assessment for People with Autism
Autism Society of North Carolina Bookstore
505 Oberlin Road, Suite 230
Raleigh, NC 27605   919-743-0204
                                            800-442-2762
                                       Fax: 919-743-0208
                                 books@autismsociety-nc.org
                                    www.autismbookstore.com

provides and introduction to functional behavior assessment
(FBA). FBA is a valuable tool that can be used by parents and
professionals to understand and address the challenging behaviors
of persons with autism spectrum disorder (ASD).

931   Handbook of Autism and Pervasive Developmental Disorders
Autism Society of North Carolina Bookstore
505 Oberlin Road, Suite 230
Raleigh, NC 27605   919-743-0204
                                            800-442-2762
                                       Fax: 919-743-0208
                                 books@autismsociety-nc.org
                                    www.autismbookstore.com

Two-volume scholarly resource presents the latest scientific research on autism spectrum disorders (ASD).

932   Healthcare for Children on the Autism Spectrum
Autism Society of North Carolina Bookstore
505 Oberlin Road, Suite 230
Raleigh, NC 27605   919-743-0204
                                            800-442-2762
                                       Fax: 919-743-0208
                                 books@autismsociety-nc.org
                                    www.autismbookstore.com

The first publication of its kind to focus on the health and medical care of children with autism spectrum disorder (ASD).

933   Helping Children with Autism Learn
Oxford University Press
2001 Evans Road
Cary, NC 27513   919-677-0977
                                            800-445-9714
                                       Fax: 919-677-1303
                                      custserv.us@oup.com
                                          www.us.oup.com

A leading authority on autism offers practical, reliable advice on
coping with learning disorders associated with autism.

2003 512 pages
ISBN: 0-195138-11-2

934   Ian's Walk: A Story About Autism
Autism Society of North Carolina Bookstore
505 Oberlin Road, Suite 230
Raleigh, NC 27605   919-743-0204
                                            800-442-2762
                                       Fax: 919-743-0208
                                 books@autismsociety-nc.org
                                    www.autismbookstore.com

In this moving fictional story, a young girl named Julie realizes
how much she cares for her brother, Ian, who has autism spectrum disorder (ASD). For readers ages 4-8.

935   Incredible 5-Point Scale
Autism Society of North Carolina Bookstore
505 Oberlin Road, Suite 230
Raleigh, NC 27605   919-743-0204
                                            800-442-2762
                                       Fax: 919-743-0208
                                 books@autismsociety-nc.org
                                    www.autismbookstore.com

Shows parents and professionals how to implement a simple
5-point scale to help students with sutism spectrum disorder
(ASD) understand and control their emotional responses and
behavior.

**936   Just Take a Bite: Easy, Effective Answers to Food Aversions
         and Eating Challenges**
Autism Society of North Carolina Bookstore
505 Oberlin Road, Suite 230
Raleigh, NC 27605   919-743-0204
                                            800-442-2762
                                       Fax: 919-743-0208
                                 books@autismsociety-nc.org
                                    www.autismbookstore.com

A much-need resource that specifically addresses the eating challenges of children who may have autism spectrum disorder
(ASD), sensory processing disorder (SPD), or other developmental delays.

937   Kids In the Syndrome Mix
Autism Society of North Carolina Bookstore
505 Oberlin Road, Suite 230
Raleigh, NC 27605   919-743-0204
                                            800-442-2762
                                       Fax: 919-743-0208
                                 books@autismsociety-nc.org
                                    www.autismbookstore.com

Children with autism spectrum disorder (ASD) often have coexisting neuropsychiatric diagnoses, and this handbook focuses on
the most common neuropsychiatric disorders and their symptoms.

938   Looking After Louis
Autism Society of North Carolina
505 Oberlin Road, Suite 230
Raleigh, NC 27605   919-743-0204
                                            800-442-2762
                                       Fax: 919-743-0208
                                 books@autismsociety-nc.org
                                    www.autismbookstore.com

Colrfully illustrated fictional story introduces readers to Louis, a
new boy in school who has autism spectrum disorder (ASD). Told
from the perspective of a female classmate, the story describes
how Louis plays and interacts with students and teachers in a
general education classroom. For readers ages 4-8.

939   Mindblindness: An Essay on Autism & Theory of Mind
MIT Press
55 Hayward Street
Cambridge, MA 02142   617-253-5646
                                            800-405-1619
                                       Fax: 617-258-6779
                                 mitpress-order-inq@mit.edu
                                     http://mitpress.mit.edu

Interpretations and research into the theory of mindblindness in
children with autism.

1995 208 pages
ISBN: 0-262023-84-9

Ellen W Faran, Director
Rebecca Schrader, Associate Director

940   Miracle to Believe In
Fawcett

A group of people from all walks of life come together and are transformed as they reach out, under the direction of the Kaufmans, to help a little boy the medical world has given up as hopeless. The heartwarming journey of loving a child back to life will not only inspire you, the reader, but presents a compelling new way to deal with life's traumas and difficulties.

1982 384 pages
ISBN: 0-449201-08-2

941   My Brother Sammy
Autism Society of North Carolina Bookstore
505 Oberlin Road, Suite 230
Raleigh, NC 27605   919-743-0204
                                                 800-442-2762
                                            Fax: 919-743-0208
                                  books@autismsociety-nc.org
                                      www.autismbookstore.com

Filled with beautiful watercolor illustrations, this book tells the fictional story of Sammy, a young boy with autism spectrum disorder (ASD). The story is told from the perspective of Sammy's older brother, who is sometimes frustrated by Sammy's behavior. For readers ages 4-8.

942   My Friend With Autism
Autism Society of North Carolina Bookstore
505 Oberlin Road, Suite 230
Raleigh, NC 27605   919-743-0204
                                                 800-442-2762
                                            Fax: 919-743-0208
                                  books@autismsociety-nc.org
                                      www.autismbookstore.com

Created for teachers and students in her son's elementary school class. The book is a valuable tool for helping typical children understand the traits and behaviors of their classmates with autism spectrum disorder (ASD). For readers ages 4-10.

943   My Social Stories Book
Autism Society of North Carolina Bookstore
505 Oberlin Road, Suite 230
Raleigh, NC 27605   919-743-0204
                                                 800-442-2762
                                            Fax: 919-743-0208
                                  books@autismsociety-nc.org
                                      www.autismbookstore.com

The Social Stones in this book are written for children with autism spectrum disorder (ASD) ages 2 to 6, and they include over 150 everyday situations that are frequently encountered in early childhood.

944   Neurobiology of Autism
Johns Hopkins University Press
2715 N Charles Street
Baltimore, MD 21218   410-516-6900
                                                 800-537-5487
                                            Fax: 410-516-6998
                                   webmaster@press.jhu.edu
                                          www.press.jhu.edu

This book discusses recent advances in scientific research that point to a neurobiological basis for autism and examines the clinical implications of this research.

2006 424 pages
ISBN: 0-801880-47-5

Alfred R Berkeley, Chairman

945   Parenting Across the Autism Spectrum
Autism Society of North Carolina Bookstore
505 Oberlin Road, Suite 230
Raleigh, NC 27605   919-743-0204
                                                 800-442-2762
                                            Fax: 919-743-0208
                                  books@autismsociety-nc.org
                                      www.autismbookstore.com

Two mothers who have children on the opposite ends of the autism spectrum wrote this poignant and insightful book, and the book also provides a look at what lies beyond the early intervention and elementary school years.

946   Positive Behavioral Strategies to Support Children & Young People with Autism

Martin Hanbury, author

Hamill Institute on Disabilities/Sage Publications
2455 Teller Road
Thousand Oaks, CA 91320   800-818-7243
                                            Fax: 800-583-2665
                                        info@sagepub.com
                                          www.sagepub.com

Offers advice on understanding and managing childrens' often challenging actions. Covering a range from birth to 19 years, this resource provides: practical advice on developing an appropriate learning environement; INSET materials for developing behavior management practices; self-audit tools for practioners; and reproducables and practical resources. Hardcover or paperback.

2007 120 pages Paperback
ISBN: 1-412929-11-0

Sara Miller McCune, Founder/Chairman
Blaise R Simqu, President/CEO
Chris Hickok, Senior Vice President/CFO

947   Preschool Issues in Autism
Plenum Publishing Corporation
233 Spring Street
New York, NY 10013   212-620-8000
                                            Fax: 212-463-0742
                                          www.springer.com

Combines some of the most important theory and data related to the early identification and intervention in autism and related disorders. Addresses clinical aspects, parental concerns and legal issues. Helps professionals understand and implement state-of-the-art services for young children and their families.

294 pages
ISBN: 0-306444-40-2

Derk Haank, CEO
Ulrich Vest, CFO
Martin Mos, COO

948   Prescription for Success
Autism Society of North Carolina Bookstore
505 Oberlin Road, Suite 230
Raleigh, NC 27605   919-743-0204
                                                 800-442-2762
                                            Fax: 919-743-0208
                                  books@autismsociety-nc.org
                                      www.autismbookstore.com

Written for medical professionals who work with patients who have autism spectrum disorder.

949   Reaching the Autistic Child: A Parent Training Program
Brookline Books/Lumen Editions
8 Trumbell Rd, Suite B-001
Northampton, MA 01060   413-584-0184
                                                 800-666-2665
                                            Fax: 413-584-6184
                                        brbooks@yahoo.com
                                      www.brooklinebooks.com

Detailed case studies of social and behavioral change in autistic children and their families show parents how to implement the principles for improved socialization and behavior.

1998 Softcover
ISBN: 1-571290-56-7

950   Riddle of Autism: A Psychological Analysis
Jason Aronson
4501 Forbes Blvd, Suite 200
Lanham, MD 20706

301-459-3366
800-462-6420
Fax: 301-429-5748
custserv@rowman.com
www.aronson.com

Dr. Victor examines the myths that cloud an understanding of this disorder and describes the meanings of its specific behavioral symptoms.

356 pages Softcover
ISBN: 1-568215-73-8

951   Social Skills Picture Book
Autism Society of North Carolina Bookstore
505 Oberlin Road, Suite 230
Raleigh, NC 27605

919-743-0204
800-442-2762
Fax: 919-743-0208
books@autismsociety-nc.org
www.autismbookstore.com

(Teaching Play, Emotions, and Communication to Children with Autism). Through photographs and conversation bubbles, the author demonstrates approximately 30 social skilld in the areas of communication, play, and emotion.

952   Solving Behavior Problems in Autism
Autism Society of North Carolina Bookstore
505 Oberlin Road, Suite 230
Raleigh, NC 27605

919-743-0204
800-442-2762
Fax: 919-743-0208
books@autismsociety-nc.org
www.autismbookstore.com

In this guide, the author explains how to use effective communication techniques to reduce problem behaviors in persons with autism spectrum disorder (ASD).

953   Son-Rise: The Miracle Continues

Describes an effective, loving and respectful method for treating children with autism. It documents the development of the Son Rise Program throught the record of Raun Kaufman's astonishing development from a lifeless, autistic, retarded child into a highly verbal, loveable youngster with no traces of his former condition. It further details Raun's extraordinary progress from the age of four into young adulthood. It also shares moving accounts of five families who successfully used the program.

1995 384 pages
ISBN: 0-915811-61-8

954   Stress and Coping in Autism
Oxford University Press
2001 Evans Road
Cary, NC 27513

919-677-0977
800-445-9714
Fax: 919-677-1303
custserv.us@oup.com
www.us.oup.com

Provides a theoretical framework for the usefukness of the stress construct in understanding and treating autism.

2006 472 pages
ISBN: 0-195182-26-X

955   Taking Autism to School
Autism Society of North Carolina Bookstore
505 Oberlin Road, Suite 230
Raleigh, NC 27605

919-743-0204
800-442-2762
Fax: 919-743-0208
books@autismsociety-nc.org
www.autismbookstore.com

A fictional story about a girl named Angel and her friendship woth Sam, a classmate who has autism spectrum disorder (ASD). From her own point of view, Angel explains how Sam thinks and behaves in school and at home. For readers ages 5-10.

956   Teaching Children with Autism to Mind-Read A Pratical Guide for Teachers & Parents
John Wiley & Sons
10475 Crosspoint Blvd
Indianapolis, IN 46256

877-762-2974
Fax: 800-597-3299
www.wiley.com

This book explains the Theory of Mind, which is the ability to infer other's mental states and then interpret their speech and actions based on this information. The author applies this theory to autistic children to help their social and communicative abnormalities.

1999 302 pages
ISBN: 0-471976-23-7

957   Teaching Coversations to Children With Autism: Scripts and Script Fading
Autism Society of North Carolina Bookstore
505 Oberlin Road, Suite 230
Raleigh, NC 27605

919-743-0204
800-442-2762
Fax: 919-743-0208
books@autismsociety-nc.org
www.autismbookstore.com

Uses the principles of Apllied Behavior Analysis (ABA) to create strategies that facilitate communication in children who have autism spectrum disorder.

958   Ten Things Every Child With Autism Wishes You Know
Autism Society of North Carolina Bookstore
505 Oberlin Road, Suite 230
Raleigh, NC 27605

919-743-0204
800-442-2762
Fax: 919-743-0208
books@autismsociety-nc.org
www.autismbookstore.com

Describes how children with autism spectrum disorder (ASD) function and what they are trying to say to the world when they cannot always express it in a conventional way.

959   The Neurology of Autism
Oxford University Press
2001 Evans Road
Cary, NC 27513

919-677-0977
800-445-9714
Fax: 919-677-1303
custserv.us@oup.com
www.us.oup.com

A valuable resource for both the latest information from basic-science research and its application to the diagnosis and treatment of autism.

2005 272 pages
ISBN: 0-195182-22-7

960   Toilet Training for Individuals with Autism and Related Disorders
Autism Society of North Carolina Bookstore
505 Oberlin Road, Suite 230
Raleigh, NC 27605

919-743-0204
800-442-2762
Fax: 919-743-0208
books@autismsociety-nc.org
www.autismbookstore.com

Comprehensive guide for parents and professionals provides over 200 toilet training tips and more than 40 helpful case examples.

961 **Treasure Chest of Behavioral Strategies for Individuals with Autism**
Autism Society of North Carolina Bookstore
505 Oberlin Road, Suite 230
Raleigh, NC 27605

919-743-0204
800-442-2762
Fax: 919-743-0208
books@autismsociety-nc.org
www.autismbookstore.com

Comprehensive resource manual provides parents and teachers with numerous behavior management strategies for individuals with autism spectrum disorder (ASD).

962 **Understanding and Treating Children with Autism**
John Wiley & Sons
10475 Crosspoint Blvd
Indianapolis, IN 46256

877-762-2974
Fax: 800-597-3299
www.wiley.com

Aimed at those concerned with the education and welfare of the children with autism, particularly at teachers in Special education and the psychologists and care professionals who work with teachers and parents of children with autism.

1995 188 pages
ISBN: 0-471958-88-3

963 **Visual Strategies for Improving Communicat ion**
Autism Society of North Carolina Bookstore
505 Oberlin Road, Suite 230
Raleigh, NC 27605

919-743-0204
800-442-2762
Fax: 919-743-0208
books@autismsociety-nc.org
www.autismbookstore.com

This how-to manual describes a communication intervention strategy for teaching persons with autism spectrum disorder (ASD) that evolved from learning style research.

964 **World of the Autistic Child**
Oxford University Press
2001 Evans Road
Cary, NC 27513

919-677-0977
800-445-9714
Fax: 919-677-1303
custserv.us@oup.com
www.us.oup.com

Comprehensive guide for parents with children diagnosed or suspected of being autistic. Includes current thinking on causes, diagnosis, and treatment, using illustrative case studies.

1998 368 pages
ISBN: 0-195119-17-7

Magazines

965 **Autism Advocate**
Autism Society of America
4340 East-West Hwy, Suite 350
Bethesda, ML 20814

301-657-0881
800-328-8476
info@autism-society.org
www.autism-society.org

Gathers a diverse collection of the latest autism news, chapter highlights, first-person accounts of families living with and growing with autism, and tips from paretns and professionals. Published 5 times a year.

James Ball, Executive Chair
Anne Holmes, Vice Chair
Lars Perner, Secretary

966 **Newslink**
Autism Society Ontario
4340 East-West Hwy, Suite 350
Bethesda, ML 20814
M6K 3C5

301-657-0881
800-328-8476
Fax: 416-246-9417
info@autism-society.org
www.autism-society.org

Covers society activities and contains information on autism. Recurring features include news of research, a calendar of events, reports of meetings, and book reviews.

10 pages

James Ball, Executive Chair
Anne Holmes, Vice Chair
Lars Perner, Secretary

Journals

967 **Focus on Autism and Other Developmental Disabilities**
Hammill Institute on Disabilities/Sage Publication
2455 Teller Road
Thousand Oaks, CA 91320

800-818-7243
Fax: 800-583-2665
journals@sagepub.com
www.sagepub.com

Practical elements of management, treatment, planning and education for persons with autism or other pervasive developmental disabilities. FOCUS publishes articles representing diverse philosophical and theoretical positions and reflecting a wide range of disciplines, inclusing, education, psychology, psychiatry, medicine, physical therapy, occupational therapy, speech/language pathology and related areas. ISSN: Print: 0885-7288; Electronic: 1538-4837

Quarterly

968 **The Journal of Positive Behavior Intervent ions**
Hamill Institute on Disabilities/Sage Publications
2455 Teller Road
Thousand Oaks, CA 91320

800-818-7243
Fax: 800-583-2665
journals@sagepub.com
www.sagepub.com

The JPBI offers sound, research-based principles of positive behavior support for use in school, home, and community settings with people with challenges in bahvior adaptations. JPBI is an official journal of the Association of Positive Behavior Support. Subscriptions: Institutional - Print Only $146, Institutional - Print & E-access $149, Individual - Print & E-access $57.

Quarterly

V Mark Durand, PhD, Co-Editor
Robert L Koegel, PhD, Co-Editor

969 **The Journal of Special Education**
Hamill Institute on Disabilities/Sage Publications
2455 Teller Road
Thousand Oaks, CA 91320

800-818-7243
Fax: 800-583-2665
journals@sagepub.com
www.sagepub.com

For four decades professionals have relied on the JSE'for timely, sound research in the area of special education. JSE provides reseach articles and scholarly review by expert authors in all subspecialties of special education for individuals with disabilities ranging from mild to severe. JSE is an official journal of the Division for Research of the CEC. Subscriptions: Institutional - Print Only $172, Institutional - Print & E-access $176, Individual - Print & E-access $57.

Quarterly

Bob Algozzine, PhD, Co-Editor
Fred Spooner, PhD, Co-Editor

Newsletters

970 Autism Research Review International
Autism Research Institute
4182 Adams Avenue
San Diego, CA 92116   619-281-7165
                                Fax: 619-563-6840
                                  www.autism.com

Discusses current research and provides information about the
causes, diagnosis, and treatment of autism and related disorders.

8 pages Quarterly

Stephen Edelson, Executive Director
Jane Johnson, Managing Director
Rebecca McKenney, Office Manager

971 MAAP Newsletter
PO Box 524
Crown Point, IN 46308   219-662-1311
                                Fax: 219-662-0638
                                 chart@netnitco.net
                                www.maapservices.org

Shares information that are not find in textbooks or read in other
sources.

Pamphlets

972 Autism Fact Sheet
NINDS
PO Box 5801
Bethesda, MD 20824   301-496-5751
                                    800-352-9424
                                 TTY: 301-468-5981
                                  www.ninds.nih.gov

Also available in Spanish.

Walter J. Koroshetz, M.D., Acting Director
Alan L. Willard, Ph.D., Acting Deputy Director
Caroline Lewis, Executive Officer

973 Facts About Autism
Indiana Institute on Disability and Community
1905 North Range Rd.
Bloomington, IN 47408   812-855-6508
                                    800-280-7010
                                Fax: 812-855-9630
                                 TTY: 812-855-9396
                                  iidc@indiana.edu
                                 www.iidc.indiana.edu

Provides concise information describing autism, diagnosis, needs
of the person with autism from diagnosis through adulthood. Information on the Autism Society of America chapters in Indiana
is listed in the back, along with a description of the Indiana Resource Center for Autism and suggested books to look for in the
local library. Also available in Spanish.

17 pages

David Mank, Director
Suzie Rimstidt
Susan Gray

974 Pervasive Developmental Disorders
National Inst. of Neurological Disorders/Stroke
31 Center Drive, MSC 2540, Building 31, Room 8A06
Bethesda, MD 20892   301-496-5751
                                    800-352-9424

Detailed booklet that describes symptoms, causes, and treatments,
with information on getting help and coping.

Camps

975 Anchor Point Camp
RBM Ministries
PO Box 128
Plainwell, MI 49080   269-342-9879
                            bobgoodenough@sbcglobal.net
                               www.rbmministries.org

Accepts mentally and physically handicapped children ages 13
and up.

Bob Goodenough, Executive Director

976 Beech Brook
3737 Lander Road
Cleveland, OH 44124   216-831-2255
                                    877-546-1225
                                Fax: 216-831-0436
                                 www.beechbrook.org

A year-round residential and day treatment center, accepts summer residents when there are openings in the regular enrollment.
The program is designed for emotionally disturbed, learning disabled and autistic children, providing therapeutically oriented
teaching and programming techniques in a camp setting.

Don Harris, Director

977 Big Crystal Camp
8533 Williams Road
DeWitt, MI 48820   517-669-9367

One week residential camp sponsored by Lansing Area Chapter
of Michigan Association for Children with Learning Disabilities.

Florence Curtis

978 Camp Buckskin
4124 Quebec Ave N, Ste 300
Minneapolis, MN 55427   763-208-4805
                                Fax: 952-938-6996
                              info@campbuckskin.com
                               www.campbuckskin.com

LD and ADD/ADHD youth have often experienced frustration
and a lack of success. Buckskin assists these individuals to realize and develop the potentials and abilities which they possess.

Thomas R Bauer, CCD, Camp Director

979 Camp Friendship
Friendship Ventures
10509 108th Street NW
Annandale, MN 55302   952-852-0101
                                    800-450-8376
                                Fax: 952-852-0123
                            info@friendshipventures.org
                             www.friendshipventures.org

Camp Friendship offers kids, teens, and adults the chance to have
the time of their lives. The program focuses on building self-esteem and independence, and practicing social skills; and we nurture each person's strengths and abilities and encourage
participation in activies at their own pace. Specially designed for
persons with developmental, physical or multiple disabilities,
special medical conditions, Down syndrome, autism or other conditions. Weekend camps and longer available.

Georgann Rumsey, Vice President, Programs
Laurie Tschetter, Program Director

980 Camp Krem
102 Brook Lane
Boulder Creek, CA 95006   510-222-6662
                                 campkrem@gmail.com
                               www.campingunlimited.com

Camp with year-around recreational activities and summer camping for children and adults with developmental disabilities.

981 Camp Lotsafun
3660 Baker Lane, Suite 103
Reno, NV 89509 775-827-3866
Fax: 775-827-0334
camp@camplotsafun.com
www.camplotsafun.com

Provides recreational, therapeutic, and educational opportunities for individuals with developmental disabilities, while providing respite care for their families.

Jill Gabel, Program Director

982 Camp Merrimack
3320 Triana Boulevard
Huntsville, AL 35805 256-534-6455
ksimari@merrimackhall.com
www.merrimackhall.com

A unique arts half-day camp for children ages 3 through 12; open to children with special needs including Cerebral Palsy, Down Syndrome, autism and others.

Ashley Dinges, Executive Director
Kim Simari, Managing Director

983 Camp New Hope
Friendship Ventures
53035 Lake Avenue
McGregor, MN 55760 952-852-0101
800-450-8376
Fax: 952-852-0123
fv@friendshipventures.org
www.friendshipventures.org

Camp New Hope is a great place for children, teens, and adults to have the time of their lives. The program provides a unique opportunity for having fun, learning skills, boosting confidence, and making friends. Services are specifically designed for persons with developmental, phyisical or multiple disabilities, special medical needs, Down syndrome, autism, or other conditions. Weekend camps and longer available. Other services available throughout the year.

Georgann Rumsey, Vice President, Programs
Laurie Tschetter, Program Director

984 Camp Nuhop
404 Hillcrest Drive
Ashland, OH 44805 419-289-2227
Fax: 419-289-2227
info@campnuhop.org
www.campnuhop.org

A summer residential program for any youngster from 6 to 18 with a learning disability, behavior disorder or Attention Deficit Disorder. Sixty two campers and 35 staff members live on site in groups of 7 campers to every 3 counselors. Activities focus on positive self-concept and behaviors and teach children to learn how to find their strengths, abilities and talents from a positive, yet realistic viewpoint.

Jerry Dunlap, Director

985 Camp Ramah in New England Tikvah Program
39 Bennett Street
Palmer, MA 01609 413-283-9771
Fax: 413-283-6661
info@campramahne.org
www.campramahne.org

The Tikvah program is one of the first summer programs for Jewish children with special needs. It continues to grow and evolve as it strives to serve campers with a wide range of special needs including, but not limited to, congitive impairments, autism, cerebral palsy and seizure disorder.

Howard Blas, Tikvah Program Director
Talya Kalender, Director, Camper Care
Benjamin Greene, Director of Education

986 Crotched Mountain School & Rehabilitation Center
1 Verney Drive
Greenfield, NH 03047 603-547-3311
800-800-966
Fax: 603-547-3232
info@crotchedmountain.org
www.cmf.org

Currently serves children ages 6-22 with multiple-handicaps including: Cerebral Palsy, Spina Bifida, visual and hearing impairments and neurological disabilities, developmental disorders, mental retardation, autism, behavioral and emotional disorders, seizure disorders, spinal cord and head injuries. Member of the National Association of Independent Schools and accredited with the NE Association of Schools and Colleges, Independent Schools of Northern NE.

Rita Phinney, Director Admissions
John Young, Registrar

987 Dallas Academy
950 Tiffany Way
Dallas, TX 75218 214-324-1481
Fax: 214-327-8537
www.dallas-academy.com

7-week summer session for students who are having difficulty in regular school classes.

Jim Richardson, Director

988 Developmental Center
6710 86th Avenue N
Pinellas Park, FL 33782 727-541-5716
Fax: 727-544-8186
infopp@centeracademy.com
www.centeracademy.com

Specifically designed for the learning disabled child and other children with difficulties in concentration, strategy, social skills, impulsivity, distractibility and study strategies. Programs offered include: attention training, visual-motor remediation, socialization skills training, relaxation training, horseback riding and more. The day camp meets weekdays from 9-3 for 3,4 or 5 week sessions.

Dr. Eric Larson

989 Eagle Hill School - Summer Program
242 Old Petersham Road, PO Box 116
Hardwick, MA 01037 413-477-6000
Fax: 413-477-6837
admission@eaglehillschool.com
www.ehs1.org

For the child, age 9-19, with a specific learning disability or Attention Deficit Disorder, this summer program offers a structured curriculum designed to build a basic foundation of academic competence. Extracurricular and outdoor activities complement the educational program.

Erin E Wynne, Dean of Admission

990 Groves Academy
3200 Highway 100 South
Saint Louis Park, MN 55416 952-920-6377
Fax: 952-920-2068
www.grovesacademy.org

A nonprofit day school in Minnesota designed especially for children with learning differences. The Center has a full day academic program from September through June, as well as an 8 week summer program. Groves also offers community services such as: psychoeducational testing for children and adults, consulting services, workshops on learning disabilities and other special learning needs, and afternoon/evening tutorial services for children and adults.

John Alexander, Head of School

991 Hill School of Fort Worth
4817 Odessa Avenue
Fort Worth, TX 817-923-9482
Fax: 817-923-4894
hillschool@hillschool.org
www.hillschool.org

Provides an alternative learning environment for students having average or above-average intelligence with learning differences. Hill school is an established leader in North Texas with a 25 year history of effectively serving LD children. Beginning in 1961 as a tutorial service, Hill became a formal school in 1973. Our mission is to help those who learn differently develop skills and strategies to succeed. We do this by developing academic/study skills, and self-discipline.

John W. Wright, Chairman
Randall Canedy, Vice Chairman
Audrey~ Boda-Davis, Executive Director

992 Kris' Camp
1132 Green Hill Trace
Tallahassee, FL 32317

801-942-1750
Fax: 877-267-9451
info@kriscamp.org
www.kriscamp.org

Therapy intensive/respite camp for children with special needs
(thus far focusing on children with autism/autistic-like challenges) and their families.

Michelle Hardy, Program Director
Leidy Van Ispelen, Assistant Director

993 Lab School of Washington Summer Program
4759 Reservoir Road NW
Washington, DC 20007

202-965-6600
Fax: 202-965-5106
alexandra.freeman@labschool.org
www.labschool.org

The Lab School 5-week summer session includes individualized
reading, spelling, writing, study skills, and math programs. A
multisensory approach addresses the needs of bright learning disabled children. Related services such as speech/language therapy
and occupational therapy are integrated into the curriculum. Ele-
mentary/Intermediate; Junior High/High School.

Sally Smith, Founder
Susan Feeley, Admissions Director

994 Maplebrook School
5142 Route 22
Amenia, NY 12501

845-373-8191
Fax: 845-373-7029
jscully@maplebrookschool.org
www.maplebrookschool.org

A coeductional boarding school for students with learning differences and ADD. A New York State registered high school servicing ages 11-18. Post secondary options offered to 18-21.

Donna M Konkolios, Head of School
Jennifer Scully, Director Admissions

995 Round Lake Camp
21 Plymouth Street
Fairfield, NJ

973-575-3333
800-776-5657
Fax: 973-575-4188
rlc@njycamps.org
www.njycamps.org

For ages 7-18, this camp provides individualized academics in
reading, language development and math for children with mild
learning disabilities, Round Lake also offers therapeutic recreation and Jewish cultural values to its participants.

Sheira Director, Asst. Director

996 Squirrel Hollow
5665 Milam Road
Fairburn, GA 30213

770-774-8001
Fax: 770-774-8005
bbox@thebedfordschool.org
www.thebedfordschool.org

A remedial summer program of The Bedford School; serves children with academic needs due to learning difficulties. For students ages 6-16 and held on the campus of The Bedford School in
Fairburn, GA. Campers participate in an individualized academic
program as well as recreational activities. Students receive the
proper academic remediation as well as specific remedial help
with physical skills, peer interaction and self-esteem.

Betsy E Box, Director
Jeff James, Assistant Director
Bonnie Sides, Administrative Secretary

997 Summer Experience
Vanguard School
PO Box 730
Paoli, PA 19301

610-296-6700
Fax: 610-640-0132
info@vanguardschool-pa.org
www.vanguardschool-pa.org

For students who are experiencing learning difficulties due to
neurological impairment, social/emotional disturbance and/or au-
tism/pervasive developmental disorder.

Susan Snyder, Admissions Director
John D Wilson, Education Director

998 Wesley Woods
1001 Fiddlersgreen Rd
Grand Valley, PA 16420

814-430-7802
Fax: 814-436-7669
www.wesleywoods.com

Exceptional children's camp for children with emotional and intellectual handicaps.

Herb West

999 Worthmore Academy
3535 Kessler Blvd East Drive
Indianapolis, IN 46220

877-700-6516
Fax: 317-251-6516
bjackson@worthmoreacademy.org
www.worthmoreacademy.org

A K-12 non-profit school for children with learning differences
providing educational assessments, alternative educational programs, academic guidance and public awareness services.

Brenda J Jackson, Director
Diana Buser, Assistant

DESCRIPTION

1000 BELL'S PALSY

Involves the following Biologic System(s):

Neurologic Disorders

Bell's palsy is the most common form of facial nerve paralysis and may affect children at any age from infancy through adolescence. The facial nerve, also known as the seventh cranial nerve, arises from a certain area of the brain (i.e., brainstem) and divides into several branches that supply (innervate) the forehead, scalp, eyelids, cheeks, jaws, and muscles of facial expression. The facial nerve also conveys taste sensations from the front two thirds of the tongue. Bell's palsy is a temporary form of facial paralysis that usually develops suddenly approximately two weeks after a widespread viral infection, such as Epstein-Barr virus, herpesvirus, or mumps virus. It is thought to represent a postinfectious demyelination of the facial nerve (neuritis) due to allergic or immune responses.

Bell's palsy typically affects one side of the face and may involve upper and lower areas on the affected side. Symptoms of Bell's palsy usually begin suddenly and reach their peak within 48 hours. Children with the condition may experience weakness or slight paralysis of the upper and lower face; drooping of the corner of the mouth; an inability to close the eye; loss of taste sensations from the front two thirds of the tongue; or abnormal sensitivity to loud sounds (hyperacusis). Because the affected eye may be overexposed to the air, some patients may develop inflammation (exposure keratitis) of the transparent, front region of the eye (cornea). In addition, saliva may dribble from the corner of the mouth and food may tend to collect between the teeth and lips.

There is no cure or standard course of treatment for Bell's palsy. Some cases are mild and do not require treatment since the symptoms usually subside on their own within 2 weeks. For others, treatment may include medications such as acyclovir, used to fight viral infections, combined with an anti-inflammatory drug such as the steroid prednisone, used to reduce inflammation and swelling. Pain medications, such as aspirin, acetaminophen, or ibuprofen may be helpful. Other treatment of children with Bell's palsy is supportive, including eye drops to lubricate the cornea, particularly at night. In over 85 percent of affected children, Bell's palsy spontaneously resolves with no remaining facial weakness. About 10 percent may have mild longstanding weakness, and approximately five percent may experience severe, permanent facial weakness.

Government Agencies

1001 NIH/National Institute of Neurological Disorders and Stroke (NINDS)

PO Box 5801
Bethesda, MD 20824

301-496-5751
800-352-9424
Fax: 301-496-0296
TTY: 301-468-5981
www.ninds.nih.gov

The mission of NINDS is to reduce the burden of neurological disease - a burden borne by every age group, by every segment of society, by people all over the world.

Walter J. Koroshetz, MD, Director

National Associations & Support Groups

1002 American Academy of Otolaryngology-Head and Neck Surgery

1650 Diagonal Road
Alexandria, VA 22314

703-836-4444
Fax: 703-683-5100
TTY: 703-519-1585
webmaster@entnet.org
www.entnet.org

The missions of the AAO-HNS and its foundation are to advance the art and science of otolaryngology-head and neck surgery through state-of-the-art education, research and learning; and to unite, serve and represent the interests of its members and their patients to the public, government, other medical specialists and related organizations. Founded in 1896, the AAO-HNS is the world's largest organization of otolaryngologist-head and neck surgeons.

11,600 Members

James L Netterville, President
Richard W Waguespack MD, President Elect
J. Gavin Setzen MD, Treasurer/Secretary

1003 American Academy of Pediatrics

141 Northwest Point Boulevard
Elk Grove Village, IL 60007

847-434-4000
800-433-9016
Fax: 847-434-8000
www.aap.org

The American Academy of Pediatrics and its member pediatricians are committed to the attainment of optimal physical, mental and social health and well-being for all infants, children, adolescents, and young adults.

Fernando Stein, MD, FAAP, President
Karen Remley, MD, CEO/Executive VP

1004 March of Dimes Foundation

1275 Mamaroneck Avenue
White Plains, NY 10605

914-997-4488
888-663-4637
Fax: 914-997-4763
answers@marchofdimes.com
www.marchofdimes.com

March of Dimes help moms have full-term pregnancies and research the problems that threaten the health of babies. The March of Dimes also acts globally: sharing best practices in perinatal health and helping improve birth outcomes where the needs are the most urgent.

Stacey D. Stewart, President

1005 National Centers for Facial Paralysis

18403 Woodfield Road, Suite D
Gaithersburg, MD 20879

301-330-3223
Fax: 301-330-9075
lgamliel@targangroup.com
www.bellspalsy.com

Strives to evaluate, inform and assist patients with past and/or current history of Facial Palsy, Bell's Palsy, Ramsey-Hunt Syndrome, or Facial Paralysis from surgery, trauma, pregnancy, Lyme disease, or other causes.

Research Centers

1006 Bell's Palsy Research Foundation

19550 Club House Road
Montgomery Village, MD 20886

301-651-9605
Fax: 301-216-2477
drtargan@erols.com
www.bellspalsy.com

An online support foundation for facial palsy patients, providing information and support to patients worldwide; also functions to educate the medical community about facial paralysis and to advance research and development in all aspects of facial palsy and facial pain.

Bob Targen, MD, Director

Conferences

1007 Annual Meeting & OTO Expo
American Academy of Otolaryngology
1650 Diagonal Road
Alexandria, VA 22314

703-836-4444
Fax: 703-683-5100
TTY: 703-519-1585
webmaster@entnet.org
www.entnet.org

Held each fall, with thousands of Academy members, non-member physicians, allied health professionals, administrators, and exhibiting companies attending. It draws more than 6,000 medical experts and professionals from around the world. The conference will feature instruction courses, miniseminars, scientific oral presentations, honorary guest lectures, and numerous scientific posters.

September

James L Netterville, President
J Gavin Setzen, Secretary/Treasurer

Web Sites

1008 American Academy of Otolaryngology Head an d Neck Surgery
www.entnet.org

Mission is to advance the art and science of otolaryngology-head and neck surgery through state-of-the-art education, research and learning.

1009 Bell's Palsy Network
www.bellspalsy.net/

Provides information on facial paralysis, Bell's Palsy, Ramsey Hunt Syndrome and other forms of facial paralysis. We were the first dedicated web portal for Bell's palsy and facial paralysis informaton and host the largest and most popular forum about bell's palsy and facial palsy information.

1010 Bell's Palsy Research Foundation
www.bellspalsyresearch.com

Online support foundation for facial palsy patients, providing information and supprt to patients worldwide.

1011 NIH/National Institute of Neurological Dis orders and Stroke (NINDS)
PO Box 5801
Bethesda, MD 20824

301-496-5751
800-352-9424
www.ninds.nih.gov

Mission is to reduce the burden of neurological disease-a burden borne by every age group, by every segment of society, by people all over the world.

Walter J. Koroshetz, MD, Director

DESCRIPTION

1012 BILIARY ATRESIA

Involves the following Biologic System(s):

Gastrointestinal Disorders

Biliary atresia is a rare condition that is present at birth (congenital) in approximately 1 in 12,500 births, and is characterized by the absence of or the abnormal or incomplete development (hypoplasia) of the bile ducts. These ducts carry bile from the liver and gallbladder into the small intestine. Bile, which is secreted by the liver, is a yellowish or greenish fluid that aids in the digestion of fats. Bile passes through the common bile duct and into the upper portion of the small intestine (duodenum). Absence or underdevelopment of the bile ducts interferes with or prevents the passage of bile into the intestine and, as a result, characteristic findings and symptoms may be noticed within the first few weeks of life.

Symptoms may include progressively darkening urine; pale stools (acholic); a persistent yellowing of the skin, eyes, and mucous membranes (jaundice); and enlargement of the liver (hepatomegaly). If untreated, additional symptoms and findings may become apparent within two or three months. These may include growth retardation, increased irritability, and itching (pruritus). A potential complication of biliary atresia involves an increase in pressure in the vein that conveys blood from the spleen, stomach, pancreas, and intestine to the liver (portal hypertension). In addition, untreated biliary atresia may result in a life-threatening condition known as biliary cirrhosis, in which the liver's function is impaired and, eventually, the liverbecomes irreversibly damaged.

Treatment for biliary atresia is often determined by the site of the obstruction and includes various surgical procedures. In some infants, surgery may be performed as a means to help postpone cirrhosis and growth retardation until liver transplantation is feasible.

National Associations & Support Groups

1013 American Academy of Pediatrics
141 Northwest Point Boulevard
Elk Grove Village, IL 60007

847-434-4000
800-433-9016
Fax: 847-434-8000
www.aap.org

The American Academy of Pediatrics and its member pediatricians are committed to the attainment of optimal physical, mental and social health and well-being for all infants, children, adolescents, and young adults.

Fernando Stein, MD, FAAP, President
Karen Remley, MD, CEO/Executive VP

1014 American Association for the Study of Liver Diseases
1001 North Fairfax Street Suite 400
Alexandria, VA 22314

703-299-9766
Fax: 703-299-9622
aasld@aasld.org
www.aasld.org

To Advance the Science and Practice of Hepatology, Liver Transplantation and Hepatobiliary Surgery, Thereby Promoting Liver Health and Optimal Care of Patients with Liver and Biliary Tract Diseases.

Anna S. Lok, MD, President
Ronald J. Sokol, MD, President Elect
Bruce A. Luxon, MD, Treasurer

1015 CHARGE Syndrome Foundation
318 Half Day Rd, #305
Buffalo Grove, IL 60089

516-684-4720
800-442-7604
Fax: 888-317-4735
info@chargesyndrome.org
www.chargesyndrome.org

The mission of the CHARGE Syndrome Foundation is to provide support to individuals with CHARGE syndrome and their families; to gather, develop, maintain and distribute information about CHARGE syndrome; and to promote awareness and research regarding its identification, cause and management.

David Wolfe, President
Sheri Stanger, Director of Outreach
Lisa Weir, Vice President

1016 Children's Liver Association for Support Services
PO Box 15061
Monaca, PA 15061

724-888-2568
info@classkids.org
www.classkids.org

CLASS is an all volunteer, nonprofit organization dedicated to serving the emotional, educational and financial needs of families coping with childhood liver disease and transplantation. Our goal is to be both a service to families and a valuable resource for the medical community.

Diane Sumner, Co-Founder
Mark Sumner, Co-Founder
Aimee Seningen, MD, Treasurer

1017 Genetic Alliance
4301 Connecticut Avenue NW, Suite 404
Washington, DC 20008

202-966-5557
800-336-4363
Fax: 202-966-8553
info@geneticalliance.org
www.geneticalliance.org

World's leading nonprofit health advocacy organization committed to transforming health through genetics and promoting an environment of openness centered on the health of individuals, families, and communities.

Sharon Terry, President/CEO
Tetyana Murza, Managing Director
Natasha Bonhomme, VP, Strategic Development

Research Centers

1018 Clinical Research Center, Pediatrics
Children's Hospital Research Foundation
3333 Burnett Avenue
Cincinnati, OH 45229

513-636-4200
800-344-2462
Fax: 513-636-7151
TTY: 513-636-4900
www.cincinnatichildrens.org

Cincinnati Children's will improve child health and transform delivery of care through fully integrated, globally recognized research, education and innovation

Michael Fisher, President and CEO
Steve Davis, COO
Margaret Hostetter, MD, Pediatrics Chair/Dir, Research Fdtn

1019 Univ. of Texas-Southwestern Med. Ctr. at D allas - Clinical Ctr. for Liver Disease
5323 Harry Hines Boulevard
Dallas, TX 75390

214-648-3111
Fax: 214-648-3715
LIVER@UTSouthwestern.edu
www.utsouthwestern.edu/about-us/contact-us.html

To achieve optimal outcomes for patients with a variety of liver disorders, including but not limited to Hepatitis B, C, and acute liver failure.

Dr. William Lee, Director
Dr Marlyn Mayo, Specialist

Conferences

1020 CHARGE Syndrome Conference
318 Half Day Rd, #305
Buffalo Grove, IL 60089
516-684-4720
800-442-7604
Fax: 888-317-4735
conference@chargesyndrome.org
www.chargesyndrome.org

Annual conference sponsored by CHARGE (Coloboma, Heart Malformations, Atresia Choanae, Retardation, Genital Abnormalities, Ear Abnormalities). Includes exhibitors, workshops, and networking for professionals, patients and parents.

July

Jackie Alshawabkeh, Development

1021 Genetic Alliance Annual Conference
Genetic Alliance
4301 Connecticut Avenue NW, Suite 404
Washington, DC 20008
202-966-5557
800-336-4363
Fax: 202-966-8553
info@geneticalliance.org
www.geneticalliance.org

Consistently inspirational and enables partnership among all stakeholders: advocates and community leaders, health and industry professionals, policymakers, and academicians.

July

Sharon Terry, President/CEO
Tetyana Murza, Managing Director
Natasha Bonhomme, VP, Strategic Development

1022 International CHARGE Syndrome Conference
CHARGE Syndrome Foundation
141 Middle Neck Rd
Sands Point, NY 11050
516-684-4720
800-442-7604
Fax: 516-883-9060
marion@chargesyndrome.org
www.chargesyndrome.org

July

Marion Norbury, Executive Director

Web Sites

1023 Children's Liver Association for Support Services
www.classkids.org

CLASS is an all volunteer, nonprofit organization dedicated to serving the emotional, educational and financial needs of families coping with childhood liver disease and transplantation. Our goal is to be both a service to families and a valuable resource for the medical community.

1024 Online Mendelian Inheritance in Man
National Library of Medicine, Building 38A
Bethesda, MD 20894
888-346-3656
info@ncbi.nlm.nih.gov
www.ncbi.nlm.nih.gov

This database is a catalog of human genes and genetic disorders.

Christine E. Seidman, M.D., Chair
David J. Lipman, M.D., Executive Secretary

Book Publishers

1025 Liver Disease in Children
Lippincott Williams & Wilkins
530 Walnut Street
Philadelphia, PA 19106
215-521-8300
Fax: 215-521-8902
www.lww.com

This is a difinitive book on pediatric liver disease, providing extensive, well-edited information that is not easily accessible or available in other textbooks. A must-have for those interested in this rapidly growing subspecialty in pediatrics.

2000 1008 pages
ISBN: 0-781720-98-2

Pamphlets

1026 Biliary Atresia
American Liver Foundation
39 Broadway, Suite 2700
New York, NY 10006
212-668-1000
Fax: 212-483-8179
www.liverfoundation.org

Pamphlet with information and symptoms on biliary atresia

Tom Nealon, Chair
David Ticker, Chief Financial Officer
Lynn Seim, Chief Operating Officer

1027 Facts on Liver Transplantation
American Liver Foundation
39 Broadway, Suite 2700
New York, NY 10006
212-668-1000
800-223-0179
Fax: 212-483-8179
www.liverfoundation.org

Provides information on liver transplantation, and the effects.

Tom Nealon, Chair
David Ticker, Chief Financial Officer
Lynn Seim, Chief Operating Officer

DESCRIPTION

1028 BIPOLAR DISORDER

Synonyms: Manic-depressive disorder, Manic-depressive illness, Manic-depressive psychosis

Involves the following Biologic System(s):

Developmental/Behavioral/Psychiatric Disorders

Bipolar disorder, also known as manic-depressive disorder, is a condition characterized by alternating depression and mania or, in rare cases, mania alone. The disorder is thought to affect less than two percent of the general population. Although bipolar disorder usually becomes apparent during the third or fourth decade of life, a significant proportion of individuals are initially affected in childhood, adolescence, or early adulthood. Individuals with bipolar disorder may initially experience either a depressive or a manic episode. In some affected children and adolescents, manic episodes may be more frequent than depressive episodes during the first years of their illness. However, as the disease progresses, episodes of depression may become more frequent than manic episodes. Bipolar disorder is often further classified as unipolar in cases in which only depression is experienced and bipolar when mania occurs, with or without depression. In addition, mixed affected states are characterized by the occurrence of depressive and manic symptoms during a single episode.

In children and adolescents with bipolar disorder, associated symptoms resemble those seen in affected adults. Depressive states usually emerge gradually and may be characterized by feelings of sadness, despair, hopelessness, and discouragement; loss of self-esteem; physical and emotional exhaustion; and lack of interest of formerly enjoyed activities. In severe cases, affected individuals may have suicidal tendencies, and hospitalization in a pediatric, general, or psychiatric facility may be essential. In such cases, consultation with child psychiatrists is important for ongoing support and decision-making regarding treatment options.

In affected children and adolescents, manic states may be characterized by overactivity (hyperactivity); excessive talking; inability to sleep (insomnia); impulsive behavior and impaired judgment that may result in reckless spending; elation that may quickly change to irritability and anger; personal neglect that may result in poor hygiene; and, in some cases, delusions of grandeur and persecution (paranoid delusions). Initial episodes of depression or mania often last approximately six months without treatment. Although most manic or depressive episodes usually cease in months, some individuals may be affected for longer periods.

Adolescents with bipolar disorder may be misdiagnosed, e.g., with a psychotic disorder characterized by disturbances in behavior, cognition, and emotional reactions (schizophrenia) or a maladjusted reaction to a stressful life event (adjustment disorder). However, most affected individuals are correctly diagnosed with bipolar disorder during adulthood. According to reports in the literature, the earlier the onset of bipolar disorder, the more susceptible affected individuals may be to frequent episodes, rapid cycling between depressive and manic states, and severe episodes that may result in suicidal tendencies. In addition, earlier onset of the disorder is often associated with an increased incidence of depression and bipolar disorder in immediate (first-degree) relatives.

The treatment of children and adolescents with bipolar disorder may include therapy with certain medications (e.g., lithium carbonate, carbamazepine) and integrated, multidisciplinary management (e.g., behavioral therapy; individual, family, or group psychodynamic therapy; etc.). In children and adolescents with the disorder, thorough patient and family histories and specific medical evaluations are typically conducted before medications are prescribed. Pretreatment evaluation for lithium may include assessment of electrolyte levels, and kidney (renal) and thyroid function. Pretreatment evaluation for tricyclic antidepressants may include a cardiovascular examination including electrocardiography. If such medications are prescribed, regular blood levels should be taken until an adequate dose is determined.

Other treatment options include antipsychotics or tranquilizers if agitation or psychotic symptoms are present, especially at the initiation of treatment when acute manic episodes are likely. Recent studies have shown that about 80% of patients treated with electroconvulsive therapy (ECT) experienced improvement, and for some, it was the only treatment that worked. The exact cause of bipolar disorder is unknown. However, many researchers agree that genetic abnormalities may play some role in the etiology of the disorder.

Government Agencies

1029 Center for Mental Health Services Knowledge Exchange Network
US Department of Health and Human Services
PO Box 42557
Washington, DC 20015

800-789-2647
Fax: 240-747-5470
TDD: 866-889-2647
www.mentalhealth.samhsa.gov

Supplies the public with responses to their commonly asked questions about mental health issues and services.

1030 NIH/National Institute of Mental Health
6001 Executive Boulevard, Room 6200, MSC 9663
Bethesda, MD 20892

301-443-4536
866-615-6464
Fax: 301-443-4279
TTY: 301-443-8431
nimhinfo@nih.gov
www.nimh.nih.gov

The mission of NIMH is to transform the understanding and treatment of mental illnesses through basic and clinical research, paving the way for prevention, recovery, and cure.

Joshua Gordon, MD, PhD, Director
Shelli Avenevoli, MD, Deputy Director

National Associations & Support Groups

1031 American Academy of Pediatrics
141 Northwest Point Boulevard
Elk Grove Village, IL 60007

847-434-4000
800-433-9016
Fax: 847-434-8000
www.aap.org

The American Academy of Pediatrics and its member pediatricians are committed to the attainment of optimal physical, mental and social health and well-being for all infants, children, adolescents, and young adults.

Fernando Stein, MD, FAAP, President
Karen Remley, MD, CEO/Executive VP

1032 American Counseling Association
6101 Stevenson Ave
Alexandria, VA 22304
703-823-9800
800-347-6647
Fax: 703-823-0252
webmaster@counseling.org
www.counseling.org

Represents professional counselors in various practice settings, and stands ready to serve more than 55,000 members with the resources they need to make a difference. From webinars, publications, and journals to Conference education sessions and legislative action alerts, ACA is where counseling professionals turn for powerful, credible content and support.

Robert L. Smith, President

1033 American Group Psychotherapy Association
25 East 21st St, 6th Floor
New York, NY 10010
212-477-2677
Fax: 212-979-6627
info@agpa.org
www.agpa.org

The American Group Psychotherapy Association is a dynamic, thriving community of mental health professionals of all disciplines dedicated to advancing knowledge and research, and providing quality training in group psychotherapy and other group interventions, consultation and direct services nationally and internationally.

Les R. Greene, Ph.D., President
Marsha S. Block, CAE, CFRE, Chief Executive Officer
Diane C. Feirman, CAE, Public Affairs Senior Director

1034 American Mental Health Counselors Association
801 N. Fairfax Street, Suite 304
Alexandria, VA 22314
703-548-6002
800-326-2642
Fax: 703-548-4775
sgiunta@troy.edu
www.amhca.org

The American Mental Health Counselors Association (AMHCA) is a national organization for licensed clinical mental health counselors. AMHCA strives to be the go-to organization for LCMHCs for education, advocacy, leadership and collaboration.

Stephen A. Giunta, Ph.D., President
Keith Mobley, Ph.D., President-Elect
Joel Miller, Executive Director/ CEO

1035 American Psychiatric Association
1000 Wilson Boulevard, Suite 1825
Arlington, VA 22209
703-907-7300
888-35-7924
apa@psych.org
www.psychiatry.org

It is a medical specialty society representing growing membership of more than 36,000 psychiatrists.

1036 American Psychiatric Nurses Association
3141 Fairview Park Drive, Suite 625
Falls Church, VA 22042
571-533-1919
855-863-2762
Fax: 855-883-2762
ncroce@apna.org
www.apna.org

The American Psychiatric Nurses Association (APNA) is a professional association organized to advance the science and education of psychiatric-mental health nursing. It is committed to the specialty practice of psychiatric-mental health nursing, health, wellness and recovery promotion through identification of mental health issues, prevention of mental health problems and the care and treatment of persons with psychiatric disorders.

Nicholas Croce, Jr., MS, Executive Director
Patricia L. Black, PhD, RN, Associate Executive Director
Lisa Deffenbaugh Nguyen, Director of Operations

1037 American Psychoanalytic Association
309 E 49th St
New York, NY 10017
212-752-0450
deankstein@apsa.org
www.apsa.org

APsaA as a professional organization for psychoanalysts, focuses on education, research and membership development.

Mark Smaller, Ph.D., President
Dean K. Stein, Executive Director
Tina Faison, Admin Assis to Executive Director

1038 American Psychological Association
750 First St. NE
Washington, DC 20002
202-336-5500
800-374-2721
TTY: 202-336-6123
www.apa.org

The mission is to advance the creation, communication and application of psychological knowledge to benefit society and improve people's lives.

Norman B. Anderson, PhD, CEO/ EVP
L. Michael Honaker, PhD, Deputy Chief Executive Officer
Ellen G. Garrison, PhD, Senior Policy Advisor

1039 Anxiety and Depression Association of America
8701 Georgia Ave., Suite #412
Silver Spring, MD 20910
240-485-1001
Fax: 240-485-1035
www.adaa.org

ADAA is a national nonprofit organization dedicated to the prevention, treatment, and cure of anxiety, depression, OCD, PTSD, and related disorders and to improving the lives of all people who suffer from them through education, practice, and research.

Mark H. Pollack, MD, President
Alies Muskin, Executive Director
Jean Kaplan Teichroew, Communications Director

1040 Association for Psychological Science
1133 15th Street, NW, Suite 1000
Washington, DC 20005
202-293-9300
Fax: 202-293-9350
www.psychologicalscience.org

The Association for Psychological Science (previously the American Psychological Society) is a nonprofit organization dedicated to the advancement of scientific psychology and its representation at the national and international level.

Nancy Eisenberg, President
Alan Kraut, Executive Director
Sarah Brookhart, Deputy Director

1041 Brain & Behavior Research Foundation
90 Park Avenue, 16th Floor
New York, NY 10016
646-681-4888
800-829-8289
info@bbrfoundation.org
bbrfoundation.org

The Brain & Behavior Research Foundation is committed to alleviating the suffering caused by mental illness by awarding grants that will lead to advances and breakthroughs in scientific research.

Steve Lieber, Chairman of the Board
Suzanne Golden, Vice President
Jeffrey Borenstein, M.D., President/ CEO

1042 Center for Psychiatric Rehabilitation
940 Commonwealth Ave. West
Boston, MA 2215
617-353-3549
Fax: 617-358-3066
psyrehab@bu.edu
cpr.bu.edu

The Center is a research, training, and service organization dedicated to improving the lives of persons who have psychiatric disabilities.

Kim T. Mueser, Executive Director
Deborah Dolan, Director of Operations
Dori Hutchinson, Director of Services

1043 College of Psychiatric and Neurologic Pharmacists
8055 O Street, Suite S113
Lincoln, NE 68510
402-476-1677
Fax: 888-551-7617
info@cpnp.org
cpnp.org

As the voice of the specialty, there mission is to advance the reach and practice of neuropsychiatric pharmacists.

Steven Burghart, DPh, MBA, BCPP, President
Ray Love, President-Elect
Julie Dopheide, PharmD, BCPP, Past President

1044 Depression and Bipolar Support Alliance
730 N Franklin Street, Suite 501
Chicago, IL 60654
800-826-3632
Fax: 312-642-7243
www.dbsalliance.org

Patient-directed organization focusing on the most prevalent mental illnesses- depression and bipolar disorder. Fosters an understanding about the impact and management of these life-threatening illnesses by providing up-to-date, scientifically-based tools and information written in language the general public can understand.

Lucinda Jewell ED. M, Chair
Rev. Cheryl T. Magrini, Ph.D., Vice Chair
Christy B. Beckmann,, Treasurer

1045 Families for Depression Awareness
395 Totten Pond Road, Suite 404
Waltham, MA 2451
781-890-0220
Fax: 781-890-2411
www.familyaware.org

Families for Depression Awareness is a national nonprofit organization helping families recognize and cope with depression and bipolar disorder to get people well and prevent suicides.

Julie Totten, Founder
Valerie Cordero, Interim Co-Executive Director
Susan Weinstein, Interim Co-Executive Director

1046 Federation of Families for Children's Mental Health
9605 Medical Center Drive, Suite 280
Rockville, MD 20850
240-403-1901
Fax: 240-403-1909
ffcmh@ffcmh.org
www.ffcmh.org

The National family run organization is dedicated exclusively to helping children with mental health needs and their families achieve a better quality of life.

Teka Dempson, President
Sherri Luthe, Vice President
Sheila Pires, Treasurer

1047 Juvenile Bipolar Research Foundation
277 Martine Avenue, Suite 226
White Plains, NY 10601
info@jbrf.org
www.jbrf.org

JBRF is a 501(c)(3) organization that actively promotes and supports scientific research focused on the cause of and treatments for bipolar disorder in children.

Charles Goldberg, Director of Development

1048 Kristin Brooks Hope Center
1250 24th Street NW, Suite 300
Washington, DC 20037
800-442-HOPE
Fax: 202-536-3206
reese@hopeline.com
www.hopeline.com

Since the suicide of his wife Kristin in April 1998, KBHC Founder Reese Butler has been on a personal crusade. His mission the past 11 years has been to offer HOPE and the option to LIVE to those in the deepest emotional pain.

H. Reese Butler II, President/ CEO
Richard Rossell, Treasurer

1049 Mental Health America
500 Montgomery Street, Ste 820
Alexandria, VA 22314
703-684-7722
800-969-6642
Fax: 703-684-5968
TTY: 800-433-5959
info@mentalhealthamerica.net
www.mentalhealthamerica.net

Addresses all aspects of mental health and mental illness. NMHA with over 340 affiliates works to improve the mental health of all Americans.

Paul Gionfriddo, President/CEO
Shavonne Carpenter, Sr Assoc., Support & Services
Mallory Pernell, Assoc. Dir, Comments/Marketing

1050 National Alliance for the Mentally Ill
3803 N. Fairfax Dr., Suite 100
Arlington, VA 22203
703-525-7600
800-950-6264
Fax: 703-524-9094
TDD: 703-516-7227
info@nami.org
www.nami.org

NAMI is a nonprofit, grassroots, self-help, support and advocacy organization of consumers, families and friends of people with severe mental illness, such as schizophrenia, bipolar disorder, major depressive disorder, obsessive compulsive disorder, anxiety disorders, autism and other severe and persistent mental illnesses that affect the brain.

Keris J,,n Myrick, President
Kevin B Sullivan, First Vice President
Jim Payne, Second Vice President

1051 National Association of State Mental Health Program Directors
66 Canal Center Plaza, Suite 302
Alexandria, VA 22314
703-739-9333
Fax: 703-548-9517
webmaster@nasmhpd.org
www.nasmhpd.org

National Association of State Mental Health Program Directors (NASMHPD) represents the $37.6 billion public mental health service delivery system serving 7.1 million people annually in all 50 states, 4 territories, and the District of Columbia.

Jay Meek, CPA, MBA, Chief Financial Officer
Robert W. Glover, PhD, Executive Director
David Miller, MPAff, Project Director

1052 National Council for Behavioral Health
1400 K Street NW, Suite 400
Washington, DC 20005
202-684-7457
Communications@TheNationalCouncil.org
www.thenationalcouncil.org

The National Council for Behavioral Health (National Council) is the unifying voice of America's community mental health and addictions treatment organizations.

Linda Rosenberg, President/ CEO
Jeannie Campbell, EVP/ COO
Heather Cobb, Vice President, Communications

1053 The Jed Foundation
1140 Broadway, Ste. 803
New York, NY 10001
212-647-7544
Fax: 212-647-7542
www.jedfoundation.org

The Jed Foundation's mission is to promote emotional health and prevent suicide among college and university students.

John MacPhee, Executive Director/ CEO
Dr. Victor Dr. Schwartz, Medical Director
Dr. Nance Roy, Clinical Director

1054 The Ryan Licht Sang Bipolar Foundation
875 N. Michigan Avenue, Suite 3100
Chicago, IL 60611
888-944-4408
www.ryanlichtsangbipolarfoundation.org

The Ryan Licht Sang Bipolar Foundation is dedicated to fostering awareness, understanding and research for early-onset Bipolar Disorder.

Joyce Licht Sang, Founder Director
Jaynee Licht Luntz, Founder Director
Joyce Licht Sang, President

State Agencies & Support Groups

1055 Center for Family Support
333 7th Avenue, #901
New York, NY 10001
Fax: 212-629-7939
Fax: 212-239-2211
svernikoff@cfsny.org
www.cfsny.org

The Center for Family (CFS) is a not-for-profit human service agency providing support and assistance to individuals with developmental disabilities and traumatic brain injuries throughout New York City, Long Island, the lower Hudson Valley region and New Jersey.

Steven Vernikoff, Executive Director
Linda Schellenberg, Director, Community Service
Barbara Greenwald, Associate Executive Director

1056 Depressive and Manic-Depressive Assocation of Mount Sinai
100 LaSalle Street, Suite 5A
New York, NY 10027
917-445-2399
jgg17@columbia.edu
www.columbia.edu/~jgg17/DMDA/PAGE_1.html

The NYC Depressive and Manic-Depressive Group is a support group for persons with mood disorders, depression and bipolar disorder, as well as their family members and friends.

Research Centers

1057 National Alliance for Research on Schizophrenia and Depression
60 Cutter Mill Road, Suite 404
Great Neck, NY 11021
516-829-0091
800-829-8289
Fax: 516-487-6930
info@bbrfoundation.org.
www.bbrfoundation.org/

NARSAD raises and distributes funds for scientific research into the causes, cures, treatments, and prevention of severe mental illnesses, primarily schizophrenia.

Steve Lieber, Chairman of the Board
Suzanne Golden, Vice President
Arthur Radin, Treasurer

Conferences

1058 DBSA National Conference
Depression and Bipolar Support Alliance
730 N Franklin Street, Suite 501
Chicago, IL 60654
800-826-3632
Fax: 312-642-7243
www.dbsalliance.org

Offers a unique peer-centered conference for individuals living with depression or bipolar disorder, as well as for family members or health care providers looking for ways to best help their loved ones, patients, or clients by partnering with them on their path to recovery. The conference consists of compelling keynote presentations, educational workshops, and pre-conference institutes.

Lucinda Jewel, Chair
Rev. Cheryl T Magrini, Vice Chair
Mike Kuhl, Secretary

1059 FFCMH Annual Conference
Federation of Families for Childrens Mental Health
9605 Medical Center Drive, Suite 280
Rockville, MD 20850
240-403-1901
Fax: 240-403-1909
ffcmh@ffcmh.org
www.ffcmh.org

Address the complex issue of trauma; the impact it has on children and families; the promotion of healing and prevention strategies; knowledge about how to address trauma through resiliency-based interventions, utilizing a familydriven, youth guided approach; and examples of how family organizations and the partners they work with are raising awareness and improving trauma-focused services and supports.

November

Teka Dempson, President
Sherri Luthe, Vice President
Sheila Pires, Treasurer

1060 NAMI Convention
National Alliance on Mental Illness
3803 N Fairfax Drive, Suite 100
Arlington, VA 22203
703-524-7600
888-999-6264
Fax: 703-524-9094
TDD: 703-516-7227
info@nami.org
www.nami.org

The NAMI Convention is packed with information, chances to network, leadership development opportunities, and lots more.

July

Keris Jan Myrik, President
Kevin B Sullivan, Vice President
Clarence Jordan, Secretary

Audio Video

1061 Families Coping with Mental Illness
Mental Illness Education Project
25 West Street
Westborough, MA 1581
USA
617-562-1111
800-343-5540
Fax: 617-779-0061
info@miepvideos.org
miepvideos.org

Ten family members share their experiences of having a family member with schizophrenia or bipolar disorder. Designed to provide insights and support to other families, the tape also profoundly conveys to professionals the needs of families when mental illness strikes. In two versions: a 22-minute version ideal for short classes and workshops, and a richer 43-minute version with more examples and details. Discounted price for families/consumers.

Video

Michael M Faenza, Executive Director

Web Sites

1062 Bipolar World
www.bipolarworld.net

A support and educational web site for individuals diagnosed with Bipolar Affective Disorder and for the families and friends who care for them.

1063 CyberPsych
www.cyberpsych.org

CyberPsych presents information about psychoanalysis, psychotherapy, and special topics such as anxiety disorder, the problematic use of alcohol, homophobia, and the traumatic effects of racism. CyberPsych is a nonprofit network which offers free web hosting and technical support for internet communication to nonprofit groups and individuals.

Carol Lindemann, Ph.D., Contact

1064 Internet Mental Health
www.mentalhealth.com

Our goal is to improve understanding, diagnosis, and treatment of mental illness throughout the world.

Phillip W. Long, M.D., Psychiatrist

1065 Mental Health Net
P.O. Box 20709
Columbus, OH 43220   614-448-4055
                                       info@centersite.net
                                       www.mentalhelp.net

We wish to provide the following: to discuss, develop and debate
in an open forum the future of the mental health field in America
and throughout the world. To help coordinate various components
of the mental health field so as to bring about greater communication between them.

1066 Planetpsych
www.planetpsych.com

                                       webmaster@planetpsych.com
                                       www.planetpsych.com

Online resource for mental health information.

Book Publishers

1067 Bipolar Disorders: A Guide to Helping Children & Adolescents
O'Reilly and Associates
1005 Gravenstein Highway N
Sebastopol, CA 95472   707-827-7019
                                       800-998-8969
                                       Fax: 707-824-8268
                                       patientguides@oreilly.com
                                       www.patientcenters.com

A million children and adolescents in the US may have child-
hood-onset bipolar disorder, including an estimated 23 percent of
those currently diagnosed with ADHD. Bipolar Disorders helps
parents and professionals recognize, treat, and cope with bipolar
disorders in children and adolescents. It covers diagnosis, family
life, medications, talk therapies, other interventions (improving
sleep patterns, diet, preventing seasonal mood swings), insurance
and school.

1999 460 pages
ISBN: 1-565926-56-0

1068 Bipolar Puzzle Solutions
Taylor & Francis
7625 Empire Drive
Florence, KT 41042   800-634-7064
                                       Fax: 800-248-4724
                                       orders@taylorandfrancis.com
                                       www.taylorandfrancis.com

187 answers to questions asked by support group members about
living with manic depressive illness.

ISBN: 1-560324-93-7

1069 Covert Modeling and Reinforcement
New Harbinger Publications
5674 Shattuck Avenue
Oakland, CA 94609   510-652-0215
                                       800-748-6273
                                       Fax: 800-652-1613
                                       customreservice@newharbinger.com
                                       www.newharbinger.com

Audio programs based on our essential book of cognitive behavioral techniques for effecting change in your life, Thoughts &
Feelings. Listeners learn step-by-step protocols for controlling
destructive behaviors such anxiety, obessional thinking, uncontrolled anger, and depression.

ISBN: 0-934986-29-0

**1070 Touched with Fire-Manic Depressive Illness & the Artistic
Temperament**
Free Press
866 3rd Avenue
New York, NY 10022
USA   212-832-2101
                                       800-323-7445
                                       Fax: 800-943-9831
                                       www.simonsays.com

Describing and discussing the markedly increased rates of severe
mood disorders and suicides among the artistically creative and
the reasons why.

384 pages
ISBN: 0-684831-83-X

Newsletters

1071 Outreach
Depression and Bipolar Support Alliance
55 E. Jackson Blvd, Suite 490
Chicago, IL 60604   800-826-3632
                                       Fax: 312-642-7243
                                       www.dbsalliance.org

Quarterly publication serving members and constituents of the organization. National DMDA educates patients, families, professionals, and the public concerning the nature of depressive and
manic-depressive illnesses as treatable medical diseases; fosters
self-help for patients and families; eliminates discrimination and
stigma; improves access to care; advocates for research toward
the elimination of these illnesses.

Cheryl T. Magrini, Chair
Allen Doederlein, President
Cindy Specht, Executive Vice President

Pamphlets

1072 Bipolar Disorder
National Institutes of Health
9000 Rockville Pike
Bethesda, MD 20892   301-443-3706
                                       Fax: 301-443-6349
                                       www.nih.gov

A short booklet offering a concise description of this disorder,
which is also called manic-depressive illness.

Francis S. Collins, Director

1073 Child and Adolescent Bipolar Disorder
Child and Adolescent Bipolar Foundation
730 N. Franklin Street, Suite 501
Chicago, IL 60654   312-642-0049
                                       Fax: 847-920-9498
                                       info@thebalancedmind.org
                                       www.thebalancedmind.org

To educate families, professsionals and the public about early onset bipolar disorder.

Julia Small, Staff Leader
Karen Cruise, Volunteer Leaders
Kathy Karle, Support Network Coordinator

1074 Mood Disorders
Center for Mental Health Services
PO Box 42557
Washington, DC 20015   800-789-2647
                                       Fax: 240-747-5470
                                       TDD: 866-889-2647
                                       nmhic-info@samhsa.hhs.gov
                                       http://mentalhealth.samhsa.gov

This fact sheet provides basic information on the symptoms, formal diagnosis, and treatment for bipolar disorder.

3 pages

DESCRIPTION

1075 BRAIN TUMORS
Involves the following Biologic System(s):
Neurologic Disorders

Brain tumors are abnormal growths in or on the brain. They may be cancerous (malignant) or noncancerous (benign), and may be classified as primary tumors that arise directly from brain tissue or as secondary tumors, which are almost always malignant and have spread or metastasized to the brain from cancers in other parts of the body. By contrast, tumors that begin in the brain or spinal cord rarely spread to other parts of the body.

All types of brain tumors, whether they are primary tumors that begin within the brain or secondary tumors that spread to the brain, originate from aberrations or mutations in the genes of a cell, causing the cell to divide and replicate itself into the large numbers of identical cells that constitute a tumor.

Space-occupying benign tumors may also present complications resulting from increasing intracranial pressure. Symptoms and characteristic findings associated with brain tumors depend upon their location as well as their size and rate of growth. However, many symptoms are common to most types of brain tumors and may include recurrent or constant headache, irregularities of vision, difficulties in balance and the coordination of voluntary movements, muscle weakness, speech difficulties, and sometimes seizures. Nausea, vomiting, fever, and fluctuations in pulse rate, breathing rate, and blood pressure may be later and more foreboding manifestations. Although there are many different types of brain tumors, children are most commonly affected by primary tumors, especially those that develop toward the back of the brain (posterior fossa tumor).

The most common of the posterior fossa tumors in children is the cerebellar astrocytoma. This type of tumor may be fluid-filled (cystic) or relatively solid and may often have a low grade of malignancy. However, cerebellar astrocytomas may sometimes invade the fibers on each side of the cerebellum that connect with other areas of the brain as well as the spinal cord (cerebellar peduncles). Symptoms and findings may include an abnormal accumulation of cerebrospinal fluid, often under increased pressure, within the skull (hydrocephalus) that is characterized by an increase in head size in infants as well as irritability, vomiting, lethargy, irregular reflex action, and leg rigidity followed by drowsiness and seizures. Older children may have a headache and may vomit, lose coordination, and exhibit deteriorating mental capabilities. Effective treatment for low-grade cerebellar astrocytoma includes surgical removal. Radiation treatment may be indicated for children with cerebellar astrocytoma of high-grade malignancy or in children who exhibit evidence of tumor growth after surgery.

Medulloblastoma is the second most common of the posterior fossa tumors in children and, in children younger than seven years of age, is the most common brain tumor. This type of malignant tumor usually grows relatively fast and spreads to other parts of the brain, the spinal cord, and sometimes other areas of the body. Symptoms associated with medulloblastoma may include headache, recurrent vomiting, and frequent falling. Diagnosis is achieved through imaging studies such as magnetic resonance imaging (MRI) or computer tomography (CT scan) which give a detailed picture of the size and extent of the tumor. Treatment may include surgical excision. In addition, children older than four years of age may receive radiation therapy, especially if the tumor is small and has not yet spread. Children who have evidence of some remaining tumor growth after surgery and those whose tumor has spread may benefit from chemotherapy in addition to further surgery and radiation therapy. Due to the possibility of adverse effects on the brain, radiation is delayed in very young children with medulloblastoma.

Craniopharyngioma is a tumor that appears most often in children and adolescents, and arises from the pituitary, an endocrine gland that is located at the base of the skull. This type of tumor may sometimes interfere with pituitary gland and other endocrine functions as well as cause compression resulting in hydrocephalus and its associated symptoms. Other findings may include headache, vomiting, irregularities in vision, and short stature resulting from hormonal irregularities. Treatment for craniopharyngioma includes surgical excision. Additional treatment with radiation may be indicated for those children whose tumor is not able to be completely removed through surgery or who experience a recurrence. Subsequent to surgery, some children may develop such hormonal abnormalities as an underactive thyroid (hypothyroidism), growth hormone deficiency, diabetes insipidus, and other problems. Evaluation for these hormonal disorders is indicated and treatment is dependent upon the particular abnormality.

Government Agencies

1076 NIH/National Cancer Institute
BG 9609 / 9609 Medical Center Drive
Bethesda, MD 20892   800-422-6237
                                      www.cancer.gov

The National Cancer Institute coordinates the National Cancer Program, which conducts and supports research, training, health information dissemination, and other programs with respect to the cause, diagnosis, prevention, and treatment of cancer, rehabilitation from cancer, and the continuing care of cancer patients and the families of cancer patients.

Douglas R. Lowy, MD, Acting Director
James Doroshow, MD, Deputy Director
Henry P. Ciolino, PhD, Acting Director, Cancer Centers

1077 NIH/National Institute of Neurological Disorders and Stroke (NINDS)
PO Box 5801
Bethesda, MD 20824   301-496-5751
                                      800-352-9424
                                      Fax: 301-496-0296
                                      TTY: 301-468-5981
                                      www.ninds.nih.gov

The mission of NINDS is to reduce the burden of neurological disease - a burden borne by every age group, by every segment of society, by people all over the world.

Walter J. Koroshetz, MD, Director

National Associations & Support Groups

1078 A Kids' Brain Tumor Cure Foundation
98 Random Farms Drive
Chappaqua, NY 10514   contact@akidsbraintumorcure.org
                             akidsbraintumorcure.org

A Kids' Brain Tumor Cure Foundation (aka The Pediatric Low Grade Astrocytoma (PLGA) Foundation) was founded in August 2007, as a 501(c)(3) organization by families and friends dedicated to giving hope to children battling the most common forms of pediatric brain tumors, by raising funds for targeted scientific and medical research.

Andrew Janower, President
John Ragnoni, Secretary
Amy Weinstein, Treasurer

1079 Accelerate Brain Cancer Cure
1717 Rhode Island Avenue, NW Suite 700
Washington, DC 20036 202-419-3140
info@abc2.org
www.abc2.org

Provides researchers with the pivotal support they need to make critical breakthroughs.

Stacey Case, Co-Founder
Steve Case, Co-Founder
Jean Case, Co-Founder

1080 American Academy of Pediatrics
141 Northwest Point Boulevard
Elk Grove Village, IL 60007 847-434-4000
800-433-9016
Fax: 847-434-8000
www.aap.org

The American Academy of Pediatrics and its member pediatricians are committed to the attainment of optimal physical, mental and social health and well-being for all infants, children, adolescents, and young adults.

Fernando Stein, MD, FAAP, President
Karen Remley, MD, CEO/Executive VP

1081 American Association for Cancer Research
615 Chestnut St., 17th Floor
Philadelphia, PA 19106 215-440-9300
866-423-3965
Fax: 215-440-9313
aacr@aacr.org
www.aacr.org

Helps prevent and cure cancer through research, education, communication, and collaboration.

Carlos L Arteaga, President
Jose Baselga, President Elect
Maragaret Foti, Chief Executive Officer

1082 American Association of Neurological Surgeons
5550 Meadowbrook Drive
Rolling Meadows, IL 60008 847-378-0500
888-566-2267
Fax: 847-378-0600
info@aans.org
www.aans.org

The AANS is dedicated to advancing the specialty of neurological surgery in order to promote the highest quality of patient care.

Robert E Harbaugh, President
H. Hunt Batjer, President Elect
Frederick A Boop, Secretary

1083 American Brain Tumor Association
8550 W. Bryn Mawr Ave. Ste 550
Chicago, IL 60631 773-577-8750
800-886-2282
Fax: 773-577-8738
info@abta.org
www.abta.org

Services include over 20 publications which address brain tumors, their treatment, and coping with the disease. Materials address brain tumors in all age groups. Provides free social service consultations; a mentorship program for new brain tumor support group leaders; a nationwide database of established support groups; the Connections pen-pal program; networking with organizations that provide services to patients and families; a resource listing of physicians offering investigative treatments

Ronald Petrocelli, M.D., Chair
Michael Cathey, Vice Chair
Brian Olson, Treasurer

1084 American Brain Tumor Association Patient Line
8550 W. Bryn Mawr Ave. Ste 550
Chicago, IL 60631 773-577-8750
800-886-2282
Fax: 773-577-8738
info@abta.org
www.abta.org

Offers emergency support, information and referrals for patients and their families.

Ronald Petrocelli, M.D., Chair
Michael Cathey, Vice Chair
Brian Olson, Treasurer

1085 American Cancer Society
Brain Tumor Support Group
8900 John W Carpenter Freeway
Dallas, TX 75247 214-819-1200
800-227-2345
Fax: 214-631-3869
www.cancer.org

Your American Cancer Society is in your corner around the clock to help you stay well and get well, to find cures, and to fight back.

Gary M Reedy, Chair of the Board
Vincent T DeVita Jr., MD, President
Pamela K Meyerhoffer, FAHP, Chair Elect

1086 American Childhood Cancer Organization (fo rmerly Candlelighters Childhood Cancer)
PO Box 498
Kensington, MD 20895 301-962-3520
855-858-2226
Fax: 310-962-3521
staff@acco.org
www.acco.org

The American Childhood Cancer Organization (ACCO) was founded in 1970 by a group of parents whose children had been diagnosed with cancer. Today, ACCO is one of the largest grassroots, national organizations dedicated to improving the lives of children and adolescents with cancer and their families.

Ruth I. Hoffman, MPH, Executive Director
Jessica DiBenedetto, Program Coordinator
Christy Perry, Director, Marketing/Communications

1087 Association for Neurologically Impaired Brain Injured Children
61-35 220th Street
Oakland Gardens, NY 11364 718-423-9550
Fax: 718-423-9838
mail@anibic.org
www.anibic.org

ANIBIc is a voluntary, multi-service organization that is dedicated to serving individuals with severe learning disabilities, neurological impairments and other developmental disabilities. Services include: residential, vocational, family support services, recreation (children and adults), respite (adult), summer day camp, counseling, and tramatic brain injury services (adults).

Michael Steward, President
Phyllis Kaye, Vice President
Helene Nieman, Vice President

1088 Beez Foundation (The)
26H World's Fair Drive
Somerset, NJ 08873 732-563-1144
www.beezfoundation.org

To raise money to support pediatric brain cancer research projects, related support activities for pediatric patients in cancer hospitals and education regarding the prevalence of pediatric brain cancer.

Joseph J. Giardina, President/Co-Founder
Gail Kurtzhals, VP/Marketing Director
Susan Giardina, Sec/Treas./Co-Founder

1089 Ben and Catherine Ivy Foundation
6710 North Scottsdale Road Suite 235
Scottsdale, AZ 85253   480-659-9621
                              Fax: 480-659-9651
                              beth@mcraeagency.com
                              www.ivyfoundation.org

At the Ivy Foundation, the long-term, ultimate goal is to cure brain cancer.

Catherine E. Ivy, Founder and Board President
Stephanie A. McRae, Secretary
Megan Edwards, Treasurer

1090 Brain Tumor Foundation - National
National Brain Tumor Foundation
22 Battery Street, Suite 612
San Francisco, CA 94111   617-924-9997
                                       800-934-2873
                              Fax: 415-834-9980
                              nbtf@braintumor.org
                              www.braintumor.org

National Brain Tumor Society is fiercely committed to finding better treatments, and ultimately a cure, for people living with a brain tumor today and anyone who will be diagnosed tomorrow. This means effecting change in the system at all levels.

Jeffrey Kolodin, Chair
Michael Nathanson, Vice Chair
Michael Corkin, Treasurer

1091 Brain Tumor Foundation for Children
6065 Roswell Road NE, Suite 505
Atlanta, GA 30328   404-252-4107
                              Fax: 404-252-4108
                              info@braintumorkids.org
                              www.braintumorkids.org

The mission of the Brain Tumor Foundation for Children is to provide financial assistance, social support, and information for families of children with brain and spinal cord tumors; fund research projects that improve treatment options and search for a cure; and raise public awareness of the disease and advocate on behalf of children who are affected.

Pamela B Ellis, President
Robert Flamini MD, Vice President
William A Guzak, Treasurer

1092 Brain Tumor Trials Collaborative
www.bttconline.org

The mission of the BTTC is to develop and perform hypothesis-based, state-of-the-art clinical trials in a collaborative and collegial environment emphasizing innovation and meticulous attention to data quality.

1093 CERN Foundation
6450 Poe Avenue, Suite 201
Dayton, OH 45414   937-264-2574
                              Fax: 937-264-7877
                              cern-foundation.org

To develop new treatments for ependymoma, improve the outcomes and care of patients, ultimately leading to a cure.

Glenn Lesser, Advisory Board
Mary Lovely, Advisory Board
Robert Jenkins, Advisory Board

1094 CancerCare
275 7th Avenue (between 25th and 26th Streets)
New York, NY 10001   212-712-8400
                                       800-813-4673
                              Fax: 212-712-8495
                              info@cancercare.org
                              www.cancercare.org

CancerCare provides free, professional support services to individuals, families, caregivers and the bereaved to help them cope with and manage the emotional and practical challenges of cancer.

Patricia J Goldsmith, CEO
John Rutigliano, Chief Operating Officer
Ahuva Morris, Children's Program Coordinator

1095 Central Brain Tumor Registry of the United States
244 East Ogden Ave Suite 116
Hinsdale, IL 60521   630-655-4786
                              Fax: 630-655-1756
                              cbtrus@aol.com
                              www.cbtrus.org

It is a not-for-profit corporation established to provide a resource for descriptive statistical data on all primary brain tumors irrespective of behavior.

Carol Kruchko, President
Steven Brem, Vice President
Donald Segal, Treasurer

1096 Childhood Brain Tumor Foundation
20312 Watkins Meadow Drive
Germantown, MD 20876   301-515-2900
                                       877-217-4166
                              Fax: 301-540-8367
                              cbtf@childhoodbraintumor.org
                              www.childhoodbraintumor.org

A major service this organization provides is the Childhood Cancer Ombudsman Program, a free service consisting of volunteers trained in the disciplines of medicine, law, and education who provide assistance in : 1) seeking second opinions, 2) access to healthcare, and 3) combating discrimination. The foundation also funds research, has a hotline and publishes a newsletter three times a year.

Jeanne P Young, President
Carol Cornman, Vice President
Kiren Day, Vice President/Secretary

1097 Childhood Brain Tumor Foundation (The)
20312 Watkins Meadow Drive
Germantown, ML 20876   301-515-2900
                                       877-217-4166
                              cbtf@childhoodbraintumor.org
                              www.childhoodbraintumor.org

It is an all-volunteer organization founded by families, friends and physicians of children with brain tumors.

Jeanne P Young, President
Carol Comman, Vice President
Kiren Day, Secretary

1098 Children's Brain Tumor Foundation
274 Madison Avenue Suite 1004
New York, NY 10016   866-228-4673
                              info@cbtf.org
                              www.cbtf.org

To improve the treatment, quality of life and the long term outlook for children with brain and spinal cord tumors through research.

Robert Budlow, President
Eric Snyder, Vice President
Miriam Barry, Secretary

1099 Cushing's Support and Research Foundation
60 Robbins Rd, #12
Plymouth, MA 02360   csrf.net

To be a resource for information and support to health care professionals.

Louise Pace, Founding President
Karen Campbell, Director
John P. Gulielmetti, Treasurer

1100 Epidermoid Brain Tumor Society
epidermoidbraintumorsociety.org

To inform, educate, and to provide a support and research organization for those affected by the epidermoid brain tumor.

1101 Glenn Garcelon Foundation
PO Box 2104
Lake Oswego, OR 97035   503-969-7651
                              glenngarcelonfoundation@msn.com
                              glenngarcelonfoundation.org

Exists to improve the quality of life of brain tumor survivors, caregivers and their families by providing emotional and financial support.

Gail Garcelon, President
Danielle Hess, Vice President
Nicole Smith, Secretary

1102 Heads Up Brain Tumor Support Group
Dominican Hospital
18300 Roscoe Boulevard
Northridge, CA 91325

818-885-5432
robert.salazar@chw.edu
www.braintumor.org/

Robert Salazar, Contact
Michael Nathanson, Vice Chair
Michael Corkin, Treasurer

1103 Healing Exchange Brain Trust
459 Broadway, Suite 302
Everett, MA 02149

877-252-8480
Fax: 617-623-0086
info@braintrust.org
www.braintrust.org

The mission of The Healing Exchange BRAIN TRUST is to improve quality of life for people living with brain tumors and related conditions TODAY.

Samantha J Scolamiero, President & Founding Director

1104 Hope for Hypothalamic Hamartomas
P. O. Box 721
Waddell, AZ 85355

admin@hopeforhh.org.
hopeforhh.org

A volunteer-based nonprofit organization founded by parents of children with hypothalamic hamartomas.

Lisa Dunn Soeby, President
Ilene Penn Miller, Vice President
Erica Webster, Secretary

1105 James S. McDonnell Foundation
1034 S. Brentwood Blvd. Suite 1850
St. Louis, MO 63117

314-721-1532
info@jsmf.org
www.jsmf.org

The Foundation has pursued his goals by supporting scientific, educational, and charitable causes locally, nationally, and internationally.

John T Bruer, President
John F. McDonnell, Board of Director
Marcella M. Stevens, Board of Director

1106 Musella Foundation for Brain Tumor Research and Information
1100 Peninsula Blvd
Hewlett, NY 11557

888-295-4740
www.virtualtrials.com

Nonprofit public charity dedicated to helping brain tumor patients through emotional and financial support, education, advocacy and raising money for brain tumor research.

Al Musella, President
Mitchell Siegel, Vice President
Neal Houslanger, Secretary

1107 National Association for Proton Therapy
1301 Highland Drive
Silver Spring, ML 20910

301-587-6100
lenarzt@proton-therapy.org
www.proton-therapy.org

The National Association for Proton Therapy (NAPT) is registered as an independent, non-profit, public benefit corporation providing education and awareness for the public, professional and governmental communities.

Leonard Arzt, Executive Director

1108 National Brain Research Association
1439 Rhode Island Avenue NW
Washington, DC 20005

202-483-6272

Also provides support groups for parents.

1109 National Brain Tumor Foundation
22 Battery Street, Suite 612
San Francisco, CA 94111

617-924-9997
800-934-2873
Fax: 510-834-9980
nbtf@braintumor.org
www.braintumor.org

NBTF is a national nonprofit health organization dedicated to providing information and support for brain tumor patients, family members, and healthcare professionals, while supporting innovative research into better treatment options and a cure for brain tumors.

Jeffrey Kolodin, Chair
Michael Nathanson, Vice Chair
Michael Corkin, Treasurer

1110 National Brain Tumor Society
124 Watertown Street, Suite 2D
Watertown, MA 02472

617-924-9997
800-770-8287
Fax: 617-924-9998
info@braintumor.org
www.braintumor.org

The Brain Tumor Society exists to find a cure for brain tumors. It strives to improve the quality of life of brain tumor patients and their families. It disseminates educational information and provides access to psychosocial support. It raises funds to advance carefully selected scientific research projects, improve clinical care and find a cure.

N Paul TonThat, Executive Director
Jeffrey Kolodin, Chair
Michael Nathanson, Vice Chair

1111 National Childhood Cancer Foundation
4600 East West Highway, Suite 600
Bethesda, MD 20814

301-718-0042
800-458-6223
Fax: 301-718-0047
info@curesearch.org
www.curesearch.org

CureSearch for Children's Cancer is a national non-profit foundation that accelerates the cure for children's cancer by driving innovation, eliminating research barriers and solving the field's most challenging problems.

Stuart Siegal MD, Chair of the Board
Timothy Harmon, Vice Chair
Mary Payne, Treasurer

1112 National Children's Cancer Society
500 North Broadway, Suite 800 St.
Louis, MO 63102

314-241-1600
Fax: 314-241-1996
www.thenccs.org

The National Children's Cancer Society (NCCS) provides emotional, financial and educational support to children with cancer, their families and survivors.

Mark Slocomb, Chairman
Maria Taxman, Vice Chairman
Mark Stolze, President

1113 National Comprehensive Cancer Network
275 Commerce Dr, Suite 300
Fort Washington, PA 19034

215-690-0300
Fax: 215-690-0280
www.nccn.org

Devoted to patient care, research, and education, is dedicated to improving the quality, effectiveness, and efficiency of cancer care so that patients can live better lives.

Samuel M. Silver, Chair
Timothy J. Eberlein, Vice Chair
Mara G. Bloom, Secretary

1114 Nevus Outreach
600 SE Delaware Ave., Suite 200
Bartlesville, OK 74003
918-331-0595
877-426-3887
ahouseal@nevus.org
www.nevus.org

Nevus Outreach is dedicated to improving awareness and providing support for people affected by congenital melanocytic nevi and finding a cure.

Anne Houseal, Chairman
Mark Beckwith, Executive Director
Michael Kushner, Secretary

1115 Pituitary Network Association
P.O. Box 1958
Thousand Oaks, CA 91358
805-499-9973
Fax: 805-480-0633
info@pituitary.org
www.pituitary.org

The PNA is an international non-profit organization for patients with pituitary tumors and disorders, their families, loved ones, and the physicians and health care providers who treat them.

Robert Knutzen, CEO / Chairman
Paula Gallegos-Maxfield, Treasurer
Christina Bourne, Board of Director

1116 Preuss Foundation
2223 Avenida de la Playa, Suite 220
La Jolla, CA 92037
858-454-0200
Fax: 858-454-4449
fari@preuss.org
www.ninds.nih.gov/find_people/voluntary_orgs/volorg2

Foundation that provides information on support groups, brochures and pamphlets.

Story C Landis, Director
Walter J Koroshetz, Deputy Director
Caroline Lewis, Executive Officer

1117 Society for NeuroOncology
PO Box 273296
Houston, TX 77277
281-554-6589
Fax: 713-583-1345
linda@soc-neuro-onc.org
www.soc-neuro-onc.org

Multi-disciplinary organization dedicated to promoting advances in neuro-oncology through research and education.

David A. Reardon, President
E. Antonio Chiocca, Vice President
Eva Galanis, Secretary/Treasurer

1118 Sontag Foundation
sontagfoundation.org
info@sontagfoundation.org
sontagfoundation.org

Our primary focus is on brain cancer, with additional support for rheumatoid arthritis.

Frederick B Sontag, President
Frederick T Sontag, Vice President
Kay W Verble, Executive Director

1119 Students Supporting Brain Tumor Research
8390 E. Via de Ventura, F-110
Scottsdale, AZ 85258
888-772-8729
admin@ssbtr.org
www.ssbtr.org

Mission is to provide education and leadership development to our youth.

1120 Tug McGraw Foundation
100 California Drive
Yountville, CA 94599
707-947-7124
707-676-4398
info@tugmcgraw.org
www.tugmcgraw.org

To provide resources and hands-on support, foster understanding, promote awareness, and stimulate research.

Tom Higgins, Chairman
Jennifer Brusstar, President & CEO
Tom McGraw, Chief Executive Officer

State Agencies & Support Groups

Alabama

1121 Pediatric Brain Tumor Support Group
Children's Hospital
1600 7th Avenue S
Birmingham, AL 35233
205-939-9090
Fax: 205-939-9010
info@braintumorkids.org
www.braintumorkids.org

Groups for parents and siblings of brain tumor patients. Related to Children's Hospital of Alabama. Babysitting available.

Pamela B Ellis, President
Robert Flamini MD, Vice President
William A Guzak, Treasurer

Arizona

1122 Brain Tumor Support Group at NovaCare Rehabilitation Institute of Tucson
2650 N Wyatt Drive
Tucson, AZ 85712
520-293-8040
www.tmcaz.com

Scott Gulbrandsen

1123 Brain Tumor Support Group at Phoenix
350 W Thomas Road
Phoenix, AZ 85013
602-873-2757
www.braintumorsupportgroup.com/hospital/children/pho

The Jaydie Lynn King Neuro-oncology Program at Phoenix Children's Hospital is the only comprehensive pediatric program of its kind in Arizona, combining the expertise of subspecialists in the Children's Neuroscience Institute and the Center for Cancer and Blood Disorders (CCBD).

Steve Westerhoff

California

1124 Brain Tumor Patient & Family Support Group
Saint Jude Medical Center
2151 N Harbor Blvd, St Jude Medical Plaza, Rm 2266
Fullerton, CA 92635
714-446-7182
www.stjudemedicalcenter.org

Periodic guest presentations.

Robert Merlino

1125 Brain Tumor Support Group at Newport Beach
301 Newport Blvd.
Newport Beach, CA 92658
949-760-2350
www.bettyclooneyfoundation.org

Speakers once a month, education materials available.

Kris O'Neal

1126 Brain Tumor Support Group at San Diego
8555 Aero Drive #340
San Diego, CA 92103
858-467-1065
www.bettyclooneyfoundation.org

Speakers once a month, education materials available.

Donna Gilpatrick RN, MS, FNP

1127 Brain Tumor Support Group at San Luis Obispo
1911 Johnson Avenue
San Luis Obispo, CA 93401
805-461-3989
www.bettyclooneyfoundation.org

Speakers once a month, education materials available.

Becky Nunez

1128   Brain Tumor Support Group at Santa Monica
2200 Colorado Boulevard
Santa Monica, CA 90404   310-453-2200
www.bettyclooneyfoundation.org

Speakers once a month, education materials available.

Michael Slater, Program Director

**1129   Brain Tumor Support Program Cedars-Sinai Neurosurgical
Inst. & Wellness Communit**
8631 W 3rd Street, Suite 800 E
Los Angeles, CA 90048   310-855-7900
Fax: 310-423-0777
www.bettyclooneyfoundation.org

Last Wednesday of month 6-7:30 pm with an RSVP.

Jennice Vilhauer, Contact

1130   Fresno Brain Tumor Support Group
7130 North Millbrook Avenue
Fresno, CA 93720   559-450-5528
Fax: 559-449-3990
karen.kennedy@samc.com
www.braintumor.org

Speakers once a month, education materials available.

Karen Kennedy, Contact
Jeffrey Kolodin, Chair
Michael Nathanson, Vice Chair

1131   Inland Empire Brain Tumor Support Group
Medical Annex Building
Riverside Community Hospital, 4445 Magnolia Avenue
Riverside, CA 92502   951-222-8090
http://events.pe.com/riverside-ca

Meets third Saturday, once a month.

Sue Melton, Contact

1132   Neuroscience Institute Brain Tumor Support Group
637 S Lucas Avenue, Suite 501
Los Angeles, CA 90017   213-977-2234
800-762-1692
www.mhmni.com/support/

The group meets the second Wednesday of every month at 6 p.m.
in the Heart & Vascular Institute, 3rd floor, conference room A.

Cherrie Valacruz, Manager

1133   Northridge Hospital: Leavey Cancer Center
18300 Roscoe Boulevard
Northridge, CA 91328   818-885-5431
www.northridgehospital.org

We are fully-accredited by the American College of Surgeons
Commission on Cancer as a Comprehensive Cancer Center since
1980.

Marylou Perelmutter, Manager

1134   Palo Alto Brain Tumor Support Group
920 Bryant Street, 2nd Floor Room B
Palo Alto, CA 94301   415-284-0208
www.pamf.org

Joanie Taylor, RN

**1135   Peninsula Support & Education Group for Parents of Children
with Brain Tumors**
3041 Olcott
Santa Clara, CA 95054   650-325-4523
www.supportforfamilies.org

Sheri Sobrato, MA, MFC

**1136   Sacramento Area Brain Tumor Support Group Lawrence J
Ellison Ambulatory Care Ctr**
UC Davis Medical Center, Camellia Cottage
4860 Y Street Suite 3740
Sacramento, CA 95817   916-734-3658
Fax: 916-703-5368
kksmith@ucdavis.edu
www.ucdmc.ucdavis.edu/neurosurg/contactus/contact_in

First Thursday of month 6:30-8:30 pm.

J. Paul . Muizelaar, M.D., Ph.D, Program Director
James E Boggan MD, Professor and Acting Chair
Kee D Kim MD, Associate Professor

1137   San Francisco Brain Tumor Support Group
UC San Francisco, Clinical Sciences Building
521 Parnassus Avenue, Room C130
San Francisco, CA 94188   415-990-4461
mary.lovely@sbcglobal.net
www.ucsfhealth.org/support_groups/neurology/

First Wednesday of each month, 7:00 - 8:30 pm

Sharon Lamb, Contact
Mary Lovely, Contact

1138   Santa Barbara Brain Tumor Support Group
Cancer Foundation of Santa Barbara
540 West Pueblo Street
Santa Barbara, CA 93105   805-682-7300
www.braintumor.org

Third Thursday of each month, 5:15-6:30 pm.

Rosario Campuzano, Contact
Jeffrey Kolodin, Chair
Michael Nathanson, Vice Chair

1139   Santa Cruz County Brain Tumor Support Group
3031 Main Street
Soquel, CA 95073   831-438-8344
www.braintumor.org

Gregory Valki-Tarsy
Jeffrey Kolodin, Chair
Michael Nathanson, Vice Chair

1140   Santa Rosa Brain Tumor Support Group
North Coast Rehab Hospital Fulton Campus Conf Room
1287 Fulton
Santa Rosa, CA 95401   415-353-2966
www.braintumor.org

Last Wednesday of each month, 6:30-8:00 pm.

Jane Rabbitt RN, Contact
Jeffrey Kolodin, Chair
Michael Nathanson, Vice Chair

1141   South Bay Brain Tumor Support Group
667 Chapman Street
San Jose, CA 95126   650-725-8630
www.braintumor.org

Genny See-Tho RN
Jeffrey Kolodin, Chair
Michael Nathanson, Vice Chair

1142   Southern California Pediatric Brain Tumor Network
UCLA Medical Center
10833 LeConte Avenue, Suite 501
Los Angeles, CA   310-825-7354
www.braintumor.org

For parents of children with brain tumors, and for teenagers with
brain tumors.

Patricia Park
Jeffrey Kolodin, Chair
Michael Nathanson, Vice Chair

1143   Support Group for Caregivers of Brain Tumor Patients
UCLA Medical Center
UCLA Medical Plaza Building
Los Angeles, CA 90052   310-206-6731
www.braintumor.org

Guest speakers on occasion.

Pamela Hoff, LCSW
Jeffrey Kolodin, Chair
Michael Nathanson, Vice Chair

1144 Support Group for Parents of Children with Brain Tumors
Oakland Children's Hospital
747 52nd Street, Auditorium Sd II
Oakland, CA 94609   510-428-3885
                                                 www.braintumor.org

Contact can be reached at extension 2161.

Trish Murphy
Jeffrey Kolodin, Chair
Michael Nathanson, Vice Chair

1145 Vital Options
4419 Coldwater Canyon Ave., Suite I
Studio City, CA 91604   818-508-5657
                                                 Fax: 818-788-5260
                                                 info@vitaloptions.org
                                                 www.vitaloptions.org

Vital Options International is a 501(c)(3) not-for-profit cancer
communications organization with a mission, to facilitate a global
cancer dialogue

Selma R Schimmel, CEO and Founder
Derek Alpert, President
Terry Merrill Wilcox, Creative Director and Supervising P

1146 Wellness Community San Francisco/East Bay
3276 McNutt Avenue
Walnut Creek, CA 94597   925-933-0107
                                                 Fax: 925-933-0249
                                                 www.twc-bayarea.org

To help people affected by cancer enhance their health and
well-being through participation in a professional program of
emotional support, education, and hope.

James R Bouquin, Executive Director
Margaret Stauffer MFT, Program Director
Amy Alanes, Development Manager

1147 West Los Angeles Brain Tumor Support Group
2716 Ocean Park Boulvard, Suite 1040
Santa Monica, CA 90405   310-314-2555
                                                 www.braintumor.org

Michael States, Program Director
Jeffrey Kolodin, Chair
Michael Nathanson, Vice Chair

Colorado

1148 Brain Tumor Patient & Family Support Group
Swedish Medical Center Conference Center
701 E Hampden Avenue #330
Englewood, CO 80113   303-806-7420
                                                 lgibson@thecni.org
                                                 www.braintumor.org

Sponsored by Colorado Neurological Institute Center for Brain
and Spinal Tumors. First Wednesday of month, 6:30-8:00 pm.

Lorre Gibson, Contact

1149 Brain Tumor Patient/Family Group
Anchutz Cancer Pavillion, University of Colorado
Fitzsimons Campus, 1635 Ursula Street
Aurora, CO 80045   303-315-6635
                                                 amy.ebert@uchsc.edu
                                                 www.braintumor.org

First Wednesday of each month, 5:00-7:00 pm. call to confirm location.

Amy Ebert, Contact
Jeffrey Kolodin, Chair
Michael Nathanson, Vice Chair

1150 Brain Tumor Support Group
Poudre Valley Hospital
1024 S Lemay, Neuroscience Floor
Ft. Collins, CO 80521   970-495-8320
                                                 ryjj@aol.com
                                                 www.braintumor.org

Second Thursday of each month at 5:00 pm. Call to confirm location.

Georgie Knaub, Contact
Jeffrey Kolodin, Chair
Michael Nathanson, Vice Chair

Connecticut

1151 Brain Tumor Support Group
Cancer Program
80 Seymour Street
Hartford, CT 06102   860-545-5000
                                                 860-545-2318
                                                 Fax: 860-545-5066
                                                 www.braintumor.org

First Thursday of each month, 5:30-7:00 pm. Call in advance to
RSVP.

Hillary Keller, Contact
Jeffrey Kolodin, Chair
Michael Nathanson, Vice Chair

1152 Connecticut Brain Tumor Support Group (Adult)
Yale New Haven Hospital, Children's Hospital
20 York Street, Room 201
New Haven, CT 06510   203-688-7528
                                                 www.braintumor.org

Second Tuesday of each month, 2:00-3:30 pm (please call to confirm date and time).

Betsy D'Andrea, Contact
Angela Thomas MSW, Contact
Michael Nathanson, Vice Chair

Delaware

1153 Pediatric Brain Tumor Support Group
1901 Rockland Road
Wilmington, DE 19803   302-995-0938
                                                 www.braintumor.org

Cathy Francisco
Jeffrey Kolodin, Chair
Michael Nathanson, Vice Chair

District of Columbia

1154 Washington DC Metropolitan Area Support Group
2121 Eye Street, NW
Washington, DC 20052   202-994-1000
                                                 www.braintumor.org

Jeffrey Kolodin, Chair
Michael Nathanson, Vice Chair

Florida

1155 Angels in the Sun Brain Tumor Support Group
3251 Proctor Road
Sarasota, FL 34231   941-364-9105
                                                 www.braintumorkids.org

Anna Browder
Jeffrey Kolodin, Chair
Michael Nathanson, Vice Chair

1156 Brain Tumor Support Group
1703 W Colonial Drive
Orlando, FL 32804
                                                 407-740-0007
                                                 www.braintumor.org

David Cox, MD
Jeffrey Kolodin, Chair
Michael Nathanson, Vice Chair

1157 Brain Tumor Support Group at Miami
Miami Children's Hospital Foundation
3000 SW 62nd Avenue, Founders Lounge
Miami, FL 33155   305-662-8386
www.braintumor.org

Call to confirm time and date.
Maria Penate RN, Contact
Jeffrey Kolodin, Chair
Michael Nathanson, Vice Chair

1158 Brain Tumor Support Group at St. Petersburg
Saint Anthony's Hospital
Saint Petersburg, FL 33730   813-825-1100
www.braintumor.org

Contact can be reached at extension 4231.
Karen McGough
Jeffrey Kolodin, Chair
Michael Nathanson, Vice Chair

1159 Brain Tumor Support Group at Tampa
12902 Magnolia Drive
Tampa, FL 33612   813-979-7258
                                    800-456-3434
www.braintumor.org

Inez Rodriquez
Jeffrey Kolodin, Chair
Michael Nathanson, Vice Chair

1160 Cancer Support Group for Children
3501 Johnson Street, 4th Floor
Hollywood, FL 33021   954-987-2000
www.ped-onc.org/resources/supportorg.html

Sub-groups for children with brain tumors and their parents. Contact at ext. 4193.
Suzanne Baxter RN

1161 South Florida Brain Tumor Association Lynn Regional Cancer Center
Boca Raton Community Hospital
800 Meadows Road, Education Center
Boca Raton, FL 33486   561-955-7100
                                    561-955-5897
www.brrh.com/Cancer_Institute.aspx

Neuropsychologist Dr. Laurence Miller and therapist Marjorie O'Sullivan are present to facilitate the meetings. Second and Fourth Thursdays of each month, 7:30-8:30 pm.

Jerry Fedele, President and Chief Executive Offic
Karen Poole, FACHE, Vice President, Chief Operating Off
Dawn P Javersack, Vice President and Chief Financial

1162 Tampa Bay Area Brain Tumor Support Group
St Joseph's Hospital, Medical Arts Building
3000 West Martin Luther King Boulevard
Tampa Bay, FL 33630   813-870-4101
www.braintumor.org

Third Tuesday of each month, 6:30-7:30 pm.
Jeffrey Kolodin, Chair
Michael Nathanson, Vice Chair
Michael Corkin, Treasurer

Georgia

1163 All Ages Support Group
1835 Savoy Drive, Suite 316
Atlanta, GA 30341   770-458-5554
btfc@bellsouth.net
www.braintumorkids.org

Contact for details.
Mary Campbell, Contact

1164 Brain Tumor Foundation for Children
6065 Roswell Road NE, Suite 505
Atlanta, GA 30328   404-252-4107
Fax: 404-252-4108
info@braintumorkids.org
www.braintumorkids.org

The mission of the Brain Tumor Foundation for Children is to provide financial assistance, social support, and information for families of children with brain and spinal cord tumors; fund research projects that improve treatment options and search for a cure; and raise public awareness of the disease and advocate on behalf of children who are affected.

Pamela B Ellis, President
Robert Flamini MD, Vice President
William A Guzak, Treasurer

1165 Brain Tumor Support Group
Emory Clinic, Neurosurgery Conference Room
1365 Clifton Road, Building B, 2nd Floor
Atlanta, GA 30341   404-778-4153
                                    404-778-3091
www.braintumor.org

First Thursday of each month, 12:30-2:30 pm. Please RSVP to attend.
Karen Shires, Contact
Linda Phillips, Contact
Jeffrey Kolodin, Chair

1166 Southeastern Brain Tumor Foundation Brain Tumor Support Group
Wellness Community, Peachtree Dunwoody Pavillion
PO Box 422471
Atlanta, GA 30342   404-843-3700
info@sbtf.org
www.sbtf.org/home.html

Second Monday of each month, 7:00-8:30 pm.
Costas G. Hadjipanayis, MD, PhD, President
Jennifer Keenan Giliberto, Vice President
Suzanne Boeren, Treasurer

Hawaii

1167 Brain Tumor Support Group
93 N Kainalu, Kailu
Oahu, HI   808-254-1989
www.braintumor.org

Chuck Rogers
Kari Rogers
Jeffrey Kolodin, Chair

Idaho

1168 Treasure Valley Brain Injury Support Group
Idaho Elks Rehabilitation Hospital
600 North Robbins Road
Boise, ID 83702   208-489-4558
bjaundalderis@elksrehab.org
www.idahoelksrehab.org

Through our expertise in rehab and uncompromising commitment to care, education and research, we help you live life to its fullest. Fourth Tuesday of each month 7:00-9:00 pm.

Bob Jaundalderis, Marketing Director
Katie McCurdy, Brain Injury Program Director

Illinois

1169 Brain Tumor Resource & Support Group
Central DuPage Hospital, Neuro-Spine Unit
25 North Winfield Road
Winfield, IL 60190   630-933-6955
debbie_brunelle@cdh.org
www.braintumor.org

Second and Fourth Wednesday of each month, 7:30-9:00 pm.

Deborah Brunelle RN, Contact
Jeffrey Kolodin, Chair
Michael Nathanson, Vice Chair

1170 Brain Tumor Support Group
303 E Superior
Chicago, IL 60611   312-908-8177
                                                www.braintumor.org

Mary Ellen Maher Deleon
Jeffrey Kolodin, Chair
Michael Nathanson, Vice Chair

1171 Brain Tumor Support Group at Northwestern Memorial Hospital
251 East Huron, Suite 3-520
Chicago, IL 60611   312-695-8143
                                                www.braintumor.org

Educational program offered at each meeting by members of the professional committee. Third Monday of each month, 5:00-6:00 pm.
Mary Ellen Maher Deleon, Contact
Jeffrey Kolodin, Chair
Michael Nathanson, Vice Chair

1172 Brain Tumor Support Group at Park Ridge
Lutheran General Hospital, Cancer Care Center
1775 Dempster St.
Park Ridge, IL 60302   847-696-5475
                                                www.braintumor.org

Third Wednesday of each month, 7:30-9:00 pm.
Syril Gilbert LCSW, Contact
Jeffrey Kolodin, Chair
Michael Nathanson, Vice Chair

1173 Parents of Children with Brain Tumors (PCBT)
Children's Memorial Hospital
2300 Children's Plaza
Chicago, IL 60614   773-880-4553
                                                www.cbtrf.org/

Monthly newsletter. Library available at meetings (at CMH). Educational speakers and family functions. Call to confirm meetings.
Teresa Berry, Contact

Indiana

1174 Benign Brain Tumor Support Group
Howard Regional Health Systems
322 North Main Street
Kokomo, IN 46901   765-455-2613
                                                www.braintumor.org

Third Wednesday of each month, 5:00-6:30 pm. Meet in southeast corner of the building, enter at set of double doors on corner of North Main and Taylor Street.
Marsha Mahoney, Contact
Jeffrey Kolodin, Chair
Michael Nathanson, Vice Chair

1175 Brain Tumor Support Group
205 E Kirkwood Avenue
Bloomington, IN 47408   812-332-4459
                                                Fax: 812-332-4479
                                                www.braintumor.org

Jean Bauer
Jeffrey Kolodin, Chair
Michael Nathanson, Vice Chair

1176 Brain Tumor Support Group at Indianapolis
Community Hospital North
Regional Cancer Center
Indianapolis, IN 46256   317-485-6616
                                                317-842-1229
                                                m.w.kempf@sbcglobal.net
                                                www.braintumor.org

Third Wednesday of each month, 6:3-7:30 pm. The Regional Cancer Center is in a building just to the south of the main hospital, across Clearvista Drive.

Lisa Peters RN, Contact
Michael Kempf, Contact
Marcia Cline, Contact

1177 Primary Brain Cancer Support Group
Women's Cancer Center at Lutheran Hospital
7910 W Jefferson Boulevard, Suite 112
Fort Wayne, IN 46804   260-435-7959
                                                www.cancercenter.com/

First Tuesday of every month, 6:00 pm.
Linda Jordan RN, Contact

Iowa

1178 Brain Tumor Support Group
University Of Iowa Hospitals
200 Hawkins Drive
Iowa City, IA 52242   319-356-4125
                                                319-356-2301
                                                suzanne-witte@uiowa.edu
                                                www.braintumor.org

First Tuesday of each month with exception of July, August, January. Meeting held at the Cancer Center Waiting Room from 7-8:30 pm.
Sue Witte, Contact
Sue May, Contact
Jeffrey Kolodin, Chair

1179 Quad Cities Brain Tumor Support Group
Genesis Medical Center
1401 W Central Park
Davenport, IA 52804   563-421-1905
                                                christyp@genesishealth.com
                                                www.braintumor.org

Fourth Monday of each month, 6:30-8:00 pm.
Pat Christy RN, Contact
Jeffrey Kolodin, Chair
Michael Nathanson, Vice Chair

Kansas

1180 Headstrong Brain Tumor Support Group
Victory in the Valley
Victory House, 3755 East Douglas,
Witchita, KS 67214   316-634-2801
                                                phyllis.jacobs@wichita.edu
                                                www.braintumor.org

Second Wednesday of each month at 7pm. Call for information.
Phyllis Jacob, Contact
Jeffrey Kolodin, Chair
Michael Nathanson, Vice Chair

Kentucky

1181 Brain Injury Support Group
2050 Versailles Road
Lexington, KY 40504   859-254-5701
                          www.braininjuryguide.org/braininjurysupportgroups.ht

First Thursday of each month at 6:00 pm. Meeting will be held in Conference Room A or B in the Center of Learning.
Tonia Wells, Contact

Louisiana

1182 Brain Injury Support And Education Group
Touro Infirmary
1401 Foucher Street
New Orleans, LA 70115   504-897-7011
                                                babies@touro.com
                                                www.touro.com

Second and fourth Wednesday and families are every Third Monday. Offers outreach programs for survivors of brain injuries as well as their family members and caregivers.

Ruth Kullman, Chair
Hugh W Long, Vice Chairman
Joy Braun, Treasurer

1183 Brain Injury Support Group
West Jefferson Medical Center
1101 Medical Center Boulevard 4th Floor Rehab
Marrero, LA 70072   504-349-6396
                                t.bordelon@wjmc.org
                                www.biala.org/support-groups-1

Second Wednesday, 2:00 pm.

Tammy , Contact

1184 Tlane Cancer Center
1430 Tulane Avenue, SL-68
New Orleans, LA 70112   504-988-6592
                                Fax: 504-988-6077
                                mcross@tulane.edu
                www.tulane.edu/som/cancer/cancer-center-history.cfm

Every other Wednesday, 6-8 pm.

Melanie N Cross, Contact

Maine

1185 Brain Tumor Support Group of Maine
22 Bramhall Street
Portland, ME 04104   207-871-4527
                                www.braintumor.org

The Brain Tumor Support Group of Maine was formed to help patients, their families, and friends deal with the consequences of being diagnosed with a brain tumor by providing: The Brain Tumor Support Group of Maine meets the second Tuesday of each month from 7:00 pm to 8:30 pm at the Maine Medical Center

Nancy Fortier LCSW, Contact
Jeffrey Kolodin, Chair
Michael Nathanson, Vice Chair

1186 Open Support Group-All Kinds of Cancer Care of Maine
489 State Street
Bangor, ME 04401   207-973-7000
                                877-366-3662
                www.emmc.org/splash_cancercareofmaine.aspx

Wednesdays at 10:30 AM - 12 Noon. For families and patients.

Liane Judd, Chair

Maryland

1187 Brain Tumor Networking Group
                                        410-832-2719

Fourth Monday of each month, 7:00-8:30 pm.

Carol Sharp, Contact

1188 Johns Hopkins Brain Tumor Education Group
Weinberg Building
Phipps Building, Room 123 600 N. Wolfe Street
Baltimore, MD 21287   410-614-1627
                                Fax: 410-502-4954
                                mlim3@jhmi.edu

First Wednesday of the month, 10:30-11:30 am. All are welcome at this group. Each meeting includes a speaker followed by discussion.

Dr Michael Lim, Contact

Massachusetts

1189 Brain Center Brain Tumor Support Group
Promontory Point
Mashpee, MA 02649   508-477-5300

Last Sunday of each month, 3:00 pm. Call to confirm.

Eleanor Grace, Contact
Dick Grace, Contact

1190 Brain Tumor Support Group
Dana Farber Cancer Center
Dana Building, 16th Floor, Room D-1635
Boston, MA 02155   617-632-3769
                                617-732-6826

First and Third Thursday of each month, 12:00-1:30 pm. Free parking is available in the Smith Garage at Dana Farber.

Nancy Olson RN, MBA, Contact
Genevieve Mason LCSW, Contact

1191 Brain Tumor Support Group at Burlington
Lahey Clinic Medical Center
Cancer Center, 3W Conference Room Lahey Hospital &
Burlington, MA 01805   781-744-8113

First and Third Monday of each month, 7:00-9:00 pm. 5 Central Clinic Conference Room.

Pam Reznick LICSW, Contact

1192 Brain Tumor Support Group at Worcester
University of Massachusetts Medical Center
Dept of Surgery Waiting Area, 55 Lake Avenue N
Worcester, MA 01655   508-334-3515

This group meets for 2 hours once a month and occasionally has speakers. Second Tuesday of every month, 6:00-8:00 pm.

Alexis Van Horn RN, Contact

1193 Brain Tumor Survivor Support Group
196 Main Street
Andover, MA 01810   617-543-1709
                                ddemella@hotmail.com

Second Saturday of the month, 10:00 am - 12 Noon. This is a Mutual Help support group that is peer led. It is an informal opportunity to share experiences, information, resources, and challenges as we learn to LIVE with brain tumors.

Debbie DeMella, Contact

1194 Parent Education/Support Group
Dana Farber Cancer Institute, Smith Family Room
44 Binney Street Yawkey 306
Boston, MA 02115   617-632-3578
                                617-632-4386

For parents of children with brain tumors. Call for details.

Kelly Birdsey, Contact
Laura Myerburg, LICSW, Contact
Nancy Bailey, RN, Contact

Michigan

1195 Brain Tumor Networking Club
Gilda's Club Metropolitan Center
Gilda's Club 3517 Rochester Road
Royal Oak, MI 48073   248-577-0800
                                Fax: 248-577-0898
                                www.gildasclubdetroit.org/

Second Monday of each month 6:00-8:00 pm.

Christin Bernat, Contact

1196 Brain Tumor Support Group
Henry Ford Hospital
6777 West Maple
West Bloomfield, MI 48322   313-916-1796

Third Saturday of each month, 10:00 am - 12 Noon. Call for location.

Sandy Remer, Contact

1197 Brain Tumor Support Group at Ann Arbor
St Joseph Mercy Hospital, Cancer Care Center
5301 E Huron River Drive
Ann Arbor, MI 48106   734-712-3658

Fourth Tuesday of each month, 7:00-8:30 pm.

Paula Nedela RN, Contact

1198   Brain Tumor Support Group for Patients & Families: University of Michigan Med Ctr
De Jong Neuro-Oncology Library, Taubman Ctr
1500 E Medical Center Dr, Reception Area C, 1st Lv
Ann Arbor, MI 48109   734-647-8906

Third Tuesday of each month, 7:00-8:30 pm.

Michaelyn Page MS RN OCN CNS, Contact

1199   Spectrum Brain Tumor Support Group
Spectrum Health East
1840 Wealthy SE
Grand Rapids, MI 49506   616-774-7278

Second Monday of each month, 7:00-9:00 pm.

Nancy Rude, Contact

1200   West Michigan Cancer Center Support Group
Lower Level Resource Room
200 North Park Street
Kalamazoo, MI 49007   269-373-7442
                                      TTY: 269-382-2500
                                      helpdesk@wmcc.org
                                      www.wmcc.org

First Thursday of each month, 2:30-4:00 pm. Call to confirm.

Linda Diane Grossheim, Contact

Minnesota

1201   Abbott Northwestern Brain Tumor Support Group at Abbott Northwestern Hospital
800 East 28th Street
Minneapolis, MN 55407   612-863-4996

Second and Fourth Thursday of each month, 5:30-8:00 pm. Call to verify time.

Kathy Gilliland RN, Contact
Margaret Callan, Contact

1202   Brain Injury Support Group at Abbott Northwestern Hospital
Abbott Northwestern Board Room 1st Floor
800 East 28th Street
Minneapolis, MN 55407   612-863-4996
                                      susan.newman@allinia.com

Second Wednesday of the month, 6:30-8:00 pm. This group has speakers that address group concerns. New members always welcome.

Sue Newman, Contact

1203   Brain Tumor Support Group at Duluth
St Mary's Medical Center
407 E 3rd Street, Michiras Room
Duluth, MN 55805   218-726-4230

Third Monday of the month at 6:30 pm.

Jan Stevens RN, Contact

1204   Brain Tumor Support Group at Robbinside
North Memorial Medical Center North Ed Ctr
3300 Oakdale Avenue N
Robbinside, MN 55422   612-520-5158

Facilitated by Radiation RN, social worker, rehab staff, chaplain and physician. Third Wednesday of each month, 7:00-8:30 pm.

Judy Zak, Contact

1205   Brain Tumor Support Group at United Hospital
St Luke's Room, Conference B & C
255 North Smith Avenue
Saint Paul, MN 55102   651-241-8575

Second Monday each month, 7:00-8:30 pm.

Kathy Maiers, Contact
Cathy Maiers RN, Contact

1206   Non-Malignant Brain Tumor Support Group
800 East 28th Street
Minneapolis, MN 55407   612-775-4681

Second Thursday, 7:00-8:30 pm.

Jerry , Contact

Missouri

1207   AMOR - A Cancer Support Group for Patients & Their Families
Brain Tumor Institute of Kansas City
2316 E Meyers Boulevard, Dining Room 3
Kansas City, MO 64132   816-235-5960

Every other Wednesday, 2:00-3:00 pm.

Peggy Smith MS, RN, Contact

1208   Brain Cancer Support Group at Mid-America Cancer Center
Saint John's Regional Health Center
2055 S Fremont, Room 116, 1st Floor
Springfield, MO 65804   417-885-3324
                                      800-432-2273
                                      Fax: 417-888-8761

Primary and metastatic brain tumors; patients, families, and friends welcome. Second and Fourth Tuesday of each month, 2:00-3:30 pm. Light refreshments provided.

Connie Zimmerman, Contact

1209   Brain Tumor Support Group
Saint Luke's Hospital of Kansas City
44th & Wornall Road, Spencer Bldg, 2nd Floor
Kansas City, MO 64141   816-932-6220

Educational materials, telephone help line, newsletter, lectures, bereavement support group. Second Tuesday of each month, 7:00-8:30 pm.

1210   Brain Tumor Support Group of Greater St Louis
The Wellness Community of Greater St Louis
Cancer Support Community, 1058 Old Des Peres Road
Saint Louis, MO 63131   314-238-2000
                                      aeilers@wellnesscommunitystl.org

Third Thursday of each month, 6:30-8:30 pm.

Amy Eilers MSW LCSW, Program Director

Nebraska

1211   Brain Tumor Support Group at the Nebraska Medical Center
981130 Nebraska Medical Center
Omaha, NE 68198   402-559-4420
                                      800-922-0000
                                      www.nebraskamed.com/neuro/brain-spine-cancer-center/

Meets monthly. Call for more information. Please contact the Social Work Department at The Nebraska Medical Center for further information regarding this monthly support group.

Sue Stensland, Contact

Nevada

1212   Southern Nevada 'Grey Matters' Valley Hospital Medical Center
Medical Executive Conference Room
620 Shadow Lane
Las Vegas, NV 89106   702-204-1907

Third Tuesday of each month, 5:30-7:00 pm.

Janet Leinen RN, Contact

New Hampshire

1213 Angels of Hope
Derry Public Library
64 East Broadway
Derry, NH 03038   603-425-2822
angelsofhope@comcast.net

Second Monday of each month, 5:30-7:00 pm. Downstairs in the
Paul Collette Conference Room A.

Urszula Mansur, Contact

New Jersey

1214 Brain Tumor Support Group
Saint Barnabas Medical Center
PO Box 221
Martinsville, NJ 08836   908-685-0917
sshrodo@optonline.net
www.njbt.org/startCNJBTSG.cfm

Third Wednesday of each month, 6:30-8:00 pm.

Stan , Contact
Virginia , Contact

**1215 Brain Tumor Support Group at Plainfield Muhlenberg
Medical Center, Neuroscience**
Saint Luke's Roman Catholic Church
300 Clinton Avenue
North Plainfield, NJ 07063   732-321-7000
sshrodo@optonline.net
www.njbt.org/startCNJBTSG.htm

First Thursday of each month, 7:00-8:30 pm.

Stan , Contact
Virginia Shrodo, Contact

New Mexico

1216 NM Alliance for the Neurologically Impaired
531 Harkle Road, Suite B
Santa Fe, NM 87505   505-992-3126
505-670-0274

traumatic brain injury program but no support group.

Terry Lucero, Contact

1217 People Living Through Cancer
3411 Candelaria Rd. NE Suite M
Albuquerque, NM 87107   505-242-3263
888-441-4439
Fax: 505-242-6756
info@pltc.org
www.pltc.org

To connect and support cancer survivors and caregivers by transforming shared individual experiences into enduring hope.

Kathleen Raskob, Executive Committee Chair/President
Nancy Hoing, Vice-President
Sara J Lynch, Treasurer

New York

1218 Brain Tumor Support Group
Albany Medical Center
47 New Scotland Avenue, D Building, Room D105
Albany, NY 12208   518-262-6696

First Monday of the month, 5:30-7:30 pm.

Susan Weaver MD, Contact

**1219 Brain Tumor Support Group at South Nassau Community
Hospital**
One Healthy Way
Oceanside, NY 11572   516-632-3310
maddybrisman@aol.com

Third Wednesday of each month at 7:00 pm. We have just started
this support group. We welcome patients, family members, and
friends to join us and share feelings, concerns, and wuestions
about brain tumors and treatments available.

Maddy Singer CSW, Contact
Kathy Garizio RN, Contact

1220 Long Island Adult Brain Tumor Support Group
Plainview-Old Bethpage Public Library
999 Old Country Road
Plainview, NY 11803   516-747-8749
bcrescenzo@lancer-ins.com

First Thursday of the month, 7:00-9:00 pm, but call for information.

Bob Crescenzo, Contact

1221 Making Headway Foundation-Family Support Program
115 King Street
Chappaqua, NY 10514   914-238-8384
Fax: 914-238-1693
info@makingheadway.org
www.makingheadway.org

Call for scheduling. Dedicated to the Care, Comfort and Cure of
Children with Brain and Spinal Cord Tumors. The program offers
free, short-term individual counseling and educational
remediational services.

Edward Manley, President
Catherine Lepone, Executive Director
Linda Mudford-Lewis, Administrator

1222 New York Brain Tumor Support Group
525 East 68th Street, Room 5-106
New York, NY 10021   212-746-3986
wem9011@nyp.org

First Wednesdady of the month, 6:00 pm. Open to patients with
brain tumors of any kind and their families, caregivers, and
friends.

Wendy Mitchell LMSW, Contact

1223 People Treated for Brain Tumors and Their Caregivers
Memorial Sloan-Kettering Cancer Center
Rockefeller Research Lab, 430 East 67th Street
New York, NY 10065   212-717-3527

Fourth Wednesday of each month, 6:00-7:30 pm.

Clarissa Potter, Contact

**1224 Support for Parents of Children with Brain Tumors, Siblings
and Young Adults**
19 E 88 Street, Suite 1D
New York, NY 10128   212-534-8877

Call for specific times.

Marcia Greenleaf MD, Contact

1225 WNY Brain Tumor Support Group
3980 Sheriddan Drive
Amherst, NY 14226   716-250-2000
cjh99@adelphia.net

Third Tuesday of the month, 6:30 pm. This group has been in existence since 2000(We also facilitate the Orchard Park, NY
group). We have at least 3 speakers a year, usually doctors, and
we focus on positive ways to sope with living with a brain tumor
or caring for a loved one with a brain tumor.

Maria Caserta, Contact

North Carolina

**1226 Brain Tumor Support Group of the Carolinas and Virginia
Cancer Services**
Wake Forest University-Baptist Medical Center
Wake Forest University Baptist Medical Center/Canc
Winston-Salem, NC 27157   336-716-4137
www.wfubmc.edu

Second Tuesday of each month, 6:30-8:00 pm.

Rayetta Johnson RN, MSN, Contact

1227 Duke Brain Tumor Support Group
Duke University Medical Center
3000 Erwin Road
Durham, NC 27710
919-681-1687
calho006@mc.duke.edu

First Wednesday of the month, 3:00-4:00 pm.

Roberta Calhoun-Eagan LCSW, Clinical Social Worker

1228 Duke Pediatric Brain Tumor Family Support Program
Duke University Medical Center
Durham, NC 27710
919-684-2913

First and Third Tuesday, Second and Fourth Thursday,
12:00-1:00 pm. Teen group meets on the 1st Thursday of the
month from 5:00-6:30 pm.

Jean Hartford-Todd, Contact

1229 Western North Carolina Brain Tumor Support Group
West Asheville Presbyterian Church
West Presbyterian Church 690 Haywood Road
Asheville, NC 28806
828-253-0726
wncbt@cs.com

Third Thursday of each month, 6:15-8:00 pm. We will have guest
speakers occasionally. This group os for adults and their care-
givers/family. Please call for location and details. Refreshments
provided.

George Plym, Contact

Ohio

1230 Brain Tumor Support Group
Cleveland Clinic Foundation
9500 Euclid Avenue, Conference Room R3-003
Cleveland, OH 44101
216-445-6910
800-223-2273
Fax: 216-444-9170

Fourth Wednesday of each month, 5:00-6:30 pm.

Kathy Lupica RN, MSN, Contact

1231 Central Ohio Brain Tumor Support Group
Arthur James Cancer Hospital & Research Institute
4918 Cooper Road
Cincinnati, OH 45242
513-791-4060
bcrawford@cancer-support.org

Call for times.

Bonnie Crawford

1232 Cleveland Brain Tumor Patient Network - Adult and Pediatric
Univ Hospitals of Cleveland, Neurosurgery Conf Rm
2065 Abington, Lakeside Room, 5218
Cleveland, OH 44101
216-932-8510
info@clevlandclinic.org
www.clevlandclinic.org

This group does not currently meet, but does offer support
through networking. Please call and leave a message.

Lynn Szakacs, Contact

1233 Southwest Ohio Brain Tumor Support Group
Kettering Hospital
3535 Southern Boulevard, Dining Room 2B
Dayton, OH 45429
937-687-3325
937-298-4331

Second Monday each month, 7:00-8:30 pm.

Darlene Carroll, Contact
Jean Ruppert, Contact

1234 Support Group for Parents of Children with a Brain Tumor
Children's Hospital Medical Center
Cincinnati, OH 45229
513-559-4726

Call for specific times.

Karen Burkett CNS, Contact
Susan Mcgee CNS, Contact

Oregon

1235 Bend Support Group
St Charles Medical Center
St. Charles Medical Center MS Support Group 2500 N
Bend, OR 97701
541-617-2617

Second Saturday of every month.

1236 Brain Tumor Education & Support Group
Comprehensive Cancer Center
1130 NW 22nd Avenue, 2nd Floor, Conference Room#21
Portland, OR 97210
503-413-7921

First and Third Wednesday of each month, 4:00-5:30 pm. Parking
is available in the garage #3-enter between NW 21st and NW
22nd on NW Marshall.

Dawn Brucker LCSW, Contact

1237 Klamath Falls Support Group
2200 Eldorado Ave
Klamath Falls, OR 97601
541-274-2696
ccoffman@skylakes.org
www.spokeunlimited.org

Third week of every month. Meets at the office, with a monthly
fliar, and focuses on traumatic brain injuries.

Cornelea Coffman, Contact

Pennsylvania

1238 Brain Tumor Support Group at Philadelphia
Hospital of University of Pennsylvania Hospital
3400 Spruce Street, 1 Rhoads Conference Room
Philadelphia, PA 19104
215-746-7742

Third Tuesday of each month, 6:30-8:00 pm.

Stacy Oppleman, Contact

1239 Brain Tumor Support Group at Pittsburgh
4117 Liberty Avenue- Bloomfield Center
Pittsburgh, PA 15224
412-522-1212
Fax: 412-622-1216
info@cancercaring.org
www.cancercaring.org

Brain tumor group offered for aduly patients and family members.

Judy Joyce, Contact

1240 Brain Tumor Support Group of the Lehigh Valley
Saint John's Lutheran Church
St. John's U.C.C. Church 139 North 4th Street
Emmaus, PA 18049
610-830-0659
info@lvbraintumor.org
www.lvbraintumor.org

Second Tuesday of each month, 7:30 pm.

Dolores Fioriglio, Contact

1241 Camelot For Children
Pediatric Cancer Foundation of the Lehigh Valley
2354 W Emmaus Ave
Allentown, PA 18103
610-791-5683
Fax: 610-791-5256
joellenm@camelotforchildren.org
www.camelotforchildren.org

Mission Statement: The mission of Camelot for Children, Inc., a
non-profit organization, is to be a gathering place for seriously,
chronically, and terminally ill, handicapped or disabled children;
to foster an environment of emotional support among these special children and their families; to provide opportunities for these
special children to interact with each other in a family/home setting; and to help to develop their physical and mental abilities.
Fourth Tuesday of each month at 6:30 pm.

Jo Ellen Moll, Executive Director
Cassie Kemmerer, Volunteer Coordinator

Shane Valles, Contact

Rhode Island

1242 Brain Tumor Support Group at Providence
Brown University Campus
Brown University Biomedical Center
Providence, RI 02940

401-789-0126
401-647-2935

First and Third Tuesday of each month, 6:30-8:00 pm.

Judy Allenson, Contact
Betty Bentley, Contact

South Carolina

1243 Newberry County Memorial Hospital Brain Tumor Support Group
2669 Kinard Street, Education Room
Newberry, SC 29108

803-276-7570
info@newberryhospital.org
www.angelfire.com/sc2/sctumor/

First Thursday of each month, 7:00-8:30 pm.

Joel S Sexton, Contact

Tennessee

1244 Memphis Regional Brain Tumor Survivors Group
Colonial Park United Methodist Church
Colonial Park United Methodist Church 5330 Park Av
Memphis, TN 38119

901-757-0806
cherrywel@earthlink.net
www.semmes-murphey.com/support_group.php

First THursday of every month at 6:30 pm.

Cherry Welborn, Contact

Texas

1245 Brain Tumor Support Group at Dallas
American Cancer Society
8900 Carpenter Freeway
Dallas, TX 75247

214-977-7969

Second Wednesday of each month, 7:00-8:30 pm.

Alice Anderson, Contact

1246 Brain Tumor Support Group at Plano
Health South Rehab Hospital
PO Box 867084
Plano, TX 75086

972-335-4948
972-867-3431
GreyMattersNorthTexas@yahoo.com
www.greymatters.us

Second Tuesday of each month, 7:00-9:00 pm.

J Hoffman, CEO
S. Kuryla, President
P Griffith, Treasurer

1247 Central Texas Brain Tumor Support Group
Health South Rehab Hospital
1215 Red River Street
Austin, TX 78701

512-479-3509
tennistoml@hotmail.com

Second Thursday of the month, 6:30 pm.

Thomas Lewman, Contact
Joam Lewman, Contact

1248 HOPE (Helping Oncology Parents Endure) Brain Tumor Foundation of the Southwest
Children's Medical Center of Dallas
1935 Motor Street
Dallas, TX 75235

214-456-6139

Call for meeting times.

1249 Houston Area Brain Tumor Network
University of Texas MD Anderson Cancer Center
Place of Wellness, 1515 Holcombe Boulevard
Houston, TX 77030

713-792-0772
800-392-1611

First Tuesday of each month, 6:00-8:00 pm.

Suki Gibson, Contact
Rebecca Savoie, Contact

Virginia

1250 Brain Tumor Support Group
Saint Mary's Hospital
5801 Bremo Road, Room 159
Richmond, VA 23226

877-284-3905
curebt@hotmail.com
www.curebt.org

Second Tuesday of the month, 7:00-9:00 pm.

Carol Roberts RN MS, Contact

Washington

1251 Adult Brain Tumor Support Group
Virginia Mason Medical Center
1201 Terry Ave, Lindeman Pavillion, 10th Floor
Seattle, WA 98101

206-341-0420

Third Tuesday of every month, 2:30-4:00 pm.

Rick Edwards, Contact

1252 Brain Tumor Support Group University of Washington Medical Center
1959 NE Pacific Street, Box 356043
Seattle, WA 98195

206-598-4108

Meets first Wednesday of each month, 5:30-7:30 pm.

Stephanie Martin MSW LICSW, Contact

Wisconsin

1253 Brain Tumor Support Group
Luther Hospital
1221 Whipple Street, Conference Rooms 2 & 3
Eau Claire, WI 54703

206-598-4108

Second Tuesday of the Month, 6:30-7:30 pm.

Karen Snoble, Contact

1254 Brain Tumor Support Group at Milwaukee
St Lukes Medical Center
2900 W Oklahoma Avenue
Milwaukee, WI 53215

414-649-7200
800-252-2990

Second Wednesday of the month, 5:00-6:30 pm.

Linda Piacentine RN, MS, CNRN

1255 Brain Tumor Support Group at Wauwatosa Froederdt Memorial Lutheran Hospital
Administrative Board Room
9200 W Wisconsin Avenue
Wauwatosa, WI 53226

414-805-2629

Third Tuesday of each month, 6:30-8:30 pm.

Celeste Volcesek, Contact

1256 John Sierzant Brain Tumor Support Group
Gunderson Lutheran Medical Center
Gundersen Lutheran Medical Center 1900 South Avenu
LaCrosse, WI 54601

608-775-2952
padavenp@gundluth.org

First Tuesday of each month, 7:00-9:00 pm.

Polly Davenport-Fortune, Contact

Research Centers

1257 Brain Research Center
Children's Hospital National Medical Center
111 Michigan Avenue NW
Washington, DC 20010
202-476-5000
800-787-0021
tbear@childrensnational.org
www.cnmc.org

Barbara Herman, Chief

1258 Brain Research Foundation
111 West Washington Street , Suite 1710
Chicago, IL 60602
312-759-5150
Fax: 312-759-5151
info@theBRF.org
www.brainresearchfdn.org

Provides support to scinetists who are working to undersatnd the functioning of the brain. It establishes and provides financial assistance for research at the Brain Research Foundation. It also funds professional and scientific education.

Nathan T. Hansen, President
Normal R Bobins, Vice President
David H Fishburn, Treasurer

Conferences

1259 Long Term Survivor Conference
Childhood Brain Tumor Foundation
20312 Watkins Meadow Drive
Germantown, MD 20876
301-515-2900
877-217-4166
Fax: 301-540-8367
cbtf@childhoodbraintumor.org
www.childhoodbraintumor.org

In collaboration with the Children's National Medical Center, includes excellent topics and speakers from the region who shared their expertise.

Jeanne Young, President

Web Sites

1260 American Brain Tumor Association
8550 W. Bryn Mawr Ave. Ste 550
Chicago, IL 60631
773-577-875
800-886-2282
Fax: 773-577-8738
info@abta.org
www.abta.org

Information about brain tumors.

Elizabeth M. Wilson, MNA, President/ CEO
Kerri Mink, Chief Operating Officer
Meg Schneider, Chief Advancement Officer

1261 CancerCare
275 Seventh Avenue
New York, NY 10001
800-813-4673
info@cancercare.org
www.cancercare.org

CancerCare is a national nonprofit, 501(c)(3) organization that provides free, professional support services to anyone affected by cancer: people with cancer, caregivers, children, loved ones, and the bereaved. CancerCare programs - including counseling and support groups, education, financial assistance and practical help - are provided by professional oncology social workers and are completely free of charge.

Patricia J Goldsmith, CEO
John Rutigliano, Chief Operating Officer
Ahuva Morris, Children's Program Coordinator

1262 Online Mendelian Inheritance in Man
National Library of Medicine, Building 38A
Bethesda, MD 20894
888-346-3656
info@ncbi.nlm.nih.gov
www.ncbi.nlm.nih.gov

This database is a catalog of human genes and genetic disorders.

Christine E. Seidman, M.D., Chair
David J. Lipman, M.D., Executive Secretary

1263 Pediatric Brain Tumor Foundation of the United States
302 Ridgefield Court
Asheville, NC 28806
800-253-6530
www.curethekids.org/events/ride-for-kids/

Our mission is in support of the efforts of the Pediatric Brian Tumor Foundation of the United States, a nonprofit chariable foundation.

Chris Hoefflin, Chair
Larry Little, Vice Chairman
Robin Boettcher, President

1264 Starting Point: To Connect with Resources Related to Pediatric Neuro-oncology
www.med.miami.edu/neurosurgery/start_intro.htm

Specializes in the management of patients with surgically treatable neurological diseases. The scope of practice includes the care of patients with disorders of the brain, spinal cord and nerves including cerebrovascular disease, intracranial and spinal tumors, disorders of the spinal cord and vertebral column, pediatric neurosurgical problems, movement disorders, medically intractable seizure disorders, and head and spinal injuries.

Illinois

1265 Caregiver Brain Tumor Support Group
www.cancercare.org/support_groups/100-brain_tumor_ca

This 15-week online support group is for people caring for a loved one with a malignant brain tumor. Fourth Wednesday of each month, 7:00-8:30 pm. Contact for location.

Book Publishers

1266 Alex's Journey: The Story of a Child with a Brain Tumor
American Brain Tumor Association
8550 W Bryn Mawr Ave. Ste 550
Chicago, IL 60631
773-577-8750
800-886-2282
Fax: 773-577-8738
info@abta.org
www.abta.org

Available in DVD or Cassette.

Elizabeth M Wilson, President/CEO
Susan Netchin Kramer, Co-Founder
Barbara Dunn, Secretary

1267 Let's Talk About Going to the Hospital
Rosen Publishing Group's PowerKids Press
29 E 21st Street
New York, NY 10010
212-777-3017
800-237-9932
Fax: 888-436-4643
rosenpub@tribeca.ios.com
www.rosenpublishing.com

If a child has to check into the hospital, chances are he or she is already upset about being ill. Knowing how a hospital functions and what the procedures are, such as when family members can visit, will help in what is already a stressful situation. Grades K-5.

24 pages
ISBN: 0-823950-36-0

1268 Let's Talk About when Kids Have Cancer
Rosen Publishing Group's PowerKids Press
29 E 21st Street
New York, NY 10010

212-777-3017
800-237-9932
Fax: 888-436-4643
customerservice@rosenpub.com
www.rosenpublishing.com

In a straightforward yet comforting way, this book explains what cancer is, what kinds of treatments surround the disease and how to cope if a child or the friend of a child has cancer.

24 pages
ISBN: 0-823951-95-2

1269 Pediatric Cancer Sourcebook
Omnigraphics
PO Box 31-1640
Detroit, MI 48231

800-234-1340
Fax: 800-875-1340
info@omnigraphics.com
omnigraphics.com

Basic consumer health information about leukemias, brain tumors, sarcomas, lymphomas and other cancers in infants, children and adolescents.

587 pages
ISBN: 0-780802-45-4

Newsletters

1270 Childhood Brain Tumor Foundation Newsletter
20312 Watkins Meadow Drive
Germantown, MD 20876

301-515-2900
877-217-4166
Fax: 301-540-8367
cbtf@childhoodbraintumor.org
www.childhoodbraintumor.org

Seeking second opinions, access to healthcare, and combating discrimination.

3x/year

Jeanne P. Young, President
Carol Cornman, Vice President
Kiren Day, Vice President

1271 Message Line
American Brain Tumor Association
8550 W. Bryn Mawr Ave. Ste 550
Chicago, IL 60631

773-577-875
800-886-2282
Fax: 773-577-8738
info@abta.org
www.abta.org

Describes research advances and announces updates to publications.

Booklet

Elizabeth M. Wilson, MNA, President/ CEO
Kerri Mink, Chief Operating Officer
Meg Schneider, Chief Advancement Officer

1272 SEARCH
National Brain Tumor Foundation
1517 North Point Street, #531
San Francisco, CA 94123

617-924-9997
800-934-2873
Fax: 617-924-9998
nbtf@braintumor.org
www.braintumor.org

Newsletter that covers topics of current interest to brain tumor survivors and their families.

Quarterly

Sally Davis, Chief Executive Officer
James Charnley, Chief Financial Officer
Mike Sachleben, Chief Technology Officer

Pamphlets

1273 A Primer of Brain Tumors
American Brain Tumor Association
8550 W. Bryn Mawr Ave. Ste 550
Chicago, IL 60631

773-577-875
800-886-2282
Fax: 773-577-8738
info@abta.org
www.abta.org

A patient's reference manual offering information on brain tumors.

Pamphlet

Elizabeth M. Wilson, MNA, President/ CEO
Kerri Mink, Chief Operating Officer
Meg Schneider, Chief Advancement Officer

1274 About Ependymoma
American Brain Tumor Association
8550 W. Bryn Mawr Ave. Ste 550
Chicago, IL 60631

773-577-875
800-886-2282
Fax: 773-577-8738
info@abta.org
www.abta.org

Pamphlet

Elizabeth M. Wilson, MNA, President/ CEO
Kerri Mink, Chief Operating Officer
Meg Schneider, Chief Advancement Officer

1275 About Glioblastoma Multiforme and Anaplastic Astrocytoma
American Brain Tumor Association
8550 W. Bryn Mawr Ave. Ste 550
Chicago, IL 60631

773-577-875
800-886-2282
Fax: 773-577-8738
info@abta.org
www.abta.org

Pamphlet

Elizabeth M. Wilson, MNA, President/ CEO
Kerri Mink, Chief Operating Officer
Meg Schneider, Chief Advancement Officer

1276 About Medulloblastoma/PNET (Medulloblastoma)
American Brain Tumor Association
8550 W. Bryn Mawr Ave. Ste 550
Chicago, IL 60631

773-577-875
800-886-2282
Fax: 773-577-8738
info@abta.org
www.abta.org

Pamphlet

Elizabeth M. Wilson, MNA, President/ CEO
Kerri Mink, Chief Operating Officer
Meg Schneider, Chief Advancement Officer

1277 About Meningioma
American Brain Tumor Association
8550 W. Bryn Mawr Ave. Ste 550
Chicago, IL 60631

773-577-875
800-886-2282
Fax: 773-577-8738
info@abta.org
www.abta.org

Pamphlet

Elizabeth M. Wilson, MNA, President/ CEO
Kerri Mink, Chief Operating Officer
Meg Schneider, Chief Advancement Officer

1278 About Metastatic Tumors to the Brain and Spine
American Brain Tumor Association
8550 W. Bryn Mawr Ave. Ste 550
Chicago, IL 60631

773-577-875
800-886-2282
Fax: 773-577-8738
info@abta.org
www.abta.org

Pamphlet

Elizabeth M. Wilson, MNA, President/ CEO
Kerri Mink, Chief Operating Officer
Meg Schneider, Chief Advancement Officer

1279 About Oligodendroglioma and Mixed Glioma
American Brain Tumor Association
8550 W. Bryn Mawr Ave. Ste 550
Chicago, IL 60631

773-577-875
800-886-2282
Fax: 773-577-8738
info@abta.org
www.abta.org

Pamphlet

Elizabeth M. Wilson, MNA, President/ CEO
Kerri Mink, Chief Operating Officer
Meg Schneider, Chief Advancement Officer

1280 About Pituitary Tumors
American Brain Tumor Association
8550 W. Bryn Mawr Ave. Ste 550
Chicago, IL 60631

773-577-875
800-886-2282
Fax: 773-577-8738
info@abta.org
www.abta.org

Pamphlet

Elizabeth M. Wilson, MNA, President/ CEO
Kerri Mink, Chief Operating Officer
Meg Schneider, Chief Advancement Officer

1281 About the American Brain Tumor Association
American Brain Tumor Association
8550 W. Bryn Mawr Ave. Ste 550
Chicago, IL 60631

773-577-875
800-886-2282
Fax: 773-577-8738
info@abta.org
www.abta.org

Pamphlet

Elizabeth M. Wilson, MNA, President/ CEO
Kerri Mink, Chief Operating Officer
Meg Schneider, Chief Advancement Officer

1282 Brain Tumors: Understanding Your Care
National Brain Tumor Foundation
1517 North Point Street, #531
San Francisco, CA 94123

617-924-9997
800-934-2873
Fax: 617-924-9998
nbtf@braintumor.org
www.braintumor.org

Easy-to-read, 24-page brochure that describes brain tumor diagnosis, surgery, radiation therapy options, chemotherapy, continuing care and adjusting to daily life.

Sally Davis, Chief Executive Officer
James Charnley, Chief Financial Officer
Mike Sachleben, Chief Technology Officer

1283 Chemotherapy of Brain Tumors
American Brain Tumor Association
8550 W. Bryn Mawr Ave. Ste 550
Chicago, IL 60631

773-577-875
800-886-2282
Fax: 773-577-8738
info@abta.org
www.abta.org

Provides information that will help you understand and participate in your chemotherapy treatment.

Elizabeth M. Wilson, MNA, President/ CEO
Kerri Mink, Chief Operating Officer
Meg Schneider, Chief Advancement Officer

1284 Clinical Trial for Brain Tumors
National Brain Tumor Foundation
1517 North Point Street, #531
San Francisco, CA 94123

617-924-9997
800-934-2873
Fax: 617-924-9998
nbtf@braintumor.org
www.braintumor.org

Lists of clinical trials by state, tumor type and/or treatment type.

Sally Davis, Chief Executive Officer
James Charnley, Chief Financial Officer
Mike Sachleben, Chief Technology Officer

1285 Conventional Radiation Therapy
American Brain Tumor Association
8550 W. Bryn Mawr Ave. Ste 550
Chicago, IL 60631

773-577-875
800-886-2282
Fax: 773-577-8738
info@abta.org
www.abta.org

Elizabeth M. Wilson, MNA, President/ CEO
Kerri Mink, Chief Operating Officer
Meg Schneider, Chief Advancement Officer

1286 Coping with Your Loved One's Brain Tumor
National Brain Tumor Foundation
1517 North Point Street, #531
San Francisco, CA 94123

617-924-9997
800-934-2873
Fax: 617-924-9998
nbtf@braintumor.org
www.braintumor.org

A 12-page brochure that describes important coping strategies for
caregivers and family members of a loved one with a brain tumor.

Sally Davis, Chief Executive Officer
James Charnley, Chief Financial Officer
Mike Sachleben, Chief Technology Officer

1287 Dictionary for Brain Tumor Patients
American Brain Tumor Association
8550 W. Bryn Mawr Ave. Ste 550
Chicago, IL 60631

773-577-875
800-886-2282
Fax: 773-577-8738
info@abta.org
www.abta.org

Offers a dictionary of terms used in the diagnosis and everyday
living with brain tumors.

128 pages

Elizabeth M. Wilson, MNA, President/ CEO
Kerri Mink, Chief Operating Officer
Meg Schneider, Chief Advancement Officer

1288 National Brain Tumor Foundation Fact Sheets
National Brain Tumor Foundation
1517 North Point Street, #531
San Francisco, CA 94123

617-924-9997
800-934-2873
Fax: 617-924-9998
nbtf@braintumor.org
www.braintumor.org

Titles include: Health Insurance Coverage and Brain Tumors,
Overview of Complementary and Alternative Medicine Therapies, How Tumors Affect the Mind, Emotion and Personality,
Healing Power of your Fork: A Brain Tumor Survivor's Eating
Plan, Pilocytic Astrocytoma in the Adult, Childhood Brain Tumors Occuring in Adults, Who Gets Brain Tumors and Why?,
How to Choose a Treatment Center and Issues to Consider, Clinical Trials for Brain Tumors and How to Get Access, and many
others.

Sally Davis, Chief Executive Officer
James Charnley, Chief Financial Officer
Mike Sachleben, Chief Technology Officer

1289 Organizing and Facilitating a Support Group
American Brain Tumor Association
8550 W. Bryn Mawr Ave. Ste 550
Chicago, IL 60631
773-577-875
800-886-2282
Fax: 773-577-8738
info@abta.org
www.abta.org

Elizabeth M. Wilson, MNA, President/ CEO
Kerri Mink, Chief Operating Officer
Meg Schneider, Chief Advancement Officer

1290 Stereotactic Radiosurgery
American Brain Tumor Association
8550 W. Bryn Mawr Ave. Ste 550
Chicago, IL 60631
773-577-875
800-886-2282
Fax: 773-577-8738
info@abta.org
www.abta.org

Elizabeth M. Wilson, MNA, President/ CEO
Kerri Mink, Chief Operating Officer
Meg Schneider, Chief Advancement Officer

1291 Understanding Glioblastoma Multiforme
National Brain Tumor Foundation
1517 North Point Street, #531
San Francisco, CA 94123
617-924-9997
800-934-2873
Fax: 617-924-9998
nbtf@braintumor.org
www.braintumor.org

A 16 page brochure to help patients and care-givers understand more about the diagnosis and treatment of the glioblastoma multiforme.

Sally Davis, Chief Executive Officer
James Charnley, Chief Financial Officer
Mike Sachleben, Chief Technology Officer

1292 What You Need to Know About Brain Tumors
National Cancer Institute
BG 9609 MSC 9760, 9609 Medical Center Drive
Bethesda, MD 20892
800-422-6237
www.cancer.gov

Offers factual information about brain tumors, possible causes, primary and secondary tumors, symptoms, diagnosis, treatment, side effects, follow up care, support and medical terms.

Harold Varmus, M.D., Director

1293 When Your Child is Ready to Return to School
American Brain Tumor Association
8550 W. Bryn Mawr Ave. Ste 550
Chicago, IL 60631
773-577-875
800-886-2282
Fax: 773-577-8738
info@abta.org
www.abta.org

Guides parents and teachers through a successful return to school when a child has had a brain tumor.

Paperback

Elizabeth M. Wilson, MNA, President/ CEO
Kerri Mink, Chief Operating Officer
Meg Schneider, Chief Advancement Officer

Camps

1294 Arizona Camp Sunrise & Sidekicks
PO Box 27872
Tempe, AZ 85285
480-382-8564
928-478-4564
melissa@azcampsunrise.org
www.azcampsunrise.org

The camp is dedicated to provide an exciting, medically safe camp program for children whose families have been affected by cancer.

Melissa Lee, Camp Director

1295 Camp Catch-A-Rainbow
American Cancer Society
1205 E Saginaw Street
Lansing, MI 48906
517-371-2920
800-227-2345
kwilson@ymcastorercamps.org
www.cancer.gov/camprainbow

Open to any child (ages 7 thru 15) who has, or has had, cancer.

Katie Wilson, Coordinator

1296 Camp Fantastic
Special Love
117 Youth Development Court
Winchester, VA 22602
703-667-3774
888-930-2707
www.specialove.org

Nonprofit organization that provides enriching programs for children with cancer, including Camp Fantastic.

Dave Smith, CEO
Angela Ashman, Program Director

1297 Camp Merry Heart/Easter Seals Easter Seal Society
21 O'Brian Road
Hackettstown, NJ 07840
908-852-3896
Fax: 908-852-9263
camp@nj.easterseals.com
www.nj.easterseals.com

An organized program of swimming, arts and crafts, boating, nature study and travel offered to the physically disabled, developmentally disabled, cerebral palsied, brain damaged and head injured children, ages 5-18, adults 19-75+. Fall and spring travel programs for adults.

Mary Ellen Ross, Camping Director

1298 Camp Sunshine Dreams
PO Box 28232
Fresno, CA 93729
contact@campsunshinedreams.com
www.campsunshinedreams.com

Summer camp for children with cancer.

Anthony Aiello, Board Member

1299 Des Moines YMCA Camp
1192 166th Drive
Boone, IA 50036
515-432-7558
Fax: 515-432-5414
ycamp@dmymca.org
www.y-camp.org

For boys and girls with cancer, diabetes, asthma, cystic fibrosis, hearing impaired and other disabilities.

David Sherry, Executive Director
Alex Kretzinger, Program Director Camps

1300 Okizu Foundation Camps
16 Digital Drive, Suite 130
Novato, CA 94949
415-382-9083
Fax: 415-382-8384
info@okizu.org
www.okizu.org

This foundation runs family camp programs for children who have cancer and their families, and for children who have or had a parent with cancer.

Lori Sparrow, Executive Director
Heather Ferrier, Camp Director of Operations

DESCRIPTION

1301 BRONCHOPULMONARY DYSPLASIA

Synonym: BPD

Involves the following Biologic System(s):

Neonatal and Infant Disorders, Respiratory Disorders

Bronchopulmonary dysplasia (BPD) is a chronic lung disease of infancy that is characterized by injury to the lung's airways, causing abnormal tissue changes, inflammation, and eventual scarring of lung tissue. BPD often affects infants who have become dependent on the long-term use of ventilators to mechanically assist their breathing. In these infants with BPD, lung injury is thought to result from prolonged breathing of high concentrations of oxygen under abnormally high pressure and volume (oxygen toxicity, barotrauma, and volutrauma). BPD affects infants who are born prior to 37 weeks of pregnancy (premature newborns) and are affected by severe respiratory distress syndrome of the newborn (RDS). RDS is characterized by insufficient production of a substance (surfactant) that is produced as the lungs mature during fetal development. Surfactant reduces the surface tension of fluids lining the air sacs (alveoli) of the lungs, enabling the air sacs to remain open between breaths. Due to insufficient surfactant in premature newborns with RDS, greater pressure is required to expand the lungs' airways and air sacs. As a result, the air sacs may collapse and the lungs may become unable to properly provide oxygenated blood to the body. Within minutes or hours after birth, newborns with RDS experience increasing difficulty breathing (dyspnea), characterized by rapid, labored, shallow breaths (tachypnea); grunting upon exhalation; drawing in of the chest wall during inhalation; and bluish discoloration of the skin and mucous membranes (cyanosis) due to lack of sufficient oxygen supply to bodily tissues (hypoxia). In infants with severe RDS, treatment typically includes prolonged support with a ventilator to keep the aveoli open (positive pressure ventilator). BPD is said to exist if lung disease persists, usually with an oxygen requirement, beyond the first month of life.

Despite receiving increasing concentrations of oxygen and other treatment measures, newborns with RDS and subsequent bronchopulmonary dysplasia continue to experience severe respiratory symptoms rather than improve as expected. These infants have ongoing respiratory distress associated with hypoxia, abnormally high levels of carbon dioxide in the blood (hypercarbia), a reduced ability of the right side of the heart to pump blood efficiently (right-sided heart failure), and continued oxygen dependency. Approximately two to three weeks after continued ventilation support, x-ray examination and other diagnostic techniques may demonstrate the abnormal tissue changes (bronchiolar metaplasia) and scarring of lung tissue associated with bronchopulmonary dysplasia.

The treatment of infants with BPD may include gradual weaning off mechanical ventilation; prescription of corticosteroid medications (e.g., dexamethasone) to reduce inflammation, administration of medications to helpexpand the airways of the lungs (bronchodilators) and drugs to promote the excretion of fluid from the body (diuretics); restriction of fluid intake; and therapies to help prevent or treat certain respiratory infections (e.g., respiratory syncytial virus). Maturation of the lungs is the most important treatment and most patients recover by approximately six to 12 months. However, these children may have an increased susceptibility to inflammation and infection of the lungs (pneumonia) or other potential complications, such as temporary growth failure. In some patients with severe BPD, prolonged hospitalization may be necessary.

Government Agencies

1302 NIH/ Eunice Kennedy Shriver National Insti tute of Child Health & Human Development

31 Center Drive, Building 31

Bethesda, MD 20892

301-496-5113

800-370-2943

Fax: 866-760-5947

TTY: 888-320-6942

nichdpress@mail.nih.gov

www.nichd.nih.gov

Established in 1962 by congress, today the institute conducts and supports laboratory research, clinical trials, and epidemiological studies that explore health processes; examines the impact of disabilities, diseases, and variations on the lives of individuals; and sponsors training programs for scientists, health care providers, and researchers to ensure that NICHD research can continue.

Diana W. Bianchi, Director

Paul Williams, Director, Communications

1303 NIH/National Heart, Lung and Blood Institu te

National Institute of Health

31 Center Dr MSC 2486, Bldg 31, Room 5A52

Bethesda, MD 20892

301-592-8573

Fax: 240-629-3246

TTY: 240-629-3255

nhlbiinfo@nhlbi.nih.gov

www.nhlbi.nih.gov

The National Heart, Lung, and Blood Institute (NHLBI) provides global leadership for a research, training, and education program to promote the prevention and treatment of heart, lung, and blood diseases and enhance the health of all individuals so that they can live longer and more fulfilling lives.

Gary H Gibbons MD, Director

Nakela Cook MD, Chief of Staff

National Associations & Support Groups

1304 American Academy of Pediatrics

141 Northwest Point Boulevard

Elk Grove Village, IL 60007

847-434-4000

800-433-9016

Fax: 847-434-8000

www.aap.org

The American Academy of Pediatrics and its member pediatricians are committed to the attainment of optimal physical, mental and social health and well-being for all infants, children, adolescents, and young adults.

Fernando Stein, MD, FAAP, President

Karen Remley, MD, CEO/Executive VP

1305 American Lung Association

55 W. Wacker Drive, Suite 1150

Chicago, IL 60601

312-801-7628

800-586-4872

info@lung.org

www.lung.org

The American Lung Association fights lung disease in all its forms, with special emphasis on asthma, tobacco control and environmental health. The American Lung Association is funded with contributions from the public, along with gifts and grants from corporations, foundations and government agencies. The association achieves its many successes through the work of thousands of committed volunteers and staff.

Harold P. Wimmer, National President & CEO

Susan Rappaport, National VP, Research/Scientific

Sue Swan, Chief Development Officer

1306 Genetic Alliance
4301 Connecticut Avenue NW, Suite 404
Washington, DC 20008
202-966-5557
800-336-4363
Fax: 202-966-8553
info@geneticalliance.org
www.geneticalliance.org

World's leading nonprofit health advocacy organization committed to transforming health through genetics and promoting an environment of openness centered on the health of individuals, families, and communities.

Sharon Terry, President/CEO
Tetyana Murza, Managing Director
Natasha Bonhomme, VP, Strategic Development

1307 March of Dimes Foundation
1275 Mamaroneck Avenue
White Plains, NY 10605
914-997-4488
888-663-4637
Fax: 914-997-4763
answers@marchofdimes.com
www.marchofdimes.com

March of Dimes help moms have full-term pregnancies and research the problems that threaten the health of babies.The March of Dimes also acts globally: sharing best practices in perinatal health and helping improve birth outcomes where the needs are the most urgent.

Stacey D. Stewart, President

Conferences

1308 Genetic Alliance Annual Conference
Genetic Alliance
4301 Connecticut Avenue NW, Suite 404
Washington, DC 20008
202-966-5557
800-336-4363
Fax: 202-966-8553
info@geneticalliance.org
www.geneticalliance.org

Consistently inspirational and enables partnership among all stakeholders: advocates and community leaders, health and industry professionals, policymakers, and academicians.

July

Sharon Terry, President/CEO
Tetyana Murza, Managing Director
Natasha Bonhomme, VP, Strategic Development

Web Sites

1309 American Lung Association
55 W. Wacker Drive, Suite 1150
Chicago, IL 60601
312-801-7628
800-LUN-USA
info@lung.org
www.lung.org

The American Lung Association fights lung disease in all its forms, with special emphasis on asthma, tobacco control and environmental health. The American Lung Association is funded with contributions from the public, along with gifts and grants from corporations, foundations and government agencies. The association achieves its many successes through the work of thousands of committed volunteers and staff.

Harold P. Wimmer, National President & CEO
Susan Rappaport, National VP, Research/Scientific
Sue Swan, Chief Development Officer

Camps

1310 VACC Camp
Nicklaus Children's Hospital
3200 SW 60th Court, Suite 203
Miami, FL 33155
305-662-8222
Fax: 786-268-1765
bela.florentin@mch.com
www.vacccamp.com

Free, week-long, overnight camp for ventilation assisted children (children needing a tracheotomy ventilator, C-PAP, BiPAP, or oxygen to support breathing) and their families. Gives families a fun oppourtinity to socialize with peers and enjoy activities not readily accessible to technology dependent children.

Bela Florentin, Camp Coordinator
Rose Ann Farrell, Volunteer Assistants Coordinator
Alyssa Garcia, Operations

DESCRIPTION

1311 BURN INJURIES

Involves the following Biologic System(s):

Dermatologic Disorders

Burn injuries account for approximately 6,000 deaths per year in the United States. Among children, it follows only automobile accidents as a leading cause of accidental fatalities. Burns may be caused by heat, chemicals, or electrical current and are classified as first degree burns, second degree burns, or third degree burns, according to the severity and depth of the injury.

First degree burns, the least severe, affect the surface of the skin (superficial) and are characterized by a sensitive or painful reddened area of skin that sometimes swells and, in some cases, peels off. These types of burns affect only the top layer of skin (epidermis), do not blister, and, in most cases, heal spontaneously with no complications.

Second degree burns affect both the upper layer of skin and varying degrees of the underlying layer (dermis). This type of burn causes blistering. Even if the burn is relatively superficial, the pain may be intense as a result of exposed nerve endings. Superficial second degree burns usually heal within one to two weeks with no residual effects. Deeper second degree burns may actually be less painful and, if kept clean and free of infection, also heal with no complications. Second degree burns that cover more than 30 percent of the body surface area are considered critical.

Third degree burns destroy the upper layer of the skin and the underlying tissues; therefore, this type of burn typically requires skin grafting or other special treatment. Third degree burns are usually characterized by either a white or charred appearance; however, the burned area may appear bright red. Third degree burns that cover more than 10 percent of the body surface area or that involve the face or extremities are considered critical.

Burns that are chracterized by significant charring and exposure of muscle and bone are sometimes referred to as fourth degree burns. Hospitalization for first and second degree burn injuries is largely determined by the amount of the body surface area that is affected. As a general rule, if there is less than 10 percent involvement, treatment may be provided at home or on an outpatient basis. Treatment may include thorough cleansing of the wounds and topical application of antibacterial ointments to small burn areas. Blister management may be provided through cream dressings. If blisters break, thorough cleansing (debridement) to prevent infection is indicated. Bandage or gauze dressings may be applied to keep the injured areas clean to avoid infection. Skin grafting may be indicated for extensive second degree burns. Other treatment may include the administration of antibiotics and analgesics, aswell as injection of a tetanus booster, if necessary.

Third degree or other severe burns may be life-threatening and usually require hospitalization. Smoke and injury due to inhalation can be severe yet go unrecognized. Facials burns should raise the suspicion that there may be damage to the respiratory tract, requiring special vigilance. Emergency intervention may include the administration of oxygen and use of a ventilator to assist in breathing. Vital signs are routinely checked. To prevent kidney failure and other serious complications such as shock, other treatment usually includes intravenous replacement of proteins, body fluids, and essential elements in the fluid portion of the blood (electrolytes such as sodium, potassium, and calcium) lost as a result of extensive injury. The wounds are meticulously cleaned and dressed, and antibiotics are usually administered intravenously to prevent infection. As with less severe burns, tetanus immunization is updated. Extreme vigilance is required in order to preserve the integrity of surrounding tissue, sometimes necessitating the surgical removal of crusted dead skin (escharotomy) that may interfere with circulation. If injured, arms or legs are elevated. In order to help avoid the tightening and contracting of skin and muscles, the limbs may be splinted. Temporary skin grafting may be performed until permanent grafting is possible. In addition, nutritional considerations may necessitate the administration of supplements or, in the case of those unable to eat or drink, insertion of a tube through the nose to deliver nutrition directly into the stomach. Burns sustained through chemical and electrical influences may involve other systems of the body and, as such, are treated symptomatically. Psychological support by a team of professionals is an extremely important element in the recovery of individuals with burn injuries. Other treatment is symptomatic and supportive.

National Associations & Support Groups

1312 American Academy of Pediatrics
141 Northwest Point Boulevard
Elk Grove Village, IL 60007
847-434-4000
800-433-9016
Fax: 847-434-8000
www.aap.org

The American Academy of Pediatrics and its member pediatricians are committed to the attainment of optimal physical, mental and social health and well-being for all infants, children, adolescents, and young adults.

Fernando Stein, MD, FAAP, President
Karen Remley, MD, CEO/Executive VP

1313 Burn Institute
8825 Aero Drive, Suite 200
San Diego, CA 92123
858-541-2277
Fax: 858-541-7179
www.burninstitute.org

A nonprofit health agency dedicated to reducing burn injuries and deaths through fire and burn prevention education, burn survivor support programs and the funding of burn care research and treatment.

Gerald S Davee, Esq., Chair
Chief David, President
Timothy O Malley PhD, Vice President Development

1314 Burn Prevention Foundation
236 N 17th Street
Allentown, PA 18104
610-969-3930
800-207-3090
Fax: 610-969-3940
info@burnprevention.org
www.burnprevention.org

The mission of the Burn Foundation is to provide burn injury prevention education and advocacy for those at greatest risk. Our primary service area is in Eastern Pennsylvania, although many of our programs and products are utilized worldwide.

Dan Dillard, Executive Director/CEO
Jessica Banks, Prevention Education Director
Susan Numbers, Administrative Assistant

1315 Burn Survivors Throughout the World
650 N Beneva Road, #305
Sarasota, FL 34232
941-364-8457
800-503-8058
Fax: 941-364-8441
info@burnsurvivorsttw.org
www.burnsurvivorsttw.org

An international nonprofit organization working to rebuild the
lives of the current and future burn survivors worldwide. Offers
membership, a peer support team, education, advocacy, medical
referrals, a free medical treatment program, medical equipment,
legal referrals, healing weekends, and public awareness for the
burn survivor community and the public worldwide.

Michael Appleman, CEO

1316 International Society for Burn Injuries
2172 US Highway 181 South
Floresville, TX 78111
617-726-3447
Fax: 617-367-8936
lizals@tgti.net
www.worldburn.org

Our society acknowledges the importance of all of these specialists in burn care and had intelligently admitted those professionals as members since its foundation. We must mention there are
very few, in fact almost no other medical societies like ours
which bring together such a number of different specialists, including nurses. One of the main purposes and aims of our society
is to disseminate knowledge and to stimulate prevention in the
field of burns.

Richard L Gamelli, MD, FACS, President
Dr. Rajeev B. Ahuja, President-Elect
William G Cioffi, M.D., FACS, Treasurer

1317 National Burn Victim Foundation
246A Madisonville Road
Basking Ridge, NJ 07920
www.nbvf.com

The National Burn Victim Foundation is a nonprofit service
agency that addresses the problems associated with burn injuries
and their prevention through consultation and education. The
NBVF also serves as an advocate for burn survivors and their
families. The foundation has provided free emergency services to
more than 3,000 New Jersey burn survivors since 1976.

1318 National Fire Protection Association
1 Batterymach Park
Quincy, MA 02169
617-770-3000
800-344-3555
Fax: 617-770-0700
custserv@nfpa.org
www.nfpa.org

The mission of the international nonprofit NFPA is to reduce the
worldwide burden of providing and advocating scientifically-based consensus codes and standards, research, training and
education.

James M Shannon, President & CEO
Nancy L. Perkins, Executive Administrator
Lisa A. Yarussi, Vice President

1319 Society for Pediatric Dermatology
8365 Keystone Crossing, Suite 107
Indianapolis, IN 46240
317-202-0224
Fax: 317-205-9481
info@pedsderm.net
www.pedsderm.net

The objective of the society is to promote, develop and advance
education, research and care of skin disease in all pediatric age
groups. The society has an international membership comprised
of physicians, scientists and professionals in training who have an
interest in pediatric skin and its diseases.

Kent Lindeman, Executive Director

Conferences

1320 Society for Pediatric Dermatology Annual Meeting
Society for Pediatric Dermatology
8365 Keystone Crossing, Suite 107
Indianapolis, IN 46240
317-202-0224
Fax: 317-205-9481
info@pedsderm.net
www.pedsderm.net

Kent Lindeman, Executive Director

Web Sites

1321 Burn Institute
8825 Aero Drive, Suite 200~
San Diego, CA 92123
858-541-2277
Fax: 858-541-7179
www.burninstitute.org

Burn prevention education, burn survivor support.

Gerald S. Davee, Chairman
David Ott, President
Bob Pfohl, Vice President

1322 Burn Prevention Foundation
236 North 17th Street
Allentown, PA 18104
610-969-3930
Fax: 610-969-3940
www.burnprevention.org

Provides burn injury prevention education and advocacy for those
at greatest risk.

Dan Dillard, Executive Director & CEO
Jessica Banks, Prevention Education Director
Meredith Casey, Coordinator

1323 Burn Survivors Throughout the World
www.burnsurvivorsttw.org

Offers a support team, e-lists, articles, stories, pictures, poems,
polls, newsletters, message boards and links, as well as weekly
scheduled, emergency, and public chats.

1324 Consumer Products Safety Commission
4330 East West Highway
Bethesda, MD 20814
301-504-7923
800-638-2772
Fax: 301-504-0124
www.cpsc.gov

The U.S. Comsumer Product Safety Commission is committed to
providing access to its web pages for individuals with disabilities.

Elliot F. Kaye, Chairman
Robert S. Adler, Commissioner
Ann Marie Buerkle, Commissioner

1325 Cool the Burn
640 Jackson Street~
St. Paul, MN 55101
651-254-3456
www.regionshospital.com

Cool the Burn is a unique resource for children whose lives have
been affected by a burn injury. Whether you, a family member or
a friend have been burned, this section will help you better understand burn unjuries.

1326 International Society for Burn Injuries
www.worldburn.org/index.cfm

Information on prevention of burn injuries.

Rajeev B. Ahuja, President

1327 National Burn Victim Foundation
www.nbvf.com

Addresses the problems associated with burn injuries and their
prevention through consultation and education.

1328 National Fire Protection Association
1 Batterymarch Park
Quincy, MA 02169   617-770-3000
                                     800-844-6058
                                     Fax: 617-770-0700
                                     www.nfpa.org

Providing and advocating scientifically-based consensus codes
and standards, research, training and education.

Ernest J. Grant, Chair
Randolph W. Tucker, 1st Vice Chair
Keith E. Williams, 2nd Vice Chair

1329 Society for Pediatric Dermatology
8365 Keystone Crossing, Suite 107
Indianapolis, IN 46240   317-202-0224
                                     Fax: 317-205-9481
                                     info@pedsderm.net
                                     www.pedsderm.net

Promotes, develop and advance education, research and care of
skin disease in all pediatric age groups.

Karen Wiss, President
Andrea Zaenglen, President-Elect
Stephanie Lander, Membership/Communications Manager

Book Publishers

1330 Burns Sourcebook
Omnigraphics
PO Box 31-1640
Detroit, MI 48231   800-234-1340
                                     Fax: 800-875-1340
                                     info@omnigraphics.com
                                     www.omnigraphics.com

Basic consumer health information on various types of burns and
scalds.

604 pages
ISBN: 0-780802-04-7

Journals

1331 Pediatric Dermatology Journal
Society for Pediatric Dermatology
8365 Keystone Crossing, Suite 107
Indianapolis, IN 46240   317-202-0224
                                     Fax: 317-205-9481
                                     info@pedsderm.net
                                     www.pedsderm.net

6 issues/yr
Kent Lindeman, Executive Director

Camps

1332 Firefighters Kids Camp Camp Concord
1000 Mount Tallac Road
South Lake Tahoe, CA 96150   916-739-8525
                                     catharine@ffburn.org
                                     www.ffburn.org

One-week program to benefit young burn survivors who are age
six to age seventeen. Our mission is to provide young burn survivors with a fun and safe camp environment that encourages healing, personal growth and character development within a natural
setting.

Catharine Shaw, Director

DESCRIPTION

1333 CELIAC DISEASE

Synonyms: CD, Celiac sprue, Gluten-sensitive enteropathy, GSE, Nontropical sprue

Involves the following Biologic System(s):

Gastrointestinal Disorders

Celiac disease (CD) is a digestive disorder in which the lining of the small intestine is damaged by gluten, a protein found in wheat, barley, rye, and oats. People with CD are thought to have an abnormal immune response to dietary gluten, resulting in the body's own immune system attacks and causes degeneration (atrophy) and flattening of the tiny projections (villi) that line the small intestine. These villi play a vital role in absorbing fats and other nutrients from food products (malabsorption). This damage to the intestinal villi seriously impairs their ability to absorb these nutrients. Although the specific cause of CD is unknown, it is thought to be multifactorial, resulting from interactions between multiple genes (polygenic) and certain environmental factors. CD may affect both children and adults. The frequency with which it occurs varies greatly among countries and among different populations, and more cases occur in Europe than in the United States. Approximately one in 10,000 infants is thought to be affected by CD in the U.S. Celiac disease is genetic, meaning it runs in families. Diagnosis is usually made by a gastroenterologist, through special blood tests and the testing of tissue from the small intestine.

The symptoms associated with celiac disease do not become apparent until gluten is introduced into the diet, and its symptoms may occur in the digestive system or elsewhere in the body. In most children with CD, symptoms begin between the ages of one to five years. Although the symptoms and findings in CD may vary, many children initially have diarrhea, and their stools become abnormally bulky, pale, frothy, and offensive smelling, the result of an abnormally increased fat content (steatorrhea). Other abnormalities in CD may include excessive gas (flatulence); a failure to grow and gain weight at the expected rate (failure to thrive), the result of a decreased intake of nutrients; lack of appetite (anorexia); hair loss; weight loss; vomiting; and swelling (distension) of the abdomen. Many children also experience muscle wasting, are unusually clingy and irritable, and have abnormally pale skin (pallor). As a result of the malabsorption of fats and other nutrients, children with this condition typically have deficiencies of certain vitamins, and some may have abnormally reduced levels of the oxygen-carrying protein hemoglobin in the blood, because of deficient intestinal absorption of iron (iron-deficiency anemia), which is an important component of hemoglobin.

The key step in treating celiac disease is eliminating gluten from the diet. Wheat and rye products must be completely eliminated, although some children with CD may be able to tolerate barley and oat products. Because gluten is widely used in various food products, parents and children may initially require assistance and guidance from an experienced dietitian in avoiding foods that contain it. Specially manufactured, gluten-free food products are available commercially, including gluten-free pasta, bread, and flour. Treatment may also include iron and vitamin supplementation as required.

National Associations & Support Groups

1334 American Academy of Pediatrics
141 Northwest Point Boulevard
Elk Grove Village, IL 60007
847-434-4000
800-433-9016
Fax: 847-434-8000
www.aap.org

The American Academy of Pediatrics and its member pediatricians are committed to the attainment of optimal physical, mental and social health and well-being for all infants, children, adolescents, and young adults.

Fernando Stein, MD, FAAP, President
Karen Remley, MD, CEO/Executive VP

1335 American Autoimmune Related Diseases Association, Inc.
22100 Gratiot Avenue
Eastpointe, MI 48021
586-776-3900
800-598-4668
Fax: 586-776-3903
aarda@aarda.org
www.aarda.org

The American Autoimmune Related Diseases Association is dedicated to the eradication of autoimmune diseases and the alleviation of suffering and the socioeconomic impact of autoimmunity through fostering and facilitating collaboration in the areas of education, public awareness, research, and patient services in an effective, ethical and efficient manner.

Virginia T. Ladd, President/Executive Director
Patricia Barber, Assistant Director
Deb Patrick, Events Specialist

1336 American Celiac Disease Alliance
americanceliac.org
feedback@americanceliac.org
americanceliac.org

In early 2003, an ad hoc group of 15 leaders in the celiac community came together to help persuade Congress to require food labels to include information about allergens.

1337 American Celiac Society
PO Box 23455
New Orleans, LA 70183
504-737-3293
Fax: 504-737-3283
americanceliacsociety@yahoo.com
www.americanceliacsociety.org

Nonprofit, tax exempt organization that supports efforts in education, research and natural support. Helps to set up support groups, sponsors conferences, seeks funding for education and research, identifies ingredients in foods and educates the public about problems facing its members.

Annette C Bentley, President
James R Bentley, VP

1338 American Celiac Society Dietary Support
www.americanceliacsociety.org
504-305-2968
www.americanceliacsociety.org

The American Celiac Society Dietary Support Coalition, a non-profit tax exempt organization, serves individuals suffering with dietary disorders.

Annette C. Bentley, President
James R. Bentley, Vice President

1339 American Dietetic Association
120 South Riverside Plaza, Suite 2000
Chicago, IL 60606
312-899-0040
800-877-1600
foundation@eatright.org
www.eatright.org

Nation's largest organization of food and nutrition professionals.

Ethan A Bergman PhD, RD, FADA, C, President
Glenna R McCollum DMOL, MPH, RD, President Elect
Patricia M Babjak, Chief Executive Officer

1340   American Society for Gastrointestinal Endoscopy
3300 Woodcreek Dr.
Downers Grove, IL 60515

630-573-0600
866-353-2743
Fax: 630-963-8332
info@asge.com
www.asge.org

ASGE has been dedicated to advancing patient care and digestive health by promoting excellence and innovation in gastrointestinal endoscopy.

Colleen M. Schmitt, President
Douglas O. Faigel, President Elect
Kenneth R. McQuaid, Secretary

1341   Association of Gastrointestinal Motility Disorders
12 Roberts Drive
Bedford, MA 01730

781-275-1300
Fax: 781-275-1304
digestive.motility@gmail.com
www.agmd-gimotility.org

AGMD is a non-profit organizations in existence with a focus on digestive motility diseases and disorders.

Thomas Abell, Advisor
Carlo Di Lorenzo, Advisor
Alex Flores, Advisor

1342   Asthma & Allergy Foundation of America
8201 Corporate Drive Suite 1000
Landover, MD 20785

800-727-8462
www.aafa.org

AAFA is a patient organization for people with asthma and allergies, and the oldest asthma and allergy patient group in the world.

Kelli Wilson, Chair
Lynn Hanessian, Immediate Past Chair
David Stukus, Secretary

1343   Catholic Celiac Society
www.catholicceliacs.org

Catholic Celiac Society's three-fold mission will be to educate Catholic celiacs about their options for Holy Communion as provided for by Canon Law and the U.S. Conference of Catholic Bishops; to inform Catholic clergy and lay ministers about the special needs of Catholic celiacs in their dioceses and parishes; and to reconcile those Catholic celiacs who have left the Church through lack of understanding, exclusion from the Eucharist, and isolation from their church community.

1344   Celiac Disease Foundation
20350 Ventura Blvd Ste 240
Woodland Hills, CA 91364

818-716-1513
Fax: 818-267-5577
cdf@celiac.org
www.celiac.org

Provides services and support to persons with celiac disease and dermatitus herpetiformis, through programs of awareness, education, advocacy and research; telephone information and referral services; medical advisory board; and special educational seminars and quarterly meetings.

Marc Riches, President
Richard Tasoff, Vice President
Christopher J. Holland, Treasurer

1345   Celiac Sprue Association/USA
PO Box 31700
Omaha, NE 68131

402-558-0600
877-272-4272
Fax: 402-643-4108
celiacs@csaceliacs.org
www.csaceliacs.org

National support organization that provides information and referral services for persons with celiac sprue and dermatitis herpetiformis and parents of celiac children. Made up of six regions in the United States, with 84 chapters and 36 resource units.

Bill Locke, President
Mary Schuluckebier, Executive Director
Clark Kolterman, Treasurer

1346   Celiac Support Association
P.O. Box 31700
Omaha, NE 68131

402-643-4101
877-272-4272
Fax: 402-643-4108
celiacs@csaceliacs.org
www.csaceliacs.org

Works to increase awareness, improve diagnosis and treatment, and help celiacs and gluten sensitive individuals to love living gluten-free.

1347   Children's National Health System
111 Michigan Avenue, NW
Washington, DC 20010

202-476-5000
888-884-2327
childrensnational.org

At Children's National, we are champions for children, with our entire team focused on pediatric care.

Kurt Newman, President & CEO
Vittorio Gallo, PhD, Chief Research Officer
Mark Batshaw, Executive VP & CAO

1348   Food Allergy Research & Education
7925 Jones Branch Dr., Suite 1100
McLean, VA 22102

703-691-3179
800-929-4040
Fax: 703-691-2713
www.foodallergy.org

FARE works on behalf of the 15 million Americans with food allergies, including all those at risk for life-threatening anaphylaxis.

Janet Atwater, Chair
Robert Nichols, Vice Chair
Sharyn T. Mann, Secretary

1349   GLC Annual Education Conference
Gluten Intolerance Group
31214 124th Ave SE
Auburn, WA 98092

253-833-6655
Fax: 206-833-6675
CustomerService@gluten.net
www.gluten.net

For individuals that are following a gluten-free diet, or want to know all you need about it.

July

David Kline, President
Joe Spancic, Vice President of Business Administ
Kim Kelly, Vice President of Programs

1350   Gluten Intolerance Group of North America (GIG)
31214 124th Ave SE
Auburn, WA 98092

253-833-6655
Fax: 206-833-6675
CustomerService@gluten.net
www.gluten.net

The mission of the Gluten Intolerance Group of North America™ is to provide support to persons with gluten intolerances, including celiac disease, dermatitis herpetiformis, and other gluten sensitivities, in order to live healthy lives.

David Kline, President
Joe Spancic, Vice President of Business Administ
Kim Kelly, Vice President of Programs

1351   Kids with Food Allergies
5049 Swamp Rd, Ste 303, PO Box 554
Fountainville, PA 18923

215-230-5394
215-340-7674
www.kidswithfoodallergies.org

Helps to mprove the day-to-day lives of families raising children with food allergies and empower them to create a safe and healthy future for their children.

Heidi Bayer, Chair
Colette Martin, Vice Chair
Amy Recob, Board of Director

1352 National Celiac Disease Society
34 Audrey Avenue, 3rd Floor
Oyster Bay, NY 11771   516-680-8873
                                      info@celiacnation.org
                                      www.celiacnation.org

It is an IRS recognized 501(c)(3) non-profit organization with a mission to raise celiac disease education and awareness.

Craig Pinto, Founder
Gary Leuis, Legal Advisor
Lawrence Baronciani, Creative Director

1353 National Foundation for Celiac Awareness
PO Box 544
Ambler, PA 19002   215-325-1306
                                 Fax: 215-643-1707
                                      www.celiaccentral.org

The National Foundation for Celiac Awareness advances widespread understanding of celiac disease as a serious genetic autoimmune condition and works to secure early diagnosis and effective management.

Wendi L. Wasik, Chair
David H. Cohen, Vice Chair
Alice Bast, President & CEO

1354 North American Society for the Study of Ce
P.O. Box 812180
Wellesley, MA 02482   781-431-8138
                                      www.nasscd.org

The NASSCD is the U.S. national society of medical, scientific and allied health professionals in the field of celiac disease.

Joseph A. Murray, President
Peter H.R. Green, President Elect
Alessio Fasano, Secretary

Conferences

1355 Annual Education Conference & Food Faire
Celiac Disease Foundation
20350 Ventura Boulevard, #240
Woodland Hills, CA 91364   818-716-1513
                                 Fax: 818-267-5577
                                      cdf@celiac.org
                                      www.celiac.org

Provides people with a greater understanding of Celiac disease, gluten sensitivity, dietary compliance, future therapies, associated conditions and the effect on family members. They networked with other people following the gluten-free lifestyle. Everyone met with exhibitors, sampled and discovered the latest gluten-free foods and services.

May

Mark Riches, President
Richard Tasoff, Vice President
Judy Thomas, Secretary

1356 CSA Annual Conference
Celiac Sprue Association
PO Box 31700
Omaha, NE 68131   402-643-4101
                                     877-272-4272
                                 Fax: 402-643-4108
                                      celiacs@csaceliacs.org
                                      www.csaceliacs.org

Invites experts from a broad spectrum of disciplines relating to celiac disease and the required gluten-free diet to share current information. Researchers, healthcare professionals, dietitians, authors, chefs, restaurant owners, and gluten-free food vendors from across the United States participate in this annual educational event.

September

Mary Schluckebier, Executive Director

Audio Video

1357 Unmarking Celiac Disease
American Celiac Society
PO Box 23455
New Orleans, LA 70183   504-737-3293
                                 Fax: 504-737-3283
                                      amerceliacsoc@onebox.com

Annette Bentley, President
James Bentley, Vice President

Web Sites

1358 Celiac Disease Foundation
20350 Ventura Boulevard, Suite 240
Woodland Hills, CA 91364   818-716-1513
                                      www.celiac.org

Provides support, information and assistance to people affected by Celiac Disease/Dermatitis Herpetiformis.

Elaine Monarch, Founder
Marc Riches, Chair
Chad Hines, Vice Chair

1359 Celiac Support Page
20350 Ventura Boulevard, Suite 240
Woodland Hills, CA 91364   818-716-1513
                                      www.celiac.com

To help as many people as possible with celiac disease get diagnosed and live happy, healthy gluten-free lives.

Elaine Monarch, Founder
Marc Riches, Chair
Chad Hines, Vice Chair

1360 Gluten-Free Page
donwiss.com

Offers links about Gluten Free Pages about the Celiac Disease/ Gluten Intolerance, gluten free food vendors, and other types of gluten free food sites.

1361 Health Answers
410 Horsham Road
Horsham, PA 19044   215-442-9017
                                      Michael.tague@healthanswers.com
                                      www.healthanswers.com

The vision was to provide a breadth of services to clients through the formation of a network of companies. Each company plays a key role in meeting out clients' needs.

Michael Tague, Managing Director

Book Publishers

1362 Digestive Diseases & Disorders Sourcebook
Omnigraphics
PO Box 625
Holmes, PA 19043   610-461-3548
                                     800-234-1340
                                 Fax: 610-532-9001
                                      info@omnigraphics.com
                                      www.omnigraphics.com

Basic consumer health information including celiac disease, Crohn's disease, diarrhea, hernias, irritable bowel syndrome and ulcers.

2000 335 pages
ISBN: 0-780803-27-2

Newsletters

1363 GIG Quarterly
Gluten Intolerance Group of North America
31214 124th Avenue SE
Auburn, WA 98092
253-833-6655
Fax: 253-833-6675
info@gluten.net
www.gluten.net

The mission of the Gluten Intolerance Group of North America™ is to provide support to persons with gluten intolerances, including celiac disease, dermatitis herpetiformis, and other gluten sensitivities, in order to live healthy lives.

Quarterly

David Kline, President
Kim Kelly, Vice President
Mark Evans, Vice President

1364 Lifeline
Celiac Sprue Association/USA
PO Box 31700
Omaha, NE 68131
402-558-0600
877-272-4272
Fax: 402-643-4108
celiacs@csaceliacs.org
www.csaceliacs.org

Quarterly newsletter for celiacs with membership forms, chapter information, resource unit information and promotion brochure.

Bruce Homstead, President
Mary A. Schluckebier, Executive Director
Jeanine Morgan, Recording Secretary

1365 Whoo's Report
PO Box 23455
New Orleans, LA 70183
504-737-3293
Fax: 504-737-3283

Provides practical assistance to members and individuals with celiac disease and information about the disease to the public.

Annette Bentley, President
James Bentley, Vice President

Pamphlets

1366 A Diet Management
Celiac Sprue Association/USA
PO Box 31700
Omaha, NE 68131
402-558-0600
877-272-4272
Fax: 402-643-4108
celiacs@csaceliacs.org
www.csaceliacs.org

A personalized chart that shows how to make your diet work.

Bruce Homstead, President
Mary A. Schluckebier, Executive Director
Jeanine Morgan, Recording Secretary

1367 A Success Story
Celiac Sprue Association/USA
PO Box 31700
Omaha, NE 68131
402-558-0600
877-272-4272
Fax: 402-643-4108
celiacs@csaceliacs.org
www.csaceliacs.org

Tells about the history of CSA. Also provides the information of how the CSA Gluten-Free Product Listing Book came about.

Bruce Homstead, President
Mary A. Schluckebier, Executive Director
Jeanine Morgan, Recording Secretary

1368 American Celiac Society
PO Box 23455
New Orleans, LA 71083
504-305-2968
Fax: 504-737-3283
info@americanceliacsociety.org
www.americanceliacsociety.org

Information package on American Celiac Society, a national support organization that provides information on celiac disease and related disorders. Provides information on local support groups throughout the US and the world.

Annette Bentley, President
James Bentley, Vice President

1369 Basics for the Gluten-free Diet
Celiac Sprue Association/USA
PO Box 31700
Omaha, NE 68131
402-558-0600; 877-272-4272
Fax: 402-643-4108
celiacs@csaceliacs.org
www.csaceliacs.org

Information sheets by the Celiac Sprue Association/USA Inc, a national support organization that provides information and referral services for persons with celiac sprue and dermatitis herpetiformis and parents of celiac children. Made up of 6 regions in the United States, with 84 chapters and 36 resource units.

Bruce Homstead, President
Mary A. Schluckebier, Executive Director
Jeanine Morgan, Recording Secretary

1370 Diet Instruction
Gluten Intolerance Group of North America
31214 124th Avenue SE
Auburn, WA 98092
253-833-6655
Fax: 253-833-6675

1371 Gluten-free Commercial Products
Celiac Sprue Association/USA
PO Box 31700
Omaha, NE 68131
402-558-0600; 877-272-4272
Fax: 402-643-4108
celiacs@csaceliacs.org
www.csaceliacs.org

Information sheets by the Celiac Sprue Association/USA.

Bruce Homstead, President
Mary A. Schluckebier, Executive Director
Jeanine Morgan, Recording Secretary

1372 Introductory Packet Brochure
Gluten Intolerance Group of North America
31214 124th Avenue SE
Auburn, WA 98092
253-833-6655
Fax: 253-833-6675

Offers facts and statistics on celiac sprue and dermatitis herpetiformis.

1373 Living a Full Life with Celiac Sprue
Celiac Sprue Association/USA
PO Box 31700
Omaha, NE 68131
402-558-0600; 877-272-4272
Fax: 402-643-4108
celiacs@csaceliacs.org
www.csaceliacs.org

Provides information on celiac-symptoms, treatments and where it was derived from.

Bruce Homstead, President
Mary A. Schluckebier, Executive Director
Jeanine Morgan, Recording Secretary

1374 Patient Packets For Celiac Disease
Gluten Intolerance Group of North America
31214 124th Avenue SE
Auburn, WA 98092
253-833-6655
Fax: 253-833-6675

Includes various brochures and research reports on celiac sprue, recipes, diet instruction and more.

DESCRIPTION

1375 CEREBRAL PALSY

Synonym: CP

Covers these related disorders: Ataxic cerebral palsy, Choreoathetoid cerebral palsy, Mixed cerebral palsy, Spastic cerebral palsy

Involves the following Biologic System(s):

Neurologic Disorders, Orthopedic and Muscle Disorders

Cerebral palsy (CP) is a nonprogressive condition characterized by stiff, rigid, and awkward movements (spasticity); involuntary, slow writhing movements (athetosis); and poor balance and coordination of voluntary movement (ataxia). Approximately two of every 1,000 infants are affected with cerebral palsy. Both premature and low birth weight infants are particularly at risk for this condition. Cerebral palsy may occur as the result of an injury to the brain during pregnancy, birth, or the early childhood years. Such brain injuries may be caused by a decrease in the supply of oxygen to the brain during the birthing period; an infection passed from the mother to the fetus during pregnancy; or an excess of bile pigment (bilirubin) in the developing fetus, usually arising from a blood incompatibility between mother and child. After birth, cerebral palsy may result from head trauma, an infection of the brain (e.g., encephalitis), an infection of the membranes surrounding the brain (meningitis), or other insult to the brain or surrounding tissue.

This condition is divided into four main types, based on the movement disorder. These include spastic, choreoathetoid, ataxic, and mixed cerebral palsy. Spastic cerebral palsy is the most common type of this condition and is characterized by stiff and weak muscles in the arms and legs on one or both sides of the body. Choreoathetoid cerebral palsy is characterized by poorly controlled, spontaneous slow movements of the muscles and accounts for approximately 20 percent of affected children. Ataxic cerebral palsy affects approximately 10 percent of all those with cerebral palsy and is characterized by poor coordination and shaky movements. Mixed cerebral palsy is a combination of two or more types of this abnormality and is characterized by the physical characteristics of the types. Although some children with cerebral palsy have below-average intelligence or are mentally retarded, others are of average or above-average intelligence.

There is no cure for cerebral palsy, but the disabilities associated with CP can be reduced. The type and extent of treatment depends upon the degree and type of disability experienced by the individual child. Medications are prescribed to reduce spasticity and abnormal movements and to prevent seizures. Surgery can also be used to reduce spasticity. Occupational and physical therapy may aid affected children with walking and muscle coordination and control. Some children may benefit from the use of braces or other orthopedic intervention. Speech therapy may be useful for improvement of speech and eating difficulties. Physical and emotional stimulation and support are very important aspects of treatment and will aid in helping children with cerebral palsy to realize their full potential.

Government Agencies

1376 NIH/ Eunice Kennedy Shriver National Insti tute of Child Health & Human Development

31 Center Drive, Building 31
Bethesda, MD 20892
301-496-5113
800-370-2943
Fax: 866-760-5947
TTY: 888-320-6942
nichdpress@mail.nih.gov
www.nichd.nih.gov

Established in 1962 by congress, today the institute conducts and supports laboratory research, clinical trials, and epidemiological studies that explore health processes; examines the impact of disabilities, diseases, and variations on the lives of individuals; and sponsors training programs for scientists, health care providers, and researchers to ensure that NICHD research can continue

Diana W. Bianchi, Director
Paul Williams, Director, Communications

1377 NIH/National Institute of Neurological Dis orders and Stroke (NINDS)

PO Box 5801
Bethesda, MD 20824
301-496-5751
800-352-9424
Fax: 301-496-0296
TTY: 301-468-5981
www.ninds.nih.gov

The mission of NINDS is to reduce the burden of neurological disease - a burden borne by every age group, by every segment of society, by people all over the world.

Walter J. Koroshetz, MD, Director

National Associations & Support Groups

1378 ADA Technical Assistance Program

401 North Washington Street, Suite 450
Rockville, MD 20805
703-448-6155
800-949-4232
Fax: 301-251-3762
TTY: 301-217-0124
adata@adata.org
www.adainfo.org/

A federally funded network of grantees which provides information, training and technical assistance to businesses and agencies with duties and responsibilities under the ADA (American with Disabilities Act) and to people with disabilities with rights under the ADA. Materials-the ADA and newsletters are available.

Marian Vessels, Director
Karen Goss, Assistant Director
Del Rae Conley, Office Manager

1379 American Academy for Cerebral Palsy and Developmental Medicine

555 E Wells Street, Suite 1100
Milwaukee, WI 53202
414-918-3014
Fax: 414-276-2146
info@aacpdm.org
www.aacpdm.org

The American Academy for Cerebral Palsy and Developmental Medicine is a multidisciplinary scientific society devoted to the study of cerebral palsy and other childhood onset disabilities, to promoting professional education for the treatment and management of these conditions, and to improving the quality of life for people with these disabilities.

Maureen O'Donnell, President
Richard Stevenson, MD, First Vice President
Darcy Fehlings, Second Vice President

1380 American Academy of Pediatrics

141 Northwest Point Boulevard
Elk Grove Village, IL 60007
847-434-4000
800-433-9016
Fax: 847-434-8000
www.aap.org

The American Academy of Pediatrics and its member pediatricians are committed to the attainment of optimal physical, mental and social health and well-being for all infants, children, adolescents, and young adults.

Fernando Stein, MD, FAAP, President
Karen Remley, MD, CEO/Executive VP

1381 American School Counselor Association
1101 King Street, Suite 310
Alexandria, VA 22314   703-683-2722
                               800-306-4722
                          Fax: 703-997-7572
                    asca@schoolcounselor.org
                     www.schoolcounselor.org

The mission of ASCA is to represent professional school counselors and to promote professionalism and ethical practices.

Richard Wong, Executive Director
Jeff Broderson, Information Technology Admin.
Kathleen M Rakestraw, Director of Communications

1382 Center for Disabilities and Development
University of Iowa Stead Family Children's Hospita
100 Hawkins Drive
Iowa City, IA 52242   319-353-6900
                               877-686-0031
                          Fax: 319-356-7700
                    cdd-webmaster@uiowa.edu
                     www.uichildrens.org/cdd/

A trusted resource for healthcare, training, research and information for people with disabilities that include: behavior disorders, brain injury, cerebral palsy, diabetes, down syndrome, learning disabilities, mental retardation, sleep disorders and spina bifida.

Dianne McBrien, MD, Medical Director

1383 Children's Neurobiological Solutions Foundation
1223 Wilshire Blvd., #937
Santa Barbara, CA 90403   310-889-8611
                               866-267-5580
                          Fax: 805-965-8838
                       info@cnsfoundation.org
                        www.cnsfoundation.org

Children's Neurobiological Solutions Foundation (CNS), is a national, nonprofit, 501(c)(3) organization, whose mission is to orchestrate cutting-edge, collaborative research with the goal of expediting the creation of effective treatments and therapies for children with neurodevelopmental abnormalities, birth injuries to the nervous system, and related neurological problems.

Carol Abrams JD, President
Fia Richmond, Founder & President, CNS
Phillip H Richmond, Co-Founder, CNS

1384 Easter Seals
233 South Wacker Drive, Suite 2400
Chicago, IL 60606   312-575-0243
                               800-221-6827
                          Fax: 312-726-1494
                          TTY: 312-726-4258
                        www.easterseals.com

Easter Seals offers a variety of services to help people with disabilities address life's challenges and achieve personal goals.

Stephen F. Rossman, Chairman
Richard W. Davidson, 1st Vice Chairman
Sandra L Bouwman, 2nd Vice Chairman

1385 Easter Seals Disability Services
233 South Wacker Drive, Suite 2400
Chicago, IL 60606   800-221-6827
                          Fax: 312-726-1494
                          TTY: 312-726-4258
                    extranetinfo@easterseals.com
                     www.extraneteasterseals.com

Easter Seals has been helping individuals with disabilities and special needs, and their families, live better lives for more then 80 years. From child development centers to physical rehabilitation and jobs training for peoplewith disabilities, Easter Seals offers a variety of services to help people with disabilities address life's challenges and achieve personal goals.

1386 Epilepsy Foundation
8301 Professional Place
Landover, MD 20785   866-330-2718
                               800-332-1000
                          Fax: 301-459-1569
                          ContactUs@efa.org
                     www.epilepsyfoundation.org

A toll free information and referral service staffed by specially trained people who will answer questions and discuss concerns about seizure disorders and their treatment. Staff will direct callers to local affiliates of the foundation and provide information about a broad range of services that respond to the needs of people with seizure disorders.

18,000 members

Phil Gattone, President and CEO
Gloria Uchegbu, Program Manager
Michele Dawson, Manager of Executive Operations

1387 Family Support Network
Tuberous Sclerosis Alliance
801 Roeder Road, Suite 750
Silver Spring, MD 20910   301-562-9890
                               800-225-6872
                          Fax: 301-562-9870
                        info@tsalliance.org
                         www.tsalliance.org

The Support Network is an organized partnership of individuals whose lives have been affected by tuberous sclerosis. Across the nation, the Support Network is providing the latest medical information, education and support to those individuals who are seeking understanding about the genetic disease and offering them words of encouragement and empowerment.

Matt Bolger, Chair
Keith Hall, Vice Chair
David Michaels, Treasurer

1388 March of Dimes Foundation
1275 Mamaroneck Avenue
White Plains, NY 10605   914-997-4488
                               888-663-4637
                          Fax: 914-997-4763
                     answers@marchofdimes.com
                       www.marchofdimes.com

March of Dimes help moms have full-term pregnancies and research the problems that threaten the health of babies.The March of Dimes also acts globally: sharing best practices in perinatal health and helping improve birth outcomes where the needs are the most urgent.

Stacey D. Stewart, President

1389 National Disability Sports Alliance
25 W Independence Way
Kingston, RI 02881   401-792-7130
                          Fax: 401-792-7132
                        info@ndsaonline.org
            www.nationaldisabilitysportsalliance.webs.com/

Nonprofit organization. Coordinates sports, recreation and fitness activities for individuals with physical disabilities. Main focus is on cerebral palsy, traumatic brain injury and stroke.

Jerry McCole, Executive Director

1390 National Dissemination Center for Children with Disabilities
1825 Connecticut Ave NW
Washington, DC 20009   202-884-8200
                               800-695-0285
                          Fax: 202-884-8441
                        nichcy@fhi360.org
                          www.nichcy.org

A national information and referral center that provides information on disabilities and disability-related issues for families, educators and other professionals.

Suzanne Ripley, Executive Director

1391 United Cerebral Palsy Associations
1825 K Street NW Suite 600
Washington, DC 20036
202-776-0406
800-872-5827
Fax: 202-776-0414
TTY: 202-973-7197
info@ucp.org
www.ucp.org

A network of approximately 119 state and local voluntary agencies which provide services, conduct public and professional education programs and support research in cerebral palsy.

Stephen Bennett, Ceo
Woody Connette, Chair
Ian Ridlon, Vice Chair

1392 WE MOVE (Worldwide Education and Advocacy for Movement Disorders)
Mt. Sinai Medical Center
5731 Mosholu Avenue
Bronx, NY 10471
212-875-8312
800-437-6682
Fax: 212-875-8389
wemove@wemove.org
www.wemove.org

WE MOVE provides movement disorder information and educational materials to physicians, patients and families, the media, and the public via its comprehensive Web sites, training courses, and more. Its goal is to make early diagnosis, up-to-date treatment and patient support a reality for all people living with movement disorders.

Susan Bressman MD, President
Mo Moadeli, Vice President
Arlene Ploshnick, Treasurer

State Agencies & Support Groups

Alabama

1393 United Cerebral Palsy of Alabama
C/O UCP of East Central Alabama
301 EA Darden Drive, Box 694
Anniston, AL 36202
256-237-8203
Fax: 256-235-2388
inda@ecaucp.org
www.ecaucp.org

United Cerebral Palsy provides information, advocacy, referral services for persons with disabilities and/or their families. UCP also operates an equipment loan program, conducts parent workshops, disseminates written literature on topics of interest to people with disabilities.

Donald Turner, Chairman of the Board
Kathy Wood, First Vice-Chairman
John Rogers, Treasurer

1394 United Cerebral Palsy of Greater Birmingham
120 Oslo Circle
Birmingham, AL 35211
205-944-3944
Fax: 205-226-9112
dlittlepage@ucpbham.com
www.ucpbham.com

United Cerebral Palsy provides information, advocacy, referral services for persons with disabilities and/or their families. UCP also operates an equipment loan program, conducts parent workshops, disseminates written literature on topics of interest to people with disabilities.

Tom Hinton, Chair
Melva Tate, Executive Vice Chair
Eddie Denaburg, Treasurer

1395 United Cerebral Palsy of Huntsville & Tennessee Valley
2075 Max Luther Drive NW
Huntsville, AL 35810
256-852-5600
256-852-5673
Fax: 256-852-6722
therapy@ucphuntsville.org
www.ucphuntsville.org

United Cerebral Palsy provides information, advocacy, referral services for persons with disabilities and/or their families. UCP also operates an equipment loan program, conducts parent workshops, disseminates written literature on topics of interest to people with disabilities.

John Jeffery, President
Cathy Scholl, President-Elect
Gretchen Jensen, Treasurer

1396 United Cerebral Palsy of Mobile
3058 Dauphin Square Connector
Mobile, AL 36607
251-479-4900
Fax: 251-479-4998
info@ucpmobile.org
www.ucpmobile.org

United Cerebral Palsy provides information, advocacy and referral services for persons with disabilities and/or their families. UCP also operates an equipment loan program, conducts parent workshops, disseminates written literature on topics of interest to people with disabilities and provides early intervention, supported employment, pre-school, therapy, and inclusive camp and adolescent services.

Allen Ladd, Chairman
Brooke Grehan, Vice Chairman
Keith Graham, Treasurer

1397 United Cerebral Palsy of Northwest Alabama
507 N. Hook Street
Tuscumbia, AL 35674
256-381-4310
Fax: 256-381-4378
alison@ucpshoals.org
www.ucpshoals.org

United Cerebral Palsy provides information, advocacy, referral services for persons with disabilities and/or their families. UCP also operates an equipment loan program, conducts parent workshops, disseminates written literature on topics of interest to people with disabilities.

Alison Isbell, Executive Director
Martha Martha, Office Manager
Gena Williams, Respite Coordinator/Billing

1398 United Cerebral Palsy of West Alabama
1100 UCP Parkway
Northport, AL 35476
205-345-3031
Fax: 205-345-3035
tfrankucp@comcast.net
www.ucpwa.org

Provides early intervention for birth through age 3, preschool services, afternoon and summer CARE services, (child and adult respite/education), Start on Success Alabama (high school transition to work program), Adult Day Habilitation Program (adults with mental retardation), UCP Miracle Riders (equestrian physical therapy program).

Nancy Rhodes, President
Brandon Stough, Vice President
Bruce Boner, Treasurer

Alaska

1399 United Cerebral Palsy of Alaska/PARENTS
4743 E Northern Lights Boulevard
Anchorage, AK 99508
907-337-7678
Fax: 907-337-7671
sanja@parentsinc.org
www.parentsinc.org

United Cerebral Palsy provides information, advocacy, referral services for persons with disabilities and/or their families. UCP also operates an equipment loan program, conducts parent workshops, disseminates written literature on topics of interest to people with disabilities.

Sanja Bolling, Executive Director

Arizona

1400 United Cerebral Palsy of Central Arizona
1802 W Parkside Lane
Phoenix, AZ 85027
602-943-5472
888-943-5472
Fax: 602-943-4936
info@ucpofcentralaz.org
www.UCPofAZ.org

United Cerebral Palsy provides information, advocacy, referral services for persons with disabilities and/or their families. UCP also operates an equipment loan program, conducts parent workshops, disseminates written literature on topics of interest to people with disabilities.

Veronica De La O, Board Chairwoman. President,
Dr. Cristina Carballo Perelman, Vice Chairman
Nathan Anspach, Treasurer

1401 United Cerebral Palsy of Southern Arizona
635 N. Craycroft Road
Tucson, AZ 85711
520-795-3108
Fax: 520-795-3196
staff@ucpsa.org
www.ucpsa.org/?contact

United Cerebral Palsy provides information, advocacy, referral services for persons with disabilities and/or their families. UCP also operates an equipment loan program, conducts parent workshops, disseminates written literature on topics of interest to people with disabilities.

Alexis Cruz, Program Manager
Sean Hammond, Program Manager
Rita Lopez, Program Manager

Arkansas

1402 United Cerebral Palsy of Central Arkansas
9720 N Rodney Parham Road
Little Rock, AR 72227
501-224-6067
800-228-6174
Fax: 501-227-5591
info@ucpcark.org
www.ucpcark.org

United Cerebral Palsy provides information, advocacy, referral services for persons with disabilities and/or their families. UCP also operates an equipment loan program, conducts parent workshops, disseminates written literature on topics of interest to people with disabilities.

Stephen Jones, Chair
Gary Wells, Vice Chair
Bill Yee, Treasurer

California

1403 United Cerebral Palsy of Central California
4224 N Cedar Avenue
Fresno, CA 93726
559-221-8272
Fax: 559-221-9347
jeffreys@ccucp.org
www.ccucp.org

United Cerebral Palsy provides information, advocacy, referral services for persons with disabilities and/or their families. UCP also operates an adult day program - the Center for Arts and Technology in Fresno, CA, and services to children and their parents in Kings County, CA.

Jeffrey Snyder, Executive Director

1404 United Cerebral Palsy of Greater Sacramento
4350 Auburn Blvd.
Sacramento, CA 95841
916-565-7700
Fax: 916-565-7773
ucp@ucpsacto.org
www.ucpsacto.org

UCP provides programs and services for people with all types of developmental disabilities. These services include: day programs for adults, an in-home respite service, transportation, independent living services, information and referral services, a toy lending library, a recreational program for children, and advocacy at the State and National levels. UCP will, upon request, furnish written literature regarding their programs and services or information regarding a variety of disabilities.

Dennis Hart md, Chair
Annie Granucci, Treasurer
Kristoffer Kalmbach, Secretary

1405 United Cerebral Palsy of Los Angeles, Ventura and Santa Barbara Counties
6430 Independence Avenue
Woodland Hills, CA 91367
818-782-2211
Fax: 818-909-9106
mail@ucpla.org
www.ucpla.org

Serving Los Angeles, Ventura and Santa Barbara counties. Serves hundreds of adults and children with disabilities every day with housing, education programs and professional and personal support for people with disabilities and their families. In addition to the high volume of people assisted, UCP is known for a caring, personal approach to each family's individual situation and choices.

Ronald Cohen, Executive Director
Ellen Kessler, President

1406 United Cerebral Palsy of Orange County
980 Roosevelt, Suite 100
Irvine, CA 92620
949-333-6400
Fax: 949-333-6440
info@ucp-oc.org
www.ucp-oc.org

United Cerebral Palsy of Orange County operaptes an infant stimulation program with physical, occupational and speech therapy consultation. Aditionally, UCP provides information and referral services for the families of children having developmental disabilities as well as an equiptment loan program, Respitality program, parent support groups and individulized support, respite/babysitter programs, and consultation/training to childcare providers.

James Corbett, President
Michele Maryott, Vice President
Thomas Quinn, Treasurer

1407 United Cerebral Palsy of San Diego County
8525 Gibbs Drive, #209
San Diego, CA 92123
858-571-7803
Fax: 858-571-0919
info@ucpsd.org
www.ucpsd.org

United Cerebral Palsy provides information, advocacy, referral services for persons with disabilities and/or their families. UCP also operates an equipment loan program, conducts parent workshops, disseminates written literature on topics of interest to people with disabilities.

Stephen Holland, President
Mike Crossley, Vice President
Greg Wells, Treasurer

1408 United Cerebral Palsy of San Joaquin, Calaveras & Amador Counties
333 W Benjamin Holt Drive, Suite 1
Stockton, CA 95207
209-956-0290
800-479-0311
Fax: 209-956-6707
rcall@ucpsj.org
www.ucpsj.org

United Cerebral Palsy provides early intervention, information, advocacy, assistive technology and referral services for persons with disabilities and/or their families. UCP also operates an equipment loan program, conducts parent workshops, disseminates written literature on topics of interest to people with disabilities.

Daniel Platt, President
Martin J. Herzog, Vice-President
Eddie Lira, Treasurer

1409 United Cerebral Palsy of San Luis Obispo
3620 Sacramento Drive, Suite 201C
San Luis Obispo, CA 93401
　　　　　　　　　　　　　　　805-543-2039
　　　　　　　　　　　　Fax: 805-543-2045
　　　　　　　　　　　　shaftmt@aol.com
　　　　　　　　　　　　www.ucp-slo.org

United Cerebral Palsy provides information, advocacy, referral services for persons with disabilities and/or their families. UCP also operates an equipment loan program, conducts parent workshops, disseminates written literature on topics of interest to people with disabilities.

Mark Shaffer, Executive Director
Jason Portugal, Technology Coordinator
Many Aslanzadeh, Youth Services

1410 United Cerebral Palsy of Santa Clara & San Mateo Counties
512 E Maude Avenue
Sunnyvale, CA 94085
　　　　　　　　　　　　　　　408-737-7112
　　　　　　　　　　　　　　　650-917-6900
　　　　　　　　　　　　Fax: 408-737-7225
　　　　　　　　　　　　ucp@ucpscsm.org
　　　　　　　　　　　　www.ucpscsm.org

United Cerebral Palsy provides information, advocacy, referral services for persons with disabilities and/or their families. UCP also operates an equipment loan program, conducts parent workshops, disseminates written literature on topics of interest to people with disabilities.

Jane Lefferdink, Executive Director

1411 United Cerebral Palsy of Stanislaus County Stanislaus
4265 Spyres Way #2
Modesto, CA 95356
　　　　　　　　　　　　　　　209-577-2122
　　　　　　　　　　　　Fax: 209-577-2392
　　　　　　　　　　　　rlonczak@ucpstan.org
　　　　　　　　　　　　www.ucpstan.org

United Cerebral Palsy provides information, advocacy, referral services for persons with disabilities and/or their families. Conducts parent workshops, disseminates written literature on topics of interest to people with disabilities.

Chris Peterson, Chair
Russ Hayward, Interim Executive Director
Michelle Gallegher, Treasurer

1412 United Cerebral Palsy of the Golden State
1970 Broadway, Suite 115
Oakland, CA 94612
　　　　　　　　　　　　　　　510-832-7430
　　　　　　　　　　　　Fax: 510-839-1329
　　　　　　　　　　　　info@ucpgg.org
　　　　　　　　　　　　www.ucpgg.org

United Cerebral Palsy provides information, advocacy, referral services for persons with disabilities and/or their families. UCP also operates an equipment loan program, conducts parent workshops, disseminates written literature on topics of interest to people with disabilities.

Barry N Gardin, President
Patricia Peck, Vice President
Henry Gusman, Treasurer

1413 United Cerebral Palsy of the Inland Empire
35-325 Date Palm Drive, Suite 139
Cathedral City, CA 92234
　　　　　　　　　　　　　　　760-321-8184
　　　　　　　　　　　　　　　877-512-2224
　　　　　　　　　　　　Fax: 760-321-8284
　　　　　　　　　　　　info@ucpie.org
　　　　　　　　　　　　www.ucpie.org

United Cerebral Palsy provides information, advocacy, referral services for persons with disabilities and/or their families. UCP conducts parent workshops, disseminates written literature on topics of interest to people with disabilities.

Greg Wetmore, President/CEO
Sofia Campos, Director of Program Services
Amber Fleming, Support Services Administrator

1414 United Cerebral Palsy of the North Bay
3835 Cypress Drive, #103
Petaluma, CA 94954
　　　　　　　　　　　　　　　707-766-9990
　　　　　　　　　　　　mchughe@sonoma.edu
　　　　　　　　　　　　www.ucpa.org

United Cerebral Palsy provides information, advocacy, referral services for persons with disabilities and/or their families. UCP also operates an equipment loan program, conducts parent workshops, disseminates written literature on topics of interest to people with disabilities.

Steve Lohrer, Board President
Elaine McHugh, Board Vice-President
Janet Hart, Treasurer

Connecticut

1415 United Cerebral Palsy of Eastern Connecticut
42 Norwich Road
Quaker Hill, CT 06375
　　　　　　　　　　　　　　　860-443-3800
　　　　　　　　　　　　Fax: 860-443-8272
　　　　　　　　　　　　mmorisson@ucpect.org
　　　　　　　　　　　　www.ucpect.org

United Cerebral Palsy provides information, advocacy, referral services for persons with disabilities and/or their families. UCP also operates an equipment loan program, conducts parent workshops, disseminates written literature on topics of interest to people with disabilities.

Margaret (Peg) Morrison, Executive Director
Jennifer Keatley, Associate Executive Director of Adm
Steven Smigiel, Financial Manager

1416 United Cerebral Palsy of Greater Hartford
80 Whitney Street
Hartford, CT 06105
　　　　　　　　　　　　　　　860-236-6201
　　　　　　　　　　　　Fax: 860-218-2454
　　　　　　　　　　　　preid@sunrisegroup.org
　　　　　　　　　　　　www.ucphartford.org/

United Cerebral Palsy provides information, advocacy, referral services for persons with disabilities and/or their families. UCP also operates an equipment loan program, conducts parent workshops, disseminates written literature on topics of interest to people with disabilities.

Pam Reid, Regional Administrator
Sarah Winiarski, Director of Development & Communica
Peter Cavanagh, Camp Coordinator

1417 United Cerebral Palsy of Southern Connecticut
94-96 South Turnpike Road (Halycon Office Park)
Wallingford, CT 06492
　　　　　　　　　　　　　　　203-269-3511
　　　　　　　　　　　　Fax: 203-269-7411
　　　　　　　　　　　　ucpasouthernct@yahoo.com
　　　　　　　　　　　　www.ucpasouthernct.com

United Cerebral Palsy provides information, advocacy, referral services for persons with disabilities and/or their families. UCP also operates an equipment loan program, conducts parent workshops, disseminates written literature on topics of interest to people with disabilities.

Arcangelo DiStefano, M.D., President
Peter DiDomizio, Vice President
Strick Woods MD, Treasurer

Delaware

1418 United Cerebral Palsy of Delaware
700A River Road
Wilmington, DE 19809
　　　　　　　　　　　　　　　302-764-2400
　　　　　　　　　　　　Fax: 302-764-8713
　　　　　　　　　　　　wmccool@ucpde.org
　　　　　　　　　　　　www.ucpde.org

United Cerebral Palsy provides information, advocacy, referral services for persons with disabilities and/or their families. UCP also operates an equipment loan program, conducts parent workshops, disseminates written literature on topics of interest to people with disabilities.

Donna M Hopkins, President
D. Bruce McClenathan, Vice President
Daniel Edgar, Treasurer

District of Columbia

1419 United Cerebral Palsy of Washington DC & Northern Virginia
3135 8th Street NE
Washington, DC 20017
202-269-1500
Fax: 202-526-0519
webmaster@ucpdc.org
www.ucpdc.org

United Cerebral Palsy provides information, advocacy, referral services for persons with disabilities and/or their families. UCP also operates an equipment loan program, conducts parent workshops, disseminates written literature on topics of interest to people with disabilities.

Mark A Simione, Board President
George Connors, 1st Vice President
Roderick Johnson, 2nd Vice President

Florida

1420 New Heights (formerly Cerebral Palsy of No rtheast Florida)
3311 Beach Boulevard
Jacksonville, FL 32207
904-396-1462
Fax: 904-396-1199
agency@cpnef.org
www.newheightsnefl.org

United Cerebral Palsy provides information, advocacy, referral services for persons with disabilities and/or their families. UCP also operates an equipment loan program, conducts parent workshops, disseminates written literature on topics of interest to people with disabilities, and provides individual and family counseling. Locations also in Kissimme, Winter Garden, Sanford and East Orange.

Sue Driscoll, President & CEO
Michelle Abner, Chief Development Officer
Joel Weaver, Secretary-Treasurer

1421 United Cerebral Palsy of Central Florida
1221 W. Colonial Dr., Ste. 300
Orlando, FL 32804
407-852-3300
Fax: 407-852-3301
iwilkins@ucpcfl.org
www.ucpcfl.org

United Cerebral Palsy provides information, advocacy, referral services for persons with disabilities and/or their families. UCP also operates an equipment loan program, conducts parent workshops, disseminates written literature on topics of interest to people with disabilities, and provides individual and family counseling. Locations also in Kissimme, Winter Garden, Sanford and East Orange.

Dr. Ilene Wilkins, CEO
Paul Brown, Chair
Lynn Fleeger, Vice-Chair

1422 United Cerebral Palsy of East Central Florida
1100 Jimmy Ann Drive
Daytona Beach, FL 32117
386-274-6474
Fax: 386-274-6532
info@ucpworc.org
www.ucpecf.org

United Cerebral Palsy provides information, advocacy, referral services for persons with disabilities and/or their families. UCP also operates an equipment loan program, conducts parent workshops, disseminates written literature on topics of interest to people with disabilities, and provides individual and family counseling. Locations also in Kissimme, Winter Garden, Sanford and East Orange.

Brooks Casey, Chair
Ed Best, Treasurer
Parker Mynchenberg, Treasurer

1423 United Cerebral Palsy of Florida
2700 W. 81 Street
Hialeah, FL 33016
305-325-9018
Fax: 850-922-1258
ucpinfo@ucpsouthflorida.org
www.ucpsouthflorida.org

United Cerebral Palsy provides information, advocacy, referral services for persons with disabilities and/or their families. UCP also operates an equipment loan program, conducts parent workshops, disseminates written literature on topics of interest to people with disabilities.

Joseph A. Aniello, Ed.D., President and CEO
Debbie Terenzio, Ed.D., Vice President & COO
Linda Gluck, CPA, Vice President & CFO

1424 United Cerebral Palsy of North Florida/ Tender Loving Care
1241 N East Avenue
Panama City, FL 32401
850-769-7960
Fax: 850-769-1060
ucpstlc@aol.com
www.ucpa.org

United Cerebral Palsy provides information, advocacy, referral services for persons with disabilities and/or their families. UCP also operates an equipment loan program, conducts parent workshops, disseminates written literature on topics of interest to people with disabilities.

1425 United Cerebral Palsy of Northwest Florida
2912 North E Street
Pensacola, FL 32501
850-432-1596
Fax: 850-432-1930
info@ucpnwfl.org
www.ucpnwfl.org

The number one service provider in Northwest Florida for individuals with cerebral palsy and other developmental disabilities, UCP provides information, advocacy and referral services for persons with disabilities and/or their families. Additionally, UCP offers individuals assistance with daily living skills training, computer training, basic education, speech, physical and occupational therapy, residential, supported living and finding long-term employment.

Brian P Bell SR, Chair
Michele W Fielder, Vice Chair
Norman Smith, Treasurer

1426 United Cerebral Palsy of Sarasota-Manatee
1090 S Tamiami Trail
Sarasota, FL 34236
941-957-3599
Fax: 941-957-3499
dwalker@sunrisegroup.org
www.ucpsarasota.org

United Cerebral Palsy provides information, advocacy, referral services for persons with disabilities and/or their families. UCP also operates an equipment loan program, conducts parent workshops, disseminates written literature on topics of interest to people with disabilities.

Barnett A Greenberg, Chairperson
Norma Israel, Executive Director

1427 United Cerebral Palsy of South Florida
2700 West 81 Street
Hialeah, FL 33016
305-325-9018
Fax: 305-325-1313
ucpinfo@ucpsouthflorida.org
www.ucpsouthflorida.org

United Cerebral Palsy provides information, advocacy, referral services for persons with disabilities and/or their families. UCP also operates an equipment loan program, conducts parent workshops, disseminates written literature on topics of interest to people with disabilities.

Joseph Aniello Ed.D, President & CEO
Linda Gluck, Vice President & CFO
Debbie Terenzio, Ed.D., Vice President & COO

1428 United Cerebral Palsy of Tampa Bay
2215 E Henry Avenue
Tampa, FL 33610
813-239-1179
800-749-5155
Fax: 813-237-3091
lwhite@ucptampa.org.
www.ucptampa.org

United Cerebral Palsy provides information, advocacy, referral services for persons with disabilities and/or their families. UCP also operates an equipment loan program, conducts parent workshops, disseminates written literature on topics of interest to people with disabilities.

Jim King, Executive Director
Dawn Gosselin, Executive Development Assistant / E
Laura White, Director of Program Development

Georgia

1429 United Cerebral Palsy of Georgia
3300 Northeast Expressway, Building 9
Atlanta, GA 30341
770-676-2000
888-827-9455
Fax: 770-455-8040
info@ucpga.org
www.ucpga.org

United Cerebral Palsy provides information, advocacy, referral services for persons with disabilities and/or their families. UCP also operates an equipment loan program, conducts parent workshops, disseminates written literature on topics of interest to people with disabilities.

Diane Wilush, Executive Director
Angela Easter, Associate Executive Director, Opera
R. Curt Harrison, Associate Executive Director, Strat

Hawaii

1430 United Cerebral Palsy of Hawaii
414 Kuwili Street, Suite 105
Honolulu, HI 96817
808-532-6744
800-606-5654
Fax: 808-532-6747
ucpa@ucpahi.org
www.ucpahi.org

United Cerebral Palsy provides information, advocacy, referral services for persons with disabilities and/or their families. UCP also operates an equipment loan program, conducts parent workshops, disseminates written literature on topics of interest to people with disabilities.

Ted Jung Jr, President
Derek Lau, Vice President
Jan Choy, Treasurer

Idaho

1431 United Cerebral Palsy of Idaho
5420 W Franklin, Suite A
Boise, ID 83705
208-377-8070
Fax: 208-322-7133
info@ucpidaho.org
www.ucpidaho.org

United Cerebral Palsy provides information, advocacy, referral services for persons with disabilities and/or their families.

Lynn Cundick, Executive Director
Kathy Griffen, Program Director

Illinois

1432 United Cerebral Palsy Land of Lincoln
101 North 16th Street
Springfield, IL 62703
217-525-6522
Fax: 217-525-9017
ucpll@ucpll.org
www.ucpll.org

United Cerebral Palsy provides information, advocacy, referral services for persons with disabilities and/or their families. UCP also operates an equipment loan program, conducts parent workshops, disseminates written literature on topics of interest to people with disabilities.

Brenda Yarnell, President
Kathy Leuelling, Chief Operating Officer
Char Fanning, Chief Financial Officer

1433 United Cerebral Palsy of Greater Chicago
7550 West 183rd Street
Tinley Park, IL 60477
708-444-8460
800-476-2836
Fax: 708-429-3981
pdulle@ucpnet.org
www.ucpnet.org

United Cerebral Palsy provides information and referral services for persons with disabilities and/or their families. UCP also operates an equipment loan program, conducts parent workshops, disseminates written literature on topics of interest to people with disabilities.

Paul Dulle, President and CEO
Peggy Childs, Executive Vice President
Mei Hong Zhang, Chief Financial Officer

1434 United Cerebral Palsy of Illinois
310 East Adams
Springfield, IL 62701
217-528-9681
Fax: 217-528-9739
ucpillinois.org
www.ucpillinois.org

United Cerebral Palsy provides information, advocacy, referral services for persons with disabilities and/or their families. UCP also operates an equipment loan program, conducts parent workshops, disseminates written literature on topics of interest to people with disabilities.

Don Moss, Executive Director

1435 United Cerebral Palsy of Southern Illinois
9 Cusumano Professional Pplaza Drive
Mt Vernon, IL 62864
618-244-2505
800-332-9745
Fax: 618-244-3568
ucpsi@onemain.com
http://home.onemain.com/~ucpsi

United Cerebral Palsy provides information, advocacy, referral services for persons with disabilities and/or their families. UCP also operates an equipment loan program, conducts parent workshops, disseminates written literature on topics of interest to people with disabilities.

Sharon Hale, Executive Director

1436 United Cerebral Palsy of Will County
311 South Reed Street
Joliet, IL 60436
815-744-3500
Fax: 815-744-3504
ucpilprairieland@ucpilprairieland.org
www.ucpilprairieland.org

United Cerebral Palsy provides information, advocacy, referral services for persons with disabilities and/or their families. UCP also operates an equipment loan program, conducts parent workshops, disseminates written literature on topics of interest to people with disabilities.

Bret Mitchell, Chair
Larry Johnson, Vice Chair - Administrative Service
Jim Keck, Vice Chair - Program Services

Indiana

1437 United Cerebral Palsy of Greater Indiana
107 N Pennsylvania St Suite 804
Indianapolis, IN 46220
317-632-3561
800-732-7620
Fax: 317-632-3338
donnar@ucpaindy.org
www.ucpaindy.org

United Cerebral Palsy provides information, advocacy, referral services for persons with Cerebal Palsy and/or their families. UCP also provides funding for equipment and operates an equipment loan program, disseminates written literature on topics of interest to people with disabilities.

Lee White, Board and Development Committee Mem
Craig Burns, Board President and Development Com
Gavin MCNAMARA, Board Treasurer and Finance Committ

1438 United Cerebral Palsy of the Wabash Valley
621 Poplar Street
Terre Haute, IN 47807

812-232-6305
Fax: 812-234-3683
info@ucpwv.org
www.ucpwv.org

United Cerebral Palsy provides information, advocacy, referral services for persons with disabilities and/or their families. UCP also operates an equipment loan program, conducts parent workshops, disseminates written literature on topics of interest to people with disabilities.

Brian Garcia, President
Anna Wetnight, First Vice-President
Pam Deady, Treasurer

Kansas

1439 United Cerebral Palsy of Greater Kansas City
3100 Broadway, Suite 330
Kansas City, MO 64111

816-531-4454
Fax: 816-531-3383
info@ucpkc.org
www.ucpkc.org

United Cerebral Palsy provides information, advocacy, referral services for persons with disabilities and/or their families. UCP also operates an equipment loan program, conducts parent workshops, disseminates written literature on topics of interest to people with disabilities.

Bruce Scott, President and CEO
Sam Switzer, Senior Vice President & Chief Finan
Bill Koch, Chairperson

1440 United Cerebral Palsy of Kansas
5111 E 21st Street N
Wichita, KS 67208

316-688-1888
Fax: 316-688-5687
davej@cprf.org
www.cprf.org

United Cerebral Palsy provides information, advocacy, referral services for persons with disabilities and/or their families. UCP also operates an equipment loan program, conducts parent workshops, disseminates written literature on topics of interest to people with disabilities.

Daniel M Carney, Chairman of the Board
Deryl K. Schuster, Vice Chairman
Daniel J Taylor, Treasurer

Louisiana

1441 United Cerebral Palsy of Baton Rouge McMains Children's Developmental Center
1805 College Drive
Baton Rouge, LA 70808

225-923-3420
Fax: 225-922-9316
cdcjanet@gmail.com
www.mcmainscdc.org

United Cerebral Palsy provides information, advocacy, referral services for persons with disabilities and/or their families. UCP also operates an equipment loan program, conducts parent workshops, disseminates written literature on topics of interest to people with disabilities.

Michael McNulty, President
Gina Dugas, Vice President
Mike Krumholt, Secretary-Treasurer

1442 United Cerebral Palsy of Greater New Orleans
2200 Veterans Memorial Boulevard, Suite 103
New Orleans, LA 70062

504-461-4266
Fax: 504-461-9976
info@ucpgno.com
www.ucpgno.org

United Cerebral Palsy provides information, advocacy, referral services for persons with disabilities and/or their families. UCP also operates an equipment loan program, conducts parent workshops, disseminates written literature on topics of interest to people with disabilities.

Tommy Freel, Chair
p.Alden kellog, Vice Chair
Jeffery Smith, Executive Vice chair

Maine

1443 United Cerebral Palsy of Northeastern Maine
700 Mount Hope Avenue, Suite 320
Bangor, ME 04401

207-941-2952
Fax: 207-941-2955
bobbijo.yeager@ucpofmaine.org
www.ucpofmaine.org

United Cerebral Palsy provides information, advocacy, referral services for persons with disabilities and/or their families. UCP also operates an equipment loan program, conducts parent workshops, disseminates written literature on topics of interest to people with disabilities.

Micheal S. Haenn, Director
Ron Cote, Vice President
Valerie Roy, Treasurer

Maryland

1444 United Cerebral Palsy of Central Maryland
1700 Reisterstown Road, Suite 226
Baltimore, MD 21208

410-484-4540
Fax: 410-486-3825
TTY: 800-451-2452
info@ucp-cm.org
www.ucp-cm.org

United Cerebral Palsy provides information, advocacy, referral services for persons with disabilities and/or their families. UCP also operates an equipment loan program, conducts parent workshops, disseminates written literature on topics of interest to people with disabilities.

Diane Coughlin, President

1445 United Cerebral Palsy of Prince Georges & Montgomery Counties
4409 Forbes Boulevard
Lanham, MD 20706

301-459-0566
Fax: 301-459-7691
TTY: 301-262-4982
ucppgmc@aol.com
www.ucppgmc.com

United Cerebral Palsy provides information, advocacy, referral services for persons with disabilities and/or their families. UCP also operates an equipment loan program, conducts parent workshops, disseminates written literature on topics of interest to people with disabilities.

Charles Mc Nelly, Manager

1446 United Cerebral Palsy of Southern Maryland
211 Chinquapin Round Road
Annapolis, MD 21401

410-280-2003
Fax: 410-269-5757
ucpinfo@ucpsm.org
www.ucpsm.org

United Cerebral Palsy provides information, advocacy, referral services for persons with disabilities and/or their families. UCP also operates an equipment loan program, conducts parent workshops, disseminates written literature on topics of interest to people with disabilities.

Massachusetts

1447 United Cerebral Palsy of Berkshire County
208 West Street
Pittsfield, MA 01201

413-442-1562
Fax: 413-499-4077
info@ucpberkshire.org
www.upcberkshire.org

United Cerebral Palsy provides information, advocacy, assistive technology, referral services for persons with disabilities and/or their families. UCP also operates an equipment loan program, conducts parent workshops, disseminates written literature on topics of interest to people with disabilities.

Anthony Hyte, President
Sarah Gaffey, 1st Vice President
Warren Buhl, 2nd Vice president

1448 United Cerebral Palsy of MetroBoston
71 Arsenal Street
Watertown, MA 02472 617-926-5480
Fax: 617-926-3059
ucpboston@ucpboston.org
www.ucpboston.org

United Cerebral Palsy provides information, advocacy, referral services for persons with disabilities and/or their families. UCP also operates an equipment loan program, conducts parent workshops, disseminates written literature on topics of interest to people with disabilities.

Richard Merson, President
Linda Cox Maguire, Vice President
Desmond Brown, Board of Director

Michigan

1449 United Cerebral Palsy Michigan
3498 Lake Lansing road Suite. 170
East Lansing, MI 48823 517-203-1200
800-828-2714
Fax: 517-203-1203
ucp@ucpmichigan.org
www.ucpmichigan.org

United Cerebral Palsy provides information, advocacy, referral services for persons with disabilities and/or their families. UCP also operates an equipment loan program, conducts parent workshops, disseminates written literature on topics of interest to people with disabilities.

Dan Vivian, President
Judy Cerano, Vice President
Jackie Doig, Chairperson

1450 United Cerebral Palsy of Metropolitan Detroit
23077 Greenfield, Suite 205
Southfield, MI 48075 248-557-5070
800-827-4843
Fax: 248-557-0224
main@ucpdetroit.org
www.ucpdetroit.org

United Cerebral Palsy provides information, advocacy, referral services for persons with disabilities and/or their families. UCP also operates an equipment loan program, conducts parent workshops, disseminates written literature on topics of interest to people with disabilities.

Leslynn R Angel, President
Thomas H. Landry, Chairman
Diann G. Dudash, 1st Vice Chair

Minnesota

1451 United Cerebral Palsy of Central Minnesota
510 25th Avenue N, Suite 8A
Saint Cloud, MN 56303 320-253-0765
Fax: 320-253-6753
info@ucpcentralmn.org
www.ucpcentralmn.org

United Cerebral Palsy provides information, advocacy, referral services for persons with disabilities and/or their families. UCP also operates an equipment loan program, conducts parent workshops, disseminates free newsletter. Computers Go Round recycles quality used computers to persons with disabilities.

Shelley Gaetz, President/Treasurer
Sue Schlosser, Vice President/Secretary
Kristin Schmidt, Treasurer

1452 United Cerebral Palsy of Minnesota
1821 University Avenue W Suite 219 South
Saint Paul, MN 55104 651-646-7588
800-328-4827
Fax: 651-646-3045
ucpmn@cpinternet.com
www.ucpmn.org

United Cerebral Palsy provides information, advocacy, referral services for persons with disabilities and/or their families. UCP also operates an equipment loan program, conducts parent workshops, disseminates written literature on topics of interest to people with disabilities.

Stacey Vogele, Executive Director

Missouri

1453 United Cerebral Palsy of Greater Kansas City
Suite 400
Kansas City, MO 64111 816-531-4454
Fax: 816-531-3383
info@ucpkc.org
www.ucpkc.org

United Cerebral Palsy provides information, advocacy, referral services for persons with disabilities and/or their families. UCP also operates an equipment loan program, conducts parent workshops, disseminates written literature on topics of interest to people with disabilities.

Bruce Scott, President/CEO
Sam Switzer, Senior Vice President
Vincent Bustamante, Vice President, community living

1454 United Cerebral Palsy of Greater St. Louis
8645 Old Bonhomme Road
Saint Louis, MO 63132 314-994-1600
Fax: 314-994-0179
forkoshr@ucpstl.org
www.ucpstl.org

Offers skill development and training programs in the areas of independent living, human relations, social and leisure activities, assistive technology, sensory and tactile stimulation, community integration, career exploration, job placement, and functional academics to individuals eighteen years of age and older with developmental disabilities.

Richard Forkosh, Executive Director

1455 United Cerebral Palsy of Northwest Missouri
3303 Frederick Avenue
Saint Joseph, MO 64506 816-364-3836
Fax: 816-390-8546
ucp@ucpnwmo.org
www.ucpnwmo.org

United Cerebral Palsy provides information, advocacy, referral services for persons with disabilities and/or their families. UCP also operates an equipment loan program, conducts parent workshops, disseminates written literature on topics of interest to people with disabilities.

Teresa Gagliano, Executive Director
Jared Brooner, President
Shawn Drew, Vice president

Nebraska

1456 United Cerebral Palsy of Nebraska
920 S. 107th Avenue, Suite 302
Omaha, NE 68114 402-502-3572
800-729-2556
Fax: 402-502-6791
ucp@ucpnebraska.org
www.ucpnebraska.org

United Cerebral Palsy provides information, advocacy, referral services for persons with disabilities and/or their families. UCP also operates an equipment loan program, conducts parent workshops, disseminates written literature on topics of interest to people with disabilities.

Carol Hahn, Executive Director
Christopher Scott, President
Dave Prough, Treasurer

New Jersey

1457 United Cerebral Palsy of Hudson County
721 Broadway
Bayonne, NJ 07002
201-436-2200
Fax: 201-436-6642
info@ucpofhudsoncounty.org
www.ucpofhudsoncounty.org

United Cerebral Palsy provides information, advocacy, referral services for persons with disabilities and/or their families. UCP also operates an equipment loan program, conducts parent workshops, disseminates written literature on topics of interest to people with disabilities.

Paul E. Venino, President
Paul Maffei, President
James Dooley, Treasurer

1458 United Cerebral Palsy of Northern, Central & Southern New Jersey
245 Main Street Suite 113
Chester, NJ 07930
908-879-2243
Fax: 908-879-8363
info@ucpncsnj.org
www.ucp.org

United Cerebral Palsy provides information, advocacy, referral services for persons with disabilities and/or their families. UCP also operates an equipment loan program, conducts parent workshops, disseminates written literature on topics of interest to people with disabilities.

Deborah Miller, Executive Director

New York

1459 Aspire of WNY
2356 N Forest Road
Getzville, NY 14068
716-505-5610
Fax: 716-894-8257
AJHoldna@aspirewny.org
www.aspirewny.org

Aspire of WNY is a provider of comprehensive programs and services for developmentally disabled children and adults in Western New York. Services areas include residential, bocational, therapeutic, clinical, habilitative and educational services among others. Aspire also offers advocacy, case management, work shops and referral services for the disabled and their families.

Nixon Peabody LLP, Chairperson
Eileen Nosek, Vice Chairperson
Leslie Wangelin, CTP, Treasurer

1460 Center for the Disabled
314 S Manning Boulevard
Albany, NY 12208
518-437-5700
Fax: 518-437-5931
www.cfdsny.org/htmlweb/CFDShome2.html

Center Health Care offers a wide variety of medical dental and therapy services provided in an outpatient practice setting, serving individuals with developmental disabilities and chronic disabling conditions. In addition, educational diagnostic and evaluation services are offered to children of different ages. parent workshops and support groups are conducted throughout the year.

Allan Krafchin, President
Donna Lamkin, Chief Program Officer
Gregory Sorrentino, Chief Financial Officer

1461 Cerebral Palsy Associations of New York State
330 West 34th Street, 15th floor
New York, NY 10001
212-947-5770
Fax: 212-594-4538
information@cpofnys.org
www.cpofnys.org

Cerebral Palsy provides information, advocacy, and services for persons with disabilities and/or their families. CP also operates an equipment loan program, conducts parent workshops, disseminates written literature on topics of interest to people with disabilities.

Susan Constantino, President & CEO
Joseph M Pancari, COO
Thomas N Mandelkow, CFO,CAO

1462 Inspire - Cerebral Palsy Center
2 Fletcher Street
Goshen, NY 10924
845-294-8806
Fax: 845-294-8650
info@inspirecp.org.
www.inspirecp.org

An affiliate of Cerebral Palsy Associations of New York, provides information, advocacy, referral services for persons with disabilities and/or their families. Inspire runs a rehabilitative clinic and special needs preschool, conducts parent workshops, disseminates written literature on topics of interest to people with disabilities.

Katharine Fitzgerald, Chairman
Suzanne Schindler, Vice-Chairman
Allen Zick, Treasurer

1463 UCP of Greater Suffolk
250 Marcus Boulevard, PO Box 18045
Hauppauge, NY 11788
631-232-0011
Fax: 631-232-4422
info@ucp-suffolk.org
www.ucp-suffolk.org

UCP Suffolk provides information, advocacy, referral services for persons with disabilities and/or their families. UCP also operates an equipment loan program, conducts parent workshops, disseminates written literature on topics of interest to people with disabilities.

Stephen H Friedman, President/CEO
Janine Klein, CFO
Colleen West-Levy, Chairperson

1464 United Cerebral Palsy of Nassau County
380 Washington Avenue
Roosevelt, NY 11575
516-378-2000
Fax: 516-378-0357
info@ucpn.org
www.ucpn.org

United Cerebral Palsy provides information, advocacy, referral services for persons with disabilities and/or their families. UCP also operates an equipment loan program, conducts parent workshops, disseminates written literature on topics of interest to people with disabilities.

Robert Masterson, President
Thomas Connolly, Executive Vice President
Anthony Galano, Vice president

1465 United Cerebral Palsy of New York City
80 Maiden Lane, 8th Floor
New York, NY 10038
212-683-6700
Fax: 212-685-8394
info@ucpnyc.org
www.ucpnyc.org

United Cerebral Palsy provides information, advocacy, referral services for persons with disabilities and/or their families. UCP also operates an equipment loan program, conducts parent workshops, disseminates written literature on topics of interest to people with disabilities.

Edward R Matthews, Ceo
Gary Geresi, President
Jerome Belsome, Chairman

Jim Rankin, Executive Director

North Carolina

1466 United Cerebral Palsy of North Carolina
2315 Myron Drive
Raleigh, NC 27607   919-863-3859
                                        800-662-7119
                                  Fax: 919-782-5486
                          info@nc.eastersealsucp.com
                          www.nc.eastersealsucp.com

United Cerebral Palsy provides information, advocacy, referral services for persons with disabilities and/or their families. UCP also operates an equipment loan program, conducts parent workshops, disseminates written literature on topics of interest to people with disabilities.

Connie Cochran, President

Ohio

1467 United Cerebral Palsy of Central Ohio
440 Industrial Mile Road
Columbus, OH 43228   614-279-0109
                                  Fax: 614-279-2527
                        gthorpe@ucpofcentralohio.org
                           www.ucpofcentralohio.org

United Cerebral Palsy provides information, advocacy, referral services for persons with disabilities and/or their families. UCP also operates an equipment loan program, conducts parent workshops, disseminates written literature on topics of interest to people with disabilities.

Kathy Streblo, Executive Director

1468 United Cerebral Palsy of Cincinnati
3601 Victory Parkway
Cincinnati, OH 45229   513-221-4606
                                  Fax: 513-872-5262
                            info@ucp-cincinnati.org
                             www.ucp-cincinnati.org

United Cerebral Palsy provides information, advocacy, referral services for persons with disabilities and/or their families. UCP also operates an equipment loan program, conducts parent workshops, disseminates written literature on topics of interest to people with disabilities.

Michael P. Folley, Chairperson
Thomas R Williams, President
Peter J. Cardullias, ll, Vice president

1469 United Cerebral Palsy of Greater Cleveland
1011 Euclid Avenue
Cleveland, OH 44115   216-791-8363
                                  Fax: 216-721-3372
                          wmorgan@ucpcleveland.org
                             www.ucpcleveland.org

United Cerebral Palsy provides information, advocacy, referral services for persons with disabilities and/or their families. UCP also operates an equipment loan program, conducts parent workshops, disseminates written literature on topics of interest to people with disabilities.

Matthew R Cox, President
Sean D. Wenger, Vice Chairperson
Jeffrey D. Minnick, Treasurer

Oklahoma

1470 United Cerebral Palsy of Oklahoma
10400 Greenbriar Place, Suite 101
Oklahoma City, OK 73159   405-759-3562
                                        800-827-2289
                                  Fax: 405-917-7082
                                    info@ucpok.org
                                     www.ucpok.org

United Cerebral Palsy provides information, advocacy, referral services for persons with disabilities and/or their families. UCP also operates an equipment loan program, disseminates written literature on topics of interest to people with disabilities.

Oregon

1471 United Cerebral Palsy of Oregon & SW Washington
305 NE 102nd Ave, Suite 100
Portland, OR 97220   503-777-4166
                                        800-473-4581
                                  Fax: 503-771-8048
                                 ucpa@ucpaorwa.org
                                   www.ucpaorwa.org

United Cerebral Palsy provides information, advocacy, referral services for persons with disabilities and/or their families. UCP also operates an equipment loan program, conducts parent workshops, disseminates written literature on topics of interest to people with disabilities.

Nancy Cicirello, President
Jerrold Pattee, Vice president
John R. Hancock, Board of Director

Pennsylvania

1472 Alleghenies United Cerebral Palsy
119 Jari Drive
Johnstown, PA 15904   814-262-9600
                                        877-371-1110
                                  Fax: 814-262-9650
                              contact-us@alucp.org
                                     www.alucp.org

United Cerebral Palsy provides information, advocacy, referral services for persons with disabilities and/or their families. UCP also operates an equipment loan program, conducts parent workshops, disseminates written literature on topics of interest to people with disabilities.

Marie Polinsky, Ceo
Mark Malzi, Chief Financial Officer
Stacey Zometsky, Executive Assistant

1473 United Cerebral Palsy Central PA
925 Linda Lane
Camp Hill, PA 17011   717-737-3477
                                        800-998-4827
                                  Fax: 717-975-3333
                          mainoffice@ucpcentralpa.org
                             www.ucpcentralpa.org

United Cerebral Palsy provides information, advocacy, referral services for persons with disabilities and/or their families. UCP also operates an equipment loan program, conducts parent workshops, disseminates written literature on topics of interest to people with disabilities.

Jeffrey W. Cooper, President/CEO
John M. Coles, Chairperson
William K. Wilkison, Vice Chairperson

1474 United Cerebral Palsy of Northeastern Pennsylvania
425 Wyoming Avenue
Scranton, PA 18503   570-347-3357
                                        877-827-8324
                                  Fax: 570-341-5308
                                  TTY: 570-347-3117
                                 ucpnepa@epix.net
                                   www.ucpnepa.com

United Cerebral Palsy provides information, advocacy, referral services for persons with disabilities and/or their families. UCP also operates an equipment loan program, conducts parent workshops, disseminates written literature on topics of interest to people with disabilities.

Daniel Ginsberg, President
Sarah A. Drob, Executive Director
Edward Karpovich, Treasurer

1475 United Cerebral Palsy of Northwestern Pennsylvania
3745 W 12th Street
Erie, PA 16505   814-836-9113
                                  Fax: 814-833-3919
                             leaton@mecaucp.com
                                   www.mecaucp.com

United Cerebral Palsy provides information, advocacy, referral services for persons with disabilities and/or their families. UCP also operates an equipment loan program, conducts parent workshops, disseminates written literature on topics of interest to people with disabilities.

1476   United Cerebral Palsy of Pennsylvania
908 North Second Street
Harrisburg, PA 17102   717-441-6049
                                              866-761-6129
                                         Fax: 717-236-2046
                                            info@ucpofpa.org
                                            www.ucpofpa.org

United Cerebral Palsy provides information, advocacy, referral services for persons with disabilities and/or their families. UCP also operates an equipment loan program, conducts parent workshops, disseminates written literature on topics of interest to people with disabilities.

Joan Martin, Executive Director

1477   United Cerebral Palsy of Philadelphia & Vicinity
102 E Mermaid Lane
Philadelphia, PA 19118   215-242-4200
                                         Fax: 215-247-4229
                                        ucpkravitz@aol.com
                                            www.ucpphila.org

United Cerebral Palsy provides information, advocacy, referral services for persons with disabilities and/or their families. UCP also operates an equipment loan program, conducts parent workshops, disseminates written literature on topics of interest to people with disabilities.

Stephen A Sheridan, Ceo

1478   United Cerebral Palsy of Pittsburgh
4638 Centre Avenue
Pittsburgh, PA 15213   412-683-7100
                                              1 8-8 9-4 24
                                         Fax: 412-683-4160
                                           info@ucpclass.org
                                           www.ucpclass.org

United Cerebral Palsy provides information, advocacy, referral services for persons with disabilities and/or their families. UCP also operates an equipment loan program, conducts parent workshops, disseminates written literature on topics of interest to people with disabilities.

Al Condelusci, Executive Director
Sally Balogh, Board Member
Shirley Biancheria, Board Member

1479   United Cerebral Palsy of South Central Pennsylvania
788 Cherry Tree Court
Hanover, PA 17331   717-632-5552
                                              1 8-0 3-3 38
                                         Fax: 717-632-2315
                                phoughton@ucpsouthcentral.org
                                        www.ucpsouthcentral.org

United Cerebral Palsy provides information, advocacy, referral services for persons with disabilities and/or their families. UCP also operates an equipment loan program, conducts parent workshops, disseminates written literature on topics of interest to people with disabilities.

Donald C McVay, President
K Scott Burns, Board Member
Scott Ganley, Board Member

1480   United Cerebral Palsy of Southwestern Pennsylvania
Washington Federal Square
190 North Main Street, Suite 306
Washington, PA 15301   724-229-0851
                                         Fax: 724-229-9252
                                          info@ucpswpa.org
                                           www.ucpswpa.org

United Cerebral Palsy provides information, advocacy, referral services for persons with disabilities and/or their families. UCP also operates an equipment loan program, conducts parent workshops, disseminates written literature on topics of interest to people with disabilities.

1481   United Cerebral Palsy of Western Pennsylvania
2904 Seminary Drive
Greensburg, PA 15601   724-832-8272
                                         Fax: 724-837-8278
                                      ucp@ucpofwesternpa.org
                                        www.ucpofwesternpa.org

United Cerebral Palsy provides information, advocacy, referral services for persons with disabilities and/or their families. UCP also operates an equipment loan program, conducts parent workshops, disseminates written literature on topics of interest to people with disabilities.

Debra Forsha, Children's Services Director

Rhode Island

1482   United Cerebral Palsy of Rhode Island
200 Main Street, Suite 210, PO Box 36
Pawtucket, RI 02862   401-728-1800
                                         Fax: 401-728-0182
                                             info@ucpri.org
                                             www.ucpri.org

United Cerebral Palsy provides information, advocacy, referral services for persons with disabilities and/or their families. UCP also operates an equipment loan program, conducts parent workshops, disseminates written literature on topics of interest to people with disabilities.

Stacey Johnson, President
Kenneth MacDonald, Vice president
Jennifer Spagnole, Treasurer

South Carolina

1483   United Cerebral Palsy of South Carolina
1101 Harbor Drive
West Columbia, SC 29169   803-926-8878
                                              888-827-7277
                                         Fax: 803-926-1272
                                            info@ucpsc.org
                                            www.ucpsc.org

United Cerebral Palsy provides information, advocacy, referral services for persons with disabilities and/or their families. UCP also operates an equipment loan program, conducts parent workshops, disseminates written literature on topics of interest to people with disabilities.

Ray E. Gentry, Chairperson
Ouida Spencer, Vice Chairperson
Diane Wilush, Executive Director

Tennessee

1484   United Cerebral Palsy of Middle Tennessee
1200 9th Avenue North Suite 110
Nashville, TN 37208   615-242-4091
                                         Fax: 615-242-3582
                                     request@ucpnashville.org
                                          www.ucpmidtn.org

United Cerebral Palsy provides information, advocacy, referral services for persons with disabilities and/or their families. UCP also operates an equipment loan program, conducts parent workshops, disseminates written literature on topics of interest to people with disabilities.

Deana Claiborne, Executive Director
Diane Dietrich,, Director of Development
Margaret Eighmy, Equipment Exchange Program Director

1485   United Cerebral Palsy of the Mid-South
3239 Players Club Parkway
Memphis, TN 38125   901-761-4277
                                         Fax: 901-761-7876
                                        ucp@ucpmemphis.org
                                         www.ucpmemphis.org

United Cerebral Palsy provides information, advocacy, referral services for persons with disabilities and/or their families. UCP also operates an equipment loan program, conducts parent workshops, disseminates written literature on topics of interest to people with disabilities.

Michael Nolen, Ceo
Clint Sidle, Chairperson
Brunetta Garner, Chair ,personal committee

Texas

1486 United Cerebral Palsy of Greater Houston
4500 Bissonet, Suite 340
Bellaire, TX 77401
713-838-9050
Fax: 713-838-9098
info@eastersealshouston.org
www.eastersealshouston.org

United Cerebral Palsy provides information, advocacy, referral services for persons with disabilities and/or their families. UCP also operates an equipment loan program, conducts parent workshops, disseminates written literature on topics of interest to people with disabilities.

Elise Hough, CEO
Wendy Dawson, President
Clark Varner, Vice President

1487 United Cerebral Palsy of Metropolitan Dallas
8802 Harry Hines Boulevard
Dallas, TX 75235
214-351-2500
800-999-1898
Fax: 214-351-2610
billknudsen@ucpdallas.org
www.ucpdallas.org

United Cerebral Palsy provides information, advocacy, referral services for persons with disabilities and/or their families. UCP also operates an equipment loan program, conducts parent workshops, disseminates written literature on topics of interest to people with disabilities.

Bill Knudsen, President
Rebecca Adams

1488 United Cerebral Palsy of Texas
1016 La Posada Drive, Suite 145
Austin, TX 78752
512-472-8696
800-798-1492
Fax: 512-472-8026
info@ucptexas.org
www.ucptexas.org

United Cerebral Palsy provides information, advocacy, referral services for persons with disabilities and/or their families. UCP also operates an equipment loan program, conducts parent workshops, disseminates written literature on topics of interest to people with disabilities.

Jean Langendorf, Executive Director

Utah

1489 United Cerebral Palsy of Utah
3550 S. 700 W
Salt Lake, UT 84119
801-266-1805
Fax: 801-266-2404
Petes@ucputah.org
www.ucputah.org

United Cerebral Palsy information, advocacy, referral services for persons with disabilities and/or their families. UCP also operates an equipment loan program, conducts parent workshops, and disseminates written literature on topics of interest to people with disabilities.

Peter M. Shingledecker, Contact

Virginia

1490 United Cerebral Palsy of Washington DC & Northern Virginia
1818 New York Avenue NE, Suite 101
Washington, DC 20002
202-526-0146
Fax: 202-526-0238
webmaster@ucpdc.org
www.ucpdc.org

United Cerebral Palsy provides information, advocacy, referral services for persons with disabilities and/or their families. UCP also operates an equipment loan program, conducts parent workshops, disseminates written literature on topics of interest to people with disabilities.

Dawn Carter, Executive Director

Washington

1491 United Cerebral Palsy of South Puget Sound
633 North Mildred Street, Suite C
Tacoma, WA 98406
253-565-1463
Fax: 253-565-0153
info@ucp-sps.org
www.ucp-sps.org

United Cerebral Palsy provides information, advocacy, referral services for persons with disabilities and/or their families. UCP also operates an equipment loan program, conducts parent workshops, disseminates written literature on topics of interest to people with disabilities.

Joan Lornez, Manager

Wisconsin

1492 United Cerebral Palsy of Greater Dane County
2801 Coho Street, Suite 300
Madison, WI 53713
608-273-4434
Fax: 608-273-3426
ucpgdc@ucpdane.org
www.ucpdane.org

United Cerebral Palsy provides information, advocacy, referral services for persons with disabilities and/or their families. UCP also conducts parent workshops and disseminates written literature on topics of interest to people with disabilities.

Wade Harrison, President
Rich Cooper, Vice President
Melanie Patterson, Treasurer

1493 United Cerebral Palsy of Southeastern Wisconsin
6102 W. Layton Avenue
Greenfield, WI 53220
414-329-4500
888-482-7739
Fax: 414-329-4510
info@ucpsew.org
www.ucpsew.org

United Cerebral Palsy provides information, advocacy, referral services for persons with disabilities and/or their families. UCP also operates an equipment loan program, conducts parent workshops, disseminates written literature on topics of interest to people with disabilities.

Scott D. Anderson, President
Sally M. Lyne, Vice President
Ryan Engelhardt, Treasurer

1494 United Cerebral Palsy of West Central Wisconsin
206 Water Street
Eau Claire, WI 54703
715-832-1782
Fax: 715-832-8203
ucp1dave@sbcglobal.net
www.ucpwcw.org

United Cerebral Palsy provides information, advocacy, referral services for persons with disabilities and/or their families. UCP also operates an equipment loan program, conducts parent workshops, disseminates written literature on topics of interest to people with disabilities.

Connie Werlein, President
Randi Johnson, Vice President
Jennifer Napolitano, Secretary

Libraries & Resource Centers

1495 National Rehabilitation Information Center
8400 Corporate Drive, Suite 500
Landover, MD 20785

301-459-5900
800-346-2742
Fax: 301-459-4263
TTY: 301-459-5984
naricinfo@heitechservices.com
www.naric.com

Committed to providing direct, personal and high quality information services to anyone interested in disability rehabilitation issues; Committed to serving consumers, researchers, family members, health professionals, educators, counselors, students, librarians and the administrators throughout the country.

Mark Odum, Director

Research Centers

1496 Orthopaedic Biomechanics Laboratory
Shriners Hospital for Crippled Children
1701 19th Avenue
San Francisco, CA 94122

415-665-1100
Fax: 415-661-3615

Offers research and studies into cerebral palsy.

Stephen R Skinner, Clinical Director

1497 United Cerebral Palsy Research and Educational Foundation
186 Princeton Hightstown Road Building 4 2nd Floor
Princeton Junction, NJ 08550

609-452-1200
800-872-5827
Fax: 609-452-1201
cpirf@cpirf.org
www.cpirf.org

Provides research grants to prevent cerebral palsy and to improve treatment, management and functioning of persons with cerebral palsy.

Glenn R Tringali, Chief Executive Officer/President
James A Blackman, M.D., M.P.H, Medical Director
Jacqueline M Carmosino, Manager of Administration

Conferences

1498 American Academy for Cerebral Palsy and Developmental Medicine Annual Meeting
555 E Wells Street, Suite 1100
Milwaukee, WI 53202

414-918-3014
Fax: 414-276-2146
info@aacpdm.org
www.aacpdm.org

October

Maureen O'Donnell, President
Richard Stevenson, Vice President
Annette Majnemer, Secretary

Audio Video

1499 Accidents of Nature
Random House
1745 Broadway
New York, NY 10019

212-782-9000
rhkidspublicity@randomhouse.com
www.randomhouse.com

About a girl who goes to a camp and has experiences that will change her life forever. Audio book feature.

2006
ISBN: 0-739335-30-8

1500 Cerebral Palsy: What Every Parent Should Know
Films for the Humanities and Sciences
132 West 31st Street
New York, NY 10001

800-257-5126
Fax: 609-275-0266
custserv@films.com
www.ffh.films.com

This program covers the causes, symptoms, and range of possible treatments of cerebral palsy, including the relationship between physical and mental handicaps, and the role of medications and physical therapy treatment.

28 minutes
ISBN: 1-421336-41-1

Web Sites

1501 American Academy for Cerebral Palsy and Developmental Medicine
555 East Wells, Suite 1100
Milwaukee, WI 53202

414-918-3014
Fax: 414-276-2146
info@aacpdm.org
www.aacpdm.org

Organization of professionals involved in the care of people with Cerebral Palsy, developmental disorders, and related diseases.

Darcy Fehlings, President
Eileen Fowler, 1st Vice President
Unni Narayanan, 2nd Vice President

1502 Children's Neurobiological Solutions Foundation
1223 Wilshire Blvd., #937
Santa Monica, CA 90403

310-889-8611
info@cnsfoundation.org
www.cnsfoundation.org

Children's Neurobiological Solutions Foundation (CNS), is a national, nonprofit, 501(c)(3) organization, whose mission is to orchestrate cutting-edge, collaborative research with the goal of expediting the creation of effective treatments and therapies for children with neurodevelopmental abnormalities, birth injuries to the nervous system, and related neurological problems.

Fia Richmond, Founder
Phill Richmond, Founder
Jeffrey D. Macklis, Board Member

1503 Easter Seals Disability Services
233 South Wacker Drive, Suite 2400
Chicago, IL 60606

800-221-6827
www.easterseals.com

For more than 80 years, Easter Seals has helped people with disabilities in communities nationwide. From creating the first national voluntary act on behalf of children with disabilities in the 1920's to leading the creation and implementation of the Americans with Disabilities Act in the 1990's. Easter Seals child development services build strong foundations for children of all abilities.

Brad Halverson, Chair
Don Young, 1st Vice Chair
Wes Blumenshine, 2nd Vice Chair

1504 Family Support Network
www.tsalliance.org

The Support Network is an organized partnership of individuals whose lives have been affected by tuberous sclerosis. Across the nation, the Support Network is providing the latest medical information, education and support to those individuals who are seeking understanding about the genetic disease and offering them words of encouragement and empowerment.

1505 Health Answers
410 Horsham Road
Horsham, PA 19044

215-442-9017
Michael.tague@healthanswers.com
www.healthanswers.com

The vision was to provide a breadth of services to clients through the formation of a network of companies. Each company plays a key role in meeting out clients' needs.

Michael Tague, Managing Director

1506 Infinitec
547 W. Jackson Street, Suite 225
Chicago, IL 60661
312-765-0419
Fax: 312-765-0503
mbettlach@ucpnet.org
www.infinitec.org

The mission of Infinitec is to advance independence and promote inclusive opportunities for children and adults with disabilities throught technology.

Mary Bettlach, Managing Director

1507 My Child Without Limits
www.mychildwithoutlimits.org

An authoritative early intervention resource for families of young children ages 0-5 with developmental delays or disabilities, and professionals looking for a single, trusted, aggregate source of information that relates to their needs and interests. All medical information is reviewed by the My Child Without Limits medical advisory board, a panel composed of doctors in the fields of developmental disability and delay.

1508 National Dissemination Center for Children with Disabilities
35 Halsey St., Fourth Floor
Newark, NJ 7102
malizo@spannj.org
www.nichcy.org

A national information and referral center that provides information on disabilities and disability-related issues for families, educators and other professionals.

Debra Jennings, Project Director
Indira Medina, Coordinator of Communication
Lisa Kupper, Product Coordinator

1509 Scope (UK)
www.scope.org.uk/

Our aim is that disabled people achieve equality: a society in which they are as valued and have the same human and civil rights as everyone else.

Andrew McDonald, Chair
John Gilbert, Treasurer
Richard Hawkes, Chief Executive

1510 United Cerebral Palsy Associations
1825 K Street NW Suite 600
Washington, DC 20006
202-776-0406
800-872-5827
www.ucp.org

The UCP is the leading source of information on cerebral palsy and is a pivitol advocate for the rights of persons with any disability. As one of the largest health charities in America, UCP's mission is to advance the independence, productivity and full citizenship of people with Cerebral Palsy and other diabilities.

Stephen Bennett, President/ CEO
Connie Garner, EVP, Public Policy
Anita Porco, VP, Affiliate Network

1511 WE MOVE (Worldwide Education and Advocacy for Movement Disorders)
www.wemove.org

WE MOVE provides movement disorder information and educational materials to physicians, patients and families, the media, and the public via its comprehensive Web sites, training courses, and more. Its goal is to make early diagnosis, up-to-date treatment and patient support a reality for all people living with movement disorders.

Book Publishers

1512 A Mother's Touch: The Tiffany Callo Story
United Cerebral Palsy Associations
1825 K Street NW, Suite 600
Washington, DC 20006
202-776-0406
800-872-5827
Fax: 202-776-0414
info@ucp.org
www.ucp.org

A vivid portrayal of a woman with cerebral palsy who faced discrimination because of her disability.

Woody Connette, Chair
Ian Ridlon, Vice Chair
Pamela Talkin, Secretary

1513 After the Tears: Parents Talk About Raising a Child with a Disability
United Cerebral Palsy Associations
1825 K Street NW, Suite 600
Washington, DC 20006
202-776-0406
800-872-5827
Fax: 202-776-0414
info@ucp.org
www.ucp.org

Book draws on stories of parents who have struggled, learned and grown in the years since their child was born with a disability.

89 pages Softcover

Woody Connette, Chair
Ian Ridlon, Vice Chair
Pamela Talkin, Secretary

1514 An Introduction to Your Child Who Has Cerebral Palsy
Medic Publishing Company
PO Box 89
Redmond, WA 98073
425-881-2883

Information and answers to questions for parents of children with cerebral palsy.

1515 Breaking Ground: Ten Families Building Opportunities Through Integration
United Cerebral Palsy Associations
1825 K Street NW, Suite 600
Washington, DC 20006
202-776-0406
800-872-5827
Fax: 202-776-0414
info@ucp.org
www.ucp.org

Gives examples of strategies families have used to integrate the children fully into their schools and communities.

75 pages Softcover

Woody Connette, Chair
Ian Ridlon, Vice Chair
Pamela Talkin, Secretary

1516 Can't You be Still?
Gemma B Publishing
101-478 River Avenue, #779
Winnipeg, Manitoba, R3L 0
Canada
204-452-7566
Fax: 204-475-9903
gempub@shaw.ca
www.gemmab.ca

This wonderfully written children's book features a heroine, Ann, with cerebral palsy who goes to school for the first time. First in a trilogy, the book is written in the first person since Ann cannot speak out loud intelligibly but has lots of words inside her head.

28 pages Softcover

Sarah Yates
Anne Allan

1517 Children With Cerebral Palsy: A Parents Guide
Peytral Publications
PO Box 1162
Minnetonka, MN 55345

952-949-8707
877-739-8725
Fax: 952-906-9777
help@peytral.com
www.peytral.com

Informative handbook for parents of children and teens; covers medical, educational, legal, family life, daily care, emotional issues and more.

470 pages

1518 Congenital Disorders Sourcebook 2nd Edition
Omnigraphics
PO Box 31-1640
Detroit, MI 48231

800-234-1340
Fax: 800-875-1340
info@omnigraphics.com
www.omnigraphics.com

Provides basic consumer health information about the most common types of nonhereditary birth defects and disorders related to prematurity, gestational injuries, congenital infections, and birth complications, including disorders of the heart, brain, gastrointestinal tract, musculoskeletal system, urinary tract, and reproductive system, craniofacial disorders, cerebral palsy, spina bifida, and fetal alcohol syndrome, and detailing the causes, diagnostic tests, and treatments for each.

650 pages
ISBN: 0-780809-45-9

1519 Connecting Students: A Guide to Thoughtful Friendship Facilitation
United Cerebral Palsy Associations
1660 L Street NW, Suite 700
Washington, DC 20036

202-776-0406
800-872-5823
Fax: 202-776-0414
info@ucp.org
www.ucp.org

Contains helpful strategies on real-life experiences on building friendships.

48 pages Softcover

Woody Connette, Chair
Ian Ridlon, Vice Chair
Pamela Talkin, Secretary

1520 Discovery Book
United Cerebral Palsy Association
1825 K Street NW, Suite 600
Washington, DC 20006

202-776-0406
800-872-5827
Fax: 202-776-0414
info@ucp.org
www.ucp.org

Created within a United Cerebral Palsy group for childern with physical disabilities, The Discovery Book is an exploration of social and psychological aspects of childhood disability. Accompanied by their artwork, children speak in their own words about important areas of life such as: What about friends?; Doctors and hospitals; Problems and challenges; and Goals, wishes & dreams.

96 pages

Woody Connette, Chair
Ian Ridlon, Vice Chair
Pamela Talkin, Secretary

1521 Each of Us Remembers: Parents of Children With Cerebral Palsy
United Cerebral Palsy Associations
1825 K Street NW, Suite 600
Washington, DC 20006

202-776-0406
800-872-5827
Fax: 202-776-0414
info@ucp.org
www.ucp.org

Parents of children with cerebral palsy answer questions that people really need to know.

Woody Connette, Chair
Ian Ridlon, Vice Chair
Pamela Talkin, Secretary

1522 Gemma B Publishing
101-478 River Avenue, Suite 779
Winnipeg, MB R3L 0
Canada

204-452-7566
Fax: 204-475-9903
gempub@shaw.ca
www.gemmab.ca

Gemma B Publishing was formed to develop literary heroines for the disabled, emphasizing their active participation in life.

Sarah Yates, Founder

1523 Handling the Young Cerebral Palsied Child at Home
United Cerebral Palsy Associations
1825 K Street NW, Suite 600
Washington, DC 20006

202-776-0406
800-872-5827
Fax: 202-776-0414
info@ucp.org
www.ucp.org

Offers chapters on bathing, feeding, dressing and play for parents of children with cerebral palsy.

337 pages Softcover

Woody Connette, Chair
Ian Ridlon, Vice Chair
Pamela Talkin, Secretary

1524 Here's What I Mean to Say
Gemma B Publishing
101-478 River Avenue, #779
Winnipeg, Manitoba, R3L 0
Canada

204-452-7566
Fax: 204-475-9903
gempub@shaw.ca
www.gemmab.ca

Third in the Ann trilogy, Ann learns to read and uncovers the magic of literacy. She uses a speech program in her computer and wonders, when she succeeds in reading, 'Is it me or is it my angel?'

24 pages
ISBN: 0-969647-72-7

Sarah Yates
Anne Allan

1525 Lucky Lou Gets Game
Gemma B Publishing
101-478 River Avenue, #779
Winnipeg, Manitoba, R3L 0
Canada

204-452-7566
Fax: 204-475-9903
gempub@shaw.ca
www.gemmab.ca

A coming of age young adult novel about 17-year old Lucky Lou who takes on a neighborhood, learns how to play baseball, and meets the boy who was never in her dreams. In this funny and insightful book, Lou gets game and the results are unexpected.

24 pages
ISBN: 0-969647-71-9

Sarah Yates, Autor
Anne Allan

1526 Natural Supports in School/Work/Community for the Severely Disabled
United Cerebral Palsy Associations
1825 K Street NW, Suite 600
Washington, DC 20006

202-776-0406
800-872-5827
Fax: 202-776-0414
info@ucp.org
www.ucp.org

Promotes the position that assistance must be defined by the needs of individuals rather than the requirements of the service systems.

361 pages Softcover

Woody Connette, Chair
Ian Ridlon, Vice Chair
Pamela Talkin, Secretary

1527 No Time for Jello: One Family's Experience
Brookline Books
8 Trumbell Rd, Suite B-001
Northampton, MA 01060

413-584-0184
Fax: 413-584-6184
brbooks@yahoo.com
http://brooklinebooks.com

One family's story of their attempts to remediate and cure the effects of cerebral palsied condition the oldest son was born with. The Bratts traveled traditional routes, through distinguished medical centers in Boston, and nontraditional routes in a search for treatments that would help their son.

Softcover
ISBN: 0-253363-65-9

1528 Nobody Knows
Gemma B Publishing
101-478 River Avenue, #779
Winnipeg, Manitoba, R3L 0
Canada

204-452-7566
Fax: 204-475-9903
gempub@shaw.ca
www.gemmab.ca

Sequel to 'Can't You Be Still,' Ann gets frustrated that nobody knows what she wants and is trying to say; they find it hard to understand her. She goes out to find someone who can understand and in the process, learns that there are many ways to communicate.

24 pages
ISBN: 0-969647-71-9

Sarah Yates
Anne Allan

1529 Opening Doors: Strategies for Including All Students in Regular Education
United Cerebral Palsy Associations
1825 K Street NW, Suite 600
Washington, DC 20006

202-776-0406
800-872-5827
Fax: 202-776-0414
info@ucp.org
www.ucp.org

Contains practical information for including and supporting all students in regular classes.

55 pages Softcover

Woody Connette, Chair
Ian Ridlon, Vice Chair
Pamela Talkin, Secretary

1530 Teaching Motor Skills to Children with Cerebral Palsy & Similar Movement Disorders
Woodbine House
6510 Bells Mill Road
Bethesda, MD 20817

301-897-3570
800-843-7323
Fax: 301-897-5838
info@woodbinehouse.com
www.woodbinehouse.com

The resource that parents, therapists, and other caregivers can consult to help children with gross motor delays learn and practice motor skills outside of therapy sessions.

2006 275 pages
ISBN: 1-890627-72-0

1531 Walk with Me
United Cerebral Palsy Associations
1825 K Sreet NW, Suite 600
Washington, DC 20006

202-776-0406
800-872-5827
Fax: 202-776-0414
info@ucp.org
www.ucp.org

A story written by eight-year-old Eric Grimm covering his thoughts on living with cerebral palsy.

Woody Connette, Chair
Ian Ridlon, Vice Chair
Pamela Talkin, Secretary

Newsletters

1532 Family Support Bulletin
United Cerebral Palsy Associations
1825 K Street NW Suite 600
Washington, DC 20006

202-776-0406
800-872-5827
Fax: 202-776-0414
info@ucp.org
www.ucp.org

A detailed quarterly journal that takes a comprehensive look at the latest policies, resources and legislative information enacted in Washington and state capitals.

Quarterly

Stephen Bennett, President/ CEO
Connie Garner, EVP, Public Policy
Anita Porco, VP, Affiliate Network

1533 My Child Without Limits Newsletter
United Cerebral Palsy
1825 K Street NW Suite 600
Washington, DC 20006

202-776-0406
800-872-5827
Fax: 202-776-0414
info@ucp.org
www.ucp.org

A monthly publication that highlights new and relevant content from the 'My Child Without Limits' web site and online community, which provides an early intervention resource for families of young children ages 0-5 with developmental delays or disabilities, and the professionals who serve them.

Stephen Bennett, President & CEO
Connie Garner, EVP, Public Policy
Anita Porco, VP, Affiliate Network

1534 Networker
United Cerebral Palsy Associations
1825 K Street NW Suite 600
Washington, DC 20006

202-776-0406
800-872-5827
Fax: 202-776-0414
info@ucp.org
www.ucp.org

Offers the latest information on the newest technology available for persons with cerebral palsy.

Quarterly

Stephen Bennett, President/ CEO
Connie Garner, EVP, Public Policy
Anita Porco, VP, Affiliate Network

1535 UCP Newsletter
United Cerebral Palsy
1825 K Street NW Suite 600
Washington, DC 20006

202-776-0406
800-872-5827
Fax: 202-776-0414
info@ucp.org
www.ucp.org

A monthly e-publication formerly known as Life Without Limits. The newsletteris not only for UCP affiliates, but also volunteers, activists and information seekers. Each issue highlights stories centered around advocacy efforts, affiliate news, information and referral sources, upcoming events, inspiring events and more.

Stephen Bennett, President & CEO
Connie Garner, EVP, Public Policy
Anita Porco, VP, Affiliate Network

1536 UCP Washington Wire
United Cerebral Palsy
1825 K Street NW Suite 600
Washington, DC 20006   202-776-0406
                                        800-872-5827
                                        Fax: 202-776-0414
                                        info@ucp.org
                                        www.ucp.org

A weekly publication that provides a comprehensive source of information on federal legislation, agency regulations, court decisions and other issues of interest to the disability community.

Stephen Bennett, President & CEO
Connie Garner, EVP, Public Policy
Anita Porco, VP, Affiliate Network

Pamphlets

1537 Cerebral Palsy-Facts & Figures
United Cerebral Palsy Associations
1825 K Street NW Suite 600
Washington, DC 20006   202-776-0406
                                        800-872-5827
                                        Fax: 202-776-0414
                                        www.ucp.org

Offers information on what cerebral palsy is, the effects, causes, types, and prevention.

Stephen Bennett, President/ CEO
Connie Garner, EVP, Public Policy
Anita Porco, VP, Affiliate Network

Camps

1538 Camp Merrimack
3320 Triana Boulevard
Huntsville, AL 35805   256-534-6455
                                        ksimari@merrimackhall.com
                                        www.merrimackhall.com

A unique arts half-day camp for children ages 3 through 12; open to children with special needs including Cerebral Palsy, Down Syndrome, autism and others.

Ashley Dinges, Executive Director
Kim Simari, Managing Director

1539 Camp Merry Heart/Easter Seals Easter Seal Society
21 O'Brian Road
Hackettstown, NJ 07840   908-852-3896
                                        Fax: 908-852-9263
                                        camp@nj.easterseals.com
                                        www.nj.easterseals.com

An organized program of swimming, arts and crafts, boating, nature study and travel offered to the physically disabled, developmentally disabled, cerebral palsied, brain damaged and head injured children, ages 5-18, adults 19-75+. Fall and spring travel programs for adults.

Mary Ellen Ross, Camping Director

1540 Camp Ramah in New England Tikvah Program
39 Bennett Street
Palmer, MA 01609   413-283-9771
                                        Fax: 413-283-6661
                                        info@campramahne.org
                                        www.campramahne.org

The Tikvah program is one of the first summer programs for Jewish children with special needs. It continues to grow and evolve as it strives to serve campers with a wide range of special needs including, but not limited to, congitive impairments, autism, cerebral palsy and seizure disorder.

Howard Blas, Tikvah Program Director
Talya Kalender, Director, Camper Care
Benjamin Greene, Director of Education

1541 Cerebral Palsy Center Summer Program
7 Sanford Avenue
Belleville, NJ   201-751-0200
                                        info@kidscamps.com
                                        www.kidscamps.com

1542 Charles Campbell Children's Camp
PO Box 23342
Billings, MT 59104   campbellcamp@msn.com
                                        www.billingslions.org

Camp for children with physical disabilities including but not limited to: sight or hearing impairment, cerebral palsy, spina bifida, amputee, gross motor skill impairments, and other disabilities.

Doug Hanson, Director

1543 Crotched Mountain School & Rehabilitation Center
1 Verney Drive
Greenfield, NH 03047   603-547-3311
                                        800-800-966
                                        Fax: 603-547-3232
                                        info@crotchedmountain.org
                                        www.cmf.org

Currently serves children ages 6-22 with multiple-handicaps including: Cerebral Palsy, Spina Bifida, visual and hearing impairments and neurological disabilities, developmental disorders, mental retardation, autism, behavioral and emotional disorders, seizure disorders, spinal cord and head injuries. Member of the National Association of Independent Schools and accredited with the NE Association of Schools and Colleges, Independent Schools of Northern NE.

Rita Phinney, Director Admissions
John Young, Registrar

1544 Easter Seals Wisconsin Camp Respite
1550 Waubeek Road
Wisconsin Dells, WI 53965   608-254-2502
                                        Fax: 608-253-0327
                                        dfourness@eastersealswisconsin.com
                                        www.eastersealswisconsin.com

Camp for individuals age 3 to adult with moderate to severe disabilities. The campers have a variety of different diagnosis such as: autism, cerebral palsy, traumatic brain injury, developmental disabilities, and behavioral issues.

Dan Fournes, Camp Director

1545 Eric RicStar Winter Music Therapy Summer Camp
4930 S Hagadorn Rd
East Lansing, MI 48823   517-353-7661
                                        Fax: 517-355-3292
                                        commusic@msu.edu
                                        www.cms.msu.edu

The purpose of this camp is to provide opportunities for musical expression, enjoyment and interaction for all people with special needs and their siblings.

Cindy Edgerton, Director
Judy Winter, Co-Chair

DESCRIPTION

1546 CHARCOT-MARIE-TOOTH DISEASE

Charcot-Marie-Tooth (CMT) disease belongs to a group of disorders known as hereditary motor-sensory neuropathies or HMSNs. The HMSNs are progressive disorders of nerves outside of the central nervous system that extend from the brain and spinal cord to particular areas of the body (peripheral nervous system). Symptoms and findings associated with these disorders are primarily the result of involvement of motor nerve fibers (those that affect motion). These nerves transmit various nerve impulses away from the brain and spinal cord to their termination (e.g., muscle tissue). As these disorders progress, affected individuals may experience some symptoms due to sensory and autonomic involvement. Sensory nerve fibers carry impulses to the brain and spinal cord. The autonomic nervous system is the portion of the peripheral nervous system that regulates involuntary functioning of particular tissues and organs.

There are different types of Charcot-Marie-Tooth disease that have varying modes of inheritance. Charcot-Marie-Tooth disease (in all its forms) is the most prevalent hereditary peripheral neuropathy, affecting approximately one in 2,500 individuals. The most common form of the disease, known as Charcot-Marie-Tooth disease type 1A or CMT1A, is inherited as an autosomal dominant trait. A disease gene for CMT1A is located on the short arm of chromosome 17.

Children with CMT type 1A usually do not have associated symptoms until late childhood or early adolescence. However, some may experience abnormalities in their manner of walking (gait disturbances) as early as the second year of life. In other, rare instances, associated symptoms may not become apparent until middle adulthood. CMT1A initially affects muscles supplied by nerves of the lower legs (peroneal and tibial nerves), causing muscle degeneration (atrophy) in the lower legs and feet. This is accompanied by muscle weakness and a distinctive stork-like contour of the legs. Bending movements of the ankles become progressively weaker, eventually resulting in footdrop, a condition in which the foot does not flex or bend upward. In addition, the arch of the foot becomes unusually increased in height (pescavus deformities). An unstable gait may develop, and children may appear clumsy, easily tripping or falling. Although muscles of both legs are affected, disease progression and associated findings usually differ slightly from one side of the body to the other.

As the disorder progresses, individuals with CMT1A also usually develop a loss of muscle tissue mass and weakness in the forearms and hands. These areas seem to be less severely affected than the lower legs. However, patients may eventually develop permanent fixation of certain joints in a bend position. This typically occurs in the fingers and wrists. Some patients also experience gradual sensory involvement, such as abnormal burning or tingling sensations (paresthesias) in the feet. Associated autonomic abnormalities may include unusual paleness (pallor) or blotching of the skin, especially of the feet. In individuals with CMT1A, specialized testing typically reveals a marked reduction in the transmission of motor and sensory nerve signals to affected muscles (reduced conduction velocities).

Although CMT1A is progressive, most affected individuals maintain the ability to walk. However, the use of special orthopedic appliances, such as stiff boots that reach to the midcalf, plastic splints, or light leg braces, are typically necessary to help stabilize the ankles. Surgical measures may be considered, such as surgical fusion of the ankles. In addition, certain medications may help to alleviate burning sensations in the feet (e.g., carbamazepine or phenytoin). Other treatment is symptomatic and supportive.

In addition to Charcot-Marie-Tooth disease type 1A, additional autosomal dominant, autosomal recessive, and X-linked forms of the disease have been identified. Specific symptoms and findings and the nature of the disorder progression may vary, depending upon the specific form of the disease.

National Associations & Support Groups

1547 American Academy of Pediatrics
141 Northwest Point Boulevard
Elk Grove Village, IL 60007
847-434-4000
800-433-9016
Fax: 847-434-8000
www.aap.org

The American Academy of Pediatrics and its member pediatricians are committed to the attainment of optimal physical, mental and social health and well-being for all infants, children, adolescents, and young adults.
Fernando Stein, MD, FAAP, President
Karen Remley, MD, CEO/Executive VP

State Agencies & Support Groups

New York

1548 CMTA Chapter - New York (Greater)
CMT Association
333 East 34th StreetSuite 1J
Manhattan, NY 10016
212-535-4314
Fax: 212-535-6392
david.younger@nyumc.org
www.cmtnyc.org

Every other month (Third Saturday from 1:00 - 3:00 p.m.) - check website
Dr David Younger, Contact

Ohio

1549 CMTA Chapter - Ohio
CMT Association
405 Wagner Avenue
Greenville, OH 45331
937-548-3963
Greenville-Ohio-CMT@who.rr.com
www.charcot-marie-tooth.org

Fourth Thursday, April - October
Dot Cain, Contact

Pennsylvania

1550 CMTA Chapter - Pennsylvania
CMT Association
PO Box 105
Glenolden, PA 19036
610-499-9264
800-606-2682
Fax: 610-499-9267
info@cmtausa.org.
www.cmtausa.org

Bi-monthly (3rd Saturday, 10:00 a.m. - 12:00 p.m.)

Herbert Beron, Chairman
Gary J Gasper, Treasurer
Elizabeth Ouellette, Secretary

Web Sites

1551 CMT Net
275 Madison Ave (corner of 40th St)~
New York, NY 10016   www.rcn.com

CMTNet is intended to provide information for both the medical and non-medical communities.

1552 Charcot-Marie-Tooth Association
PO Box 105
Glenolden, PA 19036   610-499-9264
                                      800-606-2682
                                      Fax: 610-499-9267
                                      info@cmtausa.org
                                      www.cmtausa.org

Information regarding patient support, public education, promotion of research and ultimately the treatment and cure of CMT.

Patrick A. Livney, Chief Executive Officer
Kim Magee, Director of Finance
Susan Ruediger, Director of Development

1553 Health Answers
410 Horsham Road
Horsham, PA 19044   215-442-9017
                            Michael.tague@healthanswers.com
                                      www.healthanswers.com

The vision was to provide a breadth of services to clients through the formation of a network of companies. Each company plays a key role in meeting our clients' needs.

Michael Tague, Managing Director

1554 Muscular Dystrophy Association
222 S. Riverside Plaza, Suite 1500
Chicago, IL 60606   800-572-1717
                                      mda@mdausa.org
                                      mda.org

Information regarding neuromuscular diseases through programs of worldwide research, comprehensive medical and community services, and far-reaching professional and public health education; including publications.

Steven M. Derks, President/ CEO
Valerie A. Cwik, M.D., EVP/ CMO/ CSO
Julie Faber, EVP/ CFO

Book Publishers

1555 Charcot-Marie-Tooth Disorders: A Handbook for Primary Care Physicians
Charcot-Marie-Tooth Association
PO Box 105
Glenolden, PA 19036   610-499-9264
                                      800-606-2682
                                      Fax: 610-499-9267
                                      info@cmtausa.org
                                      www.cmtausa.org

Excellent source of information about the causes, symptoms, and treatment/management of CMT.

1995 130 pages

Patrick A Livney, CEO
Patricia Dreibelbis, Director Of Program Services
Kim Magee, Director Of Finance

1556 Let's Talk About Going to the Hospital
Rosen Publishing Group's PowerKids Press
29 E 21st Street
New York, NY 10010   212-777-3017
                                      800-237-9932
                                      Fax: 888-436-4643
                                      rosenpub@tribeca.ios.com
                                      www.rosenpublishing.com

If a child has to check into the hospital, chances are he or she is already upset about being ill. Knowing how a hospital functions and what the procedures are, such as when family members can visit, will help in what is already a stressful situation. Grades K-5.

24 pages
ISBN: 0-823950-36-0

Magazines

1557 Quest Magazine
MDA Publications
222 S. Riverside Plaza, Suite 1500
Chicago, IL 60606   520-529-2000
                                      800-572-1717
                                      Fax: 520-529-5300
                                      mda@mdausa.org
                                      mda.org

A national magazine that goes out to everyone registered with MDA, MDA clinics, researchers and subscribers. It presents news related to muscular dystrophy and other neuromuscular diseases including research, personal profiles, fund raising activities, patient services, and lifestyle information including products and trends.

Bimonthly

Steven M. Derks, President/ CEO
Valerie A. Cwik, M.D., EVP/ CMO/ CSO
Julie Faber, EVP/ CFO

Newsletters

1558 CMTA Report
CMT Association
PO Box 105
Glenolden, PA 19036   610-499-9264
                                      800-606-2682
                                      Fax: 610-499-9267
                                      info@charcot-marie-tooth.org
                                      www.cmtausa.org

Contains articles on CMT topics, research news and patient profiles. Free with membership.

Bi-Monthly

Patrick A. Livney, Chief Executive Officer
Kim Magee, Director of Finance
Susan Ruediger, Director of Development

Pamphlets

1559 CMT Brochure
Charcot-Marie-Tooth Association
PO Box 105
Glenolden, PA 19036   610-499-9264
                                      800-606-2682
                                      Fax: 610-499-9267
                                      info@charcot-marie-tooth.org
                                      www.cmtausa.org

Provides a quick overview of CMT.

2005 8 pages

Patrick A. Livney, Chief Executive Officer
Kim Magee, Director of Finance
Susan Ruediger, Director of Development

1560 CMT Facts I
Charcot-Marie-Tooth Association
PO Box 105
Glenolden, PA 19036   610-499-9264
                                      800-606-2682
                                      Fax: 610-499-9267
                                      info@charcot-marie-tooth.org
                                      www.cmtausa.org

Offers information on the neurotrophic drugs, genetics and therapies for CMT, surgical options and an overview of the disorder.

1993 16 pages

Patrick A. Livney, Chief Executive Officer
Kim Magee, Director of Finance
Susan Ruediger, Director of Development

1561 CMT Facts II
Charcot-Marie-Tooth Association
PO Box 105
Glenolden, PA 19036

610-499-9264
800-606-2682
Fax: 610-499-9267
info@charcot-marie-tooth.org
www.cmtausa.org

Offers information on adaptive devices, feature specialists and the Americans with disabilities act.

1993 24 pages

Patrick A. Livney, Chief Executive Officer
Kim Magee, Director of Finance
Susan Ruediger, Director of Development

1562 CMT Facts III
Charcot-Marie-Tooth Association
PO Box 105
Glenolden, PA 19036

610-499-9264
800-606-2682
Fax: 610-499-9267
info@charcot-marie-tooth.org
www.cmtausa.org

Offers information on neurotrophic drugs, neuromuscular disorders, genetic news and doctor's questions and answers.

1995 24 pages

Patrick A. Livney, Chief Executive Officer
Kim Magee, Director of Finance
Susan Ruediger, Director of Development

1563 CMT Facts IV
Charcot-Marie-Tooth Association
PO Box 105
Glenolden, PA 19036

610-499-9264
800-606-2682
Fax: 610-499-9267
info@charcot-marie-tooth.org
www.cmtausa.org

Provides information for Charcot-Marie-Tooth patients.

1998 32 pages

Patrick A. Livney, Chief Executive Officer
Kim Magee, Director of Finance
Susan Ruediger, Director of Development

1564 CMT Facts V
Charcot-Marie-Tooth Association
PO Box 105
Glenolden, PA 19036

610-499-9264
800-606-2682
Fax: 610-499-9267
info@charcot-marie-tooth.org
www.cmtausa.org

Source for information on orthotics, pain, emotional, HNPP, physical and occupational therapy, Social Security Disability and more.

2002 56 pages

Patrick A. Livney, Chief Executive Officer
Kim Magee, Director of Finance
Susan Ruediger, Director of Development

1565 Charcot-Marie-Tooth Disorders: A Guide abo ut Genetics for Patients
Charcot-Marie-Tooth Association
PO Box 105
Glenolden, PA 19036

610-499-9264
800-606-2682
Fax: 610-499-9267
info@charcot-marie-tooth.org
www.cmtausa.org

Illustrated with easy-to-understand diagrams, this booklet outlines the basics of genetics inheritance and CMT.

2000 21 pages

Patrick A. Livney, Chief Executive Officer
Kim Magee, Director of Finance
Susan Ruediger, Director of Development

1566 Facts About Charcot-Marie-Tooth Disease an d Dejerine-Sottas
Muscular Dystrophy Association
222 S. Riverside Plaza, Suite 1500
Chicago, IL 60606

520-529-2000
800-572-1717
Fax: 520-529-5300
mda@mdausa.org
mda.org

This booklet has been prepared to give you the basic knowledge about CMT and Dejerine-Sottas disease that you'll need in order to help you prepare for changed that may offur in your future. It cover research, explaining the causes, treatments, and cures. Also available in Spanish and online.

2009 15 pages Paperback

Kristine Welker, Interim President/CEO
Valerie A. Cwik, MD, EVP, Chief Medical & Scientific
Julie Faber, EVP, CFO

1567 MDA Fact Sheet
Muscular Dystrophy Association
222 S. Riverside Plaza, Suite 1500
Chicago, IL 60606

520-529-2000
800-572-1717
Fax: 520-529-5300
mda@mdausa.org
mda.org

Provides information about the association, how it got started, and what muscular dystrophy can affect the body. Also in Spanish and online.

2008

Kristine Welker, Interim President/CEO
Valerie A. Cwik, MD, EVP, Chief Medical & Scientific
Julie Faber, EVP, CFO

DESCRIPTION

1568 CHILDHOOD DERMATOMYOSITIS

Synonym: Juvenile dermatomyositis (JDMS)

Involves the following Biologic System(s):

Connective Tissue Disorders, Dermatologic Disorders, Orthopedic and Muscle Disorders

Dermatomyositis is a connective tissue disorder characterized by inflammatory and degenerative changes of the muscles and distinctive lesions of the skin. Although the disorder may become apparent at any time, it most commonly occurs in children between five to 15 years of age or adults between the ages of 40 to 60 years. In children, the average age at onset is eight or nine years. More females than males are affected by dermatomyositis.

The cause of dermatomyositis is unknown. However, immune, genetic, and environmental factors are thought to play some role. Many researchers suggest that dermatomyositis is an autoimmune disorder resulting from abnormal immune responses directed against the body's own tissues.

The symptoms and findings associated with childhood dermatomyositis are similar to those seen in the adult form of the disease. However, involvement of the gastrointestinal (GI) tract and the development of abnormal calcium deposits (calcifications) within skin and muscle tissues are more frequent and widespread in childhood dermatomyositis. Affected children usually have widespread inflammation of small blood vessels (vasculitis) within connective tissues of the skin, muscles, tissues beneath the skin (subcutaneous tissues), and tissues underlying the nails (nail beds). In addition, cancerous growths (malignancies) occur in approximately 20 percent of affected adults; malignancies are rarely seen in those with childhood dermatomyositis.

In most patients with childhood dermatomyositis, the onset of symptoms is relatively gradual and subtle. Children initially experience slowly progressive muscle weakness affecting the upper arms, shoulders, hips, and thighs (proximal muscles) as well as the trunk. Involved muscles tend to be sore, stiff, tender, or abnormally hard. Affected children may develop an awkward manner of walking and gradually lose the ability to perform certain tasks, such as lifting the arms above the shoulders, combing their hair, dressing, climbing stairs, or rising from the floor unassisted. Involved muscles may eventually show varying degrees of degeneration (atrophy) and, in severe cases, permanent bending or extension in various fixed postures (joint contractures). Although muscles of the upper arms or legs are typically most severely affected, any muscle may become involved. In severe cases, affected muscles may include those of the roof of the mouth and those involved in respiration, resulting in a nasal quality to the voice; breathing difficulties; hyperventilation; inadvertent breathing of foreign materials into the respiratory passages (bronchial aspiration); and potentially life-threatening complications. In addition, involvement of muscles of the gastrointestinal tract may cause difficulties swallowing; abdominal pain; passage of dark, tarry stools containing digested blood (melena); and infrequent bowel movements or difficulty passing stools (constipation). In severe cases, gastrointestinal bleeding (hemorrhage) or other associated abnormalities (e.g., intestinal perforations) may cause potentially life-threatening conditions.

Patients with childhood dermatomyositis also develop characteristic skin changes, such as a reddish-purple rash of the upper eyelids (heliotrope rash); an abnormal accumulation of fluid in body tissues surrounding the eyes and in other facial areas (periorbital and facial edema); a reddish rash across the skin of the nose and cheeks (butterfly rash); and reddish-purple, raised, scaling skin lesions (papules) on the surfaces of certain joints, particularly the knuckles (Gottron's sign), elbows, and knees. These scaling lesions develop a central area of tissue loss (atrophy) that lacks color (vitiligo) or has increased pigmentation (hyperpigmentation). Patients may also have a dusky reddish rash covering the upper arms and legs and the upper trunk.

Approximately 20 to 50 percent of affected children also develop abnormal calcium deposits (calcifications) within muscle, skin, and subcutaneous tissues. These deposits may contribute to localized areas of muscle loss or the freezing of joints in permanently bent positions. Some patients may also experience additional symptoms and findings, such as a low-grade fever, joint inflammation (arthritis), enlargement of the liver and spleen (hepatosplenomegaly), or other abnormalities. In most patients, childhood dermatomyositis gradually becomes inactive over several years.

The treatment of patients with childhood dermatomyositis requires early, aggressive measures to help prevent potentially life-threatening complications. Such measures include evaluation to detect possible involvement of the respiratory or gastrointestinal systems and provision of ongoing nursing care for those with such involvement. Such care may include mechanical suctioning of the throat by way of the nose (nasopharyngeal suction), the creation of a temporary opening in the throat to ease breathing difficulties (tracheostomy), or mechanical breathing support (e.g., endotracheal intubation or respirator). In addition, the treatment of patients typically includes the use of corticosteroids (e.g., prednisone) to help suppress the inflammatory process of the disease. Blood levels of certain muscle enzymes are regularly measured to help gauge the effectiveness of such therapy. Once such enzyme levels are reduced to normal ranges, the steroid dosage may gradually be decreased to as low as possible while still being effective, owing to the numerous problems associated with prolonged administration or high-dose steroids. After about two years, such treatment may be discontinued without the reemergence of symptoms. In patients who do not respond to steroid therapy, certain immunosuppressant drugs such as methotrexate, azathioprine, or cyclosporine or, in some patients, intravenous immunoglobulin therapy may be beneficial. In addition, treatment may include surgical removal of calcium deposits. Physical therapy (e.g., passive exercises, eventual progression to active exercises) is important in helping to rebuild muscle strength and prevent permanent, disabling contractures. Splints may be required to help ensure proper positioning of certain limbs. Proper skin hygiene is also important in patients with childhood dermatomyositis.

National Associations & Support Groups

1569 American Academy of Pediatrics
141 Northwest Point Boulevard
Elk Grove Village, IL 60007

847-434-4000
800-433-9016
Fax: 847-434-8000
www.aap.org

The American Academy of Pediatrics and its member pediatricians are committed to the attainment of optimal physical, mental and social health and well-being for all infants, children, adolescents, and young adults.

Fernando Stein, MD, FAAP, President
Karen Remley, MD, CEO/Executive VP

1570 American Autoimmune Related Diseases Association
22100 Gratiot Avenue
Eastpointe, MI 48021

586-776-3900
800-598-4668
Fax: 586-776-3903
aarda@aarda.org
www.aarda.org

Dedicated to the eradiction of autoimmune diseases and the alleviation of suffering and the socio-economic impact of autoimmunity through fostering and facilitating collaboration in the areas of education, public awareness, research and patient services in an effective, ethical and efficient manner.

Virginia T. Ladd, President/Executive Director
Patricia Barber, Assistant Director
Deb Patrick, Events Specialist

1571 American Osteopathic College of Dermatology
1501 E Illinois Street, PO Box 7525
Kirksville, MO 63501

660-665-2184
800-449-2623
Fax: 660-627-2623
ExecDirector@AOCD.org
www.aocd.org

Strives to improve the standards of the practice of dermatology, to stimulate the study and extend knowledge in the field of dermatology, and to promote a more general understanding of the nature and scope of services rendered by osteopathic dermatologists to other divisions of practice, hospitals, clinics and the public.

David Grice, President
Suzanne Rozenberg, President-Elect
Rick Lin, First Vice-President

1572 Arthritis Foundation
1330 W. Peachtree Street.,Suite 100
Atlanta, GA 30309

404-872-7100
800-568-4045
Fax: 404-872-0457
www.arthritis.org

The only nonprofit organization that supports the more than 100 types of arthritis and related conditions with advocacy, programs, services and research.

Daniel T McGowan, Chair
Rowland W. Chang, Vice Chairs
Patricia Novak Nelson, Vice Chairs

1573 Juvenile Dermatomyositis
Arthritis Foundation
PO Box 7669
Atlanta, GA 30357

404-872-7100
800-283-7800
Fax: 404-872-0457
info@jdfcure.com
www.atrhritis.org

1574 Myositis Association of America
1737 King Street, Suite 600
Alexandria, VA 22314

703-299-4850
800-821-7356
Fax: 703-535-6752
tma@myositis.org
www.myositis.org

The mission of The Myositis Association is to find a cure for inflammatory and other related myopathies, while serving those affected by these diseases.

Kanneboyina Nagaraju DVM, PhD, Chair
David Fiorentino M.D., PhD, Vice Chair
Alan Pestronk M.D., Research Chair

1575 Society for Pediatric Dermatology
8365 Keystone Crossing, Suite 107
Indianapolis, IN 46240

317-202-0224
Fax: 317-205-9481
info@pedsderm.net
www.pedsderm.net

National organization dedicated to promote, develop and advance education, research and care of skin disease in all pediatric age groups.

Karen Wiss, President
Andrea Zaenglen, President Elect
Kent Lindeman, Executive Director

Libraries & Resource Centers

California

1576 University of California, San Francisco Dermatology Drug Research
515 Spruce
San Francisco, CA 94143

415-476-2001
Fax: 415-476-6014
cc.ucsf.edu/people

Conducts clinical testing of new or existing pharmalogic agents used in the treatment of skin disorders.

John Koo, MD, Director

Delaware

1577 Delaware Division of Libraries for the Blind and Physically Handicapped
43 S Dupont Highway
Dover, DE 19901

302-736-4748
800-282-8676
Fax: 302-736-6787
TDD: 302-739-4748
bedpg@lib.de.us

Braille readers receive service from Philadelphia and Pennsylvania, summer reading program, braille writer and cassettes.

Beth Landon, Librarian

Illinois

1578 Dermatology Information Network (DERMINFONET)
American Academy of Dermatology
PO Box 4014
Schaumburg, IL 60168

847-330-0230
Fax: 847-330-0050

Consists of a collection of dermatologic databases that are available to members on a subscription and/or purchase basis. These databases are designed to run on a wide variety of personal computers.

1579 National Library of Dermatologic Teaching Slides
American Academy of Dermatology
930 E Woodfield Road
Schaumburg, IL 60173

847-240-1280
866-503-7546
Fax: 847-240-1859
www.aad.org

A collection of dermatologic teaching slides offering the most comprehensive series ever assembled. Each set offers a realistic presentation of classic clinical skin conditions encountered by the dermatologist.

Dirk M Elston, President
Lisa A Garner, Vice President
Suzanne M Olbricht, Secretary/Treasurer

ISBN: 7-032994-85-0
Bob Goldberg, Executive Director

New York

1580 Laboratory of Dermatology Research
Memorial Sloan-Kettering Cancer Center
1275 York Avenue
New York, NY 10065   212-639-2000
Fax: 212-639-3576
www.mskcc.org

Specific studies on the identification of skin disorders and dermatology.
Craig B Thompson, President/CEO

1581 Rockefeller University Laboratory for Investigative Dermatology
1230 York Avenue
New York, NY 10065   212-327-7490
Fax: 212-327-7459

Research into skin disorders and the whole specialty of dermatology in general.
Barry Coller, Head

Research Centers

1582 University of California, San Francisco Dermatology Drug Research
515 Spruce Street
San Francisco, CA 94115   41 -76 -701
Fax: 415-502-4126
www.dermatology.ucsf.edu/research/areasofresearch.as

Conducts clinical testing of new or existing pharmacologic agents used in the treatment of skin disorders.
Mounira Kenaani, MBA, Department Manager
Darrell Young, Associate Director of Development
Leslie Chau, Assistant to Chair

Conferences

1583 AOCD Annual Meeting
American Osteopathic College of Dermatology
1501 E Illinois Street, PO Box 7525
Kirksville, MO 63501   660-665-2184
800-449-2623
Fax: 660-627-2623
info@aocd.org
www.aocd.org

November

Marsha Wise, Executive Director

1584 Society for Pediatric Dermatology Annual Meeting
8365 Keystone Crossing, Suite 107
Indianapolis, IN 46240   317-202-0224
Fax: 317-205-9481
info@pedsderm.net
www.pedsderm.net

Kent Lindeman, Executive Director

1585 TMA Annual Patient Conference
Myositis Association
1737 King Street, Suite 600
Alexandria, VA 22314   800-821-7356
Fax: 703-535-6752
tma@myositis.org
www.myositis.org

To meet other myositis patients, hear from TMA's medical advisors about myositis research, and benefit from the support and practical ideas of others with your disease. The Conference regularly includes sessions on research, exercise, advocacy and coping skills, and disease-specific question and answer sessions as well as new and interesting sessions each year.

Web Sites

1586 American Autoimmune Related Diseases Association
22100 Gratiot Ave.
Eastpointe, MI 48021   586-776-3900
800-598-4668
Fax: 586-776-3903
www.aarda.org

Dedicated to the eradication of autoimmune diseases and the alleviation of suffering and the socio-economic impact of autoimmunity through fostering and facilitating collaboration in the areas of education, public awareness, research and patient services in an effective, ethical and efficient manner.
Virginia T. Ladd, President/ Executive Director
Patricia Barber, Asst. Director
Eula Hoover, Exec. Assistant/ Newsletter Editor

1587 American Osteopathic College of Dermatology
2902 North Baltimore Street~~
Kirksville, MI 63501   660-665-2184
800-449-2623
Fax: 660-627-2623
www.aocd.org

Improving the standards of the practice of dermatology, to stimulate the study and extend knowledge in the field of dermatology, and to promote a more general understanding of the nature and scope of services rendered by osteopathic dermatologists to other divisions of practice, hospitals, clinics and the public.
Rick Lin, President
Karthik Krishnamurthy, 1st Vice President
Daniel Ladd, 2nd Vice President

1588 Arthritis Foundation
1330 W. Peachtree Street, Suite 100
Atlanta, GA 30309   404-872-7100
www.arthritis.org

Supports more than 100 types of arthritis and related conditions with advocacy, programs, services and research.
Ann M. Palmer, President/ CEO
Meagan Fulmer, Chief Development Officer
Wayne Guthrie, SPHR, SVP, Staff Operations

1589 Myositis Association of America
1737 King Street, Suite 600
Alexandria, VA 22314   703-299-4850
800-821-7356
Fax: 703-535-6752
TMA@myositis.org
www.myositis.org

Mission is to find a cure for inflammatory and other related myopathies, while serving those affected by these diseases.
Augie DeAugustinis, Chair
Patrick Zenner, Vice Chairman
Bob Goldberg, Executive Director

1590 Society for Pediatric Dermatology
8365 Keystone Crossing, Suite 107
Indianapolis, IN 46240   317-202-0224
Fax: 317-205-9481
info@pedsderm.net
www.pedsderm.net

Objective is to promote, develop and advance education, research and care of skin disease in all pediatric age groups.
Karen Wiss, President
Kent Lindeman, Executive Director
Stephanie Garwood, Meeting Manager

Book Publishers

1591 Let's Talk About Going to the Hospital
Rosen Publishing Group's PowerKids Press
29 E 21st Street
New York, NY 10010

212-777-3017
800-237-9932
Fax: 888-436-4643
rosenpub@tribeca.ios.com
www.rosenpublishing.com

If a child has to check into the hospital, chances are he or she is already upset about being ill. Knowing how a hospital functions and what the procedures are, such as when family members can visit, will help in what is already a stressful situation. Grades K-5.

24 pages
ISBN: 0-823950-36-0

Magazines

1592 International Journal of Dermatology
International Society of Dermatology
2323 North State Street #30
Bunnell, FL 32110

386-437-4405
Fax: 386-437-4427
info@intsocdermatol.org
www.intsocderm.org

Focuses on information for dermatologists and the whole specialty of dermatology research and education.

10 times a year
Evangeline Handog, President
Nellie Konnikov, Secretary-General
Marcia˜ Ramos-e-Silva, Assistant Secretary-General

1593 JM Companion
The Myositis Association
1737 King Street, Suite 600
Alexandria, VA 22314

703-299-4850
800-821-7356
Fax: 703-535-6752
TMA@myositis.org
www.myositis.org

Focuses on special concerns and also has an 'Ask the doctor' column with answers from leading JM physicians, a special insert for children, and clinical trial listings for JM patients.

Quarterly
Augie DeAugustinis, Chair
Patrick Zenner, Vice Chairman
Bob Goldberg, Executive Director

1594 Journal of Dermatologic Surgery and Oncology
International Society for Dermatologic Surgery
350 Main Street
Malden, MA 2148

781-388-8598
800-835-6770
Fax: 847-330-1135
cs-journals@wiley.com
onlinelibrary.wiley.com

Focuses on medical updates and information on dermatology.
Monthly

Journals

1595 Pediatric Dermatology Journal
Society for Pediatric Dermatology
8365 Keystone Crossing, Suite 107
Indianapolis, IN 46240

317-202-0224
Fax: 317-205-9481
info@pedsderm.net
www.pedsderm.net

6 issues/yr
Kent Lindeman, Executive Director

Newsletters

1596 Awareness
NAPVI
PO Box 317
Watertown, MA 2471

617-972-7441
800-562-6265
Fax: 617-972-7444
www.spedex.com/napvi

Newsletter offering regional news, sports and activities, conferences, camps, legislative updates, book reviews, audio reviews, professional question and answer column and more for the visually impaired and their families.

Quarterly

1597 DVH Quarterly
University of Arkansas at Little Rock
2801 S University Avenue
Little Rock, AR 72204

Fax: 501-663-3536

Offers information on upcoming events, conferences and workshops on and for visual disabilities. Book reviews, information on the newest resources and technology, educational programs, want ads and more.

Quarterly

Bob Brasher, Editor

1598 Dermatology Focus
Dermatology Foundation
1560 Sherman Avenue,Suite 870
Evanston, IL 60201

847-328-2256
Fax: 847-328-0509
dfgen@dermatologyfoundation.org
dermatologyfoundation.org

Includes membership activities, research articles and lists recipients of foundation awards.

Quarterly

Bruce U. Wintroub, Chairman
Michael D. Tharp, President
Stuart R. Lessin, Vice President

1599 Dermatology World
American Academy of Dermatology
P.O. Box 4014
Schaumburg, IL 60168

847-240-1280
866-503-7546
Fax: 847-240-1859
www.aad.org

Offers Academy members information outside the clinical realm. It carries news of government actions, reports of socioeconomic issues, societal trends and other events which impinge on the practice of dermatology.

Monthly

Brett M. Coldiron, MD, President
Elise A. Olsen, MD, Vice President
Mark Lebwohl, MD, President-Elect

1600 Keep In Touch (KIT) Forum
The Myositis Association
1737 King Street, Suite 600
Alexandria, VA 22314

703-299-4850
800-821-7356
Fax: 703-535-6752
TMA@myositis.org
www.myositis.org

Allows KIT leaders to share information and raise awareness. Provide a forum for members to exchange information and ideas for day-to-day living.

Augie DeAugustinis, Chair
Patrick Zenner, Vice Chairman
Bob Goldberg, Executive Director

1601 Progress in Dermatology
Dermatology Foundation
1560 Sherman Avenue, Suite 870
Evanston, IL 60201

847-328-2256
Fax: 847-328-0509
dfgen@dermatologyfoundation.org
dermatologyfoundation.org

Bulletin offering information on research reports and clinical trials.

Quarterly

Bruce U. Wintroub, Chairman
Michael D. Tharp, President
Stuart R. Lessin, Vice President

1602 The OutLook
The Myositis Association
1737 King Street, Suite 600
Alexandria, VA 22314

703-299-4850
800-821-7356
Fax: 703-535-6752
TMA@myositis.org
www.myositis.org

Newsletter featuring articles for patients with polymyositis, dermatomyositis, inclusion-body myositis, and juvenile forms of myositis.

Quarterly

Augie DeAugustinis, Chair
Patrick Zenner, Vice Chairman
Bob Goldberg, Executive Director

Pamphlets

1603 Arthritis in Children
Arthritis Foundation
1330 W. Peachtree Street, Suite 100
Atlanta, GA 30309

404-872-7100
800-568-4045
www.arthritis.org

Includes definitions of nine types of juvenile arthritis and related conditions, diagnosis, treatment options, emotional coping, school issues, federal laws and financial assistance.

28 pages

Ann M. Palmer, President/ CEO
Meagan Fulmer, Chief Development Officer
Wayne Guthrie, SPHR, SVP, Staff Operations

1604 Juvenile Dermatomyositis
Arthritis Foundation
PO Box 7669
Atlanta, GA 30357

404-872-7100
Fax: 404-872-0457
info@jdfcure.com
www.jdfcure.com

Camps

1605 Camp Discovery
American Academy of Dermatology
930 E Woodfield Road
Schaumburg, IL 60173

847-240-1280
866-503-7546
Fax: 847-240-1859
jmueller@aad.org
www.campdiscovery.org

For children with chronic skin conditions; no fee and transportation is provided. Call for locations.

David M Pariser, MD, President
Janine Mueller, Program Coordinator

DESCRIPTION

1606 CHILDHOOD SCHIZOPHRENIA

Involves the following Biologic System(s):
Developmental/Behavioral/Psychiatric Disorders

Childhood schizophrenia is characterized by disturbances in behavior, thought, and emotional reactions. These changes initially become apparent between approximately seven years of age and the onset of adolescence. Affected children may become increasingly withdrawn, have flat or blunted emotions that do not appear to change in response to environmental or external stimuli, experience episodes of unexplained silliness (hebephrenic silliness), exhibit aggressive behaviors, and have distortions in thinking. For example, some children may regularly repeat the same responses to different questions; experience sudden blockages in thought; perceive sights, sounds, or other sensations in the absence of external stimuli (hallucinations); and hold false beliefs in spite of evidence to the contrary (psychotic delusions), such as delusions of persecution (paranoid delusions). Affected children often appear to be chaotic in their emotions, thought, and behavioral patterns.

The relationship of childhood schizophrenia and adult schizophrenia remains unclear. Because schizophrenia typically becomes apparent during late adolescence or early adulthood and affects approximately one percent of the general population, only a small percentage of children exhibit symptoms that meet the criteria for a diagnosis of schizophrenia. In addition, many children who are diagnosed with schizophrenia before puberty are later diagnosed with mood disorders, such as bipolar disorder, or other conditions, such as mental retardation or a metabolic disorder. Although there is no clear relationship between childhood and adult schizophrenia, childhood symptoms that most likely predict adult psychotic disorders appear to include social withdrawal, disturbed interpersonal relationships, and blunted emotions. Though the specific underlying abnormalities that may contribute to childhood schizoid behaviors are unknown, genetic factors and certain biochemical abnormalities of the brain play some role in their development.

The treatment of children with schizoid behaviors may include therapy with certain medications known as neuroleptics to manage psychotic delusions, hallucinations, and severe agitation. In addition, an integrated, multidisciplinary approach may include individual therapy or parental training to help modify the child's behavior. In severe cases, hospitalization may be required to ensure appropriate medication adjustments, to prevent children from harming themselves, or to prevent them from hurting others if they exhibit aggressive or violent behavior.

Although certain medications can help treat children with schizoid behaviors, these drugs should be prescribed with great caution due to the potential for side effects. For example, such therapy may result in tardive dyskinesia (TD), a usually nonreversible condition characterized by tics or spasms of facial muscles and involuntary, rapid or writhing movements of the limbs (choreoathetoid movements). In other cases, therapy may cause abnormally slow movement (bradykinesis); involuntary hand movements; abnormal twisting of the neck (torticollis); drooling; and other findings.

If TD develops, treatment with other medications may be indicated and the neuroleptic medication may be decreased or discontinued.

Government Agencies

1607 Center for Mental Health Services Knowledge Exchange Network
US Department of Health and Human Services
PO Box 42557
Washington, DC 20015

800-662-4357
800-789-2647
Fax: 240-747-5470
TTY: 800-487-4889
TDD: 866-889-2647
samhsa.media@ees.hhs.gov
www.store.samhsa.gov/home

Develops national mental health policies that promote Federal/State coordination and benefit from input from consumers, family members and providers. Ensures that high quality mental health services programs are implemented to benefit seriously mentally ill populations, disasters or those involved in the criminal justice system.

Mirtha R. Beadle M.P.A., Deputy for Operations
Kana . Enomoto, M.A, Principal Deputy Administrator
Pamela S. Hyde, J.D., Administrator

1608 NIH/National Institute of Mental Health
6001 Executive Boulevard, Room 6200, MSC 9663
Bethesda, MD 20892

301-443-4536
866-615-6464
Fax: 301-443-4279
TTY: 301-443-8431
nimhinfo@nih.gov
www.nimh.nih.gov

The mission of NIMH is to transform the understanding and treatment of mental illnesses through basic and clinical research, paving the way for prevention, recovery, and cure.

Joshua Gordon, MD, PhD, Director
Shelli Avenevoli, MD, Deputy Director

National Associations & Support Groups

1609 American Academy of Pediatrics
141 Northwest Point Boulevard
Elk Grove Village, IL 60007

847-434-4000
800-433-9016
Fax: 847-434-8000
www.aap.org

The American Academy of Pediatrics and its member pediatricians are committed to the attainment of optimal physical, mental and social health and well-being for all infants, children, adolescents, and young adults.

Fernando Stein, MD, FAAP, President
Karen Remley, MD, CEO/Executive VP

1610 American Mental Health Foundation (AMHF)
PO Box 3
Riverdale, NY 10471

212-737-9027
elomke@americanmentalhealthfoundation.or
americanmentalhealthfoundation.org

Dedicated to the extensive and intensive research in the theories and techniques of treatment of emotional illness and to the implementation of reforms in the mental health system. Efforts have resulted in development of better and less expensive treatment methods. Findings are disseminated in English and other major languages.

Sister Joan Curtin. CND, Director
Evander Lomke, President & Executive Director
Eugene Gollogly, Vice President

1611 Federation of Families for Children's Mental Health
9605 Medical Center Drive, Suite 280
Rockville, MD 20850
240-403-1901
Fax: 240-403-1909
ffcmh@ffcmh.org
www.ffcmh.org

The National family run organization is dedicated exclusively to helping children with mental health needs and their families achieve a better quality of life.

Teka Dempson, President
Sherri Luthe, Vice President
Sheila Pires, Treasurer

1612 Mental Health America
500 Montgomery Street, Ste 820
Alexandria, VA 22314
703-684-7722
800-969-6642
Fax: 703-684-5968
TTY: 800-433-5959
info@mentalhealthamerica.net
www.mentalhealthamerica.net

MHA, the leading advocacy organization addressing the full spectrum of mental and substance use conditions and their effects nationwide, works to inform, advocate and enable access to quality behavioral health services for all Americans.

Paul Gionfriddo, President/CEO
Shavonne Carpenter, Sr Assoc., Support & Services
Mallory Pernell, Assoc. Dir, Comments/Marketing

1613 NADD: National Association for the Dually Diagnosed
132 Fair Street
Kingston, NY 12401
845-331-4336
800-331-5362
Fax: 845-331-4569
info@thenadd.org
www.thenadd.org

Nonprofit organization designed to promote the interests of professional and care providers for individuals who have the coexistence of mental illness and mental retardation. NADD provides conferences, educational services and training materials to professionals, parents, concerned citizens and service organizations.

Dr Robert Fletcher, CEO
Michelle Jordan, Office Manager
Edward Seliger, Project Coordinator

1614 National Alliance for Research on Schizophrenia and Depression
60 Cutter Mill Road, Suite 404
Great Neck, NY 11021
516-829-0091
800-829-8289
Fax: 516-487-6930
info@bbrfoundation.org.
www.bbrfoundation.org

Largest private 501 (c) (3) not for profit corporation and registered public charity. Raises and distributes funds for scientific research into the causes, cures, treatments and prevention of brain disorders.

Steve Lieber, Chairman of the Board
Suzanne Golden, Vice President
Anne Abramson, Director

1615 National Alliance for the Mentally Ill
3803 N. Fairfax Dr., Suite 100
Arlington, VA 22203
703-525-7600
800-950-6264
Fax: 703-524-9094
TDD: 703-516-7227
info@nami.org
www.nami.org

NAMI is a nonprofit, grassroots, self-help, support and advocacy organization of consumers, families and friends of people with severe mental illness, such as schizophrenia, bipolar disorder, major depressive disorder, obsessive compulsive disorder, anxiety disorders, autism and other severe and persistent mental illnesses that affect the brain.

Keris J,,n Myrick, President
Kevin B Sullivan, First Vice President
Jim Payne, Second Vice President

1616 National Mental Health Consumers' Self-Help Clearinghouse
1211 Chestnut Street, Suite 1207
Philadelphia, PA 19107
215-751-1810
800-553-4539
Fax: 215-636-6312
info@mhselfhelp.org
www.mhselfhelp.org

The Clearinghouse works to foster peer empowerment through our website, up-to-date news and information announcements, a directory of peer-driven services, electronic and printed publications, training packages, and individual and onsite consultation

Joseph Rogers, Executive Director & Founder
Susan Rogers, Director of Special Projects
Britani Nestel, Program Specialist

1617 North American Society for Childhood Onset Schizophrenia - NACOS
88 Briarwood Drive East
Berkeley Heights, NJ 07922
info@nascos.org
www.nascos.org

Non-profit, internet based group formed to provide a Web site devoted solely to childhood onset schizophrenia (COS). Families, caregivers and medical professionals will be able to locate and contact each other in order to access and share information related to this rare, devastating disease.

Karen Sniezek, Director
Meredith Morgan, Director
Edward Orton, Director

1618 Schizophrenics Anonymous Forum
Mental Health Association in Michigan
30233 Southfield Road, Suite 220
Southfield, MI 48076
248-647-1711
Fax: 248-647-1732
schizanon@aol.com
schizophrenia.org

Self-help organization sponsored by American Schizophrenia Association. Groups are comprised of dignosed schizophrenics who meet to share experiences, strengths and hopes in an effort to help each other cope with common problems and recover from the disease. Rehabilitation program follows the 12 principles of Alcoholics Anonymous. Publications: Newsletter, semi-annual. Monthly support group meeting.

State Agencies & Support Groups

1619 Center for Family Support
333 7th Avenue, #901
New York, NY 10001
212-629-7939
Fax: 212-239-2211
svernikoff@cfsny.org
www.cfsny.org

The Center for Family Support is committed to providing support and assistance to individuals with developmental and related disabilities, and to the family members who care for them.

Steven Vernikoff, Executive Director
Linda Schellenberg, Director, Community Service
Barbara Greenwald, Associate Executive Director

Libraries & Resource Centers

1620 National Alliance for Research on Schizophrenia and Depression
50 West Hawthorne Avenue
Valley Stream, NY 11580
516-569-6600
800-829-8289
Fax: 516-374-2261
info@narsad.org
www.pccli.org

Largest private 501 (c) (3) not for profit corporation and registered public charity. Raises and distributes funds for scientific research into the causes, cures, treatments and prevention of brain disorders.

David Schimel, President

Research Centers

1621 National Alliance for Research on Schizophrenia and Depression
60 Cutter Mill Road, Suite 404
Great Neck, NY 11021
516-829-0091
800-829-8289
Fax: 516-487-6930
info@bbrfoundation.org
www.bbrfoundation.org

Largest private 501 (c) (3) not for profit corporation and registered public charity. Raises and distributes funds for scientific research into the causes, cures, treatments and prevention of brain disorders.

Steve Lieber, Chairman of the Board
Suzanne Golden, Vice President
Anne Abramson, Director

1622 Suncoast Residential Training Center/Developmental Services Program
Goodwill Industries-Suncoast
10596 Gandy Boulevard
Saint Petersburg, FL 33702
727-523-1512
888-279-1988
Fax: 727-563-9300
TTY: 727-579-1068
www.goodwill-suncoast.org

A large group home which serves individuals diagnosed as mentally retarded with a secondary diagnosis of psychiatric difficulties as evidenced by problem behavior. Providing residential, behavioral and instructional support and services that will promote the development of adaptive, socially appropriate behavior. Each individual is assessed to determine, socialization, basic academics and recreation. The primary intervention strategy is applied behavior analysis.

Oscar J. Horton, Chair
Martin W. Gladysz, Sr. Vice Chair
Steven M Erickson, Vice Chair

Conferences

1623 FFCMH Annual Conference
Federation of Families for Childrens Mental Health
9605 Medical Center Drive, Suite 280
Rockville, MD 20850
240-403-1901
Fax: 240-403-1909
ffcmh@ffcmh.org
www.ffcmh.org

Address the complex issue of trauma; the impact it has on children and families; the promotion of healing and prevention strategies; knowledge about how to address trauma through resiliency-based interventions, utilizing a familydriven, youth guided approach; and examples of how family organizations and the partners they work with are raising awareness and improving trauma-focused services and supports.

November

Teka Dempson, President
Sherri Luthe, Vice President
Sheila Pires, Treasurer

1624 NAMI Convention
National Alliance on Mental Illness
3803 N Fairfax Drive, Suite 100
Arlington, VA 22203
703-524-7600
888-999-6264
Fax: 703-524-9094
TDD: 703-516-7227
info@nami.org
www.nami.org

The NAMI Convention is packed with information, chances to network, leadership development opportunities, and lots more

July

Keris Jan Myrick, President
Kevin B Sullivan, Vice President
Clarence Jordan, Secretary

Audio Video

1625 Bonnie Tapes
Mental Illness Education Project
25 West Street
Westborough, MA 1581
617-562-1111
800-343-5540
Fax: 617-779-0061
info@miepvideos.org
www.miepvideos.org

Bonnie's account of coping with schizophrenia will be a relevation to people whose view of mental illness has been shaped by the popular media. She and her family provide an intimate view of the frequently feared, often misrepresented and much stigmatized illness and the human side of learning to live with a psychiatric disability. Tape 1: Mental Illness in the Family (26 minutes); Tape 2: Recovering from Mental Illness (27 minutes); Tape 3: My Sister Is Mentally Ill (22 minutes) $99.95 each
1997 $143.88 for 3

1626 Families Coping with Mental Illness
Mental Illness Education Project
25 West Street
Westborough, MA 1581
617-562-1111
800-343-5540
Fax: 617-779-0061
info@miepvideos.org
miepvideos.org

10 family members share their experiences of having a family member with schizophrenia or bipolar disorder. Designed to provide insights and support to other families, the tape also profoundly conveys to professionals the needs of families when mental illness strikes. In two versions: a twenty two minute version ideal for short classes and workshops, and a richer forty three minute version with more examples and details. Discounted price for families/consumers.

Michael M Faenza, Executive Director

1627 Living with Schizophrenia
Guilford Press
370 Seventh Avenue, Suite 1200
New York, NY 10001
800-365-7006
Fax: 212-966-6708
info@guilford.com
www.guilford.com

Offers essential information and huidance for individuals and families coping with schizophrenia diagnosis. Features illuminating first-hand accounts from three people with schizophrenia and one person with schizoaffective disorder, along with commentary from treatment expert Dr Andy Campbell. Learn clear steps to take to lead fuller, more successful lives.
2006 DVD, 39 minutes
ISBN: 1-593853-86-6

1628 Pharmacotherapy of Schizophrenia
American Psychiatric Publishing
1000 Wilson Boulevard, Suite 1825
Arlington, VA 22209
703-907-7322
800-368-5777
Fax: 703-907-1091
appi@psych.org
www.appi.org

Presented by John M Kane MD, Chairman of Psychiatry at LI Jewish Medical Center, and Professor of Psychiatry at Albert Einstein College of Medicine. Illustrates the major issues and treatment considerations, and the latest findings on the effectiveness as well as on the side effects of the many and varied psychopharmacological agents are carefully illustrated and discussed. 75 minutes. ISBN # 9780880483803
1995

Robert E. Hales, Editor-in-Chief
Rebecca D. Rinehart, Publisher
John McDuffie, Associate Publisher

Web Sites

1629 CyberPsych
www.cyberpsych.org

CyberPsych presents information about psychoanalysis, psychotherapy, and special topics such as anxiety disorder, the problematic use of alcohol, homophobia, and the traumatic effects of racism. CyberPsych is a nonprofit network which offers free web hosting and technical support for internet communication to nonprofit groups and individuals.

Carol Lindemann, Ph.D., Contact

1630 Internet Mental Health
www.mentalhealth.com

Our goal is to improve understanding, diagnosis, and treatment of mental illness throughout the world.

Phillip W. Long, M.D., Psychiatrist

1631 Mental Health Net
P.O. Box 20709
Columbus, OH 43220
614-448-4055
info@centersite.net
www.mentalhelp.net

We wish to provide the following: to discuss, develope and debate in an open forum the future of the mental health field in America and throughout the world. To help coordinate various components of the mental health field so as to bring about greater communication between them. To educate the public about mental health issues, to promote active collaboration between professionals in all segments of mental health development, implementation and policy.

1632 Mental Wellness
www.choicesinrecovery.com
800-526-7736
www.choicesinrecovery.com

Mental Wellness is an online resource for bipolar disorder, schizophrenia and general mental health information.

1633 NADD: National Association for the Dually Diagnosed
www.thenadd.org

Nonprofit organization designed to promote the interests of professional and care providers for individuals who have the coexistence of mental illness and mental retardation. NADD provides conferences, educational services and training materials to professionals, parents, concerned citizens and service organizations.

Dr Robert Fletcher, CEO
Michelle Jordan, Office Manager
Edward Seliger, Project Coordinator

1634 Online Mendelian Inheritance in Man
National Library of Medicine, Building 38A
Bethesda, MD 20894
888-346-3656
info@ncbi.nlm.nih.gov
www.ncbi.nlm.nih.gov

This database is a catalog of human genes and genetic disorders.

Christine E. Seidman, M.D., Chair
David J. Lipman, M.D., Executive Secretary

1635 Planetpsych
www.planetpsych.com
webmaster@planetpsych.com
www.planetpsych.com

Planetpsych is an online resource for mental health information.

1636 Psych Central
55 Pleasant St., Suite 207
Newburyport, MA 1950
talkback@psychcentral.com
www.psychcentral.com

Offers free sinformational and educational articles sand resources on psychology, support and mental health online.

John M. Grohol, CEO & Founder

1637 Schizophrenia Support Organizations
www.members.aol.com/leonardjk/USA.htm

Contains a listing of support organizations for people with schizophrenia and their families.

1638 Schizophrenia.com
www.schizophrenia.com

Is a leading web commuity dedicated to providing high quality information, support and education to the family members, caregivers and individuals who's lives have been impacted by schizophrenia.

Brain Chiko, Executive Director
J. Megginson Hollister, Editor

1639 Schizophrenia.com Home Page
www.schizophrenia.com/discuss/Disc3.html

On-line support for patients and families.

Brain Chiko, Executive Director
J. Megginson Hollister, Editor

1640 Schizophrenia: Handbook for Families
www.mentalhealth.com/book/p40-sc01.html

This handbook is dedicated to the families and to their loved ones who carry the burden of schizophrenia, a major psychiatric disorder.

Phillip W. Long, M.D., Psychiatrist

Book Publishers

1641 Biology of Schizophrenia and Affective Disease
American Psychiatric Publishing
1000 Wilson Boulevard, Suite 1825
Arlington, VA 22209
703-907-7322
800-368-5777
Fax: 703-907-1091
appi@psych.org
www.appi.org

Provides a state-of-the-art look at the biological bases of severe mental illness from the perspective of the researchers making these exceptional discoveries. ISBN # 9780880487467

1995 560 pages

Stanley J Watson PhD MD, Author

1642 Contemporary Issues in the Treatment of Schizophrenia
American Psychiatric Press
1000 Wilson Boulevard, Suite 1825
Arlington, VA 22209
703-907-7322
800-368-5777
Fax: 703-907-1091
appi@psych.org
www.appi.org

Covers approaches to the patient by investigating biological, pharmacological, and psychological treatments. ISBN #: 9780880486811

1995 889 pages

Christian L Shriqui, MD, Editor
Henry A Nasrallah, MD, Editor

1643 Diagnosis Schizophrenia: A Comprehensive Resource
Columbia University Press
116th and Broadway
New York, NY 10027
212-854-1754
Fax: 212-459-3678
www.columbia.edu/cu/cup

Has alot of consumers' stories in the first person and sketches of their faces sprinkled throughout.

2002

Rachel Miller, Author
Susan E Mason, Author

1644 Encyclopedia of Schizophrenia and the Psychotic Disorders
Facts on File
11 Penn Plaza
New York, NY 10001   212-290-8090
                          800-322-8755
                      Fax: 212-678-3633

This volume details recent theories and research findings on schizophrenia and psychotic disorders, together with a complete overview of the field's history.

368 pages

1645 Getting Your Life Back Together When You Have Schizophrenia
New Harbinger Publications
5674 Shattuck Ave
Oakland, CA 94609   800-748-6273
                      Fax: 800-652-1613
              customerservice@newharbinger.com
                    www.newharbinger.com

Provides good information for someone who has just been diagnosed with schiophrenia.

2002
Roberta Temes PhD, Author

1646 Medical Illness and Schizophrenia
American Psychiatric Publishing
1000 Wilson Boulevard, Suite 1825
Arlington, VA 22209   703-907-7322
                          800-368-5777
                      Fax: 703-907-1091
                        appi@psych.org
                          www.appi.org

Examines the links between medical conditions and severe chronic mental illness, with a focus on the need for better medical assessment and treatment to improve outcomes in patients; links between schizophrenia and conditions such as obesity, cardiovascular disease, diabetes, HIV and hepatitis C, endocrine-related diorders, and others; the association between therapy with certain antipsychotics and adverse health outcomes; the importance of improving community health. ISBN # 9781585621064

2003 256 pages
Jonathan M Meyer MD, Author
Henry A Nasrallah MD, Author

1647 Negative Symptom and Cognitive Deficit Tre atment Response in Schizophrenia
American Psychiatric Publishing
1000 Wilson Boulevard, Suite 1825
Arlington, VA 22209   703-907-7322
                          800-368-5777
                      Fax: 703-907-1091
                        appi@psych.org
                          www.appi.org

Addresses the complex issues-issues rarely confronted in empirical studies of patients with schizophrenia-and controversial research surrounding the assessment of negative symptoms and cognitive deficits in patients with schizophrenia. ISBN # 9780880487856

2001 216 pages
Richard S E Keefe PhD, Author
Joseph P McEvoy MD, Author

1648 New Pharmacotherapy of Schizophrenia
American Psychiatric Press
1000 Wilson Boulevard, Suite 1825
Arlington, VA 22209   703-907-7322
                          800-368-5777
                      Fax: 703-907-1091
                        appi@psych.org
                          www.appi.org

Discusses the new class of antipsychotic agents that promises superior efficiency and more favorable side-effects; offers an improved understanding of how to employ exsisting pharmachotherapeutic agents. ISBN # 9780880484916

1996 264 pages

1649 Plasma Homovanillic Asid in Schhizophrenia
American Psychiatric Publishing
1000 Wilson Boulevard, Suite 1825
Arlington, VA 22209   703-907-7322
                          800-368-5777
                      Fax: 703-907-1091
                        appi@psych.org
                          www.appi.org

Provides the most comprehensive and current collection of information on plasma HVA levels to be found anywhere. Provides a consice synthesis and critique of current data as well as interesting proposals for future research. ISBN # 9780880484893

1997 216 pages
Arnold J Friedhoff MD, Author
Farooq Amin MD, Author

1650 Prenatal Exposures in Schizophrenia
American Psychiatric Press
1000 Wilson Boulevard, Suite 1825
Arlington, VA 22209   703-907-7322
                          800-368-5777
                      Fax: 703-907-1091
                        appi@psych.org
                          www.appi.org

Considers a range of epigenetic elements thought to interact with abnormal genes to produce the onset of illness. Attention to the evidence implicating obstetric complications, prenatal infection, autoimmunity and prenatal malnutrition in brain disorders. ISBN # 9780880484992

1999 296 pages Hardcover
Ezra S Susser MD, Author
Alan S Brown MD, Author
Jack M Gorman MD, Author

1651 Schizophrenia
American Psychiatric Publishing
1000 Wilson Boulevard, Suite 1825
Arlington, VA 22209   703-907-7322
                          800-368-5777
                      Fax: 703-907-1091
                        appi@psych.org
                          www.appi.org

Ideas in treating the disease, and how many patients can lead productive lives without relapse. ISBN # 9780880489508

1994 294 pages
Nancy C Andleasen MD, Author

1652 Schizophrenia Into Later Life: Treatment, Research, and Policy
American Psychiatric Publishing
1000 Wilson Boulevard, Suite 1825
Arlington, VA 22209   703-907-7322
                          800-368-5777
                      Fax: 703-907-1091
                        appi@psych.org
                          www.appi.org

Multidisciplinary reference on this important topic-a landmark work for researchers, service providers, and policy makers. ISBN # 9781585620371

2003 344 pages
Carl I Cohen MD, Author

1653 Schizophrenia Revealed: From Neurons to Social Interactions
W.W. Norton
500 Fifth Avenue
New York, NY 10110   212-354-5500
                          800-233-4830
                      Fax: 212-869-0856
                        www.wwnorton.com

Educational, informational, scientific and yet readable.

2003

1654 Schizophrenia and Comorbid Conditions Diagnosis and Treatment
American Psychiatric Publishing
1000 Wilson Boulevard, Suite 1825
Arlington, VA 22209

703-907-7322
800-368-5777
Fax: 703-907-1091
appi@psych.org
www.appi.org

Lays diagnostic oversimplification of schizophrenia to rest once and for all. Editors are criticizing the reductionist view of schizophrenia as a single unitary disorder- a view that has led many psychiatrists and mental health care professionals to overlook potentially important syndromes. ISBN # 9780880487719

2001 256 pages

1655 Scizophrenia in a Molecular Age
American Psychiatric Publishing
1000 Wilson Boulevard, Suite 1825
Arlington, VA 22209

703-907-7322
800-368-5777
Fax: 703-907-1091
appi@psych.org
www.appi.org

Reviews neuroscience mechanisms and analyzes genetic determinants. ISBN # 9780880489614

1999 204 pages

Carol A Tamminga MD, Author

1656 Surviving Schizophrenia: A Manual for Families, Consumers and Providers
Harper Collins
10 E 53rd Street
New York, NY 10022

212-207-7528
800-242-7737
Fax: 212-207-2586
orders@harpercollins.com
harpercollins.com

The third edition of this indispensable manual throughly details everything patients, families and mental health professionals need to know about one of the most widespread and misunderstood illnesses. Paperback.

464 pages
ISBN: 0-060950-76-5

1657 The American Psychiatric Publishing Text book of Schizophrenia
American Psychiatric Publishing
1000 Wilson Boulevard, Suite 1825
Arlington, VA 22209

703-907-7322
800-368-5777
Fax: 703-907-1091
appi@psych.org
www.appi.org

Offers broad coverage that encompasses the current state of knowledge the cause, nature, and treatment of schizophrenia. ISBN # 9781585621910

2006 453 pages

Jeffrey A Lieberman MD, Author
T Scott Stroup MD MPH, Author
Diana O Perkins MD MPH, Author

1658 The Complete Family Guide to Schizophrenia
Kim Mueser, Susan Gingerich, author

Guilford Press
72 Spring Street
New York, NY 10012

800-365-7006
Fax: 212-966-6708
info@guilford.com
www.guilford.com

The authors, noted therapists, deepen the reader's understanding of the illness and discuss a wide range of effective treatments. This volume walks the reader through a range of treatment and support options that can lead to a better life for the entire family.Topics include prioritizing needs, solving everyday problems, life-goals, symptoms, and the life-long journey of recovery. Hardcover, paperback, e-book.

2006 480 pages Paperback
ISBN: 1-593851-80-4

Kim T Mueser, Author
Susan Gingerich, Author

1659 The Early Stages of Schizophrenia
American Psychiatric Publishing
1000 Wilson Boulevard, Suite 1825
Arlington, VA 22209

703-907-7322
800-368-5777
Fax: 703-907-1091
appi@psych.org
www.appi.org

Divided into three major parts: Early Intervention, Epidemiology, and Natural History of Schizophrenia; Management of the Early Stages of Schizophrenia; and Neurobiological Investigations of the Early Stages of Schizophrenia. ISBN # 9780880488402

2002 280 pages

Robert B Zipursky MD, Author
S Charles Schulz MD, Author

1660 The Natural History of Mania, Depression, and Schizophrenia
American Psychiatric Publishing
1000 Wilson Boulevard, Suite 1825
Arlington, VA 22209

703-907-7322
800-368-5777
Fax: 703-907-1091
appi@psych.org
www.appi.org

Takes an unusual look at the course of mental illness, based on data from the Iowa 500 Research Project. This project involved the long-term (30-40 yrs) follow-up of patients diagnosed with schizophrenia, depression, and bipolar illness. ISBN # 9780880487269

1996 384 pages

George Winokur MD, Author
Ming T Tsuang MD PhD, Author

1661 Water Balance in Schizophrenia
American Psychiatric Publishing
1000 Wilson Boulevard, Suite 1825
Arlington, VA 22209

703-907-7322
800-368-5777
Fax: 703-907-1091
appi@psych.org
www.appi.org

Represents the first attempt to provide clinicians with a consolidated guide to polydipsia-hyponatremia, associated with schizophrenia. ISBN # 9780880484855

1996 360 pages

David B Schnur MD, Author
Darrell G Kirch MD, Author

Newsletters

1662 NADD Bulletin
NADD Press
132 Fair Street
Kingston, NY 12401

845-331-4336
800-331-5362
Fax: 845-331-4569
info@thenadd.org
www.thenadd.org

Official publication of the National Association for the Dually Diagnosed. It features articles that address clinical, programmatic, research or family oriented issues concerning mental health aspects in persons with disabilities.

20 pages Bimonthly

Dr Robert Fletcher, CEO
Michelle Jordan, Office Manager
Edward Seliger, Project Coordinator

Pamphlets

1663 Schizophrenia
National Institute of Mental Health
PO Box 5801
Bethesda, MD 20824

301-496-5751
800-352-9424
Fax: 301-443-4279
TTY: 866-415-8051
nimhinfo@nih.gov
www.nimh.nih.gov

This booklet answers many common questions about schizophrenia, one of the most chronic, severe and disabling mental disorders. Current research-based information is provided for people with schizophrenia, their family members, friends and the general public about the symptoms and diagnosis of schizophrenia, possible causes, treatments and treatment resources.

2006 28 pages

Walter J. Koroshetz, M.D., Acting Director
Alan L. Willard, Ph.D., Acting Deputy Director
Caroline Lewis, Executive Officer

1664 Schizophrenia Fact Sheet
Center for Mental Health Services
PO Box 42557
Washington, DC 20015

800-789-2647
Fax: 240-747-5470
TDD: 866-889-2647
mentalhealth.samhsa.gov

This fact sheet provides information on the symptoms, diagnosis, and treatment for schizophrenia.

2 pages

Phillip W. Long, M.D., Psychiatrist

1665 Understanding Schizophrenia
National Alliance on Mental Illness
3803 N. Fairfax Drive, Suite 100
Arlington, VA 22203

703-524-7600
800-950-6264
Fax: 703-524-9094
TDD: 703-516-7227
www.nami.org

An excellent introduction to schizophrenia. Appropriate for supprt groups, physicians offices, coventions, health fairs, and the workplace.

Jim Payne, President
Ralph E. Nelson, 1st Vice President
Marilyn Ricci, 2nd Vice President

DESCRIPTION

1666 CHOREA

Covers these related disorders: Benign familial chorea, Drug-induced chorea, Sydenham's chorea

Involves the following Biologic System(s):

Neurologic Disorders

Chorea is a neuromuscular condition characterized by irregular, rapid, jerky movements that may appear to be well coordinated but actually occur involuntarily. These movements may be simple or highly complex. In addition, the arms and legs may have abnormally diminished muscle tone (hypotonia) and therefore may be abnormally loose or slack. Choreic movements are often subtle. However, if several of these movements are present, they may essentially flow into one another, causing them to appear relatively slow, sinuous, and writhing in nature (athetosis).

The specific underlying cause of chorea is unknown. However, some researchers suspect that it may result due to overactivity of certain neurotransmitters (dopamine) in the brain. Neurotransmitters are naturally produced chemicals that regulate the transmission of messages between certain nerve cells (neurons). In some children, chorea may result from the use of particular drugs, such as certain antiseizure medications, particularly phenytoin, or antipsychotic (neuroleptic) drugs, such as haloperidol or phenothiazines. Chorea may also occur in association with certain underlying disorders, such as systemic lupus erythematosus (lupus) or Wilson's disease, a disorder of copper metabolism. In addition, chorea is a primary feature of a rare genetic disorder known as benign familial chorea in which nonprogressive chorea begins in infancy or early childhood in the absence of other neurologic abnormalities. Associated symptoms and findings include delays in attaining certain motor milestones during childhood and poorly coordinated movements of the arms and legs. Benign familial chorea is likely inherited as an autosomal dominant trait.

In addition, chorea is the dominant feature of a disorder known as Sydenham's chorea. This disorder is the most common cause of acquired chorea during childhood. Sydenham's chorea occurs in association with rheumatic fever, which is an inflammatory disease following throat infection with certain strains of streptococcal bacteria. Patients with rheumatic fever may experience fever, inflammation and swelling of one or more large joints, or inflammation of the heart (carditis), potentially causing thickening, scarring, and associated disease of heart valves. If rheumatic fever affects the nervous system, Sydenham's chorea may result. Although Sydenham's chorea previously occurred in as many as half of those with rheumatic fever, recent studies suggest that it more likely affects approximately 10 percent of rheumatic patients in the United States.

Sydenham's chorea most commonly occurs in children between ages five and 15. The condition may begin subtly and gradually, sometimes as long as several months after other symptoms associated with rheumatic fever have resolved. Patients may initially experience increasing clumsiness. As symptoms progress, involuntary movements may become prominent in the face, trunk, and arms and legs; move from one muscle group to another; and eventually affect all motor movements, including walking and speech. In some patients,

chorea may be restricted to one side of the body (hemichorea). If children have severe chorea and abnormally diminished muscle tone (hypotonia), they may become unable to dress, feed themselves, or walk. Many children with the condition also experience rapid mood swings and episodes of uncontrollable crying (emotional lability).

Sydenham's chorea is usually a self-limited disorder that subsides in weeks or months. However, in some patients, the condition may persist for up to one to two years. In approximately 20 percent of children, the condition may recur within two years of the initial episode. If patients experience mild symptoms, treatment may include symptomatic and supportive measures, including minimizing stress as much as possible. In children with more severe symptoms, treatment may be attempted with the drug diazepam.

Government Agencies

1667 NIH/National Institute of Neurological Disorders and Stroke (NINDS)

PO Box 5801
Bethesda, MD 20824

301-496-5751
800-352-9424
Fax: 301-496-0296
TTY: 301-468-5981
www.ninds.nih.gov

The mission of NINDS is to reduce the burden of neurological disease - a burden borne by every age group, by every segment of society, by people all over the world.

Walter J. Koroshetz, MD, Director

National Associations & Support Groups

1668 American Academy of Child and Adolescent Psychiatry

3615 Wisconsin Avenue NW
Washington, DC 20016

202-966-7300
Fax: 202-966-2891
communications@aacap.org
www.aacap.org

The AACAP (American Academy of Child and Adolescent Psychiatry) is the leading national professional medical association dedicated to treating and improving the quality of life for children, adolescents, and families affected by these disorders.

Martin J. Drell M.D, President
Paramjit T Joshi, M.D, President-Elect
Steven P Cuffe, M.D., Treasurer

1669 American Academy of Pediatrics

141 Northwest Point Boulevard
Elk Grove Village, IL 60007

847-434-4000
800-433-9016
Fax: 847-434-8000
www.aap.org

The American Academy of Pediatrics and its member pediatricians are committed to the attainment of optimal physical, mental and social health and well-being for all infants, children, adolescents, and young adults.

Fernando Stein, MD, FAAP, President
Karen Remley, MD, CEO/Executive VP

1670 Genetic Alliance

4301 Connecticut Avenue NW, Suite 404
Washington, DC 20008

202-966-5557
800-336-4363
Fax: 202-966-8553
info@geneticalliance.org
www.geneticalliance.org

World's leading nonprofit health advocacy organization committed to transforming health through genetics and promoting an environment of openness centered on the health of individuals, families, and communities.

Sharon Terry, President/CEO
Tetyana Murza, Managing Director
Natasha Bonhomme, VP, Strategic Development

1671 March of Dimes Foundation
1275 Mamaroneck Avenue
White Plains, NY 10605

914-997-4488
888-663-4637
Fax: 914-997-4763
answers@marchofdimes.com
www.marchofdimes.com

March of Dimes help moms have full-term pregnancies and research the problems that threaten the health of babies.The March of Dimes also acts globally: sharing best practices in perinatal health and helping improve birth outcomes where the needs are the most urgent.

Stacey D. Stewart, President

1672 Muscular Dystrophy Association
3300 E Sunrise Drive
Tucson, AZ 85718

520-529-2000
800-572-1717
Fax: 520-529-5300
mda@mdausa.org
www.mda.org

Voluntary health agency aimed at conquering nueromuscular diseases that affect more than 1,000,000 Americans. The diseases in MDA's program include nine forms of muscular dystrophy, amyotrophic lateral sclerosis (Lou Gehrig's disease), spinal muscular atrophy, Charcot-Marie-Tooth disease, and other neuromuscular conditions. With over 200 offices across the country, MDA conducts research, medical and community services, clinics, support groups, summer camps for youngsters and much more.

Jennifer Lopez, Associate Director-Health Care Svcs

1673 WE MOVE (Worldwide Education and Advocacy for Movement Disorders)
5731 Mosholu Avenue
Bronx, NY 10471

212-875-8312
800-437-6682
Fax: 212-875-8389
wemove@wemove.org
www.wemove.org

Gives the general public the knowledge that they desire regarding any disorder involving movement difficulties.

Susan Bressman MD, President
Mo Moadeli, Vice President
Arlene Ploshnick, Treasurer

Conferences

1674 AACAP & CACAP Joint Annual Meeting
American Academy of Child & Adolescent Psychiatry
3615 Wisconsin Avenue NW
Washington, DC 20016

202-966-7300
Fax: 202-966-2891
meetings@aacap.org
www.aacap.org

The world's largest gathering place for leaders in the field of child and adolescent psychiatry, children's mental health, and other allied disciplines.

Laurence Lee Greenhill MD, President

Web Sites

1675 Online Mendelian Inheritance in Man
National Library of Medicine, Building 38A
Bethesda, MD 20894

888-346-3656
info@ncbi.nlm.nih.gov
www.ncbi.nlm.nih.gov

This database is a catalog of human genes and genetic disorders.

Christine E. Seidman, M.D., Chair
David J. Lipman, M.D., Executive Secretary

Book Publishers

1676 Diagnostic and Statistical Manual of Mental Disorders
American Psychiatric Association
1000 Wilson Boulevard, Suite 1825
Arlington, VA 22209

703-907-7300
888-357-7924
apa@psych.org
www.psych.org

Includes updated information on diagnoses, etiology, and research on mental illness.

1677 Merck Manual of Diagnosis and Therapy 18th Edition
Wiley Publishers
10475 Crosspoint Boulevard
Indianapolis, IN 46256

317-572-3000
877-762-2974
Fax: 800-597-3299
consumer@wiley.com
www.wiley.com

Packed with essential information on diagnosing and treating medical disorders to help health care professionals and medical students deliver the best care.

2006
ISBN: 0-911910-18-2

1678 Neuroanatomy: Text and Atlas 3rd Edition
McGraw-Hill Medical
860 Taylor Station Road
Blacklick, OH 43004

877-833-5524
Fax: 614-759-3823
pbg.ecommerce_custserv@mcgraw-hill.com
http://books.mcgraw-hill.com

Comprehensive appraoch to neuroanatomy from both functional and regional perspective! Examines how parts of the nervous system work together to regulate body systems and produce behavior.

2003 532 pages
ISBN: 0-071381-83-X

Pamphlets

1679 Sydenham Chorea Information Page
National Inst. of Neurological Disorders/Stroke
PO Box 5801
Bethesda, MD 20824

301-496-5751
800-352-9424
TTY: 301-468-5981
www.ninds.nih.gov/disorders/sydenham/sydenham.htm

Provides information on the disease, treatment options, and the prognosis, as well as provides some research centers regarding the disease.

Walter J. Koroshetz, M.D., Acting Director
Alan L. Willard, Ph.D., Acting Deputy Director
Caroline Lewis, Executive Officer

DESCRIPTION

1680 CLEFT LIP AND CLEFT PALATE
Involves the following Biologic System(s):
Dermatologic Disorders, Orthopedic and Muscle Disorders

Cleft lip and cleft palate are birth defects that may occur together or as isolated conditions. Newborns with cleft lip have a groove in the upper lip that may be a small notch or, in more severe cases, may be deep and extend up to the nose. Cleft palate is characterized by incomplete closure of the roof of the mouth (palate). In affected newborns, an abnormal gap runs along the midline of the soft, fleshy area of the palate (soft palate) and, in some patients, extends into one or both sides of the bony, front region of the palate (hard palate). As a result, the nasal cavity may open into the palate. Cleft lip with or without cleft palate affects approximately one in 600 newborns, whereas cleft palate alone occurs in about one in 1,000 births.

In newborns with cleft lip, the defect may occur on one or both sides of the upper lip and typically affects the bony ridge of the upper jaw (upper alveolar ridge). This ridge contains the sockets in which the roots of the teeth are held (dental alveoli). As a result, affected children often experience improper development of certain teeth, potentially resulting in absent, malformed, improperly positioned, or extra teeth and increased risk of dental decay (dental caries). In addition, infants with cleft lip and cleft palate typically have feeding difficulties associated with poor suckling capability and excessive swallowing of air. Affected children with cleft palate are also prone to repeated infections of the middle ear (otitis media) that, in some cases, may contribute to associated hearing loss. Many children also experience speech defects that may be due to inadequate functioning of certain muscles of the throat and palate (pharyngeal and palatal muscles).

In affected newborns, treatment initially consists of measures to ensure improved feeding and proper intake of nutrients. In many patients, a plastic device (a prosthetic known as an obturator) may be fitted that covers the gap in the palate, thereby improving suction and intake of fluids, milk, and or formula. The obturator is typically replaced every few weeks due to rapid growth during infancy. In addition, in those with cleft palate, modified artificial nipples may help to improve feeding. In many cases, cleft lip may be surgically closed by approximately two months of age and additional corrective surgery may be performed later during childhood. If affected children do not have associated physical abnormalities, surgical correction of cleft palate may be performed before the age of one year to help improve normal speech development. However, if surgery is delayed until the age of three years or later, a device (such as a contoured speech bulb) may be used to help close off the uppermost portion of the throat (nasopharynx) during the production of certain sounds. This helps children to develop understandable speech. Treatment may also include dental procedures to correct improperly positioned teeth or to replace absent teeth (e.g., with prosthetic devices). Speech therapy may be beneficial for some affected children. Additional treatment for infants and children with cleft lip and cleft palate is symptomatic and supportive.

Cleft lip and cleft palate may occur as isolated conditions or in association with several underlying chromosomal disorders or malformation syndromes. Isolated cleft lip and/or cleft palate may potentially result due to certain environmental factors, occur randomly for unknown reasons (sporadically), or be familial. Many cases have been reported in which several individuals in multigenerational families (kindreds) have been affected by isolated cleft lip and cleft palate. In such cases, the specific modes of inheritance are not understood. The frequent association of cleft lip and cleft palate is thought to result from certain developmental abnormalities during embryonic growth.

National Associations & Support Groups

1681 AmeriFace
PO Box 751112
Las Vegas, NV 89136

702-769-9264
888-486-1209
Fax: 702-341-5351
info@ameriface.org
www.ameriface.org

Provides information, services, emotional support and educational programs for and on behalf of individuals with facial differences and their families. Working to increase understanding through public awareness and education.

3M members

Debbie Oliver, Executive Director
Robin Remele, Program Driector
Joyce Bentz, National Action Team Coordinator

1682 American Academy of Pediatrics
141 Northwest Point Boulevard
Elk Grove Village, IL 60007

847-434-4000
800-433-9016
Fax: 847-434-8000
www.aap.org

The American Academy of Pediatrics and its member pediatricians are committed to the attainment of optimal physical, mental and social health and well-being for all infants, children, adolescents, and young adults.

Fernando Stein, MD, FAAP, President
Karen Remley, MD, CEO/Executive VP

1683 Cleft Palate Foundation
1504 East Franklin Street, Suite 102
Chapel Hill, NC 27514

919-933-9044
800-242-5338
Fax: 919-933-9604
info@cleftline.org
www.cleftline.org

Provides comprehensive information to educate patients, families, and professionals; Makes referrals to cleft/craniofacial treatment teams; Funds research to learn all we can about prevention and care; Offers telephone and online counseling and support service through the Cleftline, 1-800-24-CLEFT

Nancy Smythe, Executive Director
Samantha Jennings, MSW, Director of Family Services
Emily Kiser, Foundation Administrator

1684 Craniofacial Foundation of America
975 E 3rd Street
Chattanooga, TN 37403

423-778-7000
800-418-3223
Fax: 423-778-8172
Mickey.Milita@erlanger.org
www.erlanger.org

Organization assists families with both the physical and emotional aspects, trying to make the everyday events a little easier.

Kevin Spiegel,, President/CEO
J. Britton Tabor, Senior Vice President and Chief Fin
Alana B Sullivan, Senior Vice President and Chief Com

1685 FACES: National Association for the Craniofacially Handicapped
PO Box 11082
Chattanooga, TN 37401

423-266-1632
800-332-2373
Fax: 423-267-3124
faces@faces-cranio.org
www.faces-cranio.org

Assists individuals with facial disfigurations and their families They maintain a registry of centers offering corrective surgery for craniofacial deformities and financial assistance to qualified applicants.

Lynne Mayfield, President

1686 Genetic Alliance
4301 Connecticut Avenue NW, Suite 404
Washington, DC 20008

202-966-5557
800-336-4363
Fax: 202-966-8553
info@geneticalliance.org
www.geneticalliance.org

World's leading nonprofit health advocacy organization committed to transforming health through genetics and promoting an environment of openness centered on the health of individuals, families, and communities.

Sharon Terry, President/CEO
Tetyana Murza, Managing Director
Natasha Bonhomme, VP, Strategic Development

1687 March of Dimes Foundation
1275 Mamaroneck Avenue
White Plains, NY 10605

914-997-4488
888-663-4637
Fax: 914-997-4763
answers@marchofdimes.com
www.marchofdimes.com

March of Dimes help moms have full-term pregnancies and research the problems that threaten the health of babies.The March of Dimes also acts globally: sharing best practices in perinatal health and helping improve birth outcomes where the needs are the most urgent.

Stacey D. Stewart, President

1688 Prescription Parents
45 Brentwood Circle
Needham, MA 02492

617-499-1936
www.samizdat.com/pp1.html

Organization that gives information and support to children with cleft lip and cleft palate through its educational and support materials, including its directory, newsletter and brochures.

1689 Wide Smiles
PO Box 5153
Stockton, CA 95205

209-942-2812
Fax: 209-464-1497
josmiles@yahoo.com
www.widesmiles2.org/index.html

Wide Smiles was formed to ensure that parents of cleft-affected children do not have to feel alone. We offer support, inspiration, information and networking for families everywhere who may be dealing with the challenges associated with clefting.

Joanne Green, Founding Director

Conferences

1690 Connections Conference
Cleft Palate Foundation
1504 East Franklin Street, Suite 102
Chapel Hill, NC 27514

919-933-9044
800-242-5338
Fax: 919-933-9604
info@cleftline.org
www.cleftline.org

Nancy Smythe, Executive Director
Samantha Jennings, MSW, Director of Family Services
Emily Kiser, Foundation Administrator

1691 Genetic Alliance Annual Conference
Genetic Alliance
4301 Connecticut Avenue NW, Suite 404
Washington, DC 20008

202-966-5557
800-336-4363
Fax: 202-966-8553
info@geneticalliance.org
www.geneticalliance.org

Consistently inspirational and enables partnership among all stakeholders: advocates and community leaders, health and industry professionals, policymakers, and academicians.

July

Sharon Terry, President/CEO
Tetyana Murza, Managing Director
Natasha Bonhomme, VP, Strategic Development

Web Sites

1692 AboutFace USA
1057 Steeles Ave. West
North York, ON M2R 3

416-597-2229
800-597-3223
Fax: 416-597-8494
info@aboutface.ca
www.aboutface.ca

Provides information, services, emotional support and educational programs for and on behalf of individuals with facial differences and their families. Working to increase understanding through public awareness and education.

Anna Pileggi, Executive Director
Colleen Wheatley, Manager, Programs & Services
Emily Rivers, Manager, Communications

1693 Cleft Palate/Craniofacial Birth Defects: Cleft Palate Foundation
1504 East Franklin Street, Suite 102
Chapel Hill, NC 27514

919-933-9044
800-242-5338
Fax: 919-933-9604
www.cleftline.org

The Cleft Palate Foundation operates a toll-free CLEFTLINE for parents with children born with cleft lip, palate and other craniofacial birth defects. Referrals are made to cleft palate/craniofacial healthcare teams and to parent-support groups. Free information is available to parents.

Marilyn A. Cohen, LSLP, President
Nichelle Berry Weintraub, Secretary
Emily Kiser, Administrator

1694 Craniofacial Foundation of America
www.erlanger.org/cranio

Organization assists families with both the physical and emotional aspects, trying to make the everyday events a little easier.

1695 FACES: National Association for the Craniofacially Handicapped
P.O. Box 11082
Chattanooga, TN 37401

423-266-1632
800-332-2373
faces@faces-cranio.org
www.faces-cranio.org

Assists individuals with facial disfigurations and their families They maintain a registry of centers offering corrective surgery for craniofacial deformities and financial assistance to qualified applicants.

Lynne Mayfield, President
Kim Teems, Communications & Program Director

1696 March of Dimes Birth Defects Foundation
1275 Mamaroneck Avenue
White Plains, NY 10605

914-997-4488
888-663-4637
Fax: 914-997-4763
www.marchofdimes.com

The March of Dimes Resource Center answers questions about preparing for pregnancy, pregnancy, genetic diseases, birth defects and related topics.

1697 Online Mendelian Inheritance in Man
National Library of Medicine, Building 38A
Bethesda, MD 20894
888-346-3656
info@ncbi.nlm.nih.gov
www.ncbi.nlm.nih.gov

This database is a catalog of human genes and genetic disorders.
Christine E. Seidman, M.D., Chair
David J. Lipman, M.D., Executive Secretary

1698 Prescription Parents
www.samizdat.com/pp1.html

Organization that gives information and support to children with cleft lip and cleft palate through its educational and support materials, including its directory, newsletter and brochures.

1699 Wide Smiles
P.O. Box 5153
Stockton, CA 95205
209-942-2812
Fax: 209-464-1497
josmiles@yahoo.com
www.widesmiles2.org

Wide Smiles was formed to ensure that parents of cleft-affected children do not have to feel alone. We offer support, inspiration, information and networking for families everywhere who may be dealing with the challenges associated with clefting.

Newsletters

1700 AmeriFace Newsletter
AmeriFace
PO Box 75112
Las Vegas, NV 89136
702-769-9264
888-486-1209
Fax: 702-341-5351
info@ameriface.org
www.ameriface.org

A free newsletter.
8 pages
David Reisberg, DDS, President
Christina Corsiglia, Vice President
Debbie Oliver, Executive Director

Pamphlets

1701 As You Get Older
Cleft Palate Foundation
1504 East Franklin Street, Suite 102
Chapel Hill, NC 27514
919-933-9044
800-242-5338
Fax: 919-933-9604
info@cleftline.org
www.cleftline.org

Describes medical treatment and social skills that may be necessary for teens born with clefts. There are sections on surgery, braces, speech and ear/nose/throat concerns, as well as social relationships and planning for the future.
2002 17 pages
Marilyn A. Cohen, LSLP, President
Nichelle Berry Weintraub, Secretary
Emily Kiser, Administrator

1702 CPF Teddy Bears
Cleft Palate Foundation
1504 East Franklin Street, Suite 102
Chapel Hill, NC 27514
919-933-9044
800-242-5338
Fax: 919-933-9604
info@cleftline.org
www.cleftline.org

Marilyn A. Cohen, LSLP, President
Nichelle Berry Weintraub, Secretary
Emily Kiser, Administrator

1703 Cleft Lip & Palate
March of Dimes Pregnancy & Newborn Health Edu Ctr
1275 Mamaroneck Avenue
White Plains, NY 10605
914-977-4488
888-663-4637
Fax: 914-997-4763
answers@marchofdimes.com
www.marchofdimes.com/phnec/pnhec.asp

Discusses how oral-palate clefts affect a baby's face, when and why they develop, special challenges that arise due to clefts, and repair oprtions.

1704 Cleft Surgery
Cleft Palate Foundation
1504 East Franklin Street, Suite 102
Chapel Hill, NC 27514
919-933-9044
800-242-5338
Fax: 919-933-9604
info@cleftline.org
www.cleftline.org

Provides general information about primary cleft lip and cleft palate surgeries. Complete with drawing explaining the surgical procedures and before and after photos, this brochure addresses general considerations about surgery, post-operative care, and a list of questions to ask your surgeon. Available for newborns, toddlers, preschoolers and school-aged children, teens, and adults. Available in Spanish (Preparando para la Cirug a).
2001 8 pages
Marilyn A. Cohen, LSLP, President
Nichelle Berry Weintraub, Secretary
Emily Kiser, Administrator

1705 Developing Good Speech
Cleft Palate Foundation
1504 East Franklin Street, Suite 102
Chapel Hill, NC 27514
919-933-9044
800-242-5338
Fax: 919-933-9604
info@cleftline.org
www.cleftline.org

Describes additional procedures that may be needed to improve speech in people with repaired cleft palate. Explains surgical procedures including palate lengthening, pharyngeal flap, spincter pharyngoplasty, and pharyngeal wall augmentation. Non-surgical prosthetic treatments are also described. (This information is most relevant to patients ages 4 to adult). Also available in Spanish (Desarrollando Bien el Habla).
2004 10 pages
Marilyn A. Cohen, LSLP, President
Nichelle Berry Weintraub, Secretary
Emily Kiser, Administrator

1706 Feeding Your Baby
Cleft Palate Foundation
1504 East Franklin Street, Suite 102
Chapel Hill, NC 27514
919-933-9044
800-242-5338
Fax: 919-933-9604
info@cleftline.org
www.cleftline.org

Provides information on how best to feed your baby. Intended for use by parents, caregivers, and nurses caring for infants with cleft lip and/or cleft palate, not for infants with more complicated craniofacial conditions. Also avaible in Spanish (Alimentando a su BebS).
1999 15 pages
Marilyn A. Cohen, LSLP, President
Nichelle Berry Weintraub, Secretary
Emily Kiser, Administrator

1707 Genetics and You
Cleft Palate Foundation
1504 East Franklin Street, Suite 102
Chapel Hill, NC 27514

919-933-9044
800-242-5338
Fax: 919-933-9604
info@cleftline.org
www.cleftline.org

Contains a brief overview of genetic biology and a summary of what is known about the causes of clefting. Features a graph for affected individuals, parents, and siblings, showing each group's approximate chances of having a child with a cleft. Details the steps involved i a genetic evaluation, which can help a family to determine its own particular recurrence risks. (The information presented is only applicable to patients with isolated cleft lip and/or palate).

2001 11 pages

Marilyn A. Cohen, LSLP, President
Nichelle Berry Weintraub, Secretary
Emily Kiser, Administrator

1708 Helping with Hearing
Cleft Palate Foundation
1504 East Franklin Street, Suite 102
Chapel Hill, NC 27514

919-933-9044
800-242-5338
Fax: 919-933-9604
info@cleftline.org
www.cleftline.org

Provides information on types of hearing loss, middle ear disease and its treament, and speech concerns resulting from hearing problems. Also available in Spanish (Ayuda con el Oido).

2002 9 pages

Marilyn A. Cohen, LSLP, President
Nichelle Berry Weintraub, Secretary
Emily Kiser, Administrator

1709 Information for Adults
Cleft Palate Foundation
1504 East Franklin Street, Suite 102
Chapel Hill, NC 27514

919-933-9044
800-242-5338
Fax: 919-933-9604
info@cleftline.org
www.cleftline.org

Designed to empower adults to make informed decisions about what additional treatment, if any, they want to seek out in relation to their clefts.

2000 25 pages

Marilyn A. Cohen, LSLP, President
Nichelle Berry Weintraub, Secretary
Emily Kiser, Administrator

1710 The First Year
Cleft Palate Foundation
1504 East Franklin Street, Suite 102
Chapel Hill, NC 27514

919-933-9044
800-242-5338
Fax: 919-933-9604
info@cleftline.org
www.cleftline.org

Also available in Spanish (Los Cuatro Primeros Aos).

Marilyn A. Cohen, LSLP, President
Nichelle Berry Weintraub, Secretary
Emily Kiser, Administrator

1711 The School-Aged Child
Cleft Palate Foundation
1504 East Franklin Street, Suite 102
Chapel Hill, NC 27514

919-933-9044
800-242-5338
Fax: 919-933-9604
info@cleftline.org
www.cleftline.org

Divided into two sections, one addressing the medical concerns of a school-aged child born with a cleft and other providing information about the school experience for these children. The medical section contains information about surgery, dental care, and speech providing simple diagrams of how the speech mechanism may be affected by cleft palate. Also available in Spanish (Los nios de Edad Escolar).

1995 29 pages

Marilyn A. Cohen, LSLP, President
Nichelle Berry Weintraub, Secretary
Emily Kiser, Administrator

1712 Toddlers and Preschoolers
Cleft Palate Foundation
1504 East Franklin Street, Suite 102
Chapel Hill, NC 27514

919-933-9044
800-242-5338
Fax: 919-933-9604
info@cleftline.org
www.cleftline.org

Marilyn A. Cohen, LSLP, President
Nichelle Berry Weintraub, Secretary
Emily Kiser, Administrator

DESCRIPTION

1713 CLUBFOOT

Synonym: Talipes

Covers these related disorders: Talipes equinovarus

Involves the following Biologic System(s):

Orthopedic and Muscle Disorders

The term clubfoot describes a deformity in which the foot is rotated inward and downward, rather than being in its normal position. The deformity in clubfoot is congenital or inborn, and is present at birth. It has several variants, all of which are referred to collectively under the Latin name "talipes" because they stem from structural aberrations in the anklebone, or talus, and dislocation of the ankle (i.e., talonavicular joint). In the most common type of clubfoot, known as congenital talipes equinovarus, the foot is abnormally twisted inward and the toes point downward (plantar flexion). Other deformities classified as types of clubfoot include defects in which the inner portion of the foot is raised with the sole turned inward (metatarsus varus), or the front area of the foot is raised and the heel is turned outward (talipes calcaneovalgus).

In about half of all cases of clubfoot, both feet are affected. A clubfoot tends to be smaller than an unaffected foot, and muscles of the foot and calf are typically underdeveloped, which may become more apparent with advancing age, and depending upon the severity of the deformity, the affected foot may have varying levels of stiffness and inflexibility.

Talipes equinovarus occurs in about 1 of every 1000 births, and is approximately twice as common in males as in females, and may be familiar or idiopathic, occurring as an isolated condition of unknown cause. In infants in whom the condition affects only one foot, the right side is most often involved. Familial talipes equjinovarus is thought to result from the interaction of an abnormal (mutated) gene with other genes or certain environmental factors (multifactorial inheritance). Although deformity of the ankle bone was once considered the primary abnormality in talipes, researchers speculate that a neuromuscular abnormality may be the underlying cause of the talus deformities and associated findings.

In some cases, talipes may occur in association with a neuromuscular disorder (e.g., arthrogryposis multiplex congenita) or with other underlying disorders or syndromes.

The treatment of talipes usually begins soon after birth, since failure to correct this deformity can result in walking on the edge of the foot rather than with the sole of the foot flat on the floor, and in reduced size and strength of muscles in the affected leg. Treatment typically involves the use of taping, casting, or splinting (e.g., malleable splints, serial plaster casts) to move the foot and ankle toward their normal positions. This is often done gradually and over a period of months, through successive, repeated taping, splinting, or casting procedures that each provide a small degree of correction until the proper position of the foot and ankle is achieved. The treatment may involve the use of other orthopedic appliances and corrective shoes to assist with walking. If the use of taping, splints, or casts does not result inappropriate correction, or if a clubfoot is rigid, with shortness or tightness of the Achilles tendon or other structural deformi-

ties in the connective tissues or bones of the foot and ankle, corrective surgery may be needed. This is typically delayed until at least the age of 4 months in order to allow natural growth and strengthening of these structures. Regular monitoring of children with a clubfoot is needed to ensure their continued improvement.

Although clubfoot is not always completely correctible, treatment can improve both the appearance and function of the foot, and in most cases the prognosis for children with a clubfoot is good.

Government Agencies

1714 National Center for Environmental Health

Division of Birth Defects & Developmental Disabled

1600 Clifton Road

Atlanta, GA 30333

404-639-3311

800-232-4636

TTY: 888-232-6348

www.cdc.gov

Strives to promote health and quality of life by preventing or controlling those diseases or deaths that result from interactions between people and their enviroment.

Thomas R. Frieden, MD, MPH,, Director

Ileana Arias, PhD, Principal Deputy Director of DC/ATS

Ursula E. Bauer, PhD, MPH, Director, National Center for Chron

National Associations & Support Groups

1715 American Academy of Pediatrics

141 Northwest Point Boulevard

Elk Grove Village, IL 60007

847-434-4000

800-433-9016

Fax: 847-434-8000

www.aap.org

The American Academy of Pediatrics and its member pediatricians are committed to the attainment of optimal physical, mental and social health and well-being for all infants, children, adolescents, and young adults.

Fernando Stein, MD, FAAP, President

Karen Remley, MD, CEO/Executive VP

1716 Center for Pediatric Orthopaedic Surgery

NYU Hospital for Joint Diseases

301 E 17th Street, Suite 413

New York, NY 10003

212-598-6606

Fax: 212-598-6084

A specialized sector of the Center for Children at the Hospital for Joint Diseases, offering information, consultation, and comprehensive treatment of clubfoot deformities.

Paul Gusmorino, Physician

1717 Genetic Alliance

4301 Connecticut Avenue NW, Suite 404

Washington, DC 20008

202-966-5557

800-336-4363

Fax: 202-966-8553

info@geneticalliance.org

www.geneticalliance.org

World's leading nonprofit health advocacy organization committed to transforming health through genetics and promoting an environment of openness centered on the health of individuals, families, and communities.

Sharon Terry, President/CEO

Tetyana Murza, Managing Director

Natasha Bonhomme, VP, Strategic Development

1718 March of Dimes Foundation
1275 Mamaroneck Avenue
White Plains, NY 10605   914-997-4488
                                888-663-4637
                           Fax: 914-997-4763
                  answers@marchofdimes.com
                       www.marchofdimes.com

March of Dimes help moms have full-term pregnancies and research the problems that threaten the health of babies. The March of Dimes also acts globally: sharing best practices in perinatal health and helping improve birth outcomes where the needs are the most urgent.

Stacey D. Stewart, President

Conferences

1719 Genetic Alliance Annual Conference
Genetic Alliance
4301 Connecticut Avenue NW, Suite 404
Washington, DC 20008   202-966-5557
                               800-336-4363
                          Fax: 202-966-8553
                     info@geneticalliance.org
                       www.geneticalliance.org

Consistently inspirational and enables partnership among all stakeholders: advocates and community leaders, health and industry professionals, policymakers, and academicians.
July

Sharon Terry, President/CEO
Tetyana Murza, Managing Director
Natasha Bonhomme, VP, Strategic Development

Web Sites

1720 CLIPS: Clubfoot Information and Parental Support
ixprss.com/clubfoot

A web site dedicated to providing clubfoot information and parental support, created by a parent as a resource for information, support and understanding.

1721 Children with Talipes (Clubfoot)
www.clubfoot.co.uk

Created by a parent of a child with talipes, the web site offers a first-hand account of treatment and description of clubfoot, as well as links to other sites.

1722 Johns Hopkins Department of Orthopaedic Surgery
601 North Caroline Street , JHOC #5215
Baltimore, MD 21287   443-997-2663
                      hopkinsortho@jhmi.edu
            www.hopkinsmedicine.org/orthopedicsurgery

A web site serving as a learning resource for patients and physicians alike, offering insight into the services provided by the university's professional staff members.

John V. Ingari, MD, Associate Professor
Adam S. Levin, Othopaedic Oncology
Carrol D. Morris, MD, MS, Division Chief,Othopaedic Oncology

1723 Orthoseek
www.orthoseek.com/articles/clubfoot.html

                      admin@orthoseek.com
            www.orthoseek.com/articles/clubfoot.html

A source of authoritative information on pediatric orthopedics and pediatric sports medicine.

Andrew Chong, MD, Founder

1724 TIPS: Talipes Information and Parental Support
www.clubfootaustralia.com/about-us

A support group run by parents whose children have, or had, talipes, offering comprehensive information and many web links, as well as a bi-monthly newletter, stories from parents, email correspondence, and emotional support.

1725 Virtual Children's Hospital: Treatment of Congenital Clubfoot
200 Hawkins Drive
Iowa City, IA 52242   800-777-8442
          www.vh.org/pediatric/provider/orthopaedics/clubfoot

A digital library of pediatric information committed to educating patients, healthcare providers and students for the purpose of improving patients' care, outcome and lives; uses current, authoritative, trustworthy health information created by the University of Iowa, while serving as a platform for research into the challenges facing world-wide information distribution.

Jean E. Robillard, MD, UI VP for Medical Affairs
Theresa Brennan, MD, Chief Medical Officer
Sabi Singh, MS, MA, Co-Chief Operating Officer

1726 Wheeless' Textbook of Orthopaedics
www.wheelessonline.com

Derives from a variety of sources, including journals, articles, national meetings, lectures and other textbooks.

Clifford R. Wheeless, III, M.D., Author

Pamphlets

1727 Club Foot & Other Physical Deformities
March of Dimes Pregnancy & Newborn Health Edu Ctr
1275 Mamaroneck Avenue
White Plains, NY 10605   914-977-4488
                                888-663-4637
                           Fax: 914-997-4763
                  answers@marchofdimes.com
              www.marchofdimes.com/phnec/pnhec.asp

Provides information on Club Foot and other deformities, discussing the affects on the child, diagnoses, causes, prevention, and treatment. Online.

1728 Club Foot and Other Foot Deformities
March of Dimes Resource Center
1275 Mamaroneck Avenue
White Plains, NY 10605   914-977-4488
                                888-663-4637
                           Fax: 914-997-4763
                           TTY: 914-997-4764
                   resourcecenter@modimes.org
                           www.modimes.org

Fact Sheets: one to two page review written for the general public. Also available electronically from our website www.modimes.org. Brochures: 3 panel color brochures written for the general public.

Camps

1729 Hemlocks Easter Seals Recreation
85 Jones Street
Amston, CT 06231   860-228-9496
                           800-832-4409
                      Fax: 860-228-2091
              cmerkent@eastersealsct.org
                  www.ct_easterseals.com

Accepts campers, ages 6 and under, whose major disability is orthopedic. First preference is given to Connecticut residents. A computer camp is also available.

Carl Larson

DESCRIPTION

1730 COARCTATION OF THE AORTA

Involves the following Biologic System(s):
Cardiovascular Disorders

Coarctation of the aorta is a congenital heart defect characterized by a narrowing or constriction of the body's main artery. This artery, known as the aorta, carries blood away from the heart to nourish the tissues of the body. Most of these defects are located just below the origin of the artery that supplies blood to the left arm, (left subclavian artery). Because this constriction reduces blood flow to the lower portion of the body, affected individuals may have unusually low blood pressure and weak or absent pulses in their legs. In addition, there may be higher blood pressure and strong pulses in the arms.

The severity of associated symptoms relates to the degree of pressure changes resulting from aortic narrowing. Although some children have no symptoms, others may experience dizziness, headache, weakness, fainting, nosebleeds, cold legs, and leg pain or cramps. Some affected infants may develop heart failure within the first few days or weeks of life. In some newborns, heart failure may result in decreased blood flow and abnormally high levels of acid in the blood (metabolic acidosis), sometimes accompanied by severe diarrhea and kidney (renal) failure. This life-threatening situation requires immediate treatment. Treatment of coarctation in a newborn requires surgery. (As these infants age, the narrowing may recur [restenosis] necessitating dilation or opening of the vessel through a procedure called balloon angioplasty, during which a balloon-tipped tube [catheter] is inflated inside the aorta, thus helping to expand the narrowed area of the vessel.) Correction of coarctation of the aorta through surgery or balloon catheterization may be recommended in older children with significant impairment. Because coarctation of the aorta is very often accompanied by other heart defects, early intervention is crucial. Other cardiac anomalies often associated with this defect include bicuspid aortic valve (i.e., the heart valve between the left ventricle and the aorta is composed of only two leaflets, or cusps, instead of the normal three); abnormalities of the mitral valve (located between the left atrium and the left ventricle); and an abnormal opening in the wall between the left and right ventricles (ventricular septal defect).

The cause of coarctation of the aorta is unknown. Some researchers think that it develops in the fetus in association with certain types of cardiac abnormalities. Coarctation of the aorta is more prevalent in males than in females by a ratio of about two to one.

Government Agencies

1731 NIH/ Eunice Kennedy Shriver National Institute of Child Health & Human Development
31 Center Drive, Building 31
Bethesda, MD 20892

301-496-5113
800-370-2943
Fax: 866-760-5947
TTY: 888-320-6942
nichdpress@mail.nih.gov
www.nichd.nih.gov

Established in 1962 by congress, today the institute conducts and supports laboratory research, clinical trials, and epidemiological studies that explore health processes; examines the impact of disabilities, diseases, and variations on the lives of individuals; and sponsors training programs for scientists, health care providers, and researchers to ensure that NICHD research can continue

Diana W. Bianchi, Director
Paul Williams, Director, Communications

1732 NIH/National Heart, Lung and Blood Institute
National Institute of Health
31 Center Dr MSC 2486, Bldg 31, Room 5A52
Bethesda, MD 20892

301-592-8573
Fax: 240-629-3246
TTY: 240-629-3255
nhlbiinfo@nhlbi.nih.gov
www.nhlbi.nih.gov

The National Heart, Lung, and Blood Institute (NHLBI) provides global leadership for a research, training, and education program to promote the prevention and treatment of heart, lung, and blood diseases and enhance the health of all individuals so that they can live longer and more fulfilling lives

Gary H Gibbons, MD, Director
Nakela Cook, MD, Chief of Staff

National Associations & Support Groups

1733 American Academy of Pediatrics
141 Northwest Point Boulevard
Elk Grove Village, IL 60007

847-434-4000
800-433-9016
Fax: 847-434-8000
www.aap.org

The American Academy of Pediatrics and its member pediatricians are committed to the attainment of optimal physical, mental and social health and well-being for all infants, children, adolescents, and young adults.

Fernando Stein, MD, FAAP, President
Karen Remley, MD, CEO/Executive VP

1734 American Heart Association
7272 Greenville Avenue
Dallas, TX 75231

214-373-6300
800-242-8721
Fax: 214-706-1341
inquire@amhrt.org
www.heart.org/HEARTORG/

Our mission is to build healthier lives, free of cardiovascular diseases and stroke.

Nancy Brown, CEO
Dr. Stephen Houser, President
Suzie Upton, Chief Operating Officer

1735 Genetic Alliance
4301 Connecticut Avenue NW, Suite 404
Washington, DC 20008

202-966-5557
800-336-4363
Fax: 202-966-8553
info@geneticalliance.org
www.geneticalliance.org

World's leading nonprofit health advocacy organization committed to transforming health through genetics and promoting an environment of openness centered on the health of individuals, families, and communities.

Sharon Terry, President/CEO
Tetyana Murza, Managing Director
Natasha Bonhomme, VP, Strategic Development

1736 March of Dimes Foundation
1275 Mamaroneck Avenue
White Plains, NY 10605

914-997-4488
888-663-4637
Fax: 914-997-4763
answers@marchofdimes.com
www.marchofdimes.com

March of Dimes help moms have full-term pregnancies and research the problems that threaten the health of babies. The March of Dimes also acts globally: sharing best practices in perinatal health and helping improve birth outcomes where the needs are the most urgent.

Stacey D. Stewart, President

Research Centers

1737 Children's Hospital: Academic Pediatric Surgery Department
1056 E 19th Avenue
Denver, CO 80218

303-493-8333
800-624-6553
Fax: 303-764-5997
www.chipteam.org

Strives to improve the health of children through the provision of high quality, coordinated programs of patient care, education, research and advocacy.

Emily L Dobyns

Conferences

1738 Genetic Alliance Annual Conference
Genetic Alliance
4301 Connecticut Avenue NW, Suite 404
Washington, DC 20008

202-966-5557
800-336-4363
Fax: 202-966-8553
info@geneticalliance.org
www.geneticalliance.org

Consistently inspirational and enables partnership among all stakeholders: advocates and community leaders, health and industry professionals, policymakers, and academicians.
July

Sharon Terry, President/CEO
Tetyana Murza, Managing Director
Natasha Bonhomme, VP, Strategic Development

Web Sites

1739 Congenital Heart Information Network
www.tchin.org

An international organization that provides reliable information, support services and resources to families of children with congenital heart defects and acquired heart disease, adults with congenital heart defects, and the professionals who work with them.

1740 Southern Illinois University School of Medicine
PO Box 19658
Springfield, IL 62794

217-545-8000
www.siumed.edu/peds/index.htm

Mission is to meet the health care needs of children and their families in central and Southern Illinois through provision of high quality, coordinated care of children with acute and chronic conditions with inpatient, ambulatory, and community-based programs.

1741 Yale University School of Medicine
333 Cedar St.
New Haven, CT 6510

203-737-1770
medicine.yale.edu

A site that offers information on congential heart conditions including Coarctation of the Aorta.

Peter Salovey, AB, MA, PhD, President
Richard Belitsky, MD, Deputy Dean of Education
Benjamin Polak, MA, MA, PhD, Provost

Book Publishers

1742 Congenital Disorders Sourcebook
Omnigraphics
PO Box 31-1640
Detroit, PA 48231

800-234-1340
Fax: 800-875-1340
info@omnigraphics.com
www.omnigraphics.com

Basic consumer health information on disorders aquired during gestation, including spina bifida, hydrocephalus, cerebral palsy, heart defects, craniofacial abnormalities and fetal alcohol syndrome.
650 pages
ISBN: 0-780809-45-9

DESCRIPTION

1743 COLIC

Synonyms: Infantile colic, Three-month colic

Involves the following Biologic System(s):

Gastrointestinal Disorders, Neonatal and Infant Disorders

Colic refers to a condition in which infants experience frequent episodes of abdominal pain, accompanied by irritability and intense crying. These episodes usually begin suddenly and continue for several hours. Symptoms and physical findings of colic may also include flushing of the face, swelling of the abdomen, repeated extending or flexing of the legs, and unusually cold feet.

It is suspected that colic is intestinal in origin; however, its exact cause is not known. Contributing factors may include the excessive swallowing of air during episodes of unceasing crying, overfeeding, hunger, certain foods, intestinal allergy, and environmental stress. Attacks of colic usually commence within the first few weeks of life and occur most often in the afternoon or evening. Colic often resolves spontaneously within three or four months, without residual effects.

Infants with symptoms associated with colic should be evaluated to determine if another, perhaps more serious disorder, is causing the pain and discomfort. The treatment of colic may include soothing, comforting gestures such as holding, patting, stroking, rocking, and other repetitive movements. Some affected infants may benefit from white noise or other comforting background sounds; the application of a warm wash cloth, hot water bottle, or warm heating pad under the stomach when the child is lying prone; or a ride in the car. Some episodes of colic may resolve with the passing of gas or stool. In addition, parents and caregivers may be advised to refrain from overstimulating, overfeeding, or underfeeding babies with colic. The toll colic takes on parents can be considerable. Physicians often advise that parents or caregivers try to get enough sleep as fatigue, may sometimes add to the already stressful situation.

National Associations & Support Groups

1744 American Academy of Pediatrics
141 Northwest Point Boulevard
Elk Grove Village, IL 60007

847-434-4000
800-433-9016
Fax: 847-434-8000
www.aap.org

The American Academy of Pediatrics and its member pediatricians are committed to the attainment of optimal physical, mental and social health and well-being for all infants, children, adolescents, and young adults.

Fernando Stein, MD, FAAP, President
Karen Remley, MD, CEO/Executive VP

1745 American College of Gastroenterology
6400 Goldsboro Road, Suite 200
Bethesda, MD 20817

301-263-9000
info@acg.gi.org
www.gi.org

To advance the scientific study and medical practice of diseases of the gastrointestinal tract.

1932 13,000 members
Carol A. Burke, MD, FACG, President

1746 American Medical Association
AMA Plaza, 330 North Wabash Ave., Suite 39300
Chicago, IL 60611

800-262-3211
www.ama-assn.org/ama

AMA is dedicated to ensuring sustainable physician practices that result in better health outcomes for patients.

James L. Madara, MD, CEO/ EVP
Bernard L. Hengesbaugh, Chief Operating Officer
Kenneth J. Sharigian, SVP/ Chief Strategy Officer

1747 American Pregnancy Association
1425 Greenway Drive, Suite 440
Irving, TX 75038

info@americanpregnancy.org
americanpregnancy.org

The American Pregnancy Association is a 501(c)(3) nonprofit organization committed to promoting pregnancy wellness through education, advocacy and community awareness.

1748 American Urological Association
1000 Corporate Boulevard
Linthicum, MD 21090

410-689-3700
Fax: 410-689-3800
aua@AUAnet.org
www.auanet.org

Urology is a surgical specialty which deals with diseases of the male and female urinary tract and the male reproductive organs.

1749 Digestive Disease National Coalition
507 Capitol Court NE, Suite 200
Washington, DC 20002

202-544-7497
Fax: 202-546-7105
hpayne@hmcw.org
www.ddnc.org

Advocacy organization comprised of over 30 voluntary and professional societies concerned with the many diseases of the digestive tract and liver.

Lynn Seim, Chairperson
Ralph McKibbin, President
Cathy Griffith, Vice Chairperson

1750 International Chiropractic Pediatric Assoc
icpa4kids.org

610-565-2360
icpa4kids.org

ICPA is a non-profit organization of chiropractic family practitioners dedicated to advancing public awareness and attainment of the chiropractic family wellness lifestyle.

Jeanne Ohm, Executive Director
Gabe Small, Webmaster

1751 North American Society for Pediatric Gastroenterology/Hepatology/Nutrition
714 N Bethlehem Pike, Suite 300
Ambler, PA 19002

215-641-9800
Fax: 215-641-1995
naspghan@naspghan.org
www.naspghan.org

Strives to improve the care of infants, children and adolescents with digestive disorders by promoting advances in clinical care of children with chronic abdominal pain, diarrhea, constipation, vomiting, bleeding from the GI tract, inflammatory bowel disease, liver diseases, diseases of the pancreas, poor weight gain and nutritional problems.

Margaret K Stallings, Executive Director
Kim Rose, Associate Director
Donna Murphy, Membership

Libraries & Resource Centers

1752 Family Resource Center at Lucile Packard Children's Hospital
725 Welch Road
Palo Alto, CA 94304

650-497-8102
www.lpch.org/healthLibrary

Provides hospital patients, their families and staff with access to a wide variety of information about child and maternal health and well-being. The FRC collection includes books, periodicals and pamphlets on a variety of topics from coping with chronic illness such as colic to parenting skills and child development. The Family Resource Center also maintains a large collection of recreational reading materials and video tapes.

1753 National Digestive Diseases Information Clearinghouse
9000 Rockville Pike
Bethesda, MD 20892   301-496-3583
                                          800-860-8747
                                     Fax: 301-907-8906
                                 healthinfo@niddk.nih.gov
                                      www.niddk.nih.gov

The National Institute of Diabetes and Digestive and Kidney Diseases conducts and supports research on many of the most serious diseases affecting public health. The Institute supports much of the clinical research on the diseases of internal medicine and related subspecialty fields as well as many basic science disciplines.

Dr. Griffin P. Rodgers, Director
Dr. Gregory G. Germino, Deputy Director
Camille M. Hoover, M.S.W., Executive Officer

Research Centers

1754 CRI Worldwide Pediatric Center for Excellence
CRI Worldwide
130 White Horse Pike
Clementon, NJ 08021   856-566-9000
                                     Fax: 856-566-4302
                             dkrefetz@cnsresearchinstitute.com
                                 www.cnsresearchinstitute.com

Formerly called CNS Research Institute; Psychiatrists and Child Psychologists maintains a major emphasis in the area of pediatric research. Working hard with parents and their children to educate and treat the entire family.

Dr David Krefetz, Director

1755 Central DuPage Hospital Center for Digestive Disorders
25 N Winfield Road
Winfield, IL 60190   630-933-1600
                                     Fax: 630-933-1300
                                     TTY: 630-933-4833
                                          www.cdh.org

Bringing together the best research about colic and weighed up the evidence about how to treat it.

Michael Vivoda, President/CEO
Brian Lemon, President of Delnor Hospital, Execu
Brian Lemon, President of Central DuPage Hospita

1756 Cincinnati Digestive Health Center
Cincinnati Children's Hospital Medical Center
3333 Burnet Avenue
Cincinnati, OH 45229   513-636-4200
                                          800-344-2462
                                     TTY: 513-636-4900
                                 jorge.bezerra@cchmc.org
                                 www.cincinnatichildrens.org

Promote research that will yield insights into the fundamental processes of growth and development in the digestive tract and lead to novel or improved therapies.

Michael Fisher, President/CEO
Jorge Bezerra, MD, Director, Digestive Health Center

1757 Infant Behavior, Cry and Sleep Clinic
Women & Infants Hospital of Rhode Island
50 Holden Street, 1st Floor
Providence, RI 02908   401-453-7690
                                     Fax: 401-453-7697
                              Barry_Lester@brown.edu
           www.womenandinfants.org/Services/Infant-Behavior-Cry

A clinical service developed to diagnose and treat infants with crying, sleeping, feeding and associated early behavior problems by helping parents understand and manage their infant and to adjust to the disruption caused by having an infant who has behavioral problems in the first few months of life.

Constance A. Howes, FACHE, President/CEO of Women & Infants Ho

Conferences

1758 NASPGHAN Annual Meeting and Postgraduate Course
NASPGHAN
714 N. Bethlehem Pike, Ste 300
Ambler, PA 19002   215-641-9800
                                     Fax: 215-641-1995
                                 naspghan@naspghan.org
                                      www.naspghan.org
November
Margaret K Stallings, Executive Director
Kim Rose, Associate Director
Donna Murphy, Membership

Journals

1759 Journal of Pediatric Gastroenterology and Nutrition
NASPGHAN, author

Lippincott Williams & Wilkins
Two Commerce Square, 2001 Market Street
Philadelphia, PA 19103   215-521-8300
                                     Fax: 215-521-8902
                                 www.wolterskluwerhealth.com

Publication of the North American Society for Pediatric Gastroenterolgy, Hepatology and Nutrition, which strives to improve the care of infants, children and adolescents with digestive disorders by promoting advances in clinical care of children with chronic abdominal pain, diarrhea, constipation, vomiting, bleeding from the GI tract, inflammatory bowel disease, liver diseases, diseases of the pancreas, poor weight gain and nutritional problems.

Bob Becker, President/ CEO
Susan Yules, Chief Financial Officer
Cathy Wolfe, President/ CEO, Medical Research

Newsletters

1760 NASPGHAN News
714 N. Bethlehem Pike, Ste 300
Ambler, PA 19002   215-641-9800
                                     Fax: 215-641-1995
                                 naspghan@naspghan.org
                                      www.naspgn.org

Publication of the North American Society for Pediatric Gastroenterolgy, Hepatology and Nutrition, which strives to improve the care of infants, children and adolescents with digestive disorders by promoting advances in clinical care of children with chronic abdominal pain, diarrhea, constipation, vomiting, bleeding from the GI tract, inflammatory bowel disease, liver diseases, diseases of the pancreas, poor weight gain and nutritional problems.

Margaret K Stallings, Executive Director
Kim Rose, Associate Director
Donna Murphy, Membership

DESCRIPTION

1761 CONDUCT DISORDER

Covers these related disorders: Group conduct disorder, Solitary aggressive conduct disorder, Undifferentiated conduct disorder

Involves the following Biologic System(s):

Developmental/Behavioral/Psychiatric Disorders

Conduct disorder refers to a group of distinct behavioral abnormalities characterized by the repetition of certain types of disruptive or antisocial behaviors. Children or adolescents with conduct disorder may often lie, steal, skip school, run away from home, use drugs or alcohol, hurt animals, commit arson or vandalism, engage in physical violence, use weapons, and commit other criminal acts. Those affected with solitary aggressive conduct disorder are usually selfish, rarely get along with or relate well to others, and often lack remorse for their behavior. Children and adolescents with group conduct disorder, however, may be attached and faithful to a particular clique, gang, or other group of friends while at the same time violating the rights of or displaying antisocial behavior toward those outside of the group. In some cases, affected individuals may display behavior characteristic of both solitary aggressive and group conduct disorders and, subsequently, may be diagnosed with undifferentiated conduct disorder.

Conduct disorder may be caused by a variety of factors including genetic as well as environmental influences (e.g., childrearing, etc.). In many cases, children with this type of behavioral irregularity have parents or caregivers who display similar patterns of conduct. In addition, parents or caregivers often have inconsistent parenting skills or may be overly aggressive in punishing or disciplining. Some parents or caregivers may be unsupportive of the child, or may lack other basic skills that help the child to develop a sense of self-worth, respect for others, etc. Several factors may influence whether affected children carry these characteristic patterns of behavior into adulthood. Some factors include parental or caregiver influences, the age of onset, the severity and type of behavior, the number of different types of antisocial behaviors exhibited, and whether the episodes of disruptive behavior continue to increase.

Treatment of conduct disorder may include individual, group, and family therapy, as well as parental or caregiver management training. In some cases, children with severe conduct disorder may benefit from hospitalization for psychiatric evaluation and treatment. Medication is, in most cases, not indicated for the treatment of conduct disorder; however, it is sometimes prescribed to treat other underlying disorders (e.g, depression, attention deficit hyperactivity disorder, etc.). Other treatment is supportive.

Government Agencies

1762 NIH/National Institute of Mental Health
6001 Executive Boulevard, Room 6200, MSC 9663
Bethesda, MD 20892

301-443-4536
866-615-6464
Fax: 301-443-4279
TTY: 301-443-8431
nimhinfo@nih.gov
www.nimh.nih.gov

The mission of NIMH is to transform the understanding and treatment of mental illnesses through basic and clinical research, paving the way for prevention, recovery, and cure.

Joshua Gordon, MD, PhD, Director
Shelli Avenevoli, MD, Deputy Director

National Associations & Support Groups

1763 American Academy of Pediatrics
141 Northwest Point Boulevard
Elk Grove Village, IL 60007

847-434-4000
800-433-9016
Fax: 847-434-8000
www.aap.org

The American Academy of Pediatrics and its member pediatricians are committed to the attainment of optimal physical, mental and social health and well-being for all infants, children, adolescents, and young adults.

Fernando Stein, MD, FAAP, President
Karen Remley, MD, CEO/Executive VP

1764 American Mental Health Foundation (AMHF)
PO Box 3
Riverdale,, NY 10471
USA

212-737-9027
elomke@americanmentalhealthfoundation.or
americanmentalhealthfoundation.org

Dedicated to the extensive and intensive research in the theories and techniques of treatment of emotional illness and to the implementation of reforms in the mental health system. Efforts have resulted in development of better and less expensive treatment methods. Findings are disseminated in English and other major languages.

Sister Joan Curtin. CND, Director
Evander Lomke, President/Executive Director
Eugene Gollogly, Vice President

1765 Association for Behavioral and Cognitive Therapies
305 7th Avenue, 16th Floor
New York, NY 10001

212-647-1890
Fax: 212-647-1865
membership@abct.org
www.abct.org/Home/

Formerly known as the Association for Advancement of Behavior Therapy; this organization is concerned with the application of behavioral and cognitive sciences to understanding human behavior, developing interventions to enhance the human condition, and promoting the appropriate utilization of these interventions.

Stefan G. Hofmann, Ph.D., President
Dean McKay, Ph.D, President- Elect
Denise D. Davis, Ph.D., Secretary/Treasurer

1766 Center for Disabilities and Development
University of Iowa Stead Family Children's Hospita
100 Hawkins Drive
Iowa City, IA 52242

319-353-6900
877-686-0031
Fax: 319-356-7700
cdd-webmaster@uiowa.edu
www.uichildrens.org/cdd/

A trusted resource for healthcare, training, research and information for people with disabilities that include: behavior disorders, brain injury, cerebral palsy, diabetes, down syndrome, learning disabilities, mental retardation, sleep disorders and spina bifida.

Dianne McBrien, MD, Medical Director

1767 Center for Mental Health Services Knowledge Exchange Network
US Department of Health and Human Services
PO Box 42557
Washington, DC 20015

800-662-4357
800-789-2647
Fax: 240-747-5470
TTY: 800-487-4889
TDD: 866-889-2647
samhsa.media@ees.hhs.gov
www.store.samhsa.gov/home

Develops national mental health policies that promote Federal/State coordination and benefit from input from consumers, family members and providers. Ensures that high quality mental health services programs are implemented to benefit seriously mentally ill populations, disasters or those involved in the criminal justice system.

Mirtha R. Beadle M.P.A., Deputy for Operations
Kana . Enomoto, M.A, Principal Deputy Administrator
Pamela S. Hyde, J.D., Administrator

1768 Federation of Families for Children's Mental Health
9605 Medical Center Drive, Suite 280
Rockville, MD 10205
240-403-1901
Fax: 240-403-1909
ffcmh@ffcmh.org
www.ffcmh.org

The National family run organization is dedicated exclusively to helping children with mental health needs and their families achieve a better quality of life.

Teka Dempson, President
Sherri Luthe, Vice President
Sheila Pires, Treasurer

1769 Mental Health America
500 Montgomery Street, Ste 820
Alexandria, VA 22314
703-684-7722
800-969-6642
Fax: 703-684-5968
TTY: 800-433-5959
info@mentalhealthamerica.net
www.mentalhealthamerica.net

MHA, the leading advocacy organization addressing the full spectrum of mental and substance use conditions and their effects nationwide, works to inform, advocate and enable access to quality behavioral health services for all Americans.

Paul Gionfriddo, President/CEO
Shavonne Carpenter, Sr Assoc., Support & Services
Mallory Pernell, Assoc. Dir, Comments/Marketing

1770 NADD: National Association for the Dually Diagnosed
132 Fair Street
Kingston, NY 12401
845-331-4336
800-331-5362
Fax: 845-331-4569
info@thenadd.org
www.thenadd.org

Nonprofit organization designed to promote the interests of professional and care providers for individuals who have the coexistence of mental illness and mental retardation. NADD provides conferences, educational services and training materials to professionals, parents, concerned citizens and service organizations.

Dr Robert Fletcher, CEO
Michelle Jordan, Office Manager
Edward Seliger, Project Coordinator

1771 National Alliance for the Mentally Ill
3803 N. Fairfax Dr., Suite 100
Arlington, VA 22203
703-525-7600
800-950-6264
Fax: 703-524-9094
TDD: 703-516-7227
info@nami.org
www.nami.org

NAMI is a nonprofit, grassroots, self-help, support and advocacy organization of consumers, families and friends of people with severe mental illness, such as schizophrenia, bipolar disorder, major depressive disorder, obsessive compulsive disorder, anxiety disorders, autism and other severe and persistent mental illnesses that affect the brain.

Keris J,,n Myrick, President
Kevin B Sullivan, First Vice President
Jim Payne, Second Vice President

1772 National Mental Health Consumers' Self-Help Clearinghouse
1211 Chestnut Street, Suite 1207
Philadelphia, PA 19107
215-751-1810
800-553-4539
Fax: 215-636-6312
info@mhselfhelp.org
www.mhselfhelp.org

The Clearinghouse works to foster peer empowerment through our website, up-to-date news and information announcements, a directory of peer-driven services, electronic and printed publications, training packages, and individual and onsite consultation

Joseph Rogers, Executive Director & Founder
Susan Rogers, Director of Special Projects
Britani Nestel, Program Specialist

Research Centers

1773 Menninger Child & Family Program
Menninger Clinic
2801 Gessner Drive, PO Box 809045
Houston, TX 77280
713-275-5000
800-351-9058
Fax: 713-275-5117
www.menninger.edu

Menninger's research strategies are developed through the Menninger Child & Family Program. Projects are designed to develop a better understanding of the mind in order to more effectively treat mental disorders.

Ian Aitken, Ceo

1774 National Technical Assistance Center for Children's Mental Health
Georgetown University
Center for Child and Human Development Georgetown
Washington, DC 20057
202-687-5000
Fax: 202-687-8899
TDD: 202-687-5503
gucdc@georgetown.edu
www.gucchd.georgetown.edu/67211.html

Devoted to helping states, tribes, territories, and communities discover, apply, and sustain innovative and collaborative solutions that improve the social, emotional, and behavioral well being of children and families.

James Wotring MSW, Director

1775 Research & Training Center for Children's Mental Health at University of South FL
Louis de la Parte Florida Mental Health Institute
13301 Bruce B. Downs Boulevard
Tampa, FL 33612
813-974-3154
Fax: 813-974-3078
friedman@fmhi.usf.edu
www.rtckids.fmhi.usf.edu/default.cfm

Working towards increasing the effectiveness of service systems by strengthening the empirical base for such systems through research and dissemination to key audiences. With its new, five-year research program, the Center expands its mission with an integrated research, training, and dissemination program targeted specifically at implementation issues for developing effective systems of care.

Robert M. Friedman, Ph.D, Center Director
Albert Duchnowski, Ph.D, Deputy Director
Krista Kutash, Ph.D, Deputy Director

1776 Research and Training Center on Family Support and Children's Mental Health
1600 SW 4th Avenue, Suite 900
Portland, OR 97201
503-725-4040
Fax: 503-725-4180
flemingd@pdx.edu
www.rtc.pdx.edu

Funded to pursue an integrated set of research, training, technical assistance, and dissemination activities. The center's work will focus on two related themes; community integration for children and adolescents with emotional and behavioral disorders and their families; and strengthening family and youth participation in child and adolescent mental health services.

Donna Flemming, Information Director

1777 Technical Assistance Partnership for Child and Family Mental Health
1000 Thomas Jefferson Street NW, Suite 400
Washington, DC 20007   202-403-6827
Fax: 202-342-5007
tapartnership@air.org
www.tapartnership.org

A staff of family members and professionals with extensive practice experience, grounded in an organization with vast research experience in children with serious emotional disturbance and their families.

Sharon Hunt, Deputy Director of Operations
Jeffrey Poirier, Continuous Quality Improvement
Regenia Hicks, Project Director Continuous Quality

Conferences

1778 FFCMH Annual Conference
Federation of Families for Childrens Mental Health
9605 Medical Center Drive, Suite 280
Rockville, MD 20850   240-403-1901
Fax: 240-403-1909
ffcmh@ffcmh.org
www.ffcmh.org

Address the complex issue of trauma; the impact it has on children and families; the promotion of healing and prevention strategies; knowledge about how to address trauma through resiliency-based interventions, utilizing a familydriven, youth guided approach; and examples of how family organizations and the partners they work with are raising awareness and improving trauma-focused services and supports.

November

Teka Dempson, President
Sherri Luthe, Vice President
Sheila Pires, Treausrer

1779 NADD Conference & Exhibit Show
National Association for the Dually Diagnosed
132 Fair Street
Kingston, NY 12401   845-331-4336
800-331-5362
Fax: 845-331-4569
info@thenadd.org
www.thenadd.org

Educating professionals, families and clients of services on standard and state-of-the-art information across many specialties; Enhancing specific skills required to provide maximum benefit to individuals with special or specific cognitive and/or developmental needs; Providing a forum for an exchange of ideas and information among professionals, families and those who may receive services.

November

Dr Robert Fletcher, CEO
Michelle Jordan, Office Manager
Edward Seliger, Project Coordinator

1780 NAMI Convention
National Alliance on Mental Illness
3803 N Fairfax Drive, Suite 100
Arlington, VA 22203   703-524-7600
888-999-6264
Fax: 703-524-9094
TDD: 703-516-7227
info@nami.org
www.nami.org

The NAMI Convention is packed with information, chances to network, leadership development opportunities, and lots more

July
Keris Jan Myrick, President
Kevin B Sullivan, Vice President
Clarence Jordan, Secretary

Audio Video

1781 Managing the Defiant Child
Courage To Change Publishing
PO Box 486
Wilkes-Barres, PA 18703   800-440-4003
Fax: 800-772-6499
www.couragetochange.com

An information-packed video brings to life a proven approach to behavior management. Shows clinicians, school practitioners, teachers, parents and students how enhanced parenting skills can dramatically improve the parent-child relationship.

Russell A Barkley, Editor

1782 Understanding and Treating the Hereditary Psychiatric Spectrum Disorders
Hope Press
PO Box 188
Duarte, CA 91009   818-303-0644
800-321-4039
Fax: 818-358-3520
hopepress.com

Learn with ten hours of audio tapes from a two day seminar given in May 1997 by David E Comings MD. Tapes cover: ADHD, Tourette syndrome, Obsessive-Compulsive Disorder, Conduct Disorder, Oppositional Defiant Disorder, Autism and other Hereditary Psychiatric Spectrum Disorders. Eight audio tapes.

David E Comings, MD, Presenter

1783 Understanding the Defiant Child
Courage To Change
PO Box 486
Wilkes-Barres, PA 18703   800-440-4003
Fax: 800-772-6499
www.couragetochange.com

Provides a vivid picture of what we know about Oppositional Defiant Disorder and presents real-life scenes of family interactions and commentary from parents. Illuminates the nature and causes of ODD, why it should be dealt with early, and what can be done. Ideal viewing for school practitioners, clinical child psychologists, counselors and parents coping with a defiant child.

Russell A Barkley, Editor

Web Sites

1784 Conductdisorders.com
www.conductdisorders.com

Site for parents, teachers, and family members who deal with a child with one of the defined behavioral disorders.

1785 Internet Mental Health
www.mentalhealth.com

internetmentalhealth@shaw.ca
www.mentalhealth.com

Our goal is to improve understanding, diagnosis, and treatment of mental illness throughout the world.

Phillip W. Long, M.D., Psychiatrist

1786 NADD: National Association for the Dually Diagnosed
132 Fair Street
Kingston, NY 12401   845-331-4336
800-331-5362
Fax: 845-331-4569
info@thenadd.org
www.thenadd.org

Nonprofit organization designed to promote the interests of professional and care providers for individuals who have the coexistence of mental illness and mental retardation. NADD provides conferences, educational services and training materials to professionals, parents, concerned citizens and service organizations.

Dr Robert Fletcher, CEO
Michelle Jordan, Office Manager
Edward Seliger, Project Coordinator

1787 Online Mendelian Inheritance in Man
National Library of Medicine, Building 38A
Bethesda, MD 20894
888-346-3656
info@ncbi.nlm.nih.gov
www.ncbi.nlm.nih.gov

This database is a catalog of human genes and genetic disorders.

Christine E. Seidman, M.D., Chair
David J. Lipman, M.D., Executive Secretary

1788 Planetpsych
www.planetpsych.com
webmaster@PlanetPsych.com
www.planetpsych.com

Planetpsych is an online resource for mental health information.

Book Publishers

1789 Aggression and Violence Throughout the Life Span
Sage Publications
2455 Teller Road
Thousand Oaks, CA 91320
800-818-7243
Fax: 800-583-2665
info@sagepub.com
www.sagepub.com

A unique life span developmental perspective on some of society's most perplexing and pernicious problems, aggressive and violent behaviors. Examines issues in the development of aggressive behaviors in young children, the progression of these behaviors to older children and adolescents and cause, effect and treatment of aggressive and violent behaviors in adults. Integrates empirical research with clinical applications.

360 pages Softcover
ISBN: 0-803945-51-5

Sara Miller McCune, Founder/Chairman
Blaise R Simqu, President/CEO
Chris Hickok, Senior Vice President/CFO

1790 Antisocial Behavior by Young People
Cambridge University Press
32 Avenue of the Americas
New York, NY 10013
617-264-2300
Fax: 617-264-2323
info@cambridge.com
www.cambridge.org

Written by a child psychiatrist, a criminologist and a social psychologist, this book is a major international review of research evidence on anti-social behavior. Covers all aspects of the field, including descriptions of different types of delinquency and time trends, the state of knowledge on the individuals, social-psychological and cultural factors involved and recent advances in prevention and intervention.

490 pages Paperback
ISBN: 0-521646-08-1

Michael Rutter, Editor
Ann Hagell, Editor
Henri Giller, Editor

1791 Conduct Disorders in Childhood and Adolescence
(Developmental Clinical)
Sage Publications
2455 Teller Road
Thousand Oaks, CA 91320
800-818-7243
800-818-7243
Fax: 800-583-2665
info@sagepub.com
www.sagepub.com

Conduct disorder is a clinical problem among children and adolescents that includes aggressive acts, theft, vandalism, firesetting, running away, truancy, defying authority and other antisocial behaviors. This book describes the nature of conduct disorder and what is currently known from research and clinical work. Topics include psychiatric diagnosis, parent psychopathology and child-rearing processes.

192 pages Hardcover
ISBN: 0-803971-81-8

Sara Miller McCune, Founder/Chairman
Blaise R Simqu, President/CEO
Chris Hickok, Senior Vice President/CFO

1792 Conduct Disorders in Children and Adolescents
American Psychiatric Publishing
1000 Wilson Boulevard, Suite 1825
Arlington, VA 22009
703-907-7322
800-368-5777
Fax: 703-907-1091
appi@psych.org
www.appi.org

Examines the phenomenology, etiology, and diagnosis of conduct disorders, and describes therapeutic and preventive interventions. Includes the range of treatments now available, including individual, family, group, and behavior therapy; hospitalization; and residential treatment.

1995 414 pages Hardcover
ISBN: 0-880485-17-5

G Pirooz Sholevar, MD, Editor

1793 Conduct Problem/Emotional Problem Interventions: A Holistic
Perspective
Slosson Educational Publications
PO Box 544
East Aurora, NY 14052
716-625-0930
888-756-7766
Fax: 800-655-3840
slosson@slosson.com
www.slosson.com

This innovative book is broad in scope and addresses the now what sensation that many professionals get when charged with the education or treatment of individuals with conduct disorders or emotional disturbance. Distinct intervention and screening strategies and patient involvement strategies are offered in clear and practical terms.

Edward J Kelly, Editor

1794 Difficult Child
Random House
1745 Broadway
New York, NY 10019
212-782-9000
Fax: 212-572-6066
www.randomhouse.com

One of the nation's most respected experts on children and discipline; Dr. Stanley Turecki a father of a once difficult child offers compassionate and practical advice to parents of hard-to-raise children.

320 pages Paperback

Stanley Turecki, Writer

1795 Disruptive Behavior Disorders in Children and Adolescents
Robert L Hendren, DO, author

American Psychiatric Publishing
1000 Wilson Boulevard, Suite 1825
Arlington, VA 22209
703-907-7322
800-368-5777
Fax: 703-907-1091
appi@psych.org
www.appi.org

Discusses attention deficit hyperactivity disorder, conduct disorder, substance abuse and disruptive behavior disorders. Examines the relationship between violence and mental illness in adolescence.

1999 216 pages Paperback
ISBN: 0-880489-60-7

1796 Preventing Antisocial Behavior: Interventions
Guilford Press
72 Spring Street
New York, NY 10012

212-431-9800
800-365-7006
Fax: 212-966-6708
info@guilford.com
www.guilford.com

Establishes the crucial link between theory, measurement and intervention. Brings together a collection of studies that utilize experimental approaches for evaluating intervention programs, both the feasibility, and necessity of independent evaluation. Also shows how the information obtained in such studies can be used to test and refine prevailing theories about human behavior in general, and behavior changes in particular.

1992 391 pages
ISBN: 0-898628-82-1

Joan McCord, Editor
Richard Tremblay, Editor

1797 Skills Training for Children with Behavior Disorders
Courage To Change
PO Box 486
Wilkes-Barres, PA 18703

800-440-4003
Fax: 800-772-6499
www.couragetochange.com

Designed for use by both parents and therapists, provides background information, step-by-step instructions and many useful, reproducible worksheets. Techniques offered help children with anger management, compliance and following rules, academic success, emotional well-being and self-esteem and much more.

272 pages

Michael L Bloomquist, Editor

Pamphlets

1798 Conduct Disorder in Children and Adolescents
National Mental Health Information Center
PO Box 42557
Washington, DC 20015

800-789-2647
Fax: 240-747-5470
TDD: 866-889-2647
ken@mentalhealth.org
www.mentalhealth.samhsa.gov

This fact sheet defines conduct disorder, identifies risk factors, discusses types of help available, and suggests what parents or other caregivers can do.

1997 2 pages

1799 Mental, Emotional, and Behavior Disorders in Children and Adolescents
National Mental Health Information
PO Box 42557
Washington, DC 20015

240-747-5484
800-789-2647
Fax: 240-747-5470
mentalhealth.samhsa.gov

This fact sheet describes mental, emotional, and behavioral problems that can occur during childhood and adolescence and discusses related treatment, support services, and research.

4 pages

1800 Treatment of Children with Mental Disorder
National Institute of Mental Health
PO Box 5801
Bethesda, MD 20824

301-496-5751
800-352-9424
Fax: 301-443-4279
TTY: 301-443-8431
nimhinfo@nih.gov
www.nimh.nih.gov

A short booklet that contains questions and answers about therapy for children with mental disorders. Includes a chart of mental disorders and medications used.

Walter J. Koroshetz, M.D., Acting Director
Alan L. Willard, Ph.D., Acting Deputy Director
Caroline Lewis, Executive Officer

Camps

1801 Adventure Learning Center Camp Programs
Eagle Village
4507 170th Avenue
Hersey, MI 49639

231-832-2234
800-748-0061
Fax: 231-832-1468
summercamp@eaglevillage.org
www.eaglevillage.org

Offers a variety of fun camp experiences for children, including those with emotional and/or behavioral impairments. A low staff-to-camper ratio and exciting, challenging activities make the camps rewarding experiences. As funding is available, we will offer camp scholarships to eligible participants.

Sara Kofal, Camp Director

1802 Life Adventure Center
Life Adventure Center of the Bluegrass
PO Box 447
Versailles, KY 40383

859-873-3271
Fax: 859-873-2410
www.lifeadventurecamp.org

A unique experience of discovery and development where lifelong lessons are learned. Through purposeful play, using a combination of physical and mental problem-solving exercises, participants engage in opportunities to make positive choices, gain self-confidence, improve decision making, build on group strengths and much more.

1803 Talisman Summer Camps
Talisman Schools
64 Gap Creek Road
Zirconia, NC 28790

855-588-8254
Fax: 828-669-2521
summer@talismancamps.com
www.talismansummercamp.com/

Camps for children ages 6 to 17 and young adults 18-21 with LD, ADD and ADHD, Asperger's Syndrome, and high functioning autism. Talisman has been offering such experiences since 1980 and is ACA accredited. The unique summer camps specialize in creating camps that offer not only adventure, but learning experiences, for children and teenagers with learning disabilities, attention deficit hyperactivity disorder, Asperger's syndrome and high-functioning autism.

Linda Tatsapaugh, Director
Aaron McGinley, Base Camp Program Manager

DESCRIPTION

1804 CONGENITAL ADRENAL HYPERPLASIA

Synonyms: CAH, Androgenital syndrome, Congenital virilizing adrenal hyper, 21-hydroxylase deficiency, 11-beta-hydroxylase deficiency

Involves the following Biologic System(s):

Endocrinologic Disorders

Congenital adrenal hyperplasia (CAH) refers to a group of genetic diseases that leads to the inability of the adrenal glands to make cortisol. Cortisol is a steroid hormone needed to maintain metabolism, energy, blood pressure, and a normal responses to stress or injury. There are many different steps in the production of cortisol; each step requires an enzyme for completion and as a result, a deficiency in any enzyme along the path leads to one of the forms of CAH. The inability to make cortisol leads to symptoms from both the lack of cortisol as well as from the build-up of the cortisol precursors. In CAH, male hormones (androgens) are made in excess and this will lead to exaggerated male characteristics in these patients. Some people with CAH also have deficiency in another hormone, aldosterone. Aldosterone regulates salt (sodium)levels in the body.

Symptoms of CAH can vary in girls and boys, and also may vary according to the specific type of CAH. In girls, the excess of androgens leads to masculinization of the female external genitalia (ambiguous genitalia). Symptoms in girls with milder forms of CAH include irregular menstrual periods, excessive or male pattern hair growth, or infertility. In boys, symptoms of salt-wasting CAH include adrenal crisis which typically consists of low blood pressure and sodium abnormalities. Girls can also have salt abnormalities, but are often diagnosed before an adrenal crisis because of their ambiguous external genitalia can be seen. In boys with non-salt wasting CAH, the effect of excess androgens leads to pubertal changes earlier than expected (precocious puberty).

The treatment of CAH is replacement of cortisol with glucocorticoid medications, and if needed, replacement of aldosterone with mineralocorticoid medications. It is important to remember to give extra medication (stress dose steroids during times of stress, illness, or injury because of the body's greater demand for steroids during those times.)

National Associations & Support Groups

1805 American Academy of Pediatrics
141 Northwest Point Boulevard
Elk Grove Village, IL 60007

847-434-4000
800-433-9016
Fax: 847-434-8000
www.aap.org

The American Academy of Pediatrics and its member pediatricians are committed to the attainment of optimal physical, mental and social health and well-being for all infants, children, adolescents, and young adults.

Fernando Stein, MD, FAAP, President
Karen Remley, MD, CEO/Executive VP

1806 CARES Foundation
2414 Morris Avenue, Suite 110
Union, NJ 07083

973-912-3895
866-227-3737
Fax: 973-912-8990
karenf@caresfoundation.org
www.caresfoundation.org

CARES Foundation is a nonprofit, educational organization. Its purpose is to educate the public and physicians about all forms of Congenital Adrenal Hyerplasia, its symptoms, diagnostic protocols, treatment, genetic frequency, the necessity for early intervention and benefits of newborn screening. It is also dedicated to providing support and information to affected individuals and their families.

Dina Matos, Executive Director
Cindy Rogers, Director of Finance and Operations
Karen Fountain, Program Manager

1807 MAGIC Foundation: Major Aspects of Growth in Children
4200 Cantera Drive, #106
Warrenville, IL 60555

630-836-8200
800-362-4423
Fax: 630-836-8181
ContactUs@magicfoundation.org
www.magicfoundation.org

A national nonprofit organization providing support and education regarding growth disorders in children and related adult disorders. Provides educational information, networking, a national conference, a kids' program and an extensive medical library.

10,000 members

Dianne Kremidas, Executive Director
Mary Andrews, Chief Executive Officer
Teresa Tucker, Patient Advocacy

1808 National Adrenal Diseases Foundation
505 Northern Boulevard
Great Neck, NY 11021

516-487-4992
nadfmail@aol.com
www.nadf.us/nadf/index.htm

NADF is committed to bringing information regarding adrenal diseases into the public's awareness to facilitate early diagnosis and treatment.NADF sponsors support groups across the countrty allowing for an exchange of ideas and feelings by individuals who share a common illness. NADF members receive quaterly newsletters, educational materials, and access to a library of related information.

Kalina Warren, President
Timothy Skodon, Treasurer
Paul Margulies, M.D, FACP, FACE-Medical Director

Libraries & Resource Centers

1809 University of Iowa Birth Defects and Genetic Disorders Unit
2614 JCP
Iowa City, IA 52242
James M Smith, Director

319-335-9901

Conferences

1810 Adult Endocrine Disorders/GHD Educational Convention
Magic Foundation
4200 Cantera Drive, #106
Warrenville, IL 60555

630-836-8200
800-362-4423
Fax: 630-836-8181
contactus@magicfoundation.org
www.magicfoundation.org

An educational program for adults who are affected with Growth Hormone Deficiency and/or other endocrine disorders.

June

Dianne Kremidas, Executive Director
Mary Andrews, CEO
Teresa Tucker, Patient Advocacy

Web Sites

1811 CARES Foundation
2414 Morris Ave., Suite 110
Union, NJ 7083
908-364-0272
866-227-3737
Fax: 908-686-2019
contact@caresfoundation.org
www.caresfoundation.org

Provides education to the public and physicians about all forms of Congenital Adrenal Hyerplasia — symptoms, diagnostic protocols, treatment, genetic frequency, the necessity for early intervention and benefits of newborn screening. The web site also provides support and information to affected individuals and their families.

Katherine L. Fowler, President
Chad Lapp, Vice President
Alexandra Dubois, Secretary

1812 MAGIC Foundation: Major Aspects of Growth in Children
4200 Cantera Drive, #106
Warrenville, IL 60555
630-836-8200
800-362-4423
Fax: 630-836-8181
ContactUs@magicfoundation.org
www.magicfoundation.org

Created to provide support services for the families of children afflicted with a wide variety of chronic and/or critical disorders, syndromes, and diseases that affect a child's growth.

Dianne Kremidas, Executive Director
Mary Andrews, CEO
Teresa Tucker, Patient Advocacy

1813 National Adrenal Diseases Foundation
505 Northern Boulevard
Great Neck, NY 11021
516-487-4992
nadfsupport@nadf.us
www.nadf.us

Committed to bringing information regarding rare diseases to the publics awareness to facilitate early diagnosis and treatment.

Kalina Warren, President
Melanie G. Wong, Executive Director
Paul Margulies, MD, FACP, Medical Director

Newsletters

1814 CARES Foundation Newsletter
2414 Morris Avenue, Suite 110
Union, NJ 7083
973-912-3895
866-227-3737
kelly@caresfoundation.org
www.caresfoundation.org

Provides support and information to affected individuals and their families.

3x year

Kelly R Leight, Executive Director

1815 NADF News
505 Northern Boulevard
Great Neck, NY 11021
516-487-4992
nadfsupport@nadf.us
www.nadf.us

Features important information on adrenal disorders, support groups and the latest research.

quaterly

Kalina Warren, President
Melanie G Wong, Executive Director
Paul Margulies, MD, FACP, Medical Director

DESCRIPTION

1816 CONGENITAL CATARACTS

Involves the following Biologic System(s):

Genetic/Chromosomal/Syndrome/Metabolic Disorders,
Ophthalmologic Disorders

Congenital cataracts refers to a condition in which cloudiness or opacities in the lens of the eye or eyes are present at birth. These opacities may vary in severity, with some resolving spontaneously as in cataracts of prematurity. Other congenital cataracts, if left untreated, may result in loss of transparency of the lens and subsequent visual impairment. In addition, in some newborns, remnants of other eye tissues may contribute to the formation of a stationary opacity of the cornea. In most instances , this type of stationary cloudiness does not contribute to visual impairment.

Congenital cataracts may occur as the result of many different factors (multifactorial), including genetic influences, associated metabolic and chromosomal disorders, congenital infections, and toxic exposure. If inherited as an isolated event, congenital cataracts are usually transmitted as an autosomal dominant or autosomal recessive trait. Several metabolic disorders are characterized by congenital cataracts, including galactosemia, in which an enzyme deficiency results in the inability to process the simple sugar galactose; oculocerebrorenal syndrome (Lowe's syndrome), an X-linked metabolic disorder that affects many systems of the body; certain metabolic diseases known as lyosomal storage disorders; and several other diseases related to inborn errors of metabolism. Other contributing metabolic factors may include low blood levels of calcium (hypocalcemia) or glucose (hypoglycemia). In addition, cataracts are sometimes diagnosed in newborns whose mothers have diabetes mellitus. Several chromosomal disorders are also characterized by congenital opacities including Down's syndrome (trisomy 21), trisomy 13 syndrome, Turner's syndrome (45XO), and others. Congenital cataracts are sometimes the result of maternal infections that occur during pregnancy. Such infections may include German measles (rubella), syphilis, measles, influenza, certain herpes infections, and others. Additional contributing factors may include toxic influences from drug substances taken by the mother during pregnancy.

Treatment for congenital cataracts depends upon the extent of the defect and its influence on vision. To restore lost transparency of the lens resulting from cataracts, surgery may be performed in which the cataract and lens are removed. To reestablish the ability of the eye to deflect light that was lost with lens removal, special contact lenses or implants are then fitted to the eye. In some cases, additional surgery may be indicated. Because congenital opacities of the lens are so often associated with other eye irregularities (e.g., amblyopia, glaucoma, strabismus, etc.) and in order to obtain the best outcome, treatment may also be directed toward any associated abnormalities. In addition, patients are followed carefully after surgery in order to prevent, correct, or treat any possible complications.

Government Agencies

1817 NIH/National Eye Institute
31 Center Drive MSC 2510
Bethesda, MD 20892
301-496-5248
2020@nei.nih.gov
www.nei.nih.gov

Conducts and supports research that helps prevent and treat eye diseases and other disorders of vision. This research leads to sight-saving treatments, reduces visual impairment and blindness, and improves the quality of life for people of all ages. NEI-supported research has advanced our knowledge of how the eye functions in health and disease.

Paul A Sieving M.D., Ph.D., Director

National Associations & Support Groups

1818 American Academy of Pediatrics
141 Northwest Point Boulevard
Elk Grove Village, IL 60007
847-434-4000
800-433-9016
Fax: 847-434-8000
www.aap.org

The American Academy of Pediatrics and its member pediatricians are committed to the attainment of optimal physical, mental and social health and well-being for all infants, children, adolescents, and young adults.

Fernando Stein, MD, FAAP, President
Karen Remley, MD, CEO/Executive VP

1819 American Council of the Blind
1703 N Beauregard Street, Ste 420
Alexandria, VA 22311
202-467-5081
800-424-8666
Fax: 202-467-5085
info@acb.org
www.acb.org

The American Council of the Blind strives to increase the independence, security, equality of opportunity, and quality of life, for all blind and visually-impaired people.

Eric Bridges, Executive Director
Anthony Stephens, Director, Advocacy/Govt'l Affairs
Nancy Marks-Becker, Chief Accountant

1820 Association for Education & Rehabilitation of the Blind & Visually Impaired
1703 N Beauregard Street, Suite 440
Alexandria, VA 22311
703-671-4500
877-492-2708
Fax: 703-671-6391
markr@aerbvi.org
www.aerbvi.org

The Association for Education and Rehabilitation of the Blind and Visually Impaired (AER) is the only international membership organization dedicated to rendering all possible support and assistance to the professionals who work in all phases of education and rehabilitation of blind and visually impaired children and adults. Our membership is comprised of more than 4,200 professionalswho provide services to people with visual impairment.

Lou Tutt, Executive Director
Ginger Croce, Senior Director, Marketing and Offi
Barbara James, Director, Membership and Office Ope

1821 Genetic Alliance
4301 Connecticut Avenue NW, Suite 404
Washington, DC 20008
202-966-5557
800-336-4363
Fax: 202-966-8553
info@geneticalliance.org
www.geneticalliance.org

World's leading nonprofit health advocacy organization committed to transforming health through genetics and promoting an environment of openness centered on the health of individuals, families, and communities.

Sharon Terry, President/CEO
Tetyana Murza, Managing Director
Natasha Bonhomme, VP, Strategic Development

1822 National Association for Parents of Children with Visual Impairments
175 N Beacon Street
Watertown, MA 00247
617-972-7441
800-562-6265
Fax: 617-972-7444
napvi@guildhealth.org
www.spedex.com/napvi/

NAPVI is a national organization that enables parents to find information and resources for their children who are blind or visually impaired, including those with additional disabilities. NAPVI provides leadership, support, and training to assist parents in helping children reach their potential.

Susan LaVenture, Executive Director
Julie Urban, President
Venetia Hayden, Vice President

1823 National Association for Visually Handicapped
111 East 59th Street The Sol and Lillian Goldman B
New York, NY 10022
212-821-9200
800-829-0500
Fax: 212-821-9707
TTY: 212-821-9713
info@lighthouse.org
www.lighthouse.org/navh

The only nonprofit health organization in the world solely dedicated to providing assistance to the partially sighted. Serves as a clearinghouse for information about all services available to the partially-sighted from public and private sources. Conducts self-help groups. Provides information on large print books, textbooks and educational tools.

Mark G. Ackermann, President and Chief Executive Offic
Maura J. Sweeney, Senior Vice President, Chief Operat
John Vlachos, Senior Vice President, Chief Financ

State Agencies & Support Groups

Alabama

1824 Alabama Institute for the Deaf & Blind
PO Box 698 (35161) 205 East South Street
Talladega, AL 35160
256-761-3331
Fax: 256-761-3344
www.aidb.org

Services include central directory, representatives of agencies, service providers, families, and coordinators of infant, toddler, and preschool special education programs.

Charlotte Lowry, Principal
Martha Waites, Director, Academic Department
Teresa Lacy, Director, Library and Resource Cent

Arizona

1825 National Association for Parents of the Visually Impaired
175 N Beacon Street
Watertown, MA 02472
617-972-7441
800-562-6265
Fax: 617-972-7444
napvi@guildhealth.org
www.spedex.com/napvi/

NAPVI is a national organization that enables parents to find information and resources for their children who are blind or visually impaired, including those with additional disabilities. NAPVI provides leadership, support, and training to assist parents in helping children reach their potential.

Susan LaVenture, Executive Director
Julie Urban, President
Venetia Hayden, Vice President

Ohio

1826 Region 2 of the National Association for Parents of the Visually Impaired
3910 Pocahontas Avenue
Cincinnati, OH 45227
513-561-8542
napvi@guildhealth.org
www.spedex.com/napvi

Susan LaVenture, Executive Director
Julie Urban, President
Venetia Hayden, Vice President

Pennsylvania

1827 East Central Region-Helen Keller National Center
4351 Garden City Drive
New Carrollton, MD 20785
301-459-5474
Fax: 301-459-5070
hkncreg3cl@aol.com
www.helenkeller.org

Christopher D Maher, Chairman
Richard T. Arkwright, Vice-Chairman
John R Caughey, Treasurer

South Carolina

1828 Region 4 of the National Association for Parents of the Visually Impaired
1032 Trail Road
Belton, SC 29627
864-338-9593

Washington

1829 Northwestern Region-Helen Keller National Center
1620 18th Ave Suite 201
Seattle, WA 98122
206-324-9120
Fax: 206-324-9159
TTY: 206-324-1133
nwhknc@juno.com
www.hknc.org/FieldServicesREGREPADD.htm

The Regional Representatives of HKNC are located in ten offices across the country. They are responsible for assessing the needs of individuals, communities and states within their regions; developing strategies of collaboration, coordination and cooperation to help meet those needs; advocating for those who are deaf-blind in local, state, national and international forums.

Libraries & Resource Centers

Arizona

1830 Educational Services for the Visually Impaired
PO Box 668
Little Rock, AR 72203
501-371-5710

Offers textbooks, braille books and more to the visually impaired grades K-12 in the Arkansas area.

David Beavers, Director

Arkansas

1831 Arkansas Regional Library for the Blind and Physically Handicapped
900 W Capitol, Suite 100
Little Rock, AR 72201
501-682-2053
Fax: 501-682-1533
TDD: 501-682-1002
nlsbooks@asl.lib.ar.us
www.asl.lib.ar.us/ASL_LBPH.htm

Public library books in recorded or braille format. Popular fiction and nonfiction books for all ages, books and players are on free loan, sent to patrons by mail and may be returned postage free. Anyone who cannot see well enough to read regular print with glasses on or who has a disability that makes it difficult to hold a book or turn the pages is eligible.

John D Hall, Director

California

1832 American Action Fund for Blind Children and Adults
1800 Johnson Street
Baltimore, MD 21230

410-659-9315
Fax: 818-343-3219
lucyabba@aol.com
www.actionfund.org

A lending library for the visually impaired. We send out a weekly Braille newspaper for the deaf-blind (worldwide), we also send out pocket-sized Braille calendars. Our lending library is for pre-school thru high school. All of our services are free.

Barbara Loos, President
Ramona Walhof, Vice President
Gary Mackenstadt, Secretary

1833 Blind Children's Center
4120 Marathon Street
Los Angeles, CA 90029

323-664-2153
Fax: 323-665-3828
www.blindchildrenscenter.org

Offers support and informational groups.

Midge Horton, Executive Director

1834 Braille Institute Desert Center
741 N Vermont Avenue
Los Angeles, CA 90029

323-663-1111
Fax: 323-663-0867
la@brailleinstitute.org
www.brailleinstitute.org

Dedicated to providing blind and visually impaired men, women and children with the training, programs and services they need to enjoy productive lives. Services offered include child development, youth programs, library services and adult education.

Lars Hansen, Manager

1835 Braille Institute Sight Center
741 N Vermont Avenue
Los Angeles, CA 90029

323-663-1111
Fax: 323-663-0867
la@brailleinstitute.org
www.brailleinstitute.org

Offers help, programs, services and information to the blind and visually impaired children and adults.

Les Stocker, President

1836 Braille Institute Youth Center
3450 Cahuenga Boulevard W
Los Angeles, CA 90068

213-851-5695

Offers various youth programs and services for the blind and visually impaired youngster.

1837 New Beginnings - Blind Children's Center
4120 Marathon, Street
Los Angeles, CA 90029

323-664-2153
800-222-3566
Fax: 323-665-3828

Helps children and their families become independent by creating a climate of safety and trust. Services include an infant stimulation program, educational preschool, interdisciplinary assessment services, family services, correspondence program, toll-free national hotline and a publication and research service.

1838 San Francisco Public Library for the Blind and Print Disabled
PO Box 9428327
Sacramento, CA 94237

916-654-0261
Fax: 415-557-4252
lbphmgr@sfpl.lib.ca.us
www.library.ca.us

Foreign-language books on cassette, children's books on cassettes and more.

Luis Herrera, Manager

1839 Variety Audio
PO Box 5731
San Jose, CA 95150

408-277-4839

Summer reading programs, braille writer, magnifiers, closed-circuit TV, large-print photocopier, cassette books and magazines, children's books on cassette, home visits and other reference materials on blindness and other handicaps.

Louisa Griehshammer

District of Columbia

1840 Council of Families with Visual Impairment
1155 15th Street NW
Washington, DC 20005

202-467-5081

Members are sighted parents of blind or visually impaired children. Offers a forum for support and outreach, sharing of experiences in parent-child relationships, and educational and cultural information about child development. Monitors developments in technical and legislative arenas.

Nola Webb, President

Florida

1841 Florida Bureau of Braille and Talking Book Library Services
420 Platt Street
Daytona Beach, FL 32114

386-239-6000
Fax: 386-239-6069
TDD: 800-226-6079
mike_gunde@dbs.doe.state.fl.us
www.state.fl.us/dbs/lswel.html

Discs, cassettes, closed-circuit TV, large-print photocopier, films, children's books on cassettes and more.

Michael Gunde, Librarian

1842 Talking Book Library, Jacksonville Public Library
2233 Park Avenue, Suite 402
Orange Park, FL 32073

904-278-5620
Fax: 904-278-5625
TDD: 904-768-7822
jerryr@coj.net
www.neflin.org

Discs, cassettes and reference materials on blindness and other disabilities.

Jerry Reynolds, Librarian Senior

1843 Talking Book Service - Manatee County Central Library
1112 Manatee Avenue West
Bradenton, FL 34205

941-748-4501
Fax: 941-751-7089
TDD: 941-742-5951
webmaster@mymanatee.org
www.mymanatee.org

Offers children's books on disc and cassette and more reference materials for the blind and physically handicapped.

Patricia Schubert, Librarian

Georgia

1844 Albany Library for the Blind and Physical Handicapped
300 Pine Avenue
Albany, GA 31701   229-420-3220
                                        Fax: 229-420-3215
sinquefk@mail.dougherty.public.lib.ga.us
www.docolib.org/LBPH/index.html

Offers discs, cassettes, reference materials on blindness and other handicaps, large-print photocopiers, summer reading programs, cassette books and more.

Katy Sinquefield, Manager

1845 Bainbridge Subregional Library for the Blind and Physically Handicapped
215 Sycamore Street
Decatur, GA 30030   404-370-8450
                                                800-795-2680
                                        Fax: 404-370-8469
TDD: 912-248-2665
lbph@mail.deccatur.public.lib.ga.us
www.dekalblibrary.org

Discs, cassettes, summer reading programs, closed-circuit TV, magnifiers and more.

Jon Abercrombie, Chairman
Julia H Jones, Vice Chairman
Elizabeth Joyner, Treasurer

1846 CEL Subregional Library for the Blind and Physically Handicapped
2708 Mechanics
Savannah, GA 31404   912-354-5864
                                        Fax: 912-354-5534
TDD: 912-652-3635
stokesl@cel.co.chatman.ga.us

Summer reading programs, braille writer, magnifiers, closed-circuit TV, large-print photocopier, cassette books and magazines, children's books on cassette, home visits and other reference materials on blindness and other handicaps.

Linda Stokes, Librarian

Idaho

1847 Idaho State Talking Book Library
325 W State Street
Boise, ID 83702   208-334-2150
                                                800-458-3271
                                        Fax: 208-334-4016
TDD: 800-377-1363
tblbooks@isl.state.id.us
www.lili.org/isl/tblinfo.htm

Summer reading programs, braille writer, magnifiers, closed-circuit TV, large-print photocopier, cassette books and magazines, children's books on cassette, home visits and other reference materials on blindness and other handicaps.

Sue Walker, Manager

Illinois

1848 Chicago Library Service for the Blind
1055 W Roosevelt Road
Chicago, IL 60608   312-746-9210

Summer reading programs, braille writer, magnifiers, closed-circuit TV, large-print photocopier, cassette books and magazines, children's books on cassette, home visits and other reference materials on blindness and other handicaps.

Carol Pellish, Librarian

1849 Illinois State Library, Talkng Book and Braille Service
213 State Capitol
Springfield, IL 62756   217-785-5600
                                        Fax: 217-785-4326
TDD: 800-665-5576
sruda@ilsos.net
www.cyberdriveillinois.com

Summer reading programs, braille writer, magnifiers, closed-circuit TV, large-print photocopier, cassette books and magazines, descriptive videos, children's books on cassette, home visits and other reference materials on blindness and other handicaps.

Anne Craig, Executive Director

1850 Mid Illinois Talking Book System
515 York Street
Quincy, IL 62301   217-224-6619
                                        Fax: 217-224-9818

Summer reading programs, braille writer, magnifiers, closed-circuit TV, large-print photocopier, cassette books and magazines, children's books on cassette, home visits and other reference materials on blindness and other handicaps.

1851 Mid-Illinois Talking Book Center
600 High Point Lane
East Peoria, IL 61611   309-353-4110
                                                800-426-0709
                                        Fax: 309-353-8281
hitbc@darkstar.rsa.lib.il.us
www.mitbc.org

Summer reading programs, braille writer, magnifiers, closed-circuit TV, large-print photocopier, cassette books and magazines, children's books on cassette, home visits and other reference materials on blindness and other handicaps.

Eileen Sheppard, Librarian

1852 Talking Book Center of Northwest Illinois
Ste 2
East Peoria, IL 61611   309-694-9200
                                        Fax: 309-799-7916
kodean@libby.rbls.lib.il.us
www.rbls.lib.il.us

Subregional library provides Talking Book and Braille Book programs to eligible persons unable to use standard print materials due to visual or physical disabilities. Includes cassette books and magazines; summer reading program.

Indiana

1853 Northwest Indiana Subregional Library for Blind and Physically Handicapped
1919 W Lincoln Highway
Merrillville, IN 46410   219-769-3541
                                        Fax: 219-769-0690

Summer reading programs, braille writer, magnifiers, closed-circuit TV, large-print photocopier, cassette books and magazines, children's books on cassette, home visits and other reference materials on blindness and other handicaps.

Renee Lewis

Iowa

1854 Iowa Library for the Blind and Physically Handicapped
Iowa Department for the Blind
524 4th Street
Des Moines, IA 50309   515-281-1333
                                        Fax: 515-281-1378
TDD: 515-281-1355
keninger.karen@blind.state.ia.us
www.blind.state.ia.us

Summer reading programs, magnifiers, closed-circuit TV, large-print photocopier, children's books on cassette, children's books in Braille and Print Braille, cassette magazines, home visits and reference materials on blindness and other handicaps.

Karen Keninger, Program Manager/Librarian

1855 University of Iowa Birth Defects and Genetic Disorders Unit
2614 JCP
Iowa City, IA 52242   319-335-9901
James M Smith, Director

Kansas

1856 CKLS Headquarters
PO Box 515
Northampton, MA 01061   413-268-7660
                                                   888-622-8527
                                              Fax: 316-792-5495
                                                amdf@mascular.org
                                                  www.macular.org

Summer reading programs, braille writer, magnifiers, closed-circuit TV, large-print photocopier, cassette books and magazines, children's books on cassette, home visits and other reference materials on blindness and other handicaps.

Chip Goehring, President/Treasurer
Mark E Torrey, Vice President
Paul F Gariepy, Secretary

1857 Services for the Visually Disabled
629 Poyntz Avenue
Manhattan, KS 66502   785-776-4741
                                              Fax: 785-776-1545
                                           marionr@manhattan.lib.ks.us

Summer reading programs, braille writer, magnifiers, closed-circuit TV, large-print photocopier, cassette books and magazines, children's books on cassette, home visits and other reference materials on blindness and other handicaps.

Marion Rice, Librarian

Kentucky

1858 Kentucky Library for the Blind and Physically Handicapped
PO Box 818
Frankfort, KY 40602   502-564-8300
                                                   800-372-2968
                                              Fax: 502-564-5773
                                           richard.feindel@kdla.net
                                          www.kdla.net/libserv/ktbl.htm

Large-print photocopier, cassette books and magazines, children's books on cassette, and other reference materials on blindness and other handicaps.

5,200 members

Richard Feindel, Librarian

Maryland

1859 Maryland State Library for the Blind and Physically Handicapped
415 Park Avenue
Baltimore, MD 21201   410-230-2424
                                              Fax: 410-333-2095
                                              TTY: 800-934-2541
                                              TDD: 410-333-8679
                                           recept@lbta.lib.md.us
                                              www.lbph.lib.md.us

Summer reading programs, braille writer, magnifiers, large-print photocopier, cassette books and magazines, children's books on cassette, and other reference materials on blindness and other handicaps.

Jill Lewis, Manager

1860 Prince George's County Memorial Library Talking Book Center
6530 Adelphi Road
Hyattsville, MD 20782   301-779-9330

Summer reading programs, braille writer, magnifiers, closed-circuit TV, large-print photocopier, cassette books and magazines, children's books on cassette, home visits and other reference materials on blindness and other handicaps.

Shirley Tuthill, Librarian

Massachusetts

1861 Braille and Talking Book Library Perkins School for the Blind
175 N Beacon Street
Watertown, MA 02472   617-924-3434
                                              Fax: 617-972-7315
                                                 info@perkins.org
                                                 www.perkins.org

Steven M Rothstein, President
Micheal Schnitman, Secretary
Charles C J Platt, Treasurer

Michigan

1862 Downtown Detroit Subregional Library for the Blind and Handicapped
5201 Woodward Avenue
Detroit, MI 48202   313-224-0580
                                              Fax: 313-965-1977
                                              TDD: 313-224-0584
                                          dir@detroitpubliclibrary.org
                                              www.detroit.lib.mi.us

Summer reading programs, braille writer, magnifiers, closed-circuit TV, large-print photocopier, cassette books and magazines, children's books on cassette, home visits and other reference materials on blindness and other handicaps.

Russell Bellant, President
Gregory Hicks, Vice President
Jonathan C Kinloch, Secretary

1863 Kent County Library for the Blind
775 Ball Avenue NE
Grand Rapids, MI 49503   616-336-3250
                                              Fax: 616-336-3201
                                           kdlem@lakeland.lib.mi.us

Summer reading programs, braille writer, magnifiers, closed-circuit TV, large-print photocopier, cassette books and magazines, children's books on cassette, home visits and other reference materials on blindness and other handicaps.

Claudya Muller, Librarian

1864 Library of Michigan Service for the Blind
PO Box 30007
Lansing, MI 48909   517-373-1300
                                              Fax: 517-373-5700
                                          info@sbph.libomich.lib.mi.us

Summer reading programs, braille writer, magnifiers, closed-circuit TV, large-print photocopier, cassette books and magazines, children's books on cassette, home visits and other reference materials on blindness and other handicaps.

Nancy Robertson, Manager

1865 Macomb Library for the Blind and Physically Handicapped
16480 Hall Road
Clinton Township, MI 48038   586-286-1580
                                              Fax: 586-286-0634
                                              TDD: 810-869-40
                                              macbld@libcoop.net
                                          www.macomb.lib.mi.us/macspe/

Summer reading programs, braille writer, closed-circuit TV, cassette books and magazines, children's books on cassette, reference materials on blindness and other handicaps.

Beverlee Babcock, Executive Director

1866 Mideastern Michigan Library Co-op
G-4195 W Pasadena Avenue
Flint, MI 48504   810-732-1120
                                              Fax: 810-732-1715
                                          cnash@genesse.freeret.org
                                          www.fakon.edu/gdl/talking.htm

Summer reading programs, braille writer, magnifiers, closed-circuit TV, large-print photocopier, cassette books and magazines, children's books on cassette, home visits and other reference materials on blindness and other handicaps.

Carolyn Nash, Librarian

1867 Muskegon County Library for the Blind
635 Ottawa Street
Muskegon, MI 49442
231-724-6361
Fax: 231-724-6675
TDD: 231-722-4103
www.muskcolib.org

Summer reading programs, braille typewriter, magnifiers, closed-circuit TV, large-print photocopier, cassette books and magazines, children's books on cassette, home visits and other reference materials on blindness and other handicaps, The Reading Edge, Perkins Brailler and large print books.

Linda Clapp, Librarian

1868 Upper Peninsula Library for the Blind Physically Handicapped
1615 Presque Isle Avenue
Marquette, MI 49855
906-228-7697
Fax: 906-228-5627
uproc.lib.mi.us
www.upesc.lib.mi.us/uplbph

Summer reading programs, braille writer, magnifiers, closed-circuit TV, large-print photocopier, cassette books and magazines, children's books on cassette, home visits and other reference materials on blindness and other handicaps.

Suzanne Dees, Executive Director

1869 Washtenaw County Library
PO Box 8645
Ann Arbor, MI 48107
734-994-4912
Fax: 734-663-2430
contact us@ewashtenaw.org
www.ewashtenaw.org

Summer reading programs, braille writer, magnifiers, closed-circuit TV, large-print photocopier, cassette books and magazines, children's books on cassette, home visits and other reference materials on blindness and other handicaps.

Kyeena Slater, Executive Director

1870 Washtenaw County Library for the Blind and Physically Disabled
PO Box 8645
Ann Arbor, MI 48107
734-222-4357
Fax: 734-222-6850
lbpd@co.washtennaw.mi.us
www.ewashtenaw.org

Book lovers club.adaptive technology,cassette equipment, cassette books and magazines, described videos, low vision aids reference and referral services.

Kyeena Slater, Executive Director

1871 Wayne County Regional Library for the Blind
30555 Michigan Avenue
Westland, MI 48186
734-727-7300
888-968-2737
Fax: 734-727-7333
TTY: 734-727-7330
wcrlbph@wayneregional.lib.mi.us
www.wayneregional.lib.mi.us

Summer reading programs, braille writer, magnifiers, closed-circuit TV, large-print photocopier, cassette books and magazines, children's books on cassette, home visits and other reference materials on blindness and other handicaps.

Reginald Williams, Wayne County Librarian

Minnesota

1872 Minnesota Library for the Blind & Physically Handicapped
Highway 298, PO Box 68
Fairbault, MN 55021
507-333-4828
800-722-0550
Fax: 507-333-4832
libblnd@state.mn.us
www.nfb.org/libraries for the blind

Summer reading programs, braille writer, magnifiers, closed-circuit TV, large-print photocopier, cassette, large-print books and magazines, children's books on cassette, and other reference materials on blindness and other handicaps.

Catherine A Durivage, Program Director

Missouri

1873 Adriene Resource Center for Blind Children
1445 N. Boonville Avenue
Springfield, MO 65802
417-862-2781
800-641-4310
Fax: 417-862-7566
blind@ag.org
www.gospelpublishing.com

Offers braille and cassette lending library, braille and cassette Sunday school materials for all ages, braille and cassette periodicals and resource assistance, and resources for blind children and children of blind parents.

Paul Weingariner, Director

1874 Assemblies of God National Center for the Blind
1445 N. Boonville Avenue
Springfield, MO 65802
417-862-2781
877-840-4800
Fax: 417-863-6614
info@aq.org
www.ag.org

Offers braille and cassette lending library, braille and cassette Sunday school materials for all ages, braille and cassette periodicals and resource assistance, and resources for blind children and children of blind parents.

Thomas Trask, Manager
Greg Mundis, Executive Director

1875 Wolfner Memorial Library for the Blind
PO Box 387
Jefferson City, MO 65102
573-751-8720
Fax: 573-526-2985
TDD: 800-347-1379
beckles@mail.sos.state.mo.us
www.nfb.org/libraries for the blind

Summer reading programs, braille writer, magnifiers, closed-circuit TV, large-print photocopier, cassette books and magazines, children's books on cassette, home visits and other reference materials on blindness and other handicaps.

Richard J Smith, Executive Director

Nebraska

1876 Nebraska Library Commission Talking Book & Braille Services
1200 N Street
Lincoln, NE 68508
402-471-2045
800-742-7691
Fax: 402-471-2083
TDD: 402-471-4038
david.oertli@nebraska.gov
www.nlc.nebraska.gov

Free loan of books and magazines on cartridge, cassette, and in Braille, including children's materials, along with specially designed playback equipment. Summer reading program for children, Braille embossing, closed circuit TV, large-print copier. Reference materials on blindness and other disabilities.

David Oerti, Librarian

New Jersey

1877 New Jersey State Library Talking Book and Braille Center
185 West State Street
Trenton, NJ 08625

609-278-2640
800-792-8322
Fax: 609-278-2647
TDD: 877-882-5593
njlbh@njstatelib.org
www.njstatelib.org

Free home delivery of large-print, audio, and braille books and magazines, children's books on cassettes in braille and other reference materials on blindness and other handicaps. Services are for New Jersey residents with print disabilities.

Adan Szczepaniak, Director
Anne McArthur, Head of Outreach and Audiovision

New Mexico

1878 New Mexico State Library for the Blind and Physically Handicapped
1209 Camino Carlos Ray
Santa Fe, NM 87507

505-476-9700
Fax: 505-476-9761
jbrewstr@stlib.state.nm.us
www.stlib.state.nm.us

Summer reading programs, braille writer, magnifiers, closed-circuit TV, large-print photocopier, cassette books and magazines, children's books on cassette, home visits and other reference materials on blindness and other handicaps.

Susan Overland, Manager

New York

1879 New York State Talking Book & Braille Library
National Library Service/NYS Library
Empire State Plaza, CEC
Albany, NY 12230

518-474-5935
800-342-3688
Fax: 518-486-1957
tbbl@mail.nysed.gov
www.nysl.nysed.gov/tbbl

Recorded books and players, recorded magazines, braille books, braille writers, magnifiers, closed-circuit TV, children's books on cassette, reference materials on blindness and other disabilities. Service is completely free to eligible borrowers, including loan of equipment to listen to books. Over 60,000 titles available.

Sharon B Phillips, Library Program Director

North Carolina

1880 North Carolina Library for the Blind
1811 Capital Boulevard
Raleigh, NC 27635

919-733-4376
Fax: 919-733-6910
TDD: 919-733-1462
nclbph@ncsl.der.state.nc
www.nfb.org/libraries for the blind

Summer reading programs, braille writer, magnifiers, closed-circuit TV, large-print photocopier, cassette books and magazines, children's books on cassette, home visits and other reference materials on blindness and other handicaps.

Francine Martin, Manager

Ohio

1881 American Council of Blind Parents
34400 Cedar Road, Apartment 108
University Heights, OH 44121

800-424-8666

Members are sighted parents of blind or visually impaired children. Offers a forum for support and outreach, sharing of experiences in parent-child relationships, and educational and cultural information about child development. Monitors developments in technical and legislative arenas.

Nola Webb, President

Oregon

1882 Oregon State Library, Talking Book and Braille Services
250 Winter Street NE
Salem, OR 97301

503-378-5389
800-452-0292
Fax: 503-585-8059
TDD: 503-378-4276
tbabs@sparkie.osl.state.or.us
www.tbabs.org

Cassette books and magazines, children's books on cassette, home visits and other reference materials on blindness and other handicaps.

Susan Westin, Manager

Virginia

1883 Alexandria Library Talking Book Service
5005 Duke Street
Alexandria, VA 22304

703-746-1702
Fax: 703-519-5916
TDD: 703-838-4568
emccaffr@lea.eda
www.alexandria.lib.va.us

Summer reading programs, braille writer, magnifiers, closed-circuit TV, large-print photocopier, cassette books and magazines, children's books on cassette, home visits and other reference materials on blindness and other handicaps.

Karen Russell, Manager

1884 Division for the Visually Handicapped
1920 Association Drive
Reston, VA 20191

703-620-3660

Members are teachers, college faculty members, administrators, supervisors and others concerned with the education and welfare of visually handicapped and blind children and youth. This is a division of the Council For Exceptional Children.

Dr. Kay Ferrell, President

1885 Division on Visual Impairments
Council for Exceptional Children
1110 North Glebe Road, Suite 300
Arlington, VA 22201

800-224-6830
Fax: 703-264-9494
TTY: 866-915-5000
www.ed.arizona.edu/dvi/welcome.htm; www.cec.sped.org

A division within the CEC, it handles concerns for Federal, state and local issues and policies related to education of youths, children and infants with visual impairments.

Ellyn Ross, President
Shirley J Wilson, Secretary
Phyllis T Simmons, President Elect

1886 Virginia State Library for the Visually and Physically Handicapped
1901 Roane Street
Richmond, VA 23222

804-367-0014

Summer reading programs, braille writer, magnifiers, closed-circuit TV, large-print photocopier, cassette books and magazines, children's books on cassette, home visits and other reference materials on blindness and other handicaps.

Mary Ruth Halapatz, Librarian

1887 Washington Library for the Blind and Physically Handicapped
1000 Fourth Avenue
Seattle, WA 98104
206-386-4636
Fax: 206-386-4685
wtbbl@spl.lib.wa.us
www.spl.lib.wa.us

Summer reading programs, braille writer, magnifiers, closed-circuit TV, large-print photocopier, cassette books and magazines, children's books on cassette, home visits and other reference materials on blindness and other handicaps.

Jan Ames, Librarian

West Virginia

1888 West Virginia School for the Blind
301 E Main Street
Romney, WV 26757
304-822-4801
Fax: 304-822-3370
cjohn@access.mountain.net

Summer reading programs, braille writer, magnifiers, closed-circuit TV, large-print photocopier, cassette books and magazines, children's books on cassette, home visits and other reference materials on blindness and other handicaps.

Patsy Shank, Administrator

Research Centers

1889 American Association for Pediatric Ophthalmology and Strabismus
PO Box 193832
San Francisco, CA 94119
415-561-8505
Fax: 415-561-8531
aapos@aao.org
www.aapos.org

Provides support and resources for Pediatric Ophthalmologists, Strabismologists, related personnel and their patients by way of its Internet Website.

David K. Epley MD, President
Christie L Morse, MD, Executive Vice President
Sharon F. Freedman, M.D, Vice President

1890 Center for the Partially Sighted
7462 North Figueroa Boulevard Suite 103
Los Angeles, CA 90041
310-988-1970
Fax: 310-988-1980
info@low-vision.org
www.low-vision.org

Our mission is to provide the tools and techniques that maximize the ability of partially sighted children and adults to live successful and independent lives

James Adler, Esq., Board
Steve Edwards, Board
Brenda Premo, Board

1891 Mobile Association for the Blind
2440 Gordon Smith Drive
Mobile, AL 36617
251-473-3585
877-292-5463
Fax: 251-470-8622
sales@mobile.blind.com
www.mobileblind.org

The American Foundation for the Blind removes barriers, creates solutions, and expands possibilities so people with vision loss can achieve their full potential

Jim Bullock, Executive Director

1892 New Beginnings - The Blind Children's Center
4120 Marathon Street
Los Angeles, CA 90029
213-664-2153
Fax: 323-665-3828
www.blindchildrenscenter.org/about.html

The purpose of the Center is to turn initial fears into hope. Helps children and their families become independent by creating a climate of safety and trust. Children learn to develop self confidence and to master a wide range of skills. Services include an infant stimulation program, educational preschool, interdisciplinary assessment services, family services, correspondence program, toll free national hotline and a publication and research service.

1893 Pediatric Ophathalmology and Adult Strabis mus Service Research
Indiana University
702 Rotary Circle
Indianapolis, IN 46202
317-274-2128
Fax: 317-274-2277
dplager@iupui.edu
www.iupui.edu/~ophthal/

Improve techniques and treatment modalities for children with eye and vision problems, such as cataracts, glaucoma, retinopathy of prematurity, and for both children and adults with eye muscle abnormalities.

David A Plager, MD, Director

1894 Research to Prevent Blindness
645 Madison Avenue Floor 21
New York, NY 10022
212-752-4333
800-621-0026
Fax: 212-688-6231
inforequest@rpbusa.org
www.rpbusa.org/rpb/about/overview/

Provides research grants to scientists interested in eye disease and vision disorders.

David F Weeks, Chairman Emeritus
Brian F. Hofland, PhD, President/Secretary
John I Bloomberg, Vice President

Conferences

1895 AADB National Symposium
American Association of the Deaf-Blind
PO Box 2831
Kensington, MD 20891
301-495-4403
Fax: 301-495-4404
TTY: 301-495-4402
aadb-info@aadb.org
www.aadb.org

The symposium offers a training workshop, keynote speakers, full day exhibit hall, demonstration room, awards lunch and ceremony, talent show, Walk-A-Thon, and a banquet and dance.

Jill Gaus, President
Lynn Jansen, Vice President
Debby Lieberman, Secretary

1896 AER Regional Conference
1703 N Beauregard Street, Suite 440
Alexandria, VA 22311
703-671-4500
877-492-2708
Fax: 703-671-6391
markr@aerbvi.org
www.aerbvi.org

August

Lou Tutt EdD, Executive Director
Ginger Croce, Senior Director

1897 Genetic Alliance Annual Conference
Genetic Alliance
4301 Connecticut Avenue NW, Suite 404
Washington, DC 20008
202-966-5557
800-336-4363
Fax: 202-966-8553
info@geneticalliance.org
www.geneticalliance.org

Consistently inspirational and enables partnership among all stakeholders: advocates and community leaders, health and industry professionals, policymakers, and academicians.

July

Sharon Terry, President/CEO
Tetyana Murza, Managing Director
Natasha Bonhomme, VP, Strategic Development

Audio Video

1898 Heart to Heart
Blind Children's Center
4120 Marathon Street
Los Angeles, CA 90029

323-644-2153
Fax: 323-665-3828
www.blindcntr.org

Parents of blind and partially sighted children talk about their feelings.
Videotape

1899 Let's Eat
Blind Children's Center
4120 Marathon Street
Los Angeles, CA 90029

323-664-2153
Fax: 323-665-3828
www.blindchildrenscenter.org

Teaches competent feeding skills to children with visual impairments.
Videotape

1900 See What I Feel
Britannica Film Co.
345 4th Street
San Francisco, CA 94107

415-597-5555

A blind child tells her friends about her trip to the zoo. Each experience was explained as a blind child would experience it. A teacher's guide comes with this video.
Films

Web Sites

1901 American Association for Pediatric Ophthalmology and Strabismus
P.O. Box 193832
San Francisco, CA 94119

415-561-8505
Fax: 415-561-8531
www.aapos.org

Provides support and resources for Pediatric Ophthalmologists, Strabismologists, related personnel and their patients by way of its Internet Website.

Sherwin J. Isenberg, MD, President
M. Edward Wilson, MD, Vice President
Christie L. Morse, MD, Executive Vice President

1902 Lighthouse Guild
15 West 65th Street
New York, NY 10023

212-769-6200
800-284-4422
info@lighthouseguild.org
www.lighthouseguild.org

Since 1905, Lighthouse International has led the charge in the fight against vision loss through prevention, treatment and empowerment. In 2013, it merged with Jewish Guild Healthcare to form a leading non profit vision and healthcare organization.

Alan R. Morse, President/CEO
Mark G. Ackermann, Executive VP/COO
Maura J. Sweeney, Senior VP, Programs & Services

1903 National Alliance of Blind Students
Los Angeles, CA

608-332-4147
smwhalenpsp@gmail.com
nabslink.org

The leading national advocacy and consumer organization for students in high school or college who are blind or visually impaired.

Sean Whalen, President
Karen Anderson, 1st Vice President
Gabe Cazares, 2nd Vice President

1904 National Association for Visually Handicapped
111 E 59th St
New York, NY 10022

800-284-4422
info@lighthouseguild.org
www.lighthouseguild.org

Helps to cope with the difficulties of vision impairment.

1905 Online Mendelian Inheritance in Man
National Library of Medicine, Building 38A
Bethesda, MD 20894

888-346-3656
info@ncbi.nlm.nih.gov
www.ncbi.nlm.nih.gov

This database is a catalog of human genes and genetic disorders.

Christine E. Seidman, M.D., Chair
David J. Lipman, M.D., Executive Secretary

1906 Royal National Institute of the Blind
www.rnib.org.uk

303-123-9999
helpline@rnib.org.uk
www.rnib.org.uk

Offering information, support and advice to people with sight problems.

Lesley-Anne Alexander CBE, Chief Executive
Wanda Hamilton, Group Director (Fundraising)
Sally Harvey, Managing Director (RNIB Places)

Book Publishers

1907 Children with Visual Impairments: A Parents' Guide
Peytral Publications
PO Box 1162
Minnetonka, MN 55345

952-949-8707
877-739-8725
Fax: 952-906-9777
www.peytral.com

Covers visual impairments ranging from low vision to total blindness. Offers authoritative information and empathy, parental insight on diagnosis and treatment, orientation and mobility, literacy, legal issues and more. Valuable to parents, educators and support staff.

395 pages

M Cay Holbrook PhD, Editor

1908 Ophthalmic Disorders Sourcebook
Omnigraphics Editorial Office
615 Griswold
Detroit, MI 48226

313-961-1340
800-234-1340
Fax: 313-961-1383
editorial@omnigraphics.com
www.omnigraphics.com

Basic consumer information about glaucoma, cataracts, macular degeneration, strabismus, refractive disorders and more.

1996 631 pages Hardcover
ISBN: 0-780800-81-8

Linda M Ross, Editor

Magazines

1909 Journal of Visual Impairment and Blindness
American Foundation for the Blind
2 Penn Plaza, Suite 1102
New York, NY 10121

212-502-7600
Fax: 888-545-8331
contributions@afb.net
www.afb.org

213

Published in braille, regular print and on cassette this journal contains a wide variety of subjects including rehabilitation, psychology, education, legislation, medicine, technology, employment, sensory aids and childhood development as they relate to visual impairments.

10x Year

Larry Kimbler, Chair
James H. McLaughlin, Vice Chair
Carl S. Augusto, President & CEO

1910 Reaching, Crawling, Walking - Let's Get Moving
Blind Children's Center
4120 Marathon Street
Los Angeles, CA 90029   323-664-2153
                                   Fax: 323-665-3828
                          info@blindchildrenscenter.org
                          www.blindchildrenscenter.org

Orientation and mobility for visually impaired preschool children.

24 pages

1911 Tactic
Clovernook Home and School for the Blind
7000 Hamilton Avenue
Cincinnati, OH 45231   513-522-3860
                                   Fax: 513-728-3950
                              clovernook@aol.com

Quarterly

Newsletters

1912 Gleams
Glaucoma Research Foundation
251 Post Street, Suite 600
San Francisco, CA 94108   415-986-3162
                                       800-826-6693
                                   Fax: 415-986-3763
                             question@glaucoma.org
                                www.glaucoma.org

Includes information about glaucoma, new treatments, updates on research findings, and more.

3x/year

Thomas M. Brunner, President/ CEO
Nancy Graydon, Executive Director of Development
Andrew L. Jackson, Director of Communications

1913 NAVH Update
National Association for Visually Handicapped
111 E 59th St
New York, NY 10022   212-889-3141
                                       800-284-4422
                                   Fax: 212-727-2931
                             info@lighthouseguild.org
                                    lighthouse.org

Quarterly

Alan R. Morse, JD, PhD, President/ CEO
Mark G. Ackermann, EVP/ COO
Elliot J. Hagler, CPA, EVP/ CFO

1914 National Library Service for the Blind & Physically Handicapped
Library of Congress Reference Section
1291 Taylor Street NW
Washington, DC 20542   202-707-5100
                                       800-424-8567
                                   Fax: 202-707-0712
                              TTY: 202-707-0744
                              TDD: 202-707-0744
                                     nls@loc.gov
                                www.loc.gov/nls

Provides information and advocacy resources for families and professionals, including listings of organizations focusing on more specific areas of concern to families and young adults who have disabilities. Administers a natural library service that provides recorded and braille reading materials to eligible children and adults who cannot read standard print.

12 pages Quarterly
ISSN: 1046-1663
Vicki Fitzpatrick, Editor

1915 Talking Book Topics
National Library Services for the Blind
1291 Taylor Street NW
Washington, DC 20542   202-707-5100
                                   Fax: 202-707-0712
                              TDD: 202-707-0744
                                     nls@loc.gov
                                www.loc.gov/nls

Offers hundreds of listings of books, fiction and nonfiction, for adults and children on cassette. Also offers listings on foreign language books on cassette, talking magazines and reviews.

Bimonthly

Pamphlets

1916 Dancing Cheek to Cheek
Blind Children's Center
4120 Marathon Street
Los Angeles, CA 90029   323-664-2153
                                   Fax: 323-665-3828
                          www.blindchildrenscenter.org

Discusses beginning social, play and language interactions.

33 pages

1917 Family Guide - Growth and Development of the Partially Seeing Child
National Association for Visually Handicapped
111 E 59th St
New York, NY 10022   212-889-3141
                                       800-284-4422
                                   Fax: 212-727-2931
                             info@lighthouseguild.org
                                www.lighthouseguild.org

Offers information for parents and guidelines in raising a partially seeing child.

1918 Family Guide to Vision Care
American Optometric Association
243 N Lindbergh Boulevard
Saint Louis, MO 63141   314-991-4100
                                   Fax: 314-991-4101
                                    www.aoanet.org

Offers information on the early developmental years of your vision, finding a family optometrist and how to take care of your eyesight through the learning years, the working years and the mature years.

1919 Heart to Heart
Blind Children's Center
4120 Marathon Street
Los Angeles, CA 90029   323-664-2153
                                   Fax: 323-665-3828
                          www.blindchildrenscenter.org

Parents of blind and partially sighted children talk about their feelings.

12 pages

1920 Learning to Play
Blind Children's Center
4120 Marathon Street
Los Angeles, CA 90029   323-664-2153
                                   Fax: 323-665-3828
                          www.blindchildrenscenter.org

Discusses how to present play activities to the visually impaired preschool child.

12 pages

1921 Let's Eat
Blind Children's Center
4120 Marathon Street
Los Angeles, CA 90029
323-664-2153
Fax: 323-665-3828
www.blindchildrenscenter.org

Teaches competent feeding skills to children with visual impairments.

28 pages

1922 Move with Me
Blind Children's Center
4120 Marathon Street
Los Angeles, CA 90029
323-664-2153
Fax: 323-665-3828
www.blindchildrenscenter.org

A parent's guide to movement development for visually impaired babies.

12 pages

1923 Selecting a Program
Blind Children's Center
4120 Marathon Street
Los Angeles, CA 90029
323-664-2153
Fax: 323-665-3828
www.blindchildrenscenter.org

A guide for parents of infants and preschoolers with visual impairments.

28 pages

1924 Standing on My Own Two Feet
Blind Children's Center
4120 Marathon Street
Los Angeles, CA 90029
323-664-2153
Fax: 323-665-3828
info@blindchildrenscenter.org
www.blindchildrenscenter.org

A step-by-step guide to designing and constructing simple, individually tailored adaptive mobility devices for preschool-age children who are visually impaired.

36 pages

1925 Talk to Me
Blind Children's Center
4120 Marathon Street
Los Angeles, CA 90029
323-664-2153
Fax: 323-665-3828
www.blindchildrenscenter.org

A language guide for parents of deaf children.

11 pages

1926 Talk to Me II
Blind Children's Center
4120 Marathon Street
Los Angeles, CA 90029
323-664-2153
Fax: 323-665-3828
www.blindchildrenscenter.org

A sequel to Talk To Me, available in English and Spanish.

15 pages

Camps

1927 Bloomfield
5300 Angeles Vista Boulevard
Los Angeles, CA 90043
323-295-4555
800-352-2290
Fax: 323-296-0424
info@juniorblind.org
www.juniorblind.org

This camp is dedicated to serving blind and developmentally disabled children and adults.

Miki Jordan, President

1928 Breckenridge Outdoor Education Center
PO Box 697
Breckenridge, CO 80424
970-453-6422
800-383-2632
Fax: 970-453-4676
boec@boec.org
www.boec.org

Camp with a mission to expand the potential of people with disabilities and special needs through meaningful, educational and inspiring outdoor experiences.

Tim Casey, Chair

1929 Camp Civitan
3519 East Shea Blvd # 133
Phoenix, AZ 85028
602-953-2944
Fax: 602-953-2946
info@campcivitan.org
www.campcivitan.org

A 501c3 non-profit organization, that has been providing multiple ever-changing programs to meet the needs of children and adults who are developmentally disabled.

Shannon Valenzuela, Director
Jane Armstrong, Director

1930 Camp Tushmehata
10500 Lincoln Lake Rd, PO Box 46
Greenville, MI 48838
616-754-5410
gwen@campt.org
www.campt.org

Mission is to create and foster unlimited opportunities for blind and partially sighted people throughout Michigan and the world. The camp is comprised mainly of blind adults who have a passion for blind youth. The camp gained the opportunity to implement longer camping sessions, hire a large number of blind role models and steer the camp program into a bright, determined and promising future.

Gwen Botting, Director

1931 Enchanted Hills Camp
Lighthouse
214 Van Ness Avenue
San Francisco, CA 94102
415-694-7319
Fax: 415-863-7568
TTY: 415-431-4572
afletcher@lighthouse-sf.org
www.lighthouse-sf.org

For blind, deaf/blind children and adults, ages 5 and up. This program offers a basic camping experience. Activities include music, art, dance, hiking and riding. Camperships are available to California residents.

Tony Fletcher, Camp Director

1932 Florida School-Deaf and Blind Summer Camp
207 N San Marco Avenue
Saint Augustine, FL 32084
904-827-2200
800-344-3732
info@fsdb.k12.fl.us
www.fsdb.k12.fl.us

The Florida School for the Deaf and the Blind hosts summer campers from all over teh state of Florida for a week of fun and adventure. FSDB's 80 acre campus is where campers participate in a variety of activities including rock climbing, archery, swimming, kayaking, team games, arts and crafts, dance music, and much more.

L Daniel Hutto, President
Cindy Day, Executive Director of Parent Svcs
Terri Wiseman, Administrator of Business Services

1933 Highbrook Lodge Camp
12944 Aquilla Road
Chardon, OH 44024
216-791-8118
Fax: 216-791-1101
camp@clevelandsightcenter.org
www.clevelandsightcenter.org

A summer residential camp for blind and disabled children, adults and families.

Mike Mullin, Director

1934 National Camps for Blind Children
Christian Record
4444 S 52nd Street
Lincoln, NE 68516

402-488-0981
Fax: 402-488-7582
info@christianrecord.org
www.christianrecord.org

Camps throughout the US and Canada are offered at no cost to the legally blind, ages 9-65. Activities include archery, beeper basketball, water sports, hiking and rock climbing and horseback riding.

Peggy Hansen, Director

1935 Texas Lions Camp
Lions Clubs of Texas
PO Box 290247
Kerrville, TX 78029

830-896-8500
830-896-8500
Fax: 830-896-3666
tlc@ktc.com
www.lionscamp.com

The primary purpose of Texas Lions camp is to provide, without charge, a camp for physically disabled, hearing/vision impaired and diabetic children from the State of Texas, regardless of race, religion, or national origin. Our goal is to create an atmosphere wherein campers will learn the can do philosophy and be allowed to achieve maximum personal growth and self esteem. The camp welcomes boys and girls ages 7-16.

Stephen Mabry, Executive Director
Doug Parker, Business Manager
Steven King, Program/Client Service Director

1936 VISIONS/Vacation Camp for the Blind
500 Greenwich Street, 3rd Floor
New York, NY 10013

212-625-1616
888-245-8333
Fax: 212-219-4078
info@visions.org
www.visions.org

Family programs at Vacation Camp for the Blind in Rockland County, NY for children who are blind, severely visually impaired or multi-handicapped. Parent or guardian must attend winter weekends and summer session.

Thomas M Decker, Camp Director
Nancy D Miller, Executive Director

1937 Wisconsin Lions Camp
3834 County Road A
Rosholt, WI 54473

715-677-4969
Fax: 715-677-3297
TTY: 715-677-6999
info@wisconsinlionscamp.org
www.wisconsinlionscamp.com

Serves children who have either a visual, hearing or mild cognitive disability. Many of the children also have multiple disabilities or medical conditions. Program activities include sailing, ropes course, bike and canoe trips, environmental education, swimming, camping, canoeing, outdoor living skills and handicrafts. ACA accredited, located in central Wisconsin, near Stevens Point.

Russell Link, Camp Director

DESCRIPTION

1938 CONGENITAL DIAPHRAGMATIC HERNIA

Synonym: CDH

Involves the following Biologic System(s):

Gastrointestinal Disorders, Respiratory Disorders

Congenital diaphragmatic hernia (CDH) is a birth defect characterized by projection or bulging of organs of the abdomen into the chest cavity. This occurs as a result of an abnormal opening in the diaphragm, the dome-shaped muscle that separates the abdomen from the chest and plays an essential role in breathing. Approximately one in 5,000 newborns are affected by the condition. CDH is thought to result due to failed closure of a certain area of the embryonic diaphragm (i.e., the foramen of Bochdalek) during fetal development. In some cases, disrupted development in other areas of the growing fetus may also cause CDH. This birth defect may occur as an isolated condition or, in about 20 to 30 percent of patients, in association with other abnormalities or underlying malformation syndromes, such as Down syndrome (trisomy 21), trisomy 18 syndrome, or trisomy 13 syndrome. There are reports of several infants with isolated CDH in certain families (kindreds). In such cases, the condition is thought to result from abnormal changes (mutations) of different genes, possibly in association with certain environmental factors (multifactorial inheritance).

In newborns with CDH, the diaphragmatic defect may be small or can affect up to half of the diaphragm. The left side of the diaphragm is most commonly involved. The lungs may also be unusually small and underdeveloped (pulmonary hypoplasia), and abnormalities of the blood vessels supplying the lungs may also be present. In addition, the intestines may not be positioned properly (intestinal malformation). Most newborns with CDH experience increasing difficulties breathing (respiratory distress) within the first 24 hours after birth. Associated symptoms include labored breathing (dyspnea), grunting upon exhalation, drawing in of the chest wall during inhalation, and a bluish discoloration of the skin and mucous membranes (cyanosis). These findings may potentially result in life-threatening complications. In addition, in some affected newborns, air may collect in the chest cavity, causing the lung(s) to collapse (pneumothorax). Symptoms associated with CDH may not become apparent until after the first few weeks of life. These infants may experience mild respiratory symptoms or intestinal obstruction and associated vomiting (emesis).

In newborns with CDH, immediate measures may be necessary to prevent or treat potentially life-threatening complications. Surgery to repair the diaphragmatic defect is deferred until the newborn's respiratory status has been stabilized. Ongoing supportive measures may be employed before surgery, such as use of a device known as an extracorporeal membrane oxygenator (ECMO). This device supplies oxygen to the infant's blood and returns this oxygenated blood to the body. In addition, certain medications may also be used (e.g., surfactant therapy to help improve oxygenation, etc.).

Government Agencies

1939 NIH/ Eunice Kennedy Shriver National Institute of Child Health & Human Development

31 Center Drive, Building 31

Bethesda, MD 20892

301-496-5113

800-370-2943

Fax: 866-760-5947

TTY: 888-320-6942

nichdpress@mail.nih.gov

www.nichd.nih.gov

Established in 1962 by congress, today the institute conducts and supports laboratory research, clinical trials, and epidemiological studies that explore health processes; examines the impact of disabilities, diseases, and variations on the lives of individuals; and sponsors training programs for scientists, health care providers, and researchers to ensure that NICHD research can continue.

Diana W. Bianchi, Director

Paul Williams, Director, Communications

National Associations & Support Groups

1940 American Academy of Pediatrics

141 Northwest Point Boulevard

Elk Grove Village, IL 60007

847-434-4000

800-433-9016

Fax: 847-434-8000

www.aap.org

The American Academy of Pediatrics and its member pediatricians are committed to the attainment of optimal physical, mental and social health and well-being for all infants, children, adolescents, and young adults.

Fernando Stein, MD, FAAP, President

Karen Remley, MD, CEO/Executive VP

1941 CHERUBS: Association of Congenital Diaphragmatic Hernia Research & Advocacy

3650 Rogers Rd Suite 290

Wake Forest, NC 27587

919-610-0129

866-603-1944

Fax: 815-425-9155

info@cherubs-cdh.org

www.cherubs-cdh.org

Goal is to not only help parents of children born with CDH but to lead the medical community into finding the cause and prevention of this devastating birth defect

Dawn Williamson, President/Founder

1942 Digestive Disease National Coalition

507 Capitol Court NE, Suite 200

Washington, DC 20002

202-544-7497

Fax: 202-546-7105

hpayne@hmcw.org

www.ddnc.org

Advocacy organization comprised of over 30 voluntary and professional societies concerned with the many diseases of the digestive tract and liver.

Lynn Seim, Chairperson

Ralph McKibbin, President

Cathy Griffith, Vice Chairperson

1943 Genetic Alliance

4301 Connecticut Avenue NW, Suite 404

Washington, DC 20008

202-966-5557

800-336-4363

Fax: 202-966-8553

info@geneticalliance.org

www.geneticalliance.org

World's leading nonprofit health advocacy organization committed to transforming health through genetics and promoting an environment of openness centered on the health of individuals, families, and communities.

Sharon Terry, President/CEO
Tetyana Murza, Managing Director
Natasha Bonhomme, VP, Strategic Development

1944 International CDH Conference
CHERUBS
3650 Rogers Rd Suite 290
Wake Forest, NC 27587
919-610-0129
866-603-1944
Fax: 815-425-9155
info@cherubs-cdh.org
www.cherubs-cdh.org

Designed for families of CDH survivors, grieving CDH families, adult survivors and CDH researchers.
June
Dawn Williamson, President/Founder

Libraries & Resource Centers

1945 National Digestive Diseases Information Clearinghouse
9000 Rockville Pike
Bethesda, MD 20892
301-496-3583
800-860-8747
Fax: 301-907-8906
healthinfo@niddk.nih.gov
www.niddk.nih.gov

The National Institute of Diabetes and Digestive and Kidney Diseases conducts and supports research on many of the most serious diseases affecting public health. The Institute supports much of the clinical research on the diseases of internal medicine and related subspecialty fields as well as many basic science disciplines.
Dr. Griffin P. Rodgers, Director
Dr. Gregory G. Germino, Deputy Director
Camille M. Hoover, M.S.W., Executive Officer

1946 University of Iowa Birth Defects and Genetic Disorders Unit
2614 JCP
Iowa City, IA 52242
319-335-9901
James M Smith, Director

Conferences

1947 Genetic Alliance Annual Conference
Genetic Alliance
4301 Connecticut Avenue NW, Suite 404
Washington, DC 20008
202-966-5557
800-336-4363
Fax: 202-966-8553
info@geneticalliance.org
www.geneticalliance.org

Consistently inspirational and enables partnership among all stakeholders: advocates and community leaders, health and industry professionals, policymakers, and academicians.
July
Sharon Terry, President/CEO
Tetyana Murza, Managing Director
Natasha Bonhomme, VP, Strategic Development

Web Sites

1948 Family Village
www.familyvillage.wisc.edu

A global community that integrates information, resources and communication opportunities on the Internet for persons with cognitive and other disabilities, for their families and for those that provide them services and support.

Book Publishers

1949 Digestive Diseases & Disorders Sourcebook
Omnigraphics Editorial Office
615 Griswold
Detroit, MI 48226
313-961-1340
800-234-1340
Fax: 313-961-1383
editorial@omnigraphics.com
www.omnigraphics.com

Provides basic information for the layperson about common disorders of the upper and lower digestive tract. It also includes information about medications and recommendations for maintaining a healthy digestive tract. A glossary of important terms and a directory of digestive diseases organizations are also provided.
2000 335 pages Hardcover
ISBN: 0-780803-27-2
Karen Bellenir, Editor

DESCRIPTION

1950 CONGENITAL DYSPLASIA OF THE HIP

Synonyms: CDH, Congenital dislocation of the hip, DDH, Developmental dysplasia of the hip

Covers these related disorders: Teratologic congenital dysplasia of the hip, Typical congenital dysplasia of the hip (Developmental dysplasia)

Involves the following Biologic System(s):

Neonatal and Infant Disorders, Orthopedic and Muscle Disorders

Congenital dysplasia of the hip (CDH) refers to a condition present at birth or soon thereafter in which one or both hips are dislocated. This occurs when the ball-shaped head of the upper thigh bone (femur) does not fit appropriately into the hip socket of the pelvis (acetabulum). Congenital hip dysplasia may be classified as typical, which occurs shortly after birth in infants with no underlying neurologic irregularities, or teratologic, which develops before birth. The typical form of this condition is commonly referred to as developmental dysplasia of the hip.

The cause of CDH is unknown, although it is more prevalent in newborns who were surrounded by an unusually small amount of amniotic fluid during the gestational period (oligohydramnios). Those infants who present in a breech position; those with other close family members with this condition may also be at increased risk for CDH. In addition, it is more predominant in girls than it is in boys by a ratio of nine to one. Teratologic dysplasia of the hip in the developing fetus may occur as part of a pattern of abnormalities associated with certain underlying disorders affecting the neuromuscular system such as arthrogryposis multiplex congenita and myelodysplasia.

Assessment of the hips is part of the newborn physical exam. The Ortalani and Barlow maneuvers help to detect both anterior and posterior dislocations for the femoral head. Children with certain risk factors (i.e. breech delivery) should have a hip ultrasound at 3 months.

Treatment during infancy may include manipulation of the hip joint into its proper position followed by immobilization and splinting of the thigh for a period of several months. Some infants may benefit from wearing two or three diapers at a time. In some patients, delayed detection of this birth defect may necessitate the use of traction to restore the femoral head to its correct position. However, if the dislocation is not discovered until late childhood, surgery followed by fitting with a plaster cast may be necessary to correct this condition. Delayed treatment may result in chronic difficulties with walking. Untreated dysplasia of the hip may result in degenerative changes in the joint (osteoarthritis). Approximately 4 of every 1,000 infants are affected by congenital dysplasia of the hip; however, in approximately 70 percent of these children, the dislocation corrects itself.

Government Agencies

1951 NIH/ Eunice Kennedy Shriver National Institute of Child Health & Human Development
31 Center Drive, Building 31
Bethesda, MD 20892

301-496-5113
800-370-2943
Fax: 866-760-5947
TTY: 888-320-6942
nichdpress@mail.nih.gov
www.nichd.nih.gov

Established in 1962 by congress, today the institute conducts and supports laboratory research, clinical trials, and epidemiological studies that explore health processes; examines the impact of disabilities, diseases, and variations on the lives of individuals; and sponsors training programs for scientists, health care providers, and researchers to ensure that NICHD research can continue.

Diana W. Bianchi, Director
Paul Williams, Director, Communications

1952 NIH/National Institute of Arthritis & Musculoskeletal & Skin Diseases
National Institutes of Health
1 AMS Circle
Bethesda, MD 20892

301-495-4484
877-226-4267
Fax: 301-718-6366
TTY: 301-565-2966
TDD: 301-565-2966
niamsinfo@mail.nih.gov
www.niams.nih.gov

The mission of the National Institute of Arthritis and Musculoskeletal and Skin Diseases is to support research into the causes, treatment, and prevention of arthritis and musculoskeletal and skin diseases; the training of basic and clinical scientists to carry out this research; and the dissemination of information on research progress in these diseases

Stephen I Katz, MD/Ph.D, Director
Robert H Carter MD, Deputy Director
Gahan Breithaupt, Assoc Dir. Management & Operations

National Associations & Support Groups

1953 American Academy of Pediatrics
141 Northwest Point Boulevard
Elk Grove Village, IL 60007

847-434-4000
800-433-9016
Fax: 847-434-8000
www.aap.org

The American Academy of Pediatrics and its member pediatricians are committed to the attainment of optimal physical, mental and social health and well-being for all infants, children, adolescents, and young adults.

Fernando Stein, MD, FAAP, President
Karen Remley, MD, CEO/Executive VP

1954 Genetic Alliance
4301 Connecticut Avenue NW, Suite 404
Washington, DC 20008

202-966-5557
800-336-4363
Fax: 202-966-8553
info@geneticalliance.org
www.geneticalliance.org

World's leading nonprofit health advocacy organization committed to transforming health through genetics and promoting an environment of openness centered on the health of individuals, families, and communities.

Sharon Terry, President/CEO
Tetyana Murza, Managing Director
Natasha Bonhomme, VP, Strategic Development

1955 March of Dimes Foundation
1275 Mamaroneck Avenue
White Plains, NY 10605 914-997-4488
888-663-4637
Fax: 914-997-4763
answers@marchofdimes.com
www.marchofdimes.com

Partnership of volunteers and professionals dedicated to improving the health of babies by preventing birth defects and infant mortality. Over 100 chapters are located across the country and can be located through the National Office.

Stacey D. Stewart, President

1956 National Dissemination Center for Children with Disabilities
1825 Connecticut Ave NW, PO Box 1492
Washington, DC 20009 202-884-8200
800-695-0285
Fax: 202-884-8441
nichcy@fhi360@org
www.nichcy.org

A national information and referral center that provides information on disabilities and disability-related issues for families, educators and other professionals.

Suzanne Ripley, Executive Director

Libraries & Resource Centers

1957 University of Iowa Birth Defects and Genetic Disorders Unit
2614 JCP
Iowa City, IA 52242 319-335-9901
James M Smith, Director

Conferences

1958 Genetic Alliance Annual Conference
Genetic Alliance
4301 Connecticut Avenue NW, Suite 404
Washington, DC 20008 202-966-5557
800-336-4363
Fax: 202-966-8553
info@geneticalliance.org
www.geneticalliance.org

Consistently inspirational and enables partnership among all stakeholders: advocates and community leaders, health and industry professionals, policymakers, and academicians.

July

Sharon Terry, President/CEO
Tetyana Murza, Managing Director
Natasha Bonhomme, VP, Strategic Development

Web Sites

1959 Dr. Koop
www.drkoop.com/

Information on the condition, causes, symptoms, tests and treatment.

Book Publishers

1960 Let's Talk About Going to the Hospital
Rosen Publishing Group's PowerKids Press
29 E 21st Street
New York, NY 10010 212-777-3017
800-237-9932
Fax: 888-436-4643
rosenpub@tribeca.ios.com
www.powerkidspress.com

If a child has to check into the hospital, chances are he or she is already upset about being ill. Knowing how a hospital functions and what the procedures are, such as when family members can visit, will help in what is already a stressful situation. Grades K-5.

24 pages
ISBN: 0-823950-36-0

DESCRIPTION

1961 CONGENITAL GLAUCOMA

Synonym: Infantile glaucoma

Covers these related disorders: Primary glaucoma, Secondary glaucoma

Involves the following Biologic System(s):

Ophthalmologic Disorders

Glaucoma refers to a condition in which the fluid pressure within the eyes (intraocular pressure) is abnormally elevated. This may occur as a result of the buildup of fluid (aqueous humor) due to obstruction or other problems with the eyes. Glaucoma that develops by the third year of life is referred to as congenital or infantile glaucoma, which is a very rare occurrence. Primary glaucoma refers to the condition as it relates to an irregularity in the mechanism that drains the eye. Secondary glaucoma refers to increased intraocular pressure that results from other types of irregularities that may or may not be accompanied by a drainage deficit.

Symptoms associated with congenital glaucoma may include an abnormal sensitivity to light (photophobia), involuntary, repeated squeezing and closing of the eyelids (blepharospasm), abnormal tearing, swelling and enlargement of the cornea, difficulty in seeing, and other ocular irregularities. Affected infants under three months of age are at additional risk of incurring tissue damage due to heightened sensitivity of the cornea to elevated fluid pressure within the eye. Eye irregularities may be observed by a physician upon ophthalmic examination.

Congenital glaucoma may develop subsequent to certain congenital problems such as trauma, bleeding (hemorrhage) within the eye, or tumors and inflammation. Other associated abnormalities may include the lack of transparency (opacity) of the lenses of the eye (cataracts), displacement of the lenses (ectopia lentis), partial absence of the iris (aniridia), and other abnormalities. Disorders often associated with congenital glaucoma include certain chromosomal disorders that may affect various systems of the body such as Sturge-Weber syndrome, oculocerebrorenal syndrome, neurofibromatosis, and Marfan syndrome.

Treatment for congenital glaucoma includes surgery to relieve the pressure within the eye to prevent optic nerve damage and preserve vision. In some cases, more than one surgery may be necessary and follow-up therapy may be required. Additional treatment is directed toward associated irregularities and complications.

Government Agencies

1962 NIH/National Eye Institute
31 Center Drive MSC 2510
Bethesda, MD 20892

301-496-5248
2020@nei.nih.gov
www.nei.nih.gov

Conducts and supports research that helps prevent and treat eye diseases and other disorders of vision. This research leads to sight-saving treatments, reduces visual impairment and blindness, and improves the quality of life for people of all ages. NEI-supported research has advanced our knowledge of how the eye functions in health and disease.

Paul A Sieving M.D., Ph.D., Director

National Associations & Support Groups

1963 American Academy of Pediatrics
141 Northwest Point Boulevard
Elk Grove Village, IL 60007

847-434-4000
800-433-9016
Fax: 847-434-8000
www.aap.org

The American Academy of Pediatrics and its member pediatricians are committed to the attainment of optimal physical, mental and social health and well-being for all infants, children, adolescents, and young adults.

Fernando Stein, MD, FAAP, President
Karen Remley, MD, CEO/Executive VP

1964 Children's Glaucoma Foundation
2 Longfellow Place, Suite 201
Boston, MA 02114

617-227-3011
Fax: 617-227-9538
walton.blackey@gmail.com
www.childrensglaucoma.com

A nonprofit organization dedicated to supporting programs for children with glaucoma. Serves to increase awareness of the symptoms and encourage parents and doctors to screen infants and children for glaucoma, and supports research programs.

David S Walton, MD, President

1965 Genetic Alliance
4301 Connecticut Avenue NW, Suite 404
Washington, DC 20008

202-966-5557
800-336-4363
Fax: 202-966-8553
info@geneticalliance.org
www.geneticalliance.org

A coalition of voluntary genetic support groups, consumers and professionals addressing the needs of individuals and families affected by genetic disorders from a national perspective.

Sharon Terry, President/CEO
Tetyana Murza, Managing Director
Natasha Bonhomme, VP, Strategic Development

1966 Glaucoma Research Foundation
251 Post Street, Suite 600
San Francisco, CA 94108

415-986-3162
800-826-6693
Fax: 415-986-3763
questions@glaucoma.org
www.glaucoma.org

Mission is to preserve the sight and independence of individuals with glaucoma through research and education with the ultimate goal of finding a cure.

Tom Brunner, CEO
Andrew Iwach, Executive Director
H.Allen Bouch, Vice Chair

1967 National Association for Visually Handicapped
22 W 21st Street, 6th Floor
New York, NY 10010

212-889-3141
888-205-5951
Fax: 212-727-2931
navh@navh.org
www.navh.org

The only nonprofit health organization in the world solely dedicated to providing assistance to the partially sighted. Serves as a clearinghouse for information about all services available to the partially-sighted from public and private sources. Conducts self-help groups. Provides information on large print books, textbooks and educational tools.

Lorianie Marchi, CEO

1968 Prevent Blindness America
211 West Wacker Drive, Ste 1700
Chicago, IL 60606

847-843-2020
800-331-2020
Fax: 847-843-8458
info@preventblindness.org
www.preventblindness.org

A volunteer eye health and safety organization dedicated to fighting blindness and saving sight. Focused on promoting a continuum of vision care, Prevent Blindness America touches the lives of millions of people each year through public and professional education, advocacy, certified vision screening training, community and patient service programs and research.

Pary Hugh, President
Corbett Sue, Manager
Bilazer Arzu, Creative Director

State Agencies & Support Groups

Alabama

1969 Alabama Institute for the Deaf & Blind
205 East South Street, PO Box 698
Talladega, AL 35160

256-761-3331
Fax: 256-761-3344
www.aidb.org

Services include central directory, representatives of agencies, service providers, families, and coordinators of infant, toddler, and preschool special education programs.

Dr. John Mascia, President

Arizona

1970 National Association for Parents of the Visually Impaired
PO Box 317
Watertown, MA 02471

617-972-7441
800-562-6265
Fax: 617-972-7444
napvi@guildhealth.org
www.spedex.com/napvi

Mary Ellen Simmons

Ohio

1971 Region 2 of the National Association for Parents of the Visually Impaired
3910 Pocahontas Avenue
Cincinnati, OH 45227
Victoria Gorman Miller

513-561-8542

Pennsylvania

1972 East Central Region-Helen Keller National Center
141 Middle Neck Road
Sands Point, NY 11050

516-944-8900
Fax: 516-944-7302
HKNCinfo@hknc.org
www.helenkeller.org

Christopher D Maher, Chairman
Richard T Arkwright, Vice Chairman
John R. Caughey, Treasurer

South Carolina

1973 Region 4 of the National Association for Parents of the Visually Impaired
1032 Trail Road
Belton, SC 29627

864-338-9593

Washington

1974 Northwestern Region-Helen Keller National Center
141 Middle Neck Road
Sands Point, NY 11050

516-944-8900
Fax: 516-944-7302
HKNCinfo@hknc.org
www.helenkeller.org

Christopher D Maher, Chairman
Richard T Arkwright, Vice Chairman
John R. Caughey, Treasurer

Libraries & Resource Centers

Alabama

1975 Mobile Association for the Blind
2440 Gordon Smith Drive
Mobile, AL 36617

251-473-3585
Fax: 251-470-8622
www.mobileblind.org

Offers work adjustment training, activities of daily living, mobility, communication skills and sheltered employment for adults and children who are visually impaired.

Jim Bullock, Executive Director

Arizona

1976 Educational Services for the Visually Impaired
PO Box 668
Little Rock, AR 72203

501-371-5710

Offers textbooks, braille books and more to the visually impaired grades K-12 in the Arkansas area.

David Beavers, Director

Arkansas

1977 Arkansas Regional Library for the Blind and Physically Handicapped
900 W. Capitol, Suite 100
Little Rock, AR 72201

501-682-2053
Fax: 501-682-1533
TDD: 501-682-1002
nlsbooks@asl.lib.ar.us
www.asl.lib.ar.us/ASL_LBPH.htm

Public library books in recorded or braille format. Popular fiction and nonfiction books for all ages, books and players are on free loan, sent to patrons by mail and may be returned postage free. Anyone who cannot see well enough to read regular print with glasses on or who has a disability that makes it difficult to hold a book or turn the pages is eligible.

John D Hall, Director

California

1978 American Action Fund for Blind Children and Adults
18440 Oxnard Street
Tarzana, CA 91356

818-343-2022
Fax: 818-343-3219
lucyabba@aol.com
www.actinfund.org

A lending library for the visually impaired. We send out a weekly Braille newspaper for the deaf-blind (worldwide), we also send out pocket-sized Braille calendars. Our lending library is for pre-school thru high school. All of our services are free.

Lucille Abbazia, Manager

1979 Blind Children's Center
4120 Marathon Street
Los Angeles, CA 90029   323-664-2153
Fax: 323-665-3828
www.blindchildrenscenter.org

Offers support and informational groups.

Midge Horton, Executive Director

1980 Braille Institute Desert Center
741 N Vermont Avenue
Los Angeles, CA 90029   323-663-1111
Fax: 323-663-0867
la@brailleinstitute.org
www.brailleinstitute.org

Dedicated to providing blind and visually impaired men, women and children with the training, programs and services they need to enjoy productive lives. Services offered include child development, youth programs, library services and adult education.

Lars Hansen, Manager

1981 Braille Institute Sight Center
741 N Vermont Avenue
Los Angeles, CA 90029   323-663-1111
Fax: 323-663-0867
la@brailleinstitute.org
www.brailleinstitute.org

Offers help, programs, services and information to the blind and visually impaired children and adults.

Les Stocker, President

1982 Braille Institute Youth Center
3450 Cahuenga Boulevard W
Los Angeles, CA 90068   213-851-5695

Offers various youth programs and services for the blind and visually impaired youngster.

1983 New Beginnings - Blind Children's Center
4120 Marathon, Street
Los Angeles, CA 90029   323-664-2153
800-222-3566
Fax: 323-665-3828

Helps children and their families become independent by creating a climate of safety and trust. Services include an infant stimulation program, educational preschool, interdisciplinary assessment services, family services, correspondence program, toll-free national hotline and a publication and research service.

1984 San Francisco Public Library for the Blind and Print Disabled
P.O Box 942837
Sacramento, CA 94237   415-557-4400
800-952-5666
Fax: 415-557-4252
lbphmgr@sfpl.lib.ca.us
www.library.ca.gov

Foreign-language books on cassette, children's books on cassettes and more.

Luis Herrera, Manager

1985 Variety Audio
PO Box 5731
San Jose, CA 95150   408-277-4839

Summer reading programs, braille writer, magnifiers, closed-circuit TV, large-print photocopier, cassette books and magazines, children's books on cassette, home visits and other reference materials on blindness and other handicaps.

Louisa Griehshammer

District of Columbia

1986 Council of Families with Visual Impairment
1155 15th Street NW
Washington, DC 20005   202-467-5081

Members are sighted parents of blind or visually impaired children. Offers a forum for support and outreach, sharing of experiences in parent-child relationships, and educational and cultural information about child development. Monitors developments in technical and legislative arenas.

Nola Webb, President

Florida

1987 Florida Bureau of Braille and Talking Book Library Services
421 Platt Street
Daytona Beach, FL 32114   386-239-6000
800-226-6075
Fax: 386-239-6069
TDD: 800-226-6079
mike_gunde@dbs.doe.state.fl.us
www.state.fl.us/dbs/lswel.html

Discs, cassettes, closed-circuit TV, large-print photocopier, films, children's books on cassettes and more.

Michael Gunde, Librarian

1988 Talking Book Library, Jacksonville Public Library
1755 Edgewood Avenue W, Suite 1
Jacksonville, FL 32208   904-765-5588
Fax: 904-768-7404
TDD: 904-768-7822
jerryr@coj.net
www.neflin.org/neflin/members/jackspub.html

Discs, cassettes and reference materials on blindness and other disabilities.

Jerry Reynolds, Librarian Senior

1989 Talking Book Service - Manatee County Central Library
6081 26th Street W
Bradenton, FL 34207   941-742-5914
Fax: 941-751-7089
TDD: 941-742-5951
patricia.schubert@co.manatee.fl.us
www.co.manatee.fl.us

Offers children's books on disc and cassette and more reference materials for the blind and physically handicapped.

Patricia Schubert, Librarian

Georgia

1990 Albany Library for the Blind and Physical Handicapped
300 Pine Avenue
Albany, GA 31701   229-420-3220
Fax: 229-420-3215
sinquefk@mail.dougherty.public.lib.ga.us
www.docolib.org/LBPH/index.html

Offers discs, cassettes, reference materials on blindness and other handicaps, large-print photocopiers, summer reading programs, cassette books and more.

Katy Sinquefield, Manager

1991 Bainbridge Subregional Library for the Blind and Physically Handicapped
301 S Monroe Street
Bainbridge, GA 39819   912-248-2680
800-795-2680
Fax: 912-248-2670
TDD: 912-248-2665
lbph@mail.deccatur.public.lib.ga.us
www.decatur.public.lib.ga.us/local/lbph/lbph1.htm

Discs, cassettes, summer reading programs, closed-circuit TV, magnifiers and more.

Kathy Hutchins, Librarian

1992 CEL Subregional Library for the Blind and Physically Handicapped
2708 Mechanics
Savannah, GA 31404   912-354-5864
                                  Fax: 912-354-5534
                                  TDD: 912-652-3635
                          stokesl@cel.co.chatman.ga.us

Summer reading programs, braille writer, magnifiers, closed-circuit TV, large-print photocopier, cassette books and magazines, children's books on cassette, home visits and other reference materials on blindness and other handicaps.

Linda Stokes, Librarian

Idaho

1993 Idaho State Talking Book Library
325 W State Street
Boise, ID 83702   208-334-2117
                                  Fax: 208-334-4016
                                  TDD: 800-377-1363
                            tblbooks@isl.state.id.us
                            www.lili.org/isl/tblinfo.htm

Summer reading programs, braille writer, magnifiers, closed-circuit TV, large-print photocopier, cassette books and magazines, children's books on cassette, home visits and other reference materials on blindness and other handicaps.

Sue Walker, Manager

Illinois

1994 Chicago Library Service for the Blind
1055 W Roosevelt Road
Chicago, IL 60608   312-746-9210

Summer reading programs, braille writer, magnifiers, closed-circuit TV, large-print photocopier, cassette books and magazines, children's books on cassette, home visits and other reference materials on blindness and other handicaps.

Carol Pellish, Librarian

1995 Illinois State Library, Talkng Book and Braille Service
213 State Capitol
Springfield, IL 62756   217-785-5600
                                      800-252-980
                                  Fax: 217-785-4326
                                  TDD: 800-665-5576
                                  sruda@ilsos.net
                            www.cyberdriveillinois.com

Summer reading programs, braille writer, magnifiers, closed-circuit TV, large-print photocopier, cassette books and magazines, descriptive videos, children's books on cassette, home visits and other reference materials on blindness and other handicaps.

Anne Craig, Executive Director

1996 Mid Illinois Talking Book System
515 York Street
Quincy, IL 62301   217-224-6619
                                  Fax: 217-224-9818

Summer reading programs, braille writer, magnifiers, closed-circuit TV, large-print photocopier, cassette books and magazines, children's books on cassette, home visits and other reference materials on blindness and other handicaps.

1997 Mid-Illinois Talking Book Center
600 High Point Lane
East Peoria, IL 61611   309-353-4110
                                      800-426-0709
                                  Fax: 309-353-8281
                            hitbc@darkstar.rsa.lib.il.us
                                  www.mitbc.org

Summer reading programs, braille writer, magnifiers, closed-circuit TV, large-print photocopier, cassette books and magazines, children's books on cassette, home visits and other reference materials on blindness and other handicaps.

Eileen Sheppard, Librarian
Chenoweth Rose, Director
Boucher Nancy, Reader Advisor

1998 Talking Book Center of Northwest Illinois
PO Box 125
Coal Valley, IL 61240   309-799-3137
                                      800-747-3137
                                  Fax: 309-799-7916
                            kodean@libby.rbls.lib.il.us
                                  www.rbls.lib.il.us

Subregional library provides Talking Book and Braille Book programs to eligible persons unable to use standard print materials due to visual or physical disabilities. Includes cassette books and magazines; summer reading program.

Indiana

1999 Northwest Indiana Subregional Library for Blind and Physically Handicapped
1919 W Lincoln Highway
Merrillville, IN 46410   219-769-3541
                                  Fax: 219-769-0690

Summer reading programs, braille writer, magnifiers, closed-circuit TV, large-print photocopier, cassette books and magazines, children's books on cassette, home visits and other reference materials on blindness and other handicaps.

Renee Lewis

Iowa

2000 Iowa Library for the Blind and Physically Handicapped
Iowa Department for the Blind
524 4th Street
Des Moines, IA 50309   515-281-1333
                                      800-362-2587
                                  Fax: 515-281-1263
                                  TTY: 515-281-1355
                                  TDD: 515-281-1355
                          information@blind.state.ia.us
                                www.blind.state.ia.us

Summer reading programs, magnifiers, closed-circuit TV, large-print photocopier, children's books on cassette, children's books in Braille and Print Braille, cassette magazines, home visits and reference materials on blindness and other handicaps.

Eis Karen, Program Manager/Librarian
Richard Sorey, Director
Aldini Jodi, Library Support Staff

2001 University of Iowa Birth Defects and Genetic Disorders Unit
2614 JCP
Iowa City, IA 52242   319-335-9901
James M Smith, Director

Kansas

2002 CKLS Headquarters
1409 Williams Street
Great Bend, KS 67530   620-792-4865
                                      800-362-2642
                                  Fax: 620-792-5495
                                  cenks@ink.org
                                    www.ckls.org

Summer reading programs, braille writer, magnifiers, closed-circuit TV, large-print photocopier, cassette books and magazines, children's books on cassette, home visits and other reference materials on blindness and other handicaps.

Jerri Robinson, Librarian

2003 Services for the Visually Disabled
629 Poyntz Avenue
Manhattan, KS 66502   785-776-4741
                                  Fax: 785-776-1545
                          marionr@manhattan.lib.ks.us

Summer reading programs, braille writer, magnifiers, closed-circuit TV, large-print photocopier, cassette books and magazines, children's books on cassette, home visits and other reference materials on blindness and other handicaps.

Marion Rice, Librarian

Kentucky

2004 Kentucky Library for the Blind and Physically Handicapped
PO Box 818
Frankfort, KY 40602

502-564-8300
800-372-2968
Fax: 502-564-5773
richard.feindel@kdla.net
www.kdla.net/libserv/ktbl.htm

Large-print photocopier, cassette books and magazines, children's books on cassette, and other reference materials on blindness and other handicaps.

5,200 members

Richard Feindel, Librarian

Maryland

2005 Maryland State Library for the Blind and Physically Handicapped
415 Park Avenue
Baltimore, MD 21201

410-230-2424
Fax: 410-333-2095
TTY: 800-934-2541
TDD: 410-333-8679
recept@lbta.lib.md.us
www.lbph.lib.md.us

Summer reading programs, braille writer, magnifiers, large-print photocopier, cassette books and magazines, children's books on cassette, and other reference materials on blindness and other handicaps.

Jill Lewis, Manager

2006 Prince George's County Memorial Library Talking Book Center
6530 Adelphi Road
Hyattsville, MD 20782

301-779-9330

Summer reading programs, braille writer, magnifiers, closed-circuit TV, large-print photocopier, cassette books and magazines, children's books on cassette, home visits and other reference materials on blindness and other handicaps.

Shirley Tuthill, Librarian

Massachusetts

2007 Braille and Talking Book Library Perkins School for the Blind
175 N Beacon Street
Watertown, MA 02472

617-924-3434
Fax: 617-926-2027
perkins@bpl.org
www.perkins.org

Patricia Kirk

2008 Carroll Center for the Blind
770 Centre Street
Newton, MA 02458

617-969-6200
800-852-3131
Fax: 617-969-6204
www.carroll.org

Assists blind and visually impaired adults and adolescents to adjust to loss of vision. The goal of this dynamic program is to help the person become more independent, to restore self-confidence, prepare for employment and improve the quality of life. Programs of individual counseling are offered as part of the program.

Rachel Rosenbaum, President

Michigan

2009 Downtown Detroit Subregional Library for the Blind and Handicapped
5201 Woodward Avenue
Detroit, MI 48202

313-224-0580
Fax: 313-965-1977
TDD: 313-224-0584
deveans@cms.xx.wayne.edu
www.detroit.lib.mi.us

Summer reading programs, braille writer, magnifiers, closed-circuit TV, large-print photocopier, cassette books and magazines, children's books on cassette, home visits and other reference materials on blindness and other handicaps.

Deborah Evans, Librarian
Jo Anne Mondowney, Library Director

2010 Kent County Library for the Blind
775 Ball Avenue NE
Grand Rapids, MI 49503

616-336-3250
Fax: 616-336-3201
kdlem@lakeland.lib.mi.us

Summer reading programs, braille writer, magnifiers, closed-circuit TV, large-print photocopier, cassette books and magazines, children's books on cassette, home visits and other reference materials on blindness and other handicaps.

Claudya Muller, Librarian

2011 Library of Michigan Service for the Blind
PO Box 30007
Lansing, MI 48909

517-373-1300
Fax: 517-373-5700
info@sbph.libomich.lib.mi.us
www.nfb.org/libraries for the blind

Summer reading programs, braille writer, magnifiers, closed-circuit TV, large-print photocopier, cassette books and magazines, children's books on cassette, home visits and other reference materials on blindness and other handicaps.

Nancy Robertson, Manager

2012 Macomb Library for the Blind and Physically Handicapped
16480 Hall Road
Clinton Township, MI 48038

586-286-1580
Fax: 586-286-0634
TDD: 810-869-40
macbld@libcoop.net
www.macomb.lib.mi.us/macspe/

Summer reading programs, braille writer, closed-circuit TV, cassette books and magazines, children's books on cassette, reference materials on blindness and other handicaps.

Beverlee Babcock, Executive Director

2013 Mideastern Michigan Library Co-op
G-4195 W Pasadena Avenue
Flint, MI 48504

810-732-1120
Fax: 810-732-1715
cnash@genesse.freeret.org
www.fakon.edu/gdl/talking.htm

Summer reading programs, braille writer, magnifiers, closed-circuit TV, large-print photocopier, cassette books and magazines, children's books on cassette, home visits and other reference materials on blindness and other handicaps.

Carolyn Nash, Librarian

2014 Muskegon County Library for the Blind
635 Ottawa Street
Muskegon, MI 49442

231-724-6361
Fax: 231-724-6675
TDD: 231-722-4103
www.muskcolib.org

Summer reading programs, braille typewriter, magnifiers, closed-circuit TV, large-print photocopier, cassette books and magazines, children's books on cassette, home visits and other reference materials on blindness and other handicaps, The Reading Edge, Perkins Brailler and large print books.

225

Linda Clapp, Librarian

2015 Upper Peninsula Library for the Blind Physically Handicapped
1615 Presque Isle Avenue
Marquette, MI 49855
906-228-7697
Fax: 906-228-5627
uproc.lib.mi.us
www.upesc.lib.mi.us/uplbph

Summer reading programs, braille writer, magnifiers, closed-circuit TV, large-print photocopier, cassette books and magazines, children's books on cassette, home visits and other reference materials on blindness and other handicaps.

Suzanne Dees, Executive Director

2016 Washtenaw County Library
PO Box 8645
Ann Arbor, MI 48107
734-994-4912
Fax: 734-663-2430
contact us@ewashtenaw.org
www.ewashtenaw.org

Summer reading programs, braille writer, magnifiers, closed-circuit TV, large-print photocopier, cassette books and magazines, children's books on cassette, home visits and other reference materials on blindness and other handicaps.

Kyeena Slater, Executive Director

2017 Washtenaw County Library for the Blind and Physically Disabled
PO Box 8645
Ann Arbor, MI 48107
734-994-4912
Fax: 734-663-2430
lbpd@co.washtennaw.mi.us
www.ewashtenaw.org

Book lovers club.adaptive technology,cassette equipment, cassette books and magazines, described videos, low vision aids reference and referral services.

Kyeena Slater, Executive Director

2018 Wayne County Regional Library for the Blind
30555 Michigan Avenue
Westland, MI 48186
734-727-7300
Fax: 734-727-7333
TTY: 734-727-7330
werlbph@tln.lib.mi.us
www.wayneregional.lib.mi.us

Summer reading programs, braille writer, magnifiers, closed-circuit TV, large-print photocopier, cassette books and magazines, children's books on cassette, home visits and other reference materials on blindness and other handicaps.

Reginald Williams, Wayne County Librarian

Minnesota

2019 Minnesota Library for the Blind & Physically Handicapped
Highway 298, PO Box 68
Fairbault, MN 55021
507-333-4828
800-722-0550
Fax: 507-333-4832
libblnd@state.mn.us
www.nfb.org/libraries for the blind

Summer reading programs, braille writer, magnifiers, closed-circuit TV, large-print photocopier, cassette, large print, braille books and magazines, children's books on cassette, and other reference materials on blindness and other handicaps.

Catherine A Durivage, Program Director

Missouri

2020 Adriene Resource Center for Blind Children
1445 N. Boonville Avenue
Springfield, MO 65802
417-862-2781
Fax: 417-862-7566
blind@ag.org
www.gospelpublishing.com

Offers braille and cassette lending library, braille and cassette Sunday school materials for all ages, braille and cassette periodicals and resource assistance, and resources for blind children and children of blind parents.

Paul Weingariner, Director

2021 Assemblies of God National Center for the Blind
1445 Boonville Avenue
Springfield, MO 65802
417-862-2781
Fax: 417-863-6614
blind@ag.org
www.ag.org

Offers braille and cassette lending library, braille and cassette Sunday school materials for all ages, braille and cassette periodicals and resource assistance, and resources for blind children and children of blind parents.

Thomas Trask, Manager
George O Wood, General Superintendent

2022 Wolfner Memorial Library for the Blind
PO Box 387
Jefferson City, MO 65102
573-751-8720
Fax: 573-526-2985
TDD: 800-347-1379
beckles@mail.sos.state.mo.us
www.nfb.org/libraries for the blind

Summer reading programs, braille writer, magnifiers, closed-circuit TV, large-print photocopier, cassette books and magazines, children's books on cassette, home visits and other reference materials on blindness and other handicaps.

Richard J Smith, Executive Director

Nebraska

2023 Nebraska Library Commission Talking Book & Braille Services
1200 N Street
Lincoln, NE 68508
402-471-2045
800-742-7691
Fax: 402-471-2083
TDD: 402-471-4038
david.oertli@nebraska.gov
www.nlc.nebraska.gov

Free loan of books and magazines on cartridge, cassette, and in Braille, including children's materials, along with specially designed playback equipment. Summer reading program for children, Braille embossing, closed circuit TV, large-print copier. Reference materials on blindness and other disabilities.

David Oerti, Librarian

New Jersey

2024 New Jersey State Library Talking Book and Braille Center
185 West State Street
Trenton, NJ 08625
609-278-2640
800-792-8322
Fax: 609-278-2647
TDD: 877-882-5593
njlbh@njstatelib.org
www.njstatelib.org

Free home delivery of large-print, audio, and braille books and magazines, children's books on cassettes in braille and other reference materials on blindness and other handicaps. Services are for New Jersey residents with print disabilities.

Adanrah Szczepaniak, Director
Anne McArthur, Head of Outreach and Audiovision

New Mexico

2025 New Mexico State Library for the Blind and Physically Handicapped
1209 Camino Carlos Ray
Santa Fe, NM 87507

505-476-9700
Fax: 505-476-9761
jbrewstr@stlib.state.nm.us
www.stlib.state.nm.us

Summer reading programs, braille writer, magnifiers, closed-circuit TV, large-print photocopier, cassette books and magazines, children's books on cassette, home visits and other reference materials on blindness and other handicaps.

Susan Overland, Manager

New York

2026 New York State Talking Book & Braille Library
CEC, 222 Madison Avenue
Albany, NY 12230

518-474-5935
800-342-3688
Fax: 518-474-5786
TDD: 518-474-7121
tbbl@mail.nysed.gov
www.nysl.nysed.gov/contact.htm

Books on audio cassette, cassette players, Braille books, summer reading programs, Braille writer, magnifiers, closed-circuit TV, large-print photocopier, cassette books and magazines, children's books on cassette, reference materials on blindness and other handicaps.

loretta ebert, Director
Bernard A Margolis, State Librarian

North Carolina

2027 North Carolina Library for the Blind
1841 Capital Boulevard
Raleigh, NC 27635

919-733-4376
888-388-2460
Fax: 919-733-6910
TDD: 919-733-1462
nclbph@ncdcr.gov
http://statelibrary.ncdcr.gov/lbph/

Summer reading programs, Braille writer, magnifiers, closed-circuit TV, large-print photocopier, cassette books and magazines, children's books on cassette, home visits and other reference materials on blindness and other handicaps.

Mary Boone, State Librarian

Ohio

2028 American Council of Blind Parents
14400 Cedar Road, Apartment 108
University Heights, OH 44121

216-791-8118
800-424-8666

Members are sighted parents of blind or visually impaired children. Offers a forum for support and outreach, sharing of experiences in parent-child relationships, and educational and cultural information about child development. Monitors developments in technical and legislative arenas.

Nola Webb, President

Oregon

2029 Oregon State Library, Talking Book and Braille Services
250 Winter Street NE
Salem, OR 97301

503-378-5389
800-452-0292
Fax: 503-585-8059
TDD: 503-378-4276
tbabs@sparkie.osl.state.or.us
www.tbabs.org

Cassette books and magazines, children's books on cassette, home visits and other reference materials on blindness and other handicaps.

Susan Westin, Manager

Virginia

2030 Alexandria Library Talking Book Service
5005 Duke Street
Alexandria, VA 22304

703-746-1702
Fax: 703-746-1747
TDD: 703-838-4568
rdawson@alexandria.lib.va.us
www.alexandria.lib.va.us

Summer reading programs, Braille writer, magnifiers, closed-circuit TV, large-print photocopier, cassette books and magazines, children's books on cassette, home visits and other reference materials on blindness and other handicaps.

Rose Dawson, Director
Linden Renner, Deputy Director

2031 Division for the Visually Handicapped
1920 Association Drive
Reston, VA 20191

703-620-3660
Fax: 703-264-9494
cec@cec.sped.org
www.cecp.air.org/teams/stratpart/cec.asp

Members are teachers, college faculty members, administrators, supervisors and others concerned with the education and welfare of visually handicapped and blind children and youth. This is a division of the Council For Exceptional Children.

Dr. Kay Ferrell, President

2032 Division on Visual Impairments
Council for Exceptional Children
2900 Crystal Drive Suite 1000
Arlington, VA 22202

888-233-7733
Fax: 703-264-9494
TTY: 866-915-5000
www.cec.sped.org/AM/

A division within the CEC, it handles concerns for Federal, state and local issues and policies related to education of youths, children and infants with visual impairments.

Ellyn Ross, President
Shirley J Wilson, Secretary
Phyllis T Simmons, President Elect

2033 Virginia State Library for the Visually and Physically Handicapped
395 Azalea Ave
Richmond, VA 23227

804-371-3661
800-552-7015
Fax: 804-371-3328
barbara.mccarthy@dbvi.virginia.gov
www.vdbvi.org/lrcservices.htm

Summer reading programs, Braille writer, magnifiers, closed-circuit TV, large-print photocopier, cassette books and magazines, children's books on cassette, home visits and other reference materials on blindness and other handicaps.

Barbara McCarthy, Librarian

Washington

2034 Washington Library for the Blind and Physically Handicapped
2021 9th Ave
Seattle, WA 98121

206-615-0400
800-542-0866
Fax: 206-615-0437
TTY: 206-615-0418
wtbbl@sos.wa.gov
www.wtbbl.org/

Summer reading programs, Braille writer, magnifiers, closed-circuit TV, large-print photocopier, cassette books and magazines, children's books on cassette, home visits and other reference materials on blindness and other handicaps.

Danielle Miller, Librarian

West Virginia

2035 West Virginia School for the Blind
301 E Main Street
Romney, WV 26757   304-822-4800
                                                   Fax: 304-822-3370
                                            pshank@access.k12.wv.us
                                 www.sdb2.state.k12.wv.us/About%20WVSDB.htm

Summer reading programs, Braille writer, magnifiers, closed-circuit TV, large-print photocopier, cassette books and magazines, children's books on cassette, home visits and other reference materials on blindness and other handicaps.

Patsy Shank, Administrator

Research Centers

2036 Center for the Partially Sighted
6101 W. Centinela Ave, Suite 150
Culver City, CA 90230   310-988-1970
                                                   Fax: 310-988-1980
                                                    info@low-vision.org
                                                    www.low-vision.org

Provides professional, comprehensive vision rehabilitation services to visually impaired people of all ages. For those whose sight is severely limited due to macular degeneration, diabetic retinopathy, glaucoma, retinal detachment, stroke or other conditions not correctable medically or surgically.

La Donna Ringering, President
Phillis Amaral, Director
Marc Gerberick, IT Manager

2037 Florida Ophthalmic Institute
7106 NW 11th Place Suite B
Gainesville, FL 32605   352-377-8364

Nonprofit organization that understands and treats ocular diseases including glaucoma.

Norman S Levy, Director

2038 Foundation for Glaucoma Research
251 Post Street, Suite 600
San Francisco, CA 94108   415-986-3162
                                                   Fax: 415-986-3763
                                               questions@glaucoma.org
                                                     www.glaucoma.org

Clinical and laboratory studies of glaucoma.

Tom Brunner, CEO
Andrew Iwach, Executive Director
H.Allen Bouch, Vice Chair

2039 Glaucoma Laser Trabeculoplasty Study
29275 Northwestern Highway
Southfield, MI 48034   248-493-5157

Examines the effectiveness and safety of the treatments of glaucoma.

Hugh Beckman, Chairman

2040 Glaucoma Research Foundation
251 Post Street, Suite 600
San Francisco, CA 94108   415-986-3162
                                                        800-826-6693
                                                   Fax: 415-986-3763
                                               questions@glaucoma.org
                                                     www.glaucoma.org

Conducts patient education activities, maintains eye donor network, provides multi-disciplinary seminars and conducts collaborative studies.

Tom Brunner, CEO
Andrew Iwach, Executive Director
H.Allen Bouch, Vice Chair

2041 Mobile Association for the Blind
2440 Gordon Smith Drive
Mobile, AL 36617   251-473-3585
                                                        877-292-5463
                                                   Fax: 251-470-8622
                                               sales@MobileBlind.org
                                                   www.mobileblind.org

Offers work adjustment training, activities of daily living, mobility, communication skills and sheltered employment for adults and children who are visually impaired.

Jim Bullock, Executive Director

2042 National Eye Research Foundation
910 Skokie Boulevard, Suite 207A
Northbrook, IL 60662   847-564-4652
                                                        800-621-2258
                                                   Fax: 847-564-0807
                                                        info@nerf.org
                                                        www.nerf.com

Devoted to the enhancement of care and study of eye related diseases.

Andrew Kim

2043 National Ophthalmic Research Institute
Retina Consultants of Southwest, Florida
6901 International Center Boulevard
Ft. Myers, FL 33912   239-938-1284
                                                        800-282-8281
                                                   Fax: 239-938-1270
                                                        NORI@eye.md
                                                   www.nori.md/index.htm

A physician-owned clinical research center specializing in innovative investigational treatments for ophthalmic, retinal and vitreous diseases.

Glen Wing MD, Research Director
Eileen Knips, RN, Clinical Research Coordinator
Glenn L Wing, MD, Medical Director

2044 New Beginnings - The Blind Children's Center
4120 Marathon Street
Los Angeles, CA 90029   323-664-2153
                                                   Fax: 323-665-3828
                                            www.blindchildrenscenter.org/

The purpose of the Center is to turn initial fears into hope. Helps children and their families become independent by creating a climate of safety and trust. Children learn to develop self confidence and to master a wide range of skills. Services include an infant stimulation program, educational preschool, interdisciplinary assessment services, family services, correspondence program, toll free national hotline and a publication and research service.

2045 Research to Prevent Blindness
645 Madison Avenue, Floor 21
New York, NY 10022   212-752-4333
                                                        800-621-0026
                                                   Fax: 212-688-6231
                                               inforequest@rpbusa.org
                                                     www.rpbusa.org

Provides research grants to scientists interested in eye disease and vision disorders.

Diane Swift, President
David Weeks, Chairman

Conferences

2046 AADB National Symposium
American Association of the Deaf-Blind
8630 Fenton Street, Suite 121
Silver Spring, MD 20910   301-495-4403
                                                   Fax: 301-495-4404
                                                   TTY: 301-495-4402
                                                   aadb-info@aadb.org
                                                        www.aadb.org

The symposium offers a training workshop, keynote speakers, full day exhibit hall, demonstration room, awards lunch and ceremony, talent show, Walk-A-Thon, and a banquet and dance.

Jill Gaus, President
Lynn Jansen, Vice President
Debby Lieberman, Secretary

2047 Genetic Alliance Annual Conference
Genetic Alliance
4301 Connecticut Avenue NW, Suite 404
Washington, DC 20008
202-966-5557
800-336-4363
Fax: 202-966-8553
info@geneticalliance.org
www.geneticalliance.org

Consistently inspirational and enables partnership among all stakeholders: advocates and community leaders, health and industry professionals, policymakers, and academicians.

July

Sharon Terry, President/CEO
Tetyana Murza, Managing Director
Natasha Bonhomme, VP, Strategic Development

Audio Video

2048 Heart to Heart
Blind Children's Center
4120 Marathon Street
Los Angeles, CA 90029
323-644-2153
Fax: 323-665-3828
www.blindcntr.org

Parents of blind and partially sighted children talk about their feelings.

Videotape

2049 Let's Eat
Blind Children's Center
4120 Marathon Street
Los Angeles, CA 90029
323-664-2153
Fax: 323-665-3828
www.blindchildrenscenter.org

Teaches competent feeding skills to children with visual impairments.

Videotape

2050 See What I Feel
Britannica Film Co.
345 4th Street
San Francisco, CA 94107
415-597-5555

A blind child tells her friends about her trip to the zoo. Each experience was explained as a blind child would experience it. A teacher's guide comes with this video.

Films

Web Sites

2051 Glaucoma Associates
310 East 14th Street
New York, NY 10003
212-477-7540
Fax: 212-420-8743
www.glaucoma.net

Developed to promote research into the basic causes of Glaucoma, develop new treatments for Glaucoma, and to develop public education into the treatment of Glaucoma.

2052 Glaucoma Research Foundation
251 Post Street, Suite 600
San Francisco, CA 94108
question@glaucoma.org
www.glaucoma.org

Mission is to preserve the sight and independence of individuals with glaucoma through research and education with the ultimate goal of finding a cure.

Thomas M. Brunner, President/ CEO
Nancy Graydon, Executive Director of Development
Andrew L. Jackson, Director of Communications

2053 Lighthouse Guild
15 West 65th Street
New York, NY 10023
212-769-6200
800-284-4422
info@lighthouseguild.org
www.lighthouseguild.org

Since 1905, Lighthouse International has led the charge in the fight against vision loss through prevention, treatment and empowerment. In 2013, it merged with Jewish Guild Healthcare to form a leading non profit vision and healthcare organization.

Alan R. Morse, President/CEO
Mark G. Ackermann, Executive VP/COO
Maura J. Sweeney, Senior VP, Programs & Services

2054 National Alliance of Blind Students
Los Angeles, CA
608-332-4147
smwhalenpsp@gmail.com
nabslink.org

The leading national advocacy and consumer organization for students in high school or college who are blind or visually impaired.

Sean Whalen, President
Karen Anderson, 1st Vice President
Gabe Cazares, 2nd Vice President

2055 National Association for Visually Handicapped
111 E 59th St
New York, NY 10022
800-284-4422
info@lighthouseguild.org
www.lighthouseguild.org

Helps to cope with the difficulties of vision impairment.

2056 Online Mendelian Inheritance in Man
National Library of Medicine, Building 38A
Bethesda, MD 20894
888-346-3656
info@ncbi.nlm.nih.gov
www.ncbi.nlm.nih.gov

This database is a catalog of human genes and genetic disorders.

Christine E. Seidman, M.D., Chair
David J. Lipman, M.D., Executive Secretary

2057 Royal National Institute of the Blind
www.rnib.org.uk
303-123-9999
helpline@rnib.org.uk
www.rnib.org.uk

Offering information, support and advice to over two million people with sight problems.

Lesley-Anne Alexander CBE, Chief Executive
Wanda Hamilton, Group Director (Fundraising)
Sally Harvey, Managing Director (RNIB Places)

Book Publishers

2058 Childhood Glaucoma: A Reference Guide for Families
Nat'l Assn for Parents of Children with Visual
PO Box 317
Watertown, MA 02272
617-972-7441
800-562-6265
Fax: 617-972-7444
www.spedex.com/napvi

Provides nontechnical information about childhood glaucoma and its treatment. The book also discusses educational issues and family concerns, gives a resource list, and includes a glossary.

1997 36 pages

Susan LaVenture, Editor/Executive Director

2059 Children with Visual Impairments: A Parents' Guide
Peytral Publications
PO Box 1162
Minnetonka, MN 55345
952-949-8707
877-739-8725
Fax: 952-906-9777
www.peytral.com

Covers visual impairments ranging from low vision to total blindness. Offers authoritative information and empathy, parental insight on diagnosis and treatment, orientation and mobility, literacy, legal issues and more. Valuable to parents, educators and support staff.

395 pages

M Cay Holbrook PhD, Editor

2060 Ophthalmic Disorders Sourcebook
Omnigraphics Editorial Office
615 Griswold
Detroit, MI 48226
610-461-3548
800-234-1340
Fax: 610-532-9001
editorial@omnigraphics.com
omnigraphics.com

Basic Information about glaucoma, cataracts, macular degeneration, strabismus, refractive disorders, and more.

1996 631 pages
ISBN: 0-780800-81-8

Linda M Ross, Editor

Magazines

2061 Journal of Visual Impairment and Blindness
American Foundation for the Blind
2 Penn Plaza, Suite 1102
New York, NY 10121
212-502-7600
Fax: 888-545-8331
contributions@afb.net
www.afb.org

Published in braille, regular print and on cassette this journal contains a wide variety of subjects including rehabilitation, psychology, education, legislation, medicine, technology, employment, sensory aids and childhood development as they relate to visual impairments.

10x Year

Larry Kimbler, Chair
James H. McLaughlin, Vice Chair
Carl S. Augusto, President & CEO

2062 Reaching, Crawling, Walking - Let's Get Moving
Blind Children's Center
4120 Marathon Street
Los Angeles, CA 90029
323-664-2153
Fax: 323-665-3828
info@blindchildrenscenter.org
www.blindchildrenscenter.org

Orientation and mobility for visually impaired preschool children.

24 pages

2063 Tactic
Clovernook Home and School for the Blind
7000 Hamilton Avenue
Cincinnati, OH 45231
513-522-3860
Fax: 513-728-3950
clovernook@aol.com

Quarterly

Newsletters

2064 NAVH Update
National Association for Visually Handicapped
111 E 59th St
New York, NY 10022
212-889-3141
800-284-4422
Fax: 212-727-2931
info@lighthouseguild.org
www.lighthouseguild.org

NAVH is committed to distributing its printed newsletters free in order to make certain every low-vision person has access to it's important infomation. The newsletter provides vision specific and general information in large print.

Quarterly

2065 National Library Service for the Blind & Physically Handicapped
Library of Congress Reference Section
1291 Taylor Street NW
Washington, DC 20542
202-707-5100
800-424-8567
Fax: 202-707-0712
TTY: 202-707-0744
TDD: 202-707-0744
nis@loc.gov
www.loc.gov/nls

Provides information and advocacy resources for families and professionals, including listings of organizations focusing on more specific areas of concern to families and young adults who have disabilities. Administers a natural library service that provides recorded and braille reading materials to eligible children and adults who cannot read standard print.

12 pages Quarterly
ISSN: 1046-1663

Vicki Fitzpatrick, Editor

2066 Talking Book Topics
National Library Services for the Blind
1291 Taylor Street NW
Washington, DC 20542
202-707-5100
Fax: 202-707-0712
TDD: 202-707-0744
nls@loc.gov
www.loc.gov/nls

Offers hundreds of listings of books, fiction and nonfiction, for adults and children on cassette. Also offers listings on foreign language books on cassette, talking magazines and reviews.

Bimonthly

Pamphlets

2067 Dancing Cheek to Cheek
Blind Children's Center
4120 Marathon Street
Los Angeles, CA 90029
323-664-2153
Fax: 323-665-3828
www.blindchildrenscenter.org

Discusses beginning social, play and language interactions.

33 pages

2068 Family Guide - Growth and Development of the Partially Seeing Child
National Association for Visually Handicapped
111 E 59th St
New York, NY 10022
212-889-3141
800-284-4422
Fax: 212-727-2931
info@lighthouseguild.org
www.lighthouseguild.org

Offers information for parents and guidelines in raising a partially seeing child.

2069 Family Guide to Vision Care
American Optometric Association
243 N Lindbergh Boulevard
Saint Louis, MO 63141
314-991-4100
Fax: 314-991-4101
www.aoanet.org

Offers information on the early developmental years of your vision, finding a family optometrist and how to take care of your eyesight through the learning years, the working years and the mature years.

2070 Glaucoma
Foundation for Glaucoma Research
251 Post Street, Suite 600
San Francisco, CA 94108
415-986-3162
800-826-6693
Fax: 415-986-3763
question@glaucoma.org
www.glaucoma.org

Offers information on what glaucoma is, the causes, treatments, types of glaucoma, eye exams and prevention.

Thomas M. Brunner, President/ CEO
Nancy Graydon, Executive Director of Development
Andrew L. Jackson, Director of Communications

2071 Glaucoma: The Sneak Thief of Sight
National Association for Visually Handicapped
111 E 59th St
New York, NY 10022
212-889-3141
800-284-4422
Fax: 212-727-2931
info@lighthouseguild.org
www.lighthouseguild.org

A pamphlet describing the disease, treatment and medications.

Donna A Esposito, MD, Editor

2072 Heart to Heart
Blind Children's Center
4120 Marathon Street
Los Angeles, CA 90029
323-664-2153
Fax: 323-665-3828
www.blindchildrenscenter.org

Parents of blind and partially sighted children talk about their feelings.

12 pages

2073 Learning to Play
Blind Children's Center
4120 Marathon Street
Los Angeles, CA 90029
323-664-2153
Fax: 323-665-3828
www.blindchildrenscenter.org

Discusses how to present play activities to the visually impaired preschool child.

12 pages

2074 Let's Eat
Blind Children's Center
4120 Marathon Street
Los Angeles, CA 90029
323-664-2153
Fax: 323-665-3828
www.blindchildrenscenter.org

Teaches competent feeding skills to children with visual impairments.

28 pages

2075 Move with Me
Blind Children's Center
4120 Marathon Street
Los Angeles, CA 90029
323-664-2153
Fax: 323-665-3828
www.blindchildrenscenter.org

A parent's guide to movement development for visually impaired babies.

12 pages

2076 Selecting a Program
Blind Children's Center
4120 Marathon Street
Los Angeles, CA 90029
323-664-2153
Fax: 323-665-3828
www.blindchildrenscenter.org

A guide for parents of infants and preschoolers with visual impairments.

28 pages

2077 Standing on My Own Two Feet
Blind Children's Center
4120 Marathon Street
Los Angeles, CA 90029
323-664-2153
Fax: 323-665-3828
info@blindchildrenscenter.org
www.blindchildrenscenter.org

A step-by-step guide to designing and constructing simple, individually tailored adaptive mobility devices for preschool-age children who are visually impaired.

36 pages

2078 Talk to Me
Blind Children's Center
4120 Marathon Street
Los Angeles, CA 90029
323-664-2153
Fax: 323-665-3828
www.blindchildrenscenter.org

A language guide for parents of deaf children.

11 pages

2079 Talk to Me II
Blind Children's Center
4120 Marathon Street
Los Angeles, CA 90029
323-664-2153
Fax: 323-665-3828
www.blindchildrenscenter.org

A sequel to Talk To Me, available in English and Spanish.

15 pages

Camps

2080 Bloomfield
5300 Angeles Vista Boulevard
Los Angeles, CA 90043
323-295-4555
800-352-2290
Fax: 323-296-0424
info@juniorblind.org
www.juniorblind.org

This camp is dedicated to serving blind and developmentally disabled children and adults.

Miki Jordan, President

2081 Camp Civitan
3519 East Shea Blvd # 133
Phoenix, AZ 85028
602-953-2944
Fax: 602-953-2946
info@campcivitan.org
www.campcivitan.org

A 501c3 non-profit organization, that has been providing multiple ever-changing programs to meet the needs of children and adults who are developmentally disabled.

Shannon Valenzuela, Director
Jane Armstrong, Director

2082 Enchanted Hills Camp
Lighthouse
214 Van Ness Avenue
San Francisco, CA 94102
415-694-7319
Fax: 415-863-7568
TTY: 415-431-4572
afletcher@lighthouse-sf.org
www.lighthouse-sf.org

231

For blind, deaf/blind children and adults, ages 5 and up. This program offers a basic camping experience. Activities include music, art, dance, hiking and riding. Camperships are available to California residents.

Tony Fletcher, Camp Director

2083 Florida School-Deaf and Blind Summer Camp
207 San Marco Avenue
Saint Augustine, FL 32084

904-827-2200
800-800-344
info@fsdb.k12.fl.us
www.fsdb.k12.fl.us

The Florida School for the Deaf and the Blind hosts summer campers from all over teh state of Florida for a week of fun and adventure. FSDB's 80 acre campus is where campers participate in a variety of activities including rock climbing, archery, swimming, kayaking, team games, arts and crafts, dance music, and much more.

L Daniel Hutto, President
Cindy Day, Executive Director of Parent Svcs
Terri Wiseman, Administrator of Business Services

2084 Highbrook Lodge Camp
12944 Aquilla Road
Chardon, OH 44024

216-791-8118
Fax: 216-791-1101
camp@clevelandsightcenter.org
www.clevelandsightcenter.org

A summer residential camp for blind and disabled children, adults and families.

Mike Mullin, Director

2085 National Camps for Blind Children
Christian Record
4444 S 52nd Street
Lincoln, NE 68516

402-488-0981
Fax: 402-488-7582
info@christianrecord.org
www.christianrecord.org

Camps throughout the US and Canada are offered at no cost to the legally blind, ages 9-65. Activities include archery, beeper basketball, water sports, hiking and rock climbing and horseback riding.

Peggy Hansen, Director

2086 Texas Lions Camp
Lions Clubs of Texas
PO Box 290247
Kerrville, TX 78029

830-896-8500
Fax: 830-896-3666
tlc@ktc.com
www.lionscamp.com

The primary purpose of Texas Lions camp is to provide, without charge, a camp for physically disabled, hearing/vision impaired and diabetic children from the State of Texas, regardless of race, religion, or national origin. Our goal is to create an atmosphere wherein campers will learn the can do philosophy and be allowed to achieve maximum personal growth and self esteem. The camp welcomes boys and girls ages 7-16.

Stephen Mabry, Executive Director
Doug Parker, Business Manager
Steven King, Program/Client Service Director

2087 VISIONS/Vacation Camp for the Blind
500 Greenwich Street, 3rd Floor
New York, NY 10013

212-625-1616
888-245-8333
Fax: 212-219-4078
info@visions.org
www.visions.org

Family programs at Vacation Camp for the Blind in Rockland County, NY for children who are blind, severely visually impaired or multi-handicapped. Parent or guardian must attend winter weekends and summer session.

Thomas M Decker, Camp Director
Nancy D Miller, Executive Director

2088 Wisconsin Lions Camp
3834 County Road A
Rosholt, WI 54473

715-677-4969
Fax: 715-677-3297
TTY: 715-677-6999
info@wisconsinlionscamp.org
www.wisconsinlionscamp.com

Serves children who have either a visual, hearing or mild cognitive disability. Many of the children also have multiple disabilities or medical conditions. Program activities include sailing, ropes course, bike and canoe trips, environmental education, swimming, camping, canoeing, outdoor living skills and handicrafts. ACA accredited, located in central Wisconsin, near Stevens Point.

Russell Link, Camp Director

DESCRIPTION

2089 CONJUNCTIVITIS
Synonym: Pinkeye
Covers these related disorders: Infectious conjunctivitis, Noninfectious conjunctivitis
Involves the following Biologic System(s):
Infectious Disorders, Ophthalmologic Disorders

Conjunctivitis refers to a condition characterized by acute inflammation of the delicate mucous membranes (conjunctiva) that line the inside of the eyelids and the whites of the eyes (sclerae). This condition may be caused by a virus or bacterium. Allergic reactions or exposure to certain chemicals and other environmental factors may also play a role in certain types of conjunctivitis. Neonatal conjunctivitis (also known as neonatal ophthalmia or ophthalmia neonatorum) becomes apparent during the first four weeks of life and is considered an infectious disease resulting from bacterial or viral infections carried by the mother and passed to the child during the birthing process. Bacteria responsible for neonatal conjunctivitis infections may be common disease-causing organisms (pathogens) or may include Chlamydia trachomatis, the bacteria that causes the sexually transmitted disease (STD) chlamydia or Neisseria gonorrhoeae, responsible for the STD gonorrhea. In addition, viral transmission may be caused by herpes simplex type 2 virus, which is responsible for genital herpes. In addition, bacterial contamination may occur in a hospital nursery (Pseudomonas aeruginosa) and may, in some cases, cause severe infection.

The characteristic symptoms associated with infectious neonatal conjunctivitis include redness and severe swelling of the conjunctiva, including the eyelids and whites of the eyes, and a discharge from the eyes that may or may not contain pus (purulent). Symptoms of neonatal infection resulting from transmission during the birthing process may be present at birth or may appear during the second week of life, depending on the bacterium or virus responsible. Any early conjunctival infection should be evaluated as soon as possible to determine its cause and, subsequently, the appropriate course of treatment in order to prevent complications that could potentially lead to impaired vision or blindness.

Soon after delivery, erythromycin, or tetracycline drops or ointment are routinely administered to the eyes of the newborn to prevent gonococcal (gonorrheal) conjunctivitis. The use of 1% silver nitrate drops as prophylaxis (prevention) against gonococcal ophthalmia soon after birth has reduced its incidence in the United States to less than 0.03% of infants. Although silver nitrate is effective, it also may cause a chemical conjunctival inflammation that typically resolves on its own within 48 hours. Other preventive measures are directed toward identification and treatment of pregnant women with gonococcal infection.

Treatment for bacteria-caused neonatal conjunctivitis includes the use of particular antibiotics. In addition, washing (irrigating) the eye with a solution containing salt (saline) or direct application of antibiotic ointment to the eyes is often effective in relieving itching and discomfort and clearing up the discharge. Conjunctivitis caused by viral transmission may be treated with antiviral eye drops or ointment. Sometimes the antiviral drug acyclovir may be administered to prevent viral spread.

Additional causes of conjunctivitis in children may include other viruses associated with systemic diseases such as measles, some viruses of the adenovirus family, and intestinal viruses of the enterovirus family. This type of conjunctivitis is usually characterized by a watery discharge from the eyes, is usually self-limited, and treatment is symptomatic. However, one such adenovirus may cause severe itching and burning of the eyes, sensitivity to light (photophobia), and involvement of the cornea. This type of conjunctivitis is known as keratoconjunctivitis and affects the membranes lining the eyelids as well as the corneas. This virus is transmitted by direct contact. Conjunctivitis caused by allergies is usually seasonal and is characterized by swelling, tearing, and itching. Treatment is symptomatic and may include the application of antihistamine eye drops. Certain chemicals or environmental factors may also cause noninfectious, allergic-type conjunctivitis. In addition to silver nitrate used in preventive treatment in newborns, other irritating substances may include cleaning products, different types of sprays, smoke, pollen, and other materials. Treatment is directed toward prevention and relief of symptoms.

In the United States, as mentioned, the occurrence of neonatal conjunctivitis caused by Neisseria gonorrhoeae is extremely rare, while that caused by Chlamydia trachomatis is slightly more than eight out of every 1,000 births.

Government Agencies

2090 NIH/National Eye Institute
31 Center Drive MSC 2510
Bethesda, MD 20892

301-496-5248
2020@nei.nih.gov
www.nei.nih.gov

Conducts and supports research that helps prevent and treat eye diseases and other disorders of vision. This research leads to sight-saving treatments, reduces visual impairment and blindness, and improves the quality of life for people of all ages. NEI-supported research has advanced our knowledge of how the eye functions in health and disease.

Paul A Sieving M.D., Ph.D., Director

2091 NIH/National Institute of Allergy and Infectious Diseases
5601 Fishers Lane, MSC 9806
Bethesda, MD 20892

301-496-5717
866-284-4107
Fax: 301-402-3573
TDD: 800-877-8339
ocpostoffice@niaid.nih.gov
www.niaid.nih.gov

Conducts and supports basic and applied research to better understand, treat, and ultimately prevent infectious, immunologic, and allergic diseases.

Anthony S Fauci MD, Director

National Associations & Support Groups

2092 American Academy of Pediatrics
141 Northwest Point Boulevard
Elk Grove Village, IL 60007

847-434-4000
800-433-9016
Fax: 847-434-8000
www.aap.org

The American Academy of Pediatrics and its member pediatricians are committed to the attainment of optimal physical, mental and social health and well-being for all infants, children, adolescents, and young adults.

Fernando Stein, MD, FAAP, President
Karen Remley, MD, CEO/Executive VP

2093 American Institute for Preventive Medicine
30445 Northwestern Highway, Suite 350
Farmington Hills, MI 48334
248-539-1800
800-345-2476
Fax: 248-539-1808
aipm@healthylife.com
www.healthylife.com

An internationally recognized authority on the development and implementation of health promotion, wellness, medical self-care, and disease management programs and publications.

Larry Chapman, President
Dee Edington, Director
Bill Hettler, Cofounder

2094 World Health Organization
Avenue Appia 20
Geneva, SW
Switzerland
122-791-2111
Fax: 122-791-3111
ÿerecruit@who.int.
www.who.int

WHO is the directing and coordinating authority for health within the United Nations system.

Dr Margaret Chan, Director General
Dr Anarfi Asamoa-Baah, Deputy Director General
Bruce Aylward, Assistant Director General

Web Sites

2095 American Academy of Family Physicians
11400 Tomahawk Creek Parkway
Leawood, KS 66211
913-906-6000
800-274-2237
Fax: 913-906-6075
contactcenter@aafp.org
www.aafp.org

Represents more than 94,300 family physicians, family practice residents and medical students nationwide. Its mission is to preserve and promote the science and art of family medicine and to ensure high-quality, cost effective health care for patients of all ages.

Reid B. Blackwelder, MD, FAAFP, Board Chair
Robert L. Wergin, MD, FAAFP, President
Carl R. Olden, MD, FAAFP, Director

2096 Dr. Koop
www.drkoop.com

Information on the condition, causes, symptoms, tests and treatment.

2097 LSU Health Sciences Center
433 Bolivar Street
New Orleans, LA 70112
504-568-4808
webmaster@lsuhsc.edu
www.lsuhsc.edu

An online library of resources.

Larry H. Hollier, MD, FACS, FACC, Chancellor
Evana Morales, Staff Accountant
Martha Hotard, Collections Manager

2098 MedicineNet.com
www.medicinenet.com

An online, healthcare media publishing company providing easy-to-read, in-depth, authoritative medical information for consumers via its user-friendly, interactive web site. MedicineNet.com has had a highly accomplished, uniquely experienced team of qualified executives in the fields of medicine, healthcare, internet tehnology, and business to bring you the most comprehensive, sought after healthcare information anywhere.

2099 Virtual Children's Hospital
200 Hawkins Drive
Iowa City, IA 52242
800-777-8442
www.vh.org

Mission is to educate patients, healthcare providers, and students in a free and anonymous manner, for the purpose of improving patients' care, outcome and lives.

Jean E. Robillard, MD, UI VP for Medical Affairs
Theresa Brennan, MD, Chief Medical Officer
Sabi Singh, MS, MA, Co-Chief Operating Officer

DESCRIPTION

2100 CORNELIA DE LANGE SYNDROME
Synonyms: BDLS, Brachmann-de Lange syndrome, CdLS, De Lange syndrome
Involves the following Biologic System(s):
Genetic/Chromosomal/Syndrome/Metabolic Disorders

Cornelia de Lange syndrome is a genetic disorder character-ized by growth delays before and after birth (prenatal growth retardation); delays in the acquisition of skills that require the coordination of physical and mental activities (psychomotor retardation), and mild to severe mental retardation. Character-istic physical abnormalities include delays in the maturation of bone; malformations of the head and facial (craniofacial) area that result in a distinctive facial appearance; abnormali-ties of the arms, legs, hands, and feet (limbs); or other abnor-malities. Associated symptoms and findings may vary in range and severity from case to case.

Infants with Cornelia de Lange syndrome often have feeding difficulties (e.g., projectile vomiting, regurgitation, swallow-ing difficulties); fail to grow and gain weight at the expected rate (failure to thrive); and have a weak, growling cry. Af-fected infants usually experience breathing problems, such as episodes in which there is temporary cessation of breathing (apnea), inhalation (aspiration) of food into the air passages of the lungs, and increased susceptibility to repeated respira-tory infections. Affected infants and children also typically have arched, bushy eyebrows that grow together (synophrys); unusually long, curly eyelashes; a low hair line; and general-ized excessive hair growth (hirsutism). Characteristic craniofacial abnormalities may include an abnormally promi-nent vertical groove in the center of the upper lip (philtrum); thin, downturned lips; and a small jaw (micrognathia). In ad-dition, in many affected children, the teeth may erupt later than expected and are widely spaced.

Many infants and children with Cornelia de Lange syndrome also have malformations of the upper limbs, such as small hands or abnormal positioning of the fifth fingers (clinodactyly) or thumbs. In rare cases, the forearms, hands, and fingers may be absent (phocomelia and oligodactyly). Many affected infants and children also may have abnormally small, short feet with webbing of the second and third toes (syndactyly).

In many cases, additional symptoms and findings are present. For example, in most affected males, the testes may fail to de-scend into the scrotum (cryptorchidism). Some affected in-fants may also have digestive abnormalities (e.g., gastroesophageal reflux, pyloric stenosis, bowel obstruction); heart defects (e.g., ventricular septal defects); episodes of un-controlled electrical activity in the brain (seizures); or other physical abnormalities. In addition, many affected children experience hearing loss and speech delays and may demon-strate behavioral problems, such as self-destructive tenden-cies.

Treatment of infants and children with Cornelia de Lange syndrome includes symptomatic and supportive measures, such as the prescription of certain medications to help pre-vent or control seizures (i.e., anticonvulsants); supportive therapies to ensure the proper intake of nutrients and to helpprevent or treat respiratory problems; and surgical or other appropriate methods to treat heart or digestive defects.

In most cases, Cornelia de Lange syndrome appears to occur randomly for unknown reasons. However, in a few reported cases, autosomal dominant inheritance has been suggested. The disorder is thought to affect approximately one in 10,000 newborns.

National Associations & Support Groups

2101 American Academy of Pediatrics
141 Northwest Point Boulevard
Elk Grove Village, IL 60007
847-434-4000
800-433-9016
Fax: 847-434-8000
www.aap.org

The American Academy of Pediatrics and its member pediatri-cians are committed to the attainment of optimal physical, mental and social health and well-being for all infants, children, adoles-cents, and young adults.
Fernando Stein, MD, FAAP, President
Karen Remley, MD, CEO/Executive VP

2102 Children's Craniofacial Association
13140 Colt Road, Suite 517
Dallas, TX 75240
214-570-9099
800-535-3643
Fax: 214-570-8811
contactCCA@ccakids.com
www.ccakids.com

A national, nonprofit organization dedicated to improving the quality of life for people with facial differences and their fami-lies. CCA's mission is to empower and give hope to facially dis-figured children and their families.
Charlene Smith, Executive Director
Annie Reeves, Program Director
Jill Patterson, Development Director

2103 Cornelia de Lange Syndrome Foundation
302 W Main Street, Suite 100
Avon, CT 06001
860-676-8166
800-223-8355
Fax: 860-676-8337
info@cdlsusa.org
www.cdlsusa.org

Provides a host of services that attract, educate, and unite fami-lies touched by this rare birth disorder which causes individuals to develop at a slower rate, both physically and mentally.
Liana Fresher, Executive Director
Antonie Kline MD, Medical Director
Kelley Brown, Assistant Executive Director

2104 FACES: The National Craniofacial Association
PO Box 11082
Chattanooga, TN 37401
423-266-1632
800-332-2373
faces@faces-cranio.org
www.faces-cranio.org

Serving children and adults throughout the United States with se-vere craniofacial deformities resulting from birth defects, injuries or disease. There is never a charge for any service provided by the association.

2105 Genetic Alliance
4301 Connecticut Avenue NW, Suite 404
Washington, DC 20008
202-966-5557
800-336-4363
Fax: 202-966-8553
info@geneticalliance.org
www.geneticalliance.org

A coalition of voluntary genetic support groups, consumers and professionals addressing the needs of individuals and families af-fected by genetic disorders from a national perspective.

Sharon Terry, President/CEO
Tetyana Murza, Managing Director
Natasha Bonhomme, VP, Strategic Development

2106 March of Dimes Foundation
1275 Mamaroneck Avenue
White Plains, NY 10605   914-997-4488
                                            888-663-4637
                                       Fax: 914-997-4763
                                    askus@marchofdimes.com
                                    www.marchofdimes.com

Partnership of volunteers and professionals dedicated to improving the health of babies by preventing birth defects and infant mortality. Over 100 chapters are located across the country and can be located through the National Office.

Stacey D. Stewart, President

Conferences

2107 CdLS Biennial Conference
302 W Main Street, Suite 100
Avon, CT 06001   860-676-8166
                                           800-223-8355
                                      Fax: 860-676-8337
                                       info@cdlsusa.org
                                       www.cdlsusa.org

Provides education and support to families of individuals with CdLS. Attendees receive free head-to-toe consultations with experts from a range of medical and educational fields; attend workshops on legal concerns, educational issues and medical/behaviors challenges; and have opportunities to meet other families facing similar challenges.

June

Liana Fresher, Executive Director
Gail Speers, Development/Events Coordinator
Marc Needlman, President

2108 Genetic Alliance Annual Conference
Genetic Alliance
4301 Connecticut Avenue NW, Suite 404
Washington, DC 20008   202-966-5557
                                           800-336-4363
                                      Fax: 202-966-8553
                                    info@geneticalliance.org
                                    www.geneticalliance.org

Consistently inspirational and enables partnership among all stakeholders: advocates and community leaders, health and industry professionals, policymakers, and academicians.

July

Sharon Terry, President/CEO
Tetyana Murza, Managing Director
Natasha Bonhomme, VP, Strategic Development

Web Sites

2109 Online Mendelian Inheritance in Man
National Library of Medicine, Building 38A
Bethesda, MD 20894   888-346-3656
                                    info@ncbi.nlm.nih.gov
                                    www.ncbi.nlm.nih.gov

This database is a catalog of human genes and genetic disorders.

Christine E. Seidman, M.D., Chair
David J. Lipman, M.D., Executive Secretary

Journals

2110 Facing the Challenges
Cornelia de Lange Syndrome Foundation
302 W Main Street, Suite 100
Avon, CT 6001   860-676-8166
                                           800-223-8355
                                      Fax: 860-676-8337
                                       info@cdlusa.org
                                    www.cdlsusa.org/publications

The purpose of this book is to provide emotional support and factual information to those facing the challenges of caring for a person with Cornelia de Lange Syndrome.

Robert Boneberg, Esq., President
Richard Haaland, Ph.D., Vice President
David Barnes, Esq., Treasurer

Newsletters

2111 Reaching Out
Cornelia de Lange Syndrome Foundation
302 W Main Street, Suite 100
Avon, CT 6001   860-676-8166
                                           800-223-8355
                                      Fax: 860-676-8337
                                       info@cdlusa.org
                                    www.cdlsusa.org/publications

Up-to-date on issues relevant to the syndrome and connected to a community of families who share in the joys and sorrows of CdLS.

1977 Bi-Monthly

Robert Boneberg, Esq., President
Richard Haaland, Ph.D., Vice President
David Barnes, Esq., Treasurer

DESCRIPTION

2112 CRANIOSYNOSTOSIS

Synonyms: Craniostenosis, Craniostosis

Covers these related disorders: Frontal plagiocephaly, Kleeblattschadel deformity, Scaphocephaly, Trigonocephaly, Turricephaly (oxycephaly or acrocephaly)

Involves the following Biologic System(s):
Orthopedic and Muscle Disorders

Craniosynostosis is a developmental abnormality in which early closure of one or more of the fibrous joints (sutures) between bones of the skull results in deformity of the skull and an abnormally shaped head. The severity of the deformity depends upon which fibrous joint or joints close prematurely as well as the ability of other joints in the skull to expand and compensate for the other closed joint or joints. Craniosynostosis may occur as an isolated condition or in association with certain chromosomal or malformation syndromes. In most instances of isolated craniosynostosis, the condition appears to occur randomly for unknown reasons. However, there have been reports of isolated craniosynostosis in members of several multigenerational families (kindreds), indicating autosomal dominant or autosomal recessive inheritance. Many genetic malformation syndromes have been identified in the medical literature that are associated with craniosynostosis. The specific underlying cause of craniosynostosis is not fully understood. Craniosynostosis occurs in approximately one in every 1,000 to 2,000 births and is more prevalent in males than females.

In infants with craniosynostosis, because the skull is unable to enlarge in certain directions relative to the affected fibrous joint in the skull, there is compensatory growth and enlargement in other directions at the sites of open joints. This causes deformity of the skull and an abnormally shaped head. For example, in the most common form of craniosynostosis, there is premature closure of the joint between the upper sides of the skull (sagittal suture), causing the head to appear abnormally long and narrow (scaphocephaly). Affected infants also tend to have a broad forehead and a prominent back portion of the head (occiput). This condition appears to be more common in males than females.

In the form of craniosynostosis known as frontal plagiocephaly, there is early closure of a suture between the upper sides of the head and one of the bones of the forehead (e.g., coronal suture). This results in flattening of one side of the forehead, prominence of the ear, and elevation of the eyebrow and eye on the affected side. Frontal plagiocephaly appears to affect females more commonly than males.

Trigonocephaly, another form of craniosynstosis, is characterized by premature fusion of the suture between the bones forming the forehead (metopic suture). Affected infants have a keel-shaped forehead and closely spaced eyes (hypotelorism). In infants with the form of craniosynostosis known as turricephaly (also called oxycephaly or acrocephaly), premature fusion of coronal and sagittal sutures causes the head to have an abnormally long, narrow, cone-like appearance. In addition, a rare form of craniosynostosis, known as Kleeblattschadel deformity, is characterized by premature closure of multiple cranial sutures, causing the skull to appear cloverleaf-like in shape. Affected infants have a high forehead, marked protrusion of the eyes (proptosis), abnormal prominence of the lower sides of the skull (temporal bones), and other associated abnormalities. Many affected infants also experience hydrocephalus, a condition in which obstruction or impaired absorption of the fluid surrounding the brain and spinal cord (cerebrospinal fluid) causes fluid accumulation under increasing pressure within the brain, resulting in abnormal enlargement of the brain.

In infants with craniosynostosis, premature closure of one suture is rarely associated with increased pressure within the skull or associated neurologic abnormalities, such as mental retardation. In such patients, surgery may be considered for cosmetic purposes. Premature closure of two or more sutures is more likely to cause increased pressure within the skull, potentially resulting in brain damage and associated mental retardation. Additional findings associated with increased pressure may include vomiting, headaches, and swelling of the area where the optic nerve enters the eye and joins with the nerve-rich membrane at the back of the eye (papilledema). In these infants, surgery is necessary to increase the capacity of the skull in order to prevent excessive pressure within the skull. If craniosynostosis is diagnosed before three months of age, surgery may be conducted to create artificial cranial joints in the skull, allowing skull growth and preventing abnormal shaping of the head.

National Associations & Support Groups

2113 AmeriFace
PO Box 751112
Las Vegas, NV 89136

702-769-9264
888-486-1209
Fax: 702-341-5351
info@ameriface.org
www.ameriface.org

Provides information, services, emotional support and educational programs for and on behalf of individuals with facial differences and their families. Working to increase understanding through public awareness and education.

3M members

Debbie Oliver, Executive Director

2114 American Academy of Pediatrics
141 Northwest Point Boulevard
Elk Grove Village, IL 60007

847-434-4000
800-433-9016
Fax: 847-434-8000
www.aap.org

The American Academy of Pediatrics and its member pediatricians are committed to the attainment of optimal physical, mental and social health and well-being for all infants, children, adolescents, and young adults.

Fernando Stein, MD, FAAP, President
Karen Remley, MD, CEO/Executive VP

2115 Children's Craniofacial Association
13140 Coit Road, Suite 307
Dallas, TX 75240

214-570-9099
800-535-3643
Fax: 214-570-8811
contactCCA@ccakids.com
www.ccakids.com

Devoted to the dispersion of medical knowledge of this and similar disorders, along with providing emotional support for the sufferers and their families.

Charlene Smith, Executive Director
Annie Reeves, Program Director
Jill Patterson, Development Director

2116 Craniosynostosis and Positional Plagiocephaly Support
massapequa, NY 11758
515-232-7015
888-572-5526
Fax: 516-977-3164
info@cappskids.org
www.cappskids.org/

Established by a mother whose child had Craniosynostosis to offer support and information to other families who had a child with Craniosynostosis.

Amy Galm, Director

2117 FACES: National Association for the Craniofacially Handicapped
PO Box 11082
Chattanooga, TN 37401
423-266-1632
800-332-2373
Fax: 423-267-3124
faces@faces-cranio.org
www.faces-cranio.org

Assists individuals with facial disfigurations and their families They maintain a registry of centers offering corrective surgery for craniofacial deformities and financial assistance to qualified applicants.

2118 FACES: National Craniofacial Foundation
PO Box 11082
Chattanooga, TN 37401
423-266-1632
800-332-2373
Fax: 423-267-3124
faces@faces-cranio.org
www.faces-cranio.org

A nonprofit organization serving children and adults throughout the United States with severe craniofacial deformities resulting from birth defects, injuries, or disease. There is never a charge for any service provided by the foundation.

2119 Forward Face
317 E 34th Street, Suite 901A
New York, NY 10016
212-684-5860
Fax: 212-684-5864
info@forwardface.org
www.forwardface.org

Mission is to help children and their families find immediate support to manage the medical and social effects of facial differences. Working to educate, advocate and raise public awareness.

Camille Walsh, Manager
Camille Walsh, Assistant to Executive Director

2120 Genetic Alliance
4301 Connecticut Avenue NW, Suite 404
Washington, DC 20008
202-966-5557
800-336-4363
Fax: 202-966-8553
info@geneticalliance.org
www.geneticalliance.org

A coalition of voluntary genetic support groups, consumers and professionals addressing the needs of individuals and families affected by genetic disorders from a national perspective.

Sharon Terry, President/CEO
Tetyana Murza, Managing Director
Natasha Bonhomme, VP, Strategic Development

2121 Guardians of Hydrocephalus Research Foundation
2618 Avenue Z
Brooklyn, NY 11235
718-743-4473
800-458-8655
Fax: 718-743-1171
ghrf2618@aol.com
www.ghrforg.org

Non-profit organization made up of concerned parents and dedicated volunteers. The goal of this foundation is to wipe out this top ranking birth defect.

Kathy Soriano

2122 Hydrocephalus Parent Support Group
Exceptional Family Resource Center
9245 Sky Park Court, Suite 130
San Diego, CA 92123
619-594-7416
800-281-8252
Fax: 858-268-4275
efrcproject@sdsu.edu
www.efrconline.org

Determined to provide support to the parents and relatives of the children stricken with the disorder.

Sherry Torok, Executive Director

2123 Let's Face It
University of Michigan
1011 N University
Ann Arbor, MI 48109
360-676-7325

A nonprofit network for people with facial difference, their families, friends and professionals. The mission is to advance knowledge about, by, and for people with facial differences and to promote their full and equal participation in society.

Betsy Wilson, Founder/Director

2124 March of Dimes Foundation
1275 Mamaroneck Avenue
White Plains, NY 10605
914-997-4488
888-663-4637
Fax: 914-997-4763
askus@marchofdimes.com
www.marchofdimes.com

Partnership of volunteers and professionals dedicated to improving the health of babies by preventing birth defects and infant mortality. Over 100 chapters are located across the country and can be located through the National Office.

Stacey D. Stewart, President

2125 National Foundation for Facial Reconstruction
333 East 30th Street, Lobby Unit
New York, NY 10016
212-263-6656
Fax: 212-263-7534
info@nffr.org
www.nffr.org

Created to address the plight of children with a facial disfigurement by supporting state-of-the-art treatment, innovative research, psychosocial support and medical training that inspires a new generation of pediatric doctors.

Whitney Burnett, Executive Director
Adam Conrad, Associate Executive Director
Kelly Strantz, Director of Development and Event

2126 National Hydrocephalus Foundation
12413 Centralia Road
Lakewood, CA 90715
562-924-6666
888-857-3434
nhf@earthlink.net
www.nhfonline.org

Nonprofit public service organization that assembles and disseminates information about Hydrocephalus. Promotes communication networks among those affected and their families, helps others gain a deeper understanding of those areas affected by Hydrocephalus, such as education, tax and estate planning, employment and family. Also promotes and supports research on the causes, treatment and prevention of Hydrocephalus.

Debie Fields, President/Treasurer
Debbie Fields, Executive Director

Libraries & Resource Centers

2127 University of Illinois at Chicago, Craniofacial Center
College of Medicine
808 S Wood Street
Chicago, IL 60612
312-996-7870
Fax: 312-413-1526
www.medicine.uic.edu

Richard M Novak, Director

Research Centers

2128 **Craniofacial Center at University of Illin ois, Chicago**
811 S Paulina
Chicago, IL 60612   312-996-7546
                                              Fax: 312-413-1157
                                              tkaislin@uic.edu
            uic.edu/com/surgery/plastic/craniofacial_cntr.htm
Maya Shahani, Director
Mimis Cohen, Professor of Surgery

Conferences

2129 **Genetic Alliance Annual Conference**
Genetic Alliance
4301 Connecticut Avenue NW, Suite 404
Washington, DC 20008   202-966-5557
                                                800-336-4363
                                              Fax: 202-966-8553
                                              info@geneticalliance.org
                                              www.geneticalliance.org
Consistently inspirational and enables partnership among all
stakeholders: advocates and community leaders, health and industry professionals, policymakers, and academicians.
July

Sharon Terry, President/CEO
Tetyana Murza, Managing Director
Natasha Bonhomme, VP, Strategic Development

Audio Video

2130 **Face First**
Fanlight Productions
32 Court Street, 21st Floor
Brooklyn, NY 11201   718-488-8900
                                                800-876-1710
                                              Fax: 718-488-8642
                                              info@fanlight.com
                                              www.fanlight.com

Profiles of several people born with facial deformities; they
chronicle both physical pain and the pain of rejection, as well as
the strengths that have enabled them to achieve successful adult
lives. ISBN: DVD: 1-57295-886-3; VHS: 1-572952-59-8
29 minutes DVD or VHS

Nicole Johnson, Publicity Coordinator

Web Sites

2131 **National Hydrocephalus Foundation**
www.nhfonline.org

Promotes information and educational assistance. Establishes and
facilitates a communication network and works to increase public
awareness. Promote and support research. Also has brochures,
help sheets and more. Quarterly newsletter included with annual
membership fee of $35.00.

Book Publishers

2132 **Congenital Disorders Sourcebook**
Omnigraphics
PO Box 8002
Aston, PA 19014   800-234-1340
                                              Fax: 800-875-1340
                                              info@omnigraphics.com
                                              www.omnigraphics.com

Basic consumer health information on disorders aquired during
gestation, including spina bifida, hydrocephalus, cerebral palsy,
heart defects, craniofacial abnormalities and fetal alcohol
syndrome.

650 pages
ISBN: 0-780809-45-9

Newsletters

2133 **National Hydrocephalus Foundation Newsletter**
12413 Centralia Road
Lakewood, CA 90715   562-924-6666
                                                888-598-3434
                                              Fax: 415-732-7044
                                              debbifields@nhfonline.org
                                              www.nhfonline.org

The Foundation is a national organization whose purpose is to
provide information and education, along with peer support
newsletter quarterly.
12-15 pages Quarterly

Michael Fields, President/ Treasurer
Debbie Fields, Executive Director
Jaynie Dunn, Secretary

Camps

2134 **Camp About Face**
Riley Hospital # 2514, 702 Barnhill Drive
Indianapolis, IN 46202   317-274-2489
            www.headsupfoundation.org/camp_about_face.htm
Camp designed to benefit youth ages 8-18 with craniofacial
anomalies.

DESCRIPTION

2135 CROHN'S DISEASE

Synonym: Regional enteritis

Involves the following Biologic System(s):

Gastrointestinal Disorders

Crohn's disease is an inflammatory bowel disease (IBD) characterized by chronic inflammation of any region of the digestive (gastrointestinal) tract from the mouth to the anus. The disease most commonly involves the lower region of the small intestine (ileum) and the major part of the large intestine (colon). Chronic inflammation of these areas causes thickening and scarring of the intestinal wall. The range and severity of Crohn's disease is extremely variable and depends on the intestinal region affected, the severity of symptoms and findings of inflammation, and associated complications. In children, Crohn's disease usually becomes apparent during the late teens; however, symptoms may begin during early childhood. In developed countries, inflammatory bowel disease, including Crohn's disease, is the most common cause of chronic intestinal inflammation during mid-childhood. Crohn's disease affects males and females in equal numbers. In the U.S., the disease affects approximately 30 to 100 per 100,000 individuals in the general population and occurs more frequently among Caucasians and African-Americans, (and is more common in Jewish individuals than in Hispanic-Americans and Asian-Americans. Although the exact cause of Crohn's disease is unknown, genetic, immune, and environmental factors are thought to play a role. Some researchers suspect that the disorder may result from an exaggerated immune response to an invading microorganism, such as a particular virus or bacterium.

In most children, Crohn's disease initially involves both the lower region of the small intestine and the major part of the large intestine (ileocolitis). However, initial inflammation may be restricted to the small intestine or the colon. The inflammatory process tends to be segmental in nature, and diseased regions of the intestine are often separated by apparently normal segments (skip lesions). Chronic inflammation causes thickening, ulceration, and scarring of affected areas of the intestinal walls and may lead to the development of abnormal channels (fistulas) between regions of the colon, the intestine and the urinary bladder, or the intestine and the surface of the skin. Additional complications may include the development of pus-filled pockets of infection (abscesses) or intestinal obstruction due to abnormal narrowing of certain intestinal regions.

Many children with Crohn's disease experience episodes of cramping; abdominal discomfort and pain; diarrhea that may contain blood; persistent spasms of the rectum (tenesmus); and a compelling urge to defecate. Additional symptoms and findings typically include fever, chills, easy fatigability, a general feeling of ill health (malaise), lack of appetite (anorexia), weight loss, and malnutrition due to impaired intestinal absorption of fats and nutrients (malabsorption). Many patients also develop deep grooves or cracks (fissures) in the mucous membranes of the anus. Some children have delayed bone maturation, retarded physical growth, or delayed sexual development as much as one to two years before the onset of other symptoms.

Many patients with Crohn's disease may also develop more generalized, systemic symptoms. These may include joint swelling and inflammation (arthritis); inflammation of the outermost layers of the eye's tough, white, outer coat (episcleritis); eruption of multiple, inflamed, reddish-purplish swellings on the legs and possibly the arms (erythema nodosum); and abnormal concentrations of mineral salts (calculi or stones) in the kidneys or the muscular sac (gall bladder) that stores and concentrates bile from the liver. Patients may also be prone to developing ankylosing spondylitis, a chronic, progressive, inflammatory disease that affects joints of the spine and results in pain, stiffness, and possible loss of spinal mobility. In addition, it is suspected that patients who have Crohn's disease for many years may have an increased risk of colon cancer as compared with the general population.

Symptoms typically flare up at irregular intervals throughout life. These episodes may be mild or severe and last for relatively short or prolonged periods. The treatment of Crohn's disease is directed at minimizing symptoms. Therapy may include the use of certain medication, such as sulfasalazine, azathioprine, or metronidazole. For example, azathioprine or metronidazole may be helpful in treating anal fistulas, and metronidazole has been beneficial in treating some patients who have not responded to other medications. Oral steroids may be added if needed. They are highly effective in reducing symptoms but should be used for short-term treatment only. Steroids should be tapered as soon as possible to reduce the risk of long-term side effects. In many children, treatment may include the administration of nutrients in liquid form (total parenteral nutrition) via a tube through the nose to the stomach (nasogastric tube). Some patients who experience severe, sudden episodes may require hospitalization to ensure proper intake of nutrients and fluids and to receive appropriate medical therapy. In addition, some patients may eventually require surgery to remove diseased portions of the intestine. However, such surgery is reserved for very specific indications, because the recurrence rate is high and the risk of needing additional surgery increases after such a procedure. Additional treatment is symptomatic and supportive.

National Associations & Support Groups

2136 American Academy of Pediatrics
141 Northwest Point Boulevard
Elk Grove Village, IL 60007
847-434-4000
800-433-9016
Fax: 847-434-8000
www.aap.org

The American Academy of Pediatrics and its member pediatricians are committed to the attainment of optimal physical, mental and social health and well-being for all infants, children, adolescents, and young adults.

Fernando Stein, MD, FAAP, President
Karen Remley, MD, CEO/Executive VP

2137 American Autoimmune Related Diseases Association, Inc.
22100 Gratiot Avenue
Eastpointe, MI 48021
586-776-3900
800-598-4668
Fax: 586-776-3903
aarda@aarda.org
www.aarda.org

The American Autoimmune Related Diseases Association is dedicated to the eradication of autoimmune diseases and the alleviation of suffering and the socioeconomic impact of autoimmunity through fostering and facilitating collaboration in the areas of education, public awareness, research, and patient services in an effective, ethical and efficient manner.

Virginia T. Ladd, President/Executive Director
Patricia Barber, Assistant Director
Deb Patrick, Events Specialist

2138 Crohn's & Colitis Foundation of America Hotline
Crohn's & Colitis Foundation of America
386 Park Avenue S, 17th Floor
New York, NY 10016   212-685-8707
                                            800-932-2423
                                            Fax: 212-779-4098
                                            info@ccfa.org
                                            www.ccfa.org

The mission of the Crohn's & Colitis Foundation of America
(CCFA), is to cure and prevent Crohn's disease and ulcerative colitis through research and to improve the quality of life of children and adults affected by these digestive diseases through
education and support. Known collectively as inflammatory
bowel disease (IBD), these painfaul chronic illnesses affect up to
one million Americans, including approximately 100,000 children
under the age of 18. CCFA was founded in 1967.

2139 Digestive Disease National Coalition
507 Capitol Court NE, Suite 200
Washington, DC 20002   202-544-7497
                                            Fax: 202-546-7105
                                            hpayne@hmcw.org
                                            www.ddnc.org

Advocacy organization comprised of over 30 voluntary and professional societies concerned with the many diseases of the digestive tract and liver.

Lynn Seim, Chairperson
Ralph McKibbin, President
Cathy Griffith, Vice Chairperson

2140 Genetic Alliance
4301 Connecticut Avenue NW, Suite 404
Washington, DC 20008   202-966-5557
                                            800-336-4363
                                            Fax: 202-966-8553
                                            info@geneticalliance.org
                                            www.geneticalliance.org

A coalition of voluntary genetic support groups, consumers and
professionals addressing the needs of individuals and families affected by genetic disorders from a national perspective.

Sharon Terry, President/CEO
Tetyana Murza, Managing Director
Natasha Bonhomme, VP, Strategic Development

2141 International Foundation for Bowel Dysfunction
PO Box 170864
Milwaukee, WI 53217   414-964-1799
                                            888-964-2001
                                            Fax: 414-964-7176
                                            iffgd@iffgd.org
                                            www.iffgd.org

A nonprofit education and research organization. Our mission is
to inform, assist, and support people affected by gastrointestinal
disorders.

Nancy J Norton, Founder
William Norton, VP

**2142 International Foundation for Functional Gastrointestinal
Disorders**
PO Box 170864
Milwaukee, WI 53217   414-964-1799
                                            Fax: 414-964-7176
                                            iffgd@iffgd.org
                                            www.iffgd.org

Nonprofit education and research organization founded in 1991.
IFFGD addresses the issues surrounding life with gastrointestinal
(GI) functional and mobility disorders and increases the awareness about these disorders among the general public, researchers
and the clinical care community.

Nancy J. Norton, President & Director
William Norton, Co-Founder

2143 March of Dimes Foundation
1275 Mamaroneck Avenue
White Plains, NY 10605   914-997-4488
                                            888-663-4637
                                            Fax: 914-997-4763
                                            askus@marchofdimes.com
                                            www.marchofdimes.com

Partnership of volunteers and professionals dedicated to improving the health of babies by preventing birth defects and infant
mortality. Over 100 chapters are located across the country and
can be located through the National Office.

Stacey D. Stewart, President

State Agencies & Support Groups

Alabama

**2144 Alabama/Northwest Florida Chapter of Crohn s Colitis
Foundation of America**
244 Goodwin Crest Drive, Suite 120
Birmingham, AL 35259   646-387-2149
                                            800-249-1993
                                            Fax: 205-941-1411
                                            jshugart@ccfa.org
                                            www.ccfa.org

Crohn's and Colitis Foundation of America is a nonprofit, voluntary health organization dedicated to improving the quality of life
for persons with Crohn's disease or ulcerative colitis.

Pat Talty, Executive Director
Maura Breen, Chairman

Arizona

2145 Arizona Chapter of Crohn's & Colitis Foundation of America
8098 Via de Negocio, Suite 201
Scottsdale, AZ 85258   480-246-3676
                                            877-259-2104
                                            Fax: 480-246-3679
                                            southwest@ccfa.org
                                            www.ccfa.org

Crohn's and Colitis Foundation of America is a nonprofit, voluntary health organization dedicated to improving the quality of life
for persons with Crohn's disease or ulcerative colitis.

Bridgette Haley, Executive Director
Maura Breen, Chairman

California

**2146 Greater Los Angeles/Orange County Chapter of Chron's &
Colitis Foundation**
1640 S Sepulveda Boulevard, Suite 214
Los Angeles, CA 90025   310-478-4500
                                            866-831-9157
                                            Fax: 310-478-4546
                                            losangeles@ccfa.org
                                            www.ccfa.org

Crohn's and Colitis Foundation of America is a nonprofit, voluntary health organization dedicated to improving the quality of life
for persons with Crohn's disease or ulcerative colitis.

Ronni Epstein, Executive Director
Lindsay Brown, Support Manager

**2147 Greater San Diego/Desert Chapter of Crohn' s & Colitis
Foundation of America**
7850 Mission Center Ct. Suite 100
San Diego, CA 92108   619-497-1300
                                            Fax: 619-497-1304
                                            sandiego@ccfa.org
                                            www.ccfa.org

Crohn's and Colitis Foundation of America is a nonprofit, voluntary health organization dedicated to improving the quality of life
for persons with Crohn's disease or ulcerative colitis.

Pamela Meistrell, Executive Director

2148 Northern California Chapter of Crohn's and Colitis Foundation
5 Third Street, Suite 625
San Francisco, CA 94103
415-356-2232
800-241-0758
Fax: 415-356-0880
ncal@ccfa.org
www.ccfa.org

Supports basic and clinical scientific research to find the cause of, and cure for, Crohn's disease and ulcerative colitis; provides educational programs for patients, medical professionals and the general public; offers supportive services for patients, their families and friends including support groups, information packets, education seminars, physician referral hotline and a quarterly newsletter called Rumblings.

Tamara Block, Executive Director

Colorado

2149 Rocky Mountain Chapter of Crohn's & Colitis Foundation of America
1777 S Bellaire Street, Suite 230
Denver, CO 80222
303-639-9163
800-768-2232
Fax: 303-639-9166
rockymountain@ccfa.org
www.ccfa.org

Crohn's and Colitis Foundation of America is a nonprofit, voluntary health organization dedicated to improving the quality of life for persons with Crohn's disease or ulcerative colitis.

Michele L Basche, Executive Director
Maura Breen, Chairman

Connecticut

2150 Central Connecticut Chapter of Crohn's & Colitis Foundation of America
PO Box 34
New London, CT 06320
646-499-0159
mbfecteau@ccfa.org
www.ccfa.org

Crohn's and Colitis Foundation of America is a nonprofit, voluntary health organization dedicated to improving the quality of life for persons with Crohn's disease or ulcerative colitis.

Maura Breen, Chairman

2151 Fairfield/Westchester Chapter of Crohn's & Colitis Foundation of America
200 Bloomingdale Road
White Plains, NY 10603
914-328-2874
Fax: 914-468-2133
westfield@ccfa.org
www.ccfa.org

Crohn's and Colitis Foundation of America is a nonprofit, voluntary health organization dedicated to improving the quality of life for persons with Crohn's disease or ulcerative colitis.

Russell P Girolamo, Board President
Maura Breen, Chairman

2152 Northern Connecticut Affiliate Chapter of Crohn's & Colitis Foundation of America
PO Box 370614
West Hartford, CT 06137
www.ccfa.org

Crohn's and Colitis Foundation of America is a nonprofit, voluntary health organization dedicated to improving the quality of life for persons with Crohn's disease or uilcerative colitis.

Maura Breen, Chairman

Florida

2153 Florida Chapter of Crohn's & Colitis Found ation of America
21301 Powerline Road #301
21301 Powerline Rd., Suite 301
Boca Raton, FL 33433
561-218-2929
877-664-2929
Fax: 561-218-2240
florida@ccfa.org
www.ccfa.org

Crohn's and Colitis Foundation of America is a nonprofit, voluntary health organization dedicated to improving the quality of life for persons with Crohn's disease or ulcerative colitis.

Amy Gray, Executive Director
Maura Breen, Chairman

Georgia

2154 Georgia Chapter of Crohn's & Colitis Foundation of America
2250 N Druid Hills Road, Suite 250
Atlanta, GA 30329
404-982-0616
800-472-6795
Fax: 404-982-0656
sprimm@ccfa.org
www.ccfa.org

Crohn's and Colitis Foundation of America is a nonprofit, voluntary health organization dedicated to improving the quality of life for persons with Crohn's disease or ulcerative colitis.

Marcia Greenburg, Regional Executive Director
Karen Rittenbaum, Deputy Director

Illinois

2155 Crohn's & Colitis Foundation of America Carol Fisher Chapter
2200 E Devon Avenue, Suite 351
Des Plaines, IL 60018
847-827-0404
800-886-6664
Fax: 847-827-6563
illinois@ccfa.org
www.ccfa.org

Crohn's and Colitis Foundation of America is a nonprofit, voluntary health organizaiton dedicated to finding the cause of, and cure for Crohn's disease and ulcerative colitis. The foundation is committed to conquering these devastating diseases.

$25.00 Dues

Marianne Floriano, Executive Director
Maura Breen, Chairman

Indiana

2156 Indiana Chapter of Crohn's & Colitis Found ation of America
931 e. 86th St Suite 210
Indianapolis, IN 46240
317-259-8071
800-332-6029
Fax: 317-259-8091
jbender@ccfa.org
www.ccfa.org

Provides support and education to adults, children, and families dealing with Crohn's disease and ulcerative colitis. Raises funds for research and programs. Quarterly newsletter, national magazine, award winning website. 55 chapters nationwide.

Jo Bender, Community Development Director
Maura Breen, Chairman

Iowa

2157 Iowa Chapter of Crohn's Colitis Foundation of America
8031 West Center Rd Suite 322
Omaha, NE 68124
402-505-9901
iowa@ccfa.org
www.ccfa.org

Crohn's and Colitis Foundation of America is a nonprofit, voluntary health organization dedicated to improving the quality of life for persons with Crohn's disease or ulcerative colitis.

Melissa Cupich, Development Manager
Maura Breen, Chairman

Kansas

2158   Mid-America Chapter of Crohn's & Colitis Foundation of America
1034 S. Brentwood Suite 1510
St. Louis, MO 63117

314-863-4747
800-783-8006
Fax: 314-863-4749
awillet@ccfa.org
www.ccfa.org

Crohn's and Colitis Foundation of America is a nonprofit, voluntary health organization dedicated to improving the quality of life for persons with Crohn's disease or ulcerative colitis.

Steve Skodak, Development Director
Maura Breen, Chairman

Kentucky

2159   Kentucky Chapter of Crohn's & Colitis Foundation of America
PO Box 573
Prospect, KY 40059

646-623-2620
kentucky@ccfa.org
www.ccfa.org

Crohn's and Colitis Foundation of America is a nonprofit, voluntary health organization dedicated to improving the quality of life for persons with Crohn's disease or ulcerative colitis.

Jenny Silberisen, Community Development Manager
Maura Breen, Chairman

Louisiana

2160   Louisiana/Mississippi Chapter of Crohn's & Colitis Foundation of America
8019 Maple Street
New Orleans, LA 70175

504-861-3433
866-382-2232
Fax: 504-861-3466
lams@ccfa.org
www.ccfa.org

Crohn's and Colitis Foundation of America is a nonprofit, voluntary health organization dedicated to improving the quality of life for persons with Crohn's disease or ulcerative colitis.

David Lee Thomas, Executive Director
Maura Breen, Chairman

Maryland

2161   Maryland/South Delaware Chapter of Crohn's & Colitis Foundation of America
10400 Little Patuxent Parkway, Suite 270
Columbia, MD 21044

443-276-0861
800-618-5583
Fax: 443-276-0865
maryland@ccfa.org
www.ccfa.org

Our mission is to fund research to find a cure for Crohn's disease and ulcerative colitis and to educate and provide support to patients and families with these diseases.

Allison Coffey, Community Development Director
Maura Breen, Chairman

Massachusetts

2162   New England Chapter of Crohn's & Colitis Foundation of America
280 Hillside Avenue
Needham, MA 02494

781-449-0324
800-314-3459
Fax: 781-449-0325
ne@ccfa.org
www.ccfa.org

Crohn's and Colitis Foundation of America is a nonprofit, voluntary health organization dedicated to improving the quality of life for persons with Crohn's disease or ulcerative colitis.

Craig Comins, Regional Executive Director
Maura Breen, Chairman

Michigan

2163   Michigan Chapter of Crohn's & Colitis Foundation of America
31313 Northwestern Highway, Suite 204
Farmington Hills, MI 48334

248-737-0900
Fax: 248-737-0904
michigan@ccfa.org
www.ccfa.org

Crohn's and Colitis Foundation of America is a nonprofit, voluntary health organization dedicated to improving the quality of life for persons with Crohn's disease or ulcerative colitis.

Anthonie Burke, Community Development Director
Maura Breen, Chairman

Minnesota

2164   Minnesota/Dakotas Chapter of Crohn's & Colitis Foundation of America
1885 University Avenue W, Suite 355
Saint Paul, MN 55104

651-917-2424
888-422-3266
Fax: 651-917-2425
minnesota@ccfa.org
www.ccfa.org

Voluntary health organization providing education service and support to Crohn's disease and ulcerative colitis patients and the professional community.

Danielle L Baxter, Executive Director
Ruby Lanoux, Development Coordinator

Mississippi

2165   Louisiana/Mississippi Chapter of Crohn's & Colitis Foundation of America
8019 Maple Street
New Orleans, LA 70175

504-861-3433
866-382-2232
Fax: 504-861-3466
lams@ccfa.org
www.ccfa.org

Crohn's and Colitis Foundation of America is a nonprofit, voluntary health organization dedicated to improving the quality of life for persons with Crohn's disease or ulcerative colitis. Your local chapter can supply you with a list of CCFA physician members in your area.

David Lee Thomas, Executive Director
Maura Breen, Chairman

Missouri

2166 Saint Louis Chapter of Crohn's & Colitis Foundation of America
8420 Delmar Boulevard, Suite 303
Saint Louis, MO 63124
314-997-4466
Fax: 314-991-8756
missouri@ccfa.org
www.ccfa.org

Crohn's and Colitis Foundation of America is a nonprofit, voluntary health organization dedicated to improving the quality of life for persons with Crohn's disease or ulcerative colitis.

Charise Cross, Owner
Maura Breen, Chairman

New Jersey

2167 New Jersey Chapter of Crohn's & Colitis Foundation of America
45 Wilson Avenue
Manalapan, NJ 07726
732-786-9960
Fax: 732-786-9964
newjersey@ccfa.org
www.ccfa.org

Crohn's and Colitis Foundation of America is a nonprofit, voluntary health organization dedicated to improving the quality of life for persons with Crohn's disease or ulcerative colitis.

Rosemarie Golombos, Executive Director
Maura Breen, Chairman

New Mexico

2168 Southwest Chapter of Crohn's & Colitis Foundation of America
8098 Via de Negocio, Suite 201
Scottsdale, AZ 85254
480-246-3676
877-259-2104
Fax: 480-246-3679
southwest@ccfa.org
www.ccfa.org

Crohn's and Colitis Foundation of America is a nonprofit, voluntary health organization dedicated to improving the quality of life for persons with Crohn's disease or ulcerative colitis.

Cindy Sorensen, Regional Edu. & Support Manager
Maura Breen, Chairman

New York

2169 Central New York Chapter of Crohn's & Colitis Foundation of America
2117 Buffalo Rd Suite 299
Rochester, NY 14624
585-617-4771
smassaro@ccfa.org
www.ccfa.org

Crohn's and Colitis Foundation of America is a nonprofit, voluntary health organization dedicated to improving the quality of life for persons with Crohn's disease or ulcerative colitis. Your local chapter can supply you with a list of CCFA physician members in your area.

Maura Breen, Chairman

2170 Fairfield/Westchester Chapter of Crohn's & Colitis Foundation of America
200 Bloomingdale Road
White Plains, NY 10605
914-328-2874
Fax: 914-328-2946
westfield@ccfa.org
www.ccfa.org

Crohn's and Colitis Foundation of America is a nonprofit, voluntary health organization dedicated to improving the quality of life for persons with Crohn's disease or ulcerative colitis. Your local chapter can supply you with a list of CCFA physician members in your area.

Russell P Girolamo, Board President
Maura Breen, Chairman

2171 Greater New York Chapter of Crohn's & Colitis Foundation of America
386 Park Avenue S, 14th Floor
New York, NY 10016
212-679-1570
Fax: 212-679-3567
newyork@ccfa.org
www.ccfa.org

Crohn's and Colitis Foundation of America is a nonprofit, voluntary health organization dedicated to improving the quality of life for persons with Crohn's disease or ulcerative colitis.

Stacy Clark, Manager
Maura Breen, Chairman

2172 Long Island Chapter of Crohn's & Colitis Foundation of America
585 Stewart Avenue, Suite 580
Garden City, NY 11530
516-222-5530
Fax: 516-222-5535
longisland@ccfa.org
www.ccfa.org

Crohn's and Colitis Foundation of America is a nonprofit, voluntary health organization dedicated to improving the quality of life for persons with Crohn's disease or ulcerative colitis.

Edda Ramsdell, Executive Director
Maura Breen, Chairman

2173 Rochester Chapter of Crohn's & Colitis Foundation of America
2117 Buffalo Rd Suite 299
Rochester, NY 14624
585-617-4771
smassaro@ccfa.org
www.ccfa.org

Crohn's and Colitis Foundation of America is a nonprofit, voluntary health organization dedicated to improving the quality of life for persons with Crohn's disease or ulcerative colitis.

Adam Urbanski, President
Maura Breen, Chairman

2174 Upstate/Northeast New York Chapter of Crohn's & Colitis Foundation of America
103 Patroon Dr 10
Guilderland, NY 12084
518-608-5069
upstateny@ccfa.org
www.ccfa.org

The chapter encompasses the following: Albany, Schenectady, Rensselaer, Northern Dutchess, Jefferson, Sullivan, Greene, Columbia, Schoharie, Fulton, Montgomery, Oneida, Saratoga, Ulster, Washington, Warren, Essex, Clinton, Franklin, and Herkimer counties.

Linda Winston, Community Development Director
Maura Breen, Chairman

2175 Western New York Chapter of Crohn's & Colitis Foundation of America
651 Deleware Ave Suite 214
Buffalo, NY 14202
716-362-1232
jpetri@ccfa.org
www.ccfa.org

Crohn's and Colitis Foundation of America is a nonprofit, voluntary health organization dedicated to improving the quality of life for persons with Crohn's disease or ulcerative colitis. Your local chapter can supply you with a list of CCFA physician members in your area.

Jeanenne Petri, Development Manager
Maura Breen, Chairman

North Carolina

2176 Carolinas Chapter of Crohn's & Colitis Foundation of America
2424 N. Davidson St, Suite 110
Charlotte, NC 28205
704-332-1611
Fax: 704-332-1612
jgolombos@ccfa.org
www.ccfa.org

Crohn's and Colitis Foundation of America is a nonprofit, voluntary health organization dedicated to improving the quality of life for persons with Crohn's disease or ulcerative colitis.

Joanne Colombos, National Walk Specialist
Maura Breen, Chairman

Ohio

2177 Central Ohio Chapter of Crohn's & Colitis Foundation of America
5500 Frantz Rd , Suite 155
Dublin, OH 43017
614-889-6060
Fax: 614-889-6655
centralohio@ccfa.org
www.ccfa.org

Crohn's and Colitis Foundation of America is a nonprofit, voluntary health organization dedicated to improving the quality of life for persons with Crohn's disease or ulcerative colitis.

Deborah Shub, Community Development Director
Maura Breen, Chairman

2178 Northeast Ohio Chapter of Crohn's & Colitis Foundation of America
4700 Rockside Rd. #425
Independence, OH 44131
216-524-7700
866-345-2232
Fax: 216-524-7701
neohio@aol.com
www.ccfa.org

Crohn's and Colitis Foundation of America is a nonprofit, voluntary health organization dedicated to improving the quality of life for persons with Crohn's disease or ulcerative colitis.

Lesley Hoover, Chapter Director
Maura Breen, Chairman

2179 Southwest Ohio Chapter of Crohn's & Colitis Foundation of America
8 Triangle Park Drive, Suite 800
Cincinnati, OH 45246
513-772-3550
877-283-7513
Fax: 513-772-7599
swohio@ccfa.org
www.ccfa.org

CCFA is the only national nonprofit organization dedicated to finding the cause of and cure for Crohn's disease and ulcerative colitis. We offer monthly connection and education groups, education symposium, one-on-one support through our Ambassador Program and for our children, a four day regional camp. CCFA offers free Teacher's Guides, Parent's Guide and Children's Guides to Crohn's Disease and Ulcerative Colitis. This chapter also serves Greater Dayton, Northern Kentucky and SW Indiana.

Jenny Southers, Development Director
Rachel Miller, Take Steps Walk Mgr

Oklahoma

2180 Oklahoma Chapter of Crohn's & Colitis Foundation of America
4504 E 67th Street, Suite 125
Tulsa, OK 74136
918-523-8540
Fax: 918-523-8560
oklahoma@ccfa.org
www.ccfa.org

Crohn's and Colitis Foundation of America is a nonprofit, voluntary health organization dedicated to improving the quality of life for persons with Crohn's disease or ulcerative colitis.

Mike Gramm, Board of Trustees
Maura Breen, Chairman

Pennsylvania

2181 Pennsylvania/Delaware Valley Chapter of Crohn's & Colitis Foundation of America
367 E Street Road
Trevose, PA 19053
215-396-9100
888-340-4744
Fax: 215-396-1170
philaelphia@ccfa.org
www.ccfa.org

Crohn's and Colitis Foundation of America is a nonprofit, voluntary health organization dedicated to improving the quality of life for persons with Crohn's disease and ulcerative colitis.

Barbara Berman, Executive Director
Maura Breen, Chairman

2182 Western Pennsylvania Chapter of Crohn's & Colitis Foundation of America
300 Penn Center Suite 401
Pittsburgh, PA 15235
412-823-8272
877-823-8272
Fax: 412-823-8276
wpawv@ccfa.org
www.ccfa.org

National nonprofit research-oriented voluntary health organization dedicated to improving the quality of life for people with Crohn's disease and ulcerative colitis. Our mission: support basic and clinical scientific research to find a cause and cure for Crohn's disease and ulcerative colitis, provide educational programs for patients, medical professioinals, and general public, and offer supportive services for patients, their families and friends.

600 Members

Susan Kukic, Executive Director

South Carolina

2183 South Carolina Chapter of Crohn's & Colitis Foundation of America
2424 N. Davidson St, Suite 110
Charlotte, NC 28205
704-332-1611
877-632-1611
Fax: 704-332-1612
carolinas@ccfa.org
www.ccfa.org

Crohn's and Colitis Foundation of America is a nonprofit, voluntary health organization dedicated to improving the quality of life for persons with Crohn's disease.

Kelli King, Development Director
Maura Breen, Chairman

Tennessee

2184 Tennessee Chapter of Crohn's & Colitis Foundation of America
95 White Bridge Rd Suite 209
Nashville, TN 37205
615-356-0444
866-814-2232
Fax: 615-356-0445
tennessee@ccfa.org
www.ccfa.org

Crohn's and Colitis Foundation of America is a nonprofit, voluntary health organization dedicated to improving the quality of life for persons with Crohn's disease or ulcerative colitis.

Steve Wallace, Executive Director
Maura Breen, Chairman

Texas

2185 Houston-Gulf Coast/South Texas Chapter of Crohn's & Colitis Foundation of America
5120 Woodway, Suite 8008
Houston, TX 77056
713-752-2232
800-785-2232
Fax: 713-572-2433
infohouston@ccfa.org
www.ccfa.org

Crohn's and Colitis Foundation of America is a nonprofit, voluntary health organization dedicated to cure and prevent Crohn's disease and ulcerative colitis through research and to improve the quality of life of children and adults affected by those digestive diseases through education and support.

Charles Weiss, IOM, Executive Director
Maura Breen, Chairman

2186 North Texas Chapter of Crohn's & Colitis Foundation of America
12801 N Central Expressway Suite 270
Dallas, TX 75243
972-386-0607
Fax: 972-386-0509
ntexas@ccfa.org
www.ccfa.org

Crohn's and Colitis Foundation of America is a nonprofit, voluntary health organization dedicated to improving the quality of life for persons with Crohn's disease or ulcerative colitis.

Teresa Sheffield, Executive Director
Maura Breen, Chairman

Washington

2187 Washington State Chapter of Crohn's & Colitis Foundation of America
9 Lake Bellevue Drive, Suite 203
Bellevue, WA 98005
425-451-8455
Fax: 425-451-1708
northwest@ccfa.org
www.ccfa.org

Crohn's and Colitis Foundation of America is a nonprofit, voluntary health organization dedicated to improving the quality of life for persons with Crohn's disease or ulcerative colitis.

Linda Huse, Regional Director
Maura Breen, Chairman

Wisconsin

2188 Wisconsin Chapter of Crohn's & Colitis Foundation of America
1126 S 70th Street, Suite S210A
West Allis, WI 53214
414-475-5520
877-586-5588
Fax: 414-475-5502
wisconsin@ccfa.org
www.ccfa.org

Crohn's and Colitis Foundation of America is a nonprofit, voluntary health organization dedicated to improving the quality of life for persons with Crohn's disease or ulcerative colitis.

Tyler Hillstrom, Executive Director
Maura Breen, Chairman

Libraries & Resource Centers

2189 National Digestive Diseases Information Clearinghouse
9000 Rockville Pike
Bethesda, MD 20892
301-496-3583
800-860-8747
Fax: 703-738-4929
healthinfo@niddk.nih.gov
www.niddk.nih.gov

The National Institute of Diabetes and Digestive and Kidney Diseases conducts and supports research on many of the most serious diseases affecting public health. The Institute supports much of the clinical research on the diseases of internal medicine and related subspecialty fields as well as many basic science disciplines.

Dr. Griffin P. Rodgers, Director
Dr. Gregory G. Germino, Deputy Director
Camille M. Hoover, M.S.W., Executive Officer

Research Centers

2190 Crohn's & Colitis Foundation of America
386 Park Avenue S, 17th Floor
New York, NY 10016
800-932-2423
info@ccfa.org
www.ccfa.org

Since 1967, CCFA has been the only national voluntary health agency dedicated to funding research to find a cure for Crohn's disease and ulcerative colitis. The Foundation provides educational and patient support services to both the lay and medical communities and plans to provide grants dedicated to pediatric research.

Maura Breen, Chairman

2191 Krancer Center for Inflammatory Bowel Disease Research
Hahnemann University
Broad & Vine Streets
Philadelphia, PA 19102
215-762-8618
Fax: 215-762-1998

Research into the causes and treatments of ulcerative colitis and Crohn's disease.

Harris Clearfield, Director

Conferences

2192 Genetic Alliance Annual Conference
Genetic Alliance
4301 Connecticut Avenue NW, Suite 404
Washington, DC 20008
202-966-5557
800-336-4363
Fax: 202-966-8553
info@geneticalliance.org
www.geneticalliance.org

Consistently inspirational and enables partnership among all stakeholders: advocates and community leaders, health and industry professionals, policymakers, and academicians.

July

Sharon Terry, President/CEO
Tetyana Murza, Managing Director
Natasha Bonhomme, VP, Strategic Development

2193 IFFGD Professional Symposia
Int'l Foundation for Functional Gastrointestinal
PO Box 170864
Milwaukee, WI 53217
414-964-1799
888-964-2001
Fax: 414-964-7176
iffgd@iffgd.org
www.iffgd.org

Aimed at promoting education and awareness among professionals from multiple disciplines who treat gastrointestinal disorders and incontinence.

April

Nancy J Norton, President
William Norton, Co-founder of IFFGD

Web Sites

2194 Crohn's & Colitis Foundation of America
733 Third Avenue, Suite 510
New York, NY 10017   800-932-2423
    800-932-2423
    Fax: 212-779-4098
    info@ccfa.org
    www.ccfa.org

Information regardin Crohn's disease and ulcerative colitis.

Maura Breen, Chairman
Richard Geswell, President & CEO
Judi Brown, Chief Development Officer

2195 Health Answers
410 Horsham Road
Horsham, PA 19044   215-442-9017
    Michael.tague@healthanswers.com
    www.healthanswers.com

HealthAnswers offers a breadth of services in medical education, sales force training, patient support, solutions, professional promotion and consumer solutions.

Michael Tague, Managing Director

Book Publishers

2196 Crohn's Disease and Ulcerative Colitis Fact Book
Crohn's & Colitis Foundation of America
386 Park Avenue S, 17th Floor
New York, NY 10016   212-685-3440
    800-932-2423
    Fax: 212-779-4098
    info@ccfa.org
    www.ccfa.org

Written in layman's language, this first, complete guide is helpful in understanding and coping with inflammatory bowel diseases.

2197 Digestive Diseases & Disorders Sourcebook
Omnigraphics
PO Box 625
Holmes, PA 19043   800-234-1340
    Fax: 800-875-1340
    info@omnigraphics.com
    omnigraphics.com

Basic consumer health information including celiac disease, Crohn's disease, diarrhea, hernias, irritable bowel syndrome and ulcers.

335 pages
ISBN: 0-780803-27-2

2198 Let's Talk About Going to the Hospital
Rosen Publishing Group's PowerKids Press
29 E 21st Street
New York, NY 10010   212-777-3017
    800-237-9932
    Fax: 888-436-4643
    rosenpub@tribeca.ios.com
    www.powerkidspress.com

If a child has to check into the hospital, chances are he or she is already upset about being ill. Knowing how a hospital functions and what the procedures are, such as when family members can visit, will help in what is already a stressful situation. Grades K-5.

24 pages
ISBN: 0-823950-36-0

2199 Managing Your Child's Crohn's Disease or Ulcerative Colitis
Crohn's & Colitis Foundation of America
386 Park Avenue S, 17th Floor
New York, NY 10016   212-685-3440
    800-932-2423
    Fax: 212-779-4098
    info@ccfa.org
    www.ccfa.org

This first full-length book on Crohn's disease and ulcerative colitis, specifically targeted for parents of children and teenagers, includes topics on cause and diagnosis, treatment, surgery, hospitalization, diet and nutrition, school and social issues, and resources for the patient.

$16.95 Members

2200 New People...Not Patients: a Source Book for Living with Bowel Disease
Crohn's & Colitis Foundation of America
386 Park Avenue S, 17th Floor
New York, NY 10016   212-685-3440
    800-932-2423
    Fax: 212-779-4098
    info@ccfa.org
    www.ccfa.org

This book contains the essential information you need to help you cope with Crohn's disease and ulcerative colitis after you leave the doctor's office.

2201 Treating IBD
Crohn's & Colitis Foundation of America
386 Park Avenue S, 17th Floor
New York, NY 10016   212-685-3440
    800-932-2423
    info@ccfa.org
    www.ccfa.org

A patient's guide to the medical and surgical management of Inflammatory Bowel Disease, this book gives information on treating Crohn's disease and ulcerative colitis, including drug therapies, advances in nutritional care, and recently developed surgical alternatives.

2202 Understanding Crohn Disease and Ulcerative Colitis
University Press of Mississippi
3825 Ridgewood Road, Unit 9
Jackson, MS 39211   601-432-6205
    800-737-7788
    Fax: 601-432-6246
    press@ihl.state.ms.us
    www.upress.state.ms.us

For patients and caregivers, an overview of the nature and treatments of inflammatory bowel disease.

128 pages Paperback
ISBN: 1-578062-03-9

Leila W Salisbury Director

Magazines

2203 Take Charge
Crohn's & Colitis Foundation of America
733 Third Avenue, Suite 510
New York, NY 10017   800-932-2423
    info@ccfa.org
    www.ccfa.org

Offers the most up-to-date information on IBD research, treatment, and legislative initiatives for patients, families, and friends.

Maura Breen, Chairman
Richard Geswell, President & CEO
Judi Brown, Chief Development Officer

Newsletters

2204 Under the Microscope
Crohn's & Colitis Foundation of America
733 Third Avenue, Suite 510
New York, NY 10017   800-932-2423
    800-932-2423
    Fax: 212-779-4098
    info@ccfa.org
    www.ccfa.org

Includes a variety of relevant information such as information on new research projects, clinical trials, conference notes, and breaking news about partnerships and grants.

Maura Breen, Chairman
Richard Geswell, President & CEO
Judi Brown, Chief Development Officer

Pamphlets

2205 CCFA: A Case for Support
Crohn's & Colitis Foundation of America
733 Third Avenue, Suite 510
New York, NY 10017   800-932-2423
                                        800-932-2423
                                    Fax: 212-779-4098
                                        info@ccfa.org
                                        www.ccfa.org

Reviews the work of the Crohn's and Colitis Foundation of
America, sponsors a nationally recognized research program,
which seeks to improve treatment, and ultimately find the cure for
inflammatory bowel disease.

Maura Breen, Chairman
Richard Geswell, President & CEO
Judi Brown, Chief Development Officer

2206 Coping with Crohn's and Colitis is Tough
Crohn's & Colitis Foundation of America
733 Third Avenue, Suite 510
New York, NY 10017   800-932-2423
                                        800-932-2423
                                    Fax: 212-779-4098
                                        info@ccfa.org
                                        www.ccfa.org

Offers information on the Crohn's and Colitis Association. Also
offers factual information and statistics on the diseases.

Maura Breen, Chairman
Richard Geswell, President & CEO
Judi Brown, Chief Development Officer

2207 Crohn's Disease, Ulcerative Colitis, and Your Child
Crohn's & Colitis Foundation of America
733 Third Avenue, Suite 510
New York, NY 10017   800-932-2423
                                        800-932-2423
                                    Fax: 212-779-4098
                                        info@ccfa.org
                                        www.ccfa.org

Answers questions about IBD in children, providing information
on early signs, growth and developments, treatments and special
problems in school.

Maura Breen, Chairman
Richard Geswell, President & CEO
Judi Brown, Chief Development Officer

**2208 Guide for Children and Teenagers to Crohn's
Disease/Ulcerative Colitis**
Crohn's & Colitis Foundation of America
733 Third Avenue, Suite 510
New York, NY 10017   800-932-2423
                                        800-932-2423
                                    Fax: 212-779-4098
                                        info@ccfa.org
                                        www.ccfa.org

Offers important information on these illnesses to children and
teens.

Maura Breen, Chairman
Richard Geswell, President & CEO
Judi Brown, Chief Development Officer

2209 Questions & Answers About Diet and Nutrition
Crohn's & Colitis Foundation of America
733 Third Avenue, Suite 510
New York, NY 10017   800-932-2423
                                        800-932-2423
                                    Fax: 212-779-4098
                                        info@ccfa.org
                                        www.ccfa.org

Raises important facts about how diet and nutrition affect persons
with Crohn's Disease.

2210 Questions and Answers About Complications
Crohn's & Colitis Foundation of America
733 Third Avenue, Suite 510
New York, NY 10017   800-932-2423
                                        800-932-2423
                                    Fax: 212-779-4098
                                        info@ccfa.org
                                        www.ccfa.org

Medical facts and complications from surgery.

Maura Breen, Chairman
Richard Geswell, President & CEO
Judi Brown, Chief Development Officer

**2211 Questions and Answers About Crohn's Disease & Ulcerative
Colitis**
Crohn's & Colitis Foundation of America
733 Third Avenue, Suite 510
New York, NY 10017   800-932-2423
                                        800-932-2423
                                    Fax: 212-779-4098
                                        info@ccfa.org
                                        www.ccfa.org

Offers information on the illness and answers the most frequently
asked questions about Crohn's Disease. Also includes a glossary
of IBD terms.

Maura Breen, Chairman
Richard Geswell, President & CEO
Judi Brown, Chief Development Officer

**2212 Questions and Answers About Emotional Factors In Ileitis and
Colitis**
Crohn's & Colitis Foundation of America
733 Third Avenue, Suite 510
New York, NY 10017   800-932-2423
                                        800-932-2423
                                    Fax: 212-779-4098
                                        info@ccfa.org
                                        www.ccfa.org

Answers some of the most commonly asked questions about ileitis and colitis and the role of emotional factors in their cause and
course.

Maura Breen, Chairman
Richard Geswell, President & CEO
Judi Brown, Chief Development Officer

2213 Teacher's Guide to Crohn's Disease & Ulcerative Colitis
Crohn's & Colitis Foundation of America
733 Third Avenue, Suite 510
New York, NY 10017   800-932-2423
                                        800-932-2423
                                    Fax: 212-779-4098
                                        info@ccfa.org
                                        www.ccfa.org

Maura Breen, Chairman
Richard Geswell, President & CEO
Judi Brown, Chief Development Officer

DESCRIPTION

2214 CRYPTORCHIDISM

Synonyms: Cryptorchidy, Cryptorchism

Covers these related disorders: Ectopic (maldescended) testes, True undescended testes

Involves the following Biologic System(s):

Renal and Urologic Disorders

Cryptorchidism is characterized by failure of one or both testes to descend into the pouch-like structure known as the scrotum. The testes are the paired, oval-shaped glands that produce the male reproductive cells (sperm). Early during male fetal growth, the testes develop within the abdomen near the kidneys. The testes then descend into the scrotum through a tubular canal that passes through lower muscular layers of the abdominal wall (inguinal canal). In males with cryptorchidism, one or both testes fail to complete their descent into the scrotum. Undescended testes that are located along the proper path of descent are known as true undescended testes, whereas those that have completed their descent through the inguinal canal yet have become located in areas other than the scrotum are referred to as ectopic or maldescended testes.

In most cases, one testis is affected (unilateral cryptorchidism); however, both testes may fail to descend (bilateral cryptorchidism) in up to 30 percent of affected male infants. In many cases, undescended testes may move down into the scrotum before one year of age. However, testes that fail to spontaneously descend during the first year of life typically fail to develop properly, may decrease in size, and have decreased numbers of reproductive cells. Without treatment, affected males are at an increased risk of infertility; malignant tumor development in affected testes during the third or fourth decade of life; or pain, swelling, and, in some cases, localized areas of tissue loss (necrosis).

Treatment of cryptorchidism often includes early surgery to relocate undescended testes into the scrotum (i.e., orchiopexy) and to correct inguinal hernias, which typically occur in association with true undescended testes and ectopic testes. Inguinal hernias are characterized by bulging of portions of the intestine into the inguinal canal. Surgical correction of cryptorchidism is typically recommended in the first years of life to help improve proper testicular development and fertility in adulthood.

Cryptorchidism affects about three and a half percent of full-term male newborns and increases in incidence in newborns who are born before 37 weeks of pregnancy (preterm). The condition may occur as an isolated abnormality or, in some cases, due to or in association with a number of different underlying syndromes or conditions.

Government Agencies

2215 NIH/ Eunice Kennedy Shriver National Insti tute of Child Health & Human Development
31 Center Drive, Building 31
Bethesda, MD 20892

301-496-5113
800-370-2943
Fax: 866-760-5947
TTY: 888-320-6942
nichdpress@mail.nih.gov
www.nichd.nih.gov

Established in 1962 by congress, today the institute conducts and supports research on topics related to the health of children, adults, families and populations. Some of these topics include: developmental disabilities, growth and development, infant death, reproductive health and birth defects.

Diana W. Bianchi, Director
Paul Williams, Director, Communications

National Associations & Support Groups

2216 American Academy of Pediatrics
141 Northwest Point Boulevard
Elk Grove Village, IL 60007

847-434-4000
800-433-9016
Fax: 847-434-8000
www.aap.org

The American Academy of Pediatrics and its member pediatricians are committed to the attainment of optimal physical, mental and social health and well-being for all infants, children, adolescents, and young adults.

Fernando Stein, MD, FAAP, President
Karen Remley, MD, CEO/Executive VP

2217 Genetic Alliance
4301 Connecticut Avenue NW, Suite 404
Washington, DC 20008

202-966-5557
Fax: 202-966-8553
info@geneticalliance.org
www.geneticalliance.org

A coalition of voluntary genetic support groups, consumers and professionals addressing the needs of individuals and families affected by genetic disorders from a national perspective.

Sharon Terry, President/CEO
Tetyana Murza, Managing Director
Natasha Bonhomme, VP, Strategic Development

2218 March of Dimes Foundation
1275 Mamaroneck Avenue
White Plains, NY 10605

914-997-4488
888-663-4637
Fax: 914-997-4763
info@marchofdimes.com
www.marchofdimes.com

Partnership of volunteers and professionals dedicated to improving the health of babies by preventing birth defects and infant mortality. Over 100 chapters are located across the country and can be located through the National Office.

Stacey D. Stewart, President

2219 NIH/National Institute of Mental Health
6001 Executive Boulevard, Room 6200, MSC 9663
Bethesda, MD 20892

301-443-4536
866-615-6464
Fax: 301-443-4279
TTY: 301-443-8431
nimhinfo@nih.gov
www.nimh.nih.gov

Conducts strategic planning for specific research areas as well as for the Institute as a whole.

Joshua Gordon, MD, PhD, Director
Shelli Avenevoli, MD, Deputy Director

Conferences

2220 Genetic Alliance Annual Conference
Genetic Alliance
4301 Connecticut Avenue NW, Suite 404
Washington, DC 20008

202-966-5557
800-336-4363
Fax: 202-966-8553
info@geneticalliance.org
www.geneticalliance.org

Consistently inspirational and enables partnership among all stakeholders: advocates and community leaders, health and industry professionals, policymakers, and academicians.
July

Sharon Terry, President/CEO
Tetyana Murza, Managing Director
Natasha Bonhomme, VP, Strategic Development

Web Sites

2221 European Society for Pediatric Urology
www.espu.org

025-503-8690
Fax: 025-503-2546
president@espu.org
www.espu.org

A nonprofit society whose main purpose is to promote pediatric urology, appropriate practice, education as well as exchanges between practitioners involved in the treatment of genito urinary disorders in children.

Ramnath Subramaniam, Chairman, Educational Committee
Gianantonio Manzoni, President
Dr. Emilio Merlini, Treasurer

2222 National Center for Biotechnology Information
National Library of Medicine, Building 38A
Bethesda, MD 20894

888-346-3656
info@ncbi.nlm.nih.gov
www.ncbi.nlm.nih.gov

NCBI's mission is to develop new information technologies to aid in the understanding of fundamental molecular and genetic processes that control health and disease.

Christine E. Seidman, M.D., Chair
David J. Lipman, M.D., Executive Secretary
Michael Boehnke, Ph.D., Board Member

2223 Online Mendelian Inheritance in Man
National Library of Medicine, Building 38A
Bethesda, MD 20894

888-346-3656
info@ncbi.nlm.nih.gov
www.ncbi.nlm.nih.gov

This database is a catalog of human genes and genetic disorders.

Christine E. Seidman, M.D., Chair
David J. Lipman, M.D., Executive Secretary
Michael Boehnke, Ph.D., Board Member

DESCRIPTION

2224 CUSHING'S SYNDROME

Synonyms: Cushing's basophilism, Hyperadrenocorticism, Pituitary basophilism

Involves the following Biologic System(s):

Endocrinologic Disorders

Cushing's syndrome refers to a condition characterized by excessive levels of the corticosteroid hormone, cortisol, in the blood. Cortisol is produced in the outer portion (cortex) of the adrenal glands in response to the secretion of adrenocorticotropic hormone (ACTH; corticotropin). ACTH stimulates the growth of the adrenal cortex and thus the production of cortisol. Cushing's syndrome may be caused by a variety of factors including tumors of the adrenal glands or the pituitary gland, tumors of certain other organs, and excessive intake of corticosteroid drugs. In the very young, Cushing's syndrome occurs in more girls than boys by a ratio of approximately three to one.

Because cortisol assists in the metabolism of fat, protein, and glucose, many characteristic symptoms and findings associated with this disorder are related to the levels and distribution of body fat. For example, children with Cushing's syndrome may be somewhat obese with very full cheeks, a reddish moonface appearance, double chin, and excessive fat deposits on the back of the neck. In addition, the adrenal glands may be stimulated to secrete excessive amounts of other hormones that are converted in the liver to testosterone and estrogen. Overproduction of these androgenic hormones may result in symptoms such as increased amounts of hair on the face and trunk (hypertrichosis), the development of acne, and deepening of the voice as well as other masculine traits. Other findings that may appear over a period of time include elevated blood pressure (hypertension), kidney (renal) stones, and increased vulnerability to infection. Children with Cushing's syndrome may also experience growth delays or may not achieve height (short stature). However, those children who develop masculinization symptoms may reach average or above average height. Older children may experience a delay in onset of puberty and develop purplish stretch marks (striae) on the abdomen, breasts, hips, and thighs. In addition, their skin may become thin and fragile, leading to easy tissue injury. Affected children may develop headaches and weakness, experience increasing difficulty with school work, or become depressed or experience other emotional disturbances.

Treatment of Cushing's syndrome is dependent upon the underlying cause. If the disease results from a benign or malignant tumor or enlargement of the adrenal gland, surgical removal of the tumor or the adrenal gland (adrenalectomy) may be advised. A tumor in the pituitary gland may either be surgically removed or treated with radiation. Subsequent management of surgical or other procedures often includes appropriate hormone replacement therapy. Cushing's syndrome associated with prolonged or excessive intake of corticosteroids may be re|versed by a monitored and gradual (tapered) withdrawal of the medication. Other treatment is symptomatic and supportive.

National Associations & Support Groups

2225 American Academy of Pediatrics
141 Northwest Point Boulevard
Elk Grove Village, IL 60007

847-434-4000
800-433-9016
Fax: 847-434-8000
www.aap.org

The American Academy of Pediatrics and its member pediatricians are committed to the attainment of optimal physical, mental and social health and well-being for all infants, children, adolescents, and young adults.

Fernando Stein, MD, FAAP, President
Karen Remley, MD, CEO/Executive VP

2226 American Association of Clinical Endocrinologists
245 Riverside Avenue, Suite 200
Jacksonville, FL 32202

904-353-7878
Fax: 904-353-8185
info@aace.com
www.aace.com

A professional medical organization aimed at promoting the quality of clinical epidemiologic research and improving the knowledge base for the diagnosis, prognosis, prevention and treatment of health conditions through the advancement and application of innovative methods.

Jeffrey I Mechanick, President
George Grunberger, Vice President
Jonathan D Leffert, Secretary

2227 Cushing's Support & Research Foundation
65 E India Row, Suite 22B
Boston, MA 02110

617-723-3674
Fax: 617-723-3674
cushinfo@csrf.net
www.csrf.net

To provide information and support for Cushing's Disease and Cushing's Syndrome to patients and their families to increase awareness and to educate the public about Cushing's Disease and Cushing's Syndrome. To be a resource for information and support to healthcare professionals, to raise and distribute funds for Cushing's Disease and Cushing's Syndrome research.

Louise Pace, Founding President

2228 Human Growth Foundation
997 Glen Cove Avenue, Suite 5
Glen Head, NY 11545

516-671-4041
800-451-6434
Fax: 516-671-4055
hgfl@hgfound.org
www.hgfound.org

A voluntary, nonprofit organization whose mission is to help children and adults with disorders of growth and growth hormones through research, education, support and advocacy. The foundation is dedicated to helping medical science to better understand the process of growth. It is composed of concerned parents and friends of children and adults with growth problems and interested health professionals.

Patricia D Costa, Executive Director

2229 Lawson Wilkins Pediatric Endocrine Society
6728 Old McLean Village Drive
McLean, VA 22101

703-556-9222
Fax: 703-556-8729
secretary@lwpes.org
www.lwpes.org

To promote the acquisition and dissemination of knowledge of endocrine and metabolic disorders from conception through adolescence.

Morey W Haymond, President
Karen Rubin, Treasurer
Peter A Lee, Secretary

2230 National Adrenal Diseases Foundation
505 Northern Boulevard
Great Neck, NY 11021
516-487-4992
nadfmail@aol.com
www.nadf.us

A nonprofit organization dedicated to providing support, information and education to individuals having Addison's disease as well as related diseases such as Cushing's Syndrome and Congenital Adrenal Hyperplasia. Promotes early diagnosis and treatment, and sponsors support groups and offers a quarterly newsletter, educational materials and access to a library of related information.

Kalina Warren, President
Timothy Skodon, Treasurer
Phyllis Speiser, Medical Advisor

Conferences

2231 AACE Annual Meeting and Clinical Congress
American Association of Clinical Endocrinologists
245 Riverside Avenue, Suite 200
Jacksonville, FL 32202
904-353-7878
Fax: 904-353-8185
info@aace.com
www.aace.com

April

Yehuda Handelsman, President
Donald C Jones, Chief Executive Officer

Web Sites

2232 Cushing's Support and Research Foundation
60 Robbins Road, #12
Plymouth, MA 2360
617-723-3674
Fax: 617-723-3674
cushinfo@csrf.net
csrf.net

The mission is to provide information and support for Cushing's Disease and Cushing's Syndrome patients and their families, to increase awareness and to educate the public about Cushing's Disease and Cushing's Syndrome, to be a resource for information and support to health care professionals, to raise and distribute funds for Cushing's Disease and Cushing's Syndrome research.

Louise Pace, Founding President
John P. Gulielmetti, Treasurer
Karen Campbell, Director

Book Publishers

2233 Endocrine & Metabolic Disorders Sourcebook
Omnigraphics
PO Box 8002
Aston, PA 19014
800-234-1340
Fax: 800-875-1340
info@omnigraphics.com
www.omnigraphics.com

Basic information for the lay person about pancreatic and insulin-related disorders such as pancreatitis, diabetes and hypoglycemia; adrenal gland disorders such as Cushing's syndrome, Addison's disease and congenital adrenal hyperplasia; pituitary gland disorders such as growth hormone deficiency, acromegaly and pituitary tumors; and thyroid disorders such as hypothyroidism, Grave's disease, Hashimoto's disease and goiter.

574 pages hardcover
ISBN: 0-780802-07-1

2234 Let's Talk About Going to the Hospital
Rosen Publishing Group's PowerKids Press
29 E 21st Street
New York, NY 10010
212-777-3017
800-237-9932
Fax: 888-436-4643
rosenpub@tribeca.ios.com
www.powerkidspress.com

If a child has to check into the hospital, chances are he or she is already upset about being ill. Knowing how a hospital functions and what the procedures are, such as when family members can visit, will help in what is already a stressful situation. Grades K-5.

24 pages
ISBN: 0-823950-36-0

Journals

2235 Endocrine Practice
245 Riverside Avenue, Suite 200
Jacksonville, FL 32202
904-353-7878
Fax: 904-353-8185
info@aace.com
www.aace.com

Peer-reviewed journal published six-times a year and is the official journal of the American College of Endocrinology (ACE) and the American Association of Clinical Endocrinologists (AACE).

R. Mack Harrell, MdD, FACP, FACE, President
Paulin M. Camacho, MD, FACE, Vice President
Donald C. Jones, CEO

Newsletters

2236 NADF News
National Adrenal Diseases Foundation
505 Northern Boulevard
Great Neck, NY 11021
516-487-4992
nadfsupport@nadf.us
www.nadf.us

Provides support and information to those living with adrenal diseases.

Kalina Warren, President
Melanie G. Wong, Executive Director
Edward A. Wong, Executive Director's Assistant

DESCRIPTION

2237 CYSTIC FIBROSIS
Synonyms: CF, Mucoviscidosis
Involves the following Biologic System(s):
Respiratory Disorders

Cystic fibrosis (CF) is an inherited multisystem disorder that results in the abnormal production of mucus by almost all exocrine glands, causing obstruction of those glands and ducts. Glands of the respiratory and reproductive systems as well as pancreatic glands and sweat glands are affected. CF is considered one of the most common autosomal recessive disorders affecting Caucasians. Cystic fibrosis occurs in approximately one in 2,500 to 3,000 Caucasian infants and about one in 17,000 African-American infants. It is considered extremely rare in other populations. The disorder results from abnormal changes (mutations) of a gene on the long arm (q) of chromosome 7 (7q31.2). More than 400 different mutations of the CF gene have been identified.

In infants, children, and adults with cystic fibrosis, mucus-secreting glands within the air passages of the lungs (bronchi) produce unusually thick secretions, clogging and obstructing the airways and promoting the growth of certain bacteria. As a result, affected individuals may experience chronic obstruction and infection of the airways. In addition, the pancreas lacks sufficient digestive enzymes to break down food materials (malabsorption). Other exocrine gland abnormalities may also be present. For example, the sweat glands produce secretions containing abnormally high levels of salt; glands of the neck of the uterus (cervix) in affected females may produce abnormally increased, thickened secretions of mucus; and certain ducts of the male reproductive system (e.g., epididymis, ductus [vas] deferens, seminal vesicles) may be absent (atretic).

During the first or second day of life, some newborns with cystic fibrosis may experience bloating of the abdomen (abdominal distension), vomiting (emesis), and abnormal blockage of the lower region of the small intestine with meconium (meconium ileus). Meconium is the thick, sticky, darkish green material that accumulates in the fetal intestines and forms a newborn's first stools. Infants with cystic fibrosis also usually fail to grow and gain weight at the expected rate (failure to thrive). Additional symptoms and findings may include abnormally decreased muscle mass; a protruding abdomen; and loose, foul-smelling stools that contain an excessive amount of fat (steatorrhea). Children with cystic fibrosis often have respiratory abnormalities including wheezing; a chronic cough that may be accompanied by gagging and vomiting; recurrent inflammation of the air passages (bronchiolitis); and an increased susceptibility to lower respiratory infections (e.g., pneumonia). Affected adolescents may experience abnormally slow growth and delayed sexual development (i.e., average delay of two years); in addition, affected males may be infertile due to lack of sperm development (azoospermia). As the disease progresses, individuals with cystic fibrosis tend to experience increasingly severe respiratory abnormalities that may result in life-threatening complications.

Cystic fibrosis may be diagnosed based upon characteristic physical findings (e.g., chronic obstructive pulmonary disease, exocrine pancreatic insufficiency), specialized laboratory tests (e.g., sweat testing), and a positive family history (including DNA analysis). The treatment of cystic fibrosis is symptomatic and supportive and includes early intervention, ongoing monitoring, preventive measures, the use of certain medications, and other specialized treatment techniques. Approaches to treatment may include physical therapy, a high protein, high calorie diet, pancreatic enzyme replacement therapy, vitamin supplementation, specialized respiratory therapy, medications to help clean mucus from the airways and prevent or treat respiratory infections (e.g., antibiotic therapy). Median survival is about 31 years of age.

National Associations & Support Groups

2238 American Academy of Pediatrics
141 Northwest Point Boulevard
Elk Grove Village, IL 60007
847-434-4000
800-433-9016
Fax: 847-434-8000
www.aap.org

The American Academy of Pediatrics and its member pediatricians are committed to the attainment of optimal physical, mental and social health and well-being for all infants, children, adolescents, and young adults.

Fernando Stein, MD, FAAP, President
Karen Remley, MD, CEO/Executive VP

2239 American Lung Association
55 W. Wacker Drive, Suite 1150
Chicago, IL 60601
312-801-7628
800-548-8252
info@lung.org
www.lung.org

The American Lung Association fights lung disease in all its forms, with special emphasis on asthma, tobacco control and environmental health. The American Lung Association is funded by contributions from the public, along with gifts and grants from corporations, foundations and government agencies. The association achieves its many successes through the work of thousands of committed volunteers and staff.

Harold P. Wimmer, National President & CEO
Susan Rappaport, National VP, Research/Scientific
Sue Swan, Chief Development Officer

2240 Cystic Fibrosis Foundation
6931 Arlington Road
Bethesda, MD 20814
301-951-4422
800-344-4823
Fax: 301-951-6378
info@cff.org
www.cff.org

The mission of CF Foundation is to assure the development of means to cure and control CF and to improve the quality of life for those with the disease. It funds medical research and care programs which are improving the length and quality of life for people with cystic fibrosis.

Robert J Beall, CEO

2241 Cystic Fibrosis Research, Inc.
2672 Bayshore Parkway, Suite 520
Mountain View, CA 94043
650-404-9975
855-237-4669
Fax: 650-404-9981
cfri@cfri.org
www.cfri.org

Cystic Fibrosis Research Inc.'s mission is to fund CF research, to provide educational and personal support and to spread awareness of Cystic Fibroses, a life threatening genetic disease.

Carroll P Jenkins, Executive Director
David Sohoo, Director of Program
Mary Convento, Programme Associate

2242 Genetic Alliance
4301 Connecticut Avenue NW, Suite 404
Washington, DC 20008 202-966-5557
800-336-4363
Fax: 202-966-8553
info@geneticalliance.org
www.geneticalliance.org

A coalition of voluntary genetic support groups, consumers and professionals addressing the needs of individuals and families affected by genetic disorders from a national perspective.

Sharon Terry, President/CEO
Tetyana Murza, Managing Director
Natasha Bonhomme, VP, Strategic Development

2243 March of Dimes Foundation
1275 Mamaroneck Avenue
White Plains, NY 10605 914-997-4488
888-663-4637
Fax: 914-997-4763
answers@marchofdimes.com
www.marchofdimes.com

Partnership of volunteers and professionals dedicated to improving the health of babies by preventing birth defects and infant mortality. Over 100 chapters are located across the country and can be located through the National Office.

Stacey D. Stewart, President

Libraries & Resource Centers

2244 National Digestive Diseases Information Clearinghouse
9000 Rockville Pike
Bethesda, MD 20892 301-496-3583
800-860-8747
Fax: 301-907-8906
healthinfo@niddk.nih.gov
www.niddk.nih.gov

The National Institute of Diabetes and Digestive and Kidney Diseases conducts and supports research on many of the most serious diseases affecting public health. The Institute supports much of the clinical research on the diseases of internal medicine and related subspecialty fields as well as many basic science disciplines.

Dr. Griffin P. Rodgers, Director
Dr. Gregory G. Germino, Deputy Director
Camille M. Hoover, M.S.W., Executive Officer

Research Centers

Alabama

2245 Gregory Fleming James Cystic Fibrosis Cent er
790 McCallum Basic Health Sciences Bldg
Birmingham, AL 35294 205-934-9640
Fax: 205-934-7593
sorscher@uab.edu
www.cfcenter.uab.edu

Eric J Sorscher MD, Director

Arizona

2246 Cystic Fibrosis Center: Phoenix Children's Hospital
1919 E Thomas Road
Phoenix, AZ 85016 602-546-0985
888-908-5437
www.phxchildrens.com

Wayne J Morgan MD, Director

California

2247 Brian Wesley Ray Cystic Fibrosis Center
San Bernadino County Medical Center
780 E Gilbert Street
San Bernardino, CA 92415 909-387-8111
Gerald Greene, MD

2248 Children's Hospital of Los Angeles
4650 W Sunset Boulevard
Los Angeles, CA 90027 323-660-2450
888-631-2452
webmaster@chla.usc.edu
www.chla.org
Elisabeth L Raab, Contact

2249 Children's Hospital of Orange County: Depa rtment of Pulmonology - Cystic Fibrosis
1201 W. La Veta Ave
Orange, CA 92868 714-997-3000
Fax: 714-516-4348
mail@choc.org
www.choc.org
Ivan I Kirov

2250 Children's Hospital: Pediatric Pulmonary Center
747 52nd Street
Oakland, CA 94609 510-428-3259
Kevan McCarten-Gibbs

2251 Cystic Fibrosis Center: Cedars-Sinai Medical Center
8700 Beverly Boulevard, N Tower, Fourth Floor
Los Angeles, CA 90048 800-233-2771
Fax: 310-423-1402

2252 Cystic Fibrosis Center: University of California at San Francisco
8700 Beverly Boulevard, N Tower, Fourth Floor
San Francisco, CA 94143 800-233-2771
Fax: 310-423-1402

2253 Cystic Fibrosis Research, Inc.
2672 Bayshore Parkway, Suite 520
Mountain View, CA 94043 650-404-9975
855-237-4669
Fax: 650-404-9981
cfri@cfri.org
www.cfri.org

Cystic Fibrosis Research Inc.'s mission is to fund CF research, to provide educational and personal support and to spread awareness of Cystic Fibroses, a life threatening genetic disease.

Carroll P Jenkins, Executive Director
David Sohoo, Director of Program
Mary Convento, Programme Associate

2254 Cystic Fibrosis and Pediatric Respiratory Diseases Center
University of California at Davis
2315 Stockton Boulevard
Sacramento, CA 95817 800-282-3284
Fax: 916-734-0491
children@ucdavis.edu
www.ucdmc.ucdavis.edu/children

2255 Kaiser Permanente Medical Center
Kaiser Permanente Oakland Medical Center
280 W MacArthur Boulevard
Oakland, CA 94611 510-752-1000
www.kaiserpermanente.org
Linda C Armstrong

2256 Memorial Miller Children's Hospital Cystic Fibrosis Center
2801 Atlantic Avenue
Long Beach, CA 90806 562-933-2000
Fax: 562-933-8539
www.memorialcare.org
Barry Arbuckle, President

2257 Pulmonary Care and Cystic Fibrosis Center
Lucille Packard Children's Hospital
725 Welch Road, Suite 350
Palo Alto, CA 94304
650-497-8000
Fax: 650-498-4209
www.lpch.org

Deals with children's breathing in all its aspects.

Richard B Boss MD, Director

2258 Stanford CF Center
Packard Children's Hospital At Stanford
730 Welch Road
Palo Alto, CA 94304
650-725-9302
jkirby@leland.stanford.edu
cfcenter.stanford.edu

Kim Standridge, Manager

Colorado

2259 Denver Children's Hospital
1056 E 19th Avenue
Denver, CO 80218
303-837-2680
Fax: 303-837-2924

Martin A Koyle, Pulmonology Pediatrics

Connecticut

2260 University of Connecticut Health Center
282 Washington Street
Hartford, CT 06106
860-545-9440
Fax: 860-545-9445
kdaigle@ccmckids.org

Karen Daigle MD, Pediatric Pulmonary Division

2261 Yale University Cystic Fibrosis Research Center
School of Medicine Department
333 Cedar Street, PO Box 208064
New Haven, CT 06520
203-785-4648
Fax: 203-688-7864
www.med.yale.edu

Respiratory Medicine in the Department of Pediatrics at Yale University and Yale-New Haven Hospital is a multi-disiplinary section that has developed considerably since the early 90's and continues to develop and refine its clinical and research activities. We have also reorganized our Cystic Fibrosis Care Center, increased the clinical research activities pertaining to the care of CF patients and organized a number of CF family group meetings to dissimenate new knowledge of care of patients.

Marie E Egan MD, Cystic Fibrosis Center

Florida

2262 CF & Pediatric Pulmonary Disease Center
University of Florida
PO Box 100225
Gainesville, FL 32610
352-392-3261
Fax: 352-392-0821

Eric L Olson, Director Adult CF Program

2263 Cystic Fibrosis Center - All Children's Hospital
801 6th Street S
St Petersburg, FL 33701
727-898-7451
800-456-4543

2264 Miami Children's Hospital, Division of Pulmonology
3100 SW 62nd Street
Miami, FL 33155
305-666-6511
800-432-6837
www.mch.com

Deise Granado-Villar, Director

2265 Pulmonary Wellness Program
Orlando Regional Medical Center
92 W. Miller St.
Orlando, FL 32806
321-841-4194
www.arnoldpalmerhospital.org

Our staff is trained in all diagnostic tests as well as a variety of Cystic Fibrosis therapies, including therapy vest treatments. Our professionals will work with your child and your family to create a more enriched diet including vitamin and enzyme supplements to help counteract the effects of Cystic Fibrosis. We also administer antibiotics in pill form as well as intravenously and through medicated vapors.

Georgia

2266 Department of Pediatrics, Medical College of Georgia
1120 15th Street, BT-1852
Augusta, GA 30912
706-721-2809
Fax: 706-721-7311
kcooper@ gru.edu
www.georgiahealth.edu

Tracy Chavous, Manager

2267 Egleston Cystic Fibrosis Center: Departmen t of Pediatrics
Emory University
201 Dowman
Atlanta, GA 30322
404-727-6123
Fax: 404-727-4828
www.emory.edu

Daniel Caplan MD, Director

Illinois

2268 Cystic Fibrosis Center: Children's Memoria l Hospital
Northwestern University
2300 N Children's Plaza, #43
Chicago, IL 60614
773-880-4382
cf@childrensmemorial.org
Susanna McColley MD, Head, Pulmonary Medicine

2269 Loyola University Medical Center/ Department of Pediatrics
2160 S First Avenue
Maywood, IL 60153
708-216-8563
888-584-7888
www.loyolamedicine.org

Sergio L Gonzalez, Pediatric Pulmonary

2270 Park Ridge, Cystic Fibrosis Center
Advocate Lutheran General Hospital
1775 Dempster Street
Park Ridge, IL 60068
423-622-6848
800-242-5662
www.parkridgemedicalcenter.com

Darell Moore, CEO

2271 Saint Francis Medical Center Specialty Clinics, CF Center
Hillcrest Medical Plaza
530 NE Glen Oak Avenue
Peoria, IL 61637
309-655-7171
www.childrenshospitalofil.org

2272 University of Chicago Children's Hospital, Department of Pediatrics
University of Chicago Hospitals and Clinics
5721 S Maryland Avenue
Chicago, IL 60637
773-702-6176
888-824-0200
Fax: 773-702-4753
www.uchicagokidshospital.org

Provides comperhensive, innovative medical care to children of all social and economic backgrounds. Dedicated to enhancing the health and wellness through patient care, education and research into the causes and cure of childhood diseases. Immediate access to the full resources of The University of Chicago Hospitals and to faculty of the division of Biological Sciences. The hospital sees children from the Chicago area, the Midwest and around the world who have the most complex medical problems.

Shannon Smith, Manager

Indiana

2273 Cystic Fibrosis and Chronic Pulmonary Disease Clinic
Saint Joseph's Regional Medical Center
801 E LaSalle Avenue
South Bend, IN 46617   574-239-6126
                                          800-206-0879
                                      Fax: 574-472-6067

2274 Riley Cystic Fibrosis Center
Riley Hospital for Children
702 Barnhill Drive
Indianapolis, IN 46202   317-274-5000

Iowa

2275 Blank Children's Hospital: Department of P ulmonology
1212 Pleasant Street, Suite 300
Des Moines, IA 50309   515-241-8336
                                      Fax: 515-241-6465

Carissa Schneider, Manager

2276 University of Iowa Hospitals & Clinics
Allergy and Pulmonary Division: Cystic Fibrosis Ct
200 Hawkins Drive
Iowa City, IA 52242   319-356-1616
                                      www.uihealthcare.org

Ronald Strauss, Director

Kansas

2277 Kansas University Medical Center: Departme nt of Pulmonology
Department of Pediatrics
3901 Rainbow Boulevard
Kansas City, KS 66160   913-588-5000
                                      TDD: 913-588-7963
                                          www.kumc.edu

Raymond Franklin, Manager

2278 Via Christi Specialty Clinics: Cystic Fibr osis, Adult and Pediatrics
St Joseph Campus
3600 E Harry Street
Wichita, KS 67218   316-689-5735
                                      Fax: 316-291-7963

Kentucky

2279 University of Kentucky: Pediatric Pulmonar y Medicine
Department of Pediatrics
740 S Limestone
Lexington, KY 40536   859-323-6426
                                      Fax: 859-257-7706

Michael I Anstead MD, Director

Louisiana

2280 Louisiana State University Health Sciences Center
Department of Pediatrics: Critical Care/Pulmonary
200 Henry Clay Avenue
New Orleans, LA 70118   504-896-2723
                                      Fax: 504-896-2720
                                      dhoppe@lsuhsc.edu

Robert Hopkins MD, Professor of Clinical Pediatrics

Maine

2281 Central Maine Medical Center
Department of Pediatrics
300 Main Street
Lewiston, ME 04240   207-795-0111
                                      Fax: 207-797-7241
                                          www.cmmc.org

Focuses special attention on the services that it provides to Cystic Fibrosis patients. In microbiology, for example, the lab employs a number of techniques supporting the special needs of CF patients. The CMMC pathology departments's chemistry section provides quantitative sweat analysis for the diagnosis of patients to other laboratories in the region, thereby assisting in diagnosis.

Marly L Larrabee, Special Interst: Cystic Fibrosis

2282 Eastern Maine Medical Center: Cystic Fibrosis Center
489 State Street
Bangor, ME 04401   207-973-7000
                                          www.emmc.org

Shad Deering

2283 Pediatric Cystic Fibrosis Center
Maine Medical Center: Dept. of Resp. Care
22 Bramhall Street
Portland, ME 04102   207-662-0111
                                      Fax: 207-775-6024
                                          www.mmc.org

Services offered: pediatric pulmonary consultation, flexible bronchoscopy of the pediatric airway, full pediatric and infant pulmonary function testing, including exercise testing, bronchopulmonary challenge, and accredited sleep lab. Also offered, full-time inpatient consultation service for neonates through adolesence, a bimonthly Cystic Fibrosis Clinic, and a biweekly outpatient pulmonary clinic.

Maryland

2284 John Hopkins Children's Hospital
Division of Pulmonary
600 N Wolfe Street
Baltimore, MD 21287   410-955-5089
                                      Fax: 410-955-0761
                                      www.hopkinschildren.org

Edward Chambers, Administrator

Massachusetts

2285 Baystate Medical Center
280 Chestnut Street
Springfield, MA 01199   413-794-0000
                                      Fax: 413-794-7408
                                      www.baystatehealth.com

Gordon M Saperia, Chief, Pediatric Pulmonary

2286 Children's Hospital Boston
Pulmonary and Critical Care Unit
300 Longwood Avenue
Boston, MA 02115   617-355-6000
                                          800-355-7944
                                      Fax: 617-724-9948
                                      TTY: 617-730-0152
                                      www.childrenshospital.org

James Mandell, CEO
Sandra Fenwick, President & COO
Dick Argys, Chief Administrative Officer

2287 Massachusetts General Hospital
Pulmonary and Critical Care Unit
55 Fruit Street
Boston, MA 02114
617-726-2000
TDD: 617-724-8800
www.umass.org

Mass General aims to deliver the very best health care in a safe, compassionate environment; to advance that care through innovative research and education; and to improve the health and well-being of the diverse communities we serve.

Cathy Minehan, Chair
Peter Slavin, President & Trustee
Ronald Kleinman, Physician-in-Chief, Hospital for Ch

2288 Tufts New England Medical Center Floating Hospital for Children
Division of Pulmonary, Critical Care and Sleep
755 Washington Street
Boston, MA 02111
617-636-5000
www.tuftsmedicalcenter.org

Joseph Campanelli, Chairman
Richard Freeman, Chair, Organ Transplantation
Brien Barnewolt, Chairman, Chief of Emergency Medici

Michigan

2289 Butterworth Hospital, Cystic Fibrosis Center
426 Michigan Street NE
Grand Rapids, MI 49503
616-454-1509
John Schuen, MD, Director

2290 Children's Hospital of Michigan Cystic Fibrosis Care, Teaching & Resource
Children's Hospital of Michigan
3901 Beaubien Boulevard
Detroit, MI 48201
313-745-5437
888-362-2500
www.childrensdmc.org

Herman Gray, Jr., President
Shawn Levitt, COO
Joseph Scallen, Jr., VP Finance

2291 Cystic Fibrosis Center/Pediatric Pulmonary and Sleep Medicine
330 Barclay Avenue NE, Suite 200
Grand Rapids, MI 49503
616-391-2125
Fax: 616-391-2131

John Schuen, MD, Director
Susan Millard, MD, Director

2292 Kalamazoo Center for Medical Studies
Michigan State University
1000 Oakland Drive
Kalamazoo, MI 49008
269-337-4400
www.kcms.msu.edu/

Robert Carter, CEO
Peter Ziemkowski, Family Practitioner

2293 University of Michigan, Cystic Fibrosis Center
1500 E. Medical Center Drive
Ann Arbor, MI 48109
734-936-4000
800-962-3555
Fax: 734-936-7635
www.med.umich.edu/mott/cysticfibrosiscenter/

The University of Michigan Cystic Fibrosis Program mission is to provide excellence and leadership in patient care, services, research and education.

Samya Z. Nasr, MD, Director, Cystic Fibrosis Center

Minnesota

2294 Minnesota Cystic Fibrosis Center
Fairview University Medical Center
420 Delaware Street SE, MMC 742
Minneapolis, MN 55455
612-624-0962
Fax: 612-624-0696
www.med.umn.edu/peds/cfcenter/

Comprehensive and coordinated care approach that is designed to prevent and slow the rate of disease progression. Since 1961, this care approach used by the University of Minnesota physicians has led to an increase in the average age of survival for patients with Cystic Fibrosis from 2 1/2 to 39 years.

Warren E. Regelmann, Co-Director, Ped CF Program
Carlye Tomczyk, CF Educator

Mississippi

2295 University of Mississippi Medical Center
2500 N State Street
Jackson, MS 39216
601-984-5820
www.umc.edu/

Thomas H. Fortner, Chief Public Affairs and Communicat
John E. Hall, Associate Vice Chancellor for Resea
James M. Lightsey, Chief Financial Officer

Missouri

2296 Children's Mercy Hospital, University of Missouri
Kansas City School of Medicine
2401 Gillham Road
Kansas City, MO 64108
816-234-3000
866-512-2168
TTY: 816-234-3816
webmaster@cmh.edu
www.childrensmercy.org

Ed Connolly, Jr., Chairman
Randall O'Donnell, President, CEO, and Director

2297 Cystic Fibrosis, Pediatric Pulmonary and Pediatric Gastrointestinal Center
Cardinal Glennon Memorial Hospital for Children
1465 S Grand
Saint Louis, MO 63104
314-577-5600
Anthony J Rejent, MD, Center Director

2298 University of Missouri-Columbia Cystic Fibrosis Center
University of Missouri/Department of Child Health
404 Keene Street
Columbia, MO 65203
573-875-9000
www.muhealth.org

University of Missouri Children's Hospital seves patients from every county in Missouri. With over 30 pediatric subspecialties, a pediatric ICU, adolescent unit and child life therapy, MU Children's Hospital is mid-Missouri's largest and most comprehensive pediatric health care facility.

James Ross, Chief Executive Officer
Anita Larsen, Chief Operating Officer
Jeri Doty, Chief Planning Officer

2299 Washington University Cystic Fibrosis Center
Saint Louis Children's Hospital
1 Childrens Place
Saint Louis, MO 63110
314-454-2694
888-503-2237
Fax: 314-454-2515
peds.wustl.edu/pulmonary/CysticFibrosisCenter/tabid/
Thomas Ferkol, MD, Director

Nebraska

2300 University of Nebraska at Omaha Pediatric Pulmonary/Cystic Fibrosis Center
42nd and Emile
Omaha, NE 68198
402-559-6400
Fax: 402-559-7062
www.unmc.edu/pediatrics/
John W. Sparks, MD, Chairman

Nevada

2301 Children's Lung Specialists
3820 Meadows Lane
Las Vegas, NV 89107
702-598-4411
Fax: 702-598-1988
Kris Hissung, Manager
Brian Woo, Pediatric Pulmonologist

New Hampshire

2302 New Hampshire Cystic Fibrosis Care and Teaching Center
Dartmouth Hitchcock Medical Center
1 Medical Center Drive
Lebanon, NH 03756
603-650-6244
Fax: 603-650-8601
William Boyle Jr, MD, Director

New Jersey

2303 Monmouth Medical Center, Cystic Fibrosis & Pediatric Pulmonary Center
300 Second Avenue
Long Branch, NJ 07740
732-222-5200
Fax: 908-222-4472
http://www.saintbarnabas.com/hospitals/monmouth_medi
Carol Foster, Manager

2304 New Jersey Medical School
185 S Orange Avenue
Newark, NJ 07103
973-972-4871
800-482-3627
Fax: 201-982-7597
njms.umdnj.edu
Robert Wieder, Director

New Mexico

2305 University of New Mexico School of Medicine
2400 Tucker Ne 4th Fl
Albuquerque, NM 87131
505-272-0518
Fax: 505-272-0329
somadmin@salud.unm.edu
www.som.unm.edu

The School of Medicine is committed to remain a world-leading institution in three equally valued and inter-related missions of patient care, education, and research.
Paul Roth, MD, Dean, School of Medicine
David Sklar, Emergency Medicine

New York

2306 Albany Medical College Pediatric Pulmonary & Cystic Fibrosis Center
Department of Pediatrics
47 New Scotland Avenue
Albany, NY 12208
518-262-6008
Fax: 518-262-6472
www.amc.edu
Vincent P Verdile, Exec Vp

2307 Armond V. Mascia CF Center
NY Medical College
Munger Pavillion, Room 106
Valhalla, NY 10595
914-493-7585
Fax: 914-594-4336
pedpulm@nymc.edu
www.nymc.edu/depthome/peds/pedspulm/CFCenter.asp

The mission of our CF Center is to enable our patients with cystic fibrosis to fulfill their maximal potential with the support of their families by providing state-of-the-art clinical care. To further this goal, our center is dedicated to the education of all patients, their families, healthcare professionals and the community, the pursuit of rigorous research and continuous quality improvement.
Allen Dozer, MD, Director

2308 CF & Pediatric Pulmonary Care Center
Mt. Sinai School of Medicine
5th Avenue at 100th Street
New York, NY 10029
212-241-7788
Richard J Bonforte, MD, Director

2309 CF, Pediatric Pulmonary & GI Center
Saint Vincent's Hospital & Medical Center of NY
36 7th Avenue
New York, NY 10011
212-604-8895
Joan DeGelie-Germana, MD, Director

2310 Children's Lung and Cystic Fibrosis Center
Children's Hospital of Buffalo
219 Bryant Street
Buffalo, NY 14222
716-878-7524
Fax: 716-888-3945
www.wchob.org/services/services_display.asp?PType=L

Services for infants, children and teenagers with cystic fibrosis and other chronic respiratory conditions.
Drucy Borowitz, MD, Director
David Sheehan, Medical Director

2311 Long Island College Hospital
350 Henry Street
Brooklyn, NY 11201
718-780-1071
www.futurenurselich.org/
Robert Giusti, MD, Director

2312 Pediatric Pulmonary Center
Babies Hospital & Columbia Presbyterian Med Center
750 East Adams Street
Syracuse, NY 13210
315-464-6323
Fax: 212-805-6103
Ran D Anbar, Medical Director
Mary Ann Russo, Dietician
Karen Watkins, Secretary

2313 Schneider Children's Hospital of Long Island
Albert Einstein College of Medicine
New Hyde Park, NY 14040
716-470-3250
Jack D Gorvoy, MD

2314 State University Hospital/Upstate Medical University
750 E Adams Street
Syracuse, NY 13210
315-464-8668
877-464-5540
Fax: 315-464-5158
www.upstate.edu/uh/
David Smith, President
Steven Brady, SVP Finance & Administration
Teresa Wagner, CIO

2315 University of Rochester Medical Center
Strong Memorial Hospital/Division of Pediatrics
601 Elmwood Avenue
Rochester, NY 14642
585-275-2838
www.urmc.rochester.edu/
Karen Z Voter, MD, Director

North Carolina

2316 Duke University Medical Center/ CF Center
350 Hanes House
Durham, NC 10236   919-684-3364
                                    Fax: 919-684-2292
                                    www.pediatrics.duke.edu
Marc Majure, MD, Director

2317 UNC CF Center
Department of Pediatrics
509 Burnett-Womack Building
Chapel Hill, NC 27599   919-966-1055
Gerald W Fernald, MD, Director

North Dakota

2318 Saint Alexius Medical Center/CF Center
311 N 9th Street
Bismarck, ND 58501   701-224-7500
                                    Fax: 701-224-7560
Allan Stillerman, MD, Director

Ohio

2319 Case Western Reserve University Cystic Fibrosis Center
2101 Adelbert Road
Cleveland, OH 44106   216-844-3264
                                    Fax: 216-844-5916
Pamela B Davis, MD, Director

2320 Columbus Children's Hospital, Cystic Fibrosis Center
700 Childrens Drive
Columbus, OH 43205   614-722-4766
                                    Fax: 614-722-4755
Karen S McCoy, MD, Director

2321 Lewis H. Walker, MD, Cystic Fibrosis Center
Children's Hospital Medical Center of Akron
1 Perkins Square
Akron, OH 44308   330-543-1000
                                    ÿwebmaster@chmca.org
                                    www.alchonchildrens.org

Part of the Robert T Stone Respiratory Center, one of six centers
in the state of Ohio providing comprehensive care for patients
who suffer from this disease. Caused by a defective gene, CF is
characterized by a thick, sticky mucus in the lungs, intestines and
other excretory organs that leads to severe respiratory and
digestive problems.

Robert T Stone, MD, Director

2322 Pediatric Pulmonary Center
Children's Medical Center
1 Childrens Plaza
Dayton, OH 45404   937-641-3376
                                    Fax: 937-463-5390
Michael E Steffan, MD, Director

**2323 University of Cincinnati College of Medicine/Division of
       Pediatrics**
Children's Hospital Medical Center
3333 Burnet Avenue
Cincinnati, OH 45229   513-636-0180
                                    800-344-2462
                                    TTY: 513-636-4900
                                    www.cincinnatichildrens.org
Edward Donovan, Director, Child Policy Rsch Ctr

Oklahoma

2324 University of Oklahoma Cystic Fibrosis Center
940 NW 13th Street
Oklahoma City, OK 73106   405-271-6390
                                    Fax: 405-271-7866
John E Grunow, MD, Director

Oregon

2325 Oregon Health Sciences Unit
3181 S.W. Sam Jackson Park Rd.
Portland, OR 97239   503-220-3405
Michael Heinrich, Research Director

Pennsylvania

2326 CF Center at The Children's Hospital of Philadelphia
34th & Civic Center Boulevard
Philadelphia, PA 19104   215-590-1000
                                    Fax: 215-590-4298

The CF center consists of pediatric and adult specialists who
collaorate to provide multidisciplinary care for CF patients
through their entire life span. The interdisiplinary health care
team forms the core of our Centerand meets regularly to assess
the clinical, educational and psychosocial needs of the family and
to plan and evaluate the care provided. The CF center also provides educatinal programs for health professionals and reserch focused on improved treatments.

Aaron A Chambers, Director
LeeAnn Webb CRNP, Coordinator
Thelma Gary BA, Clinical Research Specialist

2327 Cystic Fibrosis Center at Polyclinic Medical Center
Polyclinic Medical Center
2601 N 3rd Street
Harrisburg, PA 17110   717-782-4105
                                    800-334-1007
                                    Fax: 717-782-2597
Muttiah Ganeshananthan, MD, Director

2328 Pediatric Pulmonary and Cystic Fibrosis Center
Saint Christopher's Hospital For Children
Erie Avenue at Front Street
Philadelphia, PA 19134   215-427-5183
Daniel Schidlow, MD, Director

**2329 University of Pittsburgh Cystic Fibrosis Center/Children's
       Hospital**
3705 5th Avenue
Pittsburgh, PA 15213   412-692-7280
                                    www.wpahs.org
Julie R Fuchs, Director

Rhode Island

2330 Rhode Island Hospital, Cystic Fibrosis Center
CDC-APC
593 Eddy Street
Providence, RI 02903   401-444-5171
                                    Fax: 401-444-6115
Edwin N Forman, Director

South Carolina

2331 CF Center/Medical University of South Carolina
158 Rutledge Avenue
Charleston, SC 29425   803-792-3561
                                    Fax: 803-792-0732
Robert Baker, MD, Director

South Dakota

2332 Sioux Valley Hospital, South Dakota Cystic Fibrosis Center
1100 S Euclid Avenue, PO Box 5039
Sioux Falls, SD 57117   605-333-1000
Rodney Parry, MD, Director

Tennessee

2333 Memphis Cystic Fibrosis Center
LeBonheur Children's Medical Center
One Children's Plaza
Memphis, TN 38103   901-572-5222
Fax: 901-572-3337

Robert Schoumacher, MD, Director

2334 Pediatric Pulmonary Medicine
2200 Children's Way
Nashville, TN 37232   615-936-1000
Fax: 615-343-7727
www.vanderbiltchildrens.com

Texas

2335 CF Center, Pulmonary Section
Baylor College of Medicine/Dept. of Pediatrics
1 Baylor Plaza
Houston, TX 77030   713-798-4945
Peter W Hiatt, MD, Director

2336 Cook-Ft. Worth Medical Center, CF Center
801 7th Avenue
Fort Worth, TX 76104   817-885-4207
Fax: 817-885-1090
James C Cunningham, MD, Director

2337 Cystic Fibrosis Care, Teaching and Research Center
Children's Medical Center
1935 Medical District
Dallas, TX 75235   214-456-7000
www.portal.childrens.com

Claude Prestidge, MD, Director

2338 Cystic Fibrosis-Lung Disease Center Santa Rosa Children's Hospital
519 W Houston Street
San Antonio, TX 78207   210-228-2058
Fax: 210-224-2132

2339 Tri-Services Military CF Center
Brooke Army Medical Center
3851 Roger Brooke Drive
Fort Sam Houston, TX 78234   210-916-3400
bamac/home.hm
www.grmc.amed d.army.nil/

Stephen Inscore, LTC, MC, Director

Utah

2340 University of Utah Intermountain Cystic Fibrosis Center
50 N Medical Drive
Salt Lake City, UT 84132   801-581-2121
Fax: 801-581-2177
www.healthcare.utah.edu

Jeffrey R Saffle, Center Co-Director

Vermont

2341 Medical Center Hospital of Vermont
Cystic Fibrosis Center
50 Timber Lane
South Burlington, VT 05403   802-862-5529
Fax: 802-864-0294

Donald Swartz, MD, Director

Virginia

2342 Cystic Fibrosis Center/University of Virginia Health System
Department of Pediatrics
1215 Lee Street
Charlottesville, VA 22908   434-924-0211
Fax: 434-243-6618
www.healthsystem.virginia.edu

Comprehensive care for children and adults with cystic fibrosis.

Deborah K Froh, MD, Director Children's Program
Mark Robbins, MD, Director Adult Program

2343 Cystic Fibrosis Program of the Medical College of Virginia
9000 Stony Point Parkway
Richmond, VA 23235   804-786-9445
Fax: 804-560-7347

David Draper, MD, Director

2344 Eastern Virginia Medical Center
Children's Hospital of The King's Daughters
601 Childrens Lane
Norfolk, VA 23507   757-668-7243
Fax: 804-668-9767

William C Owen, Director

Washington

2345 University of Washington CF Center
4800 Sand Point Way NE
Seattle, WA 98105   206-987-2174
Fax: 206-987-2024
depts.washington.edu

Rohit K Khosla, Director

West Virginia

2346 West Virginia University Cystic Fibrosis Center
PO Box 9214
Morgantown, WV 26506   304-293-7332
Fax: 304-293-4341
Marybeth Hummel, Director

2347 West Virginia University Mountain State Cystic Fibrosis Center
PO Box 9214
Morgantown, WV 26506   304-293-7332
800-982-8242
Fax: 304-293-1216
kmoffett@hsc.wvu.edu

Marybeth Hummel, Director

Wisconsin

2348 Medical College of Wisconsin Cystic Fibrosis Center
Children's Hospital of Wisconsin
9000 W Wisconsin Avenue, MS #777A
Milwaukee, WI 53226   414-266-2412
Fax: 414-266-2653

William G Raasch, Director

2349 University of Wisconsin-Madison Cystic Fibrosis/Pulmonary Center
Clinical Science Center H4/430
600 Highland Avenue
Madison, WI 53792
608-263-6100
Fax: 608-263-0440
www.uwppc.org

Carl J Getto, Director

Conferences

2350 Genetic Alliance Annual Conference
Genetic Alliance
4301 Connecticut Avenue NW, Suite 404
Washington, DC 20008
202-966-5557
800-336-4363
Fax: 202-966-8553
info@geneticalliance.org
www.geneticalliance.org

Consistently inspirational and enables partnership among all stakeholders: advocates and community leaders, health and industry professionals, policymakers, and academicians.

July

Sharon Terry, President/CEO
Tetyana Murza, Managing Director
Natasha Bonhomme, VP, Strategic Development

2351 National Cystic Fibrosis Family Education Conference
Cystic Fibrosis Research Institute
2672 Bayshore Parkway, Suite 520
Mountain View, CA 94043
650-404-9975
855-237-4669
Fax: 650-404-9981
cfri@cfri.org
www.cfri.org

Brings together adults with cystic fibrosis, caregivers, experts and researchers for three days where a variety of CF topics are explored through presentations, panel discussions and support groups.

Carroll P Jenkins, Executive Director

Audio Video

2352 Living with Cystic Fibrosis
Aquarius Health Care Videos
5 Powderhouse Lane, PO Box 1159
Sherborn, MA 1770
508-651-2963
888-440-2963
Fax: 508-650-4216
info@aquariusproductions.com
www.aquariusproductions.com

People diagnosed with this genetic disorder are surviving longer than ever. Many patients live well into their thirties and beyond. This film looks at the hope that current research offers to those with cystic fibrosis, their caregivers and families.

Donna Kaufman

Web Sites

2353 American Lung Association of the City of New York
21 West 38th Street, 3rd Floor
New York, NY 10018
212-889-3370
800-LUN-USA
Fax: 212-889-3375
www.lungusa.org

The American Lung Association fights lung disease in all its forms, with special emphasis on asthma, tobacco control and environmental health. The American Lung Association is funded by contributions from the public, along with gifts and grants from corporations, foundations and government agencies. The association achieves its many successes through the work of thousands of committed volunteers and staff.

2354 CF Index of Online Resources
vmsb.csd.mu.edu/~541lukasr/cystic.html

2355 CF Web
cf-web.mit.edu

2356 Healing Well
www.healingwell.com
admin@healingwell.com
www.healingwell.com

An online health resource guide to medical news, chat, information and articles, newsgroups and message boards, books, disease-related web sites, medical directories, and more for patients, friends, and family coping with disabling diseases, disorders, or chronic illnesses.

Peter Waite, Founder & CEO

2357 Onhealth
www.onhealth.com

Provides over 50 links to information on cystic fibrosis.

2358 Online Mendelian Inheritance in Man
U.S. National Library of Medicine, 8600 Rockville
Bethesda, MD 20894
888-346-3656
info@ncbi.nlm.nih.gov
www.ncbi.nlm.nih.gov

This database is a catalog of human genes and genetic disorders.

Christine E. Seidman, M.D., Chair
David J. Lipman, M.D., Executive Secretary
Michael Boehnke, Ph.D., Board Member

Book Publishers

2359 Alex: The Life of a Child Rutledge Press
Frank Deford, author

7625 Empire Drive
Florence, KY 41042
800-634-7064
Fax: 800-248-4724

Paperback
ISBN: 1-558535-52-7

2360 Cystic Fibrosis
Franklin Watts
90 Old Sherman Turnpike
Danbury, CT 06816
203-797-3500
Fax: 203-797-3197
www.grolier.com

1994 128 pages
ISBN: 0-531125-52-1

2361 Cystic Fibrosis: A Guide for Patient and Family
Raven Press
1185 Avenue of the Americas
New York, NY 10036
212-930-9500

253 pages Softcover
ISBN: 0-397516-53-3

2362 Cystic Fibrosis: The Facts
Oxford University Press
2001 Evans Road
Cary, NC 27513
212-726-6000
800-445-9714
Fax: 919-677-1303
custserv.us@oup.com
www.oup-usa.org

1995 128 pages Paperback
ISBN: 0-192625-43-8

2363 Give Me One Wish
Norton Publishers
500 5th Avenue
New York, NY 10110
212-354-5500
www.scholastic.com/

This book reads like a novel because it reenacts the author's daughter's bout with cystic fibrosis.

Grades 10-12

2364 Let's Talk About Going to the Hospital
Rosen Publishing Group's PowerKids Press
29 E 21st Street
New York, NY 10010

212-777-3017
800-237-9932
Fax: 888-436-4643
rosenpub@tribeca.ios.com
www.powerkidspress.com

If a child has to check into the hospital, chances are he or she is already upset about being ill. Knowing how a hospital functions and what the procedures are, such as when family members can visit, will help in what is already a stressful situation. Grades K-5.

24 pages
ISBN: 0-823950-36-0

2365 Lung Disorders Sourcebook
Omnigraphics
PO Box 31-1640
Detroit, MI 48231

800-234-1340
Fax: 800-875-1340
info@omnigraphics.com
www.omnigraphics.com

Basic consumer health information on lung disorders including tuberculosis, asthma and cystic fibrosis.

678 pages
ISBN: 0-780803-39-6

2366 Robyn's Book: A True Diary
Scholastic
730 Broadway
New York, NY 10003

212-505-3000

This book chronicles the life of the author and her battle with cystic fibrosis.

Grades 7-12

2367 Toothpick
Holiday
40 E 49th Street
New York, NY 10017

212-688-0085

This book uses relationships between two different teenagers to parallel the life of a person with cystic fibrosis.

Grades 6-9

2368 Understanding Cystic Fibrosis
University Press of Mississippi
3825 Ridgewood Road, Unit 9
Jackson, MS 39211

601-982-6205
Fax: 601-982-6217

This book charts the progress that has been made in identifying the mutations that cause CF and understanding how these genetic errors cause a disease whose symptoms can range from mild respiratory distress to life-threatening lung infections.

128 pages Hardcover
ISBN: 0-878059-66-0

Newsletters

2369 Commitment
Cystic Fibrosis Foundation
6931 Arlington Road, 2nd Floor
Bethesda, MD 20814

301-951-4422
800-344-4823
Fax: 301-951-6378
info@cff.org
www.cff.org

Offers medical news, fund-raising features, public policy and news from across the nation on cystic fibrosis.

Catherine C. McLoud, Chair
Robert J. Beall, Ph.D., President & CEO
C. Richard Mattingly, EVP & COO

Pamphlets

2370 An Introduction to Cystic Fibrosis for Patients and Families
Cystic Fibrosis Foundation
6931 Arlington Road, 2nd Floor
Bethesda, MD 20814

301-951-4422
800-344-4823
Fax: 301-951-6378
info@cff.org
www.cff.org

Offers up-dated medical information, the latest news on assistive technology and treatments, answers to some frequently asked questions on the illness and more.

94 pages

Catherine C. McLoud, Chair
Robert J. Beall, Ph.D., President & CEO
C. Richard Mattingly, EVP & COO

2371 Consumer Fact Sheet
Cystic Fibrosis Foundation
6931 Arlington Road, 2nd Floor
Bethesda, MD 20814

301-951-4422
800-344-4823
Fax: 301-951-6378
info@cff.org
www.cff.org

Offers a brief introduction to cystic fibrosis, symptoms, causes, treatments and offers illustrations pertaining to drainage positions.

Catherine C. McLoud, Chair
Robert J. Beall, Ph.D., President & CEO
C. Richard Mattingly, EVP & COO

2372 Cystic Fibrosis: Guide for Parents
American Lung Association
55 W. Wacker Drive, Suite 1150
Chicago, IL 60601

312-801-7630
800-LUN-USA
Fax: 202-452-1805
info@lungusa.org
www.lungusa.org

Comprehensive booklet covering topics such as treatment, social aspects, inheritance, genetics and outlook for the future.

24 pages

Kathryn A. Forbes, Chair
John F. Emanuel, JD, Vice Chair
Harold Wimmer, President & CEO

2373 Here's Everything You'll Need to Save Money with the CFF Health Services
CFF Home Health & Pharmacy Services
6931 Arlington Road, 2nd Floor
Bethesda, MD 20814

301-951-4422
800-344-4823
Fax: 301-951-6378
info@cff.org
www.cff.org

Offers information on the Cystic Fibrosis Foundation's home health services.

Catherine C. McLoud, Chair
Robert J. Beall, Ph.D., President & CEO
C. Richard Mattingly, EVP & COO

2374 Here's Everything You'll Need to Start Saving Money with the CFF Pharmacy
CFF Home Health And Pharmacy Services
6931 Arlington Road, 2nd Floor
Bethesda, MD 20814

301-951-4422
800-344-4823
Fax: 301-951-6378
info@cff.org
www.cff.org

Offers information on money-saving medications and patient information for the Cystic Fibrosis Pharmacy.

Catherine C. McLoud, Chair
Robert J. Beall, Ph.D., President & CEO
C. Richard Mattingly, EVP & COO

2375 Home Line
Cystic Fibrosis Foundation
6931 Arlington Road, 2nd Floor
Bethesda, MD 20814   301-951-4422
                                  800-344-4823
                            Fax: 301-951-6378
                                  info@cff.org
                                  www.cff.org

This bimonthly newsletter offers information on services and programs offered by the Foundation.

Bimonhtly

Catherine C. McLoud, Chair
Robert J. Beall, Ph.D., President & CEO
C. Richard Mattingly, EVP & COO

2376 On the Threshold of a Cure...You Can Make the Difference!
Cystic Fibrosis Foundation
6931 Arlington Road, 2nd Floor
Bethesda, MD 20814   301-951-4422
                                  800-344-4823
                            Fax: 301-951-6378
                                  info@cff.org
                                  www.cff.org

Offers information on what Cystic Fibrosis is and what people can do to help support the foundation's research.

Catherine C. McLoud, Chair
Robert J. Beall, Ph.D., President & CEO
C. Richard Mattingly, EVP & COO

Camps

2377 Camp Funshine
PO Box 576
Pea Ridge, AR 72751   832-541-9276
                                  www.campfunshine.com

Summer camp for children with cystic fibrosis and their families.

Jeff Brown, Director

2378 Des Moines YMCA Camp
1192 166th Drive
Boone, IA 50036   515-432-7558
                            Fax: 515-432-5414
                                  ycamp@dmymca.org
                                  www.y-camp.org

For boys and girls with cancer, diabetes, asthma, cystic fibrosis, hearing impaired and other disabilities.

David Sherry, Executive Director
Alex Kretzinger, Program Director

2379 LA Lions Camp Pelican
PO Box 10235
New Orleans, LA 70181   504-466-7124
                                  800-348-6567
                            Fax: 866-295-3803
                                  campinfo@camppelican.org
                                  www.lionscamp.org

Provides residential camp for children with lung disorders.

Troy Ricard

DESCRIPTION

2380 CYTOMEGALOVIRUS
Synonyms: Child care virus, CMV, Cytomegalic inclusion disease
Involves the following Biologic System(s):
Infectious Disorders

Cytomegalovirus (CMV) is a member of the herpesvirus family. This very common, worldwide viral infection often causes no apparent disease; however, in some patients, CMV infection results in symptoms and physical findings that may range from mild to potentially life-threatening.

Cytomegalovirus may be transmitted from mother to child before birth through the placenta, during birth through genital tract secretions, or after birth through breast milk. CMV is present in the environment; therefore, infection may be acquired at virtually any age. Because this virus may be shed in the urine and saliva for months or years after infection, children and adults who work in child-care settings are especially vulnerable. This is such a common occurrence that CMV infection is sometimes called the child-care virus. CMV may also be excreted in feces or transmitted through blood transfusions and in transplanted organs such as the kidneys, heart, and bone marrow. In the case of transmission through donated organs, CMV symptoms may be particularly severe due to immune suppression that occurs with the use of immune-suppressive drugs used to prevent organ rejection. In this way, these individuals are less capable of mounting a defense against the virus. Other individuals with impaired immune systems, such as the elderly and those with acquired immunodeficiency syndrome (AIDS), are also at increased risk of potentially life-threatening complications.

Fetal infection is more common when the mother is infected by CMV for the first time as opposed to recurrent infection. The majority of CMV-infected infants have no symptoms at birth; however, approximately five to 10 percent may exhibit symptoms and physical findings involving different organs of the body. Symptomatic CMV infection in the newborn (congenital CMV) may include such characteristic findings as an unusually small head (microcephaly); accumulations of calcium salts in the tissues of the brain; enlargement of the liver and spleen (hepatosplenomegaly); yellowish discoloration of the skin, eyes, and mucous membranes (jaundice); purplish skin lesions; eye abnormalities (i.e., chorioretinitis); and other irregularities of the central nervous system that may result in loss of sight and hearing, paralysis, and mental retardation. Approximately 10 to 20 percent of asymptomatic newborns later develop similar difficulties associated with the central nervous system. Infants who contract CMV infection after birth may have enlargement of the liver and spleen, inflammation of the liver (hepatitis), or pneumonia. In addition, premature, low birth weight infants who acquire CMV infection through blood transfusion may develop inflammation of the lungs (pneumonitis), jaundice, enlargement of the liver and spleen, grayish skin coloring, and irregularities of the blood. CMV-infected children with AIDS or transplanted organs may develop potentially life-threatening conditions, including pneumonitis, inflammation of the retinas of the eyes (retinitis), and gastrointestinal abnormalities. Primary cytomegalovirus infections in children receiving transplants are more likely to have more severe symptoms than those of recurrent infection.

Older affected children and adults with cytomegalovirus infection may develop symptoms and physical findings similar to those of mononucleosis. These findings usually last about two to three weeks and may include fever, rash, headache, fatigue, muscle pain, and hepatosplenomegaly. In addition, mild CMV infections in many children and adults often subside with no treatment.

In some cases, preventive treatment for CMV infection includes administration of intravenous immunoglobulin. Although this therapy is not usually effective in preventing disease acquired through most types of organ transplantation, it may be beneficial to bone marrow recipients whose compromised immune systems may not be capable of preventing a primary CMV infection. Other preventive measures may include screening of blood and organ donors for cytomegalovirus. In addition, pregnant child-care workers are urged to practice good hygiene, including frequent and thorough handwashing. Certain antiviral drugs (e.g., gancyclovir) are sometimes used to treat symptoms associated with life-threatening disease. However, symptoms tend to recur after treatment is stopped and serious side effects associated with this type of treatment are common. Separate studies on vaccine development and the use of antiviral drugs in the treatment of congenital cytomegalovirus are ongoing. Other treatment is supportive.

Government Agencies

2381 NIH/ Eunice Kennedy Shriver National Institute of Child Health & Human Development
31 Center Drive, Building 31
Bethesda, MD 20892
301-496-5113
800-370-2943
Fax: 866-760-5947
nichdpress@mail.nih.gov
www.nichd.nih.gov

Established in 1962 by congress, today the institute conducts and supports research on topics related to the health of children, adults, families and populations. Some of these topics include: developmental disabilities, growth and development, infant death, reproductive health and birth defects.

Diana W. Bianchi, Director
Paul Williams, Director, Communications

2382 NIH/National Institute of Allergy and Infectious Diseases
5601 Fishers Lane, MSC 9806
Bethesda, MD 20892
301-496-5717
866-284-4107
Fax: 301-402-3573
TDD: 800-877-8339
ocpostoffice@niaid.nih.gov
www.niaid.nih.gov

Conducts and supports basic and applied research to better understand, treat, and ultimately prevent infectious, immunologic, and allergic diseases.

Anthony S Fauci MD, Director

National Associations & Support Groups

2383 American Academy of Pediatrics
141 Northwest Point Boulevard
Elk Grove Village, IL 60007
847-434-4000
800-433-9016
Fax: 847-434-8000
www.aap.org

The American Academy of Pediatrics and its member pediatricians are committed to the attainment of optimal physical, mental and social health and well-being for all infants, children, adolescents, and young adults.

Fernando Stein, MD, FAAP, President
Karen Remley, MD, CEO/Executive VP

2384 March of Dimes Foundation
1275 Mamaroneck Avenue
White Plains, NY 10605
914-997-4488
888-663-4637
Fax: 914-997-4763
answers@marchofdimes.com
www.marchofdimes.com

Partnership of volunteers and professionals dedicated to improving the health of babies by preventing birth defects and infant mortality. Over 100 chapters are located across the country and can be located through the National Office.

Stacey D. Stewart, President

2385 National Congenital CMV Disease Registry
Feigin Center
1102 Bates St., Suite 1150
Houston, TX 77030
832-824-4387
Fax: 832-825-4347
cvm@bcm.edu
www.bcm.edu/departments/pediatrics/

This national surveillance program tracks trends over time, identifies risk groups, and lays groundwork for evaluation of future intervention programs.

Web Sites

2386 Kid's Health
www.kidshealth.org

Kids health is the largest and most visited site on the web providing doctor-approved health information about children from before birth through adolescence. Kids health provides families with accurate, up to date and jargon free health information they can use.

Neil Izenberg, MD, Editor-in-Chief & Founder

Book Publishers

2387 Let's Talk About Going to the Hospital
Rosen Publishing Group's PowerKids Press
29 E 21st Street
New York, NY 10010
212-777-3017
800-237-9932
Fax: 888-436-4643
rosenpub@tribeca.ios.com
www.powerkidspress.com

If a child has to check into the hospital, chances are he or she is already upset about being ill. Knowing how a hospital functions and what the procedures are, such as when family members can visit, will help in what is already a stressful situation. Grades K-5.

24 pages
ISBN: 0-823950-36-0

DESCRIPTION

2388 **DENTAL CONDITIONS**

Covers these related disorders: Anodontia, Dental Caries, Discoloration of the Teeth, Malocclusion, Supernumerary Teeth

Involves the following Biologic System(s):

Dental Disorders

This chapter will discuss the following pediatric dental conditions: anodontia; dental caries; discoloration of the teeth; malocclusion; supernumerary teeth; teeth grinding.

Anodontia refers to a condition in which some or all of the teeth are missing as the result of a congenital defect or of damage sustained from disease. Ectodermal dysplasias are a group of congenital disorders characterized by abnormalities of the teeth, hair, nails, skin glands, the skin, nervous system, ears and eyes, and the membranes that line the anus and the mouth. Partial anodontia may also result from a common birth defect such as cleft palate, in which the roof of the mouth does not close completely. Partial anodontia is often a component of certain disorders or syndromes including pseudohypoparathyroidism, cleidocranial dysplasia, and other disorders affecting the face and skull. The absence of some teeth may result in malocclusion, or misalignment, of the upper and lower teeth.

Treatment of anodontia may include the use of full or partial dentures, other dental prosthetics (bridgework), and dental implants. These approaches may be delayed until underlying structural deficits, such as cleft palate, are surgically corrected.

Dental caries, or tooth decay, is a common condition characterized by the gradual destruction (erosion) of the enamel and, potentially, the dentin and interior pulp of a tooth. The main cause of dental caries is plaque, a sticky film consisting of food debris, saliva and mucus. Certain bacteria that reside in the mouth break down dietary carbohydrates within plaque, creating acids that gradually wear down the outer tooth surfaces. Dental caries initially appear as whitish spots. As loss of dental tissue progresses, the enamel is gradually destroyed. Without treatment, the dentin and pulp may erode, causing pain, infection, and eventual tooth loss. In affected infants or children, dental caries typically appear on the minute grooves on the grinding surfaces of the back molars, or on the contact surfaces between adjacent teeth.

Dental caries are thought to be caused more by the frequency of carbohydrate consumption than by the quantity of carbohydrates consumed. For example, baby bottle tooth decay, which becomes apparent between 1 and 2 years, is extensive decay due to sleeping with, and constant use of, bottles with milk, juice and other sugary liquids. The same amount of such liquids consumed during a single meal is much less likely to cause decay. The frequency of dental caries has decreased 35 to 50 percent during the past 20 years due to fluorinated water and toothpaste. Dental caries are treated by drilling out the decayed area and filling the cavity with a dental material. Treatment of advanced decay may include removal of the pulp (root canal), restoration (crown), or extraction of the tooth.

Permanent discoloration of the teeth is caused by the incorporation of particular substances into developing tooth enamel, such as taking certain antibiotic medications (e.g. tetracyclines), excessive fluoride consumption, particular pediatric conditions or disorders, or other factors. Since tetracycline medications are highly absorbed into the teeth and bones, taking such medications during the development of enamel may result in thin, deficient tooth enamel (hyypoplasia) that is permanently stained yellowish brown. The risk for this condition is from the fourth month of fetal development to 10 months for primary teeth and from four months to 16 years for secondary teeth. Risk varies with type of medication, dose, and duration of treatment. Excessive fluoride may also result in tooth discoloration known as mottling. This primarily affects children in areas with higher-than-recommended levels of fluoride in the water supply. Permanent discoloration may also result from certain vitamin deficiencies, infectious disorders, or certain pediatric conditions. The use of certain specialized dental procedures and devices may help to minimize or cover discolored teeth. Children may also experience temporary tooth staining on the surface of teeth due to certain bacteria or food dyes. These may be removed by professional tooth polishing.

Malocclusion is a dental condition in which there is improper positioning of the teeth of the upper jaw in relation to those of the lower jaw. There are three main classes of malocclusion. In proper contact of the teeth (occlusion) the front teeth of the upper jaw slightly overlap the front teeth of the lower jaw and the ridges (cusps) of the back teeth (premolars and molars) in the lower jaw interlock slightly ahead and inside the cusps of the corresponding teeth in the upper jaw. In class I malocclusion, certain upper and lower teeth do not have appropriate contact due to crowding. In class II malocclusion (retrognathism), the most common, the cusps of the back teeth in the lower jaw are positioned behind and inside the cusps of the corresponding teeth in the upper jaw. In class III malocclusion (prognathism), the cusps of the back teeth in the lower jaw are abnormally positioned in front of corresponding maxillary teeth and the front teeth of the lower jaw meet or protrude beyond the upper front teeth. Malocclusion usually occurs during childhood as the bones of the jaws grow and the teeth develop and, in most cases, is genetic. Some cases of malocclusion may result due to other dental abnormalities, such as improper development or crowding of teeth, or constant thumbsucking. Treating malocclusion may avoid strain, stiffness, or pain that may result from an abnormal bite, may improve facial appearance, and may prevent tooth decay and loss. Treatment may include a variety of measures: tooth extraction in cases of dental crowding; orthodontic appliances to correct the positioning of teeth; or, in severe cases, surgical correction of abnormal protrusion or recession of the lower jaw.

Supernumerary teeth refers to the presence of one or more teeth in excess of the normal 20 primary teeth or 32 secondary teeth. These teeth are usually abnormal in shape and size and may erupt through the gums or may remain impacted in the gums or the jaw bone. In addition, a primary or secondary tooth is typically not present to replace the supernumerary (super = "extra") tooth. In most cases, only one supernumerary tooth is present; however, instances of multiple supernumerary teeth have been reported. The presence of supernumerary teeth may cause delayed eruption, abnormal positioning, or impaction of nearby teeth. Therefore, early diagnosis is important in removal or extraction of the extra tooth, or in regular monitoring to assess the need for possible extraction. Natal teeth, which are teeth that are present at birth, may be supernumerary or primary teeth that have erupted unusually early. Natal teeth usually have little bony support or root formation and are typically loose and mobile. If natal teeth are determined to be supernumerary, they are often extracted; if they are primary teeth, attempts may be made to maintain them. Supernumerary teeth develop in different locations in the mouth, and have different names: mesiodens develop between the central front teeth in the upper jaw; paramolars form between molars in the upper jaw; disomolars, also known as retromolars, develop in the back of the third molars (widsom teeth); peridens erupt outside the dental arches, such as in the roofof the mouth. Supernumerary teeth maybe the result of abnormalities during embryonic development, and may occur with other conditions, such as cleft lip and palate. There have been reports that suggest supernumerary teeth are inherited.

Teeth grinding, or bruxism, refers to compulsive, involuntary, rhythmic, and nonfunctional grinding, clenching, or gnashing of the teeth. This habitual grinding is most evident during sleep, so the individual may be oblivious to it, but family members may notice. Affected individuals may also unconsciously grind their teeth during the day as well. Daytime teeth grinding is known as bruxomania. In some, teeth grinding may be considered a habit or habit disorder, depending upon the degree of severity and the impact upon daily functioning. Bruxism most often results from unresolved or unexpressed anger, aggression, fear, frustration, resentment, or other negative emotions. Teeth grinding that occurs during sleep exerts more force than that of normal daytime chewing or grinding. For this reason, bruxism may cause muscle pain or tightness in the jaw area, headache, earache as well as irregularities in the surface contact between the upper and lower teeth. In addition, bruxism may wear down or loosen the teeth. The goals of treatment are to reduce pain, prevent permanent damage to the teeth, and reduce clenching behaviors as much as possible.Treatment for teeth grinding may include stress management and behavior therapy. Other treatment is symptomatic, and involves a dental appliance, such as a mouthguard, worn at night to help reduce associated dental injury.

Government Agencies

2389 NIH/ Eunice Kennedy Shriver National Insti tute of Child Health & Human Development
31 Center Drive, Building 31
Bethesda, MD 20892   301-496-5113
                                     800-370-2943
                             Fax: 866-760-5947
                        nichdpress@mail.nih.gov
                            www.nichd.nih.gov

Established in 1962 by congress, today the institute conducts and supports research on topics related to the health of children, adults, families and populations. Some of these topics include: developmental disabilities, growth and development, infant death, reproductive health and birth defects.

Diana W. Bianchi, Director
Paul Williams, Director, Communications

2390 NIH/National Institute of Dental and Crani ofacial Research (NIDCR)
National Institutes of Health
31 Center Drive, MSC 2290, Building 31
Bethesda, MD 20892   301-496-4261
                                     866-232-4528
                             Fax: 301-480-4098
                          nidcrinfo@mail.nih.gov
                              www.nidcr.nih.gov

The Institute promotes the general health of the American people by improving their oral, dental and craniofacial health. The NIDCR aims to promote health, to prevent diseases and conditions, and to develop new diagonistics and therapeutics.

Dr Martha J. Somerman, Director
John W Kusiak, PhD, Acting Deputy Director
Kathleen G Stephen, Executive Officer

National Associations & Support Groups

2391 Academy for Sports Dentistry
P.O. Box 364
Farmersville, IL 62533   217-227-3431
                             Fax: 217-227-3438
                   sportsdentistry@consolidated.net
                   www.academyforsportsdentistry.org

The Academy for Sports Dentistry was founded in 1983 in San Antonio, Texas, as a forum for dentists, physicians, athletic trainers, coaches, dental technicians, and educators interested in exchanging ideas related to Sports Dentistry and the dental needs of athletes at risk to sports' injuries.

W. Robert Howarth, President
James Lovelace, President Elect
Shelly Lott, Executive Secretary

2392 Academy of General Dentistry
560 W. Lake St., Sixth Floor
Chicago, IL 60661   888-243-3368
                             Fax: 312-335-3443
                          membership@agd.org
                                 www.agd.org

The mission of the AGD is to serve the needs and represent the interests of general dentists, to promote the oral health of the public, and to foster continued proficiency of general dentists through quality continuing dental education in order to better serve the public.

John Thorner, Executive Director/ CEO
Jill Beckman, Director, Corporate Relations
George Boyle, Director, IT

2393 Academy of Operative Dentistry
P.O. Box 25637
Los Angeles, CA 90025   310-794-4387
                             Fax: 310-825-2536
               www.academyofoperativedentistry.com

The objective of the Academy of Operative Dentistry is to promote excellence in Operative Dentistry by exerting our influence in the practice of health professions, in organized dentistry.

Dan Chan, President
Michael Cochran, Vice President
Greg Smith, Secretary

2394 Academy of Osseointegration
85 W. Algonquin Road, Suite 550
Arlington Heights, IL 60005   847-439-1919
                                     800-656-7736
                             Fax: 847-439-1569
                                 www.osseo.org

The Academy of Osseointegration's dedication to the highest standards in patient care.

Joseph Gian-Grasso, President
Russell D. Nishimura, President-Elect
Alan S. Pollack,, Vice President

2395 Alpha Omega International Dental Fraternity
50 W. Edmonston Drive #206
Rockville,, MD 20852   301-738-6400
877-368-6326
Fax: 301-738-6403
headquarters@ao.org
www.ao.org

An international Jewish dental organization striving to enrich the lives of its members.

Adam Stabholz, President
Wendy Spektor, President-Elect
Gail Schupak, Secretary

2396 American Academy of Cosmetic Dentistry
402 W. Wilson Street
Madison, WI 53703   608-222-8583
800-543-9220
Fax: 608-222-9540
www.aacd.com

AACD is dedicated to advancing excellence in the art and science of comprehensive cosmetic dentistry and encouraging the highest standards of ethical conduct and responsible patient care.

S John Hanson, Chief Operating Officer
Barbara Kachelski, Executive Director
Michael DiFrisco, Chief Marketing Officer

2397 American Academy of Dental Hygiene
13 Hamilton Avenue
Stamford, CT 06902   Fax: 203-886-1001
president@aadh.org
www.aadh.org

Advancing Individual Professional Growth through Leadership, Mentorship, and Fellowship.

Lynn Southerland, President
Cynthia Koons, President Elect
Lisa Harper Mallonee, Secretary

2398 American Academy of Dental Practice Administration
1063 Whippoorwill Lane
Palatine, IL 60067   847-934-4404
executivedirector@aadpa.org
aadpa.org

Promotes leadership, life balance & success in dentistry.

Kathleen Uebel, Executive Director
Rick Roesener, Webmaster

2399 American Academy of Esthetic Dentistry
225 W. Wacker Dr., Suite 650
Chicago, IL 60606   312-981-6770
Fax: 312-265-2908
info@estheticacademy.org
www.estheticacademy.org

The American Academy of Esthetic Dentistry was formed in 1975 and has members from throughout the United States and 11 other countries. Headquartered in Chicago, Illinois the group is governed by an Executive Council.

Joseph Jackson, CAE, Executive Director
Rachel Walsh, CMP, Director of Meetings
Moira Twitty, Director of Education

2400 American Academy of Pediatric Dentistry
211 E Chicago Avenue, Suite 1600
Chicago, IL 60611   312-337-2169
Fax: 312-337-6329
www.aapd.org

The AAPD is the membership organization representing the specialty of pediatric dentistry. Our over 10,000 members serve as primary care providers for millions of children from infancy through adolescence.

4500 members

Jade Miller, D.D.S., President
John Rutkauskas, D.D.S., CEO

2401 American Academy of Pediatrics
141 Northwest Point Boulevard
Elk Grove Village, IL 60007   847-434-4000
800-433-9016
Fax: 847-434-8000
www.aap.org

The American Academy of Pediatrics and its member pediatricians are committed to the attainment of optimal physical, mental and social health and well-being for all infants, children, adolescents, and young adults.

Fernando Stein, MD, FAAP, President
Karen Remley, MD, CEO/Executive VP

2402 American Academy of Periodontology
737 N. Michigan Ave., Suite 800
Chicago, IL 60611   312-787-5518
Fax: 312-787-3670
staff@abperio.org
www.perio.org

The American Academy of Periodontology (AAP) is an 8,400-member professional organization for periodontists - specialists in the prevention, diagnosis, and treatment of diseases affecting the gums and supporting structures of the teeth, and in the placement of dental implants.

Joan Otomo-Corgel, President
Wayne A. Aldredge, President-Elect
Terrence J. Griffin, Vice President

2403 American Association for Dental Research
1619 Duke Street
Alexandria, VA 22314   703-548-0066
Fax: 703-548-1883
www.aadronline.org

The American Association for Dental Research (AADR) is headquartered in Alexandria, Va., is a non-profit organization with nearly 3,500 members in the United States. Its mission is (1) to advance research and increase knowledge for the improvement of oral health; (2) to support and represent the oral health research community; and (3) to facilitate the communication and application of research findings.

Brian H. Clarkson, President
Christopher H. Fox, Executive Director
Heidi Chapman, Executive Assistant

2404 American Association of Endodontists
211 E. Chicago Ave., Suite 1100
Chicago, IL 60611   312-266-7255
800-872-3636
Fax: 866-451-9020
info@aae.org
www.aae.org

The American Association of Endodontists is dedicated to excellence in the art and science of endodontics and to the highest standard of patient care. The Association inspires its members to pursue professional advancement and personal fulfillment through education, research, advocacy, leadership, communication and service.

Robert S. Roda, D.D.S., M.S., President
Peter Weber, M.S., CAE, Executive Director
Katherine Rouse, Executive Coordinator

2405 American Association of Oral and Maxillofacial Surgeons
9700 West Bryn Mawr Avenue
Rosemont, IL 60018   847-678-6200
800-822-6637
Fax: 847-678-6286
www.aaoms.org

The American Association of Oral and Maxillofacial Surgeons (AAOMS) represents more than 9,000 oral and maxillofacial surgeons in the United States, supporting specialized education, research and advocacy.

2406 American Association of Orthodontics
401 N Lindbergh Boulevard
Saint Louis, MO 63141
314-993-1700
800-424-2841
Fax: 314-997-1745
info@aaortho.org
www.aaomembers.org/

A professional association of educationally qualified orthodontic specialists dedicated to advancing the art and science of orthodontics and dentofacial orthopedics, improving the health of the public by promoting quality orthodontic care, and supporting the successful practice of orthodontics.

Chris Varanas, Executive Director

2407 American Association of Orthodontists
www.braces.org
314-993-1700
info@aaortho.org
www.braces.org

The American Association of Orthodontists is committed to educating the public about the need for, and benefits of, orthodontic treatment.

2408 American Association of Public Health Dentistry
3085 Stevenson Drive, Suite 200
Springfield, IL 62703
217-529-6941
Fax: 217-529-9120
info@aaphd.org
www.aaphd.org

Founded in 1937, the American Association of Public Health Dentistry (AAPHD) provides a focus for meeting the challenge to improve oral health.

Michael Monopoli, DMD, MPH, MS, President
Mary Altenberg, MS, CHES, Executive Director
David Cappelli, DMD, MPH, PhD, President-Elect

2409 American Cleft Palate-Craniofacial Association
1504 East Franklin St, Suite 102
Chapel Hill, NC 27514
919-933-9044
Fax: 919-933-9604
drhathaway54@gmail.com
www.acpa-cpf.org

The American Cleft Palate-Craniofacial Association (ACPA) is an international non-profit medical society of health care professionals who treat and/or perform research on birth defects of the head and face.

Ronald Reed Hathaway, DDS, MS, MS, President
Robert J. Havlik, MD, Vice President
Yvonne R. Gutierrez, MD, Communications Officer

2410 American College of Dentists
839J Quince Orchard Boulevard
Gaithersburg, MD 20878
301-977-3223
Fax: 301-977-3330
office@acd.org
www.acd.org

The American College of Dentists is the oldest major honorary organization for dentists.The mission of the American College of Dentists is to advance excellence, ethics, professionalism, and leadership in dentistry.

Jerome B. Miller, President
Bert W. Oettmeier, Jr., Vice President
Stephen A/ Ralls, Executive Director

2411 American Dental Assistants Association
140 N. Bloomingdale Road
Bloomingdale, IL 60108
630-994-4247
877-874-3785
Fax: 630-351-8490
www.dentalassistant.org

They work to advance the careers of dental assistants and to promote the dental assisting profession in matters of education, legislation, credentialing and professional activities which enhance the delivery of quality dental health care to the public.

Kimberly Bland, CDA EFDA M.Ed., President
Carolyn A. Regan, Vice President
Carol A. Walsh, CDA, Secretary

2412 American Dental Association
211 E Chicago Avenue
Chicago, IL 60611
312-440-2500
Fax: 312-266-9867
membership@ada.org
www.ada.org

Founded in 1859, the American Dental Association is the oldest and largest national dental society in the world.~Since then, the ADA has grown to become the leading source of oral health related information for dentists and their patients.

William Calnon, President-Elect
Raymond Gist, President
Kathleen O'Loughlin, Executive Director, COO, & Secretar

2413 American Dental Education Association
655 K Street, NW, Suite 800
Washington, DC 20001
202-289-7201
Fax: 202-289-7204
membership@adea.org
www.adea.org

The American Dental Education Association (ADEA) is The Voice of Dental Education. The mission of ADEA is to lead individuals and institutions of the dental education community to address contemporary issues influencing education, research and the delivery of oral health care for the health of the public.

Lily T. Garcia, Chair
Richard W. Valachovic, President & CEO
Robert Moran, EVP & COO

2414 American Dental Hygienists Association
444 North Michigan Avenue, Suite 3400
Chicago, IL 60611
312-440-8900
member.services@adha.net
www.adha.org

ADHA believes in helping dental hygienists achieve their full potential as they seek to improve the public's oral health. We support your goals by helping to ensure access to quality oral health care; promoting dental hygiene education, licensure, practice and research; and representing your legislative interests at the local, state and federal levels.

Kelli Swanson Jaecks, MA, RDH, President
Betty Kabel, RDH, BS, Vice President
Ann Battrell, MSDH, Executive Director

2415 American Dental Society of Anesthesiology
211 E. Chicago Avenue, Suite 780
Chicago, IL 60611
312-664-8270
adsahome@icloud.com
www.adsahome.org

The mission of the American Dental Society of Anesthesiology is to provide a forum for education, research, and recognition of achievement in order to promote safe and effective patient care for all dentists who have an interest in anesthesiology, edation and the control of anxiety and pain.

Ronald Kosinski, DMD, President
Michael Rollert, DDS, Vice President
R. Knight Charlton, Executive Director

2416 American Society for Dental Aesthetics
635 Madison Ave.
New York, NY 10022
800-454-ASDA
www.asdatoday.com

Founded in 1976,the American Society for Dental Aesthetics (ASDA) is made up of members who share a lifelong commitment to learning and providing exceptional care.

Dr. Irwin Smigel, President, Founder

2417 American Society of Forensic Odontology
PMB #121, 4414 82nd Street, Suite 212
Lubbock, TX 79424
rmetcalf@asfo.org
asfo.org

Founded in 1970, the American Society of Forensic Odontology (ASFO) was established to promote interest and research in the field of forensic odontology.

Roger Metcalf, President
Dr Jacqueline Reid, Secretary
Dr. Eric Wilson, Treasurer

2418 American Student Dental Association
211 E. Chicago Avenue, Suite 700
Chicago, IL 60611
312-440-2795
800-621-8099
Fax: 312-440-2820
Membership@ASDAnet.org
www.asdanet.org

ASDA protects and advances the rights, interests and welfare of dental students across the nation.

Christian Piers, President
Adrien Lewis, Vice President
Nancy Honeycutt, CAE, Executive Director

2419 Christian Dental Society
PO Box 296
Sumner, IA 50674
563-578-8887
cdssent@netins.net
www.christiandental.org

There mission is to show the love of Christ by offering dental relief to those in need around the world. Since its inception in 1963, CDS has provided volunteers, equipment and supplies with the objective of serving Christ.

Robert D. Meyer, DMD, President
Tina Wendel, Secretary
Robert Liebler, DMD, Treasurer

2420 Christian Medical & Dental Associations
P.O. Box 7500
Bristol, TN 37621
888-230-2637
Fax: 423-844-1005
Main@CMDA.org
cmda.org

Christian Medical & Dental Associations exists to glorify God by motivating, educating and equipping Christian healthcare professionals and students.

Richard E. Johnson, MD, President
David Stevens, MD, CEO
Gene Rudd, MD, Senior Vice President

2421 Hispanic Dental Association
3910 South IH-35., Suite # 245
Austin, TX 78704
512-904-0252
www.hdassoc.org

Founded in 1990, the history of HDA is one of inclusive nature driven by our mission. Incorporated in Texas with a national scope, the HDA's founding members shared a common commitment to improve the oral health of the Hispanic community.

Vidal Balderas, DDS, MPH, President
David Pena, Jr., CEO/ Executive Director
Frank Ramos, DDS, Treasurer

2422 Holistic Dental Association
1825 Ponce de Leon Blvd. #148
Coral Gables, FL 33134
305-356-7338
Fax: 305-468-6359
madelyn.pearson@gmail.com
holisticdental.org

Since 1978, the Holistic Dental Association has been providing support and guidance to practitioners of holistic and alternative dentistry, as well as informing the public of the benefits of holistic dentistry for their health and wellbeing. There purpose is to provide information and guidance to those persons seeking to participate in their own health care and to help in the continuing education of practitioners who have a desire to expand their knowledge and awareness.

Kevin Boehm, DDS, Chair
Madelyn Pearson, DDS, President
Roberta Glasser, Executive Director

2423 International Association for Orthodontics
750 N Lincoln Memorial Dr., #422
Milwaukee, WI 53202
414-272-2757
800-447-8770
Fax: 414-272-2754
WorldHeadquarters@iaortho.org
www.iaortho.org

The International Association for Orthodontics (IAO) was established in the United States in 1961 to promote international cooperation in the orthodontic field of dentistry. The IAO is a progressive and dynamic organization of general dentists, pediatric dentists and other dentists that provide orthodontic care to patients.

2424 International Association of Dental Research
1619 Duke Street
Alexandria, VA 22314
703-548-0066
Fax: 703-548-1883
abiko.yoshimitsu@nihon-u.ac.jp
www.iadr.com

To advance research and increase knowledge for the improvement of oral health worldwide. Through the Divisions and Sections, establish and support programs to promote oral health research and IADR activities. Regions with less developed research programs will be identified for specific support.

Yoshimitsu Abiko, President
Jukka Meurman, Vice President
Christopher H. Fox, Executive Director

2425 National Dental Association
3517 16th Street, NW
Washindton, DC 20010
202-588-1697
Fax: 202-588-1244
Cbrown2444@aol.com
ndaonline.org

The National Dental Association promotes oral health equity among people of color by harnessing the collective power of its members, advocating for the needs of and mentoring dental students of color, and raising the profile of the profession in our communities

Madge Y. Potts-Williams, D.D.S, Chairman
Carrie B. Brown, D.M.D, President
Kim Perry, D.D.S, Vice President

2426 Oral Cancer Foundation
3419 Via Lido # 205
Newport Beach, CA 92663
949-723-4400
oralcancerfoundation.org

The Oral Cancer Foundation is a national public service, non-profit entity designed to reduce suffering and save lives through prevention, education, research, advocacy, and patient support activities.

Brian Hill, Founder & Executive Director
Jamie O'Day, Director of Administration
Natalie Riggs, Dir of Special Projects

2427 Special Care Dentistry Association
330 North Wabash Avenue, Suite 2000
Chicago, IL 60611
312-527-6764
Fax: 312-673-6663
SCDA@SCDAonline.org
www.scdaonline.org

The Special Care Dentistry Association serves as a resource to all oral health care professionals who serve or are interested in serving patients with special needs through education and networking to increase access to oral healthcare for patients with special needs.

Libraries & Resource Centers

2428 University of Illinois at Chicago, Craniofacial Center
College of Medicine
1740 West Taylor Street
Chicago, IL 60612
312-996-6933
Fax: 312-355-4173
dreisber@uic.edu
www.uic.edu/com/craniofacial/

The Craniofacial Center is one of the oldest and largest facilities in the world, dedicated to the evaluation and treatment of infants, children, adolescents, and adults with cleft lip and palate and other congenital craniofacial conditions.

David J Reisberg, DDS, Medical Director

2429 University of Mississippi Medical Center
2500 N State Street
Jackson, MS 39216

601-984-5820
cporter@pubaffairs.umsmed.edu
www.umc.edu

The health sciences campus of the University of Mississippi. It houses schools of Medicine, Nursing, Health Related Professions and Dentistry.

Lawrence Hornsby, Director

Audio Video

2430 Face First
Fanlight Productions
32 Court Street, 21st Floor
Brooklyn, NY 11201

718-488-8900
800-876-1710
Fax: 718-488-8642
info@fanlight.com, orders@fanlight.com
www.fanlight.com

Profiles of several people born with facial deformities; they chronicle both physical pain and the pain of rejection, as well as the strengths that have enabled them to achieve successful adult lives. ISBN: DVD: 1-57295-886-3; VHS: 1-572952-59-8

29 minutes DVD or VHS
Nicole Johnson, Publicity Coordinator

Web Sites

2431 American Academy of Pediatric Dentistry Foundation
211 East Chicago Avenue, Suite 1600
Chicago, IL 60611

312-337-2169
Fax: 312-337-6329
www.aapd.org

Supports and promotes education, research, service and policy development that advances the oral health of infants and children through adolescence, including those with special healthcare needs.

Jade Miller, D.D.S, President
Kristi Casale, Director, Meeting Services
John S. Rutkauskas, D.D.S., M.B., CEO

2432 Dental Consumer Advisory
www.toothinfo.com/

The purpose of this site is to provide uselful and pracitcal information for the public concerning issues of dental care.

2433 Dental Resources on the Web
www.dental-resources.com

Dental sites for education, practices, laboratories, office supplies, dental care and associations.

Book Publishers

2434 Understanding Dental Health
University Press of Mississippi
3825 Ridgewood Road
Jackson, MS 39211

601-432-6205
800-737-7788
Fax: 601-432-6217
press@ihl.state.ms.us
www.upress.stat.ms.us

A user friendly manual on the basics of dental health.

128 pages Hard/Soft cover
ISBN: 1-578060-09-5

DESCRIPTION

2435 DEPRESSION

Involves the following Biologic System(s):
Developmental/Behavioral/Psychiatric Disorders

Depression refers to an emotional state characterized by exaggerated feelings of sadness, discouragement, loneliness, low self-esteem, and despair. These feelings may follow a recent loss or other tragic event. However, if feelings of depression worsen and are prolonged, or occur for no apparent reason, this may indicate a chronic (formerly called "endogenous") depressive disorder. Although clinical depression occurs more commonly among the adult population (2-3 times more common in females than in males, depression may be evident as early as infancy and is increasingly common among adolescents.

Symptoms and findings associated with depression are variable. It has a chronic course with relapses. The mood is typically depressed, irritable, and/or anxious, often accompanied by preoccupation with guilt, decreased ability to concentrate, diminished interest in usual activities (anhedonia), social withdrawal, hopelessness, and recurrent thoughts of death and suicide. Symptoms associated with depression in school-age children are similar to those seen in adults and include overwhelming feelings of sadness, crying, loss of interest in pleasurable activities, eating and sleeping irregularities, and, in some cases, suicidal thoughts (ideation). Some affected children may exhibit symptoms that belie a diagnosis of depression, such as overactivity and aggression. Adolescents with depression may have feelings of hopelessness and helplessness with no corresponding periods of happiness or well-being. However, inappropiate displays of euphoria together with such behavior as truancy, substance abuse, or other antisocial behaviors may also be symptomatic of depression. Other symptoms and findings associated with adolescent depression may include a decline in school grades, boredom, repetitive accidents, drug or alcohol abuse, absenteeism, feelings or delusions of guilt, and thoughts of suicide. Physical symptoms may sometimes include fatigue, headaches, and abdominal pain. Those who are psychotically depressed may experience delusions and hallucinations.

Depression in infants may be precipitated by such events as sudden separation from the mother or caregiver after six months of age (anaclitic depression of infancy) and may be manifested by ceaseless crying, panic, apprehension, withdrawal, and eating and sleeping disturbances. Eventually, indifference and unresponsiveness may develop and result in deficiencies in intellectual, physical, and social development. Endogenous depression may be caused by many different factors including genetic influences, hormonal disturbances, certain medications, infectious or neurologic disorders, physical conditions (i.e., stroke, etc.), certain tumors, nutritional influences, and psychosocial factors. In addition, depression may occur in association with other psychological disorders such as bipolar or other mood disorders (e.g., schizoaffective disorder).

Most persons with depression get treated as outpatients. Treatment of depression most often includes the administration of certain antidepressant medications. Most studies indicate that cognitive, interpersonal, and behavior therapy are effective, especially in combination with antidepressant medications. Electroconvulsive therapy (ECT) is effective but is usually reserved for severely depressed patients or patients who do not respond to or are not tolerant of medications. Children and adolescents with this disorder also often require individual psychotherapy and, in many cases, group and family therapy. Overall, the suicide rate is estimated at 15%. All patients with depression should be asked gently but directly about suicidal ideas or plans. All communications about self-destruction should be taken seriously.

Government Agencies

2436 NIH/National Institute of Mental Health
6001 Executive Boulevard, Room 6200, MSC 9663
Bethesda, MD 20892
301-443-4536
866-615-6464
Fax: 301-443-4279
TTY: 301-443-8431
nimhinfo@nih.gov
www.nimh.nih.gov

Conducts strategic planning for specific research areas as well as for the Institute as a whole.

Joshua Gordon, MD, PhD, Director
Shelli Avenevoli, MD, Deputy Director

National Associations & Support Groups

2437 Agency for Healthcare Research and Quality
540 Gaither Road
Rockville, MD 20850
301-427-1364
TDD: 888-586-6340
richard.kronick@ahrq.hhs.gov
www.ahrq.gov

The Agency for Healthcare Research and Quality's (AHRQ) mission is to produce evidence to make health care safer, higher quality, more accessible, equitable, and affordable, and to work within the U.S. Department of Health and Human Services and with other partners to make sure that the evidence is understood and used.

Richard Kronick, PhD., Director
Sharon B. Arnold, PhD, Deputy Director
Jeffery Toven, Director/Executive Officer

2438 American Academy of Pediatrics
141 Northwest Point Boulevard
Elk Grove Village, IL 60007
847-434-4000
800-433-9016
Fax: 847-434-8000
www.aap.org

The American Academy of Pediatrics and its member pediatricians are committed to the attainment of optimal physical, mental and social health and well-being for all infants, children, adolescents, and young adults.

Fernando Stein, MD, FAAP, President
Karen Remley, MD, CEO/Executive VP

2439 American Association of Suicidology
5221 Wisconsin Avenue
Washington, DC 20015
202-237-2280
800-273-TALK
Fax: 202-237-2282
julie.cerel@uky.edu
www.suicidology.org

AAS is a membership organization for all those involved in suicide prevention and intervention, or touched by suicide. AAS is a leader in the advancement of scientific and programmatic efforts in suicide prevention through research, education and training, the development of standards and resources, and survivor support services.

Julie Cerel, PhD, Chair
William Schmitz Jr., PsyD, President
Amy Boland, CPA, Treasurer

2440 American College Counseling Association
www.collegecounseling.org

tknappgr@scad.edu
www.collegecounseling.org

The American College Counseling Association is made up of diverse mental health professionals from the fields of counseling, psychology, and social work. Our common theme is working within higher education settings.

Tamara Knapp Grosz, President
Sylvia E. Shortt, Ed.S./ LPC, Treasurer
Ky Heinlen, PhD, LPCC-S, Secretary

2441 American College Health Association
1362 Mellon Road, Suite 180
Hanover, MD 21076
410-859-1500
Fax: 410-859-1510
contact@acha.org
www.acha.org

To serve as the principal leadership organization for advancing the health of college students and campus communities through advocacy, education, and research.

Sarah Van Orman, MD, MMM, FACHA, President
Keith Anderson, PhD, FACHA, Vice President
Doyle E. Randol, MS, Col., Executive Director

2442 American Foundation for Suicide Prevention
120 Wall Street, 29th Floor
New York, NY 10005
212-363-3500
888-333-AFSP
Fax: 212-363-6237
info@afsp.org
www.afsp.org

The American Foundation for Suicide Prevention (AFSP) is the leader in the fight against suicide. We fund research, create educational programs, advocate for public policy, and support survivors of suicide loss.

Nancy Farrell, M.P.A., Chair
Yeates Conwell, M.D., President
Robert Gebbia, CEO

2443 American Psychiatric Association
1000 Wilson Boulevard, Suite 1825
Arlington, VA 22209
703-907-7300
888-35 -7924
apa@psych.org
www.psychiatry.org

It is a medical specialty society representing growing membership of more than 36,000 psychiatrists.

2444 American Psychological Association
750 First St. NE
Washington, DC 20002
202-336-5500
800-374-2721
TTY: 202-336-6123
www.apa.org

The mission is to advance the creation, communication and application of psychological knowledge to benefit society and improve people's lives.

Norman B. Anderson, PhD, CEO/ EVP
L. Michael Honaker, PhD, Deputy Chief Executive Officer
Ellen G. Garrison, PhD, Senior Policy Advisor

2445 American Public Health Association
800 I Street, NW
Washington, DC 20001
202-777-2742
Fax: 202-777-2534
TTY: 202-777-2500
www.apha.org

APHA champions the health of all people and all communities. They aim to strengthen the public health profession and speak out for public health issues and policies backed by science.

Georges C. Benjamin, MD, Executive Director
Kemi Oluwafemi, MBA, CPA, Chief Financial Officer
Susan Polan, PhD, Associate Executive Director

2446 American School Counselor Association
1101 King Street, Suite 310
Alexandria, VA 22314
703-683-2722
800-306-4722
Fax: 703-997-7572
asca@schoolcounselor.org
www.schoolcounselor.org

The mission of ASCA is to represent professional school counselors and to promote professionalism and ethical practices.

Richard Wong, Executive Director
Jeff Broderson, Information Technology Admin.
Kathleen M Rakestraw, Director of Communications

2447 American Society of Clinical Psychopharmacology
5034-A Thoroughbred Lane
Brentwood, NJ 37027
615-649-3085
Fax: 888-417-3311
www.ascpp.org

The American Society of Clinical Psychopharmacology (ASCP) was founded in 1992 to advance the science and practice of clinical psychopharmacology. Its nearly 800 members are physicians who study and practice psychopharmacology, as well as doctoral level investigators of clinical psychopharmacology or of pharmacology. ASCP members are advocates for clinical psychopharmacology and for clinical research.

Maurizio Fava, MD, President
John M. Kane, MD, Treasurer
Leslie Citrome, MD, Board Member

2448 Anxiety Disorders Association of America
8730 Georgia Avenue, Suite 600
Silver Spring, MD 20910
240-485-1001
Fax: 240-485-1035
information@adaa.org
www.adaa.org

Offers resources and information for persons with anxiety and stress-related disorders.

Alies Muskin, Executive Director

2449 Anxiety and Depression Association of America
8701 Georgia Ave., Suite #412
Silver Spring, MD 20910
240-485-1001
Fax: 240-485-1035
www.adaa.org

ADAA is a national nonprofit organization dedicated to the prevention, treatment, and cure of anxiety, depression, OCD, PTSD, and related disorders and to improving the lives of all people who suffer from them through education, practice, and research.

Mark H. Pollack, MD, President
Alies Muskin, Executive Director
Jean Kaplan Teichroew

2450 Depression & Related Affective Disorders Association
Meyer 3-181 600 N Wolfe Street
Baltimore, MD 21287
410-955-4647
Fax: 410-614-3241
drada@jhmi.edu
www.drada.org

Provides education, information and support services for individuals with depression of bipolar illness, their families and mental health professionals.

2451 Depression and Bipolar Support Alliance
730 N Franklin Street, Suite 501
Chicago, IL 60654
800-826-3632
Fax: 312-642-7243
www.dbsalliance.org

Patient-directed organization focusing on the most prevalent mental illnesses- depression and bipolar disorder. Fosters an understanding about the impact and management of these life-threatening illnesses by providing up-to-date, scientifically-based tools and information written in language the general public can understand.

Allen Doederlein, President
Lisa Goodale, Vice President, Training
Charlene Knox, Coordinator, Human Resources

2452 Depressives Anonymous: Recovery from Depression
329 E 62nd Street
New York, NY 10065 212-689-2600

Individuals suffering from depression or anxiety. A self-help organization with meetings and sharing of experiences. Conducts research and offers classes. Disseminates information. Publications: Newsletter, three-four times a year. Brochures and pamphlets.

Dr. Helen DeRosis, Founder

2453 Families for Depression Awareness
395 Totten Pond Road, Suite 404
Waltham, 2451 781-890-0220
Fax: 781-890-2411
www.familyaware.org

Families for Depression Awareness is a national nonprofit organization helping families recognize and cope with depression and bipolar disorder to get people well and prevent suicides.

Julie Totten, Founder
Valerie Cordero, Interim Co-Executive Director
Susan Weinstein, Interim Co-Executive Director

2454 Family Service Association
6960 Mumford Road, Suite 2069
Halifax, NS NS B3 902-420-1980
888-886-5552
admin@fshalifax.com
www.fshalifax.com/index.htm

They offer professional, confidential counseling and education services to enable people to function more effectively at home, in the community and in their work environment.

Mary Clancy, Chair
Sean Reddick, Vice Chair
Valerie Bobyk, Executive Director

2455 Federation of Families for Children's Mental Health
9605 Medical Center Drive,Ste 208
Rockville, MD 20850 240-403-1901
Fax: 240-403-1909
ffcmh@ffcmh.org
www.ffcmh.org

The National family run organization is dedicated exclusively to helping children with mental health needs and their families achieve a better quality of life.

Sandra Spencer, Executive Director
Andrea Barnes, Policy and Research Assistant
Emmett Dennis, Fiscal Officer

2456 Injury Control Research Center for Suicide Prevention
43 Foundry Avenue
Waltham, MA 02453 800-273-TALK
icrc-s@edc.org
suicideprevention-icrc-s.org

The Injury Control Research Center for Suicide Prevention (ICRC-S) is a center-without-walls that promotes a public health approach to suicide prevention through a collaborative process of research, outreach, and education. There goal is to draw suicide prevention directly into the domain of public health and injury prevention and link it to complementary approaches to mental health.

Eric Caine, Md, Professor & Chair
Yeates Conwell, MD, Professor & Vice Chair
Jerry Reed,PhD, MSW, VP & Director

2457 NADD: National Association for the Dually Diagnosed
132 Fair Street
Kingston, NY 12401 845-331-4336
800-331-5362
Fax: 845-331-4569
info@thenadd.org
www.thenadd.org

NADD is the leading North American expert in providing professionals, educators, policy makers, and families with education, training, and information on mental health issues relating to persons with intellectual or developmental disabilities.

Dr Robert Fletcher, CEO
Michelle Jordan, Office Manager
Edward Seliger, Project Coordinator

2458 National Alliance for Research on Schizophrenia and Affective Disorders
60 Cutter Mill Road, Suite 404
Great Neck, NY 11021 516-829-0091
800-829-8289
Fax: 516-487-6390
info@bbrfoundation.org
www.narsad.org

Raises and distributes funds for scientific research into the causes, cures, treatments, and prevention of severe mental illness, primarily schizophrenia and affective disorders.

Stephen A Lieber, Chairman of the Board
Benita F Shobe, President & CEO
Suzanne Golden, Vice President

2459 National Alliance for the Mentally Ill
3803 N Fairfax Drive, Suite 100
Arlington, VA 22203 703-524-7600
800-950-6264
Fax: 703-524-9094
TDD: 703-516-7227
lsmith@nami.org
www.nami.org

NAMI is a nonprofit, grassroots, self-help, support and advocacy organization of consumers, families and friends of people with severe mental illness, such as schizophrenia, bipolar disorder, major depressive disorder, obsessive compulsive disorder, anxiety disorders, autism and other severe and persistent mental illnesses that affect the brain.

Liz T Smith, Director, NAMI Center for Excellenc
Benjamin Staples, Consultant with the Center for Exce

2460 National Alliance on Mental Illness
3803 N. Fairfax Drive, Suite 100
Arlington, VA 22203 703-524-7600
800-950-6264
Fax: 703-524-9094
info@nami.org
www.nami.org

Grassroots mental health organization dedicated to building better lives for the millions of Americans affected by mental illness.

Jim Payne, J.D., President
David Levy, Chief Financial Officer
Mary Giliberti, J.D., Executive Director

2461 National Anxiety Foundation
3135 Custer Drive
Lexington, KY 40517 859-272-7166
www.lexington-on-line.com/naf.html

Offers information and help to persons with panic disorders, manic and depressive disorders and mental illness.

Stephen Cox MD, President & Medical Director
Linda Vernon Blair, Vice President
C Todd Strecker, Secretary, Treasurer

2462 National Education Alliance for Borderline Personality Disorder
www.borderlinepersonalitydisorder.com

neabpd@aol.com
www.borderlinepersonalitydisorder.com

NEA.BPD National Education Alliance for Borderline Personality Disorder is a nationally recognized organization dedicated to building better lives for millions of Americans affected by Borderline Personality Disorder.

Perry D. Hoffman, PhD, President
Patricia Woodward, MAT, Secretary/ Treasurer
Alan E. Fruzzetti, PhD, Dir. Of Research

2463 National Federation of Families for Children's Mental Health
www.ffcmh.org

240-403-1901
www.ffcmh.org

The National Federation of Families for Children's Mental Health is a national family-run organization linking more than 120 chapters and state organizations focused on the issues of children and youth with emotional, behavioral, or mental health needs and their families.

Teka Dempson, President
Sherri Luthe, Vice President
Sandra Spencer, Executive Director

2464 National Foundation for Depression
2 Penn Plaza, Suite 1981
New York, NY 10121   212-268-4260
Amy Russell

2465 National Foundation for Depressive Illness
PO Box 17598
Baltimore, MD 21297   Fax: 443-782-0739
                                       info@ifred.org
                                       www.ifred.org

iFred is a 501c3 organization aiming to shed a positive light on depression throughout the world in order to prevent the onset, research causes and treatments, and rebrand the disease in a positive way.

Tom Dean, iFred President
Susan Minamyer, Secretary
Kathryn Goetzke, Founder

2466 National Multiple Sclerosis Society
www.nationalmssociety.org

The National MS Society is a collective of passionate individuals who want to do something about MS now - to move together toward a world free of multiple sclerosis. MS stops people from moving.

Eli Rubenstein, Chair
Cynthia Zagieboylo, President & CEO
Peter Porrino, Treasurer

2467 National Network of Depression Centers
2350 Green Rd., Ste 191
Ann Arbor, MI 48105   734-332-3914
                                   Fax: 734-332-3939
                                       www.nndc.org

There goal is to show the many, many people affected by depression, bipolar and other related mood illnesses. Some are people who live with depression, others are family members, co-workers, neighbors of those who do. People of all ages, races, genders, education levels, income levels, jobs, geography, etc.

John F. Greden, MD, Chair
J. Raymond Depaulo, Jr., MD, Vice Chair
Allan Tasman, MD, Treasurer

2468 National Organization for People of Color Against Suicide
4715 Sargent Road, NE
Washington, DC 20017   202-549-6039
                                       866-899-5317
                                   nopcas@onebox.com
                                       www.nopcas.org

NOPCAS promotes life-affirming strategies that will help to decrease life-threatening behaviors. It is their aim to develop prevention, intervention, and postvention support services to the families and communities impacted adversely by the effects of violence, depression, and suicide in an effort to decrease life-threatening behavior.

Donna Barnes, Executive Director

2469 National Organization for Seasonal Affective Disorder (SAD)
19217 Orbit Drive
Gaithersburg, MD 20879   301-869-5908
                                       800-548-3968
                                   Fax: 301-977-2281
                                     info@sunbox.com
                                       www.sunbox.com

A newly identified medical disorder characterized by winter symptoms which include fall and winter weight gain, carbohydrate cravings, oversleeping, decreased interest in normal activities and low mood and energy.

2470 Postpartum Progress
4920 Atlanta Highway, #316
Alpharetta, GA 3004   877-470-4877
                               wmc@postpartumprogress.org
                                   postpartumprogress.org

Postpartum Progress Inc. (PPI) is a national 501c3 non-profit focused on vastly improving awareness of perinatal mood and anxiety disorders like postpartum depression and providing peer support for the women who have them. We create innovative programs and messaging that connect women to information and treatment and support them throughout recovery to help lessen the burden of disease.

Katherine Stone, Founder & Executive Director
Becky Schroeder, Program Manager
Heather Kimg, Managing Editor

2471 Postpartum Support International
6706 SW 54th Avenue
Portland, OR 97219   503-894-9453
                                       800-944-4PPD
                                   Fax: 503-894-9452
                                   support@postpartum.net
                                       www.postpartum.net

The purpose of the organization is to increase awareness among public and professional communities about the emotional changes that women experience during pregnancy and postpartum.

Ann Smith, CNM, President
Wendy N. Davis, PhD, Executive Director
Lianne Swanson, Office Administration

2472 Recovery
802 N Dearborn Street
Chicago, IL 60610   312-337-5661
                                   Fax: 312-337-5756
                                   spot@recovery-inc.com
                                       www.recovery-inc.org

Techniques for controlling behavior, changing attitudes.

Kathleen Garcia, Executive Director

2473 Suicide Awareness Voices of Education
8120 Penn Ave. S., Suite 470
Bloomington, MN 55431   952-946-7998
                                       800-273-8255
                                       www.save.org

The mission of SAVE is to prevent suicide through public awareness and education, reduce stigma and serve as a resource to those touched by suicide.

Joseph W. Stackhouse, President
Patrick M. Klinger, VP
Daphne Fabiano, CPA, Treasurer

2474 Suicide Prevention Resource Center
43 Foundry Avenue
Waltham, MA 2453   877-438-7772
                                   Fax: 617-969-9186
                                   TTY: 617-964-5448
                                       info@sprc.org
                                       www.sprc.org

SPRC is the a federally supported resource center devoted to advancing the National Strategy for Suicide Prevention. They provide technical assistance, training, and materials to increase the knowledge and expertise of suicide prevention practitioners and other professionals serving people at risk for suicide. They also promote collaboration among a variety of organizations that play a role in developing the field of suicide prevention.

Jerry Reed, PhD, MSW, Director
Chris Miara, MS, Director of Operations & Resources
Julie Goldstein Grumet, PhD, Director of Prevention and Practice

2475 The Stanley Medical Research Institute
8401 Connecticut Avenue, Suite 200
Chevy Chase, MD 20815   301-571-0760
                                   Fax: 301-571-0769
                                   info@stanleyresearch.org
                                   www2.stanleyresearch.org

The Stanley Medical Research Institute (SMRI) is a nonprofit organization supporting research on the causes of, and treatments for, schizophrenia and bipolar disorder. Since it began in 1989, SMRI has supported more than $550 million in research in over 30 countries.

Maree J. Webster, Ph.D., Executive Director
Wendy Simmons, Research Assistant
Jana Bowcut, M.P.H., Treatment Trials Administrator

State Agencies & Support Groups

2476 Depressive and Manic-Depressive Assocation of Mount Sinai
100 LaSalle Street, Suite 5A
New York, NY 10027 917-445-2399
jgg17@columbia.edu
www.columbia.edu

The NYC Depressive and Manic-Depressive Group is a support group for persons with mood disorders, depression and bipolar disorder, as well as their family members and friends.

Research Centers

2477 National Alliance for Research on Schizophrenia & Depression
60 Cutter Mill Road, Suite 404
Great Neck, NY 11021 516-829-0091
Fax: 516-487-6930
info@bbrfoundation.org
www.narsad.org

The Brain and Behavior Research Foundation (formerly NARSAD, the National Alliance for Research on Schizophrenia and Depression) is committed to alleviating the suffering of mental illness by awarding grants that will lead to advances and breakthroughs in scientific research.

Benita Shobe, President & CEO

2478 University of Pennsylvania, Depression Research Unit
School of Medicine, Department of Psychiatry
3600 Spruce Street
Philadelphia, PA 19104 215-349-5979
Fax: 215-662-6443
www.med.upenn.edu

The mission of the Depression Research Unit (DRU) at Penn is to foster a greater understanding and knowledge of the causes, diagnosis, and treatment of mood disorders.

Adam I Rubin, Director

2479 University of Texas, Mental Health Clinical Research Center
5323 Harry Hines Boulevard
Dallas, TX 75235 214-648-2951

UT Southwestern Medical Center is home to one of the premier centers in the world for the study, diagnosis and treatment of mental health and addictive disorders.

A John Rush, MD, Director

2480 Yale University, Behavioral Medicine Clinic
Yale School of Medicine
333 Cedar Street
New Haven, CT 06510 203-785-4231

Focuses on mental disorders including schizophrenia and depression.

Henry M Rinder, Director

2481 Yale University, Ribicoff Research Facilities
CT Medical Health Center
34 Park Street
New Haven, CT 06519 203-764-9765
Fax: 203-688-2491

Clinical research in the areas of schizophrenia, depression and mental disorders.

George Heninger, MD, Director

Conferences

2482 ADAA Annual Conference
Anxiety Disorders Association of America
8701 Georgia Avenue, Suite 412
Silver Spring, MD 20910 240-485-1001
Fax: 240-485-1035
information@adaa.org
www.adaa.org

Focusing exclusively on advancing science and treatment of anxiety and related disorders in children and adults.

April

Alies Muskin, Executive Director

2483 DSBA National Conference
Depression and Bipolar Support Alliance
730 N Franklin Street, Suite 501
Chicago, IL 60654 800-826-3632
Fax: 312-642-7243
www.dbsalliance.org

Offers a unique peer-centered conference for individuals living with depression or bipolar disorder, as well as for family members or health care providers looking for ways to best help their loved ones, patients, or clients by partnering with them on their path to recovery. The conference consists of compelling keynote presentations, educational workshops, and pre-conference institutes.

May

Allen Doederlein, President
Lisa Goodale, Vice President, Training
Charlene Knox, Coordinator, Human Resources

2484 FFCMH Annual Conference
Federation of Families for Childrens Mental Health
9605 Medical Center Drive, Suite 280
Rockville, MD 20850 240-403-1901
Fax: 240-403-1909
ffcmh@ffcmh.org
www.ffcmh.org

Address the complex issue of trauma; the impact it has on children and families; the promotion of healing and prevention strategies; knowledge about how to address trauma through resiliency-based interventions, utilizing a familydriven, youth guided approach; and examples of how family organizations and the partners they work with are raising awareness and improving trauma-focused services and supports.

November

Sandra Spencer, Executive Director

2485 NADD Conference & Exhibit Show
National Association for the Dually Diagnosed
132 Fair Street
Kingston, NY 12401 845-331-4336
800-331-5362
Fax: 845-331-4569
info@thenadd.org
www.thenadd.org

November

Dr Robert Fletcher, CEO
Michelle Jordan, Office Manager
Edward Seliger, Project Coordinator

2486 NAMI Convention
National Alliance on Mental Illness
3803 N. Fairfax Dr.Suite 100
Arlington, VA 22203 703-524-7600
800-950-6264
Fax: 703-524-9094
TDD: 703-516-7227
info@nami.org
www.nami.org

The NAMI Convention is packed with information, chances to network, leadership development opportunities, and lots more

July

Suzanne Vogel-Scibilia MD, President

Audio Video

2487 Coping with Depression
New Harbinger Publications
5674 Shattuck Avenue
Oakland, CA 94609   510-652-2002
                                                 800-748-6273
                                            Fax: 510-652-1613
                              customerservice@newharbinger.com
                                             newharbinger.com

60 minute videotape that offers a powerful message of hope for
anyone struggling with depression.

ISBN: 1-879237-62-8

**2488 Cry for Help - How to Help a Friend Who is Depressed or
Suicidal**
Aquarius Health Care Videos
36 Southern Eagle Cartway
Brewster, MA 2631   508-255-4685
                                                 800-451-5006
                                            Fax: 508-255-5705
                             customerservice@paracletepress.com
                                         www.paracletepress.com

Most suicidal young people don't really want to die; they just
want their pain to end. Teen sucide is often preventable if young
people know the signs to look for and the steps to take when they
suspect a friend is suicidal. This video teaches young people to
recognize the warning signs and to take specific actions to help a
friend.

22 Minutes

Donna Kaufman

2489 Day for Night: Recognizing Teenage Depression
DRADA-Depression and Related Affective Disorders
600 N Wolfe Street
Baltimore, MD 21287   410-955-4647
                                            Fax: 410-614-3241

2490 Living with Depression and Manic Depression
New Harbinger Publications
5674 Shattuck Avenue
Oakland, CA 94609   510-652-2002
                                                 800-748-6273
                                            Fax: 510-652-1613
                              customerservice@newharbinger.com
                                             newharbinger.com

Describes a program based on years of research and hundreds of
interviews with depressed persons. Warm, helpful, and engaging,
this tape validates the feelings of people with depression while it
encourages positive change.

ISBN: 1-879237-63-6

**2491 Why Isn't My Child Happy? A Video Guide About Childhood
Depression**
ADD WareHouse
300 Northwest 70th Avenue, Suite 102
Plantation, FL 33317   954-792-8100
                                                 800-233-9273
                                            Fax: 954-792-8545
                                   websales@addwarehouse.com
                                            addwarehouse.com

The first of its kind, this new video deals with childhood depression. Informative and frank about this common problem, this
book offers helpful guidance for parents and professionals trying
to better understand childhood depression. 110 minutes.

Web Sites

2492 AACAP
3615 Wisconsin Avenue, N.W.
Washington, DC 20016   202-966-7300
                                            Fax: 202-966-2891
                                               www.aacap.org

Assisting parents and families in understanding developmental,
behavioral, emotional and mental disorders affecting children and
adolescents.

Paramjit T. Joshi, M.D., President
David G Fassler, M.D., Treasurer
Aradhana Bela Sood, M.D., Secretary

2493 Anxiety Disorders Association of America

Offers resources and information for persons with anxiety and
stress-related disorders.

2494 Dr. Ivan's Depression Central
www.psycom.net/depression.central.html

This site is the Internet's central clearinghouse for information
on all types of depressive disorders and on the most effective
tratments for individuals suffering from Major Depression, Manic
Depression (Bipolar Disorder), Cyclothymia, Dysthymia and
other mood disorders.

Ivan Goldberg, MD, Founder
Satish Reddy, M.D., Editor

2495 Internet Mental Health
www.mentalhealth.com/

                                      internetmentalhealth@shaw.ca
                                          www.mentalhealth.com/

Our goal is to improve understanding, diagnosis, and teatment of
meantal illness throughout the world.

Phillip W. Long, M.D., Psychiatrist

2496 Mental Health Net
Po Box 20709
Columbus, OH 43220   614-448-4055
                              info@centersite.net, editor@centersite.n
                                               www.mentalhelp.net

We wish to provide the following: to discuss, develop and debate
in an open forum the future of the mental health field in America
and throughout the world. To help coordinate various components of the mental health field so as to bring about greater communication between them. To educate the public about mental
health issues, to promote active collaboration between professionals in all segments of mental health development,
implementation and policy.

2497 NADD: National Association for the Dually Diagnosed
132 Fair Street
Kingston, NY 12401   845-331-4336
                                                 800-331-5362
                                            Fax: 845-331-4569
                                             info@thenadd.org
                                             www.thenadd.org

Nonprofit organization designed to promote the interests of professional and care providers for individuals who have the coexistence of mental illness and mental retardation. NADD provides
conferences, educational services and training materials to professionals, parents, concerned citizens and service organizations.

Dr Robert Fletcher, CEO
Michelle Jordan, Office Manager
Edward Seliger, Project Coordinator

2498 Online Mendelian Inheritance in Man
U.S. National Library of Medicine, 8600 Rockville
Bethesda, MD 20894   888-346-3656
                                          info@ncbi.nlm.nih.gov
                                            www.ncbi.nlm.nih.gov

This database is a catalog of human genes and genetic disorders.

Christine E. Seidman, M.D., Chair
David J. Lipman, M.D., Executive Secretary
Michael Boehnke, Ph.D., Board Member

2499 Seasonal Affective Disorder
www.alt.support.depression.seasonal

The SAD Association is a voluntary organization and registered
charity which informs the public and health professions about
SAD and supports and advises sufferers of the illness.

2500 Understanding and Treating Depression
www.couns.uiuc.edu/depression.htm

Offers an understanding of depression, causes, how to help yourself, things to do, what to avoid while in the depression state, and
treatments of the depression.

2501 Wing of Madness: A Depression Guide
www.wingofmadness.com

Is a nonprofit organization dedicated to disseminating information about depression to consumers.

Book Publishers

2502 Anxiety & Depression In Adults & Children
Sage Publications
2455 Teller Road
Newbury Park, CA 91320   805-499-0721

1994 304 pages Softcover
ISBN: 0-803970-21-8

2503 Ask the Doctor: Depression
Andrews McMeel Publishing
PO Box 419150
Kansas City, MO 64141   816-932-6700
                                 800-233-2336
                                 Fax: 212-698-7336

A look at depression, its symptoms, what causes it, and what you
can do about it. Learn the difference between mood problems and
genuine depression, and how to read warning signs such as sleep
abnormalities, nervousness, and suicidal thoughts. Information on
chemicals, genetics, and medical solutions.

128 pages Softcover
ISBN: 0-836227-11-5

2504 Coping with Depression
Rosen Publishing Group
29 E 21st Street
New York, NY 10010   800-237-9932
                                 Fax: 888-436-4643
                                 rosenpub@tribeca.ios.com
                                 www.rosenpublishing.com

With an emphasis on life's myriad difficulties, the authors help
teens find practical ways to cope with depression.

ISBN: 0-823919-51-0

2505 Dealing with Depression: Five Ways to Help
Haworth Press
10 Alice Street
Binghamton, NY 13904   607-722-8277
                                 Fax: 607-722-1424
1995
ISBN: 1-560249-33-1

2506 Depression and Its Treatment
Warner Books
1271 Avenue of the Americas
New York, NY 10020   212-522-7200

A layman's guide to help one understand and cope with America's number one mental health problem.

157 pages

2507 Depression, the Mood Disease
Johns Hopkins University Press
2715 N Charles Street
Baltimore, MD 21218   410-516-6900
                                 800-537-5487
                                 Fax: 410-516-6998
                        www.highbeam.com/doc/1G1-159331264.html

This book explores the many faces of an illness that will affect as
many as 36 million Americans at some point in their lives. Updated to reflect state-of-the-art treatment.

1993 240 pages
ISBN: 0-801851-84-X

2508 Depressive Illnesses: Treatments Bring New Hope
Superintendent of Documents
PO Box 371954
Pittsburgh, PA 15250   202-512-2250

Offers the general public an overview of the various depressive
illnesses. Topics include causes, symptoms and types of depression, clinical evaluation and treatment, helpful suggestions for
family and friends, and other sources of information.

28 pages

2509 Encyclopedia of Depression
Facts on File
Department M274, 11 Penn Plaza
New York, NY 10001   212-290-8090
                                 800-322-8755
                                 Fax: 212-678-3633

This volume defines and explains all terms and topics relating to
depression.

170 pages Hardbound

2510 Essential Guide to Psychiatric Drugs
Saint Martin's Press
175 5th Avenue
New York, NY 10010   212-674-5151
                                 800-221-7945
                                 Fax: 212-420-9314

Basic information on 123 drugs used for depression, anxiety and
bipolar illness.

2511 Everything You Need To Know About Depression
Rosen Publishing Group
29 E 21st Street
New York, NY 10010   212-777-3017
                                 800-237-9932
                                 Fax: 212-436-4643
                                 rosenpub@tribeca.ios.com
                                 www.rosenpublishing.com

An important resource for teens who are looking for help with depression.

Grades 7-12
ISBN: 0-823926-06-0

2512 Handbook of School-Based Interventions
Courage to Change
PO Box 1268
Newburgh, NY 12551   800-440-4003
                                 Fax: 800-772-6499

Comprehensive volume that describes interventions for virtually
every major problem behavior students may exhibit from K-12.
All interventions are research-based and guidance is given for
practical application of the techniques. Topics range from dishon-
esty, academic performance, procrastination and low self-esteem
to obsessive-compulsive behavior, substance abuse, AIDS and
depression.

512 pages Hardcover

2513 Help Me, I'm Sad
Penguin Putnam
PO Box 999
Bergenfield, NJ 07621   800-526-0275
                                 Fax: 800-227-9604

Helping and understanding a child with depression.

**2514 Helping Your Child Cope with Depression and Suicidal
Thoughts**
Jossey-Bass
111 River Street
Hoboken, NJ 07030   201-748-6000
                                 800-956-7739
                                 Fax: 201-748-6088
                                 www.josseybass.com

Shows parents how to learn to talk, listen, and communicate effectively with a depressed child; signs to watch for and situations which may cause a wish to commit suicide.

192 pages
ISBN: 0-787908-44-4

2515 Helping Your Depressed Child
Prima Publishing
PO Box 1260
Rocklin, CA 95677   916-624-5718

Reasuring guide to the causes and treatment of childhood and adolescent depression.

284 pages

2516 Kid Power Tactics for Dealing with Depression & Parent's Survival Guide
Childs Work/Childs Play
135 Dupont Street
Plainville, NY 11803   800-962-1141
                                        Fax: 800-262-1886
                                        info@Childswork.com
                                        www.Childswork.com

2 volume set was wriiten by a child who suffered from depression and his mother. Plain language and a wealth of information for children ages 8 and over, plus their parents and teachers.

2517 Mood Apart
Basic Books
10 E 53rd Street
New York, NY 10022   212-207-7057

An overview of depression and manic depression and the available treatments for them.

363 pages

2518 Overcoming Depression
Harper & Row
10 E 53rd Street
New York, NY 10022   212-207-7000

1987 318 pages Softcover

2519 Panic Disorder in the Medical Setting
Superintendent of Documents
PO Box 371954
Pittsburgh, PA 15250   202-512-2250

This book serves the primary care physicians as a helpful guide in recognizing and treating panic disorder in patients and in identifying those who need psychiatric consultation or referrals.

1993 135 pages

2520 Prozac Nation: Young & Depressed in America, A Memoir
Houghton Mifflin Company
222 Berkeley Street
Boston, MA 02116   617-351-3698
                                    800-225-3362

Struck with depression at 11, now 27, Wurtzel chronicles her struggle with the illness. Witty, terrifying and sometimes funny, it tells the story of a young life almost destroyed by depression.

317 pages

2521 Psychotherapy of Severe and Mild Depression
Jason Aronson
400 Keystone Industrial Park
Dunmore, PA 18521   800-782-0015
                                    Fax: 201-840-7242
                                    www.aronson.com

464 pages Softcover
ISBN: 1-568211-46-5

2522 Report of the Secretary's Task Force on Youth Suicide
Superintendent of Documents
PO Box 371954
Pittsburgh, PA 15250   202-512-2250

A comprehensive review of information about youth suicide. The task force recommendations are presented in Volume 1.

110 pages

2523 Sad Days, Glad Days
National Alliance for the Mentally Ill
PO Box 753
Waldorf, MD 20604   703-524-7600
                                     www.NIMF.org

Helps five to nine-year-olds understand a parent's depression.

1995

2524 Suicide, Why?
National Alliance for the Mentally Ill
PO Box 753
Waldorf, MD 20604   703-524-7600
                                     www.NAMI.org

An authoritative book, noting that suicide is usually caused by brain disorders.

1989

2525 Surprising Truth About Depression: Medical Breakthroughs That Can Work
Zondervan
5300 Patterson SE
Grand Rapids, MI 49530   616-698-6900
                                          Fax: 616-698-3439
                                          www.zondervan.com

1994 224 pages Softcover
ISBN: 0-310401-01-1

2526 Treating Depressed Children
New Harbinger Publications
5674 Shattuck Avenue
Oakland, CA 94609   800-748-6273
                                     Fax: 510-652-5472
                                     customerservice@newharbinger.com
                                     www.newharbinger.com

This book explains a 12-session treatment program to help children change their negative thoughts, gain confidence and recognize their emotions. These actions are achieved with the help of cartoons and role-playing games.

160 pages Hardcover
ISBN: 1-572240-61-X

Laseu Pfaff, Publicist

2527 Treating Depression
Jossey-Bass
111 River Street
Hoboken, NJ 07030   201-748-6000
                                     800-956-7739
                                     Fax: 201-748-6088
                                     www.josseybass.com

Offers guidelines and specific models for intervention in the treatment of numerous types and subtypes of depression. Also will assist you in deciding if it is appropriate to prescribe medication, if psychotherapy is the proper course of action, or if it is best to use a combination of medication and psychotherapy.

1997 223 pages
ISBN: 0-787915-85-8

2528 Understanding Depression
University Press of Mississippi
3825 Ridgewood Road
Jackson, MS 39211   601-432-6205
                                     800-737-7788
                                     Fax: 601-432-6217
                                     press@ihl.state.ms.us
                                     www.upress.state.ms.us

A clear explanation for those who know the illness personally and for those who want to understand them.

120 pages Hardcover/Ppbck
ISBN: 1-578061-68-7

2529 Understanding Your Teenager's Depression
Berkley Books
200 Madison Avenue
New York, NY 10016   212-951-8800

1994 352 pages Softcover
ISBN: 0-399518-56-8

2530 When Nothing Matters Anymore: A Survival Guide for Depressed Teens
Free Spirit Publishing
217 5th Avenue N
Minneapolis, MN 55401   612-338-2068
                                            800-735-7323
                                         Fax: 612-337-5050
                                    help4kids@freespirit.com
                                          www.freespirit.com

Written for teens with depression and those who feel despondent, dejected or alone. This powerful book offers help, hope, and potentially lifesaving facts and advice.

176 pages
ISBN: 1-575420-36-8

Penne Post, Tradesales Associate

2531 Working with Children and Adolescents in Groups
Courage to Change
PO Box 1268
Newburgh, NY 12551   800-440-4003
                                         Fax: 800-772-6499

Step-by-step guide that discusses how to effectively treat problem behavior in children and adolescents using small groups. Based on empirical research and their own work with groups, the authors show how a variety of approaches can be effectively combined to help resolve such problem behaviors as fighting and low self-esteem.

384 pages Hard Cover

2532 Yesterday's Tomorrow
Hazelden
15251 Pleasant Valley Road
Center City, MN 55012   612-257-4010
                                            800-328-9000
                                         Fax: 917-339-0325
                                          www.hazelden.org

A meditation book that shows why and how recovery works, from the author's own experiences.

432 pages Softcover
ISBN: 1-568381-60-3

Magazines

2533 EA Message
Emotions Anonymous
PO Box 4245
Saint Paul, MN 55104   651-647-9712
                                         Fax: 651-647-1593
                                 info@emotionsanonymous.org
                                    www.emotionsanonymous.org

Quarterly magazine.

Electronic

Karen Mead, Executive Director

Newsletters

2534 National Foundation for Depressive Illness
PO Box 2257
New York, NY 10116   212-268-4260
                                            800-248-4344
                                         Fax: 212-268-4434
                                          www.depression.org

Information on the myths and misconceptions surrounding the illness. Informs the public, health care providers, healthcare professionals and corporations about depression and manic depression, and provides the information about correct diagnosis and treatment and the availability of qualified doctors and support groups.

4 pages Quarterly

Amy C Russell, Editor

2535 Outreach
Depression and Bipolar Support Alliance
55 E. Jackson Blvd, Suite 490
Chicago, IL 60604   800-826-3632
                                         Fax: 312-642-7243
                                          www.dbsalliance.org

Quarterly publication serving members and constituents of the organization. National DMDA educates patients, families, professionals, and the public concerning the nature of depressive and manic-depressive illnesses as treatable medical diseases; fosters self-help for patients and families; eliminates discrimination and stigma; improves access to care; advocates for research toward the elimination of these illnesses.

Karen Kraft, Publications Manager

2536 Smooth Sailing
Depression & Related Affective Disorders Assoc.
Meyer 3-181, 600 N Wolfe Street
Baltimore, MD 21287   410-955-4647
                                         Fax: 410-614-3241
                                           drada@jhmi.edu
                                           www.drada.org

Contains a variety of information including medical, educational and first hand experiences about mood disorders. Newsletter is free with membership.

Quarterly

Pamphlets

2537 Depression Is a Treatable Illness: A Patients Guide
Department of Health & Human Services
2101 E Jefferson Street, Suite 501
Rockville, MD 20852   301-217-1245

Tells about major depressive disorder, which is only one form of depressive illness. This booklet answers important questions regarding this disorder and gives information on where to go for more help.

2538 Depression in Children and Adolescents: A Fact Sheet for Physicians
National Institute of Mental Health
6001 Executive Boulevard, Room 6200, MSC 9663
Bethesda, MD 20892   301-443-4536
                                            866-615-6464
                                         Fax: 301-443-4279
                                         TTY: 301-443-8431
                                         nimhinfo@nih.gov
                                          www.nimh.nih.gov

Discusses the scope of the problem and the screening tools used in evaluating children with depression.

8 pages

Dr. Francis S. Collins, Director

2539 Let's Talk About Depression
Superintendent of Documents
PO Box 371954
Pittsburgh, PA 15250   202-512-2250

Targeted especially for inner-city youth. The colorful design will capture attention and focus on depression in a way that young people will understand and identify with.

2540 Let's Talk Facts About Childhood Disorders
American Psychiatric Association
1400 K Street NW
Washington, DC 20005   202-682-6220

Offers information on depression and depressive disorders including the causes, symptoms, treatments, anxiety, and various other phobias.

2541 Living Without Depression & Manic Depression: A Workbook
National Alliance for the Mentally Ill
3803 N. Fairfax Drive, Suite 100
Arlington, VA 22203   703-524-7600
                                                          800-950-6264
                                                     Fax: 703-524-9094
                                                        info@nami.com
                                                         www.NAMI.org

Workbook offering checklists and helpful advice targeted for individuals whose depressive illness is stabilized.

1994

Jim Payne, J.D., President
Ralph E. Nelson, Jr., M.D., First Vice President
Marilyn Ricci, M.S., R.D., Second Vice President

2542 Major Depression in Children and Adolescents
Center for Mental Health Services
PO Box 42490
Washington, DC 20015   800-789-2647
                                                     Fax: 301-984-8796
                                                   ken@mentalhealth.org
                                                      mentalhealth.org

This fact sheet defines depression and its signs, identifies types of help available, and suggests what parents or other caregivers can do.

2 pages

2543 Now We Can Successfully Treat the Illness Called Depression
National Foundation for Depressive Illness (NAFDI)
PO Box 2257
New York, NY 10116   212-268-4260
                                                          800-248-4344
                                                     Fax: 212-268-4434
                                                     www.depression.org

Basic information on depression and manic depression, gives symptoms, encourages persons who have symptoms to seek medical treatment. Tips on managing depressive illness.

Amy C Russell, Editor

2544 Panic Disorder
National Institutes of Health
5600 Fishers Lane, Room 7C-02
Rockville, MD 20857   301-443-4707
                                                     Fax: 301-443-6000

Written for the lay public, this pamphlet contains a description of panic disorder, gives the symptoms, describes treatment methods, and encourages the person who has the symptoms to seek treatment.

2545 Plain Talk About Depression
Superintendent of Documents
PO Box 371954
Pittsburgh, PA 15250   202-512-2250

A flyer discussing types of depression, major depression; symptoms and causes.

2546 Understanding Panic Disorder
National Institutes of Health
5600 Fishers Lane, Room 7C-02
Rockville, MD 20857   301-443-4707
                                                     Fax: 301-443-6000

Offers information on what panic disorder is, symptoms, causes, treatment, medications and therapy.

2547 Useful Information on Phobias and Panic
Superintendent of Documents
PO Box 371954
Pittsburgh, PA 15250   202-512-2250

This booklet provides information on both phobias and panic. Symptoms, causes and treatments of these disorders are referred to. If you know someone who is excessively fearful, this booklet will be of great help to them in understanding their problem.

40 pages 50 copies

2548 What to Do When a Friend Is Depressed: Guide for Students
Superintendent of Documents
PO Box 371954
Pittsburgh, PA 15250   202-512-2250

Offers information on depression and its symptoms and suggests things a young person can do to guide a depressed friend in finding help.

DESCRIPTION

2549 DIABETES MELLITUS
Involves the following Biologic System(s):
Endocrinologic Disorders

Diabetes mellitis refers to an inability of the body to utilize glucose. There are two types of DM: Insulin-dependent diabetes mellitus, referred to as Type I diabetes, is a disorder in which insufficient production of insulin by the pancreas results in abnormally high levels of the sugar glucose in the blood. Insulin is a hormone that regulates and stabilizes blood glucose levels by promoting the movement of energy-rich glucose into body cells for energy production or into the liver and fat cells for storage. Type I diabetes may also cause impaired fat metabolism and long-term complications affecting certain large and small blood vessels (angiopathy), the nerve-rich membranes at the back of the eyes (retinas), skin, kidneys, nerves, or other tissues of the body. The exact cause of Type I diabetes is unknown. However, researchers speculate that certain environmental factors, such as a viral infection, may inappropriately trigger the immune system to destroy insulin-producing cells within the pancreas (beta cells), resulting in severe insulin deficiency. Genetic factors are also thought to play some role in causing a predisposition for the disorder.

Type I diabetes is the major form of diabetes affecting children. It affects 1 million patients in the United States, most often in young people, 10-14 years of age. The other major type of diabetes, Type II diabetes, may be characterized by a resistance to the effects of insulin. Although this type of diabetes may occur at any age, it most commonly becomes apparent in middle-aged or older people, but is increasingly common during childhood and adolescence. It is most common in obese patients. In some children, various forms of diabetes may occur secondary to certain genetic multisystemic disorders that affect the pancreas, such as cystic fibrosis; other endocrine disorders, such as Cushing's syndrome; the administration of particular drugs; or exposure to certain poisons.

In most children with Type I diabetes, associated symptoms and findings may appear to occur suddenly and may include excessive urine production by the kidneys, causing increased urination (polyuria) and excessive thirst (polydipsia); weight loss; and abnormally increased hunger (polyphagia). Additional abnormalities may include exhaustion, blurred vision, abnormal sensations (paresthesias) in the hands and feet, and increased irritability. Without prompt diagnosis and treatment, symptoms may rapidly progress to a metabolic condition known as ketoacidosis. Because of deficient insulin production, the body's cells begin to rely on sources of energy other than glucose, causing an excessive breakdown of fats and an abnormal accumulation of certain chemical compounds (ketones) in body tissues and fluids. Early symptoms associated with ketoacidosis may be relatively mild, including increased urination, vomiting and dehydration but, without appropriate treatment, coma and potentially life-threatening complications may occur. The treatment of ketoacidosis may include the immediate administration of intravenous fluids; replacement of electrolytes, such as sodium and potassium; initiation of intravenous insulin therapy; measures to prevent or appropriately treat increased fluid pressure within the brain; and other therapies as required.

Patients with either Type I or Type II diabetes may eventually develop certain long-term complications associated with the disease. Complications may include thickening and leaking of the walls of certain small blood vessels, narrowing of medium and large-size arteries due to plaque development (atherosclerosis), abnormally high blood pressure (hypertension), poor blood circulation, and problems affecting the eyes, kidneys, nerves, and skin. For example, kidney damage may result in impaired kidney function and kidney failure; damage to blood vessels within the nerve-rich membranes at the back of the eyes (diabetic retinopathy) may lead to visual impairment; and nerve damage may cause weakness or the loss of certain sensations, such as changes in temperature or pressure, increasing the risk of injury. In addition, impaired blood supply to certain skin areas may increase the risk of developing skin sores (ulcers). Poor wound healing and susceptibility to infected foot ulcers may lead to localized loss of tissue (necrosis), potentially requiring amputation. Diet is central to management of diabetes and must be individualized according to the patient's activity level, food preferences, and need to attain and maintain ideal weight. Regular exercise is also correlated with better glucose control. Individuals with Type I diabetes take insulin, delivered either by injection or by insulin pump. Type II diabetics can take oral blood-sugar lowering (hypoglycemic) drugs that potentiate insulin secretion. Other drugs help regulate glucose storage or release.

National Associations & Support Groups

2550 American Academy of Pediatrics
141 Northwest Point Boulevard
Elk Grove Village, IL 60007   847-434-4000
                                    800-433-9016
                               Fax: 847-434-8000
                                    www.aap.org

The American Academy of Pediatrics and its member pediatricians are committed to the attainment of optimal physical, mental and social health and well-being for all infants, children, adolescents, and young adults.

Fernando Stein, MD, FAAP, President
Karen Remley, MD, CEO/Executive VP

2551 American Association of Diabetes Educators
200 W Madison St, Suite 800
Chicago, IL 60606   312-424-2426
                                    800-338-3633
                               Fax: 312-424-2427
                                  aade@aadenet.org
                            www.diabeteseducator.org

Founded in 1973, AADE˜ is a multidisciplinary association of healthcare professionals dedicated to integrating self-management as a key outcome in the care of people with diabetes and related chronic conditions.

Donna Tomky, President
Tami Ross, Vice President
Cecilia Sauter, Treasurer

2552 American Autoimmune Related Diseases Association, Inc.
22100 Gratiot Avenue
Eastpointe, MI 48021   586-776-3900
                                    800-598-4668
                               Fax: 586-776-3903
                                   aarda@aarda.org
                                    www.aarda.org

The American Autoimmune Related Diseases Association is dedicated to the eradication of autoimmune diseases and the alleviation of suffering and the socioeconomic impact of autoimmunity through fostering and facilitating collaboration in the areas of education, public awareness, research, and patient services in an effective, ethical and efficient manner.

Virginia T. Ladd, President/Executive Director
Patricia Barber, Assistant Director
Deb Patrick, Events Specialist

2553 American Diabetes Association
1701 North Beauregard Street
Alexandria, VA 22311
703-549-1500
800-342-2383
Fax: 703-836-7439
askada@diabetes.org
www.diabetes.org

The nation's leading voluntary organization concerned with diabetes and its complications. The mission of the organization is to prevent and cure diabetes and to improve the lives of persons with diabetes. Offers a network of 52 affiliates with over 55,000 volunteers, including a professional membership of more than 10,000 physicians, social workers, nutritionists, educators and nurses.

Larry Hausner, MBA, Chief Executive Officer
Mary Vaneeda Bennett, Executive Vice President
Shereen Arent, EVP, Government Affairs & Advocacy

2554 Center for Disabilities and Development
University of Iowa Stead Family Children's Hospita
100 Hawkins Drive
Iowa City, IA 52242
319-353-6900
877-686-0031
Fax: 319-356-7700
cdd-webmaster@uiowa.edu
www.uiowa.edu

A trusted resource for healthcare, training, research and information for people with disabilities that include: behavior disorders, brain injury, cerebral palsy, diabetes, down syndrome, learning disabilities, mental retardation, sleep disorders and spina bifida.

Dianne McBrien, MD, Medical Director

2555 Juvenile Diabetes Foundation International
26 Broadway, 14th Floor
New York, NY 10004
212-785-9500
800-533-2873
Fax: 212-785-9595
info@jdrf.org
www.jdrf.org

Focuses energies on fund-raising, referrals, educational materials and information pertaining to juvenile diabetes.

Jeffrey Brewer, President & CEO
Frank Ingrassia, Chairman, Board of Directors
Mary Tyler Moore, International Chairman

2556 National Diabetes Action Network for the Blind
National Federation of the Blind
3101 NE 87th Avenue
Vancouver, WA 98662
360-576-5965
Fax: 410-685-5653
k7uij@panix.com
www.nfb.org.com

Leading support and information organization of persons losing vision due to diabetes. Provides personal contact and resource information with other blind diabetics about non-visual techniques of independently managing diabetes, monitoring glucose levels, measuring insulin and other matters concerning diabetes. Publishes Voice of the Diabetic, the leading publication about diabetes and blindness.

Michael Freeman, President

Libraries & Resource Centers

2557 National Diabetes Information Clearinghouse
1 Information Way
Bethesda, MD 20892
301-654-3327
800-860-8747
Fax: 703-738-4929
TTY: 866-569-1162
ndic@info.niddk.nih.gov
www.diabetes.niddk.nih.gov

Offers various materials, resources, books, pamphlets and more for persons and families in the area of diabetes.

Research Centers

2558 Center for the Partially Sighted
6101 W Centinela Ave, Suite 150
Culver City, CA 90230
310-988-1970
Fax: 310-458-8179
info@low-vision.org
www.low-vision.org

Provides professional, comprehensive vision rehabilitation services to visually impaired people of all ages. For those whose sight is severely limited due to macular degeneration, diabetic retinopathy, glaucoma, retinal detachment, stroke or other conditions not correctable medically or surgically.

Sidney Machtinger, Chairman
Linnae M Anderson, Secretary

2559 Joslin Diabetes Center
One Joslin Place
Boston, MA 02215
617-309-2400
800-567-5461
diabetes@joslin.harvard.edu
www.joslin.org

Joslin Diabetes Center, a teaching a research affiliate of Harvard Medical School, is a one-of-a-kind institution on the front lines of the world epidemic of diabetes - leading the battle to conquer diabetes in all of its forms through cutting-edge research and innovative approaches to clinical care and education.

John L Brooks III, President & CEO
Martin J Abrahamson, MD, Senior Vice President, Director
George L King, MD, SVP & Research Director

Audio Video

2560 Not So Sweet: Living With Diabetes
Fanlight Productions
32 Court Street, 21st Floor
Brooklyn, NY 11201
718-488-8900
800-876-1710
Fax: 718-488-8642
info@fanlight.com, orders@fanlight.com
www.fanlight.com

Exciting new approaches to the prevention and control of diabetes, and a look at its prevalence in Native American communities in particular.

47 minutes VHS

Web Sites

2561 Mediconsult
A13/5/5 One Ampang Business Avenue, Jalan Ampang U
Selangor, Ma
6- 3 -253
Fax: 6- 3 -253
info@mediconsult.com.my
www.mediconsult.com.my

We are committed to provide excellent and professional services to our business partners. Through a team approach we will develop, provide and continuously improve our knowledge and competency. We work towards the betterment of healthcare delivery systems for the community.

Sharif Lough Abdullah, Director
Dieter Nassler, Director
Nguyen Thi Dung, Director

2562 National Diabetes Information Clearinghouse
3 Information Way
Bethesda, MD 20892
800-891-5390
Fax: 703-738-4929
TTY: 866-569-1162
nkudic@info.niddk.nih.gov
www.kidney.niddk.nih.gov

The National Kidney and Urologic Diseases Information Clearinghouse is an information dissemination service of the National Institute of Diabetes and Digestive and Kidney Diseases.

Book Publishers

2563 Diabetes 101
Wiley
1 Wiley Drive
Somerset, NJ 08875
732-469-4400
800-225-5945
Fax: 732-302-2300
bookinfo@wiley.com
www.wiley.com

Revised and expanded second edition. A layman's guide to everything you need to know to live healthfully with diabetes.

175 pages
ISBN: 1-565610-24-5

2564 Diabetes Dictionary
National Diabetes Information Clearinghouse
2 Information Way
Bethesda, MD 20892
301-654-3810
Fax: 301-907-8906
nddic@info.niddk.nih.gov
www.niddk.nih.gov

Illustrated glossary of more than 300 diabetes-related terms.

2565 Diabetes Medical Nutition Therapy
American Diabetes Association
1701 North Beauregard Street
Alexandria, VA 22311
800-232-3472
Fax: 703-549-6995
www.diabetes.org

A professional guide to management and nutrition education resources. Provides in-depth coverage of nutrition assessment, goal setting, intervention, and outcome evaluation. Information is provided on specific resources and case studies are cited for practical examples.

2566 Diabetes Teaching Guide for People Who Use Insulin
Joslin Diabetes Center
1 Joslin Place
Boston, MA 02215
617-732-2400

Discusses the causes of diabetes, the role of diet and exercise, meal planning and complications. Also provides information on drawing blood, mixing and injecting insulin.

2567 Endocrine & Metabolic Disorders Sourcebook
Omnigraphics
PO Box 625
Holmes, PA 19043
800-234-1340
Fax: 800-875-1340
info@omnigraphics.com
www.omnigraphics.com

Basic information for the lay person about pancreatic and insulin-related disorders such as pancreatitis, diabetes and hypoglycemia; adrenal gland disorders such as Cushing's syndrome, Addison's disease and congenital adrenal hyperplasia; pituitary gland disorders such as growth hormone deficiency, acromegaly and pituitary tumors; and thyroid disorders such as hypothyroidism, Grave's disease, Hashimoto's disease and goiter.

574 pages
ISBN: 0-780802-07-1

2568 Even Little Kids Get Diabetes
Albert Whitman & Company
6340 Oakton Street
Morton Grove, IL 60053
847-531-0033
800-255-7675
Fax: 847-531-0039
www.albertwhitman.com

A preschooler tells how when she was only two, that she was diagnosed with this common disease and describes her daily treatment and the precautions her family must observe.

ISBN: 0-807521-58-2

Joseph Boyd, President
Joe Campbell, Customer Service

2569 Everyone Likes to Eat
Wiley
1 Wiley Drive
Somerset, NJ 08875
732-469-4400
800-225-5945
Fax: 732-302-2300
custserv@wiley.com
www.wiley.com

Revised and up-to-date second edition. How children can eat most of the foods they enjoy and still take care of their diabetes. Intended for elementary-school-age children, this guide is filled with activities, puzzles, and problem-solving exercises.

ISBN: 1-565610-26-1

2570 Grilled Cheese
American Diabetes Association
1701 North Beauregard Street
Alexandria, VA 22311
800-232-3472
Fax: 703-549-6995
www.diabetes.org

Story designed to ease children's fears and frustrations of having diabetes.

2571 If Your Child Has Diabetes: An Answer Book for Parents
Putnam Publishing Group
200 Madison Avenue
New York, NY 10016
212-951-8400

Provides information and recommendations for parents of children with diabetes on subjects such as school, recreation, medical and life insurance and employment as well as general information about diabetes.

2572 In Control: Guide for Teens with Diabetes
Wiley
1 Wiley Drive
Somerset, NJ 08875
732-469-4400
800-225-5945
Fax: 732-302-2300
custserv@wiley.com
www.wiley.com

Dispels myths and tackles the real issues that teens with diabetes face. Teaches how to care for their diabetes without letting it get in the way of their lives.

ISBN: 1-565610-61-X

Mari Baker, Former Chief Executive Officer
Jean-Lou Chameau, President

2573 Kiss the Candy Days Good-Bye
Delacorte Press
1540 Broadway
New York, NY 10036
212-354-6500

This book focuses on Jimmy who is surprised to learn he has diabetes after seeming so healthy and fit. The story contains information on symptoms and the dangers of untreated diabetes.

2574 Let's Talk About Diabetes
Rosen Publishing Group's PowerKids Press
29 E 21st Street
New York, NY 10010
212-777-3017
800-237-9932
Fax: 888-436-4643
rosenpub@tribeca.ios.com
www.powerkidspress.com

Defines diabetes and shows how a child can live a very normal life with the disease. Grades K-5.

24 pages
ISBN: 0-823951-96-0

2575 Life with Diabetes: A Series of Teaching Outlines
American Diabetes Association
1701 North Beauregard Street
Alexandria, VA 22311
800-342-2383
Fax: 703-549-6995
www.diabetes.org

Presents a comprehensive curriculum for diabetes education. Each outline includes a statement of purpose, pre-requisites for attending the session, materials needed for teaching the session, recommended teaching method, a content outline, instructor notes, and evaluation and documentation plan, and suggested readings related to each topic.

Larry Hausner, Chief Executive Officer
Shereen Arent, Executive Vice President

2576 Raising a Child with Diabetes: A Guide for Parents
American Diabetes Association
1701 North Beauregard Street
Alexandria, VA 22311
800-342-2383
Fax: 703-549-6995
www.diabetes.org

You'll learn how to help your child adjust to insulin, to allow for favorite foods, have a busy schedule and still feel healthy and strong, negotiate the twists and turns of being different, and much more.

Larry Hausner, Chief Executive Officer
Shereen Arent, Executive Vice President

Magazines

2577 Countdown
Juvenile Diabetes Foundation International
432 Park Avenue S
New York, NY 10016
212-889-7575
Fax: 212-532-7891

Offers the latest news and information in diabetes research and treatment to everyone from an international arena of diabetes investigators to parents of small children with diabetes, from physicians to school teachers, from pharmacists to corporate executives.

Sandy Dylak, Editor

2578 Diabetes Forecast
American Diabetes Association
1701 North Beauregard Street
Alexandria, VA 22311
800-342-2383
Fax: 703-549-6995
www.diabetes.org

The monthly lifestyle magazine for people with diabetes, featuring complete, in-depth coverage of all aspects of living with diabetes.

Janel Wright, JD, Chair, Anchorage,AK
David G. Marrero, PhD, President, Health Care
Suzanne Berry, MBA, CAE, Interim CEO

2579 Voice of the Diabetic
National Federation of the Blind
200 East Wells Street at Jernigan Place
Baltimore, MD 21230
410-659-9314
Fax: 410-685-5653
nfb@nfb.org
nfb.org/voice-diabetic

The leading publication in the diabetes field. Each issue addresses the problems and concerns of diabetes, with a special emphasis for those who have lost vision due to diabetes. Available in print and on cassette.

Journals

2580 Diabetes
American Diabetes Association
1701 North Beauregard Street
Alexandria, VA 22311
800-342-2383
Fax: 703-549-6995
www.diabetes.org

A peer-reviewed journal focusing on laboratory research.

Janel Wright, JD, Chair, Anchorage,AK
David G. Marrero, PhD, President, Health Care
Suzanne Berry, MBA, CAE, Interim CEO

2581 Diabetes Care
American Diabetes Association
1701 North Beauregard Street
Alexandria, VA 22311
800-342-2383
Fax: 703-549-6995
www.diabetes.org

A peer-reviewed journal emphasizing reviews, documentaries and original research on topics of interest to clinicians.

Janel Wright, JD, Chair, Anchorage,AK
David G. Marrero, PhD, President, Health Care
Suzanne Berry, MBA, CAE, Interim CEO

2582 Diabetes Spectrum: From Research to Practice
American Diabetes Association
1701 North Beauregard Street
Alexandria, VA 22311
800-342-2383
Fax: 703-549-6995
www.diabetes.org

A journal translating research into practice and focusing on diabetes education and counseling.

Janel Wright, JD, Chair, Anchorage,AK
David G. Marrero, PhD, President, Health Care
Suzanne Berry, MBA, CAE, Interim CEO

Newsletters

2583 Clinical Diabetes
American Diabetes Association
1701 North Beauregard Street
Alexandria, VA 22311
800-342-2383
Fax: 703-549-6995
www.diabetes.org

A bimonthly newsletter providing practical treatment information for primary care physicians.

Janel Wright, JD, Chair, Anchorage,AK
David G. Marrero, PhD, President, Health Care
Suzanne Berry, MBA, CAE, Interim CEO

2584 Diabetes Advisor
American Diabetes Association
1701 North Beauregard Street
Alexandria, VA 22311
800-342-2383
Fax: 703-549-6995
www.diabetes.org

Offers informative articles and research in the area of diabetes for professionals and patients. Offers facts and research on diagnosis, symptoms, technology and the newest devices for persons with diabetes, as well as referral and hotline numbers.

Janel Wright, JD, Chair, Anchorage,AK
David G. Marrero, PhD, President, Health Care
Suzanne Berry, MBA, CAE, Interim CEO

2585 Diabetes Dateline
National Diabetes Information Clearinghouse
9000 Rockville Pike
Bethesda, MD 20892
301-496-3583
Fax: 301-907-8906
nddic@info.niddk.nih.gov
www.niddk.nih.gov

Griffin P. Rodgers, MD, MACP, Director
Dr. Gregory Germino, Deputy Director
Kevin Abbott, Program Director

2586 Diabetes Educator
American Association of Diabetes Educators
444 N Michigan Avenue, Suite 1240
Chicago, IL 60611
312-424-2426
800-338-3633
Fax: 312-424-2427
www.aadenet.org

Offers information to health professionals working with persons
with diabetes.

James J Balija, Executive Director

2587 Kid's Corner
American Diabetes Association
1701 North Beauregard Street
Alexandria, VA 22311
800-342-2383
Fax: 703-549-6995
www.diabetes.org

A mini-magazine for kids that offers word searches, puzzles and
jokes-plus an encouraging story in each issue about kids with diabetes.

Janel Wright, JD, Chair, Anchorage,AK
David G. Marrero, PhD, President, Health Care
Suzanne Berry, MBA, CAE, Interim CEO

Pamphlets

2588 Children with Diabetes
9000 Rockville Pike
Bethesda, MD 20892
301-496-3583
Fax: 301-907-8906
nddic@info.niddk.nih.gov
www.niddk.nih.gov

Griffin P. Rodgers, MD, MACP, Director
Dr. Gregory Germino, Deputy Director
Kevin Abbott, Program Director

**2589 Complementary and Alternative Therapies for Diabetes
Treatment**
9000 Rockville Pike
Bethesda, MD 20892
301-496-3583
Fax: 301-907-8906
nddic@info.niddk.nih.gov
www.niddk.nih.gov

Griffin P. Rodgers, MD, MACP, Director
Dr. Gregory Germino, Deputy Director
Kevin Abbott, Program Director

2590 Diabetes Insipidus
9000 Rockville Pike
Bethesda, MD 20892
301-496-3583
Fax: 301-907-8906
nddic@info.niddk.nih.gov
www.niddk.nih.gov

Griffin P. Rodgers, MD, MACP, Director
Dr. Gregory Germino, Deputy Director
Kevin Abbott, Program Director

2591 Diabetes Overview
9000 Rockville Pike
Bethesda, MD 20892
301-496-3583
Fax: 301-907-8906
nddic@info.niddk.nih.gov
www.niddk.nih.gov

Griffin P. Rodgers, MD, MACP, Director
Dr. Gregory Germino, Deputy Director
Kevin Abbott, Program Director

2592 Diabetes in African Americans
9000 Rockville Pike
Bethesda, MD 20892
301-496-3583
Fax: 301-907-8906
nddic@info.niddk.nih.gov
www.niddk.nih.gov

Griffin P. Rodgers, MD, MACP, Director
Dr. Gregory Germino, Deputy Director
Kevin Abbott, Program Director

2593 Diabetes in Hispanic Americans
9000 Rockville Pike
Bethesda, MD 20892
301-496-3583
Fax: 301-907-8906
nddic@info.niddk.nih.gov
www.niddk.nih.gov

Griffin P. Rodgers, MD, MACP, Director
Dr. Gregory Germino, Deputy Director
Kevin Abbott, Program Director

2594 Diabetic Neuropathy: the Nerve Damage of Diabetes
9000 Rockville Pike
Bethesda, MD 20892
301-496-3583
Fax: 301-907-8906
nddic@info.niddk.nih.gov
www.niddk.nih.gov

Griffin P. Rodgers, MD, MACP, Director
Dr. Gregory Germino, Deputy Director
Kevin Abbott, Program Director

2595 Diabetics Control and Complications Trial
9000 Rockville Pike
Bethesda, MD 20892
301-496-3583
Fax: 301-907-8906
nddic@info.niddk.nih.gov
www.niddk.nih.gov

Griffin P. Rodgers, MD, MACP, Director
Dr. Gregory Germino, Deputy Director
Kevin Abbott, Program Director

2596 Financial Help for Diabetics Care
Information Clearinghouse
9000 Rockville Pike
Bethesda, MD 20892
301-496-3583
Fax: 301-907-8906
nddic@info.niddk.nih.gov
www.niddk.nih.gov

Griffin P. Rodgers, MD, MACP, Director
Dr. Gregory Germino, Deputy Director
Kevin Abbott, Program Director

2597 Gastoparesis in Diabetes
Information Clearinghouse
9000 Rockville Pike
Bethesda, MD 20892
301-496-3583
Fax: 301-907-8906
nddic@info.niddk.nih.gov
www.niddk.nih.gov

Griffin P. Rodgers, MD, MACP, Director
Dr. Gregory Germino, Deputy Director
Kevin Abbott, Program Director

2598 I Have Diabetes: How Much Should I Eat?
9000 Rockville Pike
Bethesda, MD 20892
301-496-3583
Fax: 301-907-8906
nddic@info.niddk.nih.gov
www.niddk.nih.gov

Griffin P. Rodgers, MD, MACP, Director
Dr. Gregory Germino, Deputy Director
Kevin Abbott, Program Director

2599 I Have Diabetes: What Should I Eat?
9000 Rockville Pike
Bethesda, MD 20892
301-496-3583
Fax: 301-907-8906
nddic@info.niddk.nih.gov
www.niddk.nih.gov

Griffin P. Rodgers, MD, MACP, Director
Dr. Gregory Germino, Deputy Director
Kevin Abbott, Program Director

2600 I Have Diabetes: When Should I Eat?
9000 Rockville Pike
Bethesda, MD 20892

301-496-3583
Fax: 301-907-8906
nddic@info.niddk.nih.gov
www.niddk.nih.gov

Griffin P. Rodgers, MD, MACP, Director
Dr. Gregory Germino, Deputy Director
Kevin Abbott, Program Director

2601 Kidney Disease of Diabetes
Information Clearinghouse
9000 Rockville Pike
Bethesda, MD 20892

301-496-3583
Fax: 301-907-8906
ndoc@info.niddk.nih.gov
www.niddk.nih.gov

Griffin P. Rodgers, MD, MACP, Director
Dr. Gregory Germino, Deputy Director
Kevin Abbott, Program Director

Camps

2602 American Diabetes Association
Center for Information, 1701 North Beauregard
Alexandria, VA 22311

800-342-2383
askada@diabetes.org
www.diabetes.org

The American Diabetes Association provides research, and provides information and advocacy for people with diabetes and their families. The Asssociation also provides seminars for health care professionals.

Lynne Perry

2603 Camp Discovery American Diabetes Association
1168 K-157 Highway
Junction City, KS 66441

316-684-6091
Fax: 316-941-5699
lgiles@diabetes.org
www.diabetes.org

Offers young people with diabetes a week of fun at rock springs 4-H Center. Special attention to diabetes makes Camp Discovery a safe environment for active youth while providing valuable diabetes management education. Call the American Diabetes Association-Kansas area office for more information.

Lindsay Giles, District Manager

2604 Camp Hodia
1701 N 12th St
Boise, ID 83702

208-891-1023
Fax: 208-454-2841
matt@hodia.org
www.hodia.org

Camp for children with Type 1 Diabetes. Campers learn self care, good nutrition and blood-sugar control.

Don Scott, Director

2605 Camp Joslin
The Barton Center for Diabetes Education, Inc.
150 Richardson Corner Road
Charlton, MA 01507

507-987-2056
Fax: 508-987-2002
info@bartoncenter.org
www.joslin.org

Camp Joslin's programs combine camping, sports and fun with diabetes education and support to give children with diabetes, and their families, the tools they need to live happy, healthy, balanced lives.

Michael Kasparian, Camp Director
Sarah Gorman, Camp Coordinator

2606 Camp Kudzu
5885 Glenridge Drive, Suite 160
Atlanta, GA 30328

404-250-1811
Fax: 404-250-1812
info@campkudzu.org
www.campkudzu.org

Provides education, recreation and peer-networking for Georgia's children with Type 1 Diabetes.

2607 Camp Kushtaka
801 W. Fireweed Lane, Suite 103
Anchorage, AK 99503

907-272-1428
888-342-2383
skamahele@diabetes.org
http://www.childrenwithdiabetes.com/camps/

Camp for children with diabetes and, space permitting, their siblings.

2608 Camp de los Ninos - Diabetes Society
1165 Lincoln Avenue, Ste 300
San Jose, CA 95125

408-287-3785
800-800-989
Fax: 408-287-2701
campt@diabetessociety.org
www.childrenwithdiabetes.com/camps

Since 1974, the Diabetes Society of Santa Clara Valley has sponsored Camp de los Ninos, a resident camp for children 6 through 14. This camp provides an opportunity for children with diabetes to go to camp, meet other children and gain a better understanding of their diabetes. The total experience can help campers develop more confidence in their abilities to control their diabetes effectively while enjoying the traditional camp experience.

Sharon Ogbor, Executive Director

2609 Clara Barton Camp
PO Box 356
North Oxford, MA

508-987-2056
Fax: 508-987-2002
bcdecamp@aol.com
www.bartoncenter.org

Girls, ages 6-17, with diabetes participate in a well-rounded camp program with special education in diabetes, health and safety. Activities include swimming, boating, sports, dance, music and arts and crafts. Two week adventure camp for high school girls offering camping, hiking, canoeing, etc. Also a minicamp (one week) for girls 6-12. Day camps are offered in Worcester, Boston and New York City.

Brooke Beverly, Resident Camp Director
Kerry Packard, Day Camp Director
Beth Sayers, Adventure Camp Director

2610 Des Moines YMCA Camp
1192 166th Drive
Boone, IA 50036

515-432-7558
Fax: 515-432-5414
ycamp@dmymca.org
www.y-camp.org

For boys and girls with cancer, diabetes, asthma, cystic fibrosis, hearing impaired and other disabilities.

David Sherry, Executive Director

2611 EDI
1020 Madison 9570
Fredericktown, MO 63645

chartmann@diabetes.org
www.diabetes.org

Youngsters with diabetes learn how to care for themselves while participating in a wide variety of outdoor activities and trips. The camp, managed and financed by the American Diabetes Association Greater St. Louis Affiliate, offers camperships to children from the Greater St. Louis area, ages 7-16, but nonresidents may also apply.

Fred Schaljo

2612 Easter Seal Kysoc
9810 Bluegrass Pkwy
Louisville, KY 40299   502-584-9781
                                    Fax: 502-732-0783
                                    ek1@cardinalhill.org
                                    www.cardinalhill.org

Designed for the fullest camping experience for children or adults
with physical disabilities, blind, deaf, behavior disorders, mental
retardation, diabetes and multiple handicaps, ages 7 and up.

Heide Miller, CCD, CTRS, Director

2613 Florida Camp for Children and Youth
1701 SW 16th Ave
Gainesville, FL 32608   352-334-1321
                                    Fax: 352-334-1326
                                    fccyd@floridadiabetescamp.org

An adventure camp for children and youth with diabetes.

Rhonda Rogers

2614 Floyd Rogers
PO Box 31536
Omaha, NE 68131   402-341-0866
                                    www.campfloydrogers.com

A camp for diabetic children, ages 8 to 18

Sherman Poska

2615 Hickory Hill
PO Box 1942
Columbia, MO 65205   573-698-2510
                                    camphickoryhill@gmail.com
                                    www.camphicoryhill.com

Educates diabetic children concerning diabetes and its care. In addition to daily educational sessions on some aspects of diabetes,
campers participate in swimming, sailing, arts and crafts and
overnight camping.

William Mees

2616 John Warvel
American Diabetes Association
Camp Crosley YMCA, 165 EMS T2 Land
North Webster, IN 46555   317-352-9226
                                    Fax: 317-913-1592
                                    bookorders@diabetes.org

Provides an enjoyable, safe and educational out-of-doors experience for children with insulin-dependent diabetes. A unique
learning atmosphere for children to acquire new skills in caring
for their disease. The camp experience instills confidence for the
child's self-management of diabetes. Offers one-week sessions
and can accommodate 200 campers.

Carol Helming, Executive Director

2617 Makemie Woods Camp Conference Center
PO Box 39
Barhamsville, VA 23011   757-566-1496
                                         800-566-1496
                                    Fax: 757-566-8003
                                    www.makwoods.org

Counselors serve as teachers, friends and activity leaders. The individual is important within the small group. No camper is lost in
the crowd, but is an integral partner in the group process. Residential Christian Camp and conference center. Summer camp for
children 8-18 special camp for children with diabetes.

Michelle Burcher, Director

2618 Sweeney
PO Box 918
Gainesville, TX 76241   940-665-2011
                                    Fax: 940-665-9467
                                    info@campsweeney.org
                                    www.campsweeney.org

Teaches self-care and self-reliance to children with diabetes.
Campers participate in such activities as swimming, fishing,
horseback riding, arts and crafts while learning about diabetes
and how to cope with it.

DESCRIPTION

2619 DIGEORGE SYNDROME

Synonyms: DiGeorge sequence, Thymic agenesis immunodeficiency

Involves the following Biologic System(s):

Genetic/Chromosomal/Syndrome/Metabolic Disorders, Immunologic and Rheumatologic Disorders

DiGeorge syndrome is a disorder present at birth (congenital) that is characterized by some combination of absence (aplasia) or underdevelopment (hypoplasia) of the thymus gland and the parathyroid glands, malformations of the heart and its major blood vessels (cardiovascular abnormalities), and characteristic malformations of the head and facial (craniofacial) area. Due to absence or underdevelopment of the thymus gland, affected children may have abnormalities of the immune system, causing impaired resistance to certain infections. DiGeorge syndrome occurs as the result of abnormal development of certain embryonic structures (third and fourth pharyngeal pouches) that later develop into the thymus and parathyroid glands. In some cases, other embryonic structures that are forming during the same approximate period may also be affected, resulting in certain cardiovascular, craniofacial, or other malformations. The thymus, a lymphoid tissue organ located in the upper portion of the chest, plays an essential role in the immune system beginning at approximately the 12th week of fetal development and lasts until puberty. It serves as a source of certain white blood cells (lymphocytes) before birth and then promotes the development of certain specialized lymphocytes, known as T lymphocytes, through secretion of particular hormones (e.g., thymosin). The actions of the T lymphocytes help to defend the body against certain microorganisms (i.e., cell-mediated immunity). The parathyroid glands, which are two pairs of small glands on the sides of the thyroid gland, produce parathyroid hormone, which helps to maintain normal levels of calcium in the blood.

DiGeorge syndrome usually occurs randomly and is caused by spontaneous, minute deletions of material from the long arm of chromosome 22 (22q11.2). DiGeorge syndrome may also occur in association with certain chromosomal abnormalities (e.g., chromosome 10, monosomy 10p; chromosome 22, monosomy 22q). In addition, there have been some cases in which DiGeorge syndrome affected individuals within certain families (kindreds) yet did not appear to result from known chromosome syndromes. In some familial cases, DiGeorge syndrome may have autosomal dominant inheritance. The disorder is thought to affect approximately one in 20,000 newborns.

In infants and children with DiGeorge syndrome, associated symptoms and findings may be extremely variable. Patients who have absence or severe underdevelopment of the thymus gland are prone to frequent infections from fungi, viruses, and certain bacteria (such as Pneumocystis jiroveci, previously knowns as Pneumocystis carinii). These patients often experience chronic inflammation of the mucous membranes of the nose (rhinitis), recurrent inflammation of the lungs (pneumonia), fungal infection of the mucous membranes of the mouth (oral candidiasis), recurrent diarrhea, or systemic infections in which invading microorganisms or their toxins are present inthe blood circulation (septicemia). In some cases of serious infection, life-threatening complications may result. Infants and children with mild underdevelopment (hypoplasia) of the thymus are said to have partial DiGeorge syndrome and may have little difficulty with recurring infections. Because of absence or underdevelopment of the parathyroid glands (hypoparathyroidism), many affected infants experience certain symptoms and findings during the first days of life, including abnormally low calcium levels in the blood (hypocalcemia) and muscle twitching, tremors and cramps, (neonatal tetany) and even seizures. Such symptoms and findings can be treated with calcium supplementation and are usually temporary but may recur later in life.

Some newborns with DiGeorge syndrome may also have defects of the heart and its great arteries. Some of these may be simple defects while others may be more complex, such as interrupted aortic arch, ventricular septal defects, and tetralogy of Fallot.

Infants with DiGeorge syndrome may have an unusually narrow or blind-ending esophagus (esophageal atresia) that does not form a passageway into the stomach. In addition, affected newborns may have characteristic malformations of the head and facial (craniofacial) area, such as widely spaced eyes (ocular hypertelorism); downwardly slanting eyelid folds (palpebral fissures); a small mouth; an unusually short, vertical groove in the center of the upper lip (philtrum); and low-set, notched ears. Some patients may also have mild to moderate mental retardation.

The treatment of infants and children with DiGeorge syndrome is symptomatic and supportive. Treatment measures may include the administration of calcium in those with hypoparathyroidism and hypocalcemia, therapies to help prevent and aggressively treat infections (e.g., antiviral, antifungal, and antibiotic agents) in patients with immunodeficiency, medical and surgical measures for cardiovascular malformations, or other measures as required. If patients with immunodeficiency require blood transfusions, donor blood must be exposed to high levels of radiation (irradiated) to kill the donor lymphocytes and thus prevent the occurrence of graft-versus-host disease, a serious disease caused by an immune response of donor cells against the recipient's tissues.

National Associations & Support Groups

2620 22Q and You Center
34th Street and Civic Center Boulevard
Philadelphia, PA 19104

215-590-1000
Fax: 215-590-3298
lunny@email.chop.edu
www.chop.edu/service/22q-and-you-center/home.html

Services offered by the Department of Clinical Genetics in the Children's Hospital of Philadelphia, include literature, support groups and referrals.

Beverly Emmanuel, Chief, Human Genetics
Elaine Zackai, MD, Director, Clinical Genetics
Donna McDonald-McGinn, Program Director

2621 American Academy of Pediatrics
141 Northwest Point Boulevard
Elk Grove Village, IL 60007

847-434-4000
800-433-9016
Fax: 847-434-8000
www.aap.org

The American Academy of Pediatrics and its member pediatricians are committed to the attainment of optimal physical, mental and social health and well-being for all infants, children, adolescents, and young adults.

Fernando Stein, MD, FAAP, President
Karen Remley, MD, CEO/Executive VP

2622 Genetic Alliance
4301 Connecticut Avenue NW, Suite 404
Washington, DC 20008
202-966-5557
800-336-4363
Fax: 202-966-8553
info@geneticalliance.org
www.geneticalliance.org

A coalition of voluntary genetic support groups, consumers and professionals addressing the needs of individuals and families affected by genetic disorders from a national perspective.

Sharon Terry, President/CEO
Tetyana Murza, Managing Director
Natasha Bonhomme, VP, Strategic Development

2623 Immune Deficiency Foundation
40 W Chesapeake Avenue, Suite 308
Towson, MD 21204
410-321-6647
800-296-4433
Fax: 410-321-9165
IDF@primaryimmune.org
www.primaryimmune.org

The only national charitable organization aimed at fighting the primary immune deficiency diseases. The founders included parents of children with primary immune deficiency, immunologists who treat immune deficient patients and other individuals with an interest in helping others. The Foundation's main goal is to improve the care and treatment of adults and children with primary immune deficiency diseases and to promote public education and awareness about the diseases.

Marcia Boyle, CEO
Barbara Ballard, Secretary
John Boyle, Chair

2624 March of Dimes Foundation
1275 Mamaroneck Avenue
White Plains, NY 10605
914-997-4488
888-663-4637
Fax: 914-997-4763
TDD: 914-997-4764
answers@marchofdimes.com
www.marchofdimes.com

A national not-for-profit organization that was established in 1938. The mission of the Foundation is to improve the health of babies by preventing birth defects and infant mortality.

Stacey D. Stewart, President

Conferences

2625 Genetic Alliance Annual Conference
Genetic Alliance
4301 Connecticut Avenue NW, Suite 404
Washington, DC 20008
202-966-5557
800-336-4363
Fax: 202-966-8553
info@geneticalliance.org
www.geneticalliance.org

Consistently inspirational and enables partnership among all stakeholders: advocates and community leaders, health and industry professionals, policymakers, and academicians.

July

Sharon Terry, President/CEO
Tetyana Murza, Managing Director
Natasha Bonhomme, VP, Strategic Development

2626 Immune Deficiency Foundation National Conference
Meetings Manager
40 W Chesapeake Avenue, Suite 308
Towson, MD 21204
410-321-6647
800-296-4433
Fax: 410-321-9165
info@primaryimmune.org
www.primaryimmune.org

Annual conference hosted by an organization aimed at fighting the primary immune deficiency diseases. The founders included parents of children with primary immune deficiency, immunologists who treat immune deficient patients and other individuals with an interest in helping others. The Foundation's main goal is to improve the care and treatment of adults and children with primary immune deficiency diseases and to promote public education and awareness about the diseases.

June

John Seymour, Chairman
Robert LeBien, Vice Chairman
Steve Fietek, Founder/Secretary

Web Sites

2627 International Patient Organization for Primary Immunodeficiencies
Av. Aida, Bloco 8, escritório 821
Estoril, 2765-
35- 21-407
info@ipopi.org
ipopi.org

IPOPI is an international organization whose members are national patient organizations for the primary immunodeficiencies (PID's). It was formed to benefit and serve its members and patients with expertise and resources and influence of members in order to achieve worlwide improvement in the care and treatment of patients with PID's.

Jose Drabwell, Chairman
Martine Pergent, Vice Chairman
Johan Prevot, Executive Director

2628 Jeffrey Modell Foundation
www.jmfworld.com

The foundation is dedicated to the early and precise diagnosis, meaningful treatment, and ultimate cure of Primary Immunodeficiencies.

2629 Kansas University Medical Center
www.kumc.edu/gec/support/velo.html
dcollins@kumc.edu
www.kumc.edu/gec/support/velo.html

Offers information for genetic professionals, information on genetic conditions and support groups, and genetic educational information.

Debra Collins, MS, CGC, Genetic Counselor

2630 Online Mendelian Inheritance in Man
U.S. National Library of Medicine, 8600 Rockville
Bethesda, MD 20894
888-346-3656
info@ncbi.nlm.nih.gov
www.ncbi.nlm.nih.gov

This database is a catalog of human genes and genetic disorders.

Christine E. Seidman, M.D., Chair
David J. Lipman, M.D., Executive Secretary
Michael Boehnke, Ph.D., Board Member

Book Publishers

2631 Let's Talk About Going to the Hospital
Rosen Publishing Group's PowerKids Press
29 E 21st Street
New York, NY 10010

212-777-3017
800-237-9932
Fax: 888-436-4643
rosenpub@tribeca.ios.com
www.powerkidspress.com

If a child has to check into the hospital, chances are he or she is already upset about being ill. Knowing how a hospital functions and what the procedures are, such as when family members can visit, will help in what is already a stressful situation. Grades K-5.

24 pages
ISBN: 0-823950-36-0

DESCRIPTION

2632 DOWN SYNDROME

Synonyms: Chromosome 21, trisomy 21, Trisomy 21 syndrome

Covers these related disorders: Trisomy 21 mosaicism, Trisomy 21 translocation

Involves the following Biologic System(s):
Genetic/Chromosomal/Syndrome/Metabolic Disorders

Down syndrome, also known as trisomy 21, is a chromosomal disorder that affects approximately one in 660 newborns, making it the most common genetic syndrome. Cells of the body (with the exception of reproductive cells) typically contain 23 pairs of chromosomes that are numbered from 1 to 22. The 23rd pair consists of one X chromosome from the mother and an X or Y chromosome from the father. However, in infants with Down syndrome, all or a portion of chromosome 21 is present three times rather than twice in cells of the body (trisomy). In rare cases, a certain percentage of cells contain the extra chromosome 21, whereas other cells have the normal two. This finding is known as chromosomal mosaicism.

The symptoms and physical findings associated with Down syndrome vary in range and severity and depend in part on the exact location and the percentage of body cells containing the extra chromosome 21.

Down syndrome is usually the result of errors during the division of a parent's reproductive cells. Increased maternal age (over 35) presents additional risk. The disorder may also result due to a chromosome 21 translocation that is transmitted by a parent or occurs sporadically. Translocations are chromosomal abnormalities in which pieces of two or more chromosomes break off and are rearranged, resulting in an altered set of chromosomes.

Many infants with Down syndrome have abnormally diminished muscle tone (hypotonia), a tendency to keep the mouth open, protrusion of the tongue, excessive mobility of the joints, absence of certain reflexes, and excessive skin on the back of the neck. Other abnormalities may include a small, short head, flattened facial features, upwardly slanting eyelid folds, vertical skin folds over the eyes' inner corners, a highly arched roof of the mouth, a small nose and depressed nasal bridge, and small, misshapen ears. Abnormalities of the limbs may also be present, including unusually short arms and legs; short, broad hands; improper positioning of the fifth fingers (clinodactyly); abnormal skin ridge patterns on the fingers, hands, toes, and feet (dermatoglyphics); and a wide gap between the first and second toes. Infants with Down syndrome have an increased frequency of intestinal narrowing or obstruction (atresia) at birth. Patients also tend to have relatively short stature, progressive delays in the acquisition of skills requiring the coordination of physical and mental activities (psychomotor delays), poor coordination, an awkward manner of walking (gait), and varying levels of mental retardation.

Approximately 40 percent of infants with Down syndrome have heart defects at birth (congenital heart defects). In some patients, such heart defects may require surgical repair. In addition, some individuals with Down syndrome are prone to recurrent respiratory infections and chronic inflammation of the membranes that line the eyes and eyelids (conjunctivitis) or the nasal cavity (rhinitis). Treatment of individuals with Down syndrome includes symptomatic and supportive measures, such as possible surgical correction of congenital heart defects, and special education.

Government Agencies

2633 NIH/ Eunice Kennedy Shriver National Insti tute of Child Health & Human Development
31 Center Drive, Building 31
Bethesda, MD 20892
301-496-5113
800-370-2943
Fax: 866-760-5947
nichdpress@mail.nih.gov
www.nichd.nih.gov

Established in 1962 by congress, today the institute conducts and supports research on topics related to the health of children, adults, families and populations. Some of these topics include: developmental disabilities, growth and development, infant death, reproductive health and birth defects.

Diana W. Bianchi, Director
Paul Williams, Director, Communications

National Associations & Support Groups

2634 ARC of the United States
1825 K Street, NW, Suite 1200
Washington, DC 20006
202-534-3700
800-433-5255
Fax: 202-534-3731
info@thearc.org
www.thearc.org

The ARC of the United States advocates for the rights and full participation of all children and adults with intellectual and developmental disabilities. Together with our network of members and affiliated chapters, we improve systems of supports and services; connect families; inspire communities an influence public policy.

Mohan Mehra, President
Nancy Webster, Vice President
Michael Mack, Secretary

2635 Aleh Foundation
Aleh Institutions USA
PO Box 4911
New York, NY 10185
866-717-0252
Fax: 212-517-3293
dov@aleh-israel.org
www.aleh.org

The Aleh Rehabilitation Center in Bnei Break has served as a residential facility to close to 200 children with multiple, physical and mental disabilities. These children and their families have benefitted from our wide range of services in an atmosphere of warmth and love.

Yehuda Marmorstein, Executive Director
Shlomit Grayevsky, Director, Aleh Jerusalem Center

2636 American Academy of Pediatrics
141 Northwest Point Boulevard
Elk Grove Village, IL 60007
847-434-4000
800-433-9016
Fax: 847-434-8000
www.aap.org

The American Academy of Pediatrics and its member pediatricians are committed to the attainment of optimal physical, mental and social health and well-being for all infants, children, adolescents, and young adults.

Fernando Stein, MD, FAAP, President
Karen Remley, MD, CEO/Executive VP

2637 American Association for Pediatric Opthalmology and Strabismus
655 Beach Street
San Francisco, CA 94109
415-561-8505
Fax: 415-561-8531
aapos@aao.org
www.aapos.org

AAPOS is the American Association for Pediatric Ophthalmology and Strabismus. The organization's goals are to advance the quality of children's eye care, support the training of pediatric ophthalmologists, support research activities in pediatric ophthalmology, and advance the care of adults with strabismus.

Jennifer Hull, Client Services Manager
Brooke Lyon, Client Services Coordinator
Maria A. Schweers, CO, Scientific Program Coordinator

2638 American School Counselor Association
1101 King Street, Suite 310
Alexandria, VA 22314
703-683-2722
800-306-4722
Fax: 703-997-7572
asca@schoolcounselor.org
www.schoolcounselor.org

The mission of ASCA is to represent professional school counselors and to promote professionalism and ethical practices.

Richard Wong, Executive Director
Jeff Broderson, Information Technology Admin.
Kathleen M Rakestraw, Director of Communications

2639 Arc of Montgomery County
11600 Nebel Street
Rockville, MD 20852
301-984-5777
Fax: 301-816-2429
info@arcmontmd.org
www.arcmontmd.org

Aims to provide support, advocacy and choices for people who have mental retardation and related developmental disabilities and their families.

Joyce Taylor, Executive Director
Clyde Agnew, Jr., Director, Human Resources

2640 Association for Children with Down Syndrome
4 Fern Place
Plainview, NY 11803
516-933-4700
Fax: 516-933-9524
information@acds.org
www.acds.org

Dedicated to providing lifetime resources of exceptional quality, innovation and inclusion for individuals with Down syndrome and other developmental disabilities and their families.

Michael Smith, Executive Director
Jane Shimkin, Educational Coordinator
Judith Anderson, Director of Student Services

2641 Birth Defects Research for Children
976 Lake Baldwin Lane, Suite 104
Orlando, FL 38214
407-895-0802
staff@birthdefects.org
www.birthdefects.org

An organization that provides parents and expectant parents with information about birth defects and support services for their children. BDRC has a parent-matching program that links families who have children with similar birth defects.

Betty Mekdeci, Executive Director

2642 Center for Disabilities and Development
University of Iowa Stead Family Children's Hospita
100 Hawkins Drive
Iowa City, IA 52242
319-353-6900
888-573-5437
Fax: 319-356-7700
cdd-webmaster@uiowa.edu
www.uichildrens.org

A trusted resource for healthcare, training, research and information for people with disabilities that include: behavior disorders, brain injury, cerebral palsy, diabetes, down syndrome, learning disabilities, mental retardation, sleep disorders and spina bifida.

Dianne McBrien, MD, Medical Director

2643 Down Syndrome Affiliates in Action
5010 Fountainblue Drive
Bismarck, ND 58503
701-425-7129
info@dsaia.org
www.dsaia.org

To support and advance the growth and service capabilities of the local and regional Down syndrome organizations we serve, to be the conduit of value-driven training, programs, best practices and support for our members.

Sterling Lynk, President
Amy Van Bergen, Vice President
Deanna Tharpe, Executive Director

2644 Down Syndrome Community
www.downsyndromecommunity.org
206-257-7191
contact@downsyndromecommunity.org
www.downsyndromecommunity.org

The Down Syndrome Community is a registered 501(c)(3) organization whose mission is to improve the lives of individuals with Down syndrome and their families by focusing on education, communication, and advocacy.

Linda Michael, Co-Chair
Lynne Palmisano, Co-Chair
Sean King, President

2645 Down Syndrome Guild of Greater Kansas City
10200 W 75th Street, Suite 281
Shawnee Mission, KS 66204
913-384-4848
Fax: 913-384-4949
info@kcdsg.org
www.kcdsg.org

Provides new baby/parent hospital visits, monthly newsletter, support and encouragement for individuals with Down Syndrome and their families. Bi-lingual group. Job coaching scholarships.

Amy Allison, Executive Director

2646 Down Syndrome Information Alliance
5098 Foothills Boulevard, Suite 3, #464
Roseville, CA 95747
916-658-1686
Fax: 916-914-1875
info@downsyndromeinfo.org
downsyndromeinfo.org

The Down Syndrome Information Alliance provides support and resources to empower individuals with Down syndrome, their families, and our community.

Heather Green, President
Jaoanna Heichlinger, Secretary
Trevor Stapleton, Treasurer

2647 Genetic Alliance
4301 Connecticut Avenue NW, Suite 404
Washington, DC 20008
202-966-5557
800-336-4363
Fax: 202-966-8553
info@geneticalliance.org
www.geneticalliance.org

A coalition of voluntary genetic support groups, consumers and professionals addressing the needs of individuals and families affected by genetic disorders from a national perspective.

Sharon Terry, President/CEO
Tetyana Murza, Managing Director
Natasha Bonhomme, VP, Strategic Development

2648 Global Down Syndrome Foundation
3300 East First Ave., Suite 390
Denver, CO 80206
303-321-6277
info@globaldownsyndrome.org
www.globaldownsyndrome.org

The Global Down Syndrome Foundation is dedicated to significantly improving the lives of people with Down syndrome through Research, Medical Care, Education and Advocacy.

Michelle Sie Whitten, President
David Charmatz, Senior Vice President
Martha Cronen, Project Manager

2649 International Mosaic Down Syndrome Association
PO Box 354
Trenton, OH 45067
513-988-6817
888-MDS-LINK
Fax: 775-295-9373
JACKSONC@HSC.VCU.EDU
www.imdsa.org

IMDSA is designed to support any family or individual whose life has been touched by mosaic Down syndrome by continuously pursuing research opportunities and increasing awareness in the medical, educational and public communities throughout the world

Brandy Hellard, President
Dr. Colleen Jackson-Cook, Member, Advisory Board
Lauren Vanner-Nicely,MS, Member, Advisory Board

2650 March of Dimes Foundation
1275 Mamaroneck Avenue
White Plains, NY 10605
914-997-4488
888-663-4637
Fax: 914-997-4763
answers@marchofdimes.com
www.marchofdimes.com

Partnership of volunteers and professionals dedicated to improving the health of babies by preventing birth defects and infant mortality. Over 100 chapters are located across the country and can be located through the National Office.

Stacey D. Stewart, President

2651 National Association for Child Development
549 25th Street
Ogden, UT 84401
801-621-8606
Fax: 801-621-8389
prachi@nacd.org
downsyndrome.nacd.org/index.php

NACD has created an approach to human development, the achievement of human potential, and the remediation of developmental, educational, and neurological problems that is based upon the gestalt of the individual.

Robert J. Doman Jr., Founder and Director
Laird Doman, COO/ Family Liaison
Julian Neil, Dir. Of Health

2652 National Association for Down Syndrome (NADS)
PO Box 206
Wilmette, IL 60091
630-325-9112
info@nads.org
www.nads.org

Established by parents of children with Down syndrome who felt a need to create a better environment and bring about understanding and acceptance of people with Down syndrome.

Jackie Rotondi, President
Patrick Crawford, First Vice President
Michael Walther, Treasurer

2653 National Dissemination Center for Children with Disabilities
1825 Connecticut Avenue, Suite 700
Washington, DC 20009
202-884-8200
800-695-0285
Fax: 202-884-8441
TTY: 800-695-0285
nichcy@aed.org
www.nichcy.org

A national information and referral center that provides information on disabilities and disability-related issues for families, educators and other professionals.

Suzanne Ripley, Executive Director

2654 National Down Syndrome Adoption Network
4623 Wesley Avenue, Suite A
Cincinnati, OH 45212
513-213-9615
www.ndsan.org

The mission of the NDSAN is to ensure that every child with Down syndrome has the opportunity to grow up in a loving family.

2655 National Down Syndrome Coalition
P.O. Box 725
Roseville, CA 95661
916-532-4773
Fax: 916-663-1151
heather@ndscoalition.org
ndscoalition.org

The mission is to demonstrate to society the positive impacts of Down syndrome with various forms of media, parent support groups, parent counseling, provision of resources, community outreach, and with the education and training of parents and professionals.

Heather M. Haskin, President / CEO

2656 National Down Syndrome Congress
1370 Center Drive, Suite 102
Atlanta, GA 30338
770-604-9500
800-232-6372
Fax: 770-604-9898
info@ndsccenter.org
www.ndsccenter.org

It is the mission of the National Down Syndrome Congress to be the national advocacy organization for Down syndrome and to provide leadership in all areas of concern related to persons with Down syndrome. In that capacity, NDSC will function as a major source of support and empowerment to persons with down syndrome and their families.

David Tolleson, Executive Director
Sue Joe, Resource Specialist
Betty Totten, Office Manager

2657 National Down Syndrome Society
666 Broadway, 8th Floor
New York, NY 10012
800-221-4602
Fax: 212-979-2873
info@ndss.org
www.ndss.org

The mission is to be the national advocate for the value, acceptance and inclusion of people with Down Syndrome. The NDSS envisions a world in which people with Down Syndrome have the opportunity to enhance their quality of life, realize their life aspirations, and become valued members of welcoming communities.

Jon Colman, President

2658 National Down Syndrome Society Hotline
666 Broadway, 8th Floor
New York, NY 10012
212-460-9330
800-221-4602
Fax: 212-979-2873
info@ndss.org
www.ndss.org

800-221-4602. Through its toll-free helpline and e-mail service, NDSS receives more than 32,000 requests a year for information on Down Syndrome. The professionally staffed Goodwin Family Information and Referral Center responds to questions from parents, professionals, self-advocates, and other interested individuals. Hours: 9 a.m to 5 p.m. EST, Monday thru Friday, in over 150 languages.

Jon Colman, President

2659 National Early Childhood Technical Assistance System
University of North Carolina, Chapel Hill
Campus Box 8040, UNC-CH
Chapel Hill, NC 27599
919-962-2001
Fax: 919-966-7463
TDD: 919-843-3269
nectac@unc.edu
www.nectac.org

Supports the national implementation of the early childhood provisions of the Individuals with Disabilities Education Act (IDEA). The mission is to strengthen systems at all levels to ensure that children (birth through five) with disabilities and their families receive and benefit from high quality, culturally appropriate and family centered supports and services.

Lynne Kahn, Director & Principal Investigator
Joan Danaher, Associate Director
Joicey Hurth, Associate Director Technical Assist

State Agencies & Support Groups

California

2660 Down Syndrome Association of Los Angeles
16461 Sherman Way, Suite 180
Van Nuys, CA 91406
818-786-0001
Fax: 818-786-0004
info@dsala.org
www.dsala.org

Offers information on Down syndrome, counseling, resources, facts, laws and other forms of information.

Gail Williamson, Executive Director
Jim Hodgson, Senior Director

Colorado

2661 Mile High Down Syndrome Association
3515 South Tamarac Drive, Suite 320
Denver, CO 80237
303-756-6144
Fax: 303-756-6144
info@mhdsa.org
www.mhdsa.org

Serves families of children and adults with Down syndrome, and interested professionals in the Mountain States region. Provides education, resources and support in partnership with individuals, families, professionals, and the community.

Mac Macsovits, Executive Director
Laurie Herrera, Family/Outreach Programs Director

Connecticut

2662 Connecticut Down Syndrome Congress
C/O: A.J. Pappanikou, University of Connecticut
200 Research Parkway
Meriden, CT 06450
860-563-9114
888-486-8537
manager@ctdownsyndrome.org
www.ctdownsyndrome.org/

Established as a special interest group to advocate for persons with Down syndrome in the State of Connecticut. The mission is to advocate for the realization and enhancement of the full spectrum of human and civil rights for persons with Down syndrome, gather and disseminate accurate information regarding Down syndrome, provide support to families of children with Down syndrome, and to encourage quality services for persons with Down syndrome.

Walter Glomb, President
Karen Zbierski, Executive VP
Chris McAuliffe, Secretary/Director

Florida

2663 Gold Coast Down Syndrome Organization
2255 Glades Road, 342W
Boca Raton, FL 33431
561-912-1231
Fax: 561-912-1232
gcdso@bellsouth.net
www.goldcoastdownsyndrome.com

Gold Coast Down Syndrome Organization is a private, nonprofit corporation dedicated to making the future brighter for people with Down syndrome in Palm Beach County, Florida.

Terri Harmon, Executive Director

2664 Goodwill Industries-Suncoast
10596 Gandy Boulevard
St. Petersburg, FL 33702
727-523-1512
888-279-1988
Fax: 727-563-9300
TDD: 727-579-1068
gw.marketing@goodwill-suncoast.com
www.goodwill-suncoast.org

Nonprofit organization that helps people achieve their full potential through the dignity and power of work. The agency offers a variety of employment and training services to promote self-sufficiency, and contribute to community conservation through recycling.

Lee Waits, President
R Lee Waits, President/CEO

Georgia

2665 Down Syndrome Association of Atlanta
2221 Peachtree Road NE,Ste 226
Atlanta, GA 30339
404-320-3233
Fax: 404-228-7475
contactus@atlantadsaa.org
www.atlantadsaa.org

A source of information and support to families, as well as working to promote public awareness and encouraging a better understanding of Down syndrome and individuals with Down syndrome.

Michelle Norweck, Executive Director

Hawaii

2666 Hawaii Down Syndrome Congress
419 Keoniana Street, Suite 804
Honolulu, HI 96815
808-949-1999
Conkay@AOL.com
www.hawaiidownsyndrome.com

An organization of families and professionals concerned with all aspects of Down Syndrome. We provide outreach to parents of newborns to foster fellowship and social interaction, educational opportunities and resources, public relation activities to inform the general public about Down syndrome, monthly meetings that provide emotional and psychological support, and serve as activists and advocates on behalf of children with special needs.

Connie Smith, President

Indiana

2667 Down Syndrome Association of NWI
2927 Jewett Avenue
Highland, IN 46322
219-838-3656
Fax: 219-838-6959
dsa@dsaofnwi.org
www.dsaofnwi.org

Provides informational and emotional support to parents who have a child, adolescent, or adult family member with special needs. Program offers an important connection for a parent who is seeking support for a special disability issue, by matching him or her with a trained veteran parent.

Christine Gill, President
Randy Sassano, Vice President
Dawn Weiler, Treasurer

2668 Down Syndrome Support Association of Southern Indiana (DSSASI)
1939 State Street
New Albany, IN 47150
812-725-1416
support@dssasi.org
www.dssasi.org

Provides informational and emotional support to parents who have a child, adolescent, or adult family member with special needs. Program offers an important connection for a parent who is seeking support for a special disability issue, by matching him or her with a trained veteran parent.

Kelley Jacquay, President
Michelle Engle, Vice President
Gina DeWilde, Treasurer

Maryland

2669 Parents of Children with Down Syndrome Arc of Montgomery County
PO Box 10416
Rockville, MD 20849

301-916-4985
Fax: 301-816-2429
firemom31@yahoo.com
www.downsyndromehelp.boomja.com

Aims to provide support, advocacy and choices for people who have mental retardation and related developmental disabilities and their families.

Peter Holden, Executive Director
John Slavcoff, President

Massachusetts

2670 Massachusetts Down Syndrome Congress (MDSC)
20 Burlington Mall Road, Ste 261
Burlington, MA 01803

781-221-0024
800-664-6372
Fax: 781-221-0011
mdsc@mdsc.org
www.mdsc.org

An all-volunteer, non-profit organization made up of parents, professionals and anyone interested in gaining a better understanding of Down syndrome. The mission is to enhance on a continuous basis the lives of individuals with Down syndrome through the education and support of people with Down syndrome, their families, their friends, their teachers, and the community as a whole. To ensure individuals are valued, included, and live fulfilling lives in the community.

Suzanne Boudrot Shea, President
Jonathan Fee, Vice President
Leo Hogan, Secretary

Minnesota

2671 Down Syndrome Association of Minnesota
656 Transfer Road
St. Paul, MN 55114

651-603-0720
800-511-3696
dsamn@dsamn.com
www.dsamn.org

A nonprofit organization composed of some 3,000 members; more than 900 people with Down syndrome, their families and friends, plus health-care, education and developmental professionals. We are the only organization in our region devoted exclusively to the needs of people with Down syndrome and their families.

Kathleen Forney, Executive Director
Connie Gunderson Warner, Program Coordinator
Jim Belka, Resource Coordinator

New York

2672 Center for Family Support
2811 Zulette Avenue
Bronx, NY 10461

718-518-1500
Fax: 718-518-8200
www.cfsny.org

The Center for Family Support (CFS) is a not-for-profit human service agency providing support and assistance to individuals with developmental disabilities and traumatic brain injuries throughout New York City, Long Island, the lower Hudson Valley region and New Jersey.

Steven Vernikoff, Executive Director

Ohio

2673 Miami Valley Downs Syndrome Association
1133 Edwin C Moses Boulevard, Suite 190
Dayton, OH 45408

937-222-0744
Fax: 937-222-0396
www.mvdsa.org

Informational and emotional support to parents who have a child, adolescent, or adult family member with special needs.

Tennessee

2674 Down Syndrome Association of Middle Tennessee
111 N Wilson Boulevard
Nashville, TN 37205

615-386-9002
Fax: 615-386-9754
dsamt@bellsouth.net
www.dsamt.org

A nonprofit organization that is affiliated with the National Down Syndrome Society and the National Down Syndrome Congress. DSAMT works closely with The Arc of Tennessee and other disability organizations locally and throughout the state to provide support for individuals with Down syndrome.

Sheila Moore, Executive Director

Texas

2675 Down Syndrome Guild of Dallas
701 N Central Expressway, Building I
Richardson, TX 75080

214-267-1374
dsged@sbcglobal.net
www.downsyndromedallas.org

Aims to impact the community so that everyone will acknowledge the inherent dignity and abilities of people with Down syndrome with full participation in society.

Becky Slakman, Executive Director
Kelly Drablos, Vice President
Minnie Blackwell, Membership Committee Chairperson

2676 Texas Association on Mental Retardation
PO Box 28076
Austin, TX 78755

512-349-7470
Fax: 512-349-2117
pat.holder@tamr-web.com

An organization made up of professionals, parents, consumers and advocates. The goal is to create an accessible system of services and resources which support personal choice and promotes lives of dignity and self-determination. An Annual Convention is a forum for sharing ideas and research, offering opportunities for exchanging information, and developing an understanding for other perspectives.

Pat Holder, Executive Director
Robert Welsh, President
Kimberly Littlejohn, President-Elect

Research Centers

Alabama

2677 Down Syndrome Clinic, Children's Hospital of Alabama
1600 7th Avenue S
Birmingham, AL 35233

205-368-9585
Fax: 205-975-6330
www.childrensal.org

Dr. Diane K Donley

California

2678 Children's Hospital & Research Center of Oakland
747 52nd Street
Oakland, CA 94609   510-428-3259
                                       www.childrenshospitaloakland.org

Scientific research is an important part of the work that goes on at Children's Hospital & Research Center Oakland. Researchers are making significant progress in such areas as diagnosing and treating pediatric cancers, sickle cell disease, AIDS and HIV, hemophilia, cystic fibrosis, developing prenatal techniques for diagnosing mental retardation and birth defects, and improving infant nutrition.

Kevan McCarten-Gibbs, Senior VP/Chief Medical Officer
Nancy Shibata, RN, Nursing VP
Donald Livsey, VP/Chief Information Officer

2679 Pediatric Disabilities Clinic, Down Syndrome Clinic
University of California Medical Center
400 Parnassus, Box 0374
San Francisco, CA 94143   415-476-3276
                                                 www.ucsfhealth.org
Dorothy Pang

Georgia

2680 Pediatric Neurodevelopmental Center at Marcus Institute
Marcus Institute
1920 Briarcliff Road
Atlanta, GA 30329   404-419-5300
                                            Fax: 404-419-5410
                                                 ccoles@emory.edu
                                                 www.marcus.org

Provides an array of evaluation and treatment services for individuals from infancy through adolescence. As well as providing individual evaluations, we feature a number of unique multispecialty programs. Once a child is evaluated, the proper course of treatment and/or therapy can be determined. The evaluation may result in a recommendation for further treatment at the Marcus Institute, or may involve other programs and services in the child's community.

Howard S Schub, MD, Medical Director

Illinois

2681 Adult Down Syndrome Center of Lutheran General Hospital
1999 Dempster Street
Park Ridge, IL 60068   847-318-2303
                                            Fax: 847-318-2377
                                                 www.advocatehealth.com

A comprehensive medical resource providing multidisciplinary medical and psychosocial care for adults with Down syndrome, with an emphasis on health promotion.

Brian Chicoine, MD, Medical Director
Jenny Lobough-Howard, Outreach Specialist
Ann Jonaitis, Resource Coordinator

2682 Advocate Lutheran General Children's Hospital, Pediatric Research
1775 Dempster Street
Park Ridge, IL 60068   847-318-9330
                                       denise.angst@advocatehealth.com
                                                 www.advocatehealth.com

An organization of physicians and health care professionals dedicated to serving the health needs of individuals, families and communities in Northern Illinois. Ongoing research on Pediatric disorders are being conducted and finding new procedures and medicines.

Marissa Lowenthal, Medical Director
Denise B Angst, DNSc, Research Director
Sandy Maki, MAT; CCRP, Research Operations Manager

2683 LaRabida Children's Hospital, Down Syndrome Clinic
E 65th Street @ Lake Michigan
Chicago, IL 60649   773-753-8646
                                            Fax: 773-363-7160
                                                 info@larabida.org
                                                 www.larabida.org

Recognized as a leader in the diagnosis and treatment of children with developmental disabilities and delays. La Rabida provides comprehensive care and services for children with Down syndrome. The Down syndrome program at La Rabida is designed to provide medical and developmental evaluations and be a resource for both parents and pediatricians caring for children with this chronic condition.

Paula Jaudas, Executive Director

Indiana

2684 Ann Whitehill Down Syndrome Program
Riley Hospital for Children
702 Barnhill Drive
Indianapolis, IN 46202   317-274-4846
                                            Fax: 317-274-4471
                                                 www.rileychildrenshospital.com

Brings together specialists from many areas to address the medical and psychosocial needs of children with Down Syndrome. A developmental pediatrician, pediatric nurse practitioner, pediatric social worker, pediatric occupational therapist, physical therapist and certified speech pathologist work closely with the primary care physician to help each child achieve his or her optimal potential. We also refer the family to local resources for therapy and developmental programs.

Marilyn Bell, MD

Maryland

2685 Behavioral and Developmental Pediatrics Division, University of Maryland
22 S Greene Street
Baltimore, MD 21201   410-328-2214
                                                 800-492-5538
                                            Fax: 410-328-3981
                                                 www.umm.edu

Offers comprehensive consultation, evaluation and treatment for children, birth to age 21, with developmental and behavioral problems.

Linda Grossman, MD, Associate Professor

2686 Kennedy Krieger Institute, Down Syndrome Clinic
1750 E Fairmount Avenue
Baltimore, MD 21231   443-923-9140
                                            Fax: 410-550-9292
                                                 koller@kennedykrieger.org
                                                 www.kennedykrieger.org/

Develop and conduct clinical research studies into the neurobiologic basis of cognitive impairment and co-morbid psychiatric disorders in Down syndrome; to study potential therapies for safety and efficacy; and to investigate genetic and environmental factors relevant to AV Canal defect.

George Capone, Director
Char Koller, Research Contact

Massachusetts

2687 Down Syndrome Program, Children's Hospital Boston
300 Longwood Avenue
Boston, MA 02115   617-355-6000
                                            Fax: 617-735-7429
                                            TTY: 617-730-0152
                                       CROCKER_A@A1.TCH.Harvard.edu
                                                 www.childrenshospital.org/

Medical and developmental monitoring for children from birth to 3 years of age. Evaluations are provided every 4 to 6 months by an interdisciplinary team comprised of a developmental pediatrician, physical therapist, nutritionist, audiologist, speech pathologist, and social worker. Individual support is available for families, along with information, referral, and case management assistance.

Dr. Allen Crocker, Director

Minnesota

2688 Down Syndrome Clinic of Minneapolis Children's Medical Center
2525 Chicago Avenue
Minneapolis, MN 55404

612-813-7800
Fax: 612-813-6100
dmcconn606@aol.com

Mission of the clinic is to improve the quality of life for children and adolescents with Down syndrome and to help them reach their full potentials. A multi-disciplinary team of professionals provide care to the children and adolescents who come to the clinic. Because of the full spectrum of services available, the program can provide consultation for specific medical and developmental problems, developmental assessments, management of behavioral difficulties, and family support.

Dr. Kim McConnell, Director
Mary Bergs, Social Worker

Missouri

2689 Children's Mercy Hospital, Down Syndrome Clinic
2401 Gillham Road
Kansas City, MO 64108

816-234-3041
Fax: 816-842-6107
webmaster@cmh.edu
www.childrens-mercy.org

Medical staff of nearly 600 pediatric specialists with a comprehensive range of programs and services, representing more than 40 pediatric specialities.

Erica Molitor-Kirsch, Executive Medical Director/SVP
Barbara Mueth, Community Relations VP
Davoren Tempel, Resource Development VP

2690 Down's Syndrome Medical Clinic
Washington University Medical Center
400 S Kingshighway Boulevard
Saint Louis, MO 63110

314-454-5437
800-678-5437
www.stlouischildrens.org

Dr. Arnold Strauss

New Hampshire

2691 Medical Genetics Clinic
Dartmouth-Hitchcock Medical Center
1 Medical Center Drive
Lebanon, NH 03756

603-653-6044
Fax: 603-650-8268
www.dhmc.org

Provides specialty consultations for diagnosis and treatment of suspected inherited conditions or syndromes.

John Moeschler, MD, Program Director
Mary Beth Dinulos, MD, Medical Geneticist
Susan Berg, MS, Genetic Counselor

New York

2692 Child Development Clinical Services
Westchester Institute for Human Development
Cedarwood Hallÿ
Valhalla, NY 10595

914-285-8178
Fax: 914-285-1973
info@WIHD.org
www.wihd.org

Diagnostic evaluation and treatment services are provided for children with developmental concerns, communication disorders, attention deficit disorders (including ADHD) and learning disabilities, as well as cerebral palsy and other neuromotor disorders, spina bifida, mental retardation, and autism.

Mark Bertin, MD, Director
Karen Edwards, MD, Pediatrics Director

2693 Institute for Basic Research in Developmental Disabilities
1050 Forest Hill Road
Staten Island, NY 10314

718-494-0600
Fax: 718-698-3803
ÿibr@opwdd.ny.gov
www.omr.state.ny.us

Research arm of the New York State Office of Mental Retardation and Developmental Disabilities (OMRDD). IBR conducts basic and clinical research into the causes, treatment, and prevention of mental retardation and other developmental disabilities. It also provides specialized biomedical, psychological, and laboratory services to individuals with developmental disabilities and their families, and educates the public and professionals regarding the causes, diagnosis, prevention, and treatment.

W Ted Brown, Manager

North Dakota

2694 Children's Hospital Merit Care Down Syndrome Service
737 Broadway
Fargo, ND 58102

701-234-2568
Fax: 701-234-6965

Dr. Guy Carter

Ohio

2695 Down Syndrome Clinic, Rainbow Babies and Children's Hospital
11100 Euclid Avenue
Cleveland, OH 44106

216-844-8447
888-844-844
Fax: 216-844-8444
www.uhhospitals.org/rainbow

Dr. Joanne Mortimer

2696 Jane and Richard Thomas Center for Down Syndrome
Cincinnati Children's Hospital Medical Center
3430 Burnet Avenue
Cincinnati, OH 45229

513-636-4561
800-344-2462
Fax: 513-636-7173
development@cchmc.org
www.cincinnatichildrens.org

Conducts research and offers interdisciplinary evaluations and intervention for infants, children, adolescents and young adults with Down syndrome. By providing a range of comprehensive services within one center, families can now spend less time pursuing services through multiple agencies and professionals.

Susan E. Wiley, MD, Co-Director

2697 Pediatric Clinical Trials International
10 Winthrop Square, Fifth Floor
Boston, MA 02110

617-948-5100
866-219-3440
Fax: 617-948-5101
marketing@centerwatch.com
www.centerwatch.com/

Consists of inpatient and outpatient capabilities. The inpatient facility includes research beds, a psychophysiological recording and observation/recording center. The latter, located on the neuromonitoring unit, consists of a subject testing room equipped with video cameras and psychological recording systems, and the second is the monitoring room equipped with computer programming and audio-video monitoring, etc.

Daniel R Boue, Medical Director
John P Niles, CEO
Karen Miller, RN, Affiliate Operations Manager

Pennsylvania

2698 Children's Hospital of Pittsburgh General Clinical Research Center
401 Penn Avenue
Pittsburgh, PA 15224
412-692-6438
Fax: 412-692-5723
linda.cherok@chp.edu
www.chp.edu/research

Established to increase medical knowledge about childhood diseases and to improve the management and treatment of these diseases. Participation is of great importance and value to medical research. We have a dedicated staff of physicians, nurses and health care professionals experienced in health care delivery and research who will ensure your comfort and safety as you participate in medical studies.

Pamela Murray, Program Director
Diane E Cline, Administrative Manager

2699 Children's Seashore House
Children's Hospital in Philadelphia
3405 Civic Center Boulevard
Philadelphia, PA 19104
215-590-1734
rac@email.chop.edu
www.chop.edu

Leading research institution quickly bringing scientific discoveries into the clinical setting and community to improve care. Some current research studies include: cognitive studies of the development of mathematical competence in normal children and in those with congenital defects, studies of language development in children with inherited syndromes, and development of novel strategies to prevent violence in the school setting.

Marc Yudkoff, MD, Division Chief
Nathan Blum, MD, Behavioral Pediatrics

2700 Dr. Gertrude A. Barber National Institute
100 Barber Place
Erie, PA 16507
814-45-766
Fax: 814-455-1132
BNIerie@barberinstitute.org
www.barbercenter.org

Committed to remaining on the cutting-edge of breakthrough technologies and practices. We seek out research opportunities that will enhance our services and will provide the most current proven information to present to the public.

John J Barber, President
Maureen Barber-Carey, Executive VP
Karen Hahn Berry, RN, Health Services Director

2701 International Foundation for Genetic Research/Michael Fund
4371 Northern Pike
Pittsburgh, PA 15146
412-374-0111
www.michaelfund.org

Research is directed toward preventing and treating the harmful consequences of the extra chromosome in Down's Syndrome. Also; dedicated to reversing this destructive universal trend by opening up new doors of therapy in the field of mental retardation associated with chromomal disorders such as Down Syndrome and continuing the curative research program.

Dr. Paddy Jim Baggot, Executive Director

Rhode Island

2702 Children's Neurodevelopment Center at Hasbro Children's Hospital
Rhode Island Hospital
593 Eddy Street
Providence, RI 02903
401-444-4000
Fax: 401-444-6115
sigpueschel@aol.com
www.lifespan.org/hch/services/

A site for the evaluation and treatment of children with neurological, genetic, developmental, metabolic and behavioral disorders.

Lee V Wesner, Director

Texas

2703 Down Syndrome Specialty Clinic
Children's Medical Center
1935 Medical District Dr.
Dallas, TX 75235
214-456-6388
Fax: 214-456-2567
www.childrens.com

Comprehensive care for children with Down syndrome and their families including; medical management, genetic counseling, speech and oral motor developmental evaluation and recommendations, psychosocial support, screening and referral for behavioral or psychiatric problems, and referrals to community agencies for educational intervention or therapies.

Mary Esther Carlin MD, Clinical Medical Doctor
Joanna Spahis, RN, Clinical Nurse Specialist

Washington

2704 University of Washington: Experimental Education Unit
University of Washington
Columbia Road, Gate #6
Seattle, WA 98195
206-543-2100
www.depts.washington.edu/

Provide clinical services to children and their families, and conduct interdisciplinary research.

Rick Neel, Director
Kate Ahern, Admissions Coordinator

Wisconsin

2705 Center for the Study of Bioethics
Medical College of Wisconsin
8701 Watertown Plank Road
Milwaukee, WI 53226
414-527-8191
centerbioethics@mcw.edu
www.mcw.edu/bioethics

Center for the Study of Bioethics is a leader in the field of bioethics. The Center has conscientiously served the functions of a typical institution of higher learning; research, education, and service.

Robyn S Shapiro, Director
Kristen Tym, Assistant Director

Conferences

2706 ARC Annual National Convention
The ARC
1825 K Street NW, Suite 1200
Washington, DC 20006
202-534-3700
800-433-5255
Fax: 202-534-3731
info@thearc.org
www.thearc.org

Held in cities throughout the U.S. each fall which attracts nearly 1000 people for educational sessions, business meetings and social events.

Nancy Webster, President
Ronald Brown, Vice President
Elise McMillan, Secretary

2707 Genetic Alliance Annual Conference
Genetic Alliance
4301 Connecticut Avenue NW, Suite 404
Washington, DC 20008
202-966-5557
800-336-4363
Fax: 202-966-8553
info@geneticalliance.org
www.geneticalliance.org

Consistently inspirational and enables partnership among all stakeholders: advocates and community leaders, health and industry professionals, policymakers, and academicians.

July

Sharon Terry, President/CEO
Tetyana Murza, Managing Director
Natasha Bonhomme, VP, Strategic Development

2708 NDSC Annual Convention
National Down Syndrome Congress
30 Mansel Court,Suite 108
Roswell, GA 30076

770-604-9500
800-232-6372
Fax: 770-604-9898
info@ndsccenter.org
www.ndsccenter.org

offers parents and professionals an opportunity to learn from the best speakers from around the world and share experiences with one another.

August

David Tolleson, Executive Director
Sue Joe, Resource Specialist
Betty Totten, Office Manager

2709 National Down Syndrome Society Annual National Conference
666 Broadway,8th Floor
New York, NY 10012

212-763-4365
800-221-4602
jnfo@ndss.org
www.ndss.org

The focus is on working together to improve the lives of individuals with Down syndrome, enabling them to enjoy the benefits of, and contribute to, their communities.

Jennifer Falik, Special Events Director
Elizabeth F Goodwin, Founder

Audio Video

2710 A Promising Future Together
National Down Syndrome Society
666 Broadway, 8th Floor
New York, NY 10012

800-221-4602
Fax: 212-979-2873
info@ndss.org
www.ndss.org

A guide for new and expectant parents; available in video or print.

52 pages

CAPT Robert P. Taishoff USN (ret), Chairman
Stephen Beck, Jr., Vice Chairman
Sara Weir, President

2711 A Special Love
Association for Children with Down Syndrome
2616 Martin Avenue
Bellmore, NY 11710

516-221-4700
Fax: 516-221-4311

A candid video of a ten-year-old brother playing with his six-year-old sister with Down Syndrome. The brother describes his perceptions of mental retardation and his feelings towards his sister.

4 minutes, b/w

DB Shalom, Editor

2712 Boy in the World
Fanlight Productions
32 Court Street, 21st Floor
Brooklyn, NY 11201

718-488-8900
800-876-1710
Fax: 718-488-8642
info@fanlight.com, orders@fanlight.com
www.fanlight.com

Following four-year-old Ronen, a young boy with down syndrome, this intimate documentary concretely demonstrates that inclusive preschool classrooms benefit both children with special needs and their typical peers. It examines the nuts and bolts of successful inclusion as well as the challenges of educationsl practices that help all children to learn - and find their place in the world. ISBN: DVD: 1-57295-944-4; VHS: 1-57295-488-4

44 minutes DVD of VHS

2713 Congratulations? An Introduction to Down Syndrome for Parents/Family/Friends
New Challenges
96 Ogden Avenue
White Plains, NY 10605

914-287-0723

A film for parents which addresses some of the most commonly asked questions about raising a child with Down syndrome.

57 mins.

2714 Daddy's Girl
Carle Media
110 W Main Street
Urbana, IL 61801

217-384-4838

Dina Lev, a 12-year-old actress with Down syndrome, portrays Nancy, a girl trying to deal with her divorced father's inability to accept the fact that his daughter has Down syndrome.

28 mins.

Bruce Postman, Producer
Regina Conroy, Writer/Director

2715 Educating Peter
State of the Art Production
2470 Fox Hill Road
State College, PA 16803

814-355-8004
800-458-3401
Fax: 814-355-2714
sales@resistor.com, marketing@resistor.c
www.resistor.com

Thought-provoking film follows a child with Down syndrome through a year of inclusion in a public school in Mrs. Stallings' third grade class. The film raises many questions about inclusion by honestly presenting the reactions to, and methods of, dealing with Peter's behavior problems.

30 Minutes

Thomas C Goodwin, Producer/Director
Gerardine Wurzburg, Producer/Director

2716 Infant Motor Development: A Look at the Phases
Therapy Skill Builders
San Antonio, TX 78283

732-441-0404

Shows normal infant motor development from birth to 12 months. Identifies components of movement and specific skills that are acquired during 4 phases of motor development: infantile, preparation, modification, and refinement. Transitional movement patte rns and their relationship to skill acquisition are also described.

20 Minutes

Kerry Goudy, Producer
Joan Winger, Producer

2717 New Expectations
Altschul Group Corporation
1560 Sherman Avenue, Suite 100
Evanston, IL 60201

800-421-2363
agcmedia@starnetinc.com

Focuses on the emotional and technical aspects of Down syndrome. Highlights four persons at various life stages from infancy to adulthood in the areas of education and employment.

Web Sites

2718 ARC of the United States
1825 K Street, NW, Suite 1200
Washington, DC 20006

202-534-3700
800-433-5255
Fax: 202-534-3731
tnguyen@thearc.org
www.thearc.org

The ARC is the national organization of and for people with mental retardation and related developmental disabilities and their families. Devoted to promoting and improving supports and services for people with mental retardation and their families. The association also fosters research and education regarding the prevention of mental retardation in infants and young children. The ARC was founded in 1950 by a small group of parents and other concerned individuals.

Ronald Brown, President
Elise McMillan, Vice President
Peter V. Berns, CEO

2719   Aleh Foundation
PO Box 4911
New York, NY 10185

866-717-0252
Fax: 212-517-3293
dov@aleh-israel.org
www.aleh.org

Aleh is a nonprofit organization that believes that every child, no matter how severe his/her disability, has potential. We are committed to providing severely disabled children through Israel with the high-level medical and rehabilitative care they need to grow beyond the boundaries of their prognoses.

Prof. Joehoshua Shemer, Chair, Board of Assuta
Avner Broker, Operations Manager, ALEH Negev
Dov Hirth, Marketing & Development

2720   Association for Children with Down Syndrome
4 Fern Place
Plainview, NY 11803

516-933-4700
www.acds.org

Dedicated to providing lifetime resources of exceptional quality, innovation and inclusion for individuals with Down syndrome and other developmental disabilities and their families.

Liz Lawlor Campbell, Chair, Advisory Committee
Gene Kirley, President
Thomas DeMaggio, Vice President

2721   Birth Defects Research for Children
976 Lake Baldwin Lane, Suite 104
Orlando, FL 32814

407-895-0802
staff@birthdefects.org
www.birthdefects.org

An organization that provides parents and expectant parents with information about birth defects and support services for their children. BDRC has a parent-matching program that links families who have children with similar birth defects.

2722   Down Syndrome Guild
www.downsyndromedallas.com

Provides new baby/parent hospital visits, monthly newsletter, support and encouragement for individuals with Down Syndrome and their families. Bi-lingual group. Job coaching scholarships.

2723   Health Answers
410 Horsham Road
Horsham, PA 19044

215-422-9010
Michael.tague@healthanswers.com
www.healthanswers.com

HealthAnswers offers a breadth of services in medical education, sales force training, patient support, solutions, professional promotion and consumer solutions.

Michael Tague, Managing Director

2724   National Association for Down Syndrome (NADS)
1460 Renaissance Drive, Suite #405
Park Ridge, IL 60068

630-325-9112
info@nads.org
www.nads.org

Established by parents of children with Down syndrome who felt a need to create a better environment and bring about understanding and acceptance of people with Down syndrome.

Steve Connors, President
Jeni Friedland, First Vice President
Deb Mirabelli, Second Vice President

2725   National Down Syndrome Congress
30 Mansell Court, Suite 108
Roswell, GA 30076

770-604-9500
800-232-NDSC
Fax: 770-604-9898
info@ndsccenter.org
www.ndsccenter.org

It is the mission of the National Down Syndrome Congress to be the national advocacy organization for Down syndrome and to provide leadership in all areas of concern related to persons with Down syndrome. In that capacity, NDSC will function as a major source of support and empowerment to persons with down syndrome and their families.

Marilyn Tolbert, Ed.D., President
Bret Bowerman, First Vice President
Andy Bean, Second Vice President

2726   National Down Syndrome Society
666 Broadway, 8th Floor
New York, NY 10012

800-221-4602
Fax: 212-979-2873
info@ndss.org
www.ndss.org

Our mission is to benefit people with Down Syndrome and their families through national leadership in education research and advocacy.

CAPT Robert P. Taishoff USN (ret), Chairman
Stephen Beck, Jr., Vice Chairman
Sara Weir, President

2727   Online Mendelian Inheritance in Man
U.S. National Library of Medicine, 8600 Rockville
Bethesda, MD 20894

888-346-3656
info@ncbi.nlm.nih.gov
www.ncbi.nlm.nih.gov

This database is a catalog of human genes and genetic disorders.

Christine E. Seidman, M.D., Chair
David J. Lipman, M.D., Executive Secretary
Michael Boehnke, Ph.D., Board Member

Book Publishers

2728   Adolescents with Down Syndrome
University of Victoria
3800 Finnerty Road
Victoria, BC, V8P
Canada

250-721-7211
www.uvic.ca

Adolescents with Down syndrome: International perspectives on research and programme development: Implications for parents, researchers, and practitioners.

165 pages
ISBN: 0-919955-16-9

Carey Denholm, Editor

2729   Babies with Down Syndrome
Woodbine House
6510 Bells Mill Road
Bethesda, MD 20817

301-897-3570
800-843-7323
Fax: 301-897-5838

Praised as the finest book ever written for new parents, this book covers everything they need to know about rearing these beautiful and special children in a loving environment.

340 pages Paperback
ISBN: 0-933149-64-6

Karen Stray-Gundersen, Editor

2730   Biomedical Concerns in Persons with Down's Syndrome
Brookes Publishing Company
PO Box 10624
Baltimore, MD 21285

410-337-9580
800-638-3775
Fax: 410-337-8539
www.brookespublishing.com

Written by leading authorities and spanning many disciplines and specialties, this comprehensive resource provides vital information on biomedical issues concerning individuals with Down's syndrome.

336 pages Hardcover
ISBN: 1-557660-89-1

Siegfried M Pueschel, Editor
Jeanette K Pueschel, Editor

2731 Cara: Growing with a Retarded Child
Temple University Press
1801 N.Broad Street
Philadelphia, PA 19122   215-204-8787
www.temple.edu/templepress/

Despite the fact that Cara Jablow was born with Down's syndrome, formerly known as mongolism, she was reading before she was five. Her mother, a journalist, dramatically recounts Cara's development from birth to age seven, revealing how a family reacts to the news that their baby is retarded, how they now can make use of early intervention programs, and what Cara's prospects are for the future.

210 pages Paperback
ISBN: 0-877222-69-X

Martha Moraghan Jablow, Editor

2732 Communication Skills in Children with Down Syndrome: A Guide for Parents
Woodbine House
6510 Bells Mill Road
Bethesda, MD 20817   301-468-8800
                                         800-843-7323
                                    Fax: 301-897-5838
                              info@woodbinehouse.com
                              www.woodbinehouse.com

Offers parents a chance to learn what to expect as communication skills progress from infancy through early teenage years. Discussions are included on speech and language therapy, hearing problems, school performance and intelligibility issues.

241 pages Paperback
ISBN: 0-933149-53-0

Libby Kumin, Editor

2733 Count Us In: Growing up with Down Syndrome
Harvest Book Company
185 Commerce Drive
Fort Washington, PA 19034   215-619-0307
                                         877-512-3022
                         webservice@Harvestbooks.com
                              www.harvestbooks.com/

Mitchell Levitz and Jason Kingsley share their innermost thoughts, feelings, hopes and dreams, their lifelong friendship and their experiences of growing up with Down Syndrome.

1994 208 pages Paperback
ISBN: 0-156226-60-X

Jason Kingsley, Editor
Mitchell Levitz, Editor

2734 Current Approaches to Down's Syndrome
Greenwood Publishing Group
88 Post Road W, Suite 5007
Westport, CT 06880   203-226-3571
                                    www.greenwood.com

An exploration of current initiatives relating to Down syndrome in the medical, educational and social fields.

447 pages Hardcover
ISBN: 0-275902-12-9

David Lane, Editor
Brian Stratford, Editor

2735 Differences in Common: Straight Talk on Mental Retardation/Down Syndrome & Life
Woodbine House
6510 Bells Mill Road
Bethesda, MD 20817   301-468-8800
                                         800-843-7323
                                    Fax: 301-897-5838
                              info@woodbinehouse.com
                              www.woodbinehouse.com

A collection of essays by the mother of an adult son who has Down syndrome. Focuses on mainstreaming, terminology, parent groups and advocacy.

231 pages Paperback
ISBN: 0-933149-40-9

Marilyn Trainer, Editor

2736 Down Sydrome: Living and Learning in the Community
Wiley & Sonecial Children
10475 Crosspoint Boulevard
Indianapolis, IN 46256   877-762-2974
                                    Fax: 800-597-3299
                                       www.wiley.com

Four parents' personal observations. Challenges of people with DS as they become integrated into community, family role, cognitive development and acquisition of language, education, health care, independent living arrangement.

1995 312 pages Hardcover
ISBN: 0-471022-01-2

Lynn Nadel, Editor
Donna Rosenthal, Editor

2737 Down Syndrome: Birth to Adulthood: Giving Families an Edge
Love Publishing Company
9101 E Kenyon Evenue
Denver, CO 80237   303-221-7333
                                    Fax: 303-221-7444
                              lpc@lovepublishing.com
                              www.lovepublishing.com

Provides a collection of longitudinal perspectives on experiences of individuals with Down Syndrome, from birth to adulthood.

1995 356 pages Paperback
ISBN: 0-891082-36-0

John R Rynders, Editor

2738 Down Syndrome: The Facts
Oxford University Press
2001 Evans Road
Cary, NC 27513   212-726-6000
                                         800-451-7556
                                    Fax: 919-677-1303
                                    www.oup-usa.org

A book for parents who have a child with Down Syndrome, written by a pediatrician who works with Down syndrome children.

208 pages Paperback
ISBN: 0-192626-62-0

Mark Selikowitz, Editor

2739 Let's Talk About Down Syndrome
Rosen Publishing Group's PowerKids Press
29 E 21st Street
New York, NY 10010   212-777-3017
                                         800-237-9932
                                    Fax: 888-436-4643
                              rosenpub@tribeca.ios.com
                              www.rosenpublishing.com

By stressing that children with Down syndrome are wonderful, viable members of society, this book lessens the stigma attached to this rather common genetic condition.

Ages: 4-8 24 pages Library Binding
ISBN: 0-823951-97-9

Melanie Apel Gordon, Editor

2740 Medical and Surgical Care for Children with Down Syndrome
Woodbine House
6510 Bells Mill Road
Bethesda, MD 20817
301-897-3570
800-843-7323
Fax: 301-897-5838
info@woodbinehouse.com
www.woodbinehouse.com

Provides detailed and easy-to-understand information for parents on a wide range of medical conditions and treatments including: heart disease, recurrent infections, thyroid problems, eye problems, skin conditions, ear, nose and throat problems, orthopedic conditions, leukemia, facial and dental concerns and neurological problems.

395 pages Paperback
ISBN: 0-933149-54-9

Philip Matheis, MD, Editor
Don Van Dyke, MD, Editor

2741 Our Brother Has Down's Syndrome: An Introduction for Children
Annick Press
15 Patricia Avenue
Toronto, ON, M2M
Canada
416-221-4802
Fax: 416-221-8400
www.annickpress.com

Two young sisters tell about their little brother Jai, who has Down's Syndrome. The text stresses the ways in which he is like all children, although he needs extra help to walk, use a spoon, stack blocks, etc. The color photographs show an engaging little boy going about his daily activities, often with other family members.

24 pages Paperback
ISBN: 0-920303-31-5

Shelly Cairo, Editor
Jasmine Cairo, Editor
Irene McNeil, Editor

2742 Parent's Guide to Down Syndrome: Toward a Brighter Future
Brookes Publishing Company
PO Box 10624
Baltimore, MD 21285
410-337-9580
800-638-3775
Fax: 410-337-8539
custserv@brookespublishing.com
www.brookespublishing.com

A comprehensive reference book especially for new parents, but useful and informative to seasoned parents as well. Range of topics include a history of Down syndrome, physical characteristics, developmental expectations, early intervention, feeding the young child and the school years.

352 pages Paperback
ISBN: 1-557664-52-8

Siegfried M Pueschel, Editor

2743 Perceptual-Motor Behavior in Down Syndrome
Human Kinetics Publishing
1607 N Market Street
Champaign, IL 61825
217-351-5076
800-747-4457
Fax: 217-351-2674
www.humankinetics.com

A comprehensive collection of contemporary research and provides readers a window into the life of someone with Down Syndrome.

365 pages Hardcover
ISBN: 0-880119-75-6

Daniel J Weeks, Editor
Romeo Chua, Editor
Dibgy Elliott, Editor

2744 Screening for Down Syndrome
Cambridge University Press
32 Avenue of the Americas
New York, NY 10013
212-337-5000
Fax: 212-691-3239
newyork@cambridge.org
www.cambridge.org

Summarises the recent exciting advances in screening for Down's syndrome. It addresses important clinical questions such as; risk assessment, whom to screen, when to screen, which techniques to use and the organisation of screening programmes nationally and internationally.

1995 358 pages Hardcover
ISBN: 0-521452-71-6

J G Grudzinskas, Editor
T Chard, Editor
M Chapman, Editor

2745 Shattered Dreams - Lonely Choices: Birth Parents of Babies with Disabilities
Bergin & Garvey/Greenwood Publishing
88 Post Road W, PO Box 5007
Westport, CT 06880
203-226-3571
800-225-5800
Fax: 203-222-1502
custserv@greenwood.com
www.greenwood.com

Joanne Finnegan shares her personal experience and that of several families she interviewed who, like herself, explored options other than raising their child with a disability. Parents express with candor the overwhelming pain they felt when receiving the news, the frustration when searching for options, the no-win feeling of decision making, the resolve with a final decision, and finally, life after the decision.

208 pages Hardcover
ISBN: 0-897892-86-0

Joanne Finnegan, Editor

2746 Show Me No Mercy: Compelling Story of Remarkable Courage
Abingdon Press
201 8th Avenue South, P.O. Box 801
Nashville, TN 37202
800-251-3320
orders@abingdonpress.com
www.abingdonpress.com

A father of a young adult man with Down syndrome relates the experience of his attempt to be reunited with his son after a family tragedy separates them.

144 pages Paperback
ISBN: 0-687384-35-4

Robert Perske, Editor

2747 Since Owen
Johns Hopkins University Press
2715 N Charles Street
Baltimore, MD 21218
410-516-6900
800-537-5487
Fax: 410-516-6968
webmaster@jhupress.jhu.edu
www.press.jhu.edu

A well written book displaying understanding from a veteran parent communicating with other parents of children with disabilities.

488 pages Paperback
ISBN: 0-801839-64-5

Charles R Callanan, Editor
Alfred R. Berkeley, Chairman

2748 Special Kids Make Special Friends
Association for Children with Down Syndrome
4 Fern Place
Plainview, NY 11803
516-933-4700
Fax: 516-933-9524
information@acds.org
www.acds.org

Written to assist young children, new parents, siblings, and professionals in developing a better understanding of Down syndrome. Photographs depict children in preschool, emphasizing similarities and strengths of youngsters with Down syndrome rather than their differences.

1995 Paperback
ISBN: 9-995007-64-9

Debra Shalom, Editor
Michael M. Smith, Executive Director

2749 To Give An Edge: A Guide for New Parents of Children with Down's Syndrome
Colwell Systems
1031 Mendola Heights Road
St. Paul, MN 55120   651-232-7800

A guide for new parents designed to provide information about the disorder and how other parents of children with Down syndrome have coped.

Paperback
ISBN: 9-993370-55-X

JM Horrobin, Editor

2750 Understanding Down Syndrome
Brookline Books
8 Trumbull Rd, Suite B-001
Northampton, MA 01060   413-584-0184
                                            800-666-2665
                                            Fax: 413-584-6184
                                            brbooks@yahoo.com
                                            www.brooklinebooks.com

The author provides answers and explanations to the countless questions directed to him during his twenty years' involvement with Down syndrome individuals and their families.

243 pages Paperback
ISBN: 1-571290-09-5

Cliff Cunningham, Editor

2751 Where's Chimpy?
Albert Whitman & Company
250 South Northwest Highway, Suite 320
Park Ridge, IL 60068   847-581-0033
                                            800-255-7675
                                            Fax: 847-581-0039
                                            mail@albertwhitman.com
                                            www.albertwhitman.com

Text and photographs show Misty, a little girl with Down syndrome and her father reviewing her day's activities in their search for her stuffed monkey.

32 pages Paperback
ISBN: 0-807589-27-6

Berniece Rabe, Editor
Diane Schmidt, Illustrator

Magazines

2752 Down Syndrome News
National Down Syndrome Congress
30 Mansell Court, Suite 108
Roswell, GA 30076   770-604-9500
                                            800-232-6372
                                            Fax: 770-604-9898
                                            info@ndscenter.org
                                            www.ndsccenter.org

Down Syndrome News provides advocacy news and information to parents and family members of individuals with Down syndrome and those working with them.

6x/year

Marilyn Tolbert, Ed.D., President
Bret Bowerman, First Vice President
Andy Bean, Second Vice President

2753 Upbeat
National Down Syndrome Society
666 Broadway, 8th Floor
New York, NY 10012   800-221-4602
                                            Fax: 212-979-2873
                                            info@ndss.org
                                            www.ndss.org

For and by people with Down syndrome that comes out three times a year.

CAPT Robert P. Taishoff USN (ret), Chairman
Stephen Beck, Jr., Vice Chairman
Sara Weir, President

Newsletters

2754 About NDSS
National Down Syndrome Society
666 Broadway, 8th Floor
New York, NY 10012   800-221-4602
                                            Fax: 212-979-2873
                                            info@ndss.org
                                            www.ndss.org

Offers information on the society, stats, goals, mission, activities, affiliates, and governing body.

16 pages

CAPT Robert P. Taishoff USN (ret), Chairman
Stephen Beck, Jr., Vice Chairman
Sara Weir, President

2755 Communicating Together
PO Box 6395
Columbia, MD 21045   408-253-0246
                                            Fax: 408-253-7391
                                            karen@kidsource.com
                                            www.kidsource.com

An excellent resource for parents and professionals. Each issue includes a feature article, a question and answer section and home activities.

6x/year

Dr. Libby Kumin, Editor
Karen Dillon, Media Inquiries

Pamphlets

2756 About Down Syndrome
National Down Syndrome Society
666 Broadway, 8th Floor
New York, NY 10012   800-221-4602
                                            Fax: 212-979-2873
                                            info@ndss.org
                                            www.ndss.org

An overview of Down Syndrome produced by The Goodwin Family Information & Referral Center arm of NDSS.

18 pages

CAPT Robert P. Taishoff USN (ret), Chairman
Stephen Beck, Jr., Vice Chairman
Sara Weir, President

2757 Down Syndrome
National Down Syndrome Congress
30 Mansell Court, Suite 108
Roswell, GA 30076   770-604-9500
                                            800-232-6372
                                            Fax: 770-604-9898
                                            info@ndsccenter.org
                                            www.ndsccenter.org

Pertinent information ranging from education to medicine to legal or legislative issues.

Marilyn Tolbert, Ed.D., President
Bret Bowerman, First Vice President
Andy Bean, Second Vice President

2758 Heart and Down Syndrome
National Down Syndrome Society
666 Broadway, 8th Floor
New York, NY 10012

800-221-4602
Fax: 212-979-2873
info@ndss.org
www.ndss.org

1995

CAPT Robert P. Taishoff USN (ret), Chairman
Stephen Beck, Jr., Vice Chairman
Sara Weir, President

2759 Life Planning and Down Syndrome
National Down Syndrome Society
666 Broadway, 8th Floor
New York, NY 10012

800-221-4602
Fax: 212-979-2873
info@ndss.org
www.ndss.org

CAPT Robert P. Taishoff USN (ret), Chairman
Stephen Beck, Jr., Vice Chairman
Sara Weir, President

2760 Neurology of Down Syndrome
National Down Syndrome Society
666 Broadway, 8th Floor
New York, NY 10012

800-221-4602
Fax: 212-979-2873
info@ndss.org
www.ndss.org

1995

CAPT Robert P. Taishoff USN (ret), Chairman
Stephen Beck, Jr., Vice Chairman
Sara Weir, President

2761 New Parents
Association for Children with Down Syndrome
2616 Martin Avenue
Bellmore, NY 11710

516-221-4700
Fax: 516-221-4311
info@acds.org
www.acds.org

A bibliography compiled for parents who have just given birth to a child with Down syndrome.

Liz Lawlor Campbell, Chair, Advisory Committee
Gene Kirley, President
Thomas DeMaggio, Vice President

Camps

2762 Camp Friendship
Friendship Ventures
10509 108th Street NW
Annandale, MN 55302

952-852-0101
800-450-8376
Fax: 952-852-0123
info@friendshipventures.org
www.friendshipventures.org

Camp Friendship offers kids, teens, and adults the chance to have the time of their lives. The program focuses on building self-esteem and independence, and practicing social skills; and we nurture each person's strengths and abilities and encourage participation in activies at their own pace. Specially designed for persons with developmental, physical or multiple disabilities, special medical conditions, Down syndrome, autism or other conditions. Weekend camps and longer available.

Georgann Rumsey, Vice President, Programs
Laurie Tschetter, Program Director

2763 Camp Hawkins
800 Rudeseal Road
Mt. Airy, GA 30563

706-894-1678
ksewell@gbchfm.org
www.gbchfm.org

Summer residential camp for children ages 8 to 21 with varying disabilities such as Cerebral Palsy, Down Syndrome, brain injuries and/or developmental delays.

Chris Hobbs, VP of Communications
Alice Bagley, Public Relations
Kendra Sewell, Director

2764 Camp Huntington
56 Bruceville Road
High Falls, NY 12440

845-687-7840
855-707-2267
Fax: 845-213-4313
mbednarz@camphuntington.com
www.camphuntington.com

Summer activities include recreational, academic and vocational programs for the learning disabled, neurologically impaired and mildly ADA to mild/moderately retarded. An Olympic pool, horse riding and a special work training program are featured. Programs are tailored to meet individual needs, ages 6-21, and campers may enroll for 4 to 8 weeks.

Michael Bednarz, Executive Director, MS, MBA
Alex Mellor, Program Director, MA
Dr. Bruria Bodek, Consultant, Executive Director

2765 Camp Merrimack
3320 Triana Boulevard
Huntsville, AL 35805

256-534-6455
ksimari@merrimackhall.com
www.merrimackhall.com

A unique arts half-day camp for children ages 3 through 12; open to children with special needs including Cerebral Palsy, Down Syndrome, autism and others.

Ashley Dinges, Executive Director
Kim Simari, Managing Director

2766 Camp New Hope
Friendship Ventures
53035 Lake Avenue
McGregor, MN 55760

952-852-0101
800-450-8376
Fax: 952-852-0123
fv@friendshipventures.org
www.friendshipventures.org

Camp New Hope is a great place for children, teens, and adults to have the time of their lives. The program provides a unique opportunity for having fun, learning skills, boosting confidence, and making friends. Services are specifically designed for persons with developmental, phyisical or multiple disabilities, special medical needs, Down syndrome, autism, or other conditions. Weekend camps and longer available. Other services available throughout the year.

Georgann Rumsey, Vice President, Programs
Laurie Tschetter, Program Director

2767 Camp PALS
4368 Farmington Circle
Allentown, PA 18104

215-501-7157
jenni@palsprograms.org
www.camppals.org

One-week summer camp for young adults with Down syndrome held at Cabrini College in PA.

Jason Toff, Board Chair
Jenni Newbury Ross, Executive Director
Sarah Barnes, Program Coordinator

2768 Eden Wood Center
Friendship Ventures
16165 Hillcrest Lane
Eden Prairie, MN 44346

952-852-0101
Fax: 952-934-5656
fbiw.info@gmail.com
fbiw.net/old_site/JoinIn/meetings.htm

Offers resident camp programs for children, teenagers and adults with developmental, physical or multiple disabilities, Down Syndrome, special medical conditions, Williams Syndrome, autism and/or other conditions. Fishing, creative arts, golf, sports and other activities are available. Creative Options Respite Care offers weekend camps year round for children, teenagers and adults. Ventures Travel offers guided vacations for teens and adults with developmental disabilities or other unique needs.

Vicky Miller, President
Roger Person, Vice President
Marcus Johnson, Director

DESCRIPTION

2769 DYSLEXIA

Involves the following Biologic System(s):

Neurologic Disorders

Dyslexia refers to a specific learning disability characterized by the impaired ability to process written symbols. Although individuals with dyslexia are able to see and recognize letters, this disorder impairs their ability to read, write, and spell. Affected individuals typically have no problems with the correct recognition of pictures and objects.

No definition of dyslexia is universally accepted, thus incidence is difficult to determine. An estimated 15% of public school children receive special education for reading problems of whom 3 to 5% are probably dyslexic. Young children with dyslexia may have difficulty remembering the correct names of letters and numbers. Articulating proper speech may be difficult. Some children of school age may reverse letters and words when writing. For example, affected children may substitute the letter p for q or the word was for saw, while transposing letters so that bets may become best. Children with dyslexia may also have difficulty reading due to an impaired ability to determine the sequence of letters within words and to distinguish right from left. The hallmark of this learning disability is the fact that, despite the difficulties associated with dyslexia, affected children are of average or above average intelligence as evidenced by I.Q. testing as well as their success in other scholastic achievements.

Early diagnosis of dyslexia is an important factor in treating this learning disability. Children nearing the end of first grade who exhibit difficulties with word skills or any children whose reading and writing ability is not commensurate with that of their other scholastic abilities may be tested for dyslexia. Although dyslexia is not related to eye defects, an ophthalmologic evaluation is beneficial in determining if ocular abnormalities may be eliminated as a cause of symptoms. Also, eye irregularities may be present in addition to dyslexia and, therefore, may be diagnosed and corrected at that time. Treatment for dyslexia is geared toward remedial teaching techniques specific to this disability.

Dyslexia is thought to be a familial disorder that may be inherited through an autosomal dominant trait. Boys are more frequently affected than girls.

Government Agencies

2770 NIH/ Eunice Kennedy Shriver National Insti tute of Child Health & Human Development
31 Center Drive, Building 31
Bethesda, MD 20892
301-496-5113
800-370-2943
Fax: 866-760-5947
nichdpress@mail.nih.gov
www.nichd.nih.gov

Established in 1962 by congress, today the institute conducts and supports research on topics related to the health of children, adults, families and populations. Some of these topics include: developmental disabilities, growth and development, infant death, reproductive health and birth defects.

Diana W. Bianchi, Director
Paul Williams, Director, Communications

National Associations & Support Groups

2771 American Academy of Pediatrics
141 Northwest Point Boulevard
Elk Grove Village, IL 60007
847-434-4000
800-433-9016
Fax: 847-434-8000
www.aap.org

The American Academy of Pediatrics and its member pediatricians are committed to the attainment of optimal physical, mental and social health and well-being for all infants, children, adolescents, and young adults.

Fernando Stein, MD, FAAP, President
Karen Remley, MD, CEO/Executive VP

2772 American School Counselor Association
1101 King Street, Suite 310
Alexandria, VA 22314
703-683-2722
800-306-4722
Fax: 703-997-7572
asca@schoolcounselor.org
www.schoolcounselor.org

The mission of ASCA is to represent professional school counselors and to promote professionalism and ethical practices.

Richard Wong, Executive Director
Jeff Broderson, Information Technology Admin.
Kathleen M Rakestraw, Director of Communications

2773 American Speech Language Hearing Association (ASHA)
10801 Rockville Pike
Rockville, MD 20852
301-897-5700
800-638-8255
Fax: 301-571-0457
productsales@asha.org
www.asha.org

The mission of the American Speech-Language-Hearing Association is to promote the interests of and provide the highest quality services for professionals in audiology, speech-language pathology, speech and hearing science, and to advocate for people with communication disabilities.

Arlene A Pietranton, Executive Director
Maureen E Thompson, Director Governance Operations

2774 Center for Disabilities and Development
University of Iowa Stead Family Children's Hospita
100 Hawkins Drive
Iowa City, IA 52242
319-353-6900
877-686-0031
Fax: 319-356-7700
cdd-webmaster@uiowa.edu
www.uiowa.edu

A trusted resource for healthcare, training, research and information for people with disabilities that include: behavior disorders, brain injury, cerebral palsy, diabetes, down syndrome, learning disabilities, mental retardation, sleep disorders and spina bifida.

Dianne McBrien, MD, Medical Director

2775 Davis Dyslexia Association International
1601 Bayshore Highway, Suite 245
Burlingame, CA 94010
650-692-7141
888-805-7216
Fax: 650-692-7075
info@davislearn.com
www.davislearn.com

Offers books, materials, workshops and certification in the Davis Dyslexia Correction method.

Ron Davis, Manager

2776 Genetic Alliance
4301 Connecticut Avenue NW, Suite 404
Washington, DC 20008
202-966-5557
800-336-4363
Fax: 202-966-8553
info@geneticalliance.org
www.geneticalliance.org

A coalition of voluntary genetic support groups, consumers and professionals addressing the needs of individuals and families affected by genetic disorders from a national perspective.

Sharon Terry, President/CEO
Tetyana Murza, Managing Director
Natasha Bonhomme, VP, Strategic Development

2777 International Dyslexia Association
40 York Road, Suite 400
Baltimore, MD 21204   410-296-0232
                                            800-222-3123
                                        Fax: 410-321-5069
                                         info@interdys.org
                                          www.interdys.org

Our mission is to pursue and provide the most comprehensive range of information and services that address the full scope of dyslexia and related difficulties in learning to read and write.

Steve Peregoy, Executive Director
Gerri Morris, Coordinator Information/Referral
Robert Hott, Director of Development

2778 Learning Disabilities Association of Ameri ca
4156 Library Road
Pittsburgh, PA 15234   412-341-1515
                                            888-300-6710
                                        Fax: 412-344-0224
                                    info@LDAAmerica.org
                                       www.ldaamerica.org

Helps families of the affected individual through information and referral to professionals in their area. A membership organization with affiliates across the country.

Sheila Buckley, Executive Director

2779 March of Dimes Foundation
1275 Mamaroneck Avenue
White Plains, NY 10605   914-997-4488
                                             888-663-4637
                                         Fax: 914-997-4763
                                 answers@marchofdimes.com
                                       www.marchofdimes.com

Partnership of volunteers and professionals dedicated to improving the health of babies by preventing birth defects and infant mortality. Over 100 chapters are located across the country and can be located through the National Office.

Stacey D. Stewart, President

2780 Option Institute: Son Rise Program
Autism Treatment Center of America
2080 S Undermountain Road
Sheffield, MA 01257   413-229-2100
                                             877-766-7473
                                         Fax: 413-229-3202
                                  information@son-rise.org
                                          www.son-rise.org

Describes an effective, loving and respectful method for treating children with autism. It teaches parents and healing professionals how to set up a home based program using the child's motivation to reach their special child.

Barry Neil Kaufman, Co-Founder/Co-Creator
Samahria Lyte Kaufman, Co-Founder/Co-Creator

Research Centers

2781 Dyslexia Research Institute
5746 Centerville Road
Tallahassee, FL 32309   850-893-2216
                                        Fax: 850-893-2440
                                            dri@talstar.com
                                       www.dyslexia-add.org

Searching for new and better methods to deal with the unique needs of Dyslexics.

Pat Hardman, Executive Director
Robyn A Rennick, MS, Director

Conferences

2782 ASHA Convention
American Speech-Language-Hearing Association
10801 Rockville Pike
Rockville, MD 20852   301-897-5700
                                             800-638-8255
                                        Fax: 301-571-0457
                                  productsales@asha.org
                                              www.asha.org

The premier annual professional education event for speech-language pathologists, audiologists, and speech, language, and hearing scientists. Bringing together more than 12,000 attendees, the Convention provides unparalleled opportunities to hear the latest evidence-based research and gain new skills and resources to advance your career.

November

Arlene A Pietranton, Executive Director
Maureen E Thompson, Director Governance Operations

2783 Genetic Alliance Annual Conference
Genetic Alliance
4301 Connecticut Avenue NW, Suite 404
Washington, DC 20008   202-966-5557
                                             800-336-4363
                                        Fax: 202-966-8553
                                  info@geneticalliance.org
                                     www.geneticalliance.org

Consistently inspirational and enables partnership among all stakeholders: advocates and community leaders, health and industry professionals, policymakers, and academicians.

July

Sharon Terry, President/CEO
Tetyana Murza, Managing Director
Natasha Bonhomme, VP, Strategic Development

2784 International Dyslexia Association Conference
40 York Road, Suite 400
Baltimore, MD 21204   410-296-0232
                                            800-222-3123
                                        Fax: 410-321-5069
                                         info@interdys.org
                                          www.interdys.org

Focuses on the latest advances in dyslexia, related language difficulties and related fields. Individual sessions are geared towards educators and educational administrators, educational diagnosticians and therapists, parents, speech and language pathologists and of course, individuals with dyslexia and their families.

Kristen Penczek, Conference Director
Darnella Parks, Conference Coordinator

2785 LDA Annual Conference
Learning Disabilities Association of America
4156 Library Road
Pittsburgh, PA 15234   412-341-1515
                                            888-300-6710
                                        Fax: 412-344-0224
                                    info@LDAAmerica.org
                                       www.ldaamerica.org

Meeting on learning disabilities, featuring over 200 workshops and exhibits.

February

Sheila Buckley, Executive Director

Audio Video

2786 Dyslexia
Fanlight Productions
32 Court Street, 21st Floor
Brooklyn, NY 11201   718-488-8900
                                             800-876-1710
                                        Fax: 718-488-8642
                          info@fanlight.com, orders@fanlight.com
                                            www.fanlight.com

Looks at the experiences of people with these learning disabilities as well as the potential value to society of their alternative ways of learning. Dartmouth Hitchcock Medical Center Series, The Doctor is In...

28 minutes VHS

Nicole Johnson, Publicity Coordinator

Web Sites

2787 American Speech Language Hearing Associati on (ASHA)
2200 Research Boulevard
Rockville, MD 20850
301-296-5700
800-498-2071
Fax: 301-296-8580
TTY: 301-296-5650
nsslha@asha.org
www.asha.org

An organization working to promote a better quality of life for children and adults with communication disorders. Our mission is to advance knowledge about the causes and treatment of hearing, speech, and language problems.

Judith L. Page, PhD, CCC-SLP, President
Howard Goldstein, PhD, CCC-SLP, VP for Science & Research
Arlene A. Pietranton, PhD, CAE, CEO

2788 British Dyslexia Association
Unit 8 Bracknell Beeches, Old Bracknell Lane
Bracknell, RG12
033- 40- 455
www.bdadyslexia.org.uk

The BDA offers a range of practical help for dyslexic children, dyslexic adults, parents and professionals in education.

Margaret Malpas, Chair of Trustees
Diana Baring, Vice President
Kevin Morley, Vice President

2789 Davis Dyslexia Association International Dyslexia: The Gift
1601 Bayshore Highway 260
Burlingame, CA 94010
650-692-7141
888-999-3324
Fax: 650-692-7075
ddai@dyslexia.com, orders@dyslexia.com
www.dyslexia.com

Offers information and training in methods for overcoming learning problems developed by Ron Davis, author of 'The Gift of Dyslexia,' listings of Davis Dyslexia Correction providers worldwide, a forum for networking and articles and reports on learning styles and educational approaches.

2790 International Dyslexia Association
40 York Rd., 4th Floor
Baltimore, MD 21204
410-296-0232
Fax: 410-321-5069
info@interdys.org, members@interdys.org
www.interdys.org

Dyslexia is a neurological disorder that impairs reading. If undetected in children, it can create major learning problems. Contact the IDA for free information. Publications are available for a range of fees.

Hal Malchow, President
Ben Shifrin, M.Ed., Vice President
Elsa Cÿrdenas-Hagan, Ed.D., C, Vice President

2791 Learning Disabilities Association of Ameri ca
www.ldaamerica.org

Helps families of the affected individual through information and referral to professionals in their area. A membership organization with affiliates across the country.

2792 Mental Health Net
P.O. Box 20709
Columbus, OH 43220
614-448-4055
800-232-TALK
info@centersite.net, editor@centersite.n
www.mentalhelp.net

We wish to provide the following: to discuss, develop and debate in an open forum the future of the mental health field in America and throughout the world. To help coordinate various components of the mental health field so as to bring about greater communication between them.

2793 NIH/ Eunice Kennedy Shriver National Insti tute of Child Health & Human Development
31 Center Drive, Building 31
Bethesda, MD 20892
301-496-5113
800-370-2943
Fax: 866-760-5947
TTY: 888-320-6942
nichdpress@mail.nih.gov
www.nichd.nih.gov

Established in 1962 by congress, today the institute conducts and supports research on all stages of human dveelopment to better understand the health of children, adults, families and communities. Topics of research include: birth defects, mental retardation, developmental disabilities, reproductive health, growth and development, and infant death.

Diana W. Bianchi, Director
Paul Williams, Director, Communications

2794 Option Institute
www.son-rise.org

Describes an effective, loving and respectful method for treating children with autism. It teaches parents and healing professionals how to set up a home based program using the child's motivation to reach their special child.

Barry Neil Kaufman, Co Founder/ Senior Teacher/ Trainer
Becky Damgaard, Program Teacher
Raun K. Kaufman, Program Group Facilitator

Book Publishers

2795 Let's Talk About Dyslexia

Melanie Apel Gordon, author

Rosen Publishing Group's PowerKids Press
29 E 21st Street
New York, NY 10010
212-777-3017
800-237-9932
Fax: 888-436-4643
rosenpub@tribeca.ios.com
www.powerkidspress.com

Children will learn what dyslexia is and how to tell if they have it. This book stresses that children with dyslexia are just as smart as their classmates. Tells about Albert Einstein and other well known people who were dyslexic. Grades K-5.

24 pages
ISBN: 0-823951-99-5

2796 Misunderstood Child

Larry B Silver, MD, author

Active Parenting Publishers
1220 Kennestone Circle,Suite 130
Marietta, GA 30066
770-429-0565
800-825-0060
Fax: 770-429-0334
cservice@activeparenting.com
www.activeparenting.com

The fully revised and updated must-have resource to help you become a supportive and assertive advocate for your child. The Misunderstood Child, Fourth Edition has become the go-to reference guide for families of children with learning disorders. Item #8825.

432 pages

2797   Overcoming Dyslexia in Children, Adolescents, and Adults
Dale R Jordan, author

Pro-Ed
8700 Shoal Creek Boulevard
Austin, TX 78757
                                        512-451-3246
                                        800-897-3202
                                        Fax: 800-397-7633
                                        www.proedinc.com

The third edition summarizes what science knows today about what causes the forms of dyslexia that are related to left-brain language processing. This book also discusses in detail nonverbal types of learning disabilities (LD) and social and emotional types of LD. All forms of dyslexia are described in detail with graphic illustrations of how dyslexia impacts classroom learning, social behavior, emotional maturity and development.

432 pages Softcover
ISBN: 0-890796-42-4

2798   Straight Talk about Psychological Testing for Kids
Ellen Braaten PhD, Gretcen Felopulos PhD, author

Active Parenting Publishers
1220 Kennestone Circle, Suite 130
Marietta, GA 30066
                                        770-429-0565
                                        800-825-0060
                                        Fax: 770-429-0334
                                        cservice@activeparenting.com
                                        www.activeparenting.com

This authoritative guide gives parents the inside scoop on how psychological testing works and how to use testing to get the best help for their children. Item #8670.

260 pages Softcover

Camps

2799   Camp Dunnabeck at Kildonan
425 Morse Hill Road
Amenia, NY 12501
                                        845-373-8111
                                        Fax: 845-373-2004
                                        info@kildonanadmissions.org
                                        www.kildonan.org

Specializes in helping intelligent children with specific reading, writing and spelling disablties. Provides Orton-Gillingham tutoring with camp activities, including swimming, sailing, waterskiing, horseback riding, ceramics, tennis and woodworking.

Ages 9-15

Christina Lang, Chair
Richard S. Berg, Vice Chair
Kevin F. Pendergast, Headmaster

2800   Landmark School
429 Hale Street, PO Box 227
Prides Crossing, MA 1965
                                        978-236-3010
                                        Fax: 978-927-7268
                                        admission@landmarkschool.org
                                        www.landmarkschool.org

Offers academic skill development and exciting activities for boys and girls in grades 1-12, who have been diagnosed with a language-based learning disability.

Moira M. James, Chair
Martin P. Slark, Vice Chair
Robert J. Broudo, President & Headmaster

2801   Marvelwood Summer
Marvelwood School
476 Skiff Mountain Road, PO Box 3001
Kent, CT 6757
                                        860-927-0047
                                        800-440-9107
                                        Fax: 860-927-5325
                                        summerschool@marvelwood.org
                                        www.themarvelwoodschool.com

The emphasis in this summer program is on diagnosis and remediation of individual reading, spelling, writing, mathematics and study problems. Participants are boys and girls entering grades 6-10.

Scott E Pottbecker, Head of School
Katherine Almquist, Summer Admissions

DESCRIPTION

2802 DYSTONIA

Covers these related disorders: Dopa-responsive dystonia (DRD) or Segawa syndrome, Drug-induced dystonia, Dystonia musculorum deformans (DMD) or torsion, Fecal dystonia

Involves the following Biologic System(s):
Neurologic Disorders, Orthopedic and Muscle Disorders

Dystonia is a neurologic movement disorder characterized by relatively slow, involuntary, writhing motions that may result in twisting or distorted posturing of affected muscles. The abnormal motions associated with dystonia result from unusually increased muscle rigidity due to simultaneous contractions of certain muscles termed agonists and antagonists. In unaffected individuals, when voluntary movements occur, there are usually coordinated contractions and simultaneous relaxations of several muscles. Muscles known as agonists are primarily responsible for producing a particular movement, and other muscles, called synergists, contract to assist the agonist muscles. While these muscles contract, other muscles known as antagonists normally simultaneously relax, helping to ensure smooth rather than jerky, uncoordinated motions. However, in patients with dystonia, agonist and antagonist muscles simultaneously contract, resulting in abnormally distorted movements. Depending upon the form of dystonia present, abnormal motions may vary greatly in severity and may be limited to one muscle group or may affect many muscles of the body, causing severely distorted postures and significantly interfering with activities of daily living.

Dystonias that are limited to certain specific muscle groups may be referred to as focal dystonias. Focal dystonias may be confined to muscles of the neck (cervical dystonia or spasmodic torticollis); the eyelids, causing near or complete closure of the eyelids (blepharospasm) and functional blindness; the mouth and jaw (buccomandibular dystonia); the hand (writer's cramp); or certain other areas of the body. Although such conditions are considered the most prevalent forms of dystonia, they occur much more commonly in adults than children. The main causes of dystonia during childhood include certain genetic disorders, such as dystonia musculorum deformans, dopa-responsive dystonia, Wilson disease, or Hallervorden-Spatz disease; lack of oxygen during labor, delivery, or immediately after birth (perinatal asphyxia), causing brain damage (hypoxicischemic encephalopathy); or exposure to particular medications.

The most pronounced form of dystonia is observed in a group of genetic disorders known as dystonia musculorum deformans (DMD) or torsion dystonia. One form of the disorder is thought to most commonly affect individuals of Eastern European Ashkenazi Jewish descent. Symptoms typically become apparent between the ages of six to 14 years and initially include involuntary movement or posturing of one area of the body, particularly the foot. Most patients first experience abnormal periodic bending of one foot with the toes downward (plantar flexion), potentially causing tip-toe walking. Such posturing of the foot gradually becomes constant, and muscles in other areas of the body, such as the shoulders, pelvis, and spine, begin to develop periodic, involuntary, spasmodic, twisting movements. With disease progression,

spasms become frequent and, eventually, are ongoing, causing contortion and severely distorted posturing of affected muscles. Although dystonic movements may initially subside during sleep, they may eventually be present at all times, severely restricting activities of daily living and causing a high level of functional disability. Treatment may include administration of the drug trihexyphenidyl or certain other medications, such as carbamazepine, bromocriptine, levodopa, or diazepam.

Dopa-responsive dystonia (DRD), also known as Segawa syndrome, is a genetic disorder that is thought to be transmitted as an autosomal dominant trait. The disorder more commonly affects females and usually becomes apparent between four to eight years of age. Initial symptoms often include periodic, involuntary stiffening and abnormal posturing of the foot. As the disease progresses, dystonia may also eventually affect muscles of the arms, torso, and, in some patients, the neck. Within about four to five years, all areas of the body are usually affected. Some patients may also have unusually slow movements (bradykinesia) and involuntary, rhythmic movements (tremors) of certain muscles while at rest. Symptoms usually subside with sleep and gradually worsen during the day. Administration of the medication levodopa, a biological forerunner or precursor of the neurotransmitter dopamine, typically causes a dramatic improvement of symptoms.

Wilson disease is an autosomal recessive disorder in which copper metabolism causes an abnormal accumulation of copper in the liver, brain, kidneys, corneas, and other tissues of the body. The disorder is often characterized by progressive liver disease, degenerative changes of the brain, kidney failure, and the presence of characteristic grayish-green or reddish-gold rings at the outer margins of the corneas (Kayser-Fleischer rings). Neurologic symptoms, which rarely become apparent before age 10, are thought to result from progressive involvement of a region of the brain that assists in regulating muscular movements (basal ganglia). Such symptoms usually initially include progressive dystonia that is characterized by abnormalities of muscle tone, muscle stiffness and rigidity, muscle spasms, and abnormal movement patterns and fixed postures, such as a fixed smile due to drawing back of the upper lip. Patients also experience involuntary, rhythmic, quivering movements of the extremities on one side of the body (unilateral) that eventually become generalized and disabling. The treatment of patients with Wilson disease often consists of administration of penicillamine, a medication that binds with copper and enables it to be excreted from the body; supplementation of vitamin B6; and a diet that is low in copper intake (less than one mg/day).

Hallervorden-Spatz disease is a rare autosomal recessive disorder characterized by an abnormal accumulation of iron pigment in certain areas of the brain. Symptoms usually develop during childhood and may include progressive dystonia characterized by muscle stiffness, rigidity, and relatively slow, involuntary, twisting and distorted posturing of affected muscles. By adolescence, patients may have restricted movements of certain muscles due to increased muscle rigidity (spasticity); an inability to coordinate voluntary movements (ataxia); difficulty speaking (dysarthria); and progressive confusion, disorientation, and deterioration of intellectual abilities (dementia). The treatment of patients with Hallervorden-Spatz disease is symptomatic and supportive.

In some children, the administration of certain drugs may

cause a sudden (acute) development of dystonia, such as certain antiseizure (anticonvulsant) medications or antipsychotic drugs (phenothiazines). In addition, particular medications may cause acute or chronic progressive dystonia, such as the antiseizure medications phenytoin or carbamazepine, or the antipsychotic drug haloperidol. Treatment may include the withdrawal of the offending drug and intravenous administration of the medication, diphenhydramine.

Depending upon its underlying cause or specific form, treatment measures for chronic dystonia may include the administration of certain medications (anticholinergic agents), such as trihexyphenidyl or ethopropazine. These drugs inhibit the transmission of particular nerve impulses to muscles.|In addition, focal dystonias such as dystonia limited to muscles of the neck (cervical dystiodic torticollis), are often treated with periodic injections of botulin (botulinum toxin) into affected muscles. Botulin is a bacterial toxin that blocks the release of a particular neurotransmitter (acetylcholine), resulting in temporary paralysis and thus relief from discomfort and disability associated with muscle rigidity.

Government Agencies

2803 NIH/National Institute of Neurological Dis orders and Stroke (NINDS)
PO Box 5801
Bethesda, MD 20824
301-496-5751
800-352-9424
Fax: 301-496-0296
TTY: 301-468-5981
www.ninds.nih.gov

Supports and conducts research and research training on the normal structure and function of the nervous system and on the causes, prevention, diagnosis and treatment of nervous system disorders including stroke, epilepsy, multiple sclerosis, Parkinson's disease, head and spinal cord injury, Alzheimer's disease and brain tumors.

Walter J. Koroshetz, MD, Director

National Associations & Support Groups

2804 American Academy of Pediatrics
141 Northwest Point Boulevard
Elk Grove Village, IL 60007
847-434-4000
800-433-9016
Fax: 847-434-8000
www.aap.org

The American Academy of Pediatrics and its member pediatricians are committed to the attainment of optimal physical, mental and social health and well-being for all infants, children, adolescents, and young adults.

Fernando Stein, MD, FAAP, President
Karen Remley, MD, CEO/Executive VP

2805 American Speech Language Hearing Associati on (ASHA)
2200 Research Boulevard
Rockville, MD 20852
301-296-5700
800-638-8255
Fax: 301-571-0457
pr@asha.org
www.asha.org

Works to promote a better quality of life for children and adults with communication disorders. Part of their mission is to advance knowledge about the causes and treatment of hearing, speech, and language problems.

Arlene A Pietranton, Executive Director

2806 Dystonia Medical Research Foundation
One E Wacker Drive, Suite 2810
Chicago, IL 60601
312-755-0198
800-377-3978
Fax: 312-803-0138
dystonia@dystonia-foundation.org/
www.dystonia-foundation.org

The mission of the Dystonia Medical Research Foundation is to advance research for more treatments and ultimately a cure; to promote awareness and education; and to support the needs and well being of affected individuals and families.

Janet Hieshetter, Executive Director
Art Kessler, President

2807 Genetic Alliance
4301 Connecticut Avenue NW, Suite 404
Washington, DC 20008
202-966-5557
800-336-4363
Fax: 202-966-8553
info@geneticalliance.org
www.geneticalliance.org

A coalition of voluntary genetic support groups, consumers and professionals addressing the needs of individuals and families affected by genetic disorders from a national perspective.

Sharon Terry, President/CEO
Tetyana Murza, Managing Director
Natasha Bonhomme, VP, Strategic Development

2808 March of Dimes Foundation
1275 Mamaroneck Avenue
White Plains, NY 10605
914-997-4488
888-663-4637
Fax: 914-997-4763
answers@marchofdimes.com
www.marchofdimes.com

Partnership of volunteers and professionals dedicated to improving the health of babies by preventing birth defects and infant mortality. Over 100 chapters are located across the country and can be located through the National Office.

Stacey D. Stewart, President

2809 Muscular Dystrophy Association
3300 E Sunrise Drive
Tuscon, AZ 85718
520-529-2000
800-572-1717
Fax: 520-529-5300
mda@mdausa.org
www.mda.org

Voluntary health agency aimed at conquering nueromuscular diseases that affect more than 1,000,000 Americans. The diseases in MDA's program include nine forms of muscular dystrophy, amyotrophic lateral sclerosis (Lou Gehrig's disease), spinal muscular atrophy, Charcot-Marie-Tooth disease and other neuromuscular conditions. With nearly 200 offices across the country, MDA conducts research, medical and community services, clinics, support groups, summer camp for youngsters and much more.

Jennifer Lopez, Assoc. Director of Health Care Svcs

2810 National Spasmodic Torticollis Association
9920 Talbert Avenue, Suite 233
Fountain Valley, CA 92708
714-378-9837
800-487-8385
Fax: 714-378-7830
NSTAmail@aol.com
www.torticollis.org

Nonprofit organization, providing support, referrals and information for ST patients and family members.

Justin Aqunies, Executive Director

2811 WE MOVE (Worldwide Education and Advocacy Movement Disorders)
204 W 84th Street
New York, NY 10024
212-875-8312
800-437-6682
Fax: 212-875-8389
wemove@wemove.org
www.wemove.org

WE MOVE provides movement disorder information and educational materials to physicians, patients, the media, and the public via its comprehensive Web sites training courses, and more. It's goal is to make early diagnosis, up-to-date treatment and patient support a reality for all people living with movement disorders.

Susan Bressman MD, President

Research Centers

2812 Benign Essential Blepharospasm Research Foundation
637 N 7th Street, Suite 102, PO Box 12468
Beaumont, TX 77726 409-832-0788
Fax: 409-832-0890
bebrf@blapharospasm.org
www.blepharospasm.org

The purpose of BEBRF is to undertake, promote, develop and carry on the search for the cause and a cure for benign essential blepharospace and other related disorders and infirmities of the facial musculature.

Mary Lou Thompson, President
Glynda Lucas, First Vice President

2813 Dystonia Medical Research Foundation
One E Wacker Drive, Suite 2810
Chicago, IL 60601 312-755-0198
800-377-3978
Fax: 312-803-0138
dystonia@dystonia-foundation.org/
www.dystonia-foundation.org

The mission of the Dystonia Medical Research Foundation is to advance research for more treatments and ultimately a cure; to promote awareness and education; and to support the needs and well being of affected individuals and families.

Janet Hieshetter, Executive Director
Art Kessler, President

Conferences

2814 ASHA Convention
American Speech-Language-Hearing Association
2200 Research Boulevard
Rockville, MD 20850 301-296-5700
800-638-8255
Fax: 301-571-0457
productsales@asha.org
www.asha.org

The premier annual professional education event for speech-language pathologists, audiologists, and speech, language, and hearing scientists. Bringing together more than 12,000 attendees, the Convention provides unparalleled opportunities to hear the latest evidence-based research and gain new skills and resources to advance your career.

November

Arlene A Pietranton, Executive Director
Maureen E Thompson, Director Governance Operations

2815 Genetic Alliance Annual Conference
Genetic Alliance
4301 Connecticut Avenue NW, Suite 404
Washington, DC 20008 202-966-5557
800-336-4363
Fax: 202-966-8553
info@geneticalliance.org
www.geneticalliance.org

Consistently inspirational and enables partnership among all stakeholders: advocates and community leaders, health and industry professionals, policymakers, and academicians.

July

Sharon Terry, President/CEO
Tetyana Murza, Managing Director
Natasha Bonhomme, VP, Strategic Development

2816 Jake's Ride for Dystonia Research
The Bachmann-Strauss Dystonia Parkinson Foundation
PO Box 38016
Albany, NY 12203 212-509-0995
www.dystonia-parkinsons.org

Jake's Ride for Dystonia Research began in 2007, when a young boy named Jake Silverman was diagnosed with early onset childhood dystonia. After hearing Jake's story, a neighbor and father of one of Jake's classmates, David Gardner, came up with the idea to create a bike ride that would raise awareness and needed funds for this disorder.

Web Sites

2817 American Speech Language Hearing Associati on (ASHA)
2200 Research Boulevard
Rockville, MD 20850 301-296-5700
800-498-2071
Fax: 301-296-8580
TTY: 301-296-5650
nsslha@asha.org
www.asha.org

An organization working to promote a better quality of life for children and adults with communication disorders. Our mission is to advance knowledge about the causes and treatments of hearing, speech, and language problems.

Judith L. Page, PhD, CCC-SLP, President
Howard Goldstein, PhD, CCC-SLP, VP for Science & Research
Arlene A. Pietranton, PhD, CAE, CEO

2818 Dystonia Medical Research Foundation
One East Wacker Drive, Suite 2810
Chicago, IL 60601 312-755-0198
800-377-3978
Fax: 312-803-0138
dystonia@dystonia-foundation.org
www.dystonia-foundation.org

Dedicated to serving people with dystonia, a neurological disorder. The goals of the the Foundation is to advance research into the causes of and treatments for dystonia; to build awareness of dystonia in both the medical and lay communities; and to sponsor patient and family support groups and programs.

Samuel Belzberg, Chairman/ Founder
Art Kessler, President
Richard A. Lewis, MD, VP of Science

2819 Muscular Dystrophy Association
222 S. Riverside Plaza, Suite 1500
Chicago, IL 60606 800-572-1717
mda@mdausa.org
www.mda.org

Voluntary health agency aimed at conquering nueromuscular disease that affect more than 1 million Americans.

Olin F. Morris, Chair
Christopher J. Rosa, PhD., Vice Chair
Steven M. Derks, President & CEO

2820 NIH/National Institute of Neurological Dis orders and Stroke (NINDS)
www.ninds.nih.gov

Supports and conducts research and research training on the normal structure and function of the nervous system and on the causes, prevention, diagnosis and treatment of nervous system disorders including stroke, epilepsy, multiple sclerosis, Parkinson's disease, head and spinal cord injury, Alzheimer's disease and brain tumors.

Walter J. Koroshetz, MD, Director

2821 National Spasmodic Torticollis Association
9920 Talbert Avenue
Fountain Valley, CA 92708 714-378-9837
800-487-8385
NSTAmail@aol.com
www.torticollis.org

Nonprofit organization, providing support, referrals and information for ST patients and family members.

313

Ken Price, President/ Treasurer
Diane Truong, Vice President
Justin G. Aquines, Executive Director

2822 Online Mendelian Inheritance in Man
U.S. National Library of Medicine, 8600 Rockville
Bethesda, MD 20894   888-346-3656
                                              info@ncbi.nlm.nih.gov
                                              www.ncbi.nlm.nih.gov

This database is a catalog of human genes and genetic disorders.

Christine E. Seidman, M.D., Chair
David J. Lipman, M.D., Executive Secretary
Michael Boehnke, Ph.D., Board Member

2823 WE MOVE (Worldwide Education and Advocacy Movement Disorders)
www.wemove.org

WE MOVE provides movement disorder information and educational materials to physicians, patients, the media, and the public via its comprehensive Web sites training courses, and more. It's goal is to make early diagnosis, up-to-date treatment and patient support a reality for all people living with movement disorders.

Newsletters

2824 Benign Essential Blepharospasm Research Foundation Newsletter
PO Box 12468
Beaumont, TX 77726   409-832-0788
                                              Fax: 409-832-0890
                                              bebrf@blepharospasm.org
                                              www.blepharospasm.org

BEBRF Focus for 2006: Twenty-five years of hope, and progress.

12 pages Bimonthly

Mary Lou Thompson, President
Glynda Lucas, First Vice President

2825 Dystonia Dialogue
Dystonia Medical Research Foundation
One East Wacker Drive, Suite 2810
Chicago, IL 60601   312-755-0198
                                              800-377-3978
                                              Fax: 312-803-0138
                                              dystonia@dystonia-foundation.org
                                              www.dystonia-foundation.org/

The official publication of the Dystonia Medical Research Foundation. Provides information to individuals with dystonia, their families, health care professionals, and supporters of the foundation.

Quarterly

Samuel Belzberg, Chairman/ Founder
Art Kessler, President
Richard A. Lewis, MD, VP of Science

Pamphlets

2826 DMRF/NINDS Dystonia Workshop: From Gene to Function in Dystonia
National Inst. of Neurological Disorders/Stroke
PO Box 5801
Bethesda, MD 20824   301-496-5751
                                              800-352-9424
                                              www.ninds.nih.gov

Health Disparities: Working Group-Cognitive and Emotional Health in Minority Children Workshop.

Dr. Story Landis, Director
Alan L. Wlliard, PhD, Deputy Director
Caroline Lewis, Executive Officer

2827 Dytonias: Fact Sheet
National Inst. of Neurological Disorders/Stroke
PO Box 5801
Bethesda, MD 20824   301-496-5751
                                              800-352-9424
                                              www.ninds.nih.gov

Fact Sheet listing the following contents: What are the Dystonias, What are the symptoms, How are the Dystonias classified, What do scientists know about the Dystonias, When do symptoms occur, Are their any treatments, What research is being done, Where can I get more information.

Dr. Story Landis, Director
Alan L. Wlliard, PhD, Deputy Director
Caroline Lewis, Executive Officer

2828 NINDS Seeks Patients with Generalized Dystonia
National Inst. of Neurological Disorders/Stroke
PO Box 5801
Bethesda, MD 20824   301-496-5751
                                              800-352-9424
                                              www.ninds.nih.gov

NINDS program announcements, requests for applications and clinical studies seeking patients.

Dr. Story Landis, Director
Alan L. Wlliard, PhD, Deputy Director
Caroline Lewis, Executive Officer

2829 Patients with Cervical or Focal Hand Dystonia Sought
National Inst. of Neurological Disorders/Stroke
PO Box 5801
Bethesda, MD 20824   301-496-5751
                                              800-352-9424
                                              karpb@ninds.nih.gov
                                              www.ninds.nih.gov

NINDS program announcements, requests for applications and clinical studies seeking patients.

Dr. Story Landis, Director
Alan L. Wlliard, PhD, Deputy Director
Caroline Lewis, Executive Officer

DESCRIPTION

2830 EATING DISORDERS

Synonyms: Anorexia Nervosa, Bulimia Nervosa, Binge Eating Disorder

Involves the following Biologic System(s):

Developmental/Behavioral/Psychiatric Disorders

There are two major types of eating disorders — Anorexia Nervosa and Bulimia Nervosa. A third category, according to the American Psychiatric Association (APA), is termed Eating Disorders Not Otherwise Specified (EDNOS) and includes Binge Eating Disorder. Although different in the symptoms they manifest, the three disorders are quite similar in their underlying pathology: disturbed eating patterns and dysfunctional attitudes toward food, eating, and body shape. Primary features of eating disorders are compulsive behavior, loss of control, and continuing behavior despite negative consequences. Genetic and environmental factors appear to be at the root of eating disorders, although exact mechanisms remain unknown. Eating disorders occur more frequently in females; males are also affected, but are less likely than females to be daignosed with an eating disorder. The median age range for the onset of eating disorders is between ages 8 and 21, although they can begin earlier or later in life.

There are numerous psychosocial consequences of eating disorders (e.g. problems with family, friends, school, or work; lowered perceived happiness). Eating disorders may cause grave physical damage, so treatment first involves restoring patients to a safe and healthy body weight. Once out of physical danger, patients undergo a long-term process that includes medication and psychotherapy. Fortunately, most people who undergo appropriate treatment do recover from eating disorders.

An orexia Nervosa is diagnosed when a person refuses to maintain a body weight at or above 85 percent of their normal weight. Patients have an intense fear of gaining weight or becoming fat, despite being underweight. They are disturbed by the way their body weight or shape is experienced, give it undo influence, and deny the seriousness of low body weight. Patients with anorexia nervosa may be severely depressed and may experience insomnia and irritability. In menstruating females, anorexia may disrupt normal menstrual cycles. More than 10 percent of those diagnosed with the disorder die from it. Death typically is caused by starvation, suicide, or electrolyte imbalance.

Individuals with Bulimia Nervosa eat large amounts of food in a short time. Guilt and fear then cause them to get rid of the food by vomiting (purge) or by other means, including periods of fasting, misuse of laxatives and diuretics, use of enemas, and excessive exercise. Individuals with bulimia nervosa typically are of normal or higher than normal weight. Medical consequences of bulimia nervosa include potentially dangerous fluid and electrolyte imbalances, nutritional deficiencies, menstrual and other reproductive system irregularities. Rare but potentially fatal complications include esophageal tears, gastric rupture from purging, cardiac arrhythmia, tooth decay (due to stomach acid), swollen face and throat, dizziness, blackouts, constant upset stomach, constipation, sore throat and damage to vital organs such as the liver and kidneys.

Binge Eating Disorder causes a loss of control of eating. Unlike bulimia nervosa, periods of binge eating are not followed by purging, excessive exercise, or fasting. Those affected do experience guilt, shame, and distress about their binge eating, which can lead to more binge eating. As a result, people with binge eating disorder often are over-weight or obese and are at a higher risk for developing type 2 diabetes, high blood pressure, high cholesterol, stroke, certain cancers, osteoarthritis, liver and gallbladder disease, abnormal menstrual cycles and infertility.

Related disorders include dieting and restrictive eating, which are characterized by a preoccupation with the need to lose weight. Children with these issues weigh themselves frequently, engage in fad diets, and are unreasonably restrictive about food intake. This behavior pattern is unrelated to the affected child's body weight. Being on a diet is the common denominator for those suffering from disordered eating, which, taken to the extreme, can lead to serious health problems.

The restrictive eating child is often called a picky eater, cutting out certain foods or food groups (i.e. meat). Since these children have normal appetites, their eating behavior is often considered a way of exerting control over the adults in their lives, which frequently leads to emotional struggles. Because of social pressure to be thin, parents and other adults sometimes succumb tochildren's controlling eating behavior.

Orthorexia is an unhealthy fixation on eating only healthy or pure foods. Like anorexia nervosa, orthorexia is rooted in food restriction. Orthorexics focus on the quality of food, while anorexics focus on the quantity. Orthorexics typically do not fear gaining weight in the way anorexics would, but the obsessive and progressive nature of the disorder is similar. Typical behavior is avoidance of anything processed, like white flour and sugar, food considered unpure, or food that someone else has prepared. This constant preoccupation causes an extreme amount of anxiety. Individuals suffering from orthorexia may eliminate entire groups of food from their diets in the quest for a perfectly clean, healthy diet. In severe cases, orthorexia may lead to malnourishment.

Eating disorders are a pervasive problem in our communities, states, country and around the world. They cross gender, racial, and socioeconomic barriers and the problem is worsening. In the United States approximately 10 percent of girls and women (numbering up to 10 million) and 1 million boys and men are struggling with eating disorders. According to the Journal of the American Dietetic Association, 81 percent of 10 year olds are afraid of being fat, 51 percent of 9 and 10 year old girls feel better about themselves if they are on a diet, and 35 percent of normal dieters progress to unhealthy dieting. At least 50,000 individuals will die each year as a direct resultof an eating disorder.

Prevalence studies in adolescent females show rates of 0.5 to one percent for anorexia nervosa, and one to three percent for bulimia nervosa. Binge eating disorder affects far more boys than either anorexia or bulimia; more than one-third of compulsive over eaters are men. Patients rarely seek treatment, and family members will often intervene. A multidisciplinary approach to treatment is essential. Medications, especially SSRIs (Selective Serotonin Reuptake Inhibitors), which were originally developed as antidepressants have been found to be very effective in the treatment of eating disorders. They

315

can help restore and build self-esteem, and thereby help the patient maintain a positive attitude as well as a safe and healthy body image and body weight. Because of the physical damage that eating disorders can create, nutritional counseling and monitoring is often vital to restore and maintain proper body weight. Hospitalization is often indicated in anorexia, especially if the patient is more than 20 percent below normal body weight. Restoration of fluids and chemicals in the blood (electrolytes) is critical. Outpatient management for anorxia also includes a supervised weight-gain program. The prognosis for patients with bulimia is better than that for patients with anorexia and they are more likely to seek treatment. Eating disorders are extremely complex, and patients often have conflicting psychological issues that trigger the compulsion to binge, and the morbid fear of gaining weight. Psychotherapy and cognitive behavior therapy may be required for a number of years.

Government Agencies

2831 NIH/National Institute of Mental Health Eating Disorders Program
Public Information and Communications Branch
6001 Executive Boulevard, Room 8184, MSC 9663
Bethesda, MD 20892
301-443-4513
866-615-6464
Fax: 301-443-4279
TTY: 301-443-8431
nimhinfo@nih.gov
www.nimh.nih.gov

A nonprofit organization developed to coordinate nationwide mental health screening programs and to ensure cooperation, professionalism, and accountability in mental illness screenings.

Joshua A. Gordon, MD, PhD, Director
Shelli Avenevoli, PhD, Deputy Director
Phyllis Quartey-Ampofo, Public Liaison Director

2832 National Institute of Diabetes and Digesti ve and Kiney Diseases
1 WIN Way
Bethesda, MD 20892
877-946-4627
Fax: 202-828-1028
win@info.niddk.nih.gov
www.win.niddk.nih.gov

WIN provides the general public with up-to-date, science-based information on obesity, weight control, physical activity, and related nutritional issues.

2833 Substance Abuse and Mental Health Services Administration
1 Choke Cherry Road
Rockville, MD 20857
977-726-4727
www.samhasa.gov

SAMHSA is directed by Congress to target effectively substance abuse and mental health services to the people most in need and to translate research in these areas more effectively and rapidly into the general health care system.

Pamela S. Hyde, JD, Administrator
Marla Hendrikson, MPM, Director

2834 The National Women's Health Information Ce nter
200 Independence Avenue
Washington, DC 20201
202-690-7650
800-994-9662
Fax: 202-205-2631
www.womenshealth.gov

The Office on Women's Health provides national leadership and coordination to improve the health of women and girls through policy, education and model programs.

National Associations & Support Groups

2835 Academy of Nutrition and Dietetics
120 South Riverside Plaza, Suite 2000
Chicago, IL 60606
312-899-0040
800-877-1600
amacmunn@eatright.org
www.eatright.org

The Academy of Nutrition and Dietetics is the worlds's largest organization of food and nutrition professionals. The academy is committed to improving the nation's health and advancing the profession of dietetics through research, education and advocacy.

2836 Alliance for Eating Disorder Awarenes
1649 Forum Place #2
West Palm Beach, FL 33401
561-841-0900
866-662-1235
info@allianceforeatingdisorders.com
www.allianceforeatingdisorders.com/

The Alliance is dedicated to providing programs and activities aimed at outreach and education related to health promotion, including all eating disorders, obesity, positive body image, and self-esteem.

Johanna Kandel, Founder and CEO
Joann Hendelman, Clinical Director
Sharon Glynn, Director of Programming

2837 American Academy of Pediatrics
141 Northwest Point Boulevard
Elk Grove Village, IL 60007
847-434-4000
800-433-9016
Fax: 847-434-8000
www.aap.org

The American Academy of Pediatrics and its member pediatricians are committed to the attainment of optimal physical, mental and social health and well-being for all infants, children, adolescents, and young adults.

Fernando Stein, MD, FAAP, President
Karen Remley, MD, CEO/Executive VP

2838 American Psychiatric Association
1000 Wilson Boulevard, Suite 1825
Arlington, VA 22209
703-907-7300
888-35 -7924
apa@psych.org
www.psychiatry.org

It is a medical specialty society representing growing membership of more than 36,000 psychiatrists.

2839 American Psychological Association
750 First St. NE
Washington, DC 20002
202-336-5500
800-374-2721
TTY: 202-336-6123
www.apa.org

The mission is to advance the creation, communication and application of psychological knowledge to benefit society and improve people's lives.

Norman B. Anderson, PhD, CEO/ EVP
L. Michael Honaker, PhD, Deputy Chief Executive Officer
Ellen G. Garrison, PhD, Senior Policy Advisor

2840 American Public Health Association
800 I Street, NW
Washington, DC 20001
202-777-2742
Fax: 202-777-2534
TTY: 202-777-2500
www.apha.org

APHA champions the health of all people and all communities. They aim to strengthen the public health profession and speak out for public health issues and policies backed by science.

Georges C. Benjamin, MD, Executive Director
Kemi Oluwafemi, MBA, CPA, Chief Financial Officer
Susan Polan, PhD, Associate Executive Director

2841 American School Counselor Association
1101 King Street, Suite 310
Alexandria, VA 22314
703-683-2722
800-306-4722
Fax: 703-997-7572
asca@schoolcounselor.org
www.schoolcounselor.org

The mission of ASCA is to represent professional school counselors and to promote professionalism and ethical practices.

Richard Wong, Executive Director
Jeff Broderson, Information Technology Admin.
Kathleen M Rakestraw, Director of Communications

2842 Anorexia Nervosa & Related Eating Disorders
Box 5102
Eugene, OR 97405
541-344-1144
jarinor@rio.com
www.anred.com

A national nonprofit organization that provides free and low-cost information about anorexia, bulimia, compulsive eating and compulsive exercising. Offers a free booklet as well as brochures, fact sheets and a monthly newsletter.

J Bradley Rubel, President

2843 Association for Size Diversity and Health
PO Box 3093
Redwood City, CA 94064
877-576-1102
www.sizediversityandhealth.org

The mission of the Association for Size Diversity and Health (ASDAH) is to promote education, research, and the provision of services which enhance health and well-being, and which are free from weight-based assumptions and weight discrimination.

Fall Ferguson, President
Jennifer Copeland, Vice-President
Janell Mensinger, Secretary

2844 Association of Professionals Treating Eating Disorders
www.aptedsf.org
415-771-3068
AptedSF@aol.com
www.aptedsf.org

The Association is a 501(c)(3) Non-Profit organization, designed to support prevention and recovery from eating disorders, through education, referrals, and direct service.

Pamela Brody, Board Member
Lisa Groesz, Board Member
Brittany Kipp, Board Member

2845 BeyondHunger
P.O. Box 151148
San Rafael, CA 94915
415-459-2270
info@beyondhunger.org
beyondhunger.org

Beyond Hunger is a non-profit organization dedicated to helping individuals overcome the obsession with food and weight and find a natural, loving and peaceful relationship with their food, weight, and selves.

Vikki A. Adams, Esq., Board President
Laurelee Roark, Co-founder
Cindy Soriano, Board Treasurer

2846 Binge Eating Disorder Association
637 Emerson Place
Severna Park, MD 21146
855-855-2332
Fax: 410-741-3037
bedaonline.org

It recognises the need for an organization to advocate on behalf individuals affected by binge eating disorder (BED) and the providers who treat them.

Wendy Oliver-Pyatt, Chair
Ralph Carson, Vice-Chair of Scientific Affairs
Theresa Chesnut, Board Member

2847 CEDAR Associates
67 South Bedford Road
Mount Kisco, NY 10549
914-244-1904
Fax: 914-472-4019
info@cedarassociates.com
www.cedarassociates.com

CEDAR Associates is a multi-disciplinary private group practice for the treatment of a full range of mental health issues for individuals and their family. CEDAR Associates specializes in the prevention and treatment of eating disorders and the problems that often accompany them including depression, self-harm, anxiety, relational issuel, sexual and physical trauma and body image issues.

Judy Scheel, Ph.D., LCSW, Executive Director

2848 Change for Good Coaching
Change for Good Coaching
3801 Connecticut Avenue NW, Ste 100 D
Washington, DC 20008
202-656-3801
Fax: 433-645-2420
brockhansenlcsw@aol.com
www.change-for-good.org/

Change for Good Coaching provides services to individuals that are designed to: help an individual to clarify their goals; helping an individual to craft an action plan, and, support the individual in following through to their own satisfaction. Interested individuals can contact Change for Good Coaching for a free complimentary telephone coaching session.

Brock Hansen, Owner

2849 Community Outreach for Prevention of Eating Disorders
PO BOX 128
Flagler Beach, FL 32136
www.cope-ecf.org

The mission is to eliminate eating disorders, promote widespread positive body image, and raise public awareness of how to influence both.

2850 Compulsive Eaters Anonymous
5500 E Atherton Street, Suite 227-B
Long Beach, CA 90815
562-342-9344
Fax: 562-342-9346
gso@ceahow.org
www.ceahow.org

Purpose is to stop eating compuslively and carry the message to those that still suffer.

Rosie Knieling, Manager
N Woody, President

2851 Council on Size and Weight Discrimination (CSWD)
PO Box 305
Mount Marion, NY 12456
845-679-1209
Fax: 845-679-1206
info@cswd.org
www.cswd.org

Works to influence public policy and opinion in an effort to eliminate oppression and discrimination based on body size, shape, or weight standards. Projects include International No Diet Coalition. Publications: Annotated Bibliography on Size Acceptance, Anti-Dieting, Eating Disorders and Related Issues, book. International No Diet Coalition Directory of Resources, books.

Miriam Berg, President
Lynn McAfee, Medical Advocacy Director

2852 Eating Disorder Anonymous EDA, Inc.
PO Box 55876
Phoenix, AZ 85078
info@eatingdisordersanonymous.org
www.eatingdisordersanonymous.org

Eating Disorders Anonymous is a fellowship of individuals who share their experience, strength and hope that with each other, they may solve their common problems and help others to recover from their eating disorders.

2853 Eating Disorder Hope
www.eatingdisorderhope.com
888-206-1175
www.eatingdisorderhope.com

The mission is to offer hope, information and resources to individual eating disorder sufferers, their family members and treatment providers.

Jacquelyn Ekern, Founder & Director
Baxter Ekern, Vice President
Jane McGuire, Executive Assistant

2854 Eating Disorder Recovery Support
925 Lakeville Street, Suite 217
Petaluma, CA 94952   855-588-3377
                                  www.edrs.net

Barbara Birsinger, Board Member
Bridget Whitlow, Board Member
Joe Kelly, Board Member

2855 Eating Disorders Coalition
PO Box 96503-98807
Washington, DC 20090   202-543-9570
             manager@eatingdisorderscoalition.org
             www.eatingdisorderscoalition.org

The Eating Disorders Coalition is the advocacy organization for eating disorders. We advance the recognition of eating disorders as a public health priority at the federal and state level.

Katherine Swain McClayton, Director
Ken Weiner, Director
Kitty Westin, Director

2856 Eating Disorders Group
Renfrew Center
11 East 36th Street
New York, NY 10016   800-736-3739
                                  Fax: 212-686-1865
                                  www.renfrew.org/

Women struggling to overcome anorexia, bulimia or other disordered eating patterns involving binge eating or restricting can benefit from these weekly groups. Led by experienced therapists, the sessions provide a safe, sympathetic atmosphere where group members explore what triggers their eating disorders as well as issues concerning body image, relationships, school, work and home.

Jane Fleming, Executive Director

2857 Eating Disorders Information Network
3600 Dallas Hwy, Ste 230-237
Marietta, GA 30064   404-816-3346
                                  info@myedin.org
                                  www.myedin.org

The mission is to make it easier for people with eating disorders to find help. EDIN's mission was also to reduce the stigma of eating disorders and offer hope to sufferers through stories of recovery in a monthly newsletter.

Amanda Blackmon, Board Member
Laura Glover, Board Member
Allison Powers, Board Member

2858 Eating Disorders Research Society
2111 Chestnut Ave. Suite 145
Glenview, IL 60025   847-666-5920
                                  info@edresearchsociety.org
                                  www.edresearchsociety.org

The purpose of the organization is to hold an annual scientific meeting during which the most recent research in the field can be presented and discussed.

Nadia Micali, President
Scott Crow, Secretary/Treasurer
Kathleen Pike, President - Elect

2859 Eating Disorders and Education Network
www.edenprocess.com

                                  734-476-0278
                                  edenclub@aol.com
                                  www.edenprocess.com

An eating disorder recovery group that can be accessed online or in person for those seeking healthy, positive recovery support and education from eating disorder behaviors (anorexia, bulimia, and binge/ emotional overeating).

Dwight Carlson, Chairman
Alice Grisham, President & Secretary
Lida Athearn, Vice President

2860 Focus On Recovery-United
100 Riverview Center, Suite 272
Middletown, CT 6457   860-704-0556
                                  Fax: 860-704-0767
                                  focusonrecovery@gmail.com
                                  www.focusonrecovery.org

It is a non-profit peer support program staffed entirely by paid and volunteer peers envisions a statewide network of peer-provided recovery education and support opportunities for adults (18 and older) in Connecticut.

Heather McDonald-Bellamy, Executive Director
Paul D. Acker, Assistant Executive Director
Donna Duda, Office Manager

2861 Food Addicts Anonymous
World Service Office
4623 Forest Hill Boulevard, #109-4
West Palm Beach, FL 33415   561-967-3871
                                  Fax: 561-967-9815
                                  info@foodaddictsanonymous.org
                                  www.foodaddictsanonymous.org

A 12-step fellowship of men and women who are willing to recover from the disease of food adiction. Primary purpose is to maintain abstinence from sugar, flour, and wheat. Information and referral, pen pals, online contacts, conferences. Assistance in starting groups.

Linda Closy, Manager

2862 H.O.P.E.: Helping Other People Eat
P.O. Box 2271
Orlando, FL 32802   321-231-0791
                                  AllisonKreiger@yahoo.com
                                  www.hopetolive.com

It is a 501c3 nonprofit organization focused on the prevention and awareness of eating disorders.

Allison Kreiger Walsh, Founder
Elise Kashmiry, Interim Executive Director
Deborah Kreiger, Vice President

2863 International Association of Eating Disorders Professionals
PO Box 1295
Pekin, IL 61555   309-346-3341
                                  800-800-8126
                                  Fax: 390-346-2874
                                  www.iaedp.com

The International Association of Eating Disorders Professionals provides first-quality education and high-level training standards to an international multidisciplinary group of various healthcare treatment providers and helping professions, who treat the full spectrum of eating disorder problems.

Shirley Klein, Executive Director
Emmett R Bishop, MD/CEDS, Board-Directors President
Mary Bellafatto, MA/LMHC/CEDS, Board-Directors Secretary

2864 Klaman Eating Disorders Center at McLean Hospital
McClean Hospital
115 Mill Street
Belmont, MA 02478   617-855-2000
                                  800-333-0338
                                  mcleaninfo@mclean.harvard.edu
                                  www.mclean.harvard.edu/patient/child/edc.php

Founded with the generous support of the Klarman Family Foundation, the Klarman Eating Disorders Center at Harvard-affiliated McLean Hospital provides state-of-the-art treatment for eating disorders in girls and young women ages 13 to 23. Housed in its own newly renovated building on the grounds of McLean, the Center provides a unique therapeutic environment that is conducive to recovery.

Esther Dechant, MD, Medical Director
Patricia Tarbox, LICSW, Program Director

2865 Largesse, The Network for Size Esteem
PO Box 9404
New Haven, CT 06534   203-787-1624
                                      Fax: 203-787-1624
                                 size_esteem@yahoo.com

International clearinghouse for organizations and people concerned with weight-based bias. Acts as a support and information
resource for people and groups who promote size esteem and oppose discrimination based on weight. Seeks 'the empowerment of
all women, regardless of size or shape' and develops educational
and support materials. Publications: The Fat Underground, book.
Legal Resource Kit. Room to Grow, poetry of size. Size Esteem,
periodical.

Richard K Stimson, Co-Director
Karen W Stimson, Co-Director

2866 Maudsley Parents
www.maudsleyparents.org

                               contact@maudsleyparents.org
                               www.maudsleyparents.org

We are a volunteer organization of parents who have helped our
children recover from anorexia and bulimia through the use of
Family-Based Treatment, also known as the Maudsley approach,
an evidence-based therapy for eating disorders.

Harriet Brown, Board Member
Rina Ranalli, Board Member
Ann Farine, Board Member

2867 McCallum Place
615 S New Ballas Road
Saint Louis, MO 63141   314-968-1900
                                           800-828-8158
                                      Fax: 314-968-1901
                                 www.mccallumplace.com/

McCallum Place provides comprehensive medical and psychiatric
care, specialized psychotherapies and nutritional support for patients with eating disorders. Our state-of-the-art treatment and
programs, which integrate the latest findings from eating disorders research with experienced clinical practice, are designed to
create an environment of structure and support.

Kimberli McCallum, MD, Medical Director
Lynn Stark, Program Director
Shannon Shelley, Marketing/Community Outreach

2868 Mental Fitness, Inc.
339 E. 19th Street, 2B
New York, NY 10003   www.mentalfitnessinc.org

The mission of mentalfitness, inc. is to build mental fitness in all
youth through arts-based awareness and prevention programs.

Robyn Hussa Farrell, Founder & CEO
Jamie Levine, Project Coordinator
Jacob Burman, Program Outreach Director

2869 National Association for Males with Eating Disorders (The)
164 Palm Dr. #2
Naples, FL 34112   namedinc.org

It is a nationwide professional association committed to leadership in the field of male eating disorders. We aim to provide support for males affected by eating disorders, provide access to
collective expertise, and promote the development of effective
clinical intervention and research in this population.

LEIGH COHN, President
ANDREW WALEN, Vice President
STUART MURRAY, Co-director

2870 National Association of Addiction Treatmemt Professionals
11380 ProsperityFarms Road, Suite 209A
Palm BeachGardens, FL 33410   561-429-4527
                                      Fax: 561-429-4650
                                      nkasper@naatp.org
                                           www.naatp.org

The mission is to provide leadership, advocacy, training and other
member support services to assure the continued availability and
highest quality of addiction treatment.

Nate Kasper, Director of Operations
Dwayne Beason, Board Member
Rob Waggener, Board Member

**2871 National Association of Anorexia Nervosa and Associated
Disorders (ANAD)**
750 E Diehl Road #127, PO Box 7
Naperville, IL 60563   847-831-3438
                                      Fax: 847-433-4632
                                      anadhelp@anad.org
                                           www.anad.org

Sponsors national and local programs to prevent eating disorders
and assist people with eating disorders and their families. Provides a national clearinghouse of information and is a grassroots
association for laypeople and professionals. It operates a national
network of free support groups for people with eating disorders
and their families, and provides prevention information and
education to students and lecturers.

Vivian Hanson Meehan, President

2872 National Association to Advance Fat Acceptance (NAAFA)
P.O. Box 4662,
Foster City, CA 94404   916-558-6880
                                           800-442-1214
                                      Fax: 415-863-8596
                                      naafa@naafa.org
                                              naafa.org

Nonprofit organization dedicated to improving the quality of life
for fat people. Opposes discrimination against fat people including discrimination in advertising, employment, fashion, medicine,
insurance, social acceptance, the media, schooling and public accommodations. Monitors legislative activity and litigation affecting fat people. Publications: NAAFA Newsletter, bimonthly.
Annual conference and symposium, always mid-August.

Maryanne Bodoky, Executive Director
Marilyn Wann, Activism Chair

2873 National Center for Overcoming Overeating
Old Chelsea Station, PO Box 1257
New York, NY 10113   212-875-0442
                               webmaster@overcomingovereating.com
                                      OvercomingOvereating.com

The National Center for Overcoming Overeating is an educational
and training organization working to end body hatred and dieting.
It was started in 1989 by Carol Munter and Jane Hirschmann, authors of Overcoming Overeating and When Women Stop Hating
Their Bodies.

Carol Munter, Co-Founder
Jane Hirschmann, Co-Founder

2874 National Eating Disorders Association (NED A)
603 Stewart Street, Suite 803
Seattle, WA 98101   206-382-3587
                                           800-931-2237
                               info@NationalEatingDisorders.org
                               www.nationaleatingdisorders.org

The National Eating Disorders Association (NEDA) is the largest
not-for-profit organization in the United States working to prevent eating disorders and provide treatment referrals to those suffering from anorexia, bulimia and binge eating disorder and those
concerned with body image and weight issues. Formerly known
as The American Anorexia Bulimia Association.

Lynn S Grefe, Ceo
Lynn S Grefe, Chief Executive Officer
Tonia Brown, Program Coordinator

2875 Overeaters Anonymous, World Service Office
PO Box 44020
Rio Rancho, NM 87174   505-891-2664
                                      Fax: 505-891-4320
                                           info@oa.org
                                              www.oa.org

Overeaters Anonymous is a 12-step program dealing with food
and compulsie overeating. There are no fees or dues. The only requirement for membership is the desire to stop eating compulsively. Call the World Service Office for a location near you.

Jack Finley, Chairman
Naomi Lippel, Managing Director
Sarah Armstrong, Associate Director

2876 Residential Eating Disorders Consortium
555 8th Avenue, Suite 1902
New York, NY   646-553-1340
                                    info@residentialeatingdisorders.org
                                    www.residentialeatingdisorders.org

The mission is to serve as a professional association of residential eating disorder treatment providers.

Jillian Lampert, President
Vicki Kroviak, Vice-President
Kim Dennis, Secretary

2877 Rewrite Beautiful
www.rewritebeautiful.org

                                    beautifulaction@RewriteBeautiful.org
                                    www.rewritebeautiful.org

Rewrite Beautiful creatively changes how girls see beauty in themselves for eating disorder prevention through education. We equip girls to use their creative skills to positively impact their communities.

Kate Besch, President
Rebecca Arnett, Vice President
Eileen Risbeck, Treasurer

2878 River Centre Foundation
rivercentrefoundation.org

                                    419-517-7551
                                    rivercentrefoundation.org

2879 Screening for Mental Health
One Washington Street, Suite 304
Wellesley Hills, MA 2481   781-239-0071
                                    Fax: 781-431-7447
                                    smhinfo@mentalhealthscreening.org
                                    mentalhealthscreening.org

It envisions a world where mental health is viewed and treated with the same gravity as physical health.

Douglas Jacobs, Founder & Medical Director

2880 T-FFED (Trans Folx Fighting Eating Disorders)
www.transfolxfightingeds.org

                                    TransFolxFightingEDs@gmail.com
                                    www.transfolxfightingeds.org

It is a collective of trans/gender diverse folx and allies who believe eating disorders in marginalized communities are social justice issues. The mission is to make visible, interrupt, and undermine the disproportionately high incidence of eating disorders in trans and gender-diverse individuals through radical community healing, recovery institution reform, empowerment and education.

2881 TOPS Club
4575 South 5th Street
Milwaukee, WI 53207   414-482-4620
                                    800-932-8677
                                    Fax: 414-482-1655
                                    topsinteractive@tops.org
                                    www.tops.org

Weight control self-help association using group dynamics, competition and recognition to help members lose weight. TOPS is medically oriented requiring physician-approved individual diet programs and physician-set weight goals. Publications: TOPS News, monthly, a magazine that contains member news, success stories, inspirational materials and features on diet-related subjects, chapter news, medical questions and answers. Annual International Recognition Days.

Beatrice Miller, Executive Director
Barb Cady, President/Officers
Ahmed Kissebah, MD/Ph.D/FACP, Medical Advisor

2882 The Body Positive
P.O. Box 7801
Berkeley, CA 94707   510-528-0101
                                    Fax: 510-558-0979
                                    info@thebodypositive.org
                                    www.thebodypositive.org

It teaches people how to overcome conflicts with their bodies to lead happier, more productive lives.

Adam Davis, Board Member
Jessica Diaz, Board Member
Kelle Jacobs, Board Member

2883 We Insist on Natural Shapes (WINS)
PO Box 19938
Sacramento, CA 95819   800-600-9467
                                    winsnews@aol.com
                                    winsnews.org

Nonprofit organization educates about normal, healthy shapes in recognizing that the shape of one's body is determined by one's genes. Genetic makeup determines healthy weight, whether it be thin or heavy, and a moderate amount of balanced food, with a moderate amount of exercise will allow one to achieve her/his natural, healthy shape.

June Preston, Executive Director
Mary Jane Ray, Committee Chair
Serena Ryder, RD, Board-Directors President

State Agencies & Support Groups

Connecticut

2884 Renfrew Center of Connecticut
475 Spring Lane
Philadelphia,, PA 19128   203-834-1635
                                    877-367-3383
                                    Fax: 215-482-2695
                                    info@renfrewcenter.com
                                    www.renfrewcenter.com

The Renfrew Center of Connecticut provides an Eating Disorders Group led by experienced therapists the sessions of which provide a safe, sympathetic atmosphere where group members explore what triggers their eating disorders as well as issues concerning body image, relationships, school, work and home. A therapeutic approach that allows women to recognize and confront negative thoughts and feelings about their bodies and to replace them with realistic and healthy views about themselves is used.

Douglas W Bunnell, Executive Director
Gayle Brooks, Ph.D, Clinical Director

Florida

2885 Coconut Creek Eating Disorders Support Group
Renfrew Center
7700 Renfrew Lane
Coconut Creek, FL 33073   954-698-9222
                                    800-736-3739
                                    Fax: 954-698-9007
                                    info@renfrewcenter.org
                                    www.renfrewcenter.com/locations/coconut-creek.asp

The Coconut Creek Eating Disorders Support Group at the Renfrew Center is led by experienced therapists where the sessions provide a safe, sympathetic atmosphere in which group members explore what triggers their eating disorders as well as issues concerning body image, relationships, school, work and home.

Jane Fleming, Executive Director
Gayle Brooks, Ph.D, Clinical Director

2886 Renfrew Center of Miami
151 Majorca Avenue
Coral Gables, FL 33134   800-736-3739
                                    Fax: 605-445-2779
                                    info@renfrewcenter.org
                                    www.renfrewcenter.com/locations/coral-gables.asp

The Renfrew Center of Miami provides an Eating Disorders Group led by experienced therapists the sessions of which provide a safe, sympathetic atmosphere where group members explore what triggers their eating disorders as well as issues concerning body image, relationships, school, work and home.

Jane Fleming, Executive Director
Gayle Brooks, Ph.D, Clinical Director

Illinois

2887 Academy for Eating Disorders (AED)
Ste 100
Deerfield, IL 60015
847-498-4274
Fax: 847-480-9282
info@aedweb.org
www.aedweb.org/index.cfm

The Academy for Eating Disorders is an international transdisciplinary professional organization that promotes excellence in research, treatment and prevention of eating disorders. The AED provides education, training and a forum for collaboration and professional dialogue.

Sally Finney, Executive Director
Eric Van Furth, Ph.D, President/Officers Board
Judith Banker, Treasurer

Maryland

2888 Center for Eating Disorders
Saint Josephs Medical Center
Physicians Pavilion North, Ste 300
Baltimore, MD 21204
410-938-5252
Fax: 410-938-5250
EatingDisorderInfo@sheppardpratt.org
www.eatingdisorder.org

At the Center for Eating Disorders, the staff focuses on each patient's personal needs and works with him or her to gain new confidence and coping skills. The center offers a full spectrum of services in a supportive environment.

Harry A Brandt, MD, Executive Director
Steven Crawford, MD, Associate Director
David Roth, Ph.D, Program Coordinator

Massachusetts

2889 Massachusetts Eating Disorder Association (MEDA)
92 Pearl Street
Newton, MA 02458
617-558-1881
Fax: 617-558-1771
info@medainc.com
www.medainc.org

MEDA is a non-profit organization dedicated to the prevention and treatment of eating disorders and disordered eating. MEDA's mission is to prevent the continuing spread of eating disorders through educational awareness and early detection. MEDA serves as a support network and resource for clients, loved ones, clinicians, educators and the general public.

100+ Members

Beth Mayer, Executive Director
Aiden Winslow, Assistant Director
Kristin Fabbri, Education/Outreach Director

New Jersey

2890 Eating Disorders Association of New Jersey
10 Sation Place, Suite 15
Metuchen, NJ 08840
732-549-6886
800-522-2230
Fax: 609-688-1544

Eating Disorders Association of New Jersey is dedicated to the study, prevention and treatment of eating disorders: anorexia nervosa, bulimia nervosa and binge eating disorder. We are a non-profit organization that provides education and support services in New Jersey to individuals affected by eating disorders, including sufferers, family members, friends, educators, and therapists.

Leigh Garfield, LCSW, President
Maureen Kritzer Lange, LCSW, Support Group Coordinator

2891 Renfrew Center of Northern New Jersey
174 Union Street
Ridgewood, NJ 07450
201-652-5114
Fax: 201-652-6253
info@renfrewcenter.org
www.renfrewcenter.com

A weekly group that helps women overcome compulsive overeating and make positive lifestyle changes. The group focuses on the needs of the participants and may include looking deeper at culture, family and self within a sympathetic and safe atmosphere.

Jane Fleming, Executive Director
Gayle Brooks, Ph.D, Clinical Director

New York

2892 Metro Intergroup of Overeaters Anonymous
PO Box 1235
New York, NY 10159
212-946-4599
NYOAMetroOffiice@yahoo.com
www.oanyc.org/oanyc/

Overeaters Anonymous offers a program of recovery from compulsive overeating using the Twelve Steps and Twelve Traditions of OA. Worldwide meetings and other tools provide a fellowship of experience, strength and hope where members respect one another's anonymity. OA charges no dues or fees; it is self-supporting through member contributions.

Naomi Lippel, Managing Director
Sarah Armstrong, Associate Director
Joi Young, Web Coordinator

2893 National Eating Disorders Association-Long Island (NEDA-LI)
50 Charles Lindbergh Blvd
Uniondale, NY 11553
516-237-6200

NEDA LI is a non-profit organization devoted to prevention, education and support: prevention of eating disorders, education about eating disorders and support to sufferers of eating disorders, their families and their friends. The organization is comprised of professionals who specialize in eating disorders including psychiatrists, psychologists, social workers, counselors and nutritionists.

Sondra Kronberg, MS/RD/CDN, Executive Director
Vivian Delman, MS/RD/CDN, Board-Directors President
Irene Schlagman, CEDA, Board-Directors Secretary

2894 Overeaters Anonymous Support Group
Holliswood Hospital
87-37 Palermo Street
Holliswood, NY 11423
718-776-8181
800-486-3005
Fax: 718-716-8572
HolliswoodInfo@libertymgt.com
www.holliswoodhospital.com/

The Holliswood Hospital, a 110-bed private psychiatric hospital located in a quiet residential Queens community, is a leader in providing quality, acute inpatient mental health care for adult, adolescent, geriatric and dually diagnosed patients. Services include an Overeaters Anonymous Support Group.

Alan Eskenazi, CEO
Dr. Douglas ÿ Munsey, Medical Director
Dr. John Udarbe, Adult Unit Chief

2895 Renfrew Center of New York City
11 East 36th Street
New York, NY 10016
212-685-6856
800-736-3739
Fax: 212-686-1865
info@renfrewcenter.org
www.renfrewcenter.com

Women struggling to overcome anorexia, bulimia or other disordered eating patterns involving binge eating or restricting can benefit from these weekly groups. Led by experienced therapists, the sessions provide a safe, sympathetic atmosphere where group members explore what triggers their eating disorders as well as issues concerning body image, relationships, school, work and home.

Gail Purvis, Manager
Gayle Brooks, Clinical Director

2896 Westchester Center for Eating Disorders
14 Rolling Way
New Rochelle, NY 10804   914-633-7654
                                                    Fax: 914-633-7349

Program and support group for individuals struggling with eating disorders.

Ann L Rothstein, Manager

Oregon

2897 Rainrock Treatment Center
1863 Pioneer Parkway, Suite 304 (Mailing Only)
Springfield, OR 97477   541-896-9300
                                                    Fax: 541-896-9320
                                                    mntc@montenido.com
                                                    www.montenido.com/rainrock/

Rainrock is a private residential treatment center designed and created by Annie Laughlin and Carolyn Costin to heal women suffering from anorexia, bulimia, and exercise addiction. RainRock, an affiliate of the Monte Nido Treatment Center in Malibu, California, opened in Summer 2006. It is located on four beautifully maintained acres along the McKenzie River just outside Eugene, Oregon with an ideal therapeutic environment for self-reflection, personal growth, and healing.

Carolyn Costin, LMFT, Founder/Executive Director
Annie Lauglin, Founder/Program Coordinator
Anthony Laughlin, Founder/Program Administrator

Pennsylvania

2898 Pennsylvania Chapter of the American Anorexia Bulimia Association
4200 Monument Avenue, PO Box 1287
Philadelphia, PA 19105   215-221-1864
                                                    mail.aabaphila@yahoo.com
                                                    www.aabaphila.org/

The American Anorexia / Bulimia Association of Philadelphia (American Anorexia and Bulimia (AABAP), is non-profit, providing services and programs for anyone interested in or affected by, Anorexia, Bulimia and/or related disorders. Its purpose is to aid in the education and prevention of these life threatening disorders. AABAP is a member organization of the Eating Disorders Coalition.

Samuel A Menaged, Board-Directors President EDC

2899 Pennsylvania Educational Network for Eating Disorders (PENED)
801 McKnight Rd., RM 205
Pittsburgh, PA 15237   412-215-7967
                                                    Fax: 412-487-6850
                                                    pened1@aol.com
                                                    www.pened.org/

PENED is a non-profit organization providing educational, supportive and referral services to the general and professional public on the causes, treatment, and prevention of eating disorders and related issues.

Anita Sinicrope-Maier, MSW, Executive Director

2900 Renfrew Center of Bryn Mawr
735 Old Lancaster Road
Bryn Mawr, PA 19010   800-736-3739
                                                    Fax: 610-527-9361
                                                    info@renfrewcenter.org
                                                    www.renfrewcenter.com/locations/bryn-mawr.asp

Support group for women to overcome compulsive overeating and make positive lifestyle changes. Focuses on the needs of the participants and may include looking deeper at culture, family and self within a sympathetic and safe atmosphere. Led by experienced therapists, sessions provide safe, sympathetic atmosphere where women in midlife faced with new stresses such as divorce, empty-nest syndrome,'chronic illness or career changes come together to explore what triggers their eating disorders.

Jane Fleming, Executive Director
Gayle Brooks, Clinical Director

2901 Renfrew Center of Philadelphia
475 Spring Lane
Philadelphia, PA 19128   215-482-5353
                                                    800-736-3739
                                                    Fax: 215-482-7390
                                                    info@renfrewcenter.org
                                                    www.renfrewcenter.com/locations/location.asp?id=2

Women struggling to overcome anorexia, bulimia or other disordered eating patterns involving binge eating or restricting can benefit from this weekly group. Led by experienced therapists, the sessions provide a safe, sympathetic atmosphere where group members explore what triggers their eating disorders as well as issues concerning body image, relationships, school, work and home.

Sam Menaged, President
Gayle Brooks, Clinical Director

2902 University of Pennsylvania Weight and Education Program
3535 Market Street, Suite 3108
Philadelphia, PA 19104   215-898-7314
                                                    Fax: 215-898-2878
                                                    weight@uphsnet.med.upenn.edu
                                                    www.med.upenn.edu/weight/

The Center for Weight and Eating Disorders was founded by Albert J. Stunkard, M.D., over 45 years ago to better understand the causes of weight and weight-related disorders. The Center continues to conduct a wide variety of studies on the causes and treatment of weight-related disorders. More recently, the Center for Weight and Eating Disorders has begun to offer professional services to the general public rather than only to participants in research studies.

Dr. Albert Stunkard, Founder
Thomas A Wadden, Ph.D, Director

Libraries & Resource Centers

2903 Alliance for Eating Disorders Awareness
1649 Forum Place #10
West Palm Beach, FL 33401   561-841-0900
                                                    866-662-1235
                                                    info@eatingdisorderinfo.org
                                                    www.allianceforeatingdisorders.com

The Alliance was created as a source of community outreach, education, awareness, and prevention of the various eating disorders spreading across the nation. Their aim is to share the message that recovery from these disorders is possible, and that individuals should not have to suffer or recover alone.

2904 Association of Gastrointestinal Motility Disorders
AGMD International Corporate
12 Roberts Drive
Bedford, MA 01730   781-275-1300
                                                    Fax: 781-275-1304
                                                    digestive.motility@gmail.com
                                                    www.AGMD-GIMOTILITY.org

Support and education for persons affected by digestive motility disorders. Serves as educational resource and information base for medical professionals. Physician referrals, video tapes, educational materials, networking support, symposiums, and several publications.

Mary-Angela De Grazia, President
Thomas Abell, MD, Advisory Board Member
Vijay Arya, MD, Advisory Board Member

2905 Families Empowered and Supporting Treatmen t of Eating Disorders
PO Box 331
Warrenton, VA 20188   540-227-8518
                                                    info@feast-ed.org
                                                    www.feast-ed.org

F.E.A.S.T. is an international organization of and for parents and caregivers to help loved ones recover from eating disorders by providing information and mutual support, promoting evidence-based treatment, and advocating for research and education to reduce the suffering associated with eating disorders.

2906 National Eating Disorder Association of Lo ng Island (NEDA-LI)
50 Charles Lindbergh Blvd, Suite 400
Uniondale, NY 11553   516-222-4990
Fax: 516-414-6322
www.edap.org/p.asp?WebPage_ID=717

The National Eating Disorders Association (NEDA) was formed in 2001, when Eating Disorders Awareness & Prevention (EDAP) joined forces with the American Anorexia Bulimia Association (AABA). NEDA LI is a non-profit organization devoted to prevention, education and support: prevention of eating disorders, education about eating disorders and support to sufferers of eating disorders, their families and their friends.

John Marrah, Ceo
Susan Morin, NPP, Board-Directors Vice President
Sondra Kronberg, MS/RD/CDN, Executive Director

Research Centers

2907 Center for the Research and Treatment of Anorexia Nervosa
UCLA Neuropsychiatric Institute
760 Westwood Plaza
Los Angeles, CA 90024   310-825-9822
800-825-1192
research.ucla@yahoo.com
www.wpic.pitt.edu/research/angenetics/contact.html

Appointed to the faculty of the department of psychiatry at the UCLA School of Medicine in 1975, Michael Strober, Ph.D., now holds the rank of full professor, and is director of the eating disorders program and the adolescent mood disorders program at the UCLA Neuropsychiatric Institute and Hospital. Dr. Strober's primary research activities center on the long-term course and outcome, psychopathology and genetics of eating disorders.

Michael Strober, Ph.D, Program Director

2908 Center for the Study of Anorexia and Bulimia
1841 Broadway @ 60th Street, 4th Floor
New York, NY 10023   212-333-3444
Fax: 212-333-5444
Info@csabnyc.org
www.csabnyc.org/

The Center for the Study of Anorexia and Bulimia was established as a division of the Institute for Contemporary Psychotherapy in 1979 and is the oldest non-profit eating disorders clinic in New York City. Using an eclectic approach, the professional staff and affiliates are on the cutting edge of treatment in their field. The treatment staff includes social workers, psychologists, registered nurses and nutritionists, all with special training in the treatment of eating disorders.

Jill M Pollack, LCSW/BCD, Executive Director

2909 Eating Disorders Research and Treatment Program
Michael Reese Hospital and Medical Center
4510 Executive Drive, Suite 315
San Diego,, CA 92121   858-534-8019
Fax: 858-534-6727
edresearch@ucsd.edu
www.eatingdisorders.ucsd.edu/

Michael Reese Hospital maintains a full spectrum psychiatric care for children, adolescents and adults including inpatient hospitalization for acute psychiatric cases as well as an intensive outpatient program for individuals in need of ongoing support, including that of eating disorders.

Regina Casper, Director
Enrique Beckman, MD, Chairman/CEO

2910 New York Obesity Research Center
Saint Luke's-Roosevelt Hospital
1090 Amsterdam Avenue, 14th Floor
New York, NY 10025   212-523-3622
Fax: 212-523-3571
katmarquez@chpnet.org
www.nyorc.org/

The mission of the New York Obesity Research Center is to help reduce the incidence of obesity and related diseases through leadership in basic research, clinical research, epidemiology and public health, patient care, and public education.

Dr. Xavier Pi-Sunyer, MD/MPH, Director
Richard Weil, M.Ed/CDE, Exercise Physiologist
Betty Kovac, MS/RD, Dietitian

Conferences

2911 CEA-HOW Annual Global Convention
Compulsive Eaters Anonymous
3371 Glendale Boulevard,Suite 104
Los Angeles, CA 90039   323-660-4333
Fax: 323-660-4334
gso@ceahow.org
www.ceahow.org
July

2912 FAA World Convention
Food Addicts Anonymous
529 N W Prima Vista Blvd. Suite 301 A
Port St. Lucie, FL 34983   561-967-3871
Fax: 561-967-9815
faawso@bellsouth.net
www.foodaddictsanonymous.org
September

Linda Closy, Manager

2913 IAEDP Symposium
Int'l Assoc of Eating Disorders Professionals Foun
PO Box 1295
Pekin, IL 61555   309-346-3341
800-800-8126
Fax: 390-346-2874
www.iaedp.com

Draws attendees from all corners of the globe. Geared to the needs and problems of those who work with patients in a therapeutic environment.
March

2914 NAAFA Annual Convention
National Association to Advance Fat Acceptance
PO Box 4662
Foster City, CA 94404   916-558-6880
800-442-1214
Fax: 415-863-8596
naafa@naafa.org
www.naafa.org
August

Maryanne Bodoky, Executive Director
Marilyn Wann, Activism Chair

2915 NEDA Annual Conference
National Eating Disorders Association
603 Stewart Street, Suite 803
Seattle, WA 98101   206-382-3587
800-931-2237
info@NationalEatingDisorders.org
www.nationaleatingdisorders.org

Brings together people in recovery, their families and professionals.
October

Lynn S Grefe, CEO

Audio Video

2916 Bulimia
Baxley Media Group
510 West Main Street
Urbana, IL 61801   217-384-4838
Fax: 217-384-8280
baxley@baxleymedia.com
www.baxleymedia.com/

Award-winning video presentation explores the causes and effects of bulimia. Addresses the fact that many high school and college women view this type of behavior as routine aspect of their everyday lives.

Videotape

Carolyn Baxley, President

2917 Eating Disorder Video
Library Video
PO Box 580
Wynnewood, PA 19096
610-645-4000
800-843-3620
Fax: 610-645-4040
comments@libraryvideo.com
www.libraryvideo.com

Features compelling interviews with several young people who have suffered from anorexia nervosa, bulimia and compulsive eating. Discusses the treatments, causes, and techniques for prevention with field experts.

2918 Inside Out: Stories of Bulimia
Fanlight Productions
32 Court Street, 21st Floor
Brooklyn, NY 11201
718-488-8900
800-876-1710
Fax: 718-488-8642
info@fanlight.com, orders@fanlight.com
www.fanlight.com

Bulimia can affect women and men from all walks of life, and it kills nearly 20 percent of its victims every year. This moving documentary profilesindividuals and families affected by this eating disorder. ISBN: DVD: 1-57295-856-1; VHS: 1-57295-366-7

56 minutes DVD or VHS

Ben Achtenberg, President
Sandy St. Louis, Marketing Director
Nicole Johnson, Publicity Coordinator

2919 It Only Takes One Bite: Food Allergy and Anaphylaxis
Food Allergy Network
7925 Jones Branch Dr., Suite 1100
McLean, VA 22102
703-691-3179
800-929-4040
Fax: 703-691-2713
faan@foodallergy.org
www.foodallergy.org/

Nonprofit organization dedicated to bringing about a clearer understanding of the issues surrounding food allergies and providing helpful resources. Explains food induced anaphylaxis and how to live with it. An excellent resource for training parents, teachers, caregivers and patients.

18 mins.

Janet Atwater, Chair
Robert Nichols, Vice Chair
James R. Baker, Jr., MD, CEO & Chief Medical Officer

Web Sites

2920 Anorexia Nervosa and Related Eating Disorders
www.anred.com

We are a nonprofit organization that provides information about anorexia nervosa, bulimia nervosa, binge eating disorder, and other less-well-known food and weight disorders. Our material includes self-help tips and information about recovery and prevention.

2921 Eating Disorders Online.com: 15 Styles of Distorted Thinking
www.eatingdisordersonline.com/specific/disthink.php

Reference useful for cognitive therapy.

2922 Food Allergy Network
7925 Jones Branch Dr., Suite 1100
McLean, VA 22102
703-691-3179
800-929-4040
Fax: 703-691-2713
www.foodallergy.org

Mission is to raise public awareness, to provide advocacy and education, and to advance research on behalf of all those affected by food allergies and anaphylaxis.

Janet Atwater, Chair
Robert Nichols, Vice Chair
James R. Baker, Jr., MD, CEO & Chief Medical Officer

2923 Gurze Bookstore
www.bulimia.com
888-920-1501
www.bulimia.com

Specializes in information about eating disorders including anorexia nervosa, bulimia nervosa, and binge eating, plus related topics such as body image and obesity. We offer books at discounted prices, many free articles about eating disorders, newsletters, links to treatment facilities, organizations, other websites and much more.

2924 Health Answers
410 Horsham Road
Horsham, PA 19044
215-422-9010
Michael.tague@healthanswers.com
www.healthanswers.com

HealthAnswers offers a breadth of services in medical education, sales force training, patient support, solutions, professional promotion and consumer solutions.

Michael Tague, Managing Director

2925 Mental Help Net- Eating Disorders
P.O. Box 20709
Columbus, OH 43220
614-448-4055
800-232-TALK
info@centersite.net, editor@centersite.n
www.mentalhelp.net/guide/eating.htm

We wish to provide the following: to discuss, develop and debate in an open forum the future of the mental health field in America and throughout the world. To help coordinate various components of the mental health field, so as to bring about greater communication between them and to educate the public about mental health issues.

2926 Mirror, Mirror
www.mirror-mirror.org/eatdis.htm

Helps with eating disorders, like how to get help, myths and realities, other websites, and about recovery.

Scott Mogul, Director
Dr. Lauren Muhlheim, Clinical Director
Dr. Elisha Carcieri, Editor

2927 National Association for Anorexia Nervosa and Associated Disorders (ANAD)
750 E Diehl Road #127
Naperville, IL 60563
630-577-1330
anadhelp@anad.org
www.anad.org

We provide hotline counseling, a national network of free support groups, referrals to healh care professionals, and education and prevention programs to promote self-acceptance and health lifesyles. All of our services are free of charge. ANAD also lobbies for state and national health insurance parity, undertakes and encourages advocacy campaigns to protect potential victims of eating disorders. ANAD stands with individuals and families and helps them win.

Patricia Santucci, MD, President
Kimberly Dennis, MD, Member, Scientific & Medical Board
Nomi Fredricks, MD, Member, Scientific & Medical Board

2928 Something Fishy
www.something-fishy.org

Dedicated to raising awareness, emphasizing always that Eating Disorders are NOT about food and weight, they are just the symptoms of something deeper going on, inside. We are determined to remind each and every sufferer that they are not alone, and that complete recovery is possible.

Book Publishers

2929 Anorexia Nervosa & Recovery: A Hunger for Meaning
The Haworth Press
10 Alice Street
Binghamton, NY 13904
607-771-0012
800-895-0582
getinfo@haworthpress.com
www.haworthpress.com/

Anorexia Nervosa and Recovery lets the reader hear the personal struggles of women who have fought this powerful disease. They describe how anorexia controlled their lives and how, once they overcame their obsessions with food, weight, and thinness, they were able to lead fulfilling lives.
1993 142 pages Paperback
ISBN: 0-918393-95-7

William Cohen, President/Publisher
Al Horowitz, Chief Financial Officer
Sandra Jones Sickels, VP Marketing

2930 Billy's Story
Overeaters Anonymous World Service Office
PO Box 44020
Rio Rancho, NM 87174
505-891-2664
Fax: 505-891-4320
info@oa.org
www.oa.org/

An inspirational story written for younger children suffering from eating disorders and weight problems.

Naomi Lippel, Managing Director
Sarah Armstrong, Associate Director
Rebbie Garza, Board Administrator

2931 Body Betrayed
Gurze Books
5145 B Avenida Encinas, PO Box 2238
Carlsbad, CA 92008
760-434-7533
800-756-7533
Fax: 760-434-5476
leigh@gurze.net
www.gurze.com

Covers the most important aspects of diagnosis and treatment for eating disorders. Particularly appropriate for parents and loved ones who want a deeper, more thorough understanding of eating disorders.
447 pages Paperback

Kathryn J Zerbe, Author
Leigh Cohn, Publisher
Lindsey Hall Cohn, Editor in Chief

2932 Bulimia Nervosa & Binge Eating: A Guide to Recovery
New York University Press
838 Broadway, Third Floor
New York, NY 10003
212-998-2575
800-996-6987
Fax: 212-995-3833
information@nyupress.org
www.nyupress.nyu.edu

Book offers guidance and advice for the understanding of the eating disorder bulimia and inspiring hope for change and regaining control of one's life.
1995 170 pages
ISBN: 0-814715-23-0

Steve Maikowski, Director
Ilene Kalish, Executive Editor
Eric Zinner, Editor-in-Chief

2933 Bulimia: A Guide to Recovery
Gurze Books
5145 B Avenida Encinas, PO Box 2238
Carlsbad, CA 92008
760-434-7533
800-756-7533
Fax: 760-434-5476
leigh@gurze.net
www.gurze.com

This intimate guidebook offers a complete understanding of bulimia and a plan for recovery. Contains updated information from previous editions, and has added material on men and bulimia, sexual trauma, body image, relationships and much more.
285 pages Paperback

Lindsey Hall, Author
Leigh Cohn, Author

2934 Conversation with Anorexics: A Compassionate & Hopeful Journey
Rowman & Littlefield Publisher
4501 Forbes Blvd, Suite 200
Lanham, MD 20706
301-459-3366
Fax: 301-429-5748
custserv@rowman.com
www.rowmanlittlefield.com/aronsonp/

Book is a collection of case studies on anorexia more aptly geared toward the professional as it does not provide guidance but more of an overview on the treatment of the eating disorder.
1994 238 pages Paperback
ISBN: 1-568212-61-5

Jonathan Sisk, Publisher
Christopher Anzalone, Washington Editor
Jack Meinhardt, Acquisitions Editor

2935 Coping with Eating Disorders
Rosen Publishing Group
29 East 21st Street
New York, NY 10010
212-777-3017
800-237-9932
Fax: 888-436-4643
rosenpub@tribeca.ios.com
www.rosenpublishing.com/

This book offers practical suggestions on coping with eating disorders, explaining how to set positive goals, and briefly discusses where to go for additional help.
ISBN: 0-823929-74-4

Miriam Gilbert, Sales and Marketing Director

2936 Cult of Thinness
Oxford University Press
198 Madison Avenue
New York, NY 10016
212-726-6000
800-445-9714
Fax: 919-677-1303
custserv.us@oup.com
www.oup.com/usa

Examining the testimonies of young women concerning the practice of body rituals, the author Hesse-Biber observes the extent to which these women sacrifice their bodies and minds to the pursuit of the ultra-slender ideal. Hesse-Biber provides new frameworks for envisioning femininity and personal power, overcoming body insecurity, strengthening the inner self, and changing the cultural environment itself.
1996 256 pages
ISBN: 0-195178-78-5

Joan Bossert, Psych/Behavioral Sciences Editor
Catharine Carlin, Health Psychology Editor

2937 Deadly Diet: Recovering From Anorexia and Bulimia
New Harbinger Publications
5674 Shattuck Avenue
Oakland, CA 94609
510-652-0215
800-748-6273
Fax: 800-652-1613
customerservice@newharbinger.com
www.newharbinger.com

This book provides the reader with a great discussion of the use of cognitive-behavioral therapy in the treatment of eating disorders. The author also provides the reader with a step-by-step guide to implementing this approach in his or her own life during recovery from an eating disorder.
1993 248 pages Paperback
ISBN: 1-879237-42-3

Matthew McKay, Ph.D, Publisher
Earlita Chenault, Publicist

2938 Do I Look Fat in This?: Life Doesn't Begin Five Pounds From Now
Simon & Schuster Free Press
866 3rd Avenue
New York, NY 10022
877-989-0009
Fax: 800-943-9831
www.simonsays.com

For any woman who has bonded with a stranger by complaining about how fat she feels, here is a thoughtful and inspiring guide to breaking the cycle of body criticism and creating a powerful and healthy self-image.

2006 200 pages
ISBN: 1-416913-57-2

Jack Romanos, President/CEO
David England, SVP/Chief Financial Officer
Anne Lloyd Davies, SVP/Chief Information Officer

2939 Eating Disorder Sourcebook
Gurze Books
5145 B Avenida Encinas, PO Box 2238
Carlsbad, CA 92008
760-434-7533
800-756-7533
Fax: 760-434-5476
leigh@gurze.net
www.gurze.com

This third edition is a welcomed revision and update of this popular reference guide for both the lay public and professionals.

328 pages Paperback

Carolyn Costin, Author

2940 Eating Disorders
Thomson Gale
PO Box 95501
Chicago, IL 60694
800-877-4253
Fax: 800-414-5043
gale.galeord@cengage.com
www.gale.com/lucent/index.htm

This book examines how eating disorders can be identified, who is affected by them, and how they can be treated.

1991
ISBN: 1-560061-29-4

Andrew Becker, Director
John Barnes, EVP Strategic Business Development

2941 Eating Disorders & Obesity, 2nd Ed.
Guilford Press
72 Spring Street
New York, NY 10012
212-431-9800
800-365-7006
Fax: 212-966-6708
info@guilford.com
www.guilford.com

Presents and integrates virtually all that is currently known about eating disorders and obesity in one authorative, accessible, and eminently practical volume. A comprehensive handbook for medical and social service professionals. Hard- or paperback.

2005 633 pages Paperback
ISBN: 1-593852-36-8

Robert Matloff, President
Seymoure Weingarten, Editor-in-Chief
Marian Robinson, Marketing Director

2942 Eating Disorders Resource Catalogue
Gurze Books
5145 B Avenida Encinas, PO Box 2238
Carlsbad, CA 92008
760-434-7533
800-756-7533
Fax: 760-434-5476
leigh@gurze.net
www.gurze.com/

This catalogue of resources contains over 140 books, videos, and audiotapes, lists of national organizations and treatment facilities, and basic facts about eating disorders. It is widely distributed by individuals who are suffering, their loved-ones, the health care professionals who treat them, and educators who are working towards prevention.

24 pages Annually

Lindsey Hall, Editor in Chief
Leigh Cohn, Publisher

2943 Eating Disorders: When Food Turns Against You
Franklin Watts c/o Grolier
90 Old Sherman Turnpike
Danbury, CT 06816
203-797-3500
Fax: 203-797-3197
www.grolier.com

Anorexia nervosa and bulimia are specifically examined, including a listing of the danger signals of each. A final chapter suggests places to secure help.

1993 96 pages
ISBN: 0-531111-75-0

Richard Robinson, President/Chairman/CEO
Mary Winston, EVP/Chief Financial Officer
Jeffrey Mathews, VP/Investor Relations

2944 Encyclopedia of Obesity and Eating Disorders
Facts on File
132 West 31st Street, 17th Floor
New York, NY 10001
212-967-8800
800-322-8755
Fax: 800-678-3633
custserv@factsonfile.com
www.factsonfile.com/

This revised and expanded edition includes more than 450 entries, more than 140 of them new. Complete with a history of obesity and eating disorders; chronology of key events, research, and breakthroughs; tables listing key facts and statistics; and a directory of resources and Web sites, this single-volume reference is the first stop in any serious research of these troubling health afflictions.

2006 384 pages Hardcover
ISBN: 0-816061-97-1

Laurie Katz, Publicity Director
Coreena Schultz, Library Sales Director
T J Mancini, Production Director

2945 Endorphins: Eating Disorders & Other Addictive Behavior
WW Norton & Company
500 5th Avenue
New York, NY 10110
212-354-5500
Fax: 212-869-0856
www.wwnorton.com

Dr. Huebner discusses anorexia nervosa and bulimia as addictions to endorphins, and presents a treatment model involving education about the addictive process, cognitive/behavioral strategies, and psychotherapy. He then reveals the role of endorphin addiction in other compulsive behaviors such as obsessive exercise, religious fanatacism, and cult involvement.

1993 320 pages
ISBN: 0-393701-56-5

William Drake McFeely, President

2946 Fear of Being Fat
Rowman & Littlefield Publishers
4501 Forbes Blvd, Suite 200
Lanham, MD 20706
301-459-3366
Fax: 301-429-5748
www.rowmanlittlefield.com/aronsonj/

This book, which presents one psychoanalytic approach to the treatment of anorexia nervosa, has been written by a number of authors, all members of the Psychosomatic Study Group of the Psychoanalytic Association of New York. The theoretical positions and therapeutic approaches are, consequently, conclusions based on extensive clinical experience, acquired over many years. Geared more for the professional.

366 pages
ISBN: 0-876688-99-7

Thomas Koerner, Ph.D, VP/Editorial Director
Wanda Mathews, Marketing Manager

2947 Food for Recovery
Crown Publishing Group/Random House
280 Park Avenue
New York, NY 10017
212-572-6117
Fax: 212-940-7868
crownpublicity@randomhouse.com
www.randomhouse.com/

Written for those in recovery from alcohol and drug abuse and eating disorders, this is an excellent basic book on nutrition. Beasley, director of a clinic that focuses on addictive diseases and nutritional medicine, and Knightly, a faculty member of Manhattan's Natural Gourmet Cooking School, discuss nutrition basics and explain how to select wholesome, unprocessed food.

1994 374 pages
ISBN: 0-517586-94-0

Jenny Frost, President/Publisher
Tina Constable, VP/Publicity Executive Director

2948 Getting Better Bit(e) by Bit(e)
Gurze Books
5145 B Avenida Encinas, PO Box 2238
Carlsbad, CA 92008
760-434-7533
800-756-7533
Fax: 760-434-5476
leigh@gurze.net
www.gurze.com

Written by specialists from London, the author's addresses the day-to-day problems faced by bulimia and binge eating sufferers and key behavior changes for progress.

143 pages Paperback

Ulrike Schmidt, Author
Janet Treasure, Author

2949 Group Psychotherapy for Eating Disorders
American Psychiatric Press
1000 Wilson Boulevard, Suite 1825
Arlington, VA 22209
703-907-7322
800-368-5777
Fax: 703-907-1091
appi@psych.org
www.appi.org/

The first book to fully explore the use of group therapy in the treatment of eating disorders.

353 pages Hardcover
ISBN: 0-880484-19-5

Robert E Hales, MD, Editor-in-Chief
Ron McMillen, Chief Executive Officer
John McDuffie, Editorial Director

2950 Hope and Recovery: A Mother-Daughter Story About Anorexia Nervosa & Bulimia
Franklin Watts
90 Old Sherman Turnpike
Danbury, CT 06816
800-621-1115
custserv@scholastic.com
www.scholastic.com/aboutscholastic/

Mother and daughter tell a story of a young woman's recovery from the horror of an eating disorder. This compelling account shows how anorexia and bulimia can affect an entire family.

192 pages
ISBN: 0-531111-40-7

Richard Robinson, Chairman/President/CEO
Mary A Winston, EVP/Chief Financial Officer
Lisa Holton, EVP/Book Fairs and Trade Shows

2951 How to get Your Kid to Eat...
Bull Publishing
PO Box 1377
Boulder, CO 80306
800-676-2855
Fax: 303-545-6354
bullpublishing@msn.com
www.bullpub.com

Touches on the various reasons for a child not wanting to eat, as well as continuos snacking, and not eating vegetables.

408 pages
ISBN: 0-915950-83-9

Jim Bull, Publisher

2952 I Was a Fifteen-Year-Old Blimp
Harper & Row
10 East 53rd Street
New York, NY 10022
212-207-7000
www.harpercollins.com/

This story focuses on Gabby, a teenage girl who overhears others discuss her weight and takes radical steps to become popular.

Grades 6-9

Jane Friedman, President/CEO
Lisa Herling, SVP/Corporate Communications
Brian Murray, Group President

2953 Insights in the Dynamic Psychotherapy of Anorexia And Bulimia
Rowman & Littlefield Publishers
4501 Forbes Blvd, Suite 200
Lanham, MD 20706
301-459-3366
Fax: 301-429-5748
www.rowmanlittlefield.com/

Discusses the eating disorders of anorexia and bulimia providing an overview of the dynamics in diagnosing the disease in addition to developmental and sociocultural issues, therapy and hospitalization.

320 pages Hardcover
ISBN: 0-876685-68-8

Shiela Burnett, Vice President/Marketing Director
Christopher Anzalone, Washington Editor/Director
Jack Meinhardt, Acquisitions Editor

2954 Life Beyond Your Eating Disorder
Johana S. Kandel, author

Harlequin
PO Box 5190
Buffalo, NY 14240
888-432-4879
cutomerservice@harlequin.com
www.harlequin.com

With the collaboration of professionals in the field of eating disorders, the author developed a set of practical tools to address the everyday challenges of recovery.

ISBN: 0-373892-26-6

2955 Making Peace with Food
Gurze Books
5145 B Avenida Encinas, PO Box 2238
Carlsbad, CA 92008
760-434-7533
800-756-7533
Fax: 760-434-5476
leigh@gurze.net
www.gurze.com

Filled with ideas, workbook pages, exercises, and resources, Kano's book is an excellent aid to clarifying and overcoming your personal diet/weight struggle.

224 pages Paperback

Susan Kano, Author

2956 Management of Eating Disorders and Obesity
Humana Press Scientific and Medical Publishers
999 Riverview Drive, Suite 208
Totowa, NJ 07512
973-256-1699
Fax: 973-256-8341
humana@humanapr.com
www.humanapress.com/

Stressing human physiology, treatment, and disease prevention, the authors take advantage of the new molecular understanding of the biological regulation of energy. Updated chapters review specific evidence-based and future treatment modalities, present an objective evaluation of the treatment, and identify the positives and negatives that have been seen during clinical studies, as well as cumulative data derived from clinical practice.

2004 448 pages Hardcover
ISBN: 1-588293-41-6

Paul Dolgert, Editorial Director
Ellie Shaw, Developmental Editor
Robin Weisberg, Director Editorial Services

2957 Meals Without Squeals Sense
Bull Publishing
PO Box 1377
Boulder, CO 80306
800-676-2855
Fax: 303-545-6354
bullpublishing@msn.com
www.bullpub.com

Straightforward information on childrens, growth accompanies age-specific, child-tested recipes. Explained is how common feeding problems can be solved and show ways to offer children positive experiences with food.

288 pages
ISBN: 0-923521-39-9

Jim Bull, Publisher/President

2958 Overeaters Anonymous
World Service Office
PO Box 44020
Rio Rancho, NM 87174
505-891-2664
Fax: 505-891-4320
nlippel@oa.org
www.oa.org/

World Service Office offers literature, provides information or meetings world wide. Free sample of Lifeline Magazine available.

204 pages Hardcover

Naomi Lippel, Managing Director
Sarah Armstrong, Associate Director
Rebbie Garza, Board Administrator

2959 Practice Guidelines for Eating Disorders
American Psychiatric Publishing
1000 Wilson Boulevard, Suite 1825
Arlington, VA 22209
703-907-7322
800-368-5777
Fax: 703-907-1091
appi@psych.org
www.appi.org/books.cfx

Designed for health care professionals, this guideline includes information on all aspects of anorexia nervosa and bulimia nervosa, including self-induced vomiting, use of laxatives and vigorous exercise to prevent weight gain.

38 pages Paperback
ISBN: 0-890423-00-8

Robert S Pursell, Marketing
John McDuffie, Product Information
Aimee Aponte, Technology/Webmaster

2960 Self-Starvation: from Individual to Family Therapy in the Treatment of Anorexia Ne
rvosa, author

Rowman & Littlefield Publishers
4501 Forbes Blvd, Suite 200
Lanham, MD 20706
301-459-3366
Fax: 301-429-5748
custserv@rowman.com
www.rowmanlittlefield.com/

Discusses the eating disorder anorexia nervosa and how it affects both the individual and family members alike, including information on possible treatment options.

1978 296 pages Hardcover
ISBN: 0-876683-10-3

Sheila Burnett, Marketing
Jack Meinhardt, Acquisitions Editor
Christopher Anzalone, Washington Editor/Director

2961 Starving to Death in a Sea of Objects
Rowman & Littlefield Publishers
4501 Forbes Blvd, Suite 200
Lanham, MD 20706
301-459-3366
Fax: 301-429-5748
custserv@rowan.com
www.rowmanlittlefield.com

How emancipation becomes security for anorexics.

464 pages Softcover
ISBN: 0-876684-35-5

Sheila Burnett, Marketing
Jack Meinhardt, Acquisitions Editor
Christopher Anzalone, Washington Editor/Director

2962 Surviving an Eating Disorder
Gurze Books
5145 B Avenida Encinas, PO Box 2238
Carlsbad, CA 92008
760-434-7533
800-756-7533
Fax: 760-434-5476
leigh@gurze.net
www.gurze.com

Discusses the psychological and behavioral aspects of eating disorders, pharmacology, and family therapy, with an emphasis on bringing eating disorders out in the open, seeking help, coping with anger and denial, developing a healthier relationship, and guidance for making the situation better - now.

222 pages Paperback

Michelle Siegel PhD, Author
Judith Brisman PhD, Author
Margot Weinshel PhD, Author

2963 Treating Bulimia: A Psychoeducational Approach
American Anorexia/Bulimia Association
4200 Monument Avenue
Philadelpha, PA 19131
215-877-2000
jbsmje@epix.net
www.aabaphila.org/

Book discusses the eating disorder bulimia focusing on utlizing the multifaceted treatment approach through the incorporation of education, self-monitoring, goal setting, assertion training, relaxation, and cognitive restructuring.

ISBN: 0-080323-99-5

Randi E Wirth, Ph.D, Executive Director

2964 Twelve Steps of Overeaters Anonymous
Overeaters Anonymous World Service Office
PO Box 44020
Rio Rancho, NM 87174
505-891-2664
Fax: 505-891-4320
nlippel@oa.org
www.oa.org/

The ideas expressed in the Twelve Steps, which originated in Alcoholics Anonymous, reflect practical experience and application of spiritual insights recorded by thinkers throughout the ages. Their greatest importance lies in the fact that they work! They enable compulsive overeaters and millions of other Twelve-Steppers to lead happy, productive lives. They represent the foundation upon which Overeaters Anonymous is built.

Naomi Lippel, Managing Director
Sarah Armstrong, Associate Director
Rebbie Garza, Board Administrator

2965 When Food is Love
Gurze Books
5145 B Avenida Encinas, PO Box 2238
Carlsbad, CA 92008
760-434-7533
800-756-7533
Fax: 760-434-5476
leigh@gurze.net
www.gurze.com

Roth's personal sharing in this book is both courageous and unforgettable. Explores similarities between eating and loving by exploring topics such as fantasizing, wanting the forbidden, creating drama, control issues, being strong in the broken places, and relationships.

205 pages Paperback
Geneen Roth, Author

2966 Withering Child
University of Georgia Press
320 South Jackson Street
Athens, GA 30602
404-542-2830
Fax: 706-542-6770
books@ugapress.uga.edu
www.uga.edu/ugapress

Non-fiction book of a parents' struggle with their son and his diagnosis of borderline attention deficit disorder, therapy and his eventual return to school.

1993 288 pages
ISBN: 0-820315-60-5

Nicole Mitchell, Administrative Director
Lane Stewart, Development Director
John McLeod, Marketing Director

Journals

2967 BASH Magazine
Bulimia Anorexia Self-Help/Behavior Adaptation
6125 Clayton Avenue, Suite 215
Saint Louis, MO 63139
314-567-4080
800-227-4785
www.caringonline.com/eatdis/treatment.htm

A journal of eating and mood disorders.

Monthly

2968 Internal Journal of Eating Disorders
Wiley
350 Main Street
Malden, MA 02148
781-388-8598
800-835-6770
cs-journals@wiley.com
www.onlinelibrary.wiley.com

In an effort to advance the scientific knowledge needed for understanding, treating and preventing eating disorders, the IJED publishes rigorously evaluated, high-quality manuscripts for distribution through print and electronic platforms.

2969 Journal of the American Dietetic Associati On
Elsevier Inc.
1600 John F. Kennedy Blvd. - Suite 1800
Philadelphia, PA 19103
215-239-3362
800-654-2452
Fax: 314-447-8029
journalcustomerservice-usa@elsevier.com
www.adajournal.org

The American Dietetic Association is a source for accurate, credible and timely food and nutrition information.

Newsletters

2970 AABA Newsletter
American Anorexic and Bulimia Association
PO Box 27156
Philadelphia, PA 19118
215-221-1864
mail.aabaphila@yahoo.com
www.aabaphila.org/

The American Anorexia Bulimia Association is a national, non-profit organization dedicated to the prevention and treatment of eating disorders. Publishes a monthly newsletter.
Randi E Wirth, Ph.D, Executive Director

2971 Eating Disorders Review
Gurze Books
PO Box 2238
Carlsbad, CA 92018
760-434-7533
800-756-7533
Fax: 760-434-5476
leigh@gurze.net
www.gurze.com

Presents current clinical information for the professional treating eating disorders. Review features summaries of relevant research of journals and unpublished studies

8 pages Bimonthly

Joel Yager MD, Editor-in-Chief
Leigh Hall, Co Founder
Leigh Cohn, Co Founder

2972 Food Allergy News
Food Allergy & Anaphylaxis Network
7925 Jones Branch Dr., Suite 1100
McLean, VA 22102
703-691-3179
800-929-4040
Fax: 703-691-2713
faan@foodallergy.org
www.foodallergy.org/

Contains tips for parents, including notices on ingredients in various foods, and recipes are published annually.

Bimonthly

Janet Atwater, Chair
Robert Nichols, Vice Chair
James R. Baker, Jr., MD, CEO & Chief Medical Officer

2973 Working Together
Anorexia Nervosa and Associated Disorders
750 E Diehl Road #127
Naperville, IL 60563
630-577-1330
Fax: 847-433-4632
anadhelp@anad.org
www.anad.org

Designed for individuals, families, group leaders and professionals concerned with eating disorders. Provides updates on treatments, resources, conferences, programs, articles by therapists, recovered victims, group members and leaders.

Quarterly

Patricia Santucci, MD, President
Kimberly Dennis, MD, Member, Scientific & Medical Board
Nomi Fredricks, MD, Member, Scientific & Medical Board

Pamphlets

2974 Applying New Attitudes & Directions
Anorexia Nervosa and Associated Disorders
750 E Diehl Road #127
Naperville, IL 60563
630-577-1330
Fax: 847-433-4632
anadhelp@anad.org
www.anad.org

Self-help booklet offering an eight-step program to recovery with suggestions, information and recovery stories.

Patricia Santucci, MD, President
Kimberly Dennis, MD, Member, Scientific & Medical Board
Nomi Fredricks, MD, Member, Scientific & Medical Board

2975 Body Image
ETR Associates
100 Enterprise Way, Suite G300
Scotts Valley, CA 95066
800-620-8884
Fax: 831-438-4284
customerservice@etr.org
www.etr.org

Discusses the difference between healthy and disorted body image; the link between poor body image and low self esteem; five point list to help people check out their own body image.

Dan McCormick, CEO
David Kitchen, MBA, CFO
Matt McDowell, BS, Director, Marketing

DESCRIPTION

2976 ECTODERMAL DYSPLASIAS
Synonyms: Christ-Siemens-Touraine Syndrome, Clouston Syndrome
Involves the following Biologic System(s):
Dental Disorders, Dermatologic Disorders

Ectodermal dysplasia is the term used to describe a large group of hereditary disorders in which there are defects in two or more body structures or organs derived from the body's outermost later of cells, known as the ectoderm. These body structures include the central nervous system, consisting of the brain and spinal cord, and the eyes, ears, lips, teeth, hair, sweat glands of the skin (sebaceous glands), nails, and mucous membranes that line the mouth and nose.

There are more than 150 different kinds of ectodermal dysplasia, all of which stem from aberrations or mutations in genes. Because they originate in genes, the conditions included by the term ectodermal dysplasia are typically transmitted from parents to their offspring, and inherited. However, they may also arise directly, from gene mutations occurring prenatally in an individual's own cells. Each of the various kinds of ectodermal dysplasia is present at birth, and although their effects are not usually seen in newborn infants, and may not become apparent until later in infancy or childhood, none of the different kinds of ectodermal dysplasia progresses or becomes more severe with growth. Ectodermal dysplasia may also occur as an integral part of syndromes in which it is accompanied by other disorders.

The manifestations and symptoms of a particular kinds of ectodermal dysplasia depend on the body structures it affects and the degree to which it affects them. Diminished tear flow (xerophthalmia) and conjunctivitis, diminished salivation (xerostomia), irritation and soreness of the nose and throat from deficient production of mucus, high body temperatures and fever from deficient sweat loss, cleft palate or cleft lip, missing fingers or toes, and webbings of skin between fingers and toes are among the effects of various ectodermal dysplasias and of syndromes of which these dysplasias are a part.

The two most common types of ectodermal dysplasia are X-linked recessive anhydrotic or hypohidrotic ectodermal dysplasia (Christ-Siemens-Touraine syndrome) and hidrotic ectodermal dysplasia (Clouston syndrome). The first of these syndromes is usually inherited as an X-linked recessive trait that is transmitted along with the X or female sex chromosome and is fully expressed in boys; however, some children may inherit anhidrotic or hypohidrotic ectodermal dysplasia as an autosomal recessive trait that affects boys and girls in equal numbers. This type of ectodermal dysplasia is characterized by absent (aplastic) or underdeveloped (hypoplastic) sweat glands, dental irregularities such as absent or widely-spaced, cone-shaped teeth, and sparse, light-colored hair (hypotrichosis). Facial features of this condition may include a large chin; thick lips; bulging forehead (frontal bossing); flat nasal bridge; prominent, low-set ears; and wrinkled, dark skin around the eyes. Children with this form of ectodermal dysplasia may be at increased risk for gastrointestinal infections as well as potentially life-threatening respiratory infections.

The second most common form of ectodermal dysplasia, hidrotic ectodermal dysplasia, also known as Clouston's syndrome, is inherited as an autosomal dominant trait, and is characterized by defective or absent nails, thickening of the skin on the palms of the hands and soles of the feet (palmar/plantar hyperkeratosis), and sparse hair. Other findings may include abnormally increased coloration of the skin over major joints and the development of unusually small teeth that are prone to decay. Treatment is symptomatic and supportive.

Prominent among syndromes of which ectodermal dysplasia is a part is EEC (ectrodactyly-ectodermal dysplasia-clefting) syndrome (EEC), which is inherited as an autosomal dominant trait. Symptoms and physical findings associated with this disorder are variable and may include lightly-pigmented skin, sparse hair and eyebrows, absent eyelashes, a split or opening (cleft) in the lip and palate, defective nails, tear duct irregularities, and absence of all or part of one or more fingers or toes (ectrodactyly). Other findings may include deafness and irregularities of the teeth, eyes, and urinary tract.

The treatment of ecotdermal dysplasia is focused on the structures its affects. Parents and caregivers are counseled to protect children from high environmental temperatures to avoid excessive loss of body water. Consumption of fluids and air conditioning are useful to patients who do not sweat or have deficient sweating. Artificial tears and nasal sprays may be used to ease drying of the membranes of the eyes and nose. Ointments and creams may be useful for relieving drying or scaling of the skin or scalp, as may antibiotic ointments to prevent or treat infection. Dentures and dental implants may be used to replace teeth affected by ectodermal dysplasia, and surgery may be done to correct cleft palate and deformities of the feet and hands. Genetic counseling is recommended for advising the parents of children with ectodermal dysplasia about the chance of the condition recurring in subsequent children.

Government Agencies

2977 NIH/National Institute of Arthritis and Musculoskeletal and Skin Diseases
1 AMS Circle
Bethesda, MD 20892
301-495-4484
877-226-4267
Fax: 301-718-6366
TDD: 301-565-2966
niamsinfo@mail.nih.gov
www.niams.nih.gov

The mission of the NIAMS, a part of the NIH, is to support research into the causes, treatment and prevention of arthritis and musculoskeletal and skin diseases, the training of basic and clinical scientists to carry out this research, and the dissemination of information on research progress in these diseases.

Stephen I Katz MD PhD, Director
Robert H Carter MD, Deputy Director

2978 NIH/National Institute of Dental and Crani ofacial Research (NIDCR)
National Institutes of Health
31 Center Drive, MSC 2290, Building 31
Bethesda, MD 20892
301-496-4261
Fax: 301-402-2185
nidcrinfo@mail.nih.gov
www.nidcr.nih.gov

Provides leadership for a national research program designed to understand, treat and prevent the infectious and inherited craniofacial-oral-dental diseases and disorders.

Dr Martha J. Somerman, Director
John W Kusiak, PhD, Acting Deputy Director
Kathleen G Stephen, Executive Officer

National Associations & Support Groups

2979 American Academy of Pediatrics
141 Northwest Point Boulevard
Elk Grove Village, IL 60007   847-434-4000
                                                     800-433-9016
                                                     Fax: 847-434-8000
                                                     www.aap.org

The American Academy of Pediatrics and its member pediatricians are committed to the attainment of optimal physical, mental and social health and well-being for all infants, children, adolescents, and young adults.

Fernando Stein, MD, FAAP, President
Karen Remley, MD, CEO/Executive VP

2980 American Dental Association
211 E Chicago Avenue
Chicago, IL 60611   312-266-7255
                                                     Fax: 312-266-9867
                                                     ÿinfo@aae.org
                                                     www.aae.org

Professional association of dentists committed to the public's oral health, ethics, science and professional advancement; leading a unified profession through initiatives in advocacy, education, research and the development of standards.

James Drinan, Executive Director

2981 Genetic Alliance
4301 Connecticut Avenue NW, Suite 404
Washington, DC 20008   202-966-5557
                                                     800-336-4363
                                                     Fax: 202-966-8553
                                                     info@geneticalliance.org
                                                     www.geneticalliance.org

A coalition of voluntary genetic support groups, consumers and professionals addressing the needs of individuals and families affected by genetic disorders from a national perspective.

Sharon Terry, President/CEO
Tetyana Murza, Managing Director
Natasha Bonhomme, VP, Strategic Development

2982 March of Dimes Foundation
1275 Mamaroneck Avenue
White Plains, NY 10605   914-997-4488
                                                     888-663-4637
                                                     Fax: 914-997-4763
                                                     answers@marchofdimes.com
                                                     www.marchofdimes.com

Partnership of volunteers and professionals dedicated to improving the health of babies by preventing birth defects and infant mortality. Over 100 chapters are located across the country and can be located through the National Office.

Stacey D. Stewart, President

2983 National Foundation for Ectodermal Dysplasias
410 E Main Street, PO Box 114
Mascoutah, IL 62258   618-566-2020
                                                     Fax: 618-566-4718
                                                     info@nfed.org
                                                     www.nfed.org

Seeks to enrich the lives of individuals affected by all forms of the ectodermal dysplasia syndromes.

Mary K Richter, Founder/Executive Director

2984 Society for Pediatric Dermatology
8365 Keystone Crossing, Suite 107
Indianapolis, IN 46240   317-202-0224
                                                     Fax: 317-205-9481
                                                     info@pedsderm.net
                                                     www.pedsderm.net

National organization dedicated to promote, develop and advance edcuation, research and care of skin disease in all pediatric age groups.

Kent Lindeman, Executive Director

State Agencies & Support Groups

2985 National Foundation for Ectodermal Dysplasias- Regional Office
PO Box 2069
Auburn, WA 98071   253-735-5195
                                                     Fax: 253-735-5195
                                                     TTY: 800-688-4889
                                                     nfed3@aol.com
                                                     www.nfed.org

Disseminates information on this and related disorders for people of any age to access and use in everyday life situations.

Judy Woodruff, Executive Director
Kelley Atchison, Director of Supportÿ
ÿÿGale Hoedebeck, ÿÿDirector of Administration

Libraries & Resource Centers

2986 International Center for Skeletal Dysplasia Registry
St. Joseph Hospital
7620 York Road
Townson, MD 21204   310-423-9915
                                                     Fax: 310-423-9939

Provides patient services for those with skeletal dysplasia; does s research in dwarfism.

Dr. Steven Kopitis, Director

Conferences

2987 Genetic Alliance Annual Conference
Genetic Alliance
4301 Connecticut Avenue NW, Suite 404
Washington, DC 20008   202-966-5557
                                                     800-336-4363
                                                     Fax: 202-966-8553
                                                     info@geneticalliance.org
                                                     www.geneticalliance.org

Consistently inspirational and enables partnership among all stakeholders: advocates and community leaders, health and industry professionals, policymakers, and academicians.

July

Sharon Terry, President/CEO
Tetyana Murza, Managing Director
Natasha Bonhomme, VP, Strategic Development

2988 National Foundation for Ectodermal Dysplasias Annual Conference
National Foundation for Ectodermal Dysplasias
410 E Main Street
Mascoutah, IL 62258   618-566-2020
                                                     Fax: 618-566-4718
                                                     info@nfed.org
                                                     www.nfed.org

Where individuals affected by ectodermal dysplasias and their families gather to receive information and support. Experts provide medical and dental presentations to explain the various symptoms and how to best treat them.

Mary K Richter, Founder/Executive Director

2989 Society for Pediatric Dermatology Annual M eeting
Society for Pediatric Dermatology
8365 Keystone Crossing, Suite 107
Indianapolis, IN 46240   317-202-0224
                                                     Fax: 317-205-9481
                                                     info@pedsderm.net
                                                     www.pedsderm.net

July
Kent Lindeman, Executive Director

Web Sites

2990 American Dental Association
211 East Chicago Avenue
Chicago, IL 60611   312-440-2500
affiliates@ada.org
www.ada.org

The ADA foundation enhances health by securing contributions
and providing grants for sustainable programs in dental research,
education, access to care and assistance for dentists and their
families in need.

2991 Dental Resources on the Web
www.dental-resources.com

Dental sites for education, practices, laboratories, office supplies,
dental care and associations.

2992 Online Mendelian Inheritance in Man
U.S. National Library of Medicine, 8600 Rockville
Bethesda, MD 20894   888-346-3656
info@ncbi.nlm.nih.gov
www.ncbi.nlm.nih.gov

This database is a catalog of human genes and genetic disorders.

Christine E. Seidman, M.D., Chair
David J. Lipman, M.D., Executive Secretary
Michael Boehnke, Ph.D., Board Member

Journals

2993 Pediatric Dermatology Journal
Society for Pediatric Dermatology
8365 Keystone Crossing, Suite 107
Indianapolis, IN 46240   317-202-0224
Fax: 317-205-9481
info@pedsderm.net
www.pedsderm.net

6 issues/yr
Kent Lindeman, Executive Director

DESCRIPTION

2994 ECZEMA

Synonym: Eczematous dermatitis

Covers these related disorders: Allergic contact dermatitis, Atopic dermatitis, Dyshidrosis, Irritant contact dermatitis, Seborrheic dermatitis

Involves the following Biologic System(s):
Dermatologic Disorders

Eczema is a common inflammatory condition of the skin (dermatitis) characterized by redness, itching, blistering, and oozing of affected areas. As the condition progresses, the skin often becomes abnormally dry and may scale, crust over, thicken, or develop increased or decreased areas of coloration. There are several different types of eczema that may be caused by various internal or external factors. Children are mainly affected by certain forms of the condition, including atopic dermatitis, irritant and allergic contact dermatitis, seborrheic dermatitis, or dyshidrosis.

Approximately 2-8% of children develop atopic dermatitis, which is the most common form of childhood eczema. Also known as infantile eczema when it occurs during childhood, this form of eczema is characterized by an excessive immune response to particular substances (sensitizing antigens) that the body perceives as foreign. This excessive response, known as an allergic or hypersensitivity reaction, occurs upon exposure to previously encountered, usually environmental substances (allergens). Patients with atopic dermatitis are thought to have an inherited tendency toward allergy. This may be supported by the finding that many infants and children with this type of dermatitis later develop additional conditions caused by exposure to certain allergens. These additional conditions particularly include inflammation of the mucous membranes of the nose (allergic rhinitis) and inflammation and narrowing of the airways (asthma).

Atopic dermatitis usually begins during the first year of life, and up to 90% of affected patients have symptoms by five years of age. The disorder often occurs with the introduction of particular foods into a child's diet, such as wheat, cow's milk, soy, eggs, or peanuts. Although atopic dermatitis tends to subside with advancing age, the condition may recur over a period of many years before completely disappearing. Atopic dermatitis is characterized by the development of reddish, inflamed, intensely itchy (pruritic) patches that rapidly begin to ooze and crust over. During infancy, the condition usually initially affects the skin of the cheeks and gradually extends to involve the rest of the face; the neck, abdomen, wrists, and hands; the insides of the elbows; the areas behind the knees; or other areas. In response to intense itching, infants with atopic dermatitis may rub affected areas against their cribs, clothes, or other surfaces in an attempt to obtain relief. The repeated rubbing or scratching of affected areas may lead to their infection by bacteria on the skin, on clothing, or from other sources. With the passage of time, skin areas affected by atopic dermatitis may become dry and scaly and develop changes in color. In addition, the skin may thicken, accentuating skin lines and causing an unusual, "bark-like" skin appearance (lichenification).

The treatment of atopic dermatitis may include measures to eliminate or avoid certain factors that might worsen the condition, such as certain foods, extremes of humidity and temperature, detergents or soaps, or potentially abrasive textures, such as wool. Affected children should be dressed in garments with smooth textures, such as cotton; their fingernails should be kept as short as possible to discourage scratching; and excessive bathing should be avoided. Adding bath oil to bath water and applying moisturizing lotions and creams to damp skin after bathing may help to ease some symptoms of atopic dermatitis. At locations where inflammation is severe, the application of wet dressings may reduce inflammation and associated itching. Treatment may also include the direct (topical) application of medicated skin creams and ointments, such as corticosteroid preparations, as well as medications such as oral antihistamines to help reduce itching. Bacterial infections of skin affected by atopic dermatitis are treated with appropriate antibiotics.

Contact dermatitis, another common form of eczema, is a skin inflammation that is typically confined to a particular area and may have clearly defined boundaries. This disorder is often subdivided into irritant and allergic contact dermatitis. Irritant contact dermatitis is a skin inflammation caused by repetitive or prolonged exposure to certain substances that damage the skin. Allergic contact dermatitis is an inflammatory response of the skin caused by subsequent exposure to an allergen to which the skin has previously become sensitized.

Irritant contact dermatitis may be caused by repetitive or prolonged exposure to certain soaps or detergents, citrus juices, bubble bath preparations, or other substances. In many infants, saliva from drooling may cause inflammation of the skin of the face and neck folds. Diaper dermatitis is another common form of irritant contact dermatitis. Affected infants may develop a reddish, scaling, blistering skin inflammation and secondary bacterial infections from prolonged contact with waste materials, diaper soaps, and topical skin lotions. The treatment of irritant contact dermatitis includes removal or avoidance of the responsible irritants and topical application of corticosteroid creams or ointments. Affected areas of skin should also be carefully and regularly washed with warm water and a mild soap. To help prevent diaper dermatitis, physicians may recommend frequent changing of diapers; gentle, thorough cleansing of genitals with warm water and mild soaps, and application of mild protective topical preparations during the diaper changes; or the use of disposable diapers made with absorbent materials.

Allergic contact dermatitis is characterized by a hypersensitive or allergic response to previously encountered allergens. Common causes of this form of dermatitis include metal compounds in jewelry; particular plants, such as poison ivy, poison oak, or poison sumac; medications in skin creams, such as certain antibiotic- or antihistamine-containing creams; shoes; or clothing. Patients with allergic contact dermatitis may experience intensely itchy, reddish, blistering skin inflammations, with the affected areas of skin later developing scaling, cracking, (fissuring), changes in color, or an abnormal, thickened, bark-like appearance. Treatment includes the removal or avoidance of allergens responsible for the condition and the application of cool compresses, corticosteroid ointments or oral medications, antihistamine medications, and antibiotic therapy for secondary bacterial infections.

Seborrheic dermatitis is a chronic inflammatory disorder of unknown cause that may occur at any age and may appear to follow the distribution of sebaceous glands in skin tissue. These relatively small glands, which open into hair follicles, produce an oily secretion known as sebum that helps to lubricate the hair and skin and protect the skin from drying. In children, seborrheic dermatitis most commonly occurs during infancy. Affected infants may initially develop localized or widespread crusting and scaling of the scalp, known as cradle cap. In some patients, this may be the only effect of the this form of dermatitis. Other infants may develop reddish, greasy, scaling patches that may be localized or may spread to affect most of the body. Affected areas often include the face, the regions behind the ears, the neck, the diaper region, or the armpits and underarm areas. Patients with seborrheic dermatitis may experience associated itching, hair loss, or changes in skin color. Treatment may include the use of special anti-seborrheic shampoos or the application of wet compresses or topical corticosteroid creams or ointments.

Dyshidrotic eczema, also known as dyshidrosis or pompholyx, is another form of eczema that may occur during childhood. It is a recurrent, potentially seasonal blistering condition that affects the palms of the hands and soles of the feet. The condition is initially characterized by recurrent crops of severely itchy blisters. Affected skin areas gradually become abnormally thickened and may have cracking or fissuring. Many patients with dyshidrotic eczema also experience excessive sweating (hyperhidrosis) in affected areas, and may develop secondary bacterial infections from scratching of such areas. Because dyshidrotic eczema is typically a recurrent condition, appropriate measures should be taken to protect the hands and feet of infants and children with this condition from harsh soaps, chemicals, the effects of excessive sweating or adverse weather, or other factors that may trigger the condition. Treatment of dyshidrotic eczema may include the application of wet dressings, topical corticosteroid ointments or creams, or mild topical preparations that promote skin softening and peeling (keratolytic agents), and the administration of antibiotics to treat secondary bacterial infections.

Government Agencies

2995 NIH/National Institute of Allergy and Infectious Diseases
5601 Fishers Lane, MSC 9806
Bethesda, MD 20892   301-496-5717
                                                 866-284-4107
                                            Fax: 301-402-3573
                                            TDD: 800-877-8339
                                       ocpostoffice@niaid.nih.gov
                                            www.niaid.nih.gov

Conducts and supports basic and applied research to better understand, treat, and ultimately prevent infectious, immunologic, and allergic diseases.

Anthony S Fauci MD, Director

2996 NIH/National Institute of Arthritis and Musculoskeletal and Skin Diseases
1 AMS Circle
Bethesda, MD 20892   301-495-4484
                                                 877-226-4267
                                            Fax: 301-718-6366
                                            TDD: 301-565-2966
                                       niamsinfo@mail.nih.gov
                                            www.niams.nih.gov

The mission of the NIAMS, a part of the NIH, is to support research into the causes, treatment and prevention of arthritis and musculoskeletal and skin diseases, the training of basic and clinical scientists to carry out this research, and the dissemination of information on research progress in these diseases

Stephen I Katz MD PhD, Director
Robert H Carter MD, Deputy Director

National Associations & Support Groups

2997 American Academy of Pediatrics
141 Northwest Point Boulevard
Elk Grove Village, IL 60007   847-434-4000
                                                 800-433-9016
                                            Fax: 847-434-8000
                                                 www.aap.org

The American Academy of Pediatrics and its member pediatricians are committed to the attainment of optimal physical, mental and social health and well-being for all infants, children, adolescents, and young adults.

Fernando Stein, MD, FAAP, President
Karen Remley, MD, CEO/Executive VP

2998 National Eczema Association
4460 Redwood Highway, Suite 16-D
San Rafael, CA 94903   415-499-3474
                                                 800-818-7546
                                            Fax: 415-472-5345
                                       info@nationaleczema.org
                                            www.nationaleczema.org

Works to improve the health and the quality of life of persons living with atopic dermatitis/eczema, including those who have the disease as well as their loved ones.

2999 Society for Pediatric Dermatology
8365 Keystone Crossing, Suite 107
Indianapolis, IN 46240   317-202-0224
                                            Fax: 317-205-9481
                                       info@pedsderm.net
                                            www.pedsderm.net

National organization dedicated to promote, develop and advance education, research and care of skin disease in all pediatric age groups.

Kent Lindeman, Executive Director

Libraries & Resource Centers

California

3000 University of California, San Francisco Dermatology Drug Research
515 Spruce
San Francisco, CA 94143   415-476-2001
                                            Fax: 415-476-6014
                                            cc.ucsf.edu/people

Conducts clinical testing of new or existing pharmalogic agents used in the treatment of skin disorders.

John Koo, MD, Director

Delaware

3001 Delaware Division of Libraries for the Blind and Physically Handicapped
43 S Dupont Highway
Dover, DE 19901   302-736-4748
                                                 800-282-8676
                                            Fax: 302-736-6787
                                            TDD: 302-739-4748
                                            bedpg@lib.de.us
                                   www.nfb.org/libraries-for-the-blind

Braille readers receive service from Philadelphia and Pennsylvania, summer reading program, braille writer and cassettes.

Beth Landon, Librarian

Illinois

3002 Dermatology Information Network (DERMINFONET)
American Academy of Dermatology
PO Box 4014
Schaumburg, IL 60168   847-330-0230
                                    Fax: 847-330-0050
            www.meddermsociety.org/Resource_Links.asp

Consists of a collection of dermatologic databases that are available to members on a subscription and/or purchase basis. These databases are designed to run on a wide variety of personal computers.

3003 National Library of Dermatologic Teaching Slides
American Academy of Dermatology
930 E Woodfield Road
Schaumburg, IL 60173   847-330-0230
                                    Fax: 847-330-0050
                                         www.aad.org

A collection of dermatologic teaching slides offering the most comprehensive series ever assembled. Each set offers a realistic presentation of classic clinical skin conditions encountered by the dermatologist.

New York

3004 Laboratory of Dermatology Research
Memorial Sloan-Kettering Cancer Center
1275 York Avenue
New York, NY 10065   212-639-2000
                                    Fax: 212-639-3576
                                        www.mskcc.org

Specific studies on the identification of skin disorders and dermatology.

Biijan Safai, MD, Head

3005 Rockefeller University Laboratory for Investigative Dermatology
1230 York Avenue
New York, NY 10065   212-327-8000
                                    Fax: 212-327-7459
        www.rockefeller.edu/research/faculty/labheads/JamesK

Research into skin disorders and the whole specialty of dermatology in general.

Barry Coller, Head

Research Centers

3006 University of California, San Francisco Dermatology Drug Research
515 Spruce
San Francisco, CA 94143   415-476-2001
                                    Fax: 415-221-4751

Conducts clinical testing of new or existing pharmacologic agents used in the treatment of skin disorders.

John Koo, MD, Director

Conferences

3007 Society for Pediatric Dermatology Annual M eeting
Society for Pediatric Dermatology
8365 Keystone Crossing, Suite 107
Indianapolis, IN 46240   317-202-0224
                                    Fax: 317-205-9481
                                    info@pedsderm.net
                                       www.pedsderm.net

July
Kent Lindeman, Executive Director

Audio Video

3008 National Library of Dermatologic Teaching Slides
American Academy Of Dermatology
PO Box 94020
Palatine, IL 60094   847-330-0230
                                    Fax: 847-330-0050

A collection of dermatologic teaching slides offering the most comprehensive series ever assembled. Each set offers a realistic presentation of classic clinical skin conditions encountered by the dermatologist.

Magazines

3009 International Journal of Dermatology
International Society of Dermatology
138 Palm Coast Parkway, NE No 333
Palm Coast, FL 32137   386-437-4405
                                    Fax: 386-437-4427
                                info@intsocdermatol.org
                                      www.intsocderm.org

Focuses on information for dermatologists and the whole specialty of dermatology research and education.
10 times a year

3010 Journal of Dermatologic Surgery and Oncology
International Society for Dermatologic Surgery
930 N Meachan Road
Schaumburg, IL 60173   847-330-9830
                                    Fax: 847-330-1135
           onlinelibrary.wiley.com/journal/10.1111/(ISSN)1524-4

Focuses on medical updates and information on dermatology.
Monthly

Journals

3011 Pediatric Dermatology Journal
Society for Pediatric Dermatology
8365 Keystone Crossing, Suite 107
Indianapolis, IN 46240   317-202-0224
                                    Fax: 317-205-9481
                                    info@pedsderm.net
                                       www.pedsderm.net

6 issues/yr
Kent Lindeman, Executive Director

Newsletters

3012 Awareness
NAPVI
PO Box 317
Watertown, MA 2471   617-972-7441
                                         800-562-6265
                                    Fax: 617-972-7444
                                    www.spedex.com/napvi

Newsletter offering regional news, sports and activities, conferences, camps, legislative updates, book reviews, audio reviews, professional question and answer column and more for the visually impaired and their families.
Quarterly

3013 DVH Quarterly
University of Arkansas at Little Rock
2801 S University Avenue
Little Rock, AR 72204   Fax: 501-663-3536

Offers information on upcoming events, conferences and workshops on and for visual disabilities. Book reviews, information on the newest resources and technology, educational programs, want ads and more.

Quarterly

Bob Brasher, Editor

3014 Dermatology Focus
Dermatology Foundation
1560 Sherman Avenue, Suite 870
Evanston, IL 60201
847-328-2256
Fax: 847-328-0509
dermatologyfoundation.org

Includes membership activities, research articles and lists recipients of foundation awards.

Quarterly

Bruce U. Wintroub, MD, Chair
Michael D. Tharp, MD, President
Stuart R. Lessin, MD, Vice President

3015 Dermatology World
American Academy of Dermatology
PO Box 94020
Palatine, IL 60094
847-330-0230
Fax: 847-330-0050

Offers Academy members information outside the clinical realm. It carries news of government actions, reports of socioeconomic issues, societal trends and other events which impinge on the practice of dermatology.

Monthly

3016 Progress in Dermatology
Dermatology Foundation
1560 Sherman Avenue, Suite 870
Evanston, IL 60201
847-328-2256
Fax: 847-328-0509
dermatologyfoundation.org

Bulletin offering information on research reports and clinical trials.

Quarterly

Bruce U. Wintroub, MD, Chair
Michael D. Tharp, MD, President
Stuart R. Lessin, MD, Vice President

Pamphlets

3017 Eczema/Atopic Dermatitis
American Academy of Dermatology
PO Box 4014
Schaumburg, IL 60168
847-240-1280
866-503-7546
Fax: 847-240-1859
president@aad.org
www.aad.org

Explains how to recognize and treat dermatitis.

1995

Brett M. Coldiron, MD, President
Elise A. Olsen, MD, Vice President
Suzanne M. Olbricht, MD, Secretary-Treasurer

3018 Hand Eczema
American Academy of Dermatology
PO Box 4014
Schaumburg, IL 60168
847-240-1280
866-503-7546
Fax: 847-240-1859
president@aad.org
www.aad.org

Shows examples of hand rashes, explains causes, lists protective measures and treatments.

1993

Brett M. Coldiron, MD, President
Elise A. Olsen, MD, Vice President
Suzanne M. Olbricht, MD, Secretary-Treasurer

Camps

3019 Camp Discovery
American Academy of Dermatology
930 E Woodfield Road
Schaumburg, IL 60173
847-240-1280
866-503-7546
Fax: 847-240-1859
president@aad.org
www.campdiscovery.org

A camp for young people with chronic skin conditions. There is no fee and transportation is provided. Three locations: Camp Horizon in Millville, PA, Camp Knutson in Crosslake, MN, and Camp Dermadillo in Burton, TX.

Brett M. Coldiron, MD, President
Elise A. Olsen, MD, Vice President
Suzanne M. Olbricht, MD, Secretary-Treasurer

DESCRIPTION

3020 EHLERS-DANLOS SYNDROME
Involves the following Biologic System(s):
Connective Tissue Disorders

Ehlers-Danlos syndrome is a group of hereditary connective tissue disorders characterized by abnormalities of collagen, the major structural protein in the body. At least 10 forms of the disorder have been identified based upon underlying biochemical and genetic abnormalities and associated symptoms and findings. Although such subtypes were previously indentified by Roman numerals (e.g., I to X), different classification systems have since been proposed. Most forms of Ehlers-Danlos syndrome are thought to have autosomal dominant inheritance. However, other subtypes have been identified that may be inherited as an autosomal recessive or an X-linked recessive trait. Although certain symptoms and findings are commonly associated with Ehlers-Danlos syndrome, other abnormalities may be variable in range and severity, depending upon the form of the disorder present.

Although infants with Ehlers-Danlos syndrome often appear normal at birth, associated symptoms and findings soon become apparent. The main symptoms associated with the disorder may include abnormally thin, elastic skin that is excessively fragile and unusually loose, flexible (hyperextensible) joints that may be prone to recurrent dislocation. Due to abnormal fragility of the skin, blood vessels, and other tissues, patients may be prone to tearing or splitting of the skin, be susceptible to easy bruising and bleeding, and tend to heal slowly. Healing of skin wounds may leave distinctive, cigarette paper-like scars, such as over the knees, shins, elbows, and forehead. In addition, due to abnormal accumulations of scar tissue, patients may develop small, rounded skin growths that resemble tumors (molluscoid pseudotumors). In some cases, small, round, hard lumps (calcified spheroids) may also develop under the skin.

Depending upon the form of the disorder present, affected children may have additional, variable symptoms, such as certain skeletal, blood vessel, or eye (ocular) abnormalities. Associated skeletal malformations may include front-to-back and sideways curvature of the spine (kyphoscoliosis); short, wide collarbones (clavicles); bowing of bones of the arms and legs; bone fragility; short stature; or other abnormalities. Fragility of certain blood vessels may lead to ballooning of the wall of the major artery in the body (aortic aneurysm) or spontaneous rupture of certain intermediate- or large-sized arteries, potentially causing life-threatening complications. In addition, in some patients, ocular abnormalities may include fragility of the front, transparent region of the eye (cornea); noninflammatory protrusion of the cornea (keratoconus); rupture of the cornea or the tough, fibrous, outer coating of the eye (sclera); or detachment of the nerve-rich membrane at the back of the eye (retina). Additional symptoms and findings may include diminished muscle tone (hypotonia); abnormal prominence of blood vessels under the skin; protrusion of one of the heart valves back into the left upper chamber (atrium) of the heart during contraction of the left lower heart chamber (mitral valve prolapse); severe inflammation of the tissues that surround and support the teeth (periodontitis), leading to premature tooth loss; rupture of the intestine; or other abnormalities.

The treatment of children with Ehlers-Danlos syndrome is symptomatic and supportive. Appropriate measures must be taken to avoid trauma and injuries, such as those that may occur in contact sports. Wearing protective clothing and padding may be beneficial. In addition, appropriate precautions must be taken during dental or surgical procedures.

Government Agencies

3021 NIH/National Institute of Arthritis and Musculoskeletal and Skin Diseases
1 AMS Circle
Bethesda, MD 20892

301-495-4484
877-226-4267
Fax: 301-718-6366
TDD: 301-565-2966
niamsinfo@mail.nih.gov
www.niams.nih.gov

The mission of the NIAMS, a part of the NIH, is to support research into the causes, treatment, and prevention of arthritis and musculoskeletal and skin diseases, the training of basic and clinical scientists to carry out this research, and the dissemination of information on research progress in these diseases.

Stephen I Katz MD PhD, Director
Robert H Carter MD, Deputy Director

National Associations & Support Groups

3022 American Academy of Pediatrics
141 Northwest Point Boulevard
Elk Grove Village, IL 60007

847-434-4000
800-433-9016
Fax: 847-434-8000
www.aap.org

The American Academy of Pediatrics and its member pediatricians are committed to the attainment of optimal physical, mental and social health and well-being for all infants, children, adolescents, and young adults.

Fernando Stein, MD, FAAP, President
Karen Remley, MD, CEO/Executive VP

3023 Ehlers-Danlos National Foundation
1760, Old Meadow Road, Ste 500
McLean, VG 22102

703-506-2892
Fax: 213-427-0057
ednfstaff@ednf.org
www.ednf.org

Provides emotional support and updated information to the individuals and their families who are affected by the disease. The foundation produces educational and support pamphlets, brochures, audiovisual aids, journal article reprints, newsletter, and a referral service.

Cynthia Lauren, Ceo
Edzel Lejano, Member Services Coordinator

3024 Genetic Alliance
4301 Connecticut Avenue NW, Suite 404
Washington, DC 20008

202-966-5557
800-336-4363
Fax: 202-966-8553
info@geneticalliance.org
www.geneticalliance.org

A coalition of voluntary genetic support groups, consumers and professionals addressing the needs of individuals and families affected by genetic disorders from a national perspective.

Sharon Terry, President/CEO
Tetyana Murza, Managing Director
Natasha Bonhomme, VP, Strategic Development

3025 March of Dimes Foundation
1275 Mamaroneck Avenue
White Plains, NY 10605   914-997-4488
                                                             888-663-4637
                                                        Fax: 914-997-4763
                                                 answers@marchofdimes.com
                                                    www.marchofdimes.com

Partnership of volunteers and professionals dedicated to improving the health of babies by preventing birth defects and infant mortality. Over 100 chapters are located across the country and can be located through the National Office.

Stacey D. Stewart, President

Conferences

3026 Ehlers-Danlos National Foundation Learning Conference
Ehlers-Danlos National Foundation
1760 Old Meadow Road, Suite 500
McLean, VA 22102   703-506-2892
                                                        Fax: 703-506-3266
                                                        ednstaff@ednf.org
                                                            www.ednf.org

July

Shane Robinson, Executive Director

3027 Genetic Alliance Annual Conference
Genetic Alliance
4301 Connecticut Avenue NW, Suite 404
Washington, DC 20008   202-966-5557
                                                            800-336-4363
                                                        Fax: 202-966-8553
                                                 info@geneticalliance.org
                                                    www.geneticalliance.org

Consistently inspirational and enables partnership among all stakeholders: advocates and community leaders, health and industry professionals, policymakers, and academicians.

July

Sharon Terry, President/CEO
Tetyana Murza, Managing Director
Natasha Bonhomme, VP, Strategic Development

Web Sites

3028 Wheeless' Textbook of Orthopaedics
www.wheelessonline.com

Derives from a variety of sources, including journals, articles, national meetings lectures and other textbooks.

Clifford R. Wheeless III, MD, Editor-in-Chief
James A. Nunley, II, Managing Editor
James R. Urbaniak, MD, Managing Editor

Pamphlets

3029 Ehlers-Danlos Syndrome
Arthritis Foundation
PO Box 7669
Atlanta, GA 30357   404-872-7100
                                                            800-283-7800
                                                        Fax: 404-872-0457
                                                        www.arthiritis.org

DESCRIPTION

3030 ENCEPHALOCELE

Involves the following Biologic System(s):

Neurologic Disorders

Encephalocele is an abnormality that is present at birth (congenital) and belongs to a group of birth defects known as neural tube defects. These defects develop during the early stages of pregnancy at which time a specialized layer of tissue forms and extends along the back portion of the developing embryo. As the embryo grows, this tissue, known as the neural plate, forms a groove that is bordered by folds. This groove eventually deepens and closes to form the neural tube. Later in development, the neural tube gives rise to tissue that later forms the brain and spinal cord. The neural tube is surrounded and protected by the bones of the back (vertebrae). Failure in this sequence of developmental events results in a neural tube defect.

In newborns with encephalocele, a portion of the brain protrudes through a defect in the skull. This defect may be located at the back of the head (occipital region), the forehead (frontal region), or the area of the forehead and nose (nasofrontal region). Affected children may experience visual abnormalities, mental retardation, an abnormally small head (microcephaly), and seizures. Affected newborns may also have an increase in the volume of fluid surrounding the brain (hydrocephalus), possibly resulting in increased pressure within the skull, enlargement of the head, and convulsions.

Encephalocele may occur as the result of different genetic and environmental factors (multifactorial), alone or in combination. Such factors may include vitamin deficiencies or toxic factors. Genetic transmission in some children is supported by the fact that multiple cases of this neural tube defect have been reported in some families. In addition, encephalocele may sometimes be associated with other disorders. For example, physical characteristics of Meckel-Gruber syndrome, a rare, life-threatening disorder inherited as an autosomal recessive trait, include encephalocele in the back of the head; an abnormal ridge (cleft) or opening in the lip or palate; a sloping forehead, extra fingers or toes (polydactyly); and enlarged kidneys that contain multiple cysts (polycystic kidneys).

Treatment of encephalocele may often involve a team of medical specialists working together to determine the best course of therapy or management. Such treatment may include surgery, medication, or the insertion of a tube known as a shunt into the brain. This shunt diverts fluid away from the brain into the abdominal cavity where it is harmlessly absorbed into the systemic circulation.

The risk of neural tube defects is significantly reduced when supplemental folic acid is consumed in addition to a healthful diet prior to and during the first month following conception. Women who could become pregnant, especially those at risk who may have previously delivered a child with a neural tube defect, are advised to eat foods fortified with folic acid or take a folic acid supplement in addition to eating folate-rich foods to reduce the risk of some serious birth defects.

Government Agencies

3031 NIH/ Eunice Kennedy Shriver National Institute of Child Health & Human Development
31 Center Drive, Building 31
Bethesda, MD 20892

301-496-5113
800-370-2943
Fax: 866-760-5947
nichdpress@mail.nih.gov
www.nichd.nih.gov

Established in 1962 by congress, today the institute conducts and supports research on topics related to the health of children, adults, families and populations. Some of these topics include: developmental disabilities, growth and development, infant death, reproductive health and birth defects.

Diana W. Bianchi, Director
Paul Williams, Director, Communications

National Associations & Support Groups

3032 AmeriFace
PO Box 75112
Las Vegas, NV 89130

702-301-5351
888-486-1209
Fax: 702-341-5351
info@ameriface.org
www.ameriface.org

Provides information, services, emotional support and educational programs for and on behalf of individuals with facial differences and their families. Working to increase understanding through public awareness and education.

3M members

Debbie Oliver, Executive Director

3033 American Academy of Pediatrics
141 Northwest Point Boulevard
Elk Grove Village, IL 60007

847-434-4000
800-433-9016
Fax: 847-434-8000
www.aap.org

The American Academy of Pediatrics and its member pediatricians are committed to the attainment of optimal physical, mental and social health and well-being for all infants, children, adolescents, and young adults.

Fernando Stein, MD, FAAP, President
Karen Remley, MD, CEO/Executive VP

3034 Birth Defect Research for Children
930 Woodcock Road, Suite 225
Orlando, FL 32803

407-895-0802
Fax: 407-895-0824
staff@birthdefects.org
www.birthdefects.org

Organization that helps families with free birth defect information, parent matching that links families of children with similar defects and research through the National Birth Defect Registry to discover the causes of birth defects. Support group information and newsletter on Internet.

Betty Mekdeci, Executive Director

3035 Children's Craniofacial Association
13140 Coit Road, Suite 307
Dallas, TX 75240

214-570-9099
800-535-3643
Fax: 214-570-8811
contactCCA@ccakids.com
www.ccakids.com

Devoted to the dispersion of medical knowledge of this and similar disorders, along with providing emotional support for the sufferers and their families.

Char Smith, Executive Director

3036 Fighters for Encephalocele Support Group
332 Brereton Street
Pittsburgh, PA 15219   412-261-5363

3037 Forward Face
317 E 34th Street, Suite 901A
New York, NY 10016   212-684-5860
                                           Fax: 212-684-5864
                                           info@forwardface.org
                                           www.forwardface.org

Founded in 1978 by parents of children with facial differences;
helps children and their families find immediate support to manage the medical and social effects of facial differences.

Camille Walsh, Manager

3038 Guardians of Hydrocephalus Research Foundation
2618 Avenue Z
Brooklyn, NY 11235   718-743-4473
                                           800-458-8655
                                           Fax: 718-743-1171
                                           ghrf2618@aol.com
                                           www.ghrforg.org

Nonprofit group dedicated to research into the cause and treatment of hydrocephalus. Guardians operate a laboratory in the Department of Neurology at New York University Medical Center,
in which information from clinical and research facilities is integrated to provide for better diagnosis and treatment of hydrocephalus, a frequently occuring congenital disorder that can also occur
shortly after birth. Hydrocephalus accounts for a large propotion
of adult patients with a diagnosis of dementia.

Kathy Soriano

3039 Hydrocephalus Association
4340 East West Highway, Suite 905
Bethesda, MDÿ 20814, MD 20814   301- 20- 381
                                           888-598-3789
                                           Fax: 301-202-3813
                                           info@hydroassoc.org
                                           www.hydroassoc.org

A national nonprofit organization devoted exclusively to
hydrocepahalus. We provide support, education and an extensive
range of resources to families and professionals dealing with the
complex issues of hydrocephalus, the abnormal accumulation of
cerebrospinal fluid within the brain. Our resources cover all age
groups, from prenatal to adults with normal pressure
hydrocepahalus. Our office is staffed daily from 10 AM to 4 PM
Pacific time.

Dawn Mancuso,, CEO
Randi Corey, Director of Special Events
Aisha Heath, Director of Development

3040 Hydrocephalus Support Group
9245 Sky Park Court, Suite 130
San Diego, CA 92123   619-268-8252
                                           Fax: 619-268-4275
                                           efrc@mail.sdsu.edu

Provides education and support for hydrocephalus patients and
their families. The HSG puts out a quarterly newspaper, gives
parent referrals and has a library with articles and tapes about
hydrocephalus.

3041 March of Dimes Foundation
1275 Mamaroneck Avenue
White Plains, NY 10605   914-997-4488
                                           888-663-4637
                                           Fax: 914-997-4763
                                           answers@marchofdimes.com
                                           www.marchofdimes.com

Partnership of volunteers and professionals dedicated to improving the health of babies by preventing birth defects and infant
mortality. Over 100 chapters are located across the country and
can be located through the National Office.

Stacey D. Stewart, President

3042 National Craniofacial Foundation
PO Box 11082
Chattanooga, TN 37401   800-332-2373
                                           faces@faces-cranio.org
                                           www.faces-cranio.org

Provides information to affected individuals; families of affected
individuals; the public or media and professionals. We also provide peer support; professional counseling; medical referrals; referrals for non-medical services and to local chapters or groups.
We offer pamphlets; fact sheets; newsletter; booklets; video's and
movies.

Lynne Mayfield, Director

3043 National Hydrocephalus Foundation
12413 Centralia Road
Lakewood, CA 90715   562-924-6666
                                           888-857-3434
                                           debbifields@nhfonline.org
                                           www.nhfonline.org

Promotes information and educational assistance. Establishes and
facilitates a communication network and works to increase public
awareness. Promote and support research. Also has brochures,
help sheets, and more. Quarterly newsletter with annual
membership fee of $35.00.

Debbie Fields, Executive Director
Michael Fields, President
Jaynie Dunn, Secretary

Conferences

3044 North American Craniofacial Family Confere nce
AmeriFace
PO Box 751112
Las Vegas, NV 89136   702-769-9264
                                           888-486-1209
                                           Fax: 702-341-5351
                                           info@ameriface.org
                                           www.ameriface.org

July
Debbie Oliver, Executive Director

Web Sites

3045 National Hydrocephalus Foundation
www.nhfonline.org

Promotes information and educational assistance. Establishes and
facilitates a communication network and works to increase public
awareness. Promote and support research. Also has brochures,
help sheets and more. Quarterly newsletter included with annual
membership fee of $35.00.

3046 Rare Genetic Diseases in Children (NYU)
550 First Avenue
New York, NY 10016   212-263-7300
                                           www.med.nyu.edu/rgdc/homenow.htm

We target issues arising from rare genetic diseases affecting children. Also, to assist in the endeavor to bring knowledge and hope
to those for whom there is, at present, so little.

Laurence D. Fink, Co Chair
Kenneth G. Langone, Co Chair
Robert I. Grossman, MD, Dean & CEO

Book Publishers

3047 Congenital Disorders Sourcebook
Omnigraphics
PO Box 8002
Aston, PA 19014   800-234-1340
                                           Fax: 800-875-1340
                                           info@omnigraphics.com
                                           www.omnigraphics.com

Basic consumer health information on disorders aquired during gestation, including spina bifida, hydrocephalus, cerebral palsy, heart defects, craniofacial abnormalities and fetal alcohol syndrome.

650 pages
ISBN: 0-780809-45-9

Newsletters

3048 AmeriFace Newsletter
AmeriFace
PO Box 75112
Las Vegas, NV 89136

702-769-9264
888-486-1209
Fax: 702-341-5351
info@ameriface.org
www.ameriface.org

A free newsletter.

8 pages

David Reisberg, DDS, President
Christina Corsigla, Vice President
Debbie Oliver, Executive Director

3049 National Hydrocephalus Foundation Newsletter
12413 Centralia Road
Lakewood, CA 90715

562-924-6666
888-857-3434
Fax: 415-732-7044
debbifields@nhfonline.org, info@nhfonlin
www.nhfonline.org

The Foundation is a national organization whose purpose is to provide information and education, along with peer support news-letter quarterly.

12-15 pages Quarterly

Michael Fields, President/ Treasurer
Debbie Fields, Executive Director
Jaynie Dunn, Secretary

DESCRIPTION

3050 ENCOPRESIS

Involves the following Biologic System(s):

Developmental/Behavioral/Psychiatric Disorders, Gastrointestinal Disorders

Encopresis refers to the passage of feces in inappropriate or unacceptable places by children who have no detectable disorder or organic abnormality and who are past the age when toilet training is typically completed. This type of soiling may be considered primary encopresis, in which fecal incontinence persists from birth, or secondary encopresis, a regressive form of this disorder in which fecal incontinence occurs in children who were previously toilet trained. Children with this disorder may refuse to use a commode, may soil their clothing, or may defecate in secret places. Other associated findings may include chronic constipation leading to the presence of large, hardened fecal masses in the colon or rectum (fecal impaction) that, in turn, may result in an abnormally enlarged or dilated colon (megacolon). Encopresis occurs in approximately one percent of school children and is much more common in boys than it is in girls.

The causes of encopresis may sometimes be linked to anger, defiance, resistance, or fear of toilet training and, as such, may indicate the need for psychotherapeutic intervention that includes parents or caregivers, as well as the affected child. Treatment is often supportive. For example, a reward system may be established so that the child has an incentive to cooperate. In addition, the affected child may be encouraged to use the bathroom at specific times (e.g., after meals) and for specified periods of time. Parents are advised to remain nonjudgmental and nonretaliatory, so that consequences for noncompliance are minor. Additional treatment for primary encopresis may initially include the carefully monitored, short-term use of laxatives and enemas to relieve constipation and subsequent complications. Affected children may sometimes benefit from biofeedback, during which individuals learn how to control certain involuntary physiologic functions such as, in this case, the anal sphincter muscle. In addition, the careful administration of mineral oil, together with a high fiber diet, may be effective in relieving constipation and associated complications in children with secondary encopresis. Other treatment is symptomatic and supportive.

Government Agencies

3051 NIH/ Eunice Kennedy Shriver National Institute of Child Health & Human Development
31 Center Drive, Building 31
Bethesda, MD 20892
301-496-5113
800-370-2943
Fax: 866-760-5947
nichdpress@mail.nih.gov
www.nichd.nih.gov

Established in 1962 by congress, today the institute conducts and supports research on topics related to the health of children, adults, families and populations. Some of these topics include: developmental disabilities, growth and development, infant death, reproductive health and birth defects.

Diana W. Bianchi, Director
Paul Williams, Director, Communications

National Associations & Support Groups

3052 American Academy of Pediatrics
141 Northwest Point Boulevard
Elk Grove Village, IL 60007
847-434-4000
800-433-9016
Fax: 847-434-8000
www.aap.org

The American Academy of Pediatrics and its member pediatricians are committed to the attainment of optimal physical, mental and social health and well-being for all infants, children, adolescents, and young adults.

Fernando Stein, MD, FAAP, President
Karen Remley, MD, CEO/Executive VP

3053 International Foundation for Functional Gastrointestinal Disorders
PO Box 170864
Milwaukee, WI 53217
414-964-1799
Fax: 414-964-7176
iffgd@iffgd.org
www.iffgd.org

The organization offers responses to those commonly asked questions for families and individuals whose lives have been touched with the disorder.

Nancy J. Norton, President & Director
William Norton, Co-Founder

3054 March of Dimes Foundation
1275 Mamaroneck Avenue
White Plains, NY 10605
914-997-4488
888-663-4637
Fax: 914-997-4763
answers@marchofdimes.com
www.marchofdimes.com

Partnership of volunteers and professionals dedicated to improving the health of babies by preventing birth defects and infant mortality. Over 100 chapters are located across the country and can be located through the National Office.

Stacey D. Stewart, President

Conferences

3055 IFFGD Professional Symposia
Int'l Foundation for Functional Gastrointestinal
PO Box 170864
Milwaukee, WI 53217
414-964-1799
888-964-2001
Fax: 414-964-7176
iffgd@iffgd.org
www.iffgd.org

Aimed at promoting education and awareness among professionals from multiple disciplines who treat gastrointestinal disorders and incontinence.

April

Nancy J Norton, President

Web Sites

3056 Mental Help Net
P.O. Box 20709
Columbus, OH 43220
614-448-4055
800-232-TALK
info@centersite.net, editor@centersite.n
mentalhelp.net

We wish to provide the following: to develop and debate in an open forum the future of the mental health field in America and throughout the world; to help coordinate various components of the mental health field, so as to bring about greater communication between them; also to educate the public about mental health issues.

Book Publishers

3057 What I Need to Know About Constipation
Nat'l Digestive Diseases Information Clearinghouse
31 Center Drive
Bethesda, MD 20892
301-496-3583
Fax: 301-907-8906
nddic@info.niddk.nih.gov
www.niddk.nih.gov

Defines constipation and includes a list of steps for prevention, as well as a list of additional resources

Pamphlets

3058 Constipation
NDDIC
9000 Rockville Pike
Bethesda, MD 20892
301-496-3583
800-891-5389
Fax: 301-907-8906
nddic@info.niddk.nih.gov
www.niddk.nih.gov

Includes a definition of constipation and information on how it develops, how it is diagnosed, and how it can be treated. Also provides details on misconceptions about constipation.

8 pages

Griffin P. Rodgers, MD, MACP, Director
Dr. Gregory Germino, Deputy Director
Kevin Abbott, Program Director

3059 Constipation in Children
Nat'l Digestive Diseases Information Clearinghouse
9000 Rockville Pike
Bethesda, MD 20892
301-496-3583
Fax: 301-907-8906
nddic@info.niddk.nih.gov
www.niddk.nih.gov

Griffin P. Rodgers, MD, MACP, Director
Dr. Gregory Germino, Deputy Director
Kevin Abbott, Program Director

3060 Fecal Incontinence
NDDIC
9000 Rockville Pike
Bethesda, MD 20892
301-496-3583
800-891-5389
Fax: 301-907-8906
nddic@info.niddk.nih.gov
www.niddk.nih.gov

8 pages

Griffin P. Rodgers, MD, MACP, Director
Dr. Gregory Germino, Deputy Director
Kevin Abbott, Program Director

DESCRIPTION

3061 EPIDERMOLYSIS BULLOSA

Covers these related disorders: Epidermolysis bullosa dystrophica, Epidermolysis bullosa simplex, Junctional epidermolysis bullosa

Involves the following Biologic System(s):
Dermatologic Disorders

Epidermolysis bullosa is a group of inherited diseases that are often apparent at birth (congenital) and characterized by blistering of the skin after minor injury or trauma. In addition, blistering tends to worsen in warm temperatures. These disorders vary in severity, specific features, and mode of inheritance, and are classified under one of three groupings.

Epidermolysis bullosa simplex is a relatively mild, non-scarring form of this disorder that is inherited as an autosomal dominant trait. Epidermolysis bullosa simplex is further categorized as generalized or localized. The generalized type is usually apparent at birth or soon thereafter. The blisters, also known as bullae, are usually located on areas of the body that are prone to injury such as the hands, feet, elbows, knees, etc. Blistering tendencies usually lessen with advancing age with no long-term effects or scarring. The localized form of this disorder, known as Weber-Cockayne syndrome, affects the hands and feet and may not become apparent until walking commences or, in some cases, adolescence or adulthood. Blistering may be mild, but may severely worsen with such activities as extended walking. Treatment is symptomatic and supportive and may be directed toward prevention and treatment of secondary infections.

Junctional epidermolysis bullosa is inherited as an autosomal recessive trait and is also apparent at birth or soon thereafter. Characteristic findings and symptoms associated with this|potentially life-threatening form of the disorder may include severe blistering around the mouth and on the scalp, trunk, diaper area, and legs. In addition, slow-healing lesions may develop in the mucous membranes of the respiratory, gastrointestinal, and genitourinary tracts. Affected infants are also at increased risk for infections such as septicemia, a life-threatening condition in which harmful bacteria multiply in the bloodstream. In addition, the nails may appear defective and teeth may decay easily. Other findings may include growth retardation and abnormally low levels of circulating red blood cells (anemia). Treatment for junctional epidermolysis bullosa may include the administration of antibiotics to treat infections and blood transfusions to treat anemia. In addition, nutritional supplementation may be beneficial. Other treatment is symptomatic and supportive.

Epidermolysis bullosa dystrophica may be inherited as an autosomal dominant trait, an autosomal recessive trait, or it may appear sporadically. Findings associated with autosomal dominant inheritance are less severe than those of autosomal recessive transmission. This form of epidermolysis bullosa may be further categorized as the albopapuloid Pasini variant and the Cockayne-Touraine variant. The albopapuloid Pasini variant may first appear as early as infancy or as late as adolescence and is characterized by extensive, scarring-type blistering of the skin on the joints, arms, and legs; the appearance during adolescence of flesh-colored (albopapuloid) lesions on the trunk; and involvement of certain mucuous memberanes. The Cockayne-Touraine variant of this disorder develops during infancy or early childhood and is characterized by blisters that most commonly appear on the arms and legs.

Epidermolysis bullosa dystrophica that is inherited as an autosomal recessive trait is a severe form of this disorder that may be characterized at birth by extensive blistering and erosions of the body surfaces and mucous membranes. As the lesions heal, scarring may result in deformity and limited mobility. In addition, healing of the mucous membranes of the esophagus may cause narrowing of this structure, leading to difficulties in feeding and eating. Treatment may include the implementation of a special diet or use of special feeding devices necessitated by scarring or narrowing of the esophagus. Additional treatment may be directed toward the prevention or care of associated secondary infections. Other treatment is symptomatic and supportive.

Government Agencies

3062 NIH/National Institute of Arthritis and Musculoskeletal and Skin Diseases
1 AMS Circle
Bethesda, MD 20892

301-495-4484
877-226-4267
Fax: 301-718-6366
TDD: 301-565-2966
niamsinfo@mail.nih.gov
www.niams.nih.gov

The mission of the NIAMS, a part of the NIH, is to support research into the causes, treatment, and prevention of arthritis and musculoskeletal and skin diseases, the training of basic and clinical scientists to carry out this research, and the dissemination of information on research progress in these diseases.

Stephen I Katz MD PhD, Director
Robert H Carter MD, Deputy Director

National Associations & Support Groups

3063 American Academy of Pediatrics
141 Northwest Point Boulevard
Elk Grove Village, IL 60007

847-434-4000
800-433-9016
Fax: 847-434-8000
www.aap.org

The American Academy of Pediatrics and its member pediatricians are committed to the attainment of optimal physical, mental and social health and well-being for all infants, children, adolescents, and young adults.

Fernando Stein, MD, FAAP, President
Karen Remley, MD, CEO/Executive VP

3064 DebRA: Dystrophic Epidermolysis Bullosa Research Association of America
16 East 41st Street
New York, NY 10017

212-868-1573
866-332-7276
Fax: 212-513-4099
staff@debra.org
www.debra.org

Committed to providing referrals, patient advocacy and lobbying, offers networking services, and engages in patient and professional education.

Suzanne J Cohen, Executive Director
Abby Meadows, Development Manager

3065 Genetic Alliance
4301 Connecticut Avenue NW, Suite 404
Washington, DC 20008
202-966-5557
800-336-4363
Fax: 202-966-8553
info@geneticalliance.org
www.geneticalliance.org

A coalition of voluntary genetic support groups, consumers and professionals addressing the needs of individuals and families affected by genetic disorders from a national perspective.

Sharon Terry, President/CEO
Tetyana Murza, Managing Director
Natasha Bonhomme, VP, Strategic Development

3066 March of Dimes Foundation
1275 Mamaroneck Avenue
White Plains, NY 10605
914-997-4488
888-663-4637
Fax: 914-997-4763
answers@marchofdimes.com
www.marchofdimes.com

Partnership of volunteers and professionals dedicated to improving the health of babies by preventing birth defects and infant mortality. Over 100 chapters are located across the country and can be located through the National Office.

Stacey D. Stewart, President

Conferences

3067 Genetic Alliance Annual Conference
Genetic Alliance
4301 Connecticut Avenue NW, Suite 404
Washington, DC 20008
202-966-5557
800-336-4363
Fax: 202-966-8553
info@geneticalliance.org
www.geneticalliance.org

Consistently inspirational and enables partnership among all stakeholders: advocates and community leaders, health and industry professionals, policymakers, and academicians.

July

Sharon Terry, President/CEO
Tetyana Murza, Managing Director
Natasha Bonhomme, VP, Strategic Development

Web Sites

3068 EB Medical Research Foundation
2757 Anchor Ave
Los Angeles, CA 90064
www.ebkids.org

The EBMRF is a nonprofit, whose sole purpose is dedicated to the support of medical research of epidermolysis bullosa — its causes, its cure, and the development of successful treatments.

Jerry J. Joseph, Chair
Lynn Anderson, President & Founder
Paul J. Joseph, CFO

3069 Family Village
www.familyvillage.wisc.edu

A global community that integrates information, resources and communication opportunities on the Internet for persons with cognitive and other disabilities, for their families and for those that provide them services and support.

3070 Online Mendelian Inheritance in Man
U.S. National Library of Medicine, 8600 Rockville
Bethesda, MD 20894
888-346-3656
info@ncbi.nlm.nih.gov
www.ncbi.nlm.nih.gov

This database is a catalog of human genes and genetic disorders.

Christine E. Seidman, M.D., Chair
David J. Lipman, M.D., Executive Secretary
Michael Boehnke, Ph.D., Board Member

Newsletters

3071 DebRA Currents
DebRA
75 Broad Street, Suite 300
New York, NY 10004
212-868-1573
866-332-7276
Fax: 212-868-9296
staff@deba.org
www.debra.org

Brett Kopelan, Executive Director
Rita Garson, Finance Director
Gabrielle Sedor, Program Manager

DESCRIPTION

3072 ERB'S PALSY

Synonym: Erb-Duchenne paralysis

Involves the following Biologic System(s):

Neurologic Disorders

Erb's palsy is a form of paralysis in newborns resulting from injury to certain nerves (i.e., fifth and sixth cervical nerves of upper brachial plexus) that supply specific muscles of the shoulder and arm. Nerve injury may be the result of a difficult delivery (e.g., breech presentation, delivery of an unusually large newborn, etc.). During delivery, lateral traction of the head and neck may occur and lead to stretching of these nerves, potentially resulting in such injury.

Newborns with Erb's palsy typically experience swelling and inflammation of the affected nerves and paralysis of the affected shoulder and arm muscles (e.g., deltoid, biceps, brachialis). This causes the arm to hang loosely with the elbow extended and inwardly rotated. Newborns with the condition are unable to move the affected arm away from the shoulder or rotate the arm away from the body. In addition, although they may extend the forearm, affected newborns lack a startle reflex known as Moro's reflex on the affected side. Moro's reflex, which is usually present at birth, involves stretching of the arms and legs forward and out and extension of the fingers when startled. In some severe cases, paralysis and associated loss of the muscle mass (atrophy)in the shoulder area (deltoid muscle) may cause drop shoulder, which is characterized by depression of the affected shoulder below the level of the other. Some infants may experience impairment of sensation in affected areas. Movements of the hand are typically not affected.

The effectiveness of certain treatments for Erb's palsy may vary, depending upon whether affected nerves (i.e., fifth and sixth cervical nerves) were torn or injured in a manner that allows a return of function within a few months. Treatment measures may include initial immobilization of the affected arm and shoulder with braces or splints and physical therapy including range of motion exercises, massage, and active and passive corrective exercises. Such therapy may help to improve muscle function and prevent permanent bending of affected joints in a fixed posture (flexion contractures). If paralysis continues at three to six months of age, surgical measures may be considered in some cases.

National Associations & Support Groups

3073 American Academy of Pediatrics
141 Northwest Point Boulevard
Elk Grove Village, IL 60007
847-434-4000
800-433-9016
Fax: 847-434-8000
www.aap.org

The American Academy of Pediatrics and its member pediatricians are committed to the attainment of optimal physical, mental and social health and well-being for all infants, children, adolescents, and young adults.

Fernando Stein, MD, FAAP, President
Karen Remley, MD, CEO/Executive VP

3074 Brachial Plexus Palsy Foundation
210 Springhaven Circle
Royersford, PA 19468
610-792-0974
contact@brachialplexuspalsyfoundation.or
www.brachialplexuspalsyfoundation.org

A non profit organizaztion designed to raise funds for activities in support of families with children who have suffered brachial plexus injuries. The Foundation also provides information about a brachial plexus injury ti better educate families who do not have the time or resources.

3075 March of Dimes Foundation
1275 Mamaroneck Avenue
White Plains, NY 10605
914-997-4488
888-663-4637
Fax: 914-997-4763
answers@marchofdimes.com
www.marchofdimes.com

Partnership of volunteers and professionals dedicated to improving the health of babies by preventing birth defects and infant mortality. Over 100 chapters are located across the country and can be located through the National Office.

Stacey D. Stewart, President

3076 National Brachial Plexus/Erb's Palsy Association
PO Box 23
Larsen, WI 54947
920-836-9955
Fax: 920-836-9587
erbspalsy@usa.net
www.nbpepa.org

Provides support, promotes public awareness, serves as a resource to families and professionals and provides a network of information to incearse the understanding of Brachial Pelxus injuries and to discover new and better way to treat children with the injury.

3077 United Brachial Plexus Network
1610 Kent Street
Kent, OH 44240
781-315-6161
866-877-7004
Fax: 866-877-7004
info@ubpn.org
www.ubpn.org

A registered non-profit organization devoted to providing information, support, and leadership for families and those concerned with brachial plexus injuries worldwide. Also provided is an online registry, various outreach and awareness programs and publications.

Nancy Birk, President

Libraries & Resource Centers

3078 National Rehabilitation Information Center
4200 Forbes Blvd, Suite 202
Lanham, MD 20706
301-459-5900
800-346-2742
Fax: 301-562-2401
TTY: 301-459-5984
naricinfo@heitechservices.com
www.naric.com

Committed to providing direct, personal and high quality information services to anyone interested in disability and rehabilitation issues. We are committed to serving customers, researchers, family members, health professionals, educators, counselors and students throughout the country.

Mark Odum, Director

Web Sites

3079 Texas Children's Hospital
6621 Fannin Street
Houston, TX 77030
832-824-1000
www.texaschildrenshospital.org

Is an internationally recognized full-care prediatric hospital located in the Texas Medical Center in Houston. The largest pediatric hospital in the United States, Texas Children's is nationaly ranked in the top 5 among children's hospitals.

Mark A. Wallace, President & CEO
Dr. Mark Kline, Physician-in-Chief
Dr. Charles D. Fraser, Jr., Surgeon-in-Chief

Newsletters

3080 Outreach
United Brachial Plexus Network
1610 Kent Street
Kent, OH 44240

781-315-6161
866-877-7004
Fax: 866-877-7004
info@ubpn.org
www.ubpn.org

Brachial Plexus/Erb's Palsy newsletter.

DESCRIPTION

3081 ERYTHEMA INFECTIOSUM
Synonyms: EI, Fifth disease, Sticker's disease, Parvovirus, Slapped Cheek
Involves the following Biologic System(s):
Infectious Disorders

Erythema infectiosum, or Fifth disease, is a contagious infection caused by the human parvovirus B19. It is characterized by a three-stage rash. First, there is the sudden appearance of a red rash on the face that may look as if the cheeks had been slapped. Then the rash progresses to a reddish, raised-spot, blotchy eruption that spreads to the trunk, buttocks, arms, and legs. When it begins to fade, the rash takes on a lacy-type appearance. The rash usually subsides within five to 10 days, but may reappear within a month's time, especially after exercise, stress, skin irritation, or exposure to sunlight. Transmission of this virus is through inhalation of droplets exhaled or coughed into the air by infected individuals. The incubation period for erythema infectiosum is approximately four to 14 days.

Erythema infectiosum occurs most commonly in preschool and young school-age children. The first symptoms may be low-grade fever and headache. Once the rash appears or shortly thereafter, fever and other signs of illness may be absent. However, some older children and adults may develop mild itching (pruritus), joint pain (arthralgia), and inflammation of the joints (arthritis). In addition, under certain circumstances, exposure to human parvovirus B19 may result in more severe complications. For example, individuals with certain blood disorders such as thalessemia or sickle cell anemia may develop a temporary inability to produce red blood cells, resulting in a decrease in the body's capacity to supply oxygen to the tissues of the body (anemia). Symptoms associated with severe anemia may include weakness, discomfort, pale skin (pallor), rapid breathing (tachypnea), and rapid heartbeat (tachycardia). In addition, those who have impaired immune function may experience severe consequences upon exposure to human parvovirus B19. For example, individuals undergoing certain types of chemotherapy, those with acquired immunodeficiency syndrome (AIDS), or those with certain types of primary, inherited immune defects may experience recurrent or prolonged infections, anemia, or other blood abnormalities.

Pregnant women infected with parvovirus B19 may transmit it to their unborn children, resulting, in rare cases, in miscarriage or stillbirth; however, most of those exposed in utero are born with no apparent consequences. Other viral-exposed infants may have abnormal accumulations of fluid in the tissues or cavities of the body (hydrops). If this condition is diagnosed before birth, special blood transfusions delivered by way of the umbilical vein may be of benefit to the affected fetus. Treatment for this viral infection is symptomatic.

Government Agencies

3082 NIH/National Institute of Allergy and Infectious Diseases
5601 Fishers Lane, MSC 9806
Bethesda, MD 20892
301-496-5717
866-284-4107
Fax: 301-402-3573
TDD: 800-877-8339
ocpostoffice@niaid.nih.gov
www.niaid.nih.gov

Conducts and supports basic and applied research to better understand, treat, and ultimately prevent infectious, immunologic, and allergic diseases.
Anthony S Fauci MD, Director

National Associations & Support Groups

3083 American Academy of Pediatrics
141 Northwest Point Boulevard
Elk Grove Village, IL 60007
847-434-4000
800-433-9016
Fax: 847-434-8000
www.aap.org

The American Academy of Pediatrics and its member pediatricians are committed to the attainment of optimal physical, mental and social health and well-being for all infants, children, adolescents, and young adults.
Fernando Stein, MD, FAAP, President
Karen Remley, MD, CEO/Executive VP

3084 March of Dimes Foundation
1275 Mamaroneck Avenue
White Plains, NY 10605
914-997-4488
888-663-4637
Fax: 914-997-4763
answers@marchofdimes.com
www.marchofdimes.com

Partnership of volunteers and professionals dedicated to improving the health of babies by preventing birth defects and infant mortality. Over 100 chapters are located across the country and can be located through the National Office.
Stacey D. Stewart, President

3085 World Health Organization
Avenue Appia 20
Geneva, SL
Switzerland
122-791-2111
Fax: 122-791-3111
www.who.int

WHO is the directing and coordinating authority for health within the United Nations system.
Dr Margaret Chan, Director General

Web Sites

3086 Kid's Health
kidshealth.org
Kids health is the largest and most visited site on the web providing doctor-approved health information about children from before birth through adolescence. Kids health provides families with accurate, up to date and jargon free health information they can use.
Neil Izenberg, MD, Editor-in-Chief & Founder

3087 Med Help International
www.medhelp.org
800-522-5006
www.medhelp.org

Is dedicated to helping patients find the highest quality medical information in the world today. We offer patients the tools necessary to make informed treatment decisions within the short time lines dedicated by their illness or disease.

3088 New York State Department of Health
www.medhelp.org/lib/fifth.htm

800-522-5006
www.medhelp.org/lib/fifth.htm

Information on erythema infectiosum, like how does anyone get it, what is the treatment, and what can be done to prevent this disease from occuring.

DESCRIPTION

3089 ESOPHAGEAL ATRESIA

Synonyms: Tracheo-esophageal fistula, Vacterl, Vater

Involves the following Biologic System(s):

Gastrointestinal Disorders

Esophageal atresia is a defect that is present at birth (congenital). The esophagus, which is a muscular tube, is that portion of the digestive system that connects the throat and the stomach. In infants with esophageal atresia, the channel (lumen) within the tubular esophagus fails to develop properly, resulting in an esophagus that ends in a blind pouch, failing to provide a continuous passage to the stomach. In some infants, the upper section of the esophagus may be dramatically narrowed or it may be closed at its lower end. In others, the closed-end lower portion extends upward from the stomach and there is no through connection between the two. Most affected infants also have an abnormal tube-like connection or opening between the windpipe (trachea) and either the upper or lower portion of the esophagus. This is known as a tracheoesophageal fistula. In some children, there is a double connection in which there is an abnormal passage between the trachea and part of the esophagus, as well as between the trachea and a lower region of the esophagus.

Infants with esophageal atresia cannot swallow at all and therefore salivate and regurgitate excessively. If a tracheoesophageal fistula exists between the windpipe and upper portion of the esophagus, fluid may enter the lungs, resulting in coughing, choking, a bluish discoloration (cyanosis) of the nail beds, lips, and mucous membranes, and possibly pneumonia. The presence of an abnormal passage between the trachea and the lower section of the esophagus may allow air to enter the abdomen, resulting in excessive abdominal swelling (distension) that may interfere with normal breathing. In addition, contents of the abdomen may enter the lungs and severe inflammation may occur. If esophageal atresia is present without a fistula, characteristic findings may include a boat-shaped abdomen that is devoid of air.

Treatment includes surgery to join or connect the two sections of the esophagus. This procedure is known as an esophageal anastomosis. Tracheoesophageal fistulas may be surgically corrected by ligation, a procedure in which the passageway is tied off. Before surgery, special care is taken to ensure the infants do not draw fluid (aspirate) into their lungs through the esophagus.

As many as 50 percent of infants with esophageal atresia have associated structural malformations of other organs. For example, if a tracheoesophageal fistula is present, other abnormalities of the trachea may also be apparent. In addition, approximately half of all affected infants have a complex of congenital anomalies (VACTERL syndrome) characterized by additional malformations involving the heart, skeleton, kidneys, and urinary and genital systems. Treatment for esophageal atresia includes management or correction of associated anomalies. Esophageal atresia occurs in approximately one in 3,500 births in the United States. About 33 percent of these infants are born prematurely.

National Associations & Support Groups

3090 American Academy of Pediatrics
141 Northwest Point Boulevard
Elk Grove Village, IL 60007

847-434-4000
800-433-9016
Fax: 847-434-8000
www.aap.org

The American Academy of Pediatrics and its member pediatricians are committed to the attainment of optimal physical, mental and social health and well-being for all infants, children, adolescents, and young adults.

Fernando Stein, MD, FAAP, President
Karen Remley, MD, CEO/Executive VP

3091 American College of Gastroenterology
6400 Goldsboro Road, Suite 200
Bethesda, MD 20817

301-263-9000
info@acg.gi.org
www.gi.org

Founded to advance the scientific study and medical practice of diseases of the gastrointestinal (GI) tract.

13,000 members

Carol A. Burke, MD, FACG, President

3092 Digestive Disease National Coalition
507 Capitol Court NE, Suite 200
Washington, DC 20002

202-544-7497
Fax: 202-546-7105
hpayne@hmcw.org
www.ddnc.org

Advocacy organization comprised of over 30 voluntary and professional societies concerned with the many diseases of the digestive tract and liver.

Lynn Seim, Chairperson
Ralph McKibbin, President
Cathy Griffith, Vice Chairperson

3093 International Foundation for Functional Gastrointestinal Disorders
PO Box 170864
Milwaukee, WI 53217

414-964-1799
Fax: 414-964-7176
iffgd@iffgd.org
www.iffgd.org

Nonprofit education and research organization founded in 1991. IFFGD addresses the issues surrounding life with gastrointestinal (GI) functional and mobility disorders and increases the awareness about these disorders among the general public, researchers and the clinical care community.

Nancy J. Norton, President & Director
William Norton, Co-Founder

3094 North American Society for Pediatric Gastroenterology/Hepatology/Nutrition
714 N Bethlehem Pike, Suite 300
Ambler, PA 19002

215-641-9800
Fax: 215-641-1995
naspghan@naspghan.org
www.naspghan.org

Strives to improve the care of infants, children and adolescents with digestive disorders by promoting advances in clinical care of children with chronic abdominal pain, diarrhea, constipation, vomiting, bleeding from the GI tract, inflammatory bowel disease, liver diseases, diseases of the pancreas, poor weight gain and nutritional problems.

Margaret K Stallings, Executive Director
Kim Rose, Associate Director
Donna Murphy, Membership

Libraries & Resource Centers

3095 National Digestive Diseases Information Clearinghouse
9000 Rockville Pike
Bethesda, MD 20892   301-496-3583
800-860-8747
Fax: 301-907-8906
healthinfo@niddk.nih.gov
www.niddk.nih.gov

The National Institute of Diabetes and Digestive and Kidney Diseases conducts and supports research on many of the most serious diseases affecting public health. The Institute supports much of the clinical research on the diseases of internal medicine and related subspecialty fields as well as many basic science disciplines.

Dr. Griffin P. Rodgers, Director
Dr. Gregory G. Germino, Deputy Director
Camille M. Hoover, M.S.W., Executive Officer

Conferences

3096 IFFGD Professional Symposia
Int'l Foundation for Functional Gastrointestinal
PO Box 170864
Milwaukee, WI 53217   414-964-1799
888-964-2001
Fax: 414-964-7176
iffgd@iffgd.org
www.iffgd.org

Aimed at promoting education and awareness among professionals from multiple disciplines who treat gastrointestinal disorders and incontinence.

April

Nancy J Norton, President

3097 NASPGHAN Annual Meeting and Postgraduate Course
NASPGHAN
714 N. Bethlehem Pike, Ste 300
Ambler, PA 19002   215-641-9800
Fax: 215-641-1995
naspghan@naspghan.org
www.naspghan.org

November

Margaret K Stallings, Executive Director
Kim Rose, Associate Director
Donna Murphy, Membership

Web Sites

3098 National Digestive Diseases Information Clearinghouse
9000 Rockville Pike
Bethesda, MD 20892   301-496-3583
Fax: 301-907-8906
nddic@info.niddk.nih.gov
www.digestive.niddk.nih.gov

The National Institute of Diabetes and Digestive and Kidney Diseases conducts and supports research on many of the most serious diseases affecting public health. The Institute supports much of the clinical research on the diseases of internal medicine and related subspecialty fields as well as many basic science disciplines.

Griffin P. Rodgers, MD, MACP, Director
Dr. Gregory Germino, Deputy Director
Kevin Abbott, Program Director

Journals

3099 Journal of Pediatric Gastroenterology and Nutrition
NASPGHAN, author

Lippincott Williams & Wilkins
530 Walnut Street
Philadelphia, PA 19106   215-521-8300
Fax: 215-521-8902
www.lww.com

Publication of the North American Society for Pediatric Gastroenterolgy, Hepatology and Nutrition, which strives to improve the care of infants, children and adolescents with digestive disorders by promoting advances in clinical care of children with chronic abdominal pain, diarrhea, constipation, vomiting, bleeding from the GI tract, inflammatory bowel disease, liver diseases, diseases of the pancreas, poor weight gain and nutritional problems.

Newsletters

3100 NASPGHAN News
714 N. Bethlehem Pike, Ste 300
Ambler, PA 19002   215-641-9800
Fax: 215-641-1995
naspghan@naspghan.org
www.naspgn.org

Publication of the North American Society for Pediatric Gastroenterolgy, Hepatology and Nutrition, which strives to improve the care of infants, children and adolescents with digestive disorders by promoting advances in clinical care of children with chronic abdominal pain, diarrhea, constipation, vomiting, bleeding from the GI tract, inflammatory bowel disease, liver diseases, diseases of the pancreas, poor weight gain and nutritional problems.

Margaret K Stallings, Executive Director
Kim Rose, Associate Director
Donna Murphy, Membership

3101 TEF/VATER International Support Network
9005 N Van Houten
Portland, OR 97203   301-535-7185
Fax: 301-952-9152
info@tefvater.org
www.tefvater.org

Provides support to children and adults born with esophageal atresia.

DESCRIPTION

3102 EWING'S SARCOMA

Synonym: Ewing's tumor

Involves the following Biologic System(s):

Hematologic and Oncologic Disorders, Orthopedic and Muscle Disorders

Ewing's sarcoma is a malignant tumor that typically occurs in individuals under the age of 20 years. The tumor most often arises in the long bones of the shin (tibia), thigh (femur), or upper arm (humerus) or the flat bones of the pelvis, vertebrae, or chest wall. Ewing's sarcoma often invades surrounding soft tissues and tends to spread (metastasize) to other bones, the lungs, and, less frequently, to the bone marrow or other organs. In some cases, the primary tumor may develop in soft tissue. Approximately 75 percent of these tumors occur in the legs or arms as well as the bones of the shoulders.

The most common symptoms of Ewing's sarcoma include fever, as well as pain, tenderness, and swelling in the area of the tumor. Some children may also experience weight loss, low levels of circulating red blood cells (anemia), and elevated levels of circulating white blood cells (leukocytosis). In addition, the tumor may weaken the surrounding bone and thus increase vulnerability to bone fracture. The diagnosis of Ewing's tumor is established through the use of x-rays along with examination of tissue samples obtained through biopsy. In addition, other procedures such as bone scanning, computed tomography (CT), and magnetic resonance imaging (MRI) may be used to confirm the presence of lung, bone, or other metastases.

Ewing's sarcoma develops most frequently between the ages of 10 and 20 years of age and affects boys more often than girls by a ratio of two to one. These tumors rarely occur in black children. Treatment of Ewing's sarcoma may include the use of chemotherapy and radiation. Patients are also evaluated for possible surgical removal of the tumor. Other treatment is symptomatic and supportive. Outcome (prognosis) for children with Ewing's sarcoma depends on several factors that include the extent of the disease, the size and location of the tumor, presence or absence of metastases, the tumor's response to therapy, and the age and overall health of the child. Prompt medical attention and aggressive therapy are important for the best prognosis.

Government Agencies

3103 NIH/National Cancer Institute
BG 9609 / 9609 Medical Center Drive
Bethesda, MD 20892   800-422-6237
                                           www.cancer.gov

The National Cancer Institute coordinates the National Cancer Program, which conducts and supports research, training, health information dissemination, and other programs with respect to the cause, diagnosis, prevention, and treatment of cancer, rehabilitation from cancer, and the continuing care of cancer patients and the families of cancer patients.

Douglas R. Lowy, MD, Acting Director
James Doroshow, MD, Deputy Director
Henry P. Ciolino, PhD, Acting Director, Cancer Centers

National Associations & Support Groups

3104 American Academy of Pediatrics
141 Northwest Point Boulevard
Elk Grove Village, IL 60007   847-434-4000
                                           800-433-9016
                                       Fax: 847-434-8000
                                           www.aap.org

The American Academy of Pediatrics and its member pediatricians are committed to the attainment of optimal physical, mental and social health and well-being for all infants, children, adolescents, and young adults.

Fernando Stein, MD, FAAP, President
Karen Remley, MD, CEO/Executive VP

3105 American Cancer Society
Brain Tumor Support Group
ACS Building, 8900 Carpenter Freeway
Dallas, TX 75247   214-819-1200
                                           800-227-2345
                                       Fax: 214-631-3869
                                           www.cancer.org

Attacks the support aspect of this disease from every angle including data on lowering risks to dealing with grief.

Maria Clark, Executive Director

3106 American Childhood Cancer Organization (fo rmerly Candlelighters Childhood Cancer)
PO Box 498
Kensington, MD 20895   301-962-3520
                                           800-366-2223
                                       Fax: 310-962-3521
                                           staff@acco.org
                                           www.acco.org

The Candlelighters Childhood Cancer Foundation National Office was founded in 1970 by concerned parents of children with cancer. Today our membership of over 50,000 members of the national office and more than 100,000 members across the across the country, including Candlelighters affiliate groups, includes, parents of children who are being treated or have been treated for cancer.

Ruth I. Hoffman, MPH, Executive Director
Jessica DiBenedetto, Program Coordinator
Christy Perry, Director, Marketing/Communications

3107 B.A.S.E. Camp Children's Cancer Foundation
650 North Wymore Rd, #103
Winter Park, FL 32789   407-673-5060
                                       Fax: 407-673-5095
                                           info@basecamp.org
                                           www.basecamp.org

Provides a year round base of support for children and families facing the challenge of living with cancer, hemophilia and other blood related illnesses.

Terri Jones, President
Cindy Whitaker, Program Coordinator
Rachel Perez, Office Administrator

3108 Believe In Tomorrow National Children's Fo undation
6601 Fredrick Road
Baltimore, MD 21228   410-744-1032
                                       Fax: 410-744-1984
                                           info@believeintomorrow.org
                                           www.believeintomorrow.org

Provides exceptional hospital and retreat housing services to critically ill children and their families. The Foundation also provides a unique Hands On adventures program that allows children to experience unique once in a lifetime opportunities.

Brian Morrison, Ceo

3109 CancerCare
275 7th Avenue, Floor 22
New York, NY 10001

212-712-8400
800-813-4673
Fax: 212-712-8495
info@cancercare.org
www.cancercare.org

CancerCare is a national nonprofit, 501(c)(3) organization that provides free, professional support services to anyone affected by cancer: people with cancer, caregivers, children, loved ones, and the bereaved. CancerCare programs - including counseling and support groups, education, financial assistance and practical help - are provided by professional oncology social workers and are completely free of charge.

Patricia J Goldsmith, CEO
John Rutigliano, Chief Operating Officer
Ahuva Morris, Children's Program Coordinator

3110 Hair Club for Kids: Hair Club for Men
270 Farmington Avenue, Suite 232
Farmington, CT 06032

860-674-0202
888-888-8986
Fax: 860-676-0805
www.hairclub.com/kids

If your child expresses an interest in wearing a wig, send pictures prior to hair loss with snippets of hair for a good match of original color and texture. The cost of the wig may be covered by insurance.

3111 Just In Time
PO Box 27693
Philadelphia, PA 19118

215-247-8777
Fax: 215-247-0956
www.softhats.com

100% cotton hat, turbans and caps designed for women with hair loss due to cancer, chemotherapy, alopecia or trichotillomania.

Verlay Platt, President

3112 National Childhood Cancer Foundation
4600 East West Highway, Suite 600
Bethesda, MD 20814

301-718-0042
Fax: 301-718-0047
info@curesearch.org
www.curesearch.org

CureSearch unites the world's largest childhood cancer research organization, the Children's Oncology Group, and the National Childhood Cancer Foundation through our mission to cure childhood cancer. Research is the key to the cure.

Stacy Haller, Executive Director

3113 National Coalition for Cancer Survivorship
1010 Wayne Road, Suite 770
Silver Spring, MD 20910

301-650-9127
877-622-7937
Fax: 301-565-9670
info@canceradvocacy.org
www.canceradvocacy.org

Furnishes information about legal rights and advocacy services for cancer survivors of all ages. Publications include: Health Insurance and Cancer: What You Need to Know; Working It Out: Your Employment Rights As a Cancer Survivor; and Charting the Journey: An Almanac of Practical Resources for Cancer Survivors.

Ellen Stovall, President
Michael Bergin, Chief Operating Officer

Web Sites

3114 CancerCare
275 Seventh Avenue
New York, NY 10001

212-712-8400
800-813-4673
Fax: 212-712-8495
info@cancercare.org
www.cancercare.org

CancerCare is a national nonprofit, 501(c)(3) organization that provides free, professional support services to anyone affected by cancer: people with cancer, caregivers, children, loved ones, and the bereaved. CancerCare programs - including counseling and support groups, education, financial assistance and practical help - are provided by professional oncology social workers and are completely free of charge.

Patricia J Goldsmith, CEO
John Rutigliano, Chief Operating Officer
Ahuva Morris, Children's Program Coordinator

3115 Children's Cancer Web
www.cancerindex.org/ccw

An independent nonprofit site, established to provide a directory of childhood cancer resources.

3116 Ewing's Sarcoma Support Group Resources Page
www.cureourchildren.org

310-355-6046
Fax: 310-454-9592
www.cureourchildren.org

3117 OncoLink: The University of Pennslyvania Cancer Center Resource
www.oncolink.upenn.edu

Book Publishers

3118 Let's Talk About Going to the Hospital
Rosen Publishing Group's PowerKids Press
29 E 21st Street
New York, NY 10010

212-777-3017
800-237-9932
Fax: 888-436-4643
rosenpub@tribeca.ios.com
www.powerkidspress.com

If a child has to check into the hospital, chances are he or she is already upset about being ill. Knowing how a hospital functions and what the procedures are, such as when family members can visit, will help in what is already a stressful situation. Grades K-5.

24 pages
ISBN: 0-823950-36-0

3119 Let's Talk About when Kids Have Cancer
Rosen Publishing Group's PowerKids Press
29 E 21st Street
New York, NY 10010

212-777-3017
800-237-9932
Fax: 888-436-4643
customerservice@rosenpub.com
www.powerkidspress.com

In a straightforward yet comforting way, this book explains what cancer is, what kinds of treatments surround the disease and how to cope if a child or the friend of a child has cancer.

24 pages
ISBN: 0-823951-95-2

3120 Pediatric Cancer Sourcebook
Omnigraphics
PO Box 8002
Aston, PA 19014

800-234-1340
Fax: 800-875-1340
info@omnigraphics.com
www.omnigraphics.com

Basic consumer health information about leukemias, brain tumors, sarcomas, lymphomas and other cancers in infants, children and adolescents.

587 pages
ISBN: 0-780802-45-4

Camps

3121 Arizona Camp Sunrise & Sidekicks
PO Box 27872
Tempe, AZ 85285

480-382-8564
928-478-4564
melissa@azcampsunrise.org
www.azcampsunrise.org

The camp is dedicated to provide an exciting, medically safe camp program for children whose families have been affected by cancer.

Melissa Lee, Camp Director

3122 Camp Catch-A-Rainbow
American Cancer Society
1205 E Saginaw Street
Lansing, MI 48906

248-302-8985
kwilson@ymcastorercamps.org
www.ymcastorercamps.org/ccar/camp-catch-a-rainbow/

Open to any child, ages 7 thru 15, who has, or has had, cancer.

Katie Wilson, Coordinator

3123 Camp Sunshine Dreams
PO Box 28232
Fresno, CA 93729

contact@campsunshinedreams.com
www.campsunshinedreams.com

Summer camp for children with cancer.

Anthony Aiello, Board Member

3124 Okizu Foundation Camps
16 Digital Drive, Suite 130
Novato, CA 94949

415-382-9083
Fax: 415-382-8384
info@okizu.org
www.okizu.org

This foundation runs family camp programs for children who have cancer and their families, and for children who have or had a parent with cancer.

Lori Sparrow, Executive Director
Heather Ferrier, Camp Director of Operations

DESCRIPTION

3125 FAMILIAL DYSAUTONOMIA

Synonyms: FD, HSAN-III, Riley-Day syndrome

Involves the following Biologic System(s):

Genetic/Chromosomal/Syndrome/Metabolic Disorders, Neurologic Disorders

Familial dysautonomia (FD) is a rare inherited disorder of that part of the nervous system responsible for regulating various essential involuntary functions (autonomic nervous system). This disorder is characterized in infants by feeding difficulties, including excessive salivation and poor swallowing and sucking reflexes. The breathing in of liquid or other substances into the lungs (aspiration) may lead to repeated episodes of bronchial pneumonia. Other associated symptoms and findings include skin blotching, sweating, fluctuating extremes in body temperature, and defective tear secretion (lacrimation). Affected children develop an reduced sensitivity to temperature and pain. This may lead to frequent injuries such as irritation of the corneas of the eyes. Corneal injury may also occur as the result of decreased tear production. In addition, slurred speech and drooling may become evident. Children with familial dysautonomia typically have weak reflex responses (hyporeflexia) and experience delays in walking accompanied by the inability to coordinate voluntary movements (motor incoordination). After three years of age, affected children often develop severe vomiting episodes (hyperemesis) that may occur three or four times an hour and, in some cases, may last for three days or more. These episodes may sometimes be accompanied by elevated blood pressure (hypertension), abdominal pain and swelling, increased irritability, or breathing difficulties (dyspnea). As children with this disorder reach adolescence, a sideward curvature of the spine (scoliosis) may become evident along with leg cramping and weakness. In addition, some children may experience a delay in the onset of puberty. Older children may develop emotional and behavioral changes, such as irritability and depression. Intolerance for anesthetics is a common finding among children with FD.

Treatment for familial dysautonomia is symptomatic and supportive. Artificial tears, drops, or ointments may be placed in the eyes to prevent injury to corneas. Certain medications known as antiemetics may be prescribed to help control episodes of vomiting. In addition, replacement fluids and electrolytes may be administered to prevent excessive fluid loss (dehydration) resulting from vomiting episodes. Other treatment may include surgery or the use of orthopedic aids to correct scoliosis.

Familial dysautonomia is inherited as an autosomal recessive trait and occurs most commonly among certain individuals of eastern European descent, particularly Ashkenazi Jews at a rate of one out of 10,000 to 20,000 births. The disease gene for this disorder is located on the long arm of chromosome 9 (9q31-33).

National Associations & Support Groups

3126 American Academy of Pediatrics
141 Northwest Point Boulevard
Elk Grove Village, IL 60007 847-434-4000
800-433-9016
Fax: 847-434-8000
www.aap.org

The American Academy of Pediatrics and its member pediatricians are committed to the attainment of optimal physical, mental and social health and well-being for all infants, children, adolescents, and young adults.

Fernando Stein, MD, FAAP, President
Karen Remley, MD, CEO/Executive VP

3127 Dysautonomia Foundation
315 West 39th Street, Suite 701
New York, NY 10018 212-279-1066
Fax: 212-279-2066
info@familialdysautonomia.org
www.familialdysautonomia.org

Provides parents the knowledge regarding both national and international facilities that specialize in the treatment of the disorder.

David Drenner, Executive Director

3128 Familial Dysautonomia Hope Foundation
605 5th Avenue
Conover, NC 28613 828-695-1060
Fax: 828-695-1060
info@fdhope.org
www.fdvillage.org

To find a cure and new treatment options for Familial Dysautonomia by funding relevant research programs, to provide a support network aimed at addressing the needs of patients and families and to promote Familial Dysautonomia education and awareness programs in the medical community.

3129 Genetic Alliance
4301 Connecticut Avenue NW, Suite 404
Washington, DC 20008 202-966-5557
800-336-4363
Fax: 202-966-8553
info@geneticalliance.org
www.geneticalliance.org

A coalition of voluntary genetic support groups, consumers and professionals addressing the needs of individuals and families affected by genetic disorders from a national perspective.

Sharon Terry, President/CEO
Tetyana Murza, Managing Director
Natasha Bonhomme, VP, Strategic Development

3130 March of Dimes Foundation
1275 Mamaroneck Avenue
White Plains, NY 10605 914-997-4488
888-663-4637
Fax: 914-997-4763
answers@marchofdimes.com
www.marchofdimes.com

Partnership of volunteers and professionals dedicated to improving the health of babies by preventing birth defects and infant mortality. Over 100 chapters are located across the country and can be located through the National Office.

Stacey D. Stewart, President

Conferences

3131 Genetic Alliance Annual Conference
Genetic Alliance
4301 Connecticut Avenue NW, Suite 404
Washington, DC 20008 202-966-5557
800-336-4363
Fax: 202-966-8553
info@geneticalliance.org
www.geneticalliance.org

Consistently inspirational and enables partnership among all stakeholders: advocates and community leaders, health and industry professionals, policymakers, and academicians.

July

Sharon Terry, President/CEO
Tetyana Murza, Managing Director
Natasha Bonhomme, VP, Strategic Development

Web Sites

3132 Family Village
www.familyvillage.wisc.edu

A global community that integrates information, resources and communication opportunities on the Internet for persons with cognitive and other disabilities, for their families and for those that provide them services and support.

3133 NYU

530 First Avenue
New York, 10016   212-263-7225
                                   www.med.nyu.edu/fd/fdcenter.html

Offers information about Familial Dysautonomia.

Horacio Kaufman, MD, FAAN, Director
Felicia Axelrod, MD, FAAP, Co Director
Jose Martinez, MA, Research Faculty

3134 Online Mendelian Inheritance in Man
U.S. National Library of Medicine, 8600 Rockville
Bethesda, MD 20894   888-346-3656
                                   info@ncbi.nlm.nih.gov
                                   www.ncbi.nlm.nih.gov

This database is a catalog of human genes and genetic disorders.

Christine E. Seidman, M.D., Chair
David J. Lipman, M.D., Executive Secretary
Michael Boehnke, Ph.D., Board Member

DESCRIPTION

3135 FETAL ALCOHOL SYNDROME

Synonyms: FAS, Fetal alcohol effect (FAE), Alcohol-related neurodevelopmental, Alcolol-related birth defects

Involves the following Biologic System(s):
Genetic/Chromosomal/Syndrome/Metabolic Disorders

Fetal alcohol syndrome, or FAS, is a condition that is present at birth and the result of persistent maternal alcohol consumption during pregnancy. This condition is characterized by various birth defects such as low birth weight, short birth length, and an unusually small head (microcephaly) that may be associated with slowed development of the brain. Infants with FAS may also have several abnormalities of the face and skull including an unusually short opening between the margins of the upper and lower eyelids (palpebral fissures), vertical folds of skin that extend from the inner corners of the upper eyelids to the sides of the nose (epicanthal folds), an abnormally small lower jaw (micrognathia), or a poorly developed upper jaw (maxillary hypoplasia). Additional unusual features may include an abnormal opening in the roof of the mouth (cleft palate), a prominent forehead (frontal bossing), a flattened nasal bridge, and a thin, smooth upper lip. Other characteristic findings may include heart defects, abnormalities of the limbs and joints (e.g., dislocated hip, etc.), and irregular skin crease patterns on the palms of the hands. Within the first day of life, affected newborns may also exhibit characteristic symptoms of alcohol withdrawal such as tremor, increased irritability, muscle spasms, vomiting, or other problems. The development of the brain may also be impaired resulting in moderate to severe mental retardation. Approximately 20 percent of newborns with fetal alcohol syndrome risk life-threatening symptoms and complications within the first few weeks of life.

Alcohol consumption during pregnancy affects the growth and development of the fetus within the uterus and may result not only in birth defects but, in some cases, miscarriage or stillbirth. Although it is believed that fetal alcohol syndrome results from persistent moderate or heavy drinking, no safe levels of alcohol intake during pregnancy have been established; therefore, pregnant women are counseled to avoid alcohol consumption. It has, however, been determined that the more alcohol consumed, the greater the chances of giving birth to children with associated abnormalities. Therefore, treatment is directed toward identification, counseling, and education of women at risk. Other treatment is symptomatic and supportive.

Government Agencies

3136 NIH/ Eunice Kennedy Shriver National Insti tute of Child Health & Human Development
31 Center Drive, Building 31
Bethesda, MD 20892   301-496-5113
                           800-370-2943
                           Fax: 866-760-5947
                           nichdpress@mail.nih.gov
                           www.nichd.nih.gov

Established in 1962 by congress, today the institute conducts and supports research on topics related to the health of children, adults, families and populations. Some of these topics include: developmental disabilities, growth and development, infant death, reproductive health and birth defects.

Diana W. Bianchi, Director
Paul Williams, Director, Communications

3137 NIH/National Institute of Mental Health
6001 Executive Boulevard, Room 6200, MSC 9663
Bethesda, MD 20892   301-443-4536
                           866-615-6464
                           Fax: 301-443-4279
                           TTY: 301-443-8431
                           nimhinfo@nih.gov
                           www.nimh.nih.gov

Conducts strategic planning for specific research areas as well as for the Institute as a whole.

Joshua Gordon, MD, PhD, Director
Shelli Avenevoli, MD, Deputy Director

3138 NIH/National Institute on Alcohol Abuse an d Alcoholism (NIAAA)
5635 Fishers Lane, MSC 9304
Bethesda, MD 20892   301-443-3885
                           877-266-4267
                           Fax: 301-443-7043
                           www.niaaa.nih.gov

Established in 1970, NIAAA conducts research focused on improving the treatment and prevention of alcoholism and alcohol-related problems to reduce the enormous health, social, and econmic consequences of this disease.

George F. Koob, PhD, Director
Dr Patricia Powell, Acting Deputy Director

National Associations & Support Groups

3139 ARC of the United States
1010 Wayne Avenue, Suite 650
Silver Spring, MD 20910   301-565-3842
                               Fax: 301-565-5342
                               info@thearc.org
                               www.thearc.org

The ARC is the national organization of and for people with mental retardation and related developmental disabilities and their families. Devoted to promoting and improving supports and services for people with mental retardation and their families. The association also fosters research and education regarding the prevention of mental retardation in infants and young children. The ARC was founded in 1950 by a small group of parents and other concerned individuals.

Steven M Eidelman, Ceo
Adam Aaronson, Public Inquiries Director

3140 American Academy of Pediatrics
141 Northwest Point Boulevard
Elk Grove Village, IL 60007   847-434-4000
                                   800-433-9016
                                   Fax: 847-434-8000
                                   www.aap.org

The American Academy of Pediatrics and its member pediatricians are committed to the attainment of optimal physical, mental and social health and well-being for all infants, children, adolescents, and young adults.

Fernando Stein, MD, FAAP, President
Karen Remley, MD, CEO/Executive VP

3141 American Association for Pediatric Opthalmology
655 Beach Street
San Francisco, CA 94109   415-561-8505
                               Fax: 415-561-8531
                               aapos@aao.org
                               www.aapos.org

AAPOS is the American Association for Pediatric Ophthalmology and Strabismus. The organization's goals are to advance the quality of children's eye care, support the training of pediatric ophthalmologists, support research activities in pediatric ophthalmology, and advance the care of adults with strabismus.

Jennifer Hull, Client Services Manager
Brooke Lyon, Client Services Coordinator
Maria A. Schweers, CO, Scientific Program Coordinator

3142 American Pregnancy Association
1425 Greenway Drive, Suite 440
Irving, TX 75038
info@americanpregnancy.org
americanpregnancy.org

The American Pregnancy Association is a 501(c)(3) nonprofit organization committed to promoting pregnancy wellness through education, advocacy and community awareness.

3143 Association of Reproductive Health Professionals
1330 Broadway, Suite 1100
Oakland, CA 96412
202-466-3825
ARHP@arhp.org
www.arhp.org

It is a multidisciplinary association of professionals who provide reproductive health services or education, conduct reproductive health research, or influence reproductive health policy.

Nerys Benfield, Medical Director
Alayna Florman, Associate Director of Development
Megan A. Henszey, Program Manager

3144 Families Affected by Fetal Alcohol Spectrum Disorder
P.O. Box 427
Pittsboro, NC 27312
919-360-7073
adrienne@fafasd.org
fafasd.org

It seeks to spread information, awareness, and hope for caregivers of people with FASD.

Becky Brantley, President
Janet Schanzenbach, Vice-President
Tina Andrews, Treasurer

3145 Family Empowerment Network: Supporting Families Affected by FAS/FAE
777 South Mills Street
Madison, WI 53715
608-262-6590
800-462-5254
Fax: 608-263-5813
fen@fammed.wisc.edu
www.fammed.wisc.edu/fen/index.html

Provides education, resources and referrals to families affected by Fetal Alcohol Synadrome (FAS/FAE) and other professionals involved with them.

Georgiana Wilton, PhD, Director
Patricia Cameron, BS/FAS, Family Advocacy Specialist

3146 Fetal Alcohol Education Program
7 Kent Street
Brookline, MA 02445
617-739-1424
Fax: 617-566-4019

Works to educate the professional and community on the affects of alcohol consumption during pregnancy.

3147 Fetal Alcohol Syndrome Family Resource Institute
PO Box 2525
Lynwood, WA 98036
253-531-2878
800-999-3429
Fax: 253-531-2668
vicky@fetalalcoholsyndrome.org
www.fetalalcoholsyndrome.org

Provides information packets, a statewide hotline for information, crisis and referral and a newsletter. Parents are available to give talks throughout the United States and Canada.

3148 March of Dimes Foundation
1275 Mamaroneck Avenue
White Plains, NY 10605
914-997-4488
888-663-4637
Fax: 914-997-4763
answers@marchofdimes.com
www.marchofdimes.com

Partnership of volunteers and professionals dedicated to improving the health of babies by preventing birth defects and infant mortality. Over 100 chapters are located across the country and can be located through the National Office.

Stacey D. Stewart, President

3149 Mental Health America
500 Montgomery Street, Ste 820
Alexandria, VA 22314
703-684-7722
800-969-6642
Fax: 703-684-5968
TTY: 800-433-5959
www.mentalhealthamerica.net

Addresses all aspects of mental health and mental illness. NMHA with over 340 affiliates works to improve the mental health of all Americans.

Paul Gionfriddo, President/CEO
Shavonne Carpenter, Sr Assoc., Support & Services
Mallory Pernell, Assoc. Dir, Comments/Marketing

3150 National Alliance on Mental Illness
3803 N. Fairfax Drive, Suite 100
Arlington, VA 22203
703-524-7600
800-950-6264
Fax: 703-524-9094
info@nami.org
www.nami.org

Grassroots mental health organization dedicated to building better lives for the millions of Americans affected by mental illness.

Jim Payne, J.D., President
David Levy, Chief Financial Officer
Mary Giliberti, J.D., Executive Director

3151 National Mental Health Consumers' Self-Help Clearinghouse
1211 Chestnut Street, Suite 1207
Philadelphia, PA 19107
215-751-1810
800-553-4539
Fax: 215-636-6312
info@mhselfhelp.org
www.mhselfhelp.org

Offers information, support and appropriate referrals; and promotes public and professional education. Provides networking for those with special interests related to albinism. Promotes and supports research and funding that will improve diagnosis and management of albinism and hypopigmentation.

Joseph Rogers, Executive Director & Founder

3152 National Organization on Fetal Alcohol Syndrome
200 Eton Court, NW , Third Floor
Washington, DC 20007
202-785-4585
800-666-6327
Fax: 202-466-6456
www.nofas.org

Dedicated to eliminating birth defects caused by alcohol consumption during pregnancy and to improving the quality of life for those affected individuals and families.

Tom Donaldson, President
Kathleen Tavenner Mitchell, MHS/LCADC, VP/National Spokesperson
Kelly Raiser, MPH, Program Associate

3153 National Resource Center for Prevention of Perinatal Abuse of Alcohol
CSAP Division of Communications Programs
5600 Fishers Lane, Building 2
Rockville, MD 20857
301-443-9936

Offers information and resources to pregnant women on substance abuse, alcoholism and drugs pertaining to their unborn child's health.

3154 The Arc
1825 K Street, NW, Suite 1200
Washington, DC 20006
202-534-3700
800-433-5255
Fax: 202-534-3731
tnguyen@thearc.org
www.thearc.org

An organization advocating for and serving people with intellectual and developmental disabilities and their families. They encompass all ages and all spectrums from autism, Down syndrome, Fragile X and various other developmental disabilities.

Ronald Brown, President
Elise McMillan, Vice President
M.J. Bartelmay, Jr., Secretary

Conferences

3155 ARC National Convention
1825 K Street NW, Suite 1200
Washington, DC 20006
202-534-3700
800-433-5255
Fax: 202-534-3731
info@thearc.org
www.thearc.org

Each year hundreds of members, staff, volunteers, professionals, experts, self advocates and their families gather for a dynamic convention to meet each other, learn from each other, and tackle the tough issues facing the intellectual and developmental disability (I/DD) community together.

Peter V Berns, CEO

Book Publishers

3156 Alcohol, Tobacco and Other Drugs May Harm the Unborn
National Clearinghouse for Alcohol and Drug Info.
PO Box 2345
Rockville, MD 20847
800-729-6686

Presents the most recent findings of basic research and clinical studies conducted on the effects of alcohol, drugs and tobacco on the unborn.

3157 Congenital Disorders Sourcebook
Omnigraphics
PO Box 625
Holmes, PA 19043
800-234-1340
Fax: 800-875-1340
info@omnigraphics.com
www.omnigraphics.com

Basic consumer health information on disorders aquired during gestation, including spina bifida, hydrocephalus, cerebral palsy, heart defects, craniofacial abnormalities and fetal alcohol syndrome.
650 pages
ISBN: 0-780809-45-9

3158 Drugs and Pregnancy: It's Not Worth The Risk
American Council On Drug Education
204 Monroe Street, Suite 110
Rockville, MD 20850
800-488-3784

A scientific monograph for health care providers which teaches them to identify alcohol and drug problems in their patients.
48 pages

3159 Pregnancy and Exposure to Alcohol and Other Drug Use
National Clearinghouse for Alcohol and Drug Info.
PO Box 2345
Rockville, MD 20849
800-729-6686
www.health.org

This report is for health care professionals presenting state-of-the-art information about preventing alcohol use among women of childbearing age.

3160 Prevention Resource Guide: Pregnant, Postpartum Women and Their Infants
National Clearinghouse for Alcohol and Drug Info.
PO Box 2345
Rockville, MD 20849
800-729-6686
www.health.org

This resource guide targets health care providers, prevention program planners and counselors of pregnant and postpartum women between the ages of 15 and 44.

30 pages

Pamphlets

3161 Effects of Alcohol on Pregnancy National Clearinghouse for Alcohol Information
PO Box 2345
Rockville, MD 20847
301-468-2600

Free publications are available that discuss the effects of alcohol on pregnancy: Fetal Alcohol Syndrome; and The Fact Is Alcohol and Other Drugs Can Harm an Unborn Baby.

3162 Fetal Alcohol Syndrome
Hazelden
PO Box 11
Center City, MN 55012
651-213-4200
800-257-7810
Fax: 612-257-1331
info@hazeldenbettyford.org
www.hazelden.org

A source of information about the effects of drinking while pregnant.

Mark Mishek, President & CEO
Sharon Birnbaum, Director of Human Resources
Jim Blaha, VP, CFO & CAO

3163 Fight Drug Abuse at Home, Work, School and in the Community
American Council for Drug Education
204 Monroe Street, Suite 110
Rockville, MD 20850
800-488-3784

A catalog of print and video materials pertaining to substance abuse, alcoholism and drugs.

3164 How to Take Care of Your Baby Before Birth
National Clearinghouse for Alcohol and Drug Info.
PO Box 2345
Rockville, MD 20849
800-729-6686
www.health.org

A low-literacy brochure aimed at pregnant women that describes what they should and should not do during pregnancy.

3165 Things To Avoid During Pregnancy
March of Dimes Pregnancy & Newborn Health Edu Ctr
1275 Mamaroneck Avenue
White Plains, NY 10605
914-997-4488
Fax: 914-997-4763
answers@marchofdimes.com
www.marchofdimes.com/pnhec/pnhec.asp

Information about the effects of certain drugs, stress, pets, abuse, and hazardous materials. Each topic is an online article available under the link: During Your Pregnancy.
2008

DESCRIPTION

3166 FETAL RETINOID SYNDROME

Covers these related disorders: Etretinate embryopathy, Isotretinoin embryopathy, Retinol embryopathy

Involves the following Biologic System(s):

Neonatal and Infant Disorders

Fetal retinoid syndrome is a characteristic pattern of birth defects caused by exposure to vitamin A (retinol) or its derivatives during early pregnancy. The term retinoid refers to retinol or any natural or artificially created derivative of vitamin A. In newborns with fetal retinoid syndrome, characteristic symptoms and findings include small, low-set ears or complete absence of the outer ears and external ear canals (microtia); an abnormally small head (microcephaly); enlargement of the cavities (ventricles) within the brain; and underdevelopment (hypoplasia) of the thymus, a small gland in the upper portion of the chest that functions as an essential part of the immune system during infancy and childhood.

Several studies have reported fetal retinoid syndrome in newborns as a result of maternal use of vitamin A derivatives such as isotretinoin during early pregnancy. In addition, an increasing number of studies reveal the occurrence of such birth defects due to maternal use of other vitamin A derivatives, particularly the medication etretinate, or large doses of vitamin A (e.g., greater than 15,000 units daily) during early embryonic development. Although the frequency of fetal retinoid syndrome is unknown, reported cases represent only a small percentage of actual occurrences of the syndrome. Moreover, there is ongoing concern that increasing use of high dose vitamin A preparations and of vitamin A derivatives to treat certain common skin conditions, such as cystic acne or psoriasis, may result in additional cases of fetal retinoid syndrome. The most well known retinoid is isotretinoin. Because it can cause severe birth defects, including mental retardation and physical malformations, a woman must not become pregnant while taking it. If a woman of childbearing age requests isotretinoin, her doctor will ask her to sign a detailed consent form before presribing it. If a woman accidentally becomes pregnant while taking the medication, she should immediately consult her doctor. Dosage levels and the stage of embryonic development during which retinoid exposure occurs are thought to be the major factors influencing the occurrence of fetal retinoid syndrome. The period of greatest risk may occur between approximately two to five weeks after conception. The specific underlying abnormality that causes fetal retinoid syndrome is not known. Studies indicate that retinoid exposure may cause disrupted development in the embryonic region that later becomes the brain and spinal cord (neural crest). The role that genetic influences or other environmental factors may have in contributing to fetal retinoid syndrome is unknown.

Although the symptoms and findings associated with fetal retinoid syndrome vary somewhat from case to case, affected newborns typically have a characteristic pattern of malformations. Affected newborns may have abnormalities of the head and face, including premature closure of the fibrous joint between the bones forming the forehead (metopic craniosynostosis); downslanting eyelid folds (palpebral fissures); widely spaced eyes (ocular hypertelorism) that may be abnormally small (microphthalmia); a short or broad nose; a

small jaw (micrognathia); or incomplete closure of the roof of the mouth (cleft palate) and a groove in the upper lip (cleft lip). Abnormalities of the brain and spinal cord (central nervous system) are also common and include obstruction of the flow of cerebrospinal fluid around the brain, causing the fluid to accumulate under increasing pressure within the cavities of the brain (hydrocephalus); loss of vision; or other abnormalities (e.g., holoprosencephaly [failure of the forebrain (prosencephalon) to grow as two separate hemispheres in the first few weeks of fetal life], posterior fossa cyst). Additional neurologic problems may include paralysis of the nerves that supply muscles responsible for eye movements (oculomotor paralysis) or weakness or paralysis of the nerve that supplies the forehead, scalp, eyelids, cheeks, jaws, and muscles of facial expression (facial nerve palsy).

Newborns with fetal retinoid syndrome may also have clouding of the lenses of the eyes (congenital cataracts); malformations of the heart and its major blood vessels (e.g., ventricular septal defects, hypoplastic aortic arch, transposition of the great arteries); underdevelopment (hypoplasia) of the kidneys and tubes (ureters) that carry urine from the kidneys into the bladder; and ab normalities of the liver. Many affected newborns may also have malformations of the arms, legs, hands, and feet, such as webbing or fusion of the fingers and toes (syndactyly); malformations of the bone on the thumb side of the forearm (radial defects); a defect in which the foot is twisted out of shape or position (clubfoot or talipes); or fusion of the lower legs and absence of the feet (sirenomelia). In some patients, life-threatening complications may occur soon after birth. Treatment of newborns with fetal retinoid syndrome includes symptomatic and supportive measures.

Government Agencies

3167 NIH/ Eunice Kennedy Shriver National Insti tute of Child Health & Human Development
31 Center Drive, Building 31
Bethesda, MD 20892

301-496-5113
800-370-2943
Fax: 866-760-5947
nichdpress@mail.nih.gov
www.nichd.nih.gov

Established in 1962 by congress, today the institute conducts and supports research on topics related to the health of children, adults, families and populations. Some of these topics include: developmental disabilities, growth and development, infant death, reproductive health and birth defects.

Diana W. Bianchi, Director
Paul Williams, Director, Communications

National Associations & Support Groups

3168 American Academy of Pediatrics
141 Northwest Point Boulevard
Elk Grove Village, IL 60007

847-434-4000
800-433-9016
Fax: 847-434-8000
www.aap.org

The American Academy of Pediatrics and its member pediatricians are committed to the attainment of optimal physical, mental and social health and well-being for all infants, children, adolescents, and young adults.

Fernando Stein, MD, FAAP, President
Karen Remley, MD, CEO/Executive VP

3169 Association of Children's Prosthetic/ Orthotic Clinics
6300 N River Road, Suite 727
Rosemont, IL 60018   847-698-1637
                                        Fax: 847-823-0536
                                        raymond@aaos.org
                                        www.acpoc.org

The Association of Children's Prosthetic Clinics is an association
of professionals who are involved in clinics providing prosthetic-orthotic care for children with limb loss or orthopaedic
disabilities.

Melody Raymond, Contact

3170 March of Dimes Foundation
1275 Mamaroneck Avenue
White Plains, NY 10605   914-997-4488
                                             888-663-4637
                                        Fax: 914-997-4763
                                        answers@marchofdimes.com
                                        www.marchofdimes.com

Partnership of volunteers and professionals dedicated to improving the health of babies by preventing birth defects and infant
mortality. Over 100 chapters are located across the country and
can be located through the National Office.

Stacey D. Stewart, President

3171 National Rehabilitation Information Center
4200 Forbes Blvd, Suite 202
Lanham, MD 20706   301-459-5984
                                             800-364-2742
                                        Fax: 301-459-4263
                                        TTY: 301-459-5984
                                        naricinfo@heitechservices.com
                                        www.naric.com

NARIC is a library and information center focusing in disability
and rehabilitation research. Information specialists provide quick
information and referrals free of charge. Other sevices include
customized searches of REHABDATA, the premier database of
disability and rehabilitation literature.

Mark Odum, Director

Conferences

3172 ACPOC Annual Meeting
Assoc of Children's Prosthetic-Orthotic Clinics
6300 N River Road, Suite 727
Rosemont, IL 60018   847-698-1637
                                        Fax: 847-823-0536
                                        acpoc@aaos.org
                                        www.acpoc.org

April

Web Sites

3173 Association of Children's Prosthetic/ Orthotic Clinics
9400 West Higgins Road, Suite 500
Rosemont, IL 60018   847-698-1637
                                        Fax: 847-268-9560
                                        acpoc@aaos.org
                                        www.acpoc.org

An association of professionals who are involved in clinics which
provide prosthetic-orthotic care for children with limb loss or orthopaedic disabilities.

David B. Rotter, CPO, President
Jorge Amelio Fabregas, MD, Vice President
Hank White, PT, PhD, Secretary-Treasurer

3174 March of Dimes Birth Defects Foundation
www.marchofdimes.com

Partnership of volunteers and professionals dedicated to improving the health of babies by preventing birth defects and infant
mortality. Over 100 chapters are located across the country and
can be located through the National Office.

3175 National Rehabilitation Information Center
8400 Corporate Drive, Suite 500
Landover, MD 20785   800-346-2742
                                        Fax: 301-459-4263
                                        TTY: 301-459-5984
                                        www.naric.com/naric

NARIC is a library and information center focusing in disability
and rehabilitation research. Information specialists provide quick
information and referrals free of charge. Other sevices include
customized searches of REHABDATA, the premier database of
disability and rehabilitation literature.

DESCRIPTION

3176 FRAGILE X SYNDROME

Synonyms: Marker X Syndrome, Martin-Bell Syndrome
Involves the following Biologic System(s):
Genetic/Chromosomal/Syndrome/Metabolic Disorders

Fragile X Syndrome, a disorder that results from an inherited defect of the X chromosome, is the most common cause of mental retardation in males. The disorder is thought to affect approximately one in 2,000 to 4,000 males and to be slightly less frequent in females. Although symptoms may be variable, the most common feature associated with fragile X syndrome is mental retardation.

Most males with fragile X syndrome have mild to profound mental retardation (e.g., an intelligence quotient or I.Q. ranging from approximately 30 to 55.) However, some may have an I.Q. that is considered borderline normal. Affected males with mild mental retardation may have a distinctive speech pattern characterized by rapid speech with a variable rhythm (cluttering). Those with more severe retardation typically communicate in bursts of repetitive speech. Affected males with severe or profound mental retardation may lack the ability to speak. In addition, most males with fragile X syndrome may have poor eye contact or experience emotional difficulties. Some may have poor concentration associated with hyperactivity or engage in autistic-like behaviors, such as hand biting or hand flapping.

In many cases, affected males may also have physical abnormalities. For example, many males with fragile X syndrome may have unusually large testes (macroorchidism), a finding that is most apparent after puberty; however, testicular function is normal. Affected males may also typically have characteristic facial features, such as a large head (macrocephaly) and forehead, a relatively long face and prominent jaw, thick lips, and prominent ears. Other findings may include crowding of the teeth, excessive flexibility of the finger joints, or flat feet (pes planus). In addition, approximately 50 percent of affected females have varying degrees of mental retardation or learning difficulties. In some cases, females with fragile X syndrome may also have physical abnormalities, such as irregular teeth or unusually flexible finger joints. The treatment of children with fragile X syndrome includes symptomatic and supportive measures, such as special education, speech therapy, and, in some cases, multidisciplinary techniques such as behavioral therapies to help manage hyperactivity or autistic-like behaviors.

Individuals with fragile X syndrome inherit a fragile area or site on the long arm (q) of the X chromosome (Xq27.3). Chromosomal analysis reveals that the genetic material on the end of this arm appears to be broken off. In reality, this genetic material is actually dangling from the end of the long arm. The diseased gene within this area is known as the FRAXA gene. This region (locus) of the X chromosome contains abnormally long repeats (e.g., over 200 repeats) of coded DNA instructions (CGG trinucleotide repeat expansion). Males have only one X chromosome; therefore, if they inherit a fragile X locus containing more than 200 CGG repeats, they generally express the symptoms associated with this syndrome and are typically more severely affected than females. However, because females have two X

chromosomes, certain disease traits may be masked by the presence of a normal gene on the other X chromosome, resulting in lower frequency and decreased severity of the disease among females.

Government Agencies

3177 NIH/ Eunice Kennedy Shriver National Institute of Child Health & Human Development
31 Center Drive, Building 31
Bethesda, MD 20892
301-496-5113
800-370-2943
Fax: 866-760-5947
nichdpress@mail.nih.gov
www.nichd.nih.gov

Established in 1962 by congress, today the institute conducts and supports research on topics related to the health of children, adults, families and populations. Some of these topics include: developmental disabilities, growth and development, infant death, reproductive health and birth defects.

Diana W. Bianchi, Director
Paul Williams, Director, Communications

National Associations & Support Groups

3178 ARC of the United States
1825 K Street, NW, Suite 1200
Washington, DC 20006
301-565-3842
800-433-5255
Fax: 301-565-5342
info@thearc.org
www.thearc.org

The ARC is the national organization of and for people with mental retardation and related developmental disabilities and their families. Devoted to promoting and improving supports and services for people with mental retardation and their families. The association also fosters research and education regarding the prevention of mental retardation in infants and young children. The ARC was founded in 1950 by a small group of parents and other concerned individuals.

Steven M Eidelman, Ceo
Adam Aaronson, Public Inquiries Director

3179 American Academy of Pediatrics
141 Northwest Point Boulevard
Elk Grove Village, IL 60007
847-434-4000
800-433-9016
Fax: 847-434-8000
www.aap.org

The American Academy of Pediatrics and its member pediatricians are committed to the attainment of optimal physical, mental and social health and well-being for all infants, children, adolescents, and young adults.

Fernando Stein, MD, FAAP, President
Karen Remley, MD, CEO/Executive VP

3180 FRAXA Research Foundation
10 Prince Place
Newburyport, MA 01950
978-462-1866
Fax: 978-463-9985
info@fraxa.org
www.fraxa.org

FRAXA supports research on fragile X syndrome, a genetic disorder which is the most common inherited cause of mental retardation.

2,500 members

Katie Clapp, Co-Founder & President
Megan Massey, RN, Vice President
Michael Tranfaglia, MD, Co-Founder/Medical Director

3181 Genetic Alliance
4301 Connecticut Avenue NW, Suite 404
Washington, DC 20008

202-966-5557
800-336-4363
Fax: 202-966-8553
info@geneticalliance.org
www.geneticalliance.org

A coalition of voluntary genetic support groups, consumers and professionals addressing the needs of individuals and families affected by genetic disorders from a national perspective.

Sharon Terry, President/CEO
Tetyana Murza, Managing Director
Natasha Bonhomme, VP, Strategic Development

3182 National Fragile X Foundation
1615 Bonanza Street, Suite 202
Walnut Creek, CA 94596

925-938-9300
800-688-8765
Fax: 925-938-9315
natlfx@fragilex.org
www.fragilex.org

Unites the Fragile X community with support, education, awareness, research and advocacy.

Michael Kelly, President
Robert M Miller, Executive Director

State Agencies & Support Groups

California

3183 Fragile X Association of Southern California
PO Box 6924
Burbank, CA 91510

818-754-4227
Fax: 310-276-9251
info@fraxsocal.org
www.fraxsocal.org

Promotes awareness of Fragile X syndrome with special emphasis on educators and health professionals; provides a forum for families of children with fragile X to meet and share their ideas, concerns and problems; and supports scientific research on fragile X syndrome.

Naomi Star, President
Diane Bateman, Vice President

3184 Fragile X Center of San Diego
4653 Carmel Mountain Rd, Ste 308-515
San Diego, CA 92130

760-434-6290
877-300-7143
info@fragilesandiego.org
www.fragilexsandiego.org

Provides information for families and professionals. Activities include: family support, improving awareness of fragile X syndrome, increasing the identification for affected families, promoting research into fragile X syndrome.

Nicole Schweizer, Secretary

Ohio

3185 Fragile X Alliance of Ohio
6790 Ridgecliff Drive
Solon, OH 44139

440-519-1517
Fax: 440-519-1518
fraxohio@adelphia.org
www.fragilexohio.org

Promotes awareness of Fragile X syndrome with special emphasis on educators and health professionals; provides a forum for families of children with fragile X to meet and share their ideas, concerns and problems; and supports scientific research on fragile X syndrome.

Leslie A. Bagdasarian, President

Conferences

3186 ARC Annual National Convention
The ARC
1825 K Street NW,Suite 1200
Washington, DC 20006

202-534-3700
800-433-5255
Fax: 202-534-3731
info@thearc.org
www.thearc.org

held in cities throughout the U.S. each fall which attracts nearly 1000 people for educational sessions, business meetings and social events.

Mohan Mehra, President
Nancy Webster, Vice President
Michael Mack, Secretary

3187 Genetic Alliance Annual Conference
Genetic Alliance
4301 Connecticut Avenue NW, Suite 404
Washington, DC 20008

202-966-5557
800-336-4363
Fax: 202-966-8553
info@geneticalliance.org
www.geneticalliance.org

Consistently inspirational and enables partnership among all stakeholders: advocates and community leaders, health and industry professionals, policymakers, and academicians.

July

Sharon Terry, President/CEO
Tetyana Murza, Managing Director
Natasha Bonhomme, VP, Strategic Development

Web Sites

3188 ARC of the United States
1825 K Street, NW, Suite 1200
Washington, DC 20006

202-534-3700
800-433-5255
Fax: 202-534-3731
tnguyen@thearc.org
www.thearc.org

The ARC is the national organization of and for people with mental retardation and related developmental disabilities and their families. Devoted to promoting and improving supports and services for people with mental retardation and their families. The association also fosters research and education regarding the prevention of mental retardation in infants and young children.

Ronald Brown, President
Elise McMillan, Vice President
Peter V. Berns, CEO

3189 American College of Medical Genetics
7220 Wisconsin Ave., Suite 300
Bethesda, MD 20814

301-718-9603
Fax: 301-718-9604
acmg@acmg.net
www.acmg.net

Offers information about fragile X syndrome.

3190 FRAXA Research Foundation
10 Prince Place, Suite 203
Newburyport, MA 1950

978-462-1866
info@fraxa.org
www.fraxa.org

FRAXA supports research on fragile X syndrome, a genetic disorder which is the most common inherited cause of mental retardation.

Debbie Stevenson, Chair
Katie Clapp, MS, President & Co Founder
Sasa Zorovic, PhD, Vice President

3191 National Fragile X Foundation
2100 M St., NW, Suite 170, Box 302
Washington, DC 20037
202-747-6210
800-688-8765
Fax: 202-747-6208
natlfx@fragilex.org
www.fragilex.org

Provides a wide variety data for people suffering from the disorder to acces at any time with ease.

Jennifer Silverton, President
Brian Silver, Vice President
Tony Ferlenda, CEO

Book Publishers

3192 Children With Fragile X Syndrome

Jayne Dixon Weber, author

Peytral Publications
PO Box 1162
Minnetonka, MN 55345
952-949-8707
877-739-8725
Fax: 952-906-9777
www.peytral.com

A complete, sensitive infroduction to Fragile X Syndrome, covering diagnosis, parental emotions, therapies and medications, early intervention, education, daily care, legal rights and more. Item #WP-307X.

472 pages

3193 Educating Boys with Fragile X Syndrome

Gail Spiridigliozzi, PhD, author

FRAA Research Foundation
10 Prince Place, Suite 203
Newburyport, MA 01950
978-462-1866
Fax: 978-463-9985
info@fraxa.org
www.fraxa.org

Guide for parents, teachers and therapist to give specific strategies for education.

20 pages

3194 Fragile X - A to Z: Guide for Families by Families

Sally Nantais, Mary Beth Langan, Wendy Dillworth, author

FRAA Research Foundation
10 Prince Place, Suite 203
Newburyport, MA 01950
978-462-1866
Fax: 978-463-9985
info@fraxa.org
www.fraxa.org

Intended to help families cope with many daily challenges of living with a child or adult who has fragile X syndrome.

100 pages

3195 My Brother has Fragile X

Charles Stieger, author

FRAA Research Foundation
10 Prince Place, Suite 203
Newburyport, MA 01950
978-462-1866
Fax: 978-463-9985
info@fraxa.org
www.fraxa.org

Suitable for young children and for reading in an elementary school classroom to educate children about what it's like to have fragile X.

23 pages

Newsletters

3196 FRAXA Research Foundation Newsletter
10 Prince Place, Suite 203
Newburyport, MA 1950
978-462-1866
Fax: 978-463-9985
info@fraxa.org
www.fraxa.org

FRAXA supports research on fragile X syndrome, a genetic disorder which is the most common inherited cause of mental retardation.

Quarterly

Debbie Stevenson, Chair
Katie Clapp, MS, President & Co Founder
Sasa Zorovic, PhD, Vice President

DESCRIPTION

3197 GALACTOSEMIA

Covers these related disorders: Classic galactosemia, Galactokinase deficiency, Deficiency of uridyl diphosphogalactose-4-epimerase

Involves the following Biologic System(s):

Gastrointestinal Disorders,

Genetic/Chromosomal/Syndrome/Metabolic Disorders

Galactosemia is a disorder in which the body cannot use the sugar known as galactose, which is an important component of the sugar in milk (lactose) and an important source of nutrition for infants and children. Because of this inability, this sugar accumulates in the blood, and substances produced by the partial breakdown of galactose build up in the body, where they can damage the kidneys, liver, brain, and eyes.

Galactosemia is a hereditary genetic disorder, caused by mutations in genes that carry the structural codes for three enzymes that normally break down or digest galactose. As a result, there are three forms of galactosemia, each stemming from a deficiency of one of the three galactose-digesting enzymes. The most frequent and severe form of galactosemia, named classic galatosemia, results from deficiency of galactose-1 phosphate uridyl transferase. A second form of galactosemia stems from deficiency of galactose kinase, and the third form comes from deficiency of galactose epimerase. All three forms of galactosemia are transmitted in an autosomal recessive manner, meaning that each parent of an affected child must carry a copy of the gene responsible for the same form of galactosemia.

Symptoms of galactosemia may include a yellowish discoloration of the skin, eyes, and mucous membranes (jaundice); opacity of the lenses of the eyes (cataracts); vomiting; convulsions; increased irritability; sluggishness; difficulty in feeding; and failure to gain weight. Characteristic findings may include enlargement of the liver and spleen (hepatosplenomegaly), low blood sugar (hypoglycemia), the presence of amino acids in the urine (aminoaciduria), an abnormal accumulation of fluid in the abdomen (ascites), the formation of scar tissue in the liver (cirrhosis), and mental retardation.

If infants with classic galactosemia are not treated promptly with a low-galactose diet, life-threatening complications appear within a few days after birth. Affected infants typically develop feeding difficulties, a lack of energy (lethargy), a failure to gain weight and grow (failure to thrive), yellowing of the skin and whites of the eyes (jaundice), liver damage, and bleeding. Affected children are also at increased risk of delayed development, clouding of the lens of the eye (cataract), speech difficulties, and intellectual disability. Complications of galactosemia can include severe infection and shock. Women with classic galactosemia, caused by deficiency of the enzyme galactose-1 phosphate uridyl transferase, may have disorders of the reproductive system.

The most effective treatment for galactosemia is the complete elimination of milk and milk products from the diet. Women who carry any of the three genes responsible for galactosemia should avoid lactose-containing foods during pregnancy, to prevent galactose from crossing the placenta and causing disease in the fetus. Although a completely lactose-free diet may prevent the complications of galactosemia, some affected children and adults may experience delays in growth and development, speech irregularities, and difficulties with motor function.

National Associations & Support Groups

3198 American Academy of Pediatrics
141 Northwest Point Boulevard
Elk Grove Village, IL 60007

847-434-4000
800-433-9016
Fax: 847-434-8000
www.aap.org

The American Academy of Pediatrics and its member pediatricians are committed to the attainment of optimal physical, mental and social health and well-being for all infants, children, adolescents, and young adults.

Fernando Stein, MD, FAAP, President
Karen Remley, MD, CEO/Executive VP

3199 American Liver Foundation
39 Broadway, Suite 2700
New York, NY 10006

212-668-1000
800-465-4837
Fax: 212-483-8179
info@liverfoundation.org
www.liverfoundation.org

Nonprofit, national voluntary health organization dedicated to the prevention, treatment and cure of hepatitis and other liver diseases through research, education, and advocacy on behalf of those affected by or at risk of liver disease.

Gina Parziale, Executive Director
James L Boyer MD, Chair

3200 Genetic Alliance
4301 Connecticut Avenue NW, Suite 404
Washington, DC 20008

202-966-5557
800-336-4363
Fax: 202-966-8553
info@geneticalliance.org
www.geneticalliance.org

A coalition of voluntary genetic support groups, consumers and professionals addressing the needs of individuals and families affected by genetic disorders from a national perspective.

Sharon Terry, President/CEO
Tetyana Murza, Managing Director
Natasha Bonhomme, VP, Strategic Development

3201 March of Dimes Foundation
1275 Mamaroneck Avenue
White Plains, NY 10605

914-997-4488
888-663-4637
Fax: 914-997-4763
answers@marchofdimes.com
www.marchofdimes.com

Partnership of volunteers and professionals dedicated to improving the health of babies by preventing birth defects and infant mortality. Over 100 chapters are located across the country and can be located through the National Office.

Stacey D. Stewart, President

3202 Parents of Galactosemic Children
1519 Magnolia Bluff Drive, PO Box 2401
Mandeville, LS ÿ7047

228-497-5886
ÿ86- 90- 742
president@galactosemia.org
www.galactosemia.org

National nonprofit, volunteer organization whose misssion is to provide information, support and networking opportunities to families affected by galactosemia.

Michelle Fowler, President & Treasurer
Nishkala Rao, Secretary

Libraries & Resource Centers

3203 **National Digestive Diseases Information Clearinghouse**
9000 Rockville Pike
Bethesda, MD 20892   301-496-3583
                                  800-860-8747
                                  Fax: 301-907-8906
                                  healthinfo@niddk.nih.gov
                                  www.niddk.nih.gov

The National Institute of Diabetes and Digestive and Kidney Diseases conducts and supports research on many of the most serious diseases affecting public health. The Institute supports much of the clinical research on the diseases of internal medicine and related subspecialty fields as well as many basic science disciplines.

Dr. Griffin P. Rodgers, Director
Dr. Gregory G. Germino, Deputy Director
Camille M. Hoover, M.S.W., Executive Officer

Conferences

3204 **Genetic Alliance Annual Conference**
Genetic Alliance
4301 Connecticut Avenue NW, Suite 404
Washington, DC 20008   202-966-5557
                                 800-336-4363
                                 Fax: 202-966-8553
                                 info@geneticalliance.org
                                 www.geneticalliance.org

Consistently inspirational and enables partnership among all stakeholders: advocates and community leaders, health and industry professionals, policymakers, and academicians.

July

Sharon Terry, President/CEO
Tetyana Murza, Managing Director
Natasha Bonhomme, VP, Strategic Development

Web Sites

3205 **American Liver Foundation**
39 Broadway, Suite 2700
New York, NY 10006   212-668-1000
                                 800-465-4837
                                 Fax: 212-483-8179
                                 www.liverfoundation.org

Nonprofit, national voluntary health organization dedicated to the prevention, treatment, and cure of hepatitis and other liver diseases through research, education and advocacy on behalf of those affected by or at risk of liver disease.

Thomas F. Nealon III, Chair
David Ticker, CFO
Lynn Seim, COO

3206 **Disability Information and Resource Center**
www.dircsa.org.au/pub/docs/galac.txt

DIRC provides a professional and friendly information and referral service to the people of South Australia.

3207 **Galactosemia Resources and Information**
PO Box 1512
Deerfield Beach, FL 33443   866-900-7421
                                 www.galactosemia.com

Information about galactosemia.

Scott Shepard, President
Scott Saylor, Vice President
Paul Fowler, Treasurer

3208 **Online Mendelian Inheritance in Man**
U.S. National Library of Medicine, 8600 Rockville
Bethesda, MD 20894   888-346-3656
                                 info@ncbi.nlm.nih.gov
                                 www.ncbi.nlm.nih.gov

This database is a catalog of human genes and genetic disorders.

Christine E. Seidman, M.D., Chair
David J. Lipman, M.D., Executive Secretary
Michael Boehnke, Ph.D., Board Member

3209 **Parents of Galactosemic Children**
www.galactosemia.com

National nonprofit, volunteer organization whose mission is to provide information, support and networking opportunities to families affected by galactosemia.

Scott Shepard, President
Scott Saylor, Vice President
Paul Fowler, Treasurer

3210 **Rare Genetic Diseases in Children (NYU)**
550 First Avenue
New York, NY 10016   212-263-7300
                                 www.med.nyu.edu/rgdc/homenow.htm

We target issues arising from rare genetic diseases affecting children. Also, to assist in the endeavor to bring knowledge and hope to those for whom there is, at present, so little.

Robert I. Grossman, MD, Dean & CEO
Michael T. Burke, SVP, CFO, Vice Dean
Annette Johnson, JD, PhD, SVP & Vice Dean, General Counsel

3211 **Save Babies Through Screening Foundation**
PO Box 42179
Cincinnati, OH 45242   888-454-3383
                                 email@savebabies.org
                                 www.savebabies.org

Is a national, nonprofit, public charity run by volunteers. Its mission is to improve the lives of babies by working to prevent disabilities and early death resulting from disorders detectable through newborn screening.

Jill Levy-Fisch, President
Micki Gartzke, Vice President
Anne Rugari, Treasurer

DESCRIPTION

3212 GAUCHER'S DISEASE

Synonyms: Gaucher disease, Glucosylceramide lipidosis, Glucosyl cerebroside lipidosis

Covers these related disorders: Chronic Gaucher's disease (Adult or Classic Gaucher's disease), Infantile Gaucher's disease, Juvenile Gaucher's disease

Involves the following Biologic System(s):
Genetic/Chromosomal/Syndrome/Metabolic Disorders

Gaucher's disease is an inherited metabolic disorder characterized by a deficiency of the enzyme glucocerebrosidase (glucosylceramidase), which assists in the metabolism of certain fats (lipidosis). This deficiency results in the accumulation of certain fatty substances (glucocerebroside or glucosylceramide) throughout the body. Although uncommon, Gaucher's disease is the lipidosis seen most often by physicians. Gaucher's disease is subdivided into three main types. The first, known as chronic, adult, or classic Gaucher's disease, may develop at any age from birth to 80 years old. This form of the disease is common among eastern European Jews, with an incidence rate of as many as one in 500 births. Findings associated with chronic Gaucher's disease include enlargement of the spleen (splenomegaly) or liver (hepatomegaly), or both (hepatosplenomegaly); a decrease in levels of hemoglobin in the blood (anemia); decreased numbers of circulating white blood cells (leukopenia); and abnormally low levels of circulating platelets (thrombocytopenia), which may lead to easy bruising or bleeding. Symptoms may include a brownish-pigmented skin; yellow spots in the eyes resulting from accumulation of fatty substances; and bone pain resulting from accumulations in the bone marrow. Treatment for chronic Gaucher's disease includes enzyme replacement therapy.

Infantile Gaucher's disease, a life-threatening form of this disorder, affects the central nervous system of the newborn. Symptoms and findings may include enlargement of the spleen, crossed eyes (strabismus); muscle spasms in the jaw (trismus or lockjaw); seizures; backward bending of the head; or a rigid, arched back. Additional abnormalities of the central nervous system may become apparent.

Juvenile Gaucher's disease may appear at any time during childhood. Characteristic findings may include enlargement of the liver and spleen (hepatosplenomegaly), bone abnormalities resulting in pain and swelling of the joints, anemia, and abnormally low levels of circulating white blood cells and platelets. Affected children may be pale, weak, and particularly susceptible to bleeding and recurring infection. Symptoms related to nervous system involvement include lack of motor coordination and loss of balance, inflammation of the nerves in the arms and legs accompanied by abnormal sensations and discomfort, muscle spasms, paralysis of the nerves of the eye (ophthalmoplegia), and impairment of mental function.

Enzyme replacement therapy is usually not effective in the treatment of the infantile and juvenile forms of Gaucher's disease. Alternative treatment may include removal of the spleen (splenectomy). Other treatment is symptomatic and supportive.

Gaucher's disease is inherited as an autosomal recessive trait. The gene responsible for the regulation of the enzyme glucocerebrosidase is located on the long arm of chromosome 1 (1q21-q31).

National Associations & Support Groups

3213 ARC of the United States
1010 Wayne Avenue, Suite 650
Silver Spring, MD 20910
301-565-3842
Fax: 301-565-5342
info@thearc.org
www.thearc.org

The ARC is the national organization of and for people with mental retardation and related developmental disabilities and their families. Devoted to promoting and improving supports and services for people with mental retardation and their families. The association also fosters research and education regarding the prevention of mental retardation in infants and young children. The ARC was founded in 1950 by a small group of parents and other concerned individuals.

Steven M Eidelman, Ceo
Adam Aaronson, Public Inquiries Director

3214 American Academy of Pediatrics
141 Northwest Point Boulevard
Elk Grove Village, IL 60007
847-434-4000
800-433-9016
Fax: 847-434-8000
www.aap.org

The American Academy of Pediatrics and its member pediatricians are committed to the attainment of optimal physical, mental and social health and well-being for all infants, children, adolescents, and young adults.

Fernando Stein, MD, FAAP, President
Karen Remley, MD, CEO/Executive VP

3215 National Gaucher Foundation
2227 Idlewood Road, Suite 6ÿ
Tucker, GA 30084
301-816-1515
800-504-3189
Fax: 301-816-1516
ngf@gaucherdisease.org
www.gaucherdisease.org

A nonprofit organization whose primary objective is to assist in perfecting a treatment program and discovering a cure for Gaucher disease. The Foundation supports medical research and clinical programs which enhance the current understanding of Gaucher disease.

Robin A. Ely, MD, President
Rhonda P. Buyers, Executive Director
Cyndi Frank, Director Development

3216 National Tay-Sachs and Allied Diseases Association
2001 Beacon Street, Suite 204
Boston, MA 02135
617-277-4463
800-906-8723
Fax: 617-277-0134
info@ntsad.org
www.ntsad.org

Direct, fund and promote research to develop treatments and cures; provides comprehensive support services to affected families and individuals; guides prevention, education, awareness and screening through effective grassroots collaborations with chapters and affiliates; lead advocacy efforts as the recognized authority for this family of genetic diseases.

Diana Pangonis, Interim Executive Director

Conferences

3217 Genetic Alliance Annual Conference
Genetic Alliance
4301 Connecticut Avenue NW, Suite 404
Washington, DC 20008
202-966-5557
800-336-4363
Fax: 202-966-8553
info@geneticalliance.org
www.geneticalliance.org

Consistently inspirational and enables partnership among all
stakeholders: advocates and community leaders, health and industry professionals, policymakers, and academicians.

July

Sharon Terry, President/CEO
Tetyana Murza, Managing Director
Natasha Bonhomme, VP, Strategic Development

Web Sites

3218 ARC of the United States
1825 K Street, NW, Suite 1200
Washington, DC 20006
202-534-3700
800-433-5255
Fax: 202-534-3731
tnguyen@thearc.org
www.thearc.org

The ARC is the national organization of and for people with mental retardation and related developmental disabilities and their
families. Devoted to promoting and improving supports and services for people with mental retardation and their families.

Ronald Brown, President
Elise McMillan, Vice President
Peter V. Berns, CEO

3219 Children's Gaucher Research Fund
8110 Warren Court
Granite Bay, CA 95746
916-797-3700
Fax: 916-797-3707
research@childrensgaucher.org
www.childrensgaucher.org

We are a nonprofit organization, that raises funds to coordinate
and support research to find a cure for type 2 and type 3 Gaucher
disease.

Roscoe Brady, MD, Member, Scientific Advisory Board
Gregory Grabowski, MD, Member, Scientific Advisory Board
Kondi Wong, MD, USAF, MC, Member, Scientific Advisory Board

3220 Gaucher Registry
Genzyme Corporation, 500 Kendall Street
Cambridge, MA 2142
617-591-5500
800-745-4447
help@gaucherregistry.com
www.registrynxt.com

Our goal is to significantly contribute to the medical understanding of Gaucher disease and to improve the quality of care for
Gaucher patients worldwide through active publication of Registry findings and disease management approaches.

3221 Health Answers
410 Horsham Road
Horsham, PA 19044
215-422-9010
Michael.tague@healthanswers.com
www.healthanswers.com

HealthAnswers offers a breadth of services in medical education,
sales force training, patient support, solutions, professional promotion and consumer solutions.

Michael Tague, Managing Director

3222 National Gaucher Foundation
61 Gneral Early Drive
Harpers Ferry, WV 25425
800-504-3189
ngf@gaucherdisease.org
www.gaucherdisease.org

The mission of the NGF is to find a cure for Gaucher Disease by
funding vital research programs, to meet the ever-increasing
needs of patients and families, as well as to promote commu-
nity/physician awareness and educational programs.

3223 Rare Genetic Diseases in Children (NYU)
550 First Avenue
New York, NY 10016
212-263-7300
www.med.nyu.edu/rgdc/homenow.htm

We target issues arising from rare genetic diseases affecting children. Also, to assist in the endeavor to bring knowledge and hope
to those for whom there is, at present, so little.

Robert I. Grossman, MD, Dean & CEO
Michael T. Burke, SVP, CFO, Vice Dean
Annette Johnson, JD, PhD, SVP & Vice Dean, General Counsel

Newsletters

3224 Gaucher Disease Newsletter
National Gaucher Foundation
61 Gneral Early Drive
Harpers Ferry, WV 25425
301-816-1515
800-504-3189
Fax: 301-816-1516
ngf@gaucherdisease.org
www.gaucherdisease.org

Offers information on the latest research, treatments and technology for persons affected by Gaucher Disease. Also includes legislative and medical information.

Quarterly

Robin A. Ely, MD, President
Rhonda P. Buyers, Executive Director
Cyndi Frank, Director Development

Pamphlets

3225 Gaucher Disease Fact Sheet
National Gaucher Foundation
61 Gneral Early Drive
Harpers Ferry, WV 25425
301-816-1515
800-504-3189
Fax: 301-816-1516
ngf@gaucherdisease.org
www.gaucherdisease.org

Offers information on what Gaucher Disease is, the symptoms,
risks, treatments and the workings of the National Gaucher Foundation.

Robin A. Ely, MD, President
Rhonda P. Buyers, Executive Director
Cyndi Frank, Director Development

3226 Living with Gaucher Disease
National Gaucher Foundation
61 Gneral Early Drive
Harpers Ferry, WV 25425
301-816-1515
800-504-3189
Fax: 301-816-1516
ngf@gaucherdisease.org
www.gaucherdisease.org

A guide for parents, families and relatives that teach them how to
deal with and cope with a diagnosis of Gaucher Disease.

24 pages

Robin A. Ely, MD, President
Rhonda P. Buyers, Executive Director
Cyndi Frank, Director Development

DESCRIPTION

3227 GROWTH HORMONE DEFICIENCY

Synonym: GH deficiency

Involves the following Biologic System(s):

Endocrinologic Disorders

Growth hormone deficiency is a condition characterized by deficient production or an impaired response to growth hormone (GH), resulting in growth impairment and short stature with normal proportions of the head, limbs, hands, and feet (pituitary dwarfism). Secreted by the pituitary gland in the brain, GH, also known as somatotropin, stimulates body growth and development by promoting the production of protein in cells, releasing energy through the breakdown of fats, and performing other vital functions. Also known as the master gland, the pituitary gland is connected, through a bundle of nerve fibers known as the pituitary stalk, to a region of the brain known as the hypothalamus, which controls the functioning of the pituitary gland through direct stimulation by nerves as well as through the actions of proteins known as hormone-releasing and hormone-inhibiting factors that the hypothalamus releases into the bloodstream for transport to the pituitary gland. The forward or anterior region of the pituitary gland secretes GH in response to the particular hormone-releasing factor known as growth hormone releasing factor (GHRF), which is carried by the blood from the hypothalamus to the pituitary gland.

Depending upon the underlying cause of GH deficiency, some patients with this condition may also have deficiencies of other hormones produced by the anterior pituitary gland, such as thyroid-stimulating hormone (TSH), which stimulates the production of thyroid hormones, or adrenocorticotropic hormone (ACTH), which promotes the growth and production of hormones by cells in the outer region (cortex) of the adrenal gland. Inadequate functioning of the pituitary gland is known as hypopituitarism.

GH deficiency may have many different causes, including absence, underdevelopment, or malformation of the pituitary gland or hypothalamus at birth; tumors of the anterior pituitary gland, pituitary stalk, or hypothalamus, particularly the type of pituitary tumors known as craniopharyngiomas; or radiation given for the treatment of certain cancers of the brain or other organs in the head. GH deficiency may also result from trauma affecting the pituitary gland or hypothalamus, such as injury during birth or interruption of the oxygen supplied to the brain (anoxia) by the lungs and red cells of the blood. Other causes of GH deficiency include some abnormalities affecting the genes or chromosomes that carry the structural plans for GH and the body's other substances, and some conditions that occur randomly for unknown reasons (idiopathic hypopituitarism). Moreover, some genetically caused types of hypopituitarism may result in GH deficiency alone or accompanied by deficiencies of other hormones produced by the anterior pituitary gland.

There are several genetic subtypes of isolated growth hormone deficiency (IGHD), including those that may be inherited as an autosomal recessive, autosomal dominant, or X-linked trait. Autosomal recessive IGHD may be caused by the complete absence of a gene known as the GH1 gene, located on chromosome 17. This form of IGHD is typically characterized by marked growth delays after birth and severe shortness of stature. Other types of autosomal recessive IGHD are caused by various other abnormalities (mutations) of the GH1 gene, causing varying degrees of growth failure and short stature. Some patients with autosomal dominant IGHD may also have mutations of the GH1 gene. The gene responsible for X-linked IGHD, so named because this gene is located on the X chromosome, has not yet been identified. The genetic form of growth impairment known as Laron syndrome is caused by deficient function of the pituitary gland, (hypopituitarism) and is thought to result from an impaired response to GH. This condition is characterized by abnormally increased levels of GH in the blood.

Most children with GH deficiency are of normal weight and length at birth. By the first year of life, children with severe GH deficiency or Laron syndrome may be significantly shorter than would be expected for their age and sex. Patients with less severe GH deficiency experience regular growth spurts that alternate with periods during which no growth occurs. Patients with GH deficiency may continue to experience growth beyond the age when most individuals attain their adult height. This is due to abnormal delays in the fusion of the growing ends (epiphyseal plates) and shafts of the long bones of the legs and arms. If children with GH deficiency do not receive treatment, their adult height may range from moderately to severely below the average height for a mature adult.

Children with GH deficiency typically have normally proportioned arms and legs, but they may have relatively small hands and feet. Many also have a characteristic facial appearance, including a short, broad face and relatively round head; an undeveloped upper and lower jaw; a small, saddle-shaped nose with a depressed nasal bridge; a small neck; delayed eruption and crowding of the teeth; and fine, sparse scalp hair. Because of abnormal smallness of the voice box (larynx), many patients with GH deficiency have a high-pitched voice. Other findings may include underdeveloped genitals, delayed or absent sexual development, and abnormally low concentrations of the sugar known as glucose (hypoglycemia).

Children with GH deficiency caused by tumors of the pituitary gland or hypothalamus may experience effects beyond growth deficiency, depending upon the location, nature, and growth of the tumor. In some patients, invasion and destruction of the pituitary gland cause degeneration (atrophy) of the thyroid gland, sex glands (gonads), and outer regions of the adrenal glands (adrenal cortex). Associated findings may include absence of sweating, weight loss, abnormal sensitivity to cold, delayed or absent sexual maturation, lack of response to certain stimuli (torpor), or other abnormalities. Tumors in the pituitary gland or hypothalamus may also cause total growth failure, abnormally increased urination (polyuria), vomiting, headaches, visual disturbances, episodes of abnormally increased electrical activity in the brain (seizures), and other abnormalities.

The treatment of GH deficiency depends on its underlying cause and nature. If GH deficiency is caused by a tumor, its treatment may include surgery, radiation therapy, or other appropriate measures to eliminate the tumor. Pituitary function should be carefully evaluated after such measures, in order to determine the appropriate treatment for pituitary abnormalities caused by the tumor or its treatment. The treatment of children with IGHD includes early replacement therapy with synthetic GH, which is continued until there is no further growth in response to the treatment. The maximum response usually occurs during the first year of treatment, with further treatment producing slower growth. Because such therapy may cause abnormally decreased activity of the thyroid gland (hypothyroidism), thyroid function should be regularly evaluated. Children with deficiencies of other anterior pituitary hormones in association with GH deficiency may receive additional hormone replacement therapies as required. Other treatment for GH deficiency is symptomatic and supportive.

Government Agencies

3228 NIH/ Eunice Kennedy Shriver National Institute of Child Health & Human Development
31 Center Drive, Building 31
Bethesda, MD 20892
301-496-5113
800-370-2943
Fax: 866-760-5947
nichdpress@mail.nih.gov
www.nichd.nih.gov

Established in 1962 by congress, today the institute conducts and supports research on topics related to the health of children, adults, families and populations. Some of these topics include: developmental disabilities, growth and development, infant death, reproductive health and birth defects.

Diana W. Bianchi, Director
Paul Williams, Director, Communications

National Associations & Support Groups

3229 American Academy of Pediatrics
141 Northwest Point Boulevard
Elk Grove Village, IL 60007
847-434-4000
800-433-9016
Fax: 847-434-8000
www.aap.org

The American Academy of Pediatrics and its member pediatricians are committed to the attainment of optimal physical, mental and social health and well-being for all infants, children, adolescents, and young adults.

Fernando Stein, MD, FAAP, President
Karen Remley, MD, CEO/Executive VP

3230 Dwarf Athletic Association of America
708 Gravenstein Hwy, North, #118
Sebastopol,, CA 95472
972-317-8299
888-598-3222
Fax: 972-966-0184
daaa@flash.net
www.daaa.org

The DAAA mission is to encourage people with dwarfism to participate in sports regardless of their level of skills. We promote and provide quality amateur level athletic opportunities for dwarf athletiecs in the US.

Jimmy Loyless, President
Gerry Graff, Vice President
Janet Brown, Executive Director

3231 Genetic Alliance
4301 Connecticut Avenue NW, Suite 404
Washington, DC 20008
202-966-5557
800-336-4363
Fax: 202-966-8553
info@geneticalliance.org
www.geneticalliance.org

A coalition of voluntary genetic support groups, consumers and professionals addressing the needs of individuals and families affected by genetic disorders from a national perspective.

Sharon Terry, President/CEO
Tetyana Murza, Managing Director
Natasha Bonhomme, VP, Strategic Development

3232 Human Growth Foundation
997 Glen Cove Avenue, Suite 5
Glen Head, NY 11545
516-671-4041
800-451-6434
Fax: 516-671-4055
hgfl@hgfound.org
www.hgfound.org

A nonprofit, national organization committed to expanding and accelerating research into growth and growth disorders, provides education and support to those affected by growth disorders and their families, and fosters the exchange of information with the medical community.

Patricia D Costa, Executive Director

3233 Lawson Wilkins Pediatric Endocrine Society
6728 Old McLean Village Dr.
McLean, VA ÿ2210
703-556-9222
Fax: 703-556-8729
secretary@lwpes.org
www.lwpes.org

To promote the acquisition and dissemination of knowledge of endocrine and metabolic disorders from conception through adolescence.

Kenneth Copeland, President
Ronald Rosenfield, President-Elect
John Kirkland, Treasurer

3234 Little People of America
250 El Camino Real, Suite 218
Tustin, CA 92780
714-368-3689
888-572-2001
Fax: 714-368-3367
info@lpaonline.org
www.lpaonline.org

A nonprofit organization that provides support and information to people of short stature and their families.

Gary Arnold, President
April Brazier, Senior Vice President
Jon North, Programs Director

3235 MAGIC Foundation: Major Aspects of Growth in Children
4200 Cantera Drive, #106
Warrenville, IL 60555
630-836-8200
800-362-4423
Fax: 630-836-8181
ÿContactUs@magicfoundation.org
www.magicfoundation.org

A national nonprofit organization providing support and education regarding growth disorders in children and related adult disorders. Provides educational information, networking, a national conference, a kids' program and an extensive medical library.

Dianne Kremidas, Executive Director
Mary Andrews, CEO
Teresa Tucker, Patient Advocacy

3236 March of Dimes Foundation
1275 Mamaroneck Avenue
White Plains, NY 10605
914-997-4488
888-663-4637
Fax: 914-997-4763
answers@marchofdimes.com
www.marchofdimes.com

A unique partnership of volunteers and professionals that provides leadership in the treatment and prevention of birth defects and prematurity. It is funded by voluntary contributions from individuals and a variety of organizations.

Stacey D. Stewart, President

State Agencies & Support Groups

Arkansas

3237 Little People of America - District 7
National Headquarters
250 El Camino Real, Suite 218
Tustin, CA 92780

714-368-3689
888-572-2001
Fax: 714-368-3367
info@lpaonline.org
www.lpaonline.org

District 7 of the Little People of America represents short stature individuals from the states of Arkansas, Kansas, Missouri and Oklahoma.

Chandler Crews, Director

California

3238 Little People of America - San Francisco Bay Area Chapter
National Headquarters
250 El Camino Real, Suite 218
Tustin, CA 92780

714-368-3689
888-572-2001
Fax: 714-368-3367
info@lpaonline.org
www.lpaonline.org

A nonprofit organization that provides support and information to people of short stature and their families.

Lee Uniacke, President
Keren Stronach, Co-Vice President
Caroline Jones, Co-Vice President

Colorado

3239 Little People of America - Front Range Chapter
7117 E Euclid Drive
Englewood, CO 80111

303-740-8555
ebennettebennett@netscape.net
www.curesearch.org

Little People of America, Inc. (LPA), will assist dwarfs with their physical and developmental concerns resulting from short stature. By providing medical, environmental, educational, vocational, and parental guidance, short-stature individuals and their families may enhance their lives and lifestyles with minimal limitations. Through peer support and personal example, members will be supportive of all those who reach out to LPA.

Chris & Bob Kotzian, President
Souda Bell, Vice President
Brandi VanAnne, Treasurer

Kansas

3240 Little People of America - District 7
National Headquarters
250 El Camino Real, Suite 218
Tustin, CA 92780

714-368-3689
888-572-2001
Fax: 714-368-3367
info@lpaonline.org
www.lpaonline.org

District 7 of the Little People of America represents short stature individuals from the states of Arkansas, Kansas, Missouri and Oklahoma.

Karen Shelby, Director
Jack Dohr, Vice Director
Cyndy Dohr, Treasurer

Missouri

3241 Little People of America - District 7
National Headquarters
250 El Camino Real, Suite 218
Tustin, CA 92780

714-368-3689
888-572-2001
Fax: 714-368-3367
info@lpaonline.org
www.lpaonline.org

District 7 of the Little People of America represents short stature individuals from the states of Arkansas, Kansas, Missouri and Oklahoma.

Karen Shelby, Director
Jack Dohr, Vice Director
Cyndy Dohr, Treasurer

New Jersey

3242 Little People of America - District 2
National Headquarters
250 El Camino Real, Suite 218
Tustin, CA 92780

714-368-3689
888-572-2001
Fax: 714-368-3367
info@lpaonline.org
www.lpaonline.org

A nonprofit organization that provides support and information to people of short stature and their families.

Michael Petruzzelli, District Director

New York

3243 Little People of America - District 2
National Headquarters
250 El Camino Real, Suite 218
Tustin, CA 92780

714-368-3689
888-572-2001
Fax: 714-368-3367
info@lpaonline.org
www.lpaonline.org

A nonprofit organization that provides support and information to people of short stature and their families.

Joe Zrinski, District Director
Patty Ott, Assistant District Director
Jim Davis, District Treasurer

Oklahoma

3244 Little People of America - District 7
National Headquarters
250 El Camino Real, Suite 218
Tustin, CA 92780

714-368-3689
888-572-2001
Fax: 714-368-3367
info@lpaonline.org
www.lpaonline.org

District 7 of the Little People of America represents short stature individuals from the states of Arkansas, Kansas, Missouri and Oklahoma.

Karen Shelby, Director
Jack Dohr, Vice Director
Cyndy Dohr, Treasurer

Pennsylvania

3245 Little People of America - District 2
National Headquarters
250 El Camino Real, Suite 218
Tustin, CA 92780
714-368-3689
888-572-2001
Fax: 714-368-3367
info@lpaonline.org
www.lpaonline.org

A nonprofit organization that provides support and information to people of short stature and their families.

Joe Zrinski, District Director
Patty Ott, Assistant District Director
Jim Davis, District Treasurer

Utah

3246 Little People of America - Utah Seagulls
National Headquarters
250 El Camino Real, Suite 218
Tustin, CA 92780
714-368-3689
888-572-2001
Fax: 714-368-3367
info@lpaonline.org
www.utahlittlepeople.org

A nonprofit organization that provides support and information to people of short stature and their families.

Steve Hatch, President

Research Centers

3247 Case Western Research University, Bolton Brush Growth Study Center
10900 Euclid Ave.
Cleveland, OH 44106
216-368-0592
Fax: 216-368-3204
mgh4@cwru.edu
www.case.edu

Investigations and research into the growth and development of the human body.

Kate Chapman, Manager

3248 Jackson Laboratory
600 Main Streeet
Bar Harbor, ME 04609
207-288-6000
800-474-9880
Fax: 207-288-6079
www.jax.org

Studies focusing on growth disorders and human genetics.

Rick Woychik, Executive Director

3249 New Jersey Institute of Technology Center for Biomedical Engineering
323 Martin Luther King Jr Boulevard
Fenster Hall, Sixth Floor, University Heights
Newark, NJ 07102
973-596-5268
Fax: 973-596-5222
www.njit.edu

Offers research into facial and bone disorders.

Richard Foulds, Director, Masters Program
Judith D. Redling, Coordinator, Undergraduate Program

3250 W.M. Krogman Center for Research In Child Growth and Development
University of Pennsylvania
3451 Walnut Street
Philadelphia, PA 19104
215-898-1470

Focuses research and studies on growth disorders and birth defects.

Solomon Katz, MA, PhD, Director

Conferences

3251 Genetic Alliance Annual Conference
Genetic Alliance
4301 Connecticut Avenue NW, Suite 404
Washington, DC 20008
202-966-5557
800-336-4363
Fax: 202-966-8553
info@geneticalliance.org
www.geneticalliance.org

Consistently inspirational and enables partnership among all stakeholders: advocates and community leaders, health and industry professionals, policymakers, and academicians.

July

Sharon Terry, President/CEO
Tetyana Murza, Managing Director
Natasha Bonhomme, VP, Strategic Development

3252 LPA National Conference
Little People of America
250 El Camino Real, Suite 218
Tustin, CA 92780
714-368-3689
888-572-2001
Fax: 714-368-3367
info@lpaonline.org
www.lpaonline.org

July

Leah Smith, Public Relations Director
Gary Arnold, President
April Brazier, Senior Vice President

Web Sites

3253 Alliance of Genetic Support Groups
4301 Conneticut Ave. NW, Suite 404
Washington, DC 20008
202-966-5557
Fax: 202-966-8553
www.geneticalliance.org

Is an international coalition comprised of millions of individuals with genetic conditions and more than 600 advocacy, research and health care organizations that represent their interests. As a broad-based coalition of key stakeholders, the Alliance builds partnerships to promote healthy lives for all those living with genetic condtions.

3254 Dwarf Athletic Association of America
www.daaa.org

The DAAA mission is to encourage people with dwarfism to participate in sports regardless of their level of skills. We promote and provide quality amateur level athletic opportunities for dwarf athletiecs in the US.

3255 Health Answers
410 Horsham Road
Horsham, PA 19044
215-422-9010
Michael.tague@healthanswers.com
www.healthanswers.com

HealthAnswers offers a breadth of services in medical education, sales force training, patient support solutions, professional promotion and consumer solutions.

Michael Tague, Managing Director

3256 Human Growth Foundation
www.hgfound.org

Information regarding disorders related to growth or growth hormone.

3257 Little People of America
250 El Camino Real, Suite 218
Tustin, CA 92780
www.lpaonline.org

Offers resources pertaining to dwarfism and Little People of America, medical data, instructions on how to join an e-mail discussion group, and links to numerous other dwarfism-related sites.

Gary Arnold, President
April Brazier, Senior Vice President
Jon North, Programs Director

3258 OHSU Homepage Search
www.ohsu.edu

Educates health and high-technology professionals, scienists and enviromental engineers, and it undertakes the indispendible functions of patient care, community service and biomedical research.

3259 Online Mendelian Inheritance in Man
U.S. National Library of Medicine, 8600 Rockville
Bethesda, MD 20894   888-346-3656
                                       info@ncbi.nlm.nih.gov
                                       www.ncbi.nlm.nih.gov

This database is a catalog of human genes and genetic disorders.

Christine E. Seidman, M.D., Chair
David J. Lipman, M.D., Executive Secretary
Michael Boehnke, Ph.D., Board Member

3260 Society for Endocrinology
22 Apex Court, Woodlands, Bradley Stoke
Bristol, UK BS32   145-464-2200
                                  TTY: 145-464-2210
                                       www.endocrinology.org

Aims to advance education and research in endocrinology for the public benefit.

G R Williams, Chair, Finance Committee
C J McCabe, Chair, Program Committee
D W Ray, Chair, Publications Committee

Book Publishers

3261 Endocrine & Metabolic Disorders Sourcebook
Linda M. Shin, author

Omnigraphics
PO Box 8002
Aston, PA 19014   800-234-1340
                                  Fax: 800-875-1340
                                       info@omnigraphics.com
                                       www.omnigraphics.com

Basic information for the lay person about pancreatic and insulin-related disorders such as pancreatitis, diabetes and hypoglycemia; adrenal gland disorders such as Cushing's syndrome, Addison's disease and congenital adrenal hyperplasia; pituitary gland disorders such as growth hormone deficiency, acromegaly and pituitary tumors; and thyroid disorders such as hypothyroidism, Grave's disease, Hashimoto's disease and goiter.

574 pages Hardcover
ISBN: 0-780802-07-1

3262 Growing Children: A Parent's Guide
Human Growth Foundation
977 Glen Cove Avenue, Suite 5
Glen Head, NY 11545   516-671-4041
                                       800-451-6434
                                  Fax: 516-671-4055
                                       hgfl@hgfound.org
                                       www.hgfound.org

Offers parents information on the normal pattern of their child's growth, growth charts, recognition of growth problems, evaluation of growth problems and resources for more information. Available to members.

Frank Diamond, MD, President
Emily Germain-Lee, MD, Vice President
Patricia D. Costa, Executive Director

3263 Short and OK
Patricia Rieser, Heino FL Mayer-Bahlbug, author

Human Growth Foundation
977 Glen Cove Avenue, Suite 5
Glen Head, NY 11545   516-671-4041
                                       800-451-6434
                                       www.hgfound.org

This is a guide for parents of short children offering information on behavior issues, medical issues and psychological warning signs.
54 pages

Newsletters

3264 MAGIC Foundation: Major Aspects of Growth in Children
4200 Cantera Drive, #106
Warrenville, IL 60555   630-836-8200
                                       800-362-4423
                                  Fax: 630-836-8181
                                  TTY: 123-019-99
                                       contactus@magicfoundation.org
                                       www.magicfoundation.org

A national nonprofit organization providing support and education regarding growth disorders in children and related adult disorders. Provides educational information, networking, a national conference, a kids' program and an extensive medical library.

36 pages Quarterly

Dianne Kremidas, Executive Director
Mary Andrews, Chief Executive Officer
Teresa Tucker, Patient Advocacy

3265 Orphan Disease Update
National Organization for Rare Disorders
55 Kenosia Avenue
Danbry, CT 6810   203-744-0100
                                       800-999-6673
                                  Fax: 203-798-2291
                                       orphan@rarediseases.org
                                       www.rarediseases.org

It provides updates on research, advocacy, and special events, as well as advice and sources of help for caregivers, Web sites of interest, current clinical trials, and funding opportunities.

16 pages 3/year

Sheldon M. Schuster, Chair
Peter L Saltonstall, President & CEO
Pamela Gavin, COO

Pamphlets

3266 Dental Problems with Growth Hormone Deficiency
Human Growth Foundation
997 Glen Cove Avenue, Suite 5
Glen Head, NY 11545   516-671-4041
                                       800-451-6434
                                  Fax: 516-671-4055
                                       hgfl@hgfound.org
                                       www.hgfound.org

Growth hormone has a strong effect on bone growth, including the bones of the upper and lower jaws.

Pisit (Duke) Pitukcheewanont, MD, President
Emily Germain-Lee, MD, Vice President
Patricia (Patti) D. Costa, Executive Director

3267 Growth Hormone Deficiency
Human Growth Foundation
997 Glen Cove Avenue, Suite 5
Glen Head, NY 11545   516-671-4041
                                       800-451-6434
                                  Fax: 516-671-4055
                                       hgfl@hgfound.org
                                       www.hgfound.org

Causes and control of growth hormone deficiency.

Pisit (Duke) Pitukcheewanont, MD, President
Emily Germain-Lee, MD, Vice President
Patricia (Patti) D. Costa, Executive Director

3268 Growth Hormone Testing
Human Growth Foundation
997 Glen Cove Avenue, Suite 5
Glen Head, NY 11545   516-671-4041
                                             800-454-6434
                                             Fax: 516-671-4055
                                             hgfl@hgfound.org
                                             www.hgfound.org

Describes how growth hormone testing is used, when growth hormone test is ordered, and what growth hormone test results might
mean.

Pisit (Duke) Pitukcheewanont, MD, President
Emily Germain-Lee, MD, Vice President
Patricia (Patti) D. Costa, Executive Director

3269 Intrauterine Growth Retardation
Human Growth Foundation
977 Glen Cove Avenue, Suite 5
Glen Head, NY 11545   516-671-4041
                                             800-451-6434
                                             Fax: 516-761-4055
                                             hglf@hgfound.org
                                             hgfound.org

Offers information on how to understand this growth disorder and
how to cope with it.

Pisit (Duke) Pitukcheewanont, MD, President
Emily Germain-Lee, MD, Vice President
Patricia (Patti) D. Costa, Executive Director

**3270 Most Frequently Asked Questions with Growth Hormone
Deficiency**
Human Growth Foundation
977 Glen Cove Avenue, Suite 5
Glen Head, NY 11545   516-671-4041
                                             800-451-6434
                                             Fax: 516-671-4055
                                             hgfl@hgfound.org
                                             www.hgfound.org

Discusses the consequences of growth hormone deficiency in
chidlren and adults.

Pisit (Duke) Pitukcheewanont, MD, President
Emily Germain-Lee, MD, Vice President
Patricia (Patti) D. Costa, Executive Director

DESCRIPTION

3271 GUILLAIN-BARRE SYNDROME

Synonyms: Acute ascending polyneuritis, Acute febrile polyneuritis, Acute idiopathic polyneuritis, Acute postinfectious polyneuropathy, GBS, Landry's paralysis

Involves the following Biologic System(s):

Neurologic Disorders

Guillain-Barre syndrome (GBS) (pronounced gE-Ian-ba-rA) is a progressive neurologic disorder that affects many nerves (polyneuropathy) and is characterized by unusual sensations (paresthesias) in the arms, legs, or both. GBS generally causes progressive muscle weakness over days and, in some cases, paralysis accompanied by lack of muscle tone. Guillain-Barre syndrome is thought to be an autoimmune disorder and may occur as a reaction to a previous viral infection, immunization, or bacterial infection (e.g., Lyme disease). Autoimmune disorders involve the body's inappropriate immune response to its own healthy tissues.e symptoms of GBS typically begin approximately one to three weeks following the triggering event.

Symptoms associated with Guillain-Barre syndrome range from mild to severe and may include numbness, tingling, muscle weakness, and sometimes paralysis that begins in the legs and then usually spreads upward toward the trunk, arms, muscles of the chest, and sometimes the face (ascending paralysis). Affected children may become irritable and unable or unwilling to walk. As weakness spreads to the chest and facial areas, muscles required for speech, breathing, and eating may become affected. In addition, if the nerves of the autonomic nervous system which control vital involuntary functions are affected, individuals with GBS may develop fluctuations in blood pressure and heart rate as well as other heart irregularities. A rare form of Guillain-Barreyndrome called the Miller-Fisher syndrome is characterized by paralysis of the nerves and muscles of the eyes (ophthalmoplegia), an absence of normal reflexes (areflexia), and an inability to coordinate voluntary movement (ataxia).

Most children with Guillain-Barre syndrome recover completely within two to three weeks. Some may experience ongoing muscular weakness. In addition, in rare cases, affected individuals may experience prolonged or recurring episodes of GBS that may last for months or years. These uncommon manifestations are referred to as chronic unremitting polyradiculoneuropathy and chronic relapsing polyradiculoneuropathy.

Guillain-Barre syndrome may be diagnosed through specialized tests of the fluid that surrounds the brain and spinal cord (cerebrospinal fluid) and other clinical findings. Early diagnosis and hospitalization allow for observation and monitoring of affected individuals. If the progression of muscle weakness or paralysis is very slow and limited, treatment may include observation and supportive care until recovery is complete. If, however, paralysis progresses to involve breathing and swallowing, appropriate support is necessary. Other treatment may include plasma exchange (plasmapheresis), a procedure during which blood is withdrawn and the liquid portion (plasma) removed in order to filter out harmful substances. A plasma substitute is then mixed with the blood,

and the reconstituted blood is then returned to the body. Alternative treatment may include the intravenous administration of immunoglobulin (IVIG). In some cases, certain immunosuppressive drugs or corticosteroids may be effective. Physical therapy may aid in the maintenance of joint and muscle function. Other treatment is symptomatic and supportive.

National Associations & Support Groups

3272 American Academy of Pediatrics
141 Northwest Point Boulevard
Elk Grove Village, IL 60007
847-434-4000
800-433-9016
Fax: 847-434-8000
www.aap.org

The American Academy of Pediatrics and its member pediatricians are committed to the attainment of optimal physical, mental and social health and well-being for all infants, children, adolescents, and young adults.

Fernando Stein, MD, FAAP, President
Karen Remley, MD, CEO/Executive VP

3273 American Autoimmune Related Diseases Association
22100 Gratiot Avenue
Eastpointe, MI 48021
586-776-3900
800-598-4668
Fax: 586-776-3903
aarda@aarda.org
www.aarda.org

Dedicated to the eradiction of autoimmune diseases and the alleviation of suffering and the socio-economic impact of autoimmunity through fostering and facilitating collaboration in the areas of education, public awareness, research and patient services in an effective, ethical and efficient manner.

Virginia T. Ladd, President/Executive Director
Patricia Barber, Assistant Director
Deb Patrick, Events Specialist

3274 GBS/CIDP Foundation International
Holly Bldg, 104 1/2 Forrest Avenue
Narberth, PA 19072
610-667-0131
866-224-3301
Fax: 610-667-7036
info@gbsfi.com
www.gbs-cidp.org

Provides emotional support and assistance to people affected by this rare disease. Arranges personal visits to affected individuals in hospitals and rehabilitation centers. Fosters research into the cause, treatment, and other aspects of the disorder and directs affected individuals with long-term disabilities to resources for vocational, financial, and other aspects of the disorder.

Sara Voorhees, PMP, President
Estelle L. Benson, Executive Director
Barbara Katzman, Associate Director

Web Sites

3275 American Autoimmune Related Diseases Association
22100 Gratiot Ave.
Eastpointe, MI 48021
586-776-3900
800-598-4668
Fax: 586-776-3903
www.aarda.org

Dedicated to the eradiction of autoimmune diseases and the alleviation of suffering and the socio-economic impact of autoimmunity through fostering and facilitating collaboration in the areas of education, public awareness, research and patient services in an effective, ethical and efficient manner.

Rev. Herbert G. Ford, D. Min., Chair
Stanley M. Finger, PhD, Vice Chair
Virginia T. Ladd, R.T., President & Executive Director

3276 GBS Support Group of the UK
Woodholme House, Heckingt, Li NG34

152-946-9910
080-037-4803
Fax: 152-946-9915
www.gbs.org.uk/

Objectives are to: provide emotional support to patients, families and friends; provide, when possible, personal visits by former patients to those currently in hospitals and rehabilitation centres and those recovering; supply a comprehensive short guide for patients, relatives and friends, and other literature, so that patients and their families can learn what to expect during the illness; and to educate the public and medical community about the Support Group.

Caroline Morrice, Director
Lesley Dimmick, Charity Officer
Chris Fuller, Trustee

Book Publishers

3277 Immune System Disorders Sourcebook

Joyce Brennfleck Shannon, author

Omnigraphics
PO Box 8002
Aston, PA 19014

800-234-1340
Fax: 800-875-1340
info@omnigraphics.com
www.omnigraphics.com

Basic information about lupus, multiple sclerosis, guillain-barre syndrome and more.

671 pages Hardcover
ISBN: 0-780807-48-0

Pamphlets

3278 Fact Sheet: Guillain-Barre Syndrome
National Inst. of Neurological Disorders/Stroke
PO Box 5801
Bethesda, MD 20824

301-496-5751
800-352-9424

Information about Guillain-Barren Syndrome, what causes Guillain-Barren Syndrome, how is it diagnosed and treated, etc. Also available in Spanish.

DESCRIPTION

3279 HIV INFECTION

Synonyms: Fetal AIDS, Acquired Immune Deficiency Syndrome

Involves the following Biologic System(s):

Immunologic and Rheumatologic Disorders, Infectious Disorders

HIV Infection destroys the body's ability to fight infections, resulting in Acquired Immune Deficiency, or AIDS. T-cells, which are responsible for responding to infections, are destroyed by the virus. The process is slow and silent, which means that HIV can be contracted unwittingly years before any symptoms appear. As the T-cells are destroyed, organisms that are usually defeated by a normal immune system, infect the body. Patients suffer from one infection after another. HIV is usually spread from an infected person to a non-infected person by unprotected sexual intercourse, or by sharing needles. Most young children with AIDS contract the disease through in utero transmission; however, infants may occasionally acquire the infection through mother's milk. In addition, children with hemophilia and others who may have received transfusions of blood or blood products before HIV blood-screening became standard in 1985 may have become infected by contaminated blood.

Some children with HIV infection develop symptoms in the first or second year of life, while the majority may not show signs of infection for several years. AIDS is diagnosed in about 50 percent of HIV-infected children by three years of age. Early signs may include chronic or recurrent fevers and diarrhea, rashes, swollen lymph glands (lymphadenopathy), enlarged liver and spleen (hepatosplenomegaly), and delays in growth and nervous system development. Some infants and young children are anemic, experience weight and appetite loss, decreased energy, and irregularities of the heart and kidneys. Early symptoms may include chronic or recurrent bacterial infections and uncommon viral, fungal, and other types of infections caused by microorganisms that do not ordinarily cause disease or infections. As the immune system continues to weaken, children may develop lung inflammations and potentially life-threatening pneumocystis pneumonia. Children with AIDS are also at increased risk for certain types of malignant diseases such as non-Hodgkin's lymphoma.

Most infants born to mothers with HIV show antibodies in their blood for approximately 12 to 14 months. In infants who are not infected with the virus, these passive antibodies disappear. For this reason, standardized HIV testing is not conclusive in children younger than 18 months. However, HIV infection in these children may often be detected through the use of virus cultures and a specialized DNA-copying technique called polymerase chain reaction or| PCR.

Prevention of HIV and subsequent AIDS infection in infants may be directed toward counseling of at-risk women of child-bearing age who may be advised to avoid becoming pregnant. The strictly prescribed administration of the drug AZT during the last six months of pregnancy, as well as during labor and delivery, has been shown to greatly improve the chances of an HIV-infected mother delivering an infant who is not infected with HIV. In fact, congenitally acquired HIV has been reduced dramatically in recent years. Delivery by Cesarean section may also reduce risk of transmission to the newborn. In addition, mothers with HIV should refrain from breast-feeding their infants, as there is some evidence of HIV transmission from mother to child in women who may have contracted the virus after pregnancy.

Infants and children with HIV may be treated with antibiotics to prevent pneumocystis pneumonia. Intravenous gamma globulin therapy may be used to maintain or increase the ability of the immune system to fight the effects of secondary infections. In addition, certain steroidal drugs may be administered to treat lymphoid interstitial pneumonitis, while AZT, alone or in combination, is often used to treat children and has been found to be particularly effectiv|e against neurologic irregularities. Additional therapies are also being tested in children. Other treatment is symptomatic and supportive.

Government Agencies

3280 NIH/National Institute of Allergy and Infectious Diseases
5601 Fishers Lane, MSC 9806
Bethesda, MD 20892   301-496-5717
                                       866-284-4107
                                  Fax: 301-402-3573
                                  TDD: 800-877-8339
                              ocpostoffice@niaid.nih.gov
                                   www.niaid.nih.gov

Conducts and supports basic and applied research to better understand, treat, and ultimately prevent infectious, immunologic, and allergic diseases.

Anthony S Fauci MD, Director

National Associations & Support Groups

3281 AIDS Healthcare Foundation
6255 W. Sunset Blvd. 21st Fl.
Los Angeles, CA 90028   323-860-5200
                                    info@aidshealth.org
                                     www.aidshealth.org

It is a nonprofit, tax-exempt 501(c)(3) organization, is a global organization providing cutting-edge medicine and advocacy to over 350,000 patients in 36 countries.

Michael Weinstein, President
Peter Reis, Senior Vice President
Laura Boudreau, Chief Counsel for Operations

3282 AIDS Research Alliance
1400 South Grand Avenue, Suite 701
Los Angeles, CA 90015   310-358-2423
                                  Fax: 310-358-2431
                                  info@aidsresearch.org
                                      aidsresearch.org

The mission is to develop a cure for HIV/AIDS, medical strategies to prevent new infections, and better treatments for people living with HIV.

W. David Hardy, M.D., Chairman
Cary D. Stevens, Treasurer
Kenneth "Cam" Davis, Jr., Secretary

3283 AIDS United
1424 K Street, N.W., Suite 200
Washington, DC 20005   202-408-4848
                                  Fax: 202-408-1818
                                   www.aidsunited.org

Katy Caldwell, Executive Director
Tim Armitage, Brand & Marketing Strategy
Rick Gomez, Senior Vice President, Marketing

3284 American Academy of HIV Medicine
1705 DeSales Street NW, Suite 700
Washington, DC 20036   202-659-0699
                                  Fax: 202-659-0976
                                     www.aahivm.org

3285 American Academy of Pediatrics
141 Northwest Point Boulevard
Elk Grove Village, IL 60007   847-434-4000
                                           800-433-9016
                                      Fax: 847-434-8000
                                           www.aap.org

The American Academy of Pediatrics and its member pediatricians are committed to the attainment of optimal physical, mental and social health and well-being for all infants, children, adolescents, and young adults.

Fernando Stein, MD, FAAP, President
Karen Remley, MD, CEO/Executive VP

3286 American College of Preventive Medicine
455 Massachusetts Avenue NW, Suite 200
Washington, DC 20001   202-466-2044
                                      Fax: 202-466-2662
                                           info@acpm.org
                                           www.acpm.org

The mission is to improve the health of individuals and populations through evidence-based health promotion, disease prevention, and systems-based approaches to improving health and health care.

Haydee Barno, Contact
Michael Barry, Contact
Paul Bonta, Contact

3287 American Foundation for Children with AIDS
6221 Blue Grass Avenue?
Harrisburg, PA 17112   888-683-8323
                                           info@afcaids.org
                    www.americanfoundationforchildrenwithaids.org

It is a non-profit organization providing critical support to infected and affected HIV and children and their caregivers.

Tanya Weaver, Executive Director
Michelle Miller, Executive Assistant
Betsy Dorsey, Warehouse Manager

3288 American Nurses Association
8515 Georgia Avenue, Suite 400
Silver Spring, MD 20910   800-274-4262
                                      Fax: 301-628-5001
                                           anf@ana.org
                                           www.nursingworld.org

The American Nurses Association (ANA) is the only full-service professional organization representing the interests of the nation's 3.1 million registered nurses through its constituent and state nurses associations and its organizational affiliates.

Pamela F. Cipriano, PhD, President
Marla J. Weston, PhD, RN, FAAN, Chief Executive Officer
Cindy R. Balkstra, Vice President

3289 American Psychiatric Association
1000 Wilson Boulevard, Suite 1825
Arlington, VA 22209   703-907-7300
                                           888-35 -7924
                                           apa@psych.org
                                           www.psychiatry.org

It is a medical specialty society representing growing membership of more than 36,000 psychiatrists.

3290 American Psychological Association
750 First St. NE
Washington, DC 20002   202-336-5500
                                           800-374-2721
                                      TTY: 202-336-6123
                                           www.apa.org

The mission is to advance the creation, communication and application of psychological knowledge to benefit society and improve people's lives.

Norman B. Anderson, PhD, CEO/ EVP
L. Michael Honaker, PhD, Deputy Chief Executive Officer
Ellen G. Garrison, PhD, Senior Policy Advisor

3291 American Public Health Association
800 I Street, NW
Washington, DC 20001   202-777-2742
                                      Fax: 202-777-2534
                                      TTY: 202-777-2500
                                           www.apha.org

APHA champions the health of all people and all communities. They aim to strengthen the public health profession and speak out for public health issues and policies backed by science.

Georges C. Benjamin, MD, Executive Director
Kemi Oluwafemi, MBA, CPA, Chief Financial Officer
Susan Polan, PhD, Associate Executive Director

3292 American Social Health Association
PO Box 13827
Research Triangle Park, NC 27709   919-361-8400
                                           800-783-9877
                                      Fax: 919-361-8425
                                           www.ashastd.org

Dedicated to improving the health of individuals, families, and communities with a focus on preventing sexually transmitted diseases and their harmful consequences.

Lynn Barclay, President/CEO
Deborah Arrindell, VP Health Policy
David Allen, MBA, CPA, Vice President/CFO

3293 American Society for Microbiology
1752 N Street, N.W.
Washington, DC 20036   202-737-3600
                                      Fax: 202-942-9333
                                           service@asmusa.org
                                           www.asm.org

he American Society for Microbiology is a life science membership organization. Membership has grown from 59 scientists in 1899 to more than 39,000 members today, with more than one third located outside the United States. The members represent 26 disciplines of microbiological specialization plus a division for microbiology educators.

Nancy Sansalone, Interim Executive Director
Timothy Donohue, President
Joseph M. Campos, Secretary

3294 American Society of Clinical Oncology
2318 Mill Road, Suite 800
Alexandria, VA 22314   571-483-1300
                                           www.asco.org

With the number of cancer patients projected to grow dramatically in the years ahead in the U.S. and worldwide, we must do everything possible to ensure that we are well-positioned to deliver the care they will need.

Peter Paul Yu, President
Julie M. Vose, President-Elect
Susan L. Cohn, Treasurer

3295 Association of Nurses in AIDS Care
3538 Ridgewood Road
Akron, OH 44333   330-670-0101
                                           800-260-6780
                                      Fax: 330-670-0109
                                           anac@anacnet.org
                                           www.nursesinaidscare.org

The mission of the Association is to promote the individual and collective professional development of nurses involved in the delivery of health care to persons infected or affected by the Human Immunodeficiency Virus (HIV) and to promote the health and welfare of infected persons.

Suzanne Willard, President
Jason Farley, President-Elect
Don Kurtyka, Treasurer

3296 Association of State and Territorial Health Officials
2231 Crystal Drive, Suite 450
Arlington, VA 22202   202-371-9090
                                      Fax: 571-527-3189
                                           www.astho.org

The mission is to transform public health within states and territories to help members dramatically improve health and wellness.

Jewel Mullen, President
Edward Ehlinger, President-Elect
Brenda Fitzgerald, Secretary-Treasurer

3297 Black AIDS Institute
1833 West 8th Street #200
Los Angeles, CA 90057
213-353-3610
Fax: 213-989-0181
www.blackaids.org

It is the only national HIV/AIDS think tank focused exclusively on Black people. The Institute's Mission is to stop the AIDS pandemic in Black communities by engaging and mobilizing Black institutions and individuals in efforts to confront HIV.

Grazell R. Howard, J.D, Chair
Vanessa Williams, 1st Vice Chair
Gerard McCallum II, 2nd Vice Chair

3298 Elizabeth Glazer Pediatric AIDS Foundation
1140 Connecticut Avenue, N.W, Ste 200
Washington,, DC 20036
ÿ20- 29- 916
888-499-4673
Fax: 202-296-9185
info@pedsaids.org
www.pedsaids.org

A national nonprofit organization dealing with medical problems unique to children infected with HIV/AIDS. The foundation is focused specifically on creating a future that will offer hope, finding effective therapies and issues of pregnancy and HIV. The foundation encourages students to enter the world of pediatric AIDS through a student intern program and more.

Pamela Barnes, President/CEO
Trish Carlin, Vice President Programs
Diane Thompson, VP Policy/Communications

3299 HIV Medicine Association
1300 Wilson Boulevard, ÿSuite 300
Arlington, VA 22209
703-299-1215
Fax: 703-299-8766
info@hivma.org
www.hivma.org

The HIV Medicine Association is an organization of medical professionals who practice HIV medicine.

Adaora Adimora, Chair
Carlos del Rio, Chair Elect
Wendy Armstrong, Vice Chair

3300 Hemophilia Federation of America
820 First Street NE, Suite 720
Washington, DC 20002
202-675-6984
800-230-9797
Fax: 972-616-6211
info@hemophiliafed.org
www.hemophiliafed.org

Hemophilia Federation of America (HFA) is a community based organization that serves people with bleeding disorders and their families in the USA. With a broad mission to assist and advocate, HFA provides programs, services and policy education and support through its Member Organization affiliations as well as direct to consumers.

Tracy Cleghorn, Board President
Scott Boling, Co-Vice President
Douglas Hartsough, Board Treasurer

3301 Immune Deficiency Foundation
Immune Deficiency Foundation
40 W Chesapeake Avenue, Suite 308
Towson, MD 21204
410-321-6647
800-296-4433
Fax: 410-321-9165
idf@primaryimmune.org
www.primaryimmune.org

The only national charitable organization aimed at fighting the primary immune deficiency diseases. The founders included parents of children with primary immune deficiency, immunologists who treat immune deficient patients and other individuals with an interest in helping others. The Foundation's main goal is to improve the care and treatment of adults and children with primary immune deficiency diseases and to promote public education and awareness about the diseases.

Marcia Boyle, Ceo
Katherine Antilla, Vice Chair
Carol Ann Demaret, Secretary

3302 Infectious Diseases Society of America
1300 Wilson Blvd, Suite 300
Arlington, VA 22209
703-299-0200
Fax: 703-299-0204
www.idsociety.org

The Infectious Diseases Society of America (IDSA) represents physicians, scientists and other health care professionals who specialize in infectious diseases. IDSA's purpose is to improve the health of individuals, communities, and society by promoting excellence in patient care, education, research, public health, and prevention relating to infectious diseases.

Stephen B. Calderwood, MD, FIDSA, President
Johan S. Bakken, MD, PhD, FIDSA, President-Elect
William G. Powderly, MD, FIDSA, Vice President

3303 International Antiviral Society-USA
425 California Street, Suite 1450
San Francisco, CA 94104
415-544-9400
Fax: 415-544-9401
info@iasusa.org
www.iasusa.org

TheÿIAS-USAÿis a not-for-profit professional education organization that has been sponsoring continuing medical education (CME) programs for physicians since 1992 and is accredited by the Accreditation Council for Continuing Medical Education (ACCME).

Paul A. Volberding, MD, Chair, Board of Directors
Donna M. Jacobsen, Executive Director/President
Constance A. Benson, MD, Board of Director

3304 International Association of Providers of AIDS Care
1990 M Street, NW, Suite 380
Washington, DC 20036
202-808-2754
Fax: 202-315-3651
iapac@iapac.org
www.iapac.org

IAPAC envisions a world in which people at risk for and those living with HIV/AIDS may access the best prevention, care, and treatment services delivered by clinicians and allied health workers armed with cutting-edge knowledge and expertise.

Ian Sparks, CEO
Benjamin Young, MD, PhD, SVP/ CMO
Michael S. Glass, MA, EVP/ Chief of Staff

3305 National AIDS Hotline
American Social Association
PO Box 13827
Research Triangle Park, NC 27709
919-361-8400
800-342-2437
Fax: 919-361-8425
TDD: 800-243-7889
www.ashastd.org

Information and advocacy resources for families and professionals. Includes listings of organizations providing general information and organizations focusing on more specific areas of concern to families and young adults who have disabilities.

Lynn Barclay, President/CEO
Deborah Arrindell, VP Health Policy
David Allen MBA, CPA, Vice President/CFO

3306 National Abandoned Infants Assistance Resource Center
University of California, Berkeley
1950 Addison Street, Suite 104, #7402
Berkeley, CA 94720
510-643-8390
Fax: 510-643-7019
aia@berkeley.edu
www.aia.berkeley.edu

The Center's vision is to enhance the quality of social and health services delivered to drug and HIV-affected children and their families. Its strategy is to provide state-of-the-art training, technical assistance, research, and information to professionals who serve these families. Services include a national newsletter, telephone seminars, conferences, monographs, guides and reports.

Jeanne Pietrzak, Director
Neil Gilbert PhD, Principal Investigator
Amy Price MPA, Associate Director

3307 National Alliance of State & Territorial AIDS Directors
444 North Capitol Street, NWÿÿSuite 339
Washington, DC 20001 202-434-8090
nastad@nastad.org
www.nastad.org

The National Alliance of State and Territorial AIDS Directors (NASTAD) represents the nation's chief state health agency staff who have programmatic responsibility for administering HIV/AIDS and viral hepatitis healthcare, prevention, education, and supportive service programs funded by state and federal governments. NASTAD is dedicated to reducing the incidence of HIV/AIDS and viral hepatitis infections in the U.S. and its territories, providing comprehensive, compassionate, and high-quality ca

Kevin Trotter, Manager, Operations
Lucy Slater, Director, Global Programÿ
Mark Griswold, Senior Manager, Global Program

3308 National Association of Community Health Centers
7501 Wisconsin Ave, Suite 1100W
Bethesda, MD 20814 301-347-0400
www.nachc.com

To address the widespread lack of access to basic health care, Community Health Centers serve over 23 million people at more than 9,000 sites located throughout all 50 states and U.S. territories.

Gary Wiltz, MD, Chair of the Board
Ricardo Guzman, Chair Elect
Kauilaÿ Clark, Immediate Past Chair

3309 National Association of People with AIDS
8041 Colesville Road, Suite 750
Silver Spring, MD 20910 240-247-0880
Fax: 240-247-0574
info@napwa.org
www.napwa.org

Advocates on behalf of all people with HIV and AIDS in order to end the pandemic and the human suffering caused by HIV/AIDS.

Frank Oldham, Jr, Executive Director
Vanessa Johnson, Deputy Executive Director
Andrew Spieldenner, Director Programs

3310 National Black Leadership Commission on AIDS, Inc.
215 W. 125th Street, 2ndÿFloor
New York, NY 10027 212-614-0023
Fax: 212-614-0508
info@nblca.org
www.nblca.org

The National Black Leadership Commission on AIDS, Inc. (NBLCA) is a non-profit organization in the United States. There mission is to educate, mobilize, and empower black leaders to meet the challenge of fighting HIV/AIDS and other health disparities in their local communities.

C. Virginia Fields, President and CEO
Felecia Webb, Vice President of Development
Leatrice Wactor, Program Coordinator

3311 National Medical Association
8403 Colesville Road, Suite 820
Silver Spring, MD 20910 202-347-1895
Fax: 202-347-0722
www.nmanet.org

The National Medical Association (NMA) is the collective voice of African American physicians and the leading force for parity and justice in medicine and the elimination of disparities in health.

Garfield Clunie, M.D., Chairman of the Board
Lawrence Sanders, President
Martin Hamlette, J.D., M.H.A., Executive Director

3312 National Minority AIDS Council
1931 13th Street NW
Washington, DC 20009 202-483-6622
Fax: 202-483-1135
communications@nmac.org
nmac.org

NMAC represents a coalition of faith based and community based organizations as well as AIDS Service organizations advocating and delivering HIV/AIDS services in communities of color nationwide.ÿÿ

Paul Kawata, Executive Director
Kim Ferrell, Director of Facilities Management
Kim Johnson, Director

3313 Physician's Research Network
39 West 19th Street, Suite 605
New York, NY 10011 212-924-0857
Fax: 212-924-0759
www.prn.org

The Physicians' Research Network (PRN) is a not-for-profit, peer-support and educational organization serving clinicians working in the fight against HIV/AIDS and viral hepatitis.

James F. Braun, DO, President
Edward Vladich, Office Manager

3314 Support for Children with AIDS
1222 T Street NW, Grandma's House
Washington, DC 20009 202-234-4128
Fax: 202-234-8145
terrific03@aol.com
www.grandmashouse-terrific.org

A support organization that provides service, care, and preventive education for children and adults with AIDS. It provides housing for children with AIDS (e.g. Grandma's House® in Washington, DC).

Susan McCarley, Vice President

3315 World Health Organization
Avenue Appia 20
CH-1211 Geneva 27,
Switzerland www.who.int

WHO is the directing and coordinating authority for health within the United Nations system.

Dr Margaret Chan, Director General

3316 amfAR
120 Wall Street, 13th Floor
New York, NY 10005 212-806-1600
Fax: 212-806-1601
www.amfar.org

With the freedom and flexibility to respond quickly to emerging areas of scientific promise, amfAR plays a catalytic role in accelerating the pace of HIV/AIDS research and achieving real breakthroughs.

Kenneth Cole, Chairman
Mathilde Krim, Ph.D., Founding Chairman
Wallace Sheft, C.P.A., Treasurer

Research Centers

3317 American Foundation for AIDS Research
120 Wall Street, 13th Floor
New York, NY 10005 212-806-1600
800-392-6327
Fax: 212-806-1601
www.amfar.org

Dedicated to the support of HIV/AIDS research, HIV prevention, treatment education, and the advocacy of sound AIDS related public policy.

Kevin Frost, Ceo
Deborah C. Hernan, VP Public Information
Monica S. Ruiz PhD, MPH, Acting Director, Public Policy

3318 Children's Clinical Research Center
New York Hospital, Cornell Medical Center
525 E 68th Street, Box 149
New York, NY 10065
212-746-4745
Fax: 212-746-8922
www.ccrc.med.cornell.edu

Offers research into the study of pediatric AIDS and other disorders.

Julianne Imperato-McGinley, MD, Program Director
Patricia Giardina, MD, Associate Program Director

3319 Developmental Medicine Center
Children's Hospital
300 Longwood Avenue
Boston, MA 02115
617-355-6000
800-355-7944
Fax: 617-735-7429
TTY: 617-730-0152
webteam@tch.harvard.edu
www.childrenshospital.org

The Developmental Medicine Center (DMC) at Children's Hospital Boston provides developmental evaluation and treatment services for children aged birth to adolescence with a wide range of developmental, behavioral and learning difficulties. The Center was founded for the purpose of enhancing the coordination of services for children and families with special needs.,

Leonard A. Rappaport MD, MS, Program Director

Conferences

3320 Immune Deficiency Foundation National Conference
40 West Chesapeake Avenue, Suite 308
Towson, MD 21204
410-321-6647
800-296-4433
Fax: 410-321-9165
info@primaryimmune.org
www.primaryimmune.org

Annual conference hosted by an organization aimed at fighting the primary immune deficiency diseases. The founders included parents of children with primary immune deficiency, immunologists who treat immune deficient patients and other individuals with an interest in helping others. The Foundation's main goal is to improve the care and treatment of adults and children with primary immune deficiency diseases and to promote public education and awareness about the diseases.

June

Marcia Boyle, Founder/Chairman/President
Katherine Antilla, Vice Chair
Carol Ann Demaret, Secretary

Web Sites

3321 AEGIS
10866 Washington Blvd., #309
Culver City, CA 90232
310-838-2787
info@aegis.com
www.aegis.com/

Web based reference for HIV/AIDS-related information.

Jeff Zisner, President & CEO

3322 AIDS Knowledge Base
hivinsite.ucsf.edu/InSite
415-476-9000
webdev@pubaff.ucsf.edu
hivinsite.ucsf.edu/InSite

A comprehensive, on-line textbook of HIV disease from the University of California San Francisco and San Francisco Hospital.

Sam Hawgood, MBBS, Chancellor
Daniel Lowenstein, MD, Executive Vice Chancellor & Provost
Bruce Wintroub, Interim Dean, School of Medicine

3323 American Social Health Association
www.ashastd.org

Dedicated to improving the health of individuals, families, and communities with a focus on preventing sexually transmitted diseases and their harmful consequences.

3324 Children with AIDS Project
PO Box 23778
Tempe, AZ 85285
480-774-9718
www.aidskids.org/

The mission is to transform the silence that surrounds HIV infected, children and AIDS orphans into an audible sound. This sound must be amplified until the needs are met for all children in the nation and globally affected by the AIDS epidemic.

3325 Elizabeth Glazer Pediatric AIDS Foundation
1140 Connecticut Avenue NW, Suite 200
Washington, DC 20036
202-296-9165
888-499-4673
Fax: 202-296-9185
info@pedaids.org, research@pedaids.org
www.pedaids.org/

The foundation created a future of hope for children and families worldwide by eradicating pediatric AIDS, providing care and treatment to people with HIV/AIDS, and accelerating the discovery of new treatments for other serious and life-threatening pediatric illnesses.

Russ Hagey, Chair
Charles Lyons, President & CEO
Brad Kiley, COO

3326 Food and Drug Administration
10903 New Hampshire Avenue
Silver Spring, MD 20903
301-796-8240
888-463-6332
webmail@oc.fda.gov
www.fda.gov

The FDA is responsible for protecting the public health by assuring the safety, efficacy, and security of human and veterinary drugs, biological products, medical devices, our nation's food supply, cosmetics, and products that emit radiation. The FDA is also responsible for advancing the public health by helping to speed innovations that make medicines and foods more effective, safer, and more affordable and helping the public get accurate, science-based information they need to improve health.

Margaret A. Hamburg, Commissioner
Walter S. Harris, MBA, PMP, Deputy Commissioner
James Tyler, CFO

3327 Immune Deficiency Foundation
110 West Road, Suite 300
Towson, MD 21204
800-296-4433
Fax: 410-321-9165
www.primaryimmune.org

The only national charitable organization aimed at fighting the primary immune deficiency diseases. The founders included parents of children with primary immune deficiency, immunologists who treat immune deficient patients and other individuals with an interest in helping others.

John Seymour, Phd, LMFt, Chair
Steve Fietek, Vice Chair
Marcia Boyle, President & Founder

3328 National Association of People with AIDS
8401 Colesville Road, Suite 505
Silver Spring, MD 20910
240-247-0880
866-846-9366
Fax: 240-247-0574
www.napwa.org

Advocates on behalf of all people with HIV and AIDS in order to end the pandemic and the human suffering caused by HIV/AIDS.

3329 National Pediatric & Family HIV Resource Center
www.womenchildrenhiv.org
editor@WomenChildrenHIV.org
www.womenchildrenhiv.org

The goal of this site is to contribute to an improvement in the scale and quality of international HIV/AIDS prevention care and treatment programs for women and children by increasing access to authoritative HIV/AIDS information.

Arthur Ammann, MD, President
Heather Dron, MPH, Project Manager
Robert Grey, Programmer

3330 National Pediatric AIDS Network
PO Box 1507
Nevada City, CA 95959
gary@npan.org
www.npan.org/

Is a nonprofit organization, that works collaboratively with a number of other HIV/AIDS information providers.

Gary Gale, Director

3331 Parents Helping Parents
1400 Parkmoor Ave., Suite 100
San Jose, CA 95126
408-727-5772
855-727-5775
Fax: 408-286-1116
www.php.com

Mission is to help children with special needs receive the resources, love, hope, respect, health care, education, and other services they need to reach their full potential by providing them with strong families, dedicated professionals, and responsive systems to serve them.

Hitesh Shah, Chair
Mary Ellen Peterson, MA, Executive Director/ CEO
Paul Schutz, CFO

3332 Pediatric AIDS Clinical Trials Group
pactg.s-3.com

Goals are: to optimize strategies to maintain or improve mother to infant transmission at less than 2% without long termn toxicity to exposed infants or treated pregnant women in the United States; and to enable more than 90% of children perinatally infected with HIV to achieve normal growth and development, and more than 20 years survival in the United States.

3333 Sunshine for HIV Kids
www.sunshinesite.com

Is a nonprofit tax exempt organization that identifies and raises funds for charities who directly deliver care to children afficted with HIV/AIDS and their familes.

3334 Wayne State University
42. West Warren Ave.
Detroit, MI 48202
315-577-2424
www.research.wayne.edu

Advances in therapy to prevent HIV transmission from mothers to infants have brought hope to thousands, but transmission of HIV continues to increase in developing countries. We must identify effective intervention strategies usable by all nations if we are to reduce the incidence of mother to infant HIV transmission worldwide.

Debbie Dingell, Chair
Gary S. Pollard, Vice Chair
M. Roy Wilson, President

Book Publishers

3335 AIDS Awareness Library

Anna Forbes, MSS, author

Rosen Publishing Group
29 E 21st Street
New York, NY 10010
212-777-3017
800-237-9932
Fax: 888-436-4643
info@rosenpub.com
www.rosenpublishing.com

This series of eight 24-page books for grades K-5, speaks to children in nonthreatening langauge that provides vital information without graphic detail. This series is meant to be a gentle introduction to this frightening epidemic. Titles in series: Heroes Against AIDS, Kids with AIDS, Living in a World with AIDS, Myths and Facts About AIDS, What is AIDS?, What You Can Do About AIDS, When Someone You Know Has AIDS, Where Did AIDS Come From?.

24 pages
ISBN: 0-823974-06-5

3336 AIDS and the Education of Our Children
Consumer Information Center
US Department of Education
Pueblo, CO 81009
719-948-3334
888-878-3256
www.pueblo.gsa.gov

A guide for parents and teachers offering helpful information on the topic of AIDS education.

28 pages

3337 Heroes Against AIDS
Anna Forbes, MSS, author

Rosen Publishing Group
29 E 21st Street
New York, NY 10010
212-777-3017
800-237-9932
Fax: 888-436-4643
info@rosenpub.com
www.rosenpublishing.com

Ryan White and Magic Johnson are just two of the heroes in this book who demonstrate through their courage and kindness their strength in adversity.

K-5 24 pages
ISBN: 0-823923-71-1

3338 Kids with AIDS
Anna Forbes, MSS, author

Rosen Publishing Group
29 E 21st Street
New York, NY 10010
212-777-3017
800-237-9932
Fax: 888-436-4643
info@rosenpub.com
www.rosenpublishing.com

This book is written so as not to scare kids but teach compassion for their peers who might have AIDS. It stresses the importance of eliminating blame from this disease.

K-5 24 pages
ISBN: 0-823923-72-X

3339 Let's Talk About Going to the Hospital
Rosen Publishing Group's PowerKids Press
29 E 21st Street
New York, NY 10010
212-777-3017
800-237-9932
Fax: 888-436-4643
rosenpub@tribeca.ios.com
www.powerkidspress.com

If a child has to check into the hospital, chances are he or she is already upset about being ill. Knowing how a hospital functions and what the procedures are, such as when family members can visit, will help in what is already a stressful situation. Grades K-5.

24 pages
ISBN: 0-823950-36-0

3340 Living in a World with AIDS

Anna Forbes, MSS, author

Rosen Publishing Group
29 E 21st Street
New York, NY 10010

212-777-3017
800-237-9932
Fax: 888-436-4643
info@rosenpub.com
www.rosenpublishing.com

AIDS is a reality. Kids hear about it on TV, at school, and on the streets. This introductory volume reassures kids about their basic safety and provides gentle preventative advice that is age appropriate.

K-5 24 pages
ISBN: 0-823923-67-3

3341 Myths and Facts About AIDS

Rosen Publishing Group's PowerKids Press
29 E 21st Street
New York, NY 10010

212-777-3017
800-237-9932
Fax: 888-436-4643
rosenpub@tribeca.ios.com
www.powerkidspress.com

In a simple and reassuring manner, the author demystifies this disease and puts to rest many misconceptions. Grades K-5.

K-5 24 pages
ISBN: 0-823923-66-5

3342 What Is AIDS?

Rosen Publishing Group's PowerKids Press
29 E 21st Street
New York, NY 10010

212-777-3017
800-237-9932
Fax: 888-436-4643
rosenpub@tribeca.ios.com
www.powerkidspress.com

Accessible scientific look at AIDS puts it in the context of other diseases, teaching about the human organism in an age-appropriate manner. Grades K-5.

K-5 24 pages
ISBN: 0-823923-68-1

3343 What You Can Do About AIDS

Anna Forbes, MSS, author

Rosen Publishing Group
29 E 21st Street
New York, NY 10010

212-777-3017
800-237-9932
Fax: 888-436-4643
info@rosenpub.com
www.rosenpublishing.com

It's never too early to teach kids about social responsibility. This book emphasizes community participation.

K-5 24 pages
ISBN: 0-823923-70-3

3344 When Someone You Know Has AIDS

Anna Forbes, MSS, author

Rosen Publishing Group
29 E 21st Street
New York, NY 10010

212-777-3017
800-237-9932
Fax: 888-436-4643
info@rosenpub.com
www.rosenpublishing.com

This unique volume helps kids who might know someone with AIDS to approach that person with love and compassion as one would any sick person.

K-5 24 pages
ISBN: 0-823923-69-X

3345 Where Did AIDS Come From?

Anna Forbes, MSS, author

Rosen Publishing Group
29 E 21st Street
New York, NY 10010

212-777-3017
800-237-9932
Fax: 888-436-4643
info@rosenpub.com
www.rosenpublishing.com

AIDS is frightening, especially to young children who sense the secrecy around it. This is a gentle introduction to the topic. It treats AIDS like any other epidemic.

K-5 24 pages
ISBN: 0-823923-65-7

Pamphlets

3346 Hope for Children with AIDS

Elizabeth Glazer Pediatric AIDS Foundation
1140 Connecticut Avenue NW, Suite 200
Washington, DC 20036

202-296-9165
888-499-4693
Fax: 202-296-9185
info@pedaids.org, research@pedaids.org
www.pedaids.org

The Elizabeth Glaser Pediatric AIDS Foundation creates a future of hope for children and families worldwide by eradicating pediatric AIDS, providing care and treatment to people with HIV/AIDS, and accelerating the discovery of new treatments for other serious and life-threatening pediatric illnesses. In working toward our mission the foundation is committed to ensuring that the vast majority of every dollar raised goes directly into our research education and outreach program.

Russ Hagey, Chair
Charles Lyons, President & CEO
Brad Kiley, COO

Camps

3347 Camp Heartland

1845 N Farwell Avenue, Suite 310
Milwaukee, WI 53202

414-272-1118
800-724-4673
Fax: 414-272-9916
webmaster@campheartland.org
www.campheartland.org

Set up to provide children impacted by HIV/AIDS with the best week of their lives. Provides children forever affected by the isolation and tragedy of the disease the opportunity to experience - sometimes for the first time - the pure joys of being a kid.

Neil Willenson, Founder/CEO
Jeffrey Maiken, President
Patrick Kindler, Program Manager

3348 Camp Kindle

PO Box 81147
Lincoln, NE 81147

661-257-1901
877-800-2267
Fax: 702-995-9186
info@projectkindle.org
www.campkindle.org

Camp with the purpose to enhance the overall well-being of children and young people infected with or affected by HIV and AIDS.

Eva Payne, Founder & Executive Director
Mandy Nickolite, VP & Psychosocial lead
Erin Fitzgerald, Program Coordinator

3349 Camp Kindle- Project Kindle
28245 Ave Crocker, Ste 104
Santa Clarita, CA 91355 661-257-1901
877-800-2267
Fax: 702-995-9186
info@projectkindle.org
www.campkindle.org

Camp for youth ages 7-18 who are infected with or affected by
HIV and AIDS.

Eva Payne, Founder & Executive Director
Alison Boring, Co-Camp Director

3350 Hole in the Wall Gang Camp
565 Ashford Center Road
Ashford, CT 6278 860-429-3444
Fax: 860-429-7295
ashford@holeinthewallgang.org
www.holeinthewallgang.org

Nonprofit organization that provides a recreational camp experience for children ages 7-15 with cancer, genetic blood diseases
and HIV/AIDS.

Raymond Lamontagne, Chair
James Canton, CEO
Kevin Magee, CFO

DESCRIPTION

3351 HEAD INJURIES

Synonyms: Closed head injury, Concussion, Traumatic brain injury

Involves the following Biologic System(s):
Neurologic Disorders

Head injuries describe trauma to the head that results in damage to the scalp, skull, or brain and associated membranes, nerves, or blood vessels. Every year in the United States, approximately 100,000 children require hospitalization because of head injuries. Many of these injuries are the result of motor vehicle and bicycle accidents. The risk of sustaining head or brain injury during a vehicular or bicycle accident is reduced by the proper use of restraint systems such as approved car seats, seat belts, or helmets. There are different types of head injuries, some of which are minor and, after healing, of no further significance; however, certain injuries that impact upon the brain may have severe complications and be potentially life-threatening. These include skull fractures, concussions, brain contusions and lacerations, and bleeding in the brain (e.g., subdural or epidural hematomas). Brain injury may result in mild, moderate, or severe functional disabilities, depending upon the particular area of brain tissue that is damaged or destroyed. Disabilities may affect physical, emotional, or intellectual development and include impairment in the comprehension or production of speech and language (aphasia); the inability to remember or perform certain familiar tasks requiring sequential movements (apraxia); the failure to remember past events or experiences (amnesia); the lack of ability to recognize familiar persons or objects (agnosia); and the development of episodes of uncontrolled electrical activity in the brain (posttraumatic epilepsy), usually within two years of the initial head injury.

In children with skull fractures or an open-head injury, there is an actual break in the skull bone (cranium). Many skull fractures do not interfere with normal brain function and will heal with no complications. However, in some patients, fractures may damage blood vessels or the membranes surrounding the brain (meninges), resulting in leakage of the fluid that surrounds the brain and spinal cord (cerebrospinal fluid). The break in the skull may also serve as an entry point for bacteria that may subsequently cause serious infection. A thorough evaluation is necessary to determine the extent of the injury. Surgical intervention may sometimes be necessary.

Concussions are closed-head injuries that occur as a result of a jarring of the brain within the skull. Symptoms and findings associated with this type of injury in children may include a temporary loss of consciousness, lack of muscle tone, poor or absent reflexes (areflexia), dilated pupils, blurred vision, irritability, or restlessness. These signs of concussion may be followed by rapid heartbeat (tachycardia), vomiting, listlessness, drowsiness, apathy, a pale skin color, or confusion. Treatment for concussion always involves observation. Although most children recover completely, hospitalization may be required for those whose level of consciousness continues to drop or those who appear listless, drowsy, or confused. Those who vomit excessively or experience seizures or other neurological symptoms may also require hospitalization.

Other closed-head injuries may include contusions, character-ized by bruises on the brain; lacerations, characterized by tears in the brain tissue; subdural hematomas, characterized by accumulations of blood under the outermost membrane layer surrounding the brain (dura mater); and epidural hematomas, characterized by blood between the dura mater and the skull. Hematomas may result from ruptures or lacerations in certain blood vessels. Contusions and hematomas may cause the brain to swell with an accompanying buildup of fluid (edema). Increasing pressure within the skull may result in brain damage. Symptoms and findings may include headache; seizures; altered levels of consciousness sometimes leading to coma; loss of strength; numbness; paralysis; confusion; amnesia; or life-threatening complications such as respiratory distress and heart irregularities. Treatment is aimed at the maintenance of respiratory and cardiovascular function in order to prevent further injury. If necessary, the upper spine (cervical spine) is stabilized. The monitoring and management of brain swelling and fluid accumulation may include the careful administration of intravenous fluids and medications, bed elevation, and the use of supplemental oxygen. In addition, surgical intervention may be required to relieve intracranial pressure, remove blood clots, or control bleeding around the brain. Further treatment may include medication for the control of seizures. Recovery from major head or brain trauma may be a very slow, progressive process and, as such, may require the assistance of a team of specialists who will work with the family or caregivers of the child to coordinate symptomatic and supportive care.

Government Agencies

3352 NIH/National Institute of Neurological Dis orders and Stroke (NINDS)
PO Box 5801
Bethesda, MD 20824

301-496-5751
800-352-9424
Fax: 301-496-0296
TTY: 301-468-5981
www.ninds.nih.gov

The mission of NINDS is to reduce the burden of neurological disease, a burden borne by every age group, by every segment of society, by people all over the world.

Walter J. Koroshetz, MD, Director

National Associations & Support Groups

3353 Acoustic Neuroma Association
600 Peachtree Parkway, Suite 108
Cumming, GA 30041

770-205-8211
877-200-8211
Fax: 770-205-0239
info@anausa.org
www.anausa.org

The Acoustic Neuroma Association provides information and support to patients who have been diagnosed with or experienced an acoustic neuroma or other benign problem affecting the cranial nerves. The ANA is an incorporated, nonprofit organization, and is supported by contributions from its members. The association also furnishes information on patient rehabilitation to physicians and health care personnel, promotes research on acoustic neuroma, and educates the public.

Jeffrey D. Barr, President
Alan Goldberg, VP
Steven M. Houghton, Secretary

3354 American Academy of Pediatrics
141 Northwest Point Boulevard
Elk Grove Village, IL 60007

847-434-4000
800-433-9016
Fax: 847-434-8000
www.aap.org

The American Academy of Pediatrics and its member pediatricians are committed to the attainment of optimal physical, mental and social health and well-being for all infants, children, adolescents, and young adults.

Fernando Stein, MD, FAAP, President
Karen Remley, MD, CEO/Executive VP

3355 Association for Neurologically Impaired Brain Injured Children
61-35 220th Street
Oakland Gardens, NY 11364
718-423-9550
Fax: 718-423-9838
mail@anibic.org
www.anibic.org

ANIBIC is a voluntary, multi-service organization that is dedicated to serving individuals with severe learning disabilities, neurological impairments and other developmental disabilities. Services include: residential, vocational, family support services, recreation (children and adults), respite (adult), summer day camp, counseling, and tramatic brain injury services (adults).

Michael Steward, President
Phyllis Kaye, VP
Jerry Smith, Executive Director

3356 Brain Injury Association of America Helpli ne
8201 Greensboro Drive, Suite 611
McLean, VA 22102
703-761-0750
800-444-6443
Fax: 703-761-0755
familyhelpline@biausa.org
www.biausa.org

The mission of the Brain Injury Association is to create a better future through brain injury prevention, research, education and advocacy. This national number can link people to local BIA affiliates.

Susan H Connors, President/CEO
Mary S Reitter, CAE, Executive VP/COO
Gregory J. O'Shanick, Managing Director

3357 Brain Injury Association of America Nation al Office
1608 Spring Hill Road, Suite 110
Vienna, VA 22182
703-761-0750
800-444-6443
Fax: 703-761-0755
info@biausa.org
www.biausa.org

Our mission is to create a better future through brain injury prevention, research, education and advocacy.

Susan H Connors, President/CEO
Mary S Reitter, CAE, Executive VP/COO
Gregory J. O'Shanick, Managing Director

3358 Brain Injury Association of Michigan
7305 Grand River, Suite 100
Brighton, MI 48114
810-229-5880
800-444-6443
Fax: 810-229-8947
info@biami.org
www.biami.org

The mission of BIAMI is to enhance the lives of those affected by brain injury through education, advocacy, research, and local support groups; and to reduce the incidence of brain injury through prevention.

Michael F Dabbs, President
Cheryl A Burda, VP of Operations & Programs
Helena Dinqeldey, Office Coordinator

3359 Brain Trauma Foundation
7 World Trade Center, 34th Floor, 250 Greenwich St
New York, NY 10007
212-772-0608
Fax: 212-772-0357
info@braintrauma.org
www.braintrauma.org

The Brain Trauma Foundation mission is to improve the outcome of Traumatic Brain Injury (TBI) patients nationwide.

Jamshid Ghajar, President
Alan Quasha, Chairman
Pamela J. Newman, Executive Director

3360 Center for Disabilities and Development
University of Iowa Stead Family Children's Hospita
100 Hawkins Drive
Iowa City, IA 52242
319-353-6900
877-686-0031
Fax: 319-356-7700
cdd-scheduling@uiowa.edu
www.uichildrens.org/cdd

A trusted resource for healthcare, training, research and information for people with disabilities that include: behavior disorders, brain injury, cerebral palsy, diabetes, down syndrome, learning disabilities, mental retardation, sleep disorders and spina bifida.

Dianne McBrien, MD, Medical Director

3361 Coma Recovery Association
8300 Republic Airport, Suite 106
Farmingdale, NY 11735
631-756-1826
Fax: 631-756-1827
office@comarecovery.org
www.comarecovery.org

Our purpose is to help families of coma and head injury survivors by providing information and referrals, enabling them to make informed choices regarding treatment, rehabilitation and socialization alternatives as well as support from others who struggle with similar concerns.

3362 Head Injury Hotline
212 Pioneer Building
Seattle, WA 98104
206-621-8558
Fax: 206-329-4355
brain@headinjury.com
www.headinjury.com

Sponsors public information seminars designed to bring together survivors of head injuries, their families and professionals for networking and information sharing, as well as operating a national helpline for people suffering from a head injury.

Constance Miller, MA, Founder
Paul M. Kuroiwa, PH.C., Performance management consultant
Bill Levinger, Managing Director

3363 Perspectives Network
PO Box 121012
W Melbourne, FL 32912
770-844-6898
800-685-6302
Fax: 770-844-6898
TPN@tbi.org
www.tbi.org

Primary focus is positive communication between persons with brain injury, family members, caregivers and friends of persons with brain injury, the many professionals who treat persons with brain injury and community members in order to create positive changes and enhance public awareness and knowledge of acquired and traumatic brain injury.

State Agencies & Support Groups

Alabama

3364 Alabama Head Injury Foundation
3100 Lorna Road, Suite 200
Hoover, AL 35216
205-823-3818
800-433-8002
Fax: 205-823-4544
ahif1@bellsouth.net
www.ahif.org

Our mission is to improve the quality of life for survivors of traumatic brain injury and for their families and to increase public awareness of (TBI).

Keith T. Belt, Jr., President
Kim F. Hooks, VP
Charles D Priest, Executive Director

Arizona

3365 Brain Injury Association of Arizona
5025 E Washington St., Suite 108
Phoenix, AZ 85034
602-508-8024
888-500-9165
Fax: 602-508-8285
info@biaaz.org
www.biaaz.org

A non-profit membership organiation of people with brain injuries, their families, friends and service providers working together since 1983 to provide information and referrels, education, advocacy and support for those affected by brain injury.

Lisa Counters, President
Rebecca Armendariz, VP
Mattie Cummins, Executive Director

Arkansas

3366 Brain Injury Association of Arkansas
PO Box 26236
Little Rock, AR 72221
501-374-3585
866-610-4841
Fax: 501-918-6595
info@BIA-AR.org
www.brainassociation.org

Creating a better future through brain injury prevention, research, education and advocacy.

Dana Austen, President
Kortney E Gold, VP
Tessa Davis, Secretary

California

3367 California Brain Injury Association
1800 30th St., Suite 250
Bakersfield, CA 93301
661-872-4903
888-662-4222
Fax: 661-873-2508
calbiainfo@yahoo.com
www.biacal.org

Our mission is to serve and empower the community of many thousands of persons living in California with brain injuries and to enable them to live with dignity and to access all therapy, hospitalization, long term care, and all possible means for recovery and rehabilitation and to support their families.

Paula Daoutis, Administrative Director
Ursula Pesta, Project Coordinator
Elaine Solan, Community Liaison

3368 Jodi House
1235 C Veronica Springs Road
Santa Barbara, CA 93105
805-563-2882
Fax: 805-593-3982
info@jodihouse.org

The mission of Jodi House is to create a nurturing place of order, caring, acceptance and motivation for people with acquired brain injury,and to provide opportunities for each person to discover new paths to regain responsible independence and effective interdependence to the best of our ability, in order to achieve worthwhile purposes in our community.

Jim Cook, President
Andrew Chung, VP
Tracy Cohn, Treasurer

Colorado

3369 Brain Injury Association of Colorado
1385 South Colorado Boulevard, Ste 606, Building A
Denver, CO 80204
303-355-9969
800-955-2443
Fax: 303-355-9968
informationreferralbiacolorado.org
www.biacolorado.org

The Brain Injury Association of Colorado began in April 1980. BIAC was formed by a group of family members and professionals in Denver and Colorado Springs who were concerned with the lack of support services for survivors and family members affected by head injury.The mission is to improve the quality of life for survivors of brain injury and their families, and to support programs that prevent brain injury.

Dannis Schanel, President
Helen Kellogg, Executive Director
Peggy Spaulding, Executive Director

Connecticut

3370 Brain Injury Association of Connecticut
200 Day Hill Road, Suite 250
Windsor, CT 06095
860-219-0291
800-278-8242
Fax: 860-219-0568
general@biact.org
www.biact.homestead.com

Supports persons with brain injuries and their families by promoting services to facilitate full inclusion within their local community, and to increase awareness and understanding of brain injury and its prevention through community education.

500 Members

Paul A. Slager, Esq., President
Dr. Johnny Magwood, BSME, MBA, DBA, Vice President
Julie Peters, Executive Director

3371 TBI Support Group for Families & Survivors
Gaylord Hospital Conference Room
Wallingford, CT 06492
203-284-2800
TDD: 203-284-2700

Our mission is to preserve and enhance a person's health and function. We offer people a comprehensive continuum of care ranging from our Medically Complex Program and inpatient rehabilitation programs to outpatient services and sleep services.

Delaware

3372 Brain Injury Association of Delaware
840 Walker Rd
Dover, DE 19904
302-346-2083
800-411-0505
Fax: 302-678-3183
biadresources@cavtel.net
www.biausa.org

A nonprofit organization whose mission is to advocate for and with people who survive traumatic brain injury; to secure and develop community-bases services for survivors and their families; to support research leading to better outcomes that enhance the lives of those who sustain brain injuries; and to promote prevention of brain injury through awareness, education and legislation.

Elizabeth Furber, President
Timothy J. Walker, VP
Esther J. Curtis, Executive Director

District of Columbia

3373 Brain Injury Association of Washington DC
1232 17th St, N.W.
Washington, DC 20036
202-659-0122
Fax: 202-291-5366
info@biadc.org
www.biadc.org

Provide support to survivors of brain injury and their families, education to those who are being effected by brain injury, including the general public, and advocacy, to give the many suffering from this silent epidemic a public voice.

Joseph Cammarata, President/Treasurer
Ira Sherman, VP
Michael Yochelson, M.D., Board of Director

Florida

3374 Brain Injury Association of Florida
1637 Metropolitan Blvd, Suite B
Tallahassee, FL 32308

850-410-0103
800-992-3442
Fax: 954-786-2437
admin@biaf.org
www.biaf.org

A non profit organization founded in 1985, with the mission to improve the quality of life for persons with brain injury and their families by creating a better future through brain injury prevention, research, education, suport services and advocacy.

Mark Todd, PhD, President
Elynor Kazuk, Executive Director
Marilyn Ronshausen, Admin Secretary

3375 Family/Community Support Group of the Brain Injury Association of Florida
North Broward Medical Center
201 E Sample Road
Pompano Beach, FL 33064

954-786-2400
800-992-3442
www.biaf.org

Helping individuals with traumatic brain injuries and their families find practical solutions to the difficult problems faced when living with the long-term consequences of a traumatic brain injury (TBI).

Gary Clarke, Chairman
Johny Jallad, Chair-Elect
Larry Baxter, Secretary

3376 Goodwill Industries-Suncoast: Choices for Work Program
Goodwill Industries-Suncoast
10596 Gandy Boulevard
St. Petersburg, FL 33702

727-523-1512
888-297-1988
Fax: 727-579-1068
www.goodwill-suncoast.org

Provides short-term, light-duty work options for individuals recovering from on-the-job injuries. Participants are sponsored by a referring insurance company. This service is available in Hillsborough, Pinellas, Pasco and Polk counties through Suncoast Business Solutions.

Deborah A. Passerini, President
Oscar J. Horton, Chair
Martin W. Gladysz, Vice Chair

Georgia

3377 Brain Injury Resource Foundation
1841 Montreal Road, Suite 220
Tucker, GA 30084

678-937-1555
888-334-2424
Fax: 678-937-1557
info@birf.info
www.birf.info/index.shtml

A nonprofit charitable orginazation working together with families and professionals since 1982 to provide education, advocacy and support for those effected by brain injury. Our mission is to empower individuals with brain injury by making available resources that may improve the quality of their lives.

Karen Parsley, Executive Director

Hawaii

3378 Brain Injury Association of Hawaii
420 Kuwili Street, Suite 103
Honolulu, HI 96817

808-436-8977
Fax: 808-454-1975
biahi@verizon.net
www.biausa.org/Hawaii

Dedicated to improving the quality of life of persons with brain injury and the families of such persons in Hawaii and other areas of the Pacific Basin. The goals of BIA-HI include promoting the rights of individuals experiencing disability caused by brain injury, io increase public awareness of brain injury, and to provide education for individuals who have sustained a brain injury and their families.

Mary Isley-Wilson, President
Angie Enoka, VP
Lyna Burian, Secretary

3379 Special Education Center of Hawaii
708 Palekaua Street
Honolulu, HI 96816

808-734-0233
Fax: 808-734-0391
info@secoh.org
www.secoh.org

Committed to providing individual and family supports that promote successful community living in the lifestyle of choice. Services and supports are provided to people with developmental disabilities, or acquired disabilities due to aging or head injury. Services include day care, respite care, and supported employment.

Jon McKenna, President
Douglas Inouye, VP
Debbie Hiraoka, Treasurer

Idaho

3380 Brain Injury Association of Idaho
1055 North Curtis Road, PO Box 414
Boise, ID 83706

208-367-2747
800-444-6443
Fax: 208-333-0026
info@biaid.org
www.biaid.org

A non-profit organization helping persons with brain injuryand their familiy members.

Michelle Featherson, President

Illinois

3381 Brain Injury Association of Illinois
PO Box 64420
Chicago, IL 60664

312-726-5699
800-699-6443
Fax: 312-630-4011
info@biail.org
www.biail.org

A not-for-profit statewide membership organization comprised of people with brain injuries, family members, friends and professionals, with the mission to create a better future through brain injury awareness, prevention, education and advocacy.

Ginny Lazzara, President
Philicia Deckard, Executive Director
Irene Pedersen, Founder

Indiana

3382 Brain Injury Association of Indiana
9531 Valparaiso Court, Suite A
Indianapolis, IN 46268

317-356-7722
866-854-4246
Fax: 317-808-7770
info@BIAI.org
www.biai.org

A nonprofit service organization comprised of people with brain injury, their families, and concerned stakeholders who are dedicated to creating a better future by reducing the incidence and effects of brain injury through public and professional education, advocacy, support, and by facilitating inter-agency commitment and collaboration.

Nancy Ritter, Chairman
Tom John, VP
Scott Branam, Secretary

Iowa

3383 Brain Injury Association of Iowa
7025 Hickman Road, Suite 7
Urbandale, IA 50322
319-233-3235
855-444-6443
Fax: 319-272-2109
info@biai.org
www.biaia.org

Founded in 1980, exists to support, assist, and advocate for persons with acquired brain damage and for their families; advocates for and with people with brain injury and family members by responding to their challenges and representing their concerns through legislative efforts and active support of programs created for their needs.

Jackie Preston, Manager
Geoffrey Lauer, MA, LOC, Executive Director
Natasha Retz, BS, CBIS, Director of Programs and Services

Kansas

3384 Brain Injury Association of Kansas & Greater Kansas City
6701 W. 64th St., Suite 120
Overland Park, KS 66202
913-754-8883
800-783-1356
Fax: 816-842-1531
Lliggett@biaks.org
www.biaks.org

Offers support services to individuals and their families in the greater Kansas City area and throughout the state of Kansas who are recovering from traumatic brain injury.

Terrie Price, President
Whitney Sunderland, VP
Bonnie Stephens, Secretary

Kentucky

3385 Brain Injury Association of Kentucky
7321 New LaGrange Road, Suite 100
Louisville, KY 40222
502-493-0609
800-592-1117
Fax: 502-426-2993
dir@braincenter.org
www.biak.us

Serves those affected by brain injury through advocacy, education, injury prevention, research, service and support.

Andrew Horne, President
Eileen Edlin, Treasurer
Ben Ruiz, Secretary

Louisiana

3386 Brain Injury Association of Louisiana
8325 Oak Street, PO Box 57527
New Orleans, LA 70118
504-982-0685
800-500-2026
www.biala.org

A non-profit organization that serves the needs of persons with brain injury, their families, and care providers. The focus is to create a better future for individuals who have survived brain injury through brain injury prevention awareness, promotion of research, public education, and advocacy.

Janet Clark, Chairman
Paul Genco, Vice Chairman
William E Moak, President/Executive Director

Maine

3387 Brain Injury Association of Maine
109 North State Street, Suite 2
Concord, NH 03301
603-225-8400
800-773-8400
Fax: 603-228-6749
mail@biame.org
www.biame.org

A nonprofit organization that looks to create a better future for the people of Maine, through brain injury awareness, prevention, education and advocacy.

Bev Bryant, President
John Bott, Executive Director

Maryland

3388 Brain Injury Association of Maryland
2200 Kernan Drive
Baltimore, MD 21207
410-448-2924
800-221-6443
Fax: 410-448-3541
info@biamd.org
www.biamd.org

Our mission is to create a better future through brain injury prevention, research, education and advocacy.

Diane Triplett, Executive Director
Diane Triplett, Executive Director

Massachusetts

3389 Brain Injury Association of Massachusetts
30 Lyman Street
Westborough, MA 01581
508-475-0032
800-242-0030
Fax: 508-475-0040
biama@biama.org
www.biama.org

Our mission is to serve as an information and resource center for persons with brain injury, their families and friends, and providers and professionals in the field of brain injury treatment and rehabilitation.

Teresa Hayes, President
Harold Wilkinson, Secretary
Matthew Martino, Executive Board Member

Michigan

3390 Brain Injury Association of Michigan
7305 Grand River, Suite 100
Brighton, MI 48114
810-229-5880
800-444-6443
Fax: 810-229-8947
info@biami.org
www.biami.org

The mission of BIAMI is to enhance the lives of those affected by brain injury through education, advocacy, research, and local support groups; and to reduce the incidence of brain injury through prevention.

Michael F Dabbs, President
Cheryl A Burda, VP of Operations & Programs
Helena Dinqeldey, Office Coordinator

3391 Rehabilitation Institute of Michigan
261 Mack Avenue
Detroit, MI 48201
313-745-1203
Fax: 313-745-9863
www.rimrehab.org

Providing quality patient care, academic excellence and cutting-edge research in physical medicine and rehabilitation.

Mildred Matlock, Ceo
William H. Restum, PhD, President

Minnesota

3392 Brain Injury Association of Minnesota
34 13th Avenue NE, Suite B001
Minneapolis, MN 55413

612-378-2742
800-669-6442
Fax: 612-378-2789
info@braininjurymn.org
www.braininjurymn.org

The only non-profit organization in the state devoted solely to serving the needs of the 100,000 Minnesotans who live with a disability due to brain injury. Providing hope, help and a voice for brain injured persons for over 20 years.

quaterly 20-24 pages

Ardis Sandstrom, Executive Director
Ardis Sandstrom, Executive Director

Mississippi

3393 Brain Injury Association of Mississippi
2727 Old Canton Road, Suite 191
Jackson, MS 39216

601-981-1021
800-444-6443
Fax: 601-981-1039
biaofms@aol.com
www.msbia.org

Enhances the quality of life for Traumatic Brain Injury survivors and their families, and to develop and support programs that prevent brain injury.

Lee Jenkins, Executive Director
Paul Gospodarski, EdD, Executive Director
Dana C. Pierce, Associate Director

Missouri

3394 Brain Injury Association of Missouri
2265 Schuetz Road
Saint Louis, MO 63146

314-426-4024
800-444-6443
Fax: 314-426-3290
info@biamo.org
www.biamo.org

Founded in 1982, a community based organization serving persons with brain injury, their families, caregivers, physicians, therapists, case managers, and others throught the state of Missouri.

Eric Hart, President
Scott Gee, Executive Director
Scott Gee, Executive Director

Montana

3395 Brain Injury Association of Montana
1280 S 3rd West, Suite 4
Missoula, MT 59801

406-541-6442
800-241-6442
Fax: 406-541-4360
biam@biamt.org
www.biamt.org

To create a better future through brain injury prevention, research, education and advocacy.

Kristen Morgan, Program Director
Christien Morgan, Manager
Stacy Rye, Executive Director

New Hampshire

3396 Brain Injury Association of New Hampshire
109 N State Street, Suite 2
Concord, NH 03301

800-773-8400
800-444-8400
Fax: 603-228-6749
mail@bianh.org
www.bianh.org

Founded in 1983, a private, non-profit family and consumer run organization representing over 5000 New Hamphire residents with acquired brain disorders and stroke.

Steven D. Wade, Executive Director
Laura Flashman, Ph.D, President
Amy Messer, Vice-President

New Jersey

3397 Brain Injury Association of New Jersey
825 Georges Road, Second Floor
North Brunswick, NJ 08902

732-745-0200
732-745-0211
Fax: 732-738-1132
info@bianj.org
www.bianj.org

A nonprofit organization that brings together people with brain injury, their families and friends, and concerned allied health professionals to improve the quality of life people experience after brain injury.

Edward Kim, Chairperson
Anthony G. Cuzzola, Vice-Chairperson
Michael H. Greenwald, Secretary

New Mexico

3398 Brain Injury Association of New Mexico
3232 Candelaria NE
Albuquerque, NM 87107

505-292-7414
888-292-7415
Fax: 505-271-8983
info@braininjurynm.com
www.braininjurynm.org

Actively supports progressive public policy for persons with traumatic brain injury on both state and federal levels.

John Tiwald, Board President
Clara Holguin, Executive Director

New York

3399 Brain Injury Association of New York State
10 Colvin Avenue
Albany, NY 12206

518-459-7911
800-228-8201
Fax: 518-482-5285
info@bianys.org
www.bianys.org

A statewide non-profit membership organization that advocates on behalf of individuals with brain injury and their families, and promotes prevention. Established in 1982, provides education, advocacy, and community support services that lead to improved outcomes for children and adults with brain injuries and their families.

Debbie Berenda, Manager
Judy Avner, Executive Director
Jutith Sandman, Director Membership/Development

3400 Hy Feinstein Clubhouse
Long Island Head Injury Association
300 Kennedy Drive
Hauppauge, NY 11788

631-543-2245
Fax: 631-543-2261
club@lihia.org
www.lihia.org

A non-profit organization whose primary mission is to provide a place for people with head injuries to participate in meaningful work; to have the opportunity to meet and build friendships; and ulimately seek employment within the community.

3401 Mount Sinai Traumatic Brain Injury
Mt Sinai Medical Center
5 E. 98th Street, B-15
New York, NY 10029

212-241-7911
888-241-5152
margaret.brown@mssm.edu
www.icahn.mssm.edu

Specializing not only in helping patients regain mastery over their physical environment, but also in addressing the cognitive and emotional aftermaths, including anxiety and depression, which are frequently triggered by such injuries. The program contains different treatment levels to address the very specific needs of this population.

David Vandergoot, President
Wayne A. Gordon, Director
Joshua Cantor, Co-Director

North Carolina

3402 Brain Injury Association of North Carolina
2113 Cameron Street, Bryan Bldg, Suite 242, PO Box
Raleigh, NC 27605

919-833-9634
800-377-1464
Fax: 919-833-5415
bianc@bianc.net
www.bianc.net

Founded in 1982 by families and concerned professionals. The Association is an affiliate of the Brain Injury Association of America. Today, the Association has Family and Community Support Centers in Raleigh, Greenville, and Charlotte and 29 local chapters and support groups across the state.

Marylin Lash, President
Pam Gutherie, Vice President
Karen L. McCulloch, Co-Chair Elect

North Dakota

3403 Brain Injury Association of North Dakota
Open Door Center
1225 South 12th Street
Bismarck, ND 58504

701-845-1124
877-525-2724
Fax: 701-845-1175
www.braininjurynd.com

Mary Simonson, President
Richard Ott, Executive Director
Rebecca Quinn

Ohio

3404 Brain Injury Association of Ohio
855 Grandview Avenue, Suite 225
Columbus, OH 43215

614-481-7100
800-444-6443
Fax: 614-481-7103
help@biaoh.org
www.biaoh.org

The Brain Injury Association of Ohio aims to improve community services, supports, and awareness for the life-long challenges presented by brain injury and to increase the independence of those coping with its impact. There are five core services designed to achieve this: information & resource coordination; education & training for professionals; support groups for Ohio residents; prevention initiatives; advocacy for policies and funding that address service system gaps.

Stephanie Ramsey, President
Anthon Brooks, Vice President
Julie Robbins, Vice President

Oklahoma

3405 Brain Injury Association of Oklahoma
3015 E Skelly Dr.
Tulsa, OK 74105

918-789-0406
800-765-6809
Fax: 918-712-9019
braininjuryoklahoma@gmail.com
www.braininjuryoklahoma.org

Adam Sherman, President
Mary Dobbs, Vice President
Joan Gass, Treasurer

Oregon

3406 Brain Injury Association of Oregon
Po Box 549
Molalla, OR 97038

503-413-7707
800-544-5243
Fax: 503-961-8730
biaor@biaoregon.org
www.biaoregon.org

To improve the quality of life of persons with brain injury and their families; and to prevent brain injury.

Ralph Wiser, President
Chuck McGilvrary, Vice President
Carol Altman, Treasurer

3407 Oregon Brain Injury Resource Network
345 N Monmouth Avenue, PO Box 1329
Monmouth, OR 97361

541-346-0593
877-872-7246
Fax: 541-346-0599
tbi@wou.edu
www.tr.wou.edu/tbi/

Aims to improve access to information and services for individuals with brain injuries, their families, and the professionals who serve them. The Resource Network houses information on all aspects of brain injury, from the point of initial injury throughout the life span of the individual.

Pennsylvania

3408 Pittsburgh Area Brain Injury Alliance
630 Bascom Avenue
Pittsburgh, PA 15212

412-481-0443
jp@pabia.org
www.pabia.org

Dedicated to the people recovering from Brain Injury and who live with the consequences of Traumatic Brain Injury. The purpose is to provide a forum for peer-to-peer support and to assist in the development of peer-to-peer support groups in Western Pennsylvania.

Ed Crinnion, President

Rhode Island

3409 Brain Injury Association of Rhode Island
935 Park Avenue, Suite 8, PO Box 2743
Cranston, RI 02910

401-461-6599
Fax: 401-461-6561
braininjuryctr@biaofri.org
www.biausa.org/RI

To improve the quality of life for people with brain injuries and their families, and to develop and support programs that prevent brain injuries.

Sharon Brinkworth, Executive Director
Michael L. Baker, Co-President
Jean E. Cassiere, Secretary

South Carolina

3410 Brain Injury Alliance of South Carolina
Po Box 21523
Columbia, SC 29221
803-731-9823
800-290-6461
Fax: 803-731-0589
scbraininjury@bellsouth.net
www.biausa.org/SC/

Mission is to create a better future through brain injury prevention, research, education and advocacy.

Jeremy Hertza, President
Joyce Davis, Executive Director
Lyman Whitehead, Consultant

3411 Brain Injury Association of South Carolina
5605 Bush River Road
Columbia, SC 29212
803-731-9823
877-TBI-FACT
Fax: 803-731-4804
scbraininjury@bellsouth.net
www.biausa.org/SC/

To create a better future through brain injury prevention, education, and advocacy.

Jeremy Hertza, President
Joyce Davis, Executive Director
Lyman Whitehead, Consultant

Tennessee

3412 Brain Injury Association of Tennessee
955 Woodland St
Nashville, TN 37206
615-248-2541
800-444-6443
Fax: 615-383-1176
biaoftn@yahoo.com
www.braininjurytn.com

The mission is to improve the quality of life for persons with brain injuries and their families and to reduce the incidence of brain injury.

Guynn Edwards, President
Pam Bryan, Executive Director
Brian Webb, Treasurer

Texas

3413 Brain Injury Association of Texas
316 W 12th Street, Suite 405
Austin, TX 78701
512-326-1212
800-392-0040
Fax: 512-478-3370
info@biatx.org
www.texasbia.org

A non-profit public service organization, strives to meet the urgent need to develop programs for public awareness and education, to support research and rehabilitation and to provide family guidance.

San Marcos, President
Amy Santus, Vice President
Erin Garrison, Admin Director

Utah

3414 Brain Injury Association of Utah
5280 Commerce Dr., Suite E-190
Murray, UT 84107
801-716-4993
800-281-8442
Fax: 801-716-4995
info@biau.org
www.biau.org

Created in 1984, the only non-profit organization dedicated exclusively to education and support for the issues of prevention and recovery of brain injury in the state of Utah. The mission of the Brain Injury Association of Utah is to create a better future through brain injury prevention, research, education and advocacy.

Antonietta Anna Rosso, President
Pauline Fontaine, Treasurer
Ron S. Roskos, Executive Director

Vermont

3415 Brain Injury Association of Vermont
92 South Main Street, PO Box 482
Waterbury, VT 05676
802-244-6850
877-856-1772
Fax: 802-244-4005
support1@biavt.org
www.biavt.org

To create a better future through brain injury, prevention, research, education, and advocacy.

Trevor Squirrell, Executive Director
Barb Winters, Program Manager
Christy Opuszynski, Office Administrator

Virginia

3416 Brain Injury Association of Virginia
1506 Willow Lawn Dr., Suite 212
Richmond, VA 23230
804-355-5748
800-444-6443
Fax: 804-355-6381
infoa@biav.net
www.biav.net

Nonprofit organization Creating a better future through brain injury education, awareness, advocacy, and support.

Irv Cantor, President
Anne McDonnell, Executive Director
Theresa Alonso, Data Coordinator

Washington

3417 Brain Injury Association of Washington
PO Box 3044
Seattle, WA 98114
206-388-0900
877-982-4292
Fax: 206-388-0901
admin@braininjurywa.org
www.braininjurywa.org

The mission, which begins with prevention, is to provide support to survivors of brain injury and their families, education to those who are being effected by brain injury, including the general public, and advocacy, to give the many suffering from this silent epidemic a public voice.

Mark T. Long, President
David A. Butters, Chair
Patrice Roney, Co-Chair Elect

3418 Head Injury Hotline
Brain Injury Resource Center
PO Box 84151
Seattle, WA 98124
206-621-8558
Fax: 206-624-4961
brain@headinjury.com
www.headinjury.com

Disseminates head injury information and provides referrals to facilitate adjustment to life following head injury. Organizes seminars for professionals, head injury survivors, and their families. Our intention is to help you avoid much of the greif and loss of brain injury, and perhaps to inspire you to get involved.

Constance Miller, Founder

West Virginia

3419 Brain Injury Association of West Virginia
PO Box 574
Institute, WV 25112
304-400-4506
800-356-6443
Fax: 304-205-7915
biawv@aol.com
www.biawestvirginia.org

A nonprofit agency dedicated to providing support, advocacy, education and training on behalf of survivors of brain injuries, their families and those who provide services or care for them.

Michael W Davis, President
Sharon McKenny Lord
Jennifer Rhule Stockton

Wisconsin

3420 Brain Injury Association of Wisconsin
N63 W23583 Main Street, Suite A
Sussex, WI 53089
262-790-9660
800-882-9282
Fax: 262-790-9670
lschultz@biaw.org
www.biaw.org

Established in 1980 by a group of individuals with brain injury, their families, friends, and professionals. BIAW is a chartered member affiliate of the national Brain Injury Association, Inc. BIAW provides services in these 5 core areas: information and resources, education, prevention, advocacy, and support services

Audrey Nelson, President
Lori Schultz, Executive Director
Patricia David, Operations Director

Wyoming

3421 Brain Injury Association of Wyoming
111 W 2nd Street, Suite 106
Casper, WY 82601
307-473-1767
800-643-6457
Fax: 307-237-5222
director@wybia.org
www.wybia.org

The mission is to create a better future through brain injury prevention, research, education, and advocacy.

Dorothy Cronin, Executive Director
Dorothy Cronin, Executive Director

Libraries & Resource Centers

3422 Brain Injury Association of Michigan
7305 Grand River, Suite 100
Brighton, MI 48114
810-229-5880
800-772-4323
Fax: 810-229-8947
info@biami.org
www.biami.org

The mission of BIAMI is to enhance the lives of those affected by brain injury through education, advocacy, research, and local support groups; and to reduce the incidence of brain injury through prevention.

Michael F Dabbs, President
Cheryl A Burda, VP of Operations & Programs

3423 University of Illinois at Chicago, Craniofacial Center
College of Medicine
808 S Wood Street
Chicago, IL 60612
312-996-7870
Fax: 312-413-1526
www.medicine.uic.edu

Richard M Novak, Director

Research Centers

California

3424 Brain Imaging Center at the University of California, Irvine
University of California, Irvine
Irvine, CA 92697
949-824-7872
Fax: 949-824-7873
bic@msx.hsis.uci.edu
www.bic.uci.edu

Performs clinical assessment of regional brainmetabolism for Parkinson's disease, epilepsy, brain tumor evaluation, Alzheimer'sdisease, and head injury. Other neuropsychiatric illnesses that are assessed with PETscans at UCI include stroke, psychotic disorders, and movement disorders.

Steven L Small, Director
David B. Keator, Technical Director
Jill Upton, Research Coordinator

3425 Brain Research Institute
Brain Research Institute UCLA
1506 Gonda, PO Box 951761
Los Angeles, CA 90095
310-825-5061
Fax: 310-206-5855
lmaninger@mednet.ucla.edu
www.bri.ucla.edu

An organization research unit within the School of Medicine at the University of California , Los Angeles.

Christopher J. Evans, Director
J David Jentsch, Associate Director for Research
Michael S Levine, PhD, Associate Director for Education

3426 Brain and Spinal Injury Center (BASIC) Research at University of California
UCSF Department of Neurological
505 Parnassus Avenue, Room 779 M, PO Box 0112
San Francisco, CA 94143
415-353-7500
Fax: 415-353-2889
www.neurosurgery.medschool.ucsf.edu

Established to promote collaborative basic, translational, and clinical studies on injuries to the brain and spinal cord. BASIC is a joint effort between the Departments of Neurological Surgery and Neurology. Both departments bring their particular areas of expertise to a multidisciplinary effort centered on translational research.

Mitchel S. Berger, Managing Director
Manish Aghi, Managing Director
Christopher P. Ames, Managing Director

Louisiana

3427 Tulane University, US-Japan Biomedical Research Laboratories
Herbert Research Center
6823 St. Charles Avenue
New Orleans, LA 70118
504-862-8000
Fax: 504-394-7169
pr@tulane.edu
www.tulane.edu

Focuses research efforts on neuroendocrinology and neurosciences.

Yvette M. Jones, Vice President
Michael A. Bernstein, Provost/Vice President
Benjamin P. Sachs, Senior Vice President/Dean

Massachusetts

3428   Harold Goodglass Aphasia Research Center
150 S Huntington Avenue (12A), PO Box 4817
Boston, MA 02130

617-232-9500
857-364-4774
Fax: 617-739-8926
aphasia@bu.edu
www.bu.edu/aphasia

Research done into cognitive and language impairment following brain damage and closely related topics.

Harold Goodglass, MD, Director
Martin L. Albert, Managing Director
Lena Maskowich, Managing Director

Michigan

3429   Bioengineering Center of Wayne State University
Wayne State University
818 W Hancock
Detroit, MI 48201

313-577-1345
Fax: 313-577-8333
bmeinfo@eng.wayne.edu
www.engineering.wayne.edu

A leading laboratory doing research work in the areas of impact trauma, low back pain and orthopedic biomechanics. Current projects in impact trauma include research on side impact, rear end collisions, head injury and lower extremity injuries.

Albert I King, Director
Farshad Fotouhi, Dean of Engineering
Michael A. Anderson, Research Support Officer

3430   Rehabilitation Institute of Michigan
Detroit Medical Center/Wayne State University
261 Mack Avenue
Detroit, MI 48201

313-745-1203
Fax: 313-745-9863
www.rimrehab.org

Our dedicated group of board certified physicians are committed to improving the lives of their patients by providing quality, compassionate medical care and contributing to the science of rehabilitation medicine.

Mildred Matlock, Ceo
William H. Restum, PhD, President

New York

3431   Brady Institute for Traumatic Brain Injury
Jamaica Hospital Medical Center
8900 Van Wyck Expressway
Jamaica, NY 11418

718-206-6000
hr@jhmc.org
www.jamaicahospital.org

Provides general medical, pediatric,and psychiatric emergency services, ambulatory care, on and off campus ambulatory surgery, a broad spectrum of diagnostic and treatment services, and home health services.

3432   Dana Alliance for Brain Initiatives
505 5th Avenue, 6th Floor
New York, NY 10017

212-223-4040
Fax: 212-317-8721
dabiinfo@dana.org
www.dana.org

A nonprofit organization of more than 250 pre-eminent scientists dedicated to advancing education about the progress and promise of brain research.

Edward F Rover, President
Barbara E. Gill, Vice President
Burton M. Mirsky, Vice President-Finance

3433   Rehabilitation Research and Training Center on Traumatic Brain Injury
Mt. Sinai School of Medicine, Dept. Rehabilitation
155 Washington Ave, Suite 410, PO Box 2332
New York, NY 12210

518-449-2976
Fax: 518-426-4329
TDD: 518-449-2993
wayne.gordon@mssm.edu
www.rrti.org

Research to improve mood in people with TBI; analyze the content and quality of recently published post-TBI intervention studies; development of new measures of rehabilitation outcomes that incorporates both objective and subjective perspectives on participation in home and community activities; and a capacity building program to better educate professionals in identifying, assessing and providing appropriate interventions, treatments and accommodations for people with TBI.

Jacqueline A. Negri, Interim CEO
Stacie Muscolino-Benfer, Directors of Event & Administration
Lisa Zimmermann, HRSA Program Assisstant

3434   Stroke Rehabilitation & Traumatic Brain Injury Research
Ruft Institute at NYU Medical Center
400 E 34th Street
New York, NY 10016

212-263-6519
Fax: 212-263-8510
yehuda.ben-yishay@med.nyu.edu
www.med.nyu.edu/rusk/research

Ways of improving problem-solving behavior in individual with acquired brain damage are being investigated and instruments measuring problem solving in interpersonal situations are being developed.

Joan T Gold, Medical Director

Ohio

3435   Ohio State University Laboratory of Psychobiology
225 Psychology Bldg., 1835 Neil Avenue
Columbus, OH 43210

614-292-8185
Fax: 614-292-4537
www.psy.ohio-state.edu

Studies done on recovery of function after brain damage.

Karissa Basey, Fiscal/HR Associate
Stephanie Fowler, CCBBI Business Manager
Blanche Hollingshead, Fiscal/HR Associate

Pennsylvania

3436   Institutes for Achievement of Human Potential
8801 Stenton Avenue
Wyndmoor, PA 19038

215-233-2050
800-344-8322
Fax: 215-233-9312
institutes@iahp.org
www.iahp.org

A teaching institute that focuses on home-based neurological training for brain-injured children. Commited to the significant increases of the ability of all children to perform in the physical, intellectual and social realms. Our work has led to powerful insights about the brain and, especially, about its development in the neonate and very young children. We have developed exciting concepts and practices applied by parents at home, to mulitply the intelligence of tiny children.

500 members

Janet Doman, President
Glenn Doman, Founder
Dr. Ralph Pelligra, Chairman

3437   Thomas Jefferson University Brain Injury Rehabilitation Program
Thomas Jefferson University Hospital
111 South 11th Street
Philadelphia, PA 19107

215-955-6000
www.jeffersonhealth.org

Provides coordinated, multidisciplinary acute medical and surgical care for all levels of brain injury. The program delivers care for the acute phases of injury at Jefferson and shifts follow-up care to Magee Rehabilitation Hospital.

Thomas J Lewis, Ceo

Tennessee

3438 University of Memphis Neuropsychology Lab
Department of Psychology
202 Psychology Building, Room 126
Memphis, TN 38152 901-678-2000
Fax: 901-678-2579
www.memphis.edu

Evaluation and development of assessment and treatment procedures for neurologically impaired persons.

Shirley C. Raines, President
Rosie Phillips Bingham, Vice President for Student Affairs
Linda Bonnin, Vice President for Communications,

Texas

3439 Brain Injury Research Center of the Institute for Rehabilitation & Research
1333 Moursund Avenue
Houston, TX 77030 713-799-5000
tirrreferrals@tirr.tmc.edu
www.tirr.memorialhermann.org

Brings together world-renowned researchers to study the many complicated facets of recovery from brain injury. BIRC has been able to leverage resources from the US Department of Education's National Institute for Rehabilitation and Research (NIDRR) and from NIH to conduct its research in a manner that facilitates the greatest progress in identifying effective treatments.

Carl Josehart, CEO
Gerard E. Francisco, MD/Chief Medical Officer
Mary Ann Euliarte, CNO/COO

Virginia

3440 Virginia Commonwealth University Department of Neurosurgery Research
417 North 11th Street, 6th Floor, PO Box 980631
Richmond, VA 23298 804-828-9165
Fax: 804-828-0374
www.neurosurgery.vcu.edu

Studies include work on cerebral blood flow, subarachnoid hemorrhage, vasospasm, ischemia, metabolism, cerebral edema, elevated intracranial pressure, trauma, secondary neural insults, CNS tumor biology, clinical trials for new brain tumor therapies, spinal biomechanics, computer imaging on the CNS and immunology of the nervous system.

Stuart P Adler, Research Director
Paul Dent, Vice Chair/Professor
Andrey Budanov, Asst. Professor

Conferences

3441 ANA Symposium
Acoustic Neuroma Association
600 Peachtree Parkway, Suite 108
Cumming, GA 30041 770-205-8211
877-200-8211
Fax: 770-205-0239
info@anausa.org
www.anausa.org

For pre-and post-treatment acoustic neuroma patients, family members, friends and health care professionals for a weekend of educational lectures, workshops and panel discussions-all with leading acoustic neuroma medical professionals.

June
Jeffrey D Barr, President
Alan Goldberg, Vice President
Scott Van Ells, Secretary

Audio Video

3442 Face First
Fanlight Productions
32 Court Street, 21st Floor
Brooklyn, NY 11201 718-488-8900
800-876-1710
Fax: 718-488-8642
info@fanlight.com, orders@fanlight.com
www.fanlight.com

Profiles of several people born with facial deformities; they chronicle both physical pain and the pain of rejection, as well as the strengths that have enabled them to achieve successful adult lives. ISBN: DVD: 1-57295-886-3; VHS: 1-572952-59-8

29 minutes DVD or VHS

Nicole Johnson, Publicity Coordinator

3443 Surviving Coma: the Journey Back
Brain Injury Association of Mississippi
2727 Old Canton Road
Jackson, MS 39296 601-981-1021
Fax: 601-981-1039
biaofms@aol.com

A realistic presentation about coma survival and the problems encountered during the long journey through rehabilitation.

19 Minutes

Paul Gospodarski, Ed.D, Executive Director

Web Sites

3444 Brain Injury Association
1608 Spring Hill Rd. Suite 110
Vienna, VA 22182 703-761-0750
800-444-6443
Fax: 703-761-0755
www.biausa.org

Founded in 1980, the leading national organization serving and representing individuals, families and professionals who are touched by a life-altering, often devastating, traumatic brain injury (TBI).

Daniel S. Chamberlain, Esq, Chair
Brant A. Elkind, MS, CBIST, Vice Chair
Susan H. Connors, President & CEO

3445 Brain Research Institute (BRI) School of Medicine University of California LA
PO Box 951761
Los Angeles, CA 90095 310-825-5061
Fax: 310-206-5855
bri@mednet.ucla.edu
www.bri.ucla.edu

BRI's mission is to increase understanding of how the brain works, how it dvelops, and how it responds to experience, injury and disease, and to help make UCLA the preeminent center for translating basic knowledge into medical interventions and new technologies.

Dr. Christopher Evans, Director
Rafael Romero, Asst Director for Outreach
Baljit Khakh, Assoc. Dir. For Research

3446 Centre for Neuro Skills
5215 Ashe Rd.
Bakersfield, CA 93313 661-872-3408
800-922-4994
Fax: 661-872-5150
cns@neuroskills.com, spersel@neuroskills.com
www.neuroskills.com

The TBI Resource Guide is the internet's central source of information, services, and products relating to traumatic brain injury, brain injury recovery, and post-acute rehabilitation.

Mark J. Ashley, ScD, CCM, President & CEO/ Co Founder

3447   Dana Alliance for Brain Initiatives
505 Fifth Ave., 6th Floor
New York, NY 10017

212-223-4040
Fax: 212-317-8721
www.dana.org/brainweb

Is a nonprofit organization of more then 200 neuroscientists, formed to help provide information about the personal and public benefits of brain research. Today one out of five Americans suffers from a brain-related disease or disorder, ranging from cocain addiction to learning diabilities from Alzheimer's disease to spinal cord injuries.

Edward F. Rover, Chair & President
Burton M. Mirsky, EVP, Finance
Barbara E. Gill, EVP, Public Affairs, Executive Dir.

3448   NIH/National Institute of Neurological Dis orders and Stroke (NINDS)
PO Box 5801
Bethesda, MD 20824

301-496-5751
800-352-9424
www.ninds.nih.gov

The mission of NINDS is to reduce the burden of neurological disease, a burden borne by every age group, by every segment of society, by people all over the world.

Walter J. Koroshetz, MD, Director

3449   Northeast Rehabilitation Health Network
70 Butler Street
Salem, NH 3079

603-893-2900
800-439-0183
TTY: 800-439-2370
webmaster@northeastrehab.com
www.northeastrehab.com

We provide services within a continuum of care to individuals and families whos lives have been impcated by illness or injury in order to restore stability and maximize their potential for independence, functional abilites, and quality of life. In addition, we provide services that encourage well being. Our customers include: patients, families, physicians, referrers, payers, employees and the community.

John Prochilo, CEO & Administrator

3450   Perspectives Network
www.tbi.org

It's primary focus is positive communications between persons with brain injury, family members, caregivers, friends of persons with brain injury, those many professionals who treat persons with brain injury and community members in order to create positive changes and enhance public awareness and knowledge of acquired, traumatic brain injury.

3451   Traumatic Brain Injury Model Systems Natio nal Data and Statistical Center
www.tbindc.org

tbindc@kmrrec.org
www.tbindc.org

The TBIMS program seeks to improve the lives of persons who experience traumatic brain injury, their families and their communities by creating and disseminating new knowledge about the course, treatment and outcomes relating to their condtion.

Book Publishers

3452   Children with Traumatic Brain Injury
Peytral Publications
PO Box 1162
Minnetonka, MN 55345

952-949-8707
877-739-8725
Fax: 952-949-8707
www.peytral.com

Comprehensive, must-have reference that provides parent with the support and information needed to help their child recover from a closed-head injury. Written by a team of medical specialists, therapists, educators and an attorney this publications covers medical concerns, rehabilitation, treatment, adjustment, effects on learning, thinking, language behavior and more.

482 pages

Lisa Schoenbrodt, EdD, Editor

3453   Cognitive Effects of Early Brain Injury
John's Hopkins University Press
2715 N Charles Street
Baltimore, MD 21218

410-516-6900
800-537-5487
Fax: 410-516-6968
webmaster@jhupress.jhu.edu
www.press.jhu.edu

This book offers a detailed overview of the effects of genetic, prenatal, and perinatal brain disorders on cognitive development and learning in children. Summarizing the available data as well as presenting previously unpublished research, the book provides clinicians with practical information that will aid their diagnostic and therapeutic work with children who have sustained early brain injury.

1994 336 pages Hardcover
ISBN: 0-801848-56-3

Kathleen Keane, Director
Erik A Smist, Director
Timothy D Fuller, Chief Information Officer

3454   Cognitive Rehabilitation for Persons with Traumatic Brain Injury
Paul H Brookes Publishing/Brookes
PO Box 10624
Baltimore, MD 21285

410-337-9580
800-638-3775
Fax: 410-337-8539
custserv@brookespublishing.com
www.brookespublishing.com

Virtually all persons with brain injury retain ability to learn. Cognitive rehab is a set of stategies to improve problems. Reports on theory, practices, research, consequences of brain trauma and assessment & intervention. Case studies.

1991 299 pages Hardcover
ISBN: 1-557660-71-9

Jeffrey S Kreutzer, Editor
Paul H Wehman, Editor

3455   From the Ashes
Brain Injury Resource Center
PO Box 84151
Seattle, WA 98124

206-621-8558
brain@headinjury.com
www.headinjury.com/ashesord.htm

An enduring resource for survivors, families and the professionals serving them.

1987 108 pages
ISBN: 0-963659-40-5

Constance Miller, Editor
Kay Campbell, Editor

3456   Handbook of Head Truma: Acute Care to Recovery
Springer Publishing Company
11 W 42nd Street, 15th Floor
New York, NY 10036

877-687-7476
Fax: 212-941-7842
contactus@springerpub.com
www.springerpub.com

Providing a thorough collection of information regarding clinical aspects of head injury from acute care to recovery, this treatise interrelates a variety of neural specialties and broadens the rehabilitation process to include the family

1992 472 pages
ISBN: 0-306439-47-6

Charles Long, Editor
Leslie Ross, Editor

3457 Head Injury in Children and Adolescents: A Resource and Review for School
John Wiley & Sons
10475 Crosspoint Boulevard
Indianapolis, IN 46256
877-762-2974
Fax: 800-597-3299
consumers@wiley.com
www.wiley.com

Complex nature of traumatic brain injury and its implications are examined carefully from medical, neuropsychological, rehabilitative and educational perspectives. Contents are arranged in a spiraling manner to provide the reader with a progressive and practical appreciation of traumatic brain injury and its neurobehavioral effects.

260 pages Hardcover
ISBN: 0-884220-98-2

Vivian Begali, Editor

3458 Head Trauma Sourcebook
Omnigraphics
PO Box 8002
Aston, PA 19014
800-234-1340
Fax: 800-875-1340
info@omnigraphics.com
omnigraphics.com

Basic consumer information for the layperson about open-head and closed-head injuries, treatment advances, recovery and rehabilitation.

414 pages
ISBN: 0-780802-08-X

Karen Bellenir, Editor

3459 Let's Talk About Going to the Hospital
Rosen Publishing Group's PowerKids Press
29 E 21st Street
New York, NY 10010
212-777-3017
800-237-9932
Fax: 888-436-4643
rosenpub@tribeca.ios.com
www.powerkidspress.com

If a child has to check into the hospital, chances are he or she is already upset about being ill. Knowing how a hospital functions and what the procedures are, such as when family members can visit, will help in what is already a stressful situation. Grades K-5.

24 pages
ISBN: 0-823950-36-0

3460 What To Do About Your Brain Injured Child
National Book Network
8801 Stenton Avenue
Wyndmoor, PA 19038
215-233-2050
800-344-8322
Fax: 215-233-3940
institutes@iahp.org
www.iahp.org

The author reveals life saving techniques to measure mobility, language, and manual, visual, auditory and tactile development.

318 pages
ISBN: 1-591170-23-0

Glen Doman, Editor

Magazines

3461 Brain Injury Source
Brain Injury Association of America
1608 Spring Hill Road, Suite 110
Vienna, VA 22182
703-761-0750
Fax: 703-761-0755
Publications@biausa.org
www.biausa.org

Written for and by professionals in the field. Blends professionally written articles on information and research in brain injury with a user friendly format that incorporates graphics and charts to effectively deliver the messages. Full color.

50+ pages Quarterly
Susan H Connors, President/CEO
Pat Britz, Information Director
Marianna Abashian, Director of Professional Services

Journals

3462 Journal of Head Trauma Rehabilitation
Aspen Publishers
7201 McKinney Circle
Frederick, MD 21704
301-698-7100
800-234-1660
Fax: 800-901-9075
customer.service@wolterskluwer.com
www.wklawbusiness.com

A leading, peer-reviewed resource that provides up-to-date information on the clinical management and rehabilitation of persons with traumatic brain injuries. The journal is comprised of feature articles, brief reports, pharmacological updates, legislative and public policy updates, columns on ethics, book reviews, abstracts of selected literature, and more.

Mitchell Rosenthal, MD, Editor

Newsletters

3463 American Brain Tumor Association Message Line
8550 W. Bryn Mawr Ave, Ste 550
Chicago, IL 60631
773-577-8750
800-886-2282
Fax: 773-577-8738
info@abta.org
www.abta.org

Offers association news, events, fundraising and convention news, as well as medical and legislative updates for patients and their families.

Quarterly
Jeff Fougerousse, Chair
Barbara Dunn, Vice Chair
Brian Olson, Treasurer

3464 Headlines
Brain Injury Association of Minnesota
2277 Highway 36 West, Suite 200
Roseville, MN 55113
612-378-2742
800-669-6442
Fax: 612-378-2789
info@braininjurymn.org
www.braininjurymn.org

Published for the families and professionals who are involved with brain injuries. We also have an e-mail newsletter that reaches several hundred.

Quarterly
Ardis Sandstrom, Executive Director
Brad Donaldson, Associate Director of Operations
Richard Bloom, Board Treasurer

3465 Headway
Brain Injury Association of Virginia
1506 Willow Lawn Dr., Suite 212
Richmond, VA 23230
804-355-5748
800-444-6443
Fax: 804-355-6381
biav@visi.net
www.biav.net

Information and resources for individuals with brain injury, their family members and professionals dealing with brain injury.

16 pages Quarterly
Michelle Ward, Editor
Stephen Smith, President
Steve Hicks, Director of Development

3466 TBI Challenge
Brain Injury Association of America
1608 Spring Hill Road, Suite 110
Vienna, VA 22182

703-761-0750
Fax: 703-761-0755
familyhelpline@biausa.org
www.biausa.org

Exclusively for and about persons with brain injury. Provides information to individuals with brain injury and their families. Professionals will benefit from the perspectives provided in Kid's Corner, Relatively Speaking, Ask the Lawyer, Information and Resources and Ask the Doctor.

Quarterly

Susan H Connors, President/CEO
Pat Britz, Information Director
Marianna Abashian, Director of Professional Services

3467 The Headliner
Brain Injury Association of Oregon
2145 NW Overton Street
Portland, OR 97210

503-413-7707
800-544-5243
Fax: 503-413-6849
biaor@biaoregon.org
www.biaoregon.org

To improve the quality of life of persons with brain injury and their families; and to prevent brain injury.

16 pages Quarterly

Craig Nichols, JD, President
Chuck McGilvrary, Vice President
Sherry Stock, Executive Director

Pamphlets

3468 Brain Injury Glossary
HDI Publishers
2407 Waugh Drive, PO Box 131401
Houston, TX 77219

713-526-6900
800-321-7037
Fax: 713-526-7787
sales@braininjurybooks.com
www.braininjurybooks.com

Contains special sections on terms relating to insurance, definitions relating to The Americans with Disabilities Act and descriptions of commonly prescribed medications. The Brain Injury Glossary is a must for all persons working or involved in brain injury rehabilitation.

1993 46 pages

L Don Lehmkuhl, Editor

3469 Brain Injury Update
HDI Publishers
2407 Waugh Drive, PO Box 131401
Houston, TX 77219

713-526-6900
800-321-7037
Fax: 713-526-7787
sales@braininjurybooks.com
www.braininjurybooks.com

Monthly digest of news and information from the brain injury research and rehabilitation fields. Expanded summaries of journal articles, research papers, news releases and government reports are provided in a concise, time saving format. Brain Injury Update also provides information on grant opportunities, pharmacological intervention, calls for papers, people in the news, listings of upcoming conferences and symposia, legal and legislative developments and advances in prevention.

1991 Annual

Dr. Linda Thoi, Editor-in-Chief
Nathan D Zasler, MD, Contributing Editor

Camps

3470 Camp Barefoot
Brain Injury Association of Michigan
7305 Grand River, Suite 100
Brighton, MI 48114

810-229-5880
800-772-4323
Fax: 810-229-8947
info@biami.org
www.biami.org

Primary goal of our recreational programming is to give people who have experienced a brain injury a normal camping experience. Dedicated to providing quality summer camping experiences for people who sustained a brain injury. Over six days, Camp Barefoot provides structured, enriching personal and recreational experiences for people with brain injury.

Michael F Dabbs, President
Thomas J. Constand, VP, Development and Marketing
Char Luttrell, Office Manager

3471 Camp Hickory Wood
Traumatic Brain Injury Program
425 5th Avenue N, Cordell Hull Building
Nashville, TN 37243

800-882-0611
health.state.tn.us/TBI/index.htm

Each year the TBI Program in collaboration with Easter Seals Tennessee Inc. sponsors a weekend and a weeklong camp for adult and youth survivors of brain injury. These camps focus on providing a unique social and recreational opportunity to persons with brain injury. Nestled between the banks of Old Hickory Lake and surrounded by protective woods, camp offers great outdoor fun.

3472 Crotched Mountain School & Rehabilitation Center
1 Verney Drive
Greenfield, NH 3047

603-547-3311
800-800-966
Fax: 603-547-3232
info@crotchedmountain.org
www.cmf.org

Currently serves children ages 6-22 with multiple-handicaps including: Cerebral Palsy, Spina Bifida, visual and hearing impairments and neurological disabilities, developmental disorders, mental retardation, autism, behavioral and emotional disorders, seizure disorders, spinal cord and head injuries. Member of the National Association of Independent Schools and accredited with the NE Association of Schools and Colleges, Independent Schools of Northern NE.

Kathleen C. Brittan, Vice President of Development
William Cossaboon, MS, Director of Education
W. Carl Cooley, MD, Chief Medical Officer

3473 Oklahoma Brain Injury Camp
Oklahoma Brain Injury Association
3015 E. Skelly Dr.
Tulsa, OK 74105

405-928-1647
Fax: 918-712-9019
braininjuryoklahoma@gmail.com
www.braininjuryoklahoma.org

An annual camp for brain injury survivors sponsored by the Brain Injury Association of Oklahoma. Great fun had by all with music, games, crafts, a hayride, cookout, bingo, fishing, and paddle boat rides.

Cathe Fox, Camp Director
Adam Sherman, Ph.D, President
Mary Dobbs, BSN, RN, CRRN, Vice President

DESCRIPTION

3474 HEARING IMPAIRMENT/DEAFNESS

Covers these related disorders: Conductive deafness or hearing loss, Mixed hearing loss, Sensorineural deafness or hearing loss, Noise Induced Hearing Loss

Involves the following Biologic System(s):

Neurologic Disorders

Hearing impairment may be defined as a loss of the ability to hear that is sufficient enough to impede the ability to communicate. Deafness refers to severe or profound hearing loss. Hearing loss or deafness may occur as the result of hereditary factors or birth defects. Hearing loss may also be acquired and occur after birth (e.g., from disease or physical damage to the hearing mechanism). However, genetic factors are thought to be responsible for moderate to severe hearing loss in about half of affected children. Hearing loss may be further categorized into three types: conductive, sensorineural, or mixed.

Conductive hearing loss occurs as a result of the faulty transmission of sound through the external or middle ear to the inner ear. This transmission problem may be due to infections of the middle ear (otitis media), damage to the eardrum or bones of the middle ear, the absence or the narrowing of the ear canal, impacted earwax (cerumen), foreign bodies in the ear canal, or other physical causes. In addition, conductive hearing loss is sometimes inherited as a feature of certain syndromes such as Klippel-Feil syndrome, Crouzon syndrome, osteogenesis imperfecta, and others. In children with sensorineural hearing loss, sounds are conducted to the inner ear through the external and middle ear, but are not transmitted from there to the brain. This occurs as the result of a defect in the structure of the inner ear or problems with the nerve that conveys impulses from the inner ear to the brain (auditory nerve; acoustic nerve; eighth cranial nerve). Sensorineural hearing loss that results from defects of inner ear structures is considered sensory and includes: the absence or underdevelopment of the snail shell-type tubular structure of the inner ear (cochlea); damage to hair cells or other inner ear structures from prolonged exposure to loud noise, certain drugs; viral infections or other diseases; and other irregularities.

Noise Induced Hearing Loss (NIHL) results from exposure to harmful noise levels that trigger the formation of molecules inside the ear that damage hair cells. The hair cells are small sensory cells that convert sound energy into electrical signals that travel to the brain. Damaged hair cells cannot grow back. These destructive molecules play an important role in hearing loss in children and adults who are exposed to loud noise for extended periods. Individuals of all ages, including children, can develop NIHL.

Sensorineural hearing loss that results from damage to the auditory nerve pathway is considered neural and may be due to brain lesions or tumors; childhood disorders such as German measles, mumps, inner ear infections, etc.; certain hereditary disorders (e.g., Waardenburg syndrome, Usher syndrome, etc.); diseases that affect the myelin sheath, which is the fatty, protective, insulating covering on certain nerve fibers (demyelinating diseases); or seizures. Mixed hearing loss refers to a combination of both conductive and sensorineural hearing loss.

Early screening for hearing loss is important in order to provide early intervention that will allow the best outcome for educational and social development. Treatment may require the cooperation of parents, caregivers, pediatricians, speech and language pathologists, and specialists in hearing loss (audiologists) who assess the extent of hearing loss through the use of specialized tests. Infant screening by specialists may include tests that gauge behavioral responses to noise through observation, such as a startle response to a sudden hand clap. Other tests may electronically assess hearing loss (audiometry); measure the head-turning response of an infant or toddler using animated aids in conjunction with sounds emitted through a loudspeaker (visual reinforcement audiometry or VRA); measure the lowest intensity at which certain words are heard or understood (speech recognition threshold or SRT); measure the ability of the middle ear to impede or resist sound energy (tympanometry); differentiate between sensory and neural hearing loss (auditory brain stem response); measure the integrity of the cochlea (otoacoustic emissions or OAEs).

According to the National Institute on Deafness and Other Communication Disorders, males are more likely to experience hearing loss than females. Two to three of every 1,000 children who are born deaf have hearing parents.

Treatment for conductive hearing loss may include theremoval of fluid, earwax, or foreign bodies through drainage or other means. Surgical intervention may be indicated for the correction of structural abnormalities. Children as well as infants with hearing loss may benefit from the use of certain types of hearing aids; however, repeat testing is necessary to provide more exact hearing aid specification.

In the United States, roughly 41,500 adults and 25,500 children receive cochlear implants per year. Hearing loss affects only one ear in nine out of 10 people who experience sudden deafness. Approximately 26 million Americans have Noise Induced Hearing Loss (NIHL). Recreational activities that can put someone at risk for NIHL include target shooting and hunting, snowmobile riding, woodworking and other hobbies, playing in a band, and attending rock concerts. Harmful noises at home may come from lawnmowers, leaf blowers, and shop tools.

In addition, cochlear implants are available to children with severe or profound hearing loss. Other treatment is directed toward the teaching of communication skills such as lip-reading, sign language, and speech. Cooperation and support of family, medical specialists, and educators is important in determining the best approach for the education and social development of the individual child.

Government Agencies

3475 NIH/National Institute on Deafness and Oth er Communication Disorders (NIDCD)
31 Center Dr, MSC 2320
Bethesda, MD 20892

800-241-1044
Fax: 301-770-8977
TTY: 800-241-1055
nidcdinfo@nidcd.nih.gov
www.nidcd.nih.gov

The NIDCD conducts and supports research in the normal and disordered processes of hearing, balance, tast, smell, voice, speech, and language.

James Battey, MD, PhD, Director
Judith Cooper, PhD Deputy Director, Deputy Director
Timothy J Wheeles, Executive Officer

3476 Office of Special Education and Rehabilita tion Services
400 Maryland Avenue, SW
Washington, DC 20202　　　　　　　　202-245-7468
　　　　　　　　　　　　　　　　Fax: 202-245-7636
　　　　　　　　　　　　　　　　TTY: 202-205-5637
　　　　　　　　　　　　　　　carolyn.corlett@ed.gov
　　　　　www.ed.gov/about/offices/list/osers/index.html

A service of the U.S. Department of Education, responds to people with disabilities and others who request information by conducting research and providing documents related to federal funding available for disability-related programs.

Ruth E Ryder, Assistant Secretary
Paul Steenen, Director, Communications

National Associations & Support Groups

3477 Academy of Rehabilitative Audiology
PO Box 2323
Albany, NY 12220　　　　　　　　　952-920-0484
　　　　　　　　　　　　　　　　Fax: 952-920-6098
　　　　　　　　　　　　　　　　ara@audrehab.org
　　　　　　　　　　　　　　　　www.audrehab.org

The primary purpose of ARA is to promote excellence in hearing care through the provision of comprehensive rehabilitative and habilitative services.

350 Members

Kathleen Cienkowski, President
Linda Thibodeau, President-Elect
Kristin Vasil-Dilaj, Secretary

3478 Acoustical Society of America
2 Huntington Quadrangle - Ste 1N01
Melville, NY 11747　　　　　　　　516-576-2360
　　　　　　　　　　　　　　　　Fax: 516-576-2377
　　　　　　　　　　　　　　　　asa@aip.org
　　　　　　　　　　　　　　　www.acousticalsociety.org

The ASA specializes in acoustics. They are dedicated to diffusing and increasing the knowledge of acoustics and its practical application.

3479 Alexander Graham Bell Association for the Deaf and Hearing Impaired
Alexander Graham Bell Association for the Deaf
3417 Volta Place NW
Washington, DC 20007　　　　　　　202-337-5220
　　　　　　　　　　　　　　　　800-432-7543
　　　　　　　　　　　　　　　　Fax: 202-337-8314
　　　　　　　　　　　　　　　　TTY: 202-337-5221
　　　　　　　　　　　　　　　　info@agbell.org
　　　　　　　www.listeningandspokenlanguage.org

The Alexander Graham Bell Association for the Deaf and Hard of Hearing (AG bell) is a lifelong resource,support network and advocate for listening,learning,talking and living independently with hearing loss. Through publications, advocacy,training,scholarships and financial aid,AG Bell promotes the use of spoken language and hearing technology.

Alexander T. Graham, Executive Director
Judy Harrison, Director of Programs
Robin Bailey, Programs Specialist

3480 American Academy of Audiology
11480 Commerce Park Drive, Suite 220
Reston, VA 20191　　　　　　　　　703-790-8466
　　　　　　　　　　　　　　　　800-222-2336
　　　　　　　　　　　　　　　　Fax: 703-790-8631
　　　　　　　　　　　　　　　　info@audiology.org
　　　　　　　　　　　　　　　　www.audiology.org

A professional organization dedicated to providing high quality and balanced hearing care to the public. Provides professional development, education and research and provides increased public awareness of hearing disorders and audiologic services.

Deborah Carlson, President
Bettie Borton, President-Elect
Therese Walden, AuD, Past President

3481 American Academy of Pediatrics
141 Northwest Point Boulevard
Elk Grove Village, IL 60007　　　　847-434-4000
　　　　　　　　　　　　　　　　800-433-9016
　　　　　　　　　　　　　　　　Fax: 847-434-8000
　　　　　　　　　　　　　　　　www.aap.org

The American Academy of Pediatrics and its member pediatricians are committed to the attainment of optimal physical, mental and social health and well-being for all infants, children, adolescents, and young adults.

Fernando Stein, MD, FAAP, President
Karen Remley, MD, CEO/Executive VP

3482 American Association of the Deaf-Blind
PO Box 2831
Kensington, MD 20891　　　　　　　301-495-4403
　　　　　　　　　　　　　　　　Fax: 301-495-4404
　　　　　　　　　　　　　　　　TTY: 301-495-4402
　　　　　　　　　　　　　　　　aadb-info@aadb.org
　　　　　　　　　　　　　　　　www.aadb.org

The American Association of the Deaf-Blind (AADB) is a non-profit 501(c)(3) national consumer organization, of, by, and for the deaf-blind Americans and their supporters. 'Deaf-blind' includes all types and degrees of dual vision and hearing loss. Their mission is to ensure that all deaf-blind persons achieve their maximum potential through increased independence, productivity, and integration into the community.

600 Members

Jill Gaus, President
Lynn Jansen, Vice President
Debby Lieberman, Secretary

3483 American Cochlear Implant Alliance
P.O. Box 103
McLean, VA 22101　　　　　　　　703-534-6146
　　　　　　　　　　　　　　　　info@acialliance.org
　　　　　　　　　　　　　　　　www.acialliance.org

TheÿAmerican Cochlear Implant Allianceÿis a not-for-profit membership organization created with the purpose of eliminating barriers to cochlear implantation by sponsoring research, driving heightened awareness and advocating for improved access to cochlear implants for patients of all ages across the US.

John K. Niparko, MD, Founding Chairman
Craig A. Buchman, MD FACS, Chair, Board of Director
Jill B. Firszt, PhD, Treasurer

3484 American Deafness and Rehabilitation Assoc iation (ADARA)
PO Box 480
Myersville, MD 21773　　　　　　　501-868-8850
　　　　　　　　　　　　　　　　Fax: 501-868-8812
　　　　　　　　　　　　　　　　www.adara.org

A network of professionals who serve people who are deaf or hard of hearing

Barry Critchfield, President
Michelle Niehaus, President-Elect
Doug Dittfurth, Vice President

3485 American Hearing Impaired Hockey Association
4214 W. 77th Place
Chicago, IL 60652　　　　　　　　978-922-0955
　　　　　　　　　　　　　　　　kkmm2won@aol.com
　　　　　　　　　　　　　　　　www.usadeafhockey.org

TheÿAmerican Hearing Impaired Hockey Associationÿprovides deaf and hard of hearing hockey players the opportunity to learn about and improve their hockey skills through our program. We offer these hockey players the opportunity to be coached by a coaching staff with college, national and international experience.

Jeff Sauer, Head Coach/ President
Kevin Delaney, Coach - Power Skating
Michael Drew, Coach - Current player

3486 **American Hearing Research Foundation**
8 S Michigan Avenue, Suite 1205
Chicago, IL 60603
312-726-9670
Fax: 312-726-9695
ahrf@american-hearing.org
www.american-hearing.org

As a not-profit organization, a major source of our income is through donations. We have received generous contributions from individuals, corporations, and institutions, and continue to rely on these donations to found future research.

Richard G. Muench, Chairman
Alan G. Micco, President
Mark R. Muench, Vice President

3487 **American Sign Language Teachers Association**
www.aslta.org

ASLTA is the only national organization dedicated to the improvement and expansion of the teaching of ASL and Deaf Studies at all levels of instruction. ASLTA is an individual membership organization of more than 1,000 ASL and Deaf Studies educators from elementary through graduate education as well as agencies. The mission of the American Sign Language Teachers Association (ASLTA) is to preserve the integrity of American Sign Language (ASL) and Deaf Culture.

Timothy Owens, M. Ed.ỹ, President
Arlene Gunderson, M.Ed., Vice President
Bill Newell, Ph.D., Treasurer

3488 **American Society for Deaf Children**
#2047, 800 Florida Avenue NE., PO Box 3695
Washington, DC 20002
202-644-9204
800-942-2732
Fax: 717-909-5599
asdc@deafchildren.org
www.deafchildren.org

A nonprofit parent-helping-parent organization promoting a positive attitude toward signing and deaf culture. Also provides support, encouragement, and current information about deafness to families with deaf and hard-of-hearing children.

Roger Williams, Co-President
Sherry Williams, Co-President
Diana Poeppelmeyer, Executive Secretary

3489 **American Speech Language Hearing Associati on (ASHA)**
2200 Research Boulevard
Rockville, MD 20850
301-296-5700
800-638-8255
Fax: 301-571-0457
TTY: 301-296-5650
actioncenter@asha.org
www.asha.org

ASHA is the professional, scientific and credentialling association for more than 123,000 members and affiliates who are speech-language pathologists, audiologists, and speech, language, and hearing scientitists. Their mission is to promote the interests of and provide the highest quality services for proesstionals, and to advocate for people with communication disabilities.

Patriacia A. Prelock, President
Elizabeth S. McCrea, President-Elect
Donna Fisher Smiley, Vice President

3490 **American Speech-Language-Hearing Foundatio n**
2200 Research Blvd.
Rockville, MD 20850
301-296-8700
Fax: 301-296-8567
foundation@asha.org
www.ashfoundation.org

An organization which promotes a better quality of life for children and adults with communication disorders.

3491 **American Tinnitus Association**
522 S.W. Fifth Avenue; Suite 825
Portland, OR 97204
503-248-9985
800-634-8978
Fax: 503-248-0024
tinnitus@ata.org
www.ata.org

The American Tinnitus Association exists to cure tinnitus through the development of resources that advance tinnitus research.

Thomas J. Lobl, Ph.D., Chair
Marsha Johnson, Au.D.ỹ, Treasurer
Scott C. Mitchell, J.D., Secretary

3492 **Auditory - Verbal International**
2121 Eisenhower Avenue, Suite 402
Alexandria, VA 22314
703-519-7400
Fax: 703-739-0395
TTY: 703-739-0874
audiverb@aol.com
www.rvjintl.com

Provides the choice of listening and speaking as the way of life for children and adults who are deaf or hard of hearing. Through the use of assistive technology such as digital hearing aids or cochlear implants and auditory-verbal therapy, many deaf and hard of hearing children can learn to listen and speak.

900 members

John Jones, President
Steven Rech JD, President

3493 **BEGINNINGS for Parents of Children Who Are Deaf or Hard of Hearing**
PO Box 17646
Raleigh, NC 27619
919-850-2746
800-541-HEAR
Fax: 919-715-4093
TTY: 800-541-HEAR
raleigh@ncbegin.org
www.ncbegin.com

BEGINNINGS provides emotional support and access to as a central resource for families with deaf or hard of hearing children, age birth through 21. These services are also available to deaf parents who have hearing children. Their mission is to help parents to be informed, empowered and supported as they make decisions about their child. In addition, they are committed to providing technical assistance to professionals who work with these families.

Stephanie J. Sjoblad, President
Lekita Essa, Vice President
Joni Y Alberg, Executive Director

3494 **Better Hearing Institute**
Ste 700
Washington, DC 20005
202-449-1100
800-327-9355
Fax: 703-684-6048
TTY: 703-642-0580
mail@betterhearing.org
www.betterhearing.org

A nonprofit educational organization that implements national public information programs on hearing loss and available medical, surgical, hearing aid, and rehabilitation assistance for millions with uncorrected hearing problems. Its award-winning series of television, radio, and print media public service messages include many celebrities who overcame hearing loss. BHI maintains a toll-free Hotline HelpLine telephone service that provides information on hearing loss and hearing help to callers.

Sergei Kochkin, PhD, Executive Director
Sasha Ward, Administrative Director

3495 **Center for Early Intervention of Deafness (CEID)**
1035 Grayson Street
Berkeley, CA 94710
510-848-4800
Fax: 510-848-4801
TTY: 510-848-5686
TDD: 510-527-5196
ceid@ceid.org
www.ceid.org

A non-profit organization dedicated to providing a program of intensive and comprehensive early intervention services to young children up to five years old who have hearing losses or severe speech/language delays and their families. CEID uses 'Total Communication', which includes the simultaneous use of spoken English, audition, and literal representation of sign language (SEE signing), in a play based curriculum incorporting thematic active learning strategies and total family involvement.

401

Rosalie Streett, President
Warren Wincorn, VP
Alan Gould, Treasurer

3496 Children's Legal Advocacy Program (CLA)
Alexander Graham Bell Association for the Deaf
3417 Volta Place NW
Washington, DC 20007   202-337-5220
                                        800-432-7543
                                        Fax: 202-337-8314
                                        TTY: 202-337-5221
                                        info@agbell.org
                                        www.agbell.org

Supports families of children who are deaf or hard of hearing by
providing legal representation and technical assistance to families
who need help obtaining appropriate services in their
communities.

Alexander T. Graham, Executive Director
Judy Harrison, Director of Programs
Robin Bailey, Programs Specialist

3497 Coalition for Global Hearing Health
www.coalitionforglobalhearinghealth.org
Works with the mission to promote and enhance hearing health
services in low-resourced communities.

3498 Cochlear Implant Asscociation
5335 Wisconsin Avenue NW, Suite 440
Washington, DC 20015   202-895-2781
                                        Fax: 202-895-2782
                                        C_I_A_I_info@cici.org
                                        www.cici.org

A non-profit organization dedicated to educating and supporting
cochlear implant recipients and their familiies; advocating and
promoting cochlear implants.

John McCelland, President
Lorie Singer, VP
Wayne L Roorda, Treasurer

3499 Cochlear Implant Awareness Foundation
130 South John Street
Rochester, IL 62563   info@ciafonline.org
                                    www.ciafonline.org

Connect people with the resources they need to make an educated
decision about cochlear implant surgery.

Michelle Tjelmeland, Founder and Chairwoman
Sheryl Klemm, Director
Max Klemm, Director

3500 Council of the American Instructors of the Deaf
P.O. Box 377
Bedford, TX 76095   TTY: 817-354-8414
                                    caid@swbell.net
                                    www.caid.org

The organization for all teachers, administrators, educational interpreters, residential personnel, and other concerned professionals involved in education of the deaf.

Larry Quinsland, Ph.D, President
Keith Mousley, President
Christina Yuknis, President Elect

3501 Council on Education of the Deaf
PO Box 976
North Kingstown, RI 2852   executivedirector@councilondeafed.org
                                    councilondeafed.org

The Council on Education of the Deaf (CED) is an organization
sponsored by five major national organizations dedicated to quality education for all deaf and hard of hearing students.

Joseph E. Fischgrund, Executive Director
Trina Schooley, CED Office Manager

3502 Deaf Counseling, Advocacy & Referral Agency
14895 E. 14th Street, Suite #200ÿ
San Leandro, CA 94578   510-343-6670
                                        Fax: 510-483-1790
                                        info@dcara.org
                                        www.dcara.org

Deaf, Counseling, Advocacy & Referral Agency (DCARA), is a
non-profit, community-based social service agency serving the
Deaf, Hard of Hearing, Late-Deafened and Deaf-blind
(D/HH/LD/DB)community.ÿ

Steve Longo, President
Lonnie Tanenberg, Vice President
David Martin, Treasurer

3503 Deaf REACH
3521 12th Street NE
Washington, DC 20017   202-832-6681
                                        Fax: 202-832-8454
                                        TTY: 202-832-6681
                                        www.deaf-reach.org

Nonprofit organization: our mission is to maximize the self-sufficiency of deaf adults needing special services by providing referral, education, advocacy, counseling, and housing.

Annette Riechman, President
Jon Tomar, VP
Teresa Arcarl, Secretary

3504 Dial-a-Hearing Screening Test
300 S Chester Road
Swathmore, PA 19081   610-544-7700
                                        800-222-3277
                                        Fax: 610-543-2802
                                        dahst@aol.com
                                        www.dialatest.com

National telephone hearing screening test service. Consumers receive a copy of their hearing screening test results and referral to
a hearing health care center in the Dial A Hearing Screening Test
network. Flexible participation plans for hearing health care
providers.

George Biddle, President
James Biddle, Vice President
Joseph Rago, Controller

3505 Dogs for the Deaf, Inc.
10175 Wheller Road
Central Point, OR 97502   541-826-9220
                                        800-990-3647
                                        info@dogsforthedeaf.org
                                        www.dogforthedeaf.org

This organization rescues and professionally trains dogs to assist
people with hearing loss, autism, and other challenges.

3506 EAR Foundation
Ste A
Nashville, TN 37201   615-627-2724
                                        800-545-4327
                                        Fax: 615-627-2728
                                        TDD: 615-627-2724
                                        info@earfoundation.org
                                        www.earfoundation.org

The EAR foundation has three basic purposes: to provide the general public support services promoting the integration of the hearing and balance impaired into mainstream society; to provide
practicing ear specialists continuing medical education courses
and related programs specifically regarding rehabilitation and
hearing preservation; and to educate young people and adults
about hearing preservation and early detection of hearing loss,
enabling them to prevent hearing and balance disorders.

Michael E Glasscock, III, MD, Founder and President
Steve Masie, Chair
Suzanne Wyatt, Executive Director

3507 Educational Audiology Association
700 McKnight Park Drive, Suite 708
Pittsburgh, PA 15237   800-460-7322
                                        Fax: 888-729-3489
                                        admin@edaud.org
                                        edaud.org

The Educational Audiology Association is an international organization of audiologists and related professionals who deliver a
full spectrum of hearing services to all children, particularly
those in educational settings.

Mike Sharp, AuD, CCC-A, President
Gary Pillow, President-Elect
Susan Dillmuth-Miller, Past President

3508 Episcopal Conference of the Deaf
www.ecdeaf.org

The ECD is a central clearing house concerning all aspects of work among Deaf people in the Episcopal Church. Episcopal Conference of the Deaf spreads the Gospel of Christ among Deaf people.

Marianne Stuart, President
Erich Krengel, First Vice President
Steve Holst, Treasurer

3509 Friends of Libraries for Deaf Action
2930 Craiglawn Road
Silver Spring, MD 20904   folda86@aol.com
                                 www.folda.net

The Red Notebook is a loose-leaf binder containing fact sheets, library reprints, announcements and other printed informational materials that are related to both deaf and library issues.

Alice L. Hagemeyer, MLS, President
Merrie A. Davidson, MLS, Associate
Ricardo Lopez, MS, Associate

3510 Hands & Voices National
PO Box 3093
Boulder, CO 80307   303-492-6283
                                 866-422-0422
                        parentaladvocate@handsandvoices.org
                                 www.handsandvoices.org

A nationwide non-profit organization dedicated to supporting families and their children who are deaf or hard-of-hearing as well as the professionals who serve them.

3511 Hands Organization
2501 W 103rd Street
Chicago, IL 60655   773-239-6632

Advocacy for the deaf and hard-of-hearing; information and referrals, educational events, sign language summer youth camps and newsletters.

Kate Kubey, Contact

3512 Hear Now
9745 E Hampden Avenue, Suite 300
Denver, CO 80231   303-695-7797
                                 800-648-4327
                            Fax: 303-695-7789
                            TTY: 800-648-4327
                        76350.650@compuserve.com

Committed to making technology accessible to deaf and hard-of-hearing individuals throughout the United States. Also raises funds to provide hearing aids, cochlear implants and related services to children and adults who have hearing losses but do not have financial resources to purchase their own devices.

Bernice Dinner, MA, CCC, President/Founder
Elaine Hansen

3513 Hearing Health Foundation
363 Seventh Avenue, 10th Floor
New York, NY 10001   212-257-6140
                                 866-454-3924
                    info@hearinghealthfoundation.org
                         hearinghealthfoundation.org

Hearing Health Foundation (HHF) is the largest private funder of hearing research, with a mission to prevent and cure hearing loss and tinnitus through groundbreaking research.

Shari Eberts, Chairman
Claire Schultz, CEO
Antonio Coppola, Director of Corporate Partnerships

3514 Hearing Impairments Better Hearing Institute
PO Box 1840
Washington, DC 20013   800-327-9355
                            Fax: 703-750-9302
                            TTY: 800-EAR-WELL

To educate the public and medical profession about hearing loss, its treatment and prevention.

3515 Hearing Loss Association of America
7910 Woodmont Ave, Suite 1200
Bethesda, MD 20814   301-657-2248
                            Fax: 301-913-9413
                                 www.hearingloss.org

HLAA provides assistance and resources for people with hearing loss and their families to learn how to adjust to living with hearing loss. HLAA is working to eradicate the stigma associated with hearing loss and raise public awareness about the need for prevention, treatment, and regular hearing screenings throughout life.

Anna Gilmore Hall, Executive Director
Lise Hamlin, Director of Public Policy
Nancy Macklin, Director of Events and Marketing

3516 HearingPlanet
100 Westwood Place, Suite 300
Brentwood, TN 37027   615-248-5910
                                 800-432-7669
                            Fax: 615-248-5903
                                 www.hearingplanet.com

A hearing specialist is ready to answer questions about hearing aids, hearing loss and treatments.

3517 Hearts and Homes For Youth
1320 Fenwick Lane, Suite 800
Silver Spring, MD 20910   301-589-8444
                            Fax: 301-495-0923
                        hhyinfo@heartsandhomes.org
                                 www.hh4y.org

Helps troubled children and youth who are abused, neglected or runaways, become independent, productive adults. To fulfill this mission, HHY provides a broad spectrum of educational, residential, independent living and mental health programs to a culturally diverse client population.

Rex Smith, President
Tammy O' Rourke, VP
Stephen Liggett-Creel, Administrator

3518 House Ear Institute
2100 W 3rd Street
Los Angeles, CA 90057   213-483-4431
                                 800-388-8612
                            Fax: 213-483-8789
                            TDD: 213-484-2642
                                 info@hei.org
                                 www.hei.org

A non-profit organization dedicated to advancing hearing science through research and education to improve the quality of life. HEI scientists explore the developing ear, hearing loss and ear disease at the cell and molecular level, as well as the complex relationship between the ear and the brain. They are also working to improve hearing aids and auditory implants, diagnostics, clinical treatments and intervention methods. HEI employs more than 180 staff members within 22 departments.

Catherine D. Meyer, Chair
David Z. D'Argenio, Vice Chair
William B. Witte, Treasurer

3519 International Deaf Education Association
P.O. Box 20715
Billings, MT 59104   406-656-2766
                                 info@ideadeaf.org
                                 www.ideadeaf.org

IDEA is a USA non-profit foundation that is working to educate impoverished and neglected deaf children in the Philippines.

George Dennis Drake, President / CEO
Marilouÿ Drake, CFO
Rhonda Hillabush, Sponsorship Director

3520 International Hearing Society
16880 Middlebelt Road, Suite 4
Livonia, MI 48154   734-522-7200
                                 800-521-5247
                            Fax: 734-522-0200
                                 chelms@ihsinfo.org
                                 www.ihsinfo.org

IHS is the professional association that represents Hearing Instrument Speicalists worldwide. IHS members are engaged in the practice of testing human hearing and selecting, fitting and dispensing hearing instruments. The Society continues to recognize the need for promoting and maintaining the highest possible standards for its members in the best interest of the hearing impaired it serves.

3000 members

Thomas Higgins, President
Scott Beall, President-Elect
Todd Beyer, Secretary

3521 John Tracy Clinic
806 W Adams Boulevard, PO Box 2505
Los Angeles, CA 90007

213-748-5481
800-522-4582
Fax: 213-749-1651
TTY: 213-747-2924
canguita@jtc.org
www.jtc.org

A private, non-profit education center whose mission is to offer hope, guidance and encouragement to families of infants and pre-school children with hearing loss by providing free, parent-centered services worldwide. The center has over 60 years of expertise in the spoken language option.

Michael D. Barker, Chair
Speed Fry, Vice Chair
Nihar Shah, Treasurer

3522 Junior National Association of the Deaf
8630 Fenton Street, Suite 820
Silver Spring, MD 20910

301-587-1788
Fax: 301-587-1791
TTY: 301-587-1789
nadinfo@nad.org
www.nad.org/jrnad

An organization of chapters from junior high and high schools across the United States whose motto is: Promoting the Tomorrow of All the Deaf by Working with the Deaf Youth of Today. Members learn and practice leadership, teamwork, and responsibility, and develop self-confidence.

Christopher D. Wagner, President
Melissa S. Draganac-Hawk, Vice President
Kirsten Poston, Secretary

3523 National Alliance of Black Interpreters
naobi2.org

naobiincmembershipchair@gmail.com
naobi2.org

Theÿmission of NAOBIÿis to promote excellence and empowerment among African Americans/Blacks in the profession of sign language interpreting in the context of a multi-cultural, multi-lingual environment.

3524 National Association for Hearing and Speech Action
American Speech Language Hearing Association
2200 Research Blvd., PO Box 3289
Rockville, MD 20850

301-296-5700
800-478-2071
Fax: 301-296-5777
TDD: 301-296-5650
www.asha.org

Provides general information on speech, language and hearing disorders to members and the public. Provides referrals to speech/language pathologists and audiologists.

77,346 members

Patriacia A. Prelock, President
Elizabeth S. McCrea, President-Elect
Donna Fisher Smiley, VP for Audiology Practice

3525 National Association of Parents with Children in Special Education
3642 E Sunnydale Drive
Chandler Heights, AZ 85142

800-754-4421
Fax: 800-424-0371
contact@napcse.org
www.napcse.org

NAPCSEÿis a national membership organization dedicated to rendering all possible support and assistance to parents whose children receive special education services, both in and outside of school.

Dr. George Giulianiÿ, President

3526 National Association of School Psychologists
4340 East West Highway, Suite 402
Bethesda, MD 20814

301-657-0270
866-331-NASP
Fax: 301-657-0275
www.nasponline.org

NASP empowers school psychologists by advancing effective practices to improve students' learning, behavior, and mental health.

Stephen E. Brock, President
Todd A. Savage, President-Elect
Sally Baas, Past President

3527 National Association of State Agencies of the Deaf and Hard of Hearing
4425 North Market Street
Wilmington, DE 19802

nasadhh.org

The National Association of State Agencies of the Deaf and Hard of Hearing is comprised of administrators of the state agencies serving deaf and hard of hearing.ÿ

Steve Florio, President, B.O.D.
Sherri Collins, Vice President
Virginia Moore, Treasurer

3528 National Association of the Deaf (NAD)
451 7th St. SW
Washington, DC 20410

301-587-1788
Fax: 301-587-1791
TTY: 301-587-1789
nadinfo@nad.org
www.nad.org

Established in 1880, the vision of NAD is that the language, culture, and heritage of hard of hearing Americans will be aknowledged and respected in pursuit of life, liberty and equality. There efforts to realize the vision have been in preserving, protecting, and promoting civil, human and liguitis rights of deaf and hard of hearing persons in America.

Christopher D. Wagner, President
Melissa S. Draganac-Hawk, Vice President
Kirsten Poston, Secretary

3529 National Black Deaf Advocates
P.O. Box 502658
Indianapolis, IN 46250

president@nbda.org
www.nbda.org

The National Black Deaf Advocates (NBDA) is the official advocacy organization for thousands of Black Deaf and hard of hearing people in the United States.ÿ

Patrick Robinson, President
Opeoluwa Sotonwa, Vice President
Betty Henderson, Treasurer

3530 National Captioning Institute
3725 Concorde Pkwy, Ste 100
Chantilly, VA 20151

703-917-7600
Fax: 703-917-9853
TTY: 703-917-7600
mail@ncicap.org
www.ncicap.org

NCI was established in 1979 as a non-profit corporation with the mission of ensuring that deaf and hard of hearing people, as well as others who can benefit from the same service, have access to television's entertainment and news through the technology of closed captioning. NCI employs almost 200 individuals.

Gene Chao, President
Jack Gates, President
Drake Smith, Chief Technology Officer

3531 National Catholic Office for the Deaf
www.ncod.org

info@ncod.org
www.ncod.org

There mission is to Spread God's message through the support of the Deaf and Hard of Hearing Pastoral Ministry so that we may all be one in Christ!

Kevin C. Rhoades, B.O.D.
Gregory Schott, Member at Large

3532 National Center On Deaf-Blindness
345 N. Monmouth Ave.
Monmouth, OR 97361   503-838-8754
                                    Fax: 503-838-8150
                               info@nationaldb.org
                                      nationaldb.org

NCDB works to improve the quality of life for children who are deaf-blind and their families.

Brenda Baroncelli, Administrative Assistantÿ
Robbin Bull, Project Specialist
Megan Cote, Project Specialist

3533 National Center for Hearing Assessment & Management
Utah State University, 2615 Old Main Hill
Logan, UT 84322   435-797-3584
                                  www.infanthearing.org

NCHAMÿserves as theÿNational Resource Centerÿfor the implementation and improvement of comprehensive and effective Early Hearing Detection and Intervention (EHDI) systems.

3534 National Center for Voice and Speech
University of Iowa
677 Phillips Hall
Iowa City, IA 52242   319-335-2238
                                    Fax: 319-335-8851
                               ASL-Program@uiowa.edu
                                        www.uiowa.ude

This is a consortium of the following institutions focusing on voice and speech disorders: University of Iowa, Denver Center for Performing Arts, University of Wisconsin-Madison, University of Utah. NCVS trains scientists interested in careers in voice and speech research, provides continuing education for professionals, and conducts research on voice and speech production.

Ingo Titze, PhD, Director
Cynthia Kintigh, MA

3535 National Council of Hispano Deaf and Hard of Hearing
P.O. Box 22011
Santa Fe, NM 87502   www.nchdhh.org

The mission of the National Council of Hispano Deaf and Hard of Hearing is to ensure equal access of the Hispano Deaf and Hard of Hearing community in the areas of social, recreational, cultural, educational, and vocational welfare.

Rogelio Fern ndez, Jr., President
Milmaglyn Morales, Vice President
Paolina Ramirez, Treasurer

3536 National Cued Speech Association
1300 Pennsylvania Avenue, Suite 190-713
Washington, DC 20004   216-292-6213
                                             800-459-3529
                                        TTY: 216-292-6213
                               cuedspdisc@aol.com
                                     www.cuedspeech.org

A non-profit membership organization founded in 1982 to promote and support the effective use of Cued Speech. They raise awareness of Cued Speeck and its applications, provide educational services, assist local affiliate chapters, establish standards for Cued Speech and certify Cued Speech instructors and transliterators. Their mission and goals are to promote and support the effectuve use of Cued Speech for communication, language acquistion and literacy.

Shannon Howell, President
Penny Hakim, VP
John Brubaker, VP

3537 National Family Association for Deaf-Blind
141 Middle Neck Road
Sands Point, NY 11050   800-255-0411
                                    Fax: 516-883-9060
                                    TTY: 516-944-8637
                                   nfadb@aol.com
                                       www.nfadb.org

A nonprofit, volunteer based, family association that believes individuals who are deaf-blind are valued members of society and are entitled to the same opportunity and choices as other members of the community

Susan Green, President
Debbie Ethridge, VP
Cynthia Jackson-Glenn, Treasurer

3538 National Information Center on Deafness
Gallaudet Univ. Press c/o Chicago Distrib. Center
800 Florida Avenue NE
Washington, DC 20002   202-250-2474
                                             800-995-0550
                                    Fax: 202-651-5744
                                    TTY: 202-651-5114
                         admissions.office@gallaudet.edu
                                    www.gallaudet.edu

Provides information or referrals on questions about deafness, including general information, education, research, legislation, assistive devices and more. Offers a bibliography of readings available on 30 topics relating to deafness.

Loraine DiPietro, Director
Vickie Whetstone, Executive Secretary
David King, Admissions Support

3539 National Rehabilitation Information Center
8201 Corporate Drive, Suite 600
Landover, MD 20785   301-459-5900
                                             800-346-2742
                                    Fax: 301-562-2401
                                    TTY: 301-459-5984
                         naricinfo@heitchservices.com
                                       www.naric.com

Its mission is to generate, disseminate and promote new knowledge to improve the options available to disabled persons. The ultimate goal is to allow these individuals to perform their regular activities in the community and to bolster society's ability to provide full opportunities and appropriate supports for its disabled citizens.

Mark Odum, Director

3540 National Technical Institute for the Deaf
Rochester Institute of Technology
One Lomb Memorial Drive
Rochester, NY 14623   585-475-2411
                                    Fax: 585-475-5978
                                    TTY: 585-475-6400
                                   ntidmc@rit.edu
                                         www.rit.edu

Technical college for students who are deaf or hard of hearing. Its mission is to provide these students with outstanding state-of-the-art technical and professional programs, complemented by a strong liberal arts and sciences curriculum, that prepare them to live and work in the mainstream of a rapidly changing global community and enhances their lifelong learning.

Alan Hurwitz, Vice President/Dean

3541 SEE Center for the Advancement of Deaf Chi ldren
PO Box 1181
Los Alamitos, CA 90720   562-430-1467
                                    Fax: 562-795-6614
                                    TTY: 562-430-1467
                               seecenter@seecenter.org
                                     www.seecenter.org

405

Established in 1984 as a nonprofit organization to work with parents and educators of hearing impared children. Their goals are to promote early identification and intervention; to promote development of improved English skills; to promote development and understanding of principles of Signing Exact English and its uses; to promote information to parents on deafness and related topics; and to foster the positive development of self concept in the deaf child.

Esther Zawolkow, Executive Director

3542 Self Help for Hard of Hearing People Hearing Loss Association of America
7910 Woodmont Avenue, Suite 1200
Bethesda, MD 20814
301-657-2248
Fax: 301-913-9413
TTY: 301-657-2248
info@hearingloss.org
www.hearingloss.org

The HLAA exists to open the world of communication for people with hearing loss through information, education, advocacy and support. They believe people with hearing loss can help themselves and one another to participate fully and successfully in society. HLAA promotes self-confidence; empowers individuals with skills to improve their lives; and provides an opportunity for affiliation among people with hearing loss and their friends, families, and professionals.

Barbara Kelley, Editor-In-Chief
Brenda Battat, Executive Director
Lise Hamlin, Director of Public Policy

3543 Telecommunications for the Deaf
8630 Fenton Street, Suite 604
Silver Spring, MD 20910
301-589-3786
Fax: 301-589-3797
TTY: 301-589-3006
info@tdi-online.org
www.tdi-online.org

An active national advocacy organization focusing its energies and resources to address equal access issues in telecommunications and media for four constituences in deafness and hearing loss, specifically people who are deaf, hard-of-hearing, late-deafened, or deaf-blind.

Miller Roy, President
Stout Claudd L., Executive Director
Jim House, Public Relations

3544 Telecommunications for the Deaf and Hard of Hearing
8630 Fenton Street, Suite 121
Silver Spring, MD 20910
301-563-9112
www.tdiforaccess.org

TDI (formally known as Telecommunications for the Deaf and Hard of Hearing, Inc.) was established in 1968 originally to promote further distribution of TTYs in the deaf community and to publish an annual national directory of TTY numbers.

Claude Stout, Executive Director
Don Cullens, Public Relations Director
John Skjeveland, Business Manager

Libraries & Resource Centers

3545 AbleData
8630 Fenton Street - Suite 300 B
Lexington, KY 40513
301-608-8998
800-227-0216
Fax: 301-608-8958
TTY: 301-608-8912
abledata@macrointernational.com
www.abledata.com

AbleData provides information on assistive technology and rehabilitation equipment available from international and domestic sources to consumers, professionals, organizations, and caregivers within the United States.

3546 Center for Hearing and Communication
50 Broadway - 6th Fl
New York, NY 10004
917-305-7700
Fax: 917-305-7888
TTY: 917-305-7999
www.chchearing.org

This organization provides hearing health services to people of all ages who have a hearing loss.

3547 Communication Service for the Deaf, Inc.
102 North Krohn Place
Sioux Falls, SD 57103
800-642-6410
TTY: 866-273-3323
inquiry@c-s-d.org
www.ceasd.org

CSD Relay is a telephone service which allows persons with hearing or speech disabilities to place and receive telephone calls.

3548 Dangerous Decibels Oregon Health & Science University
3181 SW Sam Jackson Park Road - NRC-04
Portland, OR 97239
503-494-0670
Fax: 503-494-0670
dd@ohsu.edu
www.dangerousdecibels.com

Through the creation of exhibits, education and research this organization helps to reduce the incidence and prevalence of Noise Induced Hearing Loss (NIHL) and tinnitus (ringing in the ear) by changing knowledge, attitudes, and behaviours of school-aged children.

3549 Hard of Hearing Advocates
245 Prospect St, PO Box 1184
Upton, MA 01701
hoha@charter.net
www.hohadvocates.org

This organization helps hard-of-hearing (HOH) people by creating and implementing programs and solutions where HOH people have undue problems.

3550 Hearing Education & Awareness for Rockers
PO Box 460847
San Francisco, CA 94146
415-409-3277
hear@hearnet.com
www.hearnet.com

H.E.A.R. is a hearing information source for musicians and music lovers.

Alabama

3551 Alabama Institute for the Deaf & Blind
PO Box 698
Talladega, AL 35161
256-761-3331
Fax: 256-761-3344
www.aidb.org

Services include central directory, representatives of agencies, service providers, families, and coordinators of infant, toddler, and preschool special education programs.

Terry Graham, President

3552 University of Alabama Speech and Hearing Center
Deparment of Communicative Disorders
166 Rose Administration Building Box 870144
Tuscaloosa, AL 35487
205-348-5320
Fax: 205-348-8320
gculton@ed.ua.edu
www.universityrelations.ua.edu

Enhancing the educational mission of the Department, the Speech and Hearing Center is further dedicated to reducing the impact of communicative disorders affecting diverse populations across a life-span.

Carl E Ferguson, Executive Director
Austin Dare, Director,Office of Design/Productio

California

3553 American Action Fund for Blind Children and Adults
18440 Oxnard Street
Tarzana, CA 91356
818-343-2022
Fax: 818-343-3219
lucyabba@aol.com
www.actinfund.org

A lending library for the visually impaired. We send out a weekly Braille newspaper for the deaf-blind (worldwide), we also send out pocket-sized Braille calendars. Our lending library is for pre-school thru high school. All of our services are free.

Lucille Abbazia, Manager

3554 Hear Center
301 E Del Mar Boulevard
Pasadena, CA 91101
626-796-2016
Fax: 626-796-2320
auditory@hearcenter.org
www.hearcenter.org

The Hear Center's mission is to help individuals with hearing loss or speech and language impairments integrate into the mainstream of the community by providing them with the means for developing auditory and oral communication skills.

Ellen Simon, Executive Director

District of Columbia

3555 Center for Auditory and Speech Sciences-Gallaudet University
800 Florida Avenue NE
Washington, DC 20002
202-651-5000
Fax: 202-651-5295
clerc.center@gallaudet.edu
www.gallaudet.edu

The Hearing and Speech Center provides comprehensive speech, language, and audiology services to Gallaudet students, faculty, staff and to clients in the Washington, D.C. area. These services include hearing and hearing aid evaluations, hearing aid dispensing, assistive devices evaluations, speech-language evaluations and therapy, communication therapy, and speech reading classes.

I King Jordan, President
Jane K Fernandes, Provost
Paul Kelly, VP Administration and Finance

3556 District of Columbia Public Library/ Librarian for the Deaf Community
901 G Street NW, Room 215
Washington, DC 20001
202-727-2142
Fax: 202-727-1129
lbphb_2000@yahoo.com
www.dclibrary.org

Offers reference services through TDD, portable TDD for public use at pay phones, signers for library programs, sign language classes, information about deafness, print and nonprint materials for persons who are deaf.

Vaneisha Denson, Manager

3557 Laurent Clerc National Deaf Education Center-Gallaudet Universty
800 Florida Avenue NE
Washington, DC 20002
202-651-5300
Fax: 202-651-5477
TTY: 202-651-5300
www.gallaudet.edu

Gallaudet University's Laurent Clerc National Deaf Education Center provides deaf and hard of hearing children through the Model Secondary School for the Deaf and the Kendall Demonstration Elementary School and also collects, evaluates and disseminates best practices in deaf education.

I King Jordan, President
Katherine Jankowski, Dean
Paul Kelly, VP Administration/Finance

3558 Volta Bureau Library
Alexander Graham Bell Association for the Deaf
3417 Volta Place NW
Washington, DC 20007
202-337-5220
866-337-5220
Fax: 202-337-8314
TTY: 202-337-5221
agbell2@aol.com
www.agbell.org

Contains one of the world's largest historical collections of publications, documents and information on deafness. In addition to the main collection, which includes books, periodicals and indexed clipping files dating from the turn of the century, the library also houses a significant archival collection dealing with the history of deafness since the 16th century. Membership dues for professionals are $50.00.

4500 members

Rebecca Parlakian, Director Member Services

Illinois

3559 Loyola University of Children, Parmly Hearing Institute
6525 N Sheridan Road
Chicago, IL 60626
773-508-2766
Fax: 773-508-2719
ssheft@luc.edu

The Parmly Hearing Institute is part of Loyola University Chicago.

Stanley Edward Sheft PhD, Director

Maine

3560 University of Maine, Conley Speech and Hearing Center
5724 Dunn Hall, Room 336
Orono, ME 04469
207-581-2006

The Madelyn E and Albert D Conley Speech, Language and Hearing Center is a center for clinical education and research as well as a facility for comprehensive state-of-the-art speech, language and hearing services. Both the Audiology Clinic and the Speech-Language Clinic provide services for individuals across the lifespan. The Speech-Language Clinic includes a Diagnostic Clinic, a Family-Based Treatment Clinic, and a Stuttering Clinic.

Susan K Riley MS, Clinic Director

Massachusetts

3561 Eaton-Peabody Laboratory of Auditory Physiology
Massachusetts Eye & Ear Institute
243 Charles Street
Boston, MA 02114
617-573-7900
Fax: 617-720-4408
TDD: 617-523-5498
www.meei.harvard.edu

A consortium between the Massachusetts Eye and Ear Infirmary, the Harvard Medical School, the Research Laboratory of Electronics at Massachusetts Institute of Technology, and the Massachusetts General Hospital. Research interests span the auditory system from peripheral to central, from normal to abnormal function, from neurophysiology to behavior, and from the molecular and genetic bases of deafness, to its treatment via hearing aids and cochlear implants.

Nelson YS Kiang, PhD, Director

Nebraska

3562 University of Nebraska, Lincoln Barkley Memorial Center
Barkley Center 301
Lincoln, NE 68583
402-472-2145
Fax: 402-472-7697
www.unl.edu.barkley/index.shtml

The University of Nebraska-Lincoln Barkley Memorial Center and Boys Town National Research Hospital have joined forces to offer an exciting future in the audiology profession.

407

John E Bernthal, Director

New York

3563 Wallace Memorial Library
Rochester Institute of Technology
90 Lomb Memorial Drive
Rochester, NY 14623   585-475-2562
www.library.rit.edu/collections/wallace.html

A multimedia resource center with a collection of more than 750,000 items. Resource materials include more than 350,000 books; 2900 print journals subscriptions; 380,000 microforms; 3,100 audio cassettes and recordings; 6,700 film and video titles. They have an extensive web-based online collection which features over 150 research databases, 7,000+ eBooks, 16,000 electronic journal subscriptions and thousands of digital images in various collections.

Melanie Norton, Reference Librarian

Oregon

3564 Regional Resource Center on Deafness
Western Oregon State University
345 N Monmouth Avenue
Monmouth, OR 97361   503-838-8444
877-877-1593
Fax: 503-838-8228
webmaster@wou.edu
www.wou.edu

Prepares professionals in the Northwest to be qualified to serve the unique communication, rehabilitation, and educational needs of deaf and hard of hearing individuals. The Center offers graduate and undergraduate degree programs for professionals entering fields that serve people who are deaf or hard of hearing, continuing education opportunities for currently practicing professionals, and consultation and community service activities designed to enhance the quality of life for all affected.

Cheryl Davis, Director
Hilda Rosselli PhD, Dean

South Carolina

3565 Described and Captioned Media Program
National Association of the Deaf
1447 E Main Street
Spartanburg, SC 29307   864-585-1778
800-237-6213
Fax: 864-585-2611
TTY: 864-585-2617
info@cfv.org
www.cfv.org

Renamed the Described and Captioned Media Program, CMP continues to provide all persons who are deaf or hard of hearing awareness of and equal access to communication and learning through the use of captioned educational media and supportive collateral materials. They also act as a captioning information and training center. Their ultimate goal is to permit media to be an integral part in the lifelong learning process for all stakeholders in the deaf and hard of hearing community.

Bill Stark, Manager

Research Centers

3566 Boston Children's Hospital Dept. of Otolaryngology & Communication
300 Longwood Ave
Boston, MA 02115   617-355-6000
TTY: 617-730-0152
www.childrenshospital.com

Provides diagnosis and surgical treatment for disorders of the head and neck.

Arkansas

3567 Arkansas Rehabilitation Research and Training Center for Deaf Persons
University of Arkansas
4601 W Markham Street
Little Rock, AR 72205   501-686-9691
Fax: 501-686-9698
TTY: 501-686-9698

The center focuses on issues affecting the employability of deaf and hard-of-hearing rehabilitation clients.

Douglas Watson, PhD, Director

Massachusetts

3568 National Temporal Bone, Hearing and Balance Pathology Resource Registry
Massachusetts Eye & Ear Infirmary
243 Charles Street, PO Box 3096
Boston, MA 02114   617-573-3711
800-822-1327
Fax: 617-573-3838
TTY: 800-439-0183
tbregistry@meei.harvard.edu
www.tbregistry.org

The Registry, established by the National Institute on Deafness and Other Communication Disorders, maintains a database of human temporal bone collections, responds to inquiries from the public and researchers interested in temporal bone donation or research, disseminates information about temporal bone collection and its importance, implements professional educational activities in the field of temporal bone and auditory brain cell stem study and implements a national acquistion network.

Nicole Pelletier, Coordinator

Michigan

3569 University of Michigan, Kresge Hearing Research Institute
1301 E Ann Street, Room 5032
Ann Arbor, MI 48109   734-763-9600
Fax: 734-764-0014
TTY: 734-764-8110

Research programs include multi-disciplinary projects in behavior, morphology, physiology, molecular biology and genetics, bioengineering, pharmacology and biochemistry. They include: the genetics of hearing and deafness, mechanisms of auditory processing, molecular otology, cochlear prosthesis and tissue bioengineering, and training.

Jochen Schacht PhD, Scientific Director
Diana Gilham, Finance
Gary Dootz, Grant Administrator

Missouri

3570 Central Institute for the Deaf
825 S Taylor Ave
Saint Louis, MO 63110   314-977-0000
888-444-4565
Fax: 314-977-0223
TTY: 314-997-0001
TDD: 314-977-0037
rfeder@cid.wustl.edu
www.cid.wustl.edu

Central Institute for the Deaf is a private, nonprofit institute composed of research laboratories in which scientists study the normal aspects as well as the disorders of hearing, language, and speech; a school for children who have hearing impairments; speech, language, and hearing clinics; and professionals with hearing impairment, and communication sciences.

Robin Feder, Ceo

Nebraska

3571 Lied Learning and Technology Center for Ch ildhood Deafness and Vision Disorders
Boys Town National Research Hospital
555 North 30th Street
Omaha, NE 68131
402-498-6511
800-448-3000
Fax: 402-498-1348
TTY: 402-498-6543
hotline@girlsandboystown.org
www.boystown.org/chlc

A not-for-profit corporation closely affiliated with the Boys Town National Research Hospital. The center houses Model Childhood Education Classrooms, a Cochlear Implant Clinic and Research Center, Educational Media Production Studios, Distance Learning and Family Outreach Center, Hearing and Vision Laboratories, Bio-informatics and Computer Center and a Communication Technology Development Center.

Patrick E Brookhouser MD, President
John K. Arch, Executive VP
Edward M. Kolb, Medical Director

New York

3572 Montifiore Medical Center
2475 St. Raymonds Avenue
Bronx, NY 10461
718-430-7300
800-636-6683
Fax: 718-741-2033
ruben@aecom.vu.edu
www.montefiore.org

Provides diagnosis, treatment and research of diseases of the ear, nose and throat.

Steven M. Safyer, MD, President/Chief Executive Officer
Philip O. Ozuah, MD, PhD, Executive Vice President/Chief Oper
Joel A. Perlman, Executive Vice President/Chief Fina

3573 State University College at Plattsburgh Auditory Research Laboratory
101 Broad Street
Plattsburgh, NY 12901
518-564-2040
888-673-0012
Fax: 518-564-2045
hamernrp@plattsburgh.edu
www.plattsburgh.edu

The Auditory Research Laboratory (ARL) is home to several laboratories, including acoustics lab, anatomy lab, auditory evoked potential lab, and otoacoustic emissions lab. Facilities include: acoustics and vibrations laboratory, otoacoustic emmissions laboratory, middle ear analysis laboratory, auditory evoked potential laboratory, and cochlear anatomy laborator.

Roger Hamernik, MD, Director

3574 Syracuse University, Institute for Sensory Research
621 Skytop Road, PO Box 5290
Syracuse, NY 13244
315-443-4164
Fax: 315-443-1184
rlsmith@syr.edu
www.isr.syr.edu

Research center dedicated to the discovery and application of knowledge of the sensory systems. Integration of engineering, life, and physical sciences, combining rigorous experimental methodology with mathematical analysis is stressed.

Robert Smith, MD, Director

Oregon

3575 Oregon Health Sciences University Research Center
3181 SW Sam Jackson Park Road, PO Box 3098
Portland, OR 97239
503-494-8311
Fax: 503-494-5656
contact@ohsuhealth.com
www.ohsuhealth.com

OSHU blends education, research, patient care and community outreach into one shared mission: to improve the well-being of people in Oregon and beyond. They incorporate the latest medical research, technology and innovation.

Michael Heinrich

Pennsylvania

3576 Temple University, Section of Auditory Research
1801 N. Broad Street
Philadelphia, PA 19122
215-707-3663
Fax: 215-707-7523
anita@ent.temple.edu
www.temple.edu

The Auditory Research Section includes the Garfied Auditory Research Laboratory, the Hearing Science Research Program and the Electrophysiology Progject.

Anita Cilea, Departmental Administrator
Kate Haney, Financial Administrator
Neil D. Theobald, President

Tennessee

3577 Bill Wilkerson Center
1211 Medical Center Drive
Nashville, TN 37232
615-322-5000
Fax: 615-936-5013
kate.carney@vanderbilt.edu
www.mc.vanderbilt.edu

The Vanderbilt Bill Wilkerson Center for Otolaryngology and Communication Sciences is dedicated to serving persons with diseases of the ear, nose, throat, head and neck, and hearing, speech, language and related disorders.

Robert H Ossoff DMD MD, Director
Fred H Bess PhD, Associate Director

Texas

3578 Houston Ear Research Foundation
7737 SW Freeway, Suite 630
Houston, TX 77074
713-771-9966
800-843-0807
Fax: 713-771-0546
TTY: 800-843-0807
info@houstoncochlear.org
www.houstoncochlear.org

The Foundation was incorporated in August, 1983 as a center to provide excellence in service dedicated to the cochlear implant.

Jan Gilden, Executive Director

Conferences

3579 AADB National Symposium
American Association of the Deaf-Blind
8630 Fenton Street, Suite 121
Silver Spring, MD 20910
301-495-4403
Fax: 301-495-4404
TTY: 301-495-4402
aadb-info@aadb.org
www.aadb.org

The symposium offers a training workshop, keynote speakers, full day exhibit hall, demonstration room, awards lunch and ceremony, talent show, Walk-A-Thon, and a banquet and dance.

Jill Gaus, President
Lynn Jansen, Vice President
Debby Lieberman, Secretary

3580 AG Bell Biennial Convention
Alexander Graham Bell Association for the Deaf
3417 Volta Place NW
Washington, DC 20007   202-337-5220
                                               800-432-7543
                                               Fax: 202-337-8314
                                               TTY: 202-337-5221
                                               info@agbell.org
                                               www.agbell.org

June

Alexander T Graham, Executive Director

3581 ANA National Symposium Acoustic Neuroma Association
600 Peachtree Pkwy, Ste 108
Cumming, GA 30041   770-205-8211
                                               877-200-8211
                                               Fax: 770-205-0239
                                               info@anausa.org
                                               www.anausa.org

Biennial national symposium for pre-and post-treatment acoustic neuroma patients, family members, friends and health care professionals for a weekend of educational lectures, workshops and panel discussions with acoustic neuroma medical professionals.

3582 ASCD Biennial Conference
American Society for Deaf Children
800 Florida Ave NE, Suite 2047
Washington, DC 20002   800-942-2732
                                               Fax: 410-795-0965
                                               asdc@deafchildren.org
                                               www.deafchildren.org

Provides families with five days of information and fun. Daytime workshops captivates parents while children participate in educational and recreational activities. Evening events bring families together, providing the opportunity to form new friendships and peer support.

June

Beth S Benedict, President

3583 ASHA Annual Convention
American Speech-Language-Hearing Association
2200 Research Boulevard
Rockville, MD 20850   301-897-5700
                                               800-638-8255
                                               Fax: 301-296-8580
                                               TTY: 301-296-5700
                                               productsales@asha.org
                                               www.asha.org

Professional education event for speech-language pathologists, audiologists, and speech, language, and hearing scientists. Provides unparalleled opportunities to hear the latest evidence-based research and gain new skills and resources to advance your career.

12,000 November

Arlene A Pietranton, Executive Director

3584 Cued Speech Conference
National Cued Speech Assocation
1300 Pennsylvania Avenue
Washington, DC 20004   800-459-3529
                                               info@cuedspeech.org
                                               www.cuedspeech.org

3585 IHS Annual Convention & Expo
International Hearing Society
16880 Middlebelt Road, Suite 4
Livonia, MI 48154   734-522-7200
                                               800-521-5247
                                               Fax: 734-522-0200
                                               chelms@ihsinfo.org
                                               www.ihsinfo.org

September

Kathleen Mennillo, Executive Director

3586 NAD Biennial Conference
National Association of the Deaf
8630 Fention Street, Suite 820
Silver Spring, MD 20910   301-587-1788
                                               Fax: 301-587-1791
                                               TTY: 301-587-1789
                                               nadinfo@nad.org
                                               www.nad.org

Held in the even numbered years, brings together deaf,hard of hearing, late-deafened, deaf-blind and hearing consumers, parents, youth, professionals, educators, organizational and corporate representatives for professional development, enrichment, training, networking, governance meetings, exhibits, receptions, and related evening.

2,000 July

Bobbie Beth Scoggins, President

Audio Video

3587 50th Anniversary Collection
Harris Communications
15155 Technology Drive
Eden Prairie, MN 55344   952-906-1180
                                               800-825-6758
                                               Fax: 952-906-1099
                                               TTY: 800-825-9187
                                               info@harriscomm.com
                                               www.harriscomm.com

Stories: A picture for Harold's Room; Corduroy; Danny and the Dinosaur; Harry the Dirty Dog; Click, clack moo, Cows that type. DVD-R, voiced; signed in ASL, no captions.

3588 A Few Errands
Modern Sign Press
10443 Los Alamitos Boulevard, PO Box 1181
Los Alamitos, CA 90720   562-596-8548
                                               800-572-7332
                                               Fax: 562-795-6614
                                               TTY: 562-493-4168
                                               modsigns@modernsignspress.com
                                               www.modernsignspress.com

Basic level videotape of signed story for Expressive and Receptive practice. Story is repeated three times for ease of use. Watch how the visual features are incorporated. Turn the sound off for receptive practice. Written script and tape use suggestions included. VHS

Esther Zawolkow, President

3589 A Lesson With Heart
American Sign Language Productions
4450 La Crosse Ave
San Diego, CA 92117   952-906-1180
                                               800-767-4461
                                               Fax: 952-906-1099
                                               TTY: 952-906-1198
                                               SignEnhancers@iCloud.com
                                               www.signenhancers.com

A skilled 4th grade teacher presents a lesson on Anatomy including the respiratory system, digestive system, and the heart that will increase your familiarity with this vocabulary and content. Improve your interpreting skills for this subject matter and grade level by accepting this assignment. You won't be alone...we provide two interpreters to demonstrate it for your. 55 minutes. DVD - $59.95; VHS - 49.95

3590 A Mother's Persepctive on the IEP Process
American Sign Language Productions
4450 La Crosse Ave
San Diego, CA 92117   952-906-1180
                                               800-767-4461
                                               Fax: 952-906-1099
                                               TTY: 952-906-1198
                                               SignEnhancers@iCloud.com
                                               www.signenhancers.com

Maxine Camvel is a parent of a Deaf daughter wanting to make it easier for other parents. She gives valuable insight into how to advocate for your children by maximizing parent input to the Individualized Education Plan (IEP) process. This program also provides an opportunity to interpret vocabulary and emotional content commonly expressed by parents. Your two team interpreters demonstrate how to interpret this sample. 1 hour. DVD - $59.95; VHS - $49.95

3591 A is for Access: Creating Full & Interacti ve Access for Students
Hands and Voices
PO Box 3093
Boulder, CO 80307

303-492-6283
866-422-0422
parentadvocate@handsandvoices.org
www.handsandvoices.org

This video is a source to generate greater awareness of communication access issues for students who are deaf or hard of hearing. DVD or VHS, captioned.

3592 ABC Stories DVD
Sign Media
4020 Blackburn Lane
Burtonsville, MD 20866

301-421-0268
800-475-4756
Fax: 301-421-0270
info@signmedia.com
www.signmedia.com

You will marvel at the skill of these Deaf performers as they use every letter of the manual alphabet, in sequence, to tell a story. To capture the creativity and genius of the stories, the videotape uses slow motion and graphic displays. 1 hour

3593 ABCs of AVT: Analyzing Auditory-Verbal Therapy
Alexander Graham Bell Association for the Deaf
3417 Volta Place NW
Washington, DC 20007

202-337-5220
800-432-7543
Fax: 202-337-8314
TTY: 202-337-5221
info@agbell.org
listeningandspokenlanguage.org

An Educational Tool for Professionals. Developed for use in university classrooms and training environments; provides an overview of Auditory-Verbal techniques and guidance on appropriate intervention for children experiencing difficulties with language development.

2005 104 pages 46 Minute video

Warren Estabrooks MEd, Author
Rhonda Schwartz MA, Co-Author
Lisa Chutjian, Chief Development Officer

3594 ASL Stories: Christmas Stories
Harris Communications
15155 Technology Drive
Eden Prairie, MN 55344

952-906-1180
800-825-6758
Fax: 952-906-1099
TTY: 800-825-9187
info@harriscomm.com
www.harriscomm.com

This video is one in a collection of videotapes featuring classic fairy tales signed by Deaf storytellers, and is a wonderful way to get into the spirit of Christmas. This video also makes a welcome gift. Stories include: The Night Before Christmas, A Christmas Carol, The First Christmas Tree, The Birth of Christ, In the Great Walled City, and The Little Match Girl. For ages 10 and over. VHS: 80 minutes; signed in ASL; no captions; voice over.

3595 ASL Stories: Fairy Tales I
Harris Communications
15155 Technology Drive
Eden Prairie, MN 55344

952-906-1180
800-825-6758
Fax: 952-906-1099
TTY: 800-825-9187
info@harriscomm.com
www.harriscomm.com

This video is one of a collection of videotapes featuring classic fairy tales signed by Deaf storytellers. Stories include Rapunzel, Snow White and Rose Red, The Frog Prince, Hansel and Gretel, and The Brave Little Tailor. For ages 10 and over. VHS: 114 minutes; signed in ASL; no captions; voice-over.

3596 ASL Stories: Fairy Tales II
Harris Communications
15155 Technology Drive
Eden Prairie, MN 55344

952-906-1180
800-825-6758
Fax: 952-906-1099
TTY: 800-825-9187
info@harriscomm.com
www.harriscomm.com

This video is one of a collection of videotapes featuring classic fairy tales signed by Deaf storytellers. Stories include Sleeping Beauty, The Golden Goose, Little Red Riding Hood, The Princess and the Pea, and The Tinder Box. For ages 10 and over. VHS: 83 minutes; signed in ASL; no captions; voice-over.

3597 Acoustics, Audition and Speech Reception

Daniel Lind OC, PhD, author

Alexander Graham Bell Association for the Deaf
3417 Volta Place NW
Washington, DC 20007

202-337-5220
202-337-8314
Fax: 202-337-8314
TTY: 203-337-5221
info@agbell.org
listeningandspokenlanguage.org

This videotape of four professionals provides viewers with an overview of the properties of speech and the ways children can get the most from their hearing aids or cochlear implants. The tape is a practical how-to guide in which team members demonstrate how speech sounds are created in the vocal tract, how distance affects the intensity of spoken language and how patterns are distorted by profound hearing loss.

Lisa Chutjian, Chief Development Officer
Emilio Alonso-Mendoza, Chief Executive Officer
Judy Harrison, Director of Programs

3598 American Sign Language Handshape Dictionar y DVD
Gallaudet University Press
800 Florida Avenue NE
Washington, DC 20002

202-651-5448
Fax: 202-651-5489
TTY: 202-651-5444
gupress@gallaudet.edu
gupress.gallaudet.edu

A perfect complement to the dictionary, this new DVD features a diverse cast of native signers forming more than 1,400 ASL signs organized by 40 basic handshapes, with a complete list of English glosses and synonyms for each sign.

Richard Tennant, Co-Producer
Marianne Gluszak Brown, Co-Producer

3599 American Sign Language Video Series
DeBee Communications/TJ Publishers
P.O. Box 702701
Dallas, TX 75370

972-416-0800
800-999-1168
Fax: 972-416-0944
TTY: 972-416-0933
customerservice@tjpublishers.com
https://www.388.safesecureweb.com/tjpublishers/store/

Learning ASL with the Deaf Robinson family. The family acts out scenes that occur in everyday life in this videotape series. Each situation is reviewed in an ASL classroom with a deaf teacher. This series also includes sections on Deaf culture and grammar, rounding off a complete and effective instructional tool. Work Day-VHS-90 minutes, School Day-VHS-90 minutes, Shopping-VHS-90 minutes, Softball Game-VHS-90 minutes. $39.95 each

3600 American Sign Language: Green Books Text a nd Tapes
Sign Media
4020 Blackburn Lane
Burtonsville, MD 20866

301-421-0268
800-475-4756
Fax: 301-421-0270
info@signmedia.com
www.signmedia.com

The classic ASL series. This unique set of texts, written by Dennis Cokely and Charlotte Baker-Shenk, is complimented by DVDs. The DVDs explain difficult concepts and offer practice situations to improve your sign language skills. The series may be ordered as a complete set of books and DVDs, a complete set of DVDs only, individual books and DVDs, or a specific DVD and book combination set. Individual DVD $44.95, DVD set & books $379.95, DVD set $233.95

3601 Ancient Greece
American Sign Language Productions
4450 La Crosse Ave
San Diego, CA 92117

952-906-1180
800-767-4461
Fax: 952-906-1099
TTY: 952-906-1198
SignEnhancers@iCloud.com
www.signenhancers.com

We often think about interpreting for Deaf children, but often need to understand the speech and thought patterns of their hearing classmates. Krisjana is a hearing child presenting a report on Ancient Greece. A great way to practice with vocabulary from the classroom before you have to sit in the hot seat. Is it all Greek to you? No need to worry. Two interpreters will show you how. 30 minutes. DVD - $59.95; VHS - $49.95

3602 Animals, Insects, School, Colors Spanish/E nglish Videos
Modern Signs Press
10443 Los Alamitos Boulevard, PO Box 1181
Los Alamitos, CA 90720

562-596-8548
800-572-7332
Fax: 562-795-6614
TTY: 562-493-4168
modsigns@modernsignspress.com
www.modernsignspress.com

Entertaining sign language instructional videos in Spanish and English. Great tool to help bridge the gap between Spanish, English and Sign Language. The videos have a split screen - Connie and Merced teach you the sign and say the word in both Spanish and English. Vocabulary words are used in sentences to reinforce the signs. There are graphics showing the vocabulary they are reviewing. 10 titles available, either alone or in a complete package.

Esther Zawolkow, President

3603 Art Show
Modern Sign Press
10443 Los Alamitos Boulevard, PO Box 1181
Los Alamitos, CA 90720

562-596-8548
800-572-7332
Fax: 562-795-6614
TTY: 562-493-4168
modsigns@modernsignspress.com
www.modernsignspress.com

Basic level videotape of signed story for Expressive and Receptive practice. Story is repeated three times for ease of use. Watch how the visual features are incorporated. Turn the sound off for receptive practice. Written script and tape use suggestions included. VHS

Esther Zawolkow, President

3604 Baby See 'n Sign
Harris Communications
15155 Technology Drive
Eden Prairie, MN 55344

952-906-1180
800-825-6758
Fax: 952-906-1099
TTY: 800-825-9187
info@harriscomm.com
www.harriscomm.com

Features American Sign Language signs and real-life images in full color. They may be used as an educational tool for effectively promoting communication with people who are autistic, have Down Syndrome, or are ESL. For parents who have decided to sign to their children, this is a great video. Over 60 basic American Sign Language signs and real-life images are presented in full-color, making it enjoyable for parents and children to watch. A parental question and answer guide is included.

6 months + DVD 45 minutes

3605 Baby See 'n Sign II
Harris Communications
15155 Technology Drive
Eden Prairie, MN 55344

952-906-1180
800-825-6758
Fax: 952-906-1099
TTY: 800-825-9187
info@harriscomm.com
www.harriscomm.com

This DVD shows over 100 real-life images that relate to your child's daily life, including animals, foods, toys and activities. Volume II has beginning abstract concepts and continues with object-word association. It is never too late to begin signing. Ages 6 months and up. DVD: 50 minutes.

3606 Baby Signing Time
Harris Communications
15155 Technology Drive
Eden Prairie, MN 55344

952-906-1180
800-825-6758
Fax: 952-906-1099
TTY: 800-825-9187
info@harriscomm.com
www.harriscomm.com

Designed specifically for babies 3-36 months old, the DVD combines sign-along songs, playful animation and the positive reinforcement of signing babies - who are all ages 2 and under - to teach you and your baby to sign the easy way. Baby Signing Time sets your baby's day to music as you learn sign and sogns for everyday events in baby's life - eating, family, pets and more.

3607 Baby Signing Time DVD 2
Harris Communications
15155 Technology Drive
Eden Prairie, MN 55344

952-906-1180
800-825-6758
Fax: 952-906-1099
TTY: 800-825-9187
info@harriscomm.com
www.harriscomm.com

This video sets your baby's day to music as you learn signs and sogns for everyday events in baby's life - eating, family, pets and more. Designed specifically for babies 3-36 months old, this DVD combines sign-along songs, playful animation and the positive reinforcement of signing babies - who are all ages 2 and under - to teach you and your baby to sign the easy way.

3608 Bachelor Father
Modern Sign Press
10443 Los Alamitos Boulevard, PO Box 1181
Los Alamitos, CA 90720

562-596-8548
800-572-7332
Fax: 562-795-6614
TTY: 562-493-4168
modsigns@modernsignspress.com
www.modernsignspress.com

Basic level videotape of signed story for Expressive and Receptive practice. Story is repeated three times for ease of use. Watch how the visual features are incorporated. Turn the sound off for receptive practice. Written script and tape use suggestions included. VHS

Esther Zawolkow, President

3609   Basic Course in American Sign Language Videotape Package
TJ Publishers
P.O. Box 702701
Dallas, TX 75370   800-999-1168
                                                          Fax: 972-416-0944
                                                          TTY: 972-416-0933
                                    customerservice@tjpublishers.com
                      https://www388.safesecureweb.com/tjpublishers/store/

This videotape features four Deaf models signing each vocabulary
word contained in all 22 lessons of the text plus the alphabet and
numbers. The tape has captions and voice which can be turned off
to sharpen visual acuity. It is ideal for classroom reinforcement
and independent home study. Available on VHS or DVD

Video

Angela K Thames, President

3610   Beginning Level Curriculum Tapes Complete Set
Modern Signs Press
10443 Los Alamitos Boulevard, PO Box 1181
Los Alamitos, CA 90720   562-596-8548
                                                                800-572-7332
                                                          Fax: 562-795-6614
                                                          TTY: 562-493-4168
                                         modsigns@modernsignspress.com
                                            www.modernsignspress.com

A good way to learn the beginning lessons of Signing Exact English with Dr. Gerilee Gustason, co-author of SEE. The full set of
tapes introduce more than 700 words and signs. There are 14 lessons with approximately 50 vocabulary items and practice sentences in each lesson. Words and sentences are presented twice
allowing time for observation and ability to imitate presenter.
Words are also shown in text form for both the individual vocabulary words and sentences to help with clarity.

VHS and DVD

Esther Zawolkow, President

3611   Beginning Reading and Sign Language Video
TJ Publishers
P.O. Box 702701
Dallas, TX 75370   972-416-0800
                                                                800-999-1168
                                                          Fax: 972-416-0944
                                                          TTY: 972-416-0933
                                    customerservice@tjpublsihers.com
                      https://www388.safesecureweb.com/tjpublishers/store/

Great for kids from 2 to 12, this video picture book feature Deaf
actress Susan Bressler signing over a hundred words at the zoos,
at home and around the community. Don't tell your kids that
learning Sign language improves reading, motor skills and visual
perception and increases language acquisition abilities. English
captions give reading practice, too. Great for hearing and Deaf
children. VHS 30 minutes.

Video
ISBN: 0-932314-00-7

Angela K Thames, President

3612   Blue's Clues: All Kinds of Signs
Harris Communications
15155 Technology Drive
Eden Prairie, MN 55344   952-906-1180
                                                                800-825-6758
                                                          Fax: 952-906-1099
                                                          TTY: 800-825-9187
                                                   info@harriscomm.com
                                                   www.harriscomm.com

Preschoolers play along with Steve and Blue with the two episodes in this video. The video uses different kinds of signs - from
directional signs to American Sign Language - to figure out
where Blue wants to eat in Where does Blue want to have her
snack?, and where she would like to go in Where does Blue want
to go? Guest appearance by Marlee Matline. Approximately 50
minutes. Closed captioned. VHS.

3613   Bold as Brianna
American Sign Language Productions
15155 Technology Drive
Eden Prairie, MN 55344   952-906-1180
                                                                800-825-6758
                                                          Fax: 952-906-1099
                                                          TTY: 800-825-9187
                                                   info@harriscomm.com
                                                   www.harriscomm.com

Elementary: 7-Year-Old Deaf Child. A Confident, articulate
seven-year-old willing and able to give you an eye-full. Precious
and precocious, Briana will entertain you as you improve your re-
ceptivity and sign-to-voice interpreting skills. Two certified interpreters provide interpretations for your to compare and
contrast to each other and your own work. 33 minutes. DVD -
$59.95; VHS - $49.95

3614   Building Cue Reading
Melanie Metzger, PhD and Earl Fleetwood, MA, author

Alexander Graham Bell Association for the Deaf
3417 Volta Place NW
Washington, DC 20007   202-337-5220
                                                                202-337-8314
                                                          Fax: 202-337-8314
                                                          TTY: 203-337-5221
                                                        info@agbell.org
                                          listeningandspokenlanguage.org

Designed for hearing individuals who already cue expressively,
this two videotape set offers lessons to develop receptive Cued
English skills. The videos comprise 15 lessons with drills and
practice exercises.

Lisa Chutjian, Chief Development Officer
Emilio Alonso-Mendoza, Chief Executive Officer
Judy Harrison, Director of Programs

3615   Communication Rules for Hard-of-Hearing People
Self Help for Hard-of-Hearing People
7910 Woodmont Avenue, Suite 1200
Bethesda, MD 20814   301-657-2248
                                                          Fax: 301-913-9413
                                                          TTY: 301-657-2249
                                                        national@shhh.org
                                                        www.hearingloss.org

For use with manual (listed separately).

1987 Open-captioned

Barbara Kelley, Editor-In-Chief
Anna Gilmore Hall, Executive Director
Lisa Hamlin, Director of Public Policy

3616   Deaf Children Signers
Harris Communications
15155 Technology Drive
Eden Prairie, MN 55344   952-906-1180
                                                                800-825-6758
                                                          Fax: 952-906-1099
                                                          TTY: 800-825-9187
                                                   info@harriscomm.com
                                                   www.harriscomm.com

This five-part collection of children signers is great for children,
teachers, parents and interpreters. Available in VHS and DVD

Bill Williams, National Sales Manager

3617   Delightful as Derek
American Sign Language Productions
4450 La Crosse Ave
San Diego, CA 92117   952-906-1180
                                                                800-767-4461
                                                          Fax: 952-906-1099
                                                          TTY: 952-906-1198
                                             SignEnhancers@iCloud.com
                                                   www.signenhancers.com

Join Derek, a bright and linguistically advanced 10-year-old, as
he shares his passion for creative projects and home schooling.
His use of ASL will delight and assist you to enhance you own
signing and voicing skills. Benefit from two certified interpreters
demonstrating how to interpret for Derek. 40 minutes. DVD -
$59.95; VHS - $49.95

413

3618 Discovering Cued Speech

Pamela H. Beck, author

Alexander Graham Bell Association for the Deaf
3417 Volta Place NW
Washington, DC 20007

202-337-5220
202-337-8314
Fax: 202-337-8314
TTY: 203-337-5221
info@agbell.org
listeningandspokenlanguage.org

Two-volume video and personal workbook are used in conjunction to make the learning and practice of Cued Speech interesting and effective. A Quick Review at the beginning of each workbook lesson lists the specific goals of that lesson. Participants will read through the lesson in the workbook, use the video instruction to learn, return to the workbook to practice, then return to the video as needed.

78 pages VHS 2:52 min

Lisa Chutjian, Chief Development Officer
Emilio Alonso-Mendoza, Chief Executive Officer
Judy Harrison, Director of Programs

3619 Economic Glitch

Modern Sign Press
10443 Los Alamitos Boulevard, PO Box 1181
Los Alamitos, CA 90720

562-596-8548
800-572-7332
Fax: 562-795-6614
TTY: 562-493-4168
modsigns@modernsignpress.com
www.modernsignpress.com

Basic level videotape of signed story for Expressive and Receptive practice. Story is repeated three times for ease of use. Watch how the visual features are incorporated. Turn the sound off for receptive practice. Written script and tape use suggestions included. VHS

Esther Zawolkow, President

3620 Family Traditions

Modern Sign Press
10443 Los Alamitos Boulevard, PO Box 1181
Los Alamitos, CA 90720

562-596-8548
800-572-7332
Fax: 562-795-6614
TTY: 562-493-4168
modsigns@modernsignpress.com
www.modernsignpress.com

Basic level videotape of signed story for Expressive and Receptive practice. Story is repeated three times for ease of use. Watch how the visual features are incorporated. Turn the sound off for receptive practice. Written script and tape use suggestions included. VHS

Esther Zawolkow, President

3621 Fantastic Videos: Colonial Times, Chocolat e, and Cars

Gallaudet University Press
800 Florida Avenue NE
Washington, DC 20002

202-651-5488
Fax: 202-651-5489
TTY: 202-651-5444
gupress@gallaudet.edu
gupress.gallaudet.edu

Young viewers visit Colonial Williamsburg in Virginia to see various crafts. Other parts show chocolate being made, and films of old cars. VHS, color, voice-over, captions.

VHS 28 minutes
ISBN: 1-563680-06-8

3622 Fantastic Videos: Dogs at Work and Play

Gallaudet University Press
800 Florida Avenue NE
Washington, DC 20002

202-651-5488
Fax: 202-651-5489
TTY: 202-651-5444
gupress@gallaudet.edu
gupress.gallaudet.edu

See how dogs are trained, including Fantastic's own hearing-ear dog, police dogs, plus puppies and dogs in space? VHS, color, voice-over, captions.

VHS 28 minutes
ISBN: 1-563680-03-3

3623 Fantastic Videos: Exciting People, Places and Things!

Gallaudet University Press
800 Florida Avenue NE
Washington, DC 20002

202-651-5488
Fax: 202-651-5489
TTY: 202-651-5444
gupress@gallaudet.edu
gupress.gallaudet.edu

In this program, Rita Corey welcomes young viewers for a trip to a crayon factory, a jump rope tournament, and mime by actor Bernard Bragg. VHS, color, voice-over captions.

VHS 28 minutes
ISBN: 1-563680-01-7

3624 Fantastic Videos: From Post Offices to Dai ry Goats!

Gallaudet University Press
800 Florida Avenue NE
Washington, DC 20002

202-651-5488
Fax: 202-651-5489
TTY: 202-651-5444
gupress@gallaudet.edu
gupress.gallaudet.edu

In this program, children follow the route of a letter from mailbox through the post office to its final destination. Also, they visit dairy goats and other animals. VHS, color, voice-over, captions

VHS 28 minutes
ISBN: 1-563680-05-X

3625 Fantastic Videos: Imagination, Actors, and 'Deaf Way!'

Gallaudet University Press
800 Florida Avenue NE
Washington, DC 20002

202-651-5488
Fax: 202-651-5489
TTY: 202-651-5444
gupress@gallaudet.edu
gupress.gallaudet.edu

Deaf clowns, mimes and actors display the wonders of imaginagion, along with performances at the international cultural celebration 'Deaf Way.' VHS, color, voice-over, captions.

VHS 28 minutes
ISBN: 1-563680-04-1

3626 Fantastic Videos: Roller Coasters, Maps, a nd Ice Cream!

Gallaudet University Press
800 Florida Avenue NE
Washington, DC 20002

202-651-5488
Fax: 202-651-5489
TTY: 202-651-5444
gupress@gallaudet.edu
gupress.gallaudet.edu

Mike Montangino leads the way on rides at Kings Dominion, and also to see how maps are drawn and how ice cream is made. VHS, color, voice-over, captions.

VHS 28 minutes
ISBN: 1-563680-07-6

3627 Fantastic Videos: Skiing, Factories, and R ace Horses

Gallaudet University Press
800 Florida Avenue NE
Washington, DC 20002

202-651-5488
Fax: 202-651-5489
TTY: 202-651-5444
gupress@gallaudet.edu
gupress.gallaudet.edu

Snow Skiing starts this program, which continues in a factory where 'who-knows-what' is made. Also, young viewers learn about horse care, and also the making of Oreos. VHS, color, voice-over, captions.

VHS 28 minutes
ISBN: 1-563680-08-4

3628 Fantastic Videos: The Wonderful Worlds of Sports and Travel
Gallaudet University Press
800 Florida Avenue NE
Washington, DC 20002

202-651-5488
Fax: 202-651-5489
TTY: 202-651-5444
gupress@gallaudet.edu
gupress.gallaudet.edu

In this program, young viewers ride on a train, watch deaf athletes compete, and see actor Bernard Bragg perform The Lion and the Mouse. VHS, color, voice-over, captions.

VHS 28 minutes
ISBN: 1-563680-02-5

3629 Fingerspelling: Expressive and Receptive Fluency
DawnSign Press
6130 Nancy Ridge Drive
San Diego, CA 92121

858-625-0600
800-549-5350
Fax: 858-625-2336
info@dawnsign.com
www.dawnsign.com

This videotape makes the elements of fingerspelling understandable to ASL students. Based on her highly successful and popular workshopes, Joyce Lindene Groode presents a variety of strategies for building and improving the skills for producing fingerspelled words. VHS.

120 minutes
ISBN: 0-915035-13-8

Joyce Linden Groode

3630 Four for You! Fables and Fairy Tales Serie s
Sign Media
4020 Blackburn Lane
Burtonsville, MD 20866

301-421-0268
800-475-4756
Fax: 301-421-0270
info@signmedia.com
www.signmedia.com

Aesop's fables and classic fairy tales performed in ASL. Stars four Sign Language performers and storytellers. Each volume contains four Aesop's fables and two classic fairy tales. The fables are presented twice - first as a straightforward rendition of the story: the second as a dramatized version using minimal sets and props. Voice-over is provided. Activity Packets include printed text of each story in the volume, crossword puzzles, word find challenges, secret message decoding and more.

5 tapes/packets

3631 From Mime to Sign
TJ Publishers
P.O. Box 702701
Dallas, TX 75370

972-416-0800
800-999-1168
Fax: 972-416-0944
TTY: 972-416-0933
customerservice@tjpublishers.com
https://www388.safesecureweb.com/tjpublishers/store/

More than 1,000 photographs illustrate how natural gestures, mime and facial expressions used every day can become the basis for learning sign language. Three videotapes accompany and enhance the text, demonstrating techniques chapter by chapter. Learn to synthesize gesture, mime, facial expression and American Sign Language to truly open the door to visual thinking. VHS or DVD.

1989

Gilbert G Eastman

3632 Generating Business
Modern Sign Press
10443 Los Alamitos Boulevard, PO Box 1181
Los Alamitos, CA 90720

562-596-8548
800-572-7332
Fax: 562-795-6614
TTY: 562-493-4168
modsigns@modernsignspress.com
www.modernsignspress.com

Basic level videotape of signed story for Expressive and Receptive practice. Story is repeated three times for ease of use. Watch how the visual features are incorporated. Turn the sound off for receptive practice. Written script and tape use suggestions included. VHS

Esther Zawolkow, President

3633 Getting Ready for the Big Date
Modern Sign Press
10443 Los Alamitos Boulevard, PO Box 1181
Los Alamitos, CA 90720

562-596-8548
800-572-7332
Fax: 562-795-6614
TTY: 562-493-4168
modsigns@modernsignspress.com
www.modernsignspress.com

Basic level videotape of signed story for Expressive and Receptive practice. Story is repeated three times for ease of use. Watch how the visual features are incorporated. Turn the sound off for receptive practice. Written script and tape use suggestions included. VHS

Esther Zawolkow, President

3634 Ghost Investigation
Modern Sign Press
10443 Los Alamitos Boulevard, PO Box 1181
Los Alamitos, CA 90720

562-596-8548
800-572-7332
Fax: 562-795-6614
TTY: 562-493-4168
modsigns@modernsignspress.com
www.modernsignspress.com

Basic level videotape of signed story for Expressive and Receptive practice. Story is repeated three times for ease of use. Watch how the visual features are incorporated. Turn the sound off for receptive practice. Written script and tape use suggestions included. VHS

Esther Zawolkow, President

3635 Governor's Campaign
Modern Sign Press
10443 Los Alamitos Boulevard, PO Box 1181
Los Alamitos, CA 90720

562-596-8548
800-572-7332
Fax: 562-795-6614
TTY: 562-493-4168
modsigns@modernsignspress.com
www.modernsignspress.com

Basic level videotape of signed story for Expressive and Receptive practice. Story is repeated three times for ease of use. Watch how the visual features are incorporated. Turn the sound off for receptive practice. Written script and tape use suggestions included. VHS

Esther Zawolkow, President

3636 Graduate School
Modern Sign Press
10443 Los Alamitos Boulevard, PO Box 1181
Los Alamitos, CA 90720

562-596-8548
800-572-7332
Fax: 562-795-6614
TTY: 562-493-4168
modsigns@modernsignspress.com
www.modernsignspress.com

Basic level videotape of signed story for Expressive and Receptive practice. Story is repeated three times for ease of use. Watch how the visual features are incorporated. Turn the sound off for receptive practice. Written script and tape use suggestions included. VHS

Esther Zawolkow, President

3637 High Five! Fables and Fairy Tales
Sign Media
4020 Blackburn Lane
Burtonsville, MD 20866

301-421-0268
800-475-4756
Fax: 301-421-0270
info@signmedia.com
www.signmedia.com

The cast of Four for You retuns with the addition of one new member for even more enjoyment. The same format is used here. Each tape includes five fables and two fairy tales. As an added bonus, two fables and one fairy tale are told twice. The first version is the traditional story, the second is how Deaf people would tell each tale. Each tape has a translated voice-over. Set of five 90 minute tapes.

3638 House Guests
Modern Sign Press
10443 Los Alamitos Boulevard, PO Box 1181
Los Alamitos, CA 90720

562-596-8548
800-572-7332
Fax: 562-795-6614
TTY: 562-493-4168
modsigns@modernsignspress.com
www.modernsignspress.com

Basic level videotape of signed story for Expressive and Receptive practice. Story is repeated three times for ease of use. Watch how the visual features are incorporated. Turn the sound off for receptive practice. Written script and tape use suggestions included. VHS

Esther Zawolkow, President

3639 Hungry Caterpillar and Goodnight Moon
Modern Signs Press
10443 Los Alamitos Boulevard, PO Box 1181
Los Alamitos, CA 90720

562-596-8548
800-572-7332
Fax: 562-795-6614
TTY: 562-493-4168
modsigns@modernsignspress.com
www.modernsignspress.com

Two favorite stories beautifully animated and signed using Signing Exact English. VHS

Esther Zawolkow, President

3640 I Remember it Well
Modern Sign Press
10443 Los Alamitos Boulevard, PO Box 1181
Los Alamitos, CA 90720

562-596-8548
800-572-7332
Fax: 562-795-6614
TTY: 562-493-4168
modsigns@modernsignspress.com
www.modernsignspress.com

Basic level videotape of signed story for Expressive and Receptive practice. Story is repeated three times for ease of use. Watch how the visual features are incorporated. Turn the sound off for receptive practice. Written script and tape use suggestions included. VHS

Esther Zawolkow, President

3641 Kudos to Kuualoha
American Sign Language Productions
4450 La Crosse Ave
San Diego, CA 92117

952-906-1180
800-767-4461
Fax: 952-906-1099
TTY: 952-906-1198
SignEnhancers@iCloud.com
www.signenhancers.com

From Hawaii, Kuuolaha, a beautiful, doe eyed child provides commentary on a number of subjects, along with the opportunity to practice reading a child's signs. Prepares you for interpreting in the middle school environment. Two certified interpreters demonstrate for you to compare, contrast and incorporate what you learn to your own skills. 30 minutes. DVD - $59.95; VHS - $49.95

3642 Let's Eat
Modern Sign Press
10443 Los Alamitos Boulevard, PO Box 1181
Los Alamitos, CA 90720

562-596-8548
800-572-7332
Fax: 562-795-6614
TTY: 562-493-4168
modsigns@modernsignspress.com
www.modernsignspress.com

Basic level videotape of signed story for Expressive and Receptive practice. Story is repeated three times for ease of use. Watch how the visual features are incorporated. Turn the sound off for receptive practice. Written script and tape use suggestions included. VHS

Esther Zawolkow, President

3643 Life in the Country
Modern Sign Press
10443 Los Alamitos Boulevard, PO Box 1181
Los Alamitos, CA 90720

562-596-8548
800-572-7332
Fax: 562-795-6614
TTY: 562-493-4168
modsigns@modernsignspress.com
www.modernsignspress.com

Basic level videotape of signed story for Expressive and Receptive practice. Story is repeated three times for ease of use. Watch how the visual features are incorporated. Turn the sound off for receptive practice. Written script and tape use suggestions included. VHS

Esther Zawolkow, President

3644 Listen Learn and Talk
Alexander Graham Bell Association for the Deaf
3417 Volta Place NW
Washington, DC 20007

202-337-5220
202-337-8314
Fax: 202-337-8314
TTY: 203-337-5221
info@agbell.org
listeningandspokenlanguage.org

Three-volume videotape and guidebook set provides general guiding theory, support materials and age-appropriate strategies for parents, families, and early interventionists who practice listening skills with young children. Videos are age specific and include the following developmental categories: 0-15 months, 16-30 months, and 31 months to school age. Softcover, spiral binding manual and three tape VHS set, 1:20 minutes.

Lisa Chutjian, Chief Development Officer
Emilio Alonso-Mendoza, Chief Executive Officer
Judy Harrison, Director of Programs

3645 Listen to This, Volume One

Warren Eastabrooks, Karen MacIver Lux, Lisa Katz, author

Alexander Graham Bell Association for the Deaf
3417 Volta Place NW
Washington, DC 20007

202-337-5220
202-337-8314
Fax: 202-337-6614
TTY: 203-337-5221
info@agbell.org
listeningandspokenlanguage.org

An Auditory-Verbal Therapy Videotape and Guidebook for Professionals and Parents designed for professionals in the fields of Auditory-Verbal therapy, auditory learning and professional education who want to enhance their service delivery of Auditory-Verbal therapy and auditory based learning and for parents of children who are participating in Auditory-Verbal therapy. Workbook - 76 pp., VHS - 47:14 minutes.

Lisa Chutjian, Chief Development Officer
Emilio Alonso-Mendoza, Chief Executive Officer
Judy Harrison, Director of Programs

3646 Listen to This, Volume Two

Warren Eastabrooks, Karen MacIver Lux, Lisa Katz, author

Alexander Graham Bell Association for the Deaf
3417 Volta Place NW
Washington, DC 20007
202-337-5220
202-337-8314
Fax: 202-337-8314
TTY: 203-337-5221
info@agbell.org
listeningandspokenlanguage.org

For health professional and parents of children with hearing loss, this interactive training resource builds upon the Auditory-Verbal therapy skills introduced in Volume 1 and chronicles the journey of Annie, a young girl who lost her hearing as an infant to meningitis. The DVD and step-by-step guidebook models more advance Auditory-Verbal therapy techniques and strategies and features the parent-professional partnership critical to guiding children with hearing loss along the path to listening.

DVD

Lisa Chutjian, Chief Development Officer
Emilio Alonso-Mendoza, Chief Executive Officer
Judy Harrison, Director of Programs

3647 Literacy, Classroom Amplification and the Brain DVD

Carol Flexer, PhD, author

Alexander Graham Bell Association for the Deaf
3417 Volta Place NW
Washington, DC 20007
202-337-5220
202-337-8314
Fax: 202-337-8314
TTY: 203-337-5221
info@agbell.org
listeningandspokenlanguage.org

This intermediate level program focuses on the essential components for enhancing classrooms to optimize the listening environment for school-age children. This video will provide educational information about sound field technology and how to create a favorable listening environment for enhanced development of learning, language and literacy.

DVD

Lisa Chutjian, Chief Development Officer
Emilio Alonso-Mendoza, Chief Executive Officer
Judy Harrison, Director of Programs

3648 Literacy, Classroom Amplification and the Brain

Carol Flexer, PhD, author

Alexander Graham Bell Association for the Deaf
3417 Volta Place NW
Washington, DC 20007
202-337-5220
202-337-8314
Fax: 202-337-8314
TTY: 203-337-5221
info@agbell.org
listeningandspokenlanguage.org

This intermediate level program focuses on the essential components for enhancing classrooms to optimize the listening environment for school-age children. This video will provide educational information about sound field technology and how to create a favorable listening environment for enhanced development of learning, language and literacy.

VHS

Lisa Chutjian, Chief Development Officer
Emilio Alonso-Mendoza, Chief Executive Officer
Judy Harrison, Director of Programs

3649 Loss & Found Hands & Voices

PO Box 3093
Boulder, CO 80307
303-492-6283
866-422-0422
parentadvocate@handsandvoices.org
www.handsandvoices.org

Advice on what to do if your baby did not pass the newborn hearing screening. DVD, voiced, captioned.

3650 Lydia's Lessons

American Sign Language Productions
4450 La Crosse Ave
San Diego, CA 92117
952-906-1180
800-767-4461
Fax: 952-906-1099
TTY: 952-906-1198
SignEnhancers@iCloud.com
www.signenhancers.com

Lydia shares her school and camp experiences along with a rare opportunity to practice receptive skills and interpreting with a 12-year-old client. Here's your stress-free chance to hone your skills for middle school interpreting. Remember, you have two team interpreters to demonstrate how to interpret for Lydia. 40 minutes. DVD - $59.95; VHS - $49.95

3651 Mercer Mayer Frog Stories

Harris Communications
15155 Technology Drive
Eden Prairie, MN 55344
952-906-1180
800-825-6758
Fax: 952-906-1099
TTY: 800-825-9187
info@harriscomm.com
www.harriscomm.com

Three classic Mercer Mayer stories on DVD-R; voiced; signed in ASL; no captions. Features: A Boy, a Dog and a Frog; Frog on His Own; and Frog, Where are You?

3652 My Baby Can Talk: First Signs

Harris Communications
15155 Technology Drive
Eden Prairie, MN 55344
952-906-1180
800-825-6758
Fax: 952-906-1099
TTY: 800-825-9187
info@harriscomm.com
www.harriscomm.com

This is the only baby sign language video that features a young baby signing all the words presented and is considered engaging for young babies. Brightly colored toys, beautiful live footage, engaging images and a young baby signing captivate your baby and as a result your baby learns to sign. This DVD was specifically developed to respect the developmental stage, attention span and intellect of babies from 10 to 24 months. Teaches elementary signs based upon ASL. Ages 10 months and up.

2004 DVD 45 minutes

3653 My Surprise

Modern Sign Press
10443 Los Alamitos Boulevard, PO Box 1181
Los Alamitos, CA 90720
562-596-8548
800-572-7332
Fax: 562-795-6614
TTY: 562-493-4168
modsigns@modernsignspress.com
www.modernsignspress.com

Basic level videotape of signed story for Expressive and Receptive practice. Story is repeated three times for ease of use. Watch how the visual features are incorporated. Turn the sound off for receptive practice. Written script and tape use suggestions included. VHS

Esther Zawolkow, President

3654 New Neighbors

Modern Sign Press
10443 Los Alamitos Boulevard, PO Box 1181
Los Alamitos, CA 90720
562-596-8548
800-572-7332
Fax: 562-795-6614
TTY: 562-493-4168
modsigns@modernsignspress.com
www.modernsignspress.com

Basic level videotape of signed story for Expressive and Receptive practice. Story is repeated three times for ease of use. Watch how the visual features are incorporated. Turn the sound off for receptive practice. Written script and tape use suggestions included. VHS

Esther Zawolkow, President

417

3655 Number Signs for Everyone: Numbering in American Sign Language

DawnSign Press
6130 Nancy Ridge Drive
San Diego, CA 92121
858-625-0600
800-549-5350
Fax: 858-625-2336
info@dawnsign.com
www.dawnsign.com

Presenter Cinnie MacDougall shows you all the different rules and handshapes for clearly and accurately communicating numbers within ASL sentences in proper context. VHS.

90 minutes
ISBN: 0-915035-32-4

Cinnie MacDougall, Presenter

3656 Opinion Section

Modern Sign Press
10443 Los Alamitos Boulevard, PO Box 1181
Los Alamitos, CA 90720
562-596-8548
800-572-7332
Fax: 562-795-6614
TTY: 562-493-4168
modsigns@modernsignspress.com
www.modernsignspress.com

Basic level videotape of signed story for Expressive and Receptive practice. Story is repeated three times for ease of use. Watch how the visual features are incorporated. Turn the sound off for receptive practice. Written script and tape use suggestions included. VHS

Esther Zawolkow, President

3657 Parent Sign Series

Sign Media
4020 Blackburn Lane
Burtonsville, MD 20866
301-421-0268
900-475-4756
Fax: 301-421-0270
info@signmedia.com
www.signmedia.com

Learn sign language within the situations that you face everyday. Rather than wasting time learning vocabulary that doesn't fit your needs, learn the signs that help you communicate quickly with your deaf child. Each tape shows conversations and interactions within a family followed by review sentences and vocabulary items. Perfect for parents to use at home or for sign language programs that offer instruction to parents and beginning signers. Comes in ten one-hour tapes.

VHS

3658 Rainbow's End

Sign Media
4020 Blackburn Lane
Burtonsville, MD 20866
301-421-0268
800-475-4756
Fax: 301-421-0270
info@signmedia.com
www.signmedia.com

It's like Sesame Street but with Deaf characters who use ASL. Designed to enhance the self-image of Deaf children, these five videotapes teach while they entertain. They encourage and lead children to acquisition of English language and reading skills. The Pot of Gold Resource Workbook contains activities and exercises and is fully reproducible. Set includes five 30 minute tapes and workbook.

3659 Rather Strange Stories

Modern Sign Press
10443 Los Alamitos Boulevard, PO Box 1181
Los Alamitos, CA 90720
562-596-8548
800-572-7332
Fax: 562-795-6614
TTY: 562-493-4168
modsigns@modernsignspress.com
www.modernsignspress.com

Created to provide practice in word groups at the intermediate level in Signing Exact English. The word groups were established by topic, and the stories created to use all the words in a given group in the shortest story possible...which is why they are Rather Strange Stories at time. 14 titles: Math/Science, Words Around the House, Prepositions, Words for People, Education/English, Body & Health, Nature, Picnic, Playacting, Sports, Grand Ball, Rabbit/Beaver, Transportation and Religion.

$15 each tape

Esther Zawolkow, President

3660 Russian Soldier

Modern Sign Press
10443 Los Alamitos Boulevard, PO Box 1181
Los Alamitos, CA 90720
562-596-8548
800-572-7332
Fax: 562-795-6614
TTY: 562-493-4168
modsigns@modernsignspress.com
www.modernsignspress.com

Basic level videotape of signed story for Expressive and Receptive practice. Story is repeated three times for ease of use. Watch how the visual features are incorporated. Turn the sound off for receptive practice. Written script and tape use suggestions included. VHS

Esther Zawolkow, President

3661 Science, Math

Modern Sign Press
10443 Los Alamitos Boulevard, PO Box 1181
Los Alamitos, CA 90720
562-596-8548
800-572-7332
Fax: 562-795-6614
TTY: 562-493-4168
modsigns@modernsignspress.com
www.modernsignspress.com

Basic level videotape of signed story for Expressive and Receptive practice. Story is repeated three times for ease of use. Watch how the visual features are incorporated. Turn the sound off for receptive practice. Written script and tape use suggestions included. VHS

Esther Zawolkow, President

3662 Sign Songs: Fun Songs to Sign and Sing

Aylmer Press/TJ Publishers
P.O. Box 702701
Dallas, TX 75370
972-416-0800
800-999-1168
Fax: 972-416-0944
TTY: 972-416-0933
customerservice@tjpublishers.com
https://www388.safesecureweb.com/tjpublishers/store/

Features performers John Kinstler, formerly with the National Theatre of the Deaf, signing along to the lyrics of the eleven kids' songs written and performed by guitarist/singer Ken Lonnquist. Songs include 'Alligator Rag,' 'One Speed Bike,' 'Nattie of the Jungle' plus eight more delightful and fun songs. Lyrics included. VHS.

29 minutes
ISBN: 0-932314-45-7

3663 Sign With Your Baby-Complete Learning Kit

Modern Sign Press
10443 Los Alamitos Boulevard, PO Box 1181
Los Alamitos, CA 90720
562-596-8548
800-572-7332
Fax: 562-795-6614
TTY: 562-493-4168
modsigns@modernsignspress.com
www.modernsignspress.com

Includes video, book and quick reference guide. The video makes learning easy with instruction, demonstrations and tips from the author and Speech-Language Pathologist. Interviews with parents and grandparents who share their experiences and footage of signing babies offers inspirational vision of the power of the system. The book is filled with anecdotes, practical guidelines and humor and offers an effective way to teach parents and infants how to communicate through sign.

VHS and DVD

Joseph Garcia, Author
Alice Stroutsos, Speech-Language Pathologist
Esther Zawolkow, President

3664 Signing Naturally
TJ Publishers
P.O. Box 702701
Dallas, TX 75370

972-416-0800
800-999-1168
Fax: 972-416-0944
TTY: 972-416-0933
customerservice@tjpublishers.com
https://www.388.safesecureweb.com/tjpublishers/store/

This series is based on the functional-notional approach to teaching sign language developed at Vista Community College at Berkeley. Signing Naturally organizes language lessons around everyday interaction. Exercises in the student workbooks coincide with exercises on the videotapes. VHS and DVD

Cheri Smith, Producer
Ella Mae Lentz, Producer
Ken Mikos, Producer

3665 Sleeping Beauty
Gallaudet University Press
800 Florida Avenue NE
Washington, DC 20002

202-651-5488
Fax: 202-651-5489
TTY: 202-651-5444
gupress@gallaudet.edu
gupress.gallaudet.edu

The Sleeping Beauty videotape features the full story in ASL and includes vocabulary and sentence structure focusing on adjectives, with a voice-over throughout. Color, 30 minutes

VHS
ISBN: 0-930323-98-X

3666 Sound & Fury
Aquarius Health Care Videos
18 N Main Street, PO Box 1159
Sherborn, MA 1770

508-650-1616
888-440-2963
Fax: 508-650-1665
info@aquariusproductions.com
www.aquariusproductions.com

This film takes viewers inside the seldom seen world of the deaf to witness a painful family struggle over a controversial medical technology called the cochlear implant. Illuminates the ongoing struggle for identity among deaf people today. Available in VHS and DVD

55 Minutes

Leslie Kusman, President/Producer

3667 Sound and Fury: Six Years Later
Aquarius Health Care Media
18 North Main Street, PO Box 1159
Sherborn, MA 1770

888-440-2963
Fax: 508-650-1665
www.aquariousproductions.com

In 2000, the first Sound & Fury captured audiences around the world and an Academy Award nomination through the riveting story of the Artinian family of Long Island. This sequel gives a new look at the family as it follows them in the next six years of their life. An excellent film for anyone dealing with issues of hearing loss. A must for both professionals and families to see. 2006 - 29 minutes, DVD

3668 Stories About Growing Up
Harris Communciations
15155 Technology Drive
Eden Prairie, MN 55344

952-906-1180
800-825-6758
Fax: 952-906-1099
TTY: 800-825-9187
info@harriscomm.com
www.harriscomm.com

DVD-R - voiced; signed in ASL; no captions. Three Scholastic stories: Leo the Late Bloomer by Robert Kraus (One day, in his own good time, Leo shows everyone how glorious it is to finally bloom); A Weekend with Wendell by Kevin Henkes (Three cheers for compromise as quiet-as-a-mouse Sophie learns to assert herself with big-mouthed Wendell), and Joey Runs Away by Jack Kent (Joey looks for another home when he doesn't like cleaning his room).

3669 The Big Test
Modern Sign Press
10443 Los Alamitos Boulevard, PO Box 1181
Los Alamitos, CA 90720

562-596-8548
800-572-7332
Fax: 562-795-6614
TTY: 562-493-4168
modsigns@modernsignspress.com
www.modernsignspress.com

Basic level videotape of signed story for Expressive and Receptive practice. Story is repeated three times for ease of use. Watch how the visual features are incorporated. Turn the sound off for receptive practice. Written script and tape use suggestions included. VHS

Esther Zawolkow, President

3670 The Driving Test
Modern Sign Press
10443 Los Alamitos Boulevard, PO Box 1181
Los Alamitos, CA 90720

562-596-8548
800-572-7332
Fax: 562-795-6614
TTY: 562-493-4168
modsigns@modernsignspress.com
www.modernsignspress.com

Basic level videotape of signed story for Expressive and Receptive practice. Story is repeated three times for ease of use. Watch how the visual features are incorporated. Turn the sound off for receptive practice. Written script and tape use suggestions included. VHS

Esther Zawolkow, President

3671 The Gossip
Modern Sign Press
10443 Los Alamitos Boulevard, PO Box 1181
Los Alamitos, CA 90720

562-596-8548
800-572-7332
Fax: 562-795-6614
TTY: 562-493-4168
modsigns@modernsignspress.com
www.modernsignspress.com

Basic level videotape of signed story for Expressive and Receptive practice. Story is repeated three times for ease of use. Watch how the visual features are incorporated. Turn the sound off for receptive practice. Written script and tape use suggestions included. VHS

Esther Zawolkow, President

3672 The Grocer and the Cook
Modern Sign Press
10443 Los Alamitos Boulevard, PO Box 1181
Los Alamitos, CA 90720

562-596-8548
800-572-7332
Fax: 562-795-6614
TTY: 562-493-4168
modsigns@modernsignspress.com
www.modernsignspress.com

Basic level videotape of signed story for Expressive and Receptive practice. Story is repeated three times for ease of use. Watch how the visual features are incorporated. Turn the sound off for receptive practice. Written script and tape use suggestions included. VHS

Esther Zawolkow, President

3673 The Memo
Modern Sign Press
10443 Los Alamitos Boulevard, PO Box 1181
Los Alamitos, CA 90720   562-596-8548
                                800-572-7332
                                Fax: 562-795-6614
                                TTY: 562-493-4168
                        modsigns@modernsignpress.com
                        www.modernsignpress.com

Basic level videotape of signed story for Expressive and Receptive practice. Story is repeated three times for ease of use. Watch how the visual features are incorporated. Turn the sound off for receptive practice. Written script and tape use suggestions included. VHS

Esther Zawolkow, President

3674 The Pet Show
Modern Sign Press
10443 Los Alamitos Boulevard, PO Box 1181
Los Alamitos, CA 90720   562-596-8548
                                800-572-7332
                                Fax: 562-795-6614
                                TTY: 562-493-4168
                        modsigns@modernsignpress.com
                        www.modernsignpress.com

Basic level videotape of signed story for Expressive and Receptive practice. Story is repeated three times for ease of use. Watch how the visual features are incorporated. Turn the sound off for receptive practice. Written script and tape use suggestions included. VHS

Esther Zawolkow, President

3675 The Race
Modern Sign Press
10443 Los Alamitos Boulevard, PO Box 1181
Los Alamitos, CA 90720   562-596-8548
                                800-572-7332
                                Fax: 562-795-6614
                                TTY: 562-493-4168
                        modsigns@modernsignpress.com
                        www.modernsignpress.com

Basic level videotape of signed story for Expressive and Receptive practice. Story is repeated three times for ease of use. Watch how the visual features are incorporated. Turn the sound off for receptive practice. Written script and tape use suggestions included. VHS

Esther Zawolkow, President

3676 The Snowman
HEAR-MORE
42 Executive Boulevard
Farmingdale, NY 11735   800-881-4327
                                Fax: 631-752-0689
                                TTY: 800-281-4327
                                www.hearmore.com

This delightful animation weaves a spell of magic enchantment as a young boy's snowman comes to life and escorts him on a fantasy dream visit to the North Pole.

3677 The Treasure Chest

Drs Michelle Anthony and Reyna Lindert, author

HEAR-MORE
42 Executive Boulevard
Farmingdale, NY 11735   800-881-4327
                                Fax: 631-752-0689
                                TTY: 800-281-4327
                                www.hearmore.com

Children of all ages will be delighted by this magical journey of discovery. Join us as we lead you and your child to a treasure trove of toys, plays, songs, and signs. The visually engaging images in the video present families with endless opportunities to make meaningful connections with their little ones. Designed for children aged 0-36 months. Running time is approximately 30 minutes. Includes more than 35 ASL signs.

DVD

3678 The World According to Pat: Reflections of Residential School Days
TJ Publishers
P.O. Box 702701
Dallas, TX 75370   972-416-0800
                                800-999-1168
                                Fax: 972-416-0944
                                TTY: 972-416-0933
                        customerservice@tjpublishers.com
            https://www.388.safesecureweb.com/tjpublishers/store/

Pat Graybill's one-man show offers humerous and touching insights into life in a residential school dormitory. Includes appearances by others who provide their own recollections of residential school days. VHS

90 minutes

3679 University Professor
Modern Sign Press
10443 Los Alamitos Boulevard, PO Box 1181
Los Alamitos, CA 90720   562-596-8548
                                800-572-7332
                                Fax: 562-795-6614
                                TTY: 562-493-4168
                        modsigns@modernsignpress.com
                        www.modernsignpress.com

Basic level videotape of signed story for Expressive and Receptive practice. Story is repeated three times for ease of use. Watch how the visual features are incorporated. Turn the sound off for receptive practice. Written script and tape use suggestions included. VHS

Esther Zawolkow, President

3680 Why We Can Hear And Speak
Alexander Graham Bell Association for the Deaf
3417 Volta Place NW
Washington, DC 20007   202-337-5220
                                202-337-8314
                                Fax: 202-337-8314
                                TTY: 203-337-5221
                                info@agbell.org
                        listeningandspokenlanguage.org

This documentary was developed to show the children of Natural Communication, Inc. at different stages of language development. Each vignette inclueds an introductory biography that briefly describes the child's diagnosis, current age, therapy history and amplification technology. The principles of Auditory-Verbal philosophy are described throughout the tape. All children featured use the Auditory-Verbal approach.

VHS 23 minutes

Lisa Chutjian, Chief Development Officer
Emilio Alonso-Mendoza, Chief Executive Officer
Judy Harrison, Director of Programs

Computer Software

3681 ASL Clip and Create Version 3
HEAR-MORE
42 Executive Boulevard
Farmingdale, NY 11735   800-881-4327
                                Fax: 631-752-0689
                                TTY: 800-281-3555
                                www.hearmore.com

Design learning materials, posters, cards, labels, postcards, and banners using over 3,500 American Sign Language pictures. Four sign-skill enhancing games. Six different templates to customize. Custom design & printing capabilities. Suggestions for learning activities and games. Minimum requirements: Windows 98 SE, Pentium II or equivalent, 64 Mb memory.

3682 **ASL Songs for Kids**
HEAR-MORE
42 Executive Boulevard
Farmingdale, NY 11735

Fax: 631-752-0689
TTY: 800-281-3555
800-881-4327
www.hearmore.com

This CD-Rom presents six songs typically learned by young children-sung and signed. The CD contains two short songs-Twinkle, Twinkle Little Star & Happy Birthday, and four songs that have multiple verses-The Ants Go Marching, Old McDonald, The Wheels on the Bus and The Greeen Grass Grows All Around. 'As the songs are sung, Paws the dog sings, and graphics convey the lyrics, as well as information about the notes and volume. The songs can be viewed with signs in English word order or in ASL.

3683 **ASL Tales and Games for Kids**
HEAR-MORE
42 Executive Boulevard
Farmingdale, NY 11735

Fax: 631-752-0689
TTY: 800-281-3555
800-881-4327
www.hearmore.com

This CD series follows Paws, the signing dog, and his friends as they explore their neighborhood. This program contains 3 community-focused stories and 10 games. The neighborhood children are deaf or hard of hearing and represent different ethnic groups. Minimum system requirements: Windows (95,98,NT,ME,2000), 166 MHz Pentium, 4x CD-ROM Drive

3684 **ASL Tales and Games for Kids 2**
HEAR-MORE
42 Executive Boulevard
Farmingdale, NY 11735

Fax: 631-752-0689
TTY: 800-281-3555
800-881-4327
www.hearmore.com

In this CD-ROM, Biscuit Boulevard focuses on events that take place on one street in Pawstown, Biscuit Boulevard. The stories are original and written to promote good English literacy, while simultaneously teaching important aspects of ASL. Each story can be viewed continuously, without the child needing to manipulate the mouse, or the child can control the story himself.

3685 **ASL Tales and Songs for Kids CD-1**
Harris Communications
15155 Technology Drive
Eden Prairie, MN 55344

952-906-1180
800-825-6758
Fax: 952-906-1099
TTY: 800-825-9187
info@harriscomm.com
www.harriscomm.com

In 'Woof, Woof Way' Paws the Dog helps children build their skills with colorful graphics. Paws, the signing dog, and the Pawstown neighborhood kids on adventures in their own community. System requirements: Windows 95, 98, NT, ME, 2000; Pentium 166MHz; 4X or more CD-ROM drive; works with most popular monochrome and color printers supported by Windows.

CD-ROM

3686 **ASL Tales and Songs for Kids CD-2**
Harris Communications
15155 Technology Drive
Eden Prairie, MN 55344

952-906-1180
800-825-6758
Fax: 952-906-1099
TTY: 800-825-9187
info@harriscomm.com
www.harriscomm.com

Paws, the signing dog, and the Pawstown neighborhood kids on adventures in their own community. In CD-2, 'Biscuit Boulevard,' Paws the Dog helps children build their skills with colorful graphics. System requirements: Windows 95, 98, NT, ME, 2000; Pentium 166MHz; 4X or more CD-ROM drive; works with most popular monochrome and color printers supported by Windows.

CD-ROM

3687 **American Sign Language V2.0**
HEAR-MORE
42 Executive Boulevard
Farmingdale, NY 11735

Fax: 631-752-0689
TTY: 800-281-3555
800-881-4327
www.hearmore.com

This updated version comes as a 5 CD-ROM set. Customize signing pace with the speed control feature. Takes you from beginner to advanced intermediate levels. Set includes SigningAvatar, HyperSign Jr, Ready! Set! Sign! Starter version, ASL Condensed Dictionary, and ASL introduction which aids children in developing essential analytical skills. System requirements: 500 MHz or faster, Windows 98/ME/XP, 128 MB RAM, 100 MB hard drive.

3688 **American Sign Language Vocabulary**
HEAR-MORE
42 Executive Boulevard
Farmingdale, NY 11735

Fax: 631-752-0689
TTY: 800-281-3555
800-881-4327
www.hearmore.com

PC requirements: Pentium 120 MHz or faster, Win 95, 98, NT4, 2000, 64 MB RAM, active movie 1.0 or higher, DirectShow 6.0 recommended, Active X Network libraries. Macintosh Requirements: PowerPC or later, 120 MHz or faster, MacOS 7+, 64 MB RAM, Quicktime 3 or higher, Quicktime mpeg extension v1.1.1 or higher.

3689 **Baby's First Book of Signs: An ASL Word Book (Volume 1-3)**
HEAR-MORE
42 Executive Boulevard
Farmingdale, NY 11735

Fax: 631-752-0689
TTY: 800-281-3555
800-881-4327
www.hearmore.com

Three sweet little electronic books depict the signs for basic words. Signs are shown in video and pictures. English equivalents, as well as concept graphics, are included. Easy to use-just click to turn each page. Volume 1 includes: Animals, Clothes, Colors, Food and Toys. Volume 2 includes: Actions, Descriptions, Feelings, When and Where. Volume 3 includes: Alphabet, Numbers, Home, Outside and People. CD-ROM

3690 **Baby's First Book of Signs: Volumes I-III**
Harris Communications
15155 Technology Drive
Eden Prairie, MN 55344

952-906-1180
800-825-6758
Fax: 952-906-1099
TTY: 800-825-9187
info@harriscomm.com
www.harriscomm.com

An ASL Word Book with Video and Audio Clips. Each CD-ROM contains an electronic flip book for basic words in video and pictures. English equivalents (in print and audio), as well as concept graphics, are included. In these three CD-ROMs, you can learn 390 words in sign language. Minimum PC requirements: Windows 98, ME, 2000, XP; 64 MB RAM, 800x600 pixels screen area; Pentium II'300 MHz; 16-bit color display; CD-ROM drive.

3691 **Cochlear Impant Auditory Training Guide**
David Sindrey, Cert. AVT, author

Alexander Graham Bell Association for the Deaf
3417 Volta Place NW
Washington, DC 20007

202-337-5220
202-337-8314
Fax: 202-337-8314
TTY: 203-337-5221
info@agbell.org
listeningandspokenlanguage.org

This second edition comes with games pieces, peg boards, and two print CDs. The manual presents easy to follow hierarchy and the CDs include a placement test, lesson plan forms, acoustic screens, and hundreds of discrimination cards and activities for single word, multiple element and broader language listening at all levels. The Wordplay product Vattier Boards has now been incorporated into this package.

Lisa Chutjian, Chief Development Officer
Emilio Alonso-Mendoza, Chief Executive Officer
Judy Harrison, Director of Programs

3692 Elf on a Shelf for Minimal Pairs: Giant CD Print Program

David Sindrey, Cert. AVT, author

Alexander Graham Bell Association for the Deaf
3417 Volta Place NW
Washington, DC 20007 202-337-5220
202-337-8314
Fax: 202-337-8314
TTY: 203-337-5221
info@agbell.org
listeningandspokenlanguage.org

Print more than 1100 English words. This program organizes effective word-pair practice into the following formats: Lotto games, Dixie Cup games, Matrix games, Fiv. Operates on any PC or MAC system.

Lisa Chutjian, Chief Development Officer
Emilio Alonso-Mendoza, Chief Executive Officer
Judy Harrison, Director of Programs

3693 Hear & Listen! Talk & Sing!

Warren Estabrooks MEd, Lois Birkenshaw-Fleming BA, author

Alexander Graham Bell Association for the Deaf
3417 Volta Place NW
Washington, DC 20007 202-337-5220
202-337-8314
Fax: 202-337-8314
TTY: 203-337-5221
info@agbell.org
listeningandspokenlanguage.org

This music book and CD integrates songs with speech sounds to enable young children with hearing loss to develop melodic, natural-sounding voices and enhance linguistic skills. Songs include sounds that are acoustically relevant to children with severe or profound hearing loss ages 18 months to 7 years. Songs are grouped in categories such as animals, weather and holidays and vary in difficulty.

Lisa Chutjian, Chief Development Officer
Emilio Alonso-Mendoza, Chief Executive Officer
Judy Harrison, Director of Programs

3694 Hearing is Believing, Volume One

Dimity Dornan, BA, author

Alexander Graham Bell Association for the Deaf
3417 Volta Place NW
Washington, DC 20007 202-337-5220
202-337-8314
Fax: 202-337-8314
TTY: 202-337-5221
info@agbell.org
listeningandspokenlanguage.org

The first volume of the Hearing is Believing distance education series on CD-ROM offers self-directed learning through four hours of lectures on the following Auditory-Verbal topics: Current Auditory-Verbal PRactice and Research, Auditory Learning, Listening for Older Children, Integration into the Mainstream School. Includes lectures within the framework of the Auditory-Verbal Curriculum, accompanying PowerPoint slides, video excerpts of Auditory-Verbal therapy sessions and transcripts.

Lisa Chutjian, Chief Development Officer
Emilio Alonso-Mendoza, Chief Executive Officer
Judy Harrison, Director of Programs

3695 Hearing is Believing, Volume Three

Dimity Dornan, BA, author

Alexander Graham Bell Association for the Deaf
3417 Volta Place NW
Washington, DC 20007 202-337-5220
202-337-8314
Fax: 202-337-8314
TTY: 202-337-5221
info@agbell.org
listeningandspokenlanguage.org

This third volume in the Hearing is Believing series provides four hours of self-directed learning on the following Auditory-Verbal topics: Teaching Spoken Language, Speech Development, Working with Parents and Infants. Includes lectures within the framework of the Auditory-Verbal curriculum, accompanying PowerPoint slides, video excerpts of Audio-Verbal therapy sessions and transcripts. A note-taking feature allows you to jot down ideas and questions as you learn.

Lisa Chutjian, Chief Development Officer
Emilio Alonso-Mendoza, Chief Executive Officer
Judy Harrison, Director of Programs

3696 Hearing is Believing, Volume Two

Judith A Marlow, PhD, author

Alexander Graham Bell Association for the Deaf
3417 Volta Place NW
Washington, DC 20007 202-337-5220
202-337-8314
Fax: 202-337-8314
TTY: 202-337-5221
info@agbell.org
listeningandspokenlanguage.org

This interactive CD-ROM, the second volume in the Hearing is Believing distance eduction series includes two hours of lectures on early detection and intervention: The Rationale for Early Detection and Current Status, Achieving Timely Evaluation and Intervention, Shifting Paradigms. Includes lectures within the framework of the Auditory-Verbal curriculum, accompanying PowerPoint slides, video excerpts of Auditory-Verbal therapy sessions and transcripts.

Lisa Chutjian, Chief Development Officer
Emilio Alonso-Mendoza, Chief Executive Officer
Judy Harrison, Director of Programs

3697 Holidays CD-ROM

Harris Communications
15155 Technology Drive
Eden Prairie, MN 55344 952-906-1180
800-825-6758
Fax: 952-906-1099
TTY: 800-825-9187
info@harriscomm.com
www.harriscomm.com

This electronic book teaches 303 basic signs for 13 holidays: New Year, Valentine's Day, Patriotic Days, St. Patrick's Day, Easter, Graduation, Jewish Holidays, Parents' Days, Halloween, Christmas, Birthdays, Weddings and Thanksgiving. Minimum PC requirements: Windows 98, ME, 2000, XP; Pentium II 300MHz; 64 MB RAM; 16-bit color display; 800x600 pixels screen area; CD-ROM drive.

3698 Holidays: An ASL Word Book

HEAR-MORE
42 Executive Boulevard
Farmingdale, NY 11735 800-881-4327
Fax: 631-752-0689
TTY: 800-281-3555
www.hearmore.com

This electronic book teaches all of the basic signs for 13 holidays. Signs are shown in video and pictures. English equivalents, as well as concept graphics, are included. Holidays covered include: New Year, Valentine's Day, Patriotic Days, St. Patrick's Day, Easter, Christmas, Jewish Holidays, Thanksgiving, Graduation, Weddings/Anniversaries, Hallowween, Birthday, and Parents' Days. Easy to use-just click to turn each page. Windows 98/ME/2000/XP, Pentium 2 300 MHz, 64 MB Ram, CD drive

3699 I Cue, U Cue
HEAR-MORE
42 Executive Boulevard
Farmingdale, NY 11735   800-881-4327
Fax: 631-752-0689
TTY: 800-281-3555
www.hearmore.com

This software provides information about Cued Speech. Cued Speech combines hand-shapes and placements with mouth movements to represent the consonants and vowels of a language. The complete American English system is taught through 14 classes, with an additional class providing extra practice. Includes guide. Windows 98SE, ME, 2000, XP; CD-ROM drive, 16X; Pentium III, 600 MHz or eqivalent; 190 MD hard drive space.

3700 Illustrated Dictionary - 3D ASL
HEAR-MORE
42 Executive Boulevard
Farmingdale, NY 11735   800-881-4327
Fax: 631-752-0689
TTY: 800-281-3555
www.hearmore.com

This CD-ROM Dictionary is designed for everyone who wants to learn American Sign Language. Choose one of nine characters with different personalities and ethnic backgrounds. Characters fidget while waiting and show emotions, like impatience or happiness. Every word in the dictionary is represented by a picture, used in a sentence and signed by your selected character. System requirements: 300 MHz PC, Windows 98/ME/NT/2000/XP, Internet Explorer 4+, CD-ROM, 1024X768 monitor, 100MB hard drive space

3701 Johnny Rock's Christmas
HEAR-MORE
42 Executive Boulevard
Farmingdale, NY 11735   800-881-4327
Fax: 631-752-0689
TTY: 800-281-3555
www.hearmore.com

This software is specially designed to enhance vocabulary development for deaf and hard of hearing students and elementary aged students with similar language needs. Teachers and Parents will love it as much as the kids will. Delightful graphics. Easy installation. Non-auditory. On-line technical support. Two 3.5 diskettes. Runs on Windows/Win95/Win98.

3702 Ling Series

Daniel Ling, PhD, author

Alexander Graham Bell Association for the Deaf
3417 Volta Place NW
Washington, DC 20007   202-337-5220
202-337-8314
Fax: 202-337-8314
TTY: 202-337-5221
info@agbell.org
listeningandspokenlanguage.org

Learn at your own pace with this CD-ROM distance education program featuring lectures from the University of Ottawa seminar in Auditory-Verbal practices. Topics include: Assessment of Spoken Language, Phonological Processes, Remediation of Deviant Speech. The CD includes the lecture, accompanying PowerPoint slides, clips of Ling's students, full lecture transcripts and a note-taking feature that allows you to jot down ideas and questions as you learn.

Lisa Chutjian, Chief Development Officer
Emilio Alonso-Mendoza, Chief Executive Officer
Judy Harrison, Director of Programs

3703 Marvin Teaches Fingerspelling
HEAR-MORE
42 Executive Boulevard
Farmingdale, NY 11735   800-881-4327
Fax: 631-752-0689
TTY: 800-281-3555
www.hearmore.com

This CD is the coolest way yet to improve your receptive fingerspelling skills. Beginners can learn to recognize the different handshapes that make up the letters of the alphabet. Signers of every ability level can practice reading many fingerspelled words at speeds varying from novice to expert. Minimum system requirements: Pentium I, Windows 95, CD drive.

3704 MyTTY Phone Messenger Software for Windows
HEAR-MORE
42 Executive Boulevard
Farmingdale, NY 11735   800-881-4327
Fax: 631-752-0689
TTY: 800-281-3555
www.hearmore.com

myTTY Phone Messenger is out-dialing software. It allows you to send pre-recorded TTY text and/or voice message to each telephone number on a customizable list. It can be used for such purposes as emergency, informational, meeting, and advertising notifications. Requires Windows 2000 or XP; 32 MB memory, Pentium Processor or compatible, CD-Rom dirve; TAPI-complieant voice modem.

3705 MyTTY for Windows 95, 98, ME, 2000, XP
HEAR-MORE
42 Executive Boulevard
Farmingdale, NY 11735   800-881-4327
Fax: 631-752-0689
TTY: 800-281-3555
www.hearmore.com

Now you can use your PC as a TTY too. myTTY is a computer program that runs under the Microsoft Windows operating system. If the computer is equipped with a voice modem, myTTY will make the computer perform like a TTY. The program allows your computer to communicate with any Baudot TTY over a telephone line. Requirements: Windows 98, SE or later (XP compatible) with Internet Explorer 4.0 or later, a Pentium processor or equivalent, CD drive, TAP compliant modem and 32 MB of memory.

3706 Paws Sign Stories
Harris Communications
15155 Technology Drive
Eden Prairie, MN 55344   952-906-1180
800-825-6758
Fax: 952-906-1099
TTY: 800-825-9187
info@harriscomm.com
www.harriscomm.com

An educational and entertaining program designed for deaf and hard of hearing children who want to learn American Sign Language. Includes 5 stories and 15 games. Click on individual words or whole sentences to have them signs and voiced. Includes video clips of a person dressed as Paws, using ASL so all information is accessible to deaf and hard of hearing children. Ages 3-7.

CD-ROM

3707 Ready! Set! Sign!
HEAR-MORE
42 Executive Boulevard
Farmingdale, NY 11735   800-881-4327
Fax: 631-752-0689
TTY: 800-281-3555
www.hearmore.com

Begin with 100 signs you already know. Then continue learning over 1,000 more using video clips, photos, animations and graphics as visual aids for learning and remembering signs. Afterwards study the topics that interest you: fingerspelling, numbers, grammar concepts, and more. Learn the vocabulary you want, when you want it. Test your current sign language knowledge by reading over 1,750 signed practice sentences, phrases, words and numbers. View one or more of twenty-three Cultural Moments.

3708 School Days
Harris Communications
15155 Technology Drive
Eden Prairie, MN 55344
                                          952-906-1180
                                          800-825-6758
                                          Fax: 952-906-1099
                                          TTY: 800-825-9187
                                          info@harriscomm.com
                                          www.harriscomm.com

An ASL Word Book with Video and Audio Clips. Prepare your
child for school with this fun electronic book of 76 basic school
vocabulary words. Each page shows the sign in both video and a
picture. English equivalents in print and audio, plus concept
graphics are included. Minimum system requirements: Windows
98, ME, 2000, XP; Pentium II 300MHz; 64MB RAM; 16-bit color
display; 800x600 pixels screen area; CD-ROM drive.

CD-ROM

3709 School Days: An ASL Word Book
HEAR-MORE
42 Executive Boulevard
Farmingdale, NY 11735
                                          800-881-4327
                                          Fax: 631-752-0689
                                          TTY: 800-281-3555
                                          www.hearmore.com

Prepare your child for school with this fun little electronic book
of basic school signs. Each page shows the sign in both video and
a picture. English equivalents (in print and audio), as well as concept graphics, are included. 76 signs in all. Easy to use-just click
to turn each page. Minimum system requirements: Windows
98/ME/2000/XP, Pentium 2 300 MHz, 64 MB Ram, 16-bit color
display, 800x600 pixels screen area, CD drive.

3710 Sign Fine - Vacations
HEAR-MORE
42 Executive Boulevard
Farmingdale, NY 11735
                                          800-881-4327
                                          Fax: 631-752-0689
                                          TTY: 800-281-3555
                                          www.hearmore.com

Join Paws, the signing dog, as he goes to 14 different travel desti-
nations. Just click on any of the items in the picture to see a video
of Paws signing the vocabulary word and an English word equivalent. This CD-Rom software for Windows has over 550 American Sign Language videos that illustrate signs and three fun
games to play. Requires Windows 98, ME, 200, XP, Pentium III,
600 MHZ or equivalent, CD-Rom drive and 90 MB of hard drive
space.

3711 Simser Series

Judith Simser, author

Alexander Graham Bell Association for the Deaf
3417 Volta Place NW
Washington, DC 20007
                                          202-337-5220
                                          202-337-8314
                                          Fax: 202-337-8314
                                          TTY: 202-337-5221
                                          info@agbell.org
                                          listeningandspokenlanguage.org

Enhance your knowledge with this interactive CD-ROM distance
education program featuring lectures from the University of
Ottowa seminar in Auditory-Verbal practices. Topics include: Au-
ditory-Verbal Techniques and Hierarchies, Ongoing Assessment,
The Why and How of Toys and Games, Goals for the Cochlear
Implant User. The CD includes the lectures, accompanying
PowerPoint slides, demonstrations of an Auditory-Verbal therapy
session, audio clips of students, and full lecture transcripts.

Lisa Chutjian, Chief Development Officer
Emilio Alonso-Mendoza, Chief Executive Officer
Judy Harrison, Director of Programs

3712 Smile

Enid G Wolf-Schein, EdD, CCC-SLP, author

Alexander Graham Bell Association for the Deaf
3417 Volta Place NW
Washington, DC 20007
                                          202-337-5220
                                          202-337-8314
                                          Fax: 202-337-8314
                                          TTY: 203-337-5221
                                          info@agbell.org
                                          listeningandspokenlanguage.org

SMILE is a multisensory program that teaches speech, reading,
and writing to children with severe language and communication
delays, including those with hearing loss, dyslexia, or autism.
Unique in its engaging yet simple focus, SMILE uses expressive
and receptive modalities to improve the reading skills of target
and general populations. Softcover manual 138 pp. CD and
five-Teacher's Guide set.

Lisa Chutjian, Chief Development Officer
Emilio Alonso-Mendoza, Chief Executive Officer
Judy Harrison, Director of Programs

3713 Snap! Kids American Sign Language
HEAR-MORE
42 Executive Boulevard
Farmingdale, NY 11735
                                          800-881-4327
                                          Fax: 631-752-0689
                                          TTY: 800-281-3555
                                          www.hearmore.com

This CD-ROM focuses on ASL basics. Especially for young read-
ers, this disc is full of interactive games and animated vocabulary
allowing kids to master new signs while having fun. 26 vocabu-
lary 'books' covering subjects from Action words to Animals;
Transportation to Telling Time. Instructional Demos featuring
Live-action video signing. ASL Games including Tic Tac Toe and
Multiple Choice. System Requirements: Processor 386 DX/33
MHz or faster, Win 3.1, 8 MB RAM, 6 MB HD, 2X CD-ROM,
Sound card

3714 Songs for Listening! Songs for Life!

Warren Estabrooks MEd, Lois Birkenshaw-Fleming BA, author

Alexander Graham Bell Association for the Deaf
3417 Volta Place NW
Washington, DC 20007
                                          202-337-5220
                                          202-337-8314
                                          Fax: 202-337-8314
                                          TTY: 203-337-5221
                                          info@agbell.org
                                          listeningandspokenlanguage.org

A song book/CD set and therapy guide. Designed to teach children with hearing loss how to listen and talk through the use of
singing and music. It includes early intervention activities as well
as resources for parents and professionals who work to develop
audition and spoken language in children with hearing loss and/or
other communicative disorders. This publication incorporates
current language-learning therapy, is presented in an easy-to-read
format, and includes technical references.

Lisa Chutjian, Chief Development Officer
Emilio Alonso-Mendoza, Chief Executive Officer
Judy Harrison, Director of Programs

3715 The Ultimate ASL Dictionary
HEAR-MORE
42 Executive Boulevard
Farmingdale, NY 11735
                                          800-881-4327
                                          Fax: 631-752-0689
                                          TTY: 800-281-3555
                                          www.hearmore.com

Over 2400 signs included. Identify words through ASL or English, Words and definitions in video clips, graphics, text and audio, variations of English words that relate to a single sign,
spell-check and parameter check.

3716 Troll In A Bowl: Games and Card Print Fact ory

David Sindrey, Cert. AVT, author

Alexander Graham Bell Association for the Deaf
3417 Volta Place NW
Washington, DC 20007

202-337-5220
202-337-8314
Fax: 202-337-8314
TTY: 203-337-5221
info@agbell.org
listeningandspokenlanguage.org

Features over 2000 articulation, minimal pair, and vocabulary cards organized by a Speech-Language Pathologist. Operates on any PC or MAC system. Includes 54 page soft-cover spiral-binding workbook, game piece and CD

Lisa Chutjian, Chief Development Officer
Emilio Alonso-Mendoza, Chief Executive Officer
Judy Harrison, Director of Programs

Book Publishers

3717 50 Freqeunty Asked Questions About Audito ry-Verbal Therapy

Warren Estabrooks, MEd, author

Alexander Graham Bell Association for the Deaf
3417 Volta Place NW
Washington, DC 20007

202-337-5220
Fax: 202-337-8314
TTY: 202-337-5221
info@agbell.org
www.agbell.org

A prolific collection of responses to most frequently asked questions about auditory-verbal therapy and its application for children who are deaf and hard of hearing. Parents, professionals and everyone concerned with deafness will welcome the guidance, encouragement and knowledge found within this collaboration of professionals who have joined both hearts and minds to provide an extraordinary, informative and invaluable worldwide resource.

213 pages Softcover

3718 A Basic Course in American Sign Lanuage, Second Edition

Tom Humphries, Carol Padden, Terrenc J O'Rourke, author

TJ Publishers
P.O Box 702701
Dallas, TX 75370

972-416-0800
800-999-1168
Fax: 972-416-0944
TTY: 972-416-0933
customerservice@tjpublishers.com
www.tjpublishers.com

Features a new introduction, which includes a section on Deaf Culture and Community, expanded dialogue introductions that incorporate cultural information, revised grammar notes and an updated bibliography.

288 pages Spiral bound
ISBN: 0-932666-42-6

3719 A Basic Vocabulary: American Sign Language for Parents and Children

Terrence J O'Rourke, author

TJ Publishers
P.O Box 702701
Dallas, TX 75370

972-416-0800
800-999-1168
Fax: 972-416-0944
TTY: 972-416-0933
customerservice@tjpublishers.com
www.tjpublishers.com

Carefully selected words and signs include those families use every day. Alphabetically organized vocabulary incorporates developmental lists helpful to both Deaf and hearing children and over 1000 clear sign language illustrations.

240 pages Softcover
ISBN: 0-932666-00-0

3720 A Book of Colors: Baby's First Sign Book

Kim Votry and Curt Waller, author

Gallaudet University Press
800 Florida Avenue NE
Washington, DC 20002

202-651-5488
Fax: 202-651-5489
gupress@gallaudet.edu
www.gupress.gallaudet.edu

Depicts the charming character with the favorite hat signing all of the primary and secondary colors - red, yellow, blue, orange green and purple - in interesting settings. The other pages display a wide variety of appealing colors, too, including pink, white, black, gray, brown, and tan, topped off with a richly rendered illustration of a rainbow.

16 pages Board book
ISBN: 1-563681-47-1

3721 A Season of Change

Lois L Hodge, author

Gallaudet University Press
800 Florida Avenue NE
Washington, DC 20002

202-651-5488
Fax: 202-651-5489
gupress@gallaudet.edu
www.gupress.gallaudet.edu

Okay, so she can't hear as well as other people, but do they believe she can't think as well? Everyone, it seems, in 13-going-on-14-year-old Biney Richmond's life treats her as though she should be wrapped in cotton and set on a shelf. Her parents act as though she can't do things for herself. The only one who seems to have any confidence in her is her best friend, Pat. When Pat's older brother, Gene-who secretly wants to date Biney-gets in trouble, Biney proves to everyone how grown up she is.

108 pages Softcover
ISBN: 0-930323-27-0

3722 ABC's of Finger Spelling

Modern Signs Press
PO Box 1181
Los Alamitos, CA 90720

562-596-8548
800-572-7332
Fax: 562-795-6614
TTY: 562-493-4168
modsigns@modernsignspress.com
www.modernsignspress.com

Helps teach upper and lower case letters of the alphabet. Includes printed letters and easy-to-follow drawings of the hand shapes.

1984 60 pages paperback

3723 ABCs of AVT: Analyzing Auditory-Verbal The rapy

Warren Estabrooks, MEd and Rhonda Schwartz, MA, author

Alexander Graham Bell Association for the Deaf
3417 Volta Place NW
Washington, DC 20007

202-337-5220
Fax: 202-337-8314
TTY: 202-337-5221
info@agbell.org
www.agbell.org

Provides an overview of Auditory-Verbal techniques and guidance on appropriate intervention for children experiencing difficulties with language development. Task analysis exercises outlined in the manual and demonstrated in the video, which contains excerpts of therapy sessions and longitudinal studies, are designed to help students and professionals of all levels of experience hone their clinical skills. Softcover/Spiral binding/manual and VHS set/Open-Captioned 46:04

104 pages Softcover

3724 ASL Babies: First Signs

Tina Jo Breindel and Michael Carter, author

Harris Communications
15155 Technology Drive
Eden Prairie, MN 55344

952-906-1180
800-825-6758
Fax: 952-906-1099
TTY: 800-825-9187
info@harriscomm.com
www.harriscomm.com

A toddler signs 14 words that first appear in a child's vocabulary: airplane, baby, bath, bed, dad, help, hot, hurt, mom, more, please, thank you, tired and toilet.

16 pages Board book

3725 ASL Babies: Let's Eat

Tina Jo Breindel and Michael Carter, author

Harris Communications
15155 Technology Drive
Eden Prairie, MN 55344

952-906-1180
800-825-6758
Fax: 952-906-1099
TTY: 800-825-9187
info@harriscomm.com
www.harriscomm.com

Food-related vocabulary words in English and American Sign Language are beautifully illustrated in this board book.

16 pages Board book

3726 AUSPLAN Auditory Speech and Language

Adeline McClatchie, LCST and MaryKay Therres, MS, author

Alexander Graham Bell Association for the Deaf
3417 Volta Place NW
Washington, DC 20007

202-337-5220
Fax: 202-337-8314
TTY: 202-337-5221
info@agbell.org
www.agbell.org

AuSpLan is a communication therapy manual for children using choclear implants or hearing aids. It addresses auditory, speech/articulation, and language skills of children between the ages of 18 months and 5 years.

212 pages Softcover

3727 Alandra's Lilacs

Tressa Bowers, author

Gallaudet University Press
800 Florida Avenue NE
Washington, DC 20002

202-651-5488
Fax: 202-651-5489
gupress@gallaudet.edu
www.gupress.gallaudet.edu

When, in 1968, 19-year-old Tressa Bowers took her baby daughter to an expert on deaf children, he pronounced that Alandra was 'stone deaf,' she most likely would never be able to talk, and she probably would not get much of an education because of her communication limitations. Tressa refused to accept this stark assessment of Alandra's prospects. Instead, she began the arduous process of starting her daughter's education.

158 pages Softcover
ISBN: 1-563680-82-3

3728 All of Us Together

Jeri Banks, author

Gallaudet University Press
800 Florida Avenue NE
Washington, DC 20002

202-651-5488
Fax: 202-651-5489
gupress@gallaudet.edu
wwwgupress.gallaudet.edu

John H. Kinzie Elementary School, in Chicago, for decades was the pride of its neighborhood until changing demographics, racial conflict, and desegregation mandates threatened its existance. Then, its new principal, James Burke, welcomed 15 classes of deaf and hard of hearing children. This is the story of the Kinzie School from 1982, when hearing and nonhearing populations were kept in separate parts of the school, to the present in which all students intermingle freely and achieve together.

212 pages Hardcover
ISBN: 1-563680-28-9

3729 Alone in the Mainstream: A Deaf Women Reme mbers Public School

Gina A Oliva, author

Gallaudet University Press
800 Florida Avenue NE
Washington, DC 20002

202-651-5488
Fax: 202-651-5489
gupress@gallaudet.edu
www.gupress.gallaudet.edu

When Gina Oliva first went to school in 1955, she didn't know that she was 'different.' If the kindergarten teacher played a tune on the piano to signal the next exercise, Olivia didn't react because she couldn't hear the music. So began her journey as a 'solitary,' her term for being the only deaf child in the entire school. Gina felt alone because she couldn't communicate easily with her classmates, but also because none of them had a hearing loss like hers.

224 pages Softcover
ISBN: 1-563683-00-8

3730 Alphabet of Animal Signs

HEAR-MORE
42 Executive Boulevard
Farmingdale, NY 11735

800-881-4327
Fax: 631-752-0689
TTY: 800-281-3555
www.hearmore.com

This book includes animal illustrations and associated signs for each letter of the alphabet.

3731 American Deaf Culture: An Anthology

Sign Media
4020 Blackburn Lane
Burtonsville, MD 20866

301-421-0268
800-475-4756
Fax: 301-421-0270
TDD: 301-421-4460
signmedia@aol.com
www.signmedia.com

Features deaf and hearing authors offering their experience and perspectives on cultural values, ASL, social interaction in the deaf community, education, folklore and more.

202 pages Paperback
ISBN: 0-932130-09-7

Barbara Olmert, Director Marketing

3732 American Sign Language Dictionary Third Ed ition

Martin L A Stemberg, author

TJ Publishers
P.O Box 702701
Dallas, TX 75370

972-416-0800
800-999-1168
Fax: 972-416-0944
TTY: 972-416-0933
customerservice@tjpublishers.com
www.tjpublishers.com

Completely updated and revised, this easy to use abridged version of the American Sign Language: A Comprehensive Dictionary has more than 500 new signs and 1500 new illustrations. It contains more than 5000 of the most widely used words, phrases, and idioms, accompanied by 8000 easy-to-follow illustrations of the hand, arm and facial movements that express each one.

772 pages Softcover
ISBN: 0-062736-34-5

3733 American Sign Language: A Student Text; Units 10-18
Sign Media
4020 Blackburn Lane
Burtonsville, MD 20866

800-475-4756
Fax: 301-421-0270
www.signmedia.com

These texts were designed to help students acquire conversational abilities in American Sign Language. Each unit targets a specific grammatical feature of ASL and presents a dialogue focusing on that grammatical feature. Dialogues are presented three times - the first is a shot of both conversational participants, the second and third presentations each focus on one of the participants. Following the dialogues are anecdotes, stories and poems.

ISBN: 0-930323-87-4

3734 American Sign Language: A Student Text; Units 1-9
Sign Media
4020 Blackburn Lane
Burtonsville, MD 20866

800-475-4756
Fax: 301-421-0270
www.signmedia.com

These texts were designed to help students acquire conversational abilities in American Sign Language. Each unit targets a specific grammatical feature of ASL and presents a dialogue focusing on that grammatical feature. Dialogues are presented three times - the first is a shot of both conversational participants, the second and third presentations each focus on one of the participants. Following the dialogues are anecdotes, stories and poems.

ISBN: 0-930323-86-6

3735 American Sign Language: A Student Text; Un its 19-27
Sign Media
4020 Blackburn Lane
Burtonsville, MD 20866

800-475-4756
Fax: 301-421-0270
www.signmedia.com

These texts were designed to help students acquire conversational abilities in American Sign Language. Each unit targets a specific grammatical feature of ASL and presents a dialogue focusing on that grammatical feature. Dialogues are presented three times - the first is a shot of both conversational participants, the second and third presentations each focus on one of the participants. Following the dialogues are anecdotes, stories and poems.

ISBN: 0-930323-88-2

3736 Animal Signs: A First Book of Sign Languag e
Debbie Slier, author

Gallaudet University Press
800 Florida Avenue NE
Washington, DC 20002

202-651-5488
Fax: 202-651-5489
gupress@gallaudet.edu
www.gupress.gallaudet.edu

Charming, full-color photographs of basic animals plus illustrations of their corresponding signs offer children ages 1 to 4 a fun way to learn their first signs and vocabulary words.

16 pages Board Book
ISBN: 1-563680-49-1

3737 Approaching Equality
TJ Publishers
P.O Box 702701
Dallas, TX 75370

972-416-0800
800-999-1168
Fax: 972-416-0944
TTY: 972-416-0933
customerservice@tjpublishers.com
www.tjpublsihers.com

Public education laws guarantee special education programs for all Deaf children, but many find the special education system confusing, or are unsure of their rights under the current law. Those with an interest in education, advocacy and the Deaf community will find this review of dramatic developments in the education of Deaf children, youth and adults most informative. Written by the former chair of the Commission on the Education of the Deaf.

1991 112 pages Softcover
ISBN: 0-932666-39-6

Frank Bowe, Author

3738 Auditory-Verbal Therapy and Practice
Alexander Graham Bell Association for the Deaf
3417 Volta Place NW
Washington, DC 20007

202-337-5220
800-432-7543
Fax: 202-337-8314
TTY: 202-337-5221
info@agbell.org
www.agbell.org

A comprehensive book introducing auditory-verbal therapy and its impact on children with hearing impairments and their families.

Warren Estabrooks MEd, Editor

3739 Baby Sign Language Basics

Monta Z Briant, author

Harris Communications
15155 Technology Drive
Eden Prairie, MN 55344

952-906-1180
800-825-6758
Fax: 952-906-1099
TTY: 800-825-9187
info@harriscomm.com
www.harriscomm.com

This is the perfect book for new parents - now, they can understand what their baby is trying to tell them. This books makes learning fun and easy, and it is small enough to take anywhere. It includes 60 baby-friendly American Sign Language signs like bird, happy, baby, and mommy, just to name a few. There are also baby-specific signing techniques, black and white photographs, songs and games.

329 pages Softcover

3740 Baby's First Signs

Kim Voltry and Curt Waller, author

Gallaudet University Press
800 Florida Avenue NE
Washington, DC 20002

202-651-5488
Fax: 202-651-5489
gupress@gallaudet.edu
www.gupress.gallaudet.edu

A durable board book, lavishly colored in bright reds, blues, greens, and yellows sure to please your child's eye. Each page features an illustration of a toddler signing a word as well as demonstrating what the sign is about. For example, on the baby page, a toddler makes the sign for baby by mimicking the cradling of a child in his arms while also smiling at his baby sister sitting beside him. The illustrations include both a diagram box that depicts how to berform the sign and English word.

16 pages Board Book
ISBN: 1-563681-14-5

3741 Be Careful
HEAR-MORE
42 Executive Boulevard
Farmingdale, NY 11735

800-881-4327
Fax: 631-752-0689
TTY: 800-281-3555
www.hearmore.com

A What-Will-Happen-Next Book of Safety, a book of cautions. It shows the child, in an amusing and dramatic manner, just what can happen to a careless or thoughtless child. Read the story aloud and sign to the child while looking at the pictures together. Let the child see your lips when you read and sign.

3742 Be Happy Not Sad
Modern Signs Press
PO Box 1181
Los Alamitos, CA 90720

562-596-8548
800-572-7332
Fax: 562-795-6614
TTY: 562-493-4168
modsigns@modersignspress.com
www.modernsignspress.com

These books help children understand hard to explain emotions through signing. Includes Be Happy Not Sad coloring workbook.

1988 2 Book Set
ISBN: 0-916708-19-5

3743 Belonging

Virginia M Scott, author

Gallaudet University Press
800 Florida Avenue NE
Washington, DC 20002

202-651-5488
Fax: 202-651-5489
gupress@gallaudet.edu
www.gupress.gallaudet.edu

Gustie is 15 when she contracts meningitis during which she loses the small amount of residual hearing she had seemed to retain, Gustie tires to pick up the pieces of her life. Her parents are unrealistic and over protective; her best friend rejects her; her teachers run the gamut from being convinced Gustie cannont function in the mainstream to being supportive...through a new boyfriend who has a deaf brother and sister-in-law, and through visits with an understanding special education teacher

176 pages Softcover
ISBN: 0-903233-35-5

3744 Children with Hearing Difficulties
Scholars International Corporation
2630 W Barry Avenue
Chicago, IL 60618

410-337-3775
800-638-3775
Fax: 410-337-8539
scholars@ameritech.net

Based on ten years of research into hearing and hearing-impaired children, this book looks at the impact of deafness on all aspects of the development and education of young children.

192 pages Softcover
ISBN: 0-304317-24-1

David Wood, Co-Author
Alec Webster, Co-Author

3745 Chris Gets Ear Tubes
Gallaudet University Press
800 Florida Avenue NE
Washington, DC 20002

202-651-5488
800-621-2736
Fax: 202-651-5489
TTY: 202-651-5488
gupress@gallaudet.edu
www.gupress.gallaudet.edu

A helpful book for parents and children to share concerning ear tubes and hospitals.

48 pages paperback
ISBN: 0-930323-36-x

3746 Chris Gets Ear Tubes: Spanish Edition
Betty Pace, author

Gallaudet University Press
800 Florida Avenue NE
Washington, DC 20002

202-651-5488
Fax: 202-651-5489
gupress@gallaudet.edu
www.gupress.gallaudet.edu

Chris Get Ear Tubes describes what happens, before, during, and after the surgery in a language a child understands. It takes away the child's natural fear of the unknown. Also available in English

48 pages Softcover
ISBN: 1-563680-93-9

3747 Classroom GOALS

Jill B Firszt, MA and Ruth M Reeder, MA, author

Alexander Graham Bell Association for the Deaf
3417 Volta Place NW
Washington, DC 20007

202-337-5220
Fax: 202-337-8314
TTY: 202-337-5221
info@agbell.org
www.agbell.org

Classroom GOALS was designed to help teachers incorporate auditory goals into academic lessons after those specific goals have been identified. Objectives accommodate students with hearing loss regardless of the degree of loss, sensory devise, grade level, mode of communication or school placement.

199 pages Softcover

3748 Classroom Notetaker

Jimmie Joan Wilson, author

Alexander Graham Bell Association for the Deaf
3417 Volta Place NW
Washington, DC 20007

202-337-5220
Fax: 202-337-8314
TTY: 202-337-5221
info@agbell.org
www.agbell.org

How to organize a program serving students with hearing impairments. Designed to help teachers incorporate auditory goals into academic lessons, after those specific goals have been identified. Objectives accommodate students with hearing loss regardless of the degree of loss, sensory device, grade level, mode of communication or school placement. This guide describes practical ways for teachers to create situations during academic instruction that encourage the use of residual hearing.

127 pages Softcover

3749 Cochlear Implant Auditory Training Guidebook
Alexander Graham Bell Association for the Deaf
3417 Volta Place NW
Washington, DC 20007

202-337-5220
800-432-7543
Fax: 202-337-8314
TTY: 202-337-5221
publications@agbell.org
www.agbell.org

Designed for parents and professionals working with children ages four and up who have cochlear implants. It includes an easy to follow hierarchy for listening goals and a quick placement test to help you find where to start. Comes with CD

236 pages

David Sindrey

3750 Cochlear Implants for Kids

Warren Estabrooks, MEd, author

Alexander Graham Bell Association for the Deaf
3417 Volta Place NW
Washington, DC 20007

202-337-5220
Fax: 202-337-8314
TTY: 202-337-5221
info@agbell.org
www.agbell.org

Written to educate parents and the professional community about cochlear implants for the pediatric population. Sections include: History and ethical issues, Surgery and programming, Habilitation, Family stories from around the world. Its accessible language and photography make this text a perfect resource for anyone interested in therapy for pre and post cochlear implantation and in the entire family experience.

404 pages Softcover

3751 Cochlear Implants in Children

John B Christiansen and Irene W Leigh, author

Alexander Graham Bell Association for the Deaf
3417 Volta Place NW
Washington, DC 20007
202-337-5220
Fax: 202-337-8314
TTY: 202-337-5221
info@agbell.org
www.agbell.org

Based on a survey of 439 parents of children who have cochlear implants, this book addresses every facet of the controversy over early implantation.

360 pages Hardcover

3752 Cochlear Implants in Children: Ethics and Choices

John B Christiansen and Irene W Leigh, author

Gallaudet University Press
800 Florida Avenue NE
Washington, DC 20002
202-651-5488
Fax: 202-651-5489
gupress@gallaudet.edu
www.gupress.gallaudet.edu

Addresses every facet of the ongoing controversy about implanting cochlear hearing devices in children as young as 12 months old and in some cases, younger. The authors analyzed the sensitive issues connected witht he procedure by reviewing 439 responses to a survey of parents with children who have cochlear implants. They followed up with interviews of the parents of children who have had a year's experience using the implants, and also the children themselves.

340 pages Hardcover
ISBN: 1-563681-16-1

3753 Cognition, Eduction, and Deafness: Directi ons for Research and Instruction

David S Martin, Editor, author

Gallaudet University Press
800 Florida Avenue NE
Washington, DC 20002
202-651-5488
Fax: 202-651-5489
gupress@gallaudet.edu
www.gupress.gallaudet.edu

This book integrates the work of 54 contributors to the 1984 symposium on cognition, education and deafness. It focuses on cognition and deaf students' growth and development, problem-solving strategies, thinking processes, language development, reading methodology, measurement of potential, and intervention programs. A synthesis of these discoveries establishes directions for new research and outlines implications for all professionals working with hearing-impaired learners.

248 pages Softcover
ISBN: 1-563681-49-8

3754 Colors

HEAR-MORE
42 Executive Boulevard
Farmingdale, NY 11735
800-881-4327
Fax: 631-752-0689
TTY: 800-281-3555
www.hearmore.com

The Early Sign Language Series: A fascinating and enjoyable way for children and adults to learn sign language. Colors presents the early concepts of color recognition. It fosters both receptive and expressive language through signs and pictures, and it is perfect for young children whether hearing impaired, hearing, pre-verbal or verbal. Reviews ten colors in bright cheery illustrations.

3755 Come Sign With Us: Sign Language Activitie s for Children

David S Martin, Editor, author

Gallaudet University Press
800 Florida Avenue NE
Washington, DC 20002
202-651-5488
Fax: 202-651-5489
gupress@gallaudet.edu
www.gupress.gallaudet.edu

Completely revised, this book now offers more follow-up activities, including many in context, to teach children sign language. The second edition of this fun, fully illustrated activities manual features more than 300 line drawings of both adults and children signing familiar words, phrases, and sentences using American Sign Language signs in English word order. Twenty lively lessons each introduce ten selected target vocabulary words in a format familiar and exciting to children.

160 pages Softcover
ISBN: 1-563680-51-3

3756 Come Sign with Us Sign Language Activities for Children

Gallaudet University Press
800 Florida Avenue NE
Washington, DC 20002
202-651-5488
800-621-2736
Fax: 202-651-5489
TTY: 202-651-5488
gupress@gallaudet.edu
www.gupress.gallaudet.edu

Revised version, offering more follow-up activities, including many in context, to teach children sign language. Features more than 300 line drawings of both adults and children signing familiar words, phrases, and sentences using ASL. Shows how to form each sign exactly and also presents the origins of ASL, facts about deafness, and the deaf community.

2002 160 pages Softcover
ISBN: 1-563680-51-3

3757 Cosmo Gets An Ear

Gary Clementine, author

Modern Signs Press
PO Box 1181
Los Alamitos, CA 90720
562-596-8548
800-572-7332
Fax: 562-795-6614
TTY: 562-493-4168
modsigns@modernsignspress.com
www.modernsignspress.com

Welcome to the world of 'Cosmo'. Once you get past the normal turmoil of his impossible room, you find a boy who needs to have the TV loud and his mother shouting at him to respond. Cosmo has a hearing problem. This story was written by a man who is hearing impaired and regretfully did not use an aid until much later in life. It is colorfully and humorously illustrated by an artist who captures the exuberance and fears of the youngster. An excellent way to help others understand what it is like.

48 pages

3758 Cued Speech Resource Book

Orin Cornett and Mary Elsie Daisey, author

Alexander Graham Bell Association for the Deaf
3417 Volta Place NW
Washington, DC 20007
202-337-5220
Fax: 202-337-8314
TTY: 202-337-5221
info@agbell.org
www.agbell.org

A fact book for parents and professionals who want to use this system of hand cues with speech to help children affected by hearing loss or auditory neuropathy learn spoken languages. Explains Cued Speech and how to use it and includes personal accounts, practice materials, and guidance. Second edition revisions describe legal rights and the mechanics of cueing. This classic text explains: Initiating communication, Language development, Reading, Speech Production, Multiple Disabilities and more.

832 pages Hardcover

3759 Dad and Me in the Morning

Patricia Lakin and Robert G steele, author

Harris Communications
15155 Technology Drive
Eden Prairie, MN 55344

952-906-1180
800-825-6758
Fax: 952-906-1099
TTY: 800-825-9187
info@harriscomm.com
www.harriscomm.com

Warm and fuzzy and beautifully illustrated! This delightful book
will provide enjoyable reading and superb pictures for a cozy,
shared reading adventure for parent and a hard of hearing child.

3760 Deaf Children in China

Alison Callaway, author

Gallaudet University Press
800 Florida Avenue NE
Washington, DC 20002

202-651-5488
Fax: 202-651-5489
gupress@gallaudet.edu
www.gupress.gallaudet.edu

Provides a striking profile of the views and attitudes of well-edu-
cated Chinese parents with preschool-age deaf children. The author's inclusion of a survey of 122 English mothers of deaf
children reveals the differences between Western and Chinese
parents, who rely upon grandparents to help them and who frequently search for medical cures. She also discovered that many
issues cross cultures and contexts, especially the problems of
achieving early diagnosis and intervention for all deaf children

256 pages Hardcover
ISBN: 1-563680-85-8

3761 Deaf Children in Public Schools: Placement , Context, and Consequences

Claire L Ramsey, author

Gallaudet University Press
800 Florida Avenue NE
Washington, DC 20002

202-651-5488
Fax: 202-651-5489
gupress@gallaudet.edu
www.gupress.gallaudet.edu

Assesses the progress of three second-grade deaf students to demonstrate the importance of placement, context, and language in
their development. The autor points out that these deaf children
were placed in two different environments, with the general population of hearing students, and separately with other deaf and hard
of hearing children. The answers found in this cohesive book offer educators and parents a remarkable stage for assessing and enhancing the education context for deaf children.

142 pages Hardcover
ISBN: 1-563680-62-9

3762 Deaf Daughter, Hearing Fahter

Richard Medugno, author

Gallaudet University Press
800 Florida Avenue NE
Washington, DC 20002

202-651-5488
Fax: 202-651-5489
gupress@gallaudet.edu
www.gupress.gallaudet.edu

A father shares practical information on many of the common
challenges faced by hearing parents. e provides a list of games
that hearing and deaf children can play together, a consideration
for many families. His enthusiasm for all possibilities, from exploring the potential of video phones to helping stage CSD musi-
cals, reveals his abiding devotion to Miranda. This has enabled
her to feel proud, confident and happy in her pursuits. Medugno
realizes that the rewards of having a deaf daughter

184 pages Softcover
ISBN: 1-563681-77-X

3763 Deaf Side Story: Deaf Sharks, Hearing Jets , and a Classic American Musical

Mark Rigney, author

Gallaudet University Press
800 Florida Avenue NE
Washington, DC 20002

202-651-5488
Fax: 202-651-5489
gupress@gallaudet.edu
www.gupress.gallaudet.edu

The 1957 classic American Musical West Side Story has been
staged by many community and school theater groups. At a small
school in Jacksonville, IL, the new drama head, determined to
add an extra element to the usual demands of putting on a show
by having deaf students perform half of the parts. The author portrays the progress of the production, including the frustrations
and triumphs of the leads, the campus and community politics,
and the clashes between the deaf cast members and hearing.

232 pages Softcover
ISBN: 1-563681-45-5

3764 Deaf Students Can Be Great Readers

Modern Signs Press
PO Box 1181
Los Alamitos, CA 90720

562-596-8548
800-572-7332
Fax: 562-795-6614
TTY: 562-493-4168
modsigns@modernsignspress.com
www.modernsignspress.com

Detailed analytical review of a case study of one deaf child. Also,
information about the place on phonological awareness in developing reading capability. Includes a comprehensive annotated
bibliography related to education of deaf and hard of hearing
children.

3765 Educating Deaf Students: Global Perspectiv es

Des Power and Greg Leigh, Editors, author

Gallaudet University Press
800 Florida Avenue NE
Washington, DC 20002

202-651-5488
Fax: 202-651-5489
gupress@gallaudet.edu
www.gupress.gallaudet.edu

The 19 chapters of this book present a select cross-section of the
issues addressed at the 19th International Congress of Education
of the Deaf. Divided into four distinct parts - Contemporary Issus
for all Learners, The Eary Years, The School Years, and Contemporary Issues in Postsecondary Education - the themes considered
here span the entire student age range. Authored by 27 different
researchers and practitioners from six different countries.

248 pages Hardcover
ISBN: 1-563683-08-3

3766 Educational Audiology for the Limited-Hear ing Infant and Preschooler

Charles C Thomas Publishers
2600 South First Street
Springfield, IL 62704

217-789-8980
800-258-8980
books@ccthomas.com
www.ccthomas.com

The third edition of this book brings up to date the material that
so many readers found helpful in the previous editions. The entire
text has been rewritten and reorganized with revised chapters focusing on current concepts and practices in audiologic screening
and evaluation, development of language, the role of parents, parent education, mainstreaming of the limited-hearing child, and
program modifications for the severely learning disabled child.
Includes 18 tables.

430 pages Softcover

3767 Educational Interpreting: How It Can Succe ed

Elizabeth A Winston, Editor, author

Gallaudet University Press
800 Florida Avenue NE
Washington, DC 20002

202-651-5488
Fax: 202-651-5489
gupress@gallaudet.edu
www.gupress.gallaudet.edu

This book explores the current state of educational interpreting and how it is failing deaf students. The contributors, all experts in their field, include former educational interpreters, teachers of deaf students, interpreter trainers, and deaf recipients of inter-preted educations. It presents the salient issues in three distinct sections. Part 1 focuses on deaf students. Part 2 raises the ques-tions about the support and training intrepreters receive. Part 3 presents possible suggestions.

224 pages Hardcover
ISBN: 1-563683-09-1

3768 Educational and Development Aspects of Deafness

Gallaudet University Press
800 Florida Avenue NE
Washington, DC 20002

202-651-5488
Fax: 202-651-5489
TTY: 202-651-5488
gupress@gallaudet.edu
www.gupress.gallaudet.edu

Book detailing the ongoing revolution in the education of deaf children.

415 pages

Donald F Moores, Editor
Kathryn P Meadow-Orlans, Editor

3769 Educational and Developmental Aspects of D eafness

Donald Moores and Kathryn Meadow-Orlans, Editors, author

Gallaudet University Press
800 Florida Avenue NE
Washington, DC 20002

202-651-5488
Fax: 202-651-5489
gupress@gallaudet.edu
www.gupress.gallaudet.edu

Details the ongoing revolution in the eduction of deaf children. More than 20 researchers contributed their discoveries in anthro-pology, education, linguistics, psychology, sociology, and other major disciplines, with special concentration upon the education of deaf children. Divided into two parts on education at home and in school, this book documents breakthroughs such as the pub-lic's interest in sign language, the increasing availability of interpreters, and other positive trends.

451 pages Hardcover
ISBN: 0-930323-52-1

3770 Fire Fighter Brown

HEAR-MORE
42 Executive Boulevard
Farmingdale, NY 11735

800-881-4327
Fax: 631-752-0689
TTY: 800-281-3555
www.hearmore.com

The Fire Fighter Brown book tells about the Fire Fighter Brown's work, the clothes he wears, and the equipment he uses in rescuing a little boy from a burning building. Use the signs when reading the book to your child, and let the child see your lips as you read and sign. This will help your child learn to associate the signs with sounds and lip shapes.

3771 First Signs at Home

HEAR-MORE
42 Executive Boulevard
Farmingdale, NY 11735

800-881-4327
Fax: 631-752-0689
TTY: 800-281-3555
www.hearmore.com

The Early Sign Language Series: A fascinating and enjoyable way for children and adults to learn sign language. First Signs present some of the very first words for parents and children.

3772 First Signs at Play

HEAR-MORE
42 Executive Boulevard
Farmingdale, NY 11735

800-881-4327
Fax: 631-752-0689
TTY: 800-281-3555
www.hearmore.com

The Early Sign Language Series: A fascinating and enjoyable way for children and adults to learn sign language. First Signs present some of the very first words for parents and children.

3773 Foundations of Spoken Language for Hearing -Impaired Children

Daniel Ling, PhD, author

Alexander Graham Bell Association for the Deaf
3417 Volta Place NW
Washington, DC 20007

202-337-5220
Fax: 202-337-8314
TTY: 202-337-5221
info@agbell.org
www.agbell.org

Emphasizes the perception of speech through residual hearing, ei-ther through the use of modern hearing aids or cochlear implants. A feature of the book is the presentation of the aspects of speech that appear in the octave bands centered on frequencies depicted in audiograms. This konowledge, in conjunction with the Six-Sound Test, allows teachers and clinicians to determine whether the frequency response charachteristics of hearing aids are adjusted to provide optimal levels of hearing.

447 pages Softcover

3774 Free Hand: Enfranchising the Education of Deaf Children

TJ Publishers
P.O Box 702701
Dallas, TX 75370

972-416-0800
800-999-1186
Fax: 972-416-0944
TTY: 972-416-0933
customerservice@tjpublishers.com
www.tjpublishers.com

Based on the proceedings of a 1990 symposium on the educa-tional uses of ASL, A Free Hand presents papers by prominent educators, researchers and linguists in the changing role of Amer-ican Sign Language in the classroom.

1992 204 pages Softcover
ISBN: 0-932666-40-X

Angela K Thames, President
Jerald Murphy, Vice President

3775 From Gesture to Language in Hearing and De af Children

Virginia Volterra and Carol J Ertling, Editors, author

Gallaudet University Press
800 Florida Avenue NE
Washington, DC 20002

202-651-5488
Fax: 202-651-5489
gupress@gallaudet.edu
www.gupress.gallaudet.edu

In 21 essays on communicative gesturing in the first two years of life, this collection demonstrates the importance of gesture in a child's transition to a linguistic system. Introductions preceding each section emphasize the parallels between the findings in these studies and the general body of scholarship devoted to the pro-cess of spoken language acquisition. Scholars contributing to this volume include Ursula Bellugi, Judy Snitzer Reilly, Susan Goldwin-Meadow, Andrew Lock, and many others.

358 pages Softcover
ISBN: 1-563680-78-5

3776 Genetics, Disability and Deafness

John Vickrey Van Cleve, Editory, author

Gallaudet University Press
800 Florida Avenue NE
Washington, DC 20002
202-651-5488
Fax: 202-651-5489
gupress@gallaudet.edu
www.gupress.gallaudet.edu

This volume brings together 13 essays from science, history, and the humanities, history and the present, to show the many ways that disability, deafness and the new genetetics interact and what that interaction means for society. Prize-winning author Louis Menand begins this volume by expressing the position shared by most authors in this wide-ranging forum—the belief in the value of human diversity and skepticism of actions that could eliminate it through modification of the human genome.

240 pages Hardcover
ISBN: 1-563683-07-5

3777 Go Togethers
HEAR-MORE
42 Executive Boulevard
Farmingdale, NY 11735
800-881-4327
Fax: 631-752-0689
TTY: 800-281-3555
www.hearmore.com

The Early Sign Language Series: A fascinating and enjoyable way for children and adults to learn sign language. Go-Togethers presents early objects and concpets that are complimentary. It fosters both receptive and expressive language through signs and pictures, and it is perfect for young children whether hearing impaired, hearing, pre-verbal or verbal. Learn 10 go-together items (20 in total).

3778 Goldilocks and the Three Bears Told in Sig ned English

Harry Bornstein and Karen L Saulnier, author

Gallaudet University Press
800 Florida Avenue NE
Washington, DC 20002
202-651-5488
Fax: 202-651-5489
gupress@gallaudet.edu
www.gupress.gallaudet.edu

Offers children ages 3-8 all of the fun their parents had when they first read about the little girl with the golden curls who turned the Bears' house upside down. In this exciting new edition, children can learn new words and the matching signs, which will help them to remember both.

48 pages
ISBN: 1-563680-57-2

3779 Good Morning Me! Hand and Voices
PO Box 3093
Boulder, CO 80307
303-492-6283
866-422-0422
parentadvocate@handsandvoices.org
www.handsandvoices.org

This book teaches your child to initial vowel/consonant combinations through fun repetition.

3780 Grandfather Moose!

Harley Hamilton, author

Modern Signs Press
PO Box 1181
Los Alamitos, CA 90720
562-596-8548
800-572-7332
Fax: 562-795-6614
TTY: 562-493-4168
modsigns@modernsignspress.com
www.modernsignspress.com

Move over 'Mother Goose'...here comes 'Grandfather Moose'! Exciting and beautifully illustrated book of rhythms, games, and chants in sign language. Hearing children enjoy the sound of rhyming words. Deaf and hard of hearing children will delight in the rythmic quality of these signing tales. Rhymes are made up of words whose signs have similar hand shapes. Games and chants provide group sign language activities for home and school.

32 pages

3781 How Children Learn Language

James McLean, PhD And Lee Snyder-McLean, PhD, author

Alexander Graham Bell Association for the Deaf
3417 Volta Place NW
Washington, DC 20007
202-337-5220
Fax: 202-337-8314
TTY: 202-337-5221
info@agbell.org
www.agbell.org

This introductory text guides professionals in nonlanguage fields and students in education/special education courses through the miracle of typical child's language development.

227 pages Softcover

3782 I Can Sign my ABCs

Susan Gibbons Chaplin, author

Harris Communications
15155 Technology Drive
Eden Prairie, MN 55344
952-906-1180
800-825-6758
Fax: 952-906-1099
TTY: 800-825-9187
info@harriscomm.com
www.harriscomm.com

In this full-color picture book, each letter's manual alphabet handshape is followed by the picture, name, and sign of an object beginning with that letter. Ideal for teaching children the English and the American Manual alphabets.

52 pages Hardcover

3783 I Can't Hear You in the Dark: How to Learn and Teach Lipreading

Betty Woerner Carter, author

Charles C Thomas Publishers
2600 South First Street
Springfield, IL 62704
217-789-8980
800-258-8980
books@ccthomas.com
www.ccthomas.com

I can't hear you in the dark, but I can lipread you in the light.' Lipreading is one of the ways that hearing-impaired people can communicate and strengthen relationships with others. Written for the beginning lipreader and the experienced, this book shows how lipreading can be taught by supplying ready-to-use lessons.

226 pages Softcover
ISBN: 0-393067-89-9

3784 I Love You Story

Walter Paul Kelly, author

Harris Communications
15155 Technology Drive
Eden Prairie, MN 55344
952-906-1180
800-825-6758
Fax: 952-906-1099
TTY: 800-825-9187
info@harriscomm.com
www.harriscomm.com

A black and white illustrated story on how love and eventually the ILY handsign in American Sign Language got started.

Hardcover

3785 I'M Deaf and It's Okay

Lorraine Aseltine, Evelyn Mueller, Nancy Tate, author

Harris Communications
15155 Technology Drive
Eden Prairie, MN 55344
952-906-1180
800-825-6758
Fax: 952-906-1099
TTY: 800-825-9187
info@harriscomm.com
www.harriscomm.com

A young boy explains how lonely and frustrated he feels because he can't hear. He dislikes the hearing aids he wears and is angered because he will never be rid of them. His feelings begin to change when he is befriended by a teenage boy who also wears hearing aids. This book is well-illustrated with sensitive line drawings done by Helen Cogancherry.

36 pages Hardcover

3786 In Our House

Carolyn Norris, author

Modern Signs Press
PO Box 1181
Los Alamitos, CA 90720
562-596-8548
800-572-7332
Fax: 562-795-6614
TTY: 562-493-4168
modsigns@modernsignspress.com
www.modernsignspress.com

This colorful picture book tells the story of Joy and Jason helping Mom and Dad around the house. Demonstrates cooking, cleaning, gardening, etc. Has a 140 word vocabulary listed in an alphabetical glossary and the manual alphabet.

3787 In Silence: Growing Up Hearing in a Deaf World

Ruth Sidransky, author

Gallaudet University Press
800 Florida Avenue NE
Washington, DC 20002
202-651-5488
Fax: 202-651-5489
gupress@gallaudet.edu
www.gupress.gallaudet.edu

This is an account of growing up as the hearing daughter of deaf Jewish parents in the Bronx and Brooklyn during the 1930s and 1940s. It reveals the challenges deaf people faced during the Depression and afterward. The author portrays her family with deep affection and honesty, and her frank account provides a living narrative of the Deaf experience in pre- and post-World War II America.

352 pages Softcover
ISBN: 1-563682-87-7

3788 Inner Lives of Deaf Children: Interviews and Analysis

Martha Sheridan, author

Gallaudet University Press
800 Florida Avenue NE
Washington, DC 20002
202-651-5488
Fax: 202-651-5489
gupress@gallaudet.edu
www.gupress.gallaudet.edu

Conducting interviews with seven deaf children between the ages of 7 and 10, the author offers a fresh look at the private thoughts and feels of deaf children. 'What does it mean to be a child who is deaf or hard of hearing?' Sheridan asks in the beginning of her study. She turns to Danny, Angie, Joe, Alex, Lisa, Mary and Pat for the answer. Footnotes, bibliography, index.

256 pages Softcover
ISBN: 1-563682-89-3

3789 Kid-Friendly Parenting with Deaf and Hard of Hearing Children

Gallaudet University Press
800 Florida Avenue NE
Washington, DC 20002
202-651-5488
Fax: 202-651-5489
TTY: 202-651-5488
gupress@gallaudet.edu
www.gupress.gallaudet.edu

A step-by-step guide offering parents hundreds of ideas and play activities for children ages three to 12.

320 pages

3790 King Midas

Robert Newby, author

Gallaudet University Press
800 Florida Avenue NE
Washington, DC 20002
202-651-5488
Fax: 202-651-5489
gupress@gallaudet.edu
www.gupress.gallaudet.edu

Now the tale of King Midas and his golden touch is retold with full-color illustrations, and key sentences shown in American Sign Language. The line drawings of the story teller (who appears in both the book and videotape) recreate 44 sentences, making this ideal for helping both hearing and deaf children to learn reading skills. The videotape shows the entire classic story performed in ASL by the storyteller accompanied by a voiceover. A perfect complement to the book. VHS, color, 30 minutes.

VHS-$39.95 72 pages Hardcover book
ISBN: 0-930323-75-0

3791 Learning Ladder: Assessing and Teaching Text Comprehension

Elisabeth H Wiig, PhD and Carolyn C Wilson, MS, author

Alexander Graham Bell Association for the Deaf
3417 Volta Place NW
Washington, DC 20007
202-337-5220
Fax: 202-337-8314
TTY: 202-337-5221
info@agbell.org
www.agbell.org

A general education program developed for students, aged 7 to 12 years, with reading comprehension difficulties. Major sections of the text include two components: assessment and interventions. The assessment component describes typical home and school social interactions. The intervention component introduces intervention options including grade-level activities, resources, and graphic organizers. The intervention component also responds to the Least Restrictive Environment provision of IDEA.

269 pages Softcover/CD

3792 Learning to See: American Sign Language as a Second Language

Gallaudet University Press
800 Florida Avenue NE
Washington, DC 20002
202-651-5488
Fax: 202-651-5489
TTY: 202-561-5488
gupress@gallaudet.edu
www.gupress.gallaudet.edu

Provides a comprehensive introduction to the history and structure of ASL to the deaf community.

160 pages
ISBN: 1-563680-59-9

3793 Legal Rights for the Deaf and Hard of Hear ing
Hearing Loss Association of America
7910 Woodmont Avenue, Suite 1200
Bethesda, MD 20814

301-657-2248
Fax: 301-913-9413
TTY: 301-657-2249
bookstore@hearingloss.org
www.hearingloss.org

A comprehensive analysis of recent laws passed to protect the rights of and guarantee equal access for people with hearing loss. In this revised, fifth edition, the book explains in layman's terminology how legislation affects individuals with disabilities in everyday life.

Softcover

Barbara Kelley, Editor-In-Chief
Brenda Battat, Executive Director

3794 Legal Rights: The Guide for Deaf and Hard of Hearing People - Fifth Edition
Gallaudet University Press
800 Florida Avenue NE
Washington, DC 20002

202-651-5488
Fax: 202-651-5489
TTY: 202-651-5488
gupress@gallaudet.edu
www.gupress.gallaudet.edu

Includes updated interpretations of legislation affecting hearing-impaired people, including chapters dealing with the ADA.

3795 Listen Little Star

Dimity Dornan, BA, author

Alexander Graham Bell Association for the Deaf
3417 Volta Place NW
Washington, DC 20007

202-337-5220
Fax: 202-337-8314
TTY: 202-337-5221
info@agbell.org
www.agbell.org

Maximize your child's auditory potential with this series of parent-child activities designed to help your baby develop listening and speaking skills using techniques based on the Auditory-Verbal approach. Designed to take approximately four-to-six months to complete. Includes:12 parent-child activities that build auditory skills, a caregiver workbook to guide you through each exercise, a note-taking section to document your child's progress, a reminder checklist, and a plush toy star.

3796 Listen with the Heart: Relationships and H earing Loss

Michael Harvey, author

Hearing Loss Association of America
7910 Woodmont Avenue, Suite 1200
Bethesda, MD 20814

301-657-2248
Fax: 301-913-9413
TTY: 301-657-2249
bookstore@hearingloss.org
www.hearingloss.org

True stories of how parents, children and spouses are transformed by helping each other heal and grow. Unique insights into the consequences of this challenge for individuals and their loved ones. Told with a deep human wisdom and touch of humor, these accounts are a genuine look at the opportunities llife gives us to listen with the heart.

Barbara Kelley, Editor-In-Chief
Brenda Battat, Executive Director

3797 Literacy and Your Deaf Child: What Every P arent Should Know

David A Steward and Bryan R Clarke, author

Gallaudet University Press
800 Florida Avenue NE
Washington, DC 20002

202-651-5488
Fax: 202-651-5489
gupress@gallaudet.edu
www.gupress.gallaudet.edu

This book begins by introducing some common concepts, among them the importance of parental involvement in a deaf child's education. It outlines how children acquire language and describes the auditory and visual links to literacy. With this information, parents can make informed decisions regarding hearing aids, cochlear implants, speechreading, and sign communication all of which can have a marked influence on their child's language development.

240 pages Softcover
ISBN: 1-563681-36-6

3798 Little Read Riding Hood: Told in Signed En lish

Harry Bornstein and Karen Luczak Saulnier, author

Gallaudet University Press
800 Florida Avenue NE
Washington, DC 20002

202-651-5488
Fax: 202-651-5489
gupress@gallaudet.edu
www.gupress.gallaudet.edu

Now one of the most beloved of all folktales, Little Red Riding Hood in a new Signed Enlish edition illustrated in full color. It presents a vivacious version of this favorite story that will intrigue and delight children. Along with the story illustrations, line drawings showing the characters and a narrator signing the story in Signed English, a system that uses American Sign Language in English grammatical order.

48 pages Hardcover
ISBN: 0-930323-63-7

3799 Living with Hearing Loss

Marcia B Dugan, author

Gallaudet University Press
800 Florida Avenue NE
Washington, DC 20002

202-651-5488
Fax: 202-651-5489
TTY: 888-630-9347
gupress@gallaudet.edu
www.gupress.gallaudet.edu

192 pages
ISBN: 1-563681-34-0

3800 Mandy

Barbara D Booth, author

Harris Communications
15155 Technology Drive
Eden Prairie, MN 55344

952-906-1180
800-825-6758
Fax: 952-906-1099
TTY: 800-825-9187
info@harriscomm.com
www.harriscomm.com

Mandy is a young deaf girl who goes searching in the woods for her grandmother's silver pin as a thunderstorm approaches. She will touch readers with her peceptions of the world and her wonder of what sound is.

32 pages Hardcover

3801 Medical Sign Language: Easily Understood D efinitions of Commonly Used Medical Term

W Joseph Garcia, author

Charles C Thomas Publishers
2600 South First Street
Springfield, IL 62704   217-789-8980
                                     800-258-8980
                                     books@ccthomas.com
                                     www.ccthomas.com

In this glossary, a multitude of medical and dental terms are accurately defined and precisely translated, through description and illustration, into American Sign Language. The book easily lends itself to use at both ends of the chain of communication that links health care professionals with their deaf patients. Includes bibliography. Comes in both hardcover and softcover

726 pages

3802 Messy Monsters Jungle Joggers and Bubble B aths

Nehama Pluznik and Rochelle Sobel, author

Alexander Graham Bell Association for the Deaf
3417 Volta Place NW
Washington, DC 20007   202-337-5220
                                     Fax: 202-337-8314
                                     TTY: 202-337-5221
                                     info@agbell.org
                                     www.agbell.org

An illustrated book of poetry for children with hearing loss. Poems are organized according to the accepted group of speechreading phonemes which are classified by their appearance on the lips. Each poem emphasizes a particular phoneme which appears in the initial, medial, or final position of the word. Four worksheets accompany each poem: About the poem, Tell me more, Speech practice, and Language activities.

97 pages Softcover

3803 Nursery Rhymes from Mother Goose: Told in Signed English

Harry Bornstein and Karen L Saulnier, author

Gallaudet University Press
800 Florida Avenue NE
Washington, DC 20002   202-651-5488
                                     Fax: 202-651-5489
                                     gupress@gallaudet.edu
                                     www.gupress.gallaudet.edu

More than a dozen favorite nursery rhymes are presented in this unique edition of Mother Goose. All of the rhymes are illustrated with full-color paintings accompanied by more than 389 drawings showing the verses in Signed English. Young readers, both hearing and deaf, will learn the special charm of rhyme while also discovering new vocabulary and new ways to experience English through signing. As they learn and memorize their favorite verses, children will also strengthen their language skills.

64 pages Hardcover
ISBN: 0-930323-99-8

3804 Operation SHHH

Self Help for Hard-of-Hearing People
7910 Woodmont Avenue, Suite 1200
Bethesda, MD 20814   301-657-2248
                                     Fax: 301-913-9413
                                     TTY: 301-657-2249
                                     info@hearingloss.org
                                     www.hearingloss.org

Features SHHHerman, the lion who does not roar. This program is designed for elementary school children. Includes video, posters, brochures and more.

Barbara Kelley, Editor-In-Chief
Brenda Battat, Executive Director

3805 Opposites

HEAR-MORE
42 Executive Boulevard
Farmingdale, NY 11735   800-881-4327
                                     Fax: 631-752-0689
                                     TTY: 800-281-4327
                                     www.hearmore.com

The Early Sign Language Series: A fascinating and enjoyable way for children and adults to learn sign language. Opposites presents the early concepts of opposite relationships. It fosters both recptive and expressive language through signs and pictures, and it is perfect for young children whether hearing impaired, hearing, pre-verbal or verbal. Reviews 10 opposite items (20 in total).

3806 Out for a Walk: Baby's First Sign Book

Kim Votry and Curt Waller, author

Gallaudet University Press
800 Florida Avenue NE
Washington, DC 20002   202-651-5488
                                     Fax: 202-651-5489
                                     gupress@gallaudet.edu
                                     www.gupress.gallaudet.edu

Offers toddlers their first look at signs for the world around them. As they follow our distinctively hatted youngster on a stroll, they encounter familiar animals and insect, among them a dog, cat, butterfly, and squirrel, and learn which ones can be pets. They'll enjoy imaginative images of senses, too - sight, smell, hearing, taste, and touch.

16 pages Board Book
ISBN: 1-563681-46-3

3807 Parent's Guide to Chochlear Implants

Patricia M Chute and Mary Ellen Nevins, author

Gallaudet University Press
800 Florida Avenue NE
Washington, DC 20002   202-651-5488
                                     Fax: 202-651-5489
                                     gupress@gallaudet.edu
                                     www.gupress.gallaudet.edu

Now, parents of deaf children have at hand a complete guide to the process of cochlear implantation. It explains in a friendly easy-to-follow style each stage of the process. Parents will discover how to have their child evaluated to determine his or her suitability for an implant. They'll learn about implant device options, how to choose an implant center, and every detail of the surgical procedure. The initial 'switch-on' is described along with counseling about device maintainance.

208 pages Softcover
ISBN: 1-563681-29-3

3808 Parents and Their Deaf Children: The Early Years
Gallaudet University Press
800 Florida Avenue NE
Washington, DC 20002   202-651-5488
                                     Fax: 202-651-5489
                                     gupress@gallaudet.edu
                                     http://gupress.gallaudet.edu

This book stems from a nationwide survey of parents with 6-7 year old deaf or hard of hearing children, followed up by interviews with 80 parents. The authors not only discuss the parents' communication choices for their children, but also provide how parents' experiences differ, especially for those whose children are hard of hearing, have additional conditions, or have cochlear implants. One chapter is devoted to minority cultures. Includes tables, figures, references and index.

272 pages Hardcover
ISBN: 1-563681-37-4

Kathryn P Meadow-Orlans, Co-Author
Donna M Mertens, Co-Author
Marilyn S Sass-Lehrer, Co-Author

3809 Police Officer Jones
HEAR-MORE
42 Executive Boulevard
Farmingdale, NY 11735

800-881-4327
Fax: 631-752-0689
TTY: 800-281-4327
www.hearmore.com

This beginning book describes a police officer and his exciting job. Use the signs when reading the book to your child and speak when you sign so the child will learn to associate the sign with sound and lip shape.

3810 Religious Signing: A Comprehensive Guide for All Faiths

Elaine Costello, author

TJ Publishers
P.O Box 702701
Dallas, TX 75370

972-416-0800
800-999-1168
Fax: 972-416-0944
TTY: 972-416-0933
customerservice@tjpublishers.com
www.tjpublishers.com

Contains over 500 religious signs and their meanings for all denominations. Clearly demonstrated and defined through illustrations that show movement of hands, body and face. Includes a special section on favorite verses, prayers and blessings.

219 pages Softcover
ISBN: 0-553342-44-4

3811 Rhode Island Test of Language Structure RITLS
Pro Ed
8700 Shoal Creed Boulevard
Austin, TX 78757

512-451-3246
800-897-3202
Fax: 800-397-7633
info@proedinc.com
www.proedinc.com

The Rhode Island Test of Language Structure (RITLS) provides a measure of English language development and assessment data. It is designed primarily for use with children who are hearing impaired, but also useful in other areas where level of language development is of concern, including mental retardation, learning disability, and bilingual programs. The RITLS focuses on syntax, unlike other tests compared with other reading, language, intelligence, and achievement tests frequently used.

1983

3812 Schedules of Development for Hearing Impaired Infants and Their Parents
Alexander Graham Bell Association for the Deaf
3417 Volta Place NW
Washington, DC 20007

202-337-5220
Fax: 202-337-8314
TTY: 202-337-5221
info@agbell.org
www.agbell.org

Written for parents and teachers, this assessment record of verbal learning will help to evaluate each child's language development.

1977 14 pages

Agnes Ling Philips PhD, Author

3813 Screening for Hearing Loss and Otitis Media in Children

Jackson Roush PhD, author

Alexander Graham Bell Association for the Deaf
3417 Volta Place NW
Washington, DC 20007

202-337-5220
Fax: 202-337-8314
TTY: 202-337-5221
info@agbell.org
www.agbell.org

Provides a concise yet comprehensive guide to hearing and middle ear screening in children. From acoustic emissions and automated ABR in newborns to hearing screening of school-age children.

245 pages Softcover

3814 Sign Language for Babies
Walter Paul Kelly, author

Harris Communications
15155 Technology Drive
Eden Prairie, MN 55344

952-906-1180
800-825-6758
Fax: 952-906-1099
TTY: 800-825-9187
info@harriscomm.com
www.harriscomm.com

A black and white illustrated story on how love and eventually the ILY handsign in American Sign Language got started.

Hardcover

3815 Sign Numbers
Nancy Bartusch, author

Modern Signs Press
PO Box 1181
Los Alamitos, CA 90720

562-596-8548
800-572-7332
Fax: 562-795-6614
TTY: 562-493-4168
modsigns@modernsignspress.com
www.modernsignspress.com

Mandy helps Handy teach manual and written numbers. Includes printed numbers and easy-to-follow drawings of the number hand shapes. Also shows words and signs for the objects counted in a picture on each page. Black and white drawings make this a coloring book, too.

60 pages

3816 Sign With Kids Supplement
Modern Signs Press
PO Box 1181
Los Alamitos, CA 90720

562-596-8548
800-572-7332
Fax: 562-795-6614
TTY: 562-493-4168
modsigns@modernsignspress.com
www.modernsignspress.com

The supplement contains easy to use illustrations for all the signs in every lesson of Sign With Kids. Both volumes together provide a comprehensive program for teaching sign language to hearing kids.

3817 Sign-Me-Fine
Gallaudet University Press
800 Florida Avenue NE
Washington, DC 20002

202-651-5488
Fax: 202-651-5489
TTY: 202-651-5488
gupress@gallaudet.edu
www.gupress.gallaudet.edu

Written for young adults, this book introduces American Sign Language and how it differs from English.

1997 120 pages paperback
ISBN: 0-930323-76-9

3818 Signing Exact English Using Affixes
Modern Signs Press
PO Box 1181
Los Alamitos, CA 90720

562-596-8548
800-572-7332
Fax: 562-795-6614
TTY: 562-493-4168
modsigns@modernsignspress.com
www.modernsignspress.com

A catalog of signed vocabulary extended by prefixes, suffixes, contractions and tenses.

3819 Signing Family: What Every Parent Should K now About Sign Communication

David A Stewart and Barbara Leutke-Stahlman, author

Gallaudet University Press
800 Florida Avenue NE
Washington, DC 20002
202-651-5488
Fax: 202-651-5489
gupress@gallaudet.edu
www.gupress.gallaudet.edu

Parents of deaf children concerned with finding the best means of communication for their family will welcome the straightforward, reader-friendly information in this book. In a style both positive and pragmatic, the authors employ common-sense reasoning to establish the importance of teach deaf children language fundamentals as early as possible. This essential book for parents continues by explaining why the visual-gestural nature of signing is generally the best languge mode for deaf children

192 pages Softcover
ISBN: 1-563680-69-6

3820 Signing Fun: American Sign Language Vocabu lary, Phrases, Games and Activities

Penny Warner and Paula Gray, author

Gallaudet University Press
800 Florida Avenue NE
Washington, DC 20002
202-651-5488
Fax: 202-651-5489
gupress@gallaudet.edu
www.gupress.gallaudet.edu

For young adults age 11 and up. Signing is visual, easy to learn, and fun to use. Offers 441 useful signs on a variety of favorite topics: activities, animals, fashion, food, holidays, home, outdoors, parties, people, places, play, emotions, school, shopping, travel, plus extra fun signs for especially popular words. Each chapter includes practice sentences using everyday phrases to help new signers learn in a fun way. Provides dozens of entertaining games and activities.

192 pages Softcover
ISBN: 1-563629-23-6

3821 Signing: How to Speak With Your Hands, Sec ond Edition

Elaine Costello, author

TJ Publishers
P.O Box 702701
Dallas, TX 75370
972-416-0800
800-999-1168
Fax: 972-416-0944
TTY: 972-416-0933
customerservice@tjpublishers.com
www.tjpublishers.com

This book presents more than 1300 signs and their descriptions. Linguistic principles are described at the beginning of each chapter giving insight into the rules which govern American Sign Language.

248 pages Softcover
ISBN: 0-553375-39-3

3822 Signs for Me

Ben Bahan and Joe Dannis, author

Harris Communications
15155 Technology Drive
Eden Prairie, MN 55344
952-906-1180
800-825-6758
Fax: 952-906-1099
TTY: 800-825-9187
info@harriscomm.com
www.harriscomm.com

Ideal for youngsters and other sign language beginners, a unique illustrated approach to presenting basic vocabulary. While the book provides a multidimentional sign vocabulary for pre-school and elementary school children, its appealing format makes it suitable for signers of all ages.

111 pages Softcover

3823 Signs for Me: Basic Sign Vocabulary for Ch ildren, Parents and Teachers

Ben Bahan and Joe Dannis, author

TJ Publishers
P.O Box 702701
Dallas, TX 75370
972-416-0800
800-999-1168
Fax: 972-416-0944
TTY: 972-416-0933
customerservice@tjpublishers.com
www.tjpublishers.com

Sign language vocabulary for preschool and elementary school children introduces household items, animals, family members, actions, emotions, safety concerns and other concepts. Over 300 vocabulary words, pictures and sign illustrations.

112 pages Softcover
ISBN: 0-915035-27-8

3824 Signs of Sharing: An Elementary Sign Language and Deaf Awareness Curriculum

Charles C Thomas Publisher
2600 S 1st Street
Springfield, IL 62704
217-789-8980
800-258-8980
Fax: 217-789-9130
books@ccthomas.com
www.ccthomas.com

A unique set of materials that provides educators whose responsibilities include the integration of hearing-impaired children, with a multifaceted tool to teach sign language and deaf awareness.

1993 380 pages
ISBN: 0-398058-51-2
Sue F V Rakow, Co-Author
Carol B Carpenter, Co-Author

3825 Silent Garden

Paul W Ogden, author

Gallaudet University Press
800 Florida Avenue NE
Washington, DC 20002
202-651-5488
Fax: 202-651-5489
gupress@gallaudet.edu
www.gupress.gallaudet.edu

This completely rewritten edition presents parents of deaf children with more crucial information enhanced by the advances made in the general understanding of what it means to be deaf and the greater possibilities afforded deaf children today. Provides parents with a firm foundation for making the difficult decisions necessary to begin their child on the road to realizing his or her full potential.

304 pages Softcover
ISBN: 1-563680-58-0

3826 Silent Observer

Christy MacKinnon, author

Gallaudet University Press
800 Florida Avenue NE
Washington, DC 20002
202-651-5488
Fax: 202-651-5489
gupress@gallaudet.edu
www.gupress.gallaudet.edu

An affectionage, poignant memoir of childhood as seen through the eyes of a vivacious young girl. Teachers, parents, and children will share in their enjoyment of this beautiful, sensitive story of a harder but wonderful time that has passed.

48 pages Hardcover
ISBN: 1-563680-22-X

3827 Simple Signs

Cindy Wheeler, author

Harris Communications
15155 Technology Drive
Eden Prairie, MN 55344

952-906-1180
800-825-6758
Fax: 952-906-1099
TTY: 800-825-9187
info@harriscomm.com
www.harriscomm.com

Children have a lot to say, whether through gestures, movement, pictures or words. American Sign Language incorporates all these natural skills. With pictures, clear diagrams, and hints, learn from these 28 signs. Ages 3-6 years.

30 pages Softcover

3828 Six-Sound Song

Warren Estabrooks MEd, author

Alexander Graham Bell Association for the Deaf
3417 Volta Place NW
Washington, DC 20007

202-337-5220
Fax: 202-337-8314
TTY: 202-337-5221
info@agbell.org
www.agbell.org

Based on the Six-Sound Tests developed by the late Daniel Ling, PhD. Used for both individual and group therapy sessions in auditory and oral environments. Children will enjoy the illustrations created by seven-year-old Hunter Jackson who received his cochlear implant while the Auditory-Verbal Centre of the Learning to Listen Foundation. Hardcover Book and CD set

3829 Songs in Sign

S Harold Collins, author

TJ Publishers
P.O Box 702701
Dallas, TX 75370

972-416-0800
800-999-1168
Fax: 972-416-0944
TTY: 972-416-0933
customerservice@tjpublishers.com
www.tjpublishers.com

Presents six songs in Signed English. The easy-to-follow illustrations enable you to sign: Twinkle, Twinkle Litt Star; The Mullberry Bush; Row, Row, Row Your Boat; If You're Happy; Bingo and The Muffin Man.

16 pages Softcover
ISBN: 0-931993-71-7

3830 Speak to Me (Second Edition)

Marcia Calhoun Forecki, author

Gallaudet University Press
800 Florida Avenue NE
Washington, DC 20002

202-651-5488
Fax: 202-651-5489
gupress@gallaudet.edu
www.gupress.gallaudet.edu

An engrossing, personal account of life with Charlie, an adorable, active, deaf seven-year-old. The story of an ordinary person confronted with an overwhelming reality - the fact that her son is deaf. Forecki's struggle as a single parent to care for her child, to find the right schools, and to establish communication with her son will strike a familiar chord in all hearing parents of deaf children. All readers will be touched by the mixture of pathos and humor in this account.

154 pages Softcover
ISBN: 0-930323-68-8

3831 Speech and the Hearing Impaired Child (Second Edition)

Daniel Ling, PhD, author

Alexander Graham Bell Association for the Deaf
3417 Volta Place NW
Washington, DC 20007

202-337-5220
Fax: 202-337-8314
TTY: 202-337-5221
info@agbell.org
www.agbell.org

An extension of the original text published by the late Daniel Ling in 1976. It looks much more closely at the development of speech in the context of spoken language. It incorporates informal strategies for promoting spoken language development that are appropriate for use with modern technology such as digital hearing aids and cochlear implants. Considerable emphasis is placed on the ongoing evaluation of speech in the context of spoken language.

440 pages Softcover

3832 Speechreading: A Way to Improve Understanding
Gallaudet University Press
800 Florida Avenue NE
Washington, DC 20002

202-651-5488
Fax: 202-651-5489
TTY: 202-651-5488
gupress@gallaudet.edu
www.gupress.gallaudet.edu

This useful guide for teachers and therapists approaches speechreading instruction with the help of context cues.
160 pages

3833 Student Study Guide to A Basic Course in American Sign Language

Frances DeCapite, author

TJ Publishers
P.O Box 702701
Dallas, TX 75370

972-416-0800
800-999-1168
Fax: 972-416-0944
TTY: 972-416-0933
customerservice@tjpublishers.com
www.tjpublishers.com

Designed to supplement the text of A Basic Course in American Sign Language, the guide provides a wide array of supplemental practice materials for student and teacher. Exercises and practice sentences allow students to practice receptive and expressive skills.

197 pages Spiral bound
ISBN: 0-932666-33-7

3834 Talking Finger Series - At Grandma's House
Modern Signs Press
PO Box 1181
Los Alamitos, CA 90720

562-596-8548
800-572-7332
Fax: 562-795-6614
TTY: 562-493-4168
modsigns@modernsignspress.com
www.modernsignspress.com

Pictures, signs and printed words tell the tale of April, a cuddly little rabbit who loves to play with her beloved Grandma. Uses 27-word vocabulary, includes manual alphabet and glossary of signs.

3835 Talking Finger Series - Little Green Monst er
Modern Signs Press
PO Box 1181
Los Alamitos, CA 90720

562-596-8548
800-572-7332
Fax: 562-795-6614
TTY: 562-493-4168
modsigns@modernsignspress.com
www.modernsignspress.com

This storybook features Becky and Barry, two playful little bears who keep you in suspense. The 45-word vocabulary in signs and printed words introduces concept of directionality (here, there, behind, etc.). Includes manual alphabet and glossary of signs.

36 pages

3836   Teach Your Tot to Sign

Stacy A Thompson and Valerie Nelson-Metlay, author

Gallaudet University Press
800 Florida Avenue NE
Washington, DC 20002   202-651-5488
                                                   Fax: 202-651-5489
                                              gupress@gallaudet.edu
                                              www.gupress.gallaudet.edu

This book provides parents and teachers the opportunity to teach more than 500 basic American Sign Language signs to their infants, toddlers, and young children. It features fundamental signs of great appeal to young children and concise instructions on how to sign, including the critical importance of facial expression. Anticipates all of the common desires and interests of young children - food, pets, planes, trains, cars and boats, games, holidays, vegetables, family - nearly everything.

232 pages Softcover
ISBN: 1-563683-11-3

3837   The Book of Choice

Hands and Voices
PO Box 3093
Boulder, CO 80307   303-492-6283
                                                   866-422-0422
                                      parentadvocate@handsandvoices.org
                                           www.handsandvoices.org

Support for parents of a child who is deaf or hard of hearing. Also available in Spanish.

3838   The Development of Deaf Children: Academic Achievement Levels and Social Processes

Kerstin Heiling, author

Gallaudet University Press
800 Florida Avenue NE
Washington, DC 20002   202-651-5488
                                                   Fax: 202-651-5489
                                              gupress@gallaudet.edu
                                              www.gupress.gallaudet.edu

This revealing volume presents the research from a videotape study of the behavior of 20 deaf children for 14 years, and a comprehensive test at age 15 to assess their development.

280 pages Hardcover
ISBN: 3-927731-58-7

3839   The Handbook of Pediatric Audiology

Sanford E Gerber, Editor, author

Gallaudet University Press
800 Florida Avenue NE
Washington, DC 20002   202-651-5488
                                                   Fax: 202-651-5489
                                              gupress@gallaudet.edu
                                              www.gupress.gallaudet.edu

Presents 14 comprehensive chapters written by expert in each discipline. Clinicians and students now can refer to specific subjects in pediatric audiology for treating children from infancy through their elementary school years. Contributors include: Yash Pal Kapur, Franklin A. Katz, Robert J. Ruben, Allen O. Diefendorf, Judith S. Gravel, Jane R. Madell, Shlomo Silman, Carol A. Silverman, Herbert Jay Gold, and Maurice Mendel. Tables, figures, references, bibliography, author and subject index

478 pages Softcover
ISBN: 1-563680-99-7

3840   The Hearing Aid Handbook: Clinician's Guid e to Client Orientation

Donna S Wayner, author

Gallaudet University Press
800 Florida Avenue NE
Washington, DC 20002   202-651-5488
                                                   Fax: 202-651-5489
                                              gupress@gallaudet.edu
                                              www.gupress.gallaudet.edu

This handbook consists of three volumes for audiologists and other clinicians to help clients learn to use hearing aids. Planned for three classes, the guide explains exactly how to conduct the initial visit, fit ear molds, clean and maintain hearing aids and adjust amplification. Clinicians will also learn to encourage the use of visual cues, speechreading, and contextual clues to ensure a high rate of success for their clients. Users Guides feature information and worksheets.

172 pages Softcover
ISBN: 0-930323-56-4

3841   The Joy of Signing Second Edition

Lottie L Riekehof, author

TJ Publishers
P.O Box 702701
Dallas, TX 75370   972-416-0800
                                                   800-999-1168
                                              Fax: 972-416-0944
                                              TTY: 972-416-0933
                                      customerservice@tjpublishers.com
                                           www.tjpublishers.com

This popular dictionary of approximately 1500 known signs makes them easier to remember. Sentences present signs in proper context. Appendix gives information about the most effective way to add signs to spoken English.

352 pages Hardcover
ISBN: 0-882435-20-5

3842   The Listener

Warren Estabrooks, MEd, author

Alexander Graham Bell Association for the Deaf
3417 Volta Place NW
Washington, DC 20007   202-337-5220
                                                   Fax: 202-337-8314
                                              TTY: 202-337-5221
                                              info@agbell.org
                                              www.agbell.org

Subject material is centered around listening, speech, language, spoken communication, and cognitive, social and psychological development of children who are deaf or hard of hearing and their families. Articles address: Making sense of complex skills lesson planning, Morphosyntax: evidence-based AVT, Your young child's newly diagnosed hearing loss: knowing how to cope, What is Auditory-Verbal Therapy?, Teachers' perceptions of the integration of children with hearing loss.

64 pages Softcover

3843   The Night Before Christmas told in Signed english

Adapted By Harry Bornstein and Karen L Saulnier, author

Gallaudet University Press
800 Florida Avenue NE
Washington, DC 20002   202-651-5488
                                                   Fax: 202-651-5489
                                              gupress@gallaudet.edu
                                              www.gupress.gallaudet.edu

Now this wonderful, seasonal poem can be enjoyed in a new way by both hearing and deaf children. Accompanying the complete verses and full-color illustrations, line drawings show this holiday favorite in Signed English, the system that uses American Sign Language signs in English word order. Uses both rhyme and signing to help children practice their vocabulary and learn English grammar. Entertains at the same time that it teaches.

64 pages Hardcover
ISBN: 1-563680-20-3

Clement C Moore, Original Author

3844   The Rising of Lotus Flowers: Self-Educating Deaf Children in Thai Boarding Schools

Charles B Reilly and Nipapon Reilly, author

Gallaudet University Press
800 Florida Avenue NE
Washington, DC 20002   202-651-5488
                                   Fax: 202-651-5489
                                 gupress@gallaudet.edu
                                www.gupress.gallaudet.edu

In developed nations around the world, residential schools for deaf students are giving way to the trend of inclusion in regular classrooms. Nonetheless, deaf education continues to lag as students struggle to communicate. In the Bua School in Thialand, however, 400 residential deaf students ranging in age from 6 to 19 have met with great success in teaching each other Thai Sign Language and a world of knowledge once thought to be lost to them.

272 pages Hardcover
ISBN: 1-563682-75-3

3845   The Young Deaf Child

David Luterman, PhD, author

Alexander Graham Bell Association for the Deaf
3417 Volta Place NW
Washington, DC 20007   202-337-5220
                                   Fax: 202-337-8314
                                   TTY: 202-337-5221
                                      info@agbell.org
                                      www.agbell.org

A valuable resource for audiologists, early interventionists and special educators who provide diagnostic or therapeutic services to parents of newborns and children with hearing loss. Discusses the history of deaf education in the United States and offers valuable information on the pros and cons of screening, elements essential to effective programming and therapy, a model for intervention centered on the parent-child connection, assistive hearing technologies and counseling techniques.

3846   Un Curso Basico de Lenguaje Americano de S enas
TJ Publishers
P.O Box 702701
Dallas, TX 75370   972-416-0800
                                        800-999-1168
                                   Fax: 972-416-0944
                                   TTY: 972-416-0933
                               customerservice@tjpublishers.com
                                   www.tjpublishers.com

Features English and Spanish translations side by side. It is designed for teachers, parents and students working with Deaf Hispanic American children and adults learning English and American Sign Language.

356 pages Spiral bound
ISBN: 0-932666-35-3

3847   We Can Hear and Speak
Alexander Graham Bell Association for the Deaf
3417 Volta Place NW
Washington, DC 20007   202-337-5220
                                   Fax: 202-337-8314
                                   TTY: 202-337-5221
                                      info@agbell.org
                                      www.agbell.org

Written by parents for families of children who are deaf or hard-of-hearing, this work describes auditory-verbal terminology and approaches and contains personal narratives written by parents and their children who are deaf or hard-of-hearing.

1998 184 pages Softcover

Carol Flexer PhD, Contributor
Catherine Richards, Contributor

3848   Winnie-the-Pooh's ABCs
HEAR-MORE
42 Executive Boulevard
Farmingdale, NY 11735   800-881-4327
                                   Fax: 631-752-0689
                                   TTY: 800-281-4327
                                      www.hearmore.com

In this special edition of Winnie-the-Pooh's ABC, both hearing and deaf children are introduced to the written and ASL alphabets, Hundred Acre Wood-Style. Inspired by A.A. Milne

32 pages

3849   Word Signs: A First Book of Sign Language

Debbie Slier, author

Gallaudet University Press
800 Florida Avenue NE
Washington, DC 20002   202-651-5488
                                   Fax: 202-651-5489
                                 gupress@gallaudet.edu
                                www.gupress.gallaudet.edu

Charming, full-cover photgraphs of basic animals plus illustrations of their corresponding signs offer children ages 1 to 4 a fun way to learn their first signs and vocabulary words.

164 pages Board book
ISBN: 1-563680-48-3

3850   You and Your Deaf Child
Gallaudet University Press
800 Florida Avenue NE
Washington, DC 20002   202-651-5488
                                   Fax: 202-651-5489
                                   TTY: 202-651-5489
                                 gupress@gallaudet.edu
                                www.gupress.gallaudet.edu

This guide for parents explores how families interact to deal with the special impact of a child who is hearing impaired.

1997 224 pages softcover
ISBN: 0-563680-60-2

3851   You and Your Deaf Child: A Self-Help Guide for Parents of Deaf and Hard of Hearing

John W Adams, author

Gallaudet University Press
800 Florida Avenue NE
Washington, DC 20002   202-651-5488
                                   Fax: 202-651-5489
                                 gupress@gallaudet.edu
                                www.gupress.gallaudet.edu

A guide for parents of deaf or hard of hearing children that explores how parents and their children interact. It examines the special impact of having a deaf child in the family. Eleven chapters focus on such topics as feelings about hearing loss, the importance of communication in the family, and effective behavior management. Many chapters contain practice activities and check their grasp of the material.

224 pages Softcover
ISBN: 1-563680-60-2

3852   Young Deaf Child
Alexander Graham Bell Association for the Deaf
3417 Volta Place NW
Washington, DC 20007   202-337-5220
                                   Fax: 202-337-8314
                                   TTY: 202-337-5221
                                      info@agbell.org
                                      www.agbell.org

With a foreward by Mark Ross, Ph.D., this book is based on experience by the three authors and outlines the best approach for the child, early intervention, maximization of technology and strong family involvment.

1999 235 pages

David Luterman PhD, Author

Magazines

3853 Auditory - Verbal International
2121 Eisenhower Avenue, Suite 402
Alexandria, VA 22314
703-739-1049
Fax: 703-739-0395
TTY: 703-739-0874
audiverb@aol.com

Magazine of the organization dedicated to helping children who have hearing losses learn to listen and speak. Promotes the Auditory-Verbal Therapy approach, which is based on the belief that the overwhelming majority of these children can hear and talk by using their residual hearing and hearing aids. Membership dues for Canada are $55, International, $60, US, $50, and students are charged $30.

Quarterly

Sara Lake, Executive Director/CEO
Mary Benson, Executive Assistant

3854 Deaf Life
c/o MSM Productions, LTD
1095 Meigs Street
Rochester, NY 14620
716-442-6370
Fax: 716-442-6371
TTY: 716-442-6370
deaflife@deaflife.com
www.deaflife.com

This magazine focuses on profiles, news, controversial issues, cultural topics and more relating to the deaf community, first published in 1988.

64 pages Monthly
ISSN: 0898-719x

Matthew Moore, Publisher

3855 Deaf USA
Eye Festival Communications
6917B Woodley Avenue
Van Nuys, CA 91406
Fax: 818-902-9840

Provides news coverage on all activities and issues of interest to deaf and hard-of-hearing readers as well as professionals and associates within this specialized market.

Monthly

David Rosenbaum, Editor

3856 Hearing Health
363 Seventh Avenue, 10th Floor
New York, NY 10001
212-257-6140
866-454-3924
Fax: 361-776-3278
info@hhf.org
hearinghealthfoundation.org/hearing-health-magazine

A publication for deaf and hard-of-hearing people, as well as hearing health care professionals, libraries, agencies, schools and organizations.

Bimonthly

Paula Bartone-Bonillas, Editor
Shari Eberts, Chairman
Robert Boucai, Principal

3857 Perspectives in Education and Deafness
Gallaudet University Press
800 Florida Avenue NE
Washington, DC 20002
202-651-5488
800-621-2736
Fax: 800-621-8476
TTY: 202-651-5444
gupress@gallaudet.edu
gupress.gallaudet.edu

A practical, reader-friendly magazine, offering help and advice in and beyond the classroom, tuned to the needs of today's students, teachers and families.

5 times a year

Mary Abrams Perica, Editor

3858 The Deaf-Blind American
American Association of the Deaf-Blind
PO Box 8064
Silver Spring, MD 20907
301-563-9064
Fax: 301-495-4404
TTY: 301-495-4402
aadb-info@aadb.org
www.aadb.org

The Deaf-Blind American (DBA), the official quarterly magazine of the AADB, is available only to its members. It contains articles of interest to deaf-blind individuals, their families, and service providers who work with people who are deaf-blind. The DBA is available in large print, Braille, disk and email.

Timothy Jackson, President
Jill Gaus, Vice President
Debby Lieberman, Secretary

3859 Volta Voices
Alexander Graham Bell Association for the Deaf
3417 Volta Place NW
Washington, DC 20007
202-337-5220
800-432-7543
Fax: 202-337-8314
TTY: 203-337-5221
info@agbell.org
listeningandspokenlanguage.org

A magazine highlighting inspirational stories from parents of children who are deaf, legislative news, technology update, and stories pertaining to speech, speech-reading, and the use of residual hearing.

Bimonthly

Brooke Rigler, Editor
Lisa Chutjian, Chief Development Officer
Emilio Alonso-Mendoza, Chief Executive Officer

Journals

3860 American Annals of the Deaf
Convention of American Instructors of the Deaf
800 Florida Avenue NE, Fowler Hall 409
Washington, DC 20002
202-651-5488
Fax: 202-651-5708
TTY: 202-651-5444
gupress@gallaudet.edu
gupress.gallaudet.edu

Scholarly journal at the forefront of research related to the education of deaf people. Annual reference Issue identifies programs and services for deaf people nationwide.

5 times a year

Donald F Moores, Editor
Mary Ellen Carew, Managing Editor

3861 Hearing Loss Magazine
Self Help for Hard-of-Hearing People
7910 Woodmont Avenue, Suite 1200
Bethesda, MD 20814
301-657-2248
Fax: 301-913-9413
TTY: 301-657-2249
www.hearingloss.org

An educational journal about hearing loss for hard-of-hearing people.

Bimonthly

Barbara Kelley, Editor-In-Chief
Anna Gilmore Hall, Executive Director
Lisa Hamlin, Director of Public Policy

3862 Journal of Speech, Language, and Hearing Research
American Speech Language Hearing Association
2200 Research Blvd
Rockville, MD 20850
301-296-5700
800-478-2071
Fax: 301-296-8580
TTY: 301-296-5650
TDD: 301-296-5650
productsales@asha.org
www.asha.org

Pertains broadly to studies of the processes and disorders of hearing, language, and speech and to the diagnosis and treatment of such disorders.

Bi-monthly

Dr Anne Smith, Editor, Speech
Dr Karla McGregor, Editor, Language
Dr Robert Schlauch, Editor, Hearing

3863 Language, Speech, and Hearing in Schools
American Speech Language Hearing Association
2200 Research Blvd
Rockville, MD 20850

301-296-5700
800-478-2071
Fax: 301-296-8580
TTY: 301-296-5650
TDD: 301-296-5650
productsales@asha.org
www.asha.org

An archival journal for research and practice in educational settings. Publishes studies and articles that pertain to speech, language, and hearing disorders and differences in children and adolescents, as well as to professional issues affecting service delivery in educational setting.

Quarterly

Dr Kenn Apel, Editor
Judith L. Page, PhD, CCC-SLP, President
Margot L. Beckerman, AuD, CCC-A, Chair

Newsletters

3864 AADB E-News
American Association of the Deaf-Blind
PO Box 8064
Silver Spring, MD 20907

301-563-9064
Fax: 301-495-4404
TTY: 301-495-4402
aadb-info@aadb.org
www.aadb.org

A free newsletter, the AADB E-News is available to anyone during the months when the DBA is not being published. It contains information about the latest events occurring within AADB and in the deaf-blind community. One does not need to be an AADB member to receive the free AADB E-News newsletter.

Timothy Jackson, President
Jill Gaus, Vice President
Debby Lieberman, Secretary

3865 Endeavor
American Society for Deaf Children
PO Box 3355
Gettysburg, PA 17325

717-334-7922
800-942-2732
Fax: 717-334-8808

Newsletter for parents of deaf children.

Quarterly

Barbara Aschembrenner, Editor

3866 Gallaudet Today
Gallaudet University Press
800 Florida Avenue NE
Washington, DC 20002

202-651-5488
800-621-2736
Fax: 800-621-8476
TTY: 202-651-5444
gupress@gallaudet.edu
gupress.gallaudet.edu

A university alumni publication with both general and special issues on deafness-related topics.

44 pages Quarterly

Roz Prickett, Publications Manager

3867 Hear
Deafness Research Foundation
15 W 39th Street
New York, NY 10018

212-768-1181

Offers information on the Foundation's activities and events, technical updates on assistive devices, legislative and medical information on the latest breakthroughs and laws for the hearing impaired, book reviews and resources.

Monte H Jacoby, Executive Director

3868 NADezine
National Association of the Deaf
8630 Fenton Street, Suite 820
Silver Spring, MD 20910

301-587-1788
Fax: 301-587-1791
TTY: 301-587-1789
nad.info@nad.org
www.nad.org

A biweekly, online web-zine providing up-to-date information about NAD advocacy, biennial conferences, workshops and training, youth happenings, community news and how you can become involved.

Internet

Christopher D. Wagner, President
Melissa S. Draganac-Hawk, Vice President
Joshua Beckman, Secretary

3869 Newsletter of American Hearing Research
American Hearing Research Foundation
275 N. York Street, Suite 401
Elmhurst, IL 60126

630-617-5079
Fax: 630-563-9181
american-hearing.org

Concerned with hearing research and education.

Richard G. Muench, Chairman
Alan G. Micco, M.D., President
Mark R. Muench, Vice President

3870 Newsline
Sertoma Foundation
1912 E Meyer Boulevard
Kansas City, MO 64132

816-333-8300
infosertoma@sertomahq.org
www.sertoma.org

Reports on activities of the Sertoma Foundation in the field of speech and hearing impairments.

David Johnson, President
Don Bartelmay, Senior Vice President
Cheryl Cherny, Junior Vice President

3871 Signs for Me: Basic Sign Vocabulary for Children, Parents, & Teachers
TJ Publishers
817 Silver Spring Avenue, Suite 206
Silver Spring, MD 20910

301-585-4440
800-999-1168
Fax: 301-585-5930
TTY: 301-585-4440
TDD: 301-585-4441
TJPubinc@aol.com

Sign language vocabulary for preschool and elementary school children introduces household items, animals, family members, actions, emotions, safety concerns and other concepts.

112 pages Softcover

3872 Speech and Deafness Newsletter
Hearing, Speech
1620 18th Avenue
Seattle, WA 98122

206-323-5770

Agency newsletter for membership and community.

8 pages

Patty Tumberg, Editor

3873 Volta Review
Alexander Graham Bell Association for the Deaf
3417 Volta Place NW
Washington, DC 20007
202-337-5220
800-432-7543
Fax: 202-337-8314
TTY: 203-337-5221
info@agbell.org
listeningandspokenlanguage.org

Offers the latest theory, research, current perspectives and practical guidance from noted specialists in education, audiology, speech and language sciences and psychology. Each issue contains a Special Focus-a group of chapters exploring a specific topic in detail.

Quarterly

Lisa Chutjian, Chief Development Officer
Emilio Alonso-Mendoza, Chief Executive Officer
Judy Harrison, Director of Programs

Pamphlets

3874 25 Ways to Promote Spoken Language in Your Child with a Hearing Loss
Alexander Graham Bell Association for the Deaf
3417 Volta Place NW
Washington, DC 20007
202-337-5220
800-432-7543
Fax: 202-337-8314
TTY: 203-337-5221
info@agbell.org
listeningandspokenlanguage.org

This pamphlet teaches twenty-five golden rules about preparing your child to listen and to speak.

1995 62 pages

Lisa Chutjian, Chief Development Officer
Emilio Alonso-Mendoza, Chief Executive Officer
Judy Harrison, Director of Programs

3875 Books for Parents of Deaf and Hard-of- Hearing Children
National Information Center on Deafness
800 Florida Avenue NE
Washington, DC 20002
202-651-5488
Fax: 202-651-5054
TTY: 202-651-5444
gupress@gallaudet.edu
gupress.gallaudet.edu

Identifies books written for parents and everday experiences of deaf and hard-of-hearing children.

3876 Can Your Baby Hear?
Alexander Graham Bell Association for the Deaf
3417 Volta Place NW
Washington, DC 20007
202-337-5220
800-432-7543
Fax: 202-337-8314
TTY: 203-337-5221
info@agbell.org
listeningandspokenlanguage.org

This simple card for parents lists risk indicators and warning signs of hearing loss in babies.

Lisa Chutjian, Chief Development Officer
Emilio Alonso-Mendoza, Chief Executive Officer
Judy Harrison, Director of Programs

3877 Care of the Ears and Hearing for Health
American Hearing Research Foundation
275 N. York Street, Suite 401
Elmhurst, IL 60126
630-617-5079
Fax: 630-563-9181
american-hearing.org

Offers information on ear infections relating to chronic progressive deafness.

Richard G. Muench, Chairman
Alan G. Micco, M.D., President
Mark R. Muench, Vice President

3878 Communicating with People who Have a Hearing Loss
Alexander Graham Bell Association for the Deaf
3417 Volta Place NW
Washington, DC 20007
202-337-5220
800-432-7543
Fax: 202-337-8314
TTY: 203-337-5221
info@agbell.org
listeningandspokenlanguage.org

This brochure describes ways to communicate more effectively with people who have hearing losses.

1994

Lisa Chutjian, Chief Development Officer
Emilio Alonso-Mendoza, Chief Executive Officer
Judy Harrison, Director of Programs

3879 Deafness: A Fact Sheet
National Information Center On Deafness
800 Florida Avenue NE
Washington, DC 20002
202-651-5488
Fax: 202-651-5054
TTY: 202-651-5444
gupress@gallaudet.edu
gupress.gallaudet.edu

3880 Developing Cognition in Young Children Who are Deaf
Hope
55 E 100 N
Logan, UT 84321
435-752-9533
Fax: 435-752-9533

Presents interesting, updated information on the importance of early cognition development in young children who are deaf. Contains many ideas for ways to promote early thinking skills, especially those that promote and enhance early communication and language development.

3881 Educating Deaf Children: An Introduction
National Information Center on Deafness
800 Florida Avenue NE
Washington, DC 20002
202-651-5488
Fax: 202-651-5054
TTY: 202-651-5444
gupress@gallaudet.edu
gupress.gallaudet.edu

Describes the different settings in which deaf children are currently educated.

3882 Hearing Alert Informational Brochures
Alexander Graham Bell Association for the Deaf
3417 Volta Place NW
Washington, DC 20007
202-337-5220
800-432-7543
Fax: 202-337-8314
TTY: 203-337-5221
info@agbell.org
listeningandspokenlanguage.org

These brochures encourage early detection of hearing loss in young children; for medical facilities, speech and hearing clinics, and schools.

Lisa Chutjian, Chief Development Officer
Emilio Alonso-Mendoza, Chief Executive Officer
Judy Harrison, Director of Programs

3883 Helping Your Hard-of-Hearing Child Succeed
Alexander Graham Bell Association for the Deaf
3417 Volta Place NW
Washington, DC 20007
202-337-5220
800-432-7543
Fax: 202-337-8314
TTY: 203-337-5221
info@agbell.org
listeningandspokenlanguage.org

Offers information on how to help children succeed in school with speech and language development.

Lisa Chutjian, Chief Development Officer
Emilio Alonso-Mendoza, Chief Executive Officer
Judy Harrison, Director of Programs

3884 How Does Your Child Hear and Talk?
American Speech Language Hearing Association
2200 Research Blvd
Rockville, MD 20850

301-296-5700
800-478-2071
Fax: 301-296-8580
TTY: 301-296-5650
TDD: 301-296-5650
productsales@asha.org
www.asha.org

Offers a chart to parents on children's growth pertaining to their hearing and speech.

Judith L. Page, PhD, CCC-SLP, President
Margot L. Beckerman, AuD, CCC-A, Chair
Barbara K. Cone, PhD, CCC-A, VP, Academic Affairs in Audiology

3885 Leading National Publications of and for Deaf People
National Information Center On Deafness
800 Florida Avenue NE
Washington, DC 20002

202-651-5488
Fax: 202-651-5054
TTY: 202-651-5444
gupress@gallaudet.edu
gupress.gallaudet.edu

Identifies publications with national circulations to deaf audiences.

3886 Listen - Hear for Parents of Hearing Impaired Children
Alexander Graham Bell Association for the Deaf
3417 Volta Place NW
Washington, DC 20007

202-337-5220
800-432-7543
Fax: 202-337-8314
TTY: 203-337-5221
info@agbell.org
listeningandspokenlanguage.org

Offers information that parents of deaf and hard-of-hearing children need to be aware of. Also includes information on hearing aids, hearing loss and the association in general.

Lisa Chutjian, Chief Development Officer
Emilio Alonso-Mendoza, Chief Executive Officer
Judy Harrison, Director of Programs

3887 National Information Center on Deafness Brochure
National Information Center on Deafness
800 Florida Avenue NE
Washington, DC 20002

202-651-5488
Fax: 202-651-5054
TTY: 202-651-5444
gupress@gallaudet.edu
gupress.gallaudet.edu

A description of services offered by NICD.

3888 Parent Packets
Alexander Graham Bell Association for the Deaf
3417 Volta Place NW
Washington, DC 20007

202-337-5220
800-432-7543
Fax: 202-337-8314
TTY: 203-337-5221
info@agbell.org
listeningandspokenlanguage.org

These educational packets for parents are specifically designed to address important age-related topics about your child with a hearing impairment.

Packet

Lisa Chutjian, Chief Development Officer
Emilio Alonso-Mendoza, Chief Executive Officer
Judy Harrison, Director of Programs

3889 Perspectives Folio: Parent-Child
Gallaudet University Press
800 Florida Avenue NE
Washington, DC 20002

202-651-5488
800-621-2736
Fax: 800-621-8476
TTY: 202-651-5444
gupress@gallaudet.edu
gupress.gallaudet.edu

Seven articles emphasizing family communication while providing important information for parents about deafness and the deaf culture.

29 pages

3890 Publications From the National Information Center on Deafness
National Information Center on Deafness
800 Florida Avenue NE
Washington, DC 20002

202-651-5488
Fax: 202-651-5054
TTY: 202-651-5444
gupress@gallaudet.edu
gupress.gallaudet.edu

Order form and explanations of NICD publications.

3891 Questions and Answers on Hearing Loss
Self Help for Hard-of-Hearing People
7910 Woodmont Avenue, Suite 1200
Bethesda, MD 20814

301-657-2248
Fax: 301-913-9413
TTY: 301-657-2249
info@hearingloss.org
www.hearingloss.org

Barbara Kelley, Editor-In-Chief
Anna Gilmore Hall, Executive Director
Lisa Hamlin, Director of Public Policy

3892 Signs for Me: Basic Sign Vocabulary for Children, Parents, & Teachers
DawnSignPress
6130 Nancy Ridge Drive
San Diego, CA 92121

858-625-0600
800-549-5350
Fax: 858-625-2336
info@dawnsign.com
www.dawnsign.com

ASL/English vocabulary primer. Young readers will associate a sign and picture with the English form of a word. Introduces more than 300 primary words arranged in thematic groupings. Captures students' interest through clearly illustrated signs and actions; includes an illustrated look at the English word for effective bilingual learning.

128 pages paperback
ISBN: 0-915035-27-8

Ben Bahan, Co-Author
Joe Dannis, Co-Author

3893 So You Have Had An Ear Operation...What Next?
American Hearing Research Foundation
275 N. York Street, Suite 401
Elmhurst, IL 60126

630-617-5079
Fax: 630-563-9181
american-hearing.org

Offers information on ear infections and surgery.

Richard G. Muench, Chairman
Alan G. Micco, M.D., President
Mark R. Muench, Vice President

3894 Speechreading: Methods and Materials
Self Help for Hard-of-Hearing People
7910 Woodmont Avenue, Suite 1200
Bethesda, MD 20814

301-657-2248
Fax: 301-913-9413
TTY: 301-657-2249
info@hearingloss.org
www.hearingloss.org

Barbara Kelley, Editor-In-Chief
Anna Gilmore Hall, Executive Director
Lisa Hamlin, Director of Public Policy

3895 Statewide Services for Deaf and Hard of Hearing People
National Information Center on Deafness
800 Florida Avenue NE
Washington, DC 20002

202-651-5488
Fax: 202-651-5054
TTY: 202-651-5444
gupress@gallaudet.edu
gupress.gallaudet.edu

A resource list of states that have established commissions and other offices to serve deaf people.

3896 World of Sound
International Hearing Society
16880 Middlebelt Road, Suite 4
Livonia, MI 48154

734-522-7200
Fax: 734-522-0200
www.hearingihs.org

The purpose of this booklet is to provide basic information for those with questions about hearing loss, hearing aids and hearing instrument specialists.

Camps

3897 Camp Civitan
12635 North 42nd Street
Phoenix, AZ 85032

602-953-2944
Fax: 602-953-2946
info@campcivitan.org
www.campcivitan.org

A 501c3 non-profit organization, that has been providing multiple ever-changing programs to meet the needs of children and adults who are developmentally disabled.

Rob Adams, Camp Director
Charlie Riggs, Camp Maintenance
Mary Kellogg, Operations

3898 Camp Emanuel
PO Box 752343
Dayton, OH 45475

973-477-5504
ginter.7@wright.edu
campemanuel.weebly.com

Camp Emanuel is a camp for children with and without disabilities. It is the only camp of its kind in southwestern Ohio. The camp is designed to promote decision-making, team building skills, self-esteem, and an understanding of acceptance between all children.

Stephanie Ackner, President
Brian Demarke, Vice President
Mary Foreman, Secretary

3899 Camp Grizzly
4708 Roseville Road, Suite 112
North Highlands, CA 95660

916-349-7500
Fax: 916-993-3048
TTY: 916-349-7500
sfarinha@norcalcenter.org
www.norcalcenter.org

A one-week residential camp program for deaf and hard of hearing youth age 7 to 17.

Sheri Farinha, CEO
Cheryl Bella, Chair
Michael D. Wilson, Vice Chair

3900 Camp Juliena
4151 Memorial Dr, Suite 103-B
Decatur, GA 30032

404-292-5312
800-541-0710
Fax: 404-299-3642
campjuliena@gmail.com
www.gachi.org

A weeklong residential summer camp for youths and teens who are deaf or hard of hearing. Through challanging, team-oriented activities, campers form lasting friendships and acquire valuable leadership, social and communication skills.

Pat Ford, President
Jeanette Lorch, Vice President
Martha Timms, Secretary

3901 Camp Shocco for the Deaf
PO Box 6569
Talladega, AL 35161

256-761-1100
campshocco@albcdeaf.org
www.campshocco.org

Camp for deaf and hard of hearing students age 8 through high school. The campers will learn about Bible stories, teamwork, and have plenty of fun with various activities during recreation time.

Chad Fleming, Camp Director
Matthew Dixon, Co-Director
Linnea Elliott, Assistant Director

3902 Central Michigan University Summer Clinics
444 Moore
Mount Pleasant, MI

517-774-3803

Designed for children, ages 6 and up, with speech, language and hearing disorders who can benefit from intensive clinical work. A wide range of recreational and social activities form part of the clinical program and promote the social use of skills learned in class.

3903 Children's Beach House
100 W, 10th Street, Suite 411
Wilmington, DE 19801

302-655-4288
Fax: 302-655-4216
childrens.beach.house@dol.net
www.cbhinc.org

Summer camp for children from Delaware of normal mental level, with speech, language and hearing disorders are accepted, ages 6-13. Activities include aquatics, art, music, nature and dramatics. Speech and language therapy are provided. Also school-year environmental education for Delaware students of all exceptionalities.

Richard T. Garrett, Executive Director
Jennifer A. Clement, Director
Nicholas Imhoff, Business Manager

3904 Des Moines YMCA Camp
1192 166th Drive
Boone, IA 50036

515-432-7558
Fax: 515-432-5414
ycamp@dmymca.org
www.y-camp.org

For boys and girls with cancer, diabetes, asthma, cystic fibrosis, hearing impaired and other disabilities.

David Sherry, Executive Director
Mike Havlik, Program Director
Alex Kretzinger, Program Director- Summer Camp

3905 Easter Seal Kysoc
2050 Versailles Road
Lexington, KY 40504

859-254-5701
800-800-888
Fax: 502-732-0783
ek1@cardinalhill.org
www.cardinalhill.org

Designed for the fullest camping experience for children or adults with physical disabilities, blind, deaf, behavior disorders, mental retardation, diabetes and multiple handicaps, ages 7 and up.

Heide Miller, CCD, CTRS, Director
Gary Payne, President/CEO

3906 Enchanted Hills Camp
Lighthouse
214 Van Ness Avenue
San Francisco, CA 94102
415-431-1481
Fax: 415-863-7568
TTY: 415-431-4572
info@lighthouse-sf.org
lighthouse-sf.org

For blind, deaf/blind children and adults, ages 5 and up. This program offers a basic camping experience. Activities include music, art, dance, hiking and riding. Camperships are available to California residents.

Joshua A. Miele, Ph.D., President
Chris Downey, 1st Vice President
Kathleen Knox, 2nd Vice President

3907 Florida School-Deaf and Blind Summer Camp
207 N. San Marco Avenue
Saint Augustine, FL 32084
904-827-2200
800-800-344
info@fsdb.k12.fl.us
www.fsdb.k12.fl.us

The Florida School for the Deaf and the Blind hosts summer campers from all over teh state of Florida for a week of fun and adventure. FSDB's 80 acre campus is where campers participate in a variety of activities including rock climbing, archery, swimming, kayaking, team games, arts and crafts, dance music, and much more.

Jeanne Glidden Prickett, President
Nancy Bloch, Executive Director, Comm & PR
Tanya Rhodes, Executive Director, Advancement

3908 Indiana Deaf Camp
100 West 86th Street
Indianapolis, IN 46260
317-846-3404
Fax: 317-844-1034
deafcamp@hotmail.com
www.indeafcamps.org

Camp dedicated to promoting the educational, social, spiritual, physical and personal development of individuals with a hearing loss, or who are related to individuals with a hearing loss.

Nunery, President

3909 Meadowood Springs Speech and Hearing Camp
PO Box 1025
Pendleton, OR 97801
541-276-2752
Fax: 541-276-7227
info@meadowoodsprings.org
www.meadowoodsprings.org

On 143 acres in the Blue Mountains of Eastern Oregon, this camp is designed to help young people who have diagnosed clinical disorders of speech, hearing or language. A full range of activities in recreational and clinical areas is available. For cabin reservations 541-566-2191.

Rosemarie Atfield, Executive Director
Marie Story, Camp Manager
Cliff Story, Camp Manager

3910 NAD Youth Leadership Camp
National Association of the Deaf
8630 Fenton Street, Suite 820
Silver Spring, MD 20910
301-587-1788
Fax: 301-587-1791
TTY: 301-587-1789
nad.info@nad.org
www.nad.org

An annual 4-week summer program designed to foster leadership and teamwork skills in deaf and hard of hearing high school students. Campers have the opportunity to build and develop their knowledge, social interaction, and leadership skills through hands-on activities focusing on literacy, and often make life-long friends here. 2009 Dates & Location: June 25 - July 22, Camp Taloali at Stayton, Oregon.

Christopher D. Wagner, President
Melissa S. Draganac-Hawk, Vice President
Joshua Beckman, Secretary

3911 Texas Lions Camp
Lions Clubs of Texas
PO Box 290247
Kerrville, TX 78029
830-896-8500
830-896-8500
Fax: 830-896-3666
tlc@ktc.com
www.lionscamp.com

The primary purpose of Texas Lions camp is to provide, without charge, a camp for physically disabled, hearing/vision impaired and diabetic children from the State of Texas, regardless of race, religion, or national origin. Our goal is to create an atmosphere wherein campers will learn the can do philosophy and be allowed to achieve maximum personal growth and self esteem. The camp welcomes boys and girls ages 7-16.

Stephen Mabry, CEO
Doug Parker, Business Manager
Steven King, Program/Client Service Director

3912 University of Iowa - Wendell Johnson Speech and Hearing Clinic
Wendell Johnson Speech And Hearing Center
Iowa City, IA 52242
319-335-1845
Fax: 319-335-8851
www.uiowa.edu

The clinic offers assessment and remediation for disordered communication in adults and children. The clinic also offers an Intensive Summer Residential Clinic for school age children needing intervention services because of speech, language, hearing and/or reading problems.

Richard Hurtig, Professor/Chair
Ann L Michael, Clinic Director

3913 Windsor Mountain Camp
One World Way
Windsor, NH 3244
603-478-3166
jake@windsormountain.org
www.windsormountain.org

Summer camp for deaf and hard of hearing students and for hearing campers who want to learn ASL.

Jake Labovitz, Director
Dianna Hahn, Student Travel Programs
Pam Butler, Administrative Assistant

3914 Wisconsin Lions Camp
3834 County Road A
Rosholt, WI 54473
715-677-4969
Fax: 715-677-3297
TTY: 715-677-6999
wlf@wlf.info
www.wisconsinlionscamp.com

Serves children who have either a visual, hearing or mild cognitive disability. Many of the children also have multiple disabilities or medical conditions. Program activities include sailing, ropes course, bike and canoe trips, environmental education, swimming, camping, canoeing, outdoor living skills and handicrafts. ACA accredited, located in central Wisconsin, near Stevens Point.

Evett J. Hartvig, Executive Director
Dale Schroeder, Facility Director
Elizabeth Shelley, Administrative Assistant

DESCRIPTION

3915   HEMANGIOMAS AND LYMPHANGIOMAS

Covers these related disorders: Capillary hemangiomas, Cavernous hemangiomas, Cystic hygromas, Disseminated hemangiomatosis, Mixed hemangiomas, Port-wine stains (or salmon patches), Kasabach-merritt syndrome

Involves the following Biologic System(s):

Dermatologic Disorders

Hemangiomas are the most common benign tumors in infants. In addition, during childhood, lymphangiomas, also known as lymphatic malformations, are the second most common benign tumor affecting vessels of the body. Hemangiomas consist of an abnormal distribution of relatively small blood vessels (e.g., capillaries) due to malformation of developing fetal tissue from which the vessels arise. Lymphangiomas consist of masses of abnormally enlarged (dilated), newly formed lymph vessels, which are the channels that transport lymphatic fluid throughout the body. Lymph, a thin bodily fluid that consists of proteins, fats, and certain white blood cells (lymphocytes), accumulates in spaces between tissue cells and flows back into the bloodstream via lymph vessels.

Hemangiomas usually affect blood vessels of the skin (cutaneous hemangiomas). They most commonly develop in the head and neck regions and are rarely fully formed at birth. These tumors, which occur more frequently in females than males, are usually single growths that occur randomly for unknown reasons. However, some multigenerational families (kindreds) have been reported in which several individuals developed isolated hemangiomas. In such cases, the condition may be transmitted as an autosomal dominant trait. In addition, in rare cases, certain forms of hemangiomas may occur in association with particular underlying syndromes.

Cutaneous hemangiomas may be superficial (capillary hemangiomas), deep (cavernous hemangiomas), or both (mixed hemangiomas). Capillary hemangiomas are considered the most common type of hemangioma, affecting approximately 60 percent of patients. These hemangiomas include port-wine stains (a form of nevus flammeus) and strawberry hemangiomas (strawberry nevi). Port-wine stains are present at birth (congenital) and are typically permanent defects. These lesions consist of mature, abnormally widened capillaries; are flat (macular) with sharply defined borders; and are usually reddish purple in color. They may vary greatly in size and typically develop on the head, face, and neck areas. As patients reach adulthood, port-wine stains may darken and form elevated (papular) areas that may occasionally bleed. Port-wine stains must be differentiated from salmon patches, which are flat, salmon-colored lesions that are typically present during infancy on certain facial areas, such as over the eyelids, on the middle of the forehead, or between the eyes. Salmon patches typically fade completely over time. Port-wine stains may be an isolated condition or may occur in association with several rare underlying syndromes (e.g., Klippel-Trenaunay-Weber syndrome, Sturge-Weber syndrome, etc.). Treatment may include a variety of measures, such as laser therapy, destruction of affected tissue through the use of extreme cold (cryosurgery), surgical removal (excision), transplantation of skin tissues (grafting), or masking with cosmetics.

Strawberry hemangiomas are dull or bright red and elevated, have clearly defined borders, and consist of immature capillaries. The lesions, which may develop as single or multiple growths, may affect any area of the body; however, they are most common on the scalp, face, chest, or back. Strawberry hemangiomas usually appear within approximately two months after birth. In most patients, the hemangiomas initially grow rapidly, cease such growth (stationary phase), and then gradually begin to regress in size (involution). After the lesions have reduced in size, approximately 10 percent of patients have residual discoloration or puckering of affected skin. In rare cases, complications associated with strawberry hemangiomas may include infection; destruction of the skin's surface, resulting in open sores and inflammation (ulceration); bleeding (hemorrhaging); or extensive growth that interferes with necessary functions, such as breathing difficulties due to tumor growth affecting the airways. Because most strawberry hemangiomas spontaneously regress, treatment typically consists of careful, ongoing observation. However, if hemangiomas rapidly grow, potentially causing tissue destruction, removal, using elastic bandages or other measures, may be recommended in selected patients. If there is rapid growth that may ultimately cause life-threatening complications, treatment may include the administration of corticosteroids by injection or| mouth or therapy with an artificial (synthetic) form of interferon (interferon alpha-2a). Interferons are natural proteins that are produced by the body's immune system in response to certain invading viruses or other stimuli. In the most severe cases, radiation therapy may be necessary. Other treatment is symptomatic and supportive.

Cavernous hemangiomas may be firm or form cysts. The skin overlying such hemangiomas is often bluish in color. However, if physicians suspect that underlying structures may be affected, specialized imaging techniques, such as CT scanning or ultrasonography, are conducted to detect and characterize such involvement. Rarely, some patients develop multiple hemangiomas. In such cases, affected children may have numerous small, red or purplish, raised hemangiomas on the skin. In addition, internal hemangiomas may be present involving certain organs, particularly the liver, lungs, brain and spinal cord, and organs of the gastrointestinal tract. In such cases, affected children are said to have disseminated hemangiomatosis. Life-threatening complications may potentially arise due to hemorrhage, tissue compression (e.g., neural tissue compression), obstruction of the airways, or an inability of the heart to effectively pump blood to the lungs and throughout the body (heart failure). In some cases, multiple internal and cutaneous hemangiomas occur in association with certain rare, underlying syndromes (e.g., macrocephaly with pseudopapilledema).

Lymphangiomas may be localized or widely distributed growths that, in some cases, may have hemangioma-like components. In almost all affected children, lymphangiomas are apparent by approximately age three. Lymphangiomas most commonly develop in the neck and facial regions, in the chest area (thorax), or under the arms (axillae). For example, some affected children may have an abnormal cystic growth consisting of dilated lymph vessels beneath the skin in the neck area (cystic hygroma). Lymphangiomas, such as cystic hygroma, may occur as isolated findings or in association with certain underlying syndromes (e.g., Noonan syndrome). Unlike hemangiomas, lymphangiomas rarely spontaneously regress. In some patients, they may expand in size and may obstruct the gastrointestinal tract or the airways, potentially causing life-threatening complications without appropriate treatment. Because most lymphangiomas are relatively widely distributed (diffuse), treatment often includes removal of the growths in several stages (staged surgical resection). Additional treatment includes symptomatic and supportive measures.

Government Agencies

3916 NIH/National Institute of Arthritis and Musculoskeletal and Skin Diseases
1 AMS Circle
Bethesda, MD 20892
301-495-4484
877-226-4267
Fax: 301-718-6366
TTY: 301-565-2966
TDD: 301-565-2966
niamsinfo@mail.nih.gov
www.niams.nih.gov

The mission of the NIAMS, a part of the NIH, is to support research into the causes, treatment, and prevention of arthritis and musculoskeletal and skin diseases, the training of basic and clinical scientists to carry out this research, and the dissemination of information on research progress in these diseases.

Stephen I Katz MD PhD, Director
Robert H Carter MD, Deputy Director

National Associations & Support Groups

3917 American Academy of Dermatology (AAD)
PO Box 4014
Schaumburg, IL 60168
866-503-7546
Fax: 847-240-1859
MRC@aad.org
www.aad.org

To promote and advance the art of medicine and surgery of the skin; promote the highest possible standards in clinical practice, education and research in dermatology and related disciplines.

Dirk M. Elston, President
Lisa A. Garner, VP
Brett M. Coldiron, President-Elect

3918 American Academy of Pediatrics
141 Northwest Point Boulevard
Elk Grove Village, IL 60007
847-434-4000
800-433-9016
Fax: 847-434-8000
www.aap.org

The American Academy of Pediatrics and its member pediatricians are committed to the attainment of optimal physical, mental and social health and well-being for all infants, children, adolescents, and young adults.

Fernando Stein, MD, FAAP, President
Karen Remley, MD, CEO/Executive VP

3919 American Skin Association
6 East 43rd Street, 28th Floor
New York, NY 10017
212-889-4858
800-499-7546
Fax: 212-889-4959
info@americanskin.org
www.americanskin.org

The American Skin Association is the only volunteer led health organization dedicated through research, education and advocacy to saving lives and alleviating human suffering caused by the full spectrum of skin disorders.

Howard P. Milstein, Chairman
George W Hambrick, Jr, President/Founder
David R Bickers, MD, Executive VP

3920 Hemangioma Support System
C/O Cynthia Schumerth
1484 Sand Acres Drive
Depere, WI 54115
920-336-9399

Provides parent-to-parent support for families with children affected by hemangiomas.
1990

3921 Society for Pediatric Dermatology
8365 Keystone Crossing, Suite 107
Indianapolis, IN 46240
317-202-0224
Fax: 317-205-9481
info@pedsderm.net
www.pedsderm.net

National organization dedicated to promote, develop and advance education, research and care of skin disease in all pediatric age groups.

Kent Lindeman, Executive Director

3922 Society for Pediatric Dermatology Annual Meeting
8365 Keystone Crossing, Suite 107
Indianapolis, IN 46240
317-202-0224
Fax: 317-205-9481
info@pedsderm.net
www.pedsderm.net
July

Kent Lindeman, Executive Director

3923 Vascular Birthmarks Foundation
PO Box 106
Latham, NY 12110
518-782-9637
877-823-4646
HVBF@aol.com
www.birthmark.org

A not for profit organization that provides support and informational resources for individuals affected by hemangiomas, port wine stains, and other vascular birthmarks and tumors.

Linda Rozell Shannon, Founder
Dr. Milton Waner, MD, Medical Chairman
Paige Salvador, Executive Director

Libraries & Resource Centers

3924 Children's Center for Cancer and Blood Disorders
University of South Carolina School of Medicine
5 Richland Memorial Park
Columbia, SC 29203
803-434-3533

Joint clinical and basic research of juvenile cancer and blood disorders.

Fauni Lowe, Manager

Conferences

3925 VBF Conference
Vascular Birthmarks Foundation
PO Box 106
Latham, NY 12110
518-782-9637
877-823-4646
HVBF@aol.com
www.birthmark.org
November

Martin Mihm Jr MD, Director

Web Sites

3926 Vascular Anomalies Center
www.hemangioma.org/

Provide the most up-to-date information to parents and patients as well as give the resources to help understand vascular anomaly.

Book Publishers

3927 Sturge-Weber Syndrome: A Resource Guide for a Reason, a Season and a Lifetime
Sturge-Weber Foundation
PO Box 418
Mt. Freedom, NJ 07970

973-895-4445
800-627-5482
Fax: 973-895-4846
swf@sturge-weber.com
www.sturge-weber.com

Covers most of the issues and concerns of parents and individuals with SWS, PWS and KT in short essays and chapters that provide practical and helpful advice

95 pages Paperback
ISBN: 0-967048-40-0

Carol Buck, Patient/Family Services Director
Lauris Partizian, Information Services Manager

Journals

3928 Pediatric Dermatology Journal
Society for Pediatric Dermatology
8365 Keystone Crossing, Suite 107
Indianapolis, IN 46240

317-202-0224
Fax: 317-205-9481
info@pedsderm.net
www.pedsderm.net

6 issues/yr
Kent Lindeman, Executive Director

DESCRIPTION

3929 **HEMOLYTIC DISEASE OF THE NEWBORN**

Synonyms: Erythroblastosis fetalis, Erythroblastosis neonatorum

Involves the following Biologic System(s):

Hematologic and Oncologic Disorders, Neonatal and Infant Disorders

Hemolytic disease of the newborn, also known as erythroblastosis neonatorum or erythroblastosis fetalis, is characterized by destruction of a newborn's red blood cells by antibodies that crossed the placenta from the mother's bloodstream during pregnancy. Antibodies are produced by certain white blood cells in response to foreign proteins (antigens) that are present in some cells and invading microorganisms. In hemolytic disease of the newborn the mother's immune system treats the baby's blood cells as foreign and makes antibodies against them. In most cases, the condition occurs when a developing fetus has Rh-positive blood (i.e., inherited from the father), but the mother has Rh-negative blood.

In approximately 85 percent of individuals, red blood cells contain an antigen called the Rh factor. Those with this antigen are said to have Rh-positive blood, whereas those without the antigen have Rh-negative blood. The blood plasma does not naturally contain antibodies to inactivate or destroy the Rh antigen (anti-Rh antibodies). However, if a fetus has Rh-positive blood and the mother is Rh negative, the presence of the Rh factor in the fetus' red blood cells causes the mother's body to produce anti-Rh antibodies. If the woman becomes pregnant again and the developing fetus has Rh-positive blood, the mother's antibodies may react with the fetus' Rh-positive cells, resulting in hemolysis (breakdown of red blood cells). In many cases, mothers who are known to have Rh-negative blood may be treated with a protein to help prevent them from producing anti-Rh antibodies (e.g., injection of human anti-D globulin), thereby lowering the risk of erythroblastosis fetalis during future pregnancies.

In infants affected by hemolytic disease of the newborn, associated symptoms and findings may vary. These may range from a mild breakdown of red blood cells to severely low levels of circulating red blood cells (anemia); paleness of the skin (pallor); tiny reddish, purplish spots on the skin (petechiae) due to abnormal bleeding under the skin's surface; enlargement of the liver and spleen (hepatosplenomegaly); or development of abnormal yellowish coloring of the mucous membranes, whites of the eyes, and skin (jaundice). In extremely severe cases, affected newborns may experience low levels of oxygen supply (hypoxia), difficulty breathing (respiratory distress), heart (cardiac) failure, severe abnormal accumulations of fluid in body tissues and cavities (hydrops), and potentially life-threatening complications. Depending upon the severity of the condition, treatment may include transfusions (e.g., partial or full exchange transfusions with Rh-negative blood) and supportive measures, such as ventilation assistance.

Hemolytic disease of the newborn may also result due to other blood type incompatibilities, primarily if the mother is type O and the developing fetus is type A or B. However, the condition develops in only about 10 percent of such cases of ABO incompatibility. In addition, the condition is typically less severe than that associated with Rh incompatibility. In cases of ABO blood type incompatibility, the development of jaundice approximately a day after birth may be the only associated symptom.

Government Agencies

3930 **NIH/ Eunice Kennedy Shriver National Institute of Child Health & Human Development**

31 Center Drive, Building 31
Bethesda, MD 20892

301-496-5113
800-370-2943
Fax: 866-760-5947
TTY: 888-320-6942
nichdpress@mail.nih.gov
www.nichd.nih.gov

Established in 1962 by congress, today the institute conducts and supports research on topics related to the health of children, adults, families and populations. Some of these topics include: developmental disabilities, growth and development, infant death, reproductive health and birth defects.

Diana W. Bianchi, Director
Paul Williams, Director, Communications

3931 **NIH/National Heart, Lung and Blood Institute**

National Institute of Health
PO Box 30105
Bethesda, MD 20824

301-592-8573
Fax: 301-592-8563
TTY: 240-629-3255
NHLBIinfo@nhlbi.nih.gov
www.nhlbi.nih.gov

Primary responsibility of this organization is the scientific investigation of heart, blood vessel, lung and blood disorders. Oversees research, demonstration, prevention, education, control and training activities in these fields and emphasizes the prevention and control of heart diseases.

Gary H Gibbons, MD, Director
Nakela Cook, MD, Chief of Staff

National Associations & Support Groups

3932 **American Academy of Pediatrics**

141 Northwest Point Boulevard
Elk Grove Village, IL 60007

847-434-4000
800-433-9016
Fax: 847-434-8000
www.aap.org

The American Academy of Pediatrics and its member pediatricians are committed to the attainment of optimal physical, mental and social health and well-being for all infants, children, adolescents, and young adults.

Fernando Stein, MD, FAAP, President
Karen Remley, MD, CEO/Executive VP

3933 **American Autoimmune Related Diseases Association**

22100 Gratiot Avenue
Eastpointe, MI 48021

586-776-3900
800-598-4668
Fax: 586-776-3903
aarda@aarda.org
www.aarda.org

Dedicated to the eradiction of autoimmune diseases and the alleviation of suffering and the socio-economic impact of autoimmunity through fostering and facilitating collaboration in the areas of education, public awareness, research and patient services in an effective, ethical and efficient manner.

Virginia T. Ladd, President/Executive Director
Patricia Barber, Assistant Director
Deb Patrick, Events Specialist

Web Sites

3934 American Autoimmune Related Diseases Association
22100 Gratiot Ave.
Eastpointe, MI 48021

586-776-3900
800-598-4668
Fax: 586-776-3903
www.aarda.org

Dedicated to the eradiction of autoimmune diseases and the alleviation of suffering and the socio-economic impact of autoimmunity through fostering and facilitating collaboration in the areas of education, public awareness, research and patient services in an effective, ethical and efficient manner.

3935 NIH/National Institutes of Health-Genetic and Rare Diseases Information Center
PO Box 8126
Gaithersburg, MD 20898

301-251-4925
888-205-2311
Fax: 301-251-4911
henrietta.hyatt-knorr@nih.gov
rarediseases.info.nih.gov/

Provides information about ORD-sponsored scientific activites, and ORD cosponsored genetic and rare disease information center, and a portal to databases that provide information on major topics of interest in rare disease research.

Henrietta Hyatt-Knorr, M.A., Task Leader/Sr Progr-Policy Analyst

3936 Online Mendelian Inheritance in Man
8600 Rockville Pike
Bethesda, MD 20894

888-346-3656
info@ncbi.nlm.nih.gov
www.ncbi.nlm.nih.gov

This database is a catalog of human genes and genetic disorders.

DESCRIPTION

3937 HEMOPHILIA

Synonyms: AHF, Antihemophilic factor deficiency, Classic hemophilia, Factor VIII deficiency, Hemophilia A

Covers these related disorders: Hemophilia A, Hemophilia B (Christmas disease; Factor IX deficiency), Von Willebrand's disease (Factor VIIIR deficiency)

Involves the following Biologic System(s):

Hematologic and Oncologic Disorders

The term hemophilia refers to a group of bleeding disorders including hemophilia A, hemophilia B, and von Willebrand's disease. Each of these diseases is characterized by the deficiency of a specific blood-clotting protein (factor). Hemophilia A, the most common form of the disease, affects approximately 80 percent of people with hemophilia and is caused by a deficiency of factor VIII. Hemophilia B, accounting for approximately 12 to 15 percent of all cases, results from a deficiency in clotting factor IX. In both forms of hemophilia, the severity of the disease and associated symptoms depend upon the level of coagulating activity of the individual clotting factors; the lower the activity of these factors, the more severe the disease. The most common symptoms, usually appearing at about 18 months when the child becomes more physically active, include easy bruising and bleeding into the joints (hemarthrosis) and muscles. Pain and swelling in the ankles, knees, and elbows may follow and eventually lead to degenerative changes and limited range of motion. Bleeding episodes may occur after injury, trauma, minor surgery, and, in some cases, for no apparent reason (spontaneously). Von Willebrand's disease involves a deficiency of factor VIIIR and is characterized by easy bruising, nose bleeds and bleeding into the gastrointestinal tract. In affected females, excessive uterine bleeding may occur during menstruation or childbirth. In some patients, blood may be present in the urine (hematuria). Unlike hemophilia A or B, bleeding into the joints is rare and the disorder seems to improve with advancing age.

Treatment of hemophilia A and B includes transfusions of appropriate clotting factor when a bleeding episode occurs. These concentrates may also be regularly self-administered to prevent bleeds. Other preventive measures may include the administration of certain clot-aiding drugs before surgery, the avoidance of certain drugs that may exacerbate bleeding problems, and avoidance of participation in contact sports or other similar activities that could provoke a bleeding episode. The treatment of von Willebrand's disease may include the infusion of DDAVP or VW protein prior to surgery or childbirth.

Hemophilia A and hemophilia B are transmitted as x-linked recessive traits and affect males almost exclusively. Approximately 10 males out of every 100,000 are born with hemophilia A, while the rate of occurrence of hemophilia B is about two males out of every 100,000. For the most part, von Willebrand's disease is inherited as an autosomal dominant disorder. In rare instances, the disease may be inherited as a recessive gene. Children with hemophilia who may have received transfusions of blood or blood products before HIV blood-screening became standard in 1985 may have

unwittingly become infected by receiving contaminated blood.

National Associations & Support Groups

3938 American Academy of Pediatrics
141 Northwest Point Boulevard
Elk Grove Village, IL 60007
847-434-4000
800-433-9016
Fax: 847-434-8000
www.aap.org

The American Academy of Pediatrics and its member pediatricians are committed to the attainment of optimal physical, mental and social health and well-being for all infants, children, adolescents, and young adults.

Fernando Stein, MD, FAAP, President
Karen Remley, MD, CEO/Executive VP

3939 Baxter Healthcare Hyland Division
One Baxter Parkway
Deerfield, IL 60015
224-948-2000
800-422-9837
Fax: 800-568-5020
www.baxter.com/

Government affairs office that monitors and selectively lobbies on issues relating to Medicare, Medicaid, orphan drugs and other subjects relating to hemophilia.

Phillip L. Batchelor, Corporate Vice President - Quality
Jean-Luc Butel, Corporate Vice President - Presiden
Robert M. Davis, Corporate Vice President - Presiden

3940 Children's Cancer & Blood Foundation
333 E 38th Street, Suite 830
New York, NY 10016
212-297-4336
Fax: 212-297-4340
info@childrenscbf.org
www.childrenscbf.org

The foundation's major emphasis is on blood diseases affecting children: leukemia, thalassemia, hemophilia, sickle cell anemia, platelet disorders. retinoblastoma and AIDS.

Drew Phillips, President
Greg Karakashian, Operations Associate

3941 Hemophilia Health Services
201 Great Circle Rd
Nashville, TN 37228
615-353-3814
866-712-5200
Fax: 800-330-0756
info@HemophiliaHealth.com
www.hemophiliahealth.com

Specializes in providing pharmaceuticals, therapeutic supplies and disease management services for people with hemophilia and related bleeding disorders.

Kyle J Callahan, President

3942 National Hemophilia Foundation
116 W 23rd Street, 11th Floor
New York, NY 10011
212-328-3700
800-424-2634
Fax: 212-328-3777
handi@hemophilia.org
www.hemophilia.org

Offers various information, articles, resources, books and more for the hemophilia and HIV/AIDS community.

Ken Trader, Chair
Jorge De La Riva, Vice Chair
Steve Helm, Secretary

State Agencies & Support Groups

Arkansas

3943 Hemophilia Center of Arkansas
Arkansas Children's Hospital
1 Children's Way, PO Box 3591
Little Rock, AR 72202   501-364-1100
TDD: 501-364-1184
www.archildrens.org

Patients with coagulation disorders can be diagnosed and evaluated by a group of physicians, physical therapists, dentists, psychologists and geneticists to provide education, prevention and continuity of care. The Hemophilia Center of Arkansas offers the latest diagnosis, prevention and treatment modalities for children and adults.

David Becton, MD, Medical Director

California

3944 Central California Chapter of the National Hemophilia Foundation
PO Box 163689
Sacramento, CA 95816   916-448-0370
Fax: 916-489-1569
hubbert@newfactor.com
www.hemophilia.org

An organization devoted to improving the quality of life for persons affected with bleeding disorders and their complications. This is accomplished through outreach development, educational programs, informational literature, support services and patient referrals.

Ken Trader, Chair
Jorge De La Riva, Vice Chair
Steve Helm, Secretary

3945 Hemophilia Association of San Diego County
3550 Camino Del Rio N, Suite 105
San Diego, CA 92108   619-325-3570
Fax: 619-325-4350
info@hasdc.org
www.hasdc.org

An organization devoted to improving the quality of life for persons affected with bleeding disorders and their complications. This is accomplished through outreach development, educational programs, informational literature, support services and patient referrals.

Michael Brown, Esq., President
Heather Masserly, Director at Large
Judy Faitek, Director at Large

3946 Hemophilia Foundation of Northern California
6400 Hollis St Suite 6
Emeryville, CA 94608   ÿ51- 65- 332
888-749-4362
Fax: 510-658-3384
execadmin@hfnconline.org
www.hemofoundation.org

An organization devoted to improving the quality of life for persons affected with bleeding disorders and their complications. This is accomplished through outreach development, educational programs, informational literature, support services and patient referrals.

Bethane Deuel, President
Ben Martin, Secretary
Hari Young, Treasurer

3947 Hemophilia Foundation of Southern California
6720 Melrose Avenue
Hollywood, CA 90038   323-525-0440
800-371-4123
Fax: 323-525-0445
hfsc@hemosocal.org
www.hemosocal.org

An organization devoted to improving the quality of life for persons affected with bleeding disorders and their complications. This is accomplished through outreach development, educational programs, informational literature, support services and patient referrals.

Tamara Kato, President
Judy Mangione, Secretary
Michael Franzen, Treasurer

Colorado

3948 Hemophilia Society of Colorado
2465 Sheridan Blvd.
Edgewater, CO 80214   720-626-1263
888-687-2568
Fax: 303-629-7035
info@cohemo.org
www.cohemo.org

An organization devoted to improving the quality of life for persons affected with bleeding disorders and their complications. This is accomplished through outreach development, educational programs, informational literature, support services and patient referrals.

Larry Hoyle, Manager
Daniel Reilly, President
Sean Perkins, Development Coordinator

Florida

3949 Florida Hemophilia Association
915 Middle River Drive, Suite 421
Ft Lauderdale, FL 33304   305-235-0717
888-880-8330
info@floridahemophilia.org
www.floridahemophilia.org

An organization devoted to improving the quality of life for persons affected with bleeding disorders and their complications. This is accomplished through outreach development, educational programs, informational literature, support services and patient referrals.

Barbie Arrebola, President
Jonathan Salk, VP
Janella Espinosa, Secretary/Treasurer

3950 Hemophilia Foundation of Greater Florida
1350 N Orange Avenue, Suite 227
Winter Park, FL 32789   407-629-0000
800-293-6527
Fax: 407-629-9600
Hemofoundation@earthlink.net
www.hemophiliaflorida.org

An organization devoted to improving the quality of life for persons affected with bleeding disorders and their complications. This is accomplished through outreach development, educational programs, informational literature, support services and patient referrals.

Alan Apte, VP
Ron Sachs, President
Mike Berkman, Secretary

Georgia

3951 Hemophilia Foundation of Georgia
8800 Roswell Road, Suite 170, PO Box 1844
Atlanta, GA 30350   770-518-8272
800-866-4366
Fax: 770-518-3310
mail@hog.org
www.hog.org

An organization devoted to improving the quality of life for persons affected with bleeding disorders and their complications. This is accomplished through outreach development, educational programs, informational literature, support services and patient referrals.

Andrew Maurer, Chief Governance Officer
Nick Blackmon, Vice CGO
Jonathan Lawrie, Secretary

Hawaii

3952 Hemophilia Foundation of Hawaii
1164 Bishop Street, Suite 1501
Honolulu, HI 96813
281-379-4600
Fax: 281-379-1450
hemophiliafoundation@hawaii.rr.com
www.bleedingdisorders.org

An organization devoted to improving the quality of life for persons affected with bleeding disorders and their complications. This is accomplished through outreach development, educational programs, informational literature, support services and patient referrals.

Rita Gonzales, President

Idaho

3953 Hemophilia Foundation of Idaho
4696 Overland Road, Suite 234
Boise, ID 83705
208-344-4476
866-453-4476
Fax: 208-344-4476
hfi@velocitus.net
www.idahoblood.org

An organization devoted to improving the quality of life for persons affected with bleeding disorders and their complications. This is accomplished through outreach development, educational programs, informational literature, support services and patient referrals.

Shane Bell, President
Ryan Hein, VP
Taryn Magrini, Executive Director

Illinois

3954 Hemophilia Foundation of Illinois
210 S. DesPlaines St, PO Box 5500
Chicago, IL 60661
312-427-1495
Fax: 312-427-1602
info@bdai.org
www.hemophiliaillinois.org

An organization devoted to improving the quality of life for persons affected with bleeding disorders and their complications. This is accomplished through outreach development, educational programs, informational literature, support services and patient referrals.

Bill Eftax, President
Eric Sary, VP
Robert Stewart, Treasurer

Indiana

3955 Hemophilia Foundation of Indiana
5172 E. 65th Street, Suite 105
Indianapolis, IN 46220
317-570-0039
800-241-2873
Fax: 317-396-0058
mrice@hemophiliaofindiana.org
www.hemophiliaofindiana.org.

An organization devoted to improving the quality of life for persons affected with bleeding disorders and their complications. This is accomplished through outreach development, educational programs, informational literature, support services and patient referrals.

Kasey Shade, President
Joseph McKamey, VP
Melissa Breedlove, Secretary

Kentucky

3956 Kentucky Hemophilia Foundation
1850 Taylor Avenue, Suite 2
Louisville, KY 40213
502-456-3233
800-582-2873
Fax: 502-456-3234
info@kyhemo.org
www.kyhemo.org

An organization devoted to improving the quality of life for persons affected with bleeding disorders and their complications. This is accomplished through outreach development, educational programs, informational literature, support services and patient referrals.

Ursela Lacer, Executive Director

Louisiana

3957 Louisiana Hemophilia Foundation
3636 S Sherwood Forest Boulevard, Suite 450
Baton Rouge, LA 70816
225-291-1675
Fax: 225-291-1679
lahemophilia@etigers.net
www.louisianahemophilia.org

An organization devoted to improving the quality of life for persons affected with bleeding disorders and their complications. This is accomplished through outreach development, educational programs, informational literature, support services and patient referrals.

Lori Keels, Executive Director
Tres Major, President

Maryland

3958 Hemophilia Foundation of Maryland
13 Class Court
Parkville, MD 21234
410-661-2307
800-964-3131
Fax: 410-661-2308
Miller8043@comcast.net
www.hfmonline.org

An organization devoted to improving the quality of life for persons affected with bleeding disorders and their complications. This is accomplished through outreach development, educational programs, informational literature, support services and patient referrals.

Harvey Gates, President
Ryan Melton, VP
Annette Maurits, Secretary

Massachusetts

3959 Massachusetts, New England Hemophilia Association
347 Washington Street, Suite 402
Dedham, MA 02026
781-326-7645
Fax: 781-329-5122
info@newenglandhemophilia.org
www.newenglandhemophilia.org

An organization devoted to improving the quality of life for persons affected with bleeding disorders and their complications. This is accomplished through outreach development, educational programs, informational literature, support services and patient referrals.

Kevin R Sorge, Executive Director
Patrick Mancini, President
William McCartney, Treasurer

Michigan

3960 Hemophilia Foundation of Michigan
1921 W Michigan Avenue
Ypsilanti, MI 48197
734-544-0015
800-482-3041
Fax: 734-544-0095
harner@hfmich.org
www.hfmich.org

An organization devoted to improving the quality of life for persons affected with bleeding disorders and their complications. This is accomplished through outreach development, educational programs, informational literature, support services and patient referrals.

Ivan Harner, Executive Director
Calvin DeKuiper, President
Amy Denton, VP

Minnesota

3961 Hemophilia Foundation of Minnesota and the Dakotas
750 S Plaza Drive, Suite 207
Mendota Heights, MN 55120
651-406-8655
800-994-4363
Fax: 651-406-8656
hemophiliafoundation@visi.com
www.hfmd.org

An organization devoted to improving the quality of life for persons affected with bleeding disorders and their complications. This is accomplished through outreach development, educational programs, informational literature, support services and patient referrals.

John Schulte, President
Mike Neubert, VP
Elizabeth Myers, Secretary

Mississippi

3962 Mississippi Hemophilia Foundation
36 Avery Circle, PO Box 13608
Jackson, MS 39236
601-957-2706
patty8501@aol.com
www.mshemophilia.com

An organization devoted to improving the quality of life for persons affected with bleeding disorders and their complications. This is accomplished through outreach development, educational programs, informational literature, support services and patient referrals.

Haley Jones, President
Leslee Londen, VP
Patty Lyons, Treasurer

Missouri

3963 Gateway Hemophilia Association of Missouri
14248 F Manchester Road, PMB#310
Manchester, MO 63011
314-482-5973
866-729-0233
Fax: 314-729-7033
hemophilia@sbcglobal.net
www.gatewayhemophilia.org

An organization devoted to improving the quality of life for persons affected with bleeding disorders and their complications. This is accomplished through outreach development, educational programs, informational literature, support services and patient referrals.

Nic Fahey, President
Brent Miller, VP
Andrea Metcalf, Treasurer

Nebraska

3964 Nebraska Chapter of the National Hemophilia Foundation
215 Centennial Mail South, Suite 512
Lincoln, NE 68508
402-742-5663
Fax: 402-742-5677
office@nebraskanhf.org
www.nebraskanhf.org

An organization devoted to improving the quality of life for persons affected with bleeding disorders and their complications. This is accomplished through outreach development, educational programs, informational literature, support services and patient referrals.

Jason Everts, President
Karie Quintana, VP
Mollie Lovell, Secretary

New York

3965 Bleeding Disorders Association of Northeas tern New York
BDANENY, PO Box 947
Rensselaer, NY 12144
518-782-9787
Fax: 518-356-5612
bdaneny@bdaneny.org
www.bdaneny.org

Formerly known as the Upper Hudson Valley Chapter of the National Hemophilia Foundation. The Association endeavors to meet the diverse needs of a geographically dispersed community through a variety of programs, including; emergency financial support, scholarships, Camp High Hopes, Double Hole in the Woods Ranch, HIV/AIDS education, outreach and support, and recreational community activities.

Deborah Huskie, Co-Executive Director
Kevin Pelletier, Co-Executive Director
David Huskie, President

3966 Hemophilia Center of Western New York
936 Delaware Avenue, Suite 300
Buffalo, NY 14209
716-896-2470
866-434-6551
Fax: 716-218-4010
www.hemophiliawny.com

A nonprofit, licensed diagnostic and treatment center. It offers a variety of services for persons with hemophilia and other herditary blood disorders ensuring that the patient is cared for at all times whether at the hospital, at home, at the center at school or on the job.

Robert Long, Chairman
Marcia Gellin, VP
Mary Haggerty, VP

3967 Mary M Gooley Hemophilia Center of the National Hemophilia Foundation
1415 Portland Avenue, Suite 500
Rochester, NY 14621
585-922-5700
Fax: 585-922-5775
Robert.Fox@viahealth.org
www.hemocenter.org

Specialized diagnostic testing, expert medical evaluation and diagnosis, personal counseling and support groups, home care treatment training, routine and urgent care, education of school and daycare personnel, research to advance knowledge, improve treatment and enhance quality of life for patients and families.

Robert Fox, President
Linda Magliocco, Sr. VP
Jennifer LaFranco, VP

North Carolina

3968 Hemophila Foundation of North Carolina
260 Town Hall Dr., Suite A
Morrisville, NC 27560
336-289-4446
880-990-5557
Fax: 336-725-4873
rbrummett@triad.rr.com
www.hemophilia-nc.org

An organization devoted to improving the quality of life for persons affected with bleeding disorders and their complications. This is accomplished through outreach development, educational programs, informational literature, support services and patient referrals.

Steven Peretti, President
Leonard Poe, VP
Kathy Register, Treasurer

Ohio

3969 Central Ohio Chapter of the National Hemophilia Foundation
PO Box 345
Worthington, OH 43085
614-457-0027
800-847-0345
steje08@aol.com
www.nhfcentralohio.org

An organization devoted to improving the quality of life for persons affected with bleeding disorders and their complications. This is accomplished through outreach development, educational programs, informational literature, support services and patient referrals.

Jeff Stewart, President
Tracy Kauffman, Treasurer
Anish Mistry, Secretary

3970 Northern Ohio Chapter of the National Hemophilia Foundation
One Independence Place
5000 Rockside Road, Suite 230
Independence, OH 44131
216-834-0051
800-554-4366
Fax: 216-834-0055
lynnecapretto@nohf.org
www.nohf.org

The mission is to enhance the quality of life for people with genetic bleeding disorders and their families, through advocacy, education, research and other constituency services.

Marlene Piatak, President
Michelle Zawadski, VP
Katey Vanderwyst, Treasurer

3971 Northwest Ohio Hemophilia Foundation
2121 Hughes Drive Harris-McIntosh Tower 2nd Floor
Toledo, OH 43606
419-291-5882
Fax: 419-479-3269
info@nwohemophilia.org
www.nwohemophilia.org

A volunteer nonprofit organization that serves the bleeding disorders community in Northwest Ohio.

Carla Wells, Executive Director
Scott Newsom, President

3972 Southwestern Ohio Chapter of the National Hemophilia Foundation
82 Elva Court, Suite B
Dayton, OH 45377
937-415-0644
Fax: 937-415-0604
SWOF@aol.com

Serving people with hemophilia and blood clotting disorders in an 11 county area. Dedicated to offering people and their families; educational opportunities about the physical, psychological and social aspects of these disorders. Workshops and seminars are regularly offered to address these issues. Offers support groups, volunteer services, telephone and walk-in education, information, counseling and referrals.

Dena M Shephard, President

3973 Tri-State Bleeding Disorders Chapter of the National Hemophilia Foundation
635 W 7th Street, Suite 407
Cincinnati, OH 45203
513-961-4366
Fax: 513-961-1740
hemophilia@fuse.net
www.tsbdf.com

Formerly known as the Greater Cincinnati/Northern Kentucky Chapter of the National Hemophilia Foundation. An organization devoted to improve the quality of life for persons affected with bleeding disorders and their complications. This is accomplished through outreach development, educational programs, informational literature, support services and patient referrals.

Lisa Raterman, Executive Director
Jeff Reichert, President
Andy Proeschel, Secretary

Oklahoma

3974 Oklahoma Chapter of the National Hemophilia Foundation
720 West Wilshire Blvd., Suite 101-B
Okhlama, OK 73116
405-463-6634
800-735-3855
Fax: 405-879-9748
ohf@dmgp.com
www.hemophilia.org

An organization devoted to improving the quality of life for persons affected with bleeding disorders and their complications. This is accomplished through outreach development, educational programs, informational literature, support services and patient referrals.

Tom Ayers, President
Kerri Crabtree, Vice President
Bob Goodley, Executive Director

Oregon

3975 Hemophilia Foundation of Oregon
10940 SW Barnes Rd #129
Portland, OR 97225
503-297-7207
Fax: 503-297-0127
info@hemophiliaoregon.org
www.hemophiliaoregon.org

An organization devoted to improving the quality of life for persons affected with bleeding disorders and their complications. This is accomplished through outreach development, educational programs, informational literature, support services and patient referrals.

Linda Charles, President
Dave Worthington, Vice President

Pennsylvania

3976 Delaware Valley Chapter of the National Hemophilia Foundation
14 E. 6th St. First Floor
Lansdale, PA 19446
215-393-3611
Fax: 215-393-9419
hemophilia@navpoint.com
www.hemophiliasupport.org

An organization devoted to improving the quality of life for persons affected with bleeding disorders and their complications. This is accomplished through outreach development, educational programs, informational literature, support services and patient referrals.

Thomas Galvin, President
William Widerman, Vice President
Jon Worthington, Treasurer

3977 Western Pennsylvania Chapter of The National Hemophilia Foundation
532 S Aiken Avenue, Suite 102
Pittsburgh, PA 15232   412-683-2231
                                      Fax: 412-683-2568
                                      wpcnhf@earthlink.net

Brings together and serves as a focal point for those segments of the community most concerned with hemophilia. They include medical and social service providers, people with hemophilia and their families, educators and the general public. This chapter combines service, education and advocacy programs.

Kerry Fatula, Executive Director
Ida McFarren, President

South Carolina

3978 Hemophilia Association of South Carolina
PO Box 3874
Sumter, SC 29151   864-350-9941
                                              888-829-4849
                                         Fax: 888-829-4849
                           information@hemophiliaofsouthcarolina.ne
                           www.hemophiliaofsouthcarolina.net

An organization devoted to improving the quality of life for persons affected with bleeding disorders and their complications. This is accomplished through outreach development, educational programs, informational literature, support services and patient referrals.

Mark Eichelberger, President
Brandy Stewart, Vice President

Tennessee

3979 Tennesse Hemophilia & Bleeding Disorders Foundation
1819 Ward Drive, Suite 102
Murfreesboro, TN 37129   615-900-1486
                                              888-703-3269
                                         Fax: 615-900-1487
                                              mail@thbdf.org
                                              www.thbdf.org

Offers a hemophilia clinic, social workers and consultants, a state hemophilia program, blood donor programs, counseling programs, genetic counseling, literature and resources, summer camp, grants and more for the hemophilia and HIV/AIDS community.

Kent Russ, President
John Snook, West-TN VP
Jerry Duntop, East-TN VP

Texas

3980 Lone Star Chapter of the National Hemophilia Foundation
10500 Northwest Freeway, Suite 226
Houston, TX 77092   713-686-6100
                                              888-LSC-NHF1
                                         Fax: 832-383-4601
                           Director@LoneStarHemophilia.org
                                      www.lonestarhemophilia.org

An organization devoted to improving the quality of life for persons affected with bleeding disorders and their complications. This is accomplished through outreach development, educational programs, informational literature, support services and patient referrals.

Nick Zasowski, President
Jennifer Borders, Vice President
Brian Crompton, Treasurer

3981 Texas Central Chapter of the National Hemophilia Foundation
12700 Hillcrest Road, Suite 191
Dallas, TX 75230   972-386-3865
                                         Fax: 214-654-9954
                                              mail@texcen.org
                                              www.texcen.org

A group of volunteers seeking solutions to the various aspects of the hemophilia problem. Supports blood drives, sponsors a summer camp for hemophiliac children, conducts educational member meetings, arranges for genetic counseling and sponsors group support meetings.

Shannon Brush, President
Jacob Banker, Vice President
David Simmons, Treasurer

Utah

3982 Utah Chapter of the National Hemophilia Foundation
772 East 3300 South, Suite 210
Salt Lake City, UT 84106   801-484-0325
                                              877-INF- VWD
                                         Fax: 801-484-2488
                                      smuir@hemophiliautah.org
                                      www.hemophiliautah.org

Offers educational information, pamphlets, fundraising events and more for persons and families affected by hemophilia.

Scott Muir, Executive Director
Reg Ecker, President
Lynn Barker, VP

Virginia

3983 Hemophilia Association of the Capital Area
10560 Main Street, Suite 419
Fairfax, VA 22030   703-267-6502
                                         Fax: 703-352-2145
                                      admin@hacacares.org
                                      www.hacacares.org

A nonprofit organization serving persons with bleeding disorders and their families in northern Virginia, Washington, DC and Montgomery and Prince George's Counties in Maryland. The mission is to improve the quality of life for persons with hemophilia and Von Willebrand's disease and their families, to educate, to act as an advocate, to provide member services and to raise money to fulfill all these purposes.

Sandi Qualley, Executive Director
Miriam Goldstein, President
Paul Brayshaw, VP

3984 United Virginia Chapter of the National Hemophilia Foundation
PO Box 188
Midlothian, VA 23113   804-740-8643
                                              800-266-8438
                                         Fax: 804-740-8643
                                      vahemophiliaed@verizon.net
                                      www.vahemophilia.org

An organization devoted to improving the qualit of life for persons affected with bleeding disorders and their complications. This is accomplished through outreach development, educational programs, informational literature, support servcies and patient referrals.

Kelly Waters, Executive Director
Kevin O'Connor, President
Erica George, President-Elect

Washington

3985 Bleeding Disorders Foundation of Washington
9639 Firdale Ave, Ste A
Edmunds, WA 98020   206-533-1660
                                         Fax: 206-533-1686
                                      general@bdfwa.org
                                      www.bdfwa.org

An organization devoted to improving the quality of life for persons affected with bleeding disorders and their complications. This is accomplished through outreach development, educational programs, informational literature, support services and patient referrals.

457

Regina Timmons, Executive Director
Reid Morgan, President
Caprice Sauter, Board President

3986 Hemophilia Foundation of Washington
PO Box 4565
West Richland, WA 99353   509-967-0203
                                       iebd4u@verizon.net

The Foundation's mission is to provide a conduit for education
and information, advocate for excellent medical care, and support
affected individuals and their families via peer outreach programs
and special events

Jill McCary, President
Debbie Campeau, Executive Director

Wisconsin

3987 Great Lakes Hemophilia Foundation
638 N 18th Street, Suite 108
Milwaukee, WI 53233   414-257-0200
                                       888-797-4543
                                       Fax: 414-257-1225
                                       info@glhf.org
                                       www.glfh.org

The only Wisconsin organization that addresses the physical,
emotional, social and financial needs of individuals affected by
hemophilia. This chapter supports high-quality, cost-effective
programs for patient care, education, research and public
awareness.

Bill Finn, President
Jeff Koopmeiners, VP
David Osswald, Secretary

Libraries & Resource Centers

Alabama

3988 Alabama Department of Rehabilitation Services
602 S Lawrence St.
Montgomery, AL 36104   334-293-7500
                                       800-441-7607
                                       Fax: 334-293-7383
                                       cboswell@rehab.state.al.us
                                       www.rehab.state.al.us

Mission is to enable children and adolescents with special health
needs and adults with hemophilia to achieve their maximum potential within a community-based, family-centered, comprehensive, culturally sensitive and coordinated system of services.

Cary Boswell, Ed.D, Director

Indiana

3989 Riley Hemophilia and Thrombophilia Center
702 Barnhill Drive, ROC 4270
Indianapolis, IN 46202   317-274-2153
                                       800-769-2848
                                       Fax: 317-278-3751
                                       anholcom@iupui.edu
                                       www.rileypeds.org

We strive to improve the health and health care of children by developing and applying best scientific evidence and methods in
health services research and informatics.

Richard Schreiner, MD, Chairman of Pediatrics
Anna Holcomb, Executive Director

Wisconsin

3990 Hemophilia Outreach Center
2060 Bellevue St
Green Bay, WI 54311   920-965-0606
                                       800-992-6026
                                       Fax: 920-965-0607
                                       info@hemophiliaoutreach.org
                                       www.hemophiliaoutreach.org

A comprehensive treatment center serving individuals and families with bleeding disorders. A facility maintained and administered through the collaboration of lay people, professionals,
medical providers, consumers and families. Offering a variety of
programs and services in a family-oriented, safe environment directed toward a holistic approach to wellness and to living a full
life, including coordinating comprehensive care, consumer
advocacy and financial and emotional support.

Katie Kralovetz, Executive Director

Research Centers

3991 Albany New York Regional Comprehensive Hemophilia
Treatment Center
Albany Medical College
43 New Scotland Avenue
Albany, NY 12208   518-262-3125
                                       800-773-7080
                                       Fax: 518-262-6320
                                       ALBANYHTC@mail.amc.edu
                                       www.amc.edu/patient/services/hemophilia

Providing comprehensive health care for patients with mild to severe hemophilia A, hemophilia B, von Willebrand's disease and
thrombophilia in the Albany, New York region.

Barbara Leckerling, Administrator
Joanne Porter, MD, Director

3992 Blood Research Institute of Saint Michael's Medical Center
Cathedral Healthcare System
111 Central Avenue
Newark, NJ 07102   973-877-5000
                                       Fax: 973-877-5466
                                       www.smmcnj.org

Dedicated to research and the treatment of blood-related disorders and cancers, the Blood Research Institute is a multi-disciplinary unit of the hematology/oncology departments.

Yale S Arkel, MD

3993 Boston Hemophilia Center
Children's Hospital Boston
300 Longwood Avenue, Fegan 7
Boston, MA 02115   617-355-4977
                                       Fax: 617-730-0641
                                       international.center@childrens.harvard.e
                                       www.childrenshosptial.org

A federally funded hemophilia treatment center, the program offers comprehensive care to people with hemophilia and their families. Services range from medical treatment, counseling and
support to discounts on clotting-factor replacement and other
products that people with hemophilia require.

Haroon Patel

3994 Cancer & Blood Diseases Institute
Cincinnati Children's Hospital Medical Center
3333 Burnet Avenue, PO Box 3026
Cincinnati, OH 45229   513-636-4200
                                       800-344-2462
                                       Fax: 513-636-4900
                                       blood@cchmc.org
                                       www.cincinnatichildrens.org

Aim is to improve the lives of children and adolescents with hemophilia and thrombophilia. This is achieved by offering compassionate, state-of-the-art clinical care to patients and their
families, advancing our understanding of the disorder through research and educating future health care providers and leaders in
the field.

Russell E. Ware, MD, PhD, Director, Divion of Hematology
John P. Perentesis, MD, Director, Division of Oncology

3995 Cardeza Foundation Hemophilia Center
Thomas Jefferson University Hospital
705 Curtis Building, 1015 Walnut Street
Philadelphia, PA 19107   215-955-8544
                                       www.jefferson.edu

Devoted to research into the causes of a wide v ariety of diseases of the blood and to the diagnosis and care of patients with blood and lvmphatic diseases. Our members have competence in all areas of hematology, with particularly well recognized depth and experience in diseases affecting blood platelets, hemorrhagic (bleeding) and thrombotic (clotting) disorders, hematologic malignancies (leukemia, Iymphoma and multiple myeloma) and other bone marrow disorders.

Jamie Siegel, MD, Director
Pamela Scruci, Admin Asst.
David Boligitz, Interim Business Manager

3996 Center for Cancer and Blood Disorders at Children's Medical Center in Dallas
1935 Medical District Drive
Dallas, TX 75235
214-456-7000
Fax: 214-456-6133
CCBDinfo@childrens.com
www.childrens.com/ccbd

Comprehensive diagnostic and treatment program for patients with disorders of blood coagulation which results in increased risk of bleeding or clotting.

George Buchanan, MD, Director

3997 Children's Center for Cancer and Blood Disorders of Palmetto Health Richland
7 Richland Medical Park Drive
Columbia, SC 29203
803-434-3533
800-775-2287
Fax: 803-434-4598
www.palmettohealth.org

Diagnosis and treatment of cancer and blood disorders. The staff includes a nurse practitioner and a patient and family educator who provide complex nursing management, treatment and navigation through the healthcare system. The multidisciplinary team also includes skilled social workers, therapists, nutritionists and child-life specialists, all of whom play an active role in each child's care.

Fauni Lowe, Manager
Beth Blackmon, Public Relations Director

3998 Children's Hospital of Philadelphia Hemophilia Program
34th Street & Civic Center Boulevard
Philadelphia, PA 19104
215-590-1000
800-879-2467
Fax: 215-426-5480
www.chop.edu

Provides multidisciplinary comprehensive care for children and adolescents with inherited bleeding disorders. Services include diagnosis, acute and chronic medical management of hemophilia and its complications, genetic counseling, physical therapy, HIV care and counseling and coordination with other services.

A Michael Broennle, Program Director
Regina B Bulter, RN, Program Nurse Coordinator

3999 Comprehensive Bleeding Disorder Center
Children's Hospital of Illinois
4727 N. Sheridan Rd.
Peoria, IL 61614
309-655-7171
Fax: 309-688-0917
CBDC@hemophilia-ctr-peoria.com
www.compbleed.com

Provides and facilitates state-of-the-art treatment for children and adults with hemophilia and related bleeding and thrombatic disorders. The staff includes a board-certified physician in pediatrics and pediatric hematology/oncology, nurses, social worker, rural outreach coordinator, reimbursement specialist/patient advocate, physical therapist and dentist.

Edward Hui, Executive Director
Sara Dill, Administration Director
John Redington, Executive Director

4000 Comprehensive Pediatric Hemophilia Treatment Center
University of Miami
1150 NW 14th Street
Miami, FL 33136
305-243-7570
www.pediatrics.med.miami.edu

Provided excellent medical and psychological care and emotional support for patients with bleeding disorders and their families since 1987. The HTC participates in national and regional research protocols dealing with various aspects of coagulation disorders. Orthopaedic and physical therapy are also offered at the monthly comprehensive clinic.

Maria Santaella, RN, Director
Steve E Lipshultz, MD, Chairman

4001 East Tennessee Comprehensive Hemophilia Center
University of Tennessee Medical Center
1924 Alcoa Highway 4 NW, Suite 180, Building E
Knoxville, TN 37920
865-454-9170
Fax: 865-544-9876
www.utmedicalcenter.org/hemophilia_services

Provides multidisciplinary comprehensive care to persons with bleeding disorders, including information, education and counseling to families affected by these disorders. The center's professional staff and consultants serve patients with hereditary bleeding disorders in Knoxville and surrounding counties.

William Rukeyser, Chairman
Renda Burkhart, Vice Chair
Bernard Bernstein, Secretary/Treasurer

4002 Eastern Michigan Hemophilia Center
Hurley Medical Center
1921 W. Michigan Avenue
Ypsilanti, MI 48197
734-544-0015
800-482-3041
Fax: 734-544-0095
www.hfmich.org/medical_resources

Provide and coordinate a broad range of treatment and prevention services provided by physicians who specialize in hematology and other relevant specialties such as orthopedics, social work, psychologists, nurses with extensive training and experience with hemophilia, genetic counselors, dentists, dental hygienists, and dieticians.

Calvin DeKuiper, President
Amy Denton, VP
Peter Deininger, Treasurer

4003 Federal Hemophilia Treatment Center Program of Los Angeles
Children's Hospital of LA
4650 Sunset Boulevard
Los Angeles, CA 90027
323-660-2450
Fax: 323-660-7128
www.chla.org

Provides continuing and comprehensive care to children and young adults with inherited bleeding disorders (in particular, hemophilia). The hemophilia treatment program is a federally funded resource which focuses on multidisciplinary management of bleeding disorders and collaborates with other programs in the United States to provide comprehensive care and teaching for patients and health care providers.

Wing-Yen Wong, MD, Director
Robert Miller, Coordinator

4004 Federal Hemophilia Treatment Center of Hawaii
Kapiolani Medical Center for Women and Children
1319 Punchou Street Pau
Honolulu, HI 96826
808-983-8551
Fax: 808-983-6000
martha.smith@kapiolani.org
www.kapiolani.org

Part of a nation-wide network established to promote comprehensive hemophilia care and to prevent hemophilia complications.

Desiree Medeiros, MD, Director
Dee Ann Omatsu, RN, Coordinator

4005 First Regional Hemophilia Center
James H Quillen College of Medicine
400 N State of Franklin Road, 1st Floor
Johnson City, TN 37604
423-433-6206
Fax: 423-433-6220

Helping patients and families to manage every aspect of living with hemophilia, from providing information about the latest medical developments to organizing support groups for parents and teens.

Sheri Miller, RN

4006 Hemophilia Center of Arkansas
Arkansas Children's Hospital
1 Children's Way, PO Box 3591
Little Rock, AR 72202
501-364-1100
Fax: 501-364-4332
TDD: 501-364-1184
www.archildrens.org/

Patients with coagulation disorders can be diagnosed and evaluated by a group of physicians, physical therapists, dentists, psychologists and geneticists to provide education, prevention and continuity of care. The Hemophilia Center of Arkansas offers the latest diagnosis, prevention and treatment modalities for children and adults.

Nikki Shock

4007 Hemophilia Center of Western New York
936 Delaware Avenue, Suite 300
Buffalo, NY 14209
716-896-2470
866-434-6551
Fax: 716-218-4010
hemoctr@pce.net
www.hemophiliawny.com

The center provides a variety of services to the hemophilia and HIV/AIDS community. Included among these services are diagnostics, registration, outpatient treatment, home care programs, home visits, school visits, dental services and counseling services. Offers an adult unit and a pediatric unit.

Thomas Long, President
Marcia Gellin, VP
Mary Haggerty, VP

4008 Hemophilia Center of Western Pennsylvania
3636 Boulevard of the Allies
Pittsburgh, PA 15213
412-209-7280
Fax: 412-683-4029
www.hcwp.net

Comprehensive care to all individuals who are diagnosed with Hemophilia residing in Western Pennsylvania.

Karen Saban, Manager
A. Kim Ritchey, MD, Vice Chair
Kim Goldby-Reffner, Co-Ordinator

4009 Hemophilia Center of the New England Medical Center
UMass Memorial Medical Center; Memorial Campus
119 Belmont Street
Worcester, MA 01605
508-334-1000
www.umassmemorial.org

Family-oriented, state-of-the-art medical and psychosocial services, education and research. Provides diagnostic and treatment services for individuals with bleeding disorders using a community-based, family centered and culturally sensitive approach. A hematologist is available 24 hours a day.

Doreen Brettler, MD, Director
Ann Forsberg, Program Administrator

4010 Hemophilia Program at Children's National Medical Center
Hematology/Oncology Department
111 Michigan Avenue NW
Washington, DC 20010
202-476-5000
www.childrensnational.org

Children's Hemophilia Program offers high quality, comprehensive care for children with hemophilia and thrombophilia. Children's is the only program in the Metropolitan DC that is supported by the National Institutes of Health. Nearly 150 patients are treated here annually.

Anne Angiolillo, MD, Director
Kurt Newman, MD

4011 Hemophilia Treatment Center at the University of Iowa
UI Health Care Department of Pediatrics
200 Hawkins Drive
Iowa City, IA 52242
319-356-1616
Fax: 319-356-3862
melinda-schultz@uiowa.edu
www.uihealthcare.com

Committed to provide the best care for individuals with bleeding disorders. To accomplish this mission we offer state of the art comprehensive clinical care, education to patients and their families and accessibility to clinical research projects that are oriented to improve the lives of people with these type of disorders.

Donna Katen-Bahensky, Ceo
Donald E McFarlane, MD, Co-Director
Mindy Schultz, Secretary

4012 Hemophilia and Coagulation Programs
Norris Cotton Cancer Center
1 Medical Center Drive
Lebanon, NH 03756
603-650-5000
Fax: 603-650-7791
www.cancer.dartmouth.edu/services/hemophilia

Provides complete clinical and laboratory diagnostic facilities for evaluation and treatment of patients with cogenital bleeding disorders and disorders of thrombosis and hemostasis.

Sophia Ouhilal, Program Director

4013 Hemophilia and Thrombosis Center at the University of Minnesota Medical Center
Phillips-Wangensteen Building, Sixth Floor, Clinic
Minneapolis, MN 55455
612-626-6455
800-688-5252
Fax: 612-625-4955
htc@fairview.org
www.uofmmedicalcenter.org

Offers a wide range of services for patients with inherited bleeding and clotting disorders. We care for patients of all ages using a team approach. Hematologists and nurse clinicians are involved and provide services including diagnostic evaluations, treatment, education, research and care coordination.

Beverly Christie, Manager
Margaret Heisel Kurth, MD, Co-Director
Shannon Fabick, Administrative Secretary

4014 Hemophilia and Thrombosis Center of Nevada
2020 W Palomino Lane, Suite 110
Las Vegas, NV 89106
702-385-2702
Fax: 702-322-0158
www.htcnevada.org

Offers diagnosis and management for persons with inherited or acquired bleeding disorders including hemophilia, von Willebrand's Disease, and platelet disorders. Comprehensive care is administered using a team approach with input from social services, physical therapy, orthopedic specialists, dentist, nursing, laboratory support, and medical services.

Nancy Sewell, Manager

4015 Indiana Hemophilia and Thrombosis Center
8402 Harcourt Road, Suite 420
Indianapolis, IN 46260
317-871-0000
888-256-8837
Fax: 317-871-0010
info@ihtc.org
www.ihtc.org

Multidisciplinary evaluation and treatment facility serving the people of Indiana who have bleeding disorders or thrombotic disease (known collectively as disorders of coagulation). The center aids local medical providers in the care of individuals of all ages with blood disorders and their families.

Phillip E. Himelstein, Founder
Ike G. Batalis, President
Edward R. Schmidt, President

4016 Kalamazoo Comprehensive Hemophilia Treatment Center
Michigan State University
1000 Oakland Drive, PO Box 8000
Kalamazoo, MI 49008
269-337-4400
webmaster@med.wmich.edu
www.kcms.msu.edu

Offers diagnosis, management, and genetic counseling for these patients, as well.

Frank J. Sardone, President/CEO
John M. Dunn, Chairman of the Board
Hal B. Jenson, Dean

4017 Louisiana Comprehensive Hemophilia Care Center
Tulane University School of Medicine
6823 St. Charles Avenue
New Orleans, LA 70118
504-865-5000
Fax: 504-988-6808
website@tulane.edu
www.tulane.edu

Provides diagnostic, evaluation and treatment services for individuals with hemophilia, von Willebrand disease and other coagulopathies throughout Louisiana and the Mississippi gulf coast. The Center provides comprehensive medical and psychosocial evaluations through a multi-disciplinary team of adult and pediatric hematologists, orthopedists, nurses, social workers, physical therapists and dentists.

Anthony Lorino, Senior Vice President for Operation
Frances Vickers, Executive Assistant to the Senior V

4018 Maine Hemophilia and Thrombosis Center
Maine Medical Center
22 Bramhall Street, PO Box 3175
Portland, ME 04102
207-662-0111
877-339-3107
Fax: 207-885-7687
TTY: 207-662-4900
www.mmc.org

Offers a wide range of services for patients with inherited bleeding and clotting disorders. We care for patients of all ages using a team approach. Hematologists and nurse clinicians are involved and provide services including diagnostic evaluations, treatment, education, research and care coordination. Also, a full-time social worker provides psychosocial assessment, counseling and resource information.

Glen Roy, RN, Contact

4019 Mayo Comprehensive Hemophilia Center
13400 E. Shea Blvd.
Scottsdale, AZ 85259
480-301-8000
800-446-2279
Fax: 507-284-0161
www.mayoclinic.org

Specializes in treating people with hemophilia and other bleeding disorders. The Center provides evaluation and care to approximately 200 patients per year. It also assists in the management and care of another 100 patients annually who come to Mayo Clinic for initial evaluation or consultation.

Denis Cortese, MD, CEO

4020 Miami Comprehensive Hemophilia Center
University of Miami, Department of Pediatrics
1601 N.W. 12th Ave
Miami, FL 33136
305-270-3400
Fax: 305-325-8387
pedsinformation@med.miami.edu
www.pediatrics.med.miami.edu

The Comprehensive Pediatric Hemophilia Treatment Center has provided excellent medical and psychological care and emotional support for patients with bleeding disorders and their families since 1987. HTC participates in national and regional research protocols dealing with various aspects of coagulation disorders. The major goal of the HTC medical team is to improve the quality of life for patients and their families coping with the stress and discomfort of living with a chronic illness.

Luis Caldera-Nieves, Medical Director

4021 Michigan State University Comprehensive Center for Bleeding Disorders
138 Service Road, Suite A-225
East Lansing, MI 48824
517-353-4920
800-759-5595
Fax: 517-353-9421
www.healthteam.msu.edu/

Offering education and information to individuals and families affected by blood clots and blood clotting disorders, and to assist with research efforts relating to all aspects of thrombosis and thrombophilia.

Gerald R Aben, Director
Roshni Kulkarni, MD, Coordinator

4022 Nebraska Regional Hemophilia Center
Nebraska Medical Center
42nd and Emile
Omaha, NE 68198
402-559-4000
800-922-0000
Fax: 402-552-2410
nmamdani@nebraskamed.com
www.unmc.edu/

Medical and educational support for those dealing with hemophilia, and their families.

Nizar Mamdani, Executive Director

4023 North Dakota Comprehensive Hemophilia and Thrombosis Treatment Center
Roger Maris Cancer Center/MeritCare Health System
820 4th Street N
Fargo, ND 58122
701-234-7544
800-437-4010
Fax: 701-234-7577
www.meritcare.com/specialties/more/hemophilia

Provides comprehensive care for people who have hemophilia, von Willebrand's disease and many other types of bleeding and clotting disorders. Using a team approach, professionals work together to provide evaluations, recommendations, treatment plans and follow-up care. They also offer a variety of services including assistance with clotting factors and home therapy.

Dr. Nathan Kobrinsky, MD, Director

4024 Northern Regional Bleeding Disorder Center
1105 6th Street
Traverse City, MI 49684
231-935-7227
800-468-6766
Fax: 231-935-6582
contact@mhc.net
www.munsonhealthcare.org

A program which cares for patients with all types of bleeding disorders from 26 northern Michigan counties. Provides specialty treatment to patients with hemophilia with the goal of minimizing complications from bleeding episodes.

Dan Wolf, Chairman
John Pelizzari, Vice Chairman
Bob Sprunk, Secretary

4025 Northwest Ohio Hemophilia Treatment Center
Toledo Childrens Hospital
2142 N Cove Boulevard
Toledo, OH 43606
419-291-5437
888-291-5437
Fax: 419-479-3258
www.promedica.org

A full range of inpatient and outpatient services is provided for children and adolescents with blood conditions and cancer. The patient care program also offers support for the psychosocial needs of patients and their families.

Ann Gilbert, RN, Director

4026 Orthopaedic Hospital's Hemophilia Treatment Center
2400 S Flower Street
Los Angeles, CA 90007
213-742-1000
Fax: 213-741-8338
info@orthohospital.org
www.orthohospital.org

Objective of the Center is the diagnosis and optimal management of bleeding disorders and their complications. Disorders treated include hemophilia A and B, von Willebrand's disease, and other inborn deficiencies of plasma clotting factors and platelets. Adolescents and adults who have acquired blood-borne infections, including chronic hepatitis and HIV infection, through prior treatment with blood products, are also treated at the Center.

Joseph Mirra, Director
Carol K Kasper, MD, Emeritus Director
James V Luck, Jr.; MD, Center's Surgeon

4027 Pediatric Hemophilia Program of Pennsylvania
Children's Hospital of Pittsburgh
4401 Penn Ave
Pittsburgh, PA 15224 412-692-5325
www.chp.edu

Provides high quality, comprehensive care for children with hemophilia and thrombophilia through research and clinical programs.

Vincent Deeney, Director
Kim Ritchey, MD, Pediatric Program Director
Melanie Finnigan, Public Affairs Director

4028 Phoenix Center for Cancer and Blood Disorders
Phoenix Children's Hospital
1919 E Thomas Road
Phoenix, AZ 85016 602-546-1000
888-908-5437
www.phoenixchildrens.com

Largest program of its kind in Arizona and is making significant difference in the quality of life for pediatric and adult hemophilia patients. It is one of only two federally funded hemophilia treatment programs in the state. The Center treats children with sickle cell disease, hemophilia and other hematologic disorders, and it is a designated center for the treatment and study of Gaucher's disease, an inherited metabolic disorder that can cause multiple medical problems.

Mark Bonsall, Chairman of the Board
Jon Hulburd, Vice Chairman
Robert L Meyer, President/CEO

4029 Puget Sound Blood Center
921 Terry Avenue
Seattle, WA 98104 206-292-6500
HumanResources@psbc.org
www.psbc.org

Puget provides all the blood and tissue services that people in our region need. It is this longstanding pledge to the community that has guided the Blood Center to more than sixty years of unparalleled success and to a leadership position in healthcare. In addition, our work in medical research is advancing medical care and making cures possible for patients around the world.

Jmaes P. AuBuchon, President/CEO
A. Kent Fisher, VP
Frederick R. Appelbaum, Executive Director

4030 Regional Hemophilia Program
Children's Hospital of Michigan
3901 Beaubien Street
Detroit, MI 48201 313-745-5437
888-362-2500
www.chmkids.org/

Clinical evaluations and recommendations by a team of experts, home treatment, training and educational programs, HIV/AIDS counceling and management, carrier detection and genetic counceling. Clinical trials provide our patients with the latest treatment modalities and in-depth surveillence of complications.

Lynne Thomas Gordon, COO
Herman Gray, MD, President

4031 Research at BloodCenter of Wisconsin
638 North 18th Street
Milwaukee, WI 53233 414-257-2424
877-232-4376
Fax: 414-937-6580
jeanne.mccabe@bcw.edu
www.bcw.edu

Through basic, clinical and applied research programs, the center's scientists are enable to continue discoveries that enables to extend continuum of care.

Jeanne McCabe, Research Administration Director

4032 Rhode Island Hemostasis and Thrombosis Center
Rhode Island Hospital
593 Eddy Street, Hasbro Lower Level
Providence, RI 02903 401-444-7731
Fax: 401-444-6104
www.rhodeislandhospital.org

Formerly known as the Rhode Island Hemophilia Treatment Center, we have expanded our services to offer to persons with clotting disorders the same cutting edge, comprehensive program that has been extremely successful for our bleeding disorders community.

Timothy J. Babineau, President/CEO
Cathy Duquette, Executive Vice President
Mamie Wakefield, Executive VP/CFO

4033 SUNY Upstate Medical University Research Development
750 E Adams Street, PO Box 2375
Syracuse, NY 13210 315-464-5540
Fax: 315-464-4318
www.upstate.edu/research

In collaboration with Upstate faculty, the Center conducts research and executes data analyses designed to guide the improvement of patient care and associated patient outcomes.

William J Hardoby, Research VP

4034 South Dakota Center For Bleeding Disorders
Sioux Valley Hospital
1600 W. 22nd St
Sioux Falls, SD 57117 605-312-1000
info@siouxvalley.org
www.glhf.org

Provides comprehensive care based on family centered/community based health care. Hemophilia specialists are available 24 hours a day.

Bill Finn, President
Jeff Koopmeiners, VP
David Osswald, Secretary

4035 South Texas Comprehensive Hemophilia and Thrombophilia Treatment Center
University of Texas Medicine
7703 Floyd Curl Drive
San Antonio, TX 78229 210-567-5200
Fax: 210-567-6921
NAVAE@UTHSCSA.EDU
www.pediatrics.uthscsa.edu

A federally funded program focusing on the evaluation, treatment, and prevention of complications from Hemophilia, Von Willebrand's disease, thrombophilia, and menorrhagia in adolescents and women.

Thomas C. Mayes, M.D., MBA, Chairman
Steven R. Neish, MD, SM, Vice Chairman
Dennis A. Conrad, MD, Associate Chairman for Continuing M

4036 Spectrum Health Research
DeVos Hospital/Spectrum Health
100 Michigan Street NE
Grand Rapids, MI 49503 616-391-9000
866-989-7999
research.department@spectrum-health.org
www.helendevoschildrens.org

Formerly known as the Cook Institute for Research and the Cook Research Department. The Spectrum Health research department has a reputation for selectively participating in clinical research that brings cutting-edge treatments to the people of West Michigan. Many of the diseases under study currently have limited or no treatment options.

David T Lock, President
Dominic Sanflippo, MD, Executive Medical Director

4037 Steele Children's Research Center
University of Arizona College of Medicine
1501 N Campbell Avenue, Suite 3301, PO Box 245073
Tucson, AZ 85724   520-626-2221
                                              Fax: 520-626-7176
                                       www.steelecenter.arizona.edu

At the University of Arizona College of Medicine, internationally
known physicians and scientists, who also are professors in the
UA Department of Pediatrics, work together to research causes
and develop cures for childhood illnesses and diseases. Our goal
is to advance medical knowledge to help improve the health of
Arizona's children and children throughout the world.

Fayez Ghishan, MD, Director
Lori Stratton, MPH, Director of Development
Darci Slaten, MA, Director of Communications and Mark

4038 Ted R. Montoya Hemophilia Program
University of New Mexico Health Sciences Center
2211 Lomas Blvd NE
Albuquerque, NM 87131   505-272-2111
                                              Fax: 505-272-6845
                                      www.hospitals.unm.edu/outpt/trmhp/

Division program provides comprehensive care to the individual
(child and adult) with hemophilia and other hereditary bleeding
disorders.

Steve Mckernan, Chief Operations Officer
Carolyn Voss, Chief Operations Officer
David Pitcher, Chief Medical Officer

4039 UCD Hemophilia Treatment Center
2315 Stockton Boulevard
Sacramento, CA 95817   916-734-2011
                                                 800-2 U- DAV
                                            TDD: 916-734-9230
                                           www.ucdmc.ucdavis.edu

Offers a variety of medical, educational and social services to
people with hemophilia or other inherited bleeding disorders and
their families across Northern California.

John Meyer, Vice Chancellor
Linda P.B. Katehi, Chancellor
Ralph Hexter, Provost and Executive Vice Chancell

4040 UCSD Hemophilia Treatment Center
Div of Hematology-Oncology, UCSD Med Ctr Hillcrest
9500 Gilman Dr., La Jolla
San Diego, CA 92093   858-534-2230
                                              Fax: 858-822-6288
                                              kdherbst@ucsd.edu
                                                  www.ucsd.edu

Part of the federal network of over 140+ specialty centers for
bleeding disorder diagnosis and management. These two HTCs
are funded, in part, by grants from the Maternal and Child Health
Bureau and Centers for Disease Control and Prevention. The purpose of the grants is to support a multidisciplinary team which
can provide comprehensive care and conduct research to prevent
hemophilia complications.

Amy Lovejoy, MD, Director
Catherine Glass, RN, Nurse Coordinator

4041 UT Southwestern Medical Center at Dallas:
Hematology-Oncology Research
5323 Harry Hines Boulevard
Dallas, TX 75390   214-648-3111
                                              Fax: 214-645-7999
                                              utsouthwestern.org
                                           www.utsouthwestern.edu

Basic science research is enhanced by the world class investigative environment at UT Southwestern that includes 4 Nobel Prize
winners and other internationally known scientists with whom hematology-oncology faculty regular collaborate. Cutting edge clinical research in hemophilia/thrombophilia and ITP are also major
commitments.

Daniel K. Podolsky, President
Robin M. Jacoby, VP/Chief of Staff

4042 United Health Services Blood Disorder Center
Wilson Regional Medical Center
33-57 Harrison Street
Johnson City, NY 13790   607-763-6000
                                              Fax: 607-763-5514
                                                  www.uhs.net/

Provides comprehensive care for those with blood disorders_from
diagnosis to treatment to home care and support services. Physicians, nurse specialists, dentists, orthopedists, physical therapists,
and social workers treat people diagnosed with hemophilia and
vWD at a dedicated site at Wilson Memorial Regional Medical
Center. They also assist family physicians throughout the region
in caring for persons with blood disorders.

Rajesh J Dave', President/CEO
Peter LoFaso, Chair
Roger Scott, Managing Director

4043 University of Cincinnati Adult Hemophilia Program
Division of Hematology & Oncology
Mail Location 11009, 3333 Burnet Avenue
Cincinnati, OH 45229   513-636-4269
                                              Fax: 513-636-5599
                                              palascje@ucmail.uc.edu
                                       www.hemophilia-information.com

Patient care, teaching, and research in the area of hematology/on-
cology. Rapidly growing in all research, clinical, and educational
components. The division participates in investigator-initiated
protocols, pharmaceutical or industry-sponsored studies, as well
as cooperative groups, such as the Southwest Oncology Group
and Radiotherapy Oncology Group.

Joseph Palascak, MD, Director
Albert Muhleman, MD, Division Director
Madeline Heffner, RN, Nurse Coordinator

4044 University of Michigan Adult Hemophilia and Coagulation
Disorders Program
1500 E Medical Center Drive, Floor B1
Ann Arbor, MI 48109   734-936-6641
                                                 800-211-8181
                                              Fax: 734-936-6666
                                     www2.med.umich.edu/healthcenters

Provides comprehensive, coordinated assessments and management services for individuals with blood disorders. Disorders
may include disorders of blood coagulation (abnormal bleeding
and clotting), hematology, hematopoietic malignancies, coagulation disorders, Von Willebrand's disease, lupus anticoagulant and
thrombosis, and hemophilia.

Christine L Holland, Director

4045 University of Tennessee Hemophilia Clinic
UT Health Science Center
920 Madison Avenue, Suite 822
Memphis, TN 38163   901-448-1751
                                              Fax: 901-448-7929
                                            TDD: 901-448-7382
                                                 www.uthsc.edu

Diagnosis, evaluation, management, and treatment. The Hemophilia Center uses a comprehensive model to deliver effective
care coordinated in the community. Emphasis is on educating
providers, educators, patients, and their families for successful
management. The center also manages a hemophilia factor
concentrate program.

Dr. Marion Dugdale, Director
Steve J. Schwab, CEO/MD

4046 University of Texas Department of Hematology Research
University of Texas Medical School at Houston
7000 Fannin, Suite 1200
Houston, TX 77030   713-500-4HSC
                                              Fax: 713-500-3026
                                               www.uthouston.edu

Major research activities include a multidisciplinary center for
vascular and thrombosis research and diversified hematologic and
oncologic research projects covering a wide scope of disciplines
from molecular biology to clinical trials.

Giuseppe N. Colasurdo, President
Kevin Dillon, Sr. VP
George M. Stancel, VP

4047 Vanderbilt Hemostasis-Thrombosis Clinic
Vanderbilt University Medical Center
2200 Children's Way, 6105 DOT, PO box 9830
Nashville, TN 37232
615-936-1765
866-372-5663
Fax: 615-936-8400
VHTCClinic@vanderbilt.edu
www.vanderbiltchildrens.com

Comprehensive health promotion; preventive medical and dental services; diagnostic testing; genetic testing and counseling; individual case management; specific and prompt treatments as needed; education and training; options for home treatment; and referrals, when necessary.

Anderson B Collier III, MD, Director
Mary G Hudson, RN, Nursing Coordinator
Kim Blittle, Administrative Assistant

4048 Vermont Regional Hemophilia Center
Fletcher Allen Health Care
UHC Campus, Old Hall Room 2106A, 1 South Prospect
Burlington, VT 05401
802-847-8041
Fax: 802-847-8041
www.hemophilia-information.com

Miriam Grant, RN
Alan Homans, MD

4049 West Central Ohio Hemophilia Center
Children's Medical Center of Dayton
1 Childrens Plaza, PO Box 1815
Dayton, OH 45404
937-641-5877
Fax: 937-641-5878
www.hemophilia-information.com

The center provides complete care for individuals and families with hemophilia and related bleeding disorders. Some of the services offered include a comprehensive clinic, emergency treatment network, consultations, diagnostic coagulation laboratory, home infusion programs, HIV/AIDS education and counseling and more.

James French III, MD, Medical Director

4050 Yale Pediatric Hematology/Oncology Research Center
Yale School of Medicine
333 Cedar Street
New Haven, CT 06510
203-785-4640
Fax: 203-737-2228
diana.beardsley@yale.edu
www.medicine.yale.edu

Oriented toward improving the lives of children with blood disorders and childhood cancer, while working toward future improved treatments and outcomes.

Diana S Beardsley, MD; PhD, Research Director
Robert J. Alpern, MD
James E. Rothman, Chairman

Conferences

4051 National Hemophilia Foundation Annual Meet ing
National Hemophilia Foundation
116 W 23rd Street, 11th Floor
New York, NY 10001
212-328-3700
800-424-2634
Fax: 212-328-3777
handi@hemophilia.org
www.hemophilia.org

A three-day conference that offers educational sessions, networking opportunities and social events for all ages.

Val Bias, CEO
Ken Trader, Chairman

Audio Video

4052 Song of Superman
National Hemophilia Foundation
116 W 32nd Street, 11th Floor
New York, NY 10001
212-328-3700
800-424-2634
Fax: 212-328-3777
handi@hemophilia.org
www.hemophilia.org

Designed to help young people with bleeding disorders come to terms with their HIV status, sexuality, and living with HIV. The video explores issues of disclosure in relationships and safer sex through dramatic scenes and frank testimonials by young people living with hemophilia and/or HIV. The companion workbook contains group exercises that follow each of the main topics of the video and serve as a bridge to discussion.

1993 33 Mins

Val Bias, CEO
John Indence, VP, Marketing & Communications
Mary Ann Ludwig, Vice President for Development

Web Sites

4053 Health Answers
410 Horsham Road
Horsham, PA 19044
215-442-9010
Michael.tague@healthanswers.com
www.healthanswers.com

HealthAnswers offers a breadth of services in medical education, sales force training, patient support solutions, professional promotion and customer solutions.

Michael Tague, Managing Director

4054 National Hemophilia Foundation
116 W 32nd Street, 11th Floor
New York, NY 10001
212-328-3700
800-424-2634
Fax: 212-328-3777
handi@hemophilia.org
www.hemophilia.org

Devoted to improving the quality of life for persons affected with bleeding disorders. This is accomplished through outreach development, educational programs, information literature, support services and patient referrals.

Val Bias, CEO
John Indence, VP, Marketing & Communications
Mary Ann Ludwig, Vice President for Development

4055 Online Mendelian Inheritance in Man
8600 Rockville Pike
Bethesda, MD 20894
888-346-3656
info@ncbi.nlm.nih.gov
www.ncbi.nlm.nih.gov

This database is a catalog of human genes and genetic disorders.

Book Publishers

4056 Adventures of Maxx
Nova Factor
1620 Century Centery Parkway, Suite 109
Memphis, TN 38137
901-385-3600
800-235-8498
Fax: 901-385-3778

An activity book for children with hemophilia, this publication is intended to be both educational and entertaining.

1991 15 pages

4057 Genetics Coloring Book
Medical College of Virginia
P.O Box 980565
Richmond, VA 23298

Fax: 804-828-9793
Fax: 804-828-5115
bodurtha@gems.vcu.edu
www.medschool.vcu.edu/

Adventures of Gene coloring book for children ages 5-9. Two coloring books, one dealing with cystic fibrosis and one with hemophilia.

1994-1995 Comic/Coloring

4058 Guide to Insurance Coverage for People With Hemophilia
Armour Pharmaceutical Company
500 Arcola Road
Collegeville, PA 19426

215-454-3720

An educational guide designed to assist with health insurance concerns.

4059 Harold Talks About How He Inherited Hemophilia
Hemophilia Foundation
1850 Taylor Avenue, Suite 2
Louisville, KY 40213

502-456-3233
800-582-2873
Fax: 502-456-3234
info@kyhemo.org
www.kyhemo.org

Children's brochure explaining hemophilia causes, symptoms and living a regular life.

4060 Harold's Secret: A Boy with Hemophilia
Bayer
400 Morgan Lane
West Haven, CT 06516

203-937-2765

A comic book for youngsters pertaining to children with hemophilia and understanding of the illness among school friends.

16 pages

4061 Hemophilia Camp Directory
National Hemophilia Foundation
116 W 32nd Street
New York, NY 10001

212-328-3700
Fax: 212-328-3777
handi@hemophilia.org
www.hemophilia.org

Lists camps in the United States for children with hemophilia and other coagulation disorders.

16 pages

4062 Hemophilia Diseases and People
Enslow Publishers
40 Industrial Road
Berkeley Heights, NJ 07922

908-771-9400
800-398-2504
Fax: 908-771-0925
CustomerService@enslow.com
www.enslow.com

An excellent resource for basic research for personal or academic use. The disease is carefully described, with effective black-and-white graphics, charts, and photos, showing blood biology and the circulatory system and the various levels of severity (depending on what clotting factors the individual is missing).

Ages: 9-12 128 pages Library Binding
ISBN: 0-766016-84-6

Edward Willet, Editor

4063 Hemophilia Handbook
Hemophilia of Georgia
8800 Roswell Road, Suite 170
Atlanta, GA 30350

770-518-8272
Fax: 770-518-3310
mail@hog.org
www.hog.org

A comprehensive, easy-to-read resource for people with hemophilia and their families. The fourth edition of this handbook, contains up-to-date information on all important topics.

1988 348 pages

Hikie Allen, Director
Arthur Herman, Director

4064 Hemophilia Nursing Handbook
National Hemophilia Foundation
116 W 32nd Street
New York, NY 10001

212-328-3700
Fax: 212-328-3777
handi@hemophilia.org
www.hemophilia.org

A revision and expansion of the 1995 Hemophilia Nursing Handbook. Now incorporating von Willebrand disease and other bleeding disorders. It is intended to provide comprehensive information as well as practical ideas to assist nurses at all levels in caring for patients with bleeding disorders. The guide is designed to be both an introduction to nurses new to coagulation and a resource for more experienced nurses.

1995 Members: $20

4065 Let's Talk About Going to the Hospital
Rosen Publishing Group's PowerKids Press
29 E 21st Street
New York, NY 10010

212-777-3017
800-237-9932
Fax: 888-436-4643
rosenpub@tribeca.ios.com
www.powerkidspress.com

If a child has to check into the hospital, chances are he or she is already upset about being ill. Knowing how a hospital functions and what the procedures are, such as when family members can visit, will help in what is already a stressful situation. Grades K-5.

24 pages
ISBN: 0-823950-36-0

4066 Passport: Global Treatment Centre Directory
World Federation of Hemophilia
1425 Rene Levesque Boulevard W, Suite 1010
Montreal, Quebec, H3G
Canada

514-875-7944
Fax: 514-875-8916
wfh@wfh.org
www.wfh.org

Lists over 900 hemophilia treatment centres and national hemophilia organizations in more than 100 countries, including contact names, telephone and fax numbers, as well as e-mail and web site addresses. It is very useful for people with hemophilia who are travelling to other countries and as a directory of hemophilia treaters around the world.

1990 188 pages Members: $6

Magazines

4067 Bloodstone Magazine
Hemophilia Health Services
1640 Century Center Parkway
Memphis, TN 38134

877-222-7336
info@hemophiliahealth.com
www.hemophiliahealth.com

A premier magazine of the bleeding disorders community. Features of community news, The Adventures of Welligan Hugsley, ProToCall, and human interest stories. A must read for anyone interested in the latest hemophilia related information.

Quarterly

Kyle J Callahan, Publisher/President
Lydia Dixon Harden, Editor-in-Chief

4068 HEMALOG
Materia Medica
208 E 51st Street, Box 234
New York, NY 10022

212-725-5151
Fax: 212-725-2794
mmca@earthlink.net
www.mmca.com

The purpose of Hemalog is to serve as a national forum for the hemophilia community, providing current news, information, opinion, and contact with others in the community. The material contained in this journal reflects the experience and opinion of a wide range of people connected with hemophilia, and encourages story and art contributions.

Quarterly

Barbara Robin Slonevsky, Publisher
Janet Spencer-King

4069 HemAware
National Hemophilia Foundation
116 W 32nd Street, 11th Floor
New York, NY 10001

212-328-3700
800-424-2634
Fax: 212-328-3777
handi@hemophilia.org
www.hemophilia.org

Packed with medical updates, analysis, professional news, and practical health information for people living with a bleeding disorder and for their care providers. This magazine showcases how custom publishing can deepen relationships within a community by providing useful information in a compelling format.

Bi-Monthly

Val Bias, CEO
John Indence, VP, Marketing & Communications
Mary Ann Ludwig, Vice President for Development

Newsletters

4070 Artery
Hemophilia Foundation of Michigan
1921 W Michigan Avenue
Ypsilanti, MI 48197

734-544-0015
800-482-3041
Fax: 734-544-0095
www.hfmich.orgs

Features articles on people in the bleeding disorders community, information and reviews on programs and services, memorials and donors.

Quarterly

Susan Lerch, Executive Director
Ann LeWalk, MA, Associate Director
Carrie McCulloch, Office Manager

4071 Big Red Factor
National Hemophilia Foundation of Nebraska
215 Centennial Mall South, Suite 512
Lincoln, NE 68508

402-742-5663
Fax: 402-742-5677
office@nebraskanhf.org
www.nebraskanhf.org

Chapter newsletter offering legislative and medical updates, technology, resources, assistive devices and more for persons affected by hemophilia and other blood disorders.

Karie Quintana, President
Mollie Lovell, Vice President
Dale Gibbs, Secretary

4072 Bloodlines
Hemophilia Association of San Diego County
3570 Camoni Del Rio N, Suite 108
San Diego, CA 92108

619-325-3570
Fax: 619-325-4350
info@hasdc.org
www.hasdc.org

Updates membership on the newest techniques and technologies on the treatment of hemophilia.

Quarterly

Teresa Ramirez, Executive Director

4073 COTT Washington Update
Committee of Ten Thousand
236 Massachusetts Avenue NE, Suite 609
Washington, DC 20002

202-543-0988
800-488-2688
Fax: 202-543-6720
cott-dc@earthlink.net
www.cott1.org

Reports monthly (when possible) on Congress, Federal policy, agencies like FDA and CDL, with regard to blood safety, hemophilia.

Quarterly

Corey Dubin, President
Mary Lou Murphy, Co-Vice President
Terry MacNeill, Co-Vice President

4074 Factor Nine News
Coalition for Hemophilia B
825 Third Avenue Suite 226
New York, NY 10022

212-520-8272
Fax: 212-554-6900
info@coalitionforhemophiliab.org
www.coalitionforhemophiliab.org

Offers information on FDA approvals, annual meetings and the latest in technology and information regarding hemophilia.

Quaterly

Kimberly Phelan, Executive Director

4075 Headline News
Great Lakes Hemophilia Foundation
638 N 18th Street, PO Box 108
Milwaukee, WI 53233

414-257-0200
Fax: 414-257-1225
info@glhf.org
www.glhf.org

Provides information on research, new treatments and support groups.

Danielle Leitner Baxter, Executive Director
Adam Haggerty, Public Ally Program Assistant
Jayne Holmes, Administrative Assistant

4076 Hemophilia Headlines
Hemophilia Foundation of Oregon
5319 SW Westgate Drive, Suite 126
Portland, OR 97204

503-297-7207
Fax: 503-297-0127
hfo@easystreet.com
www.hfo.info

Contains local, national and international news regarding bleeding disorders. It educates its readers with legislative and medical updates, as well as a current events calendar.

Quarterly

Jamie Dessellier, Editor
Dave Worthington, Vice President

4077 Infusions
Northern California Chapter of the NHF
7700 Edgewater Drive, Suite 710
Oakland, CA 94621

650-568-6243
888-749-4362
Fax: 510-568-6111

Informs members of medical, dental and orthopedic treatment advances and the latest research in the field. Helps to keep people with hemophilia and their families aware of relevant local and national meetings and includes important updates regarding research and treatment.

Bimonthly

4078 Initiatives
Philanthropic Initiative
420 Boylston Street, Floor 4
Boston, MA 2116
60
617-338-2590
Fax: 617-338-2591
www.tpi.org

Aimed at keeping patients and other interested individuals informed on important economic trends, legislation and medical issues.

Quarterly

Jane Maddox, Senior Editor
Joe Breiteneicher, President/CEO

4079 Linking Factor
Utah Hemophilia Foundation
772 East 3300 South, Suite 210
Salt Lake City, UT 84106
801-484-0325
877-463-6893
Fax: 801-746-2488
info@hemophiliautah.org
www.hemophiliautah.org

Features news pertinent to the bleeding disorders community.

Quarterly

Reg Ecker, President
Erik Rolstad, Vice President
Emmie Gardner, Secretary

4080 NEHA News
New England Hemophilia Association
347 Washington Street
Dedham, MA 2026
781-326-7645
800-228-6342
Fax: 781-329-5122
info@newenglandhemophilia.org
www.newenglandhemophilia.org

Keeps the bleeding disorders community connected and informed about NEHA's programs and events as well as relevant local and national issues affecting our community.

Quarterly

Patrick Mancini, President
William McCartney, Treasurer
Kim Lee DeAngelis, Ph.D., Secretary

4081 Newsline Eight & Nine
National Hemophilia Foundation, Florida Chapter
2176 Bent Oak Drive
Apopka, FL 32712
407-880-8330
Fax: 407-886-7649

State association news and information.

Quarterly

Pamphlets

4082 Caring For Your Child With Hemophilia
National Hemophilia Foundation
116 W 32nd Street, 11th Floor
New York, NY 10001
212-328-3700
800-424-2634
Fax: 212-328-3777
handi@hemophilia.org
www.hemophilia.org

Provides parents of children newly diagnosed with hemophilia answers to their basic questions. Many aspects are covered such as inheritance, current treatments, as well as sports, and insurance issues. The symptoms of different types of bleeding episodes are discussed explaining the severity of particular injuries. Provided are tips for babies including immunization, nutrition, and dental care. Also discussed are the social and emotional issues children with hemophilia experience.

2001 33 pages Free to Members

Val Bias, CEO
John Indence, VP, Marketing & Communications
Mary Ann Ludwig, Vice President for Development

4083 Child With A Bleeding Disorder Guidelines For Finding Childcare
National Hemophilia Foundation
116 W 32nd Street, 11th Floor
New York, NY 10001
212-328-3700
800-424-2634
Fax: 212-328-3777
handi@hemophilia.org
www.hemophilia.org

Provides a helpful guide for parents of children with bleeding disorders as they make choices about in-home care, cooperative childcare, center-based childcare and choosing a daycare center. Also included is a checklist of provider services and helpful hints for babysitters and other family caretakers.

8 pages Free to Members

Val Bias, CEO
John Indence, VP, Marketing & Communications
Mary Ann Ludwig, Vice President for Development

4084 Child With A Bleeding Disorder: First Aid For School Personnel
National Hemophilia Foundation
116 W 32nd Street, 11th Floor
New York, NY 10001
212-328-3700
800-424-2634
Fax: 212-328-3799
handi@hemophilia.org
www.hemophilia.org

Aimed at school nurses and teachers who have a student with a bleeding disorder. Descriptions of typical injuries and other incidences when bleeding occurs are discussed with proper steps that need to be followed as well as standard precautions and medications.

Val Bias, CEO
John Indence, VP, Marketing & Communications
Mary Ann Ludwig, Vice President for Development

4085 Hemophilia and Mild Hemophilia What To Expect
American Home Federation
PO Box 985
Enfield, CT 6083
800-243-4621
Fax: 860-763-7022
info@ahfinfo@.com
www.ahfinfo.com

Written in clear and easy to understand language, to provide information to those living with bleeding disorders, those who serve our children in school, and those who provide our medical care. A child or adult with mild hemophilia can live a healthy and long life. Physical activity is good and will help build strong muscles. Children and adults with mild hemophilia can do most things others can do.

1991 13 pages

4086 Hemophilia, Sports, and Exercise
National Hemophilia Foundation
116 W 32nd Street, 11th Floor
New York, NY 10001
212-328-3700
800-424-2634
Fax: 212-328-3777
handi@hemophilia.org
www.hemophilia.org

This fully revised guide presents valuable information for the person with a bleeding disorder or his/her parents considering participation in sports activities. Topics covered include conditioning, stretching and flexibility, strength, weight training, prophylaxis, and physical activities for infants, toddlers, preschoolers, and school-age children.

1996 30 pages Free to Members

Val Bias, CEO
John Indence, VP, Marketing & Communications
Mary Ann Ludwig, Vice President for Development

4087 Hemophilia: Current Medical Management
National Hemophilia Foundation
116 W 32nd Street, 11th Floor
New York, NY 10001   212-328-3700
                                      800-424-2634
                                      Fax: 212-328-3777
                                      handi@hemophilia.org
                                      www.hemophilia.org

Provides an overview of all aspects of hemophilia treatment, including prophylaxis, home therapy, inhibitors, orthopedic solutions, surgery, and dental care.

1994 30 pages

Jonathan C Goldsmith, Author
Val Bias, CEO
John Indence, VP, Marketing & Communications

4088 Inheritance of Hemophilia
National Hemophilia Foundation
116 W 32nd Street, 11th Floor
New York, NY 10001   212-328-3700
                                      800-424-2634
                                      Fax: 212-328-3777
                                      handi@hemophilia.org
                                      www.hemophilia.org

Booklet provides a sophisticated explanation of the genetic transmission of hemophilia. It also describes tests used to find out if the hemophilia gene is present, particularly in women who may carry the gene but show no signs of excessive bleeding. Reproductive choices for men and women with the hemophilia gene are reviewed.

1998 15 pages

Val Bias, CEO
John Indence, VP, Marketing & Communications
Mary Ann Ludwig, Vice President for Development

4089 Living with HIV: Talking With Your Child
National Hemophilia Foundation
116 W 32nd Street, 11th Floor
New York, NY 10001   212-328-3700
                                      800-424-2634
                                      Fax: 212-328-3777
                                      handi@hemophilia.org
                                      www.hemophilia.org

A pamphlet directed at caregivers of young children living with hemophilia and HIV disease.

1990 8 pages

Val Bias, CEO
John Indence, VP, Marketing & Communications
Mary Ann Ludwig, Vice President for Development

4090 What Is Hemophilia?
American Federation Home (AFH)
PO Box 985
Enfield, CT 6083   800-243-4621
                                      Fax: 860-763-7022
                                      info@ahfinfo.com
                                      www.ahfinfo.com

Offers information on what hemophilia is, common factors in hemophilia, the cost and treatments offered to hemophiliacs and more.

4091 What You Should Know About Bleeding Disorders
National Hemophilia Foundation
116 W 32nd Street, 11th Floor
New York, NY 10001   212-328-3700
                                      800-424-2634
                                      Fax: 212-328-3777
                                      handi@hemophilia.org
                                      www.hemophilia.org

Explains hemophilia, von Willebrand disease, blood safety issues, joint problems, HIV infection, hepatitis, special bleeding problems in women, prophylaxis, recombinant therapy, the cost of care, comprehensive care and other issues of concern to the bleeding disorders community.

1997 23 pages

Val Bias, CEO
John Indence, VP, Marketing & Communications
Mary Ann Ludwig, Vice President for Development

Camps

4092 Hole in the Wall Gang Camp
565 Ashford Center Road
Ashford, CT 6278   860-429-3444
                                      Fax: 860-429-7295
                                      ashford@holeinthewallgang.org
                                      www.holeinthewallgang.org

Nonprofit organization that provides a recreational camp experience for children ages 7-15 with cancer, genetic blood diseases and HIV/AIDS.

James Canton, CEO
Kevin M. Magee, Chief Financial Officer
Padraig Barry, Chief Program Officer

4093 NHF Camp Directory
National Hemophilia Foundation
116 W 32nd Street, 11th Floor
New York, NY 10001   212-328-3700
                                      800-424-2634
                                      Fax: 212-328-3777
                                      handi@hemophilia.org
                                      www.hemophilia.org

A comprehensive national directory of camps for the bleeding disorders community collaboratively produced by NHF. Lists camps in the United States for children with hemophilia and other coagulation disorders. Now available on web site.

16 pages

Renee LaBrew, Camp Directory Coordinator
Val Bias, CEO
John Indence, VP, Marketing & Communications

DESCRIPTION

4094 HEPATITIS

Covers these related disorders: Hepatitis A, Hepatitis B,
Hepatitis C, Hepatitis D, Hepatitis E

Involves the following Biologic System(s):

Gastrointestinal Disorders, Infectious Disorders

Hepatitis refers to an inflammatory condition of the liver that
may result from viral, bacterial, or parasitic infection; certain
blood disorders; or exposure to certain drugs, toxins, or alcohol. However, viral infection is most frequently the cause of
hepatitis. Liver inflammation may develop in association with
certain viral infections such as German measles (rubella),
chickenpox (varicella), or HIV. In addition, there are at least
five infectious agents known as hepatotropic viruses that specifically target the liver.

Hepatitis A virus is thought to be the most common cause of
hepatitis in children, with an extremely high prevalence rate
in underdeveloped countries. In addition, approximately 30
percent of adults in the United States show evidence of a previous infection with hepatitis A. This form of hepatitis is usually spread by fecal-oral contamination through drinking
water, food, or direct contact. Children under five years of
age often have no symptoms, but still acquire immunity to future hepatitis A infection. When symptoms become evident in
children, they are often mild and may include fever, weakness, general discomfort (malaise), loss of appetite (anorexia), nausea and vomiting, diarrhea, and abdominal
distress. Occasionally, some children develop a very slight
yellowing of the eyes (scleral icterus), skin, and mucous
membranes (jaundice). Hepatitis A is an acute, self-limited
form of this disease, with a return to general health typically
within one month, although relapses may occur. Life-threatening complications associated with this type of hepatitis are
extremely rare. Prevention of hepatitis A transmission is directed toward the teaching of good hygiene (e.g., frequent
hand washing) in hospitals, child-care facilities, etc. In addition, the administration of recently developed vaccines or immunoglobulin is recommended for children and adults who
plan to travel to countries with a high incidence of hepatitis
A. Young children are at risk for becoming carriers of this
disease while older travelers may be at risk for more significant disease involvement. Early administration of immunoglobulin is also recommended for children and adults who
may have been exposed to the virus. Other treatment is symptomatic and supportive.

Hepatitis B infection in children and adolescents may be
transmitted through intravenous injection of blood, blood
products, or drugs; sharing of needles or razors; ear piercing
with contaminated equipment; and other carrier-contact
modes of transmission. For example, the hepatitis B virus
may be spread by apparently healthy people who are chronic
carriers. Symptoms usually develop six to seven weeks after
exposure, persist for six to eight weeks, and are similar to
those of hepatitis A, but are often more severe. Additional
manifestations may include tenderness and enlargement of the
liver (hepatomegaly), enlargement of the spleen
(splenomegaly), swollen lymph glands (lymphadenopathy),
accumulation of fluid within the|abdomen (ascites), skin le-
sions, or joint pain (arthralgia). Newborns of infected mothers are at high risk for infection during delivery, possibly

through infected amniotic fluid, blood, or fecal material. Although infected newborns usually do not manifest symptoms,
if left untreated, most develop a chronic form of hepatitis that
may result in potentially life-threatening liver disease during
adulthood. Prevention of hepatitis B infection in newborns is
first directed toward testing for infection in pregnant women.
If a mother is positive for infection, her newborn is given a
hepatitis B immune globulin injection within the first day of
life, followed by immunization with hepatitis B vaccine. Immunizations are also recommended to anyone who may have
been exposed to hepatitis B. Treatment is symptomatic and
supportive.

Hepatitis C may be transmitted among the general population
through intravenous drug use, transfusions of blood or blood
products, sexual contact, and other, unknown causes. Although transmission from an infected mother to her infant is
possible, it is rare except in instances where the mother also
has HIV or other contributing factors. The onset of disease is
approximately seven to nine weeks after exposure and symptoms are similar to those of other types of viral hepatitis.
Hepatitis C is the most likely of all the hepatotropic viruses
to cause chronic hepatitis, a condition associated with pro-
longed inflammation of the liver that persists for six|months
or longer. Complications may also include cirrhosis and cancer of the liver, and rarely fulminant (very severe) hepatitis.
Because infection with the hepatitis C virus may occur more
than once in the same person, a preventive vaccine is not effective. Treatment is symptomatic and supportive.

The hepatitis D virus cannot replicate itself without the help
of the hepatitis B virus; therefore, hepatitis D only occurs in
people with prior or simultaneous infection with hepatitis B.
The most common mode of transmission in the United States
is through intimate contact and needle sharing; therefore, this
form of hepatitis is relatively rare in children in this country.
Symptoms and findings may be similar to but more severe
than those of hepatitis B infection. There is no vaccine for
hepatitis D; therefore, prevention is directed toward prevention of hepatitis B infection. Treatment is symptomatic and
supportive.

Hepatitis E is the cause of epidemic-associated infection and
is spread by fecal-oral transmission, usually through contaminated water or food. The symptoms and findings of this form
of disease are similar to but more severe than those
associated with hepatitis A. However, this acute, self-limited
infection may pose a life-threatening risk to pregnant women.
Hepatitis E is extremely rare in the United States, thus far
occurring only in people who have traveled to or emigrated
from indigenous countries. No vaccine is available.
Treatment is symptomatic and supportive. There are some
reports about the use of interferon, either alone or in
combination with ribavirin, another antiviral drug, in the
treatment of children with Hepatitis C. However, only a
partial antiviral response response occurred.

Government Agencies

4095 NIH/National Institute of Allergy and Infectious Diseases
5601 Fishers Lane, MSC 9806
Bethesda, MD 20892   301-496-5717
                                            866-284-4107
                                       Fax: 301-402-3573
                                      TDD: 800-877-8339
                                  ocpostoffice@niaid.nih.gov
                                        www.niaid.nih.gov

Conducts and supports basic and applied research to better understand, treat, and ultimately prevent infectious, immunologic, and allergic diseases.

Anthony S Fauci MD, Director

National Associations & Support Groups

4096 American Academy of Pediatrics
141 Northwest Point Boulevard
Elk Grove Village, IL 60007   847-434-4000
                                               800-433-9016
                                          Fax: 847-434-8000
                                               www.aap.org

The American Academy of Pediatrics and its member pediatricians are committed to the attainment of optimal physical, mental and social health and well-being for all infants, children, adolescents, and young adults.

Fernando Stein, MD, FAAP, President
Karen Remley, MD, CEO/Executive VP

4097 American Liver Foundation
39 Broadway, Suite 2700
New York, NY 10006   212-668-1000
                                               800-465-4837
                                          Fax: 212-483-8179
                                          info@liverfoundation.org
                                          www.liverfoundation.org

Nonprofit, national voluntary health organization dedicated to the prevention, treatment and cure of hepatitis and other liver diseases through research, education, and advocacy on behalf of those affected by or at risk of liver disease.

Thomas F. Nealon, Chairman
Daniel E. Weil, Treasurer
Carlo Frappolli, Secretary

4098 Hepatitis B Coalition
1573 Selby Avenue, Suite 234
Saint Paul, MN 55104   651-647-9009
                                          Fax: 651-647-9131
                                          admin@immunize.org
                                          www.immunize.org

Works to prevent transmission of hepatitis B in high risk groups, to achieve vaccination of all infants, children and adolescents and to promote education and treatment for hepatitis B carrier.

Deborah L. Wexler, MD, Founder/Executive Director
Litjen Tan, MS, PhD, Chief Strategy Officer
Diane C. Peterson, Assoc Dir Immunization Projects

4099 Hepatitis B Foundation
3805 Old Easton Road
Doylestown, PA 18902   215-489-4900
                                          Fax: 215-489-4920
                                          contact@hepb.org
                                          www.hepb.org

Dedicated to finding a cure and improving the quality of life for those affected by hepatitis B worldwide. Our commitment includes funding focused research, promoting disease awareness, supporting immunization and treatment initatives and serving as the primary source of information for patients and their families, the medical and scientific community, and the general public.

Joel Rosen, Chairman
Timothy M. Block, President
W. Thomas London, VP

4100 Hepatitis Education Project
The Maritime Building, 911 Western Ave #302
Seattle, WA 98104   206-732-0311
                                          Fax: 206-732-0312
                                          dani@hepeducation.org
                                          www.hepeducation.org

The mission of the Hepatitis Education Project is to help raise awareness amoung patients, medical personnel and the public of the facts concerning hepatitis patients and the resources available to help those who live with the disease.

Steve Graham, President
E Russell Alexander, MD, Vice President
Michael Ninburg, Executive Director

4101 Hepatitis International Foundation
504 Blick Drive
Silver Spring, MD 20904   301-879-6891
                                               800-891-0707
                                          Fax: 301-879-6890
                                          info@hepatitisfoundation.org
                                          www.hepatitisfoundation.org

Our mission is to teach the public and hepatitis patients how to prevent, diagnose and treat viral hepatitus; prevent viral hepatitis by promoting liver wellness and healthful lifestyles; serve as advocates for hepatitis patients and the related medical community worldwide; support research into prevention, treatment and cures for viral hepatitis.

Raymond Koff, Chairman
Theodre Karrison, Vice Chairman
Audrey V. Leef, Secretary

4102 March of Dimes Foundation
1275 Mamaroneck Avenue
White Plains, NY 10605   914-997-4488
                                               888-663-4637
                                          Fax: 914-997-4763
                                          answers@marchofdimes.com
                                          www.marchofdimes.com

Partnership of volunteers and professionals dedicates to improving the health of babies by preventing birth defects and infant mortality. Over 100 chapters are located across the country and can be located through the National Office.

Stacey D. Stewart, President

4103 World Health Organization
Avenue Appia 20
1211 Geneva 27,
Switzerland   www.who.int

WHO is the directing and coordinating authority for health within the United Nations system.

Dr Margaret Chan, Director General

Web Sites

4104 American Liver Foundation
39 Broadway, Suite 2700
New York, NY 10006   212-668-1000
                                               800-465-4837
                                          Fax: 212-483-8179
                                          info@liverfoundation.org
                                          www.liverfoundation.org

Nonprofit, national voluntary health organization dedicated to the prevention, treatment and cure of hepatitis and other liver diseases through research, education, and advocacy on behalf of those affected by or at risk of liver disease.

Hamilton Baiden, President
Jodi Bohr, Director
Jill Evans, R.N., M.S, Director

4105 Centers for Disease Control
1600 Clifton Road NE
Atlanta, GA 30329   404-639-3311
                                               800-232-4636
                                          TTY: 888-232-6348
                                          cdcinfo@cdc.gov
                                          www.cdc.gov

Mission is to promote health and quality of life by preventing and controlling disease, injury and disability.

Tom Frieden, Director
Ileana Arias, PhD, Principal Deputy Director
John Auerbach, Associate Director for Policy

4106 Hepatitis B Coalition
2550 University Avenue West, Suite 415 North
Saint Paul, MN 55114   651-647-9009
                                          Fax: 651-647-9131
                                          admin@immunize.org
                                          www.immunize.org

Works to prevent transmission of hepatitis B in high risk groups, to achieve vaccination of all infants, children and adolescents and to promote education and treatment for hepatitis B carrier.

Deborah L. Wexler, MD, Founder/Executive Director
Becky Payne, Assistant to Director
Diane C. Peterson, Assoc Dir Immunization Program

4107 Hepatitis B Foundation

3805 Old Easton Road
Doylestown, PA 18902

215-489-4900
Fax: 215-489-4920
contact@hepb.org
www.hepb.org

Dedicated to finding a cure and improving the quality of life for those affected by hepatitis B worldwide. Our commitment includes funding focused research, promoting disease awareness, supporting immunization and treatment initatives and serving as the primary source of information for patients and their families, the medical and scientific community, and the general public.

Joel Rosen, Esq, Chairperson
Timothy M. Block, Ph.D., President
W. Thomas London, MD, Vice President

4108 Hepatitis Education Project

The Maritime Building, 911 Western Ave #302
Seattle, WA 98104

206-732-0311
800-218-6932
www.hepeducation.org

The mission of the Hepatitis Education Project is to help raise awareness amoung patients, medical personnel and the public of the facts concerning hepatitis patients and the resources available to help those who live with the disease.

Steve Graham, President
Anne Croghan, MN ARNP, Vice President
Jeffrey R. King, CPA, Treasurer

4109 Hepatitis International Foundation

8121 Georgia Avenue, Suite 350
Silver Spring, MD 20910

301-565-9410
800-891-0707
info@hepatitisfoundation.org
www.hepfi.org

Our mission is to teach the public and hepatitis patients how to prevent, diagnose and treat viral hepatitus; prevent viral hepatitis by promoting liver wellness and healthful lifestyles; serve as advocates for hepatitis patients and the related medical community worldwide; support research into prevention, treatment and cures for viral hepatitis.

Karen Wirth, Chair
Dane R. Christiansen, BA, Vice Chair
Ivonne Perlaza Fuller, Secretary, CEO

Book Publishers

4110 Hepatitis B Prevention: A Resource Guide

National Digestive Diseases Info. Clearinghouse
2 Information Way
Bethesda, MD 20892

800-891-5389
Fax: 703-735-4929
TTY: 866-569-1162
nddic@info.niddk.nih.gov
www.digestive.niddk.nih.gov

Designed to assist health care and other professionals who work in planning or administering hepatitis B prevention programs.

252 pages

Kathy Kranzfelder, Director

4111 Hepatitis C: An Information Resource

American Liver Foundation
39 Broadway, Suite 2700
New York, NY 10006

212-668-1000
800-223-0179
Fax: 212-483-8179
info@liverfoundation.org
www.liverfoundation.org

Explains viral hepatitis, transmission, symptoms, testing and acute chronic hepatitis.

Alan P Brownstein, President/CEO
Paul D Berk, Chair

4112 Let's Talk About Going to the Hospital

Rosen Publishing Group's PowerKids Press
29 E 21st Street
New York, NY 10010

212-777-3017
800-237-9932
Fax: 888-436-4643
rosenpub@tribeca.ios.com
www.powerkidspress.com

If a child has to check into the hospital, chances are he or she is already upset about being ill. Knowing how a hospital functions and what the procedures are, such as when family members can visit, will help in what is already a stressful situation. Grades K-5.

24 pages
ISBN: 0-823950-36-0

4113 Liver Disease in Children

Lippincott Williams & Wilkins
530 Walnut Street
Philadelphia, PA 19106

215-521-8300
Fax: 215-521-8902
www.lww.com

A difinitive book on pediatric liver disease, providing extensive, well-edited information that is not easily accessible or available in other textbooks.

2000 1008 pages
ISBN: 1-556443-77-2

Newsletters

4114 American Liver Foundation

39 Broadway, Suite 2700
New York, NY 10006

212-668-1000
800-465-4837
Fax: 212-483-8179
info@liverfoundation.org
www.liverfoundation.org

Newsletter of the preeminent voluntary organization dedicated to promoting liver wellness and eradicating liver disease.

Quarterly

Hamilton Baiden, President
Jodi Bohr, Director
Jill Evans, R.N., M.S, Director

4115 Hepatitis B Coalition News

Hepatitis B Coalition
2550 University Avenue West, Suite 415 North
Saint Paul, MN 55114

612-647-9009
Fax: 651-647-9131
admin@immunize.org
www.immunize.org

Newsletter with brochures, articles, videotapes, audio-cassette tapes and manuals for different ethnic populations.

24 pages

Deborah L. Wexler, MD, Founder/Executive Director
Becky Payne, Assistant to Director
Diane C. Peterson, Assoc Dir Immunization Program

Pamphlets

4116 Chronic Viral Hepatitis Backgrounder

Centers for Disease Control
1600 Clifton Road NE
Atlanta, GA 30329

404-639-3311
800-232-4636
TTY: 888-232-6348
cdcinfo@cdc.gov
www.cdc.gov

Offers information and statistics on viral hepatitis.

Tom Frieden, Director
Ileana Arias, PhD, Principal Deputy Director
John Auerbach, Associate Director for Policy

4117 Hepatitis
National Institute of Allergy & Infectious Disease
National Institutes of Health
Bethesda, MD 20892
    301-496-4000
    Fax: 301-402-3573
    TDD: 800-877-8339
    www.3.niaid.nih.gov

A pamphlet discussing the cause, symptoms, transmission, diagnosis, tests, prevention and the latest research on hepatitis.

Anthony S. Fauci MD, Director

4118 Hepatitis B: Your Child at Risk
American Liver Foundation
1425 Pompton Avenue
Cedar Grove, NJ 7009
    973-857-2626
    800-223-0179

4119 Hepatitis Fact Sheet
Centers for Disease Control
1600 Clifton Road NE
Atlanta, GA 30329
    404-639-3311
    800-232-4636
    TTY: 888-232-6348
    cdcinfo@cdc.gov
    www.cdc.gov

Offers information on the causes, symptoms, prevention and treatments for hepatitis.

Tom Frieden, Director
Ileana Arias, PhD, Principal Deputy Director
John Auerbach, Associate Director for Policy

4120 How Many Times a Day Do You Risk Being Infected with Hepatitis B?
American Liver Foundation
39 Broadway, Suite 2700
New York, NY 10006
    212-668-1000
    800-465-4837
    Fax: 212-483-8179
    info@liverfoundation.org
    www.liverfoundation.org

A flyer emphasizing the importance of vaccination against hepatitis B.

Hamilton Baiden, President
Jodi Bohr, Director
Jill Evans, R.N., M.S, Director

4121 Q and A: Hepatitis B Prevention
SmithKline Beecham Pharmaceuticals
1 Franklin Plaza, 200 N 16th Street
Philadelphia, PA 19010
    215-751-4000
    Fax: 215-751-3400
    www.gsk.com

Informational booklet written for healthcare personnel by the manufacturer of Engerix-B vaccine, reviews hepatitis B prevention.

Jean-Pierre Garnier PhD, Chief Executive Officer

4122 Viral Hepatitis: Everybody's Problem?
American Liver Foundation
39 Broadway, Suite 2700
New York, NY 10006
    212-668-1000
    800-465-4837
    Fax: 212-483-8179
    info@liverfoundation.org
    www.liverfoundation.org

Covering a broad range of topics including: a definition of the disease, descriptions of types of infections, transmission, symptoms, treatment options and prevention.

Hamilton Baiden, President
Jodi Bohr, Director
Jill Evans, R.N., M.S, Director

4123 What Health Care Workers Should Know About Hepatitis B
Channing L Bete Company
One Community Place
South Deerfield, MA 1373-
    800-477-4776
    Fax: 800-499-6464
    custsvcs@channing-bete.com
    www.channing-bete.com

Presents information in easy-to-read, simple English for health care workers about hepatitis B.

16 pages

Mike Bete, President/CEO

DESCRIPTION

4124 HEREDITARY FRUCTOSE INTOLERANCE

Synonym: Deficiency of phosphofructaldolase

Involves the following Biologic System(s):

Genetic/Chromosomal/Syndrome/Metabolic Disorders

Hereditary fructose intolerance is a metabolic disorder characterized by a deficiency of the enzyme phosphofructaldolase (fructose-1,6-bisphosphate aldolase), resulting in the body's inability to process or metabolize fructose, a simple sugar (monosaccharide). Fructose is found in honey, certain sweet fruits, baby food and baby formula sweeteners. In combination with more complex sugars (disaccharides and polysaccharides), it is converted in the liver into glucose and is either distributed immediately for use as energy or converted into glycogen and stored in the liver, muscle, or fat for later energy use. The deficiency of the enzyme phosphofructaldolase results in the accumulation in the body of fructose-1-phosphate, a compound in the chain of fructose metabolism. This accumulation inhibits glucose production as well as the glycogen processing into energy-producing glucose.

Ingestion of fructose by affected infants may result in extremely low blood sugar (hypoglycemia), yellowing of the skin, eyes, and mucous membranes (jaundice), enlargement of the liver (hepatomegaly), bleeding from within the digestive tract, kidney involvement (i.e., proximal tubular dysfunction), vomiting, sluggishness, sweating, tremors, irritability, and seizures. Affected children have an aversion to sweets and fruits and typically do not have dental cavities (caries). However, physical findings and symptoms may be variable in their severity and manifestation.

Treatment for heredita ry fructose intolerance includes total elimination of fructose from the diet. Vigilance is extremely important in that fructose is present in many foods and medicines as an additive. Other treatment may include administration of supplemental glucose to counteract the effects of hypoglycemia.

Hereditary fructose intolerance is transmitted as an autosomal recessive trait. The defective gene for this disorder is located on the long arm of chromosome 9 (9q22). Approximately one of every 40,000 is affected with this disorder.

National Associations & Support Groups

4125 American Academy of Pediatrics
141 Northwest Point Boulevard
Elk Grove Village, IL 60007   847-434-4000
                                     800-433-9016
                                  Fax: 847-434-8000
                                       www.aap.org

The American Academy of Pediatrics and its member pediatricians are committed to the attainment of optimal physical, mental and social health and well-being for all infants, children, adolescents, and young adults.

Fernando Stein, MD, FAAP, President
Karen Remley, MD, CEO/Executive VP

4126 American College of Gastroenterology
6400 Goldsboro Road, Suite 200
Bethesda, MD 20817   301-263-9000
                                   info@acg.gi.org
                                        www.gi.org

Founded to advance the scientific study and medical practice of diseases of the gastrointestinal (GI) tract.

13,000 members

Carol A. Burke, MD, FACG, President

4127 Genetic Alliance
4301 Connecticut Avenue NW, Suite 404
Washington, DC 20008   202-966-5557
                                     800-336-4363
                                  Fax: 202-966-8553
                              info@geneticalliance.org
                               www.geneticalliance.org

A coalition of voluntary genetic support groups, consumers and professionals addressing the needs of individuals and families affected by genetic disorders from a national perspective.

Sharon Terry, President/CEO
Tetyana Murza, Managing Director
Natasha Bonhomme, VP, Strategic Development

4128 March of Dimes Foundation
1275 Mamaroneck Avenue
White Plains, NY 10605   914-997-4488
                                     888-663-4637
                                  Fax: 914-997-4763
                            answers@marchofdimes.com
                               www.marchofdimes.com

Partnership of volunteers and professionals dedicates to improving the health of babies by preventing birth defects and infant mortality. Over 100 chapters are located across the country and can be located through the National Office.

Stacey D. Stewart, President

4129 North American Society for Pediatric Gastroenterology/Hepatology/Nutrition
714 N Bethlehem Pike, Suite 300
Ambler, PA 19002   215-641-9800
                                  Fax: 215-641-1995
                               naspghan@naspghan.org
                                  www.naspghan.org

Strives to improve the care of infants, children and adolescents with digestive disorders by promoting advances in clinical care of children with chronic abdominal pain, diarrhea, constipation, vomiting, bleeding from the GI tract, inflammatory bowel disease, liver diseases, diseases of the pancreas, poor weight gain and nutritional problems.

Margaret K Stallings, Executive Director
Kim Rose, Associate Director
Donna Murphy, Membership

Libraries & Resource Centers

4130 National Digestive Diseases Information Clearinghouse
9000 Rockville Pike
Bethesda, MD 20892   301-496-3583
                                     800-860-8747
                                  Fax: 301-907-8906
                               healthinfo@niddk.nih.gov
                                   www.niddk.nih.gov

The National Institute of Diabetes and Digestive and Kidney Diseases conducts and supports research on many of the most serious diseases affecting public health. The Institute supports much of the clinical research on the diseases of internal medicine and related subspecialty fields as well as many basic science disciplines.

Dr. Griffin P. Rodgers, Director
Dr. Gregory G. Germino, Deputy Director
Camille M. Hoover, M.S.W., Executive Officer

Conferences

4131 Genetic Alliance Annual Conference
Genetic Alliance
4301 Connecticut Avenue NW, Suite 404
Washington, DC 20008

202-966-5557
800-336-4363
Fax: 202-966-8553
info@geneticalliance.org
www.geneticalliance.org

Consistently inspirational and enables partnership among all
stakeholders: advocates and community leaders, health and industry professionals, policymakers, and academicians.

July

Sharon Terry, President/CEO
Tetyana Murza, Managing Director
Natasha Bonhomme, VP, Strategic Development

4132 NASPGHAN Annual Meeting and Postgraduate Course
NASPGHAN
714 N. Bethlehem Pike, Ste 300
Ambler, PA 19002

215-641-9800
Fax: 215-641-1995
naspghan@naspghan.org
www.naspghan.org

November

Margaret K Stallings, Executive Director
Kim Rose, Associate Director
Donna Murphy, Membership

Web Sites

4133 American College of Gastroenterology
6400 Goldsboro Road, Suite 200
Bethesda, MD 20817

301-263-9000
info@acg.gi.org
www.gi.org

Founded to advance the scientific study and medical practice of
diseases of the gastrointestinal (GI) tract.

13,000 members

Carol A. Burke, MD, FACG, President

4134 National Digestive Diseases Information Clearinghouse
The National Institute of Diabetes and Digestive a
Bethesda, MD 20892

301-496-3583
Fax: 301-402-2125
germinogg@mail.nih.gov
www.niddk.nih.gov

The National Institute of Diabetes and Digestive and Kidney Diseases conducts and supports research on many of the most serious
diseases affecting public health. The Institute supports much of
the clinical research on the diseases of internal medicine and related subspecialty fields as well as many basic science
disciplines.

Griffin P. Rodgers, M.D., M.A.C.P., Director
Dr. Gregory Germino, Deputy Director

**4135 North American Society for Pediatric
Gastroenterology/Hepatology/Nutrition**
www.naspghan.org

Strives to improve the care of infants, children and adolescents
with digestive disorders by promoting advances in clinical care of
children with chronic abdominal pain, diarrhea, constipation,
vomiting, bleeding from the GI tract, inflammatory bowel disease, liver diseases, diseases of the pancreas, poor weight gain
and nutritional problems.

4136 Online Mendelian Inheritance in Man
8600 Rockville Pike
Bethesda, MD 20894

888-346-3656
info@ncbi.nlm.nih.gov
www.ncbi.nlm.nih.gov

This database is a catalog of human genes and genetic disorders.

4137 Rare Genetic Diseases in Children (NYU)
550 First Avenue
New York, NY 10016

212-263-7300
www.med.nyu.edu

We target issues arising from rare genetic diseases affecting children. Also, to assist in the endeavor to bring knowledge and hope
to those for whom there is, at present, so little.

Robert I. Grossman, MD, Dean & CEO
Steven B. Abramson, MD, Senior Vice President
Dafna Bar-Sagi, PhD, Senior Vice President

Journals

4138 Journal of Pediatric Gastroenterology and Nutrition
NASPGHAN, author

Lippincott Williams & Wilkins
Two Commerce Square, 2001 Market Street
Philadelphia, PA 19103

215-521-8300
Fax: 215-521-8902
orders@lww.com
www.lww.com

Publication of the North American Society for Pediatric
Gastroenterolgy, Hepatology and Nutrition, which strives to improve the care of infants, children and adolescents with digestive
disorders by promoting advances in clinical care of children with
chronic abdominal pain, diarrhea, constipation, vomiting, bleeding from the GI tract, inflammatory bowel disease, liver diseases,
diseases of the pancreas, poor weight gain and nutritional
problems.

Newsletters

4139 NASPGHAN News
714 N. Bethlehem Pike, Ste 300
Ambler, PA 19002

215-641-9800
Fax: 215-641-1995
naspghan@naspghan.org
www.naspghan.org

Publication of the North American Society for Pediatric
Gastroenterolgy, Hepatology and Nutrition, which strives to improve the care of infants, children and adolescents with digestive
disorders by promoting advances in clinical care of children with
chronic abdominal pain, diarrhea, constipation, vomiting, bleeding from the GI tract, inflammatory bowel disease, liver diseases,
diseases of the pancreas, poor weight gain and nutritional
problems.

Margaret K Stallings, Executive Director
Kim Rose, Associate Director
Donna Murphy, Membership

DESCRIPTION

4140 HERPES SIMPLEX

Covers these related disorders: Herpes simplex virus type 1 (HSV-1), Herpes simplex virus type 2 (HSV-2)

Involves the following Biologic System(s):

Infectious Disorders

Herpes simplex refers to a contagious infection caused by the herpes simplex virus. This infection is characterized by the formation of small, sometimes painful, fluid-filled, blister-like lesions (vesicles) on the skin and various mucous membranes. There are two strains of herpes simplex virus: type 1 (HSV-1) and type 2 (HSV-2). More than 85% of the U.S. population has evidence of infection with HSV-1, while 25% is infected with HSV-2. Although there is some overlap, HSV-1 is usually responsible for lesions of the lips such as cold sores (herpes labialis), the mouth (herpetic gingivostomatitis), and the eyes (e.g., corneal lesions, conjunctivitis, etc.). HSV-2 usually produces genital herpes and herpes associated with infections of the newborn that occur before or during birth (congenital herpes). HSV-1 is transmitted by direct contact through the saliva, while HSV-2 is generally transmitted through direct sexual contact. In addition, HSV-2 may be acquired by the fetus of an infected mother through the placenta or by direct contact during the birthing process.

Symptoms and findings associated with an initial or primary infection with herpes simplex virus usually appear in one to two weeks after contact and may range from no significant illness to the appearance of flu-like symptoms, sometimes in conjunction with blister-like lesions that usually scab and heal in a week to 10 days. Initial infection has a higher rate and longer duration of symptoms. Lesions associated with the first outbreak can be exceedingly painful. Newborns, malnourished infants, and individuals with compromised immune function may develop severe infection involving the entire body (systemic infection). After the primary infection, HSV becomes inactive but travels through the nerves that gave sensation to the affected area. Once it enters the roots of these nerves, it remains there for life. Recurrent episodes may be triggered by such factors as sun exposure, fever, physical and emotional stress, suppression of the immune system, the ingestion of certain medications or specific foods, and other factors. Such episodes may begin with mild irritation, itching, burning, tingling, or sometimes severe pain in the affected area followed a few hours or days later by the formation vesicles that often merge to form one large lesion. Associated symptoms and findings may include itching or discomfort in the affected area, fever, and swollen lymph nodes in the neck. The lesions sometimes become infected, especially in children. Typically, however, the lesions ulcerate and form a yellowish crust within a few days, with healing completed in about three weeks.

Symptoms associated with primary oral herpes infection (herpetic gingivostomatitis) usually appear suddenly and include pain, fever, excessive salivation, bad breath, and difficulty eating. Lesions may appear anywhere in the mouth, although the tongue and inside the cheeks are most frequently involved. In addition, the gums are usually inflamed and nearby lymph nodes may become enlarged. Primary episodes typically persist for about five to nine days. Lesions associated with recurrent oral herpes infection are often accompanied by itching, pain, or tingling that usually subsides within a week. Recurrent cold sore lesions sometimes precede oral herpes infections. Eye lesions may result from both primary and recurrent infections and include inflammation of the delicate mucous membranes that line the inside of the eyelids and the whites of the eyes (conjunctivitis) or inflammation and dryness involving the corneas as well as the conjunctiva.

Genital herpes most often affects adolescents and adults and is usually caused by HSV-2; however, approximately 10 to 25 percent of primary genital herpes infection results from HSV-1 through such factors as oral-genital transmission. This type of infection may be characterized by fever, painful urination, and swollen glands in the genital area. Females may develop herpetic lesions on the cervix and, less commonly, in the vagina and on the external genitalia while males typically develop lesions on the penis. Many patients exhibit few or no symptoms during a secondary episodes. However, infected individuals may unknowingly transmit the virus during this time through sexual activity or from a mother to her newborn.

Additional findings and complications associated with herpes simplex include a condition called herpetic whitlow, which is an infection of the finger resulting from transmission of HSV through a skin break. Whitlow is characterized by painful blistering and swelling at the fingertip. Eczema herpeticum is a severe condition in which patients with certain preexisting inflammatory skin conditions are infected with HSV and develop widespread blistering. Potentially life-threatening associated findings include high fever; excessive fluid loss (dehydration); decreases in the levels of essential elements known as electrolytes in the fluid portion of the blood (e.g., calcium, potassium, and sodium); spread of HSV to the brain and other organs; and bacterial infection. In addition, patients with suppressed immune systems are at risk for potentially life-threatening complications resulting from spread of disease to the liver, lungs, central nervous system, and other organs.

Treatment for herpes simplex is dependent upon the site affected as well as the severity and type of infection. For example, keeping affected areas dry is an important aspect of treatment as moisture tends to promote bacterial infection. Therefore, mild infections such as those associated with herpes of the lip may be treated by cleansing of the affected area with soap and water followed by careful drying of the lesion. Secondary bacterial infections may be treated with antibiotics. In addition, antiviral drugs such as acyclovir are often effective in treating various types of infection as well as preventing recurrences if administered during high-risk periods. Adolescents and young adults should receive counseling or training in order to reduce the risk of transmission. Other treatment is symptomatic and supportive. Patients with frequent outbreaks may benefit from suppressive therapy.

Government Agencies

4141 NIH/National Institute of Allergy and Infectious Diseases
5601 Fishers Lane, MSC 9806
Bethesda, MD 20892
301-496-5717
866-284-4107
Fax: 301-402-3573
TDD: 800-877-8339
ocpostoffice@niaid.nih.gov
www.niaid.nih.gov

Conducts and supports basic and applied research to better understand, treat, and ultimately prevent infectious, immunologic, and allergic diseases.

Anthony S Fauci MD, Director
Hugh Auchincloss, M.D., Principal Deputy Director
John J. McGowan, Ph.D., Deputy Director for Science Managem

National Associations & Support Groups

4142 American Academy of Pediatrics
141 Northwest Point Boulevard
Elk Grove Village, IL 60007
847-434-4000
800-433-9016
Fax: 847-434-8000
www.aap.org

The American Academy of Pediatrics and its member pediatricians are committed to the attainment of optimal physical, mental and social health and well-being for all infants, children, adolescents, and young adults.

Fernando Stein, MD, FAAP, President
Karen Remley, MD, CEO/Executive VP

4143 American Social Health Association
PO Box 13827
Research Triangle Park, NC 27709
919-361-8400
800-783-9877
Fax: 919-361-8425
www.ashastd.org

The American Social Health Association is dedicated to improving the health of individuals, families and communities, with a focus on preventing sexually transmitted diseases and their harmful consequences

Lynn Barclay, President/CEO
Deborah Arrindell, VP Health Policy
Dave Allen MBA, CPA, Vice President/CFO

4144 March of Dimes Foundation
1275 Mamaroneck Avenue
White Plains, NY 10605
914-997-4488
888-663-4637
Fax: 914-997-4763
answers@marchofdimes.com
www.marchofdimes.com

Partnership of volunteers and professionals dedicates to improving the health of babies by preventing birth defects and infant mortality. Over 100 chapters are located across the country and can be located through the National Office.

Stacey D. Stewart, President

4145 World Health Organization
Avenue Appia 20
CH-1211 Geneva 27,
Switzerland
www.who.int

WHO is the directing and coordinating authority for health within the United Nations system.

Dr Margaret Chan, Director General

Libraries & Resource Centers

4146 Herpes Resource Center
American Social Health Association
PO Box 13827
Research Triangle Park, NC 27709
919-361-8488
800-230-6039
www.ashastd.org

Focuses on increasing education, public awareness, and support to anyone concerned about herpes.

Lynn Barclay, President/CEO
Deborah Arrindell, VP Health Policy

Web Sites

4147 American Social Health Association
www.ashastd.org

ASHA is dedicated to improving the health of individuals, families, and communities, with a focus on preventing sexually transmitted diseases and their harmful consequences.

4148 Health Research Project (HaRP)
www.harpnet.org
harp@kmsgh.org
www.harpnet.org

A program by USAID, the project strives to improve the health status of infants, children, mothers and families through the development and research of new tools, technologies, policies and approaches.

4149 HerpeSite
www.herpesite.org

Information outlining aspects and issues relating to herpes simplex virus (HSV).

4150 Herpes.com
www.herpes.com

Purpose of this website is to fill the desperate need for herpes education, make it easier to manage herpes, inform people of ways to limit herpes reacurrences, to inform people of the beneficial products for herpes sufferers, to show the relationship between good health and herpes, to provide an opportunity for herpes sufferers to share their personal experiences and to provide communication via our live chat.

4151 International Herpes Management Forum
www.ihmf.org

Established to improve the awareness and understanding of herpes virus, and the counselling and management of people with these infections.

4152 Slack
6900 Grove Road
Thorofare, NJ 8086
856-848-1000
Fax: 856-848-6091
email@slackinc.com
www.slackinc.com

Is a leading provider of healthcare information, educational programs, and meeting and exhibit management services worldwide.

4153 Virtual Pediatric Hospital
www.virtualpediatrichospital.org

A digital library of pediatric information including resources for patients and health care professionals.

Book Publishers

4154 Understanding Herpes
Lawrence R. Stanberry MD, PhD, author

University Press of Mississippi
3825 Ridgewood Road
Jackson, MS 39211
601-432-6205
800-737-7788
Fax: 601-432-6217
press@ihl.state.ms.us
www.upress.state.ms.us

A most informative overview of herpes written for the general reader.

120 pages Hardcover/Ppbck
ISBN: 1-578060-40-0

DESCRIPTION

4155 HIRSCHSPRUNG DISEASE

Synonyms: Aganglionic megacolon, Congenital aganglionic megacolon

Involves the following Biologic System(s):

Gastrointestinal Disorders

Hirschsprung disease is a gastrointestinal disorder that is usually apparent within the first few days after birth. However, in some affected infants, symptoms may not become apparent until the first weeks of life. Hirschsprung disease is characterized by absence of groups of certain nerve cell bodies (ganglia) in the smooth muscle wall of the large intestine. In most affected infants, the affected segment begins at the ring-shaped involuntary muscle of the anus (internal anal sphincter) and extends to the lowest region of the colon (sigmoid colon). However, in other cases, this segment may extend to involve the entire colon.

In infants with Hirschsprung disease, absence of these nerve groups results in impairment or absence of rhythmic contractions that propel food through the digestive system (peristalsis). Due to impaired peristalsis, most affected newborns have inadequate or delayed passage of meconium, the thick, sticky, darkish green material that accumulates in the fetal intestines and forms a newborn's first stools. Although some affected newborns may pass meconium normally, they may subsequently experience chronic constipation. In infants with Hirschsprung disease, failure to properly pass stools results in widening of the colon (megacolon) above the affected segment and severe abdominal bloating (abdominal distension). Additional symptoms and findings may include episodes of diarrhea, nausea and vomiting, dehydration, loss of appetite (anorexia) and malnutrition, failure to grow and gain weight at the expected rate (failure to thrive), listlessness (lethargy), and other abnormalities. In addition, widening of the colon may result in deterioration of the colon's mucous membranes (mucosal barrier), potentially allowing increased reproduction of certain bacteria and associated inflammation of the colon (i.e., enterocolitis). In severe cases, severe diarrhea and potentially life-threatening complications may result.

In infants with Hirschsprung disease, treatment includes surgical removal of the affected area of the colon and rejoining of healthy areas of the colon and rectum. In some patients, before surgical correction, a temporary colostomy may be required. Colostomy is a procedure in which the lower end of the healthy region of the colon is connected to a surgically created opening in the abdominal wall.

Hirschsprung disease affects approximately one in 5,000 newborns and is considered the most common cause of lower intestinal obstruction in infants during the first month of life. The condition is about four times as common in males as females. Hirschsprung disease may occur in association with other disorders or conditions that are apparent at birth (congenital disorders) or as an isolated finding for unknown reasons (sporadic occurrence). In addition, there have been many reports of Hirschsprung disease in infants within certain families (kindreds). Researchers suggest that sporadic and familial cases may result from abnormal changes or mutations of one of several different genes expressed either alone or together (polygenic). Depending upon the specific disease gene or genes, the condition may have autosomal dominant, autosomal recessive, or polygenic inheritance.

National Associations & Support Groups

4156 American Academy of Pediatrics

141 Northwest Point Boulevard
Elk Grove Village, IL 60007

847-434-4000
800-433-9016
Fax: 847-434-8000
www.aap.org

The American Academy of Pediatrics and its member pediatricians are committed to the attainment of optimal physical, mental and social health and well-being for all infants, children, adolescents, and young adults.

Fernando Stein, MD, FAAP, President
Karen Remley, MD, CEO/Executive VP

4157 American Pseudo-Obstruction and Hirschsprung's Disease Society

158 Pleasant Street
North Andover, MA 01845

978-685-4477
Fax: 978-685-4488

Promotes public awareness of gastrointestinal motility disorders, in particular intestinal pseudo-obstruction and Hirschsprung's disease; provides education and support to individuals and families of children who have been diagnosed with these disorders through parent-to-parent contact, publications, and educational symposia; and encourages and supports medical research in the area of gastrointestinal motility disorders.

4158 Genetic Alliance

4301 Connecticut Avenue NW, Suite 404
Washington, DC 20008

202-966-5557
800-336-4363
Fax: 202-966-8553
info@geneticalliance.org
www.geneticalliance.org

A coalition of voluntary genetic support groups, consumers and professionals addressing the needs of individuals and families affected by genetic disorders from a national perspective.

Sharon Terry, President/CEO
Tetyana Murza, Managing Director
Natasha Bonhomme, VP, Strategic Development

4159 Intestinal Pseudoobstruction (IP) Support Network

8600 Rockville Pike
Bethesda, MD 20894

301-594-5983
888-346-3656
Fax: 301-402-1384
TDD: 800-735-2258
www.nlm.nih.gov

Offers peer support, matching individuals/families. Educational materials include Membership directory.

Colleen Kidder, Contact

4160 March of Dimes Foundation

1275 Mamaroneck Avenue
White Plains, NY 10605

914-997-4488
888-663-4637
Fax: 914-997-4763
answers@marchofdimes.com
www.marchofdimes.com

Partnership of volunteers and professionals dedicates to improving the health of babies by preventing birth defects and infant mortality. Over 100 chapters are located across the country and can be located through the National Office.

Stacey D. Stewart, President

4161 Pull-Thru Network

2312 Savoy Street
Hoover, AL 35226

205-978-2930
info@pullthrough.org
www.pullthrough.org

A chapter of the United Ostomy Association dedicated to the support and information needs of the families of children born with imperforate anus, cloaca, cloaca exstrophy, bladder exstrophy, VATER Syndrome, Hirschsprung's Disease and other related birth anomalies.

Bonnie McElroy, President

4162 United Ostomy Association
PO Box 512
Northfield, MN 55057
949-660-8624
800-826-0826
Fax: 949-660-9262
info@ostomy.org
www.uoaa.org

An association of affiliated, non-profit, support groups committed to improving the quality of life of people who have, or will have, an intestinal or urinary diversion.

Dave Rudzin, President
Diane Miterko, Advocacy Chair

Libraries & Resource Centers

4163 National Digestive Diseases Information Clearinghouse
9000 Rockville Pike
Bethesda, MD 20892
301-496-3583
800-860-8747
Fax: 301-907-8906
healthinfo@niddk.nih.gov
www.niddk.nih.gov

The National Institute of Diabetes and Digestive and Kidney Diseases conducts and supports research on many of the most serious diseases affecting public health. The Institute supports much of the clinical research on the diseases of internal medicine and related subspecialty fields as well as many basic science disciplines.

Dr. Griffin P. Rodgers, Director
Dr. Gregory G. Germino, Deputy Director
Camille M. Hoover, M.S.W., Executive Officer

Conferences

4164 Genetic Alliance Annual Conference
Genetic Alliance
4301 Connecticut Avenue NW, Suite 404
Washington, DC 20008
202-966-5557
800-336-4363
Fax: 202-966-8553
info@geneticalliance.org
www.geneticalliance.org

Consistently inspirational and enables partnership among all stakeholders: advocates and community leaders, health and industry professionals, policymakers, and academicians.

July

Sharon Terry, President/CEO
Tetyana Murza, Managing Director
Natasha Bonhomme, VP, Strategic Development

4165 UOAA National Conference
United Ostomy Associations of America
PO Box 512
Northfield, MN 55507
800-826-0826
info@uoaa.org
www.uoaa.org

August

Dave Rudzin, President

Web Sites

4166 NIH News Advisory
9000 Rockville Pike
Bethesda, MD 20892
301-496-4000
TTY: 301-402-9612
NIHinfo@od.nih.gov
www.nih.gov

The National Institute of Health is the steward of medical and behavioral research for the nation.

Francis S. Collins, M.D., Ph.D., Director

4167 Online Mendelian Inheritance in Man
8600 Rockville Pike
Bethesda, MD 20894
888-346-3656
info@ncbi.nlm.nih.gov
www.ncbi.nlm.nih.gov

This database is a catalog of human genes and genetic disorders.

4168 Pull-Thru Network
1705 Wintergreen Parkway
Normal, IL 61761
pullthrunetwork@gmail.com
www.pullthrunetwork.org

A chapter of the United Ostomy Association dedicated to the support and information needs of the families of children born with imperforate anus, cloaca, cloaca exstrophy, bladder exstrophy, VATER Syndrome, Hirschsprung's Disease and other related birth anomalies.

Lori Parker, Executive Director
Hollie Filce, Associate Director
Carmell Burns, Director

4169 United Ostomy Association
P.O. Box 512
Northfield, MN 55057
800-826-0826
www.ostomy.org

An association of affiliated, non-profit, support groups committed to improving the quality of life of people who have, or will have, an intestinal or urinary diversion.

Susan Burns, President
Jim Murray, 1st Vice President
Joan McGorry, 2nd Vice President

Book Publishers

4170 Online Pediatric Surgery Handbook
PO Box 10426, Caparra Heights Station
San Juan, PR 00922
787-786-3496
Fax: 787-720-6103
titolugo@coqui.net
www.home.coqui.net/titolugo/handbook.htm#IIIF

An online handbook about many different diseases and disabilities.

Newsletters

4171 Pediatric Surgery Update
PO Box 10426, Caparra Heights Station
San Juan, PR 922
787-786-3496
Fax: 787-720-6103
titolugo@coqui.net
home.coqui.net/titolugo/handbook.htm#IIIF

Periodical electronic newsletter of interest to Primary Physicians, Pediatricians, Surgeons, Residents, Medical Students, Nurses and Health-related professionals dealing with evidence-based medicine and reviews in the practice of pediatric surgery.

Humberto Lugo-Vicente MD, FACS, Editor-in-Chief

4172 Pull-Thru Network News
1705 Wintergreen Parkway
Normal, IL 61761
205-978-2930
pullthrunetwork@gmail.com
www.pullthrunetwork.org

Provides emotional support and information to patients and families of children who have had or will have pull-through surgery to correct an imperforate anus or associated malformation, Hirschsprung's disease, or other fecal incontinence problems; sponsors online discussion groups.

Lori Parker, Executive Director
Hollie Filce, Associate Director
Carmell Burns, Director

Pamphlets

4173 Hirschsprung Disease
Nat'l Digestive Diseases Information Clearinghouse
The National Institute of Diabetes and Digestive a
Bethesda, MD 20892   301-496-3583
Fax: 301-402-2125
germinogg@mail.nih.gov
www.niddk.nih.gov

Defines and explains the causes, symptoms, and treatment of
Hirschsprung's Disease. Includes a glossary of terms associated
with the condition.

Griffin P. Rodgers, M.D., M.A.C.P., Director
Dr. Gregory Germino, Deputy Director

DESCRIPTION

4174 HISTIOCYTOSIS

Synonyms: Class I histiocytosis, Langerhans cell histiocytosis, LCH

Involves the following Biologic System(s):

Hematologic and Oncologic Disorders

Histiocytosis X, also known as Langerhans cell histiocytosis, LCH, or Class I histiocytosis, refers to a group of three similar disorders called eosinophilic granuloma, Hand-Schuller-Christian disease, and Letterer-Siwe disease. These disorders are all characterized by the excessive production and accumulation of certain types of tissue cells known as histiocytes, resulting in benign growth or scar formation. Characteristic findings and symptoms are variable and depend upon the organ or organ system affected; however, approximately 80 percent of individuals with LCH have skeletal involvement. Associated bone lesions may appear in isolation or in many parts of the body. These lesions occur most often in the skull, although their appearance in other areas of the skeleton is not uncommon. Some individuals may experience complications resulting from bone involvement. For example, involvement of a certain bone near the ear (mastoid) may result in chronic ear infections and persistent drainage. Involvement of certain weight-bearing bones may result in fractures.

Letterer-Siwe disease occurs during early childhood, usually before three years of age. This disease is characterized by skin eruptions, enlargement of the liver and spleen (hepatosplenomegaly) and certain lymph nodes (lymphadenopathy), and abnormally low levels of circulating red blood cells resulting in anemia. In addition, some children may experience involvement of the lungs, sometimes resulting in lung collapse (pneumothorax). Hand-Schuller-Christian disease often appears during early childhood and is characterized by bulging of the eyeballs (exophthalmos); excessive urinary excretion (polyuria), a decrease in body fluid volume (dehydration), and excessive thirst (polydipsia); elevated cholesterol levels (hypercholesterolemia); and involvement of soft tissues and bone. Eosinophilic granulomas most often occur during the second to fourth decade of life; however, they may develop during childhood, especially between the ages of five to 10 years. Benign growths may develop in the skull, jaw, and the long bones of the arms and legs, sometimes resulting in pain and fractures. In addition, lung involvement may result in respiratory symptoms such as coughing and shortness of breath, fever, and lung collapse.

Other findings and symptoms sometimes associated with Class I histiocytoses may include growth retardation, thyroid deficiency, and other abnormalities resulting from disruption in pituitary gland function or involvement of another gland in the brain known as the hypothalamus; difficulty walking and other neurologic symptoms resulting from involvement of the central nervous system; and additional irregularities of the blood resulting from involvement of the bone marrow.

Although the exact cause of each of the disorders that comprise Class I histiocytoses is unknown, it is believed that Letterer-Siwe disease may be inherited as an autosomal recessive trait and that the diseases develop as a result of disturbanc|es within the immune system. Treatment for LCH depends upon the extent and severity of involvement. For example, if only one organ or organ system (e.g., skeletal or skin, etc.) is affected, the disease is often self-limited; therefore, treatment may be directed toward control and resolution of specific lesions through low-dose radiation therapy or removal by means of a scraping procedure (curettage). If more than one system of the body is affected, treatment may involve a chemotherapy regimen that includes the use of one or two specific drugs (i.e., etoposide and vinblastine). More resistant disease may necessitate the use of other immunosuppressive drugs, bone marrow transplantation, or experimental treatments. Other treatment is symptomatic and supportive.

Government Agencies

4175 NIH/National Cancer Institute
BG 9609 / 9609 Medical Center Drive
Bethesda, MD 20892   800-422-6237
                                          www.cancer.gov

The National Cancer Institute coordinates the National Cancer Program, which conducts and supports research, training, health information dissemination, and other programs with respect to the cause, diagnosis, prevention, and treatment of cancer, rehabilitation from cancer, and the continuing care of cancer patients and the families of cancer patients.

Douglas R. Lowy, MD, Acting Director
James Doroshow, MD, Deputy Director
Henry P. Ciolino, PhD, Acting Director, Cancer Centers

National Associations & Support Groups

4176 American Academy of Pediatrics
141 Northwest Point Boulevard
Elk Grove Village, IL 60007   847-434-4000
                                          800-433-9016
                                          Fax: 847-434-8000
                                          www.aap.org

The American Academy of Pediatrics and its member pediatricians are committed to the attainment of optimal physical, mental and social health and well-being for all infants, children, adolescents, and young adults.

Fernando Stein, MD, FAAP, President
Karen Remley, MD, CEO/Executive VP

4177 Genetic Alliance
4301 Connecticut Avenue NW, Suite 404
Washington, DC 20008   202-966-5557
                                          800-336-4363
                                          Fax: 202-966-8553
                                          info@geneticalliance.org
                                          www.geneticalliance.org

A coalition of voluntary genetic support groups, consumers and professionals addressing the needs of individuals and families affected by genetic disorders from a national perspective.

Sharon Terry, President/CEO
Tetyana Murza, Managing Director
Natasha Bonhomme, VP, Strategic Development

4178 Histiocytosis Association of America
332 North Broadway
Pitman, NJ 08071   856-589-6606
                                          800-548-2758
                                          Fax: 856-589-6614
                                          association@histio.org
                                          www.histio.org

The Histiocytosis Association of America is a global, nonprofit organization dedicated to supporting, educating, and connecting those who are fighting histiocytic disorders, and ultimately, finding a cure. It is the only organization of its kind-bringing together the patient and medical communities to grow and share knowledge; providing critical support and education to patients and families; and identifying and funding key research initiatives that will lead to a world free of these disorders.

Jeffery Toughill, President & CEO
Beth Anne Miller, COO/Director Development

4179 March of Dimes Foundation
1275 Mamaroneck Avenue
White Plains, NY 10605

914-997-4488
888-663-4637
Fax: 914-997-4763
answers@marchofdimes.com
www.marchofdimes.com

Partnership of volunteers and professionals dedicated to improving the health of babies by preventing birth defects and infant mortality. Over 100 chapters are located across the country and can be located through the National Office.

Stacey D. Stewart, President

Conferences

4180 Genetic Alliance Annual Conference
Genetic Alliance
4301 Connecticut Avenue NW, Suite 404
Washington, DC 20008

202-966-5557
800-336-4363
Fax: 202-966-8553
info@geneticalliance.org
www.geneticalliance.org

Consistently inspirational and enables partnership among all stakeholders: advocates and community leaders, health and industry professionals, policymakers, and academicians.

July

Sharon Terry, President/CEO
Tetyana Murza, Managing Director
Natasha Bonhomme, VP, Strategic Development

Web Sites

4181 National Histicytosis Organizations
332 North Broadway
Pitman, NJ 8071

856-589-6606
Fax: 856-589-6614
info@histio.org
www.histio.org/

Is an international partnership of patients, families, physicians and friends. Is is a nonprofit organization whose goals are to promote scientific research into the hitiocytoses, seeking to develop better means of control and management of the disease and ultimatley seeking to develop scientific means to prevent and cure them and to provide solutions to some of the problems which are specific to patients suffering from this disease and to offer support to such patients and their families.

James Hassan, Esq., Chairman
Robert List, Treasurer
Tracy Brown, Trustee

4182 Online Mendelian Inheritance in Man
8600 Rockville Pike
Bethesda, MD 20894

888-346-3656
info@ncbi.nlm.nih.gov
www.ncbi.nlm.nih.gov

This database is a catalog of human genes and genetic disorders.

4183 Texas Children's Cancer Center
P.O. Box 2659
Austin, TX 78768

512-474-1798
www.txcc.org

Offers innovative therapies for all forms of childhood cancer and blood disorders. The Cancer Center is working to improve the outcome for all patients afflicted with these diseases and to develop and perfect new treatment approaches that are born from only the most extraordinary scientific insights.

Geanie Morrison, President
James Frank, Vice President
Jodie Laubenberg, Secretary

Book Publishers

4184 Let's Talk About Going to the Hospital
Rosen Publishing Group's PowerKids Press
29 E 21st Street
New York, NY 10010

212-777-3017
800-237-9932
Fax: 888-436-4643
rosenpub@tribeca.ios.com
www.powerkidspress.com

If a child has to check into the hospital, chances are he or she is already upset about being ill. Knowing how a hospital functions and what the procedures are, such as when family members can visit, will help in what is already a stressful situation. Grades K-5.

24 pages
ISBN: 0-823950-36-0

DESCRIPTION

4185 HODGKIN'S DISEASE

Synonym: Hodgkin's lymphoma

Covers these related disorders: Hodgkin's disease—lymphocyte depletion type, Hodgkin's disease—lymphocyte predominance type, Hodgkin's disease—mixed cellularity type, Hodgkin's disease—nodular sclerosing type

Involves the following Biologic System(s):
Hematologic and Oncologic Disorders

Hodgkin's disease is a malignant disorder (cancer) characterized by painless, progressive enlargement of the lymph nodes, spleen, and other lymphoid tissues (lymphoma). The lymphatic system includes a network of vessels that collect a fluid known as lymph from different areas of the body and drain this fluid into the bloodstream. As lymph moves through the lymphatic system, it is filtered by a network of lymph nodes, which are small structures located along the course of the lymphatic vessels. Most lymph nodes that can be felt (palpable) are located in the neck, mouth, and groin and under the arms (axillae). Lymph nodes store certain white blood cells and are thought to play a role in producing antibodies, thus functioning as part of the body's immune system.

Malignancies of lymph tissue, known as lymphomas, are the third most common form of cancer affecting children in the United States. Approximately 13 per one million children are affected by lymphoma in the U.S. each year. There are two main categories of lymphoma, including Hodgkin's disease and non-Hodgkin's lymphoma. Although Hodgkin's disease may affect individuals of any age, it usually occurs between the ages of 15 and 35 or after age 50. In children, the disease is most common during late childhood or early adolescence and rarely affects those younger than five years of age. About 6,000 to 7,000 cases of the disease occur in the U.S. annually. Epstein-Barr virus, a member of the herpesvirus family that causes mononucleosis 35-50 percent of the time, may play some role in the disease. In addition, some familial cases have been reported, suggesting possible genetic mechanisms.

Hodgkin's disease is characterized by the presence of relatively large, abnormal white blood cells that have more than one nucleus and a distinctive appearance under a microscope. These cancerous cells, known as Reed-Sternberg cells, may be seen during the microscopic examination of small tissue samples removed from affected lymph nodes or other lymphoid tissues. Hodgkin's disease is categorized into four main subtypes based upon the number and relative proportion of such cells as well as the proportions of certain other white blood cells (e.g., plasma cells, eosinophils, macrophages, etc.). The frequency of the different subtypes varies with age. For example, nodular sclerosing type is the most common form of the disease and affects approximately 50 percent of children and up to 70 percent of adolescents with Hodgkin's disease. Another subtype, known as the mixed cellularity type, affects about 40 to 50 percent of patients, and the lymphocyte predominance type of the disease primarily occurs in males and younger patients. The fourth subtype, called lymphocyte depletion type, is the rarest and most aggressive form of the disorder and occurs in fewer than 10 percent of patients.

Hodgkin's disease usually originates in the lymphatic vessels. As the disease progresses, the malignancy may spread from lymph nodes and infiltrate certain organs, particularly the spleen, lungs, liver, and bone marrow. Most patients initially experience painless swelling of lymph nodes in the neck or, in some cases, under the arm or in the groin area. Some may gradually develop generalized symptoms including fever, night sweats, fatigue, listlessness (lethargy), generalized itching (pruritus), loss of appetite (anorexia), and weight loss. Involvement of other organs or tissues may cause varying symptoms. For example, if the lungs are affected, patients may experience coughing and shortness of breath (dyspnea). Advanced involvement of the bone marrow may result in abnormally low levels of circulating red blood cells (anemia), platelets (thrombocytopenia), or certain white blood cells (neutropenia). Advanced disease may cause progressive impairment of the body's immune system, resulting in an increased susceptibility to certain infections. In patients with severe disease progression, infection with certain microorganisms that typically cause no or only minor symptoms in healthy individuals may result in severe or potentially life-threatening complications.

Treatment of patients with the disease varies, depending on the stage of the disease and other factors. For patients in early stages who have localized disease and have obtained full growth, radiation therapy alone may be effective; the 10-year survival rate exceeds 80 percent. However, up to 15 percent of such patients may experience recurrences, requiring therapy with certain anticancer drugs (combination chemotherapy). However, combination therapy cures more than 50 percent of patients, even those with advanced-stage disease. Combination chemotherapy may include the drugs doxorubicin (Adriamycin), bleomycin, vinblastine, and dacarbazine (known as ABVD) or a combination of mechlorethamine, vincristine (Oncovin), procarbazine, and prednisone (called MOPP). Physicians who specialize in the treatment of childhood cancers (pediatric oncologists) often select alternating therapy with MOPP and ABVD in combination with low-dose radiation therapy due to this treatment's high success and a reduction in certain long-term effects potentially associated with treatment for Hodgkin's disease. For example, such combination chemotherapy/radiation therapy may help reduce the risk of potential growth defects in affected children, damage to heart and lung tissue, infertility, or the development of certain secondary malignancies later in life, such as acute myeloid leukemia (AML) or certain solid tumors. Patients should receive ongoing monitoring throughout life to ensure prompt detection and treatment of possible recurrences or secondary malignancies.

Government Agencies

4186 NIH/National Cancer Institute
BG 9609 / 9609 Medical Center Drive
Bethesda, MD 20892

800-422-6237
www.cancer.gov

The National Cancer Institute coordinates the National Cancer Program, which conducts and supports research, training, health information dissemination, and other programs with respect to the cause, diagnosis, prevention, and treatment of cancer, rehabilitation from cancer, and the continuing care of cancer patients and the families of cancer patients.

Douglas R. Lowy, MD, Acting Director
James Doroshow, MD, Deputy Director
Henry P. Ciolino, PhD, Acting Director, Cancer Centers

National Associations & Support Groups

4187 American Academy of Pediatrics
141 Northwest Point Boulevard
Elk Grove Village, IL 60007 847-434-4000
800-433-9016
Fax: 847-434-8000
www.aap.org

The American Academy of Pediatrics and its member pediatricians are committed to the attainment of optimal physical, mental and social health and well-being for all infants, children, adolescents, and young adults.

Fernando Stein, MD, FAAP, President
Karen Remley, MD, CEO/Executive VP

4188 American Childhood Cancer Organization (fo rmerly Candlelighters Childhood Cancer)
PO Box 498
Kensington, MD 20895 301-962-3520
855-858-2226
Fax: 310-962-3521
staff@acco.org
www.acco.org

The Candlelighters Childhood Cancer Foundation National Office was founded in 1970 by concerned parents of children with cancer. Today our membership of over 50,000 members of the national office and more than 100,000 members across the across the country, including Candlelighters affiliate groups, includes, parents of children who are being treated or have been treated for cancer.

Ruth I. Hoffman, MPH, Executive Director
Jessica DiBenedetto, Program Coordinator
Christy Perry, Director, Marketing/Communications

4189 Leukemia & Lymphoma Society
3 International Drive, Ste 200
Rye Brook, NY 10573 914-949-5213
Fax: 914-949-6691
www.lls.org

Largest voluntary health organization dedicated to funding blood cancer research, education and patient services.

Louis J. DeGennaro, PhD, President & CEO
Andrew Coccari, Chief Product Officer
Danielle Gee, Chief of Staff

4190 Lymphoma Research Foundation of America
115 Broadway 19th Floor, Suite 1301
New York, NY 10006 212-349-2910
800-500-9976
Fax: 212-349-2886
Helpline@lymphoma.org
www.lymphoma.org

National nonprofit organization dedicated to eradicating lymphoma and serving those touched by this disease. LRF funds research to develop safer, more effective treatments and ultimately, a cure for lymphoma. LRF delivers a comprehensive slate of educational and support programs, services, and publications for lymphoma patients and their loved ones.

Steven J. Prince, Chairman
Jerry Freundlich, Secretary
Tom Condon, Treasurer

4191 National Childhood Cancer Foundation
4600 East West Highway, Suite 600
Bethesda, MD 20814 301-718-0042
800-458-6223
Fax: 301-718-0047
info@curesearch.org
www.curesearch.org

CureSearch unites the world's largest childhood cancer research organization, the Children's Oncology Group, and the National Childhood Cancer Foundation through our mission to cure childhood cancer. Research is the key to the cure.

Stuart Siegal, Chairman
Timothy Harmon, Vice-Chair
Mary Payne, Treasurer

4192 National Foundation for Cancer Research
4600 East West Highway, Suite 525
Bethesda, MD 20814 301-654-1250
800-321-2873
Fax: 301-654-5824
info@nfcr.org
www.nfcr.org

The National Foundation for Cancer Research (NFCR) was founded in 1973 to support cancer research and public education relating to the prevention, early diagnosis, better treatments and ultimately, a cure for cancer. NFCR promotes and facilitates collaboration among scientists to accelerate the pace of discovery from bench to bedside.

Franklin C Salisbury, President
Judith P. Barnhard, Chairman
Michael Burke, Treasurer

Web Sites

4193 Children's Cancer Web
www.cancerindex.org/ccw

An independent nonprofit site, established to provide a directory of childhood cancer resources.

Book Publishers

4194 Let's Talk About Going to the Hospital
Rosen Publishing Group's PowerKids Press
29 E 21st Street
New York, NY 10010 212-777-3017
800-237-9932
Fax: 888-436-4643
rosenpub@tribeca.ios.com
www.powerkidspress.com

If a child has to check into the hospital, chances are he or she is already upset about being ill. Knowing how a hospital functions and what the procedures are, such as when family members can visit, will help in what is already a stressful situation. Grades K-5.

24 pages
ISBN: 0-823950-36-0

4195 Let's Talk About when Kids Have Cancer
Rosen Publishing Group's PowerKids Press
29 E 21st Street
New York, NY 10010 212-777-3017
800-237-9932
Fax: 888-436-4643
rosenpub@tribeca.ios.com
www.powerkidspress.com

In a straightforward yet comforting way, this book explains what cancer is, what kinds of treatments surround the disease and how to cope if a child has cancer.

24 pages
ISBN: 0-823951-95-2

4196 Living with Childhood Cancer: A Practical Guide to Help Families Cope

Leigh A. Woznick, Carol D. Goodheart EdD, author

American Psychological Association
750 1st Street
Washington, DC 20002 202-336-5500
800-374-2721
TTY: 202-336-6123
www.apa.org

This book offers information for families faced with the shattering experience of having a child with cancer.

2001 359 pages Hardcover
ISBN: 1-557988-72-2

Donald N. Bersoff,PhD, JD, President
Norman B. Anderson, PhD, Chief Executive Officer & Executive
Bonnie Markham, PhD, Treasurer

4197 Surviving Childhood Cancer: A Guide for Families
New Harbinger Publications
5674 Shattuck Avenue
Oakland, CA 94609   510-652-0215
                                           800-748-6273
                                        Fax: 800-652-1613
                          customerservice@newharbinger.com
                                       www.newharbinger.com

Cancer in a child is an overwhelming experience for a family.
This book explains common medical procedures and offers readers practical advice about how to cope with emotions and stress
during this time.

1998 215 pages
ISBN: 1-572241-02-0

Pamphlets

4198 Hodgkin's Disease and Non-Hodgkin's Lymphomas
Leukemia and Lymphoma Society
3 International Drive, Ste 200
Rye Brook, NY 10573   914-949-5213
                                           800-955-4572
                                        Fax: 914-949-6691
                                         infocenter@lls.org
                                               www.lls.org

Explanation of the disease, its symptoms, diagnosis, prognosis
and treatment, psychological responses to a confirmed diagnosis
and current research.

36 pages
Louis J. DeGennaro, Ph.D., President & CEO

DESCRIPTION

4199 HOMOCYSTINURIA

Covers these related disorders: Homocystinuria Type I (Classic homocystinuria), Homocystinuria Type II, Homocystinuria Type III

Involves the following Biologic System(s):
Genetic/Chromosomal/Syndrome/Metabolic Disorders

Homocystinuria is a metabolic disorder characterized by an inborn error in the metabolism of the amino acid methionine. There are three types of homocystinuria, each resulting from a deficiency or defect of a specific enzyme or compound that is essential in the processing of methionine.

Homocystinuria Type I (Classic homocystinuria) is caused by a deficiency of the enzyme cystathionine synthase. Although symptoms and physical findings are not apparent at birth, early symptoms may include delays in development and failure to thrive. Characteristic findings, which are often not apparent until after the age of three years, may include eye abnormalities such as dislocation of the lens of the eyes (ectopia lentis), followed by nearsightedness (myopia) and tremors of the iris (iridodonesis). Other physical findings may include skeletal abnormalities such as osteoporosis, sideways curvature of the spine (scoliosis), either a sunken or prominent chest (pectus deformity), and a condition known as genu valgum in which the legs curve inward causing the knees to touch (knock-knee) and the space between the feet to increase. Affected children often have a fair complexion, blue eyes, sparse blonde hair, and a characteristic flushed face (malar flush). In addition, there is a tendency to develop blood clots (thromboemboli) in the veins and arteries.These clots may occur at any time, and if they lodge in the brain can result in paralysis and seizures heart problems and high blood pressure may also occur. Laboratory findings may include elevated levels of both methionine and the sulfur compound homocystine in body fluids. Mental retardation is apparent in approximately 65 percent of affected people. It is estimated that about 50 percent of patients experience some form of psychiatric disorder.

Treatment for classic homocystinuria includes aggressive vitamin B6 supplementation. In addition, restriction of foods that contain methionine is recommended in conjunction with supplementation of cysteine, also a sulfur-containing amino acid. In some affected individuals who do not respond to vitamin B6 treatment, administration of betaine may be effective. Classic homocystinuria is inherited as an autosomal recessive trait and occurs in approximately one in 200,000 live births. The gene for cystathionine synthase is located on the long arm of chromosome 21 (21q22.3).

Homocystinuria Type II is transmitted as an autosomal recessive trait and results from a defect in the formation of methylcobalamin. Characteristic symptoms and findings depend on the particular underlying defect. Some children with homocystinuria type II may also have a condition called methylmalonic aciduria characterized by excessive methylmalonic acid in the urine. Symptoms usually develop in the early months of life and may include difficulty in feeding, listlessness, vomiting, diminished muscle tone (hypotonia), and delays in development. Treatment for this form of homo stinuria includes vitamin B12 supplementation (cobalamin).

Homocystinuria Type III, a very rare form of the disorder, results from a deficiency of the enzyme methylenetetrahydrofolate reductase (MTHFR), also essential to the maintenance of methionine. Symptoms and physical findings are extremely variable and depend upon the extent of the deficiency. Complete absence of this enzyme may result in life-threatening episodes of respiratory distress as well as seizure-like muscle contractions (myoclonus). A partial enzyme deficiency may cause convulsions, an abnormally small head (microcephaly), mental retardation, and muscular irregularities. Occasional findings may include psychiatric disturbances, abnormalities of certain blood vessels, and inflammation or degenerative changes of specific nerves. In addition, blood clot activity may be apparent in some affected individuals.

Treatment for homocystinuria type III may include supplementation with folic acid, vitamin B6 (pyridoxine), vitamin B12, methionine, and betaine (also known as trimethylglycine). Early intervention with betaine has a particularly effective outcome. Homocystinuria Type III is transmitted as an autosomal recessive trait. The gene for methylenetetrahydrofolate reductase is located on the short arm of chromosome 1 (1p36.3).

National Associations & Support Groups

4200 ARC of the United States
1825 K Street MW, Suite 1200
Washington, DC 20006
202-534-3700
800-433-5255
Fax: 202-534-3731
info@thearc.org
www.thearc.org

The ARC is the national organization of and for people with mental retardation and related developmental disabilities and their families. Devoted to promoting and improving supports and services for people with mental retardation and their families. The association also fosters research and education regarding the prevention of mental retardation in infants and young children. The ARC was founded in 1950 by a small group of parents and other concerned individuals.

Nancy Webster, President
Ronald Brown, VP
Elise McMillan, Secretary

4201 American Academy of Pediatrics
141 Northwest Point Boulevard
Elk Grove Village, IL 60007
847-434-4000
800-433-9016
Fax: 847-434-8000
www.aap.org

The American Academy of Pediatrics and its member pediatricians are committed to the attainment of optimal physical, mental and social health and well-being for all infants, children, adolescents, and young adults.

Fernando Stein, MD, FAAP, President
Karen Remley, MD, CEO/Executive VP

4202 Genetic Alliance
4301 Connecticut Avenue NW, Suite 404
Washington, DC 20008
202-966-5557
800-336-4363
Fax: 202-966-8553
info@geneticalliance.org
www.geneticalliance.org

A nonprofit tax exempt organization founded in 1986 as a national coalition of consumers, professionals and genetic support groups to voice the common concerns of children and adults and families living with, and at risk of, genetic conditions. The Alliance builds partnerships among consumers and professionals and the private and public sectors to promote optimum healthcare and enhanced quality of life for individuals identified with genetic conditions.

Sharon Terry, President/CEO
Tetyana Murza, Managing Director
Natasha Bonhomme, VP, Strategic Development

4203 March of Dimes Foundation
1275 Mamaroneck Avenue
White Plains, NY 10605   914-997-4488
                                      888-663-4637
                              Fax: 914-997-4763
answers@marchofdimes.com; www.marchofdimes.com

Partnership of volunteers and professionals dedicated to improving the health of babies by preventing birth defects and infant mortality. Over 100 chapters are located across the country and can be located through the National Office.

Stacey D. Stewart, President

Conferences

4204 ARC Annual National Convention
The ARC
1825 K Street NW, Suite 1200
Washington, DC 20006   202-534-3700; 800-433-5255
                                  Fax: 202-534-3731
                      info@thearc.org; www.thearc.org

held in cities throughout the U.S. each fall which attracts nearly 1000 people for educational sessions, business meetings and social events.

Nancy Webster, President
Ronald Brown, Vice President
Elise McMillan, Secretary

4205 Genetic Alliance Annual Conference
Genetic Alliance
4301 Connecticut Avenue NW, Suite 404
Washington, DC 20008   202-966-5557; 800-336-4363
                                  Fax: 202-966-8553
                  info@geneticalliance.org; www.geneticalliance.org

Consistently inspirational and enables partnership among all stakeholders: advocates and community leaders, health and industry professionals, policymakers, and academicians.

July

Sharon Terry, President/CEO
Tetyana Murza, Managing Director
Natasha Bonhomme, VP, Strategic Development

Web Sites

4206 ARC of the United States
1825 K Street, NW, Suite 1200
Washington, DC 20006   800-433-5255
                                      www.thearc.org

The ARC is the national organization of and for people with mental retardation and related developmental disabilities and their families. Devoted to promoting and improving supports and services for people with mental retardation and their families. The association also fosters research and education regarding the prevention of mental retardation in infants and young children. The ARC was founded in 1950 by a small group of parents and other concerned individuals.

Ronald Brown, President
Elise McMillan, Vice President
M.J. Bartelmay, Jr., Secretary

4207 CLIMB: Children Living with Inherited Metabolic Disorders
www.climb.org.uk

                                      800-652-3181
                                      www.climb.org.uk

Official website for the organization, committed to fighting metabolic diseases through research, awareness and support, providing advice, information and support on all metabolic diseases to children, young adults, families, carers and professionals. Includes links to other sites.

4208 Genetic Alliance
4301 Connecticut Avenue NW, Suite 404
Washington, DC 20008   202-966-5557
                                      www.geneticalliance.org

A nonprofit tax exempt organization founded in 1986 as a national coalition of consumers, professionals and genetic support groups to voice the common concerns of children and adults and families living with, and at risk of, genetic conditions. The Alliance builds partnerships among consumers and professionals and the private and public sectors to promote optimum healthcare and enhanced quality of life for individuals identified with genetic conditions.

Sharon Terry, President/CEO
Tetyana Murza, Managing Director
Natasha Bonhomme, VP, Strategic Development

4209 March of Dimes Birth Defects Foundation
1275 Mamaroneck Avenue
White Plains, NY 10605   914-997-4488
                                      www.marchofdimes.com

Partnership of volunteers and professionals dedicated to improving the health of babies by preventing birth defects and infant mortality. Over 100 chapters are located across the country and can be located through the National Office.

4210 Maryland Department of Health
201 W. Preston Street
Baltimore, MD 21201   410-767-6500; 877-463-3464
            dhmh.healthmd@maryland.gov; dhmh.maryland.gov

Our mission is to protect, promote and improve the health and well being of all Maryland citizens in a fiscally responsible way.

4211 National Center for Biotechnology Information
8600 Rockville Pike
Bethesda, MD 20894   888-346-3656
                info@ncbi.nlm.nih.gov; www.ncbi.nlm.nih.gov

A national resource for biology information, the center creates public databases, conducts research in computational biology, develops software tools for analyzing genome data, and disseminated biomedical information, all for the better understanding of molecular processes affecting human health and disease.

4212 Online Mendelian Inheritance in Man
8600 Rockville Pike
Bethesda, MD 20894   888-346-3656
                info@ncbi.nlm.nih.gov; www.ncbi.nlm.nih.gov

This database is a catalog of human genes and genetic disorders.

4213 Rare Genetic Diseases in Children (NYU)
550 First Avenue
New York, NY 10016   212-263-7300
                                      development.med.nyu.edu

We target issues arising from rare genetic diseases affecting children. Also, to assist in the endeavor to bring knowledge and hope to those for whom there is, at present, so little.

Robert I. Grossman, MD, Dean & CEO

4214 Save Babies Through Screening Foundation
P. O. Box 42197
Cincinnati, OH 45242   888-454-3383
                email@savebabies.org; www.savebabies.org

Is a national nonprofit public charity run by volunteers. Its mission is to improve the lives of babies by working to prevent disabilities and early death resulting from disorders detectable through newborn screening.

Jill Levry-Fisch, President
Micki Gartzke, Vice President
Anne Rugari, Treasurer

DESCRIPTION

4215 HYDROCEPHALUS

Synonym: Hydrocephaly

Covers these related disorders: Acute hydrocephalus, Occult tension hydrocephalus, Overt tension hydrocephalus, Communicating hydrocephalus, Non-communicating hydrocephalus, Obstructive hydrocephalus, Non-obstructive hydrocephalus

Involves the following Biologic System(s):

Neurologic Disorders

Hydrocephalus is a general term used to describe a group of conditions characterized by the accumulation of cerebrospinal fluid (CSF) around the brain. This fluid, which acts as a protective shock absorber for the brain and spinal cord, flows through the four cavities in the brain (ventricles); through the cavity containing the spinal fluid (spinal canal); and between layers of the membrane that surrounds the brain and spinal cord (subarachnoid space). Obstructed flow or impaired absorption of the CSF results in increasing fluid pressure within the brain. Hydrocephalus is thought to affect approximately one in 500 to 1,500 births. The condition may occur as a result of certain malformations that are present at birth, such as Arnold-Chiari malformation or Dandy-Walker syndrome, certain infectious diseases, head injuries, bleeding within the brain, or certain tumors.

Symptoms associated with hydrocephalus may vary, depending upon the nature of the underlying abnormality, the age of onset, and the rate and duration of increasing pressure within the brain. Hydrocephalus may be apparent at birth (congenital) or develop during the first few months or years of life. Because the fibrous joints of the skull (fontanels) have not fused or completely closed, rapid enlargement of the head may occur. The forehead appears abnormally prominent; the skin over the skull is thin with obvious scalp veins; and the face may appear relatively small. Additional symptoms and findings many include difficulties feeding, irritability, sluggishness, lack of interest in surroundings, lack of normal reflex responses, and downward turning of the eyes.
Progression of the condition without treatment may result in extreme drowsiness, episodes of uncontrolled electrical disturbances in the brain (seizures), and potentially life-threatening complications.

In other children, hydrocephalus becomes apparent after the bones of the skull are fused (i.e., after two years of age). Some children may have no apparent symptoms, whereas others may have mild, intermittent, or progressive symptoms. These symptoms may include headaches, easy distractibility, poor memory, and progressively impaired walking and balance. Others may experience an acute form of hydrocephalus in which there is rapidly increasing intracranial pressure, causing severe headache, vomiting, visual disturbances, increasing drowsiness over the period of minutes or hours, potential coma, and possibly life-threatening complications.

Treatment of infants and children with hydrocephalus depends upon the underlying cause of the condition. Therapeutic measures may include use of certain medications, such as acetazolamide and furosemide, which are diuretics ("water pills") that help to reduce the build up of cerebrospinal fluid.

Other treatment options may include surgical removal of any obstruction or surgical implantation of a specialized device known as a shunt. Shunts allow excess fluid to drain away from the brain to another part of the body for absorption into the bloodstream. After treatment, many affected children may continue to have associated impairment, such as intellectual deficits, impaired memory, and visual abnormalities. Physicians may regularly monitor affected children and suggest a variety of multidisciplinary measures.

National Associations & Support Groups

4216 American Academy of Pediatrics
141 Northwest Point Boulevard
Elk Grove Village, IL 60007
847-434-4000
800-433-9016
Fax: 847-434-8000
www.aap.org

The American Academy of Pediatrics and its member pediatricians are committed to the attainment of optimal physical, mental and social health and well-being for all infants, children, adolescents, and young adults.

Fernando Stein, MD, FAAP, President
Karen Remley, MD, CEO/Executive VP

4217 Birth Defect Research for Children
976 Lake Baldwin Lane, Suite 104
Orlando, FL 32814
407-895-0802
Fax: 407-895-0824
staff@birthdefects.org
www.birthdefects.org

Organization that helps families with free birth defect information, parent matching that links families of children with similar defects and research through the National Birth Defect Registry to discover the causes of birth defects. Support group information and newsletter on Internet.

Betty Mekdeci, Executive Director

4218 Cerebrospinal Fluid Shunt Systems for the Management of Hydrocephalus
Hydrocephalus Association
4340 East West Highway, Suite 905
Bethesda, MD 20814
415-732-7040
888-598-3789
Fax: 415-732-7044
info@hydroassoc.org
www.hydroassoc.org

The nations's largest and most repected nonprofit organization devoted exclusively to hydrocepalus. Our office is staffed daily from 10 AM to 4 PM Pacific time. We invite your inquiries.Our mission is to provide support, education and advocacy for individuals, families and professionals.

Dawn Mancuso, CEO
Randi Corey, Director
Aisha Heath, Director of Development

4219 Genetic Alliance
4301 Connecticut Avenue NW, Suite 404
Washington, DC 20008
202-966-5557
800-336-4363
Fax: 202-966-8553
info@geneticalliance.org
www.geneticalliance.org

A coalition of voluntary genetic support groups, consumers and professionals addressing the needs of individuals and families affected by genetic disorders from a national perspective.

Sharon Terry, President/CEO
Tetyana Murza, Managing Director
Natasha Bonhomme, VP, Strategic Development

4220 Guardians of Hydrocephalus Research Foundation
2618 Avenue Z
Brooklyn, NY 11235   718-743-4473
                                     800-458-8655
                                  Fax: 718-743-1171
                              GHRF2618@aol.com
                              www.ghrforg.org

Nonprofit group dedicated to research into the cause and treatment of hydrocephalus. Guardians operate a laboratory in the Department of Neurology at New York University Medical Center, in which information from clinical and research facilities is integrated to provide for better diagnosis and treatment of hydrocephalus, a frequently occuring congenital disorder that can also occur shortly after birth. Hydrocephalus accounts for a large portion of adult patients with a diagnosis of dementia.

Michael Fischette, Founder
Katherine Soriano, National Vice President

4221 Hydrocephalus Association
Hydrocephalus Association
4340 East West Highway, Suite 905
Bethesda, MD 20814   301-202-3811
                                     888-598-3789
                                  Fax: 301-202-3813
                              info@hydroassoc.org
                              www.hydroassoc.org

This is the nation's largest and most respected nonprofit organization devoted exclusively to hydrocephalus. We provide support, education and an extensive range of resources to families and professionals dealing with the complex issues of hydrocephalus, the abnormal accumulation of cerebrospinal fluid within the brain. Our resources cover all ages, from prenatal to adult normal pressure hydrocephalus. Our office is staffed daily, we invite your inquiries.

Dawn Mancuso, CEO
Randi Corey, Director
Aisha Heath, Director of Development

4222 Hydrocephalus Foundation
910 Rear Broadway, Rt. 1
Saugus, MA 01906   781-942-1161
                                  Fax: 781-231-5250
                              hyfll@nestcape.net
                              www.hydrocephalus.org

Foundation established to help assist patients and their families during the transition from their diagnosis to a resumption of their normal lifestyles. The primary focus is to contribute emotional support to patients of hydrocephalus and their families.

Dawn Mancuso, CEO
Randi Corey, Director
Aisha Heath, Director of Development

4223 March of Dimes Foundation
1275 Mamaroneck Avenue
White Plains, NY 10605   914-997-4488
                                     888-663-4637
                                  Fax: 914-997-4763
                              answers@marchofdimes.com
                              www.marchofdimes.com

Partnership of volunteers and professionals dedicated to improving the health of babies by preventing birth defects and infant mortality. Over 100 chapters are located across the country and can be located through the National Office.

Stacey D. Stewart, President

4224 National Conference on Hydrocephalus
Hydrocephalus Association
4340 East West Highway, Suite 905
Bethesda, MD 20814   415-732-7040
                                     888-598-3789
                                  Fax: 415-732-7044
                              info@hydroassoc.org
                              www.hydroassoc.org

Dawn Mancuso, CEO
Randi Corey, Director
Aisha Heath, Director of Development

4225 National Foundation for Facial Reconstruction
333 East 30th Street, Lobby Unit
New York, NY 10016   212-263-6656
                                  Fax: 212-263-7534
                              info@nffr.org
                              www.nffr.org

To enable patients with facial deformities lead productive and fulfilling lives. The NFFR lends its support to the mulidisciplinary craniofacial team at the Institute of Reconstructive Plastic Surgery at NYU Medical Center. An assembly of world-renowned surgeons, mental health professionals, research specialists and staff, give their time and expertise, using the latest techniques.

1951

Eileen Newman, President
John R. Gordon, Chairman
Yoron Cohen, VP

4226 National Hydrocephalus Foundation
12413 Centralia Road
Lakewood, CA 90715   562-924-6666
                                     888-857-3434
                              debbifields@nhfonline.org
                              www.nhfonline.org

Promotes information and educational assistance. Establishes and facilitates a communication network and works to increase public awareness. Promote and support research. Also has brochures, help sheets, and more. Quarterly newsletter with annual membership fee of $35.00.

Debbie Fields, Executive Director
Michael Fields, President
Jaynie Dunn, Secretary

State Agencies & Support Groups

Arizona

4227 Injury Prevention Center
Phoenix Children's Hospital
1919 E Thomas Road
Phoenix, AZ 85016   602-933-1000
                                     888-908-5437
                              nquay@phxchildrens.com
                              www.phoenixchildrens.com

Their mission is to promote family-directed care through education and support of children and families with hydrocephalus. Bi-annual newsletter published, yearly educational conference.

Mark Bonsall, Chairman
Robert Meyer, President/CEO
Jon Hulburd, VP

California

4228 Hydrocephalus Support Group of Southern California
412 N Coast Highway, Suite 131
Laguna Beach, CA 92651   714-389-7465
                                  Fax: 949-465-0550
                              HydroBrat@earthlink.net
                              www.hydrowoman.com

This group was formed as a group of concerned families and patients with hydrocephalus to share information and experiences in dealing with this disease, locally and nationwide.

Jason Vandriel, Manager

Florida

4229 Hydrocephalus Family Support Group of Central Florida
22 Lake Beauty Drive, Suite 204, PO Box 2010
Orlando, FL 32806   407-649-7686
                                  Fax: 407-649-7692
                              mrssm1000@aol.com
                              www.oreilly.com

Their mission is to nurture understanding and increase awareness of hydrocephalus in their community.

Jogi V Pattisapu MD
Tim O'Reilly, Founder/CEO

Michigan

4230 Hydrocephalus Support Group
Children's Hospital of Michigan
PO Box 4236
Chesterfield, MO 63006
314-532-8228
Fax: 314-995-4108
hydro@inlink.com
www.oreilly.com

Provides information to connect parents who have children with hydrocephalus in a mutual support group.

Mary Smellie-Decker RN, MSN, Clinical Nurse Specialist
Tim O'Reilly, Founder/CEO

4231 SW Michican Spina Bifida & Hydrocephalus Association
PO Box 212
Mattawan, MI 49071
269-385-3959
Fax: 269-342-9765

Provides support, education, and advocacy for families with spina bifida and/or hydrocephalus.

Richard Benthin, President

Missouri

4232 Hydrocephalus Support Group
PO Box 4236
Chesterfield, MO 63006
314-532-8228
Fax: 314-995-4108
hydro@inlink.com
www.oreilly.com

Nonprofit organization providing education and support to individuals with hydrocephalus and their families.

Debby Buffa, Founder/Director
Tim O'Reilly, Founder/CEO

New Jersey

4233 Hydrocephalus Group - Children's Hospital of New Jersey
Children's Hospital of New Jersey
201 Lyons Avenue at Osborne Terrace
Newark, NJ 07112
973-926-7000
Fax: 973-325-2078
info@sbhcs.com
www.sbhcs.com

Serves parents of infants and children in the local community and around the state.

Timothy S Yeh MD, FAAP, FAACM, Physician-in-Chief

New York

4234 New York University Medical Center Auxillary of Tisch Hospital
530 1st Avenue
New York, NY 10016
212-263-8122
www.nyukidshealth.org

Conducts national symposiums on hydrocephalus.

Ana Monteagudo, Co-President Auxillary Medical Ctr

North Carolina

4235 Lipomyelomeningocele Family Support
415 Webster Street
Cary, NC 27511
919-844-2043
Fax: 919-844-2044
bborchert@mindspring.com
www.lfsn.org

Providing support services to families and individuals affected by Occult Spinal Dysraphisms.

Bonnie Borchert, Director

Ohio

4236 Cleveland Clinic
9500 Euclid Avenue
Cleveland, OH 44195
216-444-4508
800-223-2273
Fax: 216-444-9050
www.clevelandclinic.org

Provides education about hydrocephalus using speakers and parent-to-parent information.

Gene Altus, Executive Director

Rhode Island

4237 Hydrocephalus Association of Rhode Island
PO Box 343
Valley Falls, RI 02864
401-723-6065

The mission of this Association is to provide information, support and advocacy for individuals with hydrocephalus and for friends and family members.

Gabriella Halmi, Director

Texas

4238 Hydrocephalus Association of N Texas
PO Box 670552
Dallas, TX 75367
214-528-2877
Fax: 214-528-8097

The mission is to provide information and support to parents of children with hydrocephalus in the state of Texas and neighboring states.

Jana Dransfield, Director

Washington

4239 Hydrocephalus Support Group of Seattle
Po Box 14055
Tumwater, WA 98511
206-324-4084
hydropr61@hotmail.com

The group of Seattle provides support to individuals with hydrocephalus.

Kim Anderson, Director

Wisconsin

4240 Fox Valley Hydrocephalus Support Group
W5929 Highway KK
Appleton, WI 54915
920-739-1751

The group provides referrals for parents and information to the community and throughout Wisconsin.

Donna Uitenbroek, Director

Research Centers

4241 New York University Medical Center Auxillary of Tisch Hospital
560 1st Avenue
New York, NY 10016 212-263-5800
Stevenb.Abramson@nyumc.org
www.med.nyu.edu

Conducts national symposiums on hydrocephalus.

Steven B. Abramson, Sr. VP
Dianna Jacob, VP
Ramona Batra, Business Operations Manager

4242 Seeking Techniques Advancing Research in Shunts (STARS)
33006 Seven Mile Road, Suite 113
Livonia, MI 48152 313-384-3232
www.stars-kids.org

Offers support to patients with hydrocephalus and their families.

Judy Brady, President

Conferences

4243 Genetic Alliance Annual Conference
Genetic Alliance
4301 Connecticut Avenue NW, Suite 404
Washington, DC 20008 202-966-5557
800-336-4363
Fax: 202-966-8553
info@geneticalliance.org
www.geneticalliance.org

Consistently inspirational and enables partnership among all stakeholders: advocates and community leaders, health and industry professionals, policymakers, and academicians.

July

Sharon Terry, President/CEO
Tetyana Murza, Managing Director
Natasha Bonhomme, VP, Strategic Development

Audio Video

4244 Hydrocephalus, a Neglected Disease
Guardians of Hydrocephalus Research Foundation
2618 Avenue Z
Brooklyn, NY 11235 718-748-4473
Fax: 718-743-1171
ghrf2618@aol.com
www.ghrf.homestead.com/ghrf

Information on Hydrocephalus.

Michael Fischette, Founder
Katherine Soriano, National Vice President

Web Sites

4245 Beth Israel Medical Center-Hydrocephalus
330 Brookline Avenue
Boston, MA 2215 617-667-7000
800-667-5356
TDD: 800-439-0183
custserv@bidmc.harvard.edu
www.bidmc.org

Is a full tertiary teaching hospital that was originally dedicated to serving a vulnerable population in that community.

Daniel J. Jick, Chair
Edward H. Ladd, Vice Chair
Margaret A. McKenna, Vice Chair

4246 Birth Defect Research for Children
976 Lake Baldwin Lane, Suite 104
Orlando, FL 32814 407-895-0802
staff@birthdefects.org
www.birthdefects.org

Organization that helps families with free birth defect information, parent matching that links families of children with similar defects and research through the National Birth Defect Registry to discover the causes of birth defects. Support group information and newsletter on Internet.

4247 Guardians of Hydrocephalus Research Foundation
1101 Wootton Parkway, Suite LL100
Rockville, MD 20852 240-453-8282
odphpinfo@hhs.gov
www.health.gov

Nonprofit group dedicated to research into the cause and treatment of hydrocephalus. Guardians operate a laboratory in the Department of Neurology at New York University Medical Center, in which information from clinical and research facilities is integrated to provide for better diagnosis and treatment of hydrocephalus, a frequently occuring congenital disorder that can also occur shortly after birth. Hydrocephalus accounts for a large portion of adult patients with a diagnosis of dementia.

4248 HYCEPH-L
www.geocities.com/HotSprings/Villa/2020/

The purpose of the list is to share information and support in dealing with hydrocephalus.

4249 Hydrocephalus Association
4340 East West Highway, Suite 905
Bethesda, MD 20814 301-202-3811
888-598-3789
Fax: 301-202-3813
info@hydroassoc.org
www.hydroassoc.org

Our mission is to provide support, education and advocacy for individuals families and professionals.

Aseem Chandra, Chair
Craig Brown, Senior Vice Chair
David Browdy, Vice Chair

4250 Hydrohaven Chat Room
www.geocities.com/HotSprings/Villa/2020/hydrohav

Hydrocephalus support group for patients, family and friends.

4251 National Hydrocephalus Foundation
www.nhfonline.org

Promotes information and educational assistance. Establishes and facilitates a communication network and works to increase public awareness. Promote and support research. Also has brochures, help sheets and more. Quarterly newsletter included with annual membership fee of $35.00.

4252 Online Mendelian Inheritance in Man
8600 Rockville Pike
Bethesda, MD 20894 888-346-3656
info@ncbi.nlm.nih.gov
www.ncbi.nlm.nih.gov

This database is a catalog of human genes and genetic disorders.

4253 Pediatric Neurosurgery-Hydrocephalus
710 West 168 Street
New York, NY 10032 212-305-4118
Fax: 212-305-2026
www.columbianeurosurgery.org

This site is dedicated to providing families regarding various aspects of the field of pediatric neurosurgery.

4254 Rare Genetic Diseases in Children (NYU)
550 First Avenue
New York, NY 10016 212-263-7300
www.med.nyu.edu

We target issues arising from rare genetic diseases affecting children. Also, to assist in the endeavor to bring knowledge and hope to those for whom there is, at present, so little.

Robert I. Grossman, MD, Dean & CEO
Steven B. Abramson, MD, Senior Vice President
Dafna Bar-Sagi, PhD, Senior Vice President

Book Publishers

4255 A Guide to Hydrocephalus
Spina Bifida Association of America
4590 MacArthur Boulevard NW, Suite 250
Washington, DC 20007
202-944-3285
800-621-3141
Fax: 202-944-3295
sbaa@sbaa.org
www.spinabifidaassociation.org

Information to help you understand the circumstances that surround you and make the job of advocacy an easier one.

Cindy Brownstein, President & CEO
Sara Struwe, Chief Operating Officer & Director
Christopher Vance, Director of Development

4256 Congenital Disorders Sourcebook
Omnigraphics
PO Box 8002
Aston, PA 19014
800-234-1340
Fax: 800-875-1340
info@omnigraphics.com
www.omnigraphics.com

Basic consumer health information on disorders aquired during gestation, including spina bifida, hydrocephalus, cerebral palsy, heart defects, craniofacial abnormalities and fetal alcohol syndrome.

650 pages
ISBN: 0-780809-45-9

4257 Hydrocephalus: A Guide for Patients, Families, and Friends
Chuck Toporek, Kellie Robinson, author

O'Reilly & Associates
1005 Gravenstein Highway N
Sebastopol, CA 95472
707-827-7019
800-889-8969
Fax: 707-824-8268
patientguides@oreilly.com
www.oreilly.com

This book educates families so they can select a skilled neurosurgeon, understand treatments, participate in care and know what symptoms need attention, keep records needed for follow-up treatments and make wise lifestyle choices.

1999 377 pages Softcover
ISBN: 1-565924-10-X

Tim O'Reilly, Founder & CEO

4258 Spina Bifida Association Insights into Spina Bifida
Spina Bifida Association
4590 MacArthur Boulevard NW, Suite 250
Washington, DC 20007
202-944-3285
800-621-3141
Fax: 202-944-3295
sbaa@sbaa.org
www.spinabifidaassociation.org

News on medical, legislative and education topics relevant to individuals with spina bifida

Bimonthly

Cindy Brownstein, President & CEO
Sara Struwe, Chief Operating Officer & Director
Christopher Vance, Director of Development

Newsletters

4259 G. Advocacy
Genetic Alliance
4301 Connecticut Avenue NW, Suite 404
Washington, DC 20008
202-966-5557
800-336-4363
Fax: 202-966-8553
info@geneticalliance.org
www.geneticalliance.org

Our e-newsletter features news about upcoming events, spotlights member organizations, and keeps you informed about legislation before Congress. We welcome your feedback on articles and suggestions on future topics.

Sharon F. Terry MA, President/CEO
Natasha Bonhomme, VP, Strategic Development
Ruth Evans, Director of Accounting

4260 Hydrocephalus Association Newsletter
Hydrocephalus Association
4340 East West Highway, Suite 905
Bethesda, MD 20814
301-202-3811
888-598-3789
Fax: 301-202-3813
info@hydroassoc.org
www.hydroassoc.org

Offers information on association news, conference articles, meetings, support and educational groups.

12 pages Quarterly

Aseem Chandra, Chair
Craig Brown, Senior Vice Chair
David Browdy, Vice Chair

4261 Hydrocephalus Support Group Newsletter
PO Box 4236
Chesterfield, MO 63006
314-532-8228
Fax: 314-995-4108
hydro@inlink.com

This group provides information, education and support to anyone dealing with hydrocephalus.

quarterly

Debby Buffa, Founder/Chairman

4262 LINK
Hydrocephalus Association
4340 East West Highway, Suite 905
Bethesda, MD 20814

Provides members with direct access to other families and individuals coping with the complexities of hydrocephalus with the goal being to develop a nationwide network of individuals supporting one another, sharing information and strategies which enable them to become educated and empowered advocates.

12 pages Quarterly

4263 National Hydrocephalus Foundation Newsletter
12413 Centralia Road
Lakewood, CA 90715
562-924-6666
888-857-3434
Fax: 415-732-7044
debbifields@nhfonline.org
www.nhfonline.org

The Foundation is a national organization whose purpose is to provide information and education, along with peer support newsletter quarterly.

12-15 pages Quarterly

Michael Fields, President/Treasurer
Debbie Fields, Executive Director
Jaynie Dunn, Secretary

4264 Update
Spina Bifida and Hydrocephalus Association/Canada
Suite 647-167 av. Lombard Avenue
Winnipeg, MB R3B 0
Canada

204-925-3650
800-565-9488
Fax: 204-925-3654
info@sbhac.ca
www.sbhac.ca

Newsletter dedicated to improving the quality of life of individuals with spina bifida and/or hydrocephalus and their families.

4 pages Quarterly

Colleen Talbot, President
Linda Randall, Vice President
Sarah Williams, Secretary

Pamphlets

4265 About Hydrocephalus - Book for Families
Hydrocephalus Association
4340 East West Highway, Suite 905
Bethesda, MD 20814

Booklet in either English or Spanish, detailing all aspects of hydrocephalus from diagnosis and treatment to complications and follow-up care.

36 pages Paperback

4266 Cephalic Disorders Fact Sheet
National Inst. of Neurological Disorders/Stroke
PO Box 5801
Bethesda, MD 20824

301-496-5751
800-352-9424
www.ninds.nih.gov

Fact sheet indexing the following: What are Cephalic Disorders?, What are the Different Kinds of Cephalic Disorders?, What are Other Less Common Cephalics?, What Research is Being Done?, Where Can I Get More Information?.

Walter J. Koroshetz, M.D., Acting Director
Audrey S. Penn MD, Special Advisor to the Director
Caroline Lewis, Executive Officer

4267 Cerebrospinal Fluid Shunt Systems for the Management of Hydrocephalus
Hydrocephalus Association
4340 East West Highway, Suite 905
Bethesda, MD 20814

Our resources cover hydrocephalus in all age groups from prenatal diagnosis to adult normal pressure hydrocephalus. Our office is staffed daily from 10 AM to 4 PM Pacific time. We invite your inquiries.

4268 Directory of Pediatric Neurosurgeons
Hydrocephalus Association
4340 East West Highway, Suite 905
Bethesda, MD 20814

Names and addresses of more than 200 neurosurgeons who specialize in pediatrics, listed alphabetically and geographically.

4269 Durable Power of Attorney for Health Care Decisions
Hydrocephalus Association
4340 East West Highway, Suite 905
Bethesda, MD 20814

Provided by The Hydrocephalus Association. Our resources cover hydrocephalus in all age groups from prenatal diagnosis to adult normal pressure hydrocepahlus. Our office is staffed daily from 10 AM to 4 PM Pacific time. We invite your inquiries.

4270 Endoscopic Third Ventriculoscopy
Hydrocephalus Association
4340 East West Highway, Suite 905
Bethesda, MD 20814

Provided by the Hydrocephalus Association. Our resources cover all age groups from prenatal diagnosis through normal pressure hydrocephalus in older adults. Our office is staffed daily from 10 AM to 4 PM Pacific time. We invite your inquiries.

4271 Eye Problems Associated with Hydrocephalus in Children
Hydrocephalus Association
4340 East West Highway, Suite 905
Bethesda, MD 20814

Provided by the Hydrocephalus Association. Our resources cover all age groups from prenatal diagnosis to normal pressure hydrocephalus in older adults. Our office is staffed daily from 10 AM to 4 PM Pacific time. We invite your inquiries.

4272 Fact Sheet: Hydrocephalus
Hydrocephalus Association
4340 East West Highway, Suite 905
Bethesda, MD 20814

Also available in Spanish, provided by the Hydrocephalus Association. Our resources cover all age groups from prenatal diagnosis to normal pressure hydrocephalus in older adults. Our office is staffed daily from 10 AM to 4 PM Pacific time. We invite your inquiries.

4273 Fact Sheet: Syringomyelia
National Inst. of Neurological Disorders/Stroke
PO Box 5801
Bethesda, MD 20892

301-496-5751
800-352-9424
www.ninds.nih.gov

Provided by the Hydrocephalus Association. Our resources cover all age groups, from prenatal diagnosis to normal pressure hydrocephalus in older adults. We welcome your inquiries.

Walter J. Koroshetz, M.D., Acting Director
Audrey S. Penn MD, Special Advisor to the Director
Caroline Lewis, Executive Officer

4274 Headaches and Hydrocephalus
Hydrocephalus Association
4340 East West Highway, Suite 905
Bethesda, MD 20814

Causes and tips for headache relief unique to hydrocephalus.

4275 Hospitalization Tips
Hydrocephalus Association
4340 East West Highway, Suite 905
Bethesda, MD 20814

Provided by the Hydrocephalus Association. Our resources cover all age groups, from prenatal diagnosis, to normal pressure hydrocephalus in older adults. Our office is staffed daily from 10 AM to 4 PM, Pacific time. We welcome your inquiries.

1997

4276 How to be an Assertive Member of the Treatment Team
Hydrocephalus Association
4340 East West Highway, Suite 905
Bethesda, MD 20814

Hydrocephalus information to ask involved treatment questions.

4277 Hydrocephalus: Fact Sheet
National Inst. of Neurological Disorders/Stroke
PO Box 5801
Bethesda, MD 20824

301-496-5751
800-352-9424
www.ninds.nih.gov

Our fact sheet covers all age groups, from prenatal diagnosis to normal pressure hydrocephalus in older adults. Also available in Spanish.

Walter J. Koroshetz, M.D., Acting Director
Audrey S. Penn MD, Special Advisor to the Director
Caroline Lewis, Executive Officer

4278 ID Card for Third Ventriculostomy Patients
Hydrocephalus Association
4340 East West Highway Suite 905
Bethesda, MD 20814

Patients with hydrocephalus managed by an ETV may request a free patient ID card from the Hydrocephaus Association. This card idenifies them as patients with hydrocephalus being managed by this procedure.

4279 Individualized Education Program (IEP) - Communication Skills for Parents
Hydrocephalus Association
4340 East West Highway Suite 905
Bethesda, MD 20814

Is a written education plan that describes the special education and related services a student will receive.

4280 LINK Directory Information
Hydrocephalus Association
4340 East West Highway Suite 905
Bethesda, MD 20814

A nationwide network of individuals listed in Directory format giving members direct access to others in similar circumstances.

4281 Learning Disabilities in Children with Hydrocephalus
Hydrocephalus Association
4340 East West Highway Suite 905
Bethesda, MD 20814

Also available in Spanish and English. Our offices are staffed daily from 10 AM to 4 PM, Pacific time. We welcome your inquiries.

4282 National Directory of Hydrocephalus Support Groups
Hydrocephalus Association
4340 East West Highway Suite 905
Bethesda, MD 20814

The Directory lists information on 16 hydrocephalus groups nationwide.

4283 Nonverbal Learning Disorder Syndrome
Hydrocephalus Association
4340 East West Highway Suite 905
Bethesda, MD 20814

Is a specific type of learning disability that affect's children's academic progress as well as their social and emotional development. This specific type of learning disability has been identified in some children with Hydrocephalus.

4284 Prenatal Hydrocephalus-Book for Parents
Hydrocephalus Association
4340 East West Highway Suite 905
Bethesda, MD 20814

Provides information about the diagnosis of prenatal-onset hydrocephalus.

16 pages

4285 Primary Care Needs of Children with Hydrocephalus
Hydrocephalus Association
4340 East West Highway Suite 905
Bethesda, MD 20814

Our office is staffed daily from 10 AM to 4 PM Pacific time. We welcome your inquiries.

28 pages

4286 Resource Guide
Hydrocephalus Association
4340 East West Highway Suite 905
Bethesda, MD 20814

A comprehensive listing of 450 articles on all aspects of hydrocephalus. Articles may be ordered from the Association for a small fee.

4287 Social Skills Development in Children with Hydrocephalus
Hydrocephalus Association
4340 East West Highway Suite 905
Bethesda, MD 20814

4288 Survival Skills for the Family Unit
Hydrocephalus Association
4340 East West Highway Suite 905
Bethesda, MD 20814

Our resources cover hydrocephalus in all age groups from prenatal diagnosis through normal pressure hydrocephalus in older adults.

4289 Understanding Your Child's Education Needs /Individualized Education Program Packet
Hydrocephalus Association
4340 East West Highway Suite 905
Bethesda, MD 20814

From the Hydrocephalus Association the nations largest nonprofit group devoted exclusively to this disorder. Our offices are staffed daily from 10 AM to 4 PM, Pacific time. We welcome your inquiries.

DESCRIPTION

4290 HYPERTROPHIC CARDIOMYOPATHY
Involves the following Biologic System(s):
Cardiovascular Disorders

Hypertrophic cardiomyopathy is a genetic disease that occurs because of mutations in the contraction mechanisms in the muscles of the heart. Because of this genetic abnormality, the heart muscle fibers are arranged in a disorganized fashion. This leads to enlargement of the left ventricular muscle (hypertrophy). This hypertrophic muscle may lead to variable amounts of obstruction of blood flow out of the heart into the general circulation and a spectrum of clinical manifestations. There have been several genes that have been found to be abnormal in patients with hypertrophic cardiomyopathy. Depending on the different genetic abnormality there may be different clinical findings ranging from no symptomatology to severe disease.

Hypertrophic cardiomyopathy is most commonly inherited in an autosomal dominant pattern, meaning that a child inherits a copy of the gene from one of his or her parents.aAs a result, the majority of children and adolescents who are diagnosed with the disease have a parent who also suffers from the entity. Sporadic cases are also well documented where neither parent has the disease but the child has the disease. It is presumed that in these cases, there has been a spontaneous mutation in the gene in the earliest stages of embryonic development.

Hypertrophic cardiomyopathy may become clinically evident at any time during the first two decades of life, though typically it is not diagnosed until the adolescent years. It is important to note that the hypertrophic changes that are the hallmark of the disease may not develop until as late as the teens or early twenties. As a result, in families where a parent has the disease, children should undergo repeated interval examination by a pediatric cardiologist through their adolescence.

The diagnosis is hypertrophic cardiomyopathy relies heavily on good history taking from the primary care provider. There are several important questions to ask in order to assess for risk. A family history should be taken, asking about unexplained deaths, family members with frequent episodes of fainting, or cardiac arrhythmia (abnormal heart rhythm). Patients should be questioned about episodes of shortness of breath (dyspnea) and chest pain. Any recent change in exercise tolerance should be evaluated closely. Additionally, a known history of family members with documented hypertrophic cardiomyopathy should raise the concern of disease in other family members.

There are many patients with hypertrophic cardiomyopathy who are largely asymptomatic. When patients are symptomatic they usually exhibit a slow decline in function. Often, patients may not experience symptoms until they exert themselves. Symptoms may consist of shortness of breath with exertion or when lying down, chest pain, fainting (syncope) or lightheadedness, palpitations (racing heart), and fatigue. Although it is agreed that the thickened left ventricular muscle may cause some obstruction to blood flow out of the aora (the main blood vessel leading from the left side of the

heart to the general circulation), this is not the only mechanism causing symptoms. In fact, there are some patients with a great deal of obstruction who have minimal symptoms, while other patients with minimal obstruction may have severe symptoms. Patients may also experience some of the above symptoms from decreased functioning of the heart muscle itself, or arrhythmia.

Hypertrophic cardiomyopathy is the most common cause of sudden death in young athletes who die during sports; clearly those individuals with HCM should be restricted from participating in sports.

The physical exam of patients with hypertrophic cardiomyopathy may be normal if there is no significant obstruction to blood flow. In some patients, findings may include a fourth heart sound or a systolic murmur heard best at the left lower sternal border. This murmur is often heard more easily during maneuvers that increase the amount of resistance in the body's tissues from muscular contraction, for example, when patients stand up after a sitting or squatting position, or when patients bear down (Valsalva maneuver). Additional findings may include increased carotid pulses, increased force of the heart beat felt near the left lower sternum or axilla (parasternal lift).

Patients with suspected hypertrophic cardiomyopathy should be referred to a pediatric cardiologist for further testing, which may consist of an echocardiogram (ultrasound imaging of the heart), electrocardiogram and perhaps an exercise stress test.

Treatment options are varied. Medical management may be difficult and surgical or catheter interventions may be recommended to decrease the amount of obstructing tissue in the heart. Mainstays of medical treatment include calcium channel blockers, beta blockers, and anti-arrhythmics. Most recently, the use of implantable defribrillators (small pacemaker-like devices that correct severe heart arrhythmias) have become common. It is critical that patients with confirmed hypertrophic cardiomyopathy be restricted from playing competitive sports. Additionally, patients should receive prophylactic antibiotics for prevention of endocarditis before dental or invasive procedures.

National Associations & Support Groups

4291 American Academy of Pediatrics
141 Northwest Point Boulevard
Elk Grove Village, IL 60007   847-434-4000
                                                           800-433-9016
                                                        Fax: 847-434-8000
                                                           www.aap.org

The American Academy of Pediatrics and its member pediatricians are committed to the attainment of optimal physical, mental and social health and well-being for all infants, children, adolescents, and young adults.
Fernando Stein, MD, FAAP, President
Karen Remley, MD, CEO/Executive VP

4292 American Heart Association
7272 Greenville Avenue
Dallas, TX 75231   214-373-6300
                                                           800-242-8721
                                                        Fax: 214-706-1341
                                                          inquire@amhrt.org
                                                    www.heart.org/HEARTORG/

Supports research, education and community service programs with the objective of reducing premature death and disability from cardiovascular diseases and stroke; coordinates the efforts of health professionals, and others engaged in the fight against heart and circulatory disease.

Nancy Brown, CEO
Dr. Stephen Houser, President
Suzie Upton, Chief Operating Officer

4293 Hypertrophic Cardiomyopathy Association
322 Green Pond Road, PO Box 306
Hibernia, NJ 07842   973-983-7429
Fax: 973-983-7870
support@4hcm.us
www.4hcm.org

A not-for-profit organization that provides information, support and advocacy to patients, their families and medical providers.

Lisa Salberg, Founder & President

4294 March of Dimes Foundation
1275 Mamaroneck Avenue
White Plains, NY 10605   914-997-4488
888-663-4637
Fax: 914-997-4763
answers@marchofdimes.com
www.marchofdimes.com

Partnership of volunteers and professionals dedicated to improving the health of babies by preventing birth defects and infant mortality. Over 100 chapters are located across the country and can be located through the National Office.

Stacey D. Stewart, President

Research Centers

4295 Hypertrophic Cardiomyopathy Program at St. Luke's-Roosevelt Hospital Center
University Medical Practice Associates
425 W 59th Street, Suite 9C
New York, NY 10019   212-492-5550
Fax: 212-492-5555
www.hcmny.org

We offer comprehensive diagnostic evaluation, a range of treatments and screening for relatives of affected patients.

Mark V Sherrid MD FACC FASE, Director

Web Sites

4296 American Heart Association
7272 Greenville Avenue
Dallas, TX 75231   800-242-8721
www.heart.org/HEARTORG/

Supports research, education and community service programs with the objective of reducing premature death and disability from cardiovascular diseases and stroke; coordinates the efforts of health professionals, and others engaged in the fight against heart and circulatory disease.

Nancy Brown, CEO
Dr. Stephen Houser, President
Suzie Upton, Chief Operating Officer

4297 Hypertrophic Cardiomyopathy Association
18 E. Main St - Suite 202
Denville, NJ 7834   973-983-7429
Fax: 973-983-7870
support@4hcm.org
www.4hcm.org/WCMS/

A not-for-profit organization that provides information, support and advocacy to patients, their families and medical providers.

4298 Hypertrophic Cardiomyopathy: Heart Center Online for Patients
www.heartcenteronline.com

The mission of the HeartCenterOnline is to give our premier cardiovascular patients, their families and other site visiors with the tools they need to better understand the complex nature of heart-related conditions, treatments and preventive care, and to provide services and applications that deliver value to cardiovascular practices.

4299 Implantable Defibrillators in Preventing Sudden Death
www.findarticles.com

Article from American Family Physician magazine. Search by article name.

4300 MEDLINEplus
8600 Rockville Pike
Bethesda, MD 20894 nlm.nih.gov/medlineplus/ency/article/000192.htm

MedlinePlus has extensive information from the National Institutes of Health and other trusted sources on over 650 diseases and conditions. There are also lists of hospitals and physicians, a medical encyclopedia and a medical dictionary, health information in Spanish, extensive information on perscription and nonperscription drugs, health information from the media and links to thousands of clinical trials.

Dr. Donald A.B. Lindberg, Director

4301 March of Dimes Birth Defects Foundation
1275 Mamaroneck Avenue
White Plains, NY 10605   914-997-4488
www.marchofdimes.com

Partnership of volunteers and professionals dedicated to improving the health of babies by preventing birth defects and infant mortality. Over 100 chapters are located across the country and can be located through the National Office.

Franklin Roosevelt, President

4302 Sudden Death of Young Athletes Can Be Prevented (Hypertrophic Cardiomyopathy)
www.findarticles.com

Article from USA Today. Search by article name.

Book Publishers

4303 Let's Talk About Going to the Hospital
Rosen Publishing Group's PowerKids Press
29 E 21st Street
New York, NY 10010   212-777-3017
800-237-9932
Fax: 888-436-4643
rosenpub@tribeca.ios.com
www.rosenpublishing.com

If a child has to check into the hospital, chances are he or she is already upset about being ill. Knowing how a hospital functions and what the procedures are, such as when family members can visit, will help in what is already a stressful situation. Grades K-5.

24 pages
ISBN: 0-823950-36-0

Roger Rosen, President

Newsletters

4304 HCMA - Heart Link Online
Hypertrophic Cardiomyopathy Association
18 E. Main St, Suite 202
Denville, NJ 7842   973-983-7429
Fax: 973-983-7870
support@4hcm.us
www.4hcm.org/WCMS/

A newsletter that provides information, support and advocacy to patients, their families and medical providers.

DESCRIPTION

4305 HYPOPLASTIC LEFT HEART SYNDROME
Synonym: HLHS
Involves the following Biologic System(s):
Cardiovascular Disorders

Hypoplastic Left Heart Syndrome, also referred to as HLHS, is a severe and complex form of congenital heart disease, wherein the entire left side of the heart is underdeveloped and unable to pump blood to the body. Classically, this involves underdevelopment (hypoplasia) of the: 1). mitral valve, which connects the left atrium to the left ventricle, 2). left ventricle, which is the pumping chamber that delivers oxygenated blood to the body and 3). aortic valve and aorta, the valve and blood vessel, respectively, which carry oxygenated blood from the left ventricle to the organs and the tissues of the body.

Hypoplastic Left Heart Syndrome is the 4th most common congenital heart disorder diagnosed in the first year of life and almost always in the first few days of life. Typically, infants with HLHS are full term and tend to have normal birth weights and few non-cardiac defects. In those born with the disorder, males out number female. The cause of this HLHS remains unclear, but like many of the congenital heart diseases, it likely develops in most pregnancies early in the first trimester and may very well have a genetic component.

Because of the underdevelopment of the left side of the heart, infants born with Hypoplastic Left Heart Syndrome become gravely ill soon after birth. In the fetus, a specialized blood vessel, known as the ductus arteriosus, connects the aorta and the pulmonary artery. In normal fetal heart structure, the ductus arteriosus allows the deoxy genated (blue) blood pumped by the right ventricle to the pulmonary artery to avoid going to the lungs (which in the fetus are non-functioning and filled with fluid), delivering it to the placenta for oxygenation. After birth the lungs are inflated with air and the ductus arteriosus, which is no longer necessary, begins to undergo a natural closure process. In the infant with Hypoplastic Left Heart Syndrome, the ductus arteriosus is the only source of blood flow into the aorta, as the left heart is unable to pump adequate (if any) blood forward and, therefore, crucial to the survival of the infant; without it, inadequate blood flow to the organs and tissues leads to shock. Prior to the advent of specialized medications, such as prostaglandins, that prevent the closing process of the ductus arteriosus, patients with Hypoplastic Left Heart Syndrome would not be able to survive when the ductus underwent its natural closure.

Over the last two decades, congenital heart surgery techniques have been developed to surgically alter the path of blood leaving the right heart. Surgery for Hypoplastic Left Heart Syndrome typically involves three separate operations, the first being the most difficult and complicated, occurring in the first week or two of life. The second operation usually occurs between 4 and 6 months of life and the third may be undertaken between 18 and 36 months. Alternatively, some pediatric cardiac centers have promoted heart transplant for the patient with Hypoplastic Left Heart Syndrome. Children with Hypoplastic Left Heart Syndrome require lifelong follow-up by a cardiologist for repeated checks of how their heart is working. Virtually all the children will require heart medicines. They also risk infection on the heart's valves (endocarditis) and will need antibiotics, such as amoxicillin, before dental work and certain surgeries to help prevent endocarditis.

National Associations & Support Groups

4306 American Academy of Pediatrics
141 Northwest Point Boulevard
Elk Grove Village, IL 60007

847-434-4000
800-433-9016
Fax: 847-434-8000
www.aap.org

The American Academy of Pediatrics and its member pediatricians are committed to the attainment of optimal physical, mental and social health and well-being for all infants, children, adolescents, and young adults.

Fernando Stein, MD, FAAP, President
Karen Remley, MD, CEO/Executive VP

4307 Congenital Heart Information Network
PO Box 3397
Margate City, NJ 08402

609-823-4507
Fax: 215-627-4036
mb@tchin.org
www.tchin.org

An international organization that provides reliable information, support services and resources to families of children with congenital heart defects and acquired heart disease, adults with congenital heart defects, and the professionals who work with them.

Mano Barmash, President
Stuart Berger, Associate Professor of Pedriatics
Edward L. Bove, Director

4308 The Heart Institute
Cincinnati Children's Hospital Medical Center
3333 Burnet Avenue, MLC 7020
Cincinnati, OH 45229

513-636-7058
800-344-2462
Fax: 513-636-5958
TTY: 513-636-4900
www.cincinnatichildrens.org

Cincinnati Children's Heart Center is dedicated to serving the cardiac care needs of patients, fetus through young adult, and their families in a convenient, compassionate and high quality manner. The Heart Center is committed to providing research and teaching programs in an enviroment characterized by intergrity, innovation, excellence, and respect.

Andrew Redington, MD, Exec. Co-Dir/Pediatric Cardiology
Jeffrey Robbins, PhD, Executive Co-Director
James Tweddell, MD, Executive Co-Director

State Agencies & Support Groups

Arizona

4309 Arizona HeartLight
University Medical Center
PO Box 286
Hallsville, TX 75650

903-668-2173
Fax: 903-668-3453
www.heartlightministries.org

Joe Crawford, Chairman
Jana Crawford, Chairman

Colorado

4310 Cardiac Kids/Association of Volunteers
13123 E. 16th Avenue, PO Box 465
Aurora, CO 80045

303-861-6259
abbbybee@msn.com
www.childrenscolorado.org

Mark Erickson

Florida

4311 Pediatric Heart Foundation
PO Box 540354
Lake Worth, FL 33454
561-738-4554
phfheart@aol.com
www.pediatricheartfoundation.org

Urquisa Fernandez, President
Reese Robinson
Laurie Bernat, Contact

Georgia

4312 Heart to Heart
401 S. Clairborne Rd., Suite 302
Olathe, KS 66062
913-764-5200
Fax: 913-764-0809
info@hearttoheart.org
www.hearttoheart.org

Gary Morsch, Founder/President
Jim Kerr, Board Chair
Krystal Barr, Interim CEO

Hawaii

4313 Kardiac Kids
C/O Kapi'olani Medical Center for Women & Children
1319 Punahou Street
Honolulu, HI 96826
808-983-8166
info@thekardiackids.com
www.thekardiackids.com

Lisa Rohr RN, Contact

Illinois

4314 Chilren's Heart Services
PO Box 8275
Bartlett, IL 60103
630-415-0282
CHILDHRTSVC@aol.com

4315 Heart of the Matter
4760 Highland Drive, Suite 515
Salt Lake City, UT 84117
815-469-9146
888-868-4686
CT875@aol.com
www.hotm.tv

Indiana

4316 Our Hearts
1738 N Shortridge Road
Indianapolis, IN 46219
317-322-1017
ourhearts@iquest.net

Massachusetts

4317 Heart to Heart Fund
750 Washington Street, Suite 313
Boston, MA 02111
617-636-8101
info@heart2heartfund.org

Michigan

4318 Families at Heart
100 Michigan Ave, MC117
Grand Rapids, MI 49503
616-391-4327
Rick Breon, Ceo

Minnesota

4319 Parents For Heart of Minnesota
Attention: 32-P190
2525 Chicgo Avenue S
Minneapolis, MN 55404
mailinglist@parentsforheart.org
www.parentsforheart.org

Celeste Gebauer, Contact

Missouri

4320 Heart to Heart - St. Louis
St Louis Children's Hospital
One Children's Place
St Louis, MO 63110
314-454-6000
www.heart2heartstl.com

Elaine Wear, Contact
Nan Winters, Contact

New Hampshire

4321 Families with Heart
824 High Street
Candia, NH 03034
603-483-3025
Laura Briggs, Contact

New Jersey

4322 Young Hearts
791 Fredrick Court
Wyckoff, NJ 07481
201-848-9608
Barbara Mcfadden, Contact

New York

4323 Big Hearts for Little Hearts
34 Sintsink Drive West
Port Washington, NY 11050
516-883-4080
Ruth Maszrik, Contact

4324 Cardiac Kids
PO Box 154
Fishkill, NY 12524
845-896-7321
Cindy-Jean Dennis, Contact

4325 Helping Hearts
601 Elmwood Avenue, PO Box 631
Rochester, NY 14642
716-275-6108
info@helpinghearts.org

Ohio

4326 Healing Hearts
PO Box 7890
Bonney Lake, WA 98391
253-268-0348
866-230-3463
Fax: 330-543-3084
flemings249@aol.com
www.healinghearts.org

Provides participants with an opportunity to share their emotions and concerns.

Sue Liljenberg, Founder/President
Judy Hansen, Secretary
Dan Morton, Member

Pennsylvania

4327 Fontan Friends
482 Reginald Lane
Collegeville, PA 19426
610-831-9878

Barbara Lewis, Contact

South Dakota

4328 Thumpers
HC 58, Box 26
Fairburn, SD 57738
605-255-4377
clsogge@cs.com

Tammy Sogge, Contact

Tennessee

4329 Tennessee Saving Little Hearts
5629 Barineau Lane, PO Box 52285
Knoxville, TN 37950
865-748-4605
info@savinglittlehearts.com
www.savinglittlehearts.com

Provides emotional assistance, educational information,and fun experiences for children that will help them build friendship and confidence.

Karen Coulter, President
Brad Coulter, Vice President

Texas

4330 Heart to Heart
401 S. Clairborne Rd., Suite 302
Olathe, KS 66062
913-764-5200
Fax: 913-764-0809
info@hearttoheart.org
www.hearttoheart.org

Gary Morsch, Founder/President
Jim Kerr, Board Chair
Krystal Barr, Interim CEO

4331 Texas Heart to Heart
Po Box 720072
Dallas, TX 75372
888-475-2787
www.heart-to-heart-tx.org

Offering hope, education, and support to families.

Sally Pearson, Contact

Vermont

4332 Heart to Heart
401 S. Clairborne Rd., Suite 302
Olathe, KS 66062
913-764-5200
Fax: 913-764-0809
info@hearttoheart.org
www.hearttoheart.org

Gary Morsch, Founder/President
Jim Kerr, Board Chair
Krystal Barr, Interim CEO

Virginia

4333 Precious Hearts
144 Locust Avenue
Winchester, VA 22601
540-678-0654
hurlbutK@aol.com

Washington

4334 Heart to Heart
401 S. Clairborne Rd., Suite 302
Olathe, KS 66062
913-764-5200
Fax: 913-764-0809
info@hearttoheart.org
www.hearttoheart.org

Gary Morsch, Founder/President
Jim Kerr, Board Chair
Krystal Barr, Interim CEO

Wisconsin

4335 Kids With Heart
1578 Careful Drive
Green Bay, WI 54304
920-498-0058
800-538-5390
www.kidswithheart.org

Michelle Rintamaki, President
Dean Rintamaki, VP
Melody Burkard, Secretary/Treasurer

4336 Left Hearts
250 N 6th Street
DePere, WI 54115
920-403-1154

Dyan Larmay, Contact

Web Sites

4337 Children's Heart Society
www.childrensheart.org

Reliable information and resources to families of children with congenital heart defects and acquired heart disease.

4338 Cincinnati Children's Hospital Medical Center
3333 Burnet Avenue
Cincinnati, OH 45229
513-636-4200
800-344-2462
TTY: 513-636-4900
www.cincinnatichildrens.org

Cincinnati Children's Hospital is dedicated to serving the cardiac care needs of patiens, fetus through young adult, and is committed to providing research and teaching programs.

4339 Congenital Heart Information Network
http://tchin.org

Provides reliable information, support services and resources to families of children with congenital heart defects and acquired heart disease.

4340 Yale University School of Medicine
330 Cedar St, Boardman 110. P.O. Box 208056
New Haven, CT 06520
medicine.yale.edu/intmed/cardio/

Information on congential heart conditions, including Hypoplastic Left Heart Syndrome symptoms, treatments and support.

Henry Scott Cabin, Professor of Medicine
Joseph Akar, Associate Professor of Medicine
Henry Cabin, Acting Section Chief

Book Publishers

4341 Parent's Guide to Children's Congenital Heart Defects
Random House
280 Park Avenue (11-3)
New York, NY 10017
800-733-3000
Fax: 212-940-7381
www.crownpublishing.com

A practical and useful resource for families coping with a child who has CHD. An easy to read book uses personal stories and a question and answer format on a wide range of medical and daily living issues.

ISBN: 0-609807-75-7

4342 Young People and Chronic Illness: True Stories, Help and Hope
Congenital Heart Information Network
P.O. Box 3397
Margate City, NJ 08402
609-823-4507
mb@tchin.org
www.tchin.org

Presents inspirational chapters based upon interviews of young people growing up with various chronic illnesses, including a chapter on Congenital Heart Disease.

ISBN: 1-575420-41-4

Mona Barmash, President

Pamphlets

4343 Congenital Heart Information Network
600 North 3rd Street, First Floor
Philadelphia, PA 19123

215-627-4034
Fax: 215-627-4036
http://tchin.org

Four color brochure includes information about the programs and services offered.

DESCRIPTION

4344 HYPOTHYROIDISM

Covers these related disorders: Acquired hypothyroidism, Congenital hypothyroidism, Hoishimoto's disease

Involves the following Biologic System(s):

Endocrinologic Disorders

Hypothyroidism is a condition characterized by decreased activity of the thyroid gland, an endocrine gland that consists of two lobes on either side of the windpipe (trachea). Certain specialized cells within the thyroid gland secrete the thyroid hormones thyroxine (T-4) and triiodothyronine (T-3), which assist in regulating the rate of metabolism. Metabolism refers to the chemical activities within cells that release energy from nutrients or consume energy to create certain substances. The thyroid hormones also play a vital role in the normal mental and physical development and growth of infants and children. Other specialized cells in the thyroid gland secrete the hormone calcitonin, which helps to regulate concentrations of calcium in the body by inhibiting the loss of bone.

Hypothyroidism may result from an underlying defect that is present at birth (congenital). In children with congenital hypothyroidism, associated symptoms may begin at birth or be delayed until later during childhood, depending upon the nature of the underlying abnormality. Congenital hypothyroidism may result from several underlying causes, such as abnormal development (dysplasia) or absence (aplasia) of the thyroid gland; abnormalities in the production of certain hormones due to particular biochemical defects; or fetal exposure to particular medications or therapies (e.g., radioiodine therapy) during pregnancy. In children with malformation of the thyroid gland or abnormalities in hormonal production, the condition may appear to occur randomly for unknown reasons (sporadically) or may be familial. Congenital hypothyroidism affects approximately one in 4,000 infants worldwide and is about twice as common in females as in males.

Hypothyroidism may also occur later during childhood (acquired hypothyroidism) due to an autoimmune disorder in which the immune system develops antibodies against cells of the thyroid gland (Hashimoto's disease) or in association with other underlying disorders (e.g., nephropathic cystinosis, histiocytosis). Acquired hypothyroidism may also develop due to the use of particular medications or surgical removal of all or a portion of the thyroid gland as a treatment for certain diseases or conditions (e.g., thyroid cancer, thyrotoxicosis).

In newborns and infants with congenital hypothyroidism, associated symptoms may vary in range, severity, and rate of progression, depending upon the degree of thyroid hormone deficiency. Some patients may have an abnormally enlarged thyroid gland (goiter), causing swelling in front of the neck. In addition, early symptoms may include yellowish discoloration of the skin, mucous membranes, and whites of the eyes (jaundice); sluggishness; and feeding difficulties, including choking episodes during nursing. Many patients also have a large abdomen; a weakening of the abdominal wall muscles through which an abdominal organ or fatty tissue may protrude (umbilical hernia); constipation; widely open soft spots (fontanels) under the front and back of the scalp; and respiratory difficulties, including episodes in which there is a temporary cessation of spontaneous breathing (apnea). Some patients may have progressive retardation of mental and physical development that becomes increasingly severe without early diagnosis and prompt treatment. Patients may experience delays in obtaining certain developmental milestones, such as sitting up and standing; may not learn to speak; and may be increasingly lethargic. Additional physical findings associated with severe hypothyroidism include delayed skeletal maturation; a short, thick neck; short fingers and broad hands; a thick, protruding tongue; delayed eruption of the teeth (dentition); dry, scaly skin; coarse, scanty hair; and an abnormal, progressive accumulation of fluid within body tissues and associated swelling, particularly in the genital area, eyelids, and backs of the hands (myxedema).

The symptoms and findings associated with acquired hypothyroidism may also vary, depending upon the underlying cause, the age at onset, and the degree of thyroid hormone deficiency. Children with acquired hypothyroidism may experience an abnormally decreased rate of growth, decreased energy, puffiness of the skin (myxedematous changes), constipation, cold intolerance, headaches, visual problems, or other abnormalities.

In the United States, thyroid hormone levels in the blood are routinely tested in all newborns shortly after birth. Early diagnosis and prompt treatment of congenital hypothyroidism are essential for normal brain development during infancy. Such treatment includes thyroid hormone replacement therapy (e.g., sodium-L-thyroxine by mouth). The treatment of children with acquired hypothyroidism also includes thyroid hormone replacement therapy. Additional treatment is symptomatic and supportive.

National Associations & Support Groups

4345 American Academy of Pediatrics
141 Northwest Point Boulevard
Elk Grove Village, IL 60007

847-434-4000
800-433-9016
Fax: 847-434-8000
www.aap.org

The American Academy of Pediatrics and its member pediatricians are committed to the attainment of optimal physical, mental and social health and well-being for all infants, children, adolescents, and young adults.

Fernando Stein, MD, FAAP, President
Karen Remley, MD, CEO/Executive VP

4346 American Association of Clinical Endocrinologists
1000 Riverside Avenue, Suite 205
Jacksonville, FL 32204

904-353-7878
Fax: 904-353-8185
info@aace.com
www.aace.com

A professional medical organization devoted to the enhancement of the practice of clinical endocrinology.

Donald C. Jones, CEO
Dan Kelsey, Deputy CEO
Michael Avallone, CFO

4347 Genetic Alliance
4301 Connecticut Avenue NW, Suite 404
Washington, DC 20008

202-966-5557
800-336-4363
Fax: 202-966-8553
info@geneticalliance.org
www.geneticalliance.org

A coalition of voluntary genetic support groups, consumers and professionals addressing the needs of individuals and families affected by genetic disorders from a national perspective.

Sharon Terry, President/CEO
Tetyana Murza, Managing Director
Natasha Bonhomme, VP, Strategic Development

4348 Lawson Wilkins Pediatric Endocrine Society
6728 Old McLean Village Drive
McLean, VA 22101   703-556-9222
                                              Fax: 703-556-8729
                                                info@pedsendo.org
                                                   www.lwpes.org

To promote the acquisition and dissemination of knowledge of endocrine and metabolic disorders from conception through adolescence.

Morey W. Haymond, President
Mitchell E. Geffiner, President-Elect
Karen Rubin, Treasurer

4349 March of Dimes Foundation
1275 Mamaroneck Avenue
White Plains, NY 10605   914-997-4488
                                                   888-663-4637
                                              Fax: 914-997-4763
                                          answers@marchofdimes.com
                                              www.marchofdimes.com

Partnership of volunteers and professionals dedicates to improving the health of babies by preventing birth defects and infant mortality. Over 100 chapters are located across the country and can be located through the National Office.

Stacey D. Stewart, President

4350 Thyroid Foundation of America
Ste 300
Boston, MA 02210   617-534-1500
                                                   800-832-8321
                                              Fax: 617-534-1515
                                                info@allthyroid.org
                                                  www.allthyroid.org

TFA's mission is to become the best at providing credible, unbiased information on thyroid topics using electronic, print, and voice technology for benefit of patients with thyroid disorders, their families and the general public. It is also to ensure timely diagnosis, appropriate treatment, and ongoing support for all individuals with thyroid disease.

4351 Thyroid Society for Education and Research
7515 S Main Street, Suite 545
Houston, TX 77030   713-799-9909
                                                   800-849-7643
                                              Fax: 713-799-9919
                                         help@the-thyroid-society.org
                                          www.the-thyroid-society.org

A nonprofit organization whose mission is to pursue the prevention, treatment and cure of thyroid disease.

Libraries & Resource Centers

4352 National Digestive Diseases Information Clearinghouse
9000 Rockville Pike
Bethesda, MD 20892   301-496-3583
                                                   800-860-8747
                                              Fax: 301-907-8906
                                             healthinfo@niddk.nih.gov
                                                 www.niddk.nih.govv

The National Institute of Diabetes and Digestive and Kidney Diseases conducts and supports research on many of the most serious diseases affecting public health. The Institute supports much of the clinical research on the diseases of internal medicine and related subspecialty fields as well as many basic science disciplines.

Dr. Griffin P. Rodgers, Director
Dr. Gregory G. Germino, Deputy DirectorTARY
Camille M. Hoover, M.S.W., Executive Officer

Web Sites

4353 American Association of Clinical Endocrinologists
245 Riverside Avenue Suite 200
Jacksonville,, FL 32202   904-353-7878
                                              Fax: 904-353-8185
                                                     www.aace.com

The American Association of Clinical Endocrinologists is a professional medical organization devoted to the enhancement of the practice of clinical endocrinology.

R. Mack Harrell, President
George Grunberger, President Elect
Pauline M. Camacho, Vice President

4354 Online Mendelian Inheritance in Man
8600 Rockville Pike
Bethesda, MD 20894   301-594-5983
                                                   888-346-3656
                                              Fax: 301-402-1384
                                               TDD: 800-735-2258
                                              custserv@nlm.nih.gov
                                            www.ncbi.nlm.nih.gov/omim

Is an online database catalog of human genes and genetic disorders. The database contains textual information and references. It also contains copious links to MEDLINE and sequence records in the Entrenz System, and links to additional related resources at NCBI and elsewhere.

Christine E Seidman M.D, Chairman
David J Lipman M.D, Executive Secretary
Scott Edwards, Member

4355 Thyroid Federation International
P.O. Box 471
Bath, ON K0H 1   webmaster@thyroid-fed.org
                                               www.thyroid-fed.org/

The Thyroid Federation International aims to work for the benefit of those affected by thyroid disorders throughout the world. Its objectives are to encourage and assist the formation of patient oriented thyroid organizations, to work closely with the medical professions to promote awareness and understanding of thyroid disorders and their complications, to provide through member organizations, information and moral support to those affected by thyroid disorders and to promote education.

Ashok Bhaseen, President
Beate BartSs, Secretary
Asta Tirronen, Treasurer

Book Publishers

4356 Endocrine & Metabolic Disorders Sourcebook
Omnigraphics
PO Box 8002
Aston, PA 19014   800-234-1340
                                              Fax: 800-875-1340
                                            info@omnigraphics.com
                                                  omnigraphics.com

Basic information for the lay person about pancreatic and insulin-related disorders such as pancreatitis, diabetes and hypoglycemia; adrenal gland disorders such as Cushing's syndrome, Addison's disease and congenital adrenal hyperplasia; pituitary gland disorders such as growth hormone deficiency, acromegaly and pituitary tumors; and thyroid disorders such as hypothyroidism, Grave's disease, Hashimoto's disease and goiter.

574 pages
ISBN: 0-780802-07-1

Journals

4357 Journal of Clinical Endocrinology
245 Riverside Avenue Suite 200
Jacksonville, FL 32204   904-353-7878
                                              Fax: 904-353-8185
                                                     www.aace.com

Original research and articles, visual vignettes and other clinical information spanning the science of endocrinology.

R. Mack Harrell, President
George Grunberger, President Elect
Pauline M. Camacho, Vice President

Pamphlets

4358 Congenital & Acquired Hypothyroidism
Human Growth Foundation
P.O. Box 872
Pine, CO 80470

303-400-9040
888-999-9428
Fax: 303-838-0753
jmoore@erols.com
www.genetic.org/hgf

Myra Byrd, Chair
Gary Glissman, Vice Chair
Shiela Clark, Secretary

DESCRIPTION

4359 ICHTHYOSIS

Covers these related disorders: Collodion baby, Congenital ichthyosiform erythroderma, Epidermolytic hyperkeratosis, Harlequin fetus, Ichthyosis vulgaris, X-linked ichthyosis

Involves the following Biologic System(s):
Dermatologic Disorders

Ichthyosis, literally meaning "fish skin," is a group of disorders characterized by abnormal thickening, dryness, and scaling of the skin due to abnormalities in the production of keratin, a protein that is the primary component of the skin, hair, and nails. Most forms of ichthyosis are genetic disorders that are usually apparent at birth (congenital) or during the first months of life. The genes that cause some congenital forms of ichthyosis have been mapped to particular chromosomes. Ichthyosis may also be due to other underlying genetic syndromes or may be an acquired condition due to certain nutritional deficiencies, the administration of particular drugs, or certain conditions, such as abnormally decreased activity of the thyroid gland (hypothyroidism) or Hodgkin's disease, a malignancy of the lymphatic system.

One congenital form of ichthyosis is known as harlequin fetus and may result from several different genetic abnormalities, most of which are thought to be transmitted as an autosomal recessive trait. Affected newborns may be covered with thickened, ridged, armor-like plates that confine the fingers and toes, restrict movements of the joints, and flatten the nose and ears. Additional features may include eyelids that are turned outward (ectropion), causing eyes to be indistinct; gaping lips; and absent hair and nails. Newborns with the condition may experience difficulties breathing, be susceptible to repeated skin infections, and develop life-threatening complications during the first days or weeks of life.

Another congenital form of ichthyosis, known as collodion baby, may also result from many different genetic abnormalities. Affected newborns are covered by a thick membrane that resembles an oiled parchment (collodion membrane), causing flattening of the nose and ears, abnormalities of the eyelids (ectropion), gaping of the lips, or other abnormalities. The membrane begins to crack as patients breathe and is gradually shed in large sheets. This condition is usually an early manifestation of specific genetic forms of ichthyosis (e.g., lamellar ichthyosis or congenital ichthyosiform erythroderma). Patients may develop potentially life-threatening symptoms due to skin infection, inflammation of the lungs (pneumonia), excessive loss of bodily fluids (dehydration), or other abnormalities.

Congenital ichthyosiform erythroderma is an autosomal recessive disorder that typically becomes apparent shortly after birth and may often present as collodion baby, the name given to a baby who is born encased in a skin that resembles a yellow, tight and shiny film or dried collodion (sausage skin) This form of ichthyosis is characterized by abnormal redness of the skin (erythroderma); generalized, fine, white scaling of the skin; and potentially severe itching (pruritus). Many children also have abnormally thickened skin (hyperkeratosis) on the palms of the hands and soles of the feet as well as around the knees, ankles, and elbo. Additional findings may include unusually sparse hair and abnormalities of the nails. Another form of the disorder, known as lamellar ichthyosis or nonbullous congenital ichthyosiform erythroderma, is usually inherited as an autosomal recessive trait. This form of ichthyosis becomes apparent shortly after birth and may also present as a collodion baby. After the collodion membrane is shed, the skin becomes covered with relatively large, coarse scales. Scaling often affects all surfaces of the body and may be associated with pruritus. Patients may also have thickened skin on the palms and soles, usually small ears, ectropion, and abnormally sparse, fine hair.

Another form of the disorder, known as X-linked ichthyosis, is often apparent at birth or during early infancy. Although males are primarily affected, some females who carry a single copy of the disease gene may also experience some symptoms. Patients develop prominent darkened scales on the scalp, ears, neck, arms and legs, torso, or other areas. Scaling may gradually worsen in severity and progress to affect other areas of the skin. By late childhood or adolescence, many patients develop clouding of the corneas (corneal opacities) that does not interfere with vision.

The most common form of the disorder is ichthyosis vulgaris, also known as ichthyosis simplex, an autosomal dominant disorder that affects about one in 250 to 300 children. Symptoms, which typically become apparent by the age of six months, may include slight roughness and scaling of the skin, particularly of the back and the legs. Scaling may worsen upon exposure to cold temperatures and may subside during warm months of the year. There may also be overgrowth of hair follicles (keratosis pilaris), particularly those of the thighs and upper arms, as well as abnormal thickening of the skin of the palms and soles. The condition may gradually improve or subside with age.

Another form of ichthyosis, known as epidermolytic hyperkeratosis or bullous congenital ichthyosiform erythroderma, may occur randomly for unknown reasons or be inherited as an autosomal dominant trait. This form of ichthyosis typically becomes apparent shortly after birth and is characterized by erythroderma, hyperkeratosis in certain areas, and small, rough, wart-like scales over body surfaces. Skin overgrowth may be most apparent on the neck and hips, under the arms, or at the elbows or knees and may affect the skin of the palms and soles. Recurrent blistering (bullae) may also develop, particularly on the lower legs, knees, or elbows.

The methods used to treat ichthyosis depend upon the specific disorder type as well as the severity and extent of associated symptoms. In severe neonatal forms, such as collodion baby and harlequin fetus, supportive measures may include administration of fluids to prevent dehydration; use of specialized support equipment such as an incubator that provides a heated, appropriately moisturized (humidified) environment; and use of measures to help prevent or aggressively treat infections. Treatment may also include the administration of certain vitamin A derivatives (retinoids) or emulsifying ointments or lubricants. Bathing with oils may help to moisten the skin, and the application of certain emulsifying ointments and lubricants that soften the skin may alleviate dryness and scaling. In addition, applying topical agents that promote skin softening and peeling (keratolytic agents) may facilitate the removal of scales. In some patients, the use of air conditioning in warmer months and exposure to a high-humidity environment during the colder months may also be beneficial. Additional treatment is symptomatic and supportive.

Government Agencies

4360 NIH/ Eunice Kennedy Shriver National Insti tute of Child Health & Human Development
31 Center Drive, Building 31
Bethesda, MD 20892   301-496-5113
  800-370-2943
  Fax: 866-760-5947
  TTY: 888-320-6942
  nichdpress@mail.nih.gov
  www.nichd.nih.gov

Established in 1962 by congress, today the institute conducts and supports research on topics related to the health of children, adults, families and populations. Some of these topics include: developmental disabilities, growth and development, infant death, reproductive health and birth defects.

Diana W. Bianchi, Director
Paul Williams, Director, Communications

4361 NIH/National Institute of Allergy and Infectious Diseases
5601 Fishers Lane, MSC 9806
Bethesda, MD 20892   301-496-5717
  866-284-4107
  Fax: 301-402-3573
  TDD: 800-877-8339
  ocpostoffice@niaid.nih.gov
  www.niaid.nih.gov

Conducts and supports basic and applied research to better understand, treat, and ultimately prevent infectious, immunologic, and allergic diseases.

Anthony S Fauci MD, Director

4362 NIH/National Institute of Arthritis and Musculoskeletal and Skin Diseases
1 AMS Circle
Bethesda, MD 20892   301-495-4484
  877-226-4267
  Fax: 301-718-6366
  TTY: 301-565-2966
  TDD: 301-565-2966
  niamsinfo@mail.nih.gov
  www.niams.nih.gov

The mission of the NIAMS, a part of the NIH, is to support research into the causes, treatment, and prevention of arthritis and musculoskeletal and skin diseases, the training of basic and clinical scientists to carry out this research, and the dissemination of information on research progress in these diseases.

Stephen I Katz MD PhD, Director
Robert H Carter MD, Deputy Director

National Associations & Support Groups

4363 American Academy of Pediatrics
141 Northwest Point Boulevard
Elk Grove Village, IL 60007   847-434-4000
  800-433-9016
  Fax: 847-434-8000
  www.aap.org

The American Academy of Pediatrics and its member pediatricians are committed to the attainment of optimal physical, mental and social health and well-being for all infants, children, adolescents, and young adults.

Fernando Stein, MD, FAAP, President
Karen Remley, MD, CEO/Executive VP

4364 FIRST: Foundation for Ichthyosis and Related Skin Types
2616 North Broad Street
Colmar, PA 18915   215-997-9400
  800-545-3286
  Fax: 215-997-9403
  info@firstskinfoundation.org
  www.firstskinfoundation.org

Dedicated to helping individuals and families affected by the inherited skin diseases collectively called the Ichthyoses. Provides support, information, education, and advocacy for individuals and families affected by ichthyosis.

Mike Briggs, President
Larry Silverman, CFO

4365 Genetic Alliance
4301 Connecticut Avenue NW, Suite 404
Washington, DC 20008   202-966-5557
  800-336-4363
  Fax: 202-966-8553
  info@geneticalliance.org
  www.geneticalliance.org

A coalition of voluntary genetic support groups, consumers and professionals addressing the needs of individuals and families affected by genetic disorders from a national perspective.

Sharon Terry, President/CEO
Tetyana Murza, Managing Director
Natasha Bonhomme, VP, Strategic Development

4366 March of Dimes Foundation
1275 Mamaroneck Avenue
White Plains, NY 10605   914-997-4488
  888-663-4637
  Fax: 914-997-4763
  answers@marchofdimes.com
  www.marchofdimes.com

Partnership of volunteers and professionals dedicates to improving the health of babies by preventing birth defects and infant mortality. Over 100 chapters are located across the country and can be located through the National Office.

Stacey D. Stewart, President

4367 National Registry for Ichthyosis and Related Disorders
University of Washington, Dermatology Department
Box 356524, Rm.BB1353, 1959 NE Pacific St.
Seattle, WA 98195   800-595-1265
  Fax: 206-543-2489
  info@skinregistry.org
  www.skinregistry.org

Identifies individuals in the USA who have an inherited disorder of keratinization; confirms the diagnosis by strict clinical, histiopathic and biological criteria, and by using molecular resources to assist in diagnosis, assistance with research, and a means of empowerment for affected individuals and their families.

Philip Fleckman, MD, Principal Investigator

4368 Society for Pediatric Dermatology
8365 Keystone Crossing, Suite 107
Indianapolis, IN 46240   317-202-0224
  Fax: 317-205-9481
  info@pedsderm.net
  www.pedsderm.net

National organization dedicated to promote, develop and advance education, research and care of skin disease in all pediatric age groups.

Kent Lindeman, Executive Director
Stephanie Garwood, Meeting Manager

Web Sites

4369 Family Village
www.familyvillage.wisc.edu

A global community that integrates information, resources and communication opportunities on the Internet for persons with cognitive and other disabilities, for their families and for those that provide them services and support.

4370 Ichthyosis Information
www.ichthyosis.com/

chris@ichthyosis.com
www.ichthyosis.com/

This website is to furnish users with general information.

Journals

4371 Pediatric Dermatology Journal
Society for Pediatric Dermatology
8365 Keystone Crossing, Suite 107
Indianapolis, IN 46240

317-202-0224
Fax: 317-205-9481
info@pedsderm.net
www.pedsderm.net

6 issues/yr
Kent Lindeman, Executive Director

Pamphlets

4372 Ichthyosis: An Overview
FIRST: Foundation for Ichthyosis and Related Skin
2616 N. Broad Street
Colmar, PA 18915

215-997-9400
800-545-3286
Fax: 215-619-0780
info@firstskinfoundation.org
www.firstskinfoundation.org

An overview of ichthyosis; descriptions of the primary types of ichthyosis and frequently asked questions. Available in Spanish.

18 pages

Jeff Hoerle, President
Moise Levy, Vice President
Larry Silverman, CFO

4373 Ichthyosis: The Genetics of Its Inheritance
FIRST: Foundation for Ichthyosis and Related Skin
2616 N. Broad Street
Colmar, PA 18915

215-997-9400
800-545-3286
Fax: 215-619-0780
info@firstskinfoundation.org
www.firstskinfoundation.org

A description of the genetic inheritance patterns for the different forms of ichthyosis: autosomal dominant, autosomal recessive and X-linked recessive. With illustrations. Also available in Spanish.

23 pages

Jeff Hoerle, President
Moise Levy, Vice President
Larry Silverman, CFO

DESCRIPTION

4374 INTRAVENTRICULAR HEMORRHAGE

Synonyms: IVH, germinal matrix hemorrhage, GMH,
Periventricular hemorrhage, PVH

Involves the following Biologic System(s):
Neonatal and Infant Disorders, Neurologic Disorders

Intraventricular Hemorrhage (IVH) is a disease of premature
infants in which there is bleeding inside or around the ventricles, the spaces in the brain that contain the cerebrospinal
fluid (CSF). Bleeding in the brain can put pressure on the
nerve cells and damage them. Severe damage to cells can lead
to brain injury. Intraventricular hemorrhage is most common
in premature babies, especially very low birthweight babies.
The younger the gestational age, the higher the incidence of
IVH. It is not clear why IVH occurs. Bleeding can occur because blood vessels in a premature baby's brain are very fragile and immature and easily rupture. The risk of rupture is
greatest in the first 4-5 days after birth. Abrupt changes in cerebral blood flow are thought to be one of the causes of IVH.
Symptoms of IVH include apnea (stopped breathing),
bradycardia (slow heart rate), pale or blue coloring
(cyanosis), weak suck, high-pitched cry, and seizures.

IVH is diagnosed by cranial ultrasound and graded I through
IV (IV being most severe). Infants with IVH are at higher risk
for neurological disease including seizures, developmental
delay, and hydrocephalus. Infants with IVH also have a
higher incidence of death. With higher grades of IVH, the
risk of future morbidity and mortality increases.

The treatment of IVH is supportive care. The best prevention
of IVH is to prevent premature birth. When this is unavoid-
able, the use of anti-inflammatory medication (indomethacin)
in the first 48 hours of life has been shown to decrease the
incidence of IVH.

National Associations & Support Groups

4375 American Academy of Pediatrics
141 Northwest Point Boulevard
Elk Grove Village, IL 60007
847-434-4000
800-433-9016
Fax: 847-434-8000
www.aap.org

The American Academy of Pediatrics and its member pediatricians are committed to the attainment of optimal physical, mental
and social health and well-being for all infants, children, adolescents, and young adults.

Fernando Stein, MD, FAAP, President
Karen Remley, MD, CEO/Executive VP

4376 Children's Hospital at Montefiore
3415 Bainbridge Avenue. PO Box 2940
Bronx, NY 10467
718-741-2426
Fax: 718-741-2460
montekids@montefiore.org
www.montekids.org

The Children's Hospital at Montefiore is one of the most technologically advanced hospitals for children in the world. Staffed by
the nationally renowned faclty of the Albert Einstein College of
Medicine, our pediatric specialists and caregivers are ranked
amoung the best in the nation.

Steven M. Safyer, President/CEO
Philip O. Ozuah, Executive VP
Alfredo Cabrera, Sr. VP

4377 Children's Hospital of New York Presbyterian
3959 Broadway (165th Street and Broadway)
New York, NY 10032
212-305-5437
www.childrensnyp.org

Provides a comprehensive continuum of accessible, high-quality,
family-centered children's services. Improves the health status of
children in our community and maintain a world class academic
center for children's health care services, teaching and research.

Taisha Benjamin, Executive Director

4378 IVH Parents
PO Box 56-1111
Miami, FL 33256
305-232-0381
Fax: 305-232-9890
mailto:72167.633@compuserve.com
www.familyvillage.wisc.edu

Support group for parents of children suffering from
intaventricular hemorrhage.

4379 Lucile Packard Children's Hospital
725 Welch Road
Palo Alto, CA 94304
650-497-8000
800-690-2282
Fax: 650-497-8612
www.lpch.org/index.html

Devoted entirely to the care of babies, children, adolescents and
expectant mothers. To best serve our communitites we advocate
on behalf of the children and expectant mothers, advance family
centered care, foster innovation, and educate health care
providers and leaders.

Christopher Dawes, Ceo

Web Sites

4380 Children's Hospital at Montefiore
3415 Bainbridge Avenue
Bronx, NY 10467
718-741-2426
TTY: 718-920-5027
lbank@montefiore.org
www.montekids.org

Web site of one of the most technologically advanced hospitals
with highly ranked pediatric specialists and caregivers.

Steven M Safyer, President & CEO
Philip O Ozuah, Executive Vice President
Joel A Perlman, Executive Vice President

4381 Children's Hospital of New York Presbyterian
nyp.org/kids/index.html

Provides comprehensive information for children with serious
disearse, associated with Children's Hospital of New York
Presbyterian.

4382 IVH Parents
www.familyvillage.wisc.edu

Provides support for parents of children with intaventricular hemorrhage.

4383 Yale University School of Medicine
330 Cedar St, Boardman 110, P.O. Box 208056
New Haven, CT 06520
medicine.yale.edu/intmed/cardio/

Information on heart conditions, including Intraventricular Hemorrhage — symptoms, treatments and support.

Henry Scott Cabin, Professor of Medicine
Joseph Akar, Associate Professor of Medicine
Henry Cabin, Acting Section Chief

DESCRIPTION

4384 JUVENILE RHEUMATOID ARTHRITIS

Synonym: JRA

Covers these related disorders: Pauciarticular juvenile arthritis, Systemic-onset juvenile arthritis (Still's disease), Type I polyarticular juvenile arthritis, Type II polyarticular juvenile arthritis

Involves the following Biologic System(s):

Immunologic and Rheumatologic Disorders

Juvenile rheumatoid arthritis (JRA) is a group of disorders of childhood characterized by inflammation (arthritis), tenderness, pain, and swelling of one or more joints, potentially causing impaired development, limited movements, and permanent bending or extension of affected joints in various fixed postures (contractures). The symptoms and findings associated with JRA occur as the result of inflammation of the synovial membrane of affected joints (synovitis). Synovial membranes are connective tissue membranes that line the spaces between joints and bones and secrete a thick fluid to lubricate the joints. Although the cause of JRA is unknown, researchers speculate that the disorder may be the result of infection by an unidentified microorganism, an excessive immune response to a substance that the body perceives as foreign (hypersensitivity response), or abnormal immune responses against the body's own cells or tissues (autoimmune response). Certain antibodies often present in the blood of adults with rheumatoid arthritis (e.g., rheumatoid factors) are only rarely present in children with JRA. In such cases, researchers indicate that affected children may have some genetic predisposition for certain forms of JRA. Approximately 250,000 children are thought to be affected by JRA in the United States. Females are more commonly affected than males.

There are three major categories of JRA: polyarticular (30 percent), pauciarticular (50 percent), and systemic-onset juvenile arthritis (20 percent). Polyarticular juvenile arthritis typically involves several joints. Associated symptoms and findings include inflammation, swelling, abnormal warmth, tenderness, and pain of affected joints. This form of JRA often affects joints of the elbows, wrists, fingers, knees, feet, and ankles. In addition, patients may have involvement of joints of the jaw (temporomandibular joints), causing limited opening of the mouth; the neck (cervical spine), resulting in neck pain and stiffness; and the hips, causing pain, stiffness, and limited movements. Normal growth may be delayed during periods of active disease, causing such abnormalities as unusually short fingers, small feet, or underdevelopment of the jaw (micrognathia). Some children with polyarticular juvenile arthritis may also experience more generalized symptoms, such as low-grade fever, lack of appetite (anorexia), increased irritability, a mild decrease in the level of circulating red blood cells (anemia), swelling of certain lymph nodes (lymphadenopathy), or mild enlargement of the liver and spleen (hepatosplenomegaly).

Pauciarticular juvenile arthritis is characterized by involvement of larger joints, usually four or fewer for six consecutive weeks. Type I pauciarticular juvenile arthritis primarily affects females andhas an early onset. Affected joints typically include the elbows, knees, and ankles. In addition, other joints may sometimes be affected, such as those of a single finger or toe, the wrists, the neck, or the jaw. Patients are also at risk (girls more than boys) for chronic inflammation of the colored region of the eye (iris) and its muscle (iridocyclitis). One or both eyes may be affected. Some patients may experience associated redness, sensitivity to light (photophobia), pain, or decreased clearness of vision (visual acuity). Without appropriate treatment, visual impairment or, in severe cases, blindness may result. Boys are at higher risk of arthritis of the spine. Symptoms may include a general feeling of ill health (malaise), low-grade fever, mild hepatosplenomegaly, and mild anemia. Type II pauciarticular juvenile arthritisis most common in males older than age eight. Affected joints usually include those of the hips, knees, toes, and heels. In some patients, joints of the elbows, fingers, wrists, or jaw may also be affected. In patients with this form of JRA, associated foot and hip pain may sometimes be disabling. In addition, chronic, progressive, inflammatory disease of joints of the spine (spondyloarthropathy) may develop. Symptoms may include pain, stiffness, and loss of mobility of joints of the upper and lower back (ankylosing spondylitis). In addition, some affected children may experience sudden (acute) episodes of iridocyclitis.

Systemic-onset juvenile arthritis appears to affect females and males equally. This form of JRA usually begins with generalized symptoms, such as a high, intermittent fever that rapidly returns to normal; a characteristic rash; anemia; hepatosplenomegaly; lymphadenopathy; mild liver dysfunction (hepatitis); and, in about one third of patients, inflammation of the membranous sac surrounding the heart (pericarditis) or the membrane lining the lungs and chest cavity (pleuritis). The fever associated with systemic JRA tends to rise in the evenings, although it may also be elevated in the mornings, and is often associated with shaking chills. During fever episodes, a temporary, salmon-colored rash often appears on the trunk or arms or legs (extremities), although it may appear anywhere on the body. Such a rash may also temporarily appear in association with heat exposure or stress. In patients with systemic disease, joint inflammation, swelling, stiffness, and pain may occur at disease onset or months later. Joint involvement is usually similar to that seen in patients with polyarticular juvenile arthritis. Systemic symptoms and findings typically have a self-limited course that lasts for several months. However, such findings may recur in some patients.

In approximately 75 percent of affected children, symptoms associated with JRA completely disappear with little loss of function or deformity. However, other patients, particularly those with multiple joint involvement or rheumatoid factor, may experience repeated or chronic joint inflammation and permanent stiffness, limited movement, and deformity of certain affected joints. In addition, some patients with pauciarticular juvenile arthritis may later experience additionaljoint involvement (polyarthritis) or ongoing symptoms due to progressive, inflammatory disease of joints of the spine (spondyloarthropathy).

Children with JRA should receive regular eye (e.g., slit-lamp) examinations to ensure early detection and treatment of iridocyclitis. Treatment of iridocyclitis includes the use of corticosteroid eyedrops and drugs that widen (dilate) the pupil. Joint inflammation, pain, and stiffness may be alleviated with aspirin, nonsteroidal anti-inflammatory drugs (NSAIDs), medications such as methotrexate or hydroxychloroquine, or, in extremely severe cases, corticosteroids administered by mouth (orally). Due to the potential association of aspirin and the occurrence of Reye's syndrome, NSAIDs (e.g., tolmetin, naproxen, etc.) are currently being prescribed more frequently than aspirin as a treatment for JRA. Children with JRA who do not respond to NSAIDs therapy may be treated with low-dose methotrexate. If JRA is severe and systemic or, in patients in whom iridocyclitis is uncontrolled by corticosteroid eyedrops, oral corticosteroid therapy may be prescribed. However, oral corticosteroid therapy is usually avoided in children, if possible, since such therapy may slow the growth rate and is associated with other negative side effects. Children who don't respond well to methotrexate can be offered similar medications, sometimes referred to as disease-modifying antirheumatic drugs (DMARDs). Agents being tried in therapy of JRA include sulfasalazine, intravenous immunoglobulin, and cyclosporine. Splints may be used during the day to help rest inflamed joints and at night to minimize the risk of contracture development and associated deformity. Special exercises may also be recommended to help reduce possible muscle wasting and contractures. In some patients, surgery may be required to help correct contractures. Children should also be monitored for growth abnormalities, nutritional deficiencies, and school/social impairment.

Government Agencies

4385 NIH/National Institute of Arthritis & Musculoskeletal & Skin Diseases
National Institutes of Health
1 AMS Circle. PO Box 3675
Bethesda, MD 20892
301-495-4484
877-226-4267
Fax: 301-718-6366
TTY: 301-565-2966
TDD: 301-565-2966
niamsinfo@mail.nih.gov
www.niams.nih.gov

The mission of the NIAMS, a part of the NIH, is to support research into the causes, treatment, and prevention of arthritis and musculoskeletal and skin diseases, the training of basic and clinical scientists to carry out this research, and the dissemination of information on research progress in these diseases.

Stephen I Katz MD PhD, Director
Robert H Carter MD, Deputy Director

4386 NIH/National Institute of Arthritis and Musculoskeletal and Skin Diseases
1 AMS Circle
Bethesda, MD 20892
301-495-4484
877-226-4267
Fax: 301-718-6366
TTY: 301-565-2966
TDD: 301-565-2966
niamsinfo@mail.nih.gov
www.niams.nih.gov

The mission of the NIAMS, a part of the NIH, is to support research into the causes, treatment, and prevention of arthritis and musculoskeletal and skin diseases, the training of basic and clinical scientists to carry out this research, and the dissemination of information on research progress in these diseases.

Stephen I Katz MD PhD, Director
Robert H Carter MD, Deputy Director

National Associations & Support Groups

4387 American Academy of Pediatrics
141 Northwest Point Boulevard
Elk Grove Village, IL 60007
847-434-4000
800-433-9016
Fax: 847-434-8000
www.aap.org

The American Academy of Pediatrics and its member pediatricians are committed to the attainment of optimal physical, mental and social health and well-being for all infants, children, adolescents, and young adults.

Fernando Stein, MD, FAAP, President
Karen Remley, MD, CEO/Executive VP

4388 American Juvenile Arthritis Organization
1330 West Peachtree Street Suite 100
Atlanta, GA 30309
404-872-7100
800-283-7800
Fax: 404-872-9559
info.ga@arthritis.org
www.arthritis.org

Devoted to serving the special needs of children, teens, and young adults with childhood rheumatic diseases and their families. Offers both support and information through national and local programs that serve the needs of families, friends and health professionals. Serves as a clearinghouse of information, sponsors an annual national conference, monitors and promotes legislation, sponsors research, and offers training to both parents and health professionals.

Sage Rhodes, President
Sharon Davenport

4389 Arthritis Foundation
1330 W. Peachtree Street., Suite 100
Atlanta, GA 30309
404-872-7100
800-283-7800
Fax: 404-872-0457
www.arthritis.org

The only nonprofit organization that supports the more than 100 types of arthritis and related conditions with advocacy, programs, services and research.

Daniel T. McGowan, Chair
John H. Klippel, M.D., President/CEO
Patricia Novak Nelson, Vice Chair

4390 Genetic Alliance
4301 Connecticut Avenue NW, Suite 404
Washington, DC 20008
202-966-5557
800-336-4363
Fax: 202-966-8553
info@geneticalliance.org
www.geneticalliance.org

A coalition of voluntary genetic support groups, consumers and professionals addressing the needs of individuals and families affected by genetic disorders from a national perspective.

Sharon Terry, President/CEO
Tetyana Murza, Managing Director
Natasha Bonhomme, VP, Strategic Development

4391 Kids on the Block Arthritis Programs
Arthritis Foundation
9385-C Gerwig Lane
Columbia, MD 21046
410-290-9095
800-368-5437
Fax: 410-290-9358
kob@kotb.com
www.kotb.com

State and local programs that use puppetry to help children understand what it is like for children and adults who have arthritis.

Aric Darroe, President

Research Centers

4392 Pediatric Rheumatoid Clinic
Duke Medical Center
Box 3212
Durham, NC 27710   919-684-6575

Clinical and laboratory pediatric rheumatoid studies.

Dr. Deborah Kredich, Chairman
Stacy Ardman

Web Sites

4393 Online Mendelian Inheritance in Man
8600 Rockville Pike
Bethesda, MD 20894   301-594-5983
                                                     888-346-3656
                                               Fax: 301-402-1384
                                               TDD: 800-735-2258
                                               custserv@nlm.nih.gov
                                               www.ncbi.nlm.nih.gov

This database is a catalog of human genes and genetic disorders.

Christine E Seidman M.D, Chairman
David J Lipman M.D, Executive Secretary
Scott Edwards, Member

Book Publishers

4394 Arthritis
Franklin Watts
90 Old Sherman Turnpike
Danbury, CT 06816   203-797-3500
                                                     800-724-6527
                                               Fax: 203-797-3197
                                               www.scholastic.com

This book offers a clear explanation of the various forms and effects of the disease of arthritis and what treatments are available.

96 pages Grades 7-12
ISBN: 0-531108-01-5

Dick Robinson, President & CEO

4395 Arthritis Sourcebook
Omnigraphics
PO Box 8002
Aston, PA 19014   800-234-1340
                                               Fax: 800-875-1340
                                               info@omnigraphics.com
                                               omnigraphics.com

Basic consumer health information on specific forms of arthritis
and related disorders.

550 pages Hardcover
ISBN: 0-780802-01-2

**4396 Educational Rights for Children With Arthritis: Parents
Manual**
AJAO
1330 W. Peachtree Street, Suite 100
Atlanta, GA 30309   404-872-7100
                                               Fax: 404-872-9559
                                               help@arthritis.org
                                               www.arthritis.org

A self-instructional manual helping parents to identify and obtain
school services needed by their child with arthritis. Covers laws
and special services, explores strategies for working with school
personnel and stresses good communication and advocacy
techniques.

Daniel T. McGowan, Chairman
John H. Klippel, President & CEO
Michael V. Ortman, Secretary

4397 JRA and Me
American Juvenile Arthritis Organization
PO Box 19000
Atlanta, GA 30326   800-283-7800

A workbook for school-aged children who have juvenile arthritis.
This book offers a variety of educational games, puzzles and
worksheets to teach children about their illness and how to take
care of themselves.

57 pages

4398 Living with Arthritis
Franklin Watts
90 Old Sherman Turnpike
Danbury, CT 06816   203-797-3500
                                                     800-621-1115
                                               Fax: 203-797-3197
                                               www.scholastic.com

Shows how people with arthritis can overcome their pain and lead
productive, full lives.

32 pages Grades 5-7

Dick Robinson, President & CEO

4399 Understanding Juvenile Rheumatoid Arthritis
American Juvenile Arthritis Organization
1330 W. Peachtree Street, Suite 100
Atlanta, GA 30309   404-872-7100
                                                     800-568-4045
                                               help@arthritis.org
                                               www.arthritis.org

A manual for health professionals to use in teaching children
with JRA and their families about disease management and
self-care.

372 pages

Daniel T. McGowan, Chairman
John H. Klippel, President & CEO
Michael V. Ortman, Secretary

4400 We Can: Guide for Parents of Children with Arthritis
American Juvinile Arthritis Association
1330 W. Peachtree Street, Suite 100
Atlanta, GA 30309   404-872-7100
                                                     800-568-4045
                                               Fax: 404-872-9559
                                               help@arthritis.org
                                               www.arthritis.org

Offers parents tips for daily living and practical points for helping their child toward independent adulthood.

Daniel T. McGowan, Chairman
John H. Klippel, President & CEO
Michael V. Ortman, Secretary

4401 Yard Sale Coloring Book
American Juvenile Arthritis Organization
PO Box 19000
Atlanta, GA 30326   800-283-7800

A coloring/activity book based on a Kids on the Block script,
written for third and fourth grade students. It can be used with
Kids on the Block performances, as a stand-alone piece or with a
free lesson plan packet.

Newsletters

4402 AJAO Newsletter
American Juvenile Arthritis Organization
1330 W. Peachtree Street, Suite 100
Atlanta, GA 30309   404-872-7100
                                                     800-283-7800
                                               Fax: 404-872-0457
                                               kgatmail@arthritis.org
                                               www.arthritis.org

This reliable and comprehensive newsletter for families coping with childhood arthritis and related conditions contains the latest research findings, responsible advice from pediatric specialists, practical methods to help improve quality of life, and informative updates about medications and how they affect children. Articles are written in clear understandable language. Timely medical insights and life enhancing information that provides solutions to everyday problems.

Quarterly

Michael V. Ortman, Chair
Ann M. Palmer, President & CEO
Meagan Fulmer, Chief Development Officer

Pamphlets

4403 Arthritis Information: Children
Arthritis Foundation
1330 W. Peachtree Street, Suite 100
Atlanta, GA 30309
404-872-7100
800-283-7800
Fax: 404-872-0457
www.arthritis.org

Michael V. Ortman, Chair
Ann M. Palmer, President & CEO
Meagan Fulmer, Chief Development Officer

4404 Arthritis in Children and La Artritis Infantojuvenil
American Juvenile Arthritis Organization
PO Box 7669
Atlanta, GA 30357
404-872-7100
800-568-4045

A medical information booklet about juvenile rheumatoid arthritis. This booklet is written for parents or other adults and includes details about different forms of JRA, medications, therapies and coping issues.

4405 Arthritis in Children: Resources for Children, Parents and Teachers
National Arthritis and Skin Diseases Clearinghouse
9000 Rockville Pike
Bethesda, MD 20892
301-495-4484
www.niams.nih.gov/health_info

A resource offering information on juvenile arthritis, causes, treatments and prevention.

38 pages

4406 Rheumatoid Arthritis
NAMSIC, National Institutes of Health
1 AMS Circle
Bethesda, MD 20892
301-495-4484
877-226-4267
Fax: 301-718-6366
TTY: 301-565-2966
NIAMSinfo@mail.nih.gov
www.nih.gov/niams/

Offers an introduction and definition of rheumatoid arthritis, treatments, causes, objectives, daily living, resources and medical information.

Stephen I. Katz, M.D., Ph.D., Director

4407 When Your Student Has Arthritis: Guide for Teachers
Arthritis Foundation
1330 W. Peachtree Street, Suite 100
Atlanta, GA 30309
404-872-7100
800-283-7800
Fax: 404-872-0457
www.arthritis.org

A medical information booklet written for teachers or other adults who have arthritis. The booklet describes different forms of juvenile arthritis, how arthritis might affect the child at school, and how to help the child work around these problems.

Michael V. Ortman, Chair
Ann M. Palmer, President & CEO
Meagan Fulmer, Chief Development Officer

DESCRIPTION

4408 KAWASAKI DISEASE
Synonyms: MLNS, Mucocutaneous lymph node syndrome
Involves the following Biologic System(s):
Cardiovascular Disorders, Immunologic and Rheumatologic
Disorders

Kawasaki disease is a syndrome of unknown origin that primarily affects infants and young children. The disease was initially observed in Japanese children after World War II. Kawasaki disease is becoming increasingly frequent in the United States, has been reported worldwide, and is currently considered the leading cause of acquired heart disease in children in the U.S. Although Kawasaki disease has been reported in people in all racial groups, individuals of Japanese descent appear to be most commonly affected. The disease may occur commonly in a random or an isolated manner (sporadic form) or, rarely, may suddenly affect large numbers of individuals (epidemic form). Although the cause of Kawasaki disease is unknown, researchers suspect that toxic substances produced by certain bacteria (e.g., staphylococcal toxins) may play some role. There is no evidence of transmission of the disease from one affected individual to another (person-to-person transmission).

Kawasaki disease most commonly affects children who are five years of age or younger. Affected children typically develop a sudden, sustained, high fever that is often greater than 104 degrees and unresponsive to therapy with fever-reducing (antipyretic) medications. Most patients also have inflammation of the whites of both eyes and the lining inside the eyelids (bilateral conjunctivitis), causing redness but no associated discharge; dry, red (erythematous), cracked (fissured) lips; a strawberry-red tongue; and swelling of one or several lymph nodes, particularly those of the neck (cervical lymphadenopathy). Patients also typically develop a reddish skin rash that may consist of flat, discolored spots and small, raised areas (maculopapular) or appear similar to that seen in measles (morbilliform). The trunk, the hands and feet, and the face may be affected. Patients usually experience subsequent swelling and associated pain of the hands and feet. By approximately the second to third week, affected skin may begin to peel (desquamate) from the palms of the hands, the soles of the feet, and the tips of the fingers and toes. Such peeling may also involve other affected areas, such as the trunk. In addition, children with Kawasaki disease are usually irritable and may develop joint swelling and pain (arthritis), abdominal pain, diarrhea, vomiting, coughing, inflammation of the gall bladder, or enlargement of the liver and spleen (hepatosplenomegaly). Additional symptoms and findings may include inflammation of certain muscles (myositis), nasal discharge of a thin fluid (rhinorrhea), episodes of increased electrical activity in the brain (seizures), mild inflammation of the protective membrane surrounding the brain (aseptic meningitis), or other abnormalities.

The most serious complication potentially associated with Kawasaki disease is involvement of the heart. Within the first few weeks after disease onset, approximately 25 percent of untreated patients develop inflammation of arteries that carry blood to the heart muscle (coronary arteritis) and associated widening or bulging (aneurysms) of the walls of these arteries. In rare cases, affected children, particularly those under the age of one year, may experience few early symptoms associated with the disease, yet later develop coronary arteritis. Patients with cardiac involvement may develop inflammation of heart muscle (myocarditis); deficient blood supply to heart muscle (myocardial ischemia), resulting in localized loss of tissue (infarction); and inflammation of the membranous sac surrounding the heart (pericarditis). Additional findings may include inflammation of the membrane lining the internal surfaces of the cavities of the heart (endocarditis), an inability of the heart to sufficiently pump blood to the lungs and the rest of the body (heart failure), or abnormalities of the rhythm or rate of the heartbeat (arrythmias). In some cases, without appropriate treatment, patients with severe cardiac involvement may experience potentially life-threatening complications.

All patients with diagnosed or suspected Kawasaki disease should undergo specialized diagnostic tests, such as chest x-rays, electrocardiograms, and echocardiograms. Additional testing (e.g., two-dimensional echocardiogram) may also be conducted during the first two weeks of disease. The treatment of children with Kawasaki disease should include intravenous (IV) infusion with a preparation of antibodies (immunoglobulins) obtained from plasma, the liquid portion of the blood (intravenous gammaglobulin), and therapy with high-dose aspirin (salicylate therapy). Early (within 10 days of fever onset) intravenous gammaglobulin therapy helps to alleviate fever and other associated symptoms; in addition, controlled studies have demonstrated that such therapy decreases heart involvement to some patients. Once the fever has subsided, patients may receive therapy with lower doses of aspirin. Such therapy typically continues until coronary arteritis resolves. In the rare patient with large or multiple coronary artery aneurysms, treatment may include therapy with anticlotting medications, such as warfarin or heparin. Other treatment is symptomatic and supportive. All children diagnosed with Kawasaki disease receive outpatient follow-up with a pediatric cardiologist.

Government Agencies

4409 NIH/ Eunice Kennedy Shriver National Insti tute of Child Health & Human Development
31 Center Drive, Building 31
Bethesda, MD 20892
301-496-5113
800-370-2943
Fax: 866-760-5947
TTY: 888-320-6942
nichdpress@mail.nih.gov
www.nichd.nih.gov

Established in 1962 by congress, today the institute conducts and supports research on topics related to the health of children, adults, families and populations. Some of these topics include: developmental disabilities, growth and development, infant death, reproductive health and birth defects.

Diana W. Bianchi, Director
Paul Williams, Director, Communications

4410 NIH/National Heart, Lung and Blood Institu te
National Institute of Health
Building 31, Room 5A52, 31 Center Drive MSC 2486
Bethesda, MD 20892
301-592-8573
Fax: 301-592-8563
TTY: 240-629-3255
NHLBIinfo@nhlbi.nih.gov
www.nhlbi.nih.gov

Primary responsibility of this organization is the scientific investigation of heart, blood vessel, lung and blood disorders. Oversees research, demonstration, prevention, education, control and training activities in these fields and emphasizes the prevention and control of heart diseases.

Gary H Gibbons, MD, Director
Nakela Cook, MD, Chief of Staff

4411 NIH/National Institute of Allergy and Infectious Diseases
5601 Fishers Lane, MSC 9806
Bethesda, MD 20892
301-496-5717
866-284-4107
Fax: 301-402-3573
TDD: 800-877-8339
ocpostoffice@niaid.nih.gov
www.niaid.nih.gov

Conducts and supports basic and applied research to better understand, treat, and ultimately prevent infectious, immunologic, and allergic diseases.

Anthony S Fauci MD, Director

National Associations & Support Groups

4412 American Academy of Pediatrics
141 Northwest Point Boulevard
Elk Grove Village, IL 60007
847-434-4000
800-433-9016
Fax: 847-434-8000
www.aap.org

The American Academy of Pediatrics and its member pediatricians are committed to the attainment of optimal physical, mental and social health and well-being for all infants, children, adolescents, and young adults.

Fernando Stein, MD, FAAP, President
Karen Remley, MD, CEO/Executive VP

4413 Kawasaki Disease Foundation
PO Box 45
Boxford, MA 01921
978-356-2070
Fax: 978-356-2079
info@kdfoundation.org

Raising awareness among the medical community, childcare providers, and the general public is critical to early diagnosis and treatment. Facilitating support among families is essential to helping families cope with this uncommon illness and the potentially devastating effects of heart damage. Increasing funding for research is necessary to advance diagnostic guidelines, enhance the existing treatment, improve short-term and long-term follow-up care and find a cause.

Gregory Chin, President
Anthony Olaes, VP

4414 Kawasaki Families' Network
46-111 Nahewai Place
Kaneohe, HI 96744
808-525-8053
Fax: 808-525-8055
kawasaki@compuserve.com
ourworld.compuserve.com/homepage/kawasaki

A network that works to share information on research, to share information and support through occasional mailings, and to provide links to medical literature.

DESCRIPTION

4415 KELOIDS

Synonym: Cheloids

Involves the following Biologic System(s):

Dermatologic Disorders

Keloids are firm, nodule-like overgrowths of scar tissue that occur at the sites of surgery, injury, or trauma to the skin. These overgrowths result from the formation, during the healing process, of excessive amounts of the fibrous protein collagen, which is a major structural component of connective tissue. Doctors do not understand exactly why keloids form in certain people or situations and not in others. Changes in the signals sent out by cells that control growth and proliferation may be related to the process of keloid formation, but these changes have not yet been scientifically proven. Keloids may be itchy and are usually pink in color, shiny, smooth, irregularly shaped, firm, and rubbery. Some keloids may be tender or painful. Although keloids may appear on the face, neck, earlobes, legs, or other areas, they most often occur over the breastbone (sternum) and the shoulders.

Keloid development may sometimes result following surgery, body piercing, and other types of trauma to the skin such as burns or scalds. In addition, keloids may develop in association with severe acne and occasionally with certain connective tissue disorders such as Ehlers-Danlos syndrome or skin disorders such as Touraine-Solente-Gole syndrome. In some cases, keloid development may be inherited as an autosomal recessive or autosomal dominant trait. In addition, keloids are more common in black individuals.

Without treatment, keloids tend to flatten out and become less obvious within a period of months or years. However, monthly injections of certain corticosteroid drugs directly into the lesions (intralesional) may successfully decrease their size and reduce itching, but treatment should be initiated early in their development. Treatment of large keloids may include surgical removal followed by corticosteroid injections into the lesions. Surgery alone most often results in a recurrence of the keloid. Other treatment may include laser therapy that reduces the redness of the keloid; freezing keloids (cryotherapy) may also flatten them. The direct application of silicone patches or sheeting may promote shrinkage.

Government Agencies

4416 NIH/National Institute of Arthritis and Musculoskeletal and Skin Diseases

1 AMS Circle
Bethesda, MD 20892

301-495-4484
877-226-4267
Fax: 301-718-6366
TTY: 301-565-2966
TDD: 301-565-2966
niamsinfo@mail.nih.gov
www.niams.nih.gov

The mission of the NIAMS, a part of the NIH, is to support research into the causes, treatment, and prevention of arthritis and musculoskeletal and skin diseases, the training of basic and clinical scientists to carry out this research, and the dissemination of information on research progress in these diseases.

Stephen I Katz MD PhD, Director
Robert H Carter MD, Deputy Director

National Associations & Support Groups

4417 American Academy of Dermatology (AAD)

PO Box 4014
Schaumburg, IL 60168

847-240-1280
866-503-7546
Fax: 847-240-1859
MRC@aad.org
www.aad.org

Committed to the highest quality standards in continuing medical education. Developed a platform to promote and advance the science and art of medicine and surgery related to the skin; promotes the highest possible standards in clinical practice, education and research in dermatology and related disciplines; and supports and enhances patient care and promotes the public interest relating to dermatology.

Stephen P Stone MD, President
William P Coleman III, MD, VP
David M Pariser MD, Secretary/Treasurer

4418 American Academy of Pediatrics

141 Northwest Point Boulevard
Elk Grove Village, IL 60007

847-434-4000
800-433-9016
Fax: 847-434-8000
www.aap.org

The American Academy of Pediatrics and its member pediatricians are committed to the attainment of optimal physical, mental and social health and well-being for all infants, children, adolescents, and young adults.

Fernando Stein, MD, FAAP, President
Karen Remley, MD, CEO/Executive VP

4419 American Osteopathic College of Dermatology

1501 E Illinois Street, PO Box 7525
Kirksville, MO 63501

660-665-2184
800-449-2623
Fax: 660-627-2623
info@aocd.org
www.aocd.org

Strives to improve the standards of the practice of dermatology, to stimulate the study and extend knowledge in the field of dermatology, and to promote a more general understanding of the nature and scope of services rendered by osteopathic dermatologists to other divisions of practice, hospitals, clinics and the public.

David Grice, President
Suzanne Rozenberg, President-Elect
Rick Lin, First VP

4420 American Skin Association

6 East 43rd Street, 28th Floor
New York, NY 10017

212-889-4858
800-499-7546
Fax: 212-889-4959
info@americanskin.org
www.americanskin.org

The American Skin Association is the only volunteer led health organization dedicated through research, education and advocacy to saving lives and alleviating human suffering caused by the full spectrum of skin disorders.

Howard P. Milstein, Chairman
George W. Hambrick, President/Founder
Nora M. Jordan, Vice Chair

4421 Society for Pediatric Dermatology

8365 Keystone Crossing, Suite 107
Indianapolis, IN 46240

317-202-0224
Fax: 317-205-9481
info@pedsderm.net
www.pedsderm.net

A national organization specifically dedicated to the field of pediatric dermatology, with the objective of promoting, developing, and advancing education, research and care of skin disease in all pediatric age groups. The organization holds meetings twice a year to educate physicians about advances in pediatric dermatology, help them support children with dermatological diseases and improve the care of these children.

Karen Wiss, President
Andrea Zaenglen, President-Elect
Kent Lindeman, Executive Director

Journals

4422 Pediatric Dermatology Journal
Society for Pediatric Dermatology
8365 Keystone Crossing, Suite 107
Indianapolis, IN 46240

317-202-0224
Fax: 317-205-9481
info@pedsderm.net
www.pedsderm.net

6 issues/yr
Kent Lindeman, Executive Director

DESCRIPTION

4423 KERNICTERUS

Synonym: Bilirubin encephalopathy

Involves the following Biologic System(s):

Neonatal and Infant Disorders

Kernicterus refers to a rare neurologic condition in which excessive amounts of bilirubin accumulate in the brain of affected newborns, resulting in damage to the central nervous system. Bilirubin, a reddish-yellow pigment present in bile, is derived from the breakdown of the protein in red blood cells that carries oxygen (hemoglobin). Premature infants and newborns with certain congenital disorders (e.g., erythroblastosis fetalis and Crigler-Najjar syndrome) are at risk for this life-threatening condition. In premature infants, the processes needed for bilirubin excretion may not be fully developed. Factors that put extra strain on this immature metabolic process may result in increased levels of bilirubin in the blood (hyperbilirubinemia). If these levels become excessive and are left untreated, bilirubin may be deposited in the brain. For example, in infants with erythroblastosis fetalis, antibodies from the mother's blood cross the placental barrier and destroy red blood cells of the fetus, resulting in release of excessive amounts of bilirubin. In some cases, bilirubin builds up faster than the liver is able to eliminate it, resulting in hyperbilirubinemia. Signs of this condition include a yellowing of the eyes, skin, and mucous membranes (jaundice).

Crigler-Najjar syndrome results from the deficiency of an enzyme that is required to convert bilirubin to a form that may be excreted from the body, thus causing hyperbilirubinemia. Other conditions or disorders that cause hyperbilirubinemia place the newborn, especially those who are born prematurely, at risk for kernicterus.

Symptoms of kernicterus usually become apparent within the first week of life. However, hyperbilirubinemia that occurs anytime within the first month of life may result in kernicterus. Symptoms and characteristic findings may include difficulty in feeding; vomiting; lethargy; and lack of a normal response to sudden, loud noises (Moro or startle reflex). Further signs of this condition may include breathing difficulties; severe muscle spasms resulting in a backward arching of the back and neck (opisthotonos); twitching of the arms, legs, and face; a high-pitched cry; and convulsions. In some affected infants, severe involvement of the central nervous system may cause life-threatening complications. In others, findings associated with permanent disability may be observed periodically until the third year of life when the complete neurologic picture emerges. Symptoms may include involuntary spasms of the muscles, hearing loss, eye movement irregularities, deficiencies in motor development, difficulties in speech, seizures, and mental retardation. Some infants who experience only slight kernicterus may experience mild irregularities in neuromuscular coordination, moderate deafness, and slight retardation.

Treatment of kernicterus is directed toward prevention involving the correction of hyperbilirubinemia and jaundice before kernicterus can develop. Treatment may include phototherapy in which, under careful monitoring, the infant's skin is exposed to high-intensity fluorescent light. Although phototherapy is often effective in reducing levels of bilirubin, the underlying cause of hyperbilirubinemia and jaundice must be identified and treated as well. Some infants, especially those at higher risk for kernicterus, may be effectively treated with exchange blood transfusions in which small amounts of the infant's circulating blood are repeatedly withdrawn and replaced with equal amounts of whole blood from a donor until about 80 percent of the newborn's blood has been replaced. Other treatment is symptomatic and supportive.

Government Agencies

4424 NIH/ Eunice Kennedy Shriver National Insti tute of Child Health & Human Development
31 Center Drive, Building 31
Bethesda, MD 20892
301-496-5113
800-370-2943
Fax: 866-760-5947
TTY: 888-320-6942
nichdpress@mail.nih.gov
www.nichd.nih.gov

Established in 1962 by congress, today the institute conducts and supports research on topics related to the health of children, adults, families and populations. Some of these topics include: developmental disabilities, growth and development, infant death, reproductive health and birth defects.

Diana W. Bianchi, Director
Paul Williams, Director, Communications

National Associations & Support Groups

4425 American Academy of Pediatrics
141 Northwest Point Boulevard
Elk Grove Village, IL 60007
847-434-4000
800-433-9016
Fax: 847-434-8000
www.aap.org

The American Academy of Pediatrics and its member pediatricians are committed to the attainment of optimal physical, mental and social health and well-being for all infants, children, adolescents, and young adults.

Fernando Stein, MD, FAAP, President
Karen Remley, MD, CEO/Executive VP

4426 American Liver Foundation
39 Broadway, Suite 2700
New York, NY 10006
212-668-1000
800-465-4837
Fax: 212-483-8179
info@liverfoundation.org
www.liverfoundation.org

Nonprofit, national voluntary organization dedicated to the prevention, treatment, and cure of hepatitis and other liver diseases through research, education and advocacy on behalf of those affected by or at risk of liver disease.

Thomas F. Nealon, Chairman
Daniel E. Weil, Treasurer
Carlo Frappolli, Secretary

4427 Genetic Alliance
4301 Connecticut Avenue NW, Suite 404
Washington, DC 20008
202-966-5557
800-336-4363
Fax: 202-966-8553
info@geneticalliance.org
www.geneticalliance.org

A coalition of voluntary genetic support groups, consumers and professionals addressing the needs of individuals and families affected by genetic disorders from a national perspective.

Sharon Terry, President/CEO
Tetyana Murza, Managing Director
Natasha Bonhomme, VP, Strategic Development

4428 March of Dimes Foundation
1275 Mamaroneck Avenue
White Plains, NY 10605 914-997-4488
888-663-4637
Fax: 914-997-4763
answers@marchofdimes.com
www.marchofdimes.com

Partnership of volunteers and professionals dedicates to improving the health of babies by preventing birth defects and infant mortality. Over 100 chapters are located across the country and can be located through the National Office.

Stacey D. Stewart, President

4429 United Liver Foundation
5777 W Century Boulevard
Los Angeles, CA 90045 310-670-4624
Fax: 310-670-4672
pbrady@liver411.com
www.liver411.com

A national organization that promotes research and cures for hepatitis and other liver diseases.

Pam Brady, Contact Person
Donna Gracon, Chapter Director

Libraries & Resource Centers

4430 National Digestive Diseases Information Clearinghouse
9000 Rockville Pike
Bethesda, MD 20892 301-496-3583
800-860-8747
Fax: 301-907-8906
healthinfo@niddk.nih.gov
www.niddk.nih.govv

The National Institute of Diabetes and Digestive and Kidney Diseases conducts and supports research on many of the most serious diseases affecting public health. The Institute supports much of the clinical research on the diseases of internal medicine and related subspecialty fields as well as many basic science disciplines.

Dr. Griffin P. Rodgers, Director
Dr. Gregory G. Germino, Deputy DirectorTARY
Camille M. Hoover, M.S.W., Executive Officer

Web Sites

4431 Online Mendelian Inheritance in Man
8600 Rockville Pike
Bethesda, MD 20894 301-594-5983
888-346-3656
Fax: 301-402-1384
TDD: 800-735-2258
custserv@nlm.nih.gov
www.ncbi.nlm.nih.gov

This database is a catalog of human genes and genetic disorders.

Christine E Seidman M.D, Chairman
David J Lipman M.D, Executive Secretary
Scott Edwards, Member

4432 Parents of Infants and Children with Kernicterus
www.pickonline.org

Provides information and support to families of children with kernicterus.

4433 Rare Genetic Diseases in Children (NYU)
550 First Avenue
New York, NY 10016 212-263-7300
www.med.nyu.edu

We target issues arising from rare genetic diseases affecting children. Also, to assist in the endeavor to bring knowledge and hope to those for whom there is, at present, so little.

Robert I. Grossman, MD, Dean & CEO
Steven B Abramson, Senior Vice President
Andrew W Brotman, SVP & Chief Clinical Officer

4434 Save Babies Through Screening Foundation
P. O. Box 42197
Cincinnati, OH 45242 888-454-3383
email@savebabies.org
www.savebabies.org

Is a national nonprofit public charity run by volunteers. Its mission is to improve the lives of babies by working to prevent disabilities and early death resulting from disorders detectable through newborn screening.

Jill Levy-Fisch, President
Micki Gartzke, Vice President
Laura Larks, Secretary

DESCRIPTION

4435 KLINEFELTER SYNDROME
Synonyms: Chromosome XXY, XXY syndrome
Covers these related disorders: 45,X/46,XY/47,XXY mosaicism, 46,XY/47,XXY mosaicism, 46,XY/48,XXYY mosaicism, 46,XX/47,XXY mosaicism, 48,XXXY, 49,XXXYY
Involves the following Biologic System(s):
Genetic/Chromosomal/Syndrome/Metabolic Disorders

Klinefelter syndrome is a chromosomal disorder that appears to affect approximately one in 1,000 males. Males usually have one X and one Y chromosome; however, those with Klinefelter syndrome have an extra X chromosome in cells of the body. In some patients, only a certain percentage of cells contain the XXY chromosomal abnormality. This finding is known as chromosomal mosaicism. Other cells may have the normal XY chromosomal pair or other sex chromosome abnormalities (e.g., XX, XXYY, etc.). Some males may have Klinefelter variants in which some or all cells contain more than two X chromosomes.

Because only a few or subtle symptoms may be associated with Klinefelter syndrome, the disorder is rarely diagnosed before puberty. Males with the disorder may have extremely variable I.Q.s (intelligence quotients), ranging from well above to far below average; however, most affected males have an I.Q. within average limits (mean of 85 to 90). Some children with Klinefelter syndrome may have learning problems, such as difficulties with verbal expression, reading, and spelling, potentially requiring special assistance or full-time special education classes. Children with the disorder also tend to have behavioral problems, such as immaturity, excessive shyness, anxiety, poor judgment, aggressive activity, and poor social skills. Such behavioral difficulties tend to begin when affected children begin school.

Many children with Klinefelter syndrome have slim, tall stature; long legs; and small testes and a relatively small penis (hypogenitalism). As affected males enter puberty, they may experience partial, inadequate development of secondary sexual characteristics (impaired virilization). For example, facial hair tends to be unusually sparse, the testes remain unusually small, and, in many cases, there is abnormal enlargement of the breasts (gynecomastia). In addition, many affected males experience inadequate production of the male hormone testosterone and deficient production of male reproductive cells (azoospermia), resulting in infertility. In males with deficient testosterone production, treatment may include testosterone replacement therapy beginning at approximately 11 to 12 years of age. In most cases, Klinefelter syndrome results from errors during the division of a parent's reproductive cells (meiosis). In rare cases, the disorder may result from errors during cellular division after fertilization (mitosis).

In males with XY/XXY mosaicism (i.e., a percentage of cells containing the normal XY chromosomal pair), the range and severity of associated symptoms and findings may be less severe, and there may be an increased likelihood of fertility and improved psychosocial adjustment. Affected males with Klinefelter variants (i.e., in which cells contain more than two X chromosomes) may have more severe symptoms and findings, such as a greater risk of mental retardation and impaired virilization and fertility as well as additional physical abnormalities, including malformations of the head and facial (craniofacial) areas and other skeletal abnormalities.

Government Agencies

4436 NIH/ Eunice Kennedy Shriver National Insti tute of Child Health & Human Development
31 Center Drive, Building 31
Bethesda, MD 20892
301-496-5113
800-370-2943
Fax: 866-760-5947
TTY: 888-320-6942
nichdpress@mail.nih.gov
www.nichd.nih.gov

Established in 1962 by congress, today the institute conducts and supports research on topics related to the health of children, adults, families and populations. Some of these topics include: developmental disabilities, growth and development, infant death, reproductive health and birth defects.

Diana W. Bianchi, Director
Paul Williams, Director, Communications

National Associations & Support Groups

4437 49 XXY Syndrome Association
10001 NE 74th Street
Vancouver, WA 98662
360-892-7547
kimbj@juno.com

4438 A&K Associates
7 Independence Avenue
Derry, NH 03038
603-432-5755
888-999-9428
info@akassociates911.com
www.akassociates911.com

Nonprofit organization that provides information about Klinefelter syndrome, common characteristics, and treatment. Information on current research projects and other resources.

Melissa Aylstock, Executive Director

4439 American Academy of Pediatrics
141 Northwest Point Boulevard
Elk Grove Village, IL 60007
847-434-4000
800-433-9016
Fax: 847-434-8000
www.aap.org

The American Academy of Pediatrics and its member pediatricians are committed to the attainment of optimal physical, mental and social health and well-being for all infants, children, adolescents, and young adults.

Fernando Stein, MD, FAAP, President
Karen Remley, MD, CEO/Executive VP

4440 Genetic Alliance
4301 Connecticut Avenue NW, Suite 404
Washington, DC 20008
202-966-5557
800-336-4363
Fax: 202-966-8553
info@geneticalliance.org
www.geneticalliance.org

A coalition of voluntary genetic support groups, consumers and professionals addressing the needs of individuals and families affected by genetic disorders from a national perspective.

Sharon Terry, President/CEO
Tetyana Murza, Managing Director
Natasha Bonhomme, VP, Strategic Development

Myra Byrd, Chair
Gary Glissman, Vice Chair
Shiela Clark, Secretary

4441 Klinefelter Syndrome and Associates
PO Box 872
Pine, CO 80470

916-773-2999
888-999-9428
Fax: 303-838-0753
info@genetic.org
genetic.org

Nonprofit organization.

Myra Byrd, Chair
Gary Glissman, Vive Chair
Sheila Clark, Secretary/Treasurer

4442 Klinefelter's Syndrome Association
N5879 30th Street
Pine River, WI 54965

920-987-5782

4443 Support and Educational Exchange for Klinefelter Syndrome
1417 25th Avenue, Drive W
Bradenton, FL 34205

813-750-8044

Web Sites

4444 Klinefelter Syndrome Support Group
www.klinefeltersyndrome.org/

An online support group which offers information about the group, organizations, online pharmacies, other web sites, and current research studies.

4445 NIH/National Institute of Mental Health
6001 Executive Boulevard, Room 6200, MSC 9663
Bethesda, MD 20892

301-443-4536
866-615-6464
Fax: 301-443-4279
TTY: 301-443-8431
nimhinfo@nih.gov
www.nimh.nih.gov

The mission is to reduce the burden of mental illness and behavioral disorders through research on mind, brain, and behavior. This public health mandate demands that we harness powerful scientific tools to achieve better understanding, treatment, and eventually prevention of these disabling conditions that affect millions of Americans.

Joshua Gordon, MD, PhD, Director
Shelli Avenevoli, MD, Deputy Director

Newsletters

4446 Even Exchange Newsletter
KS&A
P.O. Box 872
Pine, CO 80470

303-400-9040
888-999-9428
Fax: 303-838-0753
info@genetic.org
www.genetic.org

Information on support groups, meetings, research being conducted, book and product reviews, and ask the doctor column.

3 times a year

Myra Byrd, Chair
Gary Glissman, Vice Chair
Shiela Clark, Secretary/ Treasurer

4447 Klinefelter Syndrome Newsletter
P.O. Box 872
Pine, CO 80470

303-400-9040
888-999-9428
Fax: 303-838-0753
jmoore@erols.com
www.genetic.org

News on Klinefelter syndrome, education and support. You'll find a wealth of information on this very common, but underdiagnosed condition.

DESCRIPTION

4448 KLIPPEL-FEIL SYNDROME

Synonym: KFS

Covers these related disorders: Klippel-Feil syndrome Type I, Klippel-Feil syndrome Type II, Klippel-Feil syndrome Type III

Involves the following Biologic System(s):

Genetic/Chromosomal/Syndrome/Metabolic Disorders

Klippel-Feil syndrome (KFS) is a congenital malformation characterized by the fusion of two or more vertebrae, especially in the neck or cervical region (congenital synostosis) or by the absence of one or more cervical vertebrae. Klippel-Feil syndrome Type I involves extensive fusion of several cervical vertebrae and thoracic vertebrae located in the upper back. Type II involves fusion of a limited number of incompletely developed vertebrae (hemivertebrae) and vertebrae, fusion of the uppermost cervical vertebra with the bone at the back of the skull (occipital bone), and other irregularities. Klippel-Feil syndrome Type III is characterized by fusion of the cervical, lower thoracic, or lumbar vertebrae. Physical findings associated with Klippel-Feil syndrome may include a short neck with limited range of motion, a low hairline, and irregularities of the urinary tract and reproductive, cardiovascular, pulmonary, and nervous systems. Additional abnormalities may include curvatures of the spine (scoliosis or kyphosis), an inclination of the neck to one side (torticollis), webbing of the neck (pterygium colli) and fingers (syndactyly), and other irregularities of the bones and muscles.

Treatment of Klippel-Feil syndrome may be directed toward the particular physical findings and symptoms associated with this disorder. Such treatment may include measures to correct or halt the progression of various spinal irregularities and to correct other abnormalities as warranted. Other treatment is supportive.

In some children, Klippel-Feil syndrome is transmitted as an autosomal dominant trait, while transmission by autosomal recessive inheritance is possible in others. In addition, some affected children have no recognizable pattern of genetic transmission.

Government Agencies

4449 NIH/ Eunice Kennedy Shriver National Insti tute of Child Health & Human Development
31 Center Drive, Building 31
Bethesda, MD 20892
301-496-5113
800-370-2943
Fax: 866-760-5947
TTY: 888-320-6942
nichdpress@mail.nih.gov
www.nichd.nih.gov

Established in 1962. The institute conducts and supports research on topics related to the health of children.

Diana W. Bianchi, Director
Paul Williams, Director, Communications

4450 NIH/National Institute of Arthritis & Musculoskeletal & Skin Diseases
National Institutes of Health
1 AMS Circle, PO Box 3675
Bethesda, MD 20892
301-495-4484
877-226-4267
Fax: 301-718-6366
TTY: 301-565-2966
TDD: 301-565-2966
niamsinfo@mail.nih.gov
www.niams.nih.gov

The mission of the NIAMS, a part of the NIH, is to support research into the causes, treatment, and prevention of arthritis and musculoskeletal and skin diseases, the training of basic and clinical scientists to carry out this research, and the dissemination of information on research progress in these diseases.

Stephen I Katz MD PhD, Director
Robert H Carter MD, Deputy Director

4451 NIH/Osteoporosis and Related Bone Diseases National Resource Center
2 AMS Circle, PO Box 3676
Bethesda, MD 20892
202-223-0344
800-624-2663
Fax: 202-293-2356
TTY: 202-466-4315
NIHBoneInfo@mail.nih.gov
www.bones.nih.gov

The National Resource Center is an information service that provides general information on metabolic bone conditions.

Stephen I Katz MD, PhD, Director

National Associations & Support Groups

4452 American Academy of Pediatrics
141 Northwest Point Boulevard
Elk Grove Village, IL 60007
847-434-4000
800-433-9016
Fax: 847-434-8000
www.aap.org

The American Academy of Pediatrics and its member pediatricians are committed to the attainment of optimal physical, mental and social health and well-being for all infants, children, adolescents, and young adults.

Fernando Stein, MD, FAAP, President
Karen Remley, MD, CEO/Executive VP

4453 Klippel-Feil Syndrome Support Group
311 Bracken Avenue
Pittsburgh, PA 15227
412-884-2969

Describes congenital fusion of at least two of the seven vertebrae in the cervical-spine. In addition there may be fusion or anomalies of vertebrae in the thoracic or lumbar-spine.

4454 March of Dimes Foundation
1275 Mamaroneck Avenue
White Plains, NY 10605
914-997-4488
888-663-4637
Fax: 914-997-4763
answers@marchofdimes.com
www.marchofdimes.com

Partnership of volunteers and professionals dedicates to improving the health of babies by preventing birth defects and infant mortality. Over 100 chapters are located across the country and can be located through the National Office.

Stacey D. Stewart, President

Web Sites

4455 Online Mendelian Inheritance in Man
8600 Rockville Pike
Bethesda, MD 20894

301-594-5983
888-346-3656
Fax: 301-402-1384
TDD: 800-735-2258
custserv@nlm.nih.gov
www.ncbi.nlm.nih.gov

This database is a catalog of human genes and genetic disorders.

Christine E Seidman M.D, Chairman
David J Lipman M.D, Executive Secretary
Scott Edwards, Member

4456 Rare Genetic Diseases in Children (NYU)
550 First Avenue
New York, NY 10016

212-263-7300
www.med.nyu.edu

We target issues arising from rare genetic diseases affecting children. Also, to assist in the endeavor to bring knowledge and hope to those for whom there is, at present, so little.

Robert I. Grossman, MD, Dean & CEO
Steven B Abramson, Senior Vice President
Andrew W Brotman, SVP & Chief Clinical Officer

4457 Wheeless' Textbook of Orthopaedics
www.wheelessonline.com

410-494-4994
www.wheelessonline.com

Derives from a variety of sources, including journals, articles, national meetings lectures and other textbooks.

Clifford R. Wheeless, Editor in chief
James A Nunley, Managing Editor
James R. Urbaniak, Managing Editor

DESCRIPTION

4458 LAZY EYE

Synonym: Amblyopia

Covers these related disorders: Anisometropic Amblyopia

Involves the following Biologic System(s):

Ophthalmologic Disorders

Lazy eye, also known as amblyopia, is a condition in which the vision in one eye is impaired because the images of objects seen by the affected eye are not clearly transmitted to the brain. This visual impairment results from interference with the vision in the affected eye, such as from a cataract, or from an eye-muscle weakness. This impairment prevents the affected eye from turning normally and focusing clearly on objects.

Typically, lazy eye affects only one eye, and develops in 1 to 5% of children, usually before the age of 6 years. Its existence is not always apparent, but its symptoms may include favoring the use of one eye over another, or a tendency to miss objects in the periphery of vision, causing patients to bump into objects on the side of the affected eye. However, symptoms of this condition are not always obvious either to the patient or to others, since it neither reduces the amount of light entering the affected eye nor interferes with the vision in the unaffected eye. Thus, any adjustments made by patients seem normal to them. In many cases, persons with lazy eye discover it only through an eye examination.

If not corrected early in life, lazy eye may prevent the affected eye from ever developing clear and effective vision. Because of this, it is recommended that infants have an eye examination at the age of 6 months, and that examinations are repeated regularly and at frequent intervals, up until 6 years of age. (R)(R)Treatment of lazy eye may involve forcing the use of the amblyopic eye by applying a patch over its neighboring (good) eye, for periods ranging from weeks to months. This has been shown to strengthen the vision in the weakened eye. Eyeglasses may be prescribed to improve the visual acuity in the affected eye. In some cases surgery can repair muscles of the affected eye, thus improving its coordination with the non-affected eye in looking at and focusing on objects. Eye exercises, to strengthen the affected eye, are often used by themselves or in conjunction with surgery.

Government Agencies

4459 NIH/National Eye Institute
31 Center Drive MSC 2510, PO Box 2510
Bethesda, MD 20892

301-496-5248
2020@nei.nih.gov
www.nei.nih.gov

As part of the federal government's National Institutes of Health (NIH), the institute conducts and supports training, research, and disseminates information regarding blinding eye diseases, visual disorders, preservation of sight and mechanisms of visual function.

Paul A. Sieving MD, PhD, Director

National Associations & Support Groups

4460 American Academy of Pediatrics
141 Northwest Point Boulevard
Elk Grove Village, IL 60007

847-434-4000
800-433-9016
Fax: 847-434-8000
www.aap.org

The American Academy of Pediatrics and its member pediatricians are committed to the attainment of optimal physical, mental and social health and well-being for all infants, children, adolescents, and young adults.

Fernando Stein, MD, FAAP, President
Karen Remley, MD, CEO/Executive VP

4461 American Foundation for the Blind
2 Penn Plaza, Suite 1102
New York, NY 10121

212-502-7600
800-232-5463
Fax: 888-545-8331
afbinfo@afb.net
www.afb.org

The foundation is a national nonprofit that has been eliminating barriers that prevent people with vision loss from reaching their potential. Their priorities include broadening access to technology; elevating the quality of information and tools for professionals; and promoting healthy independent living for those with vision loss.

Kirk Adams, President & CEO
Adrianna Montague-Devaud, Chief Communications/Mkting Officer

4462 Autism, Strabismus & Amblyopia (Lazy Eye)
www.mdjunction.com

800-273-8255
www.mdjunction.com

Online support group and forum.

4463 Eye Patch Club
Prevent Blindness America
211 West Wacker Drive, Suite 1700
Chicago, IL 60606

800-331-2020
www.preventblindness.org/children/EyePatchClub.html

A supportive and fun program for families going through their children's Amblyopia patching treatment. The club kit contains a newsletter, calendar and stickers for each day of wearing the patch, member-only online content, and a pen pal form.

James E. Anderson, Chair
Marge Axelrad, Sr. VP/Editorial Director
Gary Davis, Commercial VP

4464 EyeCare America
Foundation of American Academy of Ophthalmology
PO Box 429098
San Francisco, CA 94142

877-887-6327
Fax: 415-561-8567
comm@aao.org
www.eyecareamerica.org/eyecare/conditions/amblyopia/

EyeCare America is a public service foundation of the American Academy of Ophthalmology. It is a partner in the EyeSmart campaign, offering multiple programs to help with free or reduced cost eye examinations. In addition, online educational materials are available.

Betty Lucas, Director
Gail Nyman-York, Program Manager
Allison Neves, Director, Communications

4465 Lighthouse Guild
15 West 65th Street
New York, NY 10023

212-769-6200
800-284-4422
info@lighthouseguild.org
www.lighthouseguild.org

Since 1905, Lighthouse International has led the charge in the fight against vision loss through prevention, treatment and empowerment. In 2013, it merged with Jewish Guild Healthcare to form a leading non profit vision and healthcare organization.

Alan R. Morse, President/CEO
Mark G. Ackermann, Executive VP/COO
Maura J. Sweeney, Senior VP, Programs & Services

4466 Lions Club International
300 W 22nd Street, PO Box 8842
Oak Brook, IL 60523   630-571-5466
                                                 800-747-4448
                        www.lionsclubs.org/EN/our-work/sight-programs/

Provides support for sight programs and services, including vision screenings, eye banks and eyeglass recycling. Also provides financial assistancefor eye care to individuals through local clubs.

4467 National Association for Parents of Children with Visual Impairments
Jewish Guild Healthcare, 1 North Lexington Avenue,
White Plains, NY 10601   617-972-7441
                                                 800-562-6265
                                            Fax: 617-972-7444
                                         napvi@guildhealth.org
                                         www.spedex.com/napvi/

Enables parents to find resources and information for their children who are visually impaired, blind or have additional disabilities. NAPVI provides support, leadership, and training.

Julie Urban, President
Venetia Hayden, VP
Randi Sher, Secretary

4468 Sight for Students - Vision Service Plan
www.vspglobal.com/cms

                                                 888-867-8867
                                            Fax: 916-858-5388
                                       vspglobal@vspglobal.com
                                         www.vspglobal.com/cms

Provides free vision exams and glasses to low-income uninsured children. It operates on a national level through a network of community partners who identify children in need and VSP (Vision Service Plan) network doctors who provide the eyecare services.

Rob Lynch, President/CEO

4469 Vision USA-American Optometric Association
243 North Lindbergh Blvd. Floor 1
St Louis, MO 63141   314-983-4200
                                                 800-365-2219
                                            Fax: 314-991-4101
                                            foundation@aoa.org
                                         www.aoa.org/visionusa.xml

The Vision USA program offers free eye exams to low income working families and their children. It was established by AOA (American Optometric Association) doctors of optometry who donate their services.

Dennis Holter, Chief Advancement Officer
Rebecca Hildebrand, Development Officer
Emily Stenberg, Heritage Services Specialist

Libraries & Resource Centers

4470 Talking Books - National Library Service
NLS for the Blind & Physically Handicapped
Library of Congress
Washington, DC 20542   202-707-5100
                                                 888-657-7323
                                            Fax: 202-707-0712
                                            TDD: 202-707-0744
                                                 nls@loc.gov
                                               www.loc.gov/nls

Administers a free library program of audio materials through a network of cooperating libraries to eligible borrowers in the U.S.

Karen Keninger, Director
Jane Caulton, Head, Publications & Media
Marsha Jackson, Head, Administrative Section

Research Centers

4471 Visual Systems Research Group
Cincinnati Children's Research Foundation
3333 Burnet Avenue, PO Box 3026
Cincinnati, OH 45229   513-803-2230
                                                 800-344-2462
                                            Fax: 513-636-4317
                                            TTY: 513-636-4900
                                         richard.lang@chmcc.org
                              cincinnatichildrens.org/research/divisions/

A collaboration between the Developmental Biology and Pediatric Ophthalmology divisions, the program is designed to bring basic research to Ophthalmology and to foster research efforts of the clinical faculty.

Richard Lang, PhD, Director

Web Sites

4472 3D Vision
www.vision3d.org

Learn about binocular or stereoscopic vision in a fun way.

4473 All About Amblyopia (Lazy Eye)
58 Mohonk Road
High Falls, NY 12440   www.lazyeye.org

Research and information from the National Eye Institute (part of the National Institutes of Health, NIH).

4474 All About Vision
1010 Turquoise Street, Suite 275
San Diego, CA 92109   858-454-2145
                                         www.allaboutvision.org

Lists humanitarian eye care organizations that serve the needs of those with vision challenges.

Joseph T. Barr, Advisory Board
Brian S. Boxer Wachler, Advisory Board
Michael DePaolis, Advisory Board

4475 All About Vision.Com
1010 Turquoise Street, Suite 275
San Diego, CA 92109   858-454-2145
                                         www.allaboutvision.com

Provides consumers with information resources on eye health and vision correction options.

Joseph T. Barr, Advisory Board
Brian S. Boxer Wachler, Advisory Board
Michael DePaolis, Advisory Board

4476 Attention Disorders and Eyesight
58 Mohonk Road
High Falls, NY 12440   212-923-0496
                                          www.optometrists.org

Provides information on the link between vision problems and ADD/ADHD. Articles by third-party professionals are added/updated each year.

4477 Children Special Needs-Pediatric Eye Care
58 Mohonk Road
High Falls, NY 12440   212-923-0496
                                          www.optometrists.org

Provides information on visual health including: pediatric eye doctor search; tools for parents (glossary, checklists, book list); and descriptions of vision impairments.

4478 Convergence Insufficiency
58 Mohonk Road
High Falls, NY 12440   212-923-0496
                                          www.optometrists.org

Contains an in-depth review of Convergence Insufficiency (CI) including what it is; the symptoms; how common it is; detection and diagnosis; and treatment.

4479 FamilyConnect
www.familyconnect.org

familyconnect@afb.net
www.familyconnect.org

An online, multimedia community resource for parents and guardians of children with visual impairments. 24-hour support and access to message boards, real life videos, parent blogs, and parenting articles.

4480 Lazy Eye Discussion Group
health.groups.yahoo.com/group/LazyEye/

An email list (955 members) for parents of children with amblyopia, strabismus or other conditions associated with the disorder.

4481 Optometrists Network
58 Mohonk Road
High Falls, NY 12440   212-923-0496
www.optometrists.org

Twelve education websites for patients that are free of advertisements and require no registraion. There is also a free eye doctor referral directory.

4482 Prevent Blindness America Affiliates & Divisions
211 West Wacker Drive, Suite 1700
Chicago, IL 60606   800-331-2020
www.preventblindness.org

Users will be able to find Prevent Blindness programs, services, chapters and branches by state.

Paul G. Howes, Chairman
Andy Alcorn, President
Kevin Bakewell, Senior Vice President

4483 Strabismus
58 Mohonk Road
High Falls, NY 12440   212-923-0496
www.strabismus.org

All about strabismus: what is it? who does it affect? what types exist? and how can it be treated?

4484 Vision Therapy
58 Mohonk Road
High Falls, NY 12440   212-923-0496
www.visiontherapy.org

The site provides an interview of frequently asked questions with an eye doctor who is an expert in the field of vision therapy. The effectiveness of therapy and what it involves is addressed.

4485 Vision Therapy Success Stories
58 Mohonk Road
High Falls, NY 12440   212-923-0496
www.visiontherapystories.org

Children and adult vision therapy patients express their own success stories. There are over 525 stories covering many topics.

Book Publishers

4486 All Children Have Different Eyes
Edie Glaser / Dr. Maria Burgio, author

Vidi Press
11721 Whittier Blvd, #203
Whittier, CA 90601   800-409-7170
service@vidipress.com
www.lowvisionkids.com

An illustrated book for children that models for children with visual impairment how to play and make friends competently and with confidence.

48 pages

4487 Blueberry Eyes
Monica Driscoll Beatty, author

Health Press
2920 Carlisle Blvd, NE
Albuquerque, NM 87110   505-888-1394
877-411-0707
www.healthpress.com

Children's book that addresses the different aspects of eye treatment including eye patches, eye muscle surgery, and wearing glasses. Reading level: ages 4 thru 8.

32 pages
ISBN: 0-929173-24-4

4488 My Travelin' Eye
Jenny Sue Kostecki-Shaw, author

Henry Holt & Company, Inc.
175 Fifth Avenue
New York, NY 10010   646-307-5151
Fax: 212-633-0748
customerservice@mpsvirginia.com
us.macmillan.com

Audience: pre-school- grade 3. Jenny has an eye that wanders sometimes. Although this makes her different, she is also able to see the world in a special way.

40 pages Hardcover
ISBN: 0-805081-69-0

Stefan von Holtzbrinck, Chairman, Executive Board
Klaus-Dieter Lehmann, Chairman, Supervisory Board
Sandra Dittert, Senior Vice President

4489 The Patch
Justina Chen Headley, author

Charlesbridge Publishing
85 Main Street
Watertown, MA 02472   617-926-0329
800-225-3214
Fax: 800-926-5775
books@charlesbridge.com
www.charlesbridge.com

Becca wears glasses and an eye patch. She leads the kids in her class on an imaginative adventure to explain her new fashion accessories.

32 pages
ISBN: 1-580890-49-0

Brian Walker, VP Production
Mary Ann Sabia, VP Marketing and Sales and Associat
Bob Sammartino, Sammartino

Magazines

4490 Eye on NEI
31 Center Dr, MSC 2510
Bethesda, MD 20892   301-496-5248
2020@nei.nih.gov
www.nei.nih.gov

The National Eye Institute's online news magazine is published two times a month. It features articles on vision research projects, answers to eye questions, interviews with scientists, and provides a general look into the vision research process.

Dr. Paul A. Sieving, Director
Dr. Belinda Seto, Deputy Director
Allyson T. Collins, Editor

4491 EyeWorld
American Society Cataract/Refractive Surgery-ASCRS
4000 Legato Road, Suite 700
Fairfax, VA 22033   703-591-2220
Fax: 703-591-0614
dlong@eyeworld.org
www.eyeworld.org

The monthly news magazine for the American Society of Cataract & Refractive Surgery (ASCRS).

David F. Chang, Chief Medical Editor
John A. Vukich, International Editor
Bonnie An Henderson, Cataract Editor

Journals

4492 Journal of Pediatric Health Care
Natl Assoc. of Ped. Nurse Practitioners (NAPNAP)
5 Hanover Square, Suite 1401
New York, NY 10004   917-746-8300
                                        877-662-7627
                                   Fax: 212-785-1713
                                   info@napnap.org
                                   www.napnap.org

Bi-monthly pediatric journal that contains articles about research and current developments in pediatric care.

5 pages Pub # EY-145

Felicia Taylor, MBA, BA, Director, Communications

Newsletters

4493 Awareness
NAPVI
PO Box 317
Watertown, MA 2471   800-562-6265
                                   jobs@spedex.com
                                   www.spedex.com

Quarterly newsletter of the National Association for Parents of Children with Visual Impairments. It contains regional news and announcements, notices of events and conferences, legislative updates and articles.

32 pages

Pamphlets

4494 Amblyopia
National Eye Institute (NIH)
Information Office, 31 Center Dr, MSC 2510
Bethesda, MD 20892   301-496-5248
                         catalog.nei.nih.gov/productcart/pc/

Provides a description of the causes, symptoms, diagnosis and treatment for the disorder. The information is also available in Spanish.

5 pages Pub # EY-145

DESCRIPTION

4495 LEAD POISONING

Involves the following Biologic System(s):

Developmental/Behavioral/Psychiatric Disorders, Neurologic Disorders

Children and adults exposed to lead chronically over time can develop toxic levels in their blood. Traditionally, the lead level that raises concern is 10mcg/dl or above. Lead is much more harmful to children than adults because it can affect children's developing nerves and brains. The younger the child, the more harmful lead can be. Unborn children are the most vulnerable. However, many children with these levels may be asymptomatic. There are a number of sources for lead exposure. Although paint is a common source of lead, other products that may contain lead include ceramics, crystal, gasoline, batteries, and cosmetics. In the United States, the primary sources for lead exposure include household plumbing, paint made prior to 1977, and gasoline with tetraethyl lead as an additive. Although there has been a growing movement in the US to restrict the use of lead in these products, its prior use in many products continues to pose a hazard to the general population, especially young children. Lead may be inadvertently ingested, inhaled, or absorbed through the skin. One of the most common ways small children become exposed to lead is through the ingestion of fine dust from lead based paints, by licking their hands that are coated with lead dust, or by inhaling lead dust that is then swallowed. Lead makes things taste sweet, so children are attracted to the taste of lead paint chips and especially to lead dust. Lead that enters the body gets absorbed into the blood stream. It is then deposited in soft tissue and organs, or excreted through the kidney. Most of the lead that remains in the body, though, is deposited in bones. Lead toxicity primarily involves the central nervous system and the gastrointestinal system. Although many children with lead ingestion will have asymptomatic disease, they may show increased behavioral problems, poor school performance, decreased height, and decreased cognitive function. Children with more severe lead exposure may complain of anorexia, nausea, vomiting, abdominal pain and constipation. These symptons have been reported at lead levels as low as 20 mcg/dl but more commonly seen at lead levels greater than 50 mcg/dl. Neurological symptoms may include ataxia (staggering gait), seizures, coma, and encephalopathy. Screening for lead exposure should be performed in all children under 5. A thorough history should be taken, focusing on age of the patient's home, behavioral changes, exposure to battery factories or ceramics, recent home renovations (in homes pre-1978), and history of lead poisoning in a sibling. The frequency of the blood test screening will increase based on the patient's environmental exposure. A lead level of 10 mcg/dl or greater is considered a significant exposure and warrants further evaluation. An assessment of the home should be undertaken and the patient should have repeat blood lead levels tested no later than 3 months of age. The American Academy of Pediatrics recommends repeating a lead level by 3 months. Lead exposure may in some cases also be confirmed by x-ray, studies in the abdomen and in bones (lead lines). Therapy for lead exposure/toxicity generally focuses on removing the lead from the patient's environment, diminishing hand to mouth behaviors, improving nutrition in exposed patients and removing the lead from the patient's body. Homes may be cleaned properly by professionals and old paint must be removed from environment or sealed in a fashion that will eliminate the family's exposure to paint dust and chips. Some children will need to be moved to a lead-free safehouse while this is occurring. Frequent washing of hands and toys will cut down on exposure from hand to mouth behavior exhibited by young children. Lead levels greater than 44mcg/dl are considered significant enough to warrant chelation therapy and levels greater than 70 mcg/dl should prompt referral for chelation and hospitalization. Chelation therapy involves giving patients chelating, or binding, agents which bind to the lead and make it easier to excrete from the body. This type of therapy should begin only after the source of lead in the environment has been eliminated.

National Associations & Support Groups

4496 American Academy of Pediatrics
141 Northwest Point Boulevard
Elk Grove Village, IL 60007
847-434-4000
800-433-9016
Fax: 847-434-8000
www.aap.org

The American Academy of Pediatrics and its member pediatricians are committed to the attainment of optimal physical, mental and social health and well-being for all infants, children, adolescents, and young adults.

Fernando Stein, MD, FAAP, President
Karen Remley, MD, CEO/Executive VP

4497 National Lead Information Center
8601 Georgia Avenue Suite 503
Silver Spring, MD 20910
800-424-5323
Fax: 301-585-7976
hotline.lead@epa.gov

Offers support and referrals for patients and their families. Provides testing kits, evaluation techniques, and resource materials, including publications and tapes.

State Agencies & Support Groups

4498 Connecticut Lead Poisoning Prevention Program
410 Capitol Avenue, Ms#51LED P.O. Box 340308
Hartford, CT 06134
860-509-7299
Fax: 860-509-7295

Workshops and literature on how to diagnose and prevent lead poisoning.

Web Sites

4499 Consumer Product Safety Commission Hotline
4330 East West Highway
Bethesda, MD 20814
301-504-7923
Fax: 301-504-0124
www.cpsc.gov

CPSC is an Independent Federal Regulatory Agency that works to save lives and keep families safe by reducing the risk of injuries and deaths associated with consumer products.

Elliot F. Kaye, Chairman

4500 National Conference of State Legislatures
444 North Capitol Street, N.W., Suite 515
Washington, D. 20001
202-624-5400
Fax: 202-737-1069
ncslnet-admin@ncsl.org.
www.ncsl.org

The National Conference of State Legislatures is a bipartisan organization that serves the legislators and staffs of the nation's 50 states, its commonwealths and territories. NCSL provides research, technical assistance and opportunities for policymakers to exchange ideas on the most pressing state issues. NCSL is an effective and respected advocate for the interests of state governments before Congress and federal agencies.

Senator Pamela, President
Jean Cantrel, Vice President
Tom Wright, Secretary/Treasurer

4501 Safe Drinking Water Hotline
www.epa.org/safewater/

Together with the states, tribes, and its many partners, protects public health by ensuring safe drinking water and protecting ground water. Along with EPS's ten regional drinking water programs, oversees implementation of the SAFE DRINKING WATER ACT, which is the national law safeguarding tap water in America.

DESCRIPTION

4502 LEARNING DISABILITY/READING DYSLEXIA

Synonyms: Learning Disorders, LDD

Covers these related disorders: Dyscalculia, Dyslexia, Dysgraphia

Involves the following Biologic System(s):
Developmental/Behavioral/Psychiatric Disorders

Learning Disability (LD) is a general term that refers to a group of disorders characterized by problems with learning, processing, or expressing information. When LD involves speech and language, it can affect how a person hears words (receptive language disorder), how they put thoughts into words (expressive language disorder), or how words are put together when spoken (articulation disorder).

LD can also affect academic skills. Dyscalculia is a learning disability characterized by difficulty in using mathematical symbols and understanding mathematical concepts. Dysgraphia is the difficulty in the physical process of writing letters and words. A person with dyspraxia can understand sentences in a normal way, but has difficulty putting words together into a coherent sentence. Dyslexia is characterized by the impairment in the ability to process written symbols.

Young children with dyslexia may have difficulty remembering the correct names of letters and numbers. Some school aged children may reverse letters and words when writing. For example, affected children may substitute the letter P for Q, reverse the word WAS to become SAW, or transpose letters so that BETS becomes BEST. Children with dyslexia may also have difficulty reading due to an impaired ability to determine the sequence of letters within words and to distinguish right from left. The hallmark of this learning disability is the fact that despite their difficulties, affected children are of average or above average intelligence by IQ testing and scholastic achievement.

Although learning disabilities occur in very young children, the disorders are usually not recognized until the child reaches school age. Early diagnosis of LD is an important factor in treatment. Children nearing the end of first grade who exhibit difficulties with word skills, or any children whose reading, writing, or mathematical skills are not commensurate with that of their other scholastic abilities should be tested for LD. Although LD is not related to eye defects, an ophthalmologic evaluation is beneficial in eliminating vision problems as a cause for symptoms. Treatment for LD is geared towards remedial teaching techniques specific to the disability.

LD is thought to be a familial disorder and may be inherited in an autosomal dominant fashion.

National Associations & Support Groups

4503 AVKO Dyslexia Research Foundation
3084 W Willard Road Suite W. PO Box 9404
Birch Run, MI 48415
810-686-9283
866-285-6612
Fax: 810-686-1101
webmaster@avko.org
www.avko.org

Nonprofit organization founded to help determine what dyslexia is, why traditional methods of teaching and writing fail and help most dyslexics learn to read and write.
1974
Barry Chute, President
Julie Guyette, VP
Clifford Schroeder, Treasurer

4504 American Academy of Pediatrics
141 Northwest Point Boulevard
Elk Grove Village, IL 60007
847-434-4000
800-433-9016
Fax: 847-434-8000
www.aap.org

The American Academy of Pediatrics and its member pediatricians are committed to the attainment of optimal physical, mental and social health and well-being for all infants, children, adolescents, and young adults.
Fernando Stein, MD, FAAP, President
Karen Remley, MD, CEO/Executive VP

4505 American School Counselor Association
1101 King Street, Suite 310
Alexandria, VA 22314
703-683-2722
800-306-4722
Fax: 703-997-7572
asca@schoolcounselor.org
www.schoolcounselor.org

The mission of ASCA is to represent professional school counselors and to promote professionalism and ethical practices.
Richard Wong, Executive Director
Jeff Broderson, Information Technology Admin.
Kathleen M Rakestraw, Director of Communications

4506 American Speech Language Hearing Associati on (ASHA)
2200 Research Boulevard, PO Box 3289
Rockville, MD 20850
301-296-5700
800-638-8255
Fax: 301-296-8580
TTY: 301-296-5650
nsslha@asha.org
www.asha.org

A certifying body of 123,000 professionals providing speech, language and hearing services to the public. It is an accrediting agency for college and university graduate school programs in speech-language pathology and audiology.
Patricia A. Prelock, President
Elizabeth S. McCrea, President-Elect
Donna Fisher Smiley, VP for Audiology Practice

4507 Council for Learning Disabilities
11184 Antioch Road Box 405
Overland Park, KS 66210
913-491-1011
Fax: 913-491-1012
CLDInfo@cldinternational.org
www.cldinternational.org

An international organization that promotes effective teaching and research. CDL is composed of professionals who represent diverse disciplines and who are committed to enhancing the education and life span development of individuals with learning disabilities.
Caroline Kethley, President
Silvana Watson, President-Elect
Steve Chamberlain, VP

4508 Division for Learning Disabilities
1110 N Glebe Road Suite 300
Arlington, VA 22201
703-524-0099
888-232-7733
Fax: 703-264-9494
TTY: 703-264-9446
www.teachingld.org

The Division for Learning Disabilities is a national professional organization consisting of teacher, higher education professionals, administrators, and parents. The major purpose of DLD is to promote the education and general welfare of persons with learning disabilities, provide a forum for discussion of issues facing the field of learning disabilities, and to encourage interaction amoung the many groups whose research and service efforts impact persons with learning disabilities.

Jenette Klingner, President
Erica Lembke, President-Elect
David Chard, VP

4509 Dyslexia Research Institute
5746 Centerville Road
Tallahassee, FL 32309　　　　　　　850-893-2216
　　　　　　　　　　　　　　　Fax: 850-893-2440
　　　　　　　　　　　　　　　dri@dyslexia-add.org
　　　　　　　　　　　　　　　www.dyslexia-add.org

Addresses academic, social and self-concept issues for dyslexic and ADD children and adults. College prep courses, study skills, advocacy, diagnostic testing, seminars, teachers training, day school, tutoring and adult literacy and life skills programs are available using an accredited MSLE approach.

Patricia K. Hardman, Executive Director
Robyn A Rennick MS, Assistant Director

4510 Federation for Children with Special Needs
529 Main Street, Suite 1102
Boston, MA 02129　　　　　　　617-236-7210
　　　　　　　　　　　　　　　800-331-0688
　　　　　　　　　　　　　　　Fax: 617-241-0330
　　　　　　　　　　　　　　　fcsninfo@fcsn.org
　　　　　　　　　　　　　　　www.fcsn.org

The mission of the Federation for Children with Special Needs provides information, support, and assistance to parents of children with disabilities, and encouraging full participation in community life by all people, especially those with isabilities.

Sonya Andrade, Executive Assistant
Robin Foley, Director

4511 International Dyslexia Association
40 York Road, Suite 400, 4th Floor
Baltimore, MD 21204　　　　　　　410-296-0232
　　　　　　　　　　　　　　　800-223-3123
　　　　　　　　　　　　　　　Fax: 410-321-5069
　　　　　　　　　　　　　　　info@interdys.org
　　　　　　　　　　　　　　　www.interdys.org

Our mission is to pursue and provide the most comprehensive range of information and services that address the full scope of dyslexia and related difficulties in learning to read and write.

Steve Peregoy, Executive Director
Gerri Morris, Corrdinator Information/Referral
Robert Hott, Director of Development

4512 Learning Disabilities Association of Ameri ca
4156 Library Road
Pittsburgh, PA 15234　　　　　　　412-341-1515
　　　　　　　　　　　　　　　888-300-6710
　　　　　　　　　　　　　　　Fax: 412-344-0224
　　　　　　　　　　　　　　　info@LDAAmerica.org
　　　　　　　　　　　　　　　www.ldaamerica.org

Helps families of the affected individual through information and referral to professionals in their area. A membership organization with affiliates across the country.

Sheila Buckley, Executive Director

4513 National Center For Learning Disabilities With Disabilities
381 Park Avenue S Suite 1401
New York, NY 10016　　　　　　　212-545-7510
　　　　　　　　　　　　　　　888-575-7373
　　　　　　　　　　　　　　　Fax: 212-545-9665
　　　　　　　　　　　　　　　www.ncld.org

The mission is to increase opportunities for all individuals with learning disabilities to achieve their potential.NCLD accomplishes this mission by increasing public awareness and understanding of learning disabilities, conducting educational programs and services that promote research-based knowledge, and providing national leadership in shaping public policy.

Frederic M. Poses, Chairman of the Board
Anne Ford, Chairman
John R. Langeler, Treasurer

4514 National Dissemination Center for Children with Disabilities
PO Box 1492
Washington, DC 20013　　　　　　　202-884-8200
　　　　　　　　　　　　　　　800-695-0285
　　　　　　　　　　　　　　　Fax: 202-884-8441
　　　　　　　　　　　　　　　nichcy@aed.org
　　　　　　　　　　　　　　　www.nichcy.org

Provides parents with information about special education and the rights children and youth with disabilities have under the law. NICHY can also provide parents and others with a State Resource Sheet, useful for identifying resources within their state. This sheet includes, names, addresses and phone numbers of state agencies disability organizations, and parent groups serving individuals with disabilities and their families. A variety of other publications are available upon request.

Suzanne Ripley, Executive Director

4515 New England Center for Children
33 Turnpike Road, PO Box 2108
Southborough, MA 01772　　　　　　　508-481-1015
　　　　　　　　　　　　　　　Fax: 508-485-3421
　　　　　　　　　　　　　　　info@necc.org
　　　　　　　　　　　　　　　www.necc.org

Serving students between the ages of 3 and 22 diagnosed with autism, learning disabilities, language delays, mental retardation, behavior disorders and related disabilities; educational curriculum encompasses both the teaching of functional life skills and traditional academics; communication skills are taught throughout all activities in the school, residence, and community. Tuition and fees are set by the state. Consulting services also available.

Lisel Macenka, Chairman of the Board
James C. Burling, Vice Chair of the Board
L. Vincent Strully, President

4516 Parents Helping Parents: Family Resources for Children with Special Needs
1400 Parkmoor Avenue, Suite 100
San Jose, CA 95126　　　　　　　408-727-5775
　　　　　　　　　　　　　　　855-727-5775
　　　　　　　　　　　　　　　Fax: 408-286-1116
　　　　　　　　　　　　　　　info@php.com
　　　　　　　　　　　　　　　www.php.com

Helping children with special needs receive the resources, love, hope, respect, health care, education and other services they need to achive their full potential by providing them with strong families and dedicated professional to serve them.

Suzanne Cistulli, Board Chair
Robert Badagliacco, Board Treasurer
Lisa Caywood, Board Member

Libraries & Resource Centers

4517 Berkshire Center
18 Park Street #160
Lee, MA 01238　　　　　　　413-243-2576

A postsecondary program for young adults with learning disabilities ages eighteen-twenty-six. Half the students attend Berkshire Community College part-time while others go directly into the working world. Services include vocational/adacademic preparation, tutoring, college liason, life skills instruction, driver's education, money management, psychotherapy, and more. The program is year-round with an average stay of two years.

4518 Carroll Center for the Blind
770 Centre Street
Newton, MA 02458　　　　　　　617-969-6200
　　　　　　　　　　　　　　　800-852-3131
　　　　　　　　　　　　　　　Fax: 617-969-6204
　　　　　　　　　　　　　　　www.carroll.org

Assists blind and visually impaired adults and adolescents to adjust to loss of vision. The goal of this dynamic program is to help the person become more independent, to restore self-confidence, prepare for employment and improve the quality of life. Programs of individual counseling are offered as part of the program.

Rachel Rosenbaum, President

4519 University of Kansas Center for Research on Learning
1122 West Campus Road, Room 521
Lawrence, KS 66045   785-864-4780
                                  Fax: 785-864-5728
                                       crl@ku.edu
                                      www.kucrl.org

A research center working to improve learning and performance of adolescents and adults considered to be at risk for failure in today's schools, work places, and communities. Develops products and procedures that can be used to more effectively teach these individuals. Provides support and research-validated instructional materials to an international training network that promotes system change in our schools and institutions. Newsletter for teachers containing tips and advice used in class.

Don Deshler, Director
Mike Hock, Associate Director
Julie Tollefson, Director of Communications

Audio Video

4520 How to Help Your Child Succeed in School

Sandra Rief, author

Peytral Publications
PO Box 1162
Minnetonka, MN 55345   952-949-8707
                                       877-739-8725
                                  Fax: 952-906-9777
                                    help@peytral.com
                                      www.peytral.com

Essential information needed by parents and educators. Topics include developiong reading, writing and math skills, building organization and study skills, surviving daily homework assignments and coping with learning disabilities.

56 minutes

Web Sites

4521 Children's Hospital of New York Presbyterian
nyp.org/kids/index.html

A high quality, world class center that improves the health status of children.

4522 Division for Learning Disabilities
www.teachingld.org

                          WebHelp@TeachingLD.org
                                 www.teachingld.org

Promotes the education and general welfare of persons with learning disabilities.

David Chard, President
John Lloyd, Executive Director
Jeanne Wanzek, Secretary

4523 Learning Disabilities Association of Ameri ca
www.ldaamerica.org

Helps families of the affected individual through information and referral to professionals in their area. A membership organization with affiliates across the country.

4524 National Dissemination Center for Children with Disabilities
35 Halsey St., Fourth Floor
Newark, NJ 7102   malizo@spannj.org
                                      www.nichcy.com

Provides parents with information about special education and the rights children and youth have under law. It also provides parents with a resource sheet of organizations in their state.

Debra Jennings, Project Director
Lisa K□pper, Product Development Coordinator
Myriam Alizo, Project Assistant

4525 The Parent Educational Advocacy Training C enter
100 N Washington St, Suite 234
Falls Church, VA 22046   703-923-0010
                                       800-869-6782
                                  Fax: 800-693-3514
                                  TTY: 703-923-0010
                                   partners@peatc.org
                                      www.peatc.org

Provides general research about special education and learning disabilities.

Michael Jefferson, President
Betsy McGuire, Vice President
Linda Feldstein, Secretary

Book Publishers

4526 Learning Disabilities and Challenging Beha viors

Nancy Mather PhD, Sam Goldstein PhD, author

Brooks Publishings
PO Box 10624
Baltimore, MD 21285   410-337-9850
                                       800-638-3775
                                  Fax: 410-337-8539
                          webmaster@brookespublishing.com
                              www.brookespublishing.com

A working manual for educators and others who teach children with learning disabilities. Helps readers to understand how specific developmental, behaviour, and academic problems influence school success.

416 pages

Paul H. Brookes, Chairman
Jeff Brookes, President
Melissa A. Behm, ExecutiveVice President

Magazines

4527 Get Ready to Read!
National Center for Learning Disabilities
32 Laight Street, Second Floor
New York, NY 10013   212-545-7510
                                       888-575-7373
                                  Fax: 212-545-9665
                                       hlp@ncld.org
                                       www.ncld.org

Quartely

Frederic M Poses, Chairman
Mary Kalikow, Vice Chairman
William Haney, Secretary

4528 LD Advocate
National Center for Learning Disabilities
32 Laight Street, Second Floor
New York, NY 10013   212-545-7510
                                       888-575-7373
                                  Fax: 212-545-9665
                                       help@ncld.org
                                       www.ld.org

Quarterly

Frederic M Poses, Chairman
Mary Kalikow, Vice Chairman
William Haney, Secretary

4529 LD News
National Center for Learning Disabilities
32 Laight Street, Second Floor
New York, NY 10013   212-545-7510
                                       888-575-7373
                                  Fax: 212-545-9665
                                       hlp@ncld.org
                                       www.ncld.org

Quartely

Frederic M Poses, Chairman
Mary Kalikow, Vice Chairman
William Haney, Secretary

4530 Our World
National Center for Learning Disabilities
32 Laight Street, Second Floor
New York, NY 10013

212-545-7510
888-575-7373
Fax: 212-545-9665
hlp@ncld.org
www.ncld.org

Quartely

Frederic M Poses, Chairman
Mary Kalikow, Vice Chairman
William Haney, Secretary

Journals

4531 Journal of Learning Disabilities
Hammill Institute on Disabilities/Sage Publication
2455 Teller Road
Thousand Oaks, CA 91230

800-818-7243
Fax: 800-583-2665
journals@sagepub.com
www.sagepub.com

JLD is internationally recognized as the oldest and most authoritative journal in the area of learning disabilities. The editorial board reflects the international, multidisciplinary nature of JLD, comprising researchers and practitioners in numerous fields, including education, psychology, neurology, medicine, law and counseling. ISSN: Print: 0022-2194; Electronic: 1538-4780. Avialable: Institutional - Print: $218, Institutional - Print & E-access $222, Individual - Print & E-access $71.

Bi-monthly

H Lee Swanson PhD, Editor

Newsletters

4532 Perspectives on Language and Literacy
IDA
40 York Road Suite 400
Baltimore, MD 21204

410-296-0232
800-223-3123
Fax: 410-321-5069
info@interdys.org
www.interdys.org

Features practical articles for educators and other professionals dedicated to the identification and intervention of dyslexia and other reading problems.

50-56 pages quarterly

Hal Malchow, President
Ben Shifrin, Vice President
Suzanne Carreker, Secretary

Camps

4533 Anchor Point Camp
RBM Ministries
PO Box 128
Plainwell, MI

616-342-9879

Accepts mentally and physically handicapped children ages 13 and up.

4534 Beech Brook
3737 Lander Road
Cleveland, OH

216-831-2255
877-546-1225
Fax: 216-831-0436
www.beechbrook.org

A year-round residential and day treatment center, accepts summer residents when there are openings in the regular enrollment. The program is designed for emotionally disturbed, learning disabled and autistic children, providing therapeutically oriented teaching and programming techniques in a camp setting.

Philip M. Dawson, Chair
Thomas A. Seifert, Vice Chair
Brandon R. Miller, Vice Chair

4535 Camp Buckskin
4124 Quebec Ave. N, Suite 300
Minneapolis, MN 55427

763-432- 917
Fax: 952-938-6996
info@campbuckskin.com
www.campbuckskin.com

LD and ADD/ADHD youth have often experienced frustration and a lack of success. Buckskin assists these individuals to realize and develop the potentials and abilities which they possess. Teaches a combination of academic and camp activities, so the campers experience success in many areas. By necessity fairly structured, the 1:3 staff ratio ensures the program is individualized to meet each camper's needs. Parents report that their children benefit from the experience in many ways.

Thomas R Bauer, CCD, Camp Director

4536 Camp Huntington
56 Bruceville Road
High Falls, NY 12440

845-687-7840
855-707-2267
Fax: 845-687-7211
camohtgtn@aol.com
www.camphuntington.com

Summer activities include recreational, academic and vocational programs for the learning disabled, neurologically impaired and mildly ADA to mild/moderately retarded. An Olympic pool, horse riding and a special work training program are featured. Programs are tailored to meet individual needs, ages 6-21, and campers may enroll for 4 to 8 weeks.

Dr. Bruria Falik, Director
Michael Bednarz, Executive Director
Alex Mellor, Program Director

4537 Camp Nuhop
404 Hillcrest Drive
Ashland, OH

419-289-2227
Fax: 419-289-2227
cnuhop@bright.net
www.nuhop.org

A summer residential program for any youngster from 6 to 18 with a learning disability, behavior disorder or Attention Deficit Disorder. Sixty two campers and 35 staff members live on site in groups of 7 campers to every 3 counselors. Activities focus on positive self-concept and behaviors and teach children to learn how to find their strengths, abilities and talents from a positive, yet realistic viewpoint.

Trevor Dunlap, Executive Director
Chris Clyde, Associate Director
Jerry Dunlap, Director

4538 Camp O' Fair Winds
2300 Austins Parkway
Flint, MI 48507

810-230-0244
800-482-6734
Fax: 810-230-0955
tplotz@gsfwc.org
www.gsfwc.org/camps.htm

Outdoor program for all girls, ages 7-11. Our goal is to build confidence by giving girls a chance to voice their opinions and make their own decisions. We are able to accommodate girls with diabetes, ADHD, and learning disabilities. We are willing to make special accommodations - including hiring individual assistants for girls with hearing impairments and physical disabilities.

Therese Plotz, Camp Director
Olga Recio, Camp Secretary

4539 Dallas Academy
950 Tiffany Way
Dallas, TX

214-324-1481
Fax: 214-327-8537
mail@dallas-academy.com
www.dallas-academy.com

7-week summer session for students who are having difficulty in regular school classes.

Troy Sturrock, Chair
Terrence S Welch, Vice Chair
Dallas Cothrum, Secretary

4540 Developmental Center
6710 86th Avenue N
Pinellas Park, FL
727-541-5716
Fax: 727-544-8186
NickiMaddalena@centeracademy.com
centeracademy.com

Specifically designed for the learning disabled child and other children with difficulties in concentration, strategy, social skills, impulsivity, distractibility and study strategies. Programs offered include: attention training, visual-motor remediation, socialization skills training, relaxation training, horseback riding and more. The day camp meets weekdays from 9-3 for 3,4 or 5 week sessions.

Mack R. Hicks, Chairman
Eric V. Larson, President
Andrew P. Hicks, Chief Executive Officer

4541 Eagle Hill School - Summer Program
242 Old Petersham Road
Hardwick, MA 1037
413-477-6000
Fax: 413-477-6837
admission@eaglehillschool.com
www.ehs1.org

For the child, age 9-19, with a specific learning disability or Attention Deficit Disorder, this summer program offers a structured curriculum designed to build a basic foundation of academic competence. Extracurricular and outdoor activities complement the educational program.

Jim Richardson, Chairman
Marilyn Waller, President
Alden Bianchi, Vice President

4542 Groves Academy
3200 Highway 100 South
Saint Louis Park, MN 55416
952-920-6377
Fax: 952-920-2068
www.grovesacademy.org

A nonprofit day school in Minnesota designed especially for children with learning differences. The Center has a full day academic program from September through June, as well as an 8 week summer program. Groves also offers community services such as: psychoeducational testing for children and adults, consulting services, workshops on learning disabilities and other special learning needs, and afternoon/evening tutorial services for children and adults.

Karen Sanger, Chair
Thomas Schnack, Vice Chair
Tom Sass, Secretary

4543 Hill School of Fort Worth
4817 Odessa Avenue
Fort Worth, TX 76133
817-923-9482
Fax: 817-923-4894
hillschool@hillschool.org
www.hillschool.org

Provides an alternative learning environment for students having average or above-average intelligence with learning differences. Hill school is an established leader in North Texas with a 25 year history of effectively serving LD children. Beginning in 1961 as a tutorial service, Hill became a formal school in 1973. Our mission is to help those who learn differently develop skills and strategies to succeed. We do this by developing academic/study skills, and self-discipline.

John W. Wright, Chairman
Randall Canedy, Vice Chairman
Ralph Torres, Secretary

4544 Lab School of Washington Summer Program
4759 Reservoir Road NW
Washington, DC 20007
202-965-6600
Fax: 202-965-5106
alexandra.freeman@labschool.org
www.labschool.org

The Lab School 5-week summer session includes individualized reading, spelling, writing, study skills, and math programs. A multisensory approach addresses the needs of bright learning disabled children. Related services such as speech/language therapy and occupational therapy are integrated into the curriculum. Elementary/Intermediate; Junior High/High School.

Sally Smith, Founder
Susan Feeley, Admissions Director

4545 Maplebrook School
5142 Route 22
Amenia, NY 12501
845-373-9511
Fax: 845-373-7029
mbsecho@aol.com
www.maplebrookschool.org

A coeductional boarding school for students with learning differences and ADD. A New York State registered high school servicing ages 11-18. Post secondary options offered to 18-21.

Mark J. Metzger, Chairman
Robert Audia, Vice Chairman
Charles F. Chiusano, Secretary

4546 Oakland School & Camp
128 Oakland Farm Way
Troy, VA 22974
434-293-9059
Fax: 434-296-8930
information@oaklandschool.net
www.oaklandschool.net

A highly individualized program stresses improving reading ability. Subjects taught are reading, English composition, math and word analysis. Recreational activities include horseback riding, sports, swimming, tennis, crafts, archery and camping. For girls and boys, ages 8-14.

Carol Williams, Head of School
Jamie Cato, Admissions Director

4547 Phelps School
583 Sugartown Road
Malvern, PA 19355
610-644-1754
Fax: 610-644-6679
admis@thephelpsschool.org
www.thephelpsschool.org

Phelps School is dedicated to a personalized education for the boy who seeks success academically, personally, and socially. This philosophy is accentuated by the disciplined atmosphere, small classes, and daily tutorial support. The idea which inspired Norman T. Phelps, Sr. to begin a school dedicated to the individual boy has never been more relevant that it is today. The model of educating boys according to thier interests and abilities is designed to generate success & improve self-esteem.

Norman T. Phelps, Chairman
Stephany Phelps Fahey, President
Andrew Wilmerding, Secretary

4548 Ramapo Anchorage Camp
PO Box 266, Rt. 52/Salisbury Turnpike
Rhinebeck, NY 12572
845-876-8403
Fax: 845-876-8414
www.ramapoforchildren.org

Residential program which serves children, ages 4-16, with a wide range of emotional, behavoral, and learning problems. A one-to-one ratio of counselors-to-campers enables children to build healthy relationships, increase self-esteem and improve learning skills. Character values such as honesty, concern for others, responsibility, and the courage to do one's best are encouraged. Campers demonstrate significant gains in their ability to maintain relationships, control impulses and adjust.

Teri Goldberg Horowitz, President
David Ross, Vice President
Adam Weiss, Chief Executive Officer

4549 Round Lake Camp
570 Sawkill Road
Milford, PA 18337
570-296-8596
Fax: 570-296-6381
rlc@njycamps.org
www.njycamps.org

For ages 7-18, this camp provides individualized academics in reading, language development and math for children with mild learning disabilities, Round Lake also offers therapeutic recreation and Jewish cultural values to its participants.

Sheira Director, Asst. Director

4550 Squirrel Hollow
5665 Milam Road
Fairburn, GA 30213

770-774-8001
Fax: 770-774-8005
bbox@thebedfordschool.org
www.thebedfordschool.org

A remedial summer program of The Bedford School; serves children with academic needs due to learning difficulties. For students ages 6-16 and held on the campus of The Bedford School in Fairburn, GA. Campers participate in an individualized academic program as well as recreational activities. Students receive the proper academic remediation as well as specific remedial help with physical skills, peer interaction and self-esteem.

Michael Vigil, Chairman
Betsy E Box, Director
Jeff James, Assistant Director

4551 Summer Experience
Vanguard School
PO Box 730
Paoli, PA

610-296-6700

For students who are experiencing learning difficulties due to neurological impairment, social/emotional disturbance and/or autism/pervasive developmental disorder.

Susan Snyder, Admissions Director
John D Wilson, Education Director

4552 Wesley Woods
1001 Fiddlersgreen Road
Grand Valley, PA 16420

814-430-7802
Fax: 814-436-7669
info@wesleywoods.com
www.wesleywoods.com

Exceptional children's camp for children with emotional and intellectual handicaps.

Herb West

4553 Worthmore Academy
3535 Kessler Boulevard East Drive
Indianapolis, IN 46220

317-253-5367
877-700-6516
Fax: 317-251-6516
bjackson@worthmoreacademy.org
www.worthmoreacademy.org

A center for learning disabilities providing educational assessments, alternative educational programs, academic guidance and public awareness services available as follows: full-time day school, K-8th, 1 to 1 teacher student ratio; six week summer school, K-12th, 1 to 1 teacher student ratio; after school tutoring; adult tutoring, educational assessments, counseling and educational seminars.

Brenda J Jackson, Director
Diana Buser, Assistant

DESCRIPTION

4554 LEGG-CALVE-PERTHES DISEASE
Synonyms: LCPD, Perthes disease, Avasular necrosis of femoral head
Involves the following Biologic System(s):
Orthopedic and Muscle Disorders

Legg-Calve-Perthes disease (LCPD) belongs to a group of disorders in which abnormalities of the growth centers of certain bones result in degeneration and gradual regeneration of the affected bone. This group of disorders is known as the osteochondroses. LCPD affects the growing end of the head of the thigh bone (femoral capital epiphysis). In most affected children, the thigh bone (femur) on one side of the body is affected (unilateral); however, in approximately 20 percent of patients, the disorder may eventually involve the other femur (bilateral). The age of onset and the severity and duration of the disease are variable. Legg-Calve-Perthes disease typically becomes apparent between the ages of two to 12 years, with the average age of onset approximately seven years of age. Males are affected four to five times as often as females; however, females may tend to have more severe symptoms. LCPD is thought to affect approximately one in 1,000 to 5,000 children.

Degeneration of the head of the femur is thought to occur due to insufficient blood supply (ischemia) to this area of bone, resulting in the localized loss of bone and cartilage as well as the loss of bone mass. The onset of symptoms associated with LCPD is typically slow and progressive. Many affected children initially experience muscle spasms, a limp, or mild or periodic pain that may affect the thigh, hip, knee, or groin area. As the disorder progresses, additional symptoms and findings often include delayed maturation of the thigh bone (delayed bone age); mild restriction of movements of the affected hip; potential degeneration of the front thigh muscles; abnormal positioning of the hip and thigh toward the body (internal rotation); and, in some patients, mild short stature. LCPD is considered a self-limiting disorder because, even without medical intervention, new blood supplies are eventually spontaneously reestablished (revascularization) to the femoral head, causing the formation of new bone tissue in the affected area. This may occur approximately two to four years after the onset of symptoms. In some affected children, new bony growth may be misshapen, potentially causing the affected leg to be relatively shorter than the unaffected leg, an associated limp, and an increased risk for degenerative changes of the hips, resulting in swelling, pain or tenderness, and stiffness (osteoarthritis).

Because Legg-Calve-Perthes disease is a self-limiting disorder, treatment usually is directed toward preventing deformity of the femoral head and secondary osteoarthritis. Such measures may include ongoing clinical assessment and specialized x-ray tests to monitor the progress of the disease; bed rest or special stretching exercises; the use of braces or casts; or surgery.

There is no specific cause known for LCPD and, in most cases, it is though to occur randomly for unknown reasons. However, there are some risk factors including possible links to children who are small for their age and are extremely active. Interestingly, exposure to secondhand smoke is corre-lated with LCPD. There have also been reports of several affected individuals within certain families (kindreds) that suggest autosomal dominant inheritance. Some reseachers suspect that LCPD may be caused by the interaction of several different genes, possibly in association with the involvement of certain environmental factors (multifactorial disorder). Although Legg-Calvé-Perthes disease cannot be prevented, much has been accomplished toward minimizing its effects.

Government Agencies

4555 NIH/ Eunice Kennedy Shriver National Insti tute of Child Health & Human Development
31 Center Drive, Building 31
Bethesda, MD 20892
301-496-5113
800-370-2943
Fax: 866-760-5947
TTY: 888-320-6942
nichdpress@mail.nih.gov
www.nichd.nih.gov

Established in 1962 by congress, today the institute conducts and supports research on topics related to the health of children, adults, families and populations. Some of these topics include: developmental disabilities, growth and development, infant death, reproductive health and birth defects.

Diana W. Bianchi, Director
Paul Williams, Director, Communications

4556 NIH/National Institute of Arthritis & Musculoskeletal & Skin Diseases
National Institutes of Health
1AMS Circle, PO Box 3675
Bethesda, MD 20892
301-495-4484
877-226-4267
Fax: 301-718-6366
TTY: 301-565-2966
TDD: 301-565-2966
niamsinfo@mail.nih.gov
www.niams.nih.gov

The mission of the NIAMS, a part of the NIH, is to support research into the causes, treatment, and prevention of arthritis and musculoskeletal and skin diseases, the training of basic and clinical scientists to carry out this research, and the dissemination of information on research progress in these diseases.

Stephen I Katz MD PhD, Director
Robert H Carter MD, Deputy Director

4557 NIH/National Institute of Arthritis and Musculoskeletal and Skin Diseases
1 AMS Circle
Bethesda, MD 20892
301-495-4484
877-226-4267
Fax: 301-718-6366
TTY: 301-565-2966
TDD: 301-565-2966
niamsinfo@mail.nih.gov
www.niams.nih.gov

THe mission of the NIAMS, a part of the NIH, is to support research into the causes, treatment, and prevention of arthritis and musculoskeletal and skin diseases, the training of basic and clinical scientists to carry out this research, and the dissemination of information on research progress in these diseases.

Stephen I Katz MD PhD, Director
Robert H Carter MD, Deputy Director

National Associations & Support Groups

4558 American Academy of Pediatrics
141 Northwest Point Boulevard
Elk Grove Village, IL 60007
847-434-4000
800-433-9016
Fax: 847-434-8000
www.aap.org

533

The American Academy of Pediatrics and its member pediatricians are committed to the attainment of optimal physical, mental and social health and well-being for all infants, children, adolescents, and young adults.

Fernando Stein, MD, FAAP, President
Karen Remley, MD, CEO/Executive VP

4559 March of Dimes Foundation
1275 Mamaroneck Avenue
White Plains, NY 10605   914-997-4488
                                         888-663-4637
                                         Fax: 914-428-8203
                                         answers@marchofdimes.com
                                         www.marchofdimes.com

Partnership of volunteers and professionals dedicates to improving the health of babies by preventing birth defects and infant mortality. Over 100 chapters are located across the country and can be located through the National Office.

Stacey D. Stewart, President

4560 National Information Center on Deafness
Gallaudet Univ. Press c/o Chicago Distrib. Center
800 Florida Avenue NE, PO Box 3695
Washington, DC 20002   202-651-5000
                                         800-621-2736
                                         Fax: 202-651-5109
                                         TTY: 888-630-9347
                                         clerc.center@gallaudet.edu
                                         www.gallaudet.edu

Provides information or referrals on questions about deafness, including general information, education, research, legislation, assistive devices and more. Offers a bibliography of readings available on 30 topics relating to deafness.

Loraine DiPietro, Director

Web Sites

4561 Articles on Legg-Calve-Perthes
www.orthoseek.com/articles/perthes.html

                                         admin@orthoseek.com
                                         www.orthoseek.com/articles/perthes.html

A source of authoritative information on pediatric orthopedics and pediatric information regarding your child's orthopedic condition or sports injury, and you can find useful articles that you can reproduce for yourself or others.

4562 Online Support Group
www.maxpages.com/lpsupportgroup

Provides support groups for families with children diagnosed with Legg-Perthes disease.

4563 Wheeless' Textbook of Orthopaedics
www.wheelessonline.com

                                         410-494-4994
                                         www.wheelessonline.com

Derives from a variety of sources, including journals, articles, national meetings lectures and other textbooks.

Clifford R. Wheeless, Editor in chief
James A Nunley, Managing Editor
James R. Urbaniak, Managing Editor

DESCRIPTION

4564 LEUKODYSTROPHIES

Covers these related disorders: Adrenoleukodystrophy, ALD, Adrenomyeloneuropathy, Krabbe disease, Methachromatic leukodystrophy, Pelizaeus-Merzbacher disease

Involves the following Biologic System(s):
Genetic/Chromosomal/Syndrome/Metabolic Disorders

The leukodystrophies are a group of inherited neurodegenerative diseases that affect the white (leuko) matter of the brain and are characterized by the destruction of the fatty, protective covering around the nerve fibers (myelin sheaths). The symptoms of some forms of these diseases become obvious during childhood. These diseases include adrenoleukodystrophy (ALD), adrenomyeloneuropathy, Krabbe disease, metachromatic leukodystrophy, and Pelizaeus-Merzbacher disease.

Classic adrenoleukodystrophy, or ALD, is a metabolic disorder transmitted as an X-linked recessive trait that is fully expressed in boys. This type of adrenoleukodystrophy becomes apparent between the ages of five and 15 years and is characterized by behavioral disturbances, mental deterioration, seizures, lack of coordination, and motor weakness or partial paralysis with increased muscle tone in the arms and legs accompanied by exaggerated reflex responses (spasticity). In addition, boys with ALD may have difficulty with swallowing, language development, and speech. Vision may be impaired. Other findings include insufficient adrenal gland function characterized by a darkening or tanning of the skin. Experimental treatments include bone marrow transplantation and dietary considerations. Other treatment is symptomatic and supportive. The gene for classic ALD is located on the long arm of the X chromosome (Xq28). Adrenomyeloneuropathy is considered a milder, adult form of adrenoleukodystrophy, although its onset may occur as early as late adolescence.

Neonatal adrenoleukodystrophy is inherited as an autosomal recessive trait and is characterized by seizures, severe delays in skills that involve the coordination of mental and muscular activities (psychomotor coordination), and insufficiency of the adrenal glands. Treatment is symptomatic and supportive.

Krabbe disease, sometimes called globoid cell leukodystrophy, is a rare neurodegenerative disorder that is inherited as an autosomal recessive trait. This life-threatening, progressive disease results from a deficiency of the enzyme galactocerebrosidase and is characterized during early infancy by irritability, vomiting, extremely high fevers, difficulty feeding, and failure to thrive. Seizures may develop followed by muscular rigidity, convulsions, paralysis, , loss of vision and hearing, mental deterioration, or other irregularities. Krabbe disease may sometimes have a later onset with symptoms and findings developing during childhood or adolescence. Treatment is symptomatic and supportive. The gene for Krabbe disease is located on the long arm of chromosome 14 (14q21-q31).

Metachromatic leukodystrophy (MLD) is inherited in an autosomal recessive pattern and occurs as the result of a deficiency of the enzyme sulfatase A. Late infantile MLD usually occurs in the first or second year of life and is characterized by progressive irregularities in the manner of walking (gait), frequent falling, developmental delays, seizures, diminished muscle tone in the arms and legs, and diminished deep tendon reflexes. As the disease progresses, children may be unable to stand and signs of intellectual degeneration become apparent. Additional findings include impaired speech and deteriorating visual activity or blindness. Approximately one year after symptom onset, most children are unable to sit without support and may experience swallowing and eating difficulties. Life-threatening complications such as pneumonia may develop. Juvenile MLD occurs from the ages of four to 12 years and is characterized by behavioral and intellectual deterioration followed by walking and speech difficulties, urinary incontinence, lack of coordination, impaired muscle tone, and convulsions. This form of MLD has a slower progression than that of late infantile MLD. One variant of juvenile MLD results from a deficiency of a protein that aids in the activation of cerebroside sulfatase. The gene for metachromatic leukodystrophy is located on the long arm of chromosome 22 (22q13.31-qter).

Pelizaeus-Merzbacher disease is inherited as an X-linked recessive trait. This disorder occurs during infancy or early childhood and progresses slowly into adolescence or adulthood. This life-threatening form of leukodystrophy is characterized in infancy by head-nodding and eye irregularities such as involuntary, rhythmic movement of the eyes (nystagmus). Boys with this disorder experience developmental delays followed by tremors; well-coordinated but involuntary jerky, writhing movements; a mask-like, frozen expression (parkinsonian facies); difficulty with speech; and deterioration of mental function. Treatment is symptomatic and supportive. The gene for Pelizaeus-Merzbacher disease is located on the long arm of the X chromosome (Xq22). Bone marrow transplantation is showing promise for a few of the leukodystrophies.

National Associations & Support Groups

4565 American Academy of Pediatrics
141 Northwest Point Boulevard
Elk Grove Village, IL 60007

847-434-4000
800-433-9016
Fax: 847-434-8000
www.aap.org

The American Academy of Pediatrics and its member pediatricians are committed to the attainment of optimal physical, mental and social health and well-being for all infants, children, adolescents, and young adults.

Fernando Stein, MD, FAAP, President
Karen Remley, MD, CEO/Executive VP

4566 Genetic Alliance
4301 Connecticut Avenue NW, Suite 404
Washington, DC 20008

202-966-5557
800-336-4363
Fax: 202-966-8553
info@geneticalliance.org
www.geneticalliance.org

A coalition of voluntary genetic support groups, consumers and professionals addressing the needs of individuals and families affected by genetic disorders from a national perspective.

Sharon Terry, President/CEO
Tetyana Murza, Managing Director
Natasha Bonhomme, VP, Strategic Development

4567 March of Dimes Foundation
1275 Mamaroneck Avenue
White Plains, NY 10605
914-997-4488
888-663-4637
Fax: 914-428-8203
answers@marchofdimes.com
www.marchofdimes.com

Partnership of volunteers and professionals dedicates to improving the health of babies by preventing birth defects and infant mortality. Over 100 chapters are located across the country and can be located through the National Office.

Stacey D. Stewart, President

4568 National Tay-Sachs and Allied Diseases Association
2001 Beacon Street, Suite 204
Boston, MA 02135
617-277-4463
800-906-8723
Fax: 617-277-0134
info@ntsad.org
www.ntsad.org

Direct, fund and promote research treatments and cures; provides comprehensive support services to affected families and individuals; guides prevention, education, awareness and screening through effective grassroots collaborations with chapters and affiliates; leads advocacy efforts as the recognized authority for this family of genetic diseases

Kevin Romer, President
Stewart Altman, VP
Shari Ungerleider, Executive Director

4569 Neuropathy Association
60 E 42nd Street, Suite 942
New York, NY 10165
212-692-0662
Fax: 212-692-0668
info@neuropathy.org
www.neuropathy.org

A public, nonprofit organization which was established by people with neuropathy and their families or friends to help those who suffer from disorders that affect the peripheral nerves.

James R. Gardner, Chairman
Michael Sloser, Vice Chairman/Treasurer
Thomas H. Brannagan, MD

4570 United Leukodystrophy Foundation
224 North Second Street, Suite 2
DeKalb, IL 60115
815-748-3211
800-728-5483
Fax: 815-748-0844
office@ulf.org
www.ulf.org

Organization that aids those with leukodystrophy and those who care for them.

William Kintner, President
Tim Conway, Spokesperson
Tomothy Brazeal, Executive Director

Web Sites

4571 Medical College of Wisconsin
8701 Watertown Plank Road
Milwaukee, WI 53226
414-456-8296
webmaster@mcw.edu
www.mcw.edu

Mary Ellen Stanek, Chair
Stephen Roell, Vice Chairman
Jay B Williams, President

4572 NYU
550 First Avenue
New York, NY 10016
212-263-7300
www.med.nyu.edu

Robert I. Grossman, MD
Steven B Abramson, Senior Vice President
Andrew W Brotman, Senior Vice President

4573 Neuropathy Association
110 W. 40th, Suite #1804
New York, NY 10018
212-692-0662
Fax: 212-692-0668
info@neuropathy.org
www.neuropathy.org/

Supports research into the causes and treatment of perpiheral neuropathies, provides support through education and sharing information and experiences related to pripheral neuropathy, increases the public awareness pf the nature and extent of peripheral neuropathy and the need for early intervenion and research. We encourage pharmaceutical and biotechnology companies to develop new therapies and devices for treatment of neuropathy.

James R. Gardner, Chairman
Michael Sloser, Vice Chairman
Tina M. Tockarshewsky, President

4574 Online Mendelian Inheritance in Man
8600 Rockville Pike
Bethesda, MD 20894
301-594-5983
888-346-3656
Fax: 301-402-1384
TDD: 800-735-2258
custserv@nlm.nih.gov
www.ncbi.nlm.nih.gov

This database is a catalog of human genes and genetic disorders.

Christine E Seidman M.D, Chairman
David J Lipman M.D, Executive Secretary
Scott Edwards, Member

4575 Virtual Pediatric Hospital
www.virtualpediatrichospital.org

A digital library of pediatric information including resources for patients and health care professionals.

Book Publishers

4576 Let's Talk About Going to the Hospital
Rosen Publishing Group's PowerKids Press
29 E 21st Street
New York, NY 10010
212-777-3017
800-237-9932
Fax: 888-436-4643
rosenpub@tribeca.ios.com
www.rosenpublishing.com

If a child has to check into the hospital, chances are he or she is already upset about being ill. Knowing how a hospital functions and what the procedures are, such as when family members can visit, will help in what is already a stressful situation. Grades K-5.

24 pages
ISBN: 0-823950-36-0

Roger Rosen, President

DESCRIPTION

4577 LISSENCEPHALY

Synonym: Agyria

Covers these related disorders: Isolated lissencephaly sequence, Miller-Dieker lissencephaly syndrome, Norman-Roberts lissencephaly syndrome, Walker-Warburg syndrome, X-linked lissencephaly

Involves the following Biologic System(s):

Neurologic Disorders

Lissencephaly is a developmental abnormality in which the brain's surface is relatively smooth, resulting from incomplete formation of the folds or convolutions (gyri) of its surface (cerebral cortex). In most patients, the folds may be partially developed or altogether absent. Although lissencephaly was once thought to be a rare malformation, it is now considered more common, largely because of an increase in the number of diagnosed cases resulting from the use of advanced imaging techniques.

Lissencephaly has multiple causes and may occur in isolation, or in association with several underlying syndromes. Newborns with lissencephaly typically have a small head (microcephaly); episodes of uncontrolled electrical disturbances within the brain (seizures); difficulty in swallowing; muscle spasms; deformities of the hands, fingers, or toes; and mental retardation. When an underlying syndrome is present, lissencephaly may be accompanied by additional physical abnormalities. In some patients, lissencephaly can produce life-threatening complications during infancy or childhood. Isolated lissencephaly, which is an autosomal dominant trait, is caused by mutations of a gene known as the LIS 1 gene, which is located on chromosome 17. There have also been reports of numerous cases of lissencephaly in multigenerational families caused by mutations on chromosome X, which determines the female sex when paired with another X chromosome and male sex when paired with a Y chromosome. In male infants, this condition may include seizures that do not respond to treatment (intractable), growth failure, mental retardation, absence of the thick band of nerve fibers (corpus callosum) that connects the left and right halves or hemispheres of the brain, an abnormally small penis (microphallus), and life-threatening complications shortly after birth. In affected females who inherit only a single copy of the aberrant gene (heterozygotes), abnormalities are milder, including an unusual band of brain tissue under the cerebral cortex (subcortical heterotopia) and mild mental retardation and seizures.

Lissencephaly may also occur in association with several syndromes, including Miller-Dieker syndrome and Walker-Warburg syndrome. In a third syndrome, known as Norman-Roberts syndrome, lissencephaly is inherited in an autosomal recessive manner.

Treatment of lissencephaly most often only includes symptomatic and supportive measures. The effects of lissencephaly on the structure and function of the brain are largely untreatable, depending on the severity of this malformation. Many infants with lissencephaly die before the age of 2, often from respiratory infection or other respiratory disease, while others may survive but not develop beyond 3 to 5 months of age. In some cases, infants with lissencephaly survive and experience varying limitations in development, extending to nearly normal function and growth.

Government Agencies

4578 NIH/ Eunice Kennedy Shriver National Insti tute of Child Health & Human Development

31 Center Drive, Building 31
Bethesda, MD 20892

301-496-5113
800-370-2943
Fax: 866-760-5947
TTY: 888-320-6942
nichdpress@mail.nih.gov
www.nichd.nih.gov

Established in 1962 by congress, today the institute conducts and supports research on topics related to the health of children, adults, families and populations. Some of these topics include: developmental disabilities, growth and development, infant death, reproductive health and birth defects.

Diana W. Bianchi, Director
Paul Williams, Director, Communications

National Associations & Support Groups

4579 AmeriFace

PO Box 751112
Las Vegas, NV 89136

702-769-9264
888-486-1209
Fax: 702-341-5351
info@ameriface.org
www.ameriface.org

To provide information, services, emotional support and educational programs for and on behalf of individuals with facial difference and their families. Working to increase understanding through public awareness and education.

David Reisberg, President
Christina Corsiglia, VP
Teresa Grillo, Secretary/Treasurer

4580 American Academy of Pediatrics

141 Northwest Point Boulevard
Elk Grove Village, IL 60007

847-434-4000
800-433-9016
Fax: 847-434-8000
www.aap.org

The American Academy of Pediatrics and its member pediatricians are committed to the attainment of optimal physical, mental and social health and well-being for all infants, children, adolescents, and young adults.

Fernando Stein, MD, FAAP, President
Karen Remley, MD, CEO/Executive VP

4581 Birth Defect Research for Children

976 Lake Baldwin Lane, Suite 104
Orlando, FL 32814

407-895-0802
Fax: 407-895-0824
staff@birthdefects.org
www.birthdefects.org

Organization that helps families with free birth defect information, parent matching that links families of children with similar defects and research through the National Birth Defect Registry to discover the causes of birth defects. Support group information and newsletter on Internet.

James Murphy, Associate Professor
JD Sherman, Adjunct Professor

4582 Children's Craniofacial Association

13140 Coit Road, Suite 517
Dallas, TX 75240

214-570-9099
800-535-3643
Fax: 214-570-8811
contactCCA@ccakids.com
www.ccakids.com

Devoted to the dispersion of medical knowledge of this and similar disorders, along with providing emotional support for the sufferers and their families.

Dede Dankelson, Chair
George Dale, Vice Chair
Bill Mecklenburg, Secretary

4583   FACES: National Association for the Craniofacially Handicapped
PO Box 11082
Chattanooga, TN 37401

423-266-1632
800-332-2373
Fax: 423-267-3124
faces@faces-cranio.org
www.faces-cranio.org

Assists individuals with facial disfigurations and their families They maintain a registry of centers offering corrective surgery for craniofacial deformities and financial assistance to qualified applicants.

4584   Fighters for Encephaly Support Group
332 Brereton Street
Pittsburgh, PA 15219

412-687-6437
Fax: 412-331-4365

4585   Forward Face: The Charity for Children with Craniofacial Conditions
Institute of Reconstructive Plastic Surgery
333 East 30th Street, Lobby Unit
New York, NY 10016

212-263-6656
Fax: 212-263-7534
info@forwardface.org
www.forwardface.org

Provision of data and emotional assistance to both sufferers and medical professionals.

Eileen Newman, Manager
John R. Gordon, Chairman
Richard Jennings, Treasurer

4586   Lissencephaly Network
10408 Bitterroot Court
Fort Wayne, IN 46804

260-432-4310
Fax: 260-432-4310
lissencephalyone@aol.com
www.lissencephaly.org

Lissencephaly is a genetic disorder that can be inherited from the parents or can occur during cell division. This web site is provided for the parents, siblings, physicians and therapists of children born with lissencephaly (smooth brain), and other neuronal migration disorders.

Story C. Landis, Medical Director

4587   March of Dimes Foundation
1275 Mamaroneck Avenue
White Plains, NY 10605

914-997-4488
888-663-4637
Fax: 914-428-8203
answers@marchofdimes.com
www.marchofdimes.com

Partnership of volunteers and professionals dedicates to improving the health of babies by preventing birth defects and infant mortality. Over 100 chapters are located across the country and can be located through the National Office.

Stacey D. Stewart, President

4588   National Craniofacial Foundation
7777 Forest Lane Suite C621
Dallas, TX 75230

972-566-6669
800-535-3643

4589   National Dissemination Center for Children with Disabilities
1825 Connecticut Avenue NW, Suite 700
Washington, DC 20009

202-884-8200
800-695-0285
Fax: 202-884-8441
nichcy@aed.org
www.nichcy.org

A national information and referral center that provides information on disabilities and disability-related issues for families, educators and other professionals.

Suzanne Ripley, Executive Director

4590   National Hydrocephalus Foundation
12413 Centrailia Road
Lakewood, CA 90715

562-924-6666
888-857-3434
nhf@earthlink.net
www.nhfonline.org

Promotes information and educational assistance. Establishes and facilitates a communication network and works to increase public awareness. Quarterly newsletter included with annual membership fee of $30.00.

Debbie Fields, Executive Director
Michael Fields, President/Treasurer
Jaynie Dunn, Secretary

4591   Society for the Rehabilitation of the Facially Disfigured Inc.
99 Pleasant Street
Northampton, MA 01060

413-584-1900
Fax: 413-584-1934
info@explorenorthampton.com
www.explorenorthampton.com

Rick Feldman, President
Christine Aubrey
Charles Bowles

4592   World Craniofacial Foundation
P.O. Box 515838
Dallas, TX 75251

972-566-6669
800-533-3315
Fax: 972-566-3850
info@worldcf.org
www.worldcf.org

The World Craniofacial Foundation is a nonprofit corporation, dedicated to helping children obtain the life-changing craniofacial surgery they deserve.

Kenneth E. Salyer, Founder And Chairman
Andrew Christensen, Secretary/Treasurer
Douglas Canfield, CEO

Web Sites

4593   Independent Holoprosencephaly Support Site
hpe.home.att.net

This site is home to an online support group for parents of children with HPE, or anyone who cares for a child with HPE.

4594   National Hydrocephalus Foundation
www.nhfonline.org

Promotes information and educational assistance. Establishes and facilitates a communication network and works to increase public awareness. Promote and support research. Also has brochures, help sheets and more. Quarterly newsletter included with annual membership fee of $35.00.

4595   Online Mendelian Inheritance in Man
8600 Rockville Pike
Bethesda, MD 20894

301-594-5983
888-346-3656
Fax: 301-402-1384
TDD: 800-735-2258
custserv@nlm.nih.gov
www.ncbi.nlm.nih.gov

This database is a catalog of human genes and genetic disorders.

Christine E Seidman M.D, Chairman
David J Lipman M.D, Executive Secretary
Scott Edwards, Member

4596   Rare Genetic Diseases in Children (NYU)
550 First Avenue
New York, NY 10016

212-263-7300
www.med.nyu.edu

We target issues arising from rare genetic diseases affecting children. Also, to assist in the endeavor to bring knowledge and hope to those for whom there is, at present, so little.

Robert I. Grossman, MD
Steven B Abramson, Senior Vice President
Andrew W Brotman, Senior Vice President

Book Publishers

4597 Congenital Disorders Sourcebook 2nd Edit.
Omnigraphics
PO Box 8002
Aston, PA 19014

800-234-1340
Fax: 800-875-1340
info@omnigraphics.com
www.omnigraphics.com

Basic consumer health information on disorders aquired during gestation, including spina bifida, hydrocephalus, cerebral palsy, heart defects, craniofacial abnormalities and fetal alcohol syndrome.

647 pages
ISBN: 0-780809-45-1

Peter Ruffner, Publisher
Frederick Ruffner, Jr. Chairman

4598 Let's Talk About Going to the Hospital
Rosen Publishing Group's PowerKids Press
29 E 21st Street
New York, NY 10010

212-777-3017
800-237-9932
Fax: 888-436-4643
rosenpub@tribeca.ios.com
www.rosenpublishing.com

If a child has to check into the hospital, chances are he or she is already upset about being ill. Knowing how a hospital functions and what the procedures are, such as when family members can visit, will help in what is already a stressful situation. Grades K-5.

24 pages
ISBN: 0-823950-36-0

Roger Rosen, President

Newsletters

4599 National Hydrocephalus Foundation Newsletter
12413 Centralia Road
Lakewood, CA 90715

562-924-6666
888-857-3434
Fax: 415-732-7044
debbifields@nhfonline.org
www.nhfonline.org

The Foundation is a national organization whose purpose is to provide information and education, along with peer support newsletter quarterly.

12-15 pages Quarterly

Michael Fields, President/Treasurer
Debbie Fields, Executive Director
Jaynie Dunn, Secretary

DESCRIPTION

4600 LYME DISEASE

Synonym: Deer tick disease

Covers these related disorders: Bell's palsy

Involves the following Biologic System(s):

Infectious Disorders

Lyme disease is a bacterial (Borrelia burgdorferi) infection that is transmitted by being bitten by the nymph stage of the deer tick Ixodides. It is not contagious, that is, it is not spread by contact with people or animals with Lyme disease. Lyme disease has been found in the Northeast from Maine to Virginia, the upper Midwest and on the West Coast. The most common first sign of Lyme disease is a rash at the site of the tick bite. It is a red circular rash, often with an area of central clearing (target lesion) and is called erythema migrans.

Lyme disease has three stages, early localized, early disseminated and late disease. Early localized disease is marked by the typical rash and may also include flu-like symptoms. It occurs between 7 and 10 days after the tick bite. The most common symptom of early disseminated disease is multiple erythema migrans, but patients can develop cranial nerve palsies (including Bell's palsy), meningitis, or carditis leading to heartblock on seen on an electrocardiogram (ECG). Systemic symptoms can include muscle and joint aches, fatigue and headaches. Symptoms of early disseminated disease develop from days to weeks in the untreated patient. Late Lyme disease happens weeks to months after the tick bite and is marked by arthritis of one or more large joints.

Diagnosis of Lyme disease is primarily made based on history and physical findings. Serologic testing (i.e. blood test) can be useful for diagnosis in some cases, but interpreting the immunologic tests can be difficult and it is important to utilize a high quality lab for testing. The serologic testing can not be used to assess treatment success.

Antibiotics are used to treat all stages of Lyme disease. The stage and specific symptoms determine how long treatment needs to be and whether or not the therapy can be oral or intravenous. Doxycycline is the drug of choice in patients with erythema migrans or a suspicion of Lyme disease based on clinical findings. There is no evidence supporting chronic or multiple courses of antibiotics for Lyme disease. Patients who continue to have symptoms more than six months after treatment should be evaluated for other inflammatory diseases. Prevention is important. Tick bites can be prevented by taking precautions when spending time outdoors, for instance, wearing loose fitting long sleeves and long pants; applying tick repellant; and decreasing environmental contacts with deer. A thorough search for ticks after outdoor exposure is essential. The LYMErix vaccine is no longer being manufactured, owing to its pain and at times debilitatin side effects.

National Associations & Support Groups

4601 American Academy of Pediatrics
141 Northwest Point Boulevard
Elk Grove Village, IL 60007   847-434-4000
                                             800-433-9016
                                         Fax: 847-434-8000
                                              www.aap.org

The American Academy of Pediatrics and its member pediatricians are committed to the attainment of optimal physical, mental and social health and well-being for all infants, children, adolescents, and young adults.

Fernando Stein, MD, FAAP, President
Karen Remley, MD, CEO/Executive VP

4602 American Camp Association
5000 State Road 67 North
Martinsville, IN 46151   765-342-8456
                                             800-428-2267
                                         Fax: 765-342-2065
                                          www.acacamps.org

The American Camp Association is a community of camp professionals who, for over 100 years, have joined together to share our knowledge and experience and to ensure the quality of camp programs.

Tisha Bolger, President
Rue Mapp, Vice President
Melanie Lockwood Herman, Treasurer

4603 American Lyme Disease Foundation
P.O. Box 466
Lyme, CT 06371   914-277-6970
                                             800-876-5963
                                         Fax: 914-277-6974
                                        questions@aldf.com
                                              www.aldf.com

Supports research and plays a key role in providing reliable and scientifically accurate information to the public, health care provider, and government agencies about tick-borne diseases and their potentially serious effects on our health and quality of life.

Philip J Baker, Directore Director
Thomas P. Farrell, MD
Durland Fish, Professor

4604 Center for Peripheral Neuropathy
The University of Chicago, 5841 South Maryland Ave
Chicago, IL 60637   773-702-5659
                         peripheralneuropathycenter.uchicago.edu

The Center for Peripheral Neuropathy are committed to educating the public and healthcare providers about this disease, providing state-of-the-art care to patients affected by peripheral neuropathy, and contributing to basic and clinical research in an effort to identify the causes and potential cures for these disorders.

4605 Children's Lyme Disease Network
76 Kettles Way
Queensbury, NY 12804   914-506-0890
                              www.childrenslymenetwork.org

Children's Lyme Disease Network is an all-volunteer organization consisting of parents, caregivers and family members who have seen first-hand the struggles a child can face once infected with Lyme Disease.

4606 Lyme Disease Association, Inc. (LDA)
PO Box 1438
Jackson, NJ 8527   888-366-6611
                                         Fax: 732-938-7215
                                           lymeliter@aol.com
                              www.lymediseaseassociation.org

A national organization dedicated to raising funds for Lyme and tick-borne diseases education, prevention, research and patient support. LDA has funded dozens of research projects nationally, helped endow a research center for chronic Lyme and Columbia, has a fund for children without insurance coverage and an interactive video game for kids online and free brochures.

Patricia Smith, President
Pam Lampe, Vice President

4607 Lyme Disease Foundation
Po Box 332
Tolland, CT 06084

860-525-2000
800-866-5963
Fax: 860-870-0080
info@lyme.org
www.lyme.org

Nonprofit organization dedicated to finding solutions for tick-borne disorders. Offers support to the public and medical communities.

John F Anderson, Director
Nicole Augenti, Director
Berkley Bedell, Director

4608 Lyme Disease Research Foundation
Johns Hopkins at Green Spring Station, 10755 Falls
Lutherville, MD 21093   www.lymemd.org

LymeMD, a non-profit organization, was created in 2007 by Dr. John Aucott, an infectious disease specialist, in response to the devastating toll that Lyme disease takes on previously healthy, energetic individuals. LymeMD has become a nationally recognized program attracting top collaborators around the country.

Alex Mason, President
Joseph Hardiman, Vice-President
Lawrence Macks, Vice-President

4609 Lyme Induced Autism Foundation
1771 Honors Lane
Corona, CA 92883

Fax: 951-817-1173
info@liafoundation.org
www.lymeinducedautism.com

LIA was started because parents with Lyme disease were finding that their children with autism were also testing positive for Lyme disease and experiencing symptoms of Lyme disease and associated co-infections.

4610 Lyme Research Alliance
2001 West Main Street, Suite 280
Stamford, CT 6902

203-969-1333
info@lymeresearchalliance.org
www.lymeresearchalliance.org

Lyme Research Alliance funds cutting-edge research into Lyme and other tick-borne diseases.

4611 Madisons Foundation
P.O. Box 241956
Los Angeles, CA 90024

310-264-0826
Fax: 310-264-4766
getinfo@madisonsfoundation.org
www.madisonsfoundation.org

Madisons Foundation is dedicated to improving the quality and quantity of information available to parents of children with rare, life-threatening diseases, and to facilitating effective communication among parents, physicians and medical experts.

Marcy Smith, Executive Director
Chris Barrettÿ, Board of Director
David Strybel, Board of Director

4612 NIH/National Institute of Arthritis and Musculoskeletal and Skin Diseases
1 AMS Circle
Bethesda, MD 20892

301-495-4484
877-226-4267
Fax: 301-718-6366
TTY: 301-565-2966
NIAMSinfo@mail.nih.gov
www.niams.nih.gov

The mission of the National Institute of Arthritis and Musculoskeletal and Skin Diseases is to support research into the causes, treatment, and prevention of arthritis and musculoskeletal and skin diseases; the training of basic and clinical scientists to carry out this research; and the dissemination of information on research progress in these diseases.

Stephen I. Katz, M.D., Ph.D., Executive Director

4613 National Capital Lyme Disease Association
P.O. Box 8211
McLean, VA 22106

703-821-8833
www.natcaplyme.org

The National Capital Lyme Disease Association is an all volunteer not-for-profit organization that is committed to helping patients diagnosed with tick-borne illnesses.

Monte Skall, Executive Director
Karen Weber, Executive Director
Sharon Whitehouse, Executive Director

4614 Tick-Borne Disease Alliance
244 Fifth Avenue, Suite 1450
New York, NY 10001

646-450-4882
Fax: 914-967-7744
medicalinfo@tbdalliance.org
www.tbdalliance.org

Tick-Borne Disease Alliance (TBDA) is dedicated to raising awareness, promoting advocacy, and supporting initiatives to find a cure for tick-borne diseases, including Lyme.

Staci Grodin, President
Drew Goldman, Vice President
Nan Kurzman, Vice President

Web Sites

4615 American Lyme Disease Foundation
Post Office Box 466
Lyme, CT 6371

Executivedir@aldf.com
www.aldf.com

Provides reliable and scientifically accurate information to the public about tick borne diseases and their potentially serious effects on our life.

Phillip J. Baker, Executive Director
Durland Fish, Director
Red Pfohl, Director

4616 Lyme Disease Association, Inc. (LDA)
www.lymediseaseassociation.org

A national organization dedicated to raising funds for Lyme and tick-borne diseases education, prevention, research and patient support. LDA has funded dozens of research projects nationally, helped endow a research center for chronic Lyme and Columbia, has a fund for children without insurance coverage and an interactive video game for kids online and free brochures.

4617 Lyme Disease Foundation
www.lyme.org

Nonprofit organization that works to find solutions for tick borne disorders.

Book Publishers

4618 Aspects of Lyme Borreliosis
Springer-Verlag
11 West 42nd Street 15th Floor
New York, NY 10036

212-431-4370
877-687-7476
Fax: 212-941-7842
cs@springerpub.com
www.springerpub.com

1992 384 pages hardcover
ISBN: 0-387556-28-1

Theodore C. Nardin, CEO

4619 Ecology and Enviromental Management of Lyme Disease
Rutgers University Press
100 Joyce Kilmer Avenue
Piscataway, NJ 8854

732-445-7762
800-446-9323
Fax: 732-445-7039
bksales@rci.rutgers.edu

1993 hardcover
ISBN: 0-813519-28-4

Marlie Wasserman, Director
Christina Brianik, Assistant to the Director
Molly Venezia, Director of Finance

4620 Let's Talk About Having Lyme Disease
Rosen Publishing Group
29 E 21st Street
New York, NY 10010   800-237-9932
                                    Fax: 888-436-4643
                            customerservice@rosenpub.com
                                 www.rosenpublishing.com

Discusses what Lyme disease is, how one gets it, and what to do about it.

2003 24 pages hardcover
ISBN: 0-823950-29-8

Roger Rosen, President

4621 Lyme Disease
Enslow Publishers
Box 398 40 Industrial Road,
Berkeley Heights, NJ 07922   908-771-9400
                                      800-398-2504
                                    Fax: 908-771-0925
                            customerService@enslow.com

Outlines Lyme Disease, from its discovery to current trends. The transmission of the disease from the deer tick, and its course of infection in the body are clearly discribed. Methods for protection from the disease are mixed with real life stories of patients who have contracted Lyme disease. The symptoms, diagnosis, treatment, and prevention are also covered.

104 pages hardcover
ISBN: 0-766010-52-x

Mark Enslow, President
Brian Enslow, Vice President/Publisher

4622 Lyme Disease (Deadly Diseases and Epidemics)
Chelsea House Publishing
2080 Cabot Boulevard W, Suite 201
Langhorne, PA 19047   800-848-2665
                                    Fax: 877-780-7300

110 pages

Journals

4623 Journal of Spirochetal and Tick-borne Diseases
1 Financial Plaza
Hartford, CT 6103   860-525-2000
                                    Fax: 860-525-8425
                                    lymefnd@aol.com
                                       www.jstd.org

Reviews all aspects of spirochetal or tick-borne disorders. Clinical topics may involve all medical disciplines, nursing, and pharmacy, as well as the social, ethnical and biological features of such disorders.

Quaterly

Ronald Schell PHD, Editor in Chief
Willy Burgdorfer PHD, Deputy Editor
Sam Donta, Consulting Editor

Newsletters

4624 Journal of the American Medical Association
PO Box 10946
Chicago, IL 60610   312-670-7827
                                      800-262-2350
                            subscriptions@jamanetwork.com
                                   jama.ama-assn.org

To promote the science and art of medicine and the betterment of the public health.

DESCRIPTION

4625 MACROCEPHALY

Synonyms: Macrocephalia, Megalocephaly

Covers these related disorders: Benign familial macrocephaly, Megalencephaly

Involves the following Biologic System(s):

Neurologic Disorders

Macrocephaly (macro = long; cephaly = head) is a term that is used to describe an isolated or primary condition in which an infant's or a child's head circumference is more than two standard deviations above the mean for age and sex. As a rule of thumb, a newborn's head is usually about 2 centimeters larger than the chest size. Between 6 months and 2 years, both measurements are about equal. After 2 years, the chest size becomes larger than the head.

Primary macrocephaly may be apparent at birth or during early infancy. In some affected infants and children, overgrowth of the brain results in varying degrees of mental retardation. Associated symptoms and findings may include episodes of uncontrolled electrical disturbances in the brain (seizures); unusually large or small stature; and motor abnormalities ranging from diminished muscle tone (hypotonia) to muscle rigidity and associated restrictions of movement (spasticity). Patients with overgrowth of the brain (megalencephaly) have normally sized or slightly enlarged cavities of the brain (ventricles) and no evidence of underlying conditions, such as certain metabolic disorders (metabolic megalencephaly). Although infants and children with macrocephaly may have abnormal delays in the acquisition of skills requiring the coordination of physical and mental activities (psychomotor delays), they do not experience regression of such skills, a finding that is typically associated with infantile metabolic megalencephaly or certain other underlying conditions.

Some infants and children with primary macrocephaly experience no associated mental retardation or other neurologic deficits. Several such cases have been reported in individuals within certain multigenerational families. This form of benign or nonsyndromic macrocephaly, known as benign familial macrocephaly, is thought to have autosomal dominant inheritance.

Although infants with primary macrocephaly experience increasing head size, they typically do not have symptoms and findings associated with increased cerebrospinal fluid (CSF) pressure within the brain (intracranial pressure). This is in contrast to hydrocephalus, a condition in which the brain swells due to an abnormal accumulation of CSF under increasing pressure within the brain's ventricles. However, some infants with primary macrocephaly may have a slight separation of the fibrous joints (cranial sutures) between certain bones in the skull.

Although the specific underlying cause of primary macrocephaly is not understood, overgrowth of the brain is due to the presence of abnormally large or an unusually increased number of brain cells. The outer region of the brain (cerebral cortex) appears normal in some cases; however, others have structural abnormalities.

As mentioned above, overgrowth of the brain may occur as a secondary finding associated with certain progressive infantile metabolic diseases, such as Tay-Sachs disease, or other underlying geneticdisorders, such as neurofibromatosis. The condition may also occur as a result of certain structural abnormalities of the brain, such as absence of the band of nerve fibers that joins the two cerebral hemispheres (agenesis of corpus callosum), or due to a localized accumulation of blood between the outer and middle layers of the membrane that surrounds and protects the brain and spinal cord (subdural hematoma). Infants and children with macrocephaly who experience psychomotor regression should receive thorough clinical, neurologic, metabolic, and other appropriate evaluations to rule out or confirm the presence of certain underlying disorders or conditions.

The treatment of infants and children with isolated or primary macrocephaly includes symptomatic and supportive measures. These may include the prescription of certain medications to help treat or control seizures (e.g., anticonvulsants) and physical therapy, special education, and other multidisciplinary measures to ensure that patients with motor impairments and mental retardation reach their potential. In infants and children with secondary macrocephaly, treatment includes appropriate therapies for any diagnosed, underlying causes of the condition.

Government Agencies

4626 NIH/ Eunice Kennedy Shriver National Insti tute of Child Health & Human Development
31 Center Drive, Building 31
Bethesda, MD 20892

301-496-5113
800-370-2943
Fax: 866-760-5947
TTY: 888-320-6942
nichdpress@mail.nih.gov
www.nichd.nih.gov

Established in 1962 by congress, today the institute conducts and supports research on topics related to the health of children, adults, families and populations. Some of these topics include: developmental disabilities, growth and development, infant death, reproductive health and birth defects.

Diana W. Bianchi, Director
Paul Williams, Director, Communications

National Associations & Support Groups

4627 ARC of the United States
1825 K Street MW, Suite 1200
Washington, DC 20006

202-534-3700
800-433-5255
Fax: 202-534-3731
info@thearc.org
www.thearc.org

The ARC is the national organization of and for people with mental retardation and related developmental disabilities and their families. Devoted to promoting and improving supports and services for people with mental retardation and their families. The association also fosters research and education regarding the prevention of mental retardation in infants and young children. The ARC was founded in 1950 by a small group of parents and other concerned individuals.

Nancy Webster, President
Ronald Brown, VP
Elise McMillan, Secretary

4628 American Academy of Pediatrics
141 Northwest Point Boulevard
Elk Grove Village, IL 60007

847-434-4000
800-433-9016
Fax: 847-434-8000
www.aap.org

The American Academy of Pediatrics and its member pediatricians are committed to the attainment of optimal physical, mental and social health and well-being for all infants, children, adolescents, and young adults.

Fernando Stein, MD, FAAP, President
Karen Remley, MD, CEO/Executive VP

4629 Birth Defect Research for Children
976 Lake Baldwin Lane, Suite 104
Orlando, FL 32814

407-895-0802
Fax: 407-895-0824
staff@birthdefects.org
www.birthdefects.org

Organization that helps families with free birth defect information, parent matching that links families of children with similar defects and research through the National Birth Defect Registry to discover the causes of birth defects. Support group information and newsletter on Internet.

James Murphy, Associate Professor
JD Sherman, Adjunct Professor

4630 Genetic Alliance
4301 Connecticut Avenue NW, Suite 404
Washington, DC 20008

202-966-5557
800-336-4363
Fax: 202-966-8553
info@geneticalliance.org
www.geneticalliance.org

A coalition of voluntary genetic support groups, consumers and professionals addressing the needs of individuals and families affected by genetic disorders from a national perspective.

Sharon Terry, President/CEO
Tetyana Murza, Managing Director
Natasha Bonhomme, VP, Strategic Development

4631 National Dissemination Center for Children with Disabilities
1825 Connecticut Avenue NW, Suite 700
Washington, DC 20009

202-884-8200
800-695-0285
Fax: 202-884-8441
nichcy@aed.org
www.nichcy.org

A national information and referral center that provides information on disabilities and disability-related issues for families, educators and other professionals.

Suzanne Ripley, Executive Director

Web Sites

4632 Online Mendelian Inheritance in Man
8600 Rockville Pike
Bethesda, MD 20894

301-594-5983
888-346-3656
Fax: 301-402-1384
TDD: 800-735-2258
custserv@nlm.nih.gov
www.ncbi.nlm.nih.gov

This database is a catalog of human genes and genetic disorders.

Christine E Seidman M.D, Chairman
David J Lipman M.D, Executive Secretary
Scott Edwards, Member

DESCRIPTION

4633 MAPLE SYRUP URINE DISEASE

Synonyms: Branched chain ketoaciduria, MSUD

Covers these related disorders: Classic MSUD, Mild (intermediate) MSUD, Intermittent MSUD, Thiamine-responsive MSUD

Involves the following Biologic System(s):

Genetic/Chromosomal/Syndrome/Metabolic Disorders

Maple syrup urine disease (MSUD) is a metabolic disorder characterized by the deficiency of certain enzymes of the branched-chain alpha-ketoacid dehydrogenase complex that break down (catabolize) three essential organic compounds. These compounds are known as amino acids and are the building blocks of protein. These amino acids include leucine, isoleucine, and valine. A deficiency of any enzyme within this complex results in the symptoms of MSUD and leads to encephalopathy, a condition characterized by altered brain function. There are four basic types of maple syrup urine disease.

Classic MSUD, the most severe form of this disorder, becomes apparent within the first week of life and is recognizable by a characteristic maple syrup odor of the urine and on the body. Symptoms and physical findings associated with this life-threatening form of MSUD include listlessness, drowsiness, exaggerated muscular tension (hypertonicity) and rigidity with periods of loss of muscle tone (flaccidity), severe muscle spasms resulting in a backward arching of the back and neck (opisthotonus), convulsions, and coma. Additional findings include low blood sugar (hypoglycemia) and higher-than-normal acidic levels in the blood as well as abnormally low bicarbonate levels (metabolic acidosis). In addition, severe life-threatening complications may occur following infection, surgery, or other stressful events. Such complications include an excessive accumulation of fluid around the brain (cerebral edema) and acidosis accompanied by excessive levels of certain organic compounds in the tissues and body fluids (ketosis). Many affected children experience neurologic and mental deficiencies.

Treatment for classic MSUD includes the removal of leucine, isoleucine, valine, and certain other related elements from the blood by a procedure known as peritoneal dialysis. Subsequent therapy includes a diet low in leucine, isoleucine, and valine.

Intermittent MSUD develops suddenly in children who had previously exhibited no signs of the disease. Though this form of the disease is intermittent, the characteristic findings, symptoms, severity of complications, and treatment are similar to those of classic MSUD. In addition, children with this form of the disorder may exhibit more activity of certain enzymes than those with the classic form.

Mild or intermediate MSUD is a less severe form of this disorder that usually affects children after the first month of life. Affected infants may be mildly retarded and usually emit the characteristic maple syrup odor in their urine, sweat, and earwax (cerumen).

Characteristic findings and symptoms associated with thia-mine-responsive MSUD are similar to those of intermittent or intermediate disease. The distinguishing feature is that treatment with high doses of vitamin B1 (thiamine) often results in a favorable response. Early diagnosis and dietary intervention prevent complications and may allow for normal intellectual development. Consequently, MSUD has been added to many newborn screening programs, and preliminary results indicate that asymptomatic newborns with MSUD have a better outcome compared with infants who are diagnosed after they become symptomatic.

Maple syrup urine disease is inherited as an autosomal recessive trait. Approximately one in 200,000 people in the United States is affected by this disorder.

National Associations & Support Groups

4634 ARC of the United States
1825 K Street MW, Suite 1200
Washington, DC 20006

202-534-3700
800-433-5255
Fax: 202-534-3731
info@thearc.org
www.thearc.org

The ARC is the national organization of and for people with mental retardation and related developmental disabilities and their families. Devoted to promoting and improving supports and services for people with mental retardation and their families. The association also fosters research and education regarding the prevention of mental retardation in infants and young children. The ARC was founded in 1950 by a small group of parents and other concerned individuals.

Nancy Webster, President
Ronald Brown, VP
Elise McMillan, Secretary

4635 American Academy of Pediatrics
141 Northwest Point Boulevard
Elk Grove Village, IL 60007

847-434-4000
800-433-9016
Fax: 847-434-8000
www.aap.org

The American Academy of Pediatrics and its member pediatricians are committed to the attainment of optimal physical, mental and social health and well-being for all infants, children, adolescents, and young adults.

Fernando Stein, MD, FAAP, President
Karen Remley, MD, CEO/Executive VP

4636 Association for Neuro-Metabolic Disorders
5223 Brookfield Lane
Sylvania, OH 43560

419-885-1809
volk4olks@aol.com

Nonprofit organization that serves as an advocate organization for families of patients with the following neuro-metabolic disorders: phenylketonuria, maple syrup urine disease, galactosemia, and biotinidase deficiency. Provides educational information for parents and children; provides networking information on support groups for new parents; supports scientific research into the treatments of these four neuro-metabolic disorders.

Cheryl Volk, Contact Person

4637 Genetic Alliance
4301 Connecticut Avenue NW, Suite 404
Washington, DC 20008

202-966-5557
800-336-4363
Fax: 202-966-8553
info@geneticalliance.org
www.geneticalliance.org

A coalition of voluntary genetic support groups, consumers and professionals addressing the needs of individuals and families affected by genetic disorders from a national perspective.

Sharon Terry, President/CEO
Tetyana Murza, Managing Director
Natasha Bonhomme, VP, Strategic Development

4638 MSUD:(Maple Syrup Urine Disease) Family Support Group
82 Ravine Road
Powell, OH 43065   614-389-2739
                                                    dbulcehr@aol.com
                                                    www.msud-support.org

MSUD is a nonprofit (501)(c)(3) organization for parents of children with MSUD, adults with MSUD, health-care professionals and others interested in MSUD. Dedicated to providing opportunities for support and personal contact for those with MSUD and their families, distributing information and raising public awareness of MSUD, strengthening the liaison between families and professionals and encouraging newborn screening programs and research for MSUD.

Sandy Bulcher, Director
Marcia Hubbard, Secretary
Dave Bulcher, Treasurer

4639 March of Dimes Foundation
1275 Mamaroneck Avenue
White Plains, NY 10605   914-997-4488
                                                    888-663-4637
                                                    Fax: 914-428-8203
                                                    answers@marchofdimes.com
                                                    www.marchofdimes.com

Partnership of volunteers and professionals dedicates to improving the health of babies by preventing birth defects and infant mortality. Over 100 chapters are located across the country and can be located through the National Office.

Stacey D. Stewart, President

Libraries & Resource Centers

4640 National Digestive Diseases Information Clearinghouse
9000 Rockville Pike
Bethesda, MD 20892   301-496-3583
                                                    800-860-8747
                                                    Fax: 301-907-8906
                                                    healthinfo@niddk.nih.gov
                                                    www.niddk.nih.govv

The National Institute of Diabetes and Digestive and Kidney Diseases conducts and supports research on many of the most serious diseases affecting public health. The Institute supports much of the clinical research on the diseases of internal medicine and related subspecialty fields as well as many basic science disciplines.

Dr. Griffin P. Rodgers, Director
Dr. Gregory G. Germino, Deputy Directortary
Camille M. Hoover, M.S.W., Executive Officer

Web Sites

4641 Family Village
www.familyvillage.wisc.edu

A global community that integrates information, resources and communication opportunities on the Internet for persons with cognitive and other disabilities, for their families and for those that provide them services and support.

Book Publishers

4642 Let's Talk About Going to the Hospital
Rosen Publishing Group's PowerKids Press
29 E 21st Street
New York, NY 10010   212-777-3017
                                                   800-237-9932
                                                   Fax: 888-436-4643
                                                   rosenpub@tribeca.ios.com
                                                   www.rosenpublishing.com

If a child has to check into the hospital, chances are he or she is already upset about being ill. Knowing how a hospital functions and what the procedures are, such as when family members can visit, will help in what is already a stressful situation. Grades K-5.

24 pages
ISBN: 0-823950-36-0
Roger Rosen, President

Newsletters

4643 MSUD Newsletter
MSUD Family Support Group
82 Ravine Road
Powell, OH 43065   740-548-4475
                                                   www.msud-support.org

Provides the latest information on the treatment of the disorder, reports on the latest research, current diet information, family news and related topics.

16 pages
Sandy Bulcher, Director
Dave Bulcher, Treasurer
K R Dollins, Editor

DESCRIPTION

4644 MARFAN SYNDROME
Synonym: MFS
Covers these related disorders: Neonatal or infantile Marfan syndrome
Involves the following Biologic System(s):
Cardiovascular Disorders,
Genetic/Chromosomal/Syndrome/Metabolic Disorders, Orthopedic and Muscle Disorders

Marfan syndrome is a connective tissue disorder that may result in heart (cardiac), blood vessel, skeletal, and eye (ocular) abnormalities. Children with Marfan syndrome tend to be unusually tall and slim; in some cases, this may be apparent at birth. Many affected infants also have deficiency of the layer of fat under the skin and abnormally diminished muscle tone (hypotonia) that may contribute to motor delays. In addition, in some infants with Marfan syndrome, several additional characteristic symptoms and findings may be apparent during later childhood. Neonatal or infantile Marfan syndrome is characterized by abnormal flexions (contractures), dislocations, and limited ranges of movement; an abnormally long head and face (dolichocephaly); a highly arched roof of the mouth (palate); unusually large corneas of the eyes (megalocornea); abnormal quivering movements of the colored portions of the eyes (irides); and heart defects (e.g., aortic root dilatation, mitral valve prolapse).

Older children with Marfan syndrome also tend to have an unusually long, narrow face as well as a narrow, highly arched palate and abnormal crowding of the teeth. Affected children and adults also have unusually long, thin arms and legs; a wide arm span; and long, thin fingers (arachnodactyly) with abnormally increased extension (hyperflexibility). Additional skeletal abnormalities are often present, such as unusually thin, fragile ribs; abnormal protrusion or depression of the breastbone (pectus carinatum or excavatum); and, in older children and adolescents, progressive abnormal sideways curvature (scoliosis) or front-to-back curvature (kyphosis) of the spine.

In many cases, affected children also have additional ocular abnormalities, such as dislocation (subluxation) of the lenses of the eyes (ectopia lentis); abnormal bluish coloration of the tough, outer membrane of the eyes; and severe nearsightedness (myopia). In addition, in some cases, the nerve-rich membrane at the back of the eyes (retina) may become detached.

Most individuals with Marfan syndrome also experience abnormalities of the heart and certain blood vessels (cardiovascular defects) that may be life-threatening. These may include progressive widening of the major artery of the body (aorta), causing leakage of blood through the valve between the left ventricle and the aorta (aortic regurgitation). In addition, the valve between the left ventricle and the left upper chamber (atrium) of the heart may bulge backward (prolapse) into the atrium, causing leakage of blood into the atrium.

The treatment of Marfan syndrome is directed toward preventing potential complications associated with progression of the disease. Affected children should receive regular evaluations to detect ocular defects, abnormal spinal curvatures, or cardiovascular defects. Treatment includes symptomatic and supportive measures, such as orthopedic techniques to help prevent or treat scoliosis or kyphosis; therapy with certain medications (beta-adrenergic blocking agents, e.g., propranolol) that may help to prevent or reduce the progression of certain cardiovascular abnormalities (e.g., aortic dilatation and associated complications); or surgical correction of cardiovascular defects as required. At one time, affected individuals were provided with antibiotic medications before dental visits and surgical procedures to reduce the incidence of endocarditis (an infection of the heart wall or heart valvle when bacteria enter the bloodstream). The American Heart Association no longer recommends taking routine antibiotics before certain dental procedures except for people at highest risk for bad outcomes if they develop endocarditis. Individuals with Marfan syndrome do not fall into this high-risk category.

Marfan syndrome results from abnormal changes (mutations) in a gene (fibrillin gene) located on the long arm of chromosome 15 (15q21.1). Such mutations may occur spontaneously (sporadically) for unknown reasons or may be inherited as an autosomal dominant trait. In individuals with the disease gene, the range and severity of associated symptoms and findings may vary from case to case (variable expressivity). Marfan syndrome is thought to affect about one in 10,000 individuals.

Government Agencies

4645 NIH/National Institute of Arthritis and Musculoskeletal and Skin Diseases
1 AMS Circle
Bethesda, MD 20892
301-495-4484
877-226-4267
Fax: 301-718-6366
TTY: 301-565-2966
TDD: 301-565-2966
niamsinfo@mail.nih.gov
www.niams.nih.gov

The mission of the NIAMS, a part of the NIH, is to support research into the causes, treatment, and prevention of arthritis and musculoskeletal and skin diseases, the training of basic and clinical scientists to carry out this research, and the dissemination of information on research progress in these diseases.
Stephen I Katz MD PhD, Director
Robert H Carter MD, Deputy Director

National Associations & Support Groups

4646 American Academy of Pediatrics
141 Northwest Point Boulevard
Elk Grove Village, IL 60007
847-434-4000
800-433-9016
Fax: 847-434-8000
www.aap.org

The American Academy of Pediatrics and its member pediatricians are committed to the attainment of optimal physical, mental and social health and well-being for all infants, children, adolescents, and young adults.
Fernando Stein, MD, FAAP, President
Karen Remley, MD, CEO/Executive VP

547

4647 Genetic Alliance
4301 Connecticut Avenue NW, Suite 404
Washington, DC 20008   202-966-5557
800-336-4363
Fax: 202-966-8553
info@geneticalliance.org
www.geneticalliance.org

A coalition of voluntary genetic support groups, consumers and professionals addressing the needs of individuals and families affected by genetic disorders from a national perspective.

Sharon Terry, President/CEO
Tetyana Murza, Managing Director
Natasha Bonhomme, VP, Strategic Development

4648 March of Dimes Foundation
1275 Mamaroneck Avenue
White Plains, NY 10605   914-997-4488
888-663-4637
Fax: 914-428-8203
answers@marchofdimes.com
www.marchofdimes.com

Partnership of volunteers and professionals dedicates to improving the health of babies by preventing birth defects and infant mortality. Over 100 chapters are located across the country and can be located through the National Office.

Stacey D. Stewart, President

4649 National Marfan Foundation
22 Manhasset Avenue
Port Washington, NY 11050   516-883-8712
800-862-7326
Fax: 516-883-8040
staff@marfan.org
www.marfan.org

A nonprofit voluntary health organization dedicated to saving lives and improving the quality of life for individuals and families affected by the Marfan Syndrome and related disorders.

Ray Chevallier, Chair
Mary J. Roman, Vice Chairman
Teri Dean, Treasurer

Web Sites

4650 National Marfan Foundation
22 Manhasset Avenue
Port Washington, NY 11050   516-883-8712
Fax: 516-883-8040
staff@marfan.org
www.marfan.org

A nonprofit voluntary health organization dedicated to saving lives and improving the quality of life for individuals and families affected by the Marfan Syndrome and related disorders.

Raymond Chevallier, Chair
Mary J. Roman, Vice Chair
Cory Eaves, Secretary

4651 Wheeless' Textbook of Orthopaedics
www.wheelessonline.com

410-494-4994
www.wheelessonline.com

Derives from a variety of sources, including journals, articles, national meetings lectures and other textbooks.

Clifford R. Wheeless, Editor in chief
James A Nunley, Managing Editor
James R. Urbaniak, Managing Editor

Book Publishers

4652 Let's Talk About Going to the Hospital
Rosen Publishing Group's PowerKids Press
29 E 21st Street
New York, NY 10010   212-777-3017
800-237-9932
Fax: 888-436-4643
rosenpub@tribeca.ios.com
www.rosenpublishing.com

If a child has to check into the hospital, chances are he or she is already upset about being ill. Knowing how a hospital functions and what the procedures are, such as when family members can visit, will help in what is already a stressful situation. Grades K-5.

24 pages
ISBN: 0-823950-36-0

Roger Rosen, President

Pamphlets

4653 Marfan Syndrome
March of Dimes Pregnancy & Newborn Health Edu Ctr
1275 Mamaroneck Avenue
White Plains, NY 10605   914-977-4488
888-663-4637
Fax: 914-997-4763
answers@marchofdimes.com
www.marchofdimes.org

A series of fact sheets each discussing an aspect of Marfan, inlcuding prevention, research, causes, treamtents, diagnosis, affects, eye problems, heart problems, and skeletal problems.

DESCRIPTION

4654 MCCUNE-ALBRIGHT SYNDROME

Synonyms: Albright syndrome, MAS, PFD, POFD, Polyostotic fibrous dysplasia, Precocious puberty with polyostotic

Involves the following Biologic System(s):

Endocrinologic Disorders,

Genetic/Chromosomal/Syndrome/Metabolic Disorders

McCune-Albright syndrome is a genetic disorder characterized by multiple areas of abnormal, fiber-like tissue growths (bone lesions) that replace normal bone tissue (polyostotic fibrous dysplasia); irregular, patchy areas of light brown pigmentation on the skin (cafe-au-lait spots); and abnormalities of certain hormone-producing glands that assist in regulating the body's growth, controlling the rate of metabolism, and promoting the development of secondary sexual characteristics. Although bone lesions are most common in the pelvis and the long bones of the arms and legs, other bones may be affected, including the ribs, skull and facial bones, and bones of the spinal column (vertebrae). These bone lesions may cause abnormal thickness and deformity of affected bones, susceptibility to fractures, and bone pain. In addition, lesions may cause corresponding bones to develop unevenly. For example, one leg may appear unusually short, or one side of the face may appear different from the other (facial asymmetry). Bone lesions of the skull and face may eventually result in hearing loss and visual impairment.

Many girls with McCune-Albright syndrome undergo early development of secondary sexual characteristics (precocious puberty), including early breast development and onset of menstrual cycles (menstruation). Some boys with the disorder may also experience precocious puberty, including genital development and unusually accelerated growth. In many patients, additionalendocrine abnormalities may be present. For example, some affected children may produce excessive amounts of the hormone cortisol, resulting in Cushing's syndrome. This disorder is characterized by excessive weight gain in the chest and abdominal area; a moon-shaped, rounded face; abnormal pads of fat in certain areas of the body; high blood pressure (hypertension); weakening of bones, causing increased susceptibility to fractures; thin, and fragile skin.

Some children with McCune-Albright syndrome may also produce excessive amounts of thyroid hormones (hyperthyroidism), potentially leading to heart palpitations, anxiety, heat intolerance, excessive sweating, muscle weakness, or weight loss. In addition, some affected children may be prone to developing tumors of the pituitary gland, resulting in increased secretion of growth hormone, which stimulates body growth and development. Affected children may experience enlargement of bones and soft tissues of the hands, feet, and face (acromegaly); lengthening and coarsening of the face; and enlargement of certain organs (e.g., heart). In some patients, excessive growth during childhood (gigantism) and tall stature may occur.

McCune-Albright syndrome may be obvious at birth because of unusual skin pigmentation. Alternatively, it may not be apparent until late infancy or early childhood when precocious puberty or bone lesions become apparent. The disorder is caused by spontaneous (sporadic) changes (mutations) of a gene known as the GNAS1 gene. The disease gene is located on the long arm (q) of chromosome 20 (20q13.2). Because the gene mutation is present in only some cells of the body (mosaicism), symptoms and findings may vary among affected individuals, depending upon the specific body cells affected. Treatment of McCune-Albright syndrome includes symptomatic and supportive measures. These may include drug therapy to help prevent or treat precocious puberty, surgical removal of pituitary tumors or the thyroid gland, and appropriate treatment of bone lesions and associated abnormalities.

Government Agencies

4655 NIH/ Eunice Kennedy Shriver National Insti tute of Child Health & Human Development
31 Center Drive, Building 31
Bethesda, MD 20892

301-496-5113
800-370-2943
Fax: 866-760-5947
TTY: 888-320-6942
nichdpress@mail.nih.gov
www.nichd.nih.gov

Established in 1962 by congress, today the institute conducts and supports research on topics related to the health of children, adults, families and populations. Some of these topics include: developmental disabilities, growth and development, infant death, reproductive health and birth defects.

Diana W. Bianchi, Director
Paul Williams, Director, Communications

4656 NIH/National Institute of Arthritis and Musculoskeletal and Skin Diseases
1 AMS Circle
Bethesda, MD 20892

301-495-4484
877-226-4267
Fax: 301-718-6366
TTY: 301-565-2966
TDD: 301-565-2966
niamsinfo@mail.nih.gov
www.niams.nih.gov

The mission of the NIAMS, a part of the NIH, is to support research into the causes, treatment, and prevention of arthritis and musculoskeletal and skin diseases, the training of basic and clinical scientists to carry out this research, and the dissemination of information on research progress in these diseases.

Stephen I Katz MD PhD, Director
Robert H Carter MD, Deputy Director

National Associations & Support Groups

4657 American Academy of Pediatrics
141 Northwest Point Boulevard
Elk Grove Village, IL 60007

847-434-4000
800-433-9016
Fax: 847-434-8000
www.aap.org

The American Academy of Pediatrics and its member pediatricians are committed to the attainment of optimal physical, mental and social health and well-being for all infants, children, adolescents, and young adults.

Fernando Stein, MD, FAAP, President
Karen Remley, MD, CEO/Executive VP

4658 Genetic Alliance
4301 Connecticut Avenue NW, Suite 404
Washington, DC 20008

202-966-5557
800-336-4363
Fax: 202-966-8553
info@geneticalliance.org
www.geneticalliance.org

A coalition of voluntary genetic support groups, consumers and professionals addressing the needs of individuals and families affected by genetic disorders from a national perspective.

Sharon Terry, President/CEO
Tetyana Murza, Managing Director
Natasha Bonhomme, VP, Strategic Development

4659 International Skeletal Dysplasia Registry
Medical Genetics Institute
8700 Beverly Blvd
Los Angeles, CA 90048

310-423-9915
800-233-2771
Fax: 310-423-1528
maryann.priore@cshs.org
www.cedars-sinai.edu

The International Skeletal Dysplasia Registry at Cedars-Sinai Medical Center is a referral center for research into the diagnosis; management and etiology of the skeletal dysplasias.

Lawrence B. Platt, Chair
Thomas M. Prislac, President/CEO
Vera Guerin, Vice Chair

4660 MAGIC Foundation: Major Aspects of Growth in Children
4200 Cantera Drive, #106
Warrenville, IL 60555

630-836-8200
800-362-4423
Fax: 630-836-8181
ContactUs@magicfoundation.org
www.magicfoundation.org

A national nonprofit organization providing support and education regarding growth disorders in children and related adult disorders. Provides educational information, networking, a national conference, a kids' program and an extensive medical library.

10,000 members

Dianne Kremidas, Executive Director
Mary Andrews, CEO
Teresa Tucker, Patient Advocacy

4661 March of Dimes Foundation
1275 Mamaroneck Avenue
White Plains, NY 10605

914-997-4488
888-663-4637
Fax: 914-428-8203
answers@marchofdimes.com
www.marchofdimes.com

Partnership of volunteers and professionals dedicates to improving the health of babies by preventing birth defects and infant mortality. Over 100 chapters are located across the country and can be located through the National Office.

Stacey D. Stewart, President

Web Sites

4662 Human Growth Foundation
997 Glen Cove Ave, Suite 5
Glen Head, NY 11545

800-451-6434
Fax: 516-671-4055
hgf1@hgfound.org
www.hgfound.org

Helps children and adults with growth or growth hormone related disorders through research, education, support and advocacy.

Pisit Pitukcheewanont, MD, President
Emily Germain-Lee, Vice President
Patricia Costa, Executive Director

4663 University Alabama Birmingham
1720 2nd Ave South
Birmingham, AL 35294

205-934-4011
TDD: 205-934-4642
www.uab.edu/home

Dr. Margaret A. Purcell, Executive Director
Michael A Bownes, Secretary
Linda Beasley, Assistant to Secretary

Book Publishers

4664 Let's Talk About Going to the Hospital
Rosen Publishing Group's PowerKids Press
29 E 21st Street
New York, NY 10010

212-777-3017
800-237-9932
Fax: 888-436-4643
rosenpub@tribeca.ios.com
www.rosenpublishing.com

If a child has to check into the hospital, chances are he or she is already upset about being ill. Knowing how a hospital functions and what the procedures are, such as when family members can visit, will help in what is already a stressful situation. Grades K-5.

24 pages
ISBN: 0-823950-36-0

Roger Rosen, President

DESCRIPTION

4665 MENINGITIS

Covers these related disorders: Bacterial meningitis, Chronic meningitis, Neonatal meningitis, Viral meningitis

Involves the following Biologic System(s):

Infectious Disorders, Neurologic Disorders

Meningitis is an inflammation of the protective membranes that cover the brain and spinal cord (meninges). It most often occurs from infancy to young adulthood, but can develop in persons of any age, and is most commonly caused by a viral (viral meningitis) or bacterial infection (bacterial meningitis) that reaches the meninges by way of the blood and through the cerebrospinal fluid (CSF) that surrounds the brain and spinal cord. Meningitis may also be caused by fungi and other kinds of microorganisms, by noninfectious disease, head injury, medications, and exposure to chemical substances. Cases of meningitis in which no causative infecting organism can be identified are sometimes called aseptic meningitis. However, specialized testing often reveals specific kinds of bacteria or viruses as the cause of such disease.

All types of meningitis are serious and require prompt medical attention to prevent injury to the brain, and death, but bacterial meningitis is typically more serious than viral meningitis. Bacterial meningitis most commonly affects children from 1 month to 5 years old. In children aged approximately 2 months to 12 years, bacterial meningitis is most commonly caused by two species of bacteria: *Neisseria meningitidis* (meningococcus), and *Streptococcus pneumoniae*. These bacteria are spread by the inhalation of airborne cough or sneeze droplets from infected persons, or through contact with feces or other infected body products. Viral meningitis is more common and typically less severe than bacterial meningitis, but is spread in the same way, through saliva, mucus, fecal matter, and other infected body materials.

Symptoms of meningitis include headache and stiff neck, nausea and vomiting, fever, sensitivity to light (photophobia), unnatural sleepiness, confusion, and seizures. Symptoms of meningitis in infants and young children may include irritability and loss of appetite. Meningitis that occurs within the first month of life, known as neonatal meningitis, may produce a different pattern of symptoms than that seen in older infants and children. Such meningitis affects approximately 0.2 to 0.4 in every 1,000 newborns, and is more frequent among infants born prematurely (before 37 weeks). As a result of increased fluid pressure, meningitis in newborns may cause bulging of the skull in the fontanels at the forward sides of the head, where bones of the skull have not fully fused, and enlargement of the head (hydrocephalus). Other symptoms of meningitis in children include coughing and difficulty in breathing. Without prompt treatment, these effects of meningitis can progress to coma and death.

The diagnosis of meningitis, and the type microorganism causing a particular case of infectious meningitis, is made by testing a sample of CSF from the lower back. As the treatment of meningitis proceeds, lumbar puncture and analysis of the CSF are repeated to assess the patient's response to treatment..

Prompt diagnosis and immediate treatment of bacterial meningitis are essential to help prevent brain damage and potentially life-threatening complications. Treatment requires immediate hospitalization and the intravenous administration of antibiotics, as well as careful, close monitoring and measures for reducing the increased pressure on the brain caused by fluid that passes through the inflamed meninges. Antibiotic treatment for bacterial meningitis usually lasts for a couple of weeks, but may continue after a patient is discharged from the hospital. Additional treatment of bacterial meningitis is symptomatic and supportive. Preventive antibiotic therapy may be recommended for persons who have had close contact with children or other persons who have bacterial meningitis. Currently, routine childhood immunization plays an essential role in preventing meningitis caused by the species of bacteria known as Haemophilus influenzae type b (Hib), which used to be one of the most common causes of childhood bacterial meningitis. Vaccines that can protect against some other types of meningitis are also available, such as that caused by *Streptococcus pneumoniae.*

Like bacterial meningitis, viral meningitis requires prompt medical attention, but usually disappears gradually of its own accord within a period of 2 weeks. Because they do not affect viruses, antibiotic drugs are not useful for treating this type of meningitis. Instead, treatment of viral meningitis is usually focused on relieving fever and its other symptoms, and on supporting the patient's respiration, nutrition, and movement. In more severe cases, however medications specifically directed at viruses, known as antiviral drugs, may be given to patients with viral meningitis.

Some patients with meningitis may develop fever, headache, a stiff neck, back pain, vomiting, and other symptoms that last for a month or longer. This condition, known as chronic meningitis, may result from certain bacterial, viral, or other infections, or may be due to noninfectious disorders that can affect the brain, such as sarcoidosis or multiple sclerosis; certain medications, such as some anticancer drugs; or other factors. Individuals whose immune systems have been impaired by disease or by surgical or medical treatment for disease may also be more susceptible to chronic meningitis. The treatment of chronic meningitis is based on the underlying cause of the condition.

For more information on a meningitis vaccine, see chapter on Preventable Childhood Infections.

Government Agencies

4666 NIH/National Institute of Allergy and Infectious Diseases
5601 Fishers Lane, MSC 9806
Bethesda, MD 20892

301-496-5717
866-284-4107
Fax: 301-402-3573
TDD: 800-877-8339
ocpostoffice@niaid.nih.gov
www.niaid.nih.gov

Conducts and supports basic and applied research to better understand, treat, and ultimately prevent infectious, immunologic, and allergic diseases.

Anthony S Fauci MD, Director

National Associations & Support Groups

4667 American Academy of Pediatrics
141 Northwest Point Boulevard
Elk Grove Village, IL 60007

847-434-4000

Fax: 847-434-8000

www.aap.org

The American Academy of Pediatrics and its member pediatricians are committed to the attainment of optimal physical, mental and social health and well-being for all infants, children, adolescents, and young adults.

Fernando Stein, MD, FAAP, President
Karen Remley, MD, CEO/Executive VP

4668 March of Dimes Foundation
1275 Mamaroneck Avenue
White Plains, NY 10605

914-997-4488
888-663-4637
Fax: 914-428-8203
answers@marchofdimes.com
www.marchofdimes.com

Partnership of volunteers and professionals dedicates to improving the health of babies by preventing birth defects and infant mortality. Over 100 chapters are located across the country and can be located through the National Office.

Stacey D. Stewart, President

4669 Meningitis Foundation of America
PO Box 1818
El Mirage, AZ 85335

480-270-2652
800-668-1129
Fax: 317-595-6370
support@musa.org
www.musa.org

Goals and objectives are: help support sufferers of Spinal Meningitis and their families; provide information to educate the public and medical professionals about meningitis so that its early diagnosis and treatment will save lives; and support development of vaccines and other preventions.

Daisi Pollard Sepulveda, National President
Courtney Martin, National VP
Caroline L. Petrie, National Secretary

Web Sites

4670 MGH Neurology Web Forums
www.mgh.harvard.edu/forum

4671 Maryland Department of Health
www.dhml.state.md.us

4672 Meningitis Foundation of America
P. O. Box 1818
El Mirage, AZ 85335

480-270-2652
www.musa.org

Help support sufferers of meningitis and their families and the development of vaccines and other means of treating and/or preventing meningitis.

Caroline Petrie, National Secretary
Alexander James Flatley, Board Member

4673 World Health Organization
1211 Geneva 27
Switzerland,

122-791-2111
Fax: 122-791-3111
who_reform@who.int
www.who.int/topics/meningitis/en

WHO's objective, as set out in its Constitution, is the attainment by all peoples of the highest possible level of health.

Book Publishers

4674 Let's Talk About Going to the Hospital
Rosen Publishing Group's PowerKids Press
29 E 21st Street
New York, NY 10010

212-777-3017
800-237-9932
Fax: 888-436-4643
rosenpub@tribeca.ios.com
www.rosenpublishing.com

If a child has to check into the hospital, chances are he or she is already upset about being ill. Knowing how a hospital functions and what the procedures are, such as when family members can visit, will help in what is already a stressful situation. Grades K-5.

24 pages
ISBN: 0-823950-36-0

Roger Rosen, President

DESCRIPTION

4675 MENTAL RETARDATION

Synonym: Mental deficiency

Involves the following Biologic System(s):

Developmental/Behavioral/Psychiatric Disorders, Neurologic Disorders

Mental retardation is characterized by impaired or below average intellectual functioning that results in deficits in learning ability and adaptive behaviors. The disorder is thought to affect approximately three percent of the general population. About 80 to 90 percent of patients have mild mental retardation, whereas 10 to 20 percent are affected by moderate to profound degrees of impairment.

The causes of mental retardation may be biological as well as psychosocial or sociocultural in nature. In other words, the disorder may be due to a combination of several factors and influenced both by biological abnormalities of the brain as well as the nature of a child's life experiences, such as those resulting from parent-child interactions and overall family dynamics. Biological causes of mental retardation may include fetal exposure to certain drugs, maternal infections, or radiation therapy; premature birth; or certain underlying disorders, such as inborn errors of metabolism, chromosomal abnormalities including Down syndrome and fragile X syndrome, or other genetic disorders. Mental retardation may also result from head injuries or low levels of oxygen to the brain during delivery, childhood exposure to lead, or certain infections during infancy or early childhood, such as inflammation of the protective membranes surround|ing the brain and spinal cord (meningitis). Some underlying causes may be correctable before mental retardation occurs, such as phenylketonuria (PKU), which is a metabolic disorder, or hypothyroidism, a condition characterized by decreased activity of the thyroid gland. Additional contributing factors may include malnutrition; dysfunctional interactions between caregivers and infants; or other psychosocial or sociocultural factors. In many children with mental retardation, the specific causes remain unknown. The condition may occur as the result of the interactions of several genes (polygenic inheritance), possibly in association with certain environmental influences (multifactorial).

During normal development, infants and children acquire mental, physical, and behavioral skills in certain stages known as developmental milestones. Although the particular rate of development is variable, most children acquire such skills at certain ages. However, infants and children with mental retardation typically experience delays in achieving certain developmental milestones. For example, with severe levels of mental retardation, patients may initially have delays in the acquisition of certain motor skills. With more moderate levels of retardation, children may achieve early motor milestones yet be delayed in acquiring certain skills that require the coordination of physical and mental abilities (psychomotor delays), such as delayed speech and language skills. In children with mild or borderline impairment, below average intellectual functioning may not be suspected until the early school years. Varying degrees of mental retardation are based upon the different levels of support that may be required for daily functioning as well as intelligence quotient (I.Q.), which is a standardized, age-related measure of intelligence. Mental retardation may be defined as having an I.Q. below 70 and is often subdivided into mild, moderate, severe, and profound mental retardation. Most individuals in the general population have an I.Q. between 80 and 120.

Children with what is known as borderline intellectual functioning have very mild intellectual deficits (e.g., I.Q. between 70 to 85) and minor impairments in adaptive behaviors. These behaviors include certain adaptive skills, such as social, self-care, communication, and vocational skills. Patients with mild retardation (I.Q. between 50 and 70) may develop academic skills up to the sixth grade level. In addition, with appropriate support, they may achieve social skills that enable them to function relatively independently during adulthood. Patients with moderate impairment (I.Q. between 35 and 50) may learn to communicate and tend to have only fair motor development. Although these patients rarely develop academic skills up to the second grade level, they may benefit from vocational training and achieve limited independence with appropriate supervision. Children with severe mental retardation (I.Q. between 20 and 35) typically have poor motor development and little speech or communication skills. With appropriate education and support, they may develop speech by late adolescence. In addition, with close supervision, they may learn basic hygienic skills and simple tasks by adulthood. Although children with profound impairment (I.Q. under 20) may learn some basic hygienic skills, they typically have limited psychomotor development and require close, ongoing supervision.

In infants with suspected mental retardation, a number of specialized laboratory tests may be conducted to rule out certain underlying disorders, such as fragile X syndrome or other chromosomal or genetic syndromes. The management of mental retardation is individualized for each child and may include therapeutic and special educational services as well as special social support and counseling services. Early diagnosis and the prompt development of an individualized, comprehensive intervention program is essential in helping affected children reach their potential. Prenatal screening for genetic defects, and genetic counseling for families at risk for known heritable disorders can decrease the incidence of genetically caused mental retardation. Primary care pediatricians lay an important role in consulting with specialists and other health care providers as required and developing an appropriate intervention program. As patients with mild to moderate impairment reach adolescence, specialized services may include a focus on vocational training and community living.

National Associations & Support Groups

4676 ARC of the United States
1825 K Street MW, Suite 1200
Washington, DC 20006

202-534-3700
800-433-5255
Fax: 202-534-3731
info@thearc.org
www.thearc.org

The ARC is the national organization of and for people with mental retardation and related developmental disabilities and their families. Devoted to promoting and improving supports and services for people with mental retardation and their families. The association also fosters research and education regarding the prevention of mental retardation in infants and young children. The ARC was founded in 1950 by a small group of parents and other concerned individuals.

Nancy Webster, President
Ronald Brown, VP
Elise McMillan, Secretary

4677 American Academy of Pediatrics
141 Northwest Point Boulevard
Elk Grove Village, IL 60007   847-434-4000
     800-433-9016
     Fax: 847-434-8000
     www.aap.org

The American Academy of Pediatrics and its member pediatricians are committed to the attainment of optimal physical, mental and social health and well-being for all infants, children, adolescents, and young adults.

Fernando Stein, MD, FAAP, President
Karen Remley, MD, CEO/Executive VP

4678 American Association of People with Disabilities
2013 H Street, NW, 5th Floor
Washington, DC 20006   800-840-8844
     Fax: 866-536-4461
     TTY: 202-457-0046
     www.aapd.com

It is the nation's largest disability rights organization. We promote equal opportunity, economic power, independent living, and political participation for people with disabilities.

Mark Perriello, President and CEO
Henry Claypool, Executive Vice President
TaKeisha Bobbitt, Managing Director

4679 American Association on Health and Disabilities
110 N. Washington Street, Suite 328-J
Rockville, MD 20850   301-545-6140
     Fax: 301- 54- 614
     www.aahd.us

It is dedicated to improve overall health and reduce health disparities for people with disabilities through health promotion and wellness.

Ronald G. Blankenbaker, MD, President
Roberta Carlin, MS, JD, Executive Director
E. Clarke Ross, DPA, Public Policy Director

4680 American Mental Health Foundation (AMHF)
PO Box 3
Riverdale, NY 10471
USA   212-737-9027
     elomke@americanmentalhealthfoundation.or
     www.americanmentalhealthfoundation.org

Dedicated to the extensive and intensive research in the theories and techniques of treatment of emotional illness and to the implementation of reforms in the mental health system. Efforts have resulted in development of better and less expensive treatment methods. Findings are disseminated in English and other major languages.

Sister Joan Curtin, Director
John P. Fowler, Treasurer
Eugene Gollogly, VP

4681 American Network of Community Options & Resources
1101 King Street, Suite 380,
Alexandria, VA 22314   703-535-7850
     ancor@ancor.org
     www.ancor.org

It is the advocate and resource for private community providers of services to people with disabilities.

Barbara Merrill, Chief Executive Officer
Gabrielle Sedor, Chief Operations Officer

4682 American Occupational Therapy Association
4720 Montgomery Ln Ste 200
Bethesda,, MD 20814   800-729-2682
     Fax: 240-762-5150
     www.aota.org

4683 American Public Health Association
800 I Street, NW
Washington, DC 20001   202-777-2742
     Fax: 202-777-2534
     TTY: 202-777-2500
     www.apha.org

APHA champions the health of all people and all communities. They aim to strengthen the public health profession and speak out for public health issues and policies backed by science.

Georges C. Benjamin, MD, Executive Director
Kemi Oluwafemi, MBA, CPA, Chief Financial Officer
Susan Polan, PhD, Associate Executive Director

4684 Arc (The)
1825 K Street, NW, Suite 1200
Washington, DC 20006   202-534-3700
     800-433-5255
     Fax: 202-534-3731
     tnguyen@thearc.org.
     www.thearc.org

An organization advocating for and serving people with intellectual and developmental disabilities and their families. They encompass all ages and all spectrums from autism, Down syndrome, Fragile X and various other developmental disabilities.

Ronald Brown, President
Elise McMillan, Vice President
M.J. Bartelmay, Jr., Secretary

4685 Association of Developmental Disabilities
1671 Worcester Road (Rt. 9W), Suite 201
Framingham, MA 1701   508-405-8000
     Fax: 508-405-8001
     www.addp.org

The mission is to promote and ensure the strength of the community-based provider community and its members so that our members can be successful in improving the quality, access and value of community based services.

Jean Phelps,, Chair
Chris White, Vice-Chair
Michael Andrade, Clerk

4686 Association of Professional Developmental Disabilities Administrators
www.apdda.org

The mission is to supports the continuous improvement of a comprehensive array of individual and accessible services designed to enhance the quality of life for persons with intellectual disabilities and other developmental disabilities.

David J. Thomas, President
Julene Hollenbach, President Elect

4687 Association of University Centers on Disabilities
1100 Wayne Ave., Suite 1000
Silver Spring, MD 20910   301-588-8252
     Fax: 301-588-2842
     aucdinfo@aucd.org
     www.aucd.org

The Association of University Centers on Disabilities (AUCD) is a membership organization that supports and promotes a national network of university-based interdisciplinary programs.

Andrew J. Imparato, JD, Executive Director
Abigail (Abbey) Alberico, MPH, Project Manager
Leon Barnett, MSEd, Program Specialist

4688 Bethpage Mission
4980 W 118th Street, Suite A
Omaha, NE 68137   402-896-3884
     800-628-7070
     Fax: 402-896-1511
     psanchez@bethpage.org
     www.bethpage.org

4689 Bethphage
2245 Midway Road, #300
Carrolton, TX 75006
972-866-9989
800-628-7070
Fax: 972-991-0834
hbranicki@bethphage.org
www.bethphage.org

Bethphage is an affiliate of the Evangelical Lutheran Church in America, serves and advocates for people with disabilities so that they may achieve their full potential. Bethphage provides living and vocational services to individuals with developmental disabilities, including group homes, supervised apartment living and job skills training.

4690 Center for Disabilities and Development
University of Iowa Stead Family Children's Hospita
100 Hawkins Drive
Iowa City, IA 52242
319-353-6900
877-686-0031
Fax: 319-356-7700
cdd-webmaster@uiowa.edu
www.medicine.uiowa.edu

A trusted resource for healthcare, training, research and information for people with disabilities that include: behavior disorders, brain injury, cerebral palsy, diabetes, down syndrome, learning disabilities, mental retardation, sleep disorders and spina bifida.

Dianne McBrien, MD, Medical Director

4691 Council for Exception Children - Division on Autism and Development Disabilities
daddcec.org

It is an organization composed of persons committed to enhancing the quality of life of individuals, especially children and youth, with autism, intellectual disability, and other developmental disabilities.

Dianne Zager, President
Gardner Umbarger, Treasurer

4692 Council on Quality and Leadership (The)
100 West Road, Suite 300
Towson, MD 21204
410-583-0060
info@thecouncil.org
www.c-q-l.org

CQL offers training, accreditation, consultation and certification services to organizations and systems that share our vision of dignity, opportunity and community for all people.

Cathy Ficker Terrill, President/ CEO
Kerri Melda, VP, Research and Special Projects
Tammi Watkins, VP, Operations

4693 Developmental Disabilities Nurses Association
1501 South Loop 288, Suite 104 - PMB 381
Denton, TX 76205
800-888-6733
Fax: 844-336-2329
ddna.org

Developmental Disabilities Nurses Association (DDNA) is a 501(c)(3) not-for-profit nursing specialty organization that is committed to advocacy, education, and support for nurses who provide services to persons with intellectual and developmental disabilities (IDD).

Karen Green McGowan, RN, CDDN, President
Deb Maloy, RN, CDDN, President-Elect
Wendy Herbers, RN, CDDN, QDDP, Vice-President

4694 Judge David L. Bazelon Center for Mental Health
1101 15th Street, NW, Suite 1212
Washington, DC 20005
202-467-5730
Fax: 202-223-0409
TDD: 202-467-4232
communications@bazelon.org
www.bazelon.org

The mission of the Judge David L. Bazelon Center for Mental Health Law is to protect and advance the rights of adults and children who have mental disabilities.

Robert Bernstein, President/ CEO
Ira Burnim, Director
Jennifer Mathis, Deputy Director

4695 Mosaic
4980 S. 118th St.
Omaha, NE 68137
877-3MO-SAIC
Fax: 402-896-1511
info@mosaicinfo.org
www.mosaicinfo.org

Mosaic is a faith-based organization serving people with intellectual disabilities.

Linda Timmons, President/ CEO
Raul Saldivar, Chief Operating Officer
Cindy Schroeder, Chief Financial Officer

4696 NADD: National Association for the Dually Diagnosed
132 Fair Street
Kingston, NY 12401
845-331-4336
800-331-5362
Fax: 845-331-4569
info@thenadd.org
www.thenadd.org

Nonprofit organization designed to promote the interests of professional and parent development with resources for individuals who have the coexistence of mental illness and mental retardation. Provides conferences, educational services and training materials to professionals, parents, concerned citizens and service organizations. Formerly known as the National Association for the Dually Diagnosed.

Dr Robert Fletcher, CEO
Michelle Jordan, Office Manager
Edward Seliger, Project Coordinator

4697 NYSARC
393 Delaware Ave.
Delmar, NY 12054
518-439-8311
Fax: 518-439-1893
info@nysarc.org
www.nysarc.org

NYSARC's mission is to advocate for persons with intellectual and other developmental disabilities in every manner possible. In its advocacy role, NYSARC is committed to a full quality of life for every person, as it recognizes the challenges of the present and has a clear vision for the future.

Laura J. Kennedy, President
Steven Kroll, Executive Director
Tania F. Seaburg, Esq., Chief Policy and Operations Officer

4698 National Alliance on Mental Illness
3803 N. Fairfax Drive, Suite 100
Arlington, VA 22203
703-524-7600
800-950-6264
Fax: 703-524-9094
info@nami.org
www.nami.org

Grassroots mental health organization dedicated to building better lives for the millions of Americans affected by mental illness. - See more at:
http://www.nami.org/About-NAMI#sthash.IYtjmu5h.dpuf

Jim Payne, J.D., President
David Levy, Chief Financial Officer
Mary Giliberti, J.D., Executive Director

4699 National Association for Dually Diagnosed
132 Fair Street
Kingston, NY 12401
845-331-4336
800-331-5362
Fax: 845-331-4569
rfletcher@thenadd.org
thenadd.org

NADD is a not-for-profit membership association established for professionals, care providers and families to promote understanding of and services for individuals who have developmental disabilities and mental health needs.

Robert J. Fletcher DSW, Chief Executive Officer
Donna McNelis, Ph.D., President
Michelle Jordan, Office Manager

4700 National Association of Councils on Developmental Disabilities
1825 K. Street, N.W. Suite 600
Washington, DC 20006   202-506-5813
                                        mjones@nacdd.org
                                        www.nacdd.org

The National Association of Councils on Developmental Disabilities (NACDD) is a national membership organization representing the 56 State and Territorial Councils on Developmental Disabilities.

Claire Mantonya, President
Donna A Meltzer, Chief Executive Officer
Sheryl Matney, Director

4701 National Association of QDDPs
301 Veterans Parkway
New Lenox, IL 60451   815-320-7301
                                        Fax: 815-320-7357
                                        hjanczak@qddp.org
                                        www.qddp.org

The National Association of Qualified Developmental Disability Professionals was formed in 1996 by Trinity Services staff as the result of a recognized need by QDDPs - Qualified Developmental Disability Professionals/QMRPs - Qualified Mental Retardation Professionals (also known as Case Managers) to establish a strong resource for research, networking, and addressing issues that concern QDDPs today.

Holly Janczak, Executive Director
Kevin Schaefer, Associate Director
Lori Elgas, Conference/Membership Coordinator

4702 National Association of State Directors of Developmental Disabilities Services
301 N Fairfax Street, Suite 101
Alexandria, VA 22314   703-683-4202
                                        nthaler@nasddds.org
                                        www.nasddds.org

The NASDDDS mission is to assist member state agencies in building person-centered systems of services and supports for people with intellectual and developmental disabilities and their families.

Laura L. Nuss, President
Bernard Simons, Vice President/President Elect
Nancy Thaler, Executive Director

4703 National Association of State Mental Health Program Directors
66 Canal Center Plaza, Suite 302
Alexandria, VA 22314   703-739-9333
                                        Fax: 703-548-9517
                                        webmaster@nasmhpd.org
                                        www.nasmhpd.org

Founded in 1959 and based in Alexandria, VA, the National Association of State Mental Health Program Directors (NASMHPD) represents the $37.6 billion public mental health service delivery system serving 7.1 million people annually in all 50 states, 4 territories, and the District of Columbia.

Jay Meek, CPA, MBA, Chief Financial Officer
Robert W. Glover, PhD, Executive Director
David Miller, MPAff, Project Director

4704 National Disability Rights Network
820 1st Street NE, Suite 740
Washington, DC 20002   202-408-9514
                                        Fax: 202-408-9520
                                        TTY: 220-408-9521
                                        www.ndrn.org

The National Disability Rights Network (NDRN) works to improve the lives of people with disabilities by guarding against abuse; advocating for basic rights; and ensuring accountability in health care, education, employment, housing, transportation, and within the juvenile and criminal justice systems.

Curtis L. Decker, JD, Executive Director
Janice K. Johnson Hunter, Deputy Executive Director
Eric Buehlmann, Deputy Executive Director

4705 People First International
PO Box 12642
Salem, OR 97309   503-362-0336
                                        Fax: 503-585-0287
                                        people1@people1.org
                                        www.people1.org

Developmentally disabled people joining together to learn how to speak for themselves. Offers support, information, assistance and advocacy.

Dennis L Heath, Manager

4706 Rehabilitation Research Training Center on Developmental Disabilities and Health
1640 West Roosevelt Road, M/C 626
Chicago, IL 60608   312-413-1520
                                        800-996-8845
                                        Fax: 312-996-6942
                                        TTY: 312-413-0453
                                        www.rrtcadd.org

The Rehabilitation Research and Training Center on Developmental Disabilities and Health (RRTCDD) has the following goals for people with I/DD: increase understanding of health status, health access, and health behaviors; improve health and function through health promotion interventions; and, improve health care access through integrated care practices.

Tamar Heller, PhD, Center Director
Jasmina Sisirak, PhD, MPH, Associate Director
Erika Magallanes, M.Ed., Business Manager

4707 Research and Training Center on Community Living
204 Pattee Hall, 150 Pillsbury Drive S.E.
Minneapolis, MN 55455   612-624-6328
                                        Fax: 612-625-6619
                                        rtc@umn.edu
                                        rtc.umn.edu

The Research and Training Center on Community Living provides research, evaluation, training, technical assistance and dissemination to support the aspirations of persons with developmental disabilities to live full, productive and integrated lives in their communities.

Amy Hewitt, Director

4708 VOR
836 S. Arlington Heights Rd., #351
Elk Grove Village, IL 60007   877-399-4867
                                        Fax: 847-253-0675
                                        info@vor.net
                                        www.vor.net

VOR's mission is to advocate for high quality care and human rights for all people with intellectual and developmental disabilities (I/DD).

Ann Knighton, President
Geoffrey Dubrowsky, First Vice President
Julie Huso, Executive Director

4709 Voice of the Retarded
836 S Arlington Heights Road #351
Elk Grove Village, IL 60007   847-399-4VOR
                                        Fax: 605-399-1631
                                        info@vor.net
                                        www.vor.net

Voice of the Retarded supports a full range of choices for individuals with mental retardation and their families and guardians. VOR is a national, nonprofit organization that advocates for a full continuum of quality care for persons with mental retardation.

Ann Knighton, President
Geoffrey Dubrowsky, First Vice President
Barbara Cukierski, Treasurer

State Agencies & Support Groups

4710 Center for Family Support
333 7th Avenue, #901
New York, NY 10001
212-629-7939
Fax: 212-239-2211
www.cfsny.org

The Center for Family Support (CFS) is a not-for-profit human service agency providing support and assistance to individuals with developmental disabilities and traumatic brain injuries throughout New York City, Long Island, the lower Hudson Valley region and New Jersey.

Steven Vernikoff, Executive Director
Linda Schellenberg, Director, Community Service
Barbara Greenwald, Associate Executive Director

4711 KenCrest Services
502 W Germantown Pike Suite 200
Plymouth Meeting, PA 19462
610-825-9360
Fax: 610-825-4127
www.kencrest.org

Multi-service organization with programs specifically designed for children and youth with developmental disabilities and autism, throughout Pennsylvania, Delaware, & Connecticut.

Bill Nolan, Executive Director
Jim McFalls, Executive Director
Toni McNeal, CFO

Web Sites

4712 American Association on Intellectual and Developmental Disabilities
501 3rd Street, NW Suite 200
Washington, DC 20001
202-387-1968
Fax: 202-387-2193
www.aamr.org

AAMR promotes progressive policies, sound research, effective practices, and universal human rights for people with intellectual disabilites.

Hank Bersani PhD, President
Doreen Croser, Executive Director
Danielle Webber, Manager

4713 NADD: National Association for the Dually Diagnosed
132 Fair Street
Kingston, NY 12401
845-331-4336
info@thenadd.org
www.thenadd.org

Nonprofit organization designed to promote the interests of professional and care providers for individuals who have the coexistence of mental illness and mental retardation. NADD provides conferences, educational services and training materials to professionals, parents, concerned citizens and service organizations.

Dr Robert Fletcher, CEO
Michelle Jordan, Office Manager
Edward Seliger, Project Coordinator

Book Publishers

4714 Art Projects for the Mentally Retarded Child
Ellen J Sussman, author

Charles C Thomas Publishing
2600 South First Street
Springfield, IL 62704
217-789-8980
800-258-8980
Fax: 217-789-9130
books@ccthomas.com
www.ccthomas.com

108 pages Softcover
ISBN: 0-398035-35-8

Charles Thomas, Publisher

4715 Children with Mental Retardation
Woodbine House
6510 Bells Mill Road
Bethesda, MD 20817
301-468-8800
800-843-7323
Fax: 301-897-5838
info@woodbinehouse.com
www.woodbinehouse.com

A book for parents of children with mild to moderate mental retardation, whether or not they have a diagnosed syndrome or condition. It provides a complete and compassionate introduction to their child's medical, therapeutic, and educational needs, and discusses the emotional impact on the family. New parents can rely on Children with Mental Retardation to provide the solid foundation and confidence they need to help their child reach his or her highest potential.

437 pages Softcover
ISBN: 0-933149-39-5

4716 Music Curriculum Guidelines for Moderately Retarded Adolescents
Charles C Thomas Publishing
2600 S 1st Street
Springfield, IL 62704
217-789-8980
800-258-8980
Fax: 217-789-9130
books@ccthomas.com
www.ccthomas.com

122 pages Spiral-Paper
ISBN: 0-398047-57-X

Charles Thomas, Publisher

4717 Retarded Isn't Stupid, Mom!
Sandra Z Kaufman, author

Brookes Publishing
PO Box 10624
Baltimore, MD 21285
410-337-9580
800-638-3775
Fax: 410-337-8539
webmaster@brookespublishing.com
www.brookespublishing.com

This book goes through the triumphs and sorrows of one young woman and her family and the emotions and events encountered as her daughter moves toward adulthood.

272 pages Softcover
ISBN: 1-557663-78-5

Paul Brookes, President
Jeff Brookes, President
Melissa A. Behm, Executive Vice President

Magazines

4718 American Journal on Mental Retardation
AAMR
501 3rd Street, NW Suite 200
Washington, DC 20001
202-387-1968
800-424-3688
Fax: 202-387-2193
maclean@uwyo.edu
aaidd.org

AAMR promotes progressive policies, sound research, effective practices, and universal human rights for people with intellectual and developmental disabilities.

Margaret A. Nygren, EdD, Executive Director/ CEO
Paul D. Aitken, CPA, Director, Finance & Administration
Kathleen McLane, Director, Publications Program

4719 Mental Retardation
AAMR
501 3rd Street, NW Suite 200
Washington, DC 20001
202-387-1968
Fax: 202-387-2193
staylo01@mailbox.syr.edu
www.aamr.org

Provides information on the latest program advances, current research, and information on products and services in the developmental disabilities field.

Bimonthly

Steven J Taylor, Editor

Newsletters

4720 Association for the Help of Retarded Children
83 Maiden Lane
New York, NY 10038

212-780-2500
Fax: 212-777-5893
TTY: 800-662-1220
ahrcnyc@dti.net
www.ahrcnyc.org

Developmentally disabled children and adults, their families, and interested individuals. Provides support services, training programs, clinics, schools and residential facilities to the developmentally disabled. Publications: The Chronicle, quarterly newsletter.

Biannually

Laura J Kennedy, President
Gary Lind, Executive Director
Amy West, Chief Financial Officer

4721 NADD Bulletin
132 Fair Street
Kingston, NY 12401

845-331-4336
800-331-5362
Fax: 845-331-4569
info@thenadd.org
www.thenadd.org

Official publication of the National Association for the Dually Diagnosed. It features articles that address clinical, programmatic, research or family oriented issues concerning mental health aspects in persons with disabilities.

20 pages Bimonthly

Dr Robert Fletcher, CEO
Michelle Jordan, Office Manager
Edward Seliger, Project Coordinator

Camps

4722 Camp Huntington
56 Bruceville Road
High Falls, NY 12440

845-687-7840
855-707-2267
Fax: 845-687-7211
camohtgtn@aol.com
www.camphuntington.com

Summer activities include recreational, academic and vocational programs for the learning disabled, neurologically impaired and mildly ADA to mild/moderately retarded. An Olympic pool, horse riding and a special work training program are featured. Programs are tailored to meet individual needs, ages 6-21, and campers may enroll for 4 to 8 weeks.

Dr. Bruria Falik, Director
Michael Bednarz, Executive Director
Alex Mellor, Program Director

4723 Council for Extended Care of Mentally Retarded Citizens
1600 S Hanley Road
Saint Louis, MO

314-781-4950
Fax: 314-781-3850
cecmrc@aol.com

Services are provided to adults and children with developmental disabilities. Supported living arrangements are located in St. Louis city and St. Charles County. Group home and camp services are located in Dittmer, MO. Travel program also available.

Cynthia Compton, Executive Director
Marge Lindhorst, Supported Living Director
Angela Jackson, Development Director Camp

4724 Crotched Mountain School & Rehabilitation Center
1 Verney Drive
Greenfield, NH 3047

603-547-3311
800-800-966
Fax: 603-547-3232
info@crotchedmountain.org
www.cmf.org

Currently serves children ages 6-22 with multiple-handicaps including: Cerebral Palsy, Spina Bifida, visual and hearing impairments and neurological disabilities, developmental disorders, mental retardation, autism, behavioral and emotional disorders, seizure disorders, spinal cord and head injuries. Member of the National Association of Independent Schools and accredited with the NE Association of Schools and Colleges, Independent Schools of Northern NE.

Donald L Shumway, President & CEO
Tom Zubricki, Chief Financial Officer
Michael Redmond, Senior Vice President

4725 Easter Seal Kysoc
2050 Versailles Road
Lexington, KY 40504

859-254-5701
800-233-3260
Fax: 502-732-0783
ek1@cardinalhill.org
www.cardinalhill.org

Designed for the fullest camping experience for children or adults with physical disabilities, blind, deaf, behavior disorders, mental retardation, diabetes and multiple handicaps, ages 7 and up.

Gary Payne, President & CEO
Heide Miller, CCD, CTRS, Director

4726 New Jersey Camp Jaycee
985 Livingston Avenue
North Brunswick, NJ 8902

732-246-2525
Fax: 732-214-1834
infor@campjaycee.org
www.campjaycee.org

This camp is for children and adults with mental retardation and is sponsored jointly by the New Jersey Jaycees and the ARC of New Jersey. Activities at the 185-acre Pocono Mountain camp include arts and crafts, games and sports, music, nature, swimming, boating, horseback riding and self-help skills.

Frank Pirrello, President
John O'Brien, Vice President
Patricia Rhein, Secretary

4727 Raven Rock Lutheran Camp
17912 Harbaugh Valley Road
Sabillasville, MD

717-794-2667

Christ-centered program for youth and mentally retarded adults.

Lee Sodowsky

4728 Thorpe Camp
680 Capen Hill Road
Goshen, VT 5733

802-247-6611
info@campthorpe.org
www.campthorpe.com

Summer camp for children and adults with special needs.

DESCRIPTION

4729 MICROCEPHALY

Synonyms: Microcephalia, Microcephalism, Microencephaly

Involves the following Biologic System(s):

Neurologic Disorders

Microcephaly is a developmental abnormality in which an infant's or child's head circumference is smaller than would be expected for his or her age and sex (i.e., two or three standard deviations below the mean). In most affected infants and children, underdevelopment of the brain (microencephaly) may result in varying degrees of mental retardation. Microcephaly is considered a relatively common condition, particularly among individuals affected by mental retardation.

In some affected infants and children, microcephaly occurs as an isolated genetic condition. Familial cases of isolated microcephaly have been reported that appear to have autosomal recessive or dominant inheritance. Autosomal recessive microcephaly is characterized by a narrow, sloping forehead; a flat back portion of the head (occiput); varying levels of mental retardation (although severe retardation is most common); and, in some cases, episodes of uncontrolled electrical disturbances in the brain (seizures). Autosomal dominant microcephaly may be characterized by mild slanting of the forehead, upslanting eyelid folds (palpebral fissures), prominent ears, short stature, and borderline or mild mental retardation. In others, the condition occurs in association with certain underlying genetic disorders, such as Cornelia de Lange syndrome. It may also be part of chromosomal malformation syndromes, such as trisomy 13 and trisomy 18 syndromes.

Microcephaly may also occur secondary to particular environmental factors, such as exposure before birth to radiation, certain chemical agents (e.g., alcohol), or certain maternal infections (e.g., rubella). In addition, the condition may result from particular conditions (e.g., meningitis, hyperthermia, etc.) during periods of rapid brain development after birth, particularly during the first two years of life.

When infants and children have a very small head circumference, the underlying abnormality may have begun during early embryonic or fetal development. Although the exact cause is not understood, the condition is thought to result from abnormal development of the outer region of the brain (cerebral cortex).

When infants or children are diagnosed with microcephaly, physicians typically take thorough family histories to determine whether other family members are affected or other disorders or syndromes may be present that are associated with microcephaly. The head circumference is measured periodically for a direct comparison to measurements at birth. Head circumference measurements may also be taken of both parents and any siblings. Additional testing may be undertaken to rule out potential underlying disorders or associated conditions. These tests may include advanced imaging techniques (e.g., CT scanning, MRI) of the brain, chromosomal testing (karyotyping), or certain laboratory tests to detect antibodies against certain infectious agents (e.g., rubella titers) in the child's and mother's bloodstream. Treatment of infants and children with microcephaly includes symptomatic and supportive measures, such as the prescription of certain medications to help treat or control seizures (e.g., anticonvulsants) and special education and other multidisciplinary measures to help ensure that affected children with mental retardation reach their potential. Prenatal screening for genetic defects, and genetic counseling for families at risk for known heritable disorders can decrease the incidence of genetically caused mental retardation. Primary care pediatricians lay an important role in consulting with specialists.

Government Agencies

4730 ARC of the United States
1825 K Street MW, Suite 1200
Washington, DC 20006

202-534-3700
800-433-5255
Fax: 202-534-3731
info@thearc.org
www.thearc.org

The ARC is the national organization of and for people with mental retardation and related developmental disabilities and their families. Devoted to promoting and improving supports and services for people with mental retardation and their families. The association also fosters research and education regarding the prevention of mental retardation in infants and young children. The ARC was founded in 1950 by a small group of parents and other concerned individuals.

Nancy Webster, President
Ronald Brown, VP
Elise McMillan, Secretary

4731 NIH/ Eunice Kennedy Shriver National Insti tute of Child Health & Human Development
National Institues of Health
31 Center Drive, Building 31
Bethesda, MD 20892

301-496-5113
800-370-2943
Fax: 866-760-5947
TTY: 888-320-6942
nichdpress@mail.nih.gov
www.nichd.nih.gov

Established in 1962 by congress, today the institute conducts and supports research on topics related to the health of children, adults, families and populations. These topics include: developmental disabilities, mental retardation, growth and development, infant death, reproductive health, and rehabilitation.

Diana W. Bianchi, Director
Paul Williams, Director, Communications

National Associations & Support Groups

4732 American Academy of Pediatrics
141 Northwest Point Boulevard
Elk Grove Village, IL 60007

847-434-4000
800-433-9016
Fax: 847-434-8000
www.aap.org

The American Academy of Pediatrics and its member pediatricians are committed to the attainment of optimal physical, mental and social health and well-being for all infants, children, adolescents, and young adults.

Fernando Stein, MD, FAAP, President
Karen Remley, MD, CEO/Executive VP

4733 Birth Defect Research for Children
976 Lake Baldwin Lane, Suite 104
Orlando, FL 32814

407-895-0802
Fax: 407-895-0824
staff@birthdefects.org
www.birthdefects.org

Organization that helps families with free birth defect information, parent matching that links families of children with similar defects and research through the National Birth Defect Registry to discover the causes of birth defects. Support group information and newsletter on Internet.

James Murphy, Associate Professor
JD Sherman, Adjunct Professor

4734 Genetic Alliance
4301 Connecticut Avenue NW, Suite 404
Washington, DC 20008
　　　　　　　　　　　　　　202-966-5557
　　　　　　　　　　　　　　800-336-4363
　　　　　　　　　　　　Fax: 202-966-8553
　　　　　　　　　info@geneticalliance.org
　　　　　　　　　www.geneticalliance.org

A coalition of voluntary genetic support groups, consumers and professionals addressing the needs of individuals and families affected by genetic disorders from a national perspective.

Sharon Terry, President/CEO
Tetyana Murza, Managing Director
Natasha Bonhomme, VP, Strategic Development

4735 March of Dimes Foundation
1275 Mamaroneck Avenue
White Plains, NY 10605
　　　　　　　　　　　　　　914-997-4488
　　　　　　　　　　　　　　888-663-4637
　　　　　　　　　　　　Fax: 914-428-8203
　　　　　　　　answers@marchofdimes.com
　　　　　　　　　www.marchofdimes.com

Partnership of volunteers and professionals dedicates to improving the health of babies by preventing birth defects and infant mortality. Over 100 chapters are located across the country and can be located through the National Office.

Stacey D. Stewart, President

4736 National Dissemination Center for Children with Disabilities
1825 Connecticut Avenue NW, Suite 700
Washington, DC 20009
　　　　　　　　　　　　　　202-884-8200
　　　　　　　　　　　　　　800-695-0285
　　　　　　　　　　　　Fax: 202-884-8441
　　　　　　　　　　　　nichcy@fhi360.org
　　　　　　　　　　　　www.nichcy.org

A national information and referral center that provides information on disabilities and disability-related issues for families, educators and other professionals.

Suzanne Ripley, Executive Director

Web Sites

4737 Online Mendelian Inheritance in Man
8600 Rockville Pike
Bethesda, MD 20894
　　　　　　　　　　　　　　301-594-5983
　　　　　　　　　　　　　　888-346-3656
　　　　　　　　　　　　Fax: 301-402-1384
　　　　　　　　　　　　TDD: 800-735-2258
　　　　　　　　　custserv@nlm.nih.gov
　　　　　　　　　www.ncbi.nlm.nih.gov

This database is a catalog of human genes and genetic disorders.

Christine E Seidman M.D, Chairman
David J Lipman M.D, Executive Secretary
Scott Edwards, Member

DESCRIPTION

4738 MICRODONTIA

Synonym: Microdontism

Involves the following Biologic System(s):

Dental Disorders

Microdontia is a term that refers to a developmental dental irregularity in which one or more teeth are abnormally small. This tooth abnormality often occurs in association with certain disorders, conditions, and syndromes and usually affects a single tooth or specific groups of teeth, namely the second or lateral incisors and the molars of the upper jaw. However, in rare instances, microdontia occurs in association with certain other disorders and may affect all or most of the teeth. These other disorders may include pituitary dwarfism, Down's syndrome, and certain forms of congenital heart disease.

Children with certain abnormalities of the face or skull (craniofacial defects) may often exhibit some form of microdontia. These disorders include Turner syndrome, a chromosomal disorder affecting females and characterized by various symptoms including a narrow palate and a small jaw (micrognathia); Crouzon's disease, an autosomal dominant disorder characterized by underdevelopment of the upper jaw and protrusion of the lower jaw (prognathism), a beaked nose, and other symptoms; and cleft lip, a congenital defect in which there is a split or fissure (cleft) in the upper lip. Microdontia is also manifested in several other disorders (e.g., focal dermal hypoplasia, progeria, oculomandibulodyscephaly, oculo-auriculo-vertebral anomaly, and others). Small teeth with a characteristic cone shape are often present in conjunction with missing teeth (anodontia) in certain syndromes known as ectodermal dysplasias, in which there is abnormal development of embryonic tissues that give rise to tooth enamel, hair, nails, skin glands, the outermost layer of the skin (epidermis), the nervous system, the ears and eyes, and mucous membranes of the anus and mouth. Other syndromes that involve microdontia include Williams syndrome, in which the second primary molar of the upper jaw is abnormally small. Aglossia-adactylia syndrome is characterized by partial or total absence of the tongue and missing or abnormally small incisors in the lower jaw.

Microdontia is thought to be genetically transmitted and results from an unknown factor or factors that affect the normal development of the main component of teeth (dentin) and their outermost covering (enamel). This condition is slightly more prevalent in females than males. Treatment may include oral surgery, orthodontic procedures, tooth restoration, and the use of implants or other dental appliances.

Government Agencies

4739 NIH/ Eunice Kennedy Shriver National Institute of Child Health & Human Development
31 Center Drive, Building 31
Bethesda, MD 20892
301-496-5113
800-370-2943
Fax: 866-760-5947
TTY: 888-320-6942
nichdpress@mail.nih.gov
www.nichd.nih.gov

Established in 1962 by congress, today the institute conducts and supports research on topics related to the health of children, adults, families and populations. Some of these topics include: developmental disabilities, growth and development, infant death, reproductive health and birth defects.

Diana W. Bianchi, Director
Paul Williams, Director, Communications

4740 NIH/National Institute of Dental and Craniofacial Research (NIDCR)
National Institutes of Health
31 Center Drive, MSC 2290, Building 31
Bethesda, MD 20892
301-496-4261
866-232-4528
Fax: 301-480-4098
nidcrinfo@mail.nih.gov
www.nidcr.nih.gov

Provides leadership for a national research program designed to understand, treat and prevent the infectious and inherited craniofacial-oral-dental diseases and disorders.

Dr Martha J. Somerman, Director
John W Kusiak, PhD, Acting Deputy Director
Kathleen G Stephen, Executive Officer

National Associations & Support Groups

4741 American Academy of Pediatrics
141 Northwest Point Boulevard
Elk Grove Village, IL 60007
847-434-4000
800-433-9016
Fax: 847-434-8000
www.aap.org

The American Academy of Pediatrics and its member pediatricians are committed to the attainment of optimal physical, mental and social health and well-being for all infants, children, adolescents, and young adults.

Fernando Stein, MD, FAAP, President
Karen Remley, MD, CEO/Executive VP

4742 American Dental Association
211 E Chicago Avenue
Chicago, IL 60611
312-440-2500
Fax: 312-440-7494
www.ada.org

Professional association of dentists committed to the public's oral health, ethics, science and professional advancement; leading a unified profession through initiatives in advocacy, education, research and the development of standards.

Kathleen O'Loughlin, Executive Director

Web Sites

4743 American Dental Association
211 East Chicago Ave
Chicago, IL 60611
312-440-2500
affiliates@ada.org
www.ada.org

Professional association of dentists committed to the public's oral health, ethics, science and professional advancement; leading a unified profession through initiatives in advocacy, education, research and the development of standards.

Dr. Maxine Feinberg, President
Dr. Carol Gomez Summerhays, President-Elect:
Dr. Kathleen T O'Loughlin, Executive Director

4744 Dental Consumer Advisory
toothinfo.com/

Purpose is to provide useful and practical information for the public concerning issues of dental care.

4745 Dental Resources on the Web
dental-resources.com/

Dental sites for education, practices, laboratories, office supplies, dental care and associations.

DESCRIPTION

4746 MIGRAINE HEADACHES

Covers these related disorders: Common migraine (Migraine without aura), Classic migraine (Migraine with aura)

Involves the following Biologic System(s):
Developmental/Behavioral/Psychiatric Disorders

The term migraine refers to a headache that is recurring and accompanied by three or more symptoms or findings that include the presence of certain visual, motor, or other sensations (aura or prodrome) preceding onset; head throbbing; pain on one side of the head (unilateral); nausea; vomiting; and abdominal pain. Additional associated findings include cessation of pain following sleep and a history of migraines in other family members. Migraines are the most common type of recurrent headaches that occur among children. In children younger than 10 years of age, boys are slightly more apt to develop migraines, while adolescent girls and adult females are more prone to migraines than are adolescent boys or adult men. Migraines may be caused by several different factors, alone or in combination. Such factors include genetic influences; stress-related factors; certain foods such as chocolate, citrus fruit, cheese, monosodium glutamate, etc.; red wine; stimuli such as bright lights, loud noises, etc.; medications such as birth control pills; menstruation; and other factors. Pain associated with migraines results from the narrowing and subsequent widening of the arteries that lead to the brain. This action triggers the pain receptors in that region, thus producing the characteristic pain of migraine headaches. More recent theories relate to the role played by the nervous system in the development of migraine headaches. It has been found that nerve cells in blood vessels of the migraine patient release a compound called "substance P." Substance P triggers pain and its release into the arteries is associated with the dilation of blood vessels and the release of histamine and other allergic compounds.

Migraine without aura (formerly called common migraine), is the type of migraine most likely to occur in children. Common migraine is characterized by a pounding or throbbing pain in the front or side(s) of the head. This headache may or may not be one-sided, may persist from one to 24 hours, and is usually accompanied by nausea, vomiting, and abdominal pain. Other associated symptoms may include fever, an unusual sensitivity to light (photophobia), numbness or tingling of the hands and feet, and dizziness or lightheadedness.

Migraine with aura (formerly called classic migraine), is characterized by similar symptoms and findings to those associated with common migraine; however, classic migraine is always preceded by an aura that occurs from 10 to 30 minutes before onset of the headache. This phenomenon may be characterized by visual, motor, or other sensations such as the appearance of shimmering or flashing lights (photopsia) as well as distorted images, loss of vision in part of the visual field (blind spot or scotoma), dizziness, tingling or weakness in an arm or leg, prickling or burning sensation around the mouth, and other irregularities.

In addition to the two primary types of migraine headaches, some children may develop unusual migraine headaches, called migraine variants, that may be characterized by vomiting that recurs at irregular intervals, sudden attacks of dizziness, and confusion. Children with this type of migraine, especially infants, may experience monthly episodes of severe vomiting resulting in excessive fluid loss (dehydration); the loss of essential compounds, known as electrolytes, in the fluid portion of the blood (i.e., sodium, calcium, and potassium); and associated fever, abdominal pain, and diarrhea. Children with migraine variants may at times appear disoriented, hyperactive, and nonresponsive. Other types of migraine include complicated migraine and cluster headaches. Complicated migraines refer to migraine headaches accompanied by neurologic findings that persist beyond the headache and may be further categorized as basilar migraine, ophthalmoplegic migraine, and hemiplegic migraine. These types of headaches may sometimes indicate the presence of an underlying lesion. Basilar migraine is characterized by problems with equilibrium, double or blurred vision, loss of vision in part of the visual field, lack of muscular coordination (ataxia), seizures, or other irregularities. Ophthalmoplegic migraine, which is characterized by paralysis of the eye muscles on the same side as the migraine, does not commonly occur in children. Amaurosis fugax, a variant of complicated migraine, is characterized by reversible blindness or partial blindness in one eye. Hemiplegic migraine is characterized by numbness and muscular weakness or paralysis affecting only one side of the body. It is rare for children to experience more than one hemiplegic migraine episode. Cluster headaches do not commonly occur in children.

Treatment for migraine headaches may first be directed toward prevention by identifying and removing or avoiding stimulating influences such as certain foods, medications, or underlying stress factors. Many children may benefit from simply resting in a quiet, darkened room. Treatment for pain and vomiting associated with migraine headaches may include administration of pain relievers such as acetaminophen or ibuprofen along with drugs to reduce vomiting (antiemetics). These drugs are often administered rectally in suppository form. In more severe episodes, older children and adolescents may require the administration of a preparation called ergotamine, which is most effective if taken during the early stages of the migraine episode. Ergotamine should not be administered to children with hemiplegic migraines. Some children and adolescents may benefit from behavior management therapy. Other treatment is symptomatic and supportive.

Government Agencies

4747 NIH/National Eye Institute
31 Center Drive MSC 2510
Bethesda, MD 20892

301-496-5248
2020@nei.nih.gov
www.nei.nih.gov

Conducts and supports research that helps prevent and treat eye diseases and other disorders of vision. This research leads to sight-saving treatments, reduces visual impairment and blindness, and improves the quality of life for people of all ages. NEI-supported research has advanced our knowledge of how the eye functions in health and disease.

Paul A Sieving M.D., Ph.D., Director

National Associations & Support Groups

4748 American Academy of Neurology
1080 Montreal Avenue Ste 100
Saint Paul, MN 55116

651-695-1940
800-879-1960
Fax: 651-695-2791
memberservices@aan.com
www.aan.com

Medical society established to advance the art and science of neurology, and thereby promote the best possible care for patients with neurological disorders by: ensuring appropriate access to neurological care, supporting and advocating for an environment which ensures ethical, high quality neurological care and supporting clinical and basic research in the neurosciences and related fields.

19,000 members

Catherine Rydell, CEO
Timothy A. Pedley, President
Stephen Sergay, President Elect

4749 American Academy of Pediatrics
141 Northwest Point Boulevard
Elk Grove Village, IL 60007

847-434-4000
800-433-9016
Fax: 847-434-8000
www.aap.org

The American Academy of Pediatrics and its member pediatricians are committed to the attainment of optimal physical, mental and social health and well-being for all infants, children, adolescents, and young adults.

Fernando Stein, MD, FAAP, President
Karen Remley, MD, CEO/Executive VP

4750 American Headache Society
19 Mantua Road
Mount Royal, NJ 8061

856-423-0043
Fax: 856-423-0082
ahshg@talley.com
www.americanheadachesociety.org

A professional society of health care providers dedicated to the study and treatment of headache and face pain. It was founded in 1959 and sponsors the American Council for Headache Education (ACHE), which will soon become a committee of the AHS.

Paul Winner, Chair
Linda McGillicuddy, Executive Director
Fred Sheftell, MD, President

4751 Migraine Awareness Group: National Understanding for Migraineurs (MAGNUM)
100 N Union Street, Suite B
Alexandria, VA 22314

703-349-1929
Fax: 703-739-2432
comments@migraines.org
www.migraines.org

Works to bring public awareness, utilizing the electronic, print, and artistic mediums, to the fact that Migraine is a true, biologic disease. Advocates on behalf of Migraine head pain sufferers worldwide.

Michael John Coleman, Founder/Executive Director
Terri Miller-Burchfield, Executive VP
Doug Johnson, Webmaster

4752 National Headache Foundation
820 N Orleans, Ste 217
Chicago, IL 60610

312-274-2650
888-643-5552
Fax: 312-640-9049
info@headaches.org
www.headaches.org

Nonprofit organization dedicated to the education of headache sufferers and health care professionals about the causes and treatment of headaches.

Seymour Diamond, Chairman/Founder
Roger K. Cady MD, Vice President
Edmond J. Bergeron, Treasurer

Research Centers

4753 Kennedy Krieger Institute
Pediatric Headache Program
707 N Broadway
Baltimore, MD 21205

443-923-9200
800-873-3377
webmaster@kennedykrieger.org
www.kennedykrieger.org

The Pediatric Headache Program was started in 2005 in order to facilitate the diagnosis, treatment and management of children and adolescents who suffer from persistent headaches, including migraine, tension and chronic daily.

John J Laterra, Program Clinical Coordinator
Terri Holbrook, Neurology/Nursing Staff Coordinator

Web Sites

4754 American Academy of Neurology
201 Chicago Avenue
Minneapolis, MN 55415

800-879-1960
Fax: 612-454-2746
memberservices@aan.com
www.aan.com

Medical society established to advance the art and science of neurology, and therby promote the best possible care for patients with neurological disordes by: ensuring appropriate access to neurological care, supporting and advocating for an environment which ensures ethical, high quality neurological care and supporting clinical and basic research in the neurosciences and reltated fields.

4755 Migraine Awareness Group: A National Understanding for Migraineurs
100 North Union Street, Suite B
Alexandria, VI 22314

comments@migraines.org
www.migraines.org

Brings public awareness to the fact that Migraine is a true, biological neurological disease using the electronic, print and artistic mediums of expression.

Michael John Coleman, President
Terri Miller Burchfield, Executive VP
P. Elizabeth Pirsch, General Council

4756 National Headache Foundation
820 N Orleans, Suite 411
Chicago, IL 60610

312-274-3650
888-643-5552
info@headches.com
www.headaches.org

A nonprofit organization dedicated to educating headache sufferers and healthcare professionals about headache causes and treatments.

Seymour Diamond, Executive Chairman
Arthur H. Elkind MD, President
Vincent Martin MD, Vice President

Book Publishers

4757 Freedom From Headaches
Joel Saper, author

Simon & Schuster
100 Front Street
Riverside, NJ 8075

856-461-6500
800-223-2336
Fax: 212-698-7099
www.simonandschuster.com

236 pages paperback
ISBN: 0-671254-04-9

Carolyn Reidy, President and Chief Executive Offic
Liz Perl, Senior Vice President, Marketing
Dennis Eulau, Executive Vice President, Operation

4758 Handbook of Headache
Lippincott Williams & Wilkins
351 W Camden Street
Baltimore, MD 21201
410-528-4000
800-638-3030
www.lww.com

2004 400 pages softbound
ISBN: 0-781752-23-0

Edward B. Hutton Jr., Chief Executive Officer, President
E. Passano Jr., Vice Chairman of the Board and Secr

4759 Headache Book: Prevention & Treatment for All Types of Headaches
Frank B. Minirth, author

Thomas Nelson Publishers
1 Gateway Plaza
Port Chester, NY 10573
914-937-2320
Fax: 914-937-3183
www.fsw.org

1994
ISBN: 0-785282-56-4

Susan B. Wayne, President/CEO
Geoffrey Barsky, CFO
Polly Kerrigan, Senior Vice President Program Opera

4760 Management of Headache & Headache Medications
Lawrence D. Robbins, author

Spring-Verlag
175 5th Avenue
New York, NY 10010
646-307-5151
Fax: 212-633-0748
www.us.macmillan.com

1994 294 pages
ISBN: 0-387989-44-7

Stefan von Holtzbrinck, Chairman, Executive Board
Klaus-Dieter Lehmann, Chairman, Supervisory Board
Sandra Dittert, Senior Vice President

4761 Migraine and Other Headaches: Vascular Mechanisms
Raven Press
19710 Ventura Blvd., Ste 108
Woodland Hills, CA 91364
818-888-3388
Fax: 818-888-1881
www.raven.com

Leading international experts present new concepts on the mechanisms of migraine and other vascular headaches and detail the latest strategies for diagnosis and treatment of migraine with and without aura, tension-type headaches, cluster headaches and other vascular disorders.

368 pages
ISBN: 0-881677-95-7

4762 Overcoming Headaches & Migraines
Longmeadow Press
PO Box 10218
Stamford, CT 06904
203-352-2110

1993 128 pages Paperback
ISBN: 0-681417-92-7

4763 Treating the Headache Patient
Roger K. Cady, author

Marcell Dekker, Inc.
270 Madison Avenue
New York, NY 10016
212-696-9000
Fax: 800-228-1160

1994 366 pages
ISBN: 0-824791-09-6

4764 Wolff's Headaches & Other Head Pain
Stephen D. Silberstein, author

Oxford University Press
198 Madison Avenue
New York, NY 10016
212-726-6000
800-445-9714
Fax: 919-677-1303
custserv.us@oup.com
www.us.oup.com/us

1993
ISBN: 0-195082-50-8

Newsletters

4765 Headache
American Council for Headache Education
19 Mantua Road
Mount Royal, NJ 8061
856-423-0043
Fax: 856-423-0082
achehq@talley.com
www.achenet.org

Provides valuable and current information on new treatments, as well as time-proven headache management strategies. All articles are written or reviewed by headache experts from the American Headache Society (AHS). Recent issues have included articles by headache experts on drug and nondrug treatment options and information on new treatments and research is regularly included.

12 pages Quarterly

Paul Winner, Chair
Arthur H. Elkind MD, President
Vincent Martin MD, Vice President

4766 NHF Head Lines
National Headache Foundation
820 N Orleans, Suite 411
Chicago, IL 60610
312-274-3650
888-643-5552
info@headches.com
www.headaches.org

Offers the latest information on headaches, causes and treatments. Contains news on drugs and medical forums, in-depth discussions of headaches and preventions and a question and answer section in which physicians respond to reader inquiries and support group information.

Bimonthly

Seymour Diamond, Executive Chairman
Arthur H. Elkind MD, President
Vincent Martin MD, Vice President

Pamphlets

4767 52 Proven Stress Reducers
National Headache Foundation
820 N Orleans, Suite 411
Chicago, IL 60610
312-274-3650
888-643-5552
Fax: 773-525-7357
info@headches.com
www.headaches.org

Seymour Diamond, Executive Chairman
Arthur H. Elkind MD, President
Vincent Martin MD, Vice President

4768 About Headaches
National Headache Foundation
820 N Orleans, Suite 411
Chicago, IL 60610
312-274-3650
888-643-5552
Fax: 312-640-9049
info@headches.com
www.headaches.org

Contains an in-depth look at headaches, tips on when to seek medical advice, methods of treatment and more.

16 pages

Seymour Diamond, Executive Chairman
Arthur H. Elkind MD, President
Vincent Martin MD, Vice President

4769 Analgesic Rebound Headaches-Fact Sheet
National Headache Foundation
820 N Orleans, Suite 411
Chicago, IL 60610

312-274-3650
888-643-5552
Fax: 312-640-9049
info@headaches.org
www.headaches.org

Offers information on analgesic agents or drugs used to control pain including migraine and other types of headaches.

Seymour Diamond, Executive Chairman
Arthur H. Elkind MD, President
Vincent Martin MD, Vice President

4770 Cluster Headache-Fact Sheet
National Headache Foundation
820 N Orleans, Suite 411
Chicago, IL 60610

312-274-3650
888-643-5552
Fax: 312-640-9049
info@headaches.org
www.headaches.org

Offers information on cluster headaches and the treatment available for them.

Seymour Diamond, Executive Chairman
Arthur H. Elkind MD, President
Vincent Martin MD, Vice President

4771 Diet and Headache-Fact Sheet
National Headache Foundation
820 N Orleans, Suite 411
Chicago, IL 60610

312-274-3650
888-643-5552
Fax: 312-640-9049
info@headaches.org
www.headaches.org

Offers information on what foods should be avoided, and what foods trigger headaches in all migraine sufferers.

Seymour Diamond, Executive Chairman
Arthur H. Elkind MD, President
Vincent Martin MD, Vice President

4772 Headache Facts-What Everyone Should Know
American Council for Headache Education
19 Mantua Road
Mount Royal, NJ 8061

856-423-0043
Fax: 856-423-0082
achehq@talley.com
www.achenet.org

Paul Winner, DO, Chair
Barry Baumel, Chair Of Funding Committee
John Rothrock, Journal Editor

4773 Headache Handbook
National Headache Foundation
820 N Orleans, Suite 411
Chicago, IL 60610

312-274-2650
888-643-5552
Fax: 312-640-9049
info@headaches.org
www.headaches.org

Gives information and coauses on five common types of headaches as well as treatments available.

8 pages

Arthur H. Elkind MD, President
Vincent Marin, M.D., Vice President
Chad Beste, Treasurer

4774 Headache Q & A
National Headache Foundation
820 N Orleans, Suite 411
Chicago, IL 60610

312-274-2650
888-643-5552
Fax: 312-640-9049
info@headaches.org
www.headaches.org

Handy, fact-filled card contains the most frequently asked questions and answers concerning headache triggers and treatments.

Arthur H. Elkind MD, President
Vincent Marin, M.D., Vice President
Chad Beste, Treasurer

4775 Headache in Children-Fact Sheet
National Headache Foundation
820 N Orleans, Suite 411
Chicago, IL 60610

312-274-2650
888-643-5552
Fax: 312-640-9049
info@headaches.org
www.headaches.org

Offers information on vascular headaches, tension-type headaches, traction and inflammatory headaches and treatment.

Arthur H. Elkind MD, President
Vincent Marin, M.D., Vice President
Chad Beste, Treasurer

4776 How to Talk to Your Doctor About Headaches
National Headache Foundation
820 N Orleans, Suite 411
Chicago, IL 60610

312-274-2650
888-643-5552
Fax: 312-640-9049
info@headaches.com
www.headaches.org

Learn how to keep a headache diary to pinpoint symptoms and effective diagnosis.

Arthur H. Elkind MD, President
Vincent Marin, M.D., Vice President
Chad Beste, Treasurer

4777 Impact of Migraine-A Disabling and Costly Condition
American Council for Headache Education
19 Mantua Road
Mount Royal, NJ 8061

856-423-0043
Fax: 856-423-0082
achehq@talley.com
www.achenet.org

Paul Winner, DO, Chair
Barry Baumel, Chair Of Funding Committee
John Rothrock, Journal Editor

4778 Migraine and Coexisting Conditions-Other Illnesses That May Affect Migraine
American Council for Headache Education
19 Mantua Road
Mount Royal, NJ 8061

856-423-0043
Fax: 856-423-0082
achehq@talley.com
www.achenet.org

Paul Winner, DO, Chair
Barry Baumel, Chair Of Funding Committee
John Rothrock, Journal Editor

4779 Migraine-Fact Sheet
National Headache Foundation
820 N Orleans, Suite 411
Chicago, IL 60610

312-274-2650
888-643-5552
Fax: 312-640-9049
info@headaches.com
www.headaches.org

Offers information on migraines and treatments.

Arthur H. Elkind MD, President
Vincent Marin, M.D., Vice President
Chad Beste, Treasurer

4780 Tap the Best Resource
National Headache Foundation
820 N Orleans, Suite 411
Chicago, IL 60610

312-274-2650
888-643-5552
Fax: 312-640-9049
info@headaches.org
www.headaches.org

Informational brochure offering facts and statistics on headaches.
Everything from muscle contraction, vascular headaches, sinus
headaches, TMJ, and much more.

Arthur H. Elkind MD, President
Vincent Marin, M.D., Vice President
Chad Beste, Treasurer

4781 What's the Best Medicine for My Headaches?
American Council for Headache Education
19 Mantua Road
Mount Royal, NJ 8061

856-423-0043
Fax: 856-423-0082
achehq@talley.com
www.achenet.org

Paul Winner, DO, Chair
Barry Baumel, Chair Of Funding Committee
John Rothrock, Journal Editor

**4782 When Are Opioid (Narcotic) Drugs Appropriate for
Headache?**
American Council for Headache Education
19 Mantua Road
Mount Royal, NJ 8061

856-423-0043
Fax: 856-423-0082
achehq@talley.com
www.achenet.org

Paul Winner, DO, Chair

4783 Women and Headache
American Council for Headache Education
19 Mantua Road
Mount Royal, NJ 8061

856-423-0043
Fax: 856-423-0082
achehq@talley.com
www.achenet.org

Paul Winner, DO, Chair

DESCRIPTION

4784 MILK PROTEIN ALLERGY/LACTOSE INTOLERANCE

Involves the following Biologic System(s):

Gastrointestinal Disorders

Milk protein allergy is an allergic reaction to the proteins found in cow's milk and is the most common food allergy in children. Cow's milk is a large source of nutrition for infants and children. Infant formulas are primarily composed of cow's milk proteins, and milk products are often a major source of calories, protein, vitamins, and minerals in a child's diet. Cow's milk contains proteins, sugars (carbohydrates), as well as fats. Breastmilk can also contain these proteins from the mother's diet. There are several distinct diseases entities that would fall under the category of milk allergy or intolerance.

Most infants show symptoms of cow's milk protein allergy within the first three to six months of exposure. The immune system of the infant recognizes the milk protein as foreign and reacts by making immune proteins (antibodies also known as immunoglobulins) to defend the body against the foreign protein. Milk protein allergy can be either an immediate-onset or delayed-onset allergic reaction. Immediate-onset reactions can manifest acutely with gastrointestinal (diarrhea, vomiting, abdominal pain), respiratory (asthma, wheezing), or dermatologic (eczema, hives) symptoms. Delayed-onset reactions usually manifest with chronic diarrhea that may be bloody (hematochezia). More severe disease leads to small bowel damage and poor weight gain (failure to thrive).

The diagnosis of milk protein allergy can be made by history and physical exam. Stool, blood, skin and/or milk challenge tests may also be used to aid in diagnosis. Milk protein allergy is reported in up to 4% of infants, and usually resolves by age three. Until that time, infants on formula are fed special formulas (hydrolysate formula) and breastfeeding mothers should avoid milk and milk products. Infants with cow's milk protein allergy have a higher chance of having soy milk protein allergy and therefore soy formulas are not recommended. As children get older, milk is slowly reintroduced. Fortunately, most babies outgrow their milk allergies by their second or third year.

Lactose intolerance is not an allergic reaction, but an inability to digest the primary sugar found in milk (lactose). In the small intestine there is an enzyme (lactase) that breaks lactose down into smaller sugars to be used by the body. Symptoms of lactose intolerance include abdominal cramping, bloating, diarrhea, and flatulence. There are large racial differences in the incidence of lactose intolerance; persons of Asian and African descent have a higher incidence in comparison to Caucasians.

Symptoms of lactose intolerance can occur any time after age 5 because lactase enzyme activity peaks in infancy and early childhood. One exception is congenital lactase deficiency. In this genetic disorder, infants are born without the enzyme lactase and symptoms, such as abdominal bloating and diarrhea, occur in the first week of life.

The treatment for lactose intolerance is avoidance of milk or lactase enzyme supplementation (available in pill form or added to milk products).

National Associations & Support Groups

4785 American Academy of Pediatrics
141 Northwest Point Boulevard
Elk Grove Village, IL 60007   847-434-4000
                                               800-433-9016
                                               Fax: 847-434-8000
                                               www.aap.org

The American Academy of Pediatrics and its member pediatricians are committed to the attainment of optimal physical, mental and social health and well-being for all infants, children, adolescents, and young adults.

Fernando Stein, MD, FAAP, President
Karen Remley, MD, CEO/Executive VP

4786 International Foundation for Functional Gastrointestinal Disorders (IFFGD)
PO Box 170864
Milwaukee, WI 53217   414-964-1799
                                               Fax: 414-964-7176
                                               iffgd@iffgd.org
                                               www.iffgd.org

A nonprofit education and research organization founded in 1991. IFFGD addresses the issues surrounding life with gastrointestinal functional and motility disorders and increases the awareness about these disorders among the general public, researchers, and the clinical care community.

Nancy J. Norton, President & Director
William Norton, Co-Founder
Michael Cohen, Director

4787 North American Society for Pediatric Gastroenterology/Hepatology/Nutrition
714 N Bethlehem Pike, Suite 300
Ambler, PA 19002   215-641-9800
                                               Fax: 215-641-1995
                                               naspghan@naspghan.org
                                               www.naspghan.org

Strives to improve the care of infants, children and adolescents with digestive disorders by promoting advances in clinical care of children with chronic abdominal pain, diarrhea, constipation, vomiting, bleeding from the GI tract, inflammatory bowel disease, liver diseases, diseases of the pancreas, poor weight gain and nutritional problems.

Margaret K Stallings, Executive Director
Kim Rose, Associate Director
Donna Murphy, Membership

4788 Parents of Galactosemic Children
P.O. Box 2401
Mandeville, LA 70470   228-497-5886
                                               866-900-7421
                                               president@galactosemia.org
                                               www.galactosemia.org

A nonprofit national organization founded in 1985 by a small group of mothers in New York. It offers support and educational information to galactosemic families and facilitates communication between them and professionals.

Michelle Fowler, President
Diane Flynn, Secretary
Paul Fowler, Treasurer

Web Sites

4789 Galactosemia Resources and Information
P.O. Box 1512
Deerfield Beach, FL 33443   215-233-0808
                                               866-900-7421
                                               Fax: 215-233-3939
                                               scott.shepard@galactosemia.org
                                               galactosemia.org

A repository for information about galactosemia and a jumping-off point to other places on the web.

Scott Shepard, President
Scott Saylor, Vice-President
Paul Fowler, Treasurer

4790 International Foundation for Functional Gastrointestinal Disorders (IFFGD)
PO Box 170864
Milwaukee, WI 53217
414-964-1799
Fax: 414-964-7176
iffgd@iffgd.org
www.iffgd.org

Nancy J. Norton, President & Director
William Norton, Co-Founder
Eleanor Cautley, Vice President

4791 NASPGHAN
714 N. Bethlehem Pike, Ste 300
Ambler, PA 19002
215-641-9800
Fax: 215-641-1995
naspghan@naspghan.org
www.naspghan.org

Offering information on pediatric gastroenterology, hepatology and nutrition.

Margaret K Stallings, Executive Director
Kim Rose, Associate Director
Donna Murphy, Membership

4792 Parents of Galactosemic Children
P.O. Box 1512
Deerfield Beach, FL 33443
866-900-7421
scott.shepard@galactosemia.org
galactosemia.org

Offering support and educational information to galactosemic families and interested professionals.

Scott Shepard, President
Scott Saylor, Vice-President
Paul Fowler, Treasurer

Book Publishers

4793 Raising Your Child Without Milk: Reassuring Advice and Recipes For Parent
Simon & Simon
100 Front Street
Riverside, NJ 08075
856-461-6500
800-488-4308
Fax: 800-943-9831
info@simonsays.com
www.simonandschuster.com

This book offers parents of milk-allergic or lactose intolerant children and the most up-to-date medical and nutritional information. It contains 125 dairy free recipes, and answers questions sent in from parents across the country.

384 pages Paperback

Carolyn Reidy, President/CEO
Liz Perl, Senior Vice President, Marketing
Dennis Eulau, Executive Vice President, Operation

4794 What You Need To Know About Lactose Intolerance
NIDDK Health Information Center
1 Information Way
Bethesda, MD 20892
800-860-8747
TTY: 866-569-1162
healthinfo@niddk.nih.gov
catalog.niddk.nih.gov

Defines lactose intolerance and provides information on symptoms, diagnosis and treatment.

16 pages Spanish

Griffin P. Rodgers, M.D, Director

Journals

4795 Managing Food Allergy and Intolerance
Janice Vickerstaff Joneja, PhD, author

J A Hall Publications
2401-9304 Salish Court
Burnaby, BC
Canada
604-738-9688
888-993-6133
Fax: 604-738-9425
info@hallpublications.com
www.hallpublications.com

This is a fully-referenced, extensively researched and indexed manual for health care professionals counseling those with food allergy or intolerance.

581 pages
ISBN: 0-968209-80-7

Newsletters

4796 NASPGHAN News
714 N. Bethlehem Pike, Ste 300
Ambler, PA 19002
215-641-9800
Fax: 215-641-1995
naspghan@naspghan.org
www.naspghan.org

Publication of the North American Society for Pediatric Gastroenterolgy, Hepatology and Nutrition, which strives to improve the care of infants, children and adolescents with digestive disorders by promoting advances in clinical care of children with chronic abdominal pain, diarrhea, constipation, vomiting, bleeding from the GI tract, inflammatory bowel disease, liver diseases, diseases of the pancreas, poor weight gain and nutritional problems.

Margaret K Stallings, Executive Director
Kim Rose, Associate Director
Donna Murphy, Membership

Pamphlets

4797 Lactose Intolerance
NDDIC
2 Information Way
Bethesda, MD 20892
301-496-3583
800-891-5389
Fax: 703-738-4929
nddic@info.niddk.nih.gov
www.niddk.nih.gov

8 pages

Griffin P. Rodgers, M.D., Director
Dr. Gregory Germino, Deputy Director
Kevin Abbott, Program Director

DESCRIPTION

4798 MUCOLIPIDOSES

Synonym: ML

Involves the following Biologic System(s):

Genetic/Chromosomal/Syndrome/Metabolic Disorders

The mucolipidoses (ML) are inborn errors of metabolism that belong to a group of diseases known as lysosomal storage disorders. Lysosomes are the major digestive structures within cells. Certain proteins known as enzymes break down or digest nutrients, such as particular fats or carbohydrates. The mucolipidoses are characterized by a deficiency or the abnormal functioning of certain lysosomal enzymes, causing the abnormal accumulation of complex carbohydrates (glycosaminoglycans) and fats (lipids) in cells within particular tissues. Such tissues may include those of the brain and spinal cord (central nervous system), skeleton, joints, heart, liver, spleen, or eyes. The mucolipidoses are thought to be inherited as an autosomal recessive trait.

Specific names as well as Roman numerals are used to classify the different forms of ML. Different types of mucolipidosis include I-Cell disease (ML II), pseudo-Hurler polydystrophy (ML III), and Berman syndrome (ML IV). Some forms of ML are further divided into different subtypes, such as sialidosis (ML I) types I and II, based on age of onset, associated symptoms, or other factors.

In children with mucolipidosis, associated symptoms and findings may be variable, depending upon the specific form of ML that is present. However, certain abnormalities occur in association with most forms of ML. Such findings include mild to severe coarsening of facial features, characteristic skeletal abnormalities (known as dysostosismultiplex), changes of the joints, and varying levels of mental retardation. In children with ML, skeletal malformations may include short stature; abnormal front-to-back or sideways curvature of the spine (kyphosis or scoliosis) or both; improper development of the hips (hip dysplasia); abnormally short neck; or premature fusion of the fibrous joints (sutures) between certain bones of the skull. Many affected children may develop joint stiffness and abnormal bending of certain joints in a fixed position (contractures). In addition, in some patients, neuromuscular abnormalities may be present, such as unusually decreased muscle tone (hypotonia) followed by abnormally exaggerated reflexes (hyperreflexia); shock-like contractions of certain muscles or muscle groups (myoclonus); or involuntary, rapid or writhing movements of the arms and legs (choreoathetoid movements).

Some forms of ML may also be associated with distinctive eye abnormalities, such as clouding of the corneas (corneal opacities), the development of abnormal red circular areas of the middle layer of the eyes (cherry-red spots), or other defects, causing visual impairment. Additional physical abnormalities associated with ML may include bulging of part of the intestine through a weak area in the abdominal wall (hernias), enlargement of the liver or spleen, enlargement of the heart or other heart defects, or increased susceptibility to repeated respiratory infections. Some children with these disorders may also experience delays in the acquisition of skills that require the coordination of physical and mental activities (psychomotor retardation) and may develop progressively se-

vere mental retardation. Other patients may experience mild, nonprogressive mental retardation. Some of the mucolipidoses may result in potentially life-threatening complications during childhood, adolescence, or young adulthood.

The treatment of children with mucolipidosis is symptomatic and supportive. Such measures may include therapies to help prevent or aggressively treat respiratory infections; surgical correction of joint contractures, heart abnormalities, hernias, or other defects; physical therapy; special education; or other measures as required.

National Associations & Support Groups

4799 American Academy of Pediatrics
141 Northwest Point Boulevard
Elk Grove Village, IL 60007
847-434-4000
800-433-9016
Fax: 847-434-8000
www.aap.org

The American Academy of Pediatrics and its member pediatricians are committed to the attainment of optimal physical, mental and social health and well-being for all infants, children, adolescents, and young adults.

Fernando Stein, MD, FAAP, President
Karen Remley, MD, CEO/Executive VP

4800 March of Dimes Foundation
1275 Mamaroneck Avenue
White Plains, NY 10605
914-997-4488
888-663-4637
Fax: 914-428-8203
answers@marchofdimes.com
www.marchofdimes.com

Partnership of volunteers and professionals dedicates to improving the health of babies by preventing birth defects and infant mortality. Over 100 chapters are located across the country and can be located through the National Office.

Stacey D. Stewart, President

4801 Mucolipidosis IV Foundation
719 E 17th Street
Brooklyn, NY 11230
718-434-5064
877-654-5459
www.ml4.org

Funds three major institutions comprised of the best genetic scientists recognized worldwide.

Paul Tanenholz, President
Randy Gold, VP
Paula Kutner, Secretary and Treasurer

4802 National MPS Society
PO Box 14686
Durham, NC 27709
919-806-0101
877-MPS-1001
Fax: 919-806-2055
info@mpssociety.org
www.mpssociety.org

Organization that serves as a support group for those affected by mucopolysaccharidoses and related disorders. Raises funds to promote research and increases awareness of the disorder.

Stephanie Bozarth, President
Kim Whitecotton, Vice President
Lisa Todd, Treasurer

Web Sites

4803 Healthfinder
1101 Wootton Parkway
Rockville, MD 20852
healthfinder@hhs.gov
www.healthfinder.gov

Links to carefully selected information and Web sites from over 1,500 health-related organizations.

4804 Mucolipidosis IV Foundation
3500 Piedmont Road Suite 500
Atlanta, GA 30305
877-654-5459
www.ml4.org

Funds three major institutions comprised of the best genetic scientists recognized worldwide.

Paul Tanenholz, Past President

4805 National MPS Society
PO Box 14686
Durham, NC 27709
919-806-0101
www.mpssociety.org

Shares information on the care and management of the children with Mucopolysaccharide diseases. The conference also brings in Medical Researchers reporting on advances in research related to these diseases.

Stephanie Bozarth, President
Kim Whitecotton, Vice President
Lisa Todd, Treasurer

4806 Online Mendelian Inheritance in Man
National Library of Medicine Building 38A
Bethesda, MD 20894
888-346-3656
info@ncbi.nlm.nih.gov
www.ncbi.nlm.nih.gov

This database is a catalog of human genes and genetic disorders.

Book Publishers

4807 Let's Talk About Going to the Hospital
Rosen Publishing Group's PowerKids Press
29 E 21st Street
New York, NY 10010
212-777-3017
800-237-9932
Fax: 888-436-4643
rosenpub@tribeca.ios.com
www.rosenpublishing.com

If a child has to check into the hospital, chances are he or she is already upset about being ill. Knowing how a hospital functions and what the procedures are, such as when family members can visit, will help in what is already a stressful situation. Grades K-5.

24 pages
ISBN: 0-823950-36-0

Roger Rosen, President

DESCRIPTION

4808 MUCOPOLYSACCHARIDOSES

Synonym: MPS

Involves the following Biologic System(s):

Genetic/Chromosomal/Syndrome/Metabolic Disorders

The mucopolysaccharidoses (MPS) are hereditary metabolic disorders that belong to a group of diseases known as lysosomal storage disorders. Lysosomes are the major digestive units within cells. Enzymes within lysosomes break down nutrients, such as certain fats and carbohydrates. The mucopolysaccharidoses are characterized by deficiency of certain lysosomal enzymes, causing the abnormal accumulation of complex carbohydrates in cells within particular tissues of the body. Affected tissues and organs typically include the skeleton, joints, brain and spinal cord (central nervous system), heart, liver, spleen, and eyes. The genes that encode most of these enzymes have been mapped to particular chromosomes. All of the mucopolysaccharidoses are inherited as an autosomal recessive trait, with the exception of Hunter syndrome, which has X-linked recessive inheritance. Collectively, these disorders are thought to affect approximately one in 10,000 newborns.

The various forms of MPS are typically designated by a Roman numeral and a specific name, such as Hunter syndrome (MPS II) or Sanfilippo syndrome (MPS III). In addition, some forms of MPS are divided into different subtypes, such as Hurler syndrome (MPS I H) and Hurler-Scheie syndrome (MPS I H/S), based on different changes (mutations) of the disease gene, age of onset, clinical course, or other factors. The range and severity of associated symptoms and findings may vary, depending upon the specific form of MPS that is present. However, certain findings are common to most forms of MPS, such as characteristic skeletal abnormalities (known as dysostosis multiplex), changes of the joints, growth delays, a characteristic facial appearance, and progressive mental retardation. For example, beginning in the first year of life or during later childhood, many patients develop progressively coarse facial features. Many children with MPS also experience delays in the acquisition of skills requiring the coordination of physical and mental activities (psychomotor retardation), a gradual loss of previously acquired skills (developmental regression), and progressively severe mental retardation. However, in a few forms of MPS, children may have average intelligence.

Many children with MPS also have short stature; sideways or front-to-back curvature of the spine (scoliosis or kyphosis) or both; other bone abnormalities; joint stiffness; and abnormal bending of certain joints in a fixed position (contractures). Other common findings include clouding of the corneas of the eyes and associated visual impairment, abnormal bulging of part of the intes|tine through a weak area in the abdominal wall (hernias), and enlargement of the liver and spleen (hepatosplenomegaly). Some patients also have associated abnormalities of the heart and its major blood vessels (cardiovascular defects), such as narrowing of the arteries supplying the heart; improper closure of one of the heart valves, allowing blood to leak back into the left upper chamber of the heart (mitral insufficiency); or other cardiac defects. Many of these disorders may result in potentially life-threatening complications during childhood or adolescence.

The treatment of children with MPS includes symptomatic and supportive measures, such as surgical correction of hernias, cardiovascular defects, joint contractures, or other abnormalities as required; physical therapy; or special education. In patients with some forms of MPS, enzyme replacement therapy has been shown to provide some temporary benefit. In addition, bone marrow transplantation may be effective in some patients with certain forms of mucopolysaccharidosis (e.g., Hurler syndrome).

National Associations & Support Groups

4809 American Academy of Pediatrics
141 Northwest Point Boulevard
Elk Grove Village, IL 60007

847-434-4000
800-433-9016
Fax: 847-434-8000
www.aap.org

The American Academy of Pediatrics and its member pediatricians are committed to the attainment of optimal physical, mental and social health and well-being for all infants, children, adolescents, and young adults.

Fernando Stein, MD, FAAP, President
Karen Remley, MD, CEO/Executive VP

4810 Association for Neuro-Metabolic Disorders
5223 Brookfield Lane
Sylvania, OH 43560

419-885-1809
volk4olks@aol.com

Nonprofit organization that serves as an advocate organization for families of patients with the following neuro-metabolic disorders: phenylketonuria, maple syrup urine disease, galactosemia, and biotinidase deficiency. Provides educational information for parents and children; provides networking information on support groups for new parents; supports scientific research into the treatments of these four neuro-metabolic disorders.

Cheryl Volk, Contact Person

4811 March of Dimes Foundation
1275 Mamaroneck Avenue
White Plains, NY 10605

914-997-4488
888-663-4637
Fax: 914-428-8203
answers@marchofdimes.com
www.marchofdimes.com

Partnership of volunteers and professionals dedicates to improving the health of babies by preventing birth defects and infant mortality. Over 100 chapters are located across the country and can be located through the National Office.

Stacey D. Stewart, President

4812 National MPS Society
PO Box 14686
Durham, NC 27709

919-806-0101
Fax: 919-806-2055
info@mpssociety.org
www.mpssociety.org

Organization that serves as a support group for those affected by mucopolysaccharidoses and related disorders. Raises funds to promote research and increases awareness of the disorder.

Stephan Holland, President
Stephanie Bozarth, VP
Tom Gniazdowski, Treasurer

Web Sites

4813 Canadian Society for Mucopolysaccharide & Related Diseases
Po Box 30034 RPO Parkgate
North Vancouver, BC v7h2y
canada

604-924-5130
800-667-1846
Fax: 604-924-5131
www.mpssociety.ca

Provides information and support to affected individuals and their families.

Bernie Geiss, Chair
Judy Byrne, Secretary
Brent Nichols, Treasurer

4814 Healthfinder
1101 Wootton Parkway
Rockville, MD 20852

healthfinder@hhs.gov
www.healthfinder.gov

Links to carefully selected information and Web sites from over 1,500 health-related organizations.

4815 Mucopolysaccharidoes & Related Diseases
Po Box 30034 RPO Parkgate
North Vancouver, BC v7h2y

604-924-5130
800-667-1846
Fax: 604-924-5131
www.mpssociety.ca/

Provides information and support to affected individuals and their families.

Bernie Geiss, Chair
Judy Byrne, Secretary
Brent Nichols, Treasurer

4816 National MPS Society
PO Box 14686
Durham, NC 27709

919-806-0101
www.mpssociety.org

Shares information on the care and management of the children with Mucopolysaccharide diseases. The conference also brings in Medical Researchers reporting on advances in research related to these diseases.

Stephanie Bozarth, President
Kim Whitecotton, Vice President
Lisa Todd, Treasurer

4817 Online Mendelian Inheritance in Man
National Library of Medicine Building 38A
Bethesda, MD 20894

888-346-3656
info@ncbi.nlm.nih.gov
www.ncbi.nlm.nih.gov

This database is a catalog of human genes and genetic disorders.

4818 Society for Mucopolysaccharide Diseases
MPS House, Repton Place, White Lion Road
Amersham, Bu HP7 9

345-389-9901
Fax: 345-389-9902
mps@mpssociety.org.uk
www.mpssociety.co.uk

A voluntary support group that represents from throughout the UK over 1200 children and adults suffering from mucopolysaccharide and related diseases, their families, caregivers and professionals. It is a registered charity entirely supported by voluntary donations and fundraising. It is managed by the members themselves.

Book Publishers

4819 Let's Talk About Going to the Hospital
Rosen Publishing Group's PowerKids Press
29 E 21st Street
New York, NY 10010

212-777-3017
800-237-9932
Fax: 888-436-4643
rosenpub@tribeca.ios.com
www.rosenpublishing.com

If a child has to check into the hospital, chances are he or she is already upset about being ill. Knowing how a hospital functions and what the procedures are, such as when family members can visit, will help in what is already a stressful situation. Grades K-5.

24 pages
ISBN: 0-823950-36-0

Roger Rosen, President

DESCRIPTION

4820 MUSCULAR DYSTROPHIES

Synonyms: Duchenne muscular dystrophy, Becker muscular dystrophy, Landouzy-Dejerine disease

Involves the following Biologic System(s):

Neurologic Disorders, Orthopedic and Muscle Disorders

Muscular dystrophies are a group of inherited neuromuscular disorders characterized by the progressive weakness and degeneration of muscles without accompanying nerve tissue involvement. Each of these disorders is different from the others with respect to its age of onset, clinical manifestations, severity, course, and underlying genetic defect.

Duchenne muscular dystrophy, the most common of these disorders, is transmitted as an X-linked recessive trait and, as such, is fully expressed in boys; however, on rare occasions, girls who are carriers of the disease gene may exhibit mild symptoms. The incidence rate for this disorder is about one out of every 3,600 newborn boys. Although some affected infants may exhibit signs of diminished muscle tone such as poor head control, most boys do not develop symptoms until three to seven years of age. Early symptoms may include weakness in the pelvic girdle area that may be manifested by an unusual method of moving from the supine position to the standing position (Gowers' sign). In addition, boys with this disorder may develop a waddling manner of walking (Trendelenburg gait), be prone to stumbling and falling, or having difficulty climbing stairs and standing up from a sitting position. As the disease progresses, muscles around the joints may contract resulting in the inability to fully extend the knees and elbows. In addition, the spine may develop a side-to-side curve (scoliosis) and muscles, especially of the calves, become bulky due to the enlargement (hypertrophy) of the muscle fibers, the infiltration of fat into the muscles, and the increase of connective tissue protein (collagen) in the muscles. Other findings include involvement of the heart muscle (cardiomyopathy) and intellectual impairment ranging from learning disabilities to mental retardation. Most boys with Duchenne muscular dystrophy are able to walk until the age of 10 or 12 years, at which time they may be confined to a wheelchair. Life-threatening complications such as pneumonia, respiratory failure, and congestive heart failure often occur during late adolescence or early adulthood. This disorder is believed to result from the deficiency of the essential muscle protein dystrophin. The gene for Duchenne muscular dystrophy is located on the short arm of the X chromosome (Xp21).

Duchenne muscular dystrophy is initially diagnosed through evaluation of physical findings and through tests that show increased blood levels of the enzyme creatinine kinase. Additional diagnostic screening may include the use of an electrical muscle function test called electromyography or EMG. Confirmation, however, must be determined through microscopic examination of a muscle tissue sample (biopsy). Treatment is symptomatic and supportive. For example, nutritional vigilance and immunizations against flu and other childhood diseases may help to avoid or postpone complications. The administration of digitalis medications may help to alleviate certain heart-related complications. Some children may benefit from physical therapy, exercise, or surgical intervention to aid in walking.

Becker muscular dystrophy results in symptoms similar to those of Duchenne muscular dystrophy; however, these symptoms are usually less severe, do not appear until about the age of 10 years, and follow a long course. Patients usually remain ambulatory, and most survive into their 30s and 40s. The gene for Becker muscular dystrophy is also located on the short arm of the X chromosome (Xp21); however, the essential muscle protein dystrophin is defective and dysfunctional rather than deficient.

Less common forms of muscular dystrophy include facioscapulohumeral muscular dystrophy (Landouzy-Dejerine disease), limb-girdle muscular dystrophy, and others. Facioscapulohumeral muscular dystrophy, which is an autosomal dominant disorder occurring in both males and females, is characterized by facial and shoulder muscle weakness and sometimes weakness in the lower legs. This is a relatively mild disease that usually occurs between seven years of age and early or mid-adulthood. The gene for this disorder is located on the long arm of chromosome 4 (4q35). Limb-girdle muscular dystrophy is usually transmitted as an autosomal recessive trait, although autosomal dominant inheritance has also been documented. This disorder usually occurs in late childhood or early adulthood and is characterized by the progressive weakness and degeneration of the muscles of the hips and shoulders. Treatment for these types of muscular dystrophy is symptomatic and supportive.

National Associations & Support Groups

4821 American Academy of Pediatrics
141 Northwest Point Boulevard
Elk Grove Village, IL 60007

847-434-4000
800-433-9016
Fax: 847-434-8000
www.aap.org

The American Academy of Pediatrics and its member pediatricians are committed to the attainment of optimal physical, mental and social health and well-being for all infants, children, adolescents, and young adults.

Fernando Stein, MD, FAAP, President
Karen Remley, MD, CEO/Executive VP

4822 Duchenne Parent Project Muscular Dystrophy
401 Hackensack Avenue, 9th Floor
Hackensack, NJ 07601

201-250-8440
800-714-5437
Fax: 201-250-8435
info@parentprojectmd.org
www.parentprojectmd.org

Parent Project Muscular Dystrophy is a not-for-profit organization founded in 1994 by parents of children with Duchenne and Becker muscular dystrophy. Today, the focus is on areas such as; seeking to ensure that all families, caregivers, health care professionals and others have access to state-of-the-art information about treatment and care options for children with Duchenne and Becker MD, and to ensure that the voices of people with and affected by Duchenne and Becker are heard.

Pat Furlong, Founding President/CEO
Kimberly Galberaith, Executive VP
Ryan Fischer, Office Manager

4823 Facioscapulohumeral Dystrophy Society
450 Bedford Street
Lexington, MA 02420

781-301-6060
Fax: 781-862-1116
info@fshsociety.org
www.fshsociety.org

Daniel Paul Perez, President/CEO
Nancy Van Zant, Executive Director

4824 **Muscular Dystrophy Association**
3300 E Sunrise Drive
Tucson, AZ 85718 520-529-2000
800-572-1717
Fax: 520-529-5300
mda@mdausa.org
www.mda.org

Voluntary health agency aimed at conquering neuromuscular diseases that affect more than 1,000,000 Americans. The diseases in MDA's program include nine forms of muscular dystrophy, amyotrophic lateral sclerosis (Lou Gehrig's disease), spinal muscular atrophy, Charcot-Marie-Tooth disease, and other neuromuscular conditions. With over 200 offices across the country, MDA conducts research, medical and community services, clinics, support groups, summer camps for youngsters and much more.

Jennifer Lopez, Assoc. Director of Health Care Svcs

4825 **Muscular Dystrophy Family Foundation**
1033 Third Avenue SW, Suite 108
Indianapolis, IN 46032 317-249-8488
800-544-1213
Fax: 317-853-6743
mdff@mdff.org
www.mdff.org

Provides adaptive equipment and emotional support to individuals and families affected by one of the over forty neuromuscular diseases. Established in 1958, some of the equipment provided includes: hospital beds, wheelchairs, ramps, communication devices, and lifts.

Paula McDonald, Executive Director
Hazel M Walker, Vice President

4826 **Reflex Sympathetic Dystrophy Syndrome Association**
PO Box 502
Milford, CT 06460 203-877-3790
877-662-7737
Fax: 203-882-8362
info@rsds.org
www.rsds.org

The Reflex Sympathetic Dystrophy Syndrome Association was founded in 1984 to promote public and professional awareness of Reflex Sympathetic Dystrophy Syndrome, also known as Complex Regional Pain Syndrome. Educates those afflicted with this syndrome, their family, friends, insurance and healthcare providers, on the disabling pain the syndrome causes. Publishes quarterly newsletter, clinical practice guidelines, and has a very helpful website.

James E Tyrrell Jr. Esquire, Chairman of the Board
Paul R. Charlesworth, President
Donald F. McKee, Vice President, Treasurer

Research Centers

4827 **Rusk Institute of Rehabilitation Medicine**
NYU Langone Medical Center
400 E 34th Street
New York, NY 10016 212-263-6034
Fax: 212-263-8510
gwen.treharne@nyumc.org
www.rusk.med.nyu.edu

The world's first university-affiliated facility devoted entirely to rehabilitation medicine, Rusk is among the most renowned center of its kind for the treatment of adults and children with disabilities-home to innovations and advances that have set the standard in rehabilitation care for every stage of life and for every stage of recovery.

Dr. Steven Flanagan, Professor & Chairman
Marilyn Shoo, Pediatrics Director

Minnesota

4828 **Mayo Clinic and Foundation**
200 First Street S.W.
Rochester, MN 55905 507-284-2511
800-660-4582
Fax: 507-284-0161
www.mayo.edu

Neuromuscular clinical research center with a primary research interest in neuropathies.

Julie E Hammack, CEO

New York

4829 **Columbia Presbyterian Medical Center**
Neurology Institute of NY/Research Center
630 W 168th Street
New York, NY 10032 212-305-3880
alscenter@columbia.edu
www.nyp.org

Neuromuscular clinical research center.

Steven J. Corwin, CEO
Robert E. Kelly, President

4830 **NYU Rusk Institute**
301 East 17th Street, Second Avenue
New York, NY 10003 212-263-6034
Fax: 212-263-8510
www.rusk.med.nyu.edu

Focuses on Muscular Dystrophy and related bone disorders.

Jeffrey Cohen MD, Director
Marilyn Shoo, Pediatrics Director

Ohio

4831 **Parent Project for Muscular Dystrophy Research**
401 Hackensack Avenue, 9th Floor
Hackensack, NJ 07601 201-250-8440
800-714-5437
Fax: 201-250-8435
info@parentprojectmd.org
www.parentprojectmd.org

Organization of families around the world who have children diagnosed with DMD/BMD. The goal is to invest significant amounts of money raised into medical research with clinical application.

Robert J McDonald, Chairman
John Killian, Treasurer
Daniel Garofalo, Secretary

Pennsylvania

4832 **Penn Neurological Institute**
Hospital of the University of Pennsylvania
3417 Spruce Street
Philadelphia, PA 19104 215-662-3396
800-789-7366
www.pennmedicine.org

Research program centering its efforts on finding better ways to prevent and treat neuromuscular disorders.

Michael E Selzer, Director Neuromuscular Diseases

Texas

4833 **Baylor College of Medicine**
Neuromuscular Disease Research
1 Baylor Plaza
Houston, TX 77030 713-798-4951
neurons@bcm.tmc.edu
www.bcm.edu

Offers research into biochemistry, molecular genetics and neuromuscular disorders.

Laura J Morrison, Professor And Chair
Michael Vincent Abene M.D., Assistant Professor
Farah F. Atassi, Instructor

Utah

4834 University of Utah
Eccles Institute of Human Genetics
15 N 2030 E, Room 2100
Salt Lake City, UT 84112   801-581-4422
                                        Fax: 801-581-7796
                                    efry@genetics.utah.edu
                                    www.genetics.utah.edu

John F Atkins PhD, Research Professor
Mario R. Capecchi Ph.D, Distinguished Professor & Co-Chair
Richard M. Cawthon, M.D. Ph.D., Research Associate Professor

Audio Video

4835 Muscular Dystrophy
Films for Humanities/Films Media Group
132 West 31st Street, 17th Floor
New York, NY 10001   800-322-8755
                                        Fax: 609-671-0266
                                    custserv@filsmediagroup.comm
                                            www.films.com

Muscular Dystrophy attacks muscles, so that people lose the ability to walk, talk, and in some cases, to breath. About two thirds of those affected are children, but symptoms can appear any time between birth and adolescence. This video looks at how people deal with a disease that has no cure. A young boy, a six year old girl, and a young mother are managing their disease and show us the medical interventions used to help them live more fully.

1990 VHS/DVD
ISBN: 1-421336-46-4

Web Sites

4836 Muscular Dystrophy Association
222 S. Riverside Plaza, Suite 1500
Chicago, IL 60606   800-572-1717
                                            www.mda.org

Information regarding muscular dystrophy.

Steven M. Derks, President and CEO
Valerie A. Cwik, M.D., EVP, Chief Medical & Scientific
Julie Faber, EVP, CFO

4837 Muscular Dystrophy Family Foundation
P.O. Box 776
Carmel, IN 46082   317-615-9140
                                            www.mdff.org

Provides adaptive equipment and emotional support to individuals and families affected by one of the over forty neuromuscular diseases. Established in 1958, some of the equipment provided includes: hospital beds, wheelchairs, ramps, communication devices, and lifts.

Tim Doyle, President/Chair
Emily Munson, Vice President/Vice Chair
Matthew D. Haab, Treasurer

4838 Parent Project Muscular Dystrophy
401 Hackensack Avenue, 9th Floor
Hackensack, NJ 7601   201-250-8440
                                            800-714-5437
                                        Fax: 201-250-8435
                                    info@parentprojectmd.org
                                    www.parentprojectmd.org

The Parent Project Muscular Dystrophy moblizes people in the United States and worldwide in collaborative effort to enable people with Duchenne and becker muscular dystrophy to survive, thrive and fully participate within their families and communities into adulthood and beyond.

Anessa Gaydou-Fehsenfeld, Board Chairman
Lance Hester, Board Treasurer
Daniel P. Garofalo, Board Secretary

Book Publishers

4839 Journey of Love: Parent's Guide to Duchenne Muscular Dystrophy
Muscular Dystrophy Association
222 S. Riverside Plaza, Ste 1500
Chicago, IL 60606   520-529-2000
                                            800-572-1717
                                        Fax: 520-529-5300
                                            mda@mdausa.org
                            www.mda.org/publications/journey/misc.html

Complete guide for parents with children diagnosed with DMD. Information includes explanation of the disease, treatments, research, services provided by MDA, guides to finding assistance and more. Available in paperback and online; free from a local MDA office to families with a member affected by DMD or BMD who is registered with the MDA.

1988 170 pages

Kristine Welker, Interim President/CEO
Valerie A. Cwik, MD, EVP, Chief Medical & Scientific
Julie Faber, EVP, CFO

4840 Let's Talk About Going to the Hospital
Rosen Publishing Group's PowerKids Press
29 E 21st Street
New York, NY 10010   212-777-3017
                                            800-237-9932
                                        Fax: 888-436-4643
                                    rosenpub@tribeca.ios.com
                                    www.rosenpublishing.com

If a child has to check into the hospital, chances are he or she is already upset about being ill. Knowing how a hospital functions and what the procedures are, such as when family members can visit, will help in what is already a stressful situation. Grades K-5.

24 pages
ISBN: 0-823950-36-0

Roger Rosen, President

4841 Medifocus Guidebook On Reflex Sympathetic Dystrophy
Medifocus.Com
11529 Daffodil Lane, Suite 200
Silver Spring, MD 20902   301-649-9300
                                            800-965-3002
                                        info@medifocus.com
                                        www.medifocus.com

A patient's comprehensive guide to treatment options and the latest medical advances for RSD. The book provides information about the signs and symptoms of RSD, the treatment options including drug therapy, sympathetic nerve blocks, chemical and surgical sympathectomy, physical therapy, and other methods used for controlling pain and improving quality of life. Updated regularly, purchase includes free updates for 1 year. Available online or in print; see website for details of print vs. online.

April 2009 130 pages Print

4842 Muscular Dystrophy and Allied Diseases: Im pacts on Patients, Family, and Staff

Leon I Charash, author

Center for Thanatology Research & Education
391 Atlantic Avenue
Brooklyn, NY 11217   718-858-3026
                                        Fax: 718-852-1846
                                    thanatology@pipeline.com
                                        www.thanatology.org

An Internet best-seller, it covers Duchenne Muscular Dystrophy, psychosocial aspects, anticipatory grief of parents, education issues, etc.

1988 90 pages Paper
ISBN: 0-930194-38-1

Roberta Halporn, Director

4843 Muscular Dystrophy and Other Neuromuscular Diseases
Haworth Press
711 Third Avenue
New York, NY 10017

212-216-7800
800-429-6784
Fax: 212-244-1563
getinfo@haworthpress.com
www.tandf.co.uk

A thoughtful book from professionals who assist persons afflicted
with neuromuscular disorders to help them and their families
adapt to lifestyle changes accompanying the onset of these
disorders.

1991 250 pages Hardcover
ISBN: 1-560240-77-6

4844 My Life-Melinda's Story

Melinda Lawrence, author

Children's Hospice International
1101 King Street, Suite 360
Alexandria, VA 22314

703-684-0330
800-242-4453
Fax: 703-684-0226
info@chionline.org
www.chionline.org/publications

Written by Melinda, a child with Muscular Dystrophy. This heartwarming story teaches children and their families how to cope
with the illness.

ISBN: 0-317618-38-5

Ann Armstrong-Dailey, Founding Director/CEO
Richard Larkin, Secretary/Treasurer
Rebecca Brant, Director

4845 Realities in Coping with Progressive Neuromuscular Diseases
Charles C. Thomas
2037 Chestnut Street, PO Box 15715
Philadelphia, PA 19103

215-561-2786
Fax: 215-600-1248
mailbox@charlespresspub.com
www.charlespresspub.com

248 pages Hardcover
ISBN: 0-914783-20-3

**4846 Travis:I Got Lots of Neat Stuff Children Living with Muscular
Dystrophy**

Kathy L Gordon, author

Muscular Dystrophy Association
222 S. Riverside Plaza, Ste 1500
Chicago, IL 60606

800-572-1717
publications@mdausa.org
www.mda.org/publications/travis/

Travis' mother shares his story with other children, helping them
to accept their muscular dystrophy and see the world of possibilities before them.

Online

Kristine Welker, Interim President/CEO
Valerie A. Cwik, MD, EVP, Chief Medical & Scientific
Julie Faber, EVP, CFO

Magazines

4847 MDA/ALS Newsmagazine
Muscular Dystrophy Association
222 S. Riverside Plaza, Suite 1500
Chicago, IL 60606

520-529-2000
800-322-8755
Fax: 520-529-5300
publications@mdausa.org
www.mda.org

A national magazine that goes out to everyone registered with
MDA, MDA clinics, reseacgers and subscribers. It presents news
related to ALS including research, personal profiles, fund raising
activities, patient services, and lifestyle information including
products and trends.

125,000 circ Bimonthly

Kristine Welker, Interim President/CEO
Valerie A. Cwik, MD, EVP, Chief Medical & Scientific
Julie Faber, EVP, CFO

4848 Quest Magazine
MDA Publications
222 S. Riverside Plaza, Suite 1500
Chicago, IL 60606

520-529-2000
800-322-8755
Fax: 520-529-5300
publications@mdausa.org
www.mda.org

A national magazine that goes out to everyone registered with
MDA, MDA clinics, researchers and subscribers. It presents news
related to muscular dystrophy and other neuromuscular diseases
including research, personal profiles, fund raising activities, patient services, and lifestyle information including products and
trends.

Bimonthly

Steven M. Derks, President and CEO
Valerie A. Cwik, M.D., EVP, Chief Medical & Scientific
Julie Faber, EVP, CFO

Newsletters

4849 Helping Children & Youth with RSD/CRPS Succeed in School
RSDSA
PO Box 502
Milford, CT 6460

203-877-3790
877-662-7737
Fax: 203-882-8362
info@rsds.org
www.rsds.org

This brochure is designed to help schools accoommadate the special needs of children with CRPS. Available online.

Peter Moskovitz, MD, Chairman of the Board
Francis Ludington, III, Co-President
Guy M. Tufo, Treasurer

4850 Pediatrics CRPS Tri-Fold Brochure
RSDSA
PO Box 502
Milford, CT 6460

203-877-3790
877-662-7737
Fax: 203-882-8362
info@rsds.org
www.rsds.org

This brochure offers information and resources for the family and
friends of youth with CRPS, and those who want to help.

Peter Moskovitz, MD, Chairman of the Board
Francis Ludington, III, Co-President
Guy M. Tufo, Treasurer

4851 RSDA Review
Reflex Sympathetic Dystrophy Syndrome Association
PO Box 502
Milford, CT 6460

203-877-3790
877-662-7737
Fax: 203-882-8362
info@rsds.org
www.rsds.org

Quarterly newsletter of the Reflex Sympathetic Dystrophy Syndrome Association

Peter Moskovitz, MD, Chairman of the Board
Francis Ludington, III, Co-President
Guy M. Tufo, Treasurer

Pamphlets

4852 Breathe Easy: Respiratory Care in Neuromuscular Disorders
Muscular Dystrophy Association
222 S. Riverside Plaza, Suite 1500
Chicago, IL 60606
520-529-2000
800-322-8755
Fax: 520-529-5300
publications@mdausa.org
www.mda.org/publications/breathe/

Respiratory health is a vital issue for children and adults with NMDs, which progressively weaken muscles, sometimes including those we need to breathe. A guide to respiratory care for children with muscular dystrophy. This guide is the result of efforts by a number of highly respected experts in the fileds of NMDs and children's medicine. Also available in Spanish and online.

2006

Kristine Welker, Interim President/CEO
Valerie A. Cwik, MD, EVP, Chief Medical & Scientific
Julie Faber, EVP, CFO

4853 Conference on the Cause and Treatment of Facioscapulohumeral Muscular Dystrophy
National Inst. of Neurological Disorders/Stroke
P.O. Box 5801
Bethesda, MD 20824
301-496-5751
800-352-9424
www.ninds.nih.gov

4854 Congressional Testimony on Muscular Dystrophy
National Inst. of Neurological Disorders/Stroke
P.O. Box 5801
Bethesda, MD 20824
301-496-5751
800-352-9424
www.ninds.nih.gov

Testimony by Dr. Audrey Penn, Acting Director, NINDS, from February, 2001.

4855 Everybody's Different, Nobody's Perfect
Muscular Dystrophy Association
222 S. Riverside Plaza, Suite 1500
Chicago, IL 60606
520-529-2000
800-572-1717
Fax: 520-529-5300
mda@mdausa.org
www.mda.org/publications/nobody/

Explains how muscular dystrophy affects children and describes how people are different from each other in many ways. Emphasizing fun, friendship, and caring, this booklet is ideal for heightening awareness and encouraging understanding of persons with disabilities. Pre-school edition also available; and in Spanish and online.

1999 11 pages

Kristine Welker, Interim President/CEO
Valerie A. Cwik, MD, EVP, Chief Medical & Scientific
Julie Faber, EVP, CFO

4856 Facts About Duchenne and Becker Muscular Dystrophies
Muscular Dystrophy Association
222 S. Riverside Plaza, Suite 1500
Chicago, IL 60606
520-529-2000
800-322-8755
Fax: 520-529-5300
publications@mdausa.org
www.mda.org/publications/

Describes in layman's terms Duchenne and Becker Muscular Dystrophies and addresses the most currently asked questions about these diseases, research, inheritance and treatments. Also available in Spanish or online.

2009

Kristine Welker, Interim President/CEO
Valerie A. Cwik, MD, EVP, Chief Medical & Scientific
Julie Faber, EVP, CFO

4857 Facts About Facioscapulohumeral Muscular Dystrophy
Muscular Dystrophy Association
222 S. Riverside Plaza, Suite 1500
Chicago, IL 60606
520-529-2000
800-322-8755
Fax: 520-529-5300
publications@mdausa.org
www.mda.org/publications/

Explains facioscapulohumeral muscular dystrophy (FHSD) in layman's terms and answers commonly asked questions. Also available in Spanish.

2009 20 pages Paperback

Kristine Welker, Interim President/CEO
Valerie A. Cwik, MD, EVP, Chief Medical & Scientific
Julie Faber, EVP, CFO

4858 Facts About Inflammatory Myopathies-DM, PM and IBM
Muscular Dystrophy Association
222 S. Riverside Plaza, Suite 1500
Chicago, IL 60606
520-529-2000
800-322-8755
Fax: 520-529-5300
publications@mdausa.org
www.mda.org/publications/fa-myosi.html

Outlines these forms of inflammatory myopathy. Current approaches to treatment and MDA's efforts in continued research are described. Also available in Spanish and online.

Kristine Welker, Interim President/CEO
Valerie A. Cwik, MD, EVP, Chief Medical & Scientific
Julie Faber, EVP, CFO

4859 Facts About Limb-Girdle Muscular Dystrophy
Muscular Dystrophy Association
222 S. Riverside Plaza, Suite 1500
Chicago, IL 60606
520-529-2000
800-322-8755
Fax: 520-529-5300
publications@mdausa.org
www.mda.org/publications/fa-lgmd.html

Overview of the various forms of LGMD encompassed by MDA's program. Addresses commonly asked questions and highlights MDA's research efforts aimed at finding the causes of and effective treatments for these disorders. Also available in Spanish and online.

2007 19 pages

Kristine Welker, Interim President/CEO
Valerie A. Cwik, MD, EVP, Chief Medical & Scientific
Julie Faber, EVP, CFO

4860 Facts About Metabolic Diseases of Muscle
Muscular Dystrophy Association
222 S. Riverside Plaza, Suite 1500
Chicago, IL 60606
520-529-2000
800-322-8755
Fax: 520-529-5300
www.mda.org/publications/fa-metab.html

Provides an overview of the 10 heritable metabolic diseases of muscle encompassed by MDA's program. Addresses commonly asked questions and highlights MDA's research efforts aimed at finding the causes of and effective treatments for these disorders. Also online and in Spanish.

Kristine Welker, Interim President/CEO
Valerie A. Cwik, MD, EVP, Chief Medical & Scientific
Julie Faber, EVP, CFO

4861 Facts About Mitochondrial Myopathies
Muscular Dystrophy Association
222 S. Riverside Plaza, Suite 1500
Chicago, IL 60606
520-529-2000
800-572-1717
Fax: 520-529-5300
publications@mdausa.org
www.mda.org/publications/mitchondrial_myopathies.htm

Explains Mitochondrial myopathies in layman's terms and answers the most frequently asked questions about this disease. Also available in Spanish and online.

2008 24 pages

Kristine Welker, Interim President/CEO
Valerie A. Cwik, MD, EVP, Chief Medical & Scientific
Julie Faber, EVP, CFO

4862 Facts About Muscular Dystrophy
Muscular Dystrophy Association
222 S. Riverside Plaza, Suite 1500
Chicago, IL 60606
520-529-2000
800-322-8755
Fax: 520-529-5300
www.mda.org/publications/fa-md-help.html

Answers many questions commonly asked about the forty-plus
forms of the disease encompassed by MDA's program.

Kristine Welker, Interim President/CEO
Valerie A. Cwik, MD, EVP, Chief Medical & Scientific
Julie Faber, EVP, CFO

4863 Facts About Myasthenia Gravis (MG, LEMS, & CMS)
Muscular Dystrophy Association
222 S. Riverside Plaza, Suite 1500
Chicago, IL 60606
520-529-2000
800-322-8755
Fax: 520-529-5300
publications@mdausa.org
www.mda.org/publications/fa-mg.html

Explains myasthenia gravis and Lambert-Eaton syndrome in layman's terms and answers the most frequently asked questions
about these diseases. Also available in Spanish and online.

2001 19 pages

Kristine Welker, Interim President/CEO
Valerie A. Cwik, MD, EVP, Chief Medical & Scientific
Julie Faber, EVP, CFO

4864 Facts About Myopathies
Muscular Dystrophy Association
222 S. Riverside Plaza, Suite 1500
Chicago, IL 60606
520-529-2000
800-322-8755
Fax: 520-529-5300
www.mda.org/publications/fa-myop.html

Describes the six inheritable myopathies encompassed by MDA's
program, as well as current methods for diagnosing and managing
these disorders. Also online and in Spanish.

2003

Kristine Welker, Interim President/CEO
Valerie A. Cwik, MD, EVP, Chief Medical & Scientific
Julie Faber, EVP, CFO

4865 Facts About Myotonic Muscular Dystrophy
Muscular Dystrophy Association
222 S. Riverside Plaza, Suite 1500
Chicago, IL 60606
520-529-2000
800-322-8755
Fax: 520-529-5300
publications@mdausa.org
www.mda.org/publications/fa-mmd.html

Basic knowledge about Myotonic Muscular Dystrophy, precautions, treatments, research and answers to most commonly asked
questions. Also available in Spanish and online.

2009 23 pages

Kristine Welker, Interim President/CEO
Valerie A. Cwik, MD, EVP, Chief Medical & Scientific
Julie Faber, EVP, CFO

4866 Facts About Plasmapheresis
Muscular Dystrophy Association
222 S. Riverside Plaza, Suite 1500
Chicago, IL 60606
520-529-2000
800-322-8755
Fax: 520-529-5300
publications@mdausa.org
www.mda.org/publications/fa-plasmaph.html

Describes plasmapheresis, a plasma exchange procedure often utilized as a treatment for autoimmune diseases such as myasthenia
gravis and Lambert-Eaton syndrome. Available in paperback or
online.

2005

Kristine Welker, Interim President/CEO
Valerie A. Cwik, MD, EVP, Chief Medical & Scientific
Julie Faber, EVP, CFO

4867 Facts About Rare Muscular Dystrophies
Muscular Dystrophy Association
222 S. Riverside Plaza, Suite 1500
Chicago, IL 60606
520-529-2000
800-322-8755
Fax: 520-529-5300
publications@mdausa.org
www.mda.org

This brochure gives basic facts about four forms of muscular dystrophy (congenital, distal, Emery-Dreifuss and oculopharyngeal)
and addresses commonly asked questions. Also available in
Spanish.

28 pages

Kristine Welker, Interim President/CEO
Valerie A. Cwik, MD, EVP, Chief Medical & Scientific
Julie Faber, EVP, CFO

4868 Genetics and Neuromuscular Diseases
Muscular Dystrophy Association
222 S. Riverside Plaza, Suite 1500
Chicago, IL 60606
520-529-2000
800-322-8755
Fax: 520-529-5300
publications@mdausa.org
www.mda.org

An up-to-date review of genetics information relating to
neuromatic diseases, specifically describing what a genetic disorder is, genetic testing and counseling and inheritance patterns.
Also available in Spanish and online.

19 pages

Kristine Welker, Interim President/CEO
Valerie A. Cwik, MD, EVP, Chief Medical & Scientific
Julie Faber, EVP, CFO

4869 Hey! I'm Here, Too!
Irwin M Siegel, MD, author

Muscular Dystrophy Association
222 S. Riverside Plaza, Suite 1500
Chicago, IL 60606
520-529-2000
800-322-8755
Fax: 520-529-5300
publications@mdausa.org
www.mda.org/publications/hey/

Help for siblings of boys with Duchenne muscular dystrophy. Explores how they feel about themselves, their brothers, and their
families. Also provides specific answers to some questions that
siblings may wonder about. Has the option for an introduction for
parents or for children. Available online and in Spanish.

1989

Kristine Welker, Interim President/CEO
Valerie A. Cwik, MD, EVP, Chief Medical & Scientific
Julie Faber, EVP, CFO

**4870 Learning to Live with Neuromuscular Disease: A Message for
Parents**
Muscular Dystrophy Association
222 S. Riverside Plaza, Suite 1500
Chicago, IL 60606
520-529-2000
800-322-8755
Fax: 520-529-5300
publications@mdausa.org
www.mda.org/publications/learning/

Intended to help parents and families cope with the knowledge
that their child has a neuromuscular disease and with the impact
the disease will have on everyday life. Online and in Spanish.

2006

Kristine Welker, Interim President/CEO
Valerie A. Cwik, MD, EVP, Chief Medical & Scientific
Julie Faber, EVP, CFO

4871 MDA Fact Sheet
Muscular Dystrophy Association
222 S. Riverside Plaza, Suite 1500
Chicago, IL 60606 520-529-2000
800-572-1717
Fax: 520-529-5300
publications@mdausa.org
www.mda.org/publications/

Outlines the history of MDA, the diseases included in MDA's
program, and the services available through the Association.

Kristine Welker, Interim President/CEO
Valerie A. Cwik, MD, EVP, Chief Medical & Scientific
Julie Faber, EVP, CFO

4872 MDA Services for the Individual, Family and Community
Muscular Dystrophy Association
222 S. Riverside Plaza, Suite 1500
Chicago, IL 60606 520-529-2000
800-322-8755
Fax: 520-529-5300
publications@mdausa.org
www.mda.org/publications/mdasvcs/

Contains a list of the diseases covered by MDA as well as eligibility criteria for MDA's services program, a list of MDA-spon-
sored clinics nationwide, and the services available through these
clinics. Also in Spanish and online.

2009

Kristine Welker, Interim President/CEO
Valerie A. Cwik, MD, EVP, Chief Medical & Scientific
Julie Faber, EVP, CFO

4873 MDA Summer Camp Brochure
Muscular Dystrophy Association
222 S. Riverside Plaza, Suite 1500
Chicago, IL 60606 520-529-2000
800-322-8755
Fax: 520-529-5300
www.mda.org/clinics/camp

Highlights the activities of MDA summer camps for youngsters
diagnosed with one of the more than 40 diseases in MDA's program. Shares camper and volunteer reactions. Also available in
Spanish and online.

Kristine Welker, Interim President/CEO
Valerie A. Cwik, MD, EVP, Chief Medical & Scientific
Julie Faber, EVP, CFO

4874 Neuromuscular Disease Guidebooks & Pamphlets
222 S. Riverside Plaza, Suite 1500
Chicago, IL 60606 520-529-2000
800-572-1717
Fax: 520-529-5300
publications@mdausa.org
www.mda.org/services/guidebooks-and-pamphlets

Guides to everyday living with NMD's.

Kristine Welker, Interim President/CEO
Valerie A. Cwik, M.D., EVP, Chief Medical & Scientific
Julie Faber, EVP, CFO

4875 Teacher's Guide to Neuromuscular Disease
Muscular Dystrophy Association
222 S. Riverside Plaza, Suite 1500
Chicago, IL 60606 520-529-2000
800-322-8755
Fax: 520-529-5300
publications@mdausa.org
www.mda.org/publications/tchrdmd/

A source of guidance and information to educators detailing
neuromuscular disease, how it affects school participation, and
ways that teachers can help meet the academic and social needs of
students affected by the disorder. Online and in Spanish.

2005

Kristine Welker, Interim President/CEO
Valerie A. Cwik, MD, EVP, Chief Medical & Scientific
Julie Faber, EVP, CFO

**4876 Workshop on Therapeutic Approaches for Duchenne
Muscular Dystrophy**
National Inst. of Neurological Disorders/Stroke
PO Box 5801
Bethesda, MD 20824 301-496-5751
800-352-9424
www.ninds.nih.gov/news_and_events/proceedings/

Camps

4877 MDA Summer Camp
Muscular Dystrophy Association
222 S. Riverside Plaza, Suite 1500
Chicago, IL 60606 520-529-2000
800-322-8755
Fax: 520-529-5300
mda@mdausa.org
www.mda.org/clinics/camp

With over 90 camps across the country MDA camp is a magical
place where year-round skills are developed and where a child
with a disability can just be a kid. In addition to camp and medical staff, most campers have their own 1-on-1 volunteer to help
with fun and personal care. Activites are designed for young people with limited mobility or wheelchairs, and include swimming,
boating, baseball, football, horseback riding, arts, crafts and talent shows. Free for famlies registered with MDA.

Kristine Welker, Interim President/CEO
Valerie A. Cwik, MD, EVP, Chief Medical & Scientific
Julie Faber, EVP, CFO

DESCRIPTION

4878 NARCOLEPSY

Synonyms: Gelineau's syndrome, Hypnolepsy, Paroxysmal sleep

Involves the following Biologic System(s):

Neurologic Disorders

Narcolepsy refers to a sleep disorder characterized by profound drowsiness during the day and sudden daytime attacks of sleep that may last from a few seconds to one or more hours. These episodes are sometimes accompanied by sudden loss of muscle tone (hypotonia) in response to emotional stimuli such as anger, fear, joy, or surprise (cataplexy). During a cataplectic episode, the patient remains conscious but is not able to speak or move. Some patients experience sleep paralysis and are unable to move at the onset of sleep or immediately upon waking. Hypnagogic hallucinations are disquieting occurrences that take place at onset of sleep or, less commonly, upon awakening. During these hallucinations, patients may see or hear things that are not grounded in reality. In most cases, narcolepsy begins during adolescence or early adulthood and persists throughout the life of the affected individual. Sleep attacks associated with narcolepsy may occur at any time and may take place many times during the day; however, most individuals may be easily awakened.

Very few people with narcolepsy exhibit all the symptoms associated with this disorder and, occasionally, children and adults who do not have this disorder may experience similar signs and symptoms. For this reason, diagnosis of narcolepsy may necessitate confirmation by a sleep study which uses a procedure called electroencephalography (EEG), during which electrical brain-wave activity is recorded. An EEG may demonstrate an abnormal sleep pattern in which rapid eye movement or REM-type sleep occurs at the onset of sleep. There are no pathologic changes that occur in the brain. In individuals who do not have narcolepsy, REM sleep or periods of deep sleep normally follow nonrapid eye movement sleep (NREM). The cause of narcolepsy is unknown, but researchers think that, in some cases, it may be related to genetic influences as evidenced by the tendency of this disorder to occur within families. Approximately 200,000 people in the United States are affected by narcolepsy.

Treatment for narcolepsy may include regular napping and the administration of stimulant medications to control attacks of drowsiness and sleep, while antidepressant medications may help control episodes of cataplexy. Because this disorder may increase the risk of accidents, appropriate care and caution is advised in the performance of certain tasks or jobs. Other treatment is symptomatic and supportive.

Government Agencies

4879 NIH/National Institute of Neurological Disorders and Stroke (NINDS)
PO Box 5801
Bethesda, MD 20824
301-496-5751
800-352-9424
Fax: 301-496-0296
TTY: 301-468-5981
www.ninds.nih.gov

Works to reduce the burden of neurological disease by conducting, fostering, coordinating and guiding research on the causes, prevention, diagnosis and treatment of neurological disorders and stroke, while supporting basic research in related scientific areas.

Walter J. Koroshetz, MD, Director

National Associations & Support Groups

4880 American Academy of Pediatrics
141 Northwest Point Boulevard
Elk Grove Village, IL 60007
847-434-4000
800-433-9016
Fax: 847-434-8000
www.aap.org

The American Academy of Pediatrics and its member pediatricians are committed to the attainment of optimal physical, mental and social health and well-being for all infants, children, adolescents, and young adults.

Fernando Stein, MD, FAAP, President
Karen Remley, MD, CEO/Executive VP

4881 American Academy of Sleep Medicine
2510 N Frontage Road
Darien, IL 60561
630-737-9700
Fax: 630-737-9790
inquiries@aasmnet.org
www.aasmnet.org

Provides full diagnostic and treatment services to improve the quality of care for patients with all types of sleep disorders.

Jerome A. Barrett, Executive Director
Nancy Collop, President-Elect
Timothy I. Morgenthaler, Secretary/Treasurer

4882 Association of Professional Sleep Societies
2510 N Frontage Road
Darien, IL 60561
630-737-9700
Fax: 630-737-9790
jmarkkanen@aasmnet.org
www.apss.org

A joint venture of the AASM and the Sleep Research Society. It works to facilitate the research and development of sleep disorders medically by encouraging exchange of information among members.

Jennifer Markkanen, Assistant Executive Director

4883 Florida Narcolepsy Association
2631 59th Street, PO Box 15352
Sarasota, FL 34232
941-355-5359
sleepymc@yahoo.com
www.flnarcolepsy.org

The Association is a collective of people that helps or comforts others afflicted with Narcolepsy; as well as their families, doctors and friends.

Marion L Cikovic, Vice President

4884 Genetic Alliance
4301 Connecticut Avenue NW, Suite 404
Washington, DC 20008
202-966-5557
800-336-4363
Fax: 202-966-8553
info@geneticalliance.org
www.geneticalliance.org

A coalition of voluntary genetic support groups, consumers and professionals addressing the needs of individuals and families affected by genetic disorders from a national perspective.

Sharon Terry, President/CEO
Tetyana Murza, Managing Director
Natasha Bonhomme, VP, Strategic Development

4885 NIH/National Institute of Neurological Disorders and Stroke (NINDS)
PO Box 5801
Bethesda, MD 20824
301-496-5751
800-352-9424
Fax: 301-496-0296
TTY: 301-468-5981
www.ninds.nih.gov

Information and advocacy resources for families and professionals. Includes listings of organizations providing general tips and organizations focusing on more specific areas of concern to families and young adults who have disabilities.

Walter J. Koroshetz, MD, Director

4886 Narcolepsy Institute
Montefiore Medical Center
111 E 210th Street
Bronx, NY 10467
718-920-6799
Fax: 718-654-9580
mgoswami@narcolepsyinstitute.org
www.NarcolepsyInstitute.org

The Narcolepsy Institute, at Montefiore Medical Center, provides support services to individuals who have narcolepsy and their families in New York City. Free services are provided for people who narcolepsy qualifies as a developmental disability. The Institute provides screening, counseling, case management, crisis intervention, and advocacy for affected individuals and their families.

Dr Meeta Goswami, Phd, Director

4887 Narcolepsy Network
129 Waterwheel Lane
North Kingstown, RI 02852
401-667-2523
888-292-6522
Fax: 401-633-6567
narnet@narcolepsynetwork.org
www.narcolepsynetwork.org

Nonprofit organization that serves as a resource center, to assist support groups, to educate the public, to facilitate early diagnosis, to protect the rights of those with narcolepsy, and to encourage on-going scientific research in sleep medicine.

Sara Kowalczyk, President
Sarah DiDavide, Co VP
Heidi Shilensky, Co-VP

4888 National Sleep Foundation
1010 N Glebe Road
Arlington, VA 22201
703-243-1697
Fax: 202-347-3472
nsf@sleepfoundation.org
www.sleepfoundation.org

Works to improve the quality of life for millions of Americans who suffer from sleep disorders, and to prevent the catastrophic accidents that are related to poor or disordered sleep through research, education and the dissemination of information towards the cause of the Narcolepsy Project. Seeks patients to aid new research project targeting the cause of the disorder.

David Cloud, CEO

State Agencies & Support Groups

Arizona

4889 Arizona Sleep Disorders Center
University of Arizona, College of Medicine
1501 N Campbell Avenue, PO Box 245017
Tucson, AZ 85724
520-626-4555
Fax: 520-626-6623
www.medicine.arizona.edu/centers/index.cfm

The newest addition to the University of Arizona's College of Medicine. Program and website under development at time of publication.

Steven Goldschmid, Dean
Judith DiMarco, Associate Dean

California

4890 Loma Linda University Sleep Disorders Center
11139 Anderson St.
Loma Linda, CA 92350
909-558-6344
Fax: 909-558-6343
www.llu.edu

Richard H Hart, CEO
Philip M. Gold, Medical Director
Richard E. Chinnock, MD, Medical Director

4891 Stanford University Center for Narcolepsy
450 Broadway Street, Pav B, 2nd Floor
Redwood City, CA 94063
650-721-7550
Fax: 650-721-3466
einen@stanford.edu
www.med.stanford.edu/school/psychiatry/narcolepsy/
Theodore Chen, Director

Connecticut

4892 Gaylord Hospital Sleep Medicine
Gaylord Farm Road, PO Box 400
Wallingford, CT 06492
203-284-2800
866-429-5673
TTY: 203-284-2700
TDD: 203-284-2700
lcrispino@gaylord.org
www.gaylord.org

Nadine Cartwright

District of Columbia

4893 Georgetown University Sleep Disorders Center
3800 Reservoir Road NW
Washington, DC 20007
202-444-2000
Fax: 202-444-2336
pme2@gunet.georgetown.edu
www.georgetownuniversityhospital.org

Anne O'Donnel, Chair
Raoul L Wientzen, President

Indiana

4894 Methodist Hospital Sleep Disorders Center
Rehab Centers
8701 Broadway
Merrillville, IN 46410
219-738-5500
800-909-3627
Fax: 219-738-6624
www.methodisthospitals.org

Ian E. McFadden, President/CEO
Robin Logsdon, Manager

4895 MidWest Medical Center - Sleep Disorders Center
3232 N Meridian Street
Indianapolis, IN 46208
317-927-2100
Kenneth Wiesert, MD

4896 Sleep Disorder Center, St Elizabeth Medical Center
1501 Hartford Street, PO Box 7501
Lafayette, IN 47903
766-423-6518
800-371-6011
Fax: 765-423-6525
www.glhsi.org

Dr Shahid M Ahsan, Medical Director

4897 Sleep Disorders Center-Good Samaritan Hospital
520 S 7th Street
Vincenne, IN 47591
812-885-3988
812-882-5220
gsh@gshvin.org
www.gshvin.org/goodsamaritan/

4898 Sleep/Wake Disorders Center-Community Heal th Network
1500 N Ritter Avenue, Suite 451
Indianapolis, IN 46219   317-355-1411
                                     Fax: 317-351-2785
                              sleepcenter@ecommunity.com
                              www.ecommunity.com/sleep/

Marvin E Vollmer, MD, Co-Director

Maryland

4899 Johns Hopkins University Sleep Disorders Center
Francis Scott Key Medical Center
301 Bayview Boulevard
Baltimore, MD 21224   410-550-0571
                                     Fax: 410-550-3374
                                     nschube1@jhmi.edu

Alan Schwartz, MD, Medical Director

Massachusetts

4900 Sleep Disorders Unit, Beth Israel Hospital
330 Brookline Avenue
Boston, MA 02215   617-667-7000
                                          800-439-0183
                                     Fax: 617-975-5506
                              patsite@bidmc.harvard.edu
                                         www.bidmc.org

Stephan B. Kay, Chair
Daniel Jick, First Vice Chair
Carol Anderson, Vice Chairperson

Michigan

4901 Center for Sleep Science at University of Michigan
University of Michigan Health System
2799 West Grand Boulevard Cfp3
Detroit, MI 48202   313-916-5176
                                     Fax: 313-916-5150
                                     dhudgel1@hfhs.org
                              www.med.umich.edu/umsleepscience/

The center's main goal is to advance knowledge and understanding in these three areas: the physiology of normal sleep; the diagnosis of sleep disorders; and the treatment of sleep problems.
Ronald D Chervin MD, Director
Barbara T Felts MD, Pediatrics

Minnesota

4902 Center for Sleep Diagnostics
1455 St. Frances Ave.
Shakopee, MN 55379   952-428-3000
                                     askstfrancis@allina.com
                              www.stfrancis-shakopee.com

Is dedicated to providing information, education, and support for
all your sleep needs. Our goal is to be the center of sleep information and discussion on the internet.

David Zelinsky, Chair
Kelly J. DiGrado, Vice Chairman
Lee Shimek, Secretary

New Hampshire

**4903 Dartmouth-Hitchcock Sleep Disorders Center Dartmouth
Medical Center**
One Medical Center Drive
Lebanon, NH 03756   603-650-7534
                                     Fax: 603-650-7820
                              www.dartmouth-hitchcock.org

Rocco R Addante, Director
Glen Greenough MD, Fellowship Director
Joanne MacQuarrie, BS,RPSGT,RRT, Administrator

4904 Sleep/Wake Disorders Center, Hampstead Hospital
218 East Road
Hampstead, NH 03841   603-329-5311
                                     Fax: 603-329-4746
                              www.hampsteadhospital.com

Philip Kubaik, CEO
Cynthia Gove, COO
Scott Ranks, Director support Services

New Jersey

4905 Newark Sleep Disorders Center
Newark Beth Israel Medical Center
201 Lyons Avenue
Newark, NJ 07112   973-926-7163
                                     Fax: 973-926-6672
                                     mkaretzky@sbhcs.com
                                     www.njsleephelp.com

Dr Monroe S Karetzky, Director

New York

4906 Capital Regional Sleep-Wake Disorders Center
Saint Peter's Hospital & Albany Medical Center
1220 New Scotland Road
Slingerlands, NY 12159   518-439-4326
                                     Fax: 518-439-6143
                              bwenzel@stpetershealthcare.org
                    www.capitalregionspecialsurgery.com/sleep-wake/
William Wenzel, Manager

4907 Center for Sleep Medicine of the Mount Sinai Medical Center
Box 1232, One Gustave L Levy Place
New York, NY 10029   212-241-6500
                                          800-637-4624
                                     Fax: 212-987-5584
                                     www.mountsinai.org

Kenneth L. Davis, President/CEO
Dennis S. Charney, Executive VP
Douglas Jabs, CEO

4908 Columbia Presbyterian Medical Center Sleep Disorders Center
630 West 168th St
New York, NY 10032   212-305-5371
                                     Fax: 212-305-5496
                                         www.nyp.org

Ronald E Drusin

4909 Saint Joseph's Hospital Health Center Sleep Laboratory
301 Prospect Ave.
Syracuse, NY 13203   315-448-5111
                                          888-785-6371
                                         www.sjhsyr.org

George Deptula, Chairperson
Kathryn H. Ruscitto, President
Sister Mary Obrist, Secretary

4910 Sleep Center, Community General Hospital
4900 Broad Road
Syracuse, NY 13215   315-492-5877
                                         www.chg.org

Robert Westlake, MD

**4911 Sleep Disorders Center of Western New York Millard Fillmore
Hospital**
3 Gates Circle
Buffalo, NY 14209   716-887-5337
                                     Fax: 716-887-5332
                              drifkin@kaleidahealth.org
                              www.sleepcenterwny.com

Daniel Rifkin MD, Medical Director

4912 Sleep Disorders Center, University Hospital
101 Nicolls Road
Stony Brook, NY 11794   631-444-4000
                                    Fax: 631-444-8821
                        craig.lehmann@stonybrook.edu
                www.healthtechnology.stonybrookmedicine.edu
Craig A. Lehmann, Dean
Richard W. Johnson, Associate Dean
Carol Vidal, Associate Dean for community Engage

**4913 Sleep-Wake Disorders Center, Montefiore Sleep Disorders
Center**
111 E 210th Street
Bronx, NY 10467   718-920-4841
                                    Fax: 718-798-4352
                            thorpy@aecom.yu.edu
                        www.cloud9.net/~thorpy/mmc

Center that provides diagnostic and treatment services for children with sleep disorders, such as sleep apnea, narcolepsy, insomnia, daytime sleepiness, sleepwalking, or night terrors.

Michael J Thorpy, MD, Medical Director
Karen Balaban-Gil, MD

**4914 Sleep-Wake Disorders Center, New York Presbyterian
Hospital**
Cornell Medical Center
21 Bloomingdale Road
White Plains, NY 10605   914-997-5751
                                         800-694-7533
                                    Fax: 914-682-6911
                            mmoline@med.cornell.edu
                    www.cornellphysicians.com/sleepWake/

Provides outpatient diagnostic evaluation and treatment for adults and children with problems associated with sleeping and waking. More common pediatric sleep problems include complaints of difficulty falling asleep and staying asleep, snoring, sleep apnea, sleepwalking, sleep terrors, nightmares, excessive difficulty waking up, bedwetting, and narcolepsy. Many can be successfully treated in one or several visits although some may require an overnight or daytime sleep study.

Margaret Moline, PHD, Director

4915 Unity Sleep Disorders Clinic Unity Health System
89 Genesee Street
Rochester, NY 14611   585-723-7000
                                    Fax: 585-442-6259
                            Oncall@unityhealth.org
                                www.unityhealth.org
Warren Hern, President/CEO
Annette Leahy, President
Tom Crilly, Executive VP/CFO

4916 Winthrop-University Hospital Sleep Disorders Center
1300 Franklin Avenue, Suite UL-5
Garden City, NY 11530   516-663-3907
                                    Fax: 516-663-4788
                            mweinstein@winthrop
        www.winthrop.org/departments/specialtycenters/?id=31
Charles M. Strain, Chairman
John F. Collins, President/CEO
Michael Weinstein, Medical Director

Ohio

4917 Bethesda Oak Hospital, Sleep Disorders Center
619 Oak St.
Cincinnati, OH 45206   513-569-5400
                                    Fax: 513-745-1691
                        michael_fletcher@trihealth.com
                                www.trihealth.com
Anthony P Borzotta

4918 Center for Sleep & Wake Disorders, Miami Valley Hospital
One Wyoming Street
Dayton, OH 45409   937-208-8000
                                    Fax: 937-208-2006
                            khuban@wor.rr.com
                        www.miamivalleyhospital.com

M Dallal, Manager

4919 Cleveland Clinic Foundation, Sleep Disorders Center
9500 Euclid Avenue FA20
Cleveland, OH 44195   216-444-4508
                                         800-223-2273
                                    Fax: 216-445-6205
                                foldvan@ccf.org
                            my.clevelandclinic.org
Petra Podmore, Manager

4920 Kettering Medical Center, Sleep Disorders Center
3095 Dayton-Xenia Rd
Beavercreek, OH 45439   937-458-4010
                            www.ketteringhealth.org
George G. Burton MD, Medical Director

4921 NW Ohio Sleep Disorders Center
Toledo Hospital
2121 Hughes Drive Harris-McIntosh Tower 2nd Floor
Toledo, OH 43606   419-291-5629
                                    Fax: 419-479-6954
                            pam.lang@promedica.org
                            www.nwosemsleep.org
Navin K. Jain, President
Michael Neeb, VP
James Kusina, Secretary

4922 Ohio Sleep Medicine Institute
4975 Bradenton Avenue
Dublin, OH 43017   614-766-0773
                                    Fax: 614-766-2599
                            info@sleepmedicine.com
                            www.sleepmedicine.com
Dr. Markus Schmidt, MD, President
Dr. Asim Roy, Clinic Associate

4923 Ohio State University Hospitals, Sleep Disorders Center
410 W 10th Avenue
Columbus, OH 43210   614-293-8652
                                    Fax: 614-257-2551
                            www.medicalcenter.osu.edu
Larry Anstine, CEO

4924 Saint Vincent Medical Center, Sleep Disorders Center
3829 Woodley Road Suite 1
Toledo, OH 43606   419-250-5702
                                    Fax: 419-251-0574
                                www.stvincent.org
Joseph Schaffer, PhD, Director
Gary Fammartino, Site Admin

Pennsylvania

4925 Community Medical Center, Sleep Disorders Clinic
1800 Mulberry Street
Scranton, PA 18510   570-969-8000
                            www.cmchealthsys.org
Michael Aronica, Director

4926 Crozer-Chester Medical Center
Sleep Disorders Center
Department of Neurology
Upland-Chester, PA 19013   610-447-2689
                                         800-254-3258
                            CKHSInfo@crozer.org
                            www.crozerkeystone.org
Joan Richards, President/CEO
Calvin Stafford, MD, Director

**4927 Geisinger Wyoming Valley Medical Center, Sleep Disorders
Center**
1000 E. Mountain Blvd.
Wilkes-Barre, PA 18711   570-808-7300
                                         800-275-6401
                                    Fax: 570-826-7650
                            lvender@geisinger.edu
                            www.geisinger.org
John W. McBurney, MD, Medical Director

4928 Lankenau Hospital, Sleep Disorders Center
100 Lancaster Avenue
Wynnewood, PA 19096
484-476-2000
866-CAL- MLH
Fax: 610-645-2291
pressmanm@mlhs.org
www.mainlinehealth.org

Sandra V Abramson, Director

4929 Medical College of Pennsylvania, Sleep Disorders Center
3300 Henry Avenue
Philadelphia, PA 19129
215-842-6000
Farhana Bashar, Director

4930 Mercy Hospital of Johnstown, Sleep Disorders Center
1086 Franklin Street
Johnstown, PA 15905
814-534-9000
William F Pruchnic, Director

4931 Penn Center for Sleep Disorders, Hospital of the University of Pennsylvania
3624 Market Street, Suite 201
Philadelphia, PA 19104
215-590-3703
800-789-PENN
Fax: 215-590-2632

Indira Gurubhagavatula, MD, Director

4932 Presbyterian-University Hospital, Pulmonary Sleep Evaluation Center
200 Lothrop Street
Pittsburgh, PA 15213
412-647-2345
www.upmc.com

Mark Sanders, MD, Director

4933 Thomas Jefferson University Sleep Disorders Center
Jefferson Medical College
Suite 500, 211 S 9th St
Philadelphia, PA 19107
215-955-6175
Fax: 215-923-8219
www.jeffersonhospital.org

Karl Doghramji, MD, Director

4934 Western Psychiatric Institute & Clinic, Sleep Evaluation Center
3811 O'Hara Street
Pittsburgh, PA 15213
412-624-3934
Fax: 412-246-5300

David Alan Lewis, Director

Rhode Island

4935 Sleep Disorders Center of Lifespan Hospita ls
Rhode Island Hospital
167 Point Street
Providence, RI 02903
401-444-3500
Fax: 404-431-5429
millman@lifespan.org
www.lifespan.org

Timonthy J. Babineau, President/CEO
Kenneth E. Arnold, Senior Vice-President
August Cordeiro, President

Texas

4936 Sleep Disorders Center for Children
Children's Medical Center of Dallas
1935 Medical District Dr
Dallas, TX 75235
214-456-7000
Fax: 214-456-8740
larry.brewer@childrens.com
www.childrens.com

Dr S K Naqvi, Medical Director
Dr John Herman PhD, Contact for Children

4937 Sleep Medicine Associates of Texas
5477 Glen Lakes Drive, Suite 100
Dallas, TX 75231
214-750-7776
Fax: 214-750-4621
www.sleepmed.com

Philip M Becker, President

4938 University of Texas Sleep/Wake Disorders Center
Southwestern Medical Center
5323 Harry Hines Boulevard
Dallas, TX 75235
214-648-3111
Fax: 214-648-3112

Studies sleep/wake disorders including insomnia, apnea and narcolepsy.

Howard Roffwrag, MD, Director

Research Centers

Illinois

4939 Center for Narcolepsy Research at the University of Illinois at Chicago
College of Nursing M/C 802
845 S Damen Avenue
Chicago, IL 60612
312-996-5176
Fax: 312-996-7008
CNSHR@listserv.uic.edu
www.uic.edu

David W. Carley, PhD, Director
Mary Kapella, Associate Director
Julie Law, Center Administration

Iowa

4940 Mercy Sleep Laboratory
Mercy Medical Center
1111 6th Avenue
Des Moines, IA 50314
515-358-9600
Fax: 515-643-8905
cmann@mercydesmoines.org
www.mercydesmoines.org

Sleep is an integral part of life, but it's not always a welcome or peaceful close to a busy day. Some people suffer almost unbearable torture as they toss and turn. Others find sleepiness an uncontrollable intruder. It's been estimated that 30 to 40 percent of the population suffers from a sleeping problem at some time in their lives. Mercy's Sleep Center helps patients with sleep problems.

Donald L. Burrows, MD, Medical Director

Maine

4941 Sleep Laboratory, Maine Medical Center
930 Congress Street
Portland, ME 04102
207-662-4535
Fax: 207-662-6005
www.mmc.org

Christopher W. Emmons, Chairman
Frank H. Frye, Vice-Chairman
Richard W. Peterson, President

Maryland

4942 University of Maryland Medical Center
Pediatric Sleep Disorders Center
22 S Greene Street
Baltimore, MD 21201
866-408-6885
800-492-5538
TDD: 800-735-2258
www.umm.edu

Carol J Blaisdell MD, Director

Charles A. Czeisler, PhD, MD, Chairman
Max Hirshkowitz, PhD, Vice Chairman
Joseph Ojile, MD, Secretary

Ohio

4943 Tri-State Sleep Disorders Center Center for Research in Sleep Disorders
1275 E Kemper Road
Cincinnati, OH 45246

513-671-3101
800-838-4322
Fax: 513-671-4159
web@tristatesleep.com
www.tristatesleep.com

Provides diagnostics and treatment services to thousands of people in Cincinnati and throughout the country at our state-of-the-art sleep clinic through cutting edge research efforts.

Martin B Scharf, Executive Director
Dr. David Berkowitz
Cara Zurmehly PA-C

Texas

4944 Baylor Sleep Wellness Center
Baylor Clinic
6620 Main Street
Houston, TX 77030

713-798-1000
800-229-5671
www.baylorclinic.com

A comprehensive program with a multidisciplinary approach to sleep disorders.

Sr Shyam Subramanian, Director, Sigworth
VP Rose, Clinical Psychologist

4945 University of Texas Medical Branch at Galveston, Clinical Research Center
301 University Boulevard
Galveston, TX 77555

409-772-2222
800-917-8906
Fax: 409-772-6216
public.affairs@utmb.edu
www.utmb.edu

Research focusing on sleep disorders including apnea and narcolepsy.

David L. Callender, President
Cary W. Cooper, VP/Dean
William R. Elger, Executive VP

Audio Video

4946 Narcolepsy
Fanlight Productions
32 Court Street
Brooklyn, NY 11201

718-488-8900
800-876-1710
Fax: 718-488-8642
info@fanlight.com
www.fanlight.com

Presents the experiences of three individuals whose lives and relationships have been disrupted by narcolepsy, while offering solid, comprehensive scientific information about the disorder.
ISBN: DVD: 1-57295-974-6; VHS: 1-572953-23-2

25 minutes DVD or VHS

Ben Achtenberg, President
Anthony Sweeney, Marketing Director
Nicole Johnson, Publicity Coordinator

4947 Narcolepsy: A Guide for Understanding, Dia gnosing & Treating Narcolepsy
National Sleep Foundation
1010 N. Glebe Road, Suite 310
Arlington, VA 22201

703-243-1697
nsf@sleepfoundation.org
www.sleepfoundation.org

A comprehensive PowerPoint™ , 114 slide presentation to educate health care providers about narcolepsy.

4948 Narcolepsy: Evaluation and Treatment
American Academy of Sleep Medicine
2510 North Frontage Road
Darien, IL 60561

630-737-9700
Fax: 630-737-9790
www.aasmnet.org

A 97 slide presentation designed as a foundation for a teaching curriculum on the recognition and traetment of narcolepsy.

Timothy I. Morgenthaker, MD, President
Nathaniel F. Watson, MD, President-Elect
Ronald D. Chervin, MD, MS, Secretary/Treasurer

Web Sites

4949 Narcolepsy
129 Waterwheel Lane
North Kingstown, RI 2852

401-667-2523
888-292-6522
Fax: 401-633-6567
NarNet@narcolepsynetwork.org
narcolepsynetwork.org

Narcolepsy Internet jumpstation.

4950 Online Mendelian Inheritance in Man
National Library of Medicine Building 38A
Bethesda, MD 20894

888-346-3656
info@ncbi.nlm.nih.gov
www.ncbi.nlm.nih.gov

This database is a catalog of human genes and genetic disorders.

Christine E. Seidman, M.D., Chair
David J. Lipman, Executive Secretary

4951 Sleep Disorders
http://talhost.net/sleep/narcolepsy.htm

Descriptions of certain sleep disorders and useful links.

4952 Talk About Sleep
www.talkaboutsleep.com

Sleep disorder information and resources.

Book Publishers

4953 Narcolepsy Primer
Montefiore Medical Center
111 E 210th Street
Bronx, NY 10467

718-920-4321
info@montefiore.org
www.montefiore.org

A guide for physicians, patients and their families on the affects, causes and prevention of narcolepsy.

Steven M. Safyer, MD, President/CEO
Philip O. Ozuah, Chief Operating Officer
Joel A. Perlman, Chief Financial Officer

4954 Psychosocial Aspects of Narcolepsy
Meeta Goswami, author

Haworth Press
PO BOX 8002
Aston, PA 19014

800-234-1340
Fax: 800-875-1340
info@omnigraphics.com
www.omnigraphics.com

Addresses the diagnosis, treatment and management of narcolepsy with particular emphasis on psychological and social aspects of care.

567 pages Hardcover
ISBN: 1-560242-22-1

Peter Ruffner, Publisher

4955   Sleep Disorders Sourcebook
Omnigraphics
PO Box 8002
Aston, PA 19014

800-234-1340
Fax: 800-875-1340
info@omnigraphics.com
www.omnigraphics.com

Basic consumer health information about sleep and its disorders,
including narcolepsy, insomnia, sleepwalking, sleep apnea, and
restless leg syndrome.

567 pages 2nd edition
ISBN: 0-780807-43-0

Peter Ruffner, Publisher

4956   Sleep Disorders and Psychiatry

Daniel J Buysse MD, author

American Psychiatric Publishing
1000 Wilson Boulevard, Ste 1825
Arlington, VA 22209

703-907-7322
800-368-5777
Fax: 703-907-1091
appi@psych.org
www.appi.org

Summarizes the major categories of sleep disorders including
parasomnias and narcolepsy.

2005 256 pages Paperback
ISBN: 1-585622-29-0

Robert E. Hales, M.D., Editor-in-Chief
Rebecca D. Rinehart, Publisher
John McDuffie, Editorial Director

Pamphlets

4957   Living with Narcolepsy
National Sleep Foundation
1010 N. Glebe Road, Suite 310
Arlington, VA 22201

703-243-1697
Fax: 202-347-3472
nsf@sleepfoundation.org
www.sleepfoundation.org

For people with narcolepsy and their families; defines and describes narcolepsy, as well as the effects on education, social and
family life.

packet of 25

Charles A. Czeisler, PhD, MD, Chairman
Max Hirshkowitz, PhD, Vice Chairman
Joseph Ojile, MD, Secretary

4958   Narcolepsy
American Academy of Sleep Medicine
2510 North Frontage Road
Darien, IL 60561

630-737-9700
Fax: 630-737-9790
www.aasmnet.org

Describes the causes, symptoms and treatments of a disorder
characterized by excessive sleepiness.

Lot of 50

Timothy I. Morgenthaker, MD, President
Nathaniel F. Watson, MD, President-Elect
Ronald D. Chervin, MD, MS, Secretary/Treasurer

DESCRIPTION

4959 NEONATAL HERPES SIMPLEX

Synonym: Congenital herpes

Involves the following Biologic System(s):

Infectious Disorders, Neonatal and Infant Disorders

Neonatal herpes simplex refers to an infection of the newborn caused by the herpes simplex virus (HSV) that is transmitted before birth from mother to fetus through the placenta, or more commonly, during birth as the baby passes through the birth canal. There are two strains of herpes simplex virus known as HSV-1 and HSV-2. Herpes simplex virus type 1 commonly causes infections of the skin and mucous membranes of the lips, mouth, and eyes, while type 2 typically causes genital herpes as well as approximately 75 percent of all neonatal herpes simplex infections.

Herpes simplex may be categorized as an initial (primary) infection or a recurrent infection. After an initial infection, the virus becomes inactive or latent; however, the virus may be reactivated by many different factors including stress, sun exposure, suppression of the immune system, and certain foods or drugs. Mothers with a primary genital herpes simplex virus infection have an approximately 45 percent chance of transmitting HSV-2 to their infants, while risk of transmission from a recurrent infection is less than five percent. In addition, newborns are at risk for HSV-1 transmission through such direct contact as kissing near the eyes or mouth by someone with a cold sore.

Symptoms of HSV infection transmitted through contact with infectious secretions during the birthing process may occur anywhere from one to four weeks after birth and may sometimes commence with the appearance of small, fluid-filled blisters (vesicles) on the skin or inflammation of the front part of the eyeball (cornea) and the delicate mucous membranes (conjunctiva) that line the inside of the eyelids and the whites of the eyes (keratoconjunctivitis). Other findings may include fever, drowsiness, loss of muscle tone, irritability, seizures, and inflammation of the liver (hepatitis) and brain (encephalitis), as well as other severe irregularities. If left untreated, HSV infection may cause potentially life-threatening complications. Some infants may have no skin involvement but manifest such symptoms as fluctuating temperature, listlessness, poor sucking, chills, shaking, nausea, vomiting, and diarrhea.

Transmission of the herpes simplex virus through the placenta is a rare but potentially life-threatening occurrence. This type of infection usually affects the skin, eyes, and central nervous system and is characterized by blister-type rashes and scarring, abnormally small eyes (microphthalmia) and other eye abnormalities, an abnormally small head (microcephaly), and brain and spinal cord irregularities. Some infants may also have hepatitis or lung involvement.

Prevention of neonatal herpes simplex infection may include delivery by Cesarean section, especially if the mother has a primary genital herpes infection. Treatment is directed toward early diagnosis and intervention. Such therapy may include the intravenous administration of antiviral drugs such as acyclovir in conjunction with regular testing to preclude possible associated toxic side effects related to kidney dysfunction. Eye involvement may indicate the application of antiviral ointments or drops directly into the eyes. Other treatment is symptomatic and supportive.

Government Agencies

4960 NIH/National Institute of Allergy and Infectious Diseases
5601 Fishers Lane, MSC 9806
Bethesda, MD 20892
301-496-5717
866-284-4107
Fax: 301-402-3573
TDD: 800-877-8339
ocpostoffice@niaid.nih.gov
www.niaid.nih.gov

Conducts and supports basic and applied research to better understand, treat, and ultimately prevent infectious, immunologic, and allergic diseases.

Anthony S Fauci MD, Director

National Associations & Support Groups

4961 American Academy of Pediatrics
141 Northwest Point Boulevard
Elk Grove Village, IL 60007
847-434-4000
800-433-9016
Fax: 847-434-8000
www.aap.org

The American Academy of Pediatrics and its member pediatricians are committed to the attainment of optimal physical, mental and social health and well-being for all infants, children, adolescents, and young adults.

Fernando Stein, MD, FAAP, President
Karen Remley, MD, CEO/Executive VP

4962 American Social Health Association
PO Box 13827
Research Triangle Park, NC 27709
919-361-8400
919-361-8488
Fax: 919-361-8425
info@ashastd.org
www.ashastd.org

The American Social Health Association is dedicated to improving the health of individuals, families, and communities, with a focus on preventing sexually transmitted diseases and their harmful consequences.

Lynn Barclay, President/CEO

4963 National Health Information Center: Office of Disease Preventive/Health Promotion
US Dept of Health and Human Services
PO Box 1133
Washington, DC 20013
240-453-8280
800-336-4797
Fax: 240-453-8282
info@nhif.org
www.nhic.org

The National Health Information Center is a health information referral service that links consumers and health professionals who have health questions to organizations best able to provide reiable health information.

Libraries & Resource Centers

4964 Herpes Resource Center
American Social Health Association
PO Box 13827
Research Triangle Park, NC 27709
919-361-8400
Fax: 919-361-8425
customerservice@ashastd.org
www.ashastd.org

Tom Beall, Chairman
Lynn Barclay, President and Chief Executive Offic
Deborah Arrindell, Vice President, Health Policy

Web Sites

4965 American Social Health Association
www.ashastd.org

Dedicated to improving the health of individuals, families, and communities, with a focus on preventing sexually transmitted diseases and their harmful consequences.

4966 Health Research Project (HaRP)
www.harpnet.org

harp@aimglobalhealth.org
www.harpnet.org

A program by USAID, the project strives to improve the health status of infants, children, mothers and families through the development and research of new tools, technologies, policies and approaches.

4967 HerpeSite
www.herpesite.org

800-273-8255
TTY: 800-799-4889
www.herpesite.org

Provides online personal empowerment and support; a compedium of information outlining aspects and issues relating to Herpes Simplex Virus.

4968 Herpes.com
www.herpes.com

Purpose of this website is to fill the desperate need for herpes education, make it easier to manage herpes, inform people of ways to limit herpes reoccurrences, to inform people of the beneficial products for herpes sufferers, to show the relationship between good health and herpes, to provide an opportunity for herpes sufferers to share their personal experiences and to provide communication via our live chat.

4969 Infectious Diseases in Children
6900 Grove Road
Thorofare, NJ 8086

856-848-1000
editor@healio.com
http://idinchildren.com

A leading provider of healthcare information, educational programs, and meeting and exhibit management services worldwide.

4970 International Herpes Alliance
www.herpesalliance.org

4971 Virtual Pediatric Hospital
www.virtualpediatrichospital.org

A digital library of pediatric informaion dedicated to helping patients find the highest quality medical information in the world today. Offers patients the tools necessary to make informed treatment decisions within the short time lines dictated by their illness or disease.

Book Publishers

4972 Understanding Herpes

Dr Lawrence R Stanberg, author

University Press of Mississippi
3825 Ridgewood Road
Jackson, MS 39211

601-432-6205
800-737-7788
Fax: 601-432-6217
press@ihl.state.ms.us
www.upress.state.ms.us

A most informative overview of herpes written for the general reader.

120 pages Cloth
ISBN: 1-578060-40-0

Leila W. Salisbury, Director
Cynthia Foster, Administrative Assistant
Tracey Curtis, Assistant For Development

DESCRIPTION

4973 NEONATAL JAUNDICE

Synonym: Icterus neonatorum

Involves the following Biologic System(s):

Neonatal and Infant Disorders

Neonatal jaundice refers to a condition of the newborn in which high blood levels of the reddish-orange bile pigment bilirubin cause a yellowing of the skin, eyes, and mucous membranes. Bilirubin is derived from the breakdown of the protein, hemoglobin, in red blood cells. Neonatal jaundice may be the result of many different factors including metabolic disturbances or deficiencies; certain genetic disorders; conditions associated with an increased rate of red blood cell destruction (hemolysis); conditions that affect liver function; and certain types of infections.

Blood levels of bilirubin may be somewhat elevated after the first day of life, usually peak by the fourth day, and fall to normal levels by the end of the first week. This temporary rise, frequently accompanied by jaundice, results from the increased destruction of fetal red blood cells and the inability of a still-developing metabolic mechanism to efficiently eliminate bile from the body. In addition, an enzyme present in the intestines of newborns may convert bilirubin to a form that allows it to be reabsorbed into the blood, resulting in even higher bilirubin blood levels. Premature infants are particularly at risk for jaundice. If no other underlying cause is responsible, jaundice typically resolves spontaneously along with bilirubin level stabilization.

The appearance of jaundice in a newborn is carefully evaluated for underlying causes. Factors that may indicate the presence of an underlying disorder may include jaundice within the first 24 hours of life; a higher and faster-than-expected rise in bilirubin levels; birth defects, especially those that affect the liver such as biliary atresia; a family history of diseases that cause the early destruction of red blood cells such as hemolytic disease of the newborn; or rare disorders associated with hyperbilirubinemia (e.g., Crigler-Najjar syndrome, transient familial neonatal hyperbilirubinemia, etc.). Other suspect findings may include an enlarged liver (hepatomegaly), enlarged spleen (splenomegaly), lethargy, unusual paleness, difficulty in feeding, vomiting, or excessive weight loss.

Treatment of neonatal jaundice depends upon the underlying cause. Some infants with jaundice associated with breast-feeding may benefit from phototherapy. During this treatment, which is carefully monitored, the infant's bare skin is exposed to high intensity fluorescent lights that speed up the excretion and elimination of bilirubin in the skin. Other treatment is symptomatic and supportive.

Government Agencies

4974 NIH/ Eunice Kennedy Shriver National Insti tute of Child Health & Human Development
31 Center Drive, Building 31
Bethesda, MD 20892   301-496-5113
                                      800-370-2943
                                   Fax: 866-760-5947
                                   TTY: 888-320-6942
                              nichdpress@mail.nih.gov
                                    www.nichd.nih.gov

Established in 1962 by congress, today the institute conducts and supports research on topics related to the health of children, adults, families and populations. Some of these topics include: developmental disabilities, growth and development, infant death, reproductive health and birth defects.

Diana W. Bianchi, Director
Paul Williams, Director, Communications

National Associations & Support Groups

4975 American Academy of Pediatrics
141 Northwest Point Boulevard
Elk Grove Village, IL 60007   847-434-4000
                                         800-433-9016
                                    Fax: 847-434-8000
                                         www.aap.org

The American Academy of Pediatrics and its member pediatricians are committed to the attainment of optimal physical, mental and social health and well-being for all infants, children, adolescents, and young adults.

Fernando Stein, MD, FAAP, President
Karen Remley, MD, CEO/Executive VP

4976 American College of Gastroenterology
6400 Goldsboro Road, Suite 200
Bethesda, MD 20817   301-263-9000
                                    Fax: 301-263-9025
                                       info@acg.gi.org
                                          www.gi.org

Founded to advance the scientific study and medical practice of diseases of the gastrointestinal (GI) tract.

13,000 members

Carol A. Burke, MD, FACG, President

4977 American Liver Foundation
39 Broadway, Suite 2700
New York, NY 10006   212-668-1000
                                         800-465-4837
                                    Fax: 212-483-8179
                              info@liverfoundation.org
                                 www.liverfoundation.org

Nonprofit, national, voluntary health organization dedicated to the prevention, treatment and cure of hepatitis and other liver diseases through research, education, and advocacy on behalf of those affected by or at risk of liver disease.

Thomas F. Nealon III, Chairman
Daniel E. Weil, Treasurer
Carlo Frappolli, Secretary

4978 Digestive Disease National Coalition
507 Capitol Court NE, Suite 200
Washington, DC 20002   202-544-7497
                                    Fax: 202-546-7105
                                    hpayne@hmcw.org
                                        www.ddnc.org

Advocacy organization comprised of over 30 voluntary and professional societies concerned with the many diseases of the digestive tract and liver.

Lynn Seim, Chairperson
Ralph McKibbin, President
Cathy Griffith, Vice Chairperson

4979 Greater Los Angeles Chapter
American Liver Foundation
130 N. Brand Blvd., Suite 305
Glendale, CA 91203
818-500-8636
Fax: 818-500-8638
cshort@liverfoundation.org
www.cai-glac.org/

A national organization that promotes research and cures for hepatitis and other liver diseases.

Matt D. Ober, Partner
Katy Krupp, VP
Gregg Lotane, Treasurer

4980 International Foundation for Functional Gastrointestinal Disorders
PO Box 170864
Milwaukee, WI 53217
414-964-1799
Fax: 414-964-7176
iffgd@iffgd.org
www.iffgd.org

Nonprofit education and research organization founded in 1991. IFFGD addresses the issues surrounding life with gastrointestinal (GI) functional and mobility disorders and increases the awareness about these disorders among the general public, researchers and the clinical care community.

Nancy J. Norton, President & Director
William Norton, Co-Founder
Eleanor Cautley, VP/Director

4981 March of Dimes Foundation
1275 Mamaroneck Avenue
White Plains, NY 10605
914-997-4488
888-663-4637
Fax: 914-428-8203
answers@marchofdimes.com
www.marchofdimes.com

Partnership of volunteers and professionals dedicates to improving the health of babies by preventing birth defects and infant mortality. Over 100 chapters are located across the country and can be located through the National Office.

Stacey D. Stewart, President

4982 North American Society for Pediatric Gastroenterology/Hepatology/Nutrition
714 N Bethlehem Pike, Suite 300
Ambler, PA 19002
215-641-9800
Fax: 215-641-1995
naspghan@naspghan.org
www.naspghan.org

Strives to improve the care of infants, children and adolescents with digestive disorders by promoting advances in clinical care of children with chronic abdominal pain, diarrhea, constipation, vomiting, bleeding from the GI tract, inflammatory bowel disease, liver diseases, diseases of the pancreas, poor weight gain and nutritional problems.

Margaret K Stallings, Executive Director
Kim Rose, Associate Director
Donna Murphy, Membership

Libraries & Resource Centers

4983 National Digestive Diseases Information Clearinghouse
9000 Rockville Pike
Bethesda, MD 20892
301-496-3583; 800-860-8747
Fax: 301-907-8906
healthinfo@niddk.nih.gov
www.niddk.nih.govv

The National Institute of Diabetes and Digestive and Kidney Diseases conducts and supports research on many of the most serious diseases affecting public health. The Institute supports much of the clinical research on the diseases of internal medicine and related subspecialty fields as well as many basic science disciplines.

Dr. Griffin P. Rodgers, Director
Dr. Gregory G. Germino, Deputy Directortary
Camille M. Hoover, M.S.W., Executive Officer

Web Sites

4984 American Liver Foundation
39 Broadway, Suite 2700
New York, NY 10006
212-668-1000
Fax: 212-483-8179
www.liverfoundation.org

Nonprofit, national, voluntary health organization dedicated to the prevention, treatment and cure of hepatitis and other liver diseases through research, education, and advocacy on behalf of those affected by or at risk of liver disease.

Thomas F. Nealon III, Chairman
Daniel E. Weil, Treasurer
Carlo Frappolli, Secretary

4985 Liver 411
www.liver411.com

4986 National Digestive Diseases Information Clearinghouse
www.digestive.niddk.nih.gov
301-496-3583
www.digestive.niddk.nih.gov

The National Institute of Diabetes and Digestive and Kidney Diseases conducts and supports research on many of the most serious diseases affecting public health. The Institute supports much of the clinical research on the diseases of internal medicine and related subspecialty fields as well as many basic science disciplines.

4987 Online Mendelian Inheritance in Man
National Library of Medicine Building 38A
Bethesda, MD 20894
888-346-3656
info@ncbi.nlm.nih.gov
www.ncbi.nlm.nih.gov

This database is a catalog of human genes and genetic disorders.

Journals

4988 Journal of Pediatric Gastroenterology and Nutrition
NASPGHAN, author

Lippincott Williams & Wilkins
2001 Market Street
Philadelphia, PA 19103
215-521-8300; Fax: 215-521-8902
www.lww.com

Publication of the North American Society for Pediatric Gastroenterolgy, Hepatology and Nutrition, which strives to improve the care of infants, children and adolescents with digestive disorders by promoting advances in clinical care of children with chronic abdominal pain, diarrhea, constipation, vomiting, bleeding from the GI tract, inflammatory bowel disease, liver diseases, diseases of the pancreas, poor weight gain and nutritional problems.

Newsletters

4989 NASPGHAN News
714 N. Bethlehem Pike, Ste 300
Ambler, PA 19002
215-641-9800; Fax: 215-641-1995
naspghan@naspghan.org
www.naspghan.org

Publication of the North American Society for Pediatric Gastroenterolgy, Hepatology and Nutrition, which strives to improve the care of infants, children and adolescents with digestive disorders by promoting advances in clinical care of children with chronic abdominal pain, diarrhea, constipation, vomiting, bleeding from the GI tract, inflammatory bowel disease, liver diseases, diseases of the pancreas, poor weight gain and nutritional problems.

Margaret K Stallings, Executive Director
Kim Rose, Associate Director
Donna Murphy, Membership

DESCRIPTION

4990 NEPHROTIC SYNDROME

Synonyms: Minimal change nephrotic syndrome, MCNS

Covers these related disorders: Infantile nephrotic syndrome, Primary nephrotic syndrome, Secondary nephrotic syndrome

Involves the following Biologic System(s):
Renal and Urologic Disorders

Nephrotic syndrome is characterized by an abnormality of the kidney that allows proteins to leak out of the blood and into the urine. The loss of these proteins leads to proteinuria (protein in the urine), edema (swelling) of the body, hypoproteinemia (low blood levels of protein), hyperlipidemia (high fat levels in the blood) and lipiduria (fat in the urine). Clinical examination of a patient with nephrotic syndrome will reveal swelling of the eyelids and skin around the eyes (periorbital edema), swelling of the extremities, especially feet and lower legs, and fluid in the abdomen (ascites). Laboratory examination will show large amounts of urinary protein, low serum albumin and high cholesterol.

There are three categories of nephrotic syndrome: infantile; primary; and secondary:

Infantile nephrotic syndrome is usually the result of an inherited form and symptoms occur in the first few months of life. Secondary nephrotic syndrome is nephrotic syndrome associated with another disease process. These can include infection, connective tissue disorders such as lupus erythematosus, allergen exposure and medications.

Primary nephrotic syndrome results from disease in the kidney alone. The most common form is minimal change nephrotic syndrome (MCNS), or minimal change disease. It is called minimal change because little change is seen in the kidneys when a biopsy of the kidney is examined. Minimal change nephrotic syndrome almost always responds to steroids. Although relapses are not uncommon the long-term prognosis is excellent. Other causes of primary nephrotic syndrome, such as focal segmental glomerulosclerosis, mesangial proliferative glomeruloephritis, and membranous nephropathy, may or may not improve with the steroids and generally have a worse prognosis than MCNS. These patients can be treated with immunosuppressive therapy but may progress to end-stage renal disease requiring dialysis or kidney transplant.

Children with nephrotic syndrome are at risk for several complications. These include increased risk of infection, blood clots and cardiovascular disease. Dietary management includes restriction of sodium and fluid intake. Excessive sunlight should be avoided, because sensitivity to light (photosensitivity) is common.

National Associations & Support Groups

4991 American Academy of Pediatrics
141 Northwest Point Boulevard
Elk Grove Village, IL 60007

847-434-4000
800-433-9016
Fax: 847-434-8000
www.aap.org

The American Academy of Pediatrics and its member pediatricians are committed to the attainment of optimal physical, mental and social health and well-being for all infants, children, adolescents, and young adults.

Fernando Stein, MD, FAAP, President
Karen Remley, MD, CEO/Executive VP

4992 American Kidney Fund
11921 Rockville Pike, Suite 300
Rockville, MD 20852

301-881-3052
800-638-8299
Fax: 301-881-0898
helpline@kidneyfund.org
www.akfinc.org

The American Kidney Fund is the nation's leading voluntary health organization serving people with and at risk for kidney disease through direct financial assistance, comprehensive education, clinical research and community service programs.

Timothy G. Morgan, Chair
John P. Butler, Chair-Elect
Myra A. Kleinpeter, Chair Medical Affairs

4993 National Kidney Foundation
30 E 33rd Street
New York, NY 10016

212-889-2210
855-653-2273
Fax: 212-689-9261
info@kidney.org
www.kidney.org

A major voluntary health organization, seeking to prevent kidney and urinary tract diseases, improve the health and well-being of individuals and families affected by these diseases, and increases the availability of all organs for transplant.

James Carlson, CEO
Joseph A Vassalotti MD, Chief Medical Officer

4994 NephCure Foundation
15 Waterloo Avenue
Berwyn, PA 19312

610-540-0186
866-637-4287
Fax: 610-540-0190
info@nephcure.org
www.nephcure.org

The only organization committed exclusively to support research seeking the cuses of the potentially debilitating kidney diseases, Nephrotic Syndrome and Focal Segmental Glomerulosclerosis (FSGS), improve treatment and find a cure.

Irvine Smokler, President
Ron Cohen, VP
Michael Levine, VP

Web Sites

4995 American Kidney Fund
11921 Rockville Pike, Suite 300
Rockville, MD 20852

www.akfinc.org

Providing information for people with and at risk for kidney disease such as Nephrotic Syndrome.

John P. Butler, Chair
LaVarnee A. Burton, President & Chief Executive Officer
Donald J. Roy, Jr, EVP, CFO, COO

4996 National Kidney Foundation
30 East 33rd Street
New York, NY 10016

800-622-9010
Fax: 212-689-9261
info@kidney.org
www.kidney.org

A site that offers information to prevent kidney and urinary tract diseases, improve the health and well-being of individuals and families affected by these diseases, and increases the availability of all organs for transplant.

Bruce Skyer, CEO
Joseph Vassalotti, MD, Chief Medical Officer
Petros Gregoriou, CPA, Senior Vice President & CFO

4997 NephCure Foundation
150 S. Warner Road Suite 402
King of Prussia, PA 19406   info@nephcure.org
                                        nephcure.org

The only organization committed exclusively to support research
seeking the cuses of the potentially debilitating kidney diseases,
Nephrotic Syndrome and Focal Segmental Glomerulosclerosis
(FSGS), improve treatment and find a cure.

Irving Smokler, Ph.D. ~, President
Ron Cohen ~ ~ ~, Vice President
Andrew Silverman ~, Treasurer

Book Publishers

4998 The Official Parent's Sourcebook on Childhood Nephrotic
Syndrome

James N. Parker, author

Icon Group International
9606 Tierra Grande St., Suite 205
San Diego, CA 92126   Fax: 858-635-9414
                                        orders@icongroupbooks.com
                                        www.icongrouponline.com

A comprehensive manual for anyone interested in self-directed research on childhood Nephrotic Syndrome. Fully referenced with
ample internet listings and glossary.

2002 136 pages Paperback
ISBN: 0-597832-16-1

Newsletters

4999 NephCure Now
NephCure Foundation
150 S. Warner Road, Suite 402
King of Prussia, PA 19406   610-540-0186
                                        Fax: 610-540-0190
                                        info@nephcure.org
                                        www.nephcure.org

The NephCure Foundation's newsletter that contains news and information on a variety of topics including the latest research updates, NephCure events and fundraisers and much more.

Irving Smokler, Ph.D., President
Ron Cohen ~, Vice President
Andrew Silverman, Treasurer

5000 Renalink
National Kidney Foundation
30 E 33rd Street
New York, NY 10016   212-889-2210
                                        800-622-9010
                                        Fax: 212-689-9261
                                        info@kidney.org
                                        www.kidney.org/professionals/journals/login.cfm

Renalink is the joint newsletter of the Council of Nephrology
Nurses and Technicians, the Council of Nephrology Social Work
and the Council of Renal Nutrition of the National Kidney Foundation. Renalink includes news for each Council, information vital to the renal care team and ideas that should lead to further
collaboration among allied health professionals in the renal field.

Quarterly
Bruce Skyer, CEO
Joseph Vassalotti, MD, Chief Medical Officer
Petros Gregoriou, CPA, Senior Vice President & CFO

Pamphlets

5001 Childhood Nephrotic Syndrome
Information Clearinghouse
2 Information Way
Bethesda, MD 20892   301-496-3583
                                        Fax: 301-907-8906
                                        nddic@info.niddk.nih.gov
                                        www.niddk.nih.gov

5002 Children and Kidney Disease
American Kidney Fund
30 East 33rd Street
New York, NY 10016   301-881-3052
                                        800-622-9010
                                        Fax: 212-689-9261
                                        info@kidney.org
                                        www.kidney.org

Bruce Skyer, CEO
Joseph Vassalotti, MD, Chief Medical Officer
Petros Gregoriou, CPA, Senior Vice President & CFO

5003 Financial Assistance and Insurance for People with Kidney
Disease
Information Clearinghouse
2 Information Way
Bethesda, MD 20892   301-496-3583
                                        Fax: 301-907-8906
                                        nddic@info.niddk.nih.gov
                                        www.niddk.nih.gov

5004 Kidney Disease of Diabetes
Information Clearinghouse
1 Information Way
Bethesda, MD 20892   301-496-3583
                                        Fax: 301-907-8906
                                        ndoc@info.niddk.nih.gov
                                        www.niddk.nih.gov

DESCRIPTION

5005 NEUROFIBROMATOSIS

Synonym: NF

Covers these related disorders: Neurofibromatosis type I (von Recklinghausen disease) (NF1), Neurofibromatosis type II (NF2)

Involves the following Biologic System(s):

Dermatologic Disorders, Orthopedic and Muscle Disorders

The term neurofibromatosis is often used to refer to neurofibromatosis type I (NF1), an autosomal dominant disorder that affects approximately one in 3,500 to 4,000 individuals. Neurofibromatosis type I, also known as von Recklinghausen disease, is characterized by the appearance of pale tan or light brown discolorations (macules) on the skin (cafe-au-lait spots) and multiple benign, fibrous tumors of nerves and skin (neurofibromas). A second, distinctive form of neurofibromatosis (NF), known as neurofibromatosis type II (NF2), accounts for about 10 percent of all cases of NF. Neurofibromatosis type II, also an autosomal dominant disorder, is characterized by the development of benign tumors on both acoustic nerves (bilateral acoustic neuromas), resulting in progressive hearing impairment.

In most children with neurofibromatosis type I, skin discoloration may develop by the age of one year. Such skin lesions typically increase in number and size over time, and most affected individuals have six or more spots measuring 1.5 centimeters or more in diameter after the onset of puberty. Although these cafe-au-lait spots are often distributed in various areas of the body, they are most commonly present on the trunk. In addition, after three years of age, areas of freckling, particularly under the arms (axillary) and in the groin (inguinal) area, may also be present.

In approximately 95 percent of children with NF1 over six years of age, two or more benign, tumor-like nodules, known as Lisch nodules, are present on the pigmented areas of the eyes. Benign, fibrous tumors of the skin (cutaneous neurofibromas) tend to develop during the second decade of life, typically appearing as small, soft, raised, and slightly purplish discolorations of the overlying skin. These tumors, which rarely develop before six years of age, may increase in number and size during puberty. In addition, large benign tumors composed of bundles of nerves (plexiform neurofibromas) may be apparent at birth or during early childhood. Approximately two to four percent of individuals with NF1 may develop malignant tumors (e.g., neurofibrosarcomas). Physical findings that may be associated with malignant transformation include increasing tumor size, associated pain, or various neurologic symptoms due to tumor growth. Approximately 15 percent of affected individuals may also develop tumors of the optic nerve (optic glioma), which is the cranial nerve that carries visual impulses from the back of the eye (retina) to the brain. These tumors are usually considered relatively benign and may cause no associated symptoms (asymptomatic). However, in some cases, depending upon their specific location, growth, and nature, such tumors may affect vision. In these patients, associated findings may include visual impairment; degeneration (atrophy) of the optic nerve; abnormal deviation of the eye (strabismus); or involuntary, rhythmic eye movements (nystagmus). In addition,some affected individuals may have an increased risk of developing tumors of the brain and spinal cord (e.g., astrocytomas, meningiomas, neurilemmomas, etc.).

Some individuals with NF1 may also experience associated skeletal abnormalities, such as bowing of the lower legs; improper development of a bone at the base of the skull (sphenoid wing dysplasia), potentially causing pronounced bulging of the eyes (exophthalmos); and progressive sideways curvature of the spine (scoliosis). Additional abnormalities may be present, such as mild short stature, abnormal largeness of the head (macrocephaly), and episodes of uncontrolled electrical activity in the brain (seizures). In addition, many affected children may have learning disabilities and speech abnormalities. Neurofibromatosis type I is caused by abnormal changes (mutations) of a gene located on the long arm of chromosome 17 (17q11.2). In approximately 50 percent of patients, the disease gene is inherited an an autosomal dominant trait; the remaining cases result from new (sporadic) mutations of the gene that occur for unknown reasons.

Neurofibromatosis type II (NF2) is also characterized by bilateral acoustic neuromas that are responsible for carrying sound impulses from the inner ear to the brain. Symptoms may become apparent during childhood or the second or third decades of life. These may include a facial numbness or weakness, headache, dizziness, unsteadiness, and progressive hearing loss. Individuals with NF2 may also develop clouding of the lenses of the eyes (i.e., posterior subcapsular opacities), have an increased risk of developing tumors of the brain and spinal cord (e.g., gliomas, meningiomas, schwannomas, etc.), or experience progressive visual impairment. NF2 is caused by a disease gene located on the long arm of chromosome 22 (22q12.2).

The treatment of neurofibromatosis is directed toward ensuring early detection and prompt, appropriate management of potentially associated findings or complications. Affected individuals are typically regularly monitored with complete neurologic evaluations (e.g., including visual and auditory screening) and thorough examinations to detect potential complications associated with NF. In most cases, symptoms of NF1 are mild, and patients live normal and productive lives. In some cases, however, NF1 can be severely debilitating. In some cases of NF2, the damage to nearby vital structures, such as other cranial nerves, can be life-threatening. Some tumors may be surgically removed or treated using other appropriate methods (e.g., radiation or chemotherapy for certain malignancies). Other treatment is symptomatic and supportive.

National Associations & Support Groups

5006 American Academy of Pediatrics
141 Northwest Point Boulevard
Elk Grove Village, IL 60007

847-434-4000
800-433-9016
Fax: 847-434-8000
www.aap.org

The American Academy of Pediatrics and its member pediatricians are committed to the attainment of optimal physical, mental and social health and well-being for all infants, children, adolescents, and young adults.

Fernando Stein, MD, FAAP, President
Karen Remley, MD, CEO/Executive VP

5007 Children's Tumor Foundation
95 Pine Street, 16th Floor
New York, NY 10005
212-344-6633
800-323-7938
Fax: 212-747-0004
info@ctf.org
www.ctf.org

The Children's Tumor Foundation funds research, patient support, and public awareness of the neurofibromatoses (NF1, NF2 & Schwannomatosis) genetic disorders that cause random tumor growth throughout the body.

Stuart Match Suna, Chairperson
John W Risner, President
Linda Halliday Martin, Vice Chairperson

5008 Genetic Alliance
4301 Connecticut Avenue NW, Suite 404
Washington, DC 20008
202-966-5557
800-336-4363
Fax: 202-966-8553
info@geneticalliance.org
www.geneticalliance.org

A coalition of voluntary genetic support groups, consumers and professionals addressing the needs of individuals and families affected by genetic disorders from a national perspective.

Sharon Terry, President/CEO
Tetyana Murza, Managing Director
Natasha Bonhomme, VP, Strategic Development

5009 March of Dimes Foundation
1275 Mamaroneck Avenue
White Plains, NY 10605
914-997-4488
888-663-4637
Fax: 914-428-8203
answers@marchofdimes.com
www.marchofdimes.com

Partnership of volunteers and professionals dedicates to improving the health of babies by preventing birth defects and infant mortality. Over 100 chapters are located across the country and can be located through the National Office.

Stacey D. Stewart, President

5010 National Brain Tumor Foundation
55 Chapel Street, Suite 200
Newton, MA 02458
617-924-9997
800-934-2873
Fax: 617-924-9998
info@braintumor.org
www.braintumor.org

NBTF is a national nonprofit health organization dedicated to providing information and support for brain tumor patients, family members, and healthcare professionals, while supporting innovative research into better treatment options and a cure for brain tumors.

Jeffrey Kolodin, Chair
Michael Nathanson, Vice-Chair
Michael Corkin, Treasurer

5011 Neurofibromatosis Support & Information Gr oup
Parents Helping Parents
3041 Olcott Street
Santa Clarka, CA 95054
408-727-5775
Fax: 408-727-0182
info@php.com
www.php.com

Helping children with special needs receive the resources, love, hope, respect, health care, education and other services they need to achieve their full potential by providing them with strong families and dedicated professionals to serve them.

Alexandra Cramer, Receptionist/Admin. Assistant
Carlos A. Gallegos, Kids on the Block Coordinator
Cathie Silverberg

5012 Neurofibromatosis, Inc
213 S. Wheaton Ave.
Wheaton, IL 60187
630-510-1115
800-942-6825
Fax: 630-510-8508
admin@nfnetwork.org
www.nfnetwork.org

An organization of independent state and regional chapters that provides support and services to families coping with neurofibromatosis. Works closely with clinical and research professionals who specialize in the treatment of NF. Has a newsletter and other printed materials.

Cheri Stewart, President
Rosemary Anderson, VP
Nicole Hicks, Secretary

State Agencies & Support Groups

Arizona

5013 Neurofibromatosis, Inc - Arizona Chapter
PO Box 2718
Chandler, AZ 85244
480-945-9650
info@nfarizona.org
www.nfarizona.org

Arkansas

5014 Children's Tumor Foundation-Arkansas Chapt er
1 Children's Way
Little Rock, AR 72202
501-364-1850
paws4me@cox.net
www.ctf.org/Chapters-Affiliates/Arkansas/

Julie Jarrett, Contact
Rolla Shbarou, Clinic Director
Shaneika Lewis-Williams, Clinic Coordinators

5015 Children's Tumor Foundation-Arkansas Infor www.php.com
PO Box 7262
Little Rock, AR 72217
501-920-5588
loslica@gmail.com
www.ctfarkansas.com

Lesley Oslica, Contact

California

5016 Neurofibromatosis, Inc - California Chapte r
PO Box 1234
Vacaville, CA 95696
707-469-0467
Fax: 866-571-2366
info@nfcalifornia.org
www.nfcalifornia.org

Debbie Bell, President
Dana Inigues, VP
Katie Sperring, Secretary

Colorado

5017 Children's Tumor Foundation - Colorado Cha pter
13121 E. 17th Ave.
Aurora, CO 80045
303-724-2370
ilaskey@peakpeak.com
www.ctf.org/Chapters-Affiliates/Colorado/

Mark Ebel, Chapter President
Gary Bellus, Clinic Director
Katherine Howard, Clinic Coordinators

Florida

5018 Children's Tumor Foundation - Florida Chap ter
3100 SW 62nd Avenue, Suite 301
Miami, FL 33155
305-663-8595
800-540-5721
hehrli@aol.com
www.ctf.org/Chapters-Affiliates/florida/
Hannah Erli, Chapter President
Sue Bresnahan, Office Contact
Mislen Bauer, Clinic Director

Georgia

5019 Children's Tumor Foundation - Georgia
5 Ardmore Circle
Cartersville, GA 30120
678-428-9711
ctfgeorgia@bellsouth.net
www.ctf.org/Chapters-Affiliates/Georgia/
Beth O'Brien-Burke, President
Melissa Lee, VP
Julie Santana, Patient Outreach Committee Chair

Illinois

5020 Children's Tumor Foundation - Illinois
2300 Children's Plaza
Chicago, IL 60614
773-880-4462
Fax: 217-732-8568
mmoscatello@ctf.org
www.ctf.org/Chapters-Affiliates/Illinois/

2500 members

Paul Beach, Chapter President
Joel Charrow, Clinic Co-Director
Michelle Gilats, Clinic Coordinators

5021 Children's Tumor Foundation - Illinois Cha pter
2300 Children's Plaza
Chicago, IL 60614
773-880-4462
Fax: 217-732-8568
mmoscatello@ctf.org
www.ctf.org/Chapters-Affiliates/Illinois/
Paul Beach, Chapter President
Joel Charrow, Clinic Co-Director
Michelle Gilats, Clinic Coordinators

5022 Neurofibromatosis, Inc - Illinois
213 S. Wheaton Ave
Wheaton, IL 60187
630-510-1115
800-942-6825
Fax: 630-510-8508
admin@nfnetwork.org
www.nfnetwork.org

A leading national organization advocating for the development
of local NF organizations and for federal funding for NF research

Cheri Stewart, President
Rosemary Anderson, Vice President
Mike Montgomery, Treasurer

5023 Neurofibromatosis, Inc - Illinois/Midwest
473 Dunham Rd, Suite 3
St. Charles, IL 60174
630-945-3562
800-322-6363
Fax: 630-932-8119
Diana@nfmidwest.org
www.nfmidwest.org
Diana Haberkamp, Executive Director
Jenny Perkins, Development Director
Liz Campana, Administrative Assistant

Indiana

5024 Children's Tumor Foundation - Indiana Affi liate
Suite 4700, 355 W, 16th Street
Indiannapolis, IN 46202
317-948-5450
Fax: 317-963-7533
kym1577@sbcglobal.net
www.indiananf.com
Kim Bebley, Affiliate Representative

Iowa

5025 Children's Tumor Foundation - Iowa Chapter
200 Hawkins Drive
Iowa City, IA 52242
319-356-2229
Fax: 515-277-1526
Drev@aol.com
www.ctf.org/Chapters-Affiliates/Iowa/
Sheila Drevyanko, Chapter President
Pamela Trapane, Director
Catherine Evers, Clinic Co-Coordinators

Kansas

5026 Neurofibromatosis, Inc - Kansas & Central Plains
9218 Metcalf, Ste. 335
Overland Park, KS 66212
316-669-8453
800-942-6825
nprieb@southwind.net
www.nfcentralplains.org
Nichole Servos, President
Mike Montgomery, VP
Sharon Loftspring, Secretary

Maryland

5027 Neurofibromatosis, Inc - MidAtlantic
2 Village Square., Suite #213, 5100 Falls Road
Baltimore, MD 21210
443-423-0535
Fax: 410-889-0400
info@nfmidatlantic.org
www.nfmidatlantic.org
Diana Bark, President
Lee Herman, Board of Directors
Aaron Jumani, VP

Massachusetts

5028 Children's Tumor Foundation - Northern New England
300 Longwood Ave
Boston, MA 02115
617-355-4699
888-585-5316
Fax: 617-663-4801
seburne@ctf.org
www.ctf.org/Northern-New-England
Samantha Eburne, VP, NE Development

5029 Neurofibromatosis, Inc - New England/North east
213 S. Wheaton Ave.
Wheaton, IL 60187
630-510-1115
800-942-6825
Fax: 630-510-8508
admin@nfnetwork.org
www.nfnetwork.org
Cheri Stewart, President
Rosemary Anderson, VP
Nicole Hicks, Secretary

Michigan

5030 Children's Tumor Foundation - Michigan Cha pter
6069 Brynthrop
Shelby Township, MI 48316   586-731-7811
hawkeyenf@wideopenwest.com
www.ctf.org/Chapters-Affiliates/michigan/
Peter Dingeman, Chapter President
Wendy Schaffer, Treasurer
Xia Wang, Director

Missouri

5031 Children's Tumor Foundation - Missouri Cha pter
Thompson Coburn LLP
1046 Grand Blvd.
St Louis, MO 63104   314-552-6139
Fax: 314-552-7139
dcox@thompsoncoburn.com
www.ctf.org/Chapters-Affiliates/missouri/
Thomas Geller, Director
Julie Engel, Clinic Coordinator
Annette Novak

Nevada

5032 Children's Tumor Foundation - Nevada
8351 Mountain Destiny Ave
Las Vegas, NV 89131   702-457-0745
Fax: 775-972-1885
twnsmommy@msn.com
www.ctf.org/Chapters-Affiliates/Nevada/
Jennifer Halbert, Chapter Representative
Lori Bjorkquist, Chapter Representative

Ohio

5033 Children's Tumor Foundation - Ohio
3333 Burnet Avenue
Cincinnati, OH 45229   513-636-8826
mmoscatello@ctf.org
www.ctf.org/Chapters-Affiliates/Ohio/
Elizabeth Schorry, Director
Anne Lovell, Coordinator

Oregon

5034 Children's Tumor Foundation - Oregon Suppo rt Group
Oaks Park, 7805 SE Oaks Park Way
Portland, OR 97202   503-333-6797
Fax: 503-674-9256
kellerko@ohsu.edu
www.ctf.org/Chapters-Affiliates/Oregon/
Kory Keller, Genetic Counselor

5035 Legacy Good Samaritan Hospital & Medical C enter
Neurofibromatosis Support Group
1015 NW 22nd Avenue, N-300
Portland, OR 97210   503-413-7711
800-733-9959
mflorian@lhs.org
www.legacyhealth.org
Amy Marr, Coordinator

South Carolina

5036 Children's Tumor Foundation - South Caroli na Chapter
111 Oakview Drive
Darlington, SC 29532   843-393-9672
Fax: 843-393-9673
pmchrisley@aol.com
www.ctf.org/Chapters-Affiliates/South-Carolina/
Susan Luttrell, President

Tennessee

5037 Children's Tumor Foundation - Tennessee Af filiate
3501 Central Ave.
Nashville, TN 37924   865-633-5858
Fax: 865-633-5859
www.ctf.org/Chapters-Affiliates/Tennessee/
Cynthia Hester, President

Utah

5038 Children's Tumor Foundation - Utah Chapter
Sugarhouse Park, 1500 East 2100 South
Salt Lake City, UT 84115   801-485-2801
Fax: 801-277-4042
uteNFmom@gmail.com
www.ctf.org/Chapters-Affiliates/Utah/
Kelly Carpenter, President
Andrea Davis, VP
Kelsey Richards, Secretary

Virginia

5039 Children's Tumor Foundation - MidAtlantic Region Chapter
42010 Village Center Plz Ste 180
Aldie, VA 22066   703-444-1624
bentleyaw@aol.com
www.ctf.org/Home/Chapters-Affiliates/Mid-Atlantic/
Anne Bentley

Washington

5040 Children's Tumor Foundation - Washington C hapter
12722 166th St Ct E
Puyallup, WA 98374   253-370-9509
kkaralus74@yahoo.com
www.ctf.org/Chapters-Affiliates/washington/

Provides information, support services and referrals for patients
and families affected by neurofibromatosis, while supporting
medical research toward effective treatments and a cure.

Stuart Match Suna, Chairperson
John Risner, President
Linda Halliday Martin, Vice-Chairperson

Wisconsin

5041 Children's Tumor Foundation - Wisconsin Ch apter
6562 W Glenbrook Road
Brown Deer, WI 53223   414-716-5001
Fax: 414-362-0212
epankownf@aol.com
www.ctf.org/Chapters-Affiliates/Wisconsin/
Elaine Pankow, President

Research Centers

5042 NF Clinic - University of Pittsburgh Children's Hospital
5501 Old York Road
Philadelphia, PA 19141   215-456-8722
Fax: 215-456-2356
scheida@einstein.edu
www.nfmidatlantic.org

Jennifer Berkowitz, Contact

5043 Neurofibromatosis Center at North Broward Medical Center
303 SE 17th Street
Fort Lauderdale, FL 33316   954-784-1521
www.browardhealth.org

Frank Nask, President

5044 Neuroscience Institute at Mercy Hospital
4120 W Memorial Road
Oklahoma City, OK 73120
405-302-2661
Fax: 405-302-2670
www.mercy..net

Gary Brown PhD, Contact

Web Sites

5045 Children's Tumor Foundation
120 Wall Street, 16th Floor
New York, NY 10005
212-344-6633
info@ctf.org
www.ctf.org

A nonprofit medical foundation dedicated to improving the health and well being of individuals and families affected by NF.

Linda Halliday~Martin, Chairperson
Annette Bakker, PhD, President
Colin Bryar, Vice Chairperson

5046 Neurofibromatosis, Inc
213 S. Wheaton Ave.
Wheaton, IL 60187
630-510-1115
800-942-6825
Fax: 630-510-8508
admin@nfnetwork.org
www.nfinc.org

An organization made up of independent state and regional chapters, providing support and services to NF families. In addition to assisting individuals and families, NF, Inc. works closely with clinical and research professionals who specialize in the treatment of NF.

Cheri Stewart, President
Nicole Hicks, Secretary
Mike Montgomery, Treasurer

5047 Online Mendelian Inheritance in Man
National Library of Medicine Building 38A
Bethesda, MD 20894
888-346-3656
info@ncbi.nlm.nih.gov
www.ncbi.nlm.nih.gov

This database is a catalog of human genes and genetic disorders.

Book Publishers

5048 Let's Talk About Going to the Hospital
Rosen Publishing Group's PowerKids Press
29 E 21st Street
New York, NY 10010
212-777-3017
800-237-9932
Fax: 888-436-4643
rosenpub@tribeca.ios.com
www.rosenpublishing.com

If a child has to check into the hospital, chances are he or she is already upset about being ill. Knowing how a hospital functions and what the procedures are, such as when family members can visit, will help in what is already a stressful situation. Grades K-5.

24 pages
ISBN: 0-823950-36-0

Roger Rosen, President

5049 Neurofibromatosis: A Handbook for Patients , Families and Health Care Professionals

Dr Bruce R Korf; Dr Allan E Rubenstein, author

Children's Tumor Foundation
95 Pine Street, 16th Floor
New York, NY 10005
212-344-6633
800-323-7938
Fax: 212-747-0004
info@ctf.org
www.ctf.org/patientinfo/

2005-2nd Ed 264 pages Hardbound
Stuart Match Suna, Chairperson
John Risner, President
John McCarthy, Treasurer

5050 Who Says It Has to Be Fair
Theda Schott, author

PublishAmerica
213 S. Wheaton Ave.
Wheaton, IL 60187
630-510-1115
800-942-6825
Fax: 630-510-8508
admin@nfnetwork.org
www.nfnetwork.org; www.publishamerica.com

A mother's story about raising a child with neurofibromatosis.
2006 184 pages Paperback
ISBN: 1-424118-09-3

Cheri Stewart, President
Rosemary Anderson, Vice President
Nicole Hicks, Secretary

Newsletters

5051 Neurofibromatosis Ink
Neurofibromatosis, Inc
213 S. Wheaton Ave.
Wheaton, IL 60187
630-510-1115
800-942-6825
Fax: 630-510-8508
admin@nfnetwork.org
www.nfinc.org

Cheri Stewart, President
Nicole Hicks, Secretary
Mike Montgomery, Treasurer

5052 Neurofibromatosis News
Children's Tumor Foundation
120 Wall Street, 16th Floor
New York, NY 10005
212-344-6633
800-323-7938
Fax: 212-747-0004
info@cft.org
www.ctf.org

Offers information on the newest advances in neurofibromatosis, related events and foundation activities.

Quarterly

Linda Halliday~Martin, Chairperson
Annette Bakker, PhD, President
Colin Bryar, Vice Chairperson

Pamphlets

5053 About Neurofibromatosis 1
Children's Tumor Foundation
120 Wall Street, 16th Floor
New York, NY 10005
212-344-6633
800-323-7938
Fax: 212-747-0004
info@ctf.org
www.ctf.org/patientinfo/

A pamphlet providing an introductory overview of NF1 for patients, families, and healthcare providers with the hope that readers will seek additional information about the disorder according to their own needs.

2007 36 pages

Linda Halliday~Martin, Chairperson
Annette Bakker, PhD, President
Colin Bryar, Vice Chairperson

5054 Achieving in Spite of...A Booklet on Learn ing Disabilities
Children's Tumor Foundation
120 Wall Street, 16th Floor
New York, NY 10005
212-344-6633
800-323-7938
Fax: 212-747-0004
info@ctf.org
www.ctf.org

Designed for use by parents, teachers and health professionals-information on learning disabilities and what to do about them.

34 pages

Linda Halliday~Martin, Chairperson
Annette Bakker, PhD, President
Colin Bryar, Vice Chairperson

5055 Facing Neurofibromatosis: A Guide for Teen s
Children's Tumor Foundation
120 Wall Street, 16th Floor
New York, NY 10005
212-344-6633
800-323-7938
Fax: 212-747-0004
info@ctf.org
www.ctf.org

Offers information for teenagers on how to face neurofibromatosis on a daily basis.

Linda Halliday~Martin, Chairperson
Annette Bakker, PhD, President/ Chief Scientific Officer
Colin Bryar, Vice Chairperson

5056 Neurofibromatosis Type 1: A Guide for Educ ators
Children's Tumor Foundation
120 Wall Street, 16th Floor
New York, NY 10005
212-344-6633
800-323-7938
Fax: 212-747-0004
info@ctf.org
www.ctf.org/patientinfo/

Offers concise and practical information as well as recommendations about the cognitive, physical and behavioral manifestations of the disorder. Free online PDF; English or Spanish.

12 pages

Linda Halliday~Martin, Chairperson
Annette Bakker, PhD, President
Colin Bryar, Vice Chairperson

5057 Neurofibromatosis Type 2: Information for Patients and Families
Children's Tumor Foundation
120 Wall Street, 16th Floor
New York, NY 10005
212-344-6633
800-323-7938
Fax: 212-747-0004
info@ctf.org
www.ctf.org/patientinfo/

Offers extensive information on what NF2 is and answers the most asked about questions regarding the illness. Free online PDF; English or Spanish.

2007 13 pages

Linda Halliday~Martin, Chairperson
Annette Bakker, PhD, President
Colin Bryar, Vice Chairperson

5058 Neurofibromatosis: Questions and Answers
Children's Tumor Foundation
120 Wall Street, 16th Floor
New York, NY 10005
212-344-6633
803-237-938
Fax: 212-747-0004
www.ctf.org

Information about neurofibromatosis.

Linda Halliday~Martin, Chairperson
Annette Bakker, PhD, President
Colin Bryar, Vice Chairperson

5059 The Child with NF1
Children's Tumor Foundation
120 Wall Street, 16th Floor
New York, NY 10005
212-344-6633
800-323-7938
Fax: 212-747-0004
info@ctf.org
www.ctf.org

This brochure is dedicated to the families who live with neurofibromatosis and the friends who provide support and encouragement. It's the purpose of this brochure to attempt to place mild or early NF in perspective. To some extent, NF is an unpredictable condition and uncertainty is inevitable. It is hoped, however, that access to accurate medical information will make this uncertainty easier to live with and to understand. Free online PDF.

2008 9 pages

Linda Halliday~Martin, Chairperson
Annette Bakker, PhD, President
Colin Bryar, Vice Chairperson

Camps

5060 Camp New Friends
Neurofibromatosis, Inc
213 S. Wheaton Ave.
Wheaton, IL 60187
630-510-1115
800-942-6825
Fax: 630-510-8508
admin@nfnetwork.org
www.nfinc.org

A summer camp for those affected with NF1 or NF2, between the ages of 7 and 15. Those aged 18 and over may apply as counselors or counselors-in-training. The camp is held in collaboration with Children's National Medical Center.

Cheri Stewart, President
Nicole Hicks, Secretary
Mike Montgomery, Treasurer

5061 International NF Summer Camp
Children's Tumor Foundation
120 Wall Street, 16th Floor
New York, NY 10005
212-344-6633
800-323-7938
Fax: 212-747-0004
ppanza@ctf.org
www.ctf.org

Campers have the chance to connect with other children who understand what it's like to live with NF. Held at Camp Kotsopoulos, in Emigration Canyon, Utah for the 13th year, there will be swimming, horse-back riding, fishing, canoeing, climbing wall, movie night, a day at the water park, and, of course, campfires. Campers can register for either of the two, one-week sessions. Thanks to donations, scholarships are available, and in some cases, travel assistance.

Linda Halliday~Martin, Chairperson
Annette Bakker, PhD, President
Colin Bryar, Vice Chairperson

DESCRIPTION

5062 NEUROBLASTOMA

Synonym: NB

Involves the following Biologic System(s):

Hematologic and Oncologic Disorders

Neuroblastomas are malignant tumors that account for approximately eight to 10 percent of childhood cancers. They are the most common solid tumors that develop outside the skull in children. About 500 to 600 new cases are reported each year in the United States, with males affected slightly more frequently than females. In approximately 90 percent of affected infants and children, neuroblastoma is diagnosed before age five. Neuroblastoma sometimes occurs in members of certain families (kindreds), although the specific underlying cause is unknown.

Neuroblastomas may originate in any part of the sympathetic nervous system but most commonly develop in the inner region of the adrenal gland (adrenal medulla). In other patients, neuroblastomas may arise in the chest. The sympathetic nervous system controls certain involuntary activities during times of stress, such as raising blood pressure and increasing the heart rate. The adrenal glands, two relatively small organs that curve over the top of each kidney, secrete certain hormones directly into the bloodstream.

A neuroblastoma often invades surrounding tissues and spreads to small, node-like structures located along the course of the lymphatic vessels (lymph nodes). The tumor may then spread to other parts of the body (metastasize), particularly the liver, skeleton, and bone marrow. Rarely, neuroblastomas spread to the lungs or the brain. Associated symptoms and findings are highly variable and depend upon the specific location of the tumor and the extent to which it may have spread. Many infants and children may have a hard, solid, painless lump or mass in the neck or a large mass that may be felt in the abdomen or on the back. Patients often have a general feeling of ill health (malaise) and appear pale (pallor). Those with skeletal involvement typically experience tumor-associated bone pain. In addition, because the bone marrow is a blood-producing tissue, tumor infiltration of the bone marrow may result in abnormally decreased levels of the different blood cells, including circulating red blood cells (anemia), platelets (thrombocytopenia), and certain white blood cells, (neutropenia). Due to low levels of platelets, patients may experience abnormal bleeding and easy bruising. Decreased levels of white blood cells may cause an increased susceptibility to certain infections.

Depending upon the location and potential spread of the tumor, additional symptoms and findings may occur. If a neuroblastoma spreads to the bony cavities surrounding the eyes, associated symptoms may include abnormal protrusion of the eyes (proptosis) and the appearance of bluish-purple patches (ecchymosis) around the eyes. Tumor development near the spinal cord may result in weakness or paralysis of the legs (paresis). In addition, involvement of the liver typically causes abnormal liver enlargement (hepatomegaly). Tumor growth within the adrenal glands may cause excessive secretion of the hormones epinephrine and norepinephrine, resulting in increased irritability, high blood pressure (hypertension), increased heart rate (tachycardia), flushing of the skin, severe diarrhea, and other symptoms.

Some patients may also develop Horner's syndrome, which is characterized by ptosis, absence of sweating (anhidrosis), and narrowing of the pupil of the eye (miosis). Skin abnormalities may also be present, including firm, bluish nodules under the skin or skin lesions on the scalp. Approximately four percent of patients experience a sudden onset of neuromuscular symptoms due to abnormal functioning of the cerebellum (acute cerebellar encephalopathy). The cerebellum is a region of the brain that plays an essential role in maintaining normal postures, sustaining balance, and producing coordinated movements. Neuroblastoma symptoms may include an impaired ability to coordinate voluntary movements (cerebellar ataxia); random, rapid, uncontrolled eye movements (opsoclonus); and shock-like contractions of certain muscles or muscle groups (myoclonic jerks).

In infants and children with neuroblastoma, treatment may depend upon the location of the tumor, whether it has spread, the patient's age, or other factors. If the tumor is contained and has not spread, treatment may consist of surgical removal of the tumor. When the tumor may not be removed surgically or has spread to other parts of the body, treatment measures may include the use of certain drugs (chemotherapy) or radiation therapy. Additional treatments for advanced disease may be considered.

Government Agencies

5063 NIH/National Cancer Institute
BG 9609 / 9609 Medical Center Drive
Bethesda, MD 20892
800-422-6237
www.cancer.gov

The National Cancer Institute coordinates the National Cancer Program, which conducts and supports research, training, health information dissemination, and other programs with respect to the cause, diagnosis, prevention, and treatment of cancer, rehabilitation from cancer, and the continuing care of cancer patients and the families of cancer patients.

Douglas R. Lowy, MD, Acting Director
James Doroshow, MD, Deputy Director
Henry P. Ciolino, PhD, Acting Director, Cancer Centers

National Associations & Support Groups

5064 American Academy of Pediatrics
141 Northwest Point Boulevard
Elk Grove Village, IL 60007
847-434-4000
800-433-9016
Fax: 847-434-8000
www.aap.org

The American Academy of Pediatrics and its member pediatricians are committed to the attainment of optimal physical, mental and social health and well-being for all infants, children, adolescents, and young adults.

Fernando Stein, MD, FAAP, President
Karen Remley, MD, CEO/Executive VP

5065 American Childhood Cancer Organization (fo rmerly Candlelighters Childhood Cancer)
PO Box 498
Kensington, MD 20895
301-962-3520
800-366-2223
Fax: 310-962-3521
staff@acco.org
www.acco.org

The Candlelighters Childhood Cancer Foundation National Office was founded in 1970 by concerned parents of children with cancer. Today our membership of over 50,000 members of the national office and more than 100,000 members across the across the country, including Candlelighters affiliate groups, includes, parents of children who are being treated or have been treated for cancer.

Ruth I. Hoffman, MPH, Executive Director
Jessica DiBenedetto, Program Coordinator
Christy Perry, Director, Marketing/Communications

5066 CancerCare
275 7th Avenue, Floor 22
New York, NY 10001

212-712-8400
800-813-4673
Fax: 212-712-8495
info@cancercare.org
www.cancercare.org

CancerCare is a national nonprofit, 501(c)(3) organization that provides free, professional support services to anyone affected by cancer: people with cancer, caregivers, children, loved ones, and the bereaved. CancerCare programs - including counseling and support groups, education, financial assistance and practical help - are provided by professional oncology social workers and are completely free of charge.

Patricia J Goldsmith, CEO
John Rutigliano, Chief Operating Officer
Ahuva Morris, Children's Program Coordinator

5067 Children's Wish Foundation International
8615 Roswell Road
Atlanta, GA 30350

770-393-9474
800-323-9474
Fax: 770-393-0683
wish@childrenswish.org
www.childrenswish.org

Children's Wish Foundation International is dedicated to bringing joy and hope to seeiously ill children and their families world wide by involving the public in putting children first with opportunities to experience the enhanced value and quality of life through the magic of a fulfilled wish.

Arthur Stein, President
Linda Dozoretz, Founder/Executive Director

5068 Genetic Alliance
4301 Connecticut Avenue NW, Suite 404
Washington, DC 20008

202-966-5557
800-336-4363
Fax: 202-966-8553
info@geneticalliance.org
www.geneticalliance.org

A coalition of voluntary genetic support groups, consumers and professionals addressing the needs of individuals and families affected by genetic disorders from a national perspective.

Sharon Terry, President/CEO
Tetyana Murza, Managing Director
Natasha Bonhomme, VP, Strategic Development

5069 Neuroblastoma Children's Cancer Society
PO Box 957672
Hoffman Estates, IL 60195

847-605-1245
800-532-5162
Fax: 847-605-0705
info@neuroblastomacancer.org
www.neuroblastomacancer.org

The Neuroblastoma Children's Cancer Society is a group made up of volunteers, many of whom have children or relatives who are victims or survivors of this disease. The organization is an advocate for the children who suffer from neuroblastoma and is dedicated to serving as a support center for their families.

Research Centers

5070 Children's Cancer Research Institute
University of Texas Health Science Ctr
8403 Floyd Curl Drive
San Antonio, TX 78229

210-562-9000
Fax: 210-562-9014
chessher@uthscsa.edu
ccri.uthscsa.edu

It is the mission of the institute to advance scientific knowledge relevant to childhood cancer and to accelerate the translation of knowledge into therapies.

Sharon Murphy MD, Director
Bill Chessher, Administrator

Web Sites

5071 CancerCare
275 Seventh Avenue 22nd Floor
New York, NY 10001

212-712-8400
800-813-4673
Fax: 212-712-8495
www.cancercare.org

CancerCare is a national nonprofit, 501(c)(3) organization that provides free, professional support services to anyone affected by cancer: people with cancer, caregivers, children, loved ones, and the bereaved. CancerCare programs - including counseling and support groups, education, financial assistance and practical help - are provided by professional oncology social workers and are completely free of charge.

Patricia J Goldsmith, CEO
John Rutigliano, Chief Operating Officer
Ahuva Morris, Children's Program Coordinator

5072 Children's Cancer Web
www.cancerindex.org/ccw

An independent nonprofit site, established to provide a directory of childhood cancer resources.

5073 Online Mendelian Inheritance in Man
National Library of Medicine Building 38A
Bethesda, MD 20894

888-346-3656
info@ncbi.nlm.nih.gov
www.ncbi.nlm.nih.gov

This database is a catalog of human genes and genetic disorders.

Book Publishers

5074 Let's Talk About Going to the Hospital
Rosen Publishing Group's PowerKids Press
29 E 21st Street
New York, NY 10010

212-777-3017
800-237-9932
Fax: 888-436-4643
rosenpub@tribeca.ios.com
www.rosenpublishing.com

If a child has to check into the hospital, chances are he or she is already upset about being ill. Knowing how a hospital functions and what the procedures are, such as when family members can visit, will help in what is already a stressful situation. Grades K-5.

24 pages
ISBN: 0-823950-36-0

Roger Rosen, President

5075 Let's Talk About When Kids Have Cancer

Melanie Apel Gordon, author

Rosen Publishing Group's PowerKids Press
29 E 21st Street
New York, NY 10010   212-777-3017
                                      800-237-9932
                                 Fax: 888-436-4643
                          customerservice@rosenpub.com
                             www.rosenpublishing.com

In a straightforward yet comforting way, this book explains what
cancer is, what kinds of treatments surround the disease and how
to cope if a child or the friend of a child has cancer.

24 pages Papperback
ISBN: 0-823951-95-2

Roger Rosen, President

5076 Pediatric Cancer Sourcebook

Edward J. Prucha, author

Omnigraphics
PO Box 8002
Aston, PA 19014   800-234-1340
                                 Fax: 800-875-1340
                              info@omnigraphics.com
                              www.omnigraphics.com

Basic consumer health information about leukemias, brain tumors, sarcomas, lymphomas and other cancers in infants, children
and adolescents.

1999 587 pages
ISBN: 0-780802-45-4

Peter Ruffner, Publisher

5077 Resource Survival Handbook

Neuroblastoma Children's Cancer Society
PO Box 957672
Hoffman Estates, IL 60195   847-605-0705
                                      800-532-5162
                                 Fax: 847-605-0705
                             www.neuroblastomacancer.org

An accumulation of resource information of facts about
neuroblastoma and related treatments, national and local resources for families and patients, health claim forms, pamphlets,
and other relevant forms.

Online

Jim Sexton, Chairman

5078 Surviving Childhood Cancer: A Guide for Families

New Harbinger Publications
5674 Shattuck Avenue
Oakland, CA 94609   510-652-0215
                                      800-748-6273
                                 Fax: 800-652-1613
                          customerservice@newharbinger.com
                              www.newharbinger.com

Cancer in a child is an overwhelming experience for a family.
This book explains common medical procedures and offers readers practical advice about how to cope with emotions and stress
during this time.

215 pages Paperback
ISBN: 1-572241-02-0

Journals

**5079 American Childhood Cancer Organization (fo rmerly
Candlelighters Childhood Cancer)**

PO Box 498
Kensington, MD 20895   301-962-3520
                                      855-858-2226
                                 Fax: 310-962-3521
                                      staff@acco.org
                                      www.acco.org

Provides the latest information on CCCF programs and childhood
cancer.

Quarterly

Ruth I. Hoffman, MPH, Executive Director
Jessica DiBenedetto, Program Coordinator
Christy Perry, Director, Marketing/Communications

DESCRIPTION

5080 NEUTROPENIA

Covers these related disorders: Chronic neutropenia, Transient neutropenia

Involves the following Biologic System(s):

Hematologic and Oncologic Disorders

Neutropenia is a blood condition characterized by decreased numbers of circulating white blood cells known as neutrophils. These white blood cells play an essential role in fighting bacterial infections by detecting, engulfing, and digesting invading bacteria (phagocytosis). Neutrophils mature in the bone marrow and are then released into the bloodstream, where they may circulate for approximately six to eight hours. When responding to invading microorganisms or inflammation, neutrophils may leave the blood circulation, move into affected tissues, and digest microbes or other invaders as required.

Neutropenia is specifically defined as the presence of fewer than 1,500 neutrophils per microliter of blood. The condition may result from deficient production of neutrophils by the bone marrow or abnormally increased loss of neutrophils from the blood circulation. Depending upon the nature of the condition, its underlying cause, and other factors, neutropenia may occur for only days or weeks (transient neutropenia) or be present for months or a patient's lifetime (chronic neutropenia). In addition, the findings potentially associated with neutropenia are extremely variable and may include no apparent symptoms (asymptomatic), mild infections of the mucous membranes and the skin, or, in severe cases, potentially life-threatening complications.

In children, transient neutropenia may be caused by certain viral or bacterial infections; a deficiency of folic acid or vitamin B12; or the administration of certain medications, such as a class of antipsychotic drugs (phenothiazines), penicillin preparations, nonsteroidal anti-inflammatory agents, or anticancer drugs that may suppress bone marrow production. Chronic neutropenia also has several different causes and occurs in many different forms. Benign chronic neutropenia is a condition of childhood in which patients have chronically low levels of circulating neutrophils in the blood. This may result in increased susceptibility to recurrent infections of the skin, the mouth, or other areas. The condition typically resolves on its own by age four. Patients with immune deficiency disorders that are present at birth (primary inherited immunodeficiencies) or acquired (such as acquired immune deficiency syndrome, AIDS) often develop chronic neutropenia during infancy or early childhood. These children often fail to grow and gain weight at the expected rate (failure to thrive) and may experience recurrent bacterial infections, enlargement of the liver and spleen (hepatosplenomegaly), and potentially life-threatening complications.

Other uncommon forms of childhood neutropenia include cyclic neutropenia and Kostmann's disease. In patients with cyclic neutropenia, neutropenia recurs in regular cycles (e.g., every 18 to 21 days). When circulating neutrophils are abnormally decreased, these patients may experience fever, a general feeling of ill health (malaise), and susceptibility to mouth ulcers and infections of the skin, mucous membranes, and tissues that surround and support the teeth. Cyclic neutropenia typically becomes apparent during childhood and often runs in certain families. Kostmann's disease, also known as genetic infantile agranulocytosis, is a rare, autosomal recessive disorder characterized by persistent, extremely low levels of circulating neutrophils (fewer than 200 per microliter), frequent bacterial infections, and potentially life-threatening complications by approximately age three.

Neutropenia may also occur as a component of certain genetic, multisystemic diseases, such as Shwachman syndrome and metaphyseal chondrodysplasia, or in association with certain cancers, including leukemia and lymphoma.

The treatment of children with neutropenia depends upon the condition's severity and its underlying cause. In those with mild neutropenia, treatment may not be required. If a particular medication is responsible for the condition, such drug therapy is discontinued if possible. In patients with chronic neutropenia, physicians may recommend steps to help prevent bacterial infection and institute immediate antibiotic therapy should infections occur. In severe cases of bacterial infection, hospitalization may be required. In addition, in some patients with severe neutropenia, therapies may be administered to help stimulate the bone marrow's production of neutrophils (granulocyte colony-stimulating factor [G-CSF]). In some cases, bone marrow transplantation is an option, a procedure in which healthy bone marrow is given to replace defective bone marrow.

Government Agencies

5081 NIH/ Eunice Kennedy Shriver National Insti tute of Child Health & Human Development
31 Center Drive, Building 31
Bethesda, MD 20892   301-496-5113
                                      800-370-2943
                                      Fax: 866-760-5947
                                      TTY: 888-320-6942
                                      nichdpress@mail.nih.gov
                                      www.nichd.nih.gov

Established in 1962 by congress, today the institute conducts and supports research on topics related to the health of children, adults, families and populations. Some of these topics include: developmental disabilities, growth and development, infant death, reproductive health and birth defects.

Diana W. Bianchi, Director
Paul Williams, Director, Communications

5082 NIH/National Heart, Lung and Blood Institu te
National Institute of Health
PO Box 30105
Bethesda, MD 20824   301-592-8573
                                      Fax: 301-592-8563
                                      TTY: 240-629-3255
                                      NHLBIinfo@nhlbi.nih.gov
                                      www.nhlbi.nih.gov

Primary responsibility of this organization is the scientific investigation of heart, blood vessel, lung and blood disorders. Oversees research, demonstration, prevention, education, control and training activities in these fields and emphasizes the prevention and control of heart diseases.

Gary H. Gibbons, Director
Nakela Cook, Chief of Staff

National Associations & Support Groups

5083 American Academy of Pediatrics
141 Northwest Point Boulevard
Elk Grove Village, IL 60007 — 847-434-4000
800-433-9016
Fax: 847-434-8000
www.aap.org

The American Academy of Pediatrics and its member pediatricians are committed to the attainment of optimal physical, mental and social health and well-being for all infants, children, adolescents, and young adults.

Fernando Stein, MD, FAAP, President
Karen Remley, MD, CEO/Executive VP

5084 American Autoimmune Related Diseases Association
22100 Gratiot Avenue
Eastpointe, MI 48021 — 586-776-3900
800-598-4668
Fax: 586-776-3903
aarda@aarda.org
www.aarda.org

Dedicated to the eradiction of autoimmune diseases and the alleviation of suffering and the socio-economic impact of autoimmunity through fostering and facilitating collaboration in the areas of education, public awareness, research and patient services in an effective, ethical and efficient manner.

Virginia T. Ladd, President/Executive Director
Patricia Barber, Assistant Director
Deb Patrick, Events Specialist

5085 Genetic Alliance
4301 Connecticut Avenue NW, Suite 404
Washington, DC 20008 — 202-966-5557
800-336-4363
Fax: 202-966-8553
info@geneticalliance.org
www.geneticalliance.org

A coalition of voluntary genetic support groups, consumers and professionals addressing the needs of individuals and families affected by genetic disorders from a national perspective.

Sharon Terry, President/CEO
Tetyana Murza, Managing Director
Natasha Bonhomme, VP, Strategic Development

5086 March of Dimes Foundation
1275 Mamaroneck Avenue
White Plains, NY 10605 — 914-997-4488
888-663-4637
Fax: 914-428-8203
answers@marchofdimes.com
www.marchofdimes.com

Partnership of volunteers and professionals dedicates to improving the health of babies by preventing birth defects and infant mortality. Over 100 chapters are located across the country and can be located through the National Office.

Stacey D. Stewart, President

5087 Severe Chronic Neutropenia International Registry (SCNIR)
1107 NE 45th Street, Suite 345
Seattle, WA 98105 — 206-543-9749
800-726-4463
Fax: 206-543-3668
bolyard@u.washington.edu
www.depts.washington.edu/registry

The SCNIR was established in the United States, Australia, Canada, and the European Community. The SCNIR is directed by a scientific advisory board of physicians from around the world who care for SCN patients. Our mission is to established a world-wide database of treatment and disease-related outcomes for persons diagnosed with SCN. Collection of this information will lead to improved medical care and is used for research to determine the causes of neutropenia.

Audrey Anna Bolyard, Clinical Manager

Web Sites

5088 American Autoimmune Related Diseases Association
22100 Gratiot Ave.
Eastpointe, MI 48021 — 586-776-3900
Fax: 586-776-3903
www.aarda.org

Dedicated to the eradiction of autoimmune diseases and the alleviation of suffering and the socio-economic impact of autoimmunity through fostering and facilitating collaboration in the areas of education, public awareness, research and patient services in an effective, ethical and efficient manner.

5089 National Neutropenia Network
www.neutropenianet.org

Supports general and clinical research and provides information to the families, the medical community and the general public. Also committed to helping affected families and individuals work with hospitals, physicians, nurses, and other health care professionals.

5090 Online Mendelian Inheritance in Man
National Library of Medicine Building 38A
Bethesda, MD 20894 — 888-346-3656
info@ncbi.nlm.nih.gov
www.ncbi.nlm.nih.gov

This database is a catalog of human genes and genetic disorders.

Book Publishers

5091 Let's Talk About Going to the Hospital
Rosen Publishing Group's PowerKids Press
29 E 21st Street
New York, NY 10010 — 212-777-3017
800-237-9932
Fax: 888-436-4643
rosenpub@tribeca.ios.com
www.rosenpublishing.com

If a child has to check into the hospital, chances are he or she is already upset about being ill. Knowing how a hospital functions and what the procedures are, such as when family members can visit, will help in what is already a stressful situation. Grades K-5.

24 pages
ISBN: 0-823950-36-0

Roger Rosen, President

DESCRIPTION

5092 NIGHTMARES

Involves the following Biologic System(s):
Developmental/Behavioral/Psychiatric Disorders

Nightmares are a type of sleep disturbance that occurs during the rapid eye movement (REM) phase of sleep, or deep sleep stage. Vivid, disturbing dreams often evoke feelings of extreme and inescapable fear, terror, anxiety, and distress. Nightmares are often so intense that they awaken the sleeping individual, who is then usually able to recall all or most details of the dream.

Nightmares are quite common in children, particularly in the eight to 10 year old age group. Girls are more prone to this type of sleep disturbance than boys. Precipitating factors vary and may include breathing irregularities caused by the common cold or other illnesses; violent movies or television programs, especially in younger children; separation anxiety; and other traumatic experiences or events. In addition, children with certain types of psychological disturbances (e.g., affective, mood, or anxiety disorders) may experience repeated episodes of nightmares.

It is common for most children to experience occasional nightmares and, until the anxiety or fear of the experience passes, understanding and comfort by parents or caregivers is usually helpful. However, children who experience frequent nightmares may require a careful evaluation to determine if these episodes are a manifestation of an underlying psychologic disorder or other irregularity. If this is the case, treatment may be directed toward the underlying condition. Other treatment is supportive. For example, parents and caregivers are encouraged to be reassuring, understanding, and firm but nonthreatening. Reading or other quiet or soothing activities or rituals before bedtime may also be beneficial. In addition, night lights or other reasonable accommodations may be provided to reassure or comfort affected children.

Government Agencies

5093 Center for Mental Health Services Knowledge Exchange Program

US Department of Health and Human Services
PO Box 42557
Washington, DC 20015

800-789-2647
Fax: 240-221-4295
TDD: 866-889-2647
http://mentalhealth.samhsa.gov

Supplies the public with responses to their commonly asked questions about mental health issues and services.

Kathryn Power, M.Ed., Director
Edward B. Searle M.B.A., Deputy Director
Jeffrey A. Buck, Ph.D, Associate Director

5094 NIH/National Institute of Mental Health

6001 Executive Boulevard, Room 6200, MSC 9663
Bethesda, MD 20892

301-443-4536
866-615-6464
Fax: 301-443-4279
TTY: 301-443-8431
nimhinfo@nih.govh.gov
www.nimh.nih.gov

Conducts strategic planning for specific research areas as well as for the Institute as a whole.

Joshua Gordon, MD, PhD, Director
Shelli Avenevoli, MD, Deputy Director

National Associations & Support Groups

5095 American Academy of Pediatrics

141 Northwest Point Boulevard
Elk Grove Village, IL 60007

847-434-4000
800-433-9016
Fax: 847-434-8000
www.aap.org

The American Academy of Pediatrics and its member pediatricians are committed to the attainment of optimal physical, mental and social health and well-being for all infants, children, adolescents, and young adults.

Fernando Stein, MD, FAAP, President
Karen Remley, MD, CEO/Executive VP

5096 American Academy of Sleep Medicine

2510 North Frontage Road
Darien, IL 60561

630-737-9700
Fax: 630-737-9790
www.aasmnet.org

National not-for-profit professional membership organization dedicated to the advancement of sleep medicine. The Academy's mission is to assure quality care for patients with sleep disorders, promote the advancement of sleep research and provide public and professional education. The AASM delivers programs, information and services to and through its members and advocates sleep medicine supportive policies in the medical community and the public sector.

Timothy I. Morgenthaler, MD, President
Nathaniel F. Watson, MD, President-Elect
Ronald D. Chervin, MD,, Secretary/Treasurer

5097 American Association of Sleep Technologists

2510 North Frontage Road
Darien, IL 60561

630-737-9704
Fax: 630-737-9788
coordinator@aastweb.org
www.aastweb.org

The American Association of Sleep Technologists is the leading advocate for the sleep technologist profession. Our mission is to promote and advance the profession through the continued development of educational, technical and clinical excellence in sleep disorders.

Rita Brooks, President
Laura A. Linley, President-Elect
David Gregory, Secretary

5098 American Board of Sleep Medicine

2510 North Frontage Road
Darien, IL 60561

630-737-9700
Fax: 630-737-9790
absm@absm.org
www.absm.org

The American Board of Sleep Medicine (ABSM) is an independent, nonprofit organization whose certificates are recognized throughout the world as a credential signifying a high level of competence for sleep medicine physicians, PhDs, behavioral sleep medicine specialists and sleep technologists.

Kelly Carden, MD, President
Nathaniel Watson, MD, MS, Past President
Ron Chervin, MD, Secretary-Treasurer

5099 American Mental Health Foundation (AMHF)

P.O. Box 3
Riverdale, NY 10471
USA

212-737-9027
elomke@americanmentalhealthfoundation.or
www.americanmentalhealthfoundation.org

Dedicated to the extensive and intensive research in the theories and techniques of treatment of emotional illness and to the implementation of reforms in the mental health system. Efforts have resulted in development of better and less expensive treatment methods. Findings are disseminated in English and other major languages.

Sister Joan Curtin, Director
John P. Fowler, Treasurer
Eugene Gollogly, VP

5100 American Sleep Association
1002 Lititz Pike #229
Lititz, PA 17543   www.sleepassociation.org

The American Sleep Association (ASA) is an organization dedicated to improving public awareness about sleep disorders and sleep health, promoting sleep medicine research, and providing a portal for communication between patients, physicians, healthcare professionals, corporations, and scientists.

5101 American Sleep Medicine Foundation
2510 North Frontage Road
Darien, IL 60561
                                   630-737-9700
                                   Fax: 630-737-9790
                                   asmfinfo@aasmnet.org
                                   www.discoversleep.org

The American Sleep Medicine Foundation (ASMF) promotes sleep research and education.

Merrill Wise, MD, President
Ronald D. Chervin, MD, MS, Secretary/Treasurer
Jerome A. Barrett, Executive Director

5102 Christian Horizons
PO Box 6646
Saginaw, MI 48608
                                   616-956-7063
                                   Fax: 616-956-7064
                                   info@christianhorizonsinc.org
                                   www.christianhorizonsinc.org

To share Christ's love as we equip and support Adults with developmental disabilities.

5103 Federation of Families for Children's Mental Health
9605 Medical Center Drive, Suite 280
Rockville, MD 20850
                                   240-403-1901
                                   Fax: 240-403-1909
                                   ffcmh@ffcmh.org
                                   www.ffcmh.org

The National family run organization is dedicated exclusively to helping children with mental health needs and their families achieve a better quality of life.

Teka Dempson, President
Sherri Luthe, Vice President
Josh Ross, Secretary

5104 Mental Health America
500 Montgomery Street, Ste 820
Alexandria, VA 22314
                                   703-684-7722
                                   800-969-6642
                                   Fax: 703-684-5968
                                   TTY: 800-433-5959
                                   www.mentalhealthamerica.net

Addresses all aspects of mental health and mental illness. NMHA with over 340 affiliates works to improve the mental health of all Americans.

Paul Gionfriddo, President/CEO
Shavonne Carpenter, Sr Assoc., Support & Services
Mallory Pernell, Assoc. Dir, Comments/Marketing

5105 NADD: National Association for the Dually Diagnosed
132 Fair Street
Kingston, NY 12401
                                   845-331-4336
                                   800-331-5362
                                   Fax: 845-331-4569
                                   info@thenadd.org
                                   www.thenadd.org

Nonprofit organization designed to promote the interests of professional and parent development with resources for individuals who have the coexistence of mental illness and mental retardation. Provides conferences, educational services and training materials to professionals, parents, concerned citizens and service organizations.

Dr Robert Fletcher, CEO
Michelle Jordan, Office Manager
Edward Seliger, Project Coordinator

5106 National Alliance for the Mentally Ill
3803 N Fairfax Drive, Suite 100
Arlington, VA 22203
                                   703-524-7600
                                   888-999-6264
                                   Fax: 703-524-9094
                                   TDD: 703-516-7227
                                   info@nami.org
                                   www.nami.org

NAMI is a nonprofit, grassroots, self-help, support and advocacy organization of consumers, families and friends of people with severe mental illness, such as schizophrenia, bipolar disorder, major depressive disorder, obsessive compulsive disorder, anxiety disorders, autism and other severe and persistent mental illnesses that affect the brain.

Keris J,,n Myrick, President
Kevin B. Sullivan, First Vice President
Jim Payne, Second VP

5107 National Mental Health Consumers' Self-Help Clearinghouse
1211 Chestnut Street, Suite 1207
Philadelphia, PA 19107
                                   267-507-3810
                                   800-553-4539
                                   Fax: 215-636-6312
                                   info@mhselfhelp.org
                                   www.mhselfhelp.org

Offers information, support and appropriate referrals; and promotes public and professional education. Provides networking for those with special interests related to albinism. Promotes and supports research and funding that will improve diagnosis and management of albinism and hypopigmentation.

Joseph Rogers, Executive Director & Founder
Susan Rogers, Director
Christa Burkett, Technical Assistance Coordinator

5108 National Sleep Foundation
1010 N Glebe Road
Arlington, VA 22201
                                   703-243-1697
                                   Fax: 202-347-3472
                                   nsf@sleepfoundation.org
                                   www.sleepfoundation.org

An independent, nonprofit organization dedicated to improving public health and safety by achieving public understanding of sleep and sleep disorders, and by supporting public education, sleep-related research, and advocacy. Actively collaborates with sleep centers, support groups for patients with sleep disorders and safety organizations.

David Cloud, CEO

5109 Sleep Research Society
2510 North Frontage Road
Darien, IL 60561
                                   630-737-9702
                                   Fax: 630-737-9790
                                   coordinator@srsnet.org
                                   www.sleepresearchsociety.org

The Sleep Research Society (SRS) is organization for scientific investigators who educate and research sleep and sleep disorders. The SRS serves its members and the field of sleep research through training and education, and by providing forums for the collaboration and the exchange of ideas.

Allan I. Pack, PhD, MBChB, President
Sean P.A. Drummond, PhD, President-Elect
Jerome A. Barrett, Executive Director

5110 Society of Behavioral Sleep Medicine
2510 North Frontage Road
Darien, IL 60561
                                   630-737-9706
                                   Fax: 630-737-9790
                                   membership@behavioralsleep.org
                                   www.behavioralsleep.org

Behavioral Sleep Medicine is the field of clinical practice and scientific inquiry that encompasses: the study of behavioral, psychological, and physiological factors underlying normal and disordered sleep across the life span; and, the development and application of evidence-based behavioral and psychological approaches to the prevention and treatment of sleep disorders and co-existing conditions.

Ryan G. Wetzler, PsyD, CBSM, President
Michael Scherer, PhD, CBSM, President-Elect
Valerie M. Crabtree, PhD, CBSM, Secretary/Treasurer

State Agencies & Support Groups

5111 Center for Family Support
333 7th Avenue, #901
New York, NY 10001   212-629-7939
                                              Fax: 212-239-2211
                                                 www.cfsny.org

The Center for Family (CFS) is a not-for-profit human service
agency providing support and assistance to individuals with developmental disabilities and traumatic brain injuries throughout
New York City, Long Island, the lower Hudson Valley region and
New Jersey.

Steven Vernikoff, Executive Director
Linda Schellenberg, Director, Community Service
Barbara Greenwald, Associate Executive Director

Libraries & Resource Centers

5112 American Academy of Somnology
PO Box 27077
Las Vegas, NV 89126   702-371-0947
                                           somnology@aol.com
                            www.hopperinstitute.com/aas_intro.html

Covers about 75 physicians, dentists, nurses, psychologists, technicians, and students and sponsoring organizations, including associations, institutions, and corporations, with a special interest
in sleep.

David Hopper, Director

Web Sites

5113 CyberPsych
www.cyberpsych.org

CyberPsych presents information about psychoanalysis, psychotherapy, and special topics such as anxiety disorder, the problematic use of alcohol, homophobia, and the traumatic effects of
racism. CyberPsych is a nonprofit network which offers free web
hosting and technical support for internet communication, to non
profit groups and individuals.

5114 NADD: National Association for the Dually Diagnosed
132 Fair Street
Kingston, NY 12401   845-331-4336
                                               800-331-5362
                                             Fax: 845-331-4569
                                                www.thenadd.org

Nonprofit organization designed to promote the interests of professional and care providers for individuals who have the coexistence of mental illness and mental retardation. NADD provides
conferences, educational services and training materials to professionals, parents, concerned citizens and service organizations.

Dr Robert Fletcher, CEO
Michelle Jordan, Office Manager
Edward Seliger, Project Coordinator

5115 Planetpsych
www.planetpsych.com

Planetpsych is an online resource for mental health information.

5116 Psych Central
55 Pleasant St., Suite 207
Newburyport, MA 1950   www.psychcentral.com

Offers free informational and educational articles and resources
on psychology, support and mental health online.

John M. Grohol, CEO
Rick Nauert, Ph.D., Senior News Editor
Bailey Apple, Associate Editor

5117 Sleep Disorders
http://talhost.net/sleep/parasomnia.htm

For those who have sleep disorders and have a problem sleeping.

5118 Sleepdisorders.com
www.sleepdisorders.com

Updated monthly and organized by sleep disorders with quality
links.

Book Publishers

**5119 Concise Guide to Evaluation and Management of Sleep
Disorders**
American Psychiatric Publishing
1000 Wilson Boulevard, Suite 1825
Arlington, VA 22209   703-907-7322
                                               800-368-5777
                                             Fax: 703-907-1091
                                                appi@psych.org
                                                  www.appi.org

Overview of sleep disorders medicine, sleep physiology and pathology, insomnia complaints, excessive sleepiness disorders,
parasomnias, medical and psychiatric disorders and sleep, medications with sedative-hypnotic properties, special problems and
populations.

2002 296 pages Paper 3rd Ed
ISBN: 1-585620-45-6

Robert E. Hales, M.D., Editor-in-Chief
Rebecca D. Rinehart, Publisher
John McDuffie, Editorial Director

5120 Sleep Disorders and Psychiatry
Daniel J Buysse MD, author

American Psychiatric Publishing
1000 Wilson Boulevard, Ste 1825
Arlington, VA 22209   703-907-7322
                                               800-368-5777
                                             Fax: 703-907-1091
                                                appi@psych.org
                                                  www.appi.org

Summarizes the major categories of sleep disorders including
parasomnias and narcolepsy.

2005 256 pages Paperback
ISBN: 1-585622-29-0

Robert E. Hales, M.D., Editor-in-Chief
Rebecca D. Rinehart, Publisher
John McDuffie, Editorial Director

5121 Snoring From A to Zzzz
Spencer Press
2525 NW Lovejoy Street, Suite 402
Portland, OR 97210   503-223-4959
                                             Fax: 503-223-1608
                                            dereklipman@aol.com

Covers organizations, associations, support groups, and manufacturers of sleep-related medical products relevant to sleep disorders. Discusses every aspect of snoring abd sleep apnea from
causes to cures.

256 pages Paperback
ISBN: 0-965070-81-6

Derek Lipman MD, Author/Editor

DESCRIPTION

5122 NIGHT TERRORS

Synonyms: Pavor nocturnus, Sleep-terror disorder

Involves the following Biologic System(s):

Developmental/Behavioral/Psychiatric Disorders

Night terrors is a sleep disorder characterized by episodes of sudden awakening from sleep in an extremely anxious or terrified state. This sleep disturbance occurs in from two to five children out of every hundred, and, in most cases, begins during the fourth to seventh year of life. Sleep-terror disorder more commonly affects boys than girls and often disappears before the onset of adolescence.

Episodes of night terrors usually take place during the third or fourth stage of the nonrapid eye movement or NREM phase of sleep. Each stage of NREM sleep is a successively deeper sleep leading up to rapid eye movement sleep or a deep REM during which dreams may occur. Typically, affected children awaken abruptly and may be screaming and extremely frightened. They may be in a semiconscious state and unaware of or unable to recognize people or surroundings. These children are generally inconsolable and may exhibit such physical symptoms as sweating; widening (dilation) of the pupils; elevated heart rate (tachycardia); abnormally deep, rapid breathing (hyperventilation); and violent thrashing. In about a third of patients, sleepwalking (somnambulism) may also occur. Children are usually able to fall back to sleep within minutes of these short-lived episodes and have no memory of the event when they awaken.

Night terrors are most often confused with nightmares, but unlike night terrors, a child having a nightmare is usually easily woken up and comforted. Sleep disorders such as night terrors often result from childhood fears or anxieties. For example, some young children may be apprehensive about going to bed because this actually represents a temporary separation from their parents (separation anxiety). In addition, any issues affecting the family or child (e.g., separation, divorce, death, school performance, social interactions, etc.) may translate into disturbances in normal sleep patterns. Other contributing factors may include the presence of a fever, depression, or other emotional disorders.

Although the administration of certain antianxiety and antidepressant drugs may, in some cases, be of benefit, treatment of night terrors is mainly supportive. If the precipitating cause can be determined, steps may then be taken to alleviate the fear or anxiety. In any case, parents or caregivers are encouraged to be supportive and firm, but nonjudgmental. Excitement before bedtime is discouraged; however, reading or other quiet, pleasurable activities may be beneficial.

Government Agencies

5123 Center for Mental Health Services Knowledge Exchange Program
US Department of Health and Human Services
4301 Connecticut Avenue, NW, Suite 100
Washington, DC 20008
877-871-0744
Fax: 240-747-5470
TTY: 877-871-0665
TDD: 866-889-2647
www.ncwd-youth.info/node/245

Supplies the public with responses to their commonly asked questions about mental health issues and services.

5124 NIH/National Institute of Mental Health
6001 Executive Boulevard, Room 6200, MSC 9663
Bethesda, MD 20892
301-443-4536
866-615-6464
Fax: 301-443-4279
TTY: 301-443-8431
nimhinfo@nih.govh.gov
www.nimh.nih.gov

Conducts strategic planning for specific research areas as well as for the Institute as a whole.

Joshua Gordon, MD, PhD, Director
Shelli Avenevoli, MD, Deputy Director

National Associations & Support Groups

5125 American Academy of Pediatrics
141 Northwest Point Boulevard
Elk Grove Village, IL 60007
847-434-4000
800-433-9016
Fax: 847-434-8000
www.aap.org

The American Academy of Pediatrics and its member pediatricians are committed to the attainment of optimal physical, mental and social health and well-being for all infants, children, adolescents, and young adults.

Fernando Stein, MD, FAAP, President
Karen Remley, MD, CEO/Executive VP

5126 American Academy of Sleep Medicine
2510 North Frontage Road
Darien, IL 60561
630-737-9700
Fax: 630-737-9790
www.aasmnet.org

National not-for-profit professional membership organization dedicated to the advancement of sleep medicine. The Academy's mission is to assure quality care for patients with sleep disorders, promote the advancement of sleep research and provide public and professional education. The AASM delivers programs, information and services to and through its members and advocates sleep medicine supportive policies in the medical community and the public sector.

Sam Fleishman, President
M. Safran Badr, President-Elect
Timothy I. Morgenthaler, Secretary

5127 American Mental Health Foundation (AMHF)
P.O. Box 3
Riverdale, NY 10471
USA
212-737-9027
elomke@americanmentalhealthfoundation.or
www.americanmentalhealthfoundation.org

Dedicated to the extensive and intensive research in the theories and techniques of treatment of emotional illness and to the implementation of reforms in the mental health system. Efforts have resulted in development of better and less expensive treatment methods. Findings are disseminated in English and other major languages.

Sister Joan Curtin, Director
John P. Fowler, Treasurer
Eugene Gollogly, VP

5128 Center for Disabilities and Development
University of Iowa Stead Family Children's Hospita
100 Hawkins Drive
Iowa City, IA 52242
319-353-6900
877-686-0031
Fax: 319-356-7700
cdd-webmaster@uiowa.edu
www.medicine.uiowa.edu

A trusted resource for healthcare, training, research and information for people with disabilities that include: behavior disorders, brain injury, cerebral palsy, diabetes, down syndrome, learning disabilities, mental retardation, sleep disorders and spina bifida.

Dianne McBrien, MD, Medical Director

5129 Christian Horizons
PO Box 6646
Saginaw, MI 48608

616-956-7063
Fax: 616-956-7064
info@christianhorizonsinc.org
www.christianhorizonsinc.org

To share Christ's love as we equip and support Adults with developmental disabilities.

5130 Federation of Families for Children's Mental Health
9605 Medical Center Drive, Suite 280
Rockville, MD 20850

240-403-1901
Fax: 240-403-1909
ffcmh@ffcmh.org
www.ffcmh.org

The National family run organization is dedicated exclusively to helping children with mental health needs and their families achieve a better quality of life.

Teka Dempson, President
Sherri Luthe, Vice President
Josh Ross, Secretary

5131 NADD: National Association for the Dually Diagnosed
132 Fair Street
Kingston, NY 12401

845-331-4336
800-331-5362
Fax: 845-331-4569
info@thenadd.org
www.thenadd.org

Nonprofit organization designed to promote the interests of professional and parent development with resources for individuals who have the coexistence of mental illness and mental retardation. Provides conferences, educational services and training materials to professionals, parents, concerned citizens and service organizations.

Dr Robert Fletcher, CEO
Michelle Jordan, Office Manager
Edward Seliger, Project Coordinator

5132 National Mental Health Consumers' Self-Help Clearinghouse
1211 Chestnut Street, Suite 1207
Philadelphia, PA 19107

267-507-3810
800-553-4539
Fax: 215-636-6312
info@mhselfhelp.org
www.mhselfhelp.org

Offers information, support and appropriate referrals; and promotes public and professional education. Provides networking for those with special interests related to albinism. Promotes and supports research and funding that will improve diagnosis and management of albinism and hypopigmentation.

Joseph Rogers, Executive Director & Founder
Susan Rogers, Director
Christa Burkett, Technical Assistance Coordinator

5133 National Sleep Foundation
1010 N Glebe Road
Arlington, VA 22201

703-243-1697
Fax: 202-347-3472
nsf@sleepfoundation.org
www.sleepfoundation.org

An independent, nonprofit organization dedicated to improving public health and safety by achieving public understanding of sleep and sleep disorders, and by supporting public education, sleep-related research, and advocacy. Actively collaborates with sleep centers, support groups for patients with sleep disorders and safety organizations.

David Cloud, CEO

State Agencies & Support Groups

5134 Center for Family Support
333 7th Avenue, #901
New York, NY 10001

212-629-7939
Fax: 212-239-2211
www.cfsny.org

The Center for Family (CFS) is a not-for-profit human service agency providing support and assistance to individuals with developmental disabilities and traumatic brain injuries throughout New York City, Long Island, the lower Hudson Valley region and New Jersey.

Steven Vernikoff, Executive Director
Linda Schellenberg, Director, Community Service
Barbara Greenwald, Associate Executive Director

Libraries & Resource Centers

5135 American Academy of Somnology
PO Box 27077
Las Vegas, NV 89126

702-371-0947
somnology@aol.com
www.hopperinstitute.com/aas_intro.html

Covers about 75 physicians, dentists, nurses, psychologists, technicians, and students and sponsoring organizations, including associations, institutions, and corporations, with a special interest in sleep.

David Hopper, Director

Research Centers

5136 UC Berkeley School of Social Welfare
Mental Health & Social Welfare Research Group
120 Haviland Hall #7400
Berkeley, CA 94720

510-642-4341
Fax: 510-643-6126
spsegal@berkeley.edu
www.socialwelfare.berkeley.edu

Steven P Segal, Director

Web Sites

5137 About.com on Sleep Disorders
www.sleepdisorders.about.com

Well-organized information including new developments and a chat room.

5138 CyberPsych
www.cyberpsych.org

Presents information about psychoanalysis, psychtherapy and special topics such as anxiety disorder, the problamatic use of alcohol, homophobia, and the traumatic effects of racism.

5139 NADD: National Association for the Dually Diagnosed
132 Fair Street
Kingston, NY 12401

845-331-4336
800-331-5362
Fax: 845-331-4569
www.thenadd.org

Nonprofit organization designed to promote the interests of professional and care providers for individuals who have the coexistence of mental illness and mental retardation. NADD provides conferences, educational services and training materials to professionals, parents, concerned citizens and service organizations.

Dr Robert Fletcher, CEO
Michelle Jordan, Office Manager
Edward Seliger, Project Coordinator

5140 Planetpsych
www.planetpsych.com

Online resource for mental health information.

5141 Psych Central
55 Pleasant St., Suite 207
Newburyport, MA 1950

www.psychcentral.com

Offers free informational and educational articles and resources on psychology, support and mental health online.

John M. Grohol, CEO
Rick Nauert, Ph.D., Senior News Editor
Bailey Apple, Associate Editor

5142 Sleep Disorders
http://talhost.net/sleep/parasomnia.htm

For those who have sleep disorders and have a problem sleeping.

5143 Sleepdisorders.com
www.sleepdisorders.com

Updated monthly and organized by sleep disorders with quality links.

Book Publishers

5144 Concise Guide to Evaluation and Management of Sleep Disorders
American Psychiatric Publishing
1000 Wilson Boulevard, Suite 1825
Arlington, VA 22209

703-907-7322
800-368-5777
Fax: 703-907-1091
appi@psych.org
www.appi.org

Overview of sleep disorders medicine, sleep physiology and pathology, insomnia complaints, excessive sleepiness disorders, parasomnias, medical and psychiatric disorders and sleep, medications with sedative-hypnotic properties, special problems and populations.

2002 296 pages Paper 3rd Ed
ISBN: 1-585620-45-6

Robert E. Hales, M.D., Editor-in-Chief
Rebecca D. Rinehart, Publisher
John McDuffie, Editorial Director

5145 Principles and Practice of Sleep Medicine
Elsevier Health Sciences Division
1600 John F Kennedy Blvd, Suite 1800
Philadelphia, PA 19103

215-239-3900
800-523-1649
Fax: 215-239-3990
www.us.elsevierhealth.com

Covers the recent advances in basic sciences as well as sleep pathology in adults. Encompasses developments in this rapidly advancing field and also includes topics related to psychiatry, circadian rhythms, cardiovascualr diseases and sleep apnea diagnosis and treatment. Hardcover.

2005 1552 pages 4th Edition
ISBN: 0-721607-97-7

5146 Sleep Disorders and Psychiatry
Daniel J Buysse MD, author

American Psychiatric Publishing
1000 Wilson Boulevard, Ste 1825
Arlington, VA 22209

703-907-7322
800-368-5777
Fax: 703-907-1091
appi@psych.org
www.appi.org

Summarizes the major categories of sleep disorders including parasomnias and narcolepsy.

2005 256 pages Paperback
ISBN: 1-585622-29-0

Robert E. Hales, M.D., Editor-in-Chief
Rebecca D. Rinehart, Publisher
John McDuffie, Editorial Director

5147 Snoring From A to Zzzz
Spencer Press
2525 NW Lovejoy Street, Suite 402
Portland, OR 97210

503-223-4959
Fax: 503-223-1608
dereklipman@aol.com

Covers organizations, associations, support groups, and manufacturers of sleep-related medical products relevant to sleep disorders. Discussess every aspect of snoring abd sleep apnea from causes to cures.

256 pages Paperback
ISBN: 0-965070-81-6

Derek S Lipman, MD, Author/Editor

DESCRIPTION

5148 NOCTURNAL ENURESIS

Synonym: Bed-wetting

Involves the following Biologic System(s):

Developmental/Behavioral/Psychiatric Disorders, Renal and Urologic Disorders

Nocturnal enuresis or bed-wetting refers to the discharge of urine during the night by children who have achieved urinary control during other periods of the day. It affects an estimated 5 to 7 million children in the United States. This type of bed-wetting is considered primary enuresis if nightly urinary incontinence has persisted since birth. Nocturnal enuresis that occurs in children who were previously continent during the night for a period of one year or more is considered second-ary enuresis, a regressive form of this abnormality. Bed-wet-ting is a very common problem that occurs more often in boys than in girls and tends to run in families. In most cases, enuresis resolves spontaneously. The causes of nocturnal enuresis are varied and may include delayed maturation of certain functions of the nervous system that regulate bladder control, psychological influences, spinal abnormalities (e.g., spina bifida), structural abnormalities or defects, underlying disease (e.g., diabetes mellitus), urinary tract infection, or other physical causes. Secondary enuresis may be precipitated by stressful or traumatic events such as the birth of another child, death, divorce, or other situations that impact on the normal day-to-day routine.

Children with enuresis may undergo evaluation in order to determine if the condition is caused by neurological or physi-cal problems. If this is the case, treatment is geared toward the underlying problem. Other treatment may include such supportive measures as establishing a reward system to give the child incentive to cooperate, charting the child's progress in order to offer positive reinforcement, limiting liquid intake before bedtime, having the child urinate directly before going to bed, and having affected older children take part in laun-dering soiled clothing and remaking the bed. Parents and caregivers are typically counseled to remain supportive and nonjudgmental. Additional treatment may include behavioral therapy and other counseling that involves both the parents or caregivers and the affected child. Bed-wetting alarms that de-tect small amounts of urine and certain types of medication (e.g., imipramine and desmopressin acetate nasal spray) may also be used to control enuresis. Imipramine is an antidepres-sant drug that is usually effective within two weeks; however, relapses are common after the drug is gradually stopped and, therefore, a longer course of administration may become necessary. Desmopressin acetate nasal spray reduces urine output in approximately 70 percent of affected children; however, its beneficial effect is temporary. Other treatment is supportive.

Government Agencies

5149 NIH/National Institute of Mental Health
6001 Executive Boulevard, Room 6200, MSC 9663
Bethesda, MD 20892

301-443-4536
866-615-6464
Fax: 301-443-4279
TTY: 301-443-8431
nimhinfo@nih.gov
www.nimh.nih.gov

Conducts strategic planning for specific research areas as well as for the Institute as a whole.

Joshua Gordon, MD, PhD, Director
Shelli Avenevoli, MD, Deputy Director

5150 National Kidney and Urologic Diseases Information Clearinghouse
Bldg 31, Rm 9A06, 31 Center Drive, MSC 2560
Bethesda, MD 20892

301-496-3583
800-891-5390
Fax: 703-738-4929
nkudic@info.niddk.nih.gov
www2.niddk.nih.gov

To increase knowledge and understanding about diseases of the kidneys and urologic system among people with these conditions and their families, health care professionals and the general public.

Griffin P. Rogers, Director

National Associations & Support Groups

5151 American Academy of Pediatrics
141 Northwest Point Boulevard
Elk Grove Village, IL 60007

847-434-4000
800-433-9016
Fax: 847-434-8000
www.aap.org

The American Academy of Pediatrics and its member pediatri-cians are committed to the attainment of optimal physical, mental and social health and well-being for all infants, children, adoles-cents, and young adults.

Fernando Stein, MD, FAAP, President
Karen Remley, MD, CEO/Executive VP

5152 American Urological Association Foundation
1000 Corporate Boulevard, Suite 410
Linthicum, MD 21090

410-689-3700
866-746-4282
Fax: 410-689-3800
auafoundation@auafoundation.org
www.auanet.org

Partners with physicians, researchers, healthcare professionals, patients, families, caregivers and the public to support, promote research, and patient/public education and advocacy in improving the prevention, detection, treatment and cure of urologic diseases.

Veronica Gilliard, Manager
Robert C. Flannigan MD, Secretary
William F. Gee MD, Treasurer

5153 Association for the Bladder Exstrophy Community
6737 West Washington Street, Ste 3265
West Allis, WI 53214

414-918-9002
866-300-2222
Fax: 414-918-9001
admin@bladderexstrophy.com
www.bladderexstrophy.com

The ABC is an international support network of individuals with bladder exstrophy (includes classic exstrophy, cloacal exstrophy, and epispadias), local parent-exstrophy support groups, and health care providers working with patients and families living with bladder exstrophy.

Dr. Jeffrey Niezgoda, President/Founder
Pamela Block, President
Tom Exler, Vice-President

5154 Federation of Families for Children's Mental Health
9605 Medical Center Drive, Suite 280
Rockville, MD 20850

240-403-1901
Fax: 240-403-1909
ffcmh@ffcmh.org
www.ffcmh.org

The National family run organization is dedicated exclusively to helping children with mental health needs and their families achieve a better quality of life.

Teka Dempson, President
Sherri Luthe, Vice President
Josh Ross, Secretary

5155 Mental Health America
500 Montgomery Street, Ste 820
Alexandria, VA 22314

603-684-7722
800-969-6642
Fax: 703-684-5968
TTY: 800-433-5959
www.mentalhealthamerica.net

Addresses all aspects of mental health and mental illness. NMHA with over 340 affiliates works to improve the mental health of all Americans.

Paul Gionfriddo, President/CEO
Shavonne Carpenter, Sr Assoc., Support & Services
Mallory Pernell, Assoc. Dir, Comments/Marketing

5156 National Mental Health Consumers' Self-Help Clearinghouse
1211 Chestnut Street, Suite 1207
Philadelphia, PA 19107

215-751-1810
800-553-4539
Fax: 215-636-6312
info@mhselfhelp.org
www.mhselfhelp.org

Offers information, support and appropriate referrals; and promotes public and professional education. Provides networking for those with special interests related to albinism. Promotes and supports research and funding that will improve diagnosis and management of albinism and hypopigmentation.

Joseph Rogers, Executive Director & Founder
Susan Rogers, Director
Christa Burkett, Technical Assistance Coordinator

5157 National Sleep Foundation
1010 N Glebe Road
Arlington, VA 22201

703-243-1697
Fax: 202-347-3472
nsf@sleepfoundation.org
www.sleepfoundation.org

An independent, nonprofit organization dedicated to improving public health and safety by achieving public understanding of sleep and sleep disorders, and by supporting public education, sleep-related research, and advocacy. Actively collaborates with sleep centers, support groups for patients with sleep disorders and safety organizations.

David Cloud, CEO

Web Sites

5158 American Urological Association Foundation
1000 Corporate Boulevard
Linthicum, MD 21090

410-689-3700
800-828-7866
Fax: 410-689-3998
info@urologycarefoundation.org
www.urologyhealth.org

Provides information on enuresis as well as other pediatric disorders related to the kidneys and bladder.

Richard A. Memo, MD, Chair
Steven Schlossberg, MD, MBA, Secretary/Treasurer
Martin Dineen, Member-at-Large

5159 Bedwetting Online
www.bedwetting.ferring.ca

Helps parents and children deal with Nocturnal Enuresis.

5160 Child Development Institute
500 State College, Suite 1100
Orange, CA 928 childdevelopmentinfo.com/disorders/bedwetting.shtml

Child development and parent information for learning, health and safety, as well as child disorders.

5161 Dr. Koop
750 Third Avenue, 6th Floor
New York, NY 10017

212-695-2223
Fax: 212-695-2936
www.healthcentral.com

Information on the condition, causes, symptoms, tests and treatment.

Michael Cunnion, Chief Executive Officer
Jim Curtis, Chief Revenue Officer
Rebecca Farwell, Chief Content Officer

5162 National Kidney Foundation
30 East 33rd Street
New York, NY 10016

800-622-9010
Fax: 212-689-9261
info@kidney.org
www.kidney.org/patients/bw/index.cfm

Information for parents, kids and teens, and medical professionals on bed-wetting.

Bruce Skyer, CEO
Joseph Vassalotti, MD, Chief Medical Officer
Petros Gregoriou, SVP, CFO

DESCRIPTION

5163 NON-HODGKIN'S LYMPHOMA

Synonym: NHL

Covers these related disorders: Non-Hodgkin's lymphoma, large cell type, Non-Hodgkin's lymphoma, lymphoblastic type, Non-Hodgkin's lymphoma, small noncleaved cell(SNC)

Involves the following Biologic System(s):

Hematologic and Oncologic Disorders

Non-Hodgkin's lymphoma (NHL) consists of a group of cancers of the body's lymphatic system. This specialized system consists of the spleen, thymus gland, adenoids and tonsils, lymph nodes, and lymph ducts. Together these structures carry the clear fluid known as lymph and the white blood cells known as lymphocytes, and drain fluid and waste products from the body's organs and tissues. The lymph nodes act as tiny sieves that filter invading organisms and cancerous cells from the lymph that passes through the nodes, while lymphocytes in the nodes and elsewhere in the lymphatic system attack and destroy these hostile organisms and malignant cells. Besides its presence in these lymphatic structures, lymphatic tissue is present in the skin, stomach, and small intestine.

Non-Hodgkin lymphoma (NHL) is characterized by the proliferation of either T- or B-lymphocytes (white blood cells).T-lymphocytes act directly against infecting microorganisms and body cells that have turned cancerous by coming into contact with these hostile organisms or cells and secreting substances that either kill them directly or mark them for killing by other blood cells. B-cells combat infection by secreting antibodies that target alien microorganisms for killing by other cells. Types of NHL that occur among T-cells include the diseases known as mycosis fungoides, anaplastic large cell lymphoma, and precursor T-lymphoblastic lymphoma. Most NHLs occurring in the United States are B-cell lymphomas, whichinclude chronic lymphocytic leukemia/small lymphocytic lymphoma (CLL/SLL), diffuse large B-cell lymphoma, follicular lymphoma, Burkitt's lymphoma, immunoblastic large cell lymphoma, precursor B-lymphoblastic lymphoma, and mantle cell lymphoma, as well as the condition named hairy-cell leukemia because of the hair-like projections that extend from the abnormal B-lymphocytes in this disease.

Most types of NHL arise from lymph nodes in the head and neck, the chest cavity, or the abdomen. Some types may develop in lymph nodes at other sites in the body or affect other structures of the lymphoid system or other tissues, and a close association exists between specific types of NHL and the sites at which these diseases initially occur. For example, lymphoblastic NHL, which affects the immature cells that become lymphocytes, tends to arise in the head and neck or in the front of the chest cavity (anterior mediastinum).

Besides consisting of these different diseases, NHL is classified as being either aggressive, where lymphocytes multiply rapidly, or indolent, where cells proliferate slowly. Every individual case is further classified into one of four stages, based on the degree of progression. NHL symbolized by "E" indicates that the disease exists in lymphatic structures or tissues besides or beyond the lymph nodes; "S" indicates that it exists in the spleen.

Although lymphomas can occur at any age, they are the third most common kinds of childhood cancers in the United States, affecting about 13 of every 1 million children annually. While all lymphomas originate with a genetic defect in white cells or their immature precursor cells, other factors may instigate these lymphoid cancers or increase susceptibility to them. Thus, NHL particularly affects children with impaired immune systems. These include patients with acquired immune deficiency syndrome (AIDS) or certain genetic immunodeficiency disorders that are present at birth (primary immunodeficiencies), such as Wiskott-Aldrich syndrome, a condition marked by deficiencies in the numbers of platelet cells in the blood and in the body's immune system; X-linked lymphoproliferative syndrome; or ataxia-telangiectasia. Other sources of increased risk of developing NHL include infection with Epstein-Barr virus, which causes infectious mononucleosis; a high dietary meat or fat intake; and exposure to various pesticides and other toxic substances.

The diagnosis of NHL is based on physical examination, which may reveal swelling of the lymph nodes and other telltale signs of the disease; a complete blood count (CBC) that reveals increased numbers of either T- or B-lymphocytes and possibly decreased numbers of other kinds of blood cells; a decreased content of the oxygen-carrying substance known as hemoglobin in the body's red blood cells; abnormalities in tissue specimens taken from lymph nodes or other structures of the lymphatic system or in the bone marrow where lymphocyte progenitor cells originate. Procedures used to determine the stage of NHL in a particular patient include chest X-rays, computed tomography (CT), positron emission tomography (PET), magnetic resonance imaging (MRI), and the technique known as gallium scanning, in which a minuscule quantity of the element known as gallium is injected into the body and accumulates at sites where cancerous cells are proliferating, providing images of such disease activity.

In children with NHL, initial symptoms and findings vary and depend upon the specific type of the disease, its location, and its stage, or level of involvement. Findings often include painless swelling of lymph nodes in the neck, groin, or deep within the abdominal or chest region. Tumor growth in the chest cavity area may result in abnormal accumulations of fluid (pleural effusion) between layers of the lung lining (pleura), as well as difficulty in breathing and abnormal swelling of tissues of the face, neck, and arms, causing difficulty in swallowing. Other symptoms can include nausea, vomiting, lack of appetite (anorexia), abdominal pain and swelling (distension), severe constipation, or other digestive symptoms. Some cases of NHL affect the skin, resulting in dark, thickened, itchy patches. Tumors in the bone marrow may result in decreased numbers of red blood cells (anemia) or platelets (thrombocytopenia). In advanced cases of NHL, involvement of the brain may cause increased fluid pressure around the brain, severe headache, and p aralysis of certain nerves. As it progresses, NHL may also increasingly cripple the body's immune system and impair its infection-fighting ability, leading to potentially severe or life-threatening infections.

NHL is classified into different stages, based upon the number and location of tumors, the degree that the disease has spread, and other factors. Both the prognosis or outlook for patients with NHL and their treatment depend on the stage and type of their disease.

Treatment typically involves the use of drugs that kill cancerous cells known as cytotoxic drugs; radiation therapy, in which X-rays are directed at lymph nodes and other body sites affected by disease; immunotherapy, in which substances that bolster the immune system are given to help restore its infection-fighting and other capabilities; and biotherapy, in which a drug named rituximab, belonging to a highly cell- and tissue-specific group of newer drugs known as monoclonal antibodies, is used to hone in on cancerous cells and assist the immune system in destroying them. Treatment may also include the use of bone marrow transplantation to help restore the ability of the bone marrow to generate new lymphocytes and other blood cells to replace those affected by NHL or destroyed by the drugs or radiation used to treat it. In many cases, two or more of these treatment methods are combined with one another to combat NHL. In the recent technique known as radioimmunotherapy, monoclonal antibodies that specifically hone in on cancerous cells are linked to radioactive substances that carry these substances directly to such cells and kill them.

Both chemotherapy and radiation therapy for NHL can have side effects, including nausea and vomiting, diarrhea, weight loss, hair loss, and fatigue. Some children also experience psychological depression. Most of these effects are transitory, and gradually disappear after treatment is completed. More potentially serious side effects are declines in the numbers of infection-fighting cells. Severe neutrophil deficiency, or neutropenia, can open the way to infection, and may require treatment with granulocyte colony-stimulating factor (G-CSF), which promotes the proliferation of neutrophils and thus reduces the risk of infection. In some cases, antibiotics are used to prevent and treat infection occurring in patients with NHL. Serious but infrequent complications of treatment for NHL include sterility, from radiation therapy; osteoporosis, from treatment-related damage to bone cells; and damage to the heart by some drugs used in chemotherapy for NHL.

Government Agencies

5164 NIH/National Cancer Institute
BG 9609 / 9609 Medical Center Drive
Bethesda, MD 20892
800-422-6237
www.cancer.gov

The National Cancer Institute coordinates the National Cancer Program, which conducts and supports research, training, health information dissemination, and other programs with respect to the cause, diagnosis, prevention, and treatment of cancer, rehabilitation from cancer, and the continuing care of cancer patients and the families of cancer patients.

Douglas R. Lowy, MD, Acting Director
James Doroshow, MD, Deputy Director
Henry P. Ciolino, PhD, Acting Director, Cancer Centers

National Associations & Support Groups

5165 American Academy of Pediatrics
141 Northwest Point Boulevard
Elk Grove Village, IL 60007
847-434-4000
800-433-9016
Fax: 847-434-8000
www.aap.org

The American Academy of Pediatrics and its member pediatricians are committed to the attainment of optimal physical, mental and social health and well-being for all infants, children, adolescents, and young adults.

Fernando Stein, MD, FAAP, President
Karen Remley, MD, CEO/Executive VP

5166 American Childhood Cancer Organization (fo rmerly Candlelighters Childhood Cancer)
PO Box 498
Kensington, MD 20895
301-962-3520
855-858-2226
Fax: 310-962-3521
staff@acco.org
www.acco.org

The Candlelighters Childhood Cancer Foundation National Office was founded in 1970 by concerned parents of children with cancer. Today our membership of over 50,000 members of the national office and more than 100,000 members across the across the country, including Candlelighters affiliate groups, includes, parents of children who are being treated or have been treated for cancer.

Ruth I. Hoffman, MPH, Executive Director
Jessica DiBenedetto, Program Coordinator
Christy Perry, Director, Marketing/Communications

5167 CancerCare
275 7th Avenue, Floor 22
New York, NY 10001
212-712-8400
800-813-4673
Fax: 212-712-8495
info@cancercare.org
www.cancercare.org

CancerCare is a national nonprofit, 501(c)(3) organization that provides free, professional support services to anyone affected by cancer: people with cancer, caregivers, children, loved ones, and the bereaved. CancerCare programs - including counseling and support groups, education, financial assistance and practical help - are provided by professional oncology social workers and are completely free of charge.

Patricia J Goldsmith, CEO
John Rutigliano, Chief Operating Officer
Ahuva Morris, Children's Program Coordinator

5168 Leukemia & Lymphoma Society
3 International Drive, Ste 200
Rye Brook, NY 10573
914-949-5213
Fax: 914-949-6691
www.lls.org

Large voluntary health organization dedicated to funding blood cancer research, education and patient services.

Louis J. DeGennaro, PhD, President & CEO
Andrew Coccari, Chief Product Officer
Danielle Gee, Chief of Staff

5169 Lymphoma Research Foundation
115 Broadway, Suite 1301
New York, NY 10006
212-349-2910
800-235-6848
Fax: 212-349-2886
LRF@lymphoma.org
www.lymphoma.org

Voluntary lymphoma-focused voluntary health organization devoted to funding lymphoma research and providing critical information on the disease.

Diane Blum, CEO
Kathleen Brown, Director of Research
Jen Davis, Director of Special Events

5170 National Childhood Cancer Foundation
4600 East West Highway, Suite 600
Bethesda, MD 20814
301-718-0042
800-458-6223
Fax: 301-718-0047
info@curesearch.org
www.curesearch.org

613

CureSearch unites the world's largest childhood cancer research organization, the Children's Oncology Group, and the National Childhood Cancer Foundation through our mission to cure childhood cancer. Research is the key to the cure.

Stuart Siegal, Chairman
Timothy Harmon, Vice-Chair
Mary Payne, Treasurer

5171 Wellness Community
1990 S. Bundy Dr., Suite 100
Los Angeles, CA 90025
310-314-2555
Fax: 310-314-7586
info@twc-wla.org
www.cancersupportcommunitybenjamincenter.org

Helps people with cancer and their loved ones enhance their health and well-being by providing a professional program of emotional support, education and hope.

Horald H. Benjamin, Co-Founder
Bonnie Schuman, Communications & Media Relations

Web Sites

5172 CancerCare
275 Seventh Avenue 22nd Floor
New York, NY 10001
212-712-8400
800-813-4673
Fax: 212-712-8495
www.cancercare.org

CancerCare is a national nonprofit, 501(c)(3) organization that provides free, professional support services to anyone affected by cancer: people with cancer, caregivers, children, loved ones, and the bereaved. CancerCare programs - including counseling and support groups, education, financial assistance and practical help - are provided by professional oncology social workers and are completely free of charge.

Patricia J Goldsmith, CEO
John Rutigliano, Chief Operating Officer
Ahuva Morris, Children's Program Coordinator

5173 Children's Cancer Web
www.cancerindex.org/ccw

An independent nonprofit site, established to provide a directory of childhood cancer resources.

5174 Leukemia & Lymphoma Society
3 International Drive, Suite 200
Rye Brook, NY 10573
914-949-5213
Fax: 914-949-6691
www.lls.org

Is the largest voluntary health organization dedicated to funding blood cancer research, education and patient services. The mission is to cure leukemia, lymphoma, Hodgkin's disease and myeloma, and to improve the quality of life of patients and their families.

Louis J. DeGennaro, PhD, President & CEO
Andrew Coccari, Chief Product Officer
Danielle Gee, Chief of Staff

5175 Lymphoma Innovations
www.lymphomainnovations.com

Targeted information for people with Non Hodgkins Lymphoma.

Book Publishers

5176 Let's Talk About Going to the Hospital
Rosen Publishing Group's PowerKids Press
29 E 21st Street
New York, NY 10010
212-777-3017
800-237-9932
Fax: 888-436-4643
rosenpub@tribeca.ios.com
www.rosenpublishing.com

If a child has to check into the hospital, chances are he or she is already upset about being ill. Knowing how a hospital functions and what the procedures are, such as when family members can visit, will help in what is already a stressful situation. Grades K-5.

24 pages
ISBN: 0-823950-36-0
Roger Rosen, Predident

5177 Let's Talk About When Kids Have Cancer
Melanie Apel Gordon, author

Rosen Publishing Group's PowerKids Press
29 E 21st Street
New York, NY 10010
212-777-3017
800-237-9932
Fax: 888-436-4643
customerservice@rosenpub.com
www.rosenpublishing.com

In a straightforward yet comforting way, this book explains what cancer is, what kinds of treatments surround the disease and how to cope if a child or the friend of a child has cancer.

24 pages Paperback
ISBN: 0-823951-95-2
Roger Rosen, President

5178 Pediatric Cancer Sourcebook
Omnigraphics
PO Box 8002
Aston, PA 19014
800-234-1340
Fax: 800-875-1340
info@omnigraphics.com
www.omnigraphics.com

Basic consumer health information about leukemias, brain tumors, sarcomas, lymphomas and other cancers in infants, children and adolescents.

1999 587 pages
ISBN: 0-780802-45-4
Peter Ruffner, Publisher

5179 Surviving Childhood Cancer: A Guide for Families
New Harbinger Publications
5674 Shattuck Avenue
Oakland, CA 94609
510-652-0215
800-748-6273
Fax: 800-652-1613
customerservice@newharbinger.com
www.newharbinger.com

Cancer in a child is an overwhelming experience for a family. This book explains common medical procedures and offers readers practical advice about how to cope with emotions and stress during this time.

215 pages Paperback
ISBN: 1-572241-02-0

Camps

5180 Arizona Camp Sunrise & Sidekicks
PO Box 27872
Tempe, AZ 85285
480-382-8564
928-478-4564
melissa@azcampsunrise.org
www.azcampsunrise.org

The camp is dedicated to provide an exciting, medically safe camp program for children whose families have been affected by cancer.

Melissa Lee, Camp Director

5181 Camp Catch-A-Rainbow
American Cancer Society
One Children's Plaza
Dayton, OH 45404
937-641-3000
800-228-4055
kwilson@ymcastorercamps.org
www.childrensdayton.org

Open to any child (age 7 thru 15) who has, or has had, cancer.

Katie Wilson, Coordinator

5182 Camp Sunshine Dreams
PO Box 28232
Fresno, CA 93729
contact@campsunshinedreams.com
www.campsunshinedreams.com

Summer camp for children with cancer.

Anthony Aiello, Board Member

5183 Okizu Foundation Camps
16 Digital Drive, Suite 130
Novato, CA 94949
415-382-9083
Fax: 415-382-8384
info@okizu.org
www.okizu.org

This foundation runs family camp programs for children who have cancer and their families, and for children who have or had a parent with cancer.

Lori Sparrow, Executive Director
Heather Ferrier, Camp Director of Operations

DESCRIPTION

5184 NOONAN SYNDROME

Synonyms: Female Pseudo-Turner syndrome, Male Turner syndrome, NS

Involves the following Biologic System(s):
Cardiovascular Disorders,
Genetic/Chromosomal/Syndrome/Metabolic Disorders

Noonan syndrome is a genetic disorder that is usually apparent at birth (congenital) and interferes with the normal development of various body structures and organs. The symptoms and findings associated with the disorder may be extremely variable, differing in range and severity from case to case. However, children with Noonan syndrome often have short stature, webbing of the neck (pterygium colli), and characteristic abnormalities of the head and facial (craniofacial) area, such as downwardly slanting eyelid folds (palpebral fissures), drooping of the upper eyelids (ptosis), a small jaw (micrognathia), and prominent, low-set ears that are rotated toward the back of the head. In addition, in many males with Noonan syndrome, the testes fail to descend into the scrotum (cryptorchidism) before birth or during the first year of life. Therefore, in some cases, the male reproductive cells (sperm) may fail to develop appropriately within the testes, potentially causing infertility.

The genetic mutations responsible for Noonan syndrome chiefly affect four genes, which may be inherited from a parent, or result spontaneously from mutations occurring in the embryo. Most estimates indicate that this syndrome affects one in 1,000 to 2,500 newborns, but it may be difficult to determine the true frequency of Noonan syndrome because of the wide variation in its effects.

Many children with Noonan syndrome have distinctive skeletal malformations, such as abnormal depression of the lower portion of the breastbone (pectus excavatum) and protrusion of the upper portion of the breastbone (pectus carinatum); outward deviation of the elbows upon extension (cubitus valgus); sideways curvature of the spine (scoliosis); or front-to-back curvature of the spine (kyphosis). Affected children may also have structural abnormalities of the heart that are present at birth (congenital heart defects). These include obstruction of normal blood flow from the lower right pumping chamber (ventricle) of the heart to the lungs (pulmonary valvular stenosis). During infancy, there may also be an abnormal accumulation of lymph fluid in body tissues and a consequent swelling of these tissues (lymphedema) as the result of malformations in the body's lymphatic system. Additional symptoms and findings in Noonan syndrome may include deficient functioning of the blood cells known as platelets, which play an essential role in preventing or stopping bleeding; abnormally small numbers of platelets in circulating blood (thrombocytopenia); or defects in blood clotting (coagulation factor), potentially causing abnormal bleeding and susceptibility to bruising. In some cases, children with Noonan syndrome may have mental retardation or experience delays in acquiring certain skills that require the coordination of physical and mental activities (psychomotor retardation).

The diagnosis of Noonan syndrome is based on its physical effects, such as distortions in the chest, neck, ears, or eyelids, together with ultrasound or computed tomographic (CT) scans that reveal congenital heart, or other internal organ, defects, and tests that reveal disorders in blood clotting. The severity of Noonan syndrome in an infant or child is assessed through physical, neurological, and optical examinations; studies of heart function and body development; studies of the brain, spine, and rib cage done with X-ray images and the technique known as magnetic resonance imaging (MRI); ultrasound examination of the kidneys and urinalyses to assess kidney function; hearing tests; and blood and genetic testing.

The treatment of children with Noonan syndrome depends upon its severity and may include drugs, surgery to manage or correct congenital heart defects or to move undescended testes into the scrotum (orchiopexy) in males with cryptorchidism; hormone therapy (i.e., human growth hormone therapy); administration of platelets, blood-clotting factors, and other appropriate measures for treating thrombocytopenia, platelet dysfunction, and abnormalities in blood clotting, special education; and other treatment measures as required. Genetic counseling is recommended if there is a family history of Noonan syndrome.

National Associations & Support Groups

5185 American Academy of Pediatrics
141 Northwest Point Boulevard
Elk Grove Village, IL 60007

847-434-4000
800-433-9016
Fax: 847-434-8000
www.aap.org

The American Academy of Pediatrics and its member pediatricians are committed to the attainment of optimal physical, mental and social health and well-being for all infants, children, adolescents, and young adults.

Fernando Stein, MD, FAAP, President
Karen Remley, MD, CEO/Executive VP

5186 Genetic Alliance
4301 Connecticut Avenue NW, Suite 404
Washington, DC 20008

202-966-5557
800-336-4363
Fax: 202-966-8553
info@geneticalliance.org
www.geneticalliance.org

A coalition of voluntary genetic support groups, consumers and professionals addressing the needs of individuals and families affected by genetic disorders from a national perspective.

Sharon Terry, President/CEO
Tetyana Murza, Managing Director
Natasha Bonhomme, VP, Strategic Development

5187 Human Growth Foundation
997 Glen Cove Avenue, Suite 5
Glen Head, NY 11545

516-671-4041
800-451-6434
Fax: 516-671-4055
hgfl@hgfound.org
www.hgfound.org

Nonprofit organization devoted to research and advocacy regarding people with growth and growth hormone disorders.

Pisit Pitukcheewanont, MD, President
Emily Germain-Lee, Vice President
Patricia D Costa, Executive Director

5188 MAGIC Foundation: Major Aspects of Growth in Children
4200 Cantera Drive, #106
Warrenville, IL 60555

630-836-8200
800-362-4423
Fax: 630-836-8181
mary@magicfoundation.org
www.magicfoundation.org

A national nonprofit organization providing support and education regarding growth disorders in children and related adult disorders. Provides educational information, networking, a national conference, a kids' program and an extensive medical library.

Dianne Kremidas, Executive Director
Mary Andrews, CEO

5189 March of Dimes Foundation
1275 Mamaroneck Avenue
White Plains, NY 10605   914-997-4488
                               888-663-4637
                               Fax: 914-428-8203
                               answers@marchofdimes.com
                               www.marchofdimes.com

Partnership of volunteers and professionals dedicates to improving the health of babies by preventing birth defects and infant mortality. Over 100 chapters are located across the country and can be located through the National Office.

Stacey D. Stewart, President

5190 Noonan Syndrome Support Group
PO Box 145
Upperco, MD 21155   410-374-5245
                              888-686-2224
                              info@noonansyndrome.org
                              www.noonansyndrome.org

Sharing of information and encouragement among individuals who have been affected by the syndrome. The organization offers forums where physicians and other professionals can provide information on living with the daily challenges. Offers an online newsletter.

Wanda Robinson, President
Dave Robinson, VP

Web Sites

5191 Family Village
www.familyvillage.wisc.edu

A global community that integrates information, resources and communication opportunities on the Internet for persons with cognitive and other disabilities, for their families and for those that provide them services and support.

5192 Online Mendelian Inheritance in Man
National Library of Medicine Building 38A
Bethesda, MD 20894   888-346-3656
                              info@ncbi.nlm.nih.gov
                              www.ncbi.nlm.nih.gov

This database is a catalog of human genes and genetic disorders.

Book Publishers

5193 Let's Talk About Going to the Hospital
Rosen Publishing Group's PowerKids Press
29 E 21st Street
New York, NY 10010   212-777-3017
                              800-237-9932
                              Fax: 888-436-4643
                              rosenpub@tribeca.ios.com
                              www.rosenpublishing.com

If a child has to check into the hospital, chances are he or she is already upset about being ill. Knowing how a hospital functions and what the procedures are, such as when family members can visit, will help in what is already a stressful situation. Grades K-5.

24 pages
ISBN: 0-823950-36-0

Roger Rosen, President

Newsletters

5194 Noonan Connection
Noonan Syndrome Support Group
PO Box 145
Upperco, MD 21155   410-374-5245
                              888-686-2224
                              info@noonansyndrome.org
                              www.noonansnydrome.org

Provides basic information on Noonan syndrome and related current news and events.

DESCRIPTION

5195 NYSTAGMUS

Covers these related disorders: Jerky nystagmus, Pendular nystagmus

Involves the following Biologic System(s):

Neurologic Disorders, Ophthalmologic Disorders

Nystagmus is a condition characterized by involuntary, rhythmic movements of the eyes. These movements may be vertical, horizontal, circular, or a mixture of two varieties (mixed). Nystagmus may be present at birth (congenital) or develop later in life (acquired). There are two general categories or types of nystagmus: jerky nystagmus and pendular nystagmus.

Jerky nystagmus is the most common form of the condition. It is characterized by relatively slow movements of the eyes in one direction followed by rapid, corrective movements or jerks in the opposite direction. In many patients with jerky nystagmus, head movements accompany the eye movements. These unusual head movements are thought to represent so-called compensatory posturing, that is, turning of the head to bring the eyes to a position in which the nystagmus lessens and vision is best (null positioning) In pendular nystagmus, movements of the eyes are approximately equal in rate in both directions. The different forms of nystagmus result due to abnormalities in certain mechanisms that regulate the movements and positioning of the eyes. These include conjugate gaze, fixation, and vestibular mechanisms. Conjugate gaze is the normal movement of both eyes in the same direction to bring objects into view. Fixation describes the direction of the gaze so that visual images fall on a certain area of the retina, which is the nerve-rich membrane at the back of the eye (fovea centralis). The vestibular mechanism is the balancing mechanism of the inner ear.

In some affected individuals, pendular or jerky nystagmus is present at birth or develops during early infancy or childhood. Pendular nystagmus often occurs in association with eye and visual defects (e.g., congenital glaucoma, congenital cataract, albinism, etc.). In other patients, pendular nystagmus may be an isolated finding that occurs in the absence of such conditions. Jerky nystagmus is usually unassociated with other eye or visual defects, and its cause is unknown. Familial cases of isolated pendular or jerky nystagmus are reported in which the condition appears to be transmitted as an autosomal dominant, autosomal recessive, or X-linked trait.

A specific, acquired form of pendular nystagmus, known as spasmus nutans, may also affect some infants or children. This condition typically develops at approximately four months to two years of age. In spasmus nutans, nystagmus is accompanied by head nodding and, in some children, abnormal tightness or contractions of the neck muscles, resulting in twisting of the neck and abnormal positioning of the head (torticollis). In most children with spasmus nutans, pendular nystagmus is limited to or more pronounced in one eye. Symptoms usually spontaneously resolve within months or a few years.

Some infants or children may also have a form of nystagmus in which there is repetitive jerking of the eyes toward each other or backward into the eye sockets (convergent nystag-mus). This form of nystagmus often occurs with impaired vertical gaze in association with certain underlying syndromes (e.g., Parinaud syndrome, sylvian aqueduct syndrome, etc.).

The development of persistent nystagmus later in life may occur in association with certain disorders of the nervous system (e.g., brain tumors, multiple sclerosis) or disorders affecting the balancing (vestibular) mechanism of the inner ear (labyrinthine-vestibular disease). Individuals with acquired nystagmus should receive immediate, thorough evaluations to diagnose the underlying cause and ensure prompt, appropriate treatment. Medications can cause nystagmus. Causes include excessive drinking of alcohol or use of medications such as those given for seizure control.

In infants and children with nystagmus, diagnostic evaluations typically include the use of a specialized imaging technique (electronystagmography) that records eye movements and helps to determine or confirm the type of nystagmus present. Treatment of patients with nystagmus includes appropriate therapies for any diagnosed, underlying causes of the condition. Other treatment includes symptomatic and supportive measures.

Government Agencies

5196 NIH/National Eye Institute
31 Center Drive MSC 2510
Bethesda, MD 20892
301-496-5248
2020@nei.nih.gov
www.nei.nih.gov

Conducts and supports research that helps prevent and treat eye diseases and other disorders of vision. This research leads to sight-saving treatments, reduces visual impairment and blindness, and improves the quality of life for people of all ages. NEI-supported research has advanced our knowledge of how the eye functions in health and disease.

Paul A Sieving M.D., Ph.D., Director

National Associations & Support Groups

5197 American Academy of Pediatrics
141 Northwest Point Boulevard
Elk Grove Village, IL 60007
847-434-4000
800-433-9016
Fax: 847-434-8000
www.aap.org

The American Academy of Pediatrics and its member pediatricians are committed to the attainment of optimal physical, mental and social health and well-being for all infants, children, adolescents, and young adults.

Fernando Stein, MD, FAAP, President
Karen Remley, MD, CEO/Executive VP

5198 American Nystagmus Network
303-D Beltline Place, Suite 321
Decatur, AL 35603
www.nystagmus.org

A nonprofit organization founded in 1999 to serve the needs and interests of those affected by nystagmus, and to provide information to health care providers, educators and researchers.

John D. Cranmer, President
Rick Beaudet, VP
Tony Fuhrer, Treasurer

5199 Genetic Alliance
4301 Connecticut Avenue NW, Suite 404
Washington, DC 20008
202-966-5557
800-336-4363
Fax: 202-966-8553
info@geneticalliance.org
www.geneticalliance.org

A coalition of voluntary genetic support groups, consumers and professionals addressing the needs of individuals and families affected by genetic disorders from a national perspective.

Sharon Terry, President/CEO
Tetyana Murza, Managing Director
Natasha Bonhomme, VP, Strategic Development

5200 March of Dimes Foundation
1275 Mamaroneck Avenue
White Plains, NY 10605
914-997-4488
888-663-4637
Fax: 914-428-8203
answers@marchofdimes.com
www.marchofdimes.com

Partnership of volunteers and professionals dedicates to improving the health of babies by preventing birth defects and infant mortality. Over 100 chapters are located across the country and can be located through the National Office.

Stacey D. Stewart, President

5201 National Association for Visually Handicapped
111 E 59th St
New York, NY 10022
212-889-3141
800-829-0500
Fax: 212-727-2931
staff@navh.org
www.lighthouse.org

The on only nonprofit health organization in the world solely dedicated to providing assistance to the partially sighted. Serves as a clearinghouse for information about all services available to the partially-sighted from public and private sources. Conducts self-help groups. Provides information on large print books, textbooks and educational tools.

Joseph A. Ripp, Chairman
Sarah E. Smith, Vice-Chair/Treasurer
Jonathan M. Wainwright, Vice-Chair/Secretary

State Agencies & Support Groups

Alabama

5202 Alabama Institute for the Deaf & Blind
205 East South Street
Talladega, AL 35160
256-761-3200
Fax: 256-761-3344
www.aidb.org

Services include central directory, representatives of agencies, service providers, families, and coordinators of infant, toddler, and preschool special education programs.

John Mascia, President
Frieda Meacham, VP
Mike Hubbard, Director

Arizona

5203 National Association for Parents of the Visually Impaired
2345 Commonwealth Avenue
Newton, MA 02466
617-972-7441
800-562-6265
Fax: 617-972-7444
napvi@guildhealth.org
www.spedex.com/napvi

Julie Urban, President
Venetia Hayden, VP
Randi Sher, Secretary

Ohio

5204 Region 2 of the National Association for Parents of the Visually Impaired
3910 Pocahontas Avenue
Cincinnati, OH 45227
513-561-8542
Victoria Gorman Miller

Pennsylvania

5205 East Central Region-Helen Keller National Center
141 Middle Neck Road
Sands Point, NY 11050
516-944-8900
Fax: 516-944-7302
HKNCinfo@hknc.org
www.helenkeller.org

Christopher D. Maher, Chairman
Richard T. Arkwright, Vice-Chairman
John R. Caughey, Treasurer

South Carolina

5206 Region 4 of the National Association for Parents of the Visually Impaired
1032 Trail Road
Belton, SC 29627
864-338-9593

Washington

5207 Northwestern Region-Helen Keller National Center
1620 18th Ave., Ste 201
Seattle, WA 98112
206-324-9120
Fax: 206-324-9159
TTY: 206-324-1133
dorothy.walt@hknc.org
www.khnc.org

Dorothy Walt, Regional Rep.
Taryn Hill, Administrative Assistant

Libraries & Resource Centers

Alabama

5208 Mobile Association for the Blind
2440 Gordon Smith Drive
Mobile, AL 36617
251-473-3585
Fax: 251-470-8622
www.mobileblind.org

Offers work adjustment training, activities of daily living, mobility, communication skills and sheltered employment for adults and children who are visually impaired.

Jim Bullock, Executive Director

Arizona

5209 Educational Services for the Visually Impaired
2402 Wildwood Avenue Suite 112
Sherwood, AR 72120
501-835-5448
Fax: 501-835-6840
www.esvi.org

Offers textbooks, Braille books and more to the visually impaired grades K-12 in the Arkansas area.

Angyln Young, State Coordinator
Cindy Lester, Data Management Specialist/Preschoo

Arkansas

5210 Arkansas Regional Library for the Blind and Physically Handicapped
900 W. Capitol, Suite 100
Little Rock, AR 72201
501-682-2053
Fax: 501-682-1533
TDD: 501-682-1002
nlsbooks@asl.lib.ar.us
www.library.arkansas.gov

Public library books in recorded or Braille format. Popular fiction and nonfiction books for all ages, books and players are on free loan, sent to patrons by mail and may be returned postage free. Anyone who cannot see well enough to read regular print with glasses on or who has a disability that makes it difficult to hold a book or turn the pages is eligible.

Linda Bennett, Director
Dwain Gordon, Deputy Director
Danny Koonce, Public Information Specialist

California

5211 American Action Fund for Blind Children and Adults
18440 Oxnard Street
Tarzana, CA 91356   818-343-2022
                                                            Fax: 818-343-3219
                                                          lucyabba@aol.com
                                                          www.actinfund.org

A lending library for the visually impaired. We send out a weekly Braille newspaper for the deaf-blind (worldwide), we also send out pocket-sized Braille calendars. Our lending library is for pre-school thru high school. All of our services are free.

Lucille Abbazia, Manager

5212 Blind Children's Center
4120 Marathon Street
Los Angeles, CA 90029   323-664-2153
                                                            Fax: 323-665-3828
                                                     www.blindchildrenscenter.org

Offers support and informational groups.

Scott E. Schaldenbrand, President,Executive Committee
Danette M. Jones, Vice President
Lisa D. Hansen, Secretary

5213 Braille Institute Desert Center
70-251 Ramon Road
Rancho Mirage, CA 92270   760-321-1111
                                                            Fax: 760-321-9715
                                                        dc@brailleinstitute.org
                                                        www.brailleinstitute.org

Dedicated to providing blind and visually impaired men, women and children with the training, programs and services they need to enjoy productive lives. Services offered include child development, youth programs, library services and adult education.

Lester M Sussman, Chairman
James B. Boyle Jr., Director
Thomas K. Callister, Director

5214 Braille Institute Sight Center
741 N Vermont Avenue
Los Angeles, CA 90029   323-663-1111
                                                            Fax: 323-663-0867
                                                        la@brailleinstitute.org
                                                        www.brailleinstitute.org

Offers help, programs, services and information to the blind and visually impaired children and adults.

Lester M Sussman, Chairman
James B. Boyle Jr., Director
Thomas K. Callister, Director

5215 Braille Institute Youth Center
741 N Vermont Avenue
Los Angeles, CA 90029   323-663-1111
                                                            Fax: 323-663-0867
                                                        la@brailleinstitute.org
                                                        www.brailleinstitute.org

Offers various youth programs and services for the blind and visually impaired youngster.

Lester M Sussman, Chairman
James B. Boyle Jr., Director
Thomas K. Callister, Director

5216 New Beginnings - Blind Children's Center
4120 Marathon, Street
Los Angeles, CA 90029   323-664-2153
                                                                800-222-3566
                                                            Fax: 323-665-3828

Helps children and their families become independent by creating a climate of safety and trust. Services include an infant stimulation program, educational preschool, interdisciplinary assessment services, family services, correspondence program, toll-free national hotline and a publication and research service.

5217 San Francisco Public Library for the Blind and Print Disabled
100 Larkin Street
San Francisco, CA 94102   415-557-4253
                                                            Fax: 415-557-4252
                                                              lbpd@sfpl.org
                                              www.sfpl.org/index.php?pg=0200002301

Foreign-language books on cassette, children's books on cassettes and more.

Luis Herrera, Manager

5218 Variety Audio
PO Box 5731
San Jose, CA 95150   408-277-4839

Summer reading programs, Braille writer, magnifiers, closed-circuit TV, large-print photocopier, cassette books and magazines, children's books on cassette, home visits and other reference materials on blindness and other handicaps.

Louisa Griehshammer

District of Columbia

5219 Council of Families with Visual Impairment
1155 15th Street NW
Washington, DC 20005   202-467-5081

Members are sighted parents of blind or visually impaired children. Offers a forum for support and outreach, sharing of experiences in parent-child relationships, and educational and cultural information about child development. Monitors developments in technical and legislative arenas.

Nola Webb, President

Florida

5220 Florida Bureau of Braille and Talking Book Library Services
1185 Dunn Avenue
Daytona Beach, FL 32114   386-254-3800
                                                                800-329-3801
                                                            Fax: 386-239-6107
                                                          TDD: 800-226-6079
                                                 James.Woolyhand@dbs.fldoe.org
                                              www.dbs.myflorida.com/library/

Discs, cassettes, closed-circuit TV, large-print photocopier, films, children's books on cassettes and more.

Michael Gunde, Librarian
Jim Woolyhand, District Administrator

5221 Talking Book Library, Jacksonville Public Library
303 North Laura St
Jacksonville, FL 32202   904-630-1999
                                                            Fax: 904-768-7404
                                                          TDD: 904-630-2740
                                                 JPLTBSpecialNeeds@coj.net
                                        www.jaxpubliclibrary.org/lib/talkingbooks.html

Discs, cassettes and reference materials on blindness and other disabilities.

Jerry Reynolds, Librarian Senior

5222 Talking Book Service - Manatee County Central Library
6081 26th Street W
Bradenton, FL 34207

941-742-5914
Fax: 941-751-7089
TDD: 941-742-5951
patricia.schubert@co.manatee.fl.us
www.co.manatee.fl.us

Offers children's books on disc and cassette and more reference materials for the blind and physically handicapped.

Patricia Schubert, Librarian

Georgia

5223 Albany Library for the Blind and Physical Handicapped
300 Pine Avenue
Albany, GA 31701

229-420-3220
Fax: 229-420-3215
sinquefk@mail.dougherty.public.lib.ga.us
www.docolib.org/LBPH/index.html

Offers discs, cassettes, reference materials on blindness and other handicaps, large-print photocopiers, summer reading programs, cassette books and more.

Katy Sinquefield, Manager

5224 Bainbridge Subregional Library for the Blind and Physically Handicapped
301 S Monroe Street
Bainbridge, GA 39819

229-248-2665
800-795-2680
Fax: 229-248-2670
TDD: 912-248-2665
lbph@mail.deccatur.public.lib.ga.us
www.swgrl.org

Discs, cassettes, summer reading programs, closed-circuit TV, magnifiers and more.

Kathy Hutchins, Librarian

5225 CEL Subregional Library for the Blind and Physically Handicapped
2708 Mechanics
Savannah, GA 31404

912-354-5864
Fax: 912-354-5534
TDD: 912-652-3635
stokesl@cel.co.chatman.ga.us

Summer reading programs, Braille writer, magnifiers, closed-circuit TV, large-print photocopier, cassette books and magazines, children's books on cassette, home visits and other reference materials on blindness and other handicaps.

Linda Stokes, Librarian

Idaho

5226 Idaho State Talking Book Library
325 W State Street
Boise, ID 83702

208-334-2150
Fax: 208-334-4016
TDD: 800-377-1363
tblbooks@isl.state.id.us
www.lili.org/isl/tblinfo.htm

Summer reading programs, Braille writer, magnifiers, closed-circuit TV, large-print photocopier, cassette books and magazines, children's books on cassette, home visits and other reference materials on blindness and other handicaps.

Sue Walker, Manager

Illinois

5227 Chicago Library Service for the Blind
1055 W Roosevelt Road
Chicago, IL 60608

312-746-9210

Summer reading programs, Braille writer, magnifiers, closed-circuit TV, large-print photocopier, cassette books and magazines, children's books on cassette, home visits and other reference materials on blindness and other handicaps.

Carol Pellish, Librarian

5228 Illinois State Library, Talkng Book and Braille Service
213 State Capitol
Springfield, IL 62756

217-785-3000
Fax: 217-558-4723
TDD: 800-665-5576
isltbbs@ilsos.net
www.cyberdriveillinois.com

Summer reading programs, Braille writer, magnifiers, closed-circuit TV, large-print photocopier, cassette books and magazines, descriptive videos, children's books on cassette, home visits and other reference materials on blindness and other handicaps.

Anne Craig, Executive Director

5229 Mid Illinois Talking Book System
515 York Street
Quincy, IL 62301

217-224-6619
Fax: 217-224-9818

Summer reading programs, Braille writer, magnifiers, closed-circuit TV, large-print photocopier, cassette books and magazines, children's books on cassette, home visits and other reference materials on blindness and other handicaps.

5230 Mid-Illinois Talking Book Center
600 High Point Lane #2
East Peoria, IL 61611

309-694-9200
800-426-0709
Fax: 309-799-7916
hitbc@darkstar.rsa.lib.il.us
www.mitbc.org

Summer reading programs, Braille writer, magnifiers, closed-circuit TV, large-print photocopier, cassette books and magazines, children's books on cassette, home visits and other reference materials on blindness and other handicaps.

Eileen Sheppard, Librarian
Rose Chenoweth, Director
Valerie Brandon, Administrator

5231 Talking Book Center of Northwest Illinois
600 High Point Lane #2
East Peoria, IL 61611

309-694-9200
Fax: 309-799-7916
kodean@libby.rbls.lib.il.us
www.rbls.lib.il.us

Summer reading programs, Braille writer, magnifiers, closed-circuit TV, large-print photocopier, cassette books and magazines, children's books on cassette, home visits and other reference materials on blindness and other handicaps.

Indiana

5232 Northwest Indiana Subregional Library for Blind and Physically Handicapped
1919 W 81st Street
Merrillville, IN 46410

219-769-3541
Fax: 219-756-9358

Summer reading programs, Braille writer, magnifiers, closed-circuit TV, large-print photocopier, cassette books and magazines, children's books on cassette, home visits and other reference materials on blindness and other handicaps.

Renee Lewis

Iowa

5233 Iowa Library for the Blind and Physically Handicapped
Iowa Department for the Blind
524 4th Street
Des Moines, IA 50309

515-281-1333
800-362-2587
Fax: 515-281-1263
TDD: 515-281-1355
information@blind.state.ia.us
www.blind.state.ia.us

Summer reading programs, magnifiers, closed-circuit TV, large-print photocopier, children's books on cassette, children's books in Braille and Print Braille, cassette magazines, home visits and reference materials on blindness and other handicaps.

Karen Keninger, Program Manager/Librarian

Kansas

5234 CKLS Headquarters
PO Box 515
Northampton, MA 01061

316-792-2393
888-622-8527
Fax: 316-792-5495
cenks@ink.org
www.macular.org

Summer reading programs, Braille writer, magnifiers, closed-circuit TV, large-print photocopier, cassette books and magazines, children's books on cassette, home visits and other reference materials on blindness and other handicaps.

Chip Goehring, President
Mark E. Torrey, Vice President
Paul F. Gariepy, Secretary

5235 Services for the Visually Disabled
629 Poyntz Avenue
Manhattan, KS 66502

785-776-4741
Fax: 785-776-1545
marionr@manhattan.lib.ks.us

Summer reading programs, Braille writer, magnifiers, closed-circuit TV, large-print photocopier, cassette books and magazines, children's books on cassette, home visits and other reference materials on blindness and other handicaps.

Marion Rice, Librarian

Kentucky

5236 Kentucky Library for the Blind and Physically Handicapped
300 Coffee Tree Road PO Box 537
Frankfort, KY 40602

502-564-8300
800-372-2968
Fax: 502-564-5773
richard.feindel@kdla.net
www.kdla.net/libserv/ktbl.htm

Large-print photocopier, cassette books and magazines, children's books on cassette, and other reference materials on blindness and other handicaps.

5,200 members

Richard Feindel, Librarian

Maryland

5237 Maryland State Library for the Blind and Physically Handicapped
415 Park Avenue
Baltimore, MD 21201

410-230-2424
Fax: 410-333-2095
TTY: 800-934-2541
TDD: 410-333-8679
recept@lbta.lib.md.us
www.lbph.lib.md.us

Summer reading programs, Braille writer, magnifiers, large-print photocopier, cassette books and magazines, children's books on cassette, and other reference materials on blindness and other handicaps.

Jill Lewis, Manager

5238 Prince George's County Memorial Library Talking Book Center
6532 Adelphi Road
Hyattsville, MD 20782

301-699-3500

Summer reading programs, Braille writer, magnifiers, closed-circuit TV, large-print photocopier, cassette books and magazines, children's books on cassette, home visits and other reference materials on blindness and other handicaps.

Shirley Tuthill, Librarian

Massachusetts

5239 Braille and Talking Book Library Perkins School for the Blind
175 N Beacon Street
Watertown, MA 02472

617-924-3434
Fax: 617-972-7315
info@perkins.org
www.perkins.org

Patricia Kirk

5240 Carroll Center for the Blind
770 Centre Street
Newton, MA 02458

617-969-6200
800-852-3131
Fax: 617-969-6204
www.carroll.org

Assists blind and visually impaired adults and adolescents to adjust to loss of vision. The goal of this dynamic program is to help the person become more independent, to restore self-confidence, prepare for employment and improve the quality of life. Programs of individual counseling are offered as part of the program.

Rachel Rosenbaum, President

Michigan

5241 Downtown Detroit Subregional Library for the Blind and Handicapped
121 Gratiot Avenue
Detroit, MI 48226

313-224-0580
Fax: 313-965-1977
TDD: 313-224-0584
deveans@cms.xx.wayne.edu
www.detroit.lib.mi.us

Summer reading programs, Braille writer, magnifiers, closed-circuit TV, large-print photocopier, cassette books and magazines, children's books on cassette, home visits and other reference materials on blindness and other handicaps.

Deborah Evans, Librarian

5242 Kent County Library for the Blind
775 Ball Avenue NE
Grand Rapids, MI 49503

616-336-3250
Fax: 616-336-3201
kdlem@lakeland.lib.mi.us

Summer reading programs, Braille writer, magnifiers, closed-circuit TV, large-print photocopier, cassette books and magazines, children's books on cassette, home visits and other reference materials on blindness and other handicaps.

Claudya Muller, Librarian

5243 Library of Michigan Service for the Blind
PO Box 30007
Lansing, MI 48909

517-373-5614
Fax: 517-373-5865
BTBL@michigan.gov

Summer reading programs, Braille writer, magnifiers, closed-circuit TV, large-print photocopier, cassette books and magazines, children's books on cassette, home visits and other reference materials on blindness and other handicaps.

Nancy Robertson, Manager

5244 Macomb Library for the Blind and Physically Handicapped
40900 Romeo Plank
Clinton Township, MI 48038 — 586-226-5020
Fax: 586-286-0634
TDD: 810-869-40
macbld@libcoop.net
www.cmpl.org/MLBPH/

Summer reading programs, Braille writer, closed-circuit TV, cassette books and magazines, children's books on cassette, reference materials on blindness and other handicaps.

Larry Neal, Library Director
Juliane Morian, Associate Director
Debbie Prykucki, Head of Circulation

5245 Mideastern Michigan Library Co-op
503 S Saginaw Street Suite 711
Flint, MI 48502 — 810-232-7119
800-641-6639
Fax: 810-232-6639
dhooks@mmlc.info
www.mmlc.info/

Summer reading programs, Braille writer, magnifiers, closed-circuit TV, large-print photocopier, cassette books and magazines, children's books on cassette, home visits and other reference materials on blindness and other handicaps.

Carolyn Nash, Librarian
Denise Hooks, Director
Irene Bancroft, Admin. Assistant

5246 Muskegon County Library for the Blind
4845 Airline Road
Muskegon, MI 49444 — 231-737-6310
Fax: 231-724-6675
TDD: 231-722-4103
www.muskcolib.org

Summer reading programs, Braille typewriter, magnifiers, closed-circuit TV, large-print photocopier, cassette books and magazines, children's books on cassette, home visits and other reference materials on blindness and other handicaps, The Reading Edge, Perkins Braille and large print books.

Linda Clapp, Librarian

5247 Upper Peninsula Library for the Blind Physically Handicapped
1615 Presque Isle Avenue
Marquette, MI 49855 — 906-228-7697
Fax: 906-228-5627
rruff@uproc.lib.mi.us
www.upesc.lib.mi.us/uplbph

Summer reading programs, Braille writer, magnifiers, closed-circuit TV, large-print photocopier, cassette books and magazines, children's books on cassette, home visits and other reference materials on blindness and other handicaps.

Suzanne Dees, Executive Director

5248 Washtenaw County Library
PO Box 8645
Ann Arbor, MI 48107 — 734-222-6850
Fax: 734-222-6715
mcdaniev@ewashtenaw.org
www.ewashtenaw.org

Summer reading programs, Braille writer, magnifiers, closed-circuit TV, large-print photocopier, cassette books and magazines, children's books on cassette, home visits and other reference materials on blindness and other handicaps.

Verna J. Mcdaniel, Administrator

5249 Washtenaw County Library for the Blind and Physically Disabled
PO Box 8645
Ann Arbor, MI 48107 — 734-973-4600
Fax: 734-663-2430
lbpd@co.washtennaw.mi.us
www.ewashtenaw.org

Book lovers club. adaptive technology, cassette equipment, cassette books and magazines, described videos, low vision aids reference and referral services.

Kyeena Slater, Executive Director

5250 Wayne County Regional Library for the Blind
30555 Michigan Avenue
Westland, MI 48186 — 734-727-7300
888-968-2737
Fax: 734-727-7333
TTY: 734-727-7330
werlbph@tln.lib.mi.us
www.wayneregional.lib.mi.us

Summer reading programs, Braille writer, magnifiers, closed-circuit TV, large-print photocopier, cassette books and magazines, children's books on cassette, home visits and other reference materials on blindness and other handicaps.

Vanessa Morris, RegionalLibrarian
Sue Steiger, Librarian

Minnesota

5251 Minnesota Library for the Blind & Physically Handicapped
Highway 298, PO Box 68
Fairbault, MN 55021 — 507-333-4828
800-722-0550
Fax: 507-333-4832
libblnd@state.mn.us

Summer reading programs, Braille writer, magnifiers, closed-circuit TV, large-print photocopier, cassette, large print, Braille books and magazines, children's books on cassette, and other reference materials on blindness and other handicaps.

Catherine A Durivage, Program Director

Missouri

5252 Adriene Resource Center for Blind Children
1445 Boonville Avenue
Springfield, MO 65802 — 417-831-8000
800-641-4310
Fax: 800-328-0294
blind@ag.org
www.gospelpublishing.com

Offers Braille and cassette lending library, Braille and cassette Sunday school materials for all ages, Braille and cassette periodicals and resource assistance, and resources for blind children and children of blind parents.

Paul Weingariner, Director

5253 Assemblies of God National Center for the Blind
1445 Boonville Avenue
Springfield, MO 65802 — 417-831-1964
Fax: 417-862-5120
blind@ag.org
www.radiantlife.org

Offers Braille and cassette lending library, Braille and cassette Sunday school materials for all ages, Braille and cassette periodicals and resource assistance, and resources for blind children and children of blind parents.

Thomas Trask, Manager

5254 Wolfner Memorial Library for the Blind
PO Box 387
Jefferson City, MO 65102 — 573-751-8720
Fax: 573-526-2985
TDD: 800-347-1379
wolfner@sos.mo.gov

Summer reading programs, Braille writer, magnifiers, closed-circuit TV, large-print photocopier, cassette books and magazines, children's books on cassette, home visits and other reference materials on blindness and other handicaps.

Richard J Smith, Executive Director

Nebraska

5255   Nebraska Library Commission Talking Book & Braille Services
1200 N Street
Lincoln, NE 68508

402-471-2045
800-307-2665
Fax: 402-471-2083
TDD: 402-471-4038
doertli@nlc.state.ne.us
www.nlc.state.ne.us

Free loan of books and magazines on cassette and in Braille, including children's materials, along with specially designed playback equipment. Summer reading program for children, Braille embossing, closed circuit TV, large-print copier. Reference materials on blindness and other disabilities.

David Oerti, Librarian

New Jersey

5256   New Jersey State Library Talking Book and Braille Center
185 West State Street
Trenton, NJ 08625

609-278-2640
800-792-8322
Fax: 609-278-2647
TDD: 877-882-5593
njlbh@njstatelib.org
www.njstatelib.org

Free home delivery of large-print, audio, and Braille books and magazines, children's books on cassettes in Braille and other reference materials on blindness and other handicaps. Services are for New Jersey residents with print disabilities.

Adanrah Szczepaniak, Director
Anne McArthur, Head of Outreach and Audiovision

New Mexico

5257   New Mexico State Library for the Blind and Physically Handicapped
1209 Camino Carlos Ray
Santa Fe, NM 87507

505-476-9700
Fax: 505-476-9761
jbrewstr@stlib.state.nm.us
www.stlib.state.nm.us

Summer reading programs, Braille writer, magnifiers, closed-circuit TV, large-print photocopier, cassette books and magazines, children's books on cassette, home visits and other reference materials on blindness and other handicaps.

Susan Overland, Manager

New York

5258   New York State Talking Book & Braille Library
Empire State Plaza, CEC
Albany, NY 12230

518-474-5935
Fax: 518-486-1957
TDD: 518-474-7121
tbbl@mail.nysed.gov
www.suffolk.lib.ny.us

Books on audio cassette, cassette players, Braille books, summer reading programs, Braille writer, magnifiers, closed-circuit TV, large-print photocopier, cassette books and magazines, children's books on cassette, reference materials on blindness and other handicaps.

Jane Somers, Director

North Carolina

5259   North Carolina Library for the Blind
1841 Capital Boulevard
Raleigh, NC 27635

919-733-4376
Fax: 919-733-6910
TDD: 919-733-1462
nclbph@ncder.gov

Summer reading programs, Braille writer, magnifiers, closed-circuit TV, large-print photocopier, cassette books and magazines, children's books on cassette, home visits and other reference materials on blindness and other handicaps.

Francine Martin, Manager

Ohio

5260   American Council of Blind Parents
34400 Cedar Road, Apartment 108
University Heights, OH 44121

800-424-8666

Members are sighted parents of blind or visually impaired children. Offers a forum for support and outreach, sharing of experiences in parent-child relationships, and educational and cultural information about child development. Monitors developments in technical and legislative arenas.

Nola Webb, President

Oregon

5261   Oregon State Library, Talking Book and Braille Services
250 Winter Street NE
Salem, OR 97301

503-378-5389
800-452-0292
Fax: 503-585-8059
TTY: 503-378-4334
TDD: 503-378-4276
tbabs.info@state.or.us
www.tbabs.org

Cassette books and magazines, children's books on cassette, home visits and other reference materials on blindness and other handicaps.

Susan Westin, Manager

Virginia

5262   Alexandria Library Talking Book Service
5005 Duke Street
Alexandria, VA 22304

703-746-1760
Fax: 703-519-5916
TDD: 703-838-4568
emccaffr@lea.eda
www.alexandria.lib.va.us

Summer reading programs, Braille writer, magnifiers, closed-circuit TV, large-print photocopier, cassette books and magazines, children's books on cassette, home visits and other reference materials on blindness and other handicaps.

Karen Russell, Manager

5263   Division for the Visually Handicapped
1920 Association Drive
Reston, VA 20191

703-620-3660

Members are teachers, college faculty members, administrators, supervisors and others concerned with the education and welfare of visually handicapped and blind children and youth. This is a division of the Council For Exceptional Children.

Dr. Kay Ferrell, President

5264 Division on Visual Impairments
Council for Exceptional Children
1110 North Glebe Road, Suite 300
Arlington, VA 22201   800-224-6830
                                  Fax: 703-264-9494
                                  TTY: 866-915-5000
        www.ed.arizona.edu/dvi/welcome.htm; www.cec.sped.org

A division within the CEC, it handles concerns for Federal, state and local issues and policies related to education of youths, children and infants with visual impairments.

Ellyn Ross, President
Shirley J Wilson, Secretary
Phyllis T Simmons, President Elect

5265 Virginia State Library for the Visually and Physically Handicapped
1901 Roane Street
Richmond, VA 23222   804-367-0014

Summer reading programs, Braille writer, magnifiers, closed-circuit TV, large-print photocopier, cassette books and magazines, children's books on cassette, home visits and other reference materials on blindness and other handicaps.

Mary Ruth Halapatz, Librarian

Washington

5266 Washington Library for the Blind and Physically Handicapped
1000 Fourth Ave.
Seattle, WA 98104   206-386-4636
                                  Fax: 206-386-4685
                                  wtbbl@spl.lib.wa.us
                                  www.spl.lib.wa.us

Summer reading programs, Braille writer, magnifiers, closed-circuit TV, large-print photocopier, cassette books and magazines, children's books on cassette, home visits and other reference materials on blindness and other handicaps.

Marcellus Turner, Librarian

West Virginia

5267 West Virginia School for the Blind
301 E Main Street
Romney, WV 26757   304-822-4801
                                  Fax: 304-822-3370
                                  cjohn@access.mountain.net

Summer reading programs, Braille writer, magnifiers, closed-circuit TV, large-print photocopier, cassette books and magazines, children's books on cassette, home visits and other reference materials on blindness and other handicaps.

Patsy Shank, Administrator

Research Centers

5268 Center for the Partially Sighted
6101 W Centinela Ave, Suite 150
Culver City, CA 90230   310-988-1970
                                  Fax: 310-988-1980
                                  info@low-vision.org
                                  www.low-vision.org

Provides professional, comprehensive vision rehabilitation services to visually impaired people of all ages. For those whose sight is severely limited due to macular degeneration, diabetic retinopathy, glaucoma, retinal detachment, stroke or other conditions not correctable medically or surgically.

La Donna S.Ringering, President

5269 Mobile Association for the Blind
2440 Gordon Smith Drive
Mobile, AL 36617   251-473-3585
                                  877-292-5463
                                  Fax: 251-470-8622
                                  sales@mobileblind.org
                                  www.mobileblind.org

Offers work adjustment training, activities of daily living, mobility, communication skills and sheltered employment for adults and children who are visually impaired.

James Bullock, Executive Director

5270 New Beginnings - The Blind Children's Center
4120 Marathon Street
Los Angeles, CA 90029   323-664-2153
                                  Fax: 323-665-3828
                                  www.blindchildrenscenter.org

The purpose of the Center is to turn initial fears into hope. Helps children and their families become independent by creating a climate of safety and trust. Children learn to develop self confidence and to master a wide range of skills. Services include an infant stimulation program, educational preschool, interdisciplinary assessment services, family services, correspondence program, toll free national hotline and a publication and research service.

5271 Research to Prevent Blindness
645 Madison Avenue
New York, NY 10022   212-752-4333
                                  800-621-0026
                                  Fax: 212-688-6231
                                  inforequest@rpbusa.org
                                  www.rpbusa.org

Provides research grants to scientists interested in eye disease and vision disorders.

Jules Stein, Founder
David F. Weeks, Chairman
Diane Swift, President

Audio Video

5272 Heart to Heart
Blind Children's Center
4120 Marathon Street
Los Angeles, CA 90029   323-644-2153
                                  Fax: 323-665-3828
                                  www.blindcntr.org

Parents of blind and partially sighted children talk about their feelings.

Videotape

5273 Let's Eat
Blind Children's Center
4120 Marathon Street
Los Angeles, CA 90029   213-664-2153
                                  Fax: 213-665-3828

Teaches competent feeding skills to children with visual impairments.

Videotape

5274 See What I Feel
Britannica Film Co.
345 4th Street
San Francisco, CA 94107   415-597-5555

A blind child tells her friends about her trip to the zoo. Each experience was explained as a blind child would experience it. A teacher's guide comes with this video.

Films

Web Sites

5275 American Nystagmus Network
303-D Beltline Place, #321
Decatur, AL 35603   www.nystagmus.org

Is a nonprofit organization established to serve the needs and interests of those affected by Nystagmus.

Rick Beaudet, President
Jim Conley, Vice President
Tony Fuhrer, Treasurer

5276 Lighthouse Guild
15 West 65th Street
New York, NY 10023

212-769-6200
800-284-4422
info@lighthouseguild.org
www.lighthouseguild.org

Since 1905, Lighthouse International has led the charge in the fight against vision loss through prevention, treatment and empowerment. In 2013, it merged with Jewish Guild Healthcare to form a leading non profit vision and healthcare organization.

Alan R. Morse, President/CEO
Mark G. Ackermann, Executive VP/COO
Maura J. Sweeney, Senior VP, Programs & Services

5277 National Alliance of Blind Students
www.blindstudents.org

The leading national advocacy and consumer organization for students in high school or college who are blind or visually impaired.

5278 National Association for Visually Handicapped
111 E 59th St
New York, NY 10022
www.navh.org

Serves as a clearing house for information about all services available to the partially-sighted from public and private sources. Conducts self help groups. Provides information on large print books, textbooks, and educational tools.

Rick Beaudet, President
Jim Conley, Vice President
Tony Fuhrer, Treasurer

5279 Nystagmus Network
25 Eden Way
Beckenham, KT BR3 3

29 -045-4242
shop@nystagmusnet.org
www.nystagmusnet.org

A UK-based self-help group set up to provide support for adults and children with nystagmus, their parents and teachers and foster research into the condition.

5280 Online Mendelian Inheritance in Man
National Library of Medicine Building 38A
Bethesda, MD 20894

888-346-3656
info@ncbi.nlm.nih.gov
www.ncbi.nlm.nih.gov

This database is a catalog of human genes and genetic disorders.

5281 Royal National Institute of the Blind
105 Judd Street
London, WC1H

303-123-9999
helpline@rnib.org.uk
www.rnib.org.uk

A leading UK charity offering information, support and advice to over two million people with sight problems.

Miriam Martin, Chief Executive
Wanda Hamilton, Group Director
Fazilet Hadi, Managing Director

Magazines

5282 Journal of Visual Impairment and Blindness
American Foundation for the Blind
2 Penn Plaza, Suite 1102
New York, NY 10121

212-502-7600
Fax: 212-502-7777
afbinfo@afb.net
www.afb.org

Published in braille, regular print and on cassette this journal contains a wide variety of subjects including rehabilitation, psychology, education, legislation, medicine, technology, employment, sensory aids and childhood development as they relate to visual impairments.

10x Year

Carl Augusto, President and CEO
Rick Bozeman, Chief Financial Officer
Kelly Bleach, Chief Administrative Officer

5283 NAVH Update
National Association for Visually Handicapped
111 E 59th St
New York, NY 10022

212-889-3141
800-284-4422
Fax: 212-727-2931
navh@navh.org
www.navh.org

This newsletter offers short stories, news, medical updates, assistive device information, poems, resources, crossword puzzles and more for the visually impaired.

quarterly

5284 Reaching, Crawling, Walking - Let's Get Moving
Blind Children's Center
4120 Marathon Street
Los Angeles, CA 90029

323-664-2153
Fax: 323-665-3828
info@blindchildrenscenter.org
www.blindchildrenscenter.org

Orientation and mobility for visually impaired preschool children.

24 pages

5285 Tactic
Clovernook Home and School for the Blind
400 Continental Blvd., Suite 600
El Segundo, CA 90245

310-426-2236
Fax: 513-728-3950
contact@southpawtech.com
www.southpawtech.com/tactic/

Quarterly

Newsletters

5286 National Library Service for the Blind & Physically Handicapped
Library of Congress Reference Section
1291 Taylor Street NW
Washington, DC 20542

202-707-5100
800-424-8567
Fax: 202-707-0712
TTY: 202-707-0744
TDD: 202-707-0744
nls@loc.gov
www.loc.gov/nls

Provides information and advocacy resources for families and professionals, including listings of organizations focusing on more specific areas of concern to families and young adults who have disabilities. Administers a natural library service that provides recorded and braille reading materials to eligible children and adults who cannot read standard print.

12 pages Quarterly
ISSN: 1046-1663

Vicki Fitzpatrick, Editor

5287 Talking Book Topics
National Library Services for the Blind
1291 Taylor Street NW
Washington, DC 20542

202-707-5100
Fax: 202-707-0712
TDD: 202-707-0744
www.loc.gov/nls

Offers hundreds of listings of books, fiction and nonfiction, for adults and children on cassette. Also offers listings on foreign language books on cassette, talking magazines and reviews.

Bimonthly

Pamphlets

5288 **Dancing Cheek to Cheek**
Blind Children's Center
4120 Marathon Street
Los Angeles, CA 90029
323-664-2153
Fax: 323-665-3828
www.blindchildrenscenter.org

Discusses beginning social, play and language interactions.
33 pages

5289 **Family Guide - Growth and Development of the Partially Seeing Child**
National Association for Visually Handicapped
111 E 59th St
New York, NY 10022
212-889-3141
800-284-4422
Fax: 212-727-2931
navh@navh.org
www.navh.org

Offers information for parents and guidelines in raising a partially seeing child.

5290 **Family Guide to Vision Care**
American Optometric Association
243 N Lindbergh Boulevard
Saint Louis, MO 63141
314-991-4100
Fax: 314-991-4101
www.aoanet.org

Offers information on the early developmental years of your vision, finding a family optometrist and how to take care of your eyesight through the learning years, the working years and the mature years.

5291 **Heart to Heart**
Blind Children's Center
4120 Marathon Street
Los Angeles, CA 90029
323-664-2153
Fax: 323-665-3828
www.blindchildrenscenter.org

Parents of blind and partially sighted children talk about their feelings.
12 pages

5292 **Learning to Play**
Blind Children's Center
4120 Marathon Street
Los Angeles, CA 90029
323-664-2153
Fax: 323-665-3828
www.blindchildrenscenter.org

Discusses how to present play activities to the visually impaired preschool child.
12 pages

5293 **Let's Eat**
Blind Children's Center
4120 Marathon Street
Los Angeles, CA 90029
323-664-2153
Fax: 323-665-3828
www.blindchildrenscenter.org

Teaches competent feeding skills to children with visual impairments.
28 pages

5294 **Move with Me**
Blind Children's Center
4120 Marathon Street
Los Angeles, CA 90029
323-664-2153
Fax: 323-665-3828
www.blindchildrenscenter.org

A parent's guide to movement development for visually impaired babies.

12 pages

5295 **Selecting a Program**
Blind Children's Center
4120 Marathon Street
Los Angeles, CA 90029
323-664-2153
Fax: 323-665-3828
www.blindchildrenscenter.org

A guide for parents of infants and preschoolers with visual impairments.
28 pages

5296 **Standing on My Own Two Feet**
Blind Children's Center
4120 Marathon Street
Los Angeles, CA 90029
323-664-2153
Fax: 323-665-3828
info@blindchildrenscenter.org
www.blindchildrenscenter.org

A step-by-step guide to designing and constructing simple, individually tailored adaptive mobility devices for preschool-age children who are visually impaired.
36 pages

5297 **Talk to Me**
Blind Children's Center
4120 Marathon Street
Los Angeles, CA 90029
323-664-2153
Fax: 323-665-3828
www.blindchildrenscenter.org

A language guide for parents of deaf children.
11 pages

5298 **Talk to Me II**
Blind Children's Center
4120 Marathon Street
Los Angeles, CA 90029
323-664-2153
Fax: 323-665-3828
www.blindchildrenscenter.org

A sequel to Talk To Me, available in English and Spanish.
15 pages

Camps

5299 **Bloomfield**
35375 Mullholland Highway
Malibu, CA 90065
310-457-5330
800-352-2290
Fax: 310-457-3952
smanning@juniorblind.org
www.juniorblind.org

This camp is dedicated to serving blind and developmentally disabled children and adults.

Shirley Manning, Director of Recreation
Joan Marason, Director

5300 **Florida School-Deaf and Blind Summer Camp**
207 N. San Marco Avenue
Saint Augustine, FL 32084
904-827-2200
800-344-3732
Fax: 904-245-1022
info@fsdb.k12.fl.us
www.fsdb.k12.fl.us

The Florida School for the Deaf and the Blind hosts summer campers from all over teh state of Florida for a week of fun and adventure. FSDB's 80 acre campus is where campers participate in a variety of activities including rock climbing, archery, swimming, kayaking, team games, arts and crafts, dance music, and much more.

L Daniel Hutto, President
Cindy Day, Executive Director of Parent Svcs
Terri Wiseman, Administrator of Business Services

5301 National Camps for Blind Children
Christian Record
4444 S 52nd Street
Lincoln, NE 68516
402-488-0981
Fax: 402-488-7582
info@christianrecord.org
www.christianrecord.org

Camps throughout the US and Canada are offered at no cost to the legally blind, ages 9-65. Activities include archery, beeper basketball, water sports, hiking and rock climbing and horseback riding.

Peggy Hansen, Director
Larry Pitcher, President

5302 VISIONS/Vacation Camp for the Blind
500 Greenwich Street, 3rd Floor
New York, NY 10013
212-625-1616
888-245-8333
Fax: 212-219-4078
info@visionsvcb.org
www.visionsvcb.org

Family programs at Vacation Camp for the Blind in Rockland County, NY for children who are blind, severely visually impaired or multi-handicapped. Parent or guardian must attend winter weekends and summer session.

Nancy T. Jones, President
Richard P. Simon, Vice President
Burton M. Strauss, Jr., Treasurer

DESCRIPTION

5303 OBESITY

Involves the following Biologic System(s):
Developmental/Behavioral/Psychiatric Disorders, Endocrinologic Disorders

Obesity refers to a condition in which there is an excessive accumulation of fat in subcutaneous (below the skin) and other tissues of the body. Being obese and being overweight are not necessarily synonymous, as people who are overweight may have an increased body size as a result of increased muscle or skeletal tissue mass. Obesity in children may develop at any age, but peak development periods occur during the first 12 months of life, between the ages of five and six years, and during the adolescent years. The obesity epidemic is especially evident in industrialized nations where many people live sedentary lives and eat more convenience foods, which are typically high in calories and low in nutritional value, and is becoming an epidemic in the western hemisphere. Obesity may result from an increase in the actual number of fat cells or from an increase in the size of the individual fat cells. Researchers believe that fat cells increase in number in proportion to caloric intake increase and that this increase is particularly evident in the first 12 months of life. As children grow, increases in fat cell populations continue at a slower rate. Because the number of fat cells cannot be decreased, except surgically, later weight loss must result from the reduction of fat in individual cells.

Obesity usually results when caloric intake exceeds the energy demands of the body, thus increasing the storage of body fat. Fat accumulation is usually a progressive process, resulting from repeated episodes of food intake exceeding the body's demand for energy (calories). Many factors may influence appetite or obesity. Such factors may include environmental influences; psychologic disturbances that may be induced by stress or emotional upset or trauma; brain lesions that may involve certain areas of the brain such as the hypothalamus or the pituitary gland (both essential to hormone production); an overabundance of insulin in the body (hyperinsulinism); and genetic influences. In addition, in rare instances, obesity may be a feature of certain genetic disorders.

Complications of childhood obesity may include respiratory difficulties such as shortness of breath and increased cardiovascular risk factors such as high blood pressure, elevated total cholesterol levels as well as increased bad or LDL cholesterol and decreased good or HDL cholesterol, and increased levels of fatty acid and glycerol compounds (triglycerides). In addition, childhood obesity may be associated with a resistance to the hormone insulin that aids in the metabolism of glucose, fats, carbohydrates, and proteins. This resistance may lead to excessive levels of circulating insulin in the body (hyperinsulinism); however, the body is not able to appropriately use insulin and Type 2 Diabetes Mellitus results. The symptoms associated with insulin resistance may include hunger, weight loss, sweating, and tremor.

The diagnosis of obesity in children and adolescents is usually determined through the use of certain screening methods such as measurement of the body mass index (BMI) as well as the triceps skinfold thickness. In addition, special consideration may be given to certain criteria in determining differential diagnosis and possible treatment. These criteria may include elevated blood pressure; high total cholesterol levels; regular and consecutive increases in annual body mass index screenings; psychologic or emotional weight concerns; and a family history of heart disease, elevated cholesterol levels, and diabetes.

Patterns of behavior that may lead to obesity may be established as early as infancy. For example, if parents or caregivers persistently use a bottle to pacify a crying baby, the baby may learn that food is equivalent to relief of stress. Treatment for childhood and adolescent obesity should include the cooperation and support of the entire family and may be directed toward psychologic considerations, as well as proper exercise and nutrition to avoid complications. Treatment for psychologic and emotional needs may include behavior modification, as well as individual and family counseling.

For more information on binge eating, see chapter on Eating Disorders.

National Associations & Support Groups

5304 Action for Healthy Kids
600 West Van Buren Street, Suite #720
Chicago, IL 60607   800-416-5136
                                Fax: 312-212-0098
                     trainings@ActionforHealthyKids.org
                          www.actionforhealthykids.org

Action for Healthy Kidsr fights childhood obesity, undernourishment and physical inactivity by helping schools become healthier places so kids can live healthier lives.
Loren Fisher-Coleman, Director of Communications
Rob Bisceglie, M.A., Chief Executive Officer
Jill Camber Davidson, School Program Manager

5305 African American Collaborative Obesity Research Network
www.aacorn.org

                     skumanyi@mail.med.upenn.edu
                                www.aacorn.org

AACORN is a collaboration of U.S. researchers, scholars-in-training, and community-based research partners.
Shiriki K. Kumanyika, PhD, MPH, Founder & Chair
Vikki C. Lassiter, MS, Executive Director

5306 Alliance for a Healthier Generation
606 SE 9th Ave
Portland, OR 97214   888-KID-HLTH
                          www.healthiergeneration.org

The Alliance for a Healthier Generation is a catalyst for children's health. They work with schools, companies, community organizations, healthcare professionals and families to transform the conditions and systems that lead to healthier kids.
Dr. Howell Wechsler, Chief Executive Officer

5307 American Academy of Pediatrics
141 Northwest Point Boulevard
Elk Grove Village, IL 60007   847-434-4000
                                      800-433-9016
                                 Fax: 847-434-8000
                                        www.aap.org

The American Academy of Pediatrics and its member pediatricians are committed to the attainment of optimal physical, mental and social health and well-being for all infants, children, adolescents, and young adults.
Fernando Stein, MD, FAAP, President
Karen Remley, MD, CEO/Executive VP

5308   American Beverage Association
1101 Sixteenth St. NW
Washington, DC 20036
202-463- 673
Fax: 202-659-5349
info@ameribev.org
www.ameribev.org

The American Beverage Association (ABA) is the trade association that represents America's non-alcoholic beverage industry.

Susan K. Neely, President/ CEO
Mark Hammond, SVP/ CFO
William Dermody, Vice President, Policy

5309   American Medical Association
AMA Plaza, 330 North Wabash Ave., Suite 39300
Chicago, IL 60611
800-262-3211
www.ama-assn.org/ama

AMA is dedicated to ensuring sustainable physician practices that result in better health outcomes for patients.

James L. Madara, MD, CEO/ EVP
Bernard L. Hengesbaugh, Chief Operating Officer
Kenneth J. Sharigian, SVP/ Chief Strategy Officer

5310   American Obesity Treatment Association
117 Anderson Court Suite 1
Dothan, AL 36303
334-403-4057
info@americanobesity.org
www.americanobesity.org

AOTA was formed to bring together individuals who are facing the often life-long struggle with obesity.

Cesar Cuneo, President/ Founder
Gonzalo Tovar, Vice President
Connie Pillares, Fundraising

5311   American Psychological Association
750 First St. NE
Washington, DC 20002
202-336-5500
800-374-2721
TTY: 202-336-6123
www.apa.org

The mission is to advance the creation, communication and application of psychological knowledge to benefit society and improve people's lives.

Norman B. Anderson, PhD, CEO/ EVP
L. Michael Honaker, PhD, Deputy Chief Executive Officer
Ellen G. Garrison, PhD, Senior Policy Advisor

5312   American School Counselor Association
1101 King Street, Suite 310
Alexandria, VA 22314
703-683-2722
800-306-4722
Fax: 703-997-7572
asca@schoolcounselor.org
www.schoolcounselor.org

The mission of ASCA is to represent professional school counselors and to promote professionalism and ethical practices.

Richard Wong, Executive Director
Jeff Broderson, Information Technology Admin.
Kathleen M Rakestraw, Director of Communications

5313   American Society for Metabolic and Bariatric Surgery
100 SW 75th Street, Suite 201
Gainesville, FL 32607
352-331-4900
Fax: 352-331-4975
info@asmbs.org
asmbs.org

The vision of the Society is to improve public health and well being by lessening the burden of the disease of obesity and related diseases throughout the world.

Georgeann Mallory, RD, Executive Director
Kristie Kaufman, Director of Operations
Kim Carmichael, Financial Manager

5314   American Society for Nutrition
9650 Rockville Pike
Bethesda, MD 20814
301-634-7050
Fax: 301-634-7894
www.nutrition.org

The American Society for Nutrition (ASN) is a non-profit organization dedicated to bringing together the world's top researchers, clinical nutritionists and industry to advance our knowledge and application of nutrition for the sake of humans and animals.

Simin Nikbin Meydani, DVM, PhD, President
Gwen Twillman, VP, Education & Professional Dev
John E. Courtney, PhD, Executive Officer

5315   American Society of Bariatric Physicians
2821 S. Parker Road, Ste. 625
Aurora, CO 80014
303-770-2526
Fax: 303-779-4834
www.asbp.org

The American Society of Bariatric Physiciansr (ASBPr) is the leading association for physicians and other health care providers dedicated to the comprehensive medical treatment of patients affected by obesity and associated conditions. Many ASBP-member physicians also hold certification from the American Board of Obesity Medicine.

Eric C. Westman, MD, MHS, President
Wendy Scinta, MD, MS, Vice President
Craig Primack, MD, FAAP, FACP, Secretary/Treasurer

5316   American Society of Clinical Oncology
2318 Mill Road, Suite 800
Alexandria, VA 22314
571-483-1300
www.asco.org

ASCO was founded in 1964 by a small group of physician members of the American Association of Cancer Research (AACR) who recognized the need for the creation of a separate society dedicated to issues unique to clinical oncology.

Peter Paul Yu, MD, FACP, FASCO, President
Allen S. Lichter, MD, FASCO, ASCO CEO and CCF CEO (ex-officio)
Richard L. Schilsky,, Chief Medical Officer

5317   American Thoracic Society
25 Broadway
New York, NY 10004
212-315-8600
Fax: 212-315-6498
ATSInfo@Thoracic.org
www.thoracic.org

The American Thoracic Society improves global health by advancing research, patient care, and public health in pulmonary disease, critical illness, and sleep disorders. Founded in 1905 to combat TB, the ATS has grown to tackle asthma, COPD, lung cancer, sepsis, acute respiratory distress, and sleep apnea, among other diseases.

Thomas W. Ferkol, MD, President
Atul Malhotra, MD, President-elect
Stephen C. Crane, PhD, MPH, Executive Director

5318   CHEF - Comprehensive Health Education Foun dation
159 S Jackson Street Suite 510
Seattle, WA 98104
206-824-2907
800-323-2433
Fax: 206-824-3072
TTY: 800-833-6388
info@chef.org
www.chef.org

Addresses issues that are pertinent to the health and well-being of today's society. A leader in prevention education, provider of skills and information and resources.

Scott Bozman, Chairman
Rudy Vasquez, Vice-Chair
Rick Mockler, Treasurer

5319   Child Care Aware of America
1515 N. Courthouse Rd, 11th fl
Arlington, VA 22201
703-341-4100
Fax: 703-341-4101
jobs@usa.childcareaware.org
usa.childcareaware.org

They work with state and local Child Care Resource and Referral agencies (CCR&Rs) and other community partners to ensure that all families have access to quality, affordable child care.

L. Carol Scott, Ph.D., President
Sandy Myers, Vice President
Lynette M. Fraga, Ph.D., Executive Director

5320 Children's Hospital Association
600 13th Street, NW, Suite 500
Washington, DC 20005   202-753-5500
                                   Fax: 202-347-5147
                               www.childrenshospitals.net

Representing more than 220 children's hospitals, the Association is the voice of children's hospitals nationally. The Association champions public policies that enable hospitals to better serve children and is the premier resource for pediatric data and analytics, driving improved clinical and operational performance of member hospitals.

Mark Wietecha, President/ CEO
Amy Knight, SVP/ COO
David Bertoch, VP, Informatics Services

5321 Compulsive Eaters Anonymous
3371 Glendale Boulevard, Suite 104
Los Angeles, CA 90039   323-660-4333
                                   Fax: 323-660-4334
                                   gso@ceahow.org
                                   www.ceahow.org

A twelve-step program, with the primary purpose of, to stop eating compulsively.

K Pamela, President
N Woody, Vice-President
M David, Treasurer

5322 Food Research and Action Center
1200 18th Street NW, Suite 400
Washington, DC 20036   202-986-2200
                                   Fax: 202-986-2525
                                   frac.org

RAC works with hundreds of national, state and local nonprofit organizations, public agencies, corporations and labor organizations to address hunger, food insecurity, and their root cause, poverty.

James D. Weill, President
Mike Ambrose, Web Communications Coordinator
Colleen Barton Sutton, Communications Director

5323 National Collaborative on Childhood Obesity Research
nccor.org
                                   202-884-8313
                                   tphillips@fhi360.org
                                   nccor.org

NCCOR focuses on efforts that have the potential to benefit children, teens, and their families, and the communities in which they live.

5324 National Eating Disorders Association (NED A)
165 West 46th St.
New York, NY 10036   212-575-6200
                                   800-931-2237
                                   Fax: 212-575-1650
                           info@NationalEatingDisorders.org
                           www.nationaleatingdisorders.org

Formed in 2001 when Eating Disorders Awareness & Prevention (EDAP) and the American Anorexia Bulimia Association (AABA) joined forces. It works to eliminate eating disorders through prevention efforts, education, referral and support services, advocacy, training, and research.

Bob Kovarik, Chairman
Deborah Q. Belfatto, Vice Chair
Phoeba Megna, Secretary

5325 National Obesity Foundation
10921 Wilshire Blvd, #1114
Los Angeles, CA 90024   800-663-9300
                                   info@nofusa.org
                                   nofusa.org

A non-profit organization created to help Americans who are struggling with obesity and its related diseases.

Isaac Verbukh, MD, Founding Director/ President
Fira Verbukh, Director
Gedion Ismael, Humanitarian Awards Program Dir

5326 National Resource Center for Health & Safety in Child Care & Early Education
13120 E. 19th Ave., Mail Stop F541, PO Box 6511
Aurora, CO 80045   800-598-5437
                                   Fax: 303-724-0960
                                   info@nrckids.org
                                   nrckids.org

Works to improve the quality of child care and early education programs by supporting child care providers and early educators, families, health professionals, early childhood comprehensive systems, state child care regulatory agencies, state and local health departments, and policy makers in their efforts to identify and promote healthy and safe child care and early education programs.

5327 Obesity Action Coalition
4511 North Himes Avenue, Suite 250
Tampa, FL 33614   800-717-3117
                                   www.obesityaction.org

The Obesity Action Coalition (OAC) is a nearly 50,000 member-strong 501(c)(3) National non-profit organization dedicated to giving a voice to the individual affected by the disease of obesity and helping individuals along their journey toward better health through education, advocacy and support.

Joseph Nadglowski, President/ Chief Executive Officer
Kristy Kuna, VP, Programs and Operations
James Zervios, VP, Marketing and Communications

5328 Partnership for a Healthier America
ahealthieramerica.org
                                   info@ahealthieramerica.org
                                   ahealthieramerica.org

The Partnership for a Healthier America (PHA) is devoted to working with the private sector to ensure the health of our nation's youth by solving the childhood obesity crisis.

Lawrence A. Soler, President/ Chief Executive Officer

5329 Rudd Center for Food Policy & Obesity
University of Connecticut (UConn), One Constitutio
Hartford, CT 6103   860-380-1000
                                   rudd.center@uconn.edu
                                   www.yaleruddcenter.org

The Rudd Center for Food Policy & Obesity is a non-profit research and public policy organization devoted to improving the world's diet, preventing obesity, and reducing weight stigma.

Marlene B. Schwartz, PhD, Director
Rebecca M. Puhl, PhD, Deputy Director
Roberta R. Friedman, ScM, Director of Public Policy

5330 Shape Up America
www.shapeup.org

Founded in 1994, Shape Up America!r is a 501(c)3 not-for-profit organization committed to raising awareness of obesity as a health issue and to providing responsible information on healthy weight management.

Barbara J. Moore, PhD, President/ Chief Executive Officer
Adrienne Forman, MS, RD, Director of Nutrition Comm.
Alex Colcord, MA, CTO/ Director of Content

5331 The Campaign to End Obesity
805 15th Street, N.W., Suite 650
Washington, DC 20005   202-466-8100
                                   www.obesitycampaign.org

By bringing together leaders from across industry, academia and public health with policymakers and their advisors, the Campaign provides the information and guidance that decision-makers need to make policy changes that will reverse one of the nation's costliest and most prevalent diseases.

Stephanie Silverman, Cofounder
Drew Littman, Director, Policy
Chris Fox, Director, External Affairs

5332 The Obesity Society
8757 Georgia Avenue, Suite 1320
Silver Spring, MD 20910
301-563-6526
800-974-3084
Fax: 301-563-6595
fdea@obesity.org
www.obesity.org

The Obesity Society is the leading professional society dedicated to better understanding, preventing and treating obesity.

Francesca M. Dea, CAE, Executive Director
Julia Strachan, Governance and Executive Assistant
Kathie Cleary, Senior Director, Finance and Admin

Libraries & Resource Centers

5333 National Digestive Diseases Information Clearinghouse
9000 Rockville Pike
Bethesda, MD 20892
301-496-3583
800-860-8747
Fax: 703-738-4929
healthinfo@niddk.nih.gov
www.niddk.nih.govv

The National Institute of Diabetes and Digestive and Kidney Diseases conducts and supports research on many of the most serious diseases affecting public health. The Institute supports much of the clinical research on the diseases of internal medicine and related subspecialty fields as well as many basic science disciplines.

Dr. Griffin P. Rodgers, Director
Dr. Gregory G. Germino, Deputy Directortary
Camille M. Hoover, M.S.W., Executive Officer

Research Centers

5334 New York Obesity Research Center
Saint Luke's-Roosevelt Hospital Center
1111 Amsterdam Avenue, 14th Floor, Babcock 10
New York, NY 10025
212-523-4161
Fax: 212-523-4830
katmarquez@chpnet.org
www.nyorc.org

Dr F Xavier Pi-Sunyer, Co-Director
Dr. Rudolph Leibel, Co-Director
Rudolf L. Leibel, Core Director

5335 University of Chicago-Department of Psychi atry
5841 S Maryland Avenue. MC 3077, Rm W-413
Chicago, IL 60637
773-834-1007
Fax: 773-702-9929
eaccurso@uchicago.edu
www.psychiatry.uchicago.edu

Emil F. Coccaro, Chairman
Jean Harris, Secretary
Robert Naclerio, Research Administrator

Audio Video

5336 Reality Matters - Obesity & Nutrition
Discovery Education
PO Box 2284
South Burlington, VT 5407
888-892-3484
education_info@discovery.com
store.discoveryeduction.com

Teenagers have always been drawn to junk food, but more than ever, today's teens are suffering at the hands of less active lifestyles and unhealthy eating habits. Explore America's culture of obesity and its contributing factors-along with ways to help kids make healthy choices.

DVD/VHS 30 minutes

Web Sites

5337 American Anorexia Bulimia Association of P hiladelphia
PO Box 27156
Philadelphia, PA 19118
www.aabaphila.org

Support for sufferers friends and family.

5338 Gurze Books
5145 B Avenida Encinas
Carlsbad, CA 92008
800-756-7533
www.gurze.com

Specializes in information about eating disorders including anorexia nervosa, bulimia nervosa, and binge eating, plus related topics such as body image and obesity. Books are offered at discounted prices, many free articles about eating disorders, newsletters, links to treatment facilities, organizations, other websites and much more.

5339 Obesity Online
www.obesity-online.com/

Is a multi-disciplinary forum for research and treatment of massive obesity, including plastics, psychiatry, endocrinology nutrition, nursing, dietetics and allied health.

Book Publishers

5340 Feed Your Kids Well: How to Help Your Child Lose Weight and Get Healthy
Fred Pescatore MD, author

Wiley Publishing, Inc
10475 Crosspoint Boulevard
Indianapolis, IN 46256
317-572-3000
877-762-2974
Fax: 800-597-3299
consumer@wiley.com
www.wiley.com

Aimed toward parents, this book offers advice and tips to help their children lose excess weight. It also examines the popular fat-free diet fads and advises diets containing the small amounts of fat that are crucial to human growth.

1999 304 pages Paperback
ISBN: 0-471349-63-1

Peter B. Wiley, Chairman
Stephen M. Smith, President & CEO
Ellis E. Cousens, Executive Vice President, Chief Fin

5341 Let's Talk About Being Overweight
Melanie Apel Gordon, author

Rosen Publishing Group's PowerKids Press
29 E 21st Street
New York, NY 10010
212-777-3017
800-237-9932
Fax: 888-436-4643
rosenpub@tribeca.ios.com
www.rosenpublishing.com

Reminds kids that everyone's body is different and assures them that it is okay. Readers will also learn that they will feel better if they eat right and get regular exercise. Grades K-5.

2000 24 pages
ISBN: 0-823954-13-7

Roger Rosen, President

5342 Making Peace with Food
Gurze Books
5145 B Avenida Encinas, PO Box 2238
Carlsbad, CA 92008
760-434-7533
800-756-7533
Fax: 760-434-5476
leigh@gurze.net
www.gurze.com

Filled with ideas, workbook pages, exercises, and resources, an excellent aid to clarifying and overcoming your personal diet/weight struggle.

224 pages Paperback

Suan Kano, Author

5343 Obesity Sourcebook
Omnigraphics
PO Box 625
Holmes, PA 19043   800-234-1340
                                              Fax: 800-875-1340
                                              info@omnigraphics.com
                                              www.omnigraphics.com

Basic consumer health information about diseases and other problems associated with obesity, including risk factors, prevention and management.

2001 376 pages
ISBN: 0-780803-33-7

Peter Ruffner, Publisher

5344 Overeaters Anonymous Lifeline Sampler
World Service Office
6075 Zenith Court NE, PO Box 44020
Rio Rancho, NM 87144   505-891-2664
                                              Fax: 505-891-4320
                                              info@overeatersanonymous.org
                                              www.overeatersanonymous.org

A selection of articles from Lifeline magazine. Issues and topics include: relationships in recovery, food and weight, relapse, spiritual insights, abstinent living and traditions and steps.

448 pages

5345 Twelve Steps and Twelve Traditions of Over eaters Anonymous
World Service Office
6075 Zenith Court NE, PO Box 44020
Rio Rancho, NM 87144   505-891-2664
                                              Fax: 505-891-4320
                                              info@overeatersanonymous.org
                                              www.overeatersanonymous.org

Provides a detailed exploration of how the 12 traditions help members recover and how the Fellowship functions as a whole.

240 pages Softcover

5346 Understanding Childhood Obesity

J Clinton Smith MD, author

University Press of Mississippi
3825 Ridgewood Road
Jackson, MS 39211   601-432-6205
                                              800-737-7788
                                              Fax: 601-432-6217
                                              press@ihl.state.ms.us
                                              www.upress.state.ms.us

A clear explanation of causes, diagnosis, and treatment of childhood obesity. A comprehensive guide that covers nearly every field of obesity research.

120 pages Paper
ISBN: 1-578061-34-2

5347 When Food is Love

Geneen Roth, author

Gurze Books
PO Box 2238
Carlsbad, CA 92018   760-434-7533
                                              800-756-7533
                                              Fax: 760-434-5467
                                              mylo@gurze.net
                                              www.gurze.com

Drawing on her own personal experience, Roth explores similarities between eating and loving such as fantasizing, wanting the forbidden, creating drama, control issues, and the experience of relationship.

1991 205 pages Paperback
ISBN: 0-452268-18-4

Leigh Cohn, Publisher & Marketing
Lindsey Hall Cohn, Editor-in-Chief

Pamphlets

5348 Media-Smart Youth: Eat, Think, and Be Acti ve Fact Sheet
Natl Institute of Child Health & Human Development
P.O. Box 3006
Rockvill, MD 20852   301-496-5133
                                              800-370-2943
                                              Fax: 866-760-5947
                                              TTY: 888-320-6942
                                              NICHDInformationResourceCenter@mail.nih.
                                              www.nichd.nih.gov

Free government information on an interactive after-school education program that helps young people between the ages of 11 and 13 understand how physical activity and nutrition can influence their health.

2005 2 pages

Alan E. Guttmacher, Director

Camps

5349 Camp Shane
302 Harris Road
Ferndale, NY 12734   845-292-4644
                                              Fax: 845-292-8636
                                              office@campshane.com
                                              www.campshane.com

Camp dedicated to weight loss.

David Ettenberg, Director

5350 Camp Shane Arizona
1000 Orme Road
Mayer, AZ 86333   928-227-3883
                                              office@campshanearizona.com
                                              www.campshanearizona.com

Camp dedicated to weight loss.

Vanessa Stiller, Director
Jessica Gray, Nutritionist
Andrea Crandell, Sports and Crafts

5351 Camp Shane California
60 W Olsen Rd
Thousand Oaks, CA 91360   805-259-3366
                                              office@campshanecalifornia.com
                                              www.campshanecalifornia.com

Camp dedicated to weight loss.

David Ruales, Camp Director
Camryn Kruger, Assistant Director
Erika Smith, Program Guru

5352 Camp Shining Stars
Barton College
Wilson, NC 27893   919-246-4865
                                              866-644-2709
                                              ira@campshiningstars.org
                                              www.campshiningstars.org

Camp Shining Stars will help children lose weight, raise their self esteem, and learn the tools and habits necessary to lead a healthy lifestyle and reduce their risks for developing chronic diseases later in life.

Ira Green, Director

5353 Kingsmont
893 West Street
Amherst, MA 1002   703-288-0047
                                              877-348-2267
                                              Fax: 703-288-0075
                                              info@campkingsmont.com
                                              www.campkingsmont.com

A non-profit organization dedicated to eliminating childhood obesity by promoting proper nutrition, physical activity and emotional well-being. The camp is dedicated to providing children with the tools needed to make fundamental changes in their lives.

Meghan Roman, Director
Danny Heisler, Programming Director
Katie Roman, Administrative Director

5354 New Image Camps
PO Box 417
Norwood, NJ 7648

201-750-1557
800-365-0556
tsparber@aol.com
www.newimagecamp.com

Weight loss camp that features private lakefronts at 2 outstanding camps where kids, ages 7-19, have fun, lose weight & gain self-esteem. With separate facilities for boys and girls including two swimming pools, about 30 kids in a given age group, and roughly a 4 to 1 counselor-to-camper ratio, your child will form healthy, age-appropriate friendships, with a guidance they need for a fun and successful summer.

Tony Sparber, Owner
Dale Sparber, Owner

5355 Wellspring Camps
42675 Road 44
Reedley, CA 93654

866-364-0808
www.wellspringcamps.com

Wellspring is the leading organization of weight loss camps for kids, teens, young adults and women. The scientific Wellspring Plan trains campers on the self-regulatory skills they need to return to a healthy weight, and ofers families a simple and sustainable solution to supporting their child at home. Locations in La Jolla, Texas, New York, North Carolina, Wisconsin, Pennsylvania, and Florida.

Eliza Kingsford, MA, Executive Director
Jessie Dean, Director of Operations
Michaela Clinton, Director of Admissions

DESCRIPTION

5356 OBSESSIVE-COMPULSIVE DISORDER

Synonyms: Obsessive-compulsive neurosis, OCD

Involves the following Biologic System(s):
Developmental/Behavioral/Psychiatric Disorders

Obsessive-compulsive disorder (OCD) is characterized by the performance of repetitive actions, rituals, or compulsions in response to recurrent, persistent thoughts or obsessions. These actions and thoughts may cause significant anxiety and interfere with personal, social, or occupational functioning. OCD may affect approximately two to three percent of the general population worldwide. In most cases, the onset of OCD is gradual and typically becomes apparent during adolescence or early adulthood. However, onset of the disorder during childhood is not rare. Males and females are thought to be affected equally.

Many children have minor compulsions that result in little or no distress, such as avoiding cracks while walking on the sidewalk. Most such compulsions typically subside later in life. However, some rituals may continue through adulthood, such as repeatedly checking that the stove is turned off. Children who develop obsessive-compulsive disorder may initially have repetitive, persistent thoughts that constantly invade their consciousness. They may conduct a repetitive action or a series of actions during certain situations, particularly during times of stress, such as preparing to go to school. Performing compulsive actions or rituals may temporarily relieve a feeling of anxiety, whereas resisting such compulsions may serve to increase their tension. Obsessions may consist of certain ideas, phrases, or strong images; impulses to perform objectionable acts; or impulses to perform objectionable acts; or impulses to repeatedly analyze certain acts before carrying them out. Some obsessions may concern bodily secretions or wastes or a need for routine or sameness. Compulsions often include repetitive hand washing, touching certain objects in a particular sequence, or checking and rechecking door locks. Attempts may be made to involve parents or other family members in the performance of certain compulsive actions or rituals. Children with OCD are usually aware of the irrationality of their obsessive thoughts and compulsive behaviors but are unable to control them. The symptoms associated with OCD often periodically decrease or increase in intensity over time. However, in some patients, a progressive worsening of the condition may result in gradual deterioration of personal and social functioning. First-line treatment of OCD may include antidepressant medications, such as fluoxetine, fluvoxamine, or clomipramine.Behavioral therapy, including gradually increased exposure to situations that typically trigger compulsive behaviors, may be helpful. Relaxation therapy has also demonstrated some benefit.

OCD may occur as an isolated condition or in association with other underlying disorders or conditions, such as Tourette syndrome, epilepsy, or anorexia nervosa. Although the exact cause of obsessive-compulsive disorder is not known, studies suggest that the disorder may result from biochemical abnormalities affecting particular areas of the brain. There are also reports of multiple cases of isolated OCD in a multigenerational family (kindred), suggesting autosomal dominant inheritance in these patients. In addition, the occurrence of OCD in several kindreds affected by Tourette syndrome also indicates that changes (mutations) of certain genes may result in or contribute to OCD.

Government Agencies

5357 Center for Mental Health Services Knowledge Exchange Network
US Department of Health and Human Services
1 Choke Cherry Road
Rockville, MD 20857
877-SAM-HSA7
800-789-2647
Fax: 240-747-5470
TDD: 866-889-2647
www.mentalhealth.samhsa.gov

Supplies the public with responses to their commonly asked questions about mental health issues and services.

5358 NIH/National Institute of Mental Health
6001 Executive Boulevard, Room 6200, MSC 9663
Bethesda, MD 20892
301-443-4536
866-615-6464
Fax: 301-443-4279
TTY: 301-443-8431
nimhinfo@nih.gov
www.nimh.nih.gov

Conducts strategic planning for specific research areas as well as for the Institute as a whole.

Joshua Gordon, MD, PhD, Director
Shelli Avenevoli, MD, Deputy Director

National Associations & Support Groups

5359 American Academy of Pediatrics
141 Northwest Point Boulevard
Elk Grove Village, IL 60007
847-434-4000
800-433-9016
Fax: 847-434-8000
www.aap.org

The American Academy of Pediatrics and its member pediatricians are committed to the attainment of optimal physical, mental and social health and well-being for all infants, children, adolescents, and young adults.

Fernando Stein, MD, FAAP, President
Karen Remley, MD, CEO/Executive VP

5360 Anxiety Disorders Association of America
8730 Georgia Avenue, Suite 600
Silver Spring, MD 20910
240-485-1001
Fax: 240-485-1035
information@adaa.org
www.adaa.org

Offers resources and information for persons with anxiety and stress-related disorders.

Alies Muskin, Executive Director

5361 Awareness Foundation for OCD and Related D isorders
PO Box 1795
Soquel, CA 95073
831-684-9684
afocd@sbcglobal.net
www.afocd.ors

Combines the expertise and experience of dynamic workshop speakers with the emotional impact of film to increase professional, educational, and public understanding of OCD and related disorders. Speakers are available for consulting and workshops in school functions, for parents and students, and family and support groups.

James Callner MA, Founder/President
Michael Morris, Secretary
Renee Fuqua, Treasurer

5362 Federation of Families for Children's Mental Health
9605 Medical Center Drive, Suite 280
Rockville, MD 20850   240-403-1901
                                                  Fax: 240-403-1909
                                                   ffcmh@ffcmh.org
                                                    www.ffcmh.org

The National family run organization is dedicated exclusively to helping children with mental health needs and their families achieve a better quality of life.

Teka Dempson, President
Sherri Luthe, VP
Sheila Pires, Treasurer

5363 Genetic Alliance
4301 Connecticut Avenue NW, Suite 404
Washington, DC 20008   202-966-5557
                                                   800-336-4363
                                              Fax: 202-966-8553
                                          info@geneticalliance.org
                                            www.geneticalliance.org

A coalition of voluntary genetic support groups, consumers and professionals addressing the needs of individuals and families affected by genetic disorders from a national perspective.

Sharon Terry, President/CEO
Tetyana Murza, Managing Director
Natasha Bonhomme, VP, Strategic Development

5364 Mental Health America
500 Montgomery Street, Ste 820
Alexandria, VA 22314   703-684-7722
                                                   800-969-6642
                                              Fax: 703-684-5968
                                              TTY: 800-433-5959
                                           www.mentalhealthamerica.net

Addresses all aspects of mental health and mental illness. NMHA with over 340 affiliates works to improve the mental health of all Americans.

Paul Gionfriddo, President/CEO
Shavonne Carpenter, Sr Assoc., Support & Services
Mallory Pernell, Assoc. Dir, Comments/Marketing

5365 NADD: National Association for the Dually Diagnosed
132 Fair Street
Kingston, NY 12401   845-331-4336
                                                   800-331-5362
                                              Fax: 845-331-4569
                                                 info@thenadd.org
                                                  www.thenadd.org

Nonprofit organization designed to promote the interests of professional and parent development with resources for individuals who have the coexistence of mental illness and mental retardation. Provides conferences, educational services and training materials to professionals, parents, concerned citizens and service organizations.

Dr Robert Fletcher, CEO
Michelle Jordan, Office Manager
Edward Seliger, Project Coordinator

5366 National Alliance for the Mentally Ill
3803 N Fairfax Drive, Suite 100
Arlington, VA 22203   703-524-7600
                                                   888-999-6264
                                              Fax: 703-524-9094
                                              TDD: 703-516-7227
                                                   info@nami.org
                                                    www.nami.org

NAMI is a nonprofit, grassroots, self-help, support and advocacy organization of consumers, families and friends of people with severe mental illness, such as schizophrenia, bipolar disorder, major depressive disorder, obsessive compulsive disorder, anxiety disorders, autism and other severe and persistent mental illnesses that affect the brain.

Keris J,,n Myrick, President
Kevin B. Sullivan, First Vice President
Jim Payne, Second VP

5367 National Anxiety Foundation
3135 Custer Drive
Lexington, KY 40517   859-281-0003
                                          www.lexington-on-line.com/naf.html

A volunteer nonprofit organization. Its goal is to educate the public and health professionals about anxiety and anxiety disorders (such as panic disorder and obsessive-compulsive disorder) through printed materials and electronic media.

Stephen Cox MD, President & Medical Director
Linda Vernon Blair, Vice President
C. Todd Strecker, Treasurer

5368 National Mental Health Consumers' Self-Help Clearinghouse
1211 Chestnut Street, Suite 1207
Philadelphia, PA 19107   267-507-3810
                                                   800-553-4539
                                              Fax: 215-636-6312
                                              info@mhselfhelp.org
                                               www.mhselfhelp.org

Offers information, support and appropriate referrals; and promotes public and professional education. Provides networking for those with special interests related to albinism. Promotes and supports research and funding that will improve diagnosis and management of albinism and hypopigmentation.

Joseph Rogers, Executive Director & Founder
Susan Rogers, Director
Britani Nestel, Program Specialist

5369 Obsessive Compulsive Anonymous
PO Box 215
New Hyde Park, NY 11040   516-739-0662
                                         howardsedlitz@gmail.com
                                      www.obsessivecompulsiveanonymous.org

A fellowship of individuals dedicated to sharing their experience, strength and hope with one another to enable them to solve their common problems and help others recover from OCD. The Twelve Steps are adapted for OCA, to help obtain relief from obsessions and compulsions. Consisting of approximately 1,000 members and 50 chapters, OCA is not allied with any sect, denomination or organization.

5370 Obsessive Compulsive Foundation
PO Box 961029
Boston, MA 02196   617-973-5801
                                              Fax: 617-973-5803
                                              info@ocfoundation.org
                                               www.ocfoundation.org

Provides vital support to educate the public and professional communities about OCD and related disorders, provides assistance to individuals with OCD and related disorders, their families and friends. The foundation also funds research into the causes and effective treatments of OCD and related disorders.

Denise Egan Stack, President
Susan B. Dailey, VP
Michael J. Stack, Treasurer

5371 Suncoast Residential Training Center/Developmental Services Program
Goodwill Industries-Suncoast
10596 Gandy Boulevard
Saint Petersburg, FL 33702   727-523-1512
                                                   888-279-1988
                                              Fax: 727-563-9300
                                              TTY: 727-579-1068
                                            www.goodwill-suncoast.org

A large group home which serves individuals diagnosed as mentally retarded with a secondary diagnosis of psychiatric difficulties as evidenced by problem behavior. Providing residential, behavioral and instructional support and services that will promote the development of adaptive, socially appropriate behavior, each individual is assessed to determine socialization, basic academics and recreation. The primary intervention strategy is applied behavior analysis.

Oscar J. Horton, Chairman
Martin W. Gladysz, Sr. Vice Chair
Steven M. Erickson, Vice Chair

State Agencies & Support Groups

5372 Center for Family Support
333 7th Avenue, #901
New York, NY 10001   212-629-7939
                                              Fax: 212-239-2211
                                                  www.cfsny.org

The Center for Family (CFS) is a not-for-profit human service
agency providing support and assistance to individuals with developmental disabilities and traumatic brain injuries throughout
New York City, Long Island, the lower Hudson Valley region and
New Jersey.

Steven Vernikoff, Executive Director
Linda Schellenberg, Director, Community Service
Barbara Greenwald, Associate Executive Director

5373 Obsessive Compulsive Foundation of Metropo litan Chicago
2300 Lincoln Park West
Chicago, IL 60614   773-661-9530
                                              Fax: 773-661-9535
                                               info@ocfchicago.org
                                               www.ocdchicago.org

Serves adults and children with OCD, their families, and the mental health professionals who treat them. The only Chicago area organization dedicated to OCD.

Ellen Sawyer, Executive Director

Research Centers

**5374 National Alliance for Research on Schizophrenia and
Depression**
60 Cutter Mill Road, Suite 404
Great Neck, NY 11021   516-829-0091
                                                  800-829-8289
                                              Fax: 516-487-6930
                                             info@bbrfoundation.org
                                             www.bbrfoundation.org

NARSAD raises and distributes funds for scientific research into
the causes, cures, treatments, and prevention of severe mental illnesses, primarily schizophrenia.

Steve Lieber, Chairman
Suzzane Golden, VP
John B. Hollister, Secretary

Audio Video

5375 Hope and Solutions for OCD
ADD WareHouse
300 NW 70th Avenue, Suite 102
Plantation, FL 33317   954-792-8100
                                                  800-233-9273
                                              Fax: 954-792-8545
                                            sales@addwarehouse.com
                                              www.addwarehouse.com

A video series about obsessive compulsive disorder with some
straight forward solutions and advice for individuals with OCD,
their families, doctors, and school personnel. Viewers will learn
what OCD is and how to treat it. Discusses how OCD can affect
students in school and the impact on the family life.

85 Minutes
ISBN: 1-886941-37-8

5376 It's Not Me...It's My OCD: A Look at Behav ioral Therapy
Aquarius Health Care Videos
3435 Main Street, Bldg. 28
Buffalo, NY 14214   716-829-5744
                                                  888-440-2963
                                              Fax: 508-650-1665
                                             emro.lib.buffalo.edu

1997 28 Minutes
ISBN: 1-581403-38-0

Lori Widzinski, Editor
Oksana Dykyj, Associate Editor
Angela Davis, Social Network Coordinator

5377 Touching Tree
Awareness Films, author

Pyramid Media
3200 Airport Ave, Ste 19
Santa Monica, CA 90405   310-398-6149
                                                  800-421-2304
                                              Fax: 310-398-7869
                                             info@pyramidmedia.com
                                              www.pyramidmedia.com

Chronicles of a young boy trapped in the pain of OCD; how he
faces his fears and begins the slow recovery with professional
help. A film ideal for teaching the need for sensitivity when dealing with special children and their differences.

38 Minutes

Web Sites

5378 Anxiety Disorders Association of America

Offers resources and information for persons with anxiety and
stress-related disorders.

5379 CyberPsych
www.cyberpsych.org

CyberPsych presents information about psychoanalysis, psychotherapy, and special topics such as anxiety disorder, the problematic use of alcohol, homophobia, and the traumatic effects of
racism. CyberPsych is a nonprofit network which offers free web
hosting and technical support for internet communication, to
nonprofit groups and individuals.

5380 Guidelines for Families Coping with OCD
4901 NW 17th Way, Suite 101
Fort Lauderdale, FL 33309   954-962-6662
                                              Fax: 954-962-6164
                                          www.ocdhope.com/gdlines.htm

Offers 19 guidelines for families coping with OCD.

Dr. Bruce Hyman, Founder & Director
Dr. Stacy Sanders Shaup, Associate
Dr. Jennifer Hochman, Associate

5381 NADD: National Association for the Dually Diagnosed
132 Fair Street
Kingston, NY 12401   845-331-4336
                                                  800-331-5362
                                              Fax: 845-331-4569
                                                  www.thenadd.org

Nonprofit organization designed to promote the interests of professional and care providers for individuals who have the coexistence of mental illness and mental retardation. NADD provides
conferences, educational services and training materials to professionals, parents, concerned citizens and service organizations.

Dr Robert Fletcher, CEO
Michelle Jordan, Office Manager
Edward Seliger, Project Coordinator

5382 National Anxiety Foundation
www.lexington-on-line.com/naf.html

Nonprofit organization that provides education to the public and
professionals about anxiety through printed and electronic media.

Stephen Cox, MD, President
Linda Vernon Blair, Vice-President
C. Todd Strecker, Secretary-Treasurer

5383 National Mental Health Consumers' Self-Help Clearinghouse
www.mhselfhelp.org

637

A consumer run national technical assistance center serving the mental health consumer movement. We help connect individuals to self-help and advocacy resources, and we offer expertise to self-help groups, and other peer-run services for mental health consumers.

Joseph Rogers, Executive Director
Susan Rogers, Director
Christa Burkett, Technical Assistance Coordinator

5384 Obsessive Compulsive Disorder (OCD)
6001 Executive Boulevard
Rockville, MD 20852   NIMHinfo@mail.nih.gov
                    www.nimh.nih.gov/healthinformation/ocdmenu.cfm

Discusses the diagnosis of obsessive-compulsive disorder, its prevalence among both children and adults. Descibes types of treatment including pharmacotherapy. Gives sources of information for both the individual who has OCD and the family.

5385 Obsessive Compulsive Foundation
P.O. Box 961029
Boston, MA 2196   617-973-5801
                         Fax: 617-973-5803
                         info@iocdf.org
                         iocdf.org

An international nonprofit organization composed of people with obsessive compulsive disorder and related disorders, their families, friends, professionals, and other concerned individuals.

Denise Egan Stack, LMHC, President
Susan B. Dailey, Vice President
Michael J Stack, CFA, Treasurer

5386 Planetpsych
www.planetpsych.com

Planetpsych is an online resource for mental health information.

5387 Psych Central
55 Pleasant St., Suite 207
Newburyport, MA 1950   www.psychcentral.com

Offers free informational and educational articles and resources on psychology, support and mental health online.

John M. Grohol, CEO
Rick Nauert, Senior News Editor
Bailey Apple, Associate Editor

Book Publishers

5388 Boy Who Couldn't Stop Washing: The Experience and Treatment of OCD

Judith L Rapoport, author

Penguin Group
375 Hudson Street
New York, NY 10014   212-366-2372
                     Fax: 212-366-2933
                     online@us.penguingroup.com
                     us.penguingroup.com

A comprehensive treatment of obsessive-compulsive disorder that summarizes evidence that the disorder is neurobiological. It also describes the effect of medication combined with behavioral therapy.

1991 304 pages Paperback
ISBN: 0-451172-02-0

John Makinson, CHAIRMAN
Coram Williams, CFO
David Shanks, CEO

5389 Brain Lock: Free Yourself from Obsessive Compulsive Behavior

Jeffrey M Schwartz, author

Harper Collins
10 E 53rd Street
New York, NY 10022   212-207-7000
                     800-242-7737
                     Fax: 212-207-7901
                     feedback2@harpercollins.com
                     www.harpercollins.com

A simple four-step method for overcoming OCD that is so effective, it's now used in academic treatment centers throughout the world. Proven by brain-imaging tests to actually alter the brain's chemistry, this method doesn't rely on psychopharmaceuticals but cognitive self-therapy and behavior modification to develop new patterns of response. Offers real-life stories of actual patients.

1997 256 pages Paperback
ISBN: 0-060987-11-1

5390 Brief Strategic Solution-Oriented Therapy of Phobic and Obsessive Disorders

Giorgio Nardone, author

Jason Aronson Publishers
4501 Forbes Boulevard, Suite 200
Lanham, MD 20706   301-459-3366
                     800-462-6420
                     Fax: 301-429-5748
                     www.aronson.com

1996 188 pages Cloth
ISBN: 1-568218-04-4

5391 Childhood Obsessive Compulsive Disorder

Greta Francis, author

Sage Publications
2455 Teller Road
Thousand Oaks, CA 91320   800-818-7243
                     800-818-7243
                     Fax: 800-583-2665
                     supplements@sagepub.com.
                     www.sagepub.com

1996 120 pages
ISBN: 0-803959-22-2

Sara Miller McCune, Chairman
Blaise R. Simqu, President & CEO
Chris Hickok, Senior Vice President & Chief Finan

5392 Freeing Your Child from Obsessive-Compulsi ve Disorder

Tamar E Chansky PhD, author

Crown Publishing Group/Random House
280 Park Avenue
New York, NY 10017   212-940-7381
                     800-733-3000
                     www.crownpublishing.com

ISBN: 0-812931-17-4

5393 It's Nobody's Fault-New Hope and Help for Difficult Children and Their Parents
ADD WareHouse
300 NW 70th Avenue, Suite 102
Plantation, FL 33317   954-792-8100
                     800-233-9273
                     Fax: 954-792-8545
                     www.addwarehouse.com

This book explains that neither the parents nor children are causes of mental disorders and related problems.

1997 320 pages Paperback
ISBN: 0-812929-21-7

5394 Obsessive Compulsive Disorder: Helping Children and Adolescents

Mitzi Waltz, author

O'Reilly Media
1005 Gravenstein Highway N
Sebastopol, CA 95472   707-827-7019
                                         800-889-8969
                                    Fax: 707-829-0104
                                    www.oreilly.com

This book helps parents secure an accurate and complete diagnosis, and live with OCD children using effective parenting techniques. Offers support systems, medical interventions and explores therapeutic and other interventions, such as cognitive therapy; helps to secure care with an existing health plan even with no coverage of mental disorders, navigate the special education system and find resources.

2000 404 pages
ISBN: 1-565927-58-3

Tim O'Reilly, Founder & CEO

5395 Obsessive-Compulsive Disorder in Children and Adolescents

American Psychiatric Publishing
1000 Wilson Boulevard, Suite 1825
Arlington, VA 22209   703-907-7322
                                         800-368-5777
                                    Fax: 703-907-1091
                                      appi@psych.org
                                        www.appi.org

Examines the early development of obsessive-compulsive disorder and describes effective treatments.

1989 368 pages Hardcover
ISBN: 0-880482-82-0

Robert E. Hales, M.D, Editor-in-Chief
Rebecca D. Rinehart, Publisher
John McDuffie, Editorial Director

5396 School Personnel: A Critical Link in the Identification and Management of OCD

Gail B Adams, author

Obsessive Compulsive Foundation
18 Tremont Street, Suite 903
Boston, MA 02108   617-973-5801
                                    Fax: 617-973-5803
                                info@ocfoundation.org
                                 www.ocfoundation.org

Recognizing OCD in the school setting, current treatments, the role of school personnel in identification, assessment, and educational interventions are thoroughly covered in this brief, but informative booklet especially targeted to educators and guidance counselors.

2003 32 pages Booklet

Denise Egan Stack, President
Susan B. Dailey, Vice President
Diane Davey, Secretary

5397 Talking Back to OCD: The Program That Help Kids & Teens Say No Way

John March W/ Christine Benton, author

Guilford Publications
72 Spring Street
New York, NY 10012   212-431-9800
                                         800-365-7006
                                    Fax: 212-966-6708
                                     info@guilford.com
                                     www.guilford.com

Dr March's 8-step program to empower young people overcome OCD. Each chapter begins with a section that helps young readers zero in on specific problems and develop skills they can use to tune out the obsessions and resist compulsions. Filled with tips for parents to seperate the disorder from the child and to encourage their child in recovery. Hard- or paperback.

2007 276 pages Paperback
ISBN: 1-593853-55-6

Bob Matloff, President
Seymour Weingarten, Editor-in-Chief

5398 Teaching the Tiger
Hope Press
PO Box 188
Duarte, CA 91009   800-321-4039
                                    Fax: 626-358-3520
                                 dcomings@earthlink.net
                                     www.hopepress.com

A handbook for individuals involved in the education of students with Attention Deficit Disorder, Tourette Syndrome, or Obsessive Compulsive Disorder.

ISBN: 1-878267-34-5

David E Comings MD, Presenter

Newsletters

5399 Key Update
National Mental Health Consumer's Self-Help Clrhs.
1211 Chestnut Street, Suite 1207
Philadelphia, PA 19107   215-751-1810
                                         800-553-4539
                                    Fax: 215-636-6312
                                   info@mhselfhelp.org
                                     www.mhselfhelp.org

A monthly e-newsletter that provides timely news and notes on important mental health issues, details on upcoming events, and recent publications on policy issues. Topics addressed in the newsletter include self-advocacy, self-care, community integration, human rights and mental health treatments and services.

Monthly

Joseph Rogers, Executive Director
Susan Rogers, Director
Christa Burkett, Technical Assistance Coordinator

5400 OCD Newsletter
Obsessive Compulsive Foundation
P.O. Box 961029
Boston, MA 2196   617-973-5801
                                    Fax: 617-973-5803
                                       info@iocdf.org
                                          iocdf.org

For sufferers of obsessive-compulsive disorder and their families and friends.

16-20 pages 6 times/yr

Denise Egan Stack, LMHC, President
Susan B. Dailey, Vice President
Michael J Stack, CFA, Treasurer

Pamphlets

5401 Children and Adolescents
Madison Institute of Medicine
7617 Mineral Point Road, Suite 300
Madison, WI 53717   608-827-2470
                                    Fax: 608-827-2479
                                      mim@miminc.org
                                       www.miminc.org

Literature packet: diagnosis, treatment and other information on OCD in young children and adolescents.

5402 Obsessive Compulsive Disorder General Pack et
Madison Institute of Medicine
7617 Mineral Point Road, Suite 300
Madison, WI 53717   608-827-2470
                                    Fax: 608-827-2479
                                      mim@miminc.org
                                       www.miminc.org

Literature packet: overview of OCD, including information on prevalence, diagnosis and treatment.

5403 Obsessive-Compulsive Disorder, A Real Illness
National Institute of Mental Health
Public Info, 6001 Executive Blvd, Rm 8184
Rockville, MD 20852

301-443-4513
866-615-6464
Fax: 301-443-4279
TTY: 301-443-8431
NIMHinfo@mail.nih.gov
www.nimh.nih.gov

Easy-to read booklet on OCD, explaining what it is, when it starts, how long it lasts and how to get help. The booklet also includes a self-test.

Camps

5404 Tourette Syndrome Camp Organization
6933 N Kedzie, #816
Chicago, IL 60640

773-465-7536
info@tourettecamp.com
www.tourettecamp.com

Dedicated to promoting camping opportunities for children with Tourette Syndrome and its assocaited disorders, Obsessive Compulsive Disorder (OCD) and Attention Deficit/Hyperactivity Disorder (ADD/ADHD).

Monica Newman, Camp Director
Marleen Martinez, Assistant Director
Sarah Matchen, Director

DESCRIPTION

5405 OMPHALOCELE

Involves the following Biologic System(s):

Gastrointestinal Disorders, Neonatal and Infant Disorders

An omphalocele is a birth defect characterized by bulging or protrusion of a portion of the intestines through an abnormal opening in the abdominal wall near the navel, the region where the umbilical cord meets the abdomen during fetal growth and development. The bulging area of the intestines is covered by a thin, membrane-like sac consisting of part of the amnion and peritoneum. The amnion is the inner layer of membrane that forms the amniotic sac, the fluid-filled sac within which a fetus grows and develops. The peritoneum is the thin membrane that lines the abdominal cavity and covers the internal abdominal organs.

Depending upon the size of the abdominal wall defect in an affected newborn, varying amounts of intestine or, in severe cases, other abdominal organs, may protrude through the navel. Associated complications may include rupture of the protruding, membranous sac, damage to body tissues due to drying, or onset of infection. Because these complications may be life-threatening, an omphalocele is usually surgically repaired immediately after birth.

An omphalocele is thought to affect approximately one in 4,000 newborns. Prenatal ultrasounds often identify infants with an omphalocele before birth. Otherwise, physical examination of the infant is sufficient to diagnose this condition. In many infants, omphaloceles occur in association with other birth defects, such as abnormalities of the urinary and reproductive systems, central nervous system, or cardiovascular system. This condition may also occur in association with certain rare malformation syndromes that are apparent at birth. These include Beckwith-Wiedemann syndrome, also known as exomphalos-macroglossia-gigantism, and Shprintzen omphalocele syndrome, also called pharynx and larynx hypoplasia with omphalocele.

In other cases, omphaloceles may occur as isolated findings for unknown reasons. Omphaloceles are repaired with surgery, although not always immediately; complete recovery is expected. There have been reports of multiple cases of isolated omphaloceles within certain families (kindreds). In these families, the condition may be caused by abnormal changes (mutations) in a gene or genes that may be inherited as an autosomal recessive or X-linked trait. It is also possible that the interaction of several different genes in association with certain environmental factors (multifactorial inheritance) may play a role in the development of some omphaloceles.

Government Agencies

5406 Division of Birth Defects & Developmental Disabilities
1600 Clifton Road
Atlanta, GA 30333

404-639-3311
800-232-4636
Fax: 404-639-3534
TTY: 888-232-6348
www.cdc.gov

Information and advocacy resources for families and professionals dealing with children with birth defects and developmental disabilities.

National Associations & Support Groups

5407 American Academy of Pediatrics
141 Northwest Point Boulevard
Elk Grove Village, IL 60007

847-434-4000
800-433-9016
Fax: 847-434-8000
www.aap.org

The American Academy of Pediatrics and its member pediatricians are committed to the attainment of optimal physical, mental and social health and well-being for all infants, children, adolescents, and young adults.

Fernando Stein, MD, FAAP, President
Karen Remley, MD, CEO/Executive VP

5408 American College of Gastroenterology
6400 Goldsboro Road, Suite 200
Bethesda, MD 20817

301-263-9000
info@acg.gi.org
www.gi.org

Founded to advance the scientific study and medical practice of diseases of the gastrointestinal (GI) tract.

13,000 members

Carol A. Burke, MD, FACG, President

5409 March of Dimes Foundation
1275 Mamaroneck Avenue
White Plains, NY 10605

914-997-4488
888-663-4637
Fax: 914-428-8203
answers@marchofdimes.com
www.marchofdimes.com

Partnership of volunteers and professionals dedicates to improving the health of babies by preventing birth defects and infant mortality. Over 100 chapters are located across the country and can be located through the National Office.

Stacey D. Stewart, President

5410 North American Society for Pediatric Gastroenterology/Hepatology/Nutrition
714 N Bethlehem Pike, Suite 300
Ambler, PA 19002

215-641-9800
Fax: 215-641-1995
naspghan@naspghan.org
www.naspghan.org

Strives to improve the care of infants, children and adolescents with digestive disorders by promoting advances in clinical care of children with chronic abdominal pain, diarrhea, constipation, vomiting, bleeding from the GI tract, inflammatory bowel disease, liver diseases, diseases of the pancreas, poor weight gain and nutritional problems.

Margaret K Stallings, Executive Director
Kim Rose, Associate Director
Donna Murphy, Membership

Libraries & Resource Centers

5411 National Digestive Diseases Information Clearinghouse
9000 Rockville Pike
Bethesda, MD 20892

301-496-3583
800-860-8747
Fax: 703-738-4929
healthinfo@niddk.nih.gov
www.niddk.nih.govv

The National Institute of Diabetes and Digestive and Kidney Diseases conducts and supports research on many of the most serious diseases affecting public health. The Institute supports much of the clinical research on the diseases of internal medicine and related subspecialty fields as well as many basic science disciplines.

Dr. Griffin P. Rodgers, Director
Dr. Gregory G. Germino, Deputy Directortary
Camille M. Hoover, M.S.W., Executive Officer

Web Sites

5412 Mothers of Omphaloceles
www.omphalocele.com

Support and Webring.

5413 National Digestive Diseases Information Clearinghouse
www.digestive.niddk.nih.gov

The National Institute of Diabetes and Digestive and Kidney Diseases conducts and supports research on many of the most serious diseases affecting public health. The Institute supports much of the clinical research on the diseases of internal medicine and related subspecialty fields as well as many basic science disciplines.

5414 Online Mendelian Inheritance in Man
National Library of Medicine Building 38A
Bethesda, MD 20894   888-346-3656
                                         info@ncbi.nlm.nih.gov
                                         www.ncbi.nlm.nih.gov

This database is a catalog of human genes and genetic disorders.

5415 Pediatric Surgery Update
P.O. Box 10426
San Juan, PR 922   home.coqui.net/titolugo/PSU11.htm#1152

An online handbook about many differnt diseases and disablilies.

Journals

5416 Journal of Pediatric Gastroenterology and Nutrition
NASPGHAN, author

Lippincott Williams & Wilkins
2700 Lake Cook~Road
Riverwoods, IL 60015   847-580-5000
                                              Fax: 215-521-8902
                                                     www.lww.com

Publication of the North American Society for Pediatric Gastroenterolgy, Hepatology and Nutrition, which strives to improve the care of infants, children and adolescents with digestive disorders by promoting advances in clinical care of children with chronic abdominal pain, diarrhea, constipation, vomiting, bleeding from the GI tract, inflammatory bowel disease, liver diseases, diseases of the pancreas, poor weight gain and nutritional problems.

Newsletters

5417 NASPGHAN News
714 N. Bethlehem Pike, Ste 300
Ambler, PA 19002   215-641-9800
                                              Fax: 215-641-1995
                                          naspghan@naspghan.org
                                                www.naspghan.org

Publication of the North American Society for Pediatric Gastroenterolgy, Hepatology and Nutrition, which strives to improve the care of infants, children and adolescents with digestive disorders by promoting advances in clinical care of children with chronic abdominal pain, diarrhea, constipation, vomiting, bleeding from the GI tract, inflammatory bowel disease, liver diseases, diseases of the pancreas, poor weight gain and nutritional problems.

Margaret K Stallings, Executive Director
Kim Rose, Associate Director
Donna Murphy, Membership

DESCRIPTION

5418 OPPOSITIONAL DEFIANT DISORDER

Synonym: ODD

Involves the following Biologic System(s):

Developmental/Behavioral/Psychiatric Disorders

Oppositional Defiant Disorder (ODD) is a disruptive behavioral disorder along with conduct disorder. It is marked by an ongoing pattern of negativistic, argumentative, and hostile behaviors when interacting with some or all authority figures. The symptoms are usually seen in multiple settings, but may be more noticeable at home or at school. Five to fifteen percent of all school-age children have ODD. This disorder is usually apparent before age eight. Although it is more common in boys in the pre-pubertal years, the sex ratio evens out post puberty. The causes of ODD are unknown, but many parents report that their child with ODD was more rigid and demanding than the child's siblings from an early age. Biological and environmental factors may have a role. ODD can also be a precursor to conduct disorder later in life. Children with ODD also have a higher risk of other conditions, including ADHD (attention deficit hyperactivity disorder), anxiety and depression.

ODD is diagnosed by the presence of at least six months of hostile, negative and defiant behavior that is more frequent and intense than expected for a child's age. The behavior must cause significant functional impairment, either socially, academically or occupationally. ODD can not be diagnosed in patients who are actively psychotic or who meet criteria for conduct disorder or antisocial personality disorder.

Treatment for ODD centers upon evaluating the child's physical and psychosocial environment, ruling out or treating co-morbid conditions and assisting parents in anticipating and modifying behavior. Problems in the family or environment that may be driving the behaviors also need to be addressed. Many children with ODD will respond to the positive parenting techniques. A child with ODD can be very difficult for parents who need support and understanding. Older school age children and adolescents with ODD are more likely to benefit from an intensive intervention program.

National Associations & Support Groups

5419 American Academy of Child and Adolescent Psychiatry
3615 Wisconsin Avenue NW
Washington, DC 20016   202-966-7300
                                         Fax: 202-966-2891
                                    clinical@aacap.org
                                         www.aacap.org

The AACAP (American Academy of Child and Adolescent Psychiatry) is the leading national professional medical association dedicated to treating and improving the quality of life for children, adolescents, and families affected by these disorders. The AACAP is a 501 (c)(3) nonprofit organization established in 1953.

Elizabeth Hughes, Asst. Director of Education & Recer
Quentin Bernhard III, CME Coordinator
Alan Ezagui, Deputy Director of Development

5420 American Academy of Pediatrics
141 Northwest Point Boulevard
Elk Grove Village, IL 60007   847-434-4000
                                              800-433-9016
                                         Fax: 847-434-8000
                                              www.aap.org

The American Academy of Pediatrics and its member pediatricians are committed to the attainment of optimal physical, mental and social health and well-being for all infants, children, adolescents, and young adults.

Fernando Stein, MD, FAAP, President
Karen Remley, MD, CEO/Executive VP

Audio Video

5421 Explosive Child

Ross W Greene PhD, author

HarperCollins Publishers
1350 Avenue of the Americas
New York, NY 10019   212-261-6500
                                              800-242-7737
                                    www.harpercollins.com

A new approach for understanding and parenting easily frustrated, cronically inflexible children. Dr Greene offers help for you and your child. Now updated with new practical information, The Explosive Child lays out a sensitive, practical approach to helping your child at home and school.

1999 Audio Cassette
ISBN: 0-694521-90-6

Brian Murray, President and CEO
Chantal Restivo-Alessi, Chief Digital Officer
Janet Gervasio, SVP & CFO

Web Sites

5422 American Academy of Child and Adolescent Psychiatry
3615 Wisconsin Avenue, N.W.
Washington, DC 20016   202-966-7300
                                         Fax: 202-966-2891
                                              www.aacap.org

Information on treating and improving the quality of life for children, adolescents, and families affected by such disorders as Oppositional Defiant.

Book Publishers

5423 Disruptive Behavior Disorders in Children and Adolescents

Robert L Hendren, DO, author

American Psychiatric Publishing
1000 Wilson Boulevard, Suite 1825
Arlington, VA 22209   703-907-7322
                                              800-368-5777
                                         Fax: 703-907-1091
                                         appi@psych.org
                                              www.appi.org

Comprehensively reviews current research and clinical observations on this timely topic. The authors look at three subtypes of attention-deficit/hyperactivity disorder (ADHD), conduct disorder, and oppositional defiant disorder, all of which are common among youths and often share similar symptoms of impulse control problems.

1999 216 pages Paperback
ISBN: 0-880489-60-7

Robert E. Hales, M.D., Editor-in-Chief
Rebecca D. Rinehart, Publisher
John McDuffie, Editorial Director

5424 Explosive Child

Ross W Greene PhD, author

HarperCollins Publishers
10 East 53rd Street
New York, NY 10022
212-207-7000
800-242-7737
Fax: 212-207-7901
feedback2@harpercollins.com
www.harpercollins.com

A new approach for understanding and parenting easily frustrated, cronically inflexible children. Dr Greene offers help for you and your child. Now updated with new practical information, The Explosive Child lays out a sensitive, practical approach to helping your child at home and school.

2005 334 pages Paperbcak
ISBN: 0-060931-02-7

5425 Helping the Noncompliant Child

Robert McMahon, Rex Forehand, author

Guilford Press
72 Spring Street
New York, NY 10012
212-431-9800
800-365-7006
Fax: 212-966-6708
info@guilford.com
www.guilford.com

An empirically proven program for teaching parents to manage non-compliance in 3- to 8- year olds. Practitioners are provided step-by-step guidelines for child and family assessment, detailed descriptions of parent training procedures, effective adjunctive treatment strategies, and complete protocols for conducting the program. Hard- or soft-cover.

2005 264 pages Paperback
ISBN: 1-593852-41-2

Bob Matloff, President
Seymour Weingarten, Editor-in-Chief

5426 New Strong-Willed Child

James C Dobson, author

Tyndale House Publishers
351 Executive Drive
Carol Stream, IL 60188
800-323-9400
Fax: 800-684-0247
www.tyndale.com

A complete update of The Strong-Willed Child for a new generation of parents and teachers. It offers practical advice on raising difficult-to-handle children and incorporates the latest research.

2004 270 pages Hardcover
ISBN: 0-842336-22-2

Magazines

5427 EHealth

UAB Health System
1802 6th Avenue South
Birmingham, AL 35233
205-934-4011
800-822-8816
Fax: 205-934-9991
www.uabmedicine.org

A health and fitness publication packed with all the latest news and health tips from the UAB Health System.

Quarterly

Journals

5428 Official Journal of the American Academy of Child and Adolescent Psychiatry

Lippincott Williams & Wilkins
351 West Camden Street
Baltimore, MD 21201
410-528-4200
800-638-3030
Fax: 410-528-8557
www.jaacap.com

The journal is recognized as THE major journal focusing exclusively on today's psychiatric research and treatment of the child and adolescent.

12x a year

Mina K Dulcan MD, Editor
Sara Tiner, Editorial Coordinator

Newsletters

5429 AACAP News

American Academy of Child & Adolescent Psychiatry
3615 Wisconsin Avenue NW
Washington, DC 20016
202-966-7300
Fax: 202-966-2891
www.aacap.org

Official membership publication; provides the latest information on issues that directly affect child and adolescent psychiatrists.

6400 48 pages Bi-monthly

Paramjit T. Joshi, M.D, President
Gregory K. Fritz, M.D., President-Elect
Aradhana Sood, M.D., Secretary

5430 DevelopMentor

American Academy of Child & Adolescent Psychiatry
3615 Wisconsin Avenue NW
Washington, DC 20016
202-966-7300
Fax: 202-966-2891
www.aacap.org

Introduces medical students and residens to the clinical, academic, and research opportunities in child and adolescent psychiatry. Ideal for training directors.

Semi-annual

Paramjit T. Joshi, M.D, President
Gregory K. Fritz, M.D., President-Elect
Aradhana Sood, M.D., Secretary

DESCRIPTION

5431 OSTEOGENESIS IMPERFECTA

Synonyms: Brittle bone disease, OI

Covers these related disorders: Osteogenesis imperfecta Type I (OI Type I), Osteogenesis imperfecta Type II (OI Type II), Osteogenesis imperfecta Type III (OI Type III), Osteogenesis imperfecta Type IV (OI Type IV)

Involves the following Biologic System(s):

Genetic/Chromosomal/Syndrome/Metabolic Disorders, Orthopedic and Muscle Disorders

Osteogenesis imperfecta (OI) is an inherited genetic disorder characterized by abnormally brittle, fragile bones that are prone to fracture. The genetic abnormality responsible for OI produces defects in collagen, a protein that forms connective tissue such as bone, and is essential to normal bone growth and development.

Eight types of OI have been recognized, with each type having specific characteristics. The most common forms of OI are Types I through VI. Types VII and VIII of OI are recently recognized forms of the disease, of which only a few cases have so far been identified. Symptoms of OI, and how the disease is acquired, vary according to Type.

Of the eight types of OI, Type I is the least severe and most frequent. It occurs in approximately one in every 30,000 live births, and is inherited in an autosomal dominant manner, meaning that the defective gene that causes it can be inherited from only one parent, who will also have OI because of its dominant nature. Although the bones of infants and children with Type I are fragile and easily broken, and their teeth may be predisposed to cavities and breakage, there is little deformity of the bones. Other characteristics associated with Type I include flat feet, short stature, and a blue, purple, or gray coloration of the whites of the eyes. As children with this type of OI reach adolescence, they may experience bone fractures much less often than when they were younger.

OI Type II is the most severe form of the disease. Infants with Type II typically have a low birth weight, skeletal abnormalities of the limbs, ribs, and face, and frequent breakage of bones in prenatal fetuses. As many as half of births with OI of Type II are stillbirths, and many infants born with Type II die soon after birth from defects in the rib cage, resulting respiratory problems. Approximately one in 60,000 infants is affected with OI Type II. Both Types I and II are inherited as an autosomal dominant trait, or an recessive trait. The disease can also be caused by a genetic mutation, occurring only in the individual in whom the disease develops.

OI Type III is inherited as an autosomal recessive trait or as the result of a new mutation in affected offspring. It is a progressive form of the condition, characterized by multiple fractures and severely fragile bones in newborns, followed by deformity of the skeleton and skull. Other features of children with this type of OI include a triangular-shaped face, curvature of the spine, a barrel-shaped rib cage, diminished muscle development in the arms and legs, and short stature. Although many children with this type of OI reach adolescence, most do not reach adulthood.

OI Type IV, inherited as an autosomal dominant trait, is characterized by a reduced density of bones (osteoporosis) that causes them to be easily broken, and by shortness of stature. Bone fractures may be present at birth or at any time up to adulthood. As in Type I, curvature of thespine is likely to occur in Type IV, as is a barrel-shaped rib cage and triangular shape of the face, as well as brittleness of the teeth.

Type V is inherited in an autosomal dominant manner, and resembles Type IV, with the added symptom of calluses that develop at sites of bone fractures or surgical procedures. In many cases, the characteristics and symptoms of Type VI resemble those of Type IV, but it is not yet known whether this type of OI is inherited in a dominant or recessive manner. Type VII has so far been identified in only a small number of cases, some similar to Type IV, while others resembling the severe Type II, with surviving infants having short arm and leg bones, a short stature, a round face, and a small head. Type VIII OI resembles Type II or Type III, but surviving infants have seriously deficient growth and bones with a deficient mineral content.

OI is often detected as the result of a bone fracture, which then prompts further studies of an infant or child. Because of its effects on bone structure, OI can often be detected before birth by ultrasound examination, in which high-frequency sound waves are reflected by the bones and organs of a fetus in such a way as to permit a detailed examination of their structure. In some cases, laboratory tests can reveal the specific genetic defects responsible for OI.

OI cannot be completely cured or corrected. Treatment for most types and cases of the disease is medical and orthopedic, involving the use of drugs that reduce bone loss and others that promote growth of the body; casts and splints to repair fractures; and either braces or spinal fusion, in which bones of the spine are joined or fused to one another, to ease curvature of the spine and improve its supportive strength. Depending on the type and severity of OI, surgery may be done to treat fractures or to insert metal rods into the long bones of the arms and legs to strengthen and straighten them during growth. Physical therapy and exercise, including swimming, are used to build muscle, aid bone development, and strengthen the body.

Government Agencies

5432 NIH/ Eunice Kennedy Shriver National Insti tute of Child Health & Human Development
National Institutes of Health
31 Center Drive, Building 31
Bethesda, MD 20892

301-496-5113
800-370-2943
Fax: 866-760-5947
nichdpress@mail.nih.gov
www.nichd.nih.gov

Supports several basic and clinical research projects on osteogenesis imperfecta.

Diana W. Bianchi, Director
Paul Williams, Director, Communications

5433 NIH/Osteoporosis and Related Bone Diseases National Resource Center
2 AMS Circle
Bethesda, MD 20892
202-223-0344
800-624-2663
Fax: 202-293-2356
TTY: 202-466-4315
NIAMSBoneinfo@mail.nih.gov
www.bones.nih.gov

The National Resource Center is an information service that provides general information on metabolic bone conditions including osteoporosis, osteogenesis imperfecta, and Paget's disease of bone.

Stephen I Katz MD, PhD, Director

National Associations & Support Groups

5434 American Academy of Pediatrics
141 Northwest Point Boulevard
Elk Grove Village, IL 60007
847-434-4000
800-433-9016
Fax: 847-434-8000
www.aap.org

The American Academy of Pediatrics and its member pediatricians are committed to the attainment of optimal physical, mental and social health and well-being for all infants, children, adolescents, and young adults.

Fernando Stein, MD, FAAP, President
Karen Remley, MD, CEO/Executive VP

5435 Genetic Alliance
4301 Connecticut Avenue NW, Suite 404
Washington, DC 20008
202-966-5557
800-336-4363
Fax: 202-966-8553
info@geneticalliance.org
www.geneticalliance.org

A coalition of voluntary genetic support groups, consumers and professionals addressing the needs of individuals and families affected by genetic disorders from a national perspective.

Sharon Terry, President/CEO
Tetyana Murza, Managing Director
Natasha Bonhomme, VP, Strategic Development

5436 Little People of America
250 El Camino Real, Suite 218
Tustin, CA 92780
714-368-3689
888-572-2001
Fax: 714-368-3367
info@lpaonline.org
www.lpaonline.org

A nonprofit organization that provides support and information to people of short stature and their families.

Lois Gerage-Lamb, President
Bill Bradford, Senior Vice President
Jon North, Vice President, Finance

5437 March of Dimes Foundation
1275 Mamaroneck Avenue
White Plains, NY 10605
914-997-4488
888-663-4637
Fax: 914-428-8203
answers@marchofdimes.com
www.marchofdimes.com

Partnership of volunteers and professionals dedicates to improving the health of babies by preventing birth defects and infant mortality. Over 100 chapters are located across the country and can be located through the National Office.

Stacey D. Stewart, President

5438 National Dissemination Center for Children with Disabilities
1825 Connecticut Avenue NW, Suite 700
Washington, DC 20009
202-884-8200
800-695-0285
Fax: 202-884-8441
nichcy@aed.org
www.nichcy.org

A national information and referral center for families, educators and other professionals on: disabilities in children and youth; programs and services; IDEA, the nation's special education law; and research-based information on effective practices.

Suzanne Ripley, Executive Director

5439 Osteogenesis Imperfecta Foundation
804 W Diamond Avenue
Gaithersburg, MD 20878
301-947-0083
800-981-2663
Fax: 301-947-0456
bonelink@oif.org
www.oif.org

This foundation serves the needs of people affected by osteogenesis imperfecta, a brittle bone disorder. Offers information, resources, support and a biannual conference.

Tracy Hart, Ceo
Mary Beth Huber, Information/Resource Director

State Agencies & Support Groups

Arkansas

5440 Little People of America - District 7
National Headquarters
250 El Camino Real, Suite 218
Tustin, CA 92780
714-368-3689
888-572-2001
Fax: 714-368-3367
info@lpaonline.org
www.lpaonline.org

District 7 of the Little People of America represents short stature individuals from the states of Arkansas, Kansas, Missouri and Oklahoma.

Karen Shelby, Director
Jack Dohr, Vice Director
Cyndy Dohr, Treasurer

California

5441 Little People of America - San Francisco Bay Area Chapter
National Headquarters
250 El Camino Real, Suite 218
Tustin, CA 92780
714-368-3689
888-572-2001
Fax: 714-368-3367
info@lpaonline.org
www.lpabayarea.org

A nonprofit organization that provides support and information to people of short stature and their families.

Lee Uniacke, President
Keren Stronach, Co-Vice President
Caroline Jones, Co-Vice President

Colorado

5442 Little People of America - Front Range Chapter
7117 E Euclid Drive
Englewood, CO 80111
303-740-8555
ebennettebennett@netscape.net
http://frontrangelpa26.org

Little People of America, Inc. (LPA), will assist dwarfs with their physical and developmental concerns resulting from short stature. By providing medical, environmental, educational, vocational, and parental guidance, short-stature individuals and their families may enhance their lives and lifestyles with minimal limitations. Through peer support and personal example, members will be supportive of all those who reach out to LPA.

Chris & Bob Kotzian, President
Souda Bell, Vice President
Brandi VanAnne, Treasurer

Kansas

5443 Little People of America - District 7
National Headquarters
250 El Camino Real, Suite 218
Tustin, CA 92780

714-368-3689
888-572-2001
Fax: 714-368-3367
info@lpaonline.org
www.lpaonline.org

District 7 of the Little People of America represents short stature individuals from the states of Arkansas, Kansas, Missouri and Oklahoma.

Karen Shelby, Director
Jack Dohr, Vice Director
Cyndy Dohr, Treasurer

Missouri

5444 Little People of America - District 7
National Headquarters
250 El Camino Real, Suite 218
Tustin, CA 92780

714-368-3689
888-572-2001
Fax: 714-368-3367
info@lpaonline.org
www.lpaonline.org

District 7 of the Little People of America represents short stature individuals from the states of Arkansas, Kansas, Missouri and Oklahoma.

Karen Shelby, Director
Jack Dohr, Vice Director
Cyndy Dohr, Treasurer

New Jersey

5445 Little People of America - District 2
National Headquarters
250 El Camino Real, Suite 218
Tustin, CA 92780

714-368-3689
888-572-2001
Fax: 714-368-3367
info@lpaonline.org
www.lpaonline.org

A nonprofit organization that provides support and information to people of short stature and their families.

Joe Zrinski, District Director
Patty Ott, Assistant District Director
Jim Davis, District Treasurer

New York

5446 Little People of America - District 2
National Headquarters
250 El Camino Real, Suite 218
Tustin, CA 92780

714-368-3689
888-572-2001
Fax: 714-368-3367
info@lpaonline.org
www.lpaonline.org

A nonprofit organization that provides support and information to people of short stature and their families.

Joe Zrinski, District Director
Patty Ott, Assistant District Director
Jim Davis, District Treasurer

Oklahoma

5447 Little People of America - District 7
National Headquarters
250 El Camino Real, Suite 218
Tustin, CA 92780

714-368-3689
888-572-2001
Fax: 714-368-3367
info@lpaonline.org
www.lpaonline.org

District 7 of the Little People of America represents short stature individuals from the states of Arkansas, Kansas, Missouri and Oklahoma.

Karen Shelby, Director
Jack Dohr, Vice Director
Cyndy Dohr, Treasurer

Pennsylvania

5448 Little People of America - District 2
National Headquarters
250 El Camino Real, Suite 218
Tustin, CA 92780

714-368-3689
888-572-2001
Fax: 714-368-3367
info@lpaonline.org
www.lpaonline.org

A nonprofit organization that provides support and information to people of short stature and their families.

Joe Zrinski, District Director
Patty Ott, Assistant District Director
Jim Davis, District Treasurer

Utah

5449 Little People of America - Utah Seagulls
National Headquarters
250 El Camino Real, Suite 218
Tustin, CA 92780

714-368-3689
888-572-2001
Fax: 714-368-3367
info@lpaonline.org
www.utahlittlepeople.org

A nonprofit organization that provides support and information to people of short stature and their families.

Steve Hatch, President

Libraries & Resource Centers

5450 NIH/Osteoporosis and Related Bone Diseases National Resource Center
2 AMS Circle
Bethesda, MD 20892

202-223-0344
800-624-2663
Fax: 202-293-2356
TTY: 202-466-4315
NIHBoneInfo@mail.nih.gov
www.niams.nih.gov/bone/

Devoted to the dissemination of knowledge regarding the disease along with several helpful medias to explore.

Stephen I Katz MD, PhD, Director

Conferences

5451 LPA National Conference
Little People of America
250 El Camino Real, Suite 218
Tustin, CA 92780

714-368-3689
888-572-2001
Fax: 714-368-3367
info@lpaonline.org
www.lpaonline.org

July

Leah Smith, Public Relations Director
Gary Arnold, President
April Brazier, Senior Vice President

5452 National Conference on OI
Osteogenesis Imperfecta Foundation
804 W Diamond Avenue, Suite 210
Gaithersburg, MD 20878

301-947-0083
800-981-2663
Fax: 301-947-0456
bonelink@oif.org
www.oif.org

Annual conference that allows the Foundation to build on important advocacy efforts while providing an exciting conference.

Sharon Trahan, President
Mark Birdwhistell, Vice President
Tracy Smith Hart, Chief Executive Officer

Audio Video

5453 Plan for Success: Educator's Guide to Students with Osteogenesis Imperfecta
Osteogenesis Imperfecta Foundation
804 W Diamond Avenue, Suite 210
Gaithersburg, MD 20878

301-947-0083
844-889-7579
Fax: 301-947-0456
bonelink@oif.org
www.oif.org

Information for parents and educators on planning steps that will help children with osteogenesis imperfecta to fully particapate in school activities.

15 minutes

Heller An Shapiro, Executive Director
Mary Beth Huber, Information/Resource Director

Web Sites

5454 Little People of America
250 El Camino Real, Suite 218
Tustin, CA 92780

714-368-3689
888-LPA-2001
Fax: 714-368-3367
www.lpaonline.org

Offers resources pertaining to dwarfism and Little People of America, medical data, instructions on how to join an e-mail discussion group, and links to numerous other dwarfism-related sites.

Gary Arnold, President
April Brazier, Senior Vice President
Jon North, Programs Director

5455 Online Mendelian Inheritance in Man
National Library of Medicine Building 38A
Bethesda, MD 20894

888-346-3656
info@ncbi.nlm.nih.gov
www.ncbi.nlm.nih.gov

This database is a catalog of human genes and genetic disorders.

5456 Osteogenesis Imperfecta Foundation
804 W Diamond Avenue, Suite 210
Gaithersburg, MD 20878

301-947-0083
844-889-7579
Fax: 301-947-0456
www.oif.org

Is the only voluntary national health organization dedicated to helping people cope with the problems associated with osteogenesis imperfecta. The foundations mission is to improve the quality of life for individuals affected by OI through research to find treatments and a cure, education, awareness, and mutual support.

5457 Osteoporosis and Related Bone Diseases - National Resource Center
2 AMS Circle
Bethesda, DC

202-223-0344
800-624-2663
Fax: 202-293-2356
TTY: 202-466-4315
NIHBoneInfo@mail.nih.gov
www.niams.nih.gov/bone/

The National Resource Center is dedicated to increasing the awareness, knowledge and understanding of physicians, health professionals, patients, underserves and at-risk populations and the general public about the prevention, early detection and treatment of osteoperosis and related bone diseases.

5458 Shriner's Hospital Research Study Report
www.shrinershq.org

Provides patients, health professionals, and the public with an important link to resources and information on metabolic bone disease, including osteoporosis, Paget's disease of the bone, osteogenesis imperfecta, and hyperparathyroidism. It is dedicated to increasing the underserved and at-risk populations and the general public about the prevention, early detection and treatment of osteoporosis and related bone disease.

5459 Wheeless' Textbook of Orthopaedics
www.wheelessonline.com

Derives from a variety of sources, including journals, articles, national meetings lectures and other textbooks.

Clifford R. Wheeless III, MD, Editor-in-Chief
James A. Nunley, II, MD, Managing Editor
James R. Urbaniak, MD, Managing Editor

Book Publishers

5460 Children with Osteogenesis Imperfecta: Str ategies to Enhance Performance
Osteogenesis Imperfecta Foundation
804 W Diamond Avenue
Gaithersburg, MD 20878

301-947-0083
Fax: 301-947-0456
BoneLink@oif.org
www.oif.org

A guide to fitness and exercise for children and teens who have OI. It focuses on practical strategies designed to maximize mobility and function, and prevent some of the complications related to immobility.

2005 270 pages Paperback
ISBN: 0-964218-95-0

Sharon Trahan, President
Mark Birdwhistell, Vice President
Tracy Smith Hart, Chief Executive Officer

5461 Growing Up with OI: Guide for Children
Osteogenesis Imperfecta Foundation
804 W Diamond Avenue, Suite 210
Gaithersburg, MD 20878

301-947-0083
800-981-2663
Fax: 301-947-0456
bonelink@oif.org
www.oif.org

Tips and experiences from families of people who have osteogenesis imperfecta.

2001 122 pages Paperback
ISBN: 0-964218-92-5

Sharon Trahan, President
Mark Birdwhistell, Vice President
Tracy Smith Hart, Chief Executive Officer

5462 Growing Up with OI: Guide for Families and Caregivers
Osteogenesis Imperfecta Foundation
804 W Diamond Avenue, Suite 210
Gaithersburg, MD 20878   301-947-0083
800-981-2663
Fax: 301-947-0456
bonelink@oif.org
www.oif.org

Tips and experiences from families of people who have
Osteogenesis Imperfecta.

2001 295 pages Paperback
ISBN: 0-964218-91-7

Sharon Trahan, President
Mark Birdwhistell, Vice President
Tracy Smith Hart, Chief Executive Officer

5463 Jason's First Day!
Osteogenesis Imperfecta Foundation
804 W Diamond Avenue
Gaithersburg, MD 20878   301-947-0083
Fax: 301-947-0456
BoneLink@oif.org
www.oif.org

This picture book tells the story of the first day of school for a
child with OI. It can be read to preschool, kindergarten and first
grade children. The book includes a teacher's guide and resources
for educators to make the transition to school easier for children
with OI or other mobility impairing disabilities.

2004 43 pages Paperback
ISBN: 0-964218-94-1

Sharon Trahan, President
Mark Birdwhistell, Vice President
Tracy Smith Hart, Chief Executive Officer

5464 Let's Talk About Going to the Hospital
Rosen Publishing Group's PowerKids Press
29 E 21st Street
New York, NY 10010   212-777-3017
800-237-9932
Fax: 888-436-4643
rosenpub@tribeca.ios.com
www.rosenpublishing.com

If a child has to check into the hospital, chances are he or she is
already upset about being ill. Knowing how a hospital functions
and what the procedures are, such as when family members can
visit, will help in what is already a stressful situation. Grades
K-5.

24 pages
ISBN: 0-823950-36-0

Roger Rosen, President

5465 Managing Osteogenesis Imperfecta: a Medical Manual
Osteogenesis Imperfecta Foundation
804 W Diamond Avenue, Suite 210
Gaithersburg, MD 20878   301-947-0083
800-981-2663
Fax: 301-947-0456
bonelink@oif.org
www.oif.org

The manual is designed for physicians, physical and occupational
therapists, orthopedic technologists, early intervention providers
and others who come in contact with persons with OI. It covers a
broad range of topics including genetics, diagnosis, pregnancy,
arthritis, and osteoperosis.

1997

Sharon Trahan, President
Mark Birdwhistell, Vice President
Tracy Smith Hart, Chief Executive Officer

5466 Osteogenesis Imperfecta: A Guide for Nurse s
Osteogenesis Imperfecta Foundation
804 W Diamond Avenue
Gaithersburg, MD 20878   301-947-0083
Fax: 301-947-0456
BoneLink@oif.org
www.oif.org

A comprehensive guide to assist nursing professionals as they
come into contact with people who have OI of all ages. Topics include diagnosis, family education, standard treatments, emergencies and medical procedures. It is intended for nursing
professionals, nursing students and familes.

2003 64 pages Paperback

Sharon Trahan, President
Mark Birdwhistell, Vice President
Tracy Smith Hart, Chief Executive Officer

Newsletters

5467 Breakthrough
Osteogenesis Imperfecta Foundation
804 W Diamond Avenue
Gaithersburg, MD 20878   301-947-0083
844-889-7579
Fax: 301-947-0456
bonelink@oif.org
www.oif.org

Newsletter of the Osteogenesis Imperfecta Foundation that provides information on current research and OIF fundraising activities as well as support features. Free within the United States.

24 pages Quarterly

Heller An Shapiro, Executive Director
Mary Beth Huber, Information/Resource Director

Pamphlets

5468 Caring for Infants and Children with Osteogenesis Imperfecta
Osteogenesis Imperfecta Foundation
804 W Diamond Avenue
Gaithersburg, MD 20878   301-947-0083; 844-889-7579
Fax: 301-947-0456
BoneLink@oif.org
www.oif.org

Presents information on caring for a babies and toddlers with OI.
Available in Spanish.

17 pages

5469 Osteogenesis Imperfecta: A Guide for Medical Professionals, Ind. & Families
Osteogenesis Imperfecta Foundation
804 W Diamond Avenue
Gaithersburg, MD 20878   301-947-0083; 844-889-7579
Fax: 301-947-0456
BoneLink@oif.org
www.oif.org

Briefly describes osteogenesis imperfecta, its diagnosis and treatment.

10 pages Paperback

5470 Therapeutic Strategies for OI: A Guide for Physical and Occupational Therapists
Osteogenesis Imperfecta Foundation
804 W Diamond Avenue
Gaithersburg, MD 20878   301-947-0083; 844-889-7579
Fax: 301-947-0456
BoneLink@oif.org
www.oif.org

It covers the role of physical and occupational therapy in managing OI. Topics include safe handling of children and adults with
OI and strategies for safe, successful therapy.

14 pages Paperback

Heller An Shapiro, Executive Director
Mary Beth Huber, Information/Resource Director

DESCRIPTION

5471 OTITIS MEDIA

Synonym: Tympanitis

Covers these related disorders: Acute otitis media, Chronic otitis media, Secretory otitis media

Involves the following Biologic System(s):

Infectious Disorders

Otitis media refers to an infection or inflammation of the middle ear, the irregularly-shaped cavity that lies in the temporal bone on each side of the skull, and contains structures essential to hearing. Otitis media is one of the most common disorders of childhood, especially in children from the ages of 6 months to 3 years.

Acute otitis media usually occurs in conjunction with or as a complication of upper respiratory tract infections such as the common cold. Infections of the respiratory tract can extend to the middle ear and cause otitis media by way of the eustachian tube, a narrow canal that extends from the rear of the nasal area to the middle ear and helps to maintain normal air pressure in the middle ear. Infants and young children are especially vulnerable to otitis media because they have a short and narrow eustachian tube that is positioned somewhat horizontally, making them more susceptible to the backward flow of infectious secretions from the nasal area and into the middle ear. Further increasing the risk of otitis media during colds and other respiratory infections in infants and young children is swelling of the lymph nodes known as the adenoids, which are located at the back of the throat, near the opening of the eustachian tube that extends to each ear, and which can block these tubes and limit their ability to drain infected secretions out of the middle ear.

Symptoms of acute otitis media often develop soon after the onset of a respiratory tract infection, and include sudden and severe ear pain (otalgia), ringing in the ears (tinnitus), fever, temporary hearing loss, and discomfort. Infants and young children with otitis media may exhibit the following symptoms: irritability; pulling at the infected ear; fluid draining from the infected ear; nausea; vomiting; and diarrhea. The eardrum (tympanic membrane) of the infected ear may rupture, thus releasing fluid, which usually relieves the pain in an infected ear. The eardrum may then heal within a short period, but if healing does not occur, this rupture can result in a permanent impairment of hearing, leading to difficulties in speech. Symptoms such as dizziness, headache, sudden and significant hearing loss or deafness, chills, and fever may suggest complications that may result from otitis media or which may occur in conjunction with it, including inflammation of the membranes surrounding the brain and spinal cord (meningitis), infection of the inner ear canals (labyrinthitis), or infection in the mastoid bone behind the ear (mastoiditis).

Otitis media can be detected with an otoscope, an instrument that allows examination of the eardrum to see whether it is inflamed or swollen, thus reflecting an infection of the middle ear, located behind the eardrum. A pneumatic otoscope is used to deliver a puff of air onto the eardrum to check for flexibility or swelling. A microphone can also be used to hear the sound that the air makes.

Treatment of acute otitis media depends upon its cause. If the infection causing an episode of otitis media is bacterial, antibiotics may be given. Some children may require a surgical procedure known as myringotomy, in which an incision is made in the eardrum to relieve pressure and allow the release of pus and other secretions, or through tympanocentesis, a procedure in which the eardrum is surgically punctured to release fluid. Other treatment of otitis media is symptomatic and supportive, with pain relievers, antihistamines, nasal decongestants, and other medications.

Some children with otitis media develop secretory otitis media, which sometimes follows blockage of the eustachian tube, or the successful treatment of acute otitis media. This is characterized by the escape of thin (serous), thick (mucoid), or pus-like fluid from the ear. Symptoms associated with secretory otitis media may include dizziness and tinnitus. Although this condition may resolve spontaneously, its treatment is often indicated to prevent possible hearing loss and subsequent difficulties in the acquisition of speech and language. This may be accomplished through surgical incision and the insertion of tubes into the eardrum to allow the drainage of fluid. Children who do not respond to such treatment may benefit by having their adenoids removed surgically (adenoidectomy) to drain fluids from the eustachian tubes and allow a normal flow of air through them.

An infection of the middle ear that persists beyond the usually course of acute otitis media is known as chronic otitis media Such infection is much less common than acute otitis media, but its symptoms, being less severe, may persist for varying periods without being noticed. This can impair hearing, learning, and speech. Chronic otitis media may, for example, result in small growths (polyps) in the ear and damage to the small bones (ossicles) of the middle ear, impairing the ability of the ear to conduct sound. Chronic otitis media may be treated by the continued administration of antibiotics for a longer period than for the acute condition, as well as by drainage of the ear and the other procedures used in acute otitis media, and by the surgical repair of a ruptured eardrum (tympanoplasty). Tympanoplasty may also be used to restore the mechanism by which the middle ear transmits sound, which involves three small bones known as the malleus, incus, and stapes. The incus transmits vibrations it receives from the malleus to the stapes, which in turn sends the vibrations through a membrane and into the fluid-filled canal of the inner ear, where the vibrations are transformed into nerve signals that travel to the hearing centers of the brain for sensing and comprehension.

Government Agencies

5472 NIH/National Institute of Allergy and Infectious Diseases
5601 Fishers Lane, MSC 9806
Bethesda, MD 20892

301-496-5717
866-284-4107
Fax: 301-402-3573
TDD: 800-877-8339
ocpostoffice@niaid.nih.gov
www.niaid.nih.gov

Conducts and supports basic and applied research to better understand, treat, and ultimately prevent infectious, immunologic, and allergic diseases.

Anthony S Fauci MD, Director

National Associations & Support Groups

5473 American Academy of Audiology
11480 Commerce Park Drive, Ste 220
Reston, VA 20191
703-790-8466
800-222-2336
Fax: 703-790-8631
info@audiology.org
www.audiology.org

A professional organization dedicated to providing high quality and balanced hearing care to the public. Provides professional development, education and research and provides increased public awareness of hearing disorders and audiologic services.
ISSN: 1050-0545

Allison Grimes, President
Sydney Hawthorne Davis, Director Communications

5474 American Academy of Pediatrics
141 Northwest Point Boulevard
Elk Grove Village, IL 60007
847-434-4000
800-433-9016
Fax: 847-434-8000
www.aap.org

The American Academy of Pediatrics and its member pediatricians are committed to the attainment of optimal physical, mental and social health and well-being for all infants, children, adolescents, and young adults.

Fernando Stein, MD, FAAP, President
Karen Remley, MD, CEO/Executive VP

5475 American Hearing Research Foundation
8 S Michigan Avenue, Suite 1205
Chicago, IL 60603
312-726-9670
Fax: 312-726-9695
ahrf@american-hearing.org
www.american-hearing.org

Funds medical research and education into the causes, prevention, and cures of hearing losses, and balance disorders. Also keeps physicians and the public informed of the latest developments in hearing research and education.

Richard G. Muench, Chairman
Alan G. Micco, President
Mark R. Muench, Vice President

5476 March of Dimes Foundation
1275 Mamaroneck Avenue
White Plains, NY 10605
914-997-4488
888-663-4637
Fax: 914-428-8203
answers@marchofdimes.com
www.marchofdimes.com

Partnership of volunteers and professionals dedicates to improving the health of babies by preventing birth defects and infant mortality. Over 100 chapters are located across the country and can be located through the National Office.

Stacey D. Stewart, President

5477 World Health Organization
Avenue Appia 20
CH-1211 Geneva 27, SL
Switzerland
122-791-2111
Fax: 122-791-3111
www.who.int

WHO is the directing and coordinating authority for health within the United Nations system.

Dr Margaret Chan, Director General

Web Sites

5478 Baylor College of Medicine-Pathology & Pathogenesis of Otitis Media
One Baylor Plaza
Houston, TX 77030
713-798-4951
www.bcm.edu

Paul Klotman, M.D., President/ CEO & Executive Dean
William T. Butler, M.D., Chancellor Emeritus
Alicia Monroe, M.D., Provost/ SVP

5479 Indiana State University School of Medicine
340 West 10th Street, Suite 6200
Indianapolis, IN 46202
317-274-8157
medicine.iu.edu

Provides a presentation of the disease including signs, symptoms and illustrations.

Jay L. Hess, M.D., Vice President
Stephen P. Bogdewic, PhD, Executive Vice Dean
Diane Iseminger, Chief of Staff

5480 PDR.net
5 Paragon Drive
Montvale, NJ 7645
888-227-6469
PDRnet@pdr.net
www.pdr.net

Offers integrated medical information and education tools. Updated frequently, this site contains the drug information resources needed daily by its prescriber user base arranged together in one site for convenience and ease-of-use.

5481 University of Texas Medical Branch
301 University Boulevard
Galveston, TX 77555
www.utmb.edu/oto/
David L. Callender, President
Danny O. Jacobs, MD, Executive Vice President
Carolee King, JD, Senior Vice President

Book Publishers

5482 Let's Talk About Going to the Hospital
Rosen Publishing Group's PowerKids Press
29 E 21st Street
New York, NY 10010
212-777-3017
800-237-9932
Fax: 888-436-4643
rosenpub@tribeca.ios.com
www.rosenpublishing.com

If a child has to check into the hospital, chances are he or she is already upset about being ill. Knowing how a hospital functions and what the procedures are, such as when family members can visit, will help in what is already a stressful situation. Grades K-5.

24 pages
ISBN: 0-823950-36-0

Roger Rosen, President

5483 Living with Hearing Loss
Marcia B Dugan, author

Gallaudet University Press
800 Florida Avenue NE
Washington, DC 20002
202-651-5488; Fax: 202-651-5489
TTY: 888-630-9347
gupress@gallaudet.edu
gupress.gallaudet.edu

192 pages
ISBN: 1-563681-34-0

5484 Screening for Hearing Loss and Other Otitis Media
Jackson Roush PhD, author

AGB Association for the Deaf and Hard of Hearing
3417 Volta Place NW
Washington, DC 20007
202-337-5220; 800-432-7543
Fax: 202-337-8314
TTY: 202-337-5221
info@agbell.org
www.listeningandspokenlanguage.org

2001 245 pages Softcover
ISBN: 0-769300-00-6

Donald M. Goldberg, President
Alexander T. Graham, Executive Director/CEO
Ted A. Meyer, MD, Ph.D. (SC), Secretary-Treasurer

DESCRIPTION

5485 PASSIVE-AGGRESSIVE BEHAVIOR
Involves the following Biologic System(s):
Developmental/Behavioral/Psychiatric Disorders

Passive-aggressive behavior refers to a type of disruptive conduct that is apparent in approximately 20 percent of children and adolescents. Although seemingly compliant, affected individuals usually harbor negative, aggressive, or hostile feelings, but are unable to directly express them. These negative, hostile feelings are typically manifested indirectly and nonviolently through procrastination, forgetfulness, inefficiency, pouting or sullenness, stubbornness, obstructionism, and resistance to requests or demands. When infants and toddlers, passive-aggressive children and adolescents may have manifested their negativistic personalities through difficulties with feeding and toilet training.

Passive-aggressive individuals may be unaware that they are using their behavior to counteract or offset certain frustrations (e.g., feelings of inadequacy). They may persist in these behaviors in an attempt to regain control of a situation or to punish and retaliate. These stubbornly compliant behaviors are apparent in other situations that typically provoke direct displays of assertiveness, hostility, or other forms of aggression. Parents may be overly, but inconsistently, demanding and critical; conversely, affected individuals may, in some cases, be reared by parents or caregivers who are overly permissive and tolerant.

Treatment for passive-aggressive behavior includes the cooperation of parents or caregivers who are often in the best position to provide motivation for children to learn to appropriately express their assertiveness. Such motivation may be further supported by the establishment of firm rules and guidelines, the setting of realistic goals, and the prioritizing of responsibilities. Some parents or caregivers may benefit from direct management training that teaches the necessary skills to facilitate proper behavior and other social skills. Individual, group, and family psychotherapy may also be indicated. Other treatment is supportive.

Government Agencies

5486 NIH/National Institute of Mental Health
6001 Executive Boulevard, Room 6200, MSC 9663
Bethesda, MD 20892

301-443-4536
866-615-6464
Fax: 301-443-4279
TTY: 301-443-8431
nimhinfo@nih.gov
www.nimh.nih.gov

Conducts strategic planning for specific research areas as well as for the Institute as a whole.

Joshua Gordon, MD, PhD, Director
Shelli Avenevoli, MD, Deputy Director

National Associations & Support Groups

5487 American Academy of Pediatrics
141 Northwest Point Boulevard
Elk Grove Village, IL 60007

847-434-4000
800-433-9016
Fax: 847-434-8000
www.aap.org

The American Academy of Pediatrics and its member pediatricians are committed to the attainment of optimal physical, mental and social health and well-being for all infants, children, adolescents, and young adults.

Fernando Stein, MD, FAAP, President
Karen Remley, MD, CEO/Executive VP

5488 American Mental Health Foundation (AMHF)
PO Box 3
Riverdale, NY 10471
USA

212-737-9027
elomke@americanmentalhealthfoundation.or
americanmentalhealthfoudnation.org

Dedicated to the extensive and intensive research in the theories and techniques of treatment of emotional illness and to the implementation of reforms in the mental health system. Efforts have resulted in development of better and less expensive treatment methods. Findings are disseminated in English and other major languages.

Evander Lomke, President/Executive Director

5489 Christian Horizons
25 Sportsworld Crossing Road
Kitchener, MI N2P 0

519-650-0966
866-362-6810
Fax: 519-650-8984
info@christian-horizons.org
www.christian-horizons.org

To share Christ's love as we equip and support Adults with developmental disabilities.

5490 Federation of Families for Children's Mental Health
9605 Medical Center Drive, Suite 280
Rockville, MD 20850

240-403-1901
Fax: 240-403-1909
ffcmh@ffcmh.org
www.ffcmh.org

The National family run organization is dedicated exclusively to helping children with mental health needs and their families achieve a better quality of life.

Sandra Spencer, Executive Director

5491 Mental Health America
500 Montgomery Street, Ste 820
Alexandria, VA 22314

703-684-7722
800-969-6642
Fax: 703-684-5968
TTY: 800-433-5959
www.mentalhealthamerica.net

Addresses all aspects of mental health and mental illness. NMHA with over 340 affiliates works to improve the mental health of all Americans.

Paul Gionfriddo, President/CEO
Shavonne Carpenter, Sr Assoc., Support & Services
Mallory Pernell, Assoc. Dir, Comments/Marketing

5492 NADD: National Association for the Dually Diagnosed
132 Fair Street
Kingston, NY 12401

845-331-4336
800-331-5362
Fax: 845-331-4569
info@thenadd.org
www.thenadd.org

Nonprofit organization designed to promote the interests of professional and parent development with resources for individuals who have the coexistence of mental illness and mental retardation. Provides conferences, educational services and training materials to professionals, parents, concerned citizens and service organizations.

Dr Robert Fletcher, CEO
Michelle Jordan, Office Manager
Edward Seliger, Project Coordinator

5493 National Alliance for the Mentally Ill
3803 N Fairfax Drive, Suite 100
Arlington, VA 22203

703-524-7600
888-999-6264
Fax: 703-524-9094
TDD: 703-516-7227
info@nami.org
www.nami.org

NAMI is a nonprofit, grassroots, self-help, support and advocacy organization of consumers, families and friends of people with severe mental illness, such as schizophrenia, bipolar disorder, major depressive disorder, obsessive compulsive disorder, anxiety disorders, autism and other severe and persistent mental illnesses that affect the brain.

Suzanne Vogel-Scibilia MD, President

5494 National Mental Health Consumers' Self-Help Clearinghouse
1211 Chestnut Street, Suite 1207
Philadelphia, PA 19107

215-751-1810
800-553-4539
Fax: 215-636-6312
info@mhselfhelp.org
www.mhselfhelp.org

Offers information, support and appropriate referrals; and promotes public and professional education. Provides networking for those with special interests related to albinism. Promotes and supports research and funding that will improve diagnosis and management of albinism and hypopigmentation.

Joseph Rogers, Executive Director & Founder

State Agencies & Support Groups

5495 Center for Family Support
2811 Zulettey Avenue
Bronx, NY 10461

718-518-1500
Fax: 718-518-8200
svernikoff@cfsny.org
www.cfsny.org

The Center for Family (CFS) is a not-for-profit human service agency providing support and assistance to individuals with developmental disabilities and traumatic brain injuries throughout New York City, Long Island, the lower Hudson Valley region and New Jersey.

Steven Vernikoff, Executive Director
Barbara Greenwald, Associate Executive Director

Web Sites

5496 Borderline Personality Disorder Sanctuary
borderlinepersonality.ca/bpdlinks.htm

Offers a bookstore, resources, articles, hotlines and answers questions about mental health.

5497 CyberPsych
www.cyberpsych.org

CyberPsych presents information about psychoanalysis, psychotherapy, and special topics such as anxiety disorder, the problematic use of alcohol, homophobia, and the traumatic effects of racism. CyberPsych is a nonprofit network which offers free web hosting and technical support for internet communicatios, to nonprofit groups and individuals.

5498 Dual Diagnosis
1050 Hull Street
Baltimore, MD 21230

410-209-6799
877-438-8623
Fax: 410-244-5042
www.toad.net/~arcturus/dd/papd.htm

Review of personality disorders including PAPD.

5499 El Rolphe Center
members.aol.com/elrolphe/PassiveAggressive.html

Description and overview of the Passive/Aggressive Personality by Dr Sidney Langston.

5500 I.D. Weeks Library
414 E. Clark St.
Vermillion, SD 57069

www.usd.edu/library/

5501 NADD: National Association for the Dually Diagnosed
132 Fair Street
Kingston, NY 12401

845-331-4336
800-331-5362
Fax: 845-331-4569
www.thenadd.org

Nonprofit organization designed to promote the interests of professional and care providers for individuals who have the coexistence of mental illness and mental retardation. NADD provides conferences, educational services and training materials to professionals, parents, concerned citizens and service organizations.

Dr Robert Fletcher, CEO
Michelle Jordan, Office Manager
Edward Seliger, Project Coordinator

5502 National Anxiety Foundation
www.lexington-on-line.com/naf.html

Offers information and help to persons with panic disorders, manic and depressive disorders and mental illness.

Stephen Cox, MD, President
Linda Vernon Blair, Vice-President
C. Todd Strecker, Secretary

5503 New York Online Access to Health
National Library of Medicine Building 38A
Bethesda, MD 20894

888-346-3656
info@ncbi.nlm.nih.gov
www.ncbi.nlm.nih.gov

Provides access to high quality full-text consumer health information that is accurate, timely, relevant and unbiased.

5504 Planetpsych
www.planetpsych.com

webmaster@planetpsych.com
www.planetpsych.com

Planetpsych is an online resource for mental health information.

5505 Psych Central
55 Pleasant St., Suite 207
Newburyport, MA 1950

talkback@psychcentral.com
www.psychcentral.com

Offers free informational and educational articles and resources on psychology, support and mental health online.

John M. Grohol, Psy.D., CEO & Founder
Holly R. Counts, Psy.d., Clinical Psychologist
Marie˜ Hartwell-Walker, Ed.D., Psychologist/ Therapist

Book Publishers

5506 Challenging Behaviour

Eric Emerson, author

Cambridge University Press
32 Avenue of the Americas
New York, NY 10013

212-924-3900
800-872-7423
Fax: 212-691-3239
information@cup.org
www.cup.org

Analysis and intervention in people with severe intellectual disabilities

2nd Edition 232 pages Paperback
ISBN: 0-521794-44-7

5507 Clinical Assessment and Management of Severe Personality Disorders

American Psychiatric Press
1000 Wilson Boulevard, Suite 1825
Arlington, VA 22209

703-907-7322
800-368-5777
Fax: 703-907-1091
appi@psych.org
www.appi.org

Focuses on issues relevant to the clinician in private practice, including the diagnosis of a wide range of personality disorders and alternative management approaches.

1996 250 pages Hardcover
ISBN: 0-880484-88-6

Robert E. Hales, M.D, Editor-in-Chief
Rebecca D. Rinehart, Publisher
John McDuffie, Editorial Director

5508 Personality and Psychopathology

American Psychiatric Press
1000 Wilson Boulevard, Suite 1825
Arlington, VA 22209

703-907-7322
800-368-5777
Fax: 703-907-1091
appi@psych.org
www.appi.org

Compiles the most recent findings from more than 30 internationally recognized experts. Analyzes the association between personality and psychopathology from several interlocking perspectives: descriptive, developmental, etiological, and theraputic.

1999 544 pages Hardcover
ISBN: 0-880489-23-2

Robert E. Hales, M.D, Editor-in-Chief
Rebecca D. Rinehart, Publisher
John McDuffie, Editorial Director

DESCRIPTION

5509 PATENT DUCTUS ARTERIOSUS

Synonym: PDA

Involves the following Biologic System(s):

Cardiovascular Disorders

Patent ductus arteriosus is characterized by the persistence of a fetal vessel that maintains a passageway between the major artery that carries oxygen-rich blood to the tissues of the body (descending aorta) and the artery that carries deoxygenated blood to the lungs (pulmonary artery). Before birth, fetal blood receives oxygen from the mother's blood rather than from its own lungs, making it unnecessary for fetal blood to pass from the right side of the heart to the lungs to be oxygenated. To accommodate this fetal blood flow, blood passes through an opening (foramen ovale) in the wall (septum) between the two upper chambers of the heart (atria). Fetal blood is diverted away from the lungs through a vessel known as the ductus arteriosus that connects the pulmonary artery and the aorta. Normally, both the foramen ovale and ductus arteriosus close soon after birth. The persistence of the opening (patency) of the ductus arteriosus causes some blood from the aorta to flow into the pulmonary artery to the lungs instead of moving away from the heart to nourish the tissues of the body.

Symptoms and physical findings associated with patent ductus arteriosus depend upon the size of the opening and the volume of the diverted blood. A small defect may result in no symptoms while a larger opening may result in difficulty in breathing (dyspnea), rapid heartbeat (tachycardia), failure to gain weight, inflammation of the lining of the heart (bacterial endocarditis), and inefficient pumping by the heart (heart failure). Physical findings may include enlargement of the heart (cardiomegaly); characteristic heart sounds; a machinery-like heart murmur; and, if left untreated, abnormally high pressure in the lung's circulatory system (pulmonary hypertension).

Premature infants may require early intervention through restriction of fluid intake, certain drug therapy, or surgery to prevent malfunctioning of the heart or lungs. However, if no immediate surgical or medicinal intervention is required or administered, this defect may spontaneously close in many premature newborns.

In full-term infants and children, a patent ductus arteriosus may require intervention (surgical or catheter closure). Such treatment may be helpful in preventing or alleviating associated complications. The exact cause of patent ductus arteriosus in the full-term infant is unknown. It is thought to result from different genetic and environmental factors (multifactorial). For example, this irregularity may be associated with maternal German measles (rubella) infection. In addition, patent ductus arteriosus is often accompanied by other congenital heart defects. This defect appears in approximately 60 of 100,000 births and is more prevalent in females than males by a ratio of about two to one. The patent ductus arteriosus is non routinely closed in a non-surgical, outpatient catheter procedure in otherwise healthy children.

Government Agencies

5510 NIH/ Eunice Kennedy Shriver National Insti tute of Child Health & Human Development

31 Center Drive, Building 31
Bethesda, MD 20892

301-496-5113
800-370-2943
Fax: 866-760-5947
nichdpress@mail.nih.gov
www.nichd.nih.gov

Established in 1962 by congress, today the institute conducts and supports research on topics related to the health of children, adults, families and populations. Some of these topics include: developmental disabilities, growth and development, infant death, reproductive health and birth defects.

Diana W. Bianchi, Director
Paul Williams, Director, Communications

5511 NIH/National Heart, Lung and Blood Institu te

National Institute of Health
31 Center Dr MSC 2486, Bldg 31, Room 5A52
Bethesda, MD 20892

301-592-8573
Fax: 240-629-3246
TTY: 240-629-3255
NHLBIinfo@nhlbi.nih.gov
www.nhlbi.nih.gov

Primary responsibility of this organization is the scientific investigation of heart, blood vessel, lung and blood disorders. Oversees research, demonstration, prevention, education, control and training activities in these fields and emphasizes the prevention and control of heart diseases.

Gary H Gibbons, MD, Director
Nakela Cook, MD, Chief of Staff

National Associations & Support Groups

5512 American Academy of Pediatrics

141 Northwest Point Boulevard
Elk Grove Village, IL 60007

847-434-4000
800-433-9016
Fax: 847-434-8000
www.aap.org

The American Academy of Pediatrics and its member pediatricians are committed to the attainment of optimal physical, mental and social health and well-being for all infants, children, adolescents, and young adults.

Fernando Stein, MD, FAAP, President
Karen Remley, MD, CEO/Executive VP

5513 American Heart Association

7272 Greenville Avenue
Dallas, TX 75231

214-373-6300
800-242-8721
Fax: 214-706-1341
review.personal.info@heart.org
www.heart.org/HEARTORG/

Supports research, education and community service programs with the objective of reducing premature death and disability from cardiovascular diseases and stroke; coordinates the efforts of health professionals, and others engaged in the fight against heart and circulatory disease.

Nancy Brown, CEO
Dr. Stephen Houser, President
Suzie Upton, Chief Operating Officer

5514 Genetic Alliance

4301 Connecticut Avenue NW, Suite 404
Washington, DC 20008

202-966-5557
800-336-4363
Fax: 202-966-8553
info@geneticalliance.org
www.geneticalliance.org

A coalition of voluntary genetic support groups, consumers and professionals addressing the needs of individuals and families affected by genetic disorders from a national perspective.

Sharon Terry, President/CEO
Tetyana Murza, Managing Director
Natasha Bonhomme, VP, Strategic Development

5515 March of Dimes Foundation
1275 Mamaroneck Avenue
White Plains, NY 10605
914-997-4488
888-663-4637
Fax: 914-428-8203
answers@marchofdimes.com
www.marchofdimes.com

Partnership of volunteers and professionals dedicates to improving the health of babies by preventing birth defects and infant mortality. Over 100 chapters are located across the country and can be located through the National Office.

Stacey D. Stewart, President

Web Sites

5516 Congenital Heart Information Network
www.tchin.org

An international organization that provides reliable information, support services and resources to families of children with congenital heart defects and acquired heart disease, adults with congenital heart defects, and the professionals who work with them.

5517 Southern Illinois University School of Medicine
P.O.Box 19658
Springfield, IL 62794
217-545-8000
www.siumed.edu/peds/index.htm

Mission is to assist the people of central and southern Illinois in meeting their present and future health care needs through education, clinical service and research.

5518 Yale University School of Medicine
333 Cedar Street
New Haven, CT 6510
203-737-1770
medicine.yale.edu

A helpful site that explains the causes, symptoms and treatments for Patent Ductus Arteriosus.

Peter Salovey, President
Richard Belitsky, Deputy Dean
Benjamin Polak, Provost

Book Publishers

5519 Congenital Disorders Sourcebook
Omnigraphics
PO Box 625
Holmes, PA 19043
800-234-1340
Fax: 800-875-1340
info@omnigraphics.com
www.omnigraphics.com

Basic consumer health information on disorders aquired during gestation, including spina bifida, hydrocephalus, cerebral palsy, heart defects, craniofacial abnormalities and fetal alcohol syndrome.

650 pages
ISBN: 0-780809-45-9

Peter Ruffner, Publisher

DESCRIPTION

5520 PEMPHIGUS

Involves the following Biologic System(s):

Dermatologic Disorders

Pemphigus refers to a group of chronic skin disorders that are characterized by the appearance of blisters on the skin and delicate mucous membranes that line the mouth, for example. Pemphigus most often occurs amoung the adult population, but may appear at any age. Associated findings include a phenomenon known as Nikolsky's sign, characterized by the tendency of the upper layer of the skin to separate or slough off from the lower layer upon rubbing or other minor trauma. Pemphigus is thought to result from an autoimmune reaction during which the body mistakenly attacks healthy cells. In this case, antibodies attack the cells that glue skin together, resulting in disruptions in contact between the cells.

Benign familial pemphigus is a relatively mild form of this disorder that is inherited as an autosomal dominant trait and is characterized by the persistent and recurrent formation of blisters mainly in the groin area, the armpit (axillary) region, the sides of the neck, and on the bending surfaces of the arms and legs. These localized or widespread lesions rupture, erode, and then crust over and heal. This form of pemphigus is also known as Hailey-Hailey disease.

Pemphigus foliaceus is a rare, usually mild form of the disorder that is characterized by small blisters that are usually localized and rupture easily, erode, and then heal by crusting over or scaling. These lesions most commonly appear on the scalp, neck, face, and trunk. The blisters may cause itching, pain, or burning in the affected areas. Affected individuals may also experience the sloughing off of the upper skin layer (Nikolsky's sign). Some affected individuals may develop a more generalized pattern of eruptions characterized by excessive shedding or peeling of the skin. Treatment for pemphigus foliaceus may include therapy with corticosteriod drugs. In some cases, topical application of corticosteroid ointments, salves, or creams proves beneficial.

Pemphigus vulgaris is a very severe form of disease that is manifested by eruptions of painful, ulcerative lesions in the delicate mucous membranes that line the mouth. Later findings include the appearance of large blisters on previously unaffected areas of the face, chest, abdomen, armpit region, groin area, and the various pressure points of the body. These lesions enlarge and rupture, leaving raw areas that may partially crust over, but have little or no tendency to heal. These raw or denuded areas sometimes give rise to wart-like granulations that emit a strong, offensive odor. This stage of pemphigus vulgaris is sometimes referred to as pemphigus vegetans. The folds of the skin are particularly susceptible to the development of these wart-like lesions. Individuals with pemphigus vulgaris also exhibit Nikolsky's sign. Life-threatening complications associated with pemphigus vulgaris may include secondary bacterial infections such as sepsis or debilitating conditions such as malnutrition and the loss of essential elements, known as electrolytes, in the fluid portion of the blood (e.g., sodium, potassium, and calcium). For this reason, early diagnosis and treatment of pemphigus vulgaris is essential to its successful management. Positive diagnosis may be determined through microscopic examination of a skin sample, obtained through biopsy, that indicates the presence of certain antibody deposits. Initial treatment may include high-dose corticosteroid therapy, followed by long-term administration of corticosteroid or other immunosuppressive drugs to control the disease. Antibiotic therapy may be indicated for treatment of skin or secondary bacterial infections.

Neonatal pemphigus vulgaris develops in the unborn fetus of an affected mother by transmission of the mother's antibodies through the placenta. In most cases, the severity of disease in the fetus is related to the severity of the mother's disease. If the mother is severely affected, the placental transmission of antibodies may potentially threaten the life of the unborn child.

Government Agencies

5521 NIH/ Eunice Kennedy Shriver National Insti tute of Child Health & Human Development

31 Center Drive, Building 31
Bethesda, MD 20892

301-496-5113
800-370-2943
Fax: 866-760-5947
nichdpress@mail.nih.gov
www.nichd.nih.gov

Established in 1962 by congress, today the institute conducts and supports research on topics related to the health of children, adults, families and populations. Some of these topics include: developmental disabilities, growth and development, infant death, reproductive health and birth defects.

Diana W. Bianchi, Director
Paul Williams, Director, Communications

5522 NIH/National Institute of Arthritis and Musculoskeletal and Skin Diseases

1 AMS Circle
Bethesda, MD 20892

301-495-4484
877-226-4267
Fax: 301-718-6366
TDD: 301-565-2966
niamsinfo@mail.nih.gov
www.niams.nih.gov

The mission of the NIAMS, a part of the NIH, is to support research into the causes, treatment, and prevention of arthritis and musculoskeletal and skin diseases, the training of basic and clinical scientists to carry out this research, and the dissemination of information on research progress in these diseases.

Stephen I Katz MD PhD, Director
Robert H Carter MD, Deputy Director

National Associations & Support Groups

5523 American Academy of Pediatrics

141 Northwest Point Boulevard
Elk Grove Village, IL 60007

847-434-4000
800-433-9016
Fax: 847-434-8000
www.aap.org

The American Academy of Pediatrics and its member pediatricians are committed to the attainment of optimal physical, mental and social health and well-being for all infants, children, adolescents, and young adults.

Fernando Stein, MD, FAAP, President
Karen Remley, MD, CEO/Executive VP

5524 American Autoimmune Related Diseases Association

22100 Gratiot Avenue
Eastpointe, MI 48021

586-776-3900
800-598-4668
Fax: 586-776-3903
aarda@aarda.org
www.aarda.org

Dedicated to the eradication of autoimmune diseases and the alleviation of suffering and the socio-economic impact of autoimmunity through fostering and facilitating collaboration in the areas of education, public awareness, research and patient services in an effective, ethical and efficient manner.

Virginia T. Ladd, President/Executive Director
Patricia Barber, Assistant Director
Deb Patrick, Events Specialist

5525 Genetic Alliance
4301 Connecticut Avenue NW, Suite 404
Washington, DC 20008   202-966-5557
                                        800-336-4363
                                   Fax: 202-966-8553
                               info@geneticalliance.org
                               www.geneticalliance.org

A coalition of voluntary genetic support groups, consumers and professionals addressing the needs of individuals and families affected by genetic disorders from a national perspective.

Sharon Terry, President/CEO
Tetyana Murza, Managing Director
Natasha Bonhomme, VP, Strategic Development

5526 International Pemphigus Foundation
1331 Garden Highway, Ste 100
Sacramento, CA 95833   916-922-1298
                                   Fax: 916-922-1458
                               pemphigus@pemphigus.org
                               www.pemphigus.org

A nonprofit organization with these goals: to increase awareness of pemphigus and pemphigold among the public and the medical community; to provide information and emotional support to pemphigus and pemphigold patients and caregivers; to provide referrals to specialists and to support research into advanced treatments and a cure.

Molly Stuart, CEO
David A Sirois PhD, President
Will Zrnchik, Director Development/Communications

5527 March of Dimes Foundation
1275 Mamaroneck Avenue
White Plains, NY 10605   914-997-4488
                                        888-663-4637
                                   Fax: 914-428-8203
                               answers@marchofdimes.com
                               www.marchofdimes.com

Partnership of volunteers and professionals dedicates to improving the health of babies by preventing birth defects and infant mortality. Over 100 chapters are located across the country and can be located through the National Office.

Stacey D. Stewart, President

5528 Society for Pediatric Dermatology
8365 Keystone Crossing, Suite 107
Indianapolis, IN 46240   317-202-0224
                                   Fax: 317-205-9481
                               info@pedsderm.net
                               www.pedsderm.net

Objective is to promote, develop and advance education, research and care of skin disease in all pediatric age groups.

Kent Lindeman, Executive Director

State Agencies & Support Groups

California

5529 International Pemphigus Foundation: Southern California Support Group

                                        310-559-5462
                                   lynntg@prodigy.net

Lynn Glick

Maryland

5530 International Pemphigus Foundation: Baltimore Support Group

                                        410-750-1618
                                   byrnete@comcast.net

Erica Byrne

Massachusetts

5531 International Pemphigus Foundation: Massachusetts Support Group

                                        978-463-0965
                                   alppy@comcast.net

Alan Papert

New York

5532 International Pemphigus Foundation: New York Support Group
Valley Stream, NY   516-825-4594
                                   mayykoe@aol.com

Matt Koenig

South Carolina

5533 International Pemphigus Foundation: South Carolina Support Group
Gray Court, SC 29645   864-386-1620
                                   bubba2coggins@juno.com

Cheryl Jordan

Texas

5534 International Pemphigus Foundation
2701 Cottage Way #16
Sacramento, CA 95825   916-922-1298
                                   Fax: 916-922-1458
                               pemphigus@pemphigus.org
                               www.pemphigus.org

A nonprofit organization with these goals: to increase awareness of pemphigus and pemphigold among the public and the medical community; to provide information and emotional support to pemphigus and pemphigold patients and caregivers; to provide referrals to specialists and to support research into advanced treatments and a cure.

Molly Stuart, CEO
David A Sirois PhD, President
Will Zrnchik, Director Development/Communications

5535 International Pemphigus Foundation Dallas Support Group

                                        817-557-9642
                                   angela.bob@netzero.net

Angela Vickers

5536 International Pemphigus Foundation: Houston Support Group
5231 Kinglet Street
Houston, TX 77035   713-723-5647
                                   Fax: 713-726-0286
                               richardm@hal-pc.org

Richard M Schwartz

Audio Video

5537 International Pemphigus Foundation Promotional Video
International Pemphigus Foundation
1331 Garden Highway, Ste 100
Sacramento, CA 95833
916-922-1298
info@pemphigus.org
www.pemphigus.org

Promotional video available ($5.00 S/H).

Free 15 Minutes

Victoria Werth, M.D., Chair
Sergei Grando, M.D., Ph.D., Vice Chair
Badri Rengarajan, M.D., President

Web Sites

5538 American Autoimmune Related Diseases Association
22100 Gratiot Ave.
Eastpointe, MI 48021
586-776-3900
Fax: 586-776-3903
www.aarda.org

Dedicated to the eradiction of autoimmune diseases and the alleviation of suffering and the socio-economic impact of autoimmunity through fostering and facilitating collaboration in the areas of education, public awareness, research and patient services in an effective, ethical and efficient manner.

5539 Pemphigus FAQ
www.pemphigus.org.uk

Offers information about pemphigus.

Journals

5540 Pediatric Dermatology Journal
Society for Pediatric Dermatology
8365 Keystone Crossing, Suite 107
Indianapolis, IN 46240
317-202-0224
Fax: 317-205-9481
info@pedsderm.net
www.pedsderm.net

6 issues/yr

Kent Lindeman, Executive Director

Newsletters

5541 IPF Quarterly
1331 Garden Highway, Ste 100
Sacramento, CA 95833
916-922-1298
pemphigus@pemphigus.org
www.pemphigus.org

The International Pemphigus Foundation's newsletter. Dedicated exclusively to the subject of pemphigus and pemphigoid, providing the latest medical research news and reports on treatment, drugs and events.

12 pages Quarterly

Victoria Werth, M.D., Chair
Sergei Grando, M.D., Ph.D., Vice Chair
Badri Rengarajan, M.D., President

Pamphlets

5542 An Introduction to Pemphigus
1331 Garden Highway, Ste 100
Sacramento, CA 95833
916-922-1298
Fax: 916-922-1458
pemphigus@pemphigus.org
www.pemphigus.org/pubs.html

An overview of pemphigus

14 pages Handbook

Victoria Werth, M.D., Chair
Sergei Grando, M.D., Ph.D., Vice Chair
Badri Rengarajan, M.D., President

5543 Pemphigus and Pemphigoid At a Glance
1331 Garden Highway, Ste 100
Sacramento, CA 95833
916-922-1298
Fax: 916-922-1458
pemphigus@pemphigus.org
www.pemphigus.org/pubs.html

An introductory brochure designed for the doctors office. It provides a helpful overview of each disease.

2 pages Brochure

Victoria Werth, M.D., Chair
Sergei Grando, M.D., Ph.D., Vice Chair
Badri Rengarajan, M.D., President

DESCRIPTION

5544 PHENYLKETONURIA (PKU)

Synonyms: Classic phenylketonuria, PKU

Involves the following Biologic System(s):

Genetic/Chromosomal/Syndrome/Metabolic Disorders

Phenylketonuria (PKU) is an inherited metabolic disorder characterized by the absence or deficiency of phenylalanine hydroxylase (PAH), an enzyme that assists in processing or metabolizing the amino acid known as phenylalanine — which is present in almost all foods — so that cells can use it for various purposes. The role of PAH is to convert phenylalanine into another amino acid named tyrosine. An absence or deficiency of PAH results in the accumulation of excessive phenylalanine in the blood. This may lead to severe mental retardation that is frequently accompanied by seizures and other neurologic problems.

Phenylketonuria gets its name from the appearance in the urine of abnormally large quantities of byproducts of phenylalanine known as phenylketones, which give an unpleasant odor to the sweat and urine of infants and children with PKU.

Phenylketonuria is transmitted as an autosomal recessive trait, meaning that both parents must carry and transmit the mutated genes for their child develop PKU. The mutations that cause the disease occur in the genes that carry instructions for making PAH. In the United States, approximately one in 16,000 infants is affected by PKU. All infants born in hospitals in the United States are now routinely screened for PKU. This procedure, known as the Guthrie or PKU test, takes a small sample of blood from an infant's heel and examining it for phenylalanine.

Initially, most newborns with PKU have no symptoms. Early symptoms may include severe vomiting and poor eating. As they increase in age, children with untreated PKU may have an abnormally small head, irregularities of the teeth and upper jaw (maxilla), abnormalities in the structure and function of the heart, and mental retardation that develops slowly but progressively and may become apparent within the first few months of life. Other effects of untreated PKU include unusual paleness of the skin, accompanied by skin disorders such as eczema, behavioral abnormalities, and neuromuscular irregularities such as involuntary, continuous, slow movements of the arms and legs (athetosis). Other findings may include seizures and hyperactivity, sometimes accompanied by rhythmic behaviors such as rocking; light-colored skin, blonde hair, and blue eyesand an eczema-type rash that disappears with age.

Treatment for PKU is aimed toward reducing dietary intake of phenylalanine in order to prevent or reduce damage to the brain. The most effective treatment consists of a special diet of foods that help control the amount of PAH consumed (some PAH is needed for normal growth and development). The diet is begun as soon after birth as PKU is identified, and is monitored under close supervision. It consists of fruits and vegetables, breads, pastas, and cereals with a low protein content, since proteins contain relatively large quantities of phenylalanine. The diet does not contain high-protein foods such as eggs, cheeses, meat, milk, or nuts. People with PKU who are on this diet from birth or shortly thereafter develop normally and often have no symptoms of PKU. It is recommended that pregnant women with PKU or affected women who are planning to become pregnant maintain a low phenylalanine diet to avoid the risk of miscarriage. Infants born to women with PKU and are not on a special diet are at high risk of experiencing serious effects of the disease.

National Associations & Support Groups

5545 American Academy of Pediatrics
141 Northwest Point Boulevard
Elk Grove Village, IL 60007

847-434-4000
800-433-9016
Fax: 847-434-8000
www.aap.org

The American Academy of Pediatrics and its member pediatricians are committed to the attainment of optimal physical, mental and social health and well-being for all infants, children, adolescents, and young adults.

Fernando Stein, MD, FAAP, President
Karen Remley, MD, CEO/Executive VP

5546 Children's PKU Network
3306 Bumann Rd
Encinitas, CA 92024

858-509-0767
800-377-6677
Fax: 858-509-0768
pkunetwork@aol.com
www.pkunetwork.org

Provides support services and treatment products to families affected by phenylketonuria (PKU). Services include referral, newborn express packages, digital scale sales and crises intervention aid.

Cindy Neptune, Executive Director

5547 March of Dimes Foundation
1275 Mamaroneck Avenue
White Plains, NY 10605

914-997-4488
888-663-4637
Fax: 914-428-8203
answers@marchofdimes.com
www.marchofdimes.com

Partnership of volunteers and professionals dedicates to improving the health of babies by preventing birth defects and infant mortality. Over 100 chapters are located across the country and can be located through the National Office.

Stacey D. Stewart, President

State Agencies & Support Groups

5548 PKU Organization of Illinois
PO Box 102
Palatine, IL 60078

630-415-2219
Fax: 208-978-8963
info@pkuil.org
www.pkuil.org

Resource for families in Illinois and around the world dealing with phenylketonuria. Founded in 1969 for the benefit of patients and families.

Joseph Annunzio, President
Lisa Irgang, VP
Christine Davis, Treasurer

Web Sites

5549 National Human Genome Research Institute
biotech.law.lsu.edu/research/fed/tfgt/appendix5.htm

Report on the history of phenylketonuria screening in newborns in the U.S.

Diane B. Paul, Author

5550 National Society for Phenylketonuria (UK)
PO Box 3143
Purley, CR 89DD
303-040-1090
Fax: 845-004-8341
info@nspku.org
www.nspku.org

Helps and supports people with PKU, their families and care-givers. The NSPKU actively promotes the care and treatment of PKU and works closely with medical professionals in the UK.

Eric Lange, Chair
Iain Williamson, Secretary
Lisa Lee, Treasurer

5551 Online Mendelian Inheritance in Man
National Library of Medicine, Building 38A
Bethesda, MD 20894
888-346-3656
info@ncbi.nlm.nih.gov
www.ncbi.nlm.nih.gov

This database is a catalog of human genes and genetic disorders.

5552 PKU Kid Zone
www.pkuil.org/kidzone.htm

Provides activities for chidren to have fun online.

5553 PKU Mailing List
PO Box 3143
Purley, CR 89DD
303-040-1090
Fax: 845-004-8341
info@nspku.org
www.nspku.org/listserve

Worldwide mailing list making communication between families dealing with PKU easier.

Eric Lange, Chair
Iain Williamson, Secretary
Lisa Lee, Treasurer

5554 PKU Organization of Illinois
PO Box 102
Palatine, IL 60078
630-344-9758
pkuillinois@gmail.com
www.pkuil.org

Committed to the support of appropriate research initiatives to better understand PKU and eventually find a cure. Support services include: get togethers for kids and parents to express their concerns and share ways of coping with the disease, annual picnics throughout the state and family camp to get to know other PKU families, and activities on both state and national levels in protecting the interests of PKU families.

5555 Star-G: Screening, Technology and Research in Genetics
741 Sunset Avenue
Honolulu, HI 96816
808-733-9039
Fax: 808-733-9068
lianne@hawaiigenetics.org
www.newbornscreening.info

General and newborn screening information for amino acid disorders including PKU.

Newsletters

5556 National PKU News
6869 Woodland Avenue NE, Suite 116
Seattle, WA 98115
206-525-8140
Fax: 206-525-5023
schuett@pkunews.org
www.pkunews.org

Nonprofit organization dedicated to providing up-to-date, accurate news and information to families and professionals dealing with phenylketonuria through this newsletter.

2000+ 3 issues/year

Virginia Schuett, Director/Editor

5557 PKU Press
PKU Organization of Illinois
PO Box 102
Palatine, IL 60078
630-344-9758
Fax: 208-978-8963
pkuillinois@gmail.com
www.pkuil.org

Provides information, support, and highlights achievements for the benefit of the PKU community.

20 pages 3x/year

Joseph Annunzio, President
Lisa Irgang, VP
Christine Davis, Treasurer

Pamphlets

5558 Phenylketonuria (PKU) Information Sheet
March of Dimes Pregnancy & Newborn Health Edu Ctr
1275 Mamaroneck Avenue
White Plains, NY 10605
914-997-4488
Fax: 914-997-4763
answers@marchofdimes.com
www.marchofdimes.org/pregnancy.aspx

Defines and discusses the implications and causes of PKU, as well as testing, treatment, prevention and research.

DESCRIPTION

5559 PHOBIAS

Involves the following Biologic System(s):

Developmental/Behavioral/Psychiatric Disorders

A phobia is a persistent, exaggerated, unreasonable fear or dread of certain activities, situations, objects, or events. Exposure to the activity, situation, or object that arouses fear typically elicits signs of anxiety or panic reaction. Such symptoms may include nausea, abdominal pain, irregular pulsation or racing of the heart (palpitations), sweating, and dizziness. In contrast to adults, children, especially younger one, don't see their fear as excessive or unreasonable. Most children are fearful of particular things as they reach certain age plateaus. For example, young children are often afraid of monsters or of being alone in the dark. Older children may be fearful of death or other distressing situations. Children may become fearful of events or situations that they view on television. Others may have fear or dread related to conflicts in the home. These fears are not unusual and may often be alleviated by reassurances and comforting by parents and caregivers. However, a fear or phobia that interferes with normal, day-to-day functioning is considered pathologic.

Simple or specific phobias include fear of certain animals and insects or particular situations (e.g., fear of flying, etc.). Social phobias, often appearing in late childhood or adolescence, include fear and avoidance of certain social situations such as using public bathroom facilities or eating, speaking, performing, or writing in public. Researchers believe that some simple phobias may result from an associated, traumatic childhood experience or from the existence of a similar fear in a parent or caregiver. More complicated specific phobias (e.g., fear of attending school, etc.) may be associated with such conflicts as a hostile-dependent relationship between the parent or caregiver and the child.

Treatment for phobias is dependent upon the specific fear, the extent of the fear, and the effect of the phobias on day-to-day living. Parents or caregivers are counseled to remain calm and patient when confronted with a phobic episode. Behavioral therapy, including relaxation therapy for older children, may be indicated and may include the training of parents or caregivers in the use of supportive measures and techniques. Slow and orderly exposure to the activity, situation, or object of fear (desensitization) may help to alleviate the fear. Older children and adolescents with social phobias may learn to overcome their particular fear through social skills training. Other treatment is symptomatic and supportive.

Government Agencies

5560 Center for Mental Health Services Knowledge Exchange Program

US Department of Health and Human Services
PO Box 42557
Washington, DC 20015

800-789-2647
Fax: 240-747-5470
TDD: 866-889-2647
http://mentalhealth.samhsa.gov

Supplies the public with expert responses to commonly asked questions about various mental health disorders, and directs the caller to appropriate resources.

5561 NIH/National Institute of Mental Health

6001 Executive Boulevard, Room 6200, MSC 9663
Bethesda, MD 20892

301-443-4536
866-615-6464
Fax: 301-443-4279
TTY: 301-443-8431
nimhinfo@nih.gov
www.nimh.nih.gov

Conducts strategic planning for specific research areas as well as for the Institute as a whole.

Joshua Gordon, MD, PhD, Director
Shelli Avenevoli, MD, Deputy Director

National Associations & Support Groups

5562 Agoraphobics in Motion

P.O. Box 725363
Berkley, MI 48072

248-547-0400
anny@ameritech.net
www.aimforrecovery.com

A.I.M. has been helping people with anxiety disorders since 1983.

James Fortune, President
Robert Diedrich, Vice President
Mary Ann Gogoleski, SWT, Director

5563 American Academy of Pediatrics

141 Northwest Point Boulevard
Elk Grove Village, IL 60007

847-434-4000
800-433-9016
Fax: 847-434-8000
www.aap.org

The American Academy of Pediatrics and its member pediatricians are committed to the attainment of optimal physical, mental and social health and well-being for all infants, children, adolescents, and young adults.

Fernando Stein, MD, FAAP, President
Karen Remley, MD, CEO/Executive VP

5564 American Counseling Association

6101 Stevenson Ave
Alexandria, VA 22304

703-823-9800
800-347-6647
Fax: 703-823-0252
webmaster@counseling.org
www.counseling.org

Represents professional counselors in various practice settings, and stands ready to serve more than 55,000 members with the resources they need to make a difference. From webinars, publications, and journals to Conference education sessions and legislative action alerts, ACA is where counseling professionals turn for powerful, credible content and support.

Robert L. Smith, President

5565 American Mental Health Foundation (AMHF)

PO Box 3
Riverdale, NY 10028

212-737-9027
elomke@americanmentalhealthfoundation.or
americanmentalhealthfoudnation.org

Dedicated to the extensive and intensive research in the theories and techniques of treatment of emotional illness and to the implementation of reforms in the mental health system. Efforts have resulted in development of better and less expensive treatment methods. Findings are disseminated in English and other major languages.

Monroe W Spero, MD
Evander Lomke, Executive Director

5566 American Psychiatric Association

1000 Wilson Boulevard, Suite 1825
Arlington, VA 22209

703-907-7300
888-35-7924
apa@psych.org
www.psychiatry.org

It is a medical specialty society representing growing membership of more than 36,000 psychiatrists.

5567 American Psychological Association
750 First St. NE
Washington, DC 20002   202-336-5500
                                    800-374-2721
                                    TTY: 202-336-6123
                                    www.apa.org

The mission is to advance the creation, communication and application of psychological knowledge to benefit society and improve people's lives.

Norman B. Anderson, PhD, CEO/ EVP
L. Michael Honaker, PhD, Deputy Chief Executive Officer
Ellen G. Garrison, PhD, Senior Policy Advisor

5568 American School Counselor Association
1101 King Street, Suite 310
Alexandria, VA 22314   703-683-2722
                                    800-306-4722
                                    Fax: 703-997-7572
                                    asca@schoolcounselor.org
                                    www.schoolcounselor.org

The mission of ASCA is to represent professional school counselors and to promote professionalism and ethical practices.

Richard Wong, Executive Director
Jeff Broderson, Information Technology Admin.
Kathleen M Rakestraw, Director of Communications

5569 Anxiety Disorders Association of America
8730 Georgia Avenue, Suite 600
Silver Spring, MD 20910   240-485-1001
                                    Fax: 240-485-1035
                                    information@adaa.org
                                    www.adaa.org

Offers resources and information for persons with anxiety and stress-related disorders.

Alies Muskin, Executive Director

5570 Anxiety Disorders Institute
1 Dunwoody Park Suite 112
Atlanta, GA 30338   770-395-6845

Provides support, training, and services for those suffering from anxiety disorders, and their families.

5571 Anxiety and Depression Association of America
8701 Georgia Ave., Suite #412
Silver Spring, MD 20910   240-485-1001
                                    Fax: 240-485-1035
                                    www.adaa.org

ADAA is a national nonprofit organization dedicated to the prevention, treatment, and cure of anxiety, depression, OCD, PTSD, and related disorders and to improving the lives of all people who suffer from them through education, practice, and research.

Mark H. Pollack, MD, President
Alies Muskin, Executive Director
Jean Kaplan Teichroew

5572 Anxiety and Phobia Treatment Center
Whire Plains Hospital Center
Davis Avenue & East Post Road
White Plains, NY 10601   914-681-1038
                                    Fax: 914-681-2284
                                    jchessa@wphospital.org
                                    phobia-anxiety.com

Treatment groups for individuals suffering from phobias. Deals with fears through contextual therapy, a treatment and study of the phobia in the actual setting in which the phobic reactions occur. Conducts Intensive Courses, Phobia Self-Help Groups, 8-week Phobia Clinics and individual treatment. Publications: PM Newsletter, bimonthly. Articles and papers. Annual conference.

Fredrick J Neumen, MD, Director

5573 Federation of Families for Children's Mental Health
9605 Medical Center Drive, Suite 280
Rockville, MD 20850   240-403-1901
                                    Fax: 240-403-1909
                                    ffcmh@ffcmh.org
                                    www.ffcmh.org

The National family run organization is dedicated exclusively to helping children with mental health needs and their families achieve a better quality of life.

Sandra Spencer, Executive Director

5574 Freedom From Fear
308 Seaview Avenue
Staten Island, NY 10305   718-351-1717
                                    Fax: 718-667-8893
                                    help@freedomfromfear.org
                                    www.freedomfromfear.org

The mission of Freedom From Fear is to aid and counsel individuals and their families who suffer from anxiety and depressive illness.

Mary Guardino, Founder

5575 Mental Health America
500 Montgomery Street, Ste 820
Alexandria, VA 22314   703-684-7722
                                    800-969-6642
                                    Fax: 703-684-5968
                                    TTY: 800-433-5959
                                    www.mentalhealthamerica.net

Addresses all aspects of mental health and mental illness. NMHA with over 340 affiliates works to improve the mental health of all Americans.

Paul Gionfriddo, President/CEO
Shavonne Carpenter, Sr Assoc., Support & Services
Mallory Pernell, Assoc. Dir, Comments/Marketing

5576 National Alliance for the Mentally Ill
3803 N Fairfax Drive, Suite 100
Arlington, VA 22203   703-524-7600
                                    888-999-6264
                                    Fax: 703-524-9094
                                    TDD: 703-516-7227
                                    info@nami.org
                                    www.nami.org

NAMI is a nonprofit, grassroots, self-help, support and advocacy organization of consumers, families and friends of people with severe mental illness, such as schizophrenia, bipolar disorder, major depressive disorder, obsessive compulsive disorder, anxiety disorders, autism and other severe and persistent mental illnesses that affect the brain.

Suzanne Vogel-Scibilia MD, President

5577 National Alliance on Mental Illness
3803 N. Fairfax Drive, Suite 100
Arlington, VA 22203   703-524-7600
                                    800-950-6264
                                    Fax: 703-524-9094
                                    info@nami.org
                                    www.nami.org

Grassroots mental health organization dedicated to building better lives for the millions of Americans affected by mental illness. - See more at:
http://www.nami.org/About-NAMI#sthash.lYtjmu5h.dpuf

Jim Payne, J.D., President
David Levy, Chief Financial Officer
Mary Giliberti, J.D., Executive Director

5578 National Anxiety Foundation
3135 Custer Drive
Lexington, KY 40517   859-281-0003
                                    www.lexington-on-line.com/naf.html

Nonprofit organization that provides education to the public and professionals about anxiety through printed and electronic media.

Stephen Cox MD, President & Medical Director

5579 National Mental Health Consumers' Self-Help Clearinghouse
1211 Chestnut Street, Suite 1207
Philadelphia, PA 19107
215-751-1810
800-553-4539
Fax: 215-636-6312
info@mhselfhelp.org
www.mhselfhelp.org

Offers information, support and appropriate referrals; and promotes public and professional education. Provides networking for those with special interests related to albinism. Promotes and supports research and funding that will improve diagnosis and management of albinism and hypopigmentation.

Joseph Rogers, Executive Director & Founder

5580 Phobia Society of America
133 Rollins Avenue, Suite 4B
Rockville, MD 20852
301-231-9350
Fax: 301-231-7392
www.adaa.org

Offers support for those suffering from phobia and panic attacks.

5581 Phobics Anonymous
PO Box 1180
Palm Springs, CA 92263
706-327-2148

Twelve-step program for panic disorders and anxiety. Publications available.

Marily Gellis PhD, Contact

5582 Selective Mutism Foundation
PO Box 25972
Tamarac, FL 33320
305-748-7714
Fax: 305-748-7714
www.selectivemutismfoundation.org

Promotes awareness and understanding for individuals and families affected by selective mutism, an inherited anxiety disorder in which children with normal or deficient language skills are unable to speak in school or social situations. SM is often mistaken for normal shyness and may go undetected for as long as two years. Encourages research and treatment. Maintains speakers' bureau. Publications: Let's Talk, annual newsletter. Selective Mutism, A Silent Cry for Help, brochure.

Sue Newman, Co-Founder & Director

5583 Social Anxiety Association
socialphobia.org

The Social Anxiety Association is a non-profit organization founded in 1997 to meet the growing needs of people with social anxiety.

Thomas A. Richards, Ph.D., President

5584 Special Interest Group on Phobias and Related Anxiety Disorders (SIGPRAD)
245 E 87th Street
New York, NY 10128
212-860-5560
Fax: 212-744-5751
lindy@interport.net
www.cyberpsych.org

For psychologists, psychiatrists, social workers and other individuals interested in treatment of anxiety disorders. Objectives are to increase knowledge, facilitate communication, and support research and treatment of phobias and related anxiety disorders. Conducts programs at professional meetings. Affiliated with the Association for Advancement of Behavior Therapy. Periodic symposiums and workshops.

Carol Lindemann, PhD, CEO

5585 Territorial Apprehensiveness (TERRAP) Programs
932 Evelyn Street
Menlo Park, CA 94025
800-274-6242

To disseminate information concerning the recognition, causes, and treatment of anxieties, fears and phobias especially agoraphobia. Provides information and counseling for those with phobias. Sponsors service centers and training for psychotherapists and counselors. Publications: TERRAP Manual, audiotapes, booklets, monographs, and videos.

Crucita V Hardy, Director

State Agencies & Support Groups

5586 Center for Family Support
333 7th Avenue, #901
New York, NY 10001
212-629-7939
Fax: 212-239-2211
www.cfsny.org

The Center for Family (CFS) is a not-for-profit human service agency providing support and assistance to individuals with developmental disabilities and traumatic brain injuries throughout New York City, Long Island, the lower Hudson Valley region and New Jersey.

Steven Vernikoff, Executive Director
Linda Schellenberg, Director, Community Service
Barbara Greenwald, Associate Executive Director

Research Centers

5587 UC Berkeley School of Social Welfare
Mental Health & Social Welfare Research Group
120 Haviland Hall #7400
Berkeley, CA 94720
510-642-4341
spsegal@berkeley.edu
socialwelfare.berkeley.edu/mhswrg/mhswrg.html
Steven P Segal, Director

Audio Video

5588 Acquiring Courage: Audio Cassette Program for the Rapid Treatment of Phobias
New Harbinger Publications
5674 Shattuck Avenue
Oakland, CA 94609
510-652-2002
800-748-6273
Fax: 510-652-5472
customerservice@newharbinger.com
newharbinger.com

ISBN: 1-879237-03-2

5589 Anxiety Disorders
American Counseling Association
6101 Stevenson Ave.
Alexandria, VA 22304
703-823-9800
800-347-6647
Fax: 703-823-0252
webmaster@counseling.org
counseling.org

Increase your awareness of anxiety disorders, their symptoms, and effective treatments. Learn the effect these disorders can have on life and how treatment can change the quality of life for people presently suffering from these disorders. Includes 6 audiotapes and a study guide.

Robert L. Smith, Ph.D., NCC, FPPR, President
Brain Canfield, Treasurer
Richard Yep, Chief Executive Officer

5590 Fear of Illness
New Harbinger Publications
5674 Shattuck Avenue
Oakland, CA 94609
510-652-2002
800-748-6273
Fax: 510-652-5472
customerservice@newharbinger.com
newharbinger.com

120 minute videotape that reduces fears arising from unexplained pain or symptoms; learn to relax while you desensitize to strange body sensations.

ISBN: 1-572240-15-6

5591 Flying
New Harbinger Publications
5674 Shattuck Avenue
Oakland, CA 94609   510-652-2002
                                                     800-748-6273
                                                Fax: 510-652-5472
                           customerservice@newharbinger.com
                                              newharbinger.com

120 minute videotape that reduces fear to the point where you can take longer and longer flights; desensitize to the sensations of flying.

ISBN: 1-879237-90-3

5592 Heights
New Harbinger Publications
5674 Shattuck Avenue
Oakland, CA 94609   510-652-2002
                                                     800-748-6273
                                                Fax: 510-652-5472
                           customerservice@newharbinger.com
                                              newharbinger.com

120 minute videotape that makes you feel more comfortable in high - rise buildings, on bridges, and on mountain roads.

ISBN: 1-879237-91-1

Web Sites

5593 Answers to Your Questions about Panic Disorder
750 First St. NE
Washington, DC 20002   202-336-5500
                                                     800-374-2721
                                    www.apa.org/pubinfo/panic.html

The objects of the APA shall be to advance psychology as a science and profession and as a means of promoting health, education, and human welfare by: encouragement of psychology in all its branches in the broadest and most liberal manner, the promotion of research in psychology and the improvement fo research methods and conditions, and the improvement of the qualifications and usefulness of psychologists through high standards of ethics, conduct, education, and achievement.

Barry S. Anton, PhD, President
Bonnie Markham, Treasurer
Norman B. Anderson, CEO & VP

5594 Anxiety Disorders Association of America

Offers resources and information for persons with anxiety and stress-related disorders.

5595 Anxiety Panic Internet Resource
www.algy.com/anxiety/

It is the web's first and still best self-help resource for those with anxiety disorders, Panic attacks, phobias, extreme shyness, obsessive-compulsive behaviors, and generalized anxiety disrupt the lives of an estimated 15% of the population. It is a free grass-root website dedicated to providing information, relief, and support for those recovering from debilitating anxiety.

5596 Basic Guided Relaxation: Advanced Technique
1258 Eagle Crest Dr.
Oak Harbor, WA 98277   360-593-3833
                                          wellness@dstress.com
                                      www.dstress.com/guided.htm

A guide to relaxation.

L. John Mason, Founder

5597 Causes of Anxiety and Panic Attacks
www.algy.com/anxiety/files/barlow.html

Provides information concerning phobias, what they are, the symptoms, and the effects of phobias.

5598 CyberPsych
www.cyberpsych.org

CyberPsych presents information about psychoanalysis, psychotherapy, and special topics such as anxiety disorder, the problematic use of alcohol, homophobia, and the traumatic effects of racism. CyberPsych is a nonprofit network which offers free web hosting and technical support for internet communication, to nonprofit groups and individuals.

5599 National Anxiety Foundation
3135 Custer Dr.
Lexington, KY 40517   www.lexington-on-line.com/naf.html

Endeavours to educate the public and professionals about anxiety through printed and electronic media. A volunteer, nonprofit entity.

Stephen Cox, President
Linda Vermon Blair, Vice-President
C. Todd Strecker, Secretary-Treasurer

5600 National Panic/Anxiety Disorder Newsletter
www.npadnews.com

                                          editor@npadnews.com
                                             www.npadnews.com

We provide the most up to date material which is gathered from many resourced and contributors form all corners of the globe.

5601 Panic Disorder, Separation, Anxiety Disorder
www.klis.com/chandler/pamphlet/panic

Provides information about panic attacks and more, about what can be done and what medican treatments there are.

5602 Planetpsych
www.planetpsych.com

                                      webmaster@planetpsych.com
                                           www.planetpsych.com

Planetpsych is an online resource for mental health information.

5603 Recovery Panic Anxiety
www.alt.recovery.panic.anxiety.self-help

An online support group t talk about anxiety recovery.

Book Publishers

5604 An End to Panic: Breakthrough Techniques for Overcoming Panic Disorder

Elke Zuercher-White, author

New Harbinger Publications
5674 Shattuck Avenue
Oakland, CA 94609   510-652-2002
                                                     800-748-6273
                                                Fax: 510-652-5472
                                           TTY: 800-652-1613
                           customerservice@newharbinger.com
                                          www.newharbinger.com

A state of the art treatment program covers breathing retraining, taking charge of fear-fueling thoughts, overcoming the fear of physical symptoms, coping with phobic situations, avoiding relapse, and living in the here and now.

232 pages Paperback
ISBN: 1-572241-13-6

5605 Anxiety & Phobia Workbook

Edmund J Bourne, author

New Harbinger Publications
5674 Shattuck Avenue
Oakland, CA 94609   510-652-2002
                                                     800-748-6273
                                                Fax: 510-652-5472
                                           TTY: 800-652-1613
                           customerservice@newharbinger.com
                                          www.newharbinger.com

This comprehensive guide is recommended to those struggling with anxiety disorders. Includes step-by-step instructions for the crucial cognitive-behavioral techniques that have given real help to hundreds of thousands of readers struggling with anxiety disorders.

448 pages 4th Edition
ISBN: 1-572244-13-5

5606 Anxiety Cure: An Eight-Step Program for Getting Well
John Wiley & Sons
10475 Crosspoint Boulevard
Indianapolis, IN 46256   877-762-2974
                                              Fax: 800-597-3299
                                                  www.wiley.com

A practical guide, written by a father and his two daughters, featuring a step-by-step program for curing the six main kinds of anxiety.

272 pages 2nd Edition
ISBN: 0-471464-87-2

Peter B. Wiley, Chairman
Stephen M. Smith, President & CEO
Ellis E. Cousens, Executive Vice President, Chief Fin

5607 Anxiety Disorders
Cambridge University Press
40 W 20th Street
New York, NY 10011   212-924-3900
                                               800-872-7423
                                              Fax: 914-937-4712
                                             marketing@cup.org
                                                       cup.org

This comprehensive text covers all the anxiety disorders found in the latest DSM and ICD classifications. Provides detailed information about seven principal disorders, including anxiety in the medically ill. For each disorder, the book covers diagnosis criteria, epidemiology, etiology and pathogenesis, clinical features, natural history and different diagnoses. Describes treatment approaches, both psychological and pharmacological.

354 pages

5608 Anxiety Disorders: Practioner's Guide
John Wiley & Sons
605 3rd Avenue
New York, NY 10058   212-850-6000
                                              Fax: 212-850-6008
                                                info@wiley.com
                                                     wiley.com

210 pages
ISBN: 0-471931-12-8

Peter B. Wiley, Chairman
Stephen M. Smith, President & CEO
Ellis E. Cousens, Executive Vice President, Chief Fin

5609 Encyclopedia of Phobias, Fears, and Anxieties
Facts on File
11 Penn Plaza, Room M274
New York, NY 10001   212-290-8090
                                               800-322-8755

500 pages

5610 Helping Your Anxious Child
New Harbinger Publications
5674 Shattuck Avenue
Oakland, CA 94609   510-652-2002
                                               800-748-6273
                                              Fax: 510-652-5472
                                             TTY: 800-652-1613
                              customerservice@newharbinger.com
                                          www.newharbinger.com

Step-by-step guide for parents of anxious children to help them overcome their fears and anxieties. Detailed strategies and techniques.

168 pages Paperback
ISBN: 1-572241-91-8

5611 It's Nobody's Fault: New Hope and Help for Difficult Children and Their Parents
ADD WareHouse
300 NW 70th Avenue
Plantation, FL 33317   954-792-8944
                                               800-233-9273
                                              Fax: 954-792-8545
                                              addwarehouse.com

This book explains that neither the parents nor children are causes of mental disorders and related problems.

184 pages

5612 Perfectionism: What's Bad About Being Too Good
Free Spirit Pub

With help for superkids, workaholics, type A's, straight A's, procrastinators, overacheivers, and caring adults, this book explains the differance between healthy ambition and unhealthy perfectionism and gives straight strategies for getting out of the perfectionist trap- from recognizing the symptoms to rewarding yourself for who you are, not what you do. It explains why some people become perfectionists, what it does to the body, and why girls are more prone to it, and more.

1999 144 pages

Miriam Adderholt, PhD, Author
Miriam Elliot, Author
Judy Galbraith, Author

5613 Psychological Trauma
American Psychiatric Press
1400 K Street, NW
Washington, DC 20005   202-682-6262
                                               800-368-5777
                                              Fax: 202-789-2648
                                                order@appi.org
                                                  www.appi.org

Epidemiology of trauma and post-tramatic stress disorder. Evaluation, neuroimaging, neuroendocrinology and pharmacology.

1998 206 pages

Robert E. Hales M.D, Editor-in-Chief
Rebecca D. Rinehart, Publisher
John McDuffie, Editorial Director

5614 Shy Children, Phobic Adults: Nature and Treatment of Social Phobia
American Psychological Press
1400 K Street, NW
Washington, DC 20005   202-682-6262
                                               800-368-5777
                                              Fax: 202-789-2648
                                               orders@appi.org
                                                  www.appi.org

Describes the simuliarities and differences in the syndrome across all ages. Draws from the clinical, social and developmental literatures, as well as from extensive clinical experience. Illustrates the impact of developmental stage on phenomenology, diagnosis and assessment and treatment of social phobia.

1998 321 pages

Robert E. Hales M.D. Editor-in-Chief
Rebecca D. Rinehart, Publisher
John McDuffie, Editorial Director

Pamphlets

5615 5 Smart Steps to Less Stress
ETR Associates
PO Box 1830
Santa Cruz, CA 95061   831-438-4060
                                               800-321-4407
                                              Fax: 800-435-8433

Steps to managing stress include: know what stresses you, manage your stress, take care of your body, take care of your feelings, ask for help.

5616 Anxiety Disorders
National Institute of Mental Health
6001 Executive Boulevard, Room 6200
Bethesda, MD 20892   301-443-4513
                                      866-615-6464
                                 Fax: 301-443-4279
                                 TTY: 301-443-8431
                                 nimhinfo@nih.gov
                                 www.nimh.nih.gov

This brochure helps to identify the symptoms of anxiety disorders, explains the role of research in understanding the causes of these conditions, describes effective treatments, helps you learn how to obtain treatment and work with a doctor or therapist, and suggests ways to make treatment more effective.

Francis Collins, M.D., Director
Tom Insel, Director

5617 Anxiety Disorders Fact Sheet
Center for Mental Health Services
PO Box 42490
Washington, DC 20015   800-789-2647
                                 Fax: 301-984-8796
                                 ken@mentalhealth.org
                                 mentalhealth.org

This fact sheet presents basic information on the symptoms, formal diagnosis, and treatment for generalized anxiety disorder, panic disorders, phobias, and post traumatic stress disorder.

3 pages

5618 Anxiety Disorders in Children and Adolescents
Center for Mental Health Services
PO Box 42490
Washington, DC 20015   800-789-2647
                                 Fax: 301-984-8796
                                 ken@mentalhealth.org
                                 mentalhealth.org

This fact sheet defines anxiety disorders, identifies warning signs, discusses risk factors, describes types of help available, and suggests what parents or other caregivers can do.

3 pages

5619 Families Can Help Children Cope with Fear, Anxiety
Center for Mental Health Services
PO Box 42490
Washington, DC 20015   800-789-2647
                                 Fax: 301-984-8796
                                 ken@mentalhealth.org
                                 mentalhealth.org

This fact sheet defines conduct disorder, identifies risk factors, discusses types of help available, and suggests what parents or other caregivers responses should be to common signs of fear and anxiety.

5620 Panic Attacks
ETR Associates
PO Box 1830
Santa Cruz, CA 95061   831-438-4060
                                      800-321-4407
                                 Fax: 800-435-8433

Describes causes of panic attacks, including genetics, stress, and drug use; prevention and treatment, and how to stop a panic attack in its tracks.

DESCRIPTION

5621 PHOTOSENSITIVITY

Covers these related disorders: Photoallergic reaction, Phototoxic reaction

Involves the following Biologic System(s):
Dermatologic Disorders

Photosensitivity, sometimes referred to as sun allergy, is an abnormal reaction of the skin to sunlight or artificial light that is usually characterized by the rapid development of redness, swelling, tenderness, peeling, blistering, hives, or other skin irregularities. The skin reactions associated with photosensitivity are often induced by the interaction of light and certain substances known as photosensitizers that are ingested or applied directly to the skin. Such photosensitizers may include antibiotics, antifungal agents, and other drugs as well as some perfumes, soaps, dyes, and plants (e.g., buttercups, parsley, parsnips, mustard, etc.).

Particular wavelengths of light interact with photosensitizers to produce skin inflammations (dermatitis) that may be considered photoallergic or phototoxic. A photoallergic reaction is a delayed immune or allergic response of the skin that results from having been previously exposed to a photosensitizer and light. Such photosensitizers may include barbiturates, certain antibiotics such as tetracycline, and other medications as well as certain topical agents such as coal tar derivatives, perfume oils such as bergamot, etc. A phototoxic reaction is a nonimmune response to the accumulation of certain chemicals in the skin. This type of skin reaction may be similar in appearance to a severe sunburn; some individuals may develop hives or blisters. The initial inflammation is usually followed by abnormally increased skin pigmentation (hyperpigmentation). Phototoxic reactions result from high doses of certain photosensitizers that may cause photoallergic reactions in lower doses, as well as from additional chemical substances. Treatment includes the withdrawal of offending medications and other photosensitizers and sunlight avoidance. In addition, administration of antihistamines and topical corticosteroids may be effective in eliminating associated itching (pruritus).

Photosensitivity is also associated with certain disorders in children. Such disorders may include congenital erythropoietic porphyria (EPP), an autosomal recessive disorder that results from a deficiency of an enzyme. This particular enzyme is necessary for the synthesis of heme, which is the oxygen-carrying component of a certain protein (hemoprotein) found in the tissues of the body. Congenital erythropoietic porphyria develops within a few months of birth and is characterized by a severe sensitivity to light that may cause blistering eruptions on the skin, leading to severe scarring, abnormally increased skin pigmentation, and other skin irregularities. Children with this disorder may also have numerous other abnormalities. Erythropoietic protoporphyria is an autosomal dominant disorder that results from a deficiency of an enzyme that is also essential to the proper synthesis of heme. This disorder appears during early childhood and is characterized by pain, tingling, and a burning feeling upon exposure to sunlight. The skin may redden, swell, and form blisters or hives. In addition to having nail irregularities, children may develop fever and chills. Repeated exposure to sunlight may result in skin thickening and other chronic associated irregularities; however, some children experience improvement during their preadolescent years. Treatment for these types of disorders includes the avoidance of direct sunlight and the use of protective clothing and appropriate sunscreens. In addition, the administration of sufficient quantities of beta-carotene to cause a light yellowing of the skin may be effective in reducing sensitivity to sunlight. Photosensitivity is a feature of many other disorders that may include Cockayne syndrome, xeroderma pigmentosum, hydroa vacciniforme, Rothmund-Thomson syndrome, and other diseases.

Occasionally, some individuals experience an unusual photosensitive reaction to sunlight in the absence of any apparent photosensitizer or associated disease. This type of photosensitivity is called polymorphous light eruption and is one of the most common sun-related skin problems. It is characterized by the appearance of hives or other itchy, rash-type reactions on exposed areas. Polymorphous light eruption usually occurs after a prolonged initial sun exposure in the spring or summer. The eruption may occur within hours or days of the exposure and may remain for hours, days, or weeks. Treatment may include oral or topical corticosteroid therapy. In addition, susceptible people are counseled to avoid the sun, wear protective clothing, and use sunscreen.

Individuals with certain types of photosensitivity may benefit from the cautious administration of photosensitizing drugs that enhance pigmentation of the skin (psoralens). In addition, certain types of phototherapy may be effective. Other treatment is symptomatic and supportive.

Government Agencies

5622 NIH/ Eunice Kennedy Shriver National Institute of Child Health & Human Development
31 Center Drive, Building 31
Bethesda, MD 20892
301-496-5113
800-370-2943
Fax: 866-760-5947
nichdpress@mail.nih.gov
www.nichd.nih.gov

Established in 1962 by congress, today the institute conducts and supports research on topics related to the health of children, adults, families and populations. Some of these topics include: developmental disabilities, growth and development, infant death, reproductive health and birth defects.

Diana W. Bianchi, Director
Paul Williams, Director, Communications

5623 NIH/National Eye Institute
31 Center Drive MSC 2510
Bethesda, MD 20892
301-496-5248
2020@nei.nih.gov
www.nei.nih.gov

Conducts and supports research that helps prevent and treat eye diseases and other disorders of vision. This research leads to sight-saving treatments, reduces visual impairment and blindness, and improves the quality of life for people of all ages. NEI-supported research has advanced our knowledge of how the eye functions in health and disease.

Paul A Sieving M.D., Ph.D., Director

5624 NIH/National Institute of Arthritis and Musculoskeletal and Skin Diseases
1 AMS Circle
Bethesda, MD 20892
301-495-4484
877-226-4267
Fax: 301-718-6366
TDD: 301-565-2966
niamsinfo@mail.nih.gov
www.niams.nih.gov

The mission of the NIAMS, a part of the NIH, is to support research into the causes, treatment, and prevention of arthritis and musculoskeletal and skin diseases, the training of basic and clinical scientists to carry out this research, and the dissemination of information on research progress in these diseases.

Stephen I Katz MD PhD, Director
Robert H Carter MD, Deputy Director

National Associations & Support Groups

5625 American Academy of Pediatrics
141 Northwest Point Boulevard
Elk Grove Village, IL 60007
847-434-4000
800-433-9016
Fax: 847-434-8000
www.aap.org

The American Academy of Pediatrics and its member pediatricians are committed to the attainment of optimal physical, mental and social health and well-being for all infants, children, adolescents, and young adults.

Fernando Stein, MD, FAAP, President
Karen Remley, MD, CEO/Executive VP

5626 Genetic Alliance
4301 Connecticut Avenue NW, Suite 404
Washington, DC 20008
202-966-5557
800-336-4363
Fax: 202-966-8553
info@geneticalliance.org
www.geneticalliance.org

A coalition of voluntary genetic support groups, consumers and professionals addressing the needs of individuals and families affected by genetic disorders from a national perspective.

Sharon Terry, President/CEO
Tetyana Murza, Managing Director
Natasha Bonhomme, VP, Strategic Development

5627 March of Dimes Foundation
1275 Mamaroneck Avenue
White Plains, NY 10605
914-997-4488
888-663-4637
Fax: 914-428-8203
answers@marchofdimes.com
www.marchofdimes.com

Partnership of volunteers and professionals dedicates to improving the health of babies by preventing birth defects and infant mortality. Over 100 chapters are located across the country and can be located through the National Office.

Stacey D. Stewart, President

5628 Society for Pediatric Dermatology
8365 Keystone Crossing, Suite 107
Indianapolis, IN 46240
317-202-0224
Fax: 317-205-9481
info@pedsderm.net
www.pedsderm.net

Objective is to promote, develop and advance education, research and care of skin disease in all pediatric age groups.

Kent Lindeman, Executive Director

Libraries & Resource Centers

California

5629 University of California, San Francisco Dermatology Drug Research
515 Spruce Street
San Francisco, CA 94115
415-476-4701
Fax: 415-502-4126
cc.ucsf.edu/people

Conducts clinical testing of new or existing pharmalogic agents used in the treatment of skin disorders.

John Koo, MD, Director

Delaware

5630 Delaware Division of Libraries for the Blind and Physically Handicapped
121 Duke of York Street
Dover, DE 19901
302-736-4748
800-282-8676
Fax: 302-736-6787
TDD: 302-739-4748
bedpg@lib.de.us

Braille readers receive service from Philadelphia and Pennsylvania, summer reading program, Braille writer and cassettes.

Beth Landon, Librarian

Illinois

5631 Dermatology Information Network (DERMINFONET)
American Academy of Dermatology
PO Box 4014
Schaumburg, IL 60168
847-330-0230
Fax: 847-330-0050

Consists of a collection of dermatologic databases that are available to members on a subscription and/or purchase basis. These databases are designed to run on a wide variety of personal computers.

5632 National Library of Dermatologic Teaching Slides
American Academy of Dermatology
930 E. Woodfield Road
Shaumburg, IL 60173
847-240-1280
866-503-7546
Fax: 847-240-1859
www.aad.org

A collection of dermatologic teaching slides offering the most comprehensive series ever assembled. Each set offers a realistic presentation of classic clinical skin conditions encountered by the dermatologist.

New York

5633 Laboratory of Dermatology Research
Memorial Sloan-Kettering Cancer Center
1275 York Avenue
New York, NY 10065
212-639-2000
Fax: 212-639-3576
www.mskcc.org

Specific studies on the identification of skin disorders and dermatology.

Biijan Safai, MD, Head

5634 Rockefeller University Laboratory for Investigative Dermatology
1230 York Avenue
New York, NY 10065
212-327-8000
Fax: 212-327-7974

Research into skin disorders and the whole specialty of dermatology in general.

Barry Coller, Head

Research Centers

5635 University of California, San Francisco Dermatology Drug Research
515 Spruce Street
San Francisco, CA 94115
415-476-4701
Fax: 415-502-4126
cc.ucsf.edu/people

Conducts clinical testing of new or existing pharmalogic agents used in the treatment of skin disorders.

John Koo, MD, Director

Magazines

5636 International Journal of Dermatology
International Society of Dermatology
2323 North State Street #30
Bunnell, FL 32110
386-437-4405
Fax: 386-437-4427
info@intsocderm.org
www.intsocderm.org

Focuses on information for dermatologists and the whole specialty of dermatology research and education.

10 times a year

Evangeline~ Handog, MD, President
Luca Borradori, Vice President
Paulo Rowilson Cunha, Vice President

5637 Journal of Dermatologic Surgery and Oncology
International Society for Dermatologic Surgery
930 N Meachan Road
Schaumburg, IL 60173
847-330-9830
Fax: 847-330-1135

Focuses on medical updates and information on dermatology.

Monthly

Journals

5638 Pediatric Dermatology Journal
Society for Pediatric Dermatology
8365 Keystone Crossing, Suite 107
Indianapolis, IN 46240
317-202-0224
Fax: 317-205-9481
info@pedsderm.net
www.pedsderm.net

6 issues/yr

Kent Lindeman, Executive Director

Newsletters

5639 Awareness
NAPVI
PO Box 317
Watertown, MA 2471
617-972-7441
800-562-6265
Fax: 617-972-7444
www.spedex.com/napvi

Newsletter offering regional news, sports and activities, conferences, camps, legislative updates, book reviews, audio reviews, professional question and answer column and more for the visually impaired and their families.

Quarterly

5640 DVH Quarterly
University of Arkansas at Little Rock
2801 S University Avenue
Little Rock, AR 72204
Fax: 501-663-3536

Offers information on upcoming events, conferences and workshops on and for visual disabilities. Book reviews, information on the newest resources and technology, educational programs, want ads and more.

Quarterly

Bob Brasher, Editor

5641 Dermatology Focus
Dermatology Foundation
1560 Sherman Avenue, Suite 870
Evanston, IL 60201
847-328-2256
Fax: 847-328-0509
dfgen@dermatologyfoundation.org
dermatologyfoundation.org

Includes membership activities, research articles and lists recipients of foundation awards.

Quarterly

Bruce U. Wintroub, Chairman
Michael D. Tharp, M.D., President
Staurt R. Lessin, M.D., Vice President

5642 Dermatology World
American Academy of Dermatology
930 E. Woodfield Road
Schaumburg, IL 60173
847-240-1280
866-503-7546
Fax: 847-240-1859
www.aad.org/dw

Offers Academy members information outside the clinical realm. It carries news of government actions, reports of socioeconomic issues, societal trends and other events which impinge on the practice of dermatology.

Monthly

Brett M.~ Coldiron, MD, President
Elise A.~ Olsen, MD, Vice President
Suzanne M.~ Olbricht, MD, Secretary-Treasurer

5643 Progress in Dermatology
Dermatology Foundation
1560 Sherman Avenue, Suite 870
Evanston, IL 60201
847-328-2256
Fax: 847-328-0509
dfgen@dermatologyfoundation.org
dermatologyfoundation.org

Bulletin offering information on research reports and clinical trials.

Quarterly

Bruce U. Wintroub, Chairman
Michael D. Tharp, M.D., President
Staurt R. Lessin, M.D., Vice President

Camps

5644 Camp Discovery
American Academy of Dermatology
930 E Woodfield Road
Schaumburg, IL 60173
847-240-1280
866-503-7546
Fax: 847-240-1859
jmueller@aad.org
www.aad.org/dermatology-a-to-z/for-kids/camp-discove

A camp for young people with chronic skin conditions. There is no fee and transportation is provided. Three locations: Camp Horizon in Millville, PA, Camp Knutson in Crosslake, MN, and Camp Dermadillo in Burton, TX.

Brett M.~ Coldiron, MD, President
Elise A.~ Olsen, MD, Vice President
Suzanne M.~ Olbricht, MD, Secretary-Treasurer

DESCRIPTION

5645 PHYSICAL & SEXUAL ABUSE
Involves the following Biologic System(s):
Developmental/Behavioral/Psychiatric Disorders

Child abuse is a pervasive societal disease that has been gaining increasing recognition in the last 40 years. Maltreatment of children includes neglect, physical abuse and sexual abuse. In 1996, one million children were confirmed by protective US agencies as having been abused. Reporting figures since that time have been on the rise.

Neglect is the most common form of abuse, and covers a wide range of irresponsible behaviors that negatively impact the growth and well being of a child. Inadequate supervision may result in injury from falling, usage of a dangerous object such as a knife, scissors or other tools, or ingestion of toxic products and medications. Neglect may also include providing insufficient food, clothing and shelter for a child, which carries a high risk of malnutrition, illness, and poor emotional development. Parents or guardians who do not ensure proper medical care for their children are also negligent, particularly for children with chronic serious medical illnesses.

Physical abuse encompasses a wide range of symptoms but always involves purposeful injury inflicted on a child. Physical abuse can be difficult to identify, especially in toddlers, because children are prone to accidents and receive bruises and cuts as routine events. One key element in the diagnosis is ascertaining whether the injury could have happened the way it was reported. Another important clue is whether the child at a given developmental stage, could have performed the reported event. For example, a report of a six-month old who "fell" and broke his femur (thigh bone) should raise suspicion as a six-month old infant is too young to walk. Common abusive injuries include bruises from belts, hands or cords, burns from cigarettes or hot water immersion, fractures or brain injury from vigorous shaking and internal abdominal injuries from trauma to the back and abdomen. It is important for health care providers, or friends and family members, to record all injuries as a pattern may develop that will help diagnose the situation.

Sexual abuse occurs when a child is involved in sexual activities that he/she cannot fully comprehend, he/she cannot give consent to, or that violate societal norms. Common ages of abuse are between 9 and 12 years. Approximately 25 percent of women and 12 percent of men report histories of being sexually abused as children. Normal sexual play between children of similar age and developmental level can be distinguished from abuse by assessing disparity of age/development and the level of coercion involved. Abusive acts include fondling, intercourse, oral-genital and anal-genital contact, as well as voyeurism, exhibitionism and pornography. Perpetrators are more commonly male adults and adolescents, although women have been known to commit these crimes as well. This type of abuse is often very difficult to recognize because there are frequently no physical signs or symptoms and victims are reluctant and embarrassed to disclose the information. There is often a trusting and/or fearful relationship between the perpetrator and victim that binds the victim to secrecy. Certain telltale signs include inappropriate sexualized behaviors and language, and sexually transmitted diseases such as gonorrhea and chlamydia or symptoms such as discharge or bleeding. Physical evidence may include abrasions, hymenal tears, bruising, foul discharge or even pregnancy.

Professionals working with children, including teachers, social workers and health care providers are all mandated reporters, which means that if abuse is suspected they must report the family to the local protective service agency. It is critical to note that the burden of proof does not lie with the reporter, so even if there is a degree of uncertainty, one is required to act upon his or her concern.

Government Agencies

5646 Administration for Children & Families-Child Abuse and Neglect Prevention
Department of Health & Human Services
330 C Street SW, Room 2422
Washington, DC 20201   202-205-8618
                                        Fax: 202-205-8221
                                        www.acf.hhs.gov/programs/cb
Wade F Horn PhD, Assistant Secretary

National Associations & Support Groups

5647 AMT Children of Hope Foundation
c/o Nassau County Police Department
1490 Franklin Avenue
Mineola, NY 11501   516-781-3511
                                        877-796-4673
                                        Fax: 516-781-0691
                                        www.amtchildrenofhope.com

Safe infant abandonment, nationwide, 24-hour crisis line. Confidential referrals to 'safe havens' and professional services.
Timothy Jaccard, Founder & President

5648 American Academy of Pediatrics
141 Northwest Point Boulevard
Elk Grove Village, IL 60007   847-434-4000
                                        800-433-9016
                                        Fax: 847-434-8000
                                        www.aap.org

The American Academy of Pediatrics and its member pediatricians are committed to the attainment of optimal physical, mental and social health and well-being for all infants, children, adolescents, and young adults.
Fernando Stein, MD, FAAP, President
Karen Remley, MD, CEO/Executive VP

5649 American Professional Society on the Abuse of Children
350 Poplar Avenue, PO Box 30669
Elmhurst,, IL 60126   843-764-2905
                                        877-402-7722
                                        Fax: 803-753-9823
                                        apsac@comcast.net
                                        www.apsac.org

Dedicated to providing professional education which promotes effective, culturally sensitive and interdisciplinary approaches to the identification, intervention, treatment and prevention of child abuse and neglect.
Daphne Wright, National Operations Manager

5650 Child Abuse Prevention Association
503 E 23rd Street
Independence, MO 64055   816-252-8388
                                        Fax: 816-252-1337
                                        capa@childabuseprevention.org
                                        www.childabuseprevention.org

Mission is to prevent and treat all forms of child abuse by creating changes in individuals, families and society which strengthen relationships and promote healing.

Jenatta Issa, CEO
Tamara Tucker, Program Director
Diana Castillo, Resource/Communications Dierctor

5651 Child Welfare League of America
1726 M Street NW, Suite 500
Washington, DC 20036   202-688-4200
                                   Fax: 202-833-1689
                                        www.cwla.org

National nonprofit organization dedicated to developing and promoting policies and programs to protect America's children from
harm and strengthen America's families.

Shay Bilchik, President/CEO
Joyce Johnson, Public Relations

5652 Childhelp
Childhelp National Headquarters
15757 N 78th Street
Scottsdale, AZ 85260   480-922-8212
                                   Fax: 480-922-7061
                                   TDD: 800-2AC-HILD
                                        www.childhelp.org

Dedicated to meeting the physical, emotional and spiritual needs
of abused and neglected children through focusing its efforts and
resources upon treatment, prevention and research.

Sara O'Mara, CEO
Yvonne Federson, Co-Founder/President
John Rteid, Executive Director

5653 Childhelp National Child Abuse Hotline
15757 N. 78th Street, Ste B
Scottsdale,, AZ 85260   480-922-8212
                                        800-4AC-HILD
                                   Fax: 480-922-7061
                                   TDD: 800-2AC-HILD
                                        www.childhelp.org
                                        www.childhelp.org

Abuse crisis counseling and referral services available 24/7 with
assistance in over 140 languages.

5654 Children's Defense Fund
25 E Street NW
Washington, DC 20001   202-628-8787
                                        800-233-1200
                                   Fax: 202-662-3510
                                   cdfinfo@childrensdefense.org
                                        www.childrensdefense.org

Mission is to ensure every child a healthy start, a head start, a fair
start, a safe start and a moral start in life.

Mariane Wright-Edelman, President
DD Eisenberg, Child Advocate/Commissioner

5655 IVAT: Institute on Violence, Abuse and Tra uma
10065 Old Grove Road
San Diego, CA 92131   858-527-1860
                                   Fax: 858-527-1743
                                        www.ivatcenters.org

Formerly the Family Violence & Sexual Assault Institute. Shares
and disseminates vital information, improves networking among
professionals, and assists with program evaluation, consultation
and training that promotes violence-free living.

Robert Geffner PhD, President
Dawn Alley PhD, Community Relations & Outreach
Sandi C Morrison, Executive President

5656 KidsPeace National Centers/Hospital
5300 KidsPeace Drive
Orefield, PA 18069   610-799-8471
                                        800-854-3123
                                   admissions@kidspeace.org
                                        www.kidspeace.org

Counseling, info and referral services for children and youth in
crisis.

Richard Zelko, Executive Director

5657 KlaasKids Foundation for Children
PO Box 925
Sausalito, CA 94966   415-331-6867
                                   Fax: 415-331-5633
                                   info@klaaskids.org
                                        www.klaaskids.org

Established in 1994 to give meaning to the death of
twelve-year-old kidnap and murder victim Polly Hannah
Klaas and to create a legacy in her name that would be protective of
children for generations to come. The Foundation's mission is to
stop crimes against children.

Marc Klaas, President

5658 National Center for Missing & Exploited Children
Charles B Wang International Children's Building
699 Prince Street
Alexandria, VA 22314   703-224-2150
                                        800-843-5678
                                   Fax: 703-224-2122
                                        www.missingkids.com

Private, nonprofit organization, co-founded in 1984 by John
Walsh, whose son Adam was abducted and murdered. NCMEC
serves as a focal point in providing assistance to parents, children, law enforcement, schools and the community in recovering
missing children and raising public awareness about ways to help
prevent child abduction, molestation and sexual exploitation.
NCMEC spends 94 cents of every dollar directly on programs and
services.

Ernie Allen, CEO

**5659 National Center for Missing and Exploited Children: 24-hour
Hotline**
                                        800-843-5678
                                        800-THE-LOST

The primary means by which NCMEC serves as an information
clearinghouse and delivers technical assistance.

5660 National Child Pornography Tipline and Cyber Tipline
www.cybertipline.com
                                        703-224-2150
                                        800-843-5678
                                   Fax: 703-224-2122
                                        www.cybertipline.com

The National Center for Missing and Exploited Children, in conjunction with the US Postal Inspection Service, US Customs Service and the Federal Bureau of Investigation, serves as the
tipline, handling calls from individuals reporting the sexual exploitation of children through the production and distribution of
pornography. For online reporting visit the website.

5661 National Children's Advocacy Center
210 Pratt Avenue
Huntsville, AL 35801   256-533-5437
                                   Fax: 256-534-6883
                                   prevention@nationalcac.org
                                        www.nationalcac.org

A non profit organization that provides training, prevention, intervention and treatment services to fight child abuse and neglect.

Deborah Callins, Executive Director
JoAnn Jaco Plucker, Federal Programs Director

5662 National Children's Alliance
516 C Street NE
Washington, DC 20002   202-548-0090
                                        800-239-9950
                                   Fax: 202-548-0099
                                   info@nca-online.org
                                        www.nca-online.org

Nationwide nonprofit membership organization which promotes
and supports communities in providing a coordinated investigation and response to victims of severe child abuse.

Janet Fine, Executive Director
Julie Pape, Director Programs
Benjamin Murray, Director Member Services

5663 National Exchange Club Foundation
3050 Central Avenue
Toledo, OH 43606

419-535-3232
800-924-2643
Fax: 419-535-1989
ÿÿÿinfo@nationalexchangeclub.org
www.nationalexchangeclub.org

Committed to making a difference in the lives of children, families and communities through its national project, the prevention of child abuse.

Dave Nershi, VP

5664 Prevent Child Abuse America
228 S Wabash Avenue
Chicago, IL 60604

312-663-3520
Fax: 312-939-8962
mailbox@preventchildabuse.org
www.preventchildabuse.org

Mission is to prevent the abuse and neglect of the nation's children. Supports education and research.

Jim Hmurovich, President

5665 Project Cuddle
2973 Harbor Boulevard, # 326
Costa Mesa, CA 92626

714-432-9681
888-628-3353
Fax: 714-433-6815
info@projectcuddle.org
www.projectcuddle.org

Safe infant abandonment, nationwide, 24-hour crisis line. All calls are confidential. Help in finding a safe, legal alternative to abandonment.

Debbe Magnusen, Owner

5666 Rape, Abuse and Incest National Network (RAINN)
1220 L Street, NW, Ste 505
Washington, DC 20036

202-544-3064
800-656-HOPE
Fax: 202-544-3556
info@rainn.org
www.rainn.org

Operates a 24 hour national sexual assault hotline and carries out programs to prevent sexual assault, help victims and ensure that rapists are brought to justice.

Darcey West, Communications Manager
Chelsea Bowers, Membership Information

5667 Safe Place for Newborns
120 S 6th Street, Suite 1150
Minneapolis, MN 55402

414-447-3030
877-440-2229
Fax: 612-317-2899
safeplace@safeplacefornewborns.com
www.safeplacefornewborns.com

Crisis line. Will provide a list of hospitals in Minnesota and Wisconsin which accept healthy babies up to three days old with no questions asked. Will provide information on other states with 'safe place' programs.

Laure Krupp, Executive Director

5668 Stop It Now! (DBA Child Sex Abuse Preventi on & Protection
351 Pleasant Street, Suite B-319
Northampton, MA 01060

413-587-3500
888-773-8368
Fax: 413-587-3505
info@stopitnow.org
www.stopitnow.org

Deborah Donoran Rice, Executive Director

5669 The Kempe Center: For the Prevention & Tre atment of Child Abuse and Neglect
13123 E 16th Avenue B390
Aurora, CO 80045

303-864-5300
Fax: 303-837-2599
questions@kempe.org
http://kempecenter.org

Provides education, clinical services and research on child abuse and neglect. Can provide referrals to local agencies.

Rob Clyman, Executive Director
Gene Liffick, Operations Director
Lindsey Zimmerman, Communications Director

5670 Youth Crisis Hotline
Youth Development International
PO Box 178408
San Diego, CA 92177

800-843-5200
http://hometown.aol.com/garnierlaw/hithome.html

Services for runaway/homeless youth, referrals to resources for abuse and crisis counseling.

State Agencies & Support Groups

Alaska

5671 Rid Alaska of Child Abuse
PO Box 35595
Juneau, AK 99803

800-478-4444
Help@RIDAlaskaOfChildAbuse
www.ridalaskaofchildabuse.org

Nonprofit organization dedicated to providing resources and information, raising public awareness of the occurrence of child abuse, lessening the stigma placed on child sexual abuse victims/survivors, promoting child safety and abuse prevention programs, researching and posting safety tips and maintaining a website.

Debra Gerrish, President/State Coordinator
Tia M Holley, VP
Patti Fay Hickox, Treasurer/Secretary

Arizona

5672 Crisis Nursery
2334 East Polk Street
Phoenix, AZ 85006

602-273-7363
Fax: 602-244-1316
cninfo1@crisisnurseryphx.com
www.crisisnurseryphx.org

Offers hope and support, through prevention and protection, to children in our community threatened with abuse and neglect. Since 1977, over 13,000 children have found a safe refuge at Crisis Nursery. Its mission is to provide a last resort for parents and families who are simply overwhelmed, a safe and healthy place for children who can no longer remain with their families, a temporary home for children who haven't one to call their own and a transitional placement with follow up for services.

Marsha Porter, Executive Director

California

5673 Child Sexual Abuse Treatment Program (Giar retto)
EMQ Children & Family Services
232 E Gish Road
San Jose, CA 95112

408-453-7616
csc@emq.org
www.emq.org

Sexual abuse treatment center

F Jerome Doyle, CEO
Kristine Austin, Director Public Relations

Georgia

5674 Prevent Child Abuse Georgia
PO Box 3995
Atlanta, GA 30302

404-413-1281
800-244-5373
Fax: 404-413-1299
feedback@pcageorgia.org
www.preventchildabusega.org

Private, statewide, community-based nonprofit organization with the sole mission of preventing child abuse and neglect.

Doug Middleton, Executive Director
Sonda Abernathy, College Facilities Manager
Frances Marine, Director of Communications

Illinois

5675 Prevent Child Abuse Illinois
528 S 5th Street, Suite 211
Springfield, IL 62701   217-522-1129
                                   Fax: 217-522-0655
                  rharley@preventchildabuseillinois.org
                        www.preventchildabuseillinois.org
Roy Harley, Executive Director

Indiana

5676 Prevent Child Abuse Indiana
3833 N Meridian Suite 101
Indianapolis, IN 46208   317-775-6439
                                        888-542-7064
                                   Fax: 317-775-6420
                  Generalinfo.pcain@villages.org
                                    www.pcain.org
Sandy Runkle, Manager

Iowa

5677 Prevent Child Abuse Iowa
505 Fifth Avenue, Suite 900
Des Moines, IA 50309   515-244-2200
                                   Fax: 515-280-7835
                            sscott@pcaiowa.org
                                  www.pcaiowa.org
Stephen Scott, Executive Director

New York

5678 Child Abuse Prevention Project: Be'ad HaYeled (For the Sake of the Child)
Board of Jewish Education of Greater New York
135 West 50th Street
New York, NY 10020   212-582-9100
                                   Fax: 646-472-5421
                              admin@jbfcs.org
                                   www.bjeny.org

Be'ad HaYeled was created in 1995 specifically for the Jewish community by the Board of Jewish Education of Greater New York and the Jewish Board of Family and Children's Services. Training workshops give educators, parents and communal workers the skills needed to recognize signs of abuse and to intervene in an effective and appropriate manner Halachically, clinically and legally. Additional programs deal with parenting methods, communication skills and other relevant family issues.

Martin Haber, President

5679 Prevent Child Abuse New York
33 Elk Street Suite 201
Albany, NY 12207   518-445-1273
                                   Fax: 518-436-5889
                  cdeyss@preventchildabuseny.org
                        www.preventchildabuseny.org

Not-for-profit agency whose singular mission is to prevent child abuse in all its forms. Prevent Child Abuse New York is a chartered state chapter of Prevent Child Abuse America.

Christine Deyss, Executive Director
Jennifer Matrazzo, Associate Executive Director

North Carolina

5680 Prevent Child Abuse North Carolina
3701 National Drive, Suite 211
Raleigh, NC 27612   919-829-8009
                                   Fax: 919-832-0308
                  info@preventchildabusenc.org
                        www.prventchildabusenc.org

Statewide not-for-profit organization with the mission of ending child abuse in the state of North Carolina.

Rosie Allen, CEO

Virginia

5681 Childhelp Children's Center of Virginia
11230 Waples Mill Road #105
Fairfax, VA 22030   703-208-1500
                                   Fax: 703-208-1540
                            mail@childhelpva.org
                  www.childhelpusa.org/regional/virginia2

Dedicated to meeting the physical, emotional and spiritual needs of abused and neglected children through focusing its efforts and resources upon treatment, prevention and research.

Stanley D Beder

Libraries & Resource Centers

5682 Child Welfare Information Gateway
Children's Burea/ACYF
1250 Maryland Avenue SW, 8th Floor
Washington, DC 20024   703-385-7565
                                        800-394-3366
                                   Fax: 703-385-3206
                            info@childwelfare.gov
                                  www.childwelfare.gov

The National Clearinghouse on Child Abuse and Neglect Information and the National Adoption Information Clearinghouse have consolidated and expanded to create the Child Welfare Information Gateway. It is a service of the US DHHS and provides access to information and resources to help protect children and strengthen families.

Research Centers

5683 National Center on Child Abuse Prevention Research
228 S Wabash Avenue
Chicago, IL 60604   312-663-3520
                                   Fax: 312-939-8962
                  ÿmailbox@preventchildabuse.org
                        www.preventchildabuse.org

Established with the support of the Skillman Foundation to increase understanding of the complex causes of child maltreatment, to evaluate the effectiveness of prevention programs, and to disseminate this information out into the field and public.

Gregory Hilton, Owner

Conferences

5684 Annual New York State Child Abuse Prevention Conference
33 Elk Street, Suite 201
Albany, NY 12207   518-445-1273
                                        800-244-5373
                                   Fax: 518-436-5889
                  rreyes@preventchildabuseny.org
                        www.preventchildabuseny.org/conf06/

Presented by Prevent Child Abuse New York, a not-for-profit agency whose singular mission is to prevent child abuse in all its forms. PCANY is a chartered state chapter of Prevent Child Abuse America. Conference attendees include those who work in home-based and center-based family support programs, child abuse prevention and child protective services, intervention and treatment, health care and mental health, schools, religious and civic organizations, and parents, themselves.

Christine Deyss, Executive Director
Robin Christenson, President
Dean Geesler, Vice President

Audio Video

5685 Break the Silence: Kids Against Child Abuse
The Health Connection
55 W Oak Ridge Drive
Hagerstown, MD 21740

301-393-3270
800-765-6955
Fax: 888-294-8405
www.adventistbookcenter.com/resources/health-connect

Jane Seymore explains physical abuse, sexual abuse and neglect. Animation illustrates each story. All the stories end happily, and the main point is that children should tell a trusted adult. 28 minutes. Grades 1-5.

1994

5686 I Am the Boss of My Body: Preventing Child Sexual Abuse
The Health Connection
55 W Oak Ridge Drive
Hagerstown, MD 21740

301-393-3270
800-765-6955
Fax: 888-294-8405
www.adventistbookcenter.com/resources/health-connect

Children feel empowered when they see this video and learn that they have the authority and the right to say no to any touch that makes them feel strange. Grades 1-4.

1999 18 Minutes

Web Sites

5687 American Professional Society on the Abuse of Children
1706 E. Broad Street
Columbus, OH 43203

614-827-1321
877-402-7722
Fax: 614-251-6005
apsac@apsac.org
www.apsac.org

Dedicated to providing professional education which promotes effective, culturally sensitive and interdisciplinary approaches to the identification, intervention, treatment and prevention of child abuse and neglect.

Frank E. Vandevort, President
Tricia Gardner, Vice President
Michael L. Haney, Ph.D., Executive Director

5688 Bikers Against Child Abuse
www.bacausa.com

Has the intent to create a safer environment for abused children. An established, united body of bikers in a stand to empower children to not feel afraid of the world in which they live. They work in conjunction with local officials who are already in place to protect children.

Scootr , President
Pipes , Vice President

5689 Child Abuse Legislation
www.childabuse.com/legislat.htm

Prevention through education and awareness.

5690 Child Abuse Prevention Network
child-abuse.com

For professionals in the field of child abuse and neglect. Child maltreatment, physical abuse, psychological maltreatment, neglect, sexual abuse and emotional abuse and neglect are the key areas of concern. Provides unique and powerful tools for all workers to support the identification, investigation, treatment, adjudication and prevention of child abuse and neglect.

5691 Child Abuse Quilts: Revealing and Healing the Pain of Child Abuse
mbgoodman.tripod.com/caq/caq1.html

Site shows 28 quilts made dealing with the subject of child abuse, child abuse prevention and violence against children. Some of the quiltmakers knew the pain of abuse first hand, others knew it through the eyes of others, often close family members. Quilts are displayed in the hope that each person who sees them will leave re-awakened to the tragedy of child abuse and resolved to prevent it.

5692 Child Abuse.com
1231 W. Northern Lights Blvd, STE 458
Anchorage, AL 99503

www.childabuse.com

Comprehensive resource bringing awareness and education in preventing child abuse and related issues. The site was created to inform, support and encourage those dealing with any aspect of child abuse, in a positive non-threatening environment.

5693 Child Trauma Academy
www.childtraumaacademy.com

Provides information on free online courses that offer creative and practical approaches to understanding and working with maltreated children.

5694 Children's Bureau
1250 Maryland Avenue, SW Eighth Floor
Wasington, DC 20024

www.acf.hhs.gov/programs/cb

Is responsible for programs that promote the economic and social well-being of families, chidren, individuals, and communities. Programs aim to achieve the following: families and individuals empowered to increase their own economic independence and productivity, and strong healthy, supportive commuities that have a positive impact on the quality of life and the development of children.

Joe Bock, Director/Commissioner

5695 Children's House
child-abuse.com/childhouse/

An interactive resource center and meeting place for the exchange of information that serves the well-being of children.

5696 Connect for Kids
Benton Foundation
P.O. Box 45372
Westlake, OH 44145

440-250-5563
info@connectingforkids.org
www.connectforkids.org

Family-friendly politics and information on how to connect with hundreds of groups working on behalf of children.

Kathy Nash, President
Andrea Campesino, Secretary
Rebecca Baker, Treasurer

5697 Intrafamilial (Incest) Abuse Resources
www.vachss.com/help_text/incest.html

Many resources on the subject of child abuse, both physical and sexual.

5698 KidsPeace
4085 Independence Drive
Schnecksville, PA 18078

800-257-3223
kpinfo@KidsPeace.org
www.kidspeace.org

Counseling, info and referral services for children and youth in crisis.

L. Richard Plunkett, Chairman
Larry Bell, Vice Chairman
William R. Isemann, President/ CEO

5699 Making Daughters Safe Again
mdsa-online.org

Is the only organization in the world specializing in mother-daughter sexual abuse. We are also distinguished by the innovative online group experience we provide for survivors.

5700 National Council on Child Abuse & Family Violence
1025 Connecticut Avenue NW, Suite 1000
Washington, DC 20036   202-429-6695
Fax: 202-521-3479
info@nccafv.org
www.nccafv.org

Providing intergenerational violence prevention services since 1984.

5701 Pandora's Box
www.prevent-abuse-now.com

Offers more than 270 pages of resource information on child abuse prevention and child protection.

5702 Prevent Child Abuse America
228 South Wabash Avenue, 10th Floor
Chicago, IL 60604   312-663-3520
800-244-5373
Fax: 312-939-8962
mailbox@preventchildabuse.org
www.preventchildabuse.org

Providing and inspiring hope to everyone involved in the effort to prevent the abuse and neglect of our nations children. Working with 40 statewide chapters to provide leadership in promoting and implementing prevention efforts at both the national and local levels.

Fred M. Riley, Chair
David Rudd, Vice Chair
James Hmurovich, President/ CEO

5703 Prevent Child Abuse California
P.O. Box 6400
Columbia, MD 21045   410-381-0911
Fax: 410-381-0924
www.pca.org

Mission is to prevent child abuse in all its forms by maximizing resources throughout the state of California.

Caren Cooper, President
Thomas Gorsuch, Vice President
Cindy Jacisin, Secretary

5704 Rape, Abuse and Incest National Network (RAINN)
1220 L Street, NW, Suite 505
Washington, DC 20005   202-544-3064
Fax: 202-544-3556
info@rainn.org
www.rainn.org

Operates a 24 hour national sexual assault hotline and carries out programs to prevent sexual assault, help victims and ensure that rapists are brought to justice.

Regan Burke, Chairperson
Scott Berkowitz, President and Founder
Cybele Daley, Treasurer

5705 Sibling Abuse Survivors' Information & Adv ocacy Network
www.sasian.org

Provides information about problems associated with domestic sibling incest abuse.

5706 Stop Child Abuse Now
www.efn.org/~scan/scan.html

Is a nonprofit organization dedicated to stopping child abuse of all forms, and improving the lives of survivors of all types of abuse and loss. By speaking out about abuse, we increase the public's awareness of the prevalence of abuse. Our goal is to join with other organizations and individuals who wish to ultimately put a stop to child abuse.

Book Publishers

5707 A Child Called It: One Child's Courage to Survive
Dave Pelzer, author

Health Communications, Inc (HCI)
3201 SW 15th Street
Deerfield Beach, FL 33442   954-360-0909
800-441-5569
Fax: 954-360-0034
www.hci-online.com

The author's true story of abuse he suffered as a child.
ISBN: 1-558743-66-9

5708 Body Language of the Abused Child
Jacqueline A Rankin, author

Rankin File/Signature Book Printing
8041 Cessna Avenue
Gaithersburg, MD 20879   301-258-8353
Fax: 301-670-4147
book@sbpbooks.com
www.signaturebook.com/Books/rankin.htm

Uses body language to identify a suspected victim.
1999 271 pages Paperback
ISBN: 1-887711-06-6

5709 It's My Body
Lory Freeman, author

Parenting Press
PO Box 75267
Seattle, WA 98175   206-364-2900
800-992-6657
Fax: 206-364-0702
www.parentingpress.com

Helps adults and preschool children talk about sexual abuse together. Introduces touching codes children can use for their protection. Ages 3-8.

32 pages Paperback
ISBN: 1-403408-96-3

5710 My Body is Mine, My Feelings are Mine
Susan Hoke, author

YouthLight
714 Cove Trail, PO Box 115
Chapin, SC 29036   800-209-9774
Fax: 803-345-0888
yl@sc.rr.com
www.youthlightbooks.com

For K-5th grade. First part to be read to children, the second part teaches adults how to educate children about body safety. Sexual victimization can be prevented through explanation of how to identify inappropriate touching and what to do about it.

77 pages Paperback

5711 Out of Harm's Way: A Parent's Guide to Pro tecting Young Children from Sexual Abuse
Janie Hart-Rossi, author

Parenting Press
PO Box 75267
Seattle, WA 98175   206-364-2900
800-992-6657
Fax: 206-364-0702
office@parentingpress.com
www.parentingpress.com

An authoritative and objective look at child sexual abuse, which can be used at home and in school, or as a complement to existing school safety curricula. It describes how community members or extended family members might groom a child for abuse, as well as how to watch for such grooming and how to discuss it with children.

32 pages Paperback

Homer J Henderson, Operations Manager

5712   Something Happened and I'm Scared to Tell

Patricia Kehoe PhD, author

Parenting Press
PO Box 75267
Seattle, WA 98175

206-364-2900
800-992-6657
Fax: 206-364-0702
www.parentingpress.com

With the help of a friendly lion, a young sexual abuse victim is able to talk about sexual abuse and recover self-esteem. A gentle and positive approach to reassure children. Ages 3-7.

32 pages Paperback
ISBN: 0-943990-28-9

5713   Soul Murder Revisited

Leonard Shengold, author

Yale University Press
PO Box 209040
New Haven, CT 06520

203-432-0960
800-405-1619
Fax: 203-432-0948
marketing@yale.edu.
yalepress.yale.edu/yupbooks

Further reflections on how abuse occurs and its consequences. Discusses the psychopathology of soul murder and appropriate therapy for victims.

2000 336 pages Paperback
ISBN: 0-300086-99-7

John Donatich, Director

5714   Treating Abused and Traumatized Children

Eliana Gil, author

Guilford Press
72 Spring Street
New York, NY 10012

800-365-7006
Fax: 212-966-6708
info@guilford.com
www.guilford.com

The author presents a program combining play, art, and expressive therapies, with strategies from cognitave-behvior therapy and family therapy, as she demonstrates how to tailor the treatment to the needs of each child. Paperback or e-book.

2006 254 pages Paperback
ISBN: 1-593853-34-1

Bob Matloff, President
Seymour Weingarten, Editor-in-Chief

5715   Trouble with Secrets

Karen Johnson, author

Parenting Press
PO Box 75267
Seattle, WA 98175

206-364-2900
800-992-6657
Fax: 206-364-0702
www.parentingpress.com

Helps children distinguish between secrets that should be kept and those that shouldn't.

32 pages Paperback
ISBN: 0-943990-22-X

Newsletters

5716   APSAC Advisor

American Profess. Society on the Abuse of Children
1706 E. Broad Street
Columbus, OH 43203

614-827-1321
877-402-7722
Fax: 614-251-6005
apsac@apsac.org
www.apsac.org

News journal for professionals in the field of child abuse and neglect. It provides succint, data-based articles that keep professionals informed of the latest developments in policy and practice in the field of child maltreatment.

Frank E. Vandevort, President
Tricia Gardner, Vice President
Michael L. Haney, Ph.D., Executive Director

5717   Lookin' Up

Prevent Child Abuse America
228 South Wabash Avenue, 10th Floor
Chicago, IL 60604

312-663-3520
800-244-5373
Fax: 312-939-8962
mailbox@preventchildabuse.org
www.preventchildabuse.org

Newsletter of Prevent Child Abuse America.

Quarterly

Fred M. Riley, Chair
David Rudd, Vice Chair
James Hmurovich, President/ CEO

Pamphlets

5718   Understanding SBS/Shaken Impact Syndrome B rochure

National Center on Shaken Baby Syndrome
1433 N 1075 W Ste 110
Farmington, UT 84025

801-447-9360
888-273-0071
Fax: 801-447-9364
mail@dontshake.com
www.dontshake.com

Information brochure on shaken baby syndrome.

Jill Moore, Chairperson
Lori Frasier, Vice Chairperson
Ryan Steinbeigle, Executive Director

DESCRIPTION

5719 PICA

Involves the following Biologic System(s):
Developmental/Behavioral/Psychiatric Disorders

Pica is a type of eating disorder characterized by the recurrent or chronic ingestion of nonfood or nonnutritive substances such as dirt, flaking paint or plaster, clay, charcoal, ashes, wool, and other nonfoods. Although this psychological disorder usually commences during the first or second year of life, some children are affected during infancy. The pattern should last at least one month to fit the diagnosis of pica. Pica is often self-limiting with resolution occurring during the childhood years; however, sometimes it may persist into adolescence or adulthood. If the symptoms associated with pica occur initially in older children or adults (e.g., pregnant women), this is usually indicative of a nutritional deficiency, such as iron or zinc, rather than a psychological disorder.

Children who are mentally retarded are particularly susceptible to development of this unusual disorder. Other factors that may influence the evolution of pica include environmental influences such as family discord, lack of or ineffective nurturing, and nutritional and emotional neglect. In addition, pica is sometimes associated with certain psychiatric disorders.

Children who eat nonfood or nonnutritive substances may be at risk of developing certain types of parasitic infections. For example, the ingestion of dirt (geophagia) may result in toxocariasis, an infection resulting from the spread of the larvae of the common roundworm (Toxocara canis) throughout the body. Symptoms of toxocariasis are often mild and may include fever, weakness, and discomfort. Other children may develop a cough, wheezing, enlarged liver (hepatomegaly), and eye lesions. In addition, another parasitic infection known as toxoplasmosis may develop from dirt ingestion. This common parasitic infection is caused by Toxoplasma gondii and may produce no symptoms or may sometimes be characterized by rash, fever, and other mononucleosis-type symptoms. In individuals with compromised immune systems, toxoplasmosis may result in more serious, widespread disease. Children who eat paint, paint dust, or paint flakes are at risk of developing lead poisoning that may damage the central nervous system, red blood cells, and digestive system.

Any nutritional deficiencies and other medical problems, such as lead toxicity, should be addressed. Treatment emphasizes psychosocial, environmental, and family education approaches. Nutritional supplements may be considered.

National Associations & Support Groups

5720 American Academy of Pediatrics
141 Northwest Point Boulevard
Elk Grove Village, IL 60007

847-434-4000
800-433-9016
Fax: 847-434-8000
www.aap.org

The American Academy of Pediatrics and its member pediatricians are committed to the attainment of optimal physical, mental and social health and well-being for all infants, children, adolescents, and young adults.

Fernando Stein, MD, FAAP, President
Karen Remley, MD, CEO/Executive VP

5721 International Association of Eating Disorders Professionals Foundation
PO Box 1295
Pekin, IL 61555

309-346-3341
800-800-8126
Fax: 775-239-1597
iaedpmembers@earthlink.net
www.iaedp.com

Well-known for providing first-quality education and high-level training standards to an international multidisciplinary group of healthcare treatment providers who treat the full spectrum of eating disorder problems.

Emmett R Bishop MD, President
Bonnie Harken, Managing Director

5722 Mental Health America
500 Montgomery Street, Ste 820
Alexandria, VA 22314

703-684-7722
800-969-6642
Fax: 703-684-5968
TTY: 800-433-5959
www.mentalhealthamerica.net

Addresses all aspects of mental health and mental illness. NMHA with over 340 affiliates works to improve the mental health of all Americans.

Paul Gionfriddo, President/CEO
Shavonne Carpenter, Sr Assoc., Support & Services
Mallory Pernell, Assoc. Dir, Comments/Marketing

5723 NIH/National Institute of Mental Health Eating Disorders Program
6001 Executive Boulevard, Room 8184
Bethesda, MD 20892

301-443-4513
Fax: 301-443-4279

5724 National Alliance for the Mentally Ill
3803 N Fairfax Drive, Suite 100
Arlington, VA 22203

703-524-7600
888-999-6264
Fax: 703-524-9094
TDD: 703-516-7227
info@nami.org
www.nami.org

NAMI is a nonprofit, grassroots, self-help, support and advocacy organization of consumers, families and friends of people with severe mental illness, such as schizophrenia, bipolar disorder, major depressive disorder, obsessive compulsive disorder, anxiety disorders, autism and other severe and persistent mental illnesses that affect the brain.

Suzanne Vogel-Scibilia MD, President

5725 National Eating Disorders Association (NED A)
603 Stewart Street, Suite 803
Seattle, WA 98101

206-382-3587
800-931-2237
Fax: 206-829-8501
info@NationalEatingDisorders.org
www.nationaleatingdisorders.org

Dedicated to the elimination of eating disorders through prevention efforts, education, referral and support services, advocacy, training and research. Offers free information and referrals as well as educational curriculum and materials for sale. A toll free information & referral helpline is also available, linking more than 1,200 callers per month to vital information and life-saving treatment.

Lynn S Grefe, CEO
Lynn S Grefe, Chief Executive Officer
Tracy Kahlo, Chief Operating Officer

5726 National Mental Health Consumers' Self-Help Clearinghouse
1211 Chestnut Street, Suite 1207
Philadelphia, PA 19107

215-751-1810
800-553-4539
Fax: 215-636-6312
info@mhselfhelp.org
www.mhselfhelp.org

Offers information, support and appropriate referrals; and promotes public and professional education. Provides networking for those with special interests related to albinism. Promotes and supports research and funding that will improve diagnosis and management of albinism and hypopigmentation.

Joseph Rogers, Executive Director & Founder

Web Sites

5727 Eating Disorder Referrals
www.eating-disorder-referral.com/pica.php

866-690-7238
www.eating-disorder-referral.com/pica.php

A free referral resource with listings across the nation. Can also access by phone, toll free at 866-323-5608

5728 KidsHealth for Parents
kidshealth.org/parent/emotions/behavior/pica.html

General overview of pica.

Neil Izenberg, MD, Editor-in-Chief & Founder

5729 Pica Information Page
archive.tobacco.org/resources/health/pica

A small group of citizens that seeks to alert the public about a new category of hazardous waste.

DESCRIPTION

5730 PINWORM (ENTEROBIUS VERMICULARIS)
Synonyms: Enterobiasis, Oxyuriasis, Threadworm
Involves the following Biologic System(s):
Infectious Disorders

Pinworm infection (enterobiasis) refers to a common condition in which small, white, parasitic worms (Enterobius vermicularis) infect the human intestinal tract. Such infection results from ingestion of parasitic eggs. The eggs hatch in the stomach, and the larvae then typically migrate to and grow within the upper part of the large intestine (cecum). On rare occasions, pinworms may migrate to the vagina of affected girls, potentially causing such symptoms as vaginal irritation or itching. Pinworms can also cause appendicitis, cystitis (infection of the urinary tract), and diverticulitis (inflammation from out-pouchings in the colon (large intestinal tract).

At night, pinworms migrate from the intestines to the anal region where they deposit their eggs, potentially causing itching (pruritus), irritation, and sleeplessness. Scratching often results in reinfestation from ingestion of eggs that become imbedded under the fingernails and are inadvertently deposited in the mouth. Parasitic eggs are also often deposited from the anal area onto clothing, bedding, furniture, or toys, where they may then be transferred from the fingers to the mouth, causing reinfection or infection of others. In addition, in some cases, eggs may be inhaled from the air and swallowed. Parasitic eggs may remain viable for up to three weeks at regular room temperature.

The diagnosis of enterobiasis is made by detecting parasitic eggs or pinworms. The eggs or worms may be obtained by pressing sticky tape against the perianal region of affected children during early morning hours before the children awaken. The tape is then examined under a microscope to verify the presence of pinworms or eggs. In addition, pinworms may sometimes be detected by the naked eye. Treatment may include the administration of drugs that destroy pinworms (anthelmintic drugs), such as pyrantel pamoate or mebendazole, and, in some patients, topical anti-itch ointments that help relieve itching and irritation. Anthelmintic medications should also be given to all other members of the household. Handwashing after going to the bathroom and before meals is critical. Linens should be washed thoroughly.

Enterobiasis is a very common infection that may occur in individuals of all ages. However, children between the ages of five to 14 years are most commonly affected.

Government Agencies

5731 NIH/ Eunice Kennedy Shriver National Insti tute of Child Health & Human Development
31 Center Drive, Building 31
Bethesda, MD 20892   301-496-5113
                                          800-370-2943
                                    Fax: 866-760-5947
                              nichdpress@mail.nih.gov
                                      www.nichd.nih.gov

Established in 1962 by congress, today the institute conducts and supports research on topics related to the health of children, adults, families and populations. Some of these topics include: developmental disabilities, growth and development, infant death, reproductive health and birth defects.

Diana W. Bianchi, Director
Paul Williams, Director, Communications

5732 NIH/National Institute of Allergy and Infectious Diseases
5601 Fishers Lane, MSC 9806
Bethesda, MD 20892   301-496-5717
                                          866-284-4107
                                    Fax: 301-402-3573
                                    TDD: 800-877-8339
                            ocpostoffice@niaid.nih.gov
                                      www.niaid.nih.gov

Conducts and supports basic and applied research to better understand, treat, and ultimately prevent infectious, immunologic, and allergic diseases.

Anthony S Fauci MD, Director

National Associations & Support Groups

5733 American Academy of Pediatrics
141 Northwest Point Boulevard
Elk Grove Village, IL 60007   847-434-4000
                                          800-433-9016
                                    Fax: 847-434-8000
                                            www.aap.org

The American Academy of Pediatrics and its member pediatricians are committed to the attainment of optimal physical, mental and social health and well-being for all infants, children, adolescents, and young adults.

Fernando Stein, MD, FAAP, President
Karen Remley, MD, CEO/Executive VP

5734 World Health Organization
Avenue Appia 20
CH-1211 Geneva 27,
Switzerland   www.who.int

WHO is the directing and coordinating authority for health within the United Nations system.

Dr Margaret Chan, Director General

Web Sites

5735 KidsHealth for Parents
www.kidshealth.org

Signs, symptoms, doagnosis, and treatment of pinworms.

Neil Izenberg, MD, Editor-in-Chief & Founder

5736 MayoClinic.com
www.mayoclinic.com/health/pinworm/DS00687

Introduction, risk factors, prevention and treatment of pinworms.

Pamphlets

5737 Pinworm Infection
CDC
13400 E. Shea Blvd.
Scottsdale, AZ 85259   480-301-8000
                                          800-446-2279
                          www.mayoclinic.org/about-mayo-clinic

Pinworm infection factsheet provided by the CDC.

DESCRIPTION

5738 PITYRIASIS ROSEA

Involves the following Biologic System(s):

Dermatologic Disorders, Infectious Disorders

Pityriasis rosea is an inflammatory skin condition that may develop at any age but mostly commonly affects children and young adults. In some cases, the onset of the condition may be preceded by certain generalized symptoms, such as fever, inflammation of the throat (pharyngitis), and muscle and joint pain (myalgia and arthralgia). Pityriasis rosea typically begins with the development of a single oval or round patch known as a herald patch. This patch is usually red, pink, or light brown with a raised border and is covered with fine scales. A herald patch varies in diameter from one to 10 centimeters and may occur anywhere on the body. About five to 10 days after the appearance of the herald patch, there is a widespread eruption of similar, smaller patches (lesions), particularly on the torso and upper arms and thighs. These lesions, which are less than one centimeter in diameter, are usually slightly raised, oval or round, and red, pink, or light brown. In addition, they may be scaly and tend to peel. Lesions may continue to appear over several days and develop on other areas of the body, such as the forearms and calves, face, and scalp. The lesions are typically distributed along the subtle lines in the skin that indicate the direction of skin fibers (Langer's or cleavage lines). Some individuals with the condition may experience no associated symptoms (asymptomatic). Others may experience mild to severe itching (pruritus). Pityriasis rosea is a self-limited condition that has a duration of approximately two to 12 weeks, with an average of approximately four to five weeks. As skin lesions heal, affected areas may have abnormally increased or diminished pigmentation (postinflammatory hyperpigmentation or hypopigmentation) that gradually resolves after several weeks or months.

If individuals with pityriasis rosea experience no associated symptoms, treatment may not be necessary. Those with widespread lesions and scaling may benefit from using a cream that softens the skin (emollient). Associated itching may be relieved by lubricating lotions that contain the natural compounds camphor or menthol or medicated skin creams, such as a nonfluorinated topical corticosteroid. Certain medications taken by mouth such as oral antihistamines may help those who experience bothersome itching while attempting to sleep. Antihistamines, which are medications that often induce drowsiness, reduce the effects of histamine, a chemical that is released during allergic inflammatory reactions.

The cause of pityriasis rosea is unknown. However, many researchers speculate that the condition results from infection with a viral agent.

Government Agencies

5739 NIH/National Institute of Arthritis and Musculoskeletal and Skin Diseases
1 AMS Circle
Bethesda, MD 20892

301-495-4484
877-226-4267
Fax: 301-718-6366
TDD: 301-565-2966
niamsinfo@mail.nih.gov
www.niams.nih.gov

The mission of the NIAMS, a part of the NIH, is to support research into the causes, treatment, and prevention of arthritis and musculoskeletal and skin diseases, the training of basic and clinical scientists to carry out this research, and the dissemination of information on research progress in these diseases.

Stephen I Katz MD PhD, Director
Robert H Carter MD, Deputy Director

National Associations & Support Groups

5740 American Academy of Dermatology (AAD)
930 E. Woodfield Roa, PO Box 4014
Schaumburg, IL 60173

847-240-1280
866-503-7546
Fax: 847-240-1859
mrc@aad.org
www.aad.org

Dedicated to achieving high quality dermatologic care for everyone which encompasses: responsiveness, unification and representation of the specialty, and excellence in patient care, education and research.

Ronald Moy MD, President
Suzanne Connolly, VP
Robert Greenberg, Secretary/Treasurer

5741 American Academy of Pediatrics
141 Northwest Point Boulevard
Elk Grove Village, IL 60007

847-434-4000
800-433-9016
Fax: 847-434-8000
www.aap.org

The American Academy of Pediatrics and its member pediatricians are committed to the attainment of optimal physical, mental and social health and well-being for all infants, children, adolescents, and young adults.

Fernando Stein, MD, FAAP, President
Karen Remley, MD, CEO/Executive VP

5742 Society for Pediatric Dermatology
8365 Keystone Crossing, Suite 107
Indianapolis, IN 46240

317-202-0224
Fax: 317-205-9481
info@pedsderm.net
www.pedsderm.net

Objective is to promote, develop and advance education, research and care of skin disease in all pediatric age groups.

Kent Lindeman, Executive Director

Web Sites

5743 DermNet NZ: The Dermatology Resource
www.dermnetnz.org

Information about the skin from the New Zealand Dermatological Society.

Marius Rademaker, Chairperson
Anthony Young, Secretary
Sandra Winhoven, Treasurer

Journals

5744 Pediatric Dermatology Journal
Society for Pediatric Dermatology
8365 Keystone Crossing, Suite 107
Indianapolis, IN 46240

317-202-0224
Fax: 317-205-9481
info@pedsderm.net
www.pedsderm.net

6 issues/yr

Kent Lindeman, Executive Director

Pamphlets

5745 Pityriasis Rosea
American Academy of Dermatology
PO Box 4014
Schaumburg, IL 60168

847-240-1280
866-503-7546
Fax: 847-240-1859
mrc@aad.org
www.aad.org

Discusses the appearance, symptoms, and causes of this common rash. Diagnosis and treatment are also explained.

Pkgs of 50

Brett M.~ Coldiron, President
Elise A. Olsen, MD, Vice President
Suzanne M.~ Olbricht, Secretary-Treasurer

DESCRIPTION

5746 PNEUMONIA

Involves the following Biologic System(s):

Infectious Disorders, Respiratory Disorders

Pneumonia refers to a group of disorders characterized by an acute inflammation of the lungs. The causes of pneumonia are many and may include infection by certain bacteria, viruses, bacteria-like organisms, fungi, yeasts, and protozoa. In addition, noninfectious causes include the inhalation (aspiration) of food or other substances into the airway and lungs, an abnormal response of the immune system to certain substances (hypersensitivity reaction), and an inflammatory response to radiation or certain drugs. Pneumonia may also result as a complication of surgery or injury, due to the impaired ability to cough, breathe deeply, or expel mucus.

Pneumonia in very young children is most commonly caused by certain respiratory viruses, such as RSV, or respiratory syncytial virus; influenza; parainfluenza (the virus that causes croup); and adenoviruses. Symptoms and findings associated with this type of pneumonia in infants and young children may include cough, nasal discharge, fever, rapid breathing (tachypnea), or a bluish color to the skin and mucous membranes (cyanosis). Antibiotics do not treat viral infections, though some viruses are susceptible to new antiviral therapies. Most infants and children recover from viral pneumonia with no complications. However, some may develop subsequent lung irregularities.

Although bacterial pneumonia is not common among children, certain conditions (e.g., viral respiratory illnesses, immune deficiency disorders, certain congenitaldefects, blood irregularities, etc.) may put them at increased risk for developing this type of pneumonia. The most common types of bacteria that cause pneumonia in children include Streptococcus pneumoniae (pneumococcus), Streptococcus pyogenes, Staphylococcus aureus, and Haemophilus influenzae type b. Symptoms associated with bacterial pneumonia vary according to age, type of bacteria involved, and other factors. Infants and young children may develop a stuffy nose and other signs of upper respiratory infection, loss of appetite, sudden onset of fever, restlessness, respiratory distress, and cyanosis. In addition, infants with Staphylococcus aureus infection, a more serious type of disease, may develop lethargy, increased irritability, difficulty breathing (dyspnea), vomiting, or diarrhea. Abscesses may form in the lungs and may lead to the development of air-containing cysts (pneumatoceles). Accumulation of pus, or empyema, may occur in the space surrounding the lungs. Older children and adolescents with bacterial pneumonia may develop symptoms commonly associated with mild upper respiratory tract infection followed by chills, shaking, fever, drowsiness, rapid breathing, coughing, or chest pain. Treatment for bacterial pneumonia includes the use of appropriate antibiotics. In the case of Staphylococcus aureus infection, drainage of pus accumulations may be indicated. Other treatment is symptomatic and supportive. Vaccination is important for preventing pneumonia in children. Vaccinations against Haemophilus influenzae and Streptococcus pneumoniae in the first year of life have greatly reduced their role in pneumonia in children.

Atypical pneumonias include those resulting from infection by bacteria-like microorganisms such as Mycoplasma pneumoniae and Chlamydia pneumoniae. Symptoms associated with these types of infections include fatigue, sore throat, cough, joint pain, or rash. Treatment may include the use of certain antibiotics.

Children with compromised immune systems are at risk for developing certain types of pneumonia infections caused by fungi (e.g., histoplasmosis, coccidioidomycosis, cryptococcosis, etc.) and other common organisms such as Pneumocystis carinii. Pneumocystis pneumonia is particularly prevalent among individuals with AIDS. Choice of drug therapy relates to the appropriate identification of the causative organism. Other treatment is symptomatic and supportive.

Government Agencies

5747 NIH/National Institute of Allergy and Infectious Diseases
5601 Fishers Lane, MSC 9806
Bethesda, MD 20892
301-496-5717
866-284-4107
Fax: 301-402-3573
TDD: 800-877-8339
ocpostoffice@niaid.nih.gov
www.niaid.nih.gov

Conducts and supports basic and applied research to better understand, treat, and ultimately prevent infectious, immunologic, and allergic diseases.

Anthony S Fauci MD, Director

National Associations & Support Groups

5748 American Academy of Pediatrics
141 Northwest Point Boulevard
Elk Grove Village, IL 60007
847-434-4000
800-433-9016
Fax: 847-434-8000
www.aap.org

The American Academy of Pediatrics and its member pediatricians are committed to the attainment of optimal physical, mental and social health and well-being for all infants, children, adolescents, and young adults.

Fernando Stein, MD, FAAP, President
Karen Remley, MD, CEO/Executive VP

5749 March of Dimes Foundation
1275 Mamaroneck Avenue
White Plains, NY 10605
914-997-4488
888-663-4637
Fax: 914-428-8203
answers@marchofdimes.com
www.marchofdimes.com

Partnership of volunteers and professionals dedicates to improving the health of babies by preventing birth defects and infant mortality. Over 100 chapters are located across the country and can be located through the National Office.

Stacey D. Stewart, President

5750 World Health Organization
Avenue Appia 20
CH-1211 Geneva 27,
Switzerland
www.who.int

WHO is the directing and coordinating authority for health within the United Nations system.

Dr Margaret Chan, Director General

683

Research Centers

5751 National Jewish Medical & Research Center
1400 Jackson Street
Denver, CO 80206   303-388-4461
877-225-5654
www.njc.org

National Jewish is a nonsectarian, nonprofit independent clinical research, medical center that focuses on respiratory, immunologic, allergic, and infectious diseases.

Russell P Bowler, President/CEO
J Verne Singleton, COO
Gary Cott MD, Medical & Clinical Services

Web Sites

5752 American Lung Association
55 W. Wacker Drive, Suite 1150
Chicago, IL 60601   312-801-7628
info@lung.org
www.lung.org

Information regarding lung disease in all its forms, with special emphasis on asthma, tobacco control and environmental health. Includes information and a fact sheet on pneumonia.

Harold P. Wimmer, National President & CEO
Susan Rappaport, National VP, Research/Scientific
Sue Swan, Chief Development Officer

5753 Department of Health and Human Services
540 Gaither Road
Rockville, MD 20850   301-427-1364
www.ahrq.gov

Pneumonia research findings for consumers.

5754 Kid's Health
kidshealth.org/parent/infections/

Kids health is the largest and most visited site on the web providing doctor-approved health information about children from before birth through adolescence. Kids health provides families with accurate, up to date and jargon free health information they can use.

Neil Izenberg, MD, Editor-in-Chief & Founder

5755 Mayo Clinic
13400 E. Shea Blvd.
Scottsdale, AZ 85259   480-301-8000
800-446-2279
www.mayoclinic.com/health/pneumonia/DS00135

5756 National Jewish Medical & Research Center
1400 Jackson St.
Denver, CO 80206   877-225-5654
www.nationaljewish.org

National Jewish is a nonsectarian, nonprofit independent clinical research, medical center. Focusing on respiratory, immunologic, allergic, and infectious diseases. The Center's mission is to develop and provide innovative clinical programs for treating and rehabilitating patients of all ages and for preventing disease, discovering knowledge to enhance prevention, treatment and cures through an integrated program of basic and clinical research, and educating professionals and the public.

Michael Salem, MD, FACS, President & CEO

Book Publishers

5757 Let's Talk About Going to the Hospital
Rosen Publishing Group's PowerKids Press
29 E 21st Street
New York, NY 10010   212-777-3017
800-237-9932
Fax: 888-436-4643
rosenpub@tribeca.ios.com
www.rosenpublishing.com

If a child has to check into the hospital, chances are he or she is already upset about being ill. Knowing how a hospital functions and what the procedures are, such as when family members can visit, will help in what is already a stressful situation. Grades K-5.

24 pages
ISBN: 0-823950-36-0

Roger Rosen, President

DESCRIPTION

5758 POLYDACTYLY

Synonyms: Polydactylia, Polydactylism

Involves the following Biologic System(s):
Genetic/Chromosomal/Syndrome/Metabolic Disorders, Orthopedic and Muscle Disorders

Poldactyly refers to an abnormality that is present at birth (congenital) in which an infant has more than the usual number of fingers or toes. Defects associated with this abnormality may range from simple skin tags or stumps of flesh to extra fingers or toes that are completely developed. In some families polydactyly is passed from generation to generation.

Polydactyly involving the toes occurs in approximately two out of every 1,000 births. Although the fifth toe is the digit most often duplicated, polydactyly sometimes affects the great or big toe. Careful evaluation is indicated so that treatment of possible associated abnormalities may be appropriately coordinated. However, if the extra digit is small or rudimentary, it may be tied off (ligated) at birth or soon thereafter. This method allows for the digit to spontaneously detach itself after a period of time. In those cases where the digit is jointed, treatment usually involves surgical amputation of the extra digit and repair of other associated structures and tissues. Surgical intervention of this type is usually performed at approximately one year of age.

Duplication of a finger usually appears near the small finger (pinky) or thumb. As in polydactyly of the toes, small, rudimentary digits may be tied off, while more complex deformities typically require surgical intervention at about one year of age.

Polydactyly may also occur in association with several genetic disorders. These disordersinclude acrocephalopolysyndactyly type II (Carpenter's syndrome), characterized by mental retardation and irregularities involving the head, hand, and genitalia; trisomy 13 syndrome (Patau's syndrome), characterized by cleft lip and palate, polydactyly, mental retardation, and irregularities of the central nervous system, heart, genitalia, and internal organs; chondroectodermal dysplasia (Ellis-van Creveld syndrome), a bone growth disorder characterized by short stature, cardiac defects, polydactyly, and developmental defects of the teeth, and nails (hypoplastic). The efficacy of treating polydactyly associated with these and other disorders depends upon the exact nature of the disorder in question.

Government Agencies

5759 NIH/ Eunice Kennedy Shriver National Insti tute of Child Health & Human Development
31 Center Drive, Building 31
Bethesda, MD 20892   301-496-5113
                                                  800-370-2943
                                             Fax: 866-760-5947
                                       nichdpress@mail.nih.gov
                                              www.nichd.nih.gov

Established in 1962 by congress, today the institute conducts and supports research on topics related to the health of children, adults, families and populations. Some of these topics include: developmental disabilities, growth and development, infant death, reproductive health and birth defects.

Diana W. Bianchi, Director
Paul Williams, Director, Communications

5760 NIH/National Institute of Arthritis and Musculoskeletal and Skin Diseases
1 AMS Circle
Bethesda, MD 20892   301-495-4484
                                                  877-226-4267
                                             Fax: 301-718-6366
                                             TDD: 301-565-2966
                                         niamsinfo@mail.nih.gov
                                                 www.niams.nih.gov

The mission of the NIAMS, a part of the NIH, is to support research into the causes, treatment, and prevention of arthritis and musculoskeletal and skin diseases, the training of basic and clinical scientists to carry out this research, and the dissemination of information on research progress in these diseases.

Stephen I Katz MD PhD, Director
Robert H Carter MD, Deputy Director

National Associations & Support Groups

5761 American Academy of Pediatrics
141 Northwest Point Boulevard
Elk Grove Village, IL 60007   847-434-4000
                                                  800-433-9016
                                             Fax: 847-434-8000
                                                   www.aap.org

The American Academy of Pediatrics and its member pediatricians are committed to the attainment of optimal physical, mental and social health and well-being for all infants, children, adolescents, and young adults.

Fernando Stein, MD, FAAP, President
Karen Remley, MD, CEO/Executive VP

5762 CHERUB-Association of Families and Friends of Children with Limb Disorders
Children's Hospital of Buffalo
936 Delaware Avenue
Buffalo, NY 14209   716-762-9997
                                                  888-881-0805
                                               pffdvsg@ohio.net
                                                   www.ohio.net

Offers support to families of juveniles diagnosed with a limb disorder.

Sandra Richenberg
Kathy Gura

5763 Genetic Alliance
4301 Connecticut Avenue NW, Suite 404
Washington, DC 20008   202-966-5557
                                                  800-336-4363
                                             Fax: 202-966-8553
                                        info@geneticalliance.org
                                             www.geneticalliance.org

A coalition of voluntary genetic support groups, consumers and professionals addressing the needs of individuals and families affected by genetic disorders from a national perspective.

Sharon Terry, President/CEO
Tetyana Murza, Managing Director
Natasha Bonhomme, VP, Strategic Development

5764 March of Dimes Foundation
1275 Mamaroneck Avenue
White Plains, NY 10605   914-997-4488
                                                  888-663-4637
                                             Fax: 914-428-8203
                                       answers@marchofdimes.com
                                             www.marchofdimes.com

Partnership of volunteers and professionals dedicates to improving the health of babies by preventing birth defects and infant mortality. Over 100 chapters are located across the country and can be located through the National Office.

Stacey D. Stewart, President

5765 Shriners Hospitals for Children
Headquarters
12502 USF Pine Drive
Tampa, FL 33607

813-972-2250
800-237-5055
Fax: 813-975-7125
aargiz-lyons@shrinenet.org
www.shrinershospitalsforchildren.org

Network of 22 hospitals that provide expert, no-cost orthopedic
and burn care to children under 18.

Peter F Armstrong, VP

Web Sites

5766 On The Other Hand
www.ontheotherhand.org

Provides information, support, and suggestions for parents, relatives. and friends of children with hand anomalies.

5767 Polydactyly
www.eatonhand.com/hw/hw024.htm

Explanation and general overview of the disorder.

DESCRIPTION

5768 PORPHYRIA

Synonyms: EPP, Erythrohepatic protoporphyria, Ferrochelatase deficiency, Protoporphyria

Involves the following Biologic System(s):

Hematologic and Oncologic Disorders

Porphyria is a rare group of hereditary metabolic disorders characterized by enzyme deficiencies that result in the abnormal accumulation of chemicals known as porphyrins in certain tissues of the body. Porphyrins are formed during the manufacture of heme, the pigmented, iron-containing component of hemoglobin, which is the oxygen-carrying protein in red blood cells. The porphyrias may be classified as erythropoietic or hepatic porphyrias. The erythropoietic porphyrias are characterized by overproduction of porphyrins in the blood-forming tissue of the bone marrow. In individuals with hepatic porphyrias, there is abnormally increased production of porphyrins in the liver. The range and severity of associated symptoms and the age at onset are variable and depend on the underlying enzyme deficiency and the form of porphyria present. Erythropoietic protoporphyria is the most common form of porphyria and is thought to affect approximately one in 5,000 to 10,000 individuals.

In patients with erythropoietic protoporphyria, also known as EPP, deficiency of the enzyme ferrochelatase results in excessive accumulation of protoporphyrin in red blood cells and the fluid portion of the blood (plasma). Excessive protoporphyrin is also concentrated in a liquid secreted by the liver (bile) and is eliminated in the feces. In some patients, abnormal accumulations of protoporphyrin also become deposited within the liver itself.

Symptoms associated with EPP usually begin in childhood before age 10. The most common symptom is an abnormal sensitivity of the skin to sunlight and certain forms of artificial light (photosensitivity). Affected children typically experience pain, burning, and itching of the skin within an hour of exposure to sunlight. Such symptoms are often followed hours later by redness and inflammation of the skin and abnormal accumulation of fluid (edema) beneath the skin in affected areas. However, abnormal burning sensations of the skin may occur in the absence of associated redness or fluid accumulation. Rarely, if sun exposure is prolonged, fluid-filled blisters (vesicles) may develop or there may be bleeding in the skin or mucous membranes, appearing as pinpoint purplish spots (petechiae) or small bluish-purple patches (purpura). Such blistering or bruising may persist for several days after exposure to the sun. In addition, prolonged, repeated sun exposure may cause mild scarring, abnormal thickening of the skin in certain areas, or an abnormality of the nails in which the nails become separated from the nail beds (onycholysis). Although symptoms associated with photosensitivity typically become apparent during infancy or early childhood, the condition sometimes does not occur until adolescence or adulthood.

Many patients with EPP may also develop lumps of solid matter in the gall bladder (gallstones or cholelithiasis) at an unusually early age. The gall bladder is a small, muscular sac under the liver that stores and concentrates bile from the liver. In addition, uncommonly, there may be mildly de-

creased levels of circulating red blood cells (anemia). Rarely, patients may develop progressive liver damage that may lead to liver failure.

EPP is caused by changes (mutations) in the gene that regulates the production of the enzyme ferrochelatase. This gene is located on the long arm of chromosome 18 (18q21.3). Several different mutations of the gene have been identified in individuals with the disorder. In most cases, EPP has autosomal dominant inheritance. However, there have been reports in which patients inherited two different mutations of the gene, one from each parent. In addition, some individuals who inherit one copy of the disease gene may have slightly elevated levels of protoporphyrin, yet do not experience symptoms associated with the disease.

Patients with EPP benefit from avoiding sunlight, using topical sunscreens, and wearing protective clothing, such as sunglasses, hats, long sleeves, and double layers. Administration of beta-carotene by mouth may help improve tolerance to sunlight. Therapy with cholestyramine, a medication that acts upon the liver's bile acids, may help to alleviate skin symptoms and liver disease. Additional treatment is symptomatic and supportive.

Government Agencies

5769 NIH/ Eunice Kennedy Shriver National Insti tute of Child Health & Human Development

31 Center Drive, Building 31
Bethesda, MD 20892

301-496-5113
800-370-2943
Fax: 866-760-5947
nichdpress@mail.nih.gov
www.nichd.nih.gov

Established in 1962 by congress, today the institute conducts and supports research on topics related to the health of children, adults, families and populations. Some of these topics include: developmental disabilities, growth and development, infant death, reproductive health and birth defects.

Diana W. Bianchi, Director
Paul Williams, Director, Communications

National Associations & Support Groups

5770 American Academy of Pediatrics

141 Northwest Point Boulevard
Elk Grove Village, IL 60007

847-434-4000
800-433-9016
Fax: 847-434-8000
www.aap.org

The American Academy of Pediatrics and its member pediatricians are committed to the attainment of optimal physical, mental and social health and well-being for all infants, children, adolescents, and young adults.

Fernando Stein, MD, FAAP, President
Karen Remley, MD, CEO/Executive VP

5771 American Porphyria Foundation

4900 Woodway, Suite 780, PO Box 22712
Houston, TX 77056

713-266-9617
866-273-3635
Fax: 713-840-9552
porphyrus@aol.com
www.porphyriafoundation.com

Dedicated to improving the health and wellness of individuals and families affected by porphyria through enhanced public awareness; support of research; and development of educational programs and educational material.

Desiree Lyon Howe, Executive Director

5772 Erythropoietic Protoporphyria Research & Education Fund
Brigham & Women's Hospital
Channing Laboratory, 181 Longwood Avenue
Boston, MA 02115 617-525-8249
Fax: 617-731-1541
mmmathroth@rics.bwh.harvard.edu
www.brighamandwomens.org/eppref

A support group for patients with Erythropoietic Protoporphyria and their families and their physicians, providing information on this disease and publishing a bi-annual newsletter available online on the website.

Micheline Mathews Roth, MD, Medical Director

5773 Genetic Alliance
4301 Connecticut Avenue NW, Suite 404
Washington, DC 20008 202-966-5557
800-336-4363
Fax: 202-966-8553
info@geneticalliance.org
www.geneticalliance.org

A coalition of voluntary genetic support groups, consumers and professionals addressing the needs of individuals and families affected by genetic disorders from a national perspective.

Sharon Terry, President/CEO
Tetyana Murza, Managing Director
Natasha Bonhomme, VP, Strategic Development

5774 March of Dimes Foundation
1275 Mamaroneck Avenue
White Plains, NY 10605 914-997-4488
888-663-4637
Fax: 914-428-8203
answers@marchofdimes.com
www.marchofdimes.com

Partnership of volunteers and professionals dedicates to improving the health of babies by preventing birth defects and infant mortality. Over 100 chapters are located across the country and can be located through the National Office.

Stacey D. Stewart, President

Libraries & Resource Centers

5775 National Digestive Diseases Information Clearinghouse
9000 Rockville Pike
Bethesda, MD 20892 301-496-3583
800-860-8747
Fax: 703-738-4929
healthinfo@niddk.nih.gov
www.niddk.nih.govv

The National Institute of Diabetes and Digestive and Kidney Diseases conducts and supports research on many of the most serious diseases affecting public health. The Institute supports much of the clinical research on the diseases of internal medicine and related subspecialty fields as well as many basic science disciplines.

Dr. Griffin P. Rodgers, Director
Dr. Gregory G. Germino, Deputy Directortary
Camille M. Hoover, M.S.W., Executive Officer

Newsletters

5776 APF Newsletter
American Porphyria Foundation
4900 Woodway, Suite 780
Houston, TX 77056 713-266-9617
866-APF-3635
Fax: 713-840-9552
porphyrus@aol.com
www.porphyriafoundation.com

The newsletter provides updates on treatment and reserach, as well as informative articles on patients and specialists who treat porphyria.

Quarterly
James V. Young, Chairman
Desiree H. Lyon, Executive Director
Dr. William McCutchen, Board Member

Pamphlets

5777 Porphyria Fact Sheet
Nat'l Digestive Diseases Information Clearinghouse
2 Information Way
Bethesda, MD 20892 301-496-3583
800-891-5389
Fax: 703-738-4929
nddic@info.niddk.nih.gov
www.niddk.nih.gov

Griffin P. Rodgers, M.D., Director

DESCRIPTION

5778 POST-TRAUMATIC STRESS DISORDER
Synonym: PTSD
Involves the following Biologic System(s):
Developmental/Behavioral/Psychiatric Disorders

Traumatic events can stay with children for a long time. Such events can range from the rare and horrific, such as severe torture, to more common events such as an automobile accident or a violent crime. With immediate media coverage of violence in our world, children are often exposed to the violent acts of war and terror through the television. Moreover, children may be directly or indirectly affected by events of terror and violence that now pervade our society. Effects of some childhood experiences can last well into adulthood. When the after-effects of a traumatic event are so severe and so persistent that they impair normal childhood functioning, behavior or development, professional help should be considered.

Post-Traumatic Stress Disorder, or PTSD, is a diagnosis made to describe the psychological and physiological symptoms that arise from experiencing, witnessing or participating in a traumatic event. PTSD in a child may result from exposure to a traumatic event which the child experienced or witnessed. It may occur if the child was confronted by death or serious injury, or a threat to the physical integrity of self or others. Studies indicate that 15 to 43% of girls and 14 to 43% of boys have experienced at least one traumatic event in their lifetime. Of those children and adolescents who have experienced a trauma, 3 to 15% of girls and 1 to 6% of boys meet criteria for PTSD. Researchers and clinicians are beginning to recognize that PTSD may not present itself in children in the same way as it does in adults. The classical triad of symptoms includes re-experiencing, numbing of responsiveness, and hyperarousal. Other symptoms include regression, bedwetting, separation anxiety and new fears previously not expressed. Children are also more likely to exhibit their 're-experience' in play. Very young children may present with few PTSD symptoms. Instead, young children may report more generalized fears such as stranger or separation anxiety, avoidance of situations that may or may not be related to the trauma, sleep disturbances, and a preoccupation with words or symbols that may or may not be related to the trauma. Elementary school-aged children may be unable to recall the sequence of the events related to the trauma or believe that there were warning signs that predicted the trauma. PTSD in adolescents may begin to more closely resemble PTSD in adults. Adolescents are more likely to engage in traumatic reenactment in which they incorporate aspects of the trauma into their daily lives. In addition, adolescents are more likely than younger children or adults to exhibit impulsive and aggressive behaviors. Response to traumatic events can also vary from child to child. Some characteristics, however, are common among all children with PTSD. If a child has survived a life-threatening event, there may be a profound sense of guilt, particularly if others did not survive the event. These guilt feelings may be exacerbated if the child had to do extraordinary things to survive. In other cases, a child with PTSD may complain of physical symptoms that have no discernible anatomic or physiological explanation, but which are manifestations of psychic distress; these are known as somatic complaints. The child with PTSD is also liable to experience a range of feelings that make it difficult or impossible for him or her to carry on with life in a normal fashion. They may feel that the trauma they experienced damaged them permanently and irreparably. Children who suffer from PTSD may also experience depression, Obsessive-Compulsive Disorder, social phobia or in the adolescent population, substance abuse.

Therapies include medication and/or psychotherapy. Behavior therapy focuses on helping the child recognize the thought processes that result in traumatic stress reactions. Behavior therapy may involve exposing the patient in a safe and controlled environment to stimuli that prompt a stress reaction; through repeated exposures, the child slowly is desensitized and in time will be able to experience the stimuli without having a stress reaction. As with many psychiatric disorders, treatment often involves some combination of therapy and medication.

Early intervention with skilled providers is vital for successful treatment of children with PTSD.

Government Agencies

5779   National Center for PTSD
www.ptsd.va.gov

802-296-6300
ncptsd@va.gov
www.ptsd.va.gov

A special center within the US Department of Veterans Affairs, which advances clinical care and social welfare through research, education, training and diagnosis.

National Associations & Support Groups

5780   American Academy of Pediatrics
141 Northwest Point Boulevard
Elk Grove Village, IL 60007

847-434-4000
800-433-9016
Fax: 847-434-8000
www.aap.org

The American Academy of Pediatrics and its member pediatricians are committed to the attainment of optimal physical, mental and social health and well-being for all infants, children, adolescents, and young adults.

Fernando Stein, MD, FAAP, President
Karen Remley, MD, CEO/Executive VP

5781   American Counseling Association
6101 Stevenson Ave
Alexandria, VA 22304

703-823-9800
800-347-6647
Fax: 703-823-0252
webmaster@counseling.org
www.counseling.org

Represents professional counselors in various practice settings, and stands ready to serve more than 55,000 members with the resources they need to make a difference. From webinars, publications, and journals to Conference education sessions and legislative action alerts, ACA is where counseling professionals turn for powerful, credible content and support.

Robert L. Smith, President

5782   American Psychological Association
750 First St. NE
Washington, DC 20002

202-336-5500
800-374-2721
TTY: 202-336-6123
www.apa.org

The mission is to advance the creation, communication and application of psychological knowledge to benefit society and improve people's lives.

Norman B. Anderson, PhD, CEO/ EVP
L. Michael Honaker, PhD, Deputy Chief Executive Officer
Ellen G. Garrison, PhD, Senior Policy Advisor

5783 Anxiety Disorders Association of America
8730 Georgia Avenue, Suite 600
Silver Spring, MD 20910
240-485-1001
Fax: 240-485-1035
information@adaa.org
www.adaa.org

Offers resources and information for persons with anxiety and stress-related disorders.

Alies Muskin, Executive Director

5784 Association of Traumatic Stress Specialists
88 Pompton Avenue
Verona, NJ 07044
973-559-9200
800-991-2877
Fax: 973-227-7169
admin@atss.info
www.atss.info

An international membership organization which develops standards of service and education for qualified individuals who provide services, intervention and treatment in the field of traumatic stress.

Mike Garone, CEO
Barbara Maurer, Vice President

5785 CEDAR Associates
39 Smith Ave.
Mount Kisco, NY 10549
914-224-1904
info@cedarassociates.com
www.cedarassociates.com

CEDAR Associates is a multi-disciplinary private group practice for the treatment of a full range of mental health issues for individuals and their family. CEDAR Associates specializes in the prevention and treatment of eating disorders and the problems that often accompany them including depression, self-harm, anxiety, relational issuel, sexual and physical trauma and body image issues.

Judy Scheel, Ph.D., LCSW, Executive Director

5786 International Critical Incident Stress Foundation
3290 Pine Orchard Lane, Suite 106
Ellicott City, MD 21042
410-750-9600
410-750-9601
Fax: 410-750-9601
info@icisf.org
www.icisf.org

Nonprofit, open membership foundation dedicated to the prevention and mitigation of disabling stress by education, training and support services for all emergency service professionals; Continuing education and training in emergency mental health services for psychologists, psychiatrists, social workers and licensed professional counselors.

Donald Howell, Executive Director
Stephanie Beam, General Information

5787 National Child Traumatic Stress Network NCCTS - University of California, LA
11150 W Olympic Blvd., Suite 650
Los Angeles, CA 90064
310-235-2633
Fax: 310-235-2612
www.nctsnet.org

The mission is to raise the standard of care and improve access to services for traumatized children, their families and communities throughout the United States.

Robert S Pynoos, Co-Director
Alan Steinberg, Associate Director
Jenifer Maze, Co-Managing Director

5788 Traumatic Incident Reduction Association
5145 Pontiac Trail
Ann Arbor, MI 48105
734-761-6268
800-499-2751
Fax: 734-663-6861
info@tir.org
www.tir.org

Devoted to reducing the effects of traumatic incidents and providing education on how to deal with traumatic events.

Marian Volkman, President
Ragnhild Malnati, VP

Research Centers

5789 International Society for Traumatic Stress Studies
111 Deer Lake Road Suite 100
Deerfield, IL 60015
847-480-9028
Fax: 847-480-9282
istss@istss.org
www.istss.org

Provides a forum for sharing research, clinical strategies, public policy concerns and theoretical formulation on trauma in the US and worldwide. Dedicated to discovery and dissemination of knowledge and to the stimulation of policy, program and service initiatives that seek to reduce traumatic stressors and their permanent and long-term consequences. Members include psychiatrists, psychologists, social workers, nurses, counselors, researchers, administrators, advocates, and others.

Marylene Cloitre PhD, President
Karestan C Koenen PhD, Vice President
Dean G Kilpatrick PhD, Treasurer

Audio Video

5790 Complex PTSD in Children
Sidran Institute
PO Box 436
Brooklandville, MD 21022
410-825-8888
888-825-8249
Fax: 410-560-0134
help@sidran.org
www.sidran.org

Tape I: Etiology, Assessment, Advocacy; Tape II: Therapeutic Interventions

VHS 41 Minutes

Esther Giller, President and Director
Sheila~ Giller, Secretary/Treasurer
Tracy Howard, Book Sales/ Office Manager

5791 PTSD in Children: Move in the Rhythm of th e Child
Sidran Institute
PO Box 436
Brooklandville, MD 21022
410-825-8888
888-825-8249
Fax: 410-560-0134
help@sidran.org
www.sidran.org

Trauma experts explain the circumstances, symptoms and therapy techniques for PTSD in children and the effect on our communities. Primarily for use by mental health professionals, it is an excellent resource for any who work with children.

VHS 58 Minutes

Esther Giller, President and Director
Sheila~ Giller, Secretary/Treasurer
Tracy Howard, Book Sales/ Office Manager

5792 Significant Event Childhood Trauma
Sidran Institute
PO Box 436
Brooklandville, MD 21022
410-825-8888
888-825-8249
Fax: 410-560-0134
help@sidran.org
www.sidran.org

Topics discussed inlude: effects; targeting resources; in the classroom; single parents; divorce; violence; addiction; and intervention.

DVD

Esther Giller, President and Director
Sheila˜ Giller, Secretary/Treasurer
Tracy Howard, Book Sales/ Office Manager

Web Sites

5793 Association of Traumatic Stress Specialists
5000 Old Buncombe Road, Suite 27-11
Greenville, SC 29617   864-294-4337
                                               www.atss.info

An international membership organization which develops standards of service and education for qualified individuals who provide services, intervention and treatment in the field of traumatic stress.

Chrys Harris, President
Bill Mc Dermott, Vice President
Linda Hood, Secretary

5794 David Baldwin's Trauma Information Pages
www.trauma-pages.com

Brief summary of what is known about traumatic symptoms and responses including PTSD and coping strategies. Pages include additional links to more detailed references, online articles and web resources.

5795 Facts for Health: PTSD
ptsd.factsforhealth.org

5796 Helping Kids Cope With a New Threat
750 First St. NE
Washington, DC 20002   202-336-5500
                                               800-374-2721
                   www.apa.org/monitor/apr02/helpingkids.html

An online article about the issues of traumatic stress in children in particular after the September 11 attacks.

Barry S. Anton, PhD, President
Bonnie Markham, Treasurer
Linda Frye Campbell, Member

5797 International Critical Incident Stress Foundation
3290 Pine Orchard Lane, Suite 106
Ellicott City, MD 21042   410-750-9600
                                               www.icisf.org

Nonprofit, open membership foundation dedicated to the prevention and mitigation of disabling stress by education, training and support services for all emergency service professionals; Continuing education and training in emergency mental health services for psychologists, psychiatrists, social workers and licensed professional counselors.

Becky Stoll, Chair
Lisa Joubert, Secretary
Richard Bloch, Counsel

5798 Madison Institute of Medicine
www.miminc.org

Disseminates innovative approaches to the education of professionals and the general public on many mental health topics such as PTSD, OCD, depression, SAD and others.

5799 PTSD Alliance
www.ptsdalliance.org

A group of professional and advocacy organizaions that have joined forces to provide educational resources to individuals diagnosed wth PTSD and their loves ones; those at risk for developing PTSD; and medical, healthcare and other frontline professionals.

5800 Sidran Institute - Traumatic Stress Educat ion & Advocacy
PO Box 436
Brooklandville, MD 21022   410-825-8888
                                               888-825-8249
                                          Fax: 410-560-0134
                                               help@sidran.org
                                               www.sidran.org

Provides education, resources, information and advocacy, publications, training and consulting on traumatic stress.

Esther Giller, President and Director
Sheila˜ Giller, Secretary/Treasurer
Tracy Howard, Book Sales/ Office Manager

Book Publishers

5801 Coping with Post-Traumatic Stress Disorder
Rosen Publishing Group
29 E 21st Street
New York, NY 10010   800-237-9932
                                          Fax: 888-436-4643
                                               www.rosenpublishing.com

Revised 2002 192 pages
Roger Rosen, President

5802 Effective Treatments for PTSD, 2nd Ed
Foa, Keane, Friedman, & Cohen, author

Guilford Press
72 Spring Street
New York, NY 10012   800-365-7006
                                          Fax: 212-966-6708
                                               info@guilford.com
                                               www.guilford.com

Represents the collaborative work of experts across a range of theoretical orientations and professional backgrounds. Addresses general treatment considerations and methodological issues, reviews and evaluates literature on treatment approaches for children, adolescents and adults.

2008 604 pages Paperback
ISBN: 1-606230-01-5
Bob Matloff, President
Seymour Weingarten, Editor-in-Chief

**5803 Helping Kids Heal - 75 Activities to Help Children Recover
from Trauma & Loss**
Rebecca Carman CSW, author

Sidran Institute
PO Box 436
Brooklandville, MD 21022   410-825-8888
                                               888-825-8249
                                          Fax: 410-560-0134
                                               info@sidran.org
                                               www.sidran.org

75 activities to use with school-aged children after traumatic events. Broken down into 13 sections that follow the natural sequence of recovery.

117 pages Paperback
Esther Giller, President & Director
Sheila Giller, Secretary/Treasurer
Ruta Mazelis, Editor

5804 PTSD Workbook
Courage to Change
PO Box 486
Wilkes-Barre, PA 18703   800-440-4003
                                          Fax: 800-772-6499
                                               www.couragetochange.com

Outlines simple and effective techniques employed by PTSD experts for trauma survivors in order to conquer their most distressing symptoms. Readers learn to evaluate their type of trauma and then learn the most effective strategies to overcome them.

5805 Post Traumatic Stress Disorder Sourcebook

Glenn R Schiraldi, author

McGraw Hill Publishers
860 Taylor Station Road
Blacklick, 43004

877-833-5524
877-833-5524
Fax: 614-759-3823
pbg.ecommerce_custserv@mcgraw-hill.com
www.mhprofessional.com

Offers help and hope for lasting recovery. A guide for sufferers and theor loved ones.

446 pages Paperback
ISBN: 0-737302-65-8

Lloyd G. Waterhouse, President & CEO
Patrick Milano, CFO
David Stafford, Senior Vice President

5806 Posttraumatic Stress Disorder in Children and Adolescents

Raul R Silva MD, author

Sidran Institute
PO Box 436
Brooklandville, MD 21022

410-825-8888
888-825-8249
Fax: 410-560-0134
info@sidran.org
www.sidran.org

An expert guide to the most importatnt issues pertaining to PTSD, trauma, stress and concurrent conditions. Includes 15 chapters that address different aspects of childhood and adolescent trauma.

384 pages Paperback

Esther Giller, President & Director
Sheila Giller, Secretary/Treasurer
Ruta Mazelis, Editor

5807 Treating Psychological Trauma and PTSD

John Wilson et al, author

Sidran Institute
PO Box 436
Brooklandville, MD 21022

410-825-8888
888-825-8249
Fax: 410-560-0134
info@sidran.org
www.sidran.org

Identifies 65 PTSD symptoms contained within five symptom clusters, and then addresses 80 target objectives for treatment, which can be treated by 11 different psychotherapeutic approaches.

443 pages Paperback

Esther Giller, President & Director
Sheila Giller, Secretary/Treasurer
Ruta Mazelis, Editor

5808 Treating Trauma & Traumatic Grief in Child ren and Adolescents

J Cohen, A Mannarino, E Deblinger, author

Guilford Press
72 Spring Street
New York, NY 10012

800-365-7006
Fax: 212-966-6708
info@guilford.com
www.guilford.com

The book presents a systematic treatment approach, grounded in CBT, for traumatized children and their families. Provides a comprehensive frameworkl for assessing PTSD, depression, anxiety, and other symptoms; assists in developing a flxible, patient-specific treatment plan to work with the children and parents in building core skills. Includes age and culture specific treatment components. Print or e-book.

2006 256 pages
ISBN: 1-593853-08-2

Bob Matloff, President
Seymour Weingarten, Editor-in-Chief

Pamphlets

5809 Helping Children and Adolescents Cope with Violence and Disasters

National Institute of Mental Health
6001 Executive Boulevard, Room 6200
Bethesda, MD 20892

301-443-4513
866-615-6464
Fax: 301-443-4279
TTY: 301-443-8431
nimhinfo@nih.gov
www.nimh.nih.gov

Booklet that discusses children and adolescents' reactions to violence and disasters, emphasizing the wide range of responses and the role that parents, teachers and therapists can play in the healing process.

Francis Collins, M.D., Director
Tom Insel, Director

5810 Post Traumatic Stress Disorder: A Guide

Madison Institute of Medicine
www.miminc.org/shop/store/

Comprehensive overview, diagnosis and treatment of PTSD.

2000 69 pages

5811 Post-Traumatic Stress Disorder, A Real Ill ness

National Institute of Mental Health
6001 Executive Boulevard, Room 6200
Bethesda, MD 20892

301-443-4513
866-615-6464
Fax: 301-443-4279
TTY: 301-443-8431
nimhinfo@nih.gov
www.nimh.nih.gov

An easy-to-read pamphlet of simple information about what it is, when it starts, how long it lasts and how to get help.

9 pages

Francis Collins, M.D., Director
Tom Insel, Director

5812 What Is Post Traumatic Stress Disorder?

Sidran Institute
PO Box 436
Brooklandville, MD 21022

410-825-8888
888-825-8249
Fax: 410-560-0134
help@sidran.org
www.sidran.org

Provides an introduction of PTSD as well as symptoms, possible treatment, and other helpful resources.

Esther Giller, President and Director
Sheila Giller, Secretary/Treasurer
Tracy Howard, Book Sales/ Office Manager

DESCRIPTION

5813 PRADER-WILLI SYNDROME

Synonym: PWS

Involves the following Biologic System(s):

Endocrinologic Disorders,

Genetic/Chromosomal/Syndrome/Metabolic Disorders

Prader-Willi syndrome is a genetic disorder characterized by severely diminished muscle tone (hypotonia) during early infancy, short stature, unusually small hands and feet, obesity, genital abnormalities, and mental retardation. The disorder is thought to affect approximately one in 15,000 individuals. In most cases of Prader-Willi syndrome, there is decreased fetal activity during the last months of pregnancy. After birth, most affected infants experience hypotonia, have feeding difficulties due to decreased swallowing and sucking reflexes, and fail to grow and gain weight at the expected rate (failure to thrive). Starting at approximately six months to six years of age, affected infants or children begin to have an excessive appetite (polyphagia), become obsessed with eating, or lack a sense of satisfaction after a meal and often engage in binge-type eating. As a result, patients develop an abnormally increased body weight (progressive obesity) due to an excessive accumulation of body fat, particularly over the thighs, buttocks, and lower abdomen.

Infants and children with Prader-Willi syndrome also may have characteristic abnormalities of the head and face (craniofacial area), such as almond-shaped eyes, upslanting eyelid folds (palpebral fissures), abnormal deviation of one eye in relation to the other (strabismus), a thin, tented upper lip, and full cheeks. In addition, affected males and females may have insufficient secretion of certain hormones that stimulate the gonads (hypogonadotropic hypogonadism). The gonads are the reproductive glands, such as the testes or ovaries, within which the reproductive cells (sperm or ova) are produced. Affected males typically have an abnormally small penis (micropenis) and undescended testes (cryptorchidism), potentially delayed or incomplete development of secondary sexual characteristics, insufficient production of the male sex hormone testosterone, decreased or absent sperm production, and infertility. Affected females often have abnormally small underdeveloped external genitalia (i.e., hypoplastic labia minor and clitoris), absence or abnormal cessation of menstrual cycles (primary or secondary amenorrhea), and infertility. Development of female secondary sexual characteristics may be normal or incomplete. Most children with Prader-Willi syndrome also have mild to moderate mental retardation; however, in some cases, severe mental retardation may be present. Many affected children experience difficulties with speech articulation and may have an abnormally high-pitched, nasal voice. Children with Prader-Willi syndrome may have behavioral problems that become apparent during later childhood, including outbursts of anger, rage-like episodes, and stubbornness.

Some individuals with Prader-Willi syndrome may develop diabetes mellitus during or soon after puberty. Diabetes mellitus is characterized by impaired fat, protein, and carbohydrate metabolism due to insufficient production of the hormone insulin or the body's inability to appropriately utilize insulin. Associated symptoms may include excessive thirst (polydipsia) and urination (polyuria). In addition, adolescents and young adults may be prone to experiencing cardiac insufficiency, potentially resulting in life-threatening complications during the second or third decade of life.

In children with Prader-Willi syndrome, treatment typically includes measures to help prevent progressive obesity or to ensure strict weight control, such as a low-calorie diet and a proper exercise program under a physician's direction. Nutritional behavioral modification methods may be implemented that require the cooperation and support of all family members, such as ensuring regular feeding habits (e.g., having meals at the same time and location on a daily basis) and the inaccessibility of food between meals. In young males with Prader-Willi syndrome, testosterone replacement therapy may result in enlargement of micropenis; in addition, testosterone therapy during adolescence or young adulthood may have beneficial effects on the development of secondary sexual characteristics. Treatment of children with Prader-Willi syndrome also may include special education and behavioral therapies to help manage behavioral problems.

Prader-Willi syndrome is caused by deletion or disruption of certain genes (contiguous gene syndrome) located on the long arm of chromosome 15 (15q11-13). Most affected individuals have missing genetic material or deletion of 15q11-13 that affects the chromosome received from the father (paternally derived chromosome).

Government Agencies

5814 NIH/ Eunice Kennedy Shriver National Institute of Child Health & Human Development
National Institutes of Health
31 Center Drive, Building 31
Bethesda, MD 20892

301-496-5113
800-370-2943
Fax: 866-760-5947
nichdpress@mail.nih.gov
www.nichd.nih.gov

Offers reprints, articles and various information on Prader-Willi Syndrome in children and adults.

Diana W. Bianchi, Director
Paul Williams, Director, Communications

National Associations & Support Groups

5815 American Academy of Pediatrics
141 Northwest Point Boulevard
Elk Grove Village, IL 60007

847-434-4000
800-433-9016
Fax: 847-434-8000
www.aap.org

The American Academy of Pediatrics and its member pediatricians are committed to the attainment of optimal physical, mental and social health and well-being for all infants, children, adolescents, and young adults.

Fernando Stein, MD, FAAP, President
Karen Remley, MD, CEO/Executive VP

5816 Foundation for Prader-Willi Research
6407 Bardstown Road, Suite 252
Louisville, KY 40291

502-384-8405
Fax: 502-749-9388
www.fpwr.org

Dedicated to the advancement of research on PWS. The Foundation chooses projects that are highly relevant for individuals with PWS and their families and that are scientifically sound.

Rachel Tugon, Executive Director
Alice Viroslav, President
Kathryn McGhee, Membership

693

5817 Genetic Alliance
4301 Connecticut Avenue NW, Suite 404
Washington, DC 20008
202-966-5557
800-336-4363
Fax: 202-966-8553
info@geneticalliance.org
www.geneticalliance.org

A coalition of voluntary genetic support groups, consumers and professionals addressing the needs of individuals and families affected by genetic disorders from a national perspective.

Sharon Terry, President/CEO
Tetyana Murza, Managing Director
Natasha Bonhomme, VP, Strategic Development

5818 March of Dimes Foundation
1275 Mamaroneck Avenue
White Plains, NY 10605
914-997-4488
888-663-4637
Fax: 914-428-8203
answers@marchofdimes.com
www.marchofdimes.com

Partnership of volunteers and professionals dedicates to improving the health of babies by preventing birth defects and infant mortality. Over 100 chapters are located across the country and can be located through the National Office.

Stacey D. Stewart, President

5819 Prader-Willi Syndrome Association
8588 Potter Park Drive, Suite 500ÿ
Sarasota, FL 34238
941-312-0400
800-926-4797
Fax: 941-312-0142
info@pwsausa.org
www.pwsausa.org

Provides educational materials, support, and advocacy for parents, caregivers, medical professionals, educators and all others involved with persons in PWS community.

Evan Farrar, Acting Executive Director
Sharon Middleton, Business Manager
Jodi O'Sullivan, Director Community Development

State Agencies & Support Groups

Alaska

5820 Prader-Willi Northwest Association
3706 29th Avenue W
Seattle, WA 98199
206-285-7679
jlunderwood@juno.com

Joane Underwood, Co-President

Arizona

5821 Prader-Willi Syndrome Arizona Association
13839 N Bentwater Drive
Tucson, AZ 85737
520-297-7025
p.penta@comcast.net

Tammie Penta, President

California

5822 Prader-Willi California Foundation
514 N. Prospect Avenue, Ste 110, Lower Level
Redondo Beach, CA 90277
310-372-5053
800-400-9994
Fax: 310-316-3730
PWCF1@aol.com
www.pwcf.org

Willi Prader, Owner

Colorado

5823 Prader-Willi Colorado Association
PWSA
8290 South Yukon Way
Littleton, CO 80128
303-973-4780
hosler@dynamicssolutions.com

Lynette Hosler, President

Connecticut

5824 Prader-Willi Connecticut Association
PWSA
35 Ansonia Drive
North Haven, CT 06473
860-204-9386
pwsactchapter@yahoo.com
www.angelfire.com/ct/pwsctchapter/

Eileen Fletcher
Vicki Knopf

Delaware

5825 Prader-Willi Delaware Association
PWSA
300 Bethel Circle Millwood
Middletown, DE 19709
302-378-7385
swede455@aol.com

Karen Swanson, President

Florida

5826 PWSA Florida Chapter
PWSA
694 SE Ashley Oak Way
Stuart, FL 34997
772-287-2587
pwfa2000@aol.com
http://members.aol.com/delchert/pwsa2.htm

Dan Krauer, President

Georgia

5827 PWSA of Georgia
562 Lakeland Plaza #327
Cumming, GA 30040
770-886-2334
877-886-2334
Fax: 770-886-2335
pwsaga@earthlink.net
www.pwsaga.org

Debbie Lange, Executive Director

Hawaii

5828 Prader-Willi Northwest Association
3706 29th Avenue W
Seattle, WA 98199
206-285-7679
jlunderwood@juno.com

Joane Underwood, Co-President

Idaho

5829 Prader-Willi Northwest Association-Idaho
550 Lodgepole Road
Athol, ID 83801
208-683-2993
idaho4ts@aol.com

Gene Todhunter, Contact

Illinois

5830 PWSA of Illinois
PWSA
505 Drexel Avenue
Glencoe, IL 60022
847-242-9082
contact@pwsaillinois.org
www.pwsausa.org/IL/
Ron Bruns, President

Indiana

5831 PWSA of Indiana
Prader-Willi Syndrome Association
7536 Moonbeam Drive
Indianapolis, IN 46259
317-527-9173
amypfeiffer@comcast.net
www.pwsausa.org/IN/
Jaque McGuire

Iowa

5832 PWSA of Iowa
15554 226th Street
Zwingle, IA 52079
319-686-4270
Ktcaedav@netins.net
www.pwsaiowa.org

Tammy Davis, President

Kansas

5833 Prader-Willi Syndrome Advocates
14 NE Bayview Drive
Lees Summit, MO 64064
816-350-1375
Teri Douglas
Barry Douglas

Kentucky

5834 PWSA of Kentucky
Prader-Willi Syndrome Association
9213 Reigate Ct
Louisville,ÿ, KY 40222
502-339-7872
frankandannette@fuse.net
Frank Beck, President

Maine

5835 Prader-Willi Association of New England (Maine, Mass, RI, NH, VT)
2 Ernest Street
Webster, MA 01570
508-943-1400
sunsetrock@comcast.net
www.pwsane.org

Eileen Rullo, President
Mary Raymond, Vice President

Maryland

5836 PWSA of Maryland, Virginia & DC
Prader-Willi Syndrome Association
547 Varndell Road
Grantsville,ÿ, MD 21536
301- 89- 416
ÿlisa@varndellengineering.com
www.pwsausa.org/MD/

Linda Keder, President
Susaie Wood, Maryland Contact

Massachusetts

5837 Prader-Willi Association of New England (Maine, Mass, RI, NH, VT)
2 Ernest Street
Webster, MA 01570
508-943-1400
www.pwsane.org

Eileen Rullo, President
Mary Raymond, Vice President

Michigan

5838 PWSA of Michigan
Prader-Willi Syndrome Association
10756 Woodbushe
Lowell, MI 49331
734-998-3507
Fax: 941-313-0142
info@pwsami.org
www.pwsausa.org/MI/

Jon Hendrick
Chris Hendrick

Minnesota

5839 PWSA Chapter - Minnesota
Prader-Willi Syndrome Association
7691 Iverson Avenue S
Cottage Grove, MN 55016
651-768-0045
dwestenfield@datalink.com
www.pwsausa.org/MN/

Denise Westenfield, President
Kymm Salwasser, Treasurer

Missouri

5840 PWSA Missouri Chapter
Prader-Willi Syndrome Missouri Association
3233 Hedgetree Lane Street, PO Box 410252
Creve Coeur, MO 63141
314-935-9358
Fax: 314-935-7461
whitmanb@slu.edu
www.pwsausa.org/MO/

Judy O'Leary, President

Montana

5841 Prader-Willi Northwest Association
3706 29th Avenue W
Seattle, WA 98199
206-285-7679
jlunderwood@juno.com
Joane Underwood, Co-President

Nebraska

5842 PWSA of Nebraska
Prader-Willi Syndrome Association
302 S 49th Avenue
Omaha, NE 68132
402-551-9168
jvarner@cox.net
www.pwsausa.org

Jennifer Varner, Contact

Nevada

5843 PWSA Las Vegas/Nevada Support Group
PWS NV S.H.A.R.E.
www.pwsnv.org

702-526-0630
pwsnv.org@gmail.com
www.pwsnv.org

New Jersey

5844 PWSA - New Jersey Chapter
Prader-Willi Syndrome Association
514 Gatewood Road
Cherry Hill, NJ 08003   856-795-4229
                                          pwsa.nj@gmail.com
                                          www.pwsausa.org/NJ/

Sybil Cohen, President

New Mexico

5845 PWS Project for New Mexico

                                          505-332-6700
                                          claroque@arc-a.org

New York

5846 Prader-Willi Alliance of New York
PWSA NY Chapter
2224 Agnew Ter
The Villages, FL 32162   585-442-1655
                                            800-442-1655
                                          alliance@prader-willi.org
                                          www.prader-willi.org

Hon. Daniel D Angiolillo, President
Rachel ÿÿÿÿ Johnson , Vice President

North Carolina

5847 PWSA of North Carolina
PWSA
4627 Mt Sinai Road
Durham, NC 27705   919-332-0621
Mary Jones Patterson

Ohio

5848 PWSA of Ohio
State Office
1087 Dover Drive
Medina, OH 44256   440-716-0552
                                          pwsaohio@aol.com
                                          www.pwsaohio.org

Jennifer Bolander, President

5849 Prader-Willi Families of Ohio
4075 West 226 Street
Fairview Park, OH ÿ4412   440-716-0552
                                          pwfohio@aol.com
                                          www.pwsaohio.org/

Johanna Costello, President

Oklahoma

5850 PWSA of Oklahoma
Prader-Willi Syndrome Association
3820 SE 89th Street
Oklahoma City, OK 73135   405-677-8089
                                          Fax: 405-522-6256
                                          Rdmosley@swbell.net
                                          www.pwsausa.org

Daphne Mosley, President
Curt Shacklett, Chairman

Oregon

5851 PWSA of Oregon
Prader-Willi Syndrome Association
456 Horn Lane
Eugene, OR 97404   360-609-5197
                                          wade175@juno.com
                                          www.pwsausa.org

Lennae Elkington, President

Pennsylvania

5852 PWSA of Pennsylvania
Prader-Willi Syndrome Association
2415 Maryland Drive
Pittsburgh, PA 15241   412-854-8885
                                          pwsa_pa@verizon.net
                                          www.pwsausa.org

Donn & John Forster, Co-Presidents

South Carolina

5853 PWSA - South Carolina
Prader-Willi Syndrome Association
912 Lake Spur Lane
Chapin, SC 29036   803-345-1379
                                          rleazer8@cs.com
                                          www.pwsausa.org

Rhett Eleazer, Contact

Tennessee

5854 PWSA - Tennessee
Prader-Willi Syndrome Association
105 Foxwood Lane
Franklin, TN 37069   615-790-6659
                                          Tcbo333@aol.com
                                          www.pwsausa.org

Terry Bolander

Texas

5855 Texas Prader-Willi Syndrome Association
PO Box 1542
Whitehouse, TX 75791   903-363-8680
                                          info@texaspwsa.com
                                 www.pwsausa.org; www.texaspwsa.com

Derek Snitker

Utah

5856 Prader-Willi Utah Association
Prader-Willi Syndrome Association
2652 E Nottingham Way
Salt Lake City, UT 84108   801-556-8012
                                          Fax: 801-768-3924
                                          sidlisathornton@aol.com
                                          www.pwsausa.org/UT/

Lisa Thornton, President

Virginia

5857 PWSA of Maryland, Virginia & DC
Prader-Willi Syndrome Association
2601 Chriswell Place
Herndon, VA 20171   703-716-4189
                                          pwsamd@pwsausa.org
                                          www.pwsausa.org/MD/

Linda Keder, President
Sherri Planton, Virginia Contact

Wisconsin

5858 PWSA of Wisconsin
Prader-Willi Syndrome Association
2701 N Alexander Street
Appleton, WI 54911   920-882-6371
                                       866-797-2947
                              wisonsin@pwsausa.org
                              www.pwsausa.org/wi/

Mary Lynn Larson, Manager

Research Centers

5859 Foundation for Prader-Willi Research
5455 Wilshire Blvd, Suite 2020,
Los Angeles, CA 90036   760-536-3027
                                       888-322-5487
                                  Fax: 502-749-9388
                                       www.fpwr.org

Dedicated to the advancement of research on PWS. The Foundation chooses projects that are highly relevant for individuals with PWS and their families and that are scientifically sound.

Rachel Tugon, Executive Director
Alice Viroslav, President
Kathryn McGhee, Membership

Audio Video

5860 A Deadly Hunger
Prader-Willi Syndrome Association
8588 Potter Park Drive, Suite 500
Sarasota, FL 34238   941-312-0400
                                       800-926-4797
                                  Fax: 941-312-0142
                                   info@pwsausa.org
                                   www.pwsausa.org

A five part series of news segments that spotlight PWS. Overview of syndrome and stresses problems associated with appetite, obesity, and behavior.

DVD

Michelle˜ Torbert, Chair
James Koerber, Vice Chair
Ken Smith, Executive Director

5861 A Tribute to PWS Children from Around the World
Prader-Willi Syndrome Association
8588 Potter Park Road, Suite 500
Sarasota, FL 34238   941-312-0400
                                       800-926-4797
                                  Fax: 941-312-0142
                                   info@pwsausa.org
                                   www.pwsausa.org

A video of children with PWS of all ages. The presentation is set to music.

10 Minutes

Michelle˜ Torbert, Chair
James Koerber, Vice Chair
Ken Smith, Executive Director

5862 Food, Behavior and Beyond
Prader-Willi Syndrome Association
8588 Potter Park Drive, Suite 500
Sarasota, FL 34238   941-312-0400
                                       800-926-4797
                                  Fax: 941-312-0142
                                   info@pwsausa.org
                                   www.pwsausa.org

Suggestions on nutrition, food and behavior, cognitive and behavioral traits and medications.

DVD

Michelle˜ Torbert, Chair
James Koerber, Vice Chair
Ken Smith, Executive Director

5863 Maribel
Prader-Willi Syndrome Association
8588 Potter Park Drive, Suite 500
Sarasota, FL 34238   941-312-0400
                                       800-926-4797
                                  Fax: 941-312-0142
                                   info@pwsausa.org
                                   www.pwsausa.org

Chronicles a family's struggle with their adult daughter with PWS. Helpful for families with replacement needs who need to show dramatic impact.

2004 DVD/VHS

Michelle˜ Torbert, Chair
James Koerber, Vice Chair
Ken Smith, Executive Director

5864 PWS - The Early Years
Prader-Willi Syndrome Association
8588 Potter Park Drive, Suite 500
Sarasota, FL 34238   941-312-0400
                                       800-926-4797
                                  Fax: 941-312-0142
                                   info@pwsausa.org
                                   www.pwsausa.org

Practical suggestions for families with a young child newly diagnosed with PWS. Includes family interviews.

2002 Video 42 Mins

Michelle˜ Torbert, Chair
James Koerber, Vice Chair
Ken Smith, Executive Director

5865 Prader-Willi Syndrome - An Overview for He alth Professionals
Prader-Willi Syndrome Association
8588 Potter Park Drive, Suite 500
Sarasota, FL 34238   941-312-0400
                                       800-926-4797
                                  Fax: 941-312-0142
                                   info@pwsausa.org
                                   www.pwsausa.org

A medical overview of PWS for health care professionals. It handles all the major genetics and health care issues of the child with PWS.

2004 35 Minutes

Michelle˜ Torbert, Chair
James Koerber, Vice Chair
Ken Smith, Executive Director

Web Sites

5866 International Prader-Willi Syndrome Organi zation (IPWSO)
www.ipwso.org

                                   info@ipwso.org
                                   www.ipwso.org

5867 Online Mendelian Inheritance in Man
National Library of Medicine, Building 38A
Bethesda, MD 20894   888-346-3656
                              info@ncbi.nlm.nih.gov
                              www.ncbi.nlm.nih.gov

This database is a catalog of human genes and genetic disorders.

5868 Prader-Willi Alliance of New York
244 5th˜Avenue, Suite D-110
New York, NY 10001   718-846-6606
                                       800-442-1655
                                   www.prader-willi.org

A chapter of the PWSA, it represents the interests of individuals in New York State with Prader-Willi Syndrome, their families, and the professionals who provide services to the Prader-Willi population.

Rachel Johnson, President
Nancy Finegold, Vice President
Tammy Reals, Vice President

5869 Prader-Willi Syndrome Association
8588 Potter Park Drive, Suite 500
Sarasota, FL 34238   941-312-0400
                                         800-926-4797
                                         Fax: 941-312-0142
                                         info@pwsausa.org
                                         www.pwsausa.org

Dedicated to serving individuals affected by Prader-Willi Syndrome, their families, and interested professionals. To provide information, education, and support services to its members. PWSA offers a toll free telephone number for informationand referrals, a bimonthly newsletter, publications and audiovisual presentations about PWS, an annual national conference for families and professionals and a nationwide network of local chapters, parents, and professionals.

Michelle~ Torbert, Chair
James Koerber, Vice Chair
Ken Smith, Executive Director

Book Publishers

5870 Cookbook for the PWS Diet
Prader-Willi Syndrome Association
8588 Potter Park Drive, Suite 500
Sarasota, FL 34238   941-312-0400
                                         800-926-4797
                                         Fax: 941-312-0142
                                         info@pwsausa.org
                                         www.pwsausa.org

Filled with low-fat, low-sugar recipes designed to be used by the whole family. Great substitution list, fun snack recipes, mealtime tips, full nutritional values calculated for each recipe. Can be used by anyone wanting to lose weight while eating nutritious, interesting food.

2003

John Heybach, Co-Chair
Ken Smith, Co-Chair
Dale Cooper, Interim Executive Directo

5871 Growth Hormone and Prader-Willi Syndrome
Linda Keder, author

Prader-Willi Syndrome Association
8588 Potter Park Drive, Suite 500
Sarasota, FL 34238   941-312-0400
                                         800-926-4797
                                         Fax: 941-312-0142
                                         info@pwsausa.org
                                         www.pwsausa.org

Reference for families and care givers.

2001 52 pages Softcover

John Heybach, Co-Chair
Ken Smith, Co-Chair
Dale Cooper, Interim Executive Directo

5872 Management of Prader-Willi Syndrome
Prader-Willi Syndrome Association
8588 Potter Park Drive, Suite 500
Sarasota, FL 34238   941-312-0400
                                         800-926-4797
                                         Fax: 941-312-0142
                                         info@pwsausa.org
                                         www.pwsausa.org

Latest edition of the only comprehensive textbook on PWS in print. Excellent reference tool for professionals and service providers.

550 pages 3rd Edition

John Heybach, Co-Chair
Ken Smith, Co-Chair
Dale Cooper, Interim Executive Directo

5873 Nutitional Care for Children with PWS, Inf ants and Toddlers
Prader-Willi Syndrome Association
8588 Potter Park Drive, Suite 500
Sarasota, FL 34238   941-312-0400
                                         800-926-4797
                                         Fax: 941-312-0142
                                         info@pwsausa.org
                                         www.pwsausa.org

Provides answers to frequently asked questions about nutrition and feeding of infants and toddlers with PWS.

Revised 2004 62 pages Softcover

John Heybach, Co-Chair
Ken Smith, Co-Chair
Dale Cooper, Interim Executive Directo

5874 Overview of the Prader-Willi Syndrome
Prader-Willi Syndrome Association
8588 Potter Park Drive, Suite 500
Sarasota, FL 34232   941-312-0400
                                         800-926-4797
                                         Fax: 941-312-0142
                                         info@pwsausa.org
                                         www.pwsausa.org

A short introduction to the syndrome for professionals and parents.

13 pages Softcover

John Heybach, Co-Chair
Ken Smith, Co-Chair
Dale Cooper, Interim Executive Directo

5875 Prader-Willi Syndrome is What I Have Not W ho I Am!
Prader-Willi Syndrome Association
8588 Potter Park Drive, Suite 500
Sarasota, FL 34238   941-312-0400
                                         800-926-4797
                                         Fax: 941-312-0142
                                         info@pwsausa.org
                                         www.pwsausa.org

A book of feelings written by children and young adults with PWS. This book gives an important insight into lives and thoughts of our people dealing with PWS on a daily basis. A portion of the book opens the door to journal writing and an opportunity for the reader with PWS to share their feelings.

2005 70 pages softcover

John Heybach, Co-Chair
Ken Smith, Co-Chair
Dale Cooper, Interim Executive Directo

5876 Sometimes I'm Mad, Sometimes I'm Glad - A Sibling Booklet
Prader-Willi Syndrome Association
8588 Potter Park Drive, Suite 500
Sarasota, FL 34238   941-312-0400
                                         800-926-4797
                                         Fax: 941-312-0142
                                         info@pwsausa.org
                                         www.pwsausa.org

It is in the voice of a sibling of someone with PWS. Recognizes the range of feelings that arise in having a brother or sister with the syndrome.

Revised 2005

John Heybach, Co-Chair
Ken Smith, Co-Chair
Dale Cooper, Interim Executive Directo

5877 Teacher's Handbook for the Student with PW S (Educator's Resource)
Prader-Willi Syndrome Association
8588 Potter Park Drive, Suite 500
Sarasota, FL 34238   941-312-0400
                                         800-926-4797
                                         Fax: 941-312-0142
                                         info@pwsausa.org
                                         www.pwsausa.org

A resource book for educators. Important for all who work with these students to gain knowledge about this disorder as well as the many factors that influence their learning. This manual will provide teachers with valuable information to assist in working with students of all abilities.

2003

John Heybach, Co-Chair
Ken Smith, Co-Chair
Dale Cooper, Interim Executive Directo

5878 Tool Box of Hope - For When Your Body Does n't Feel Good
Prader-Willi Syndrome Association
8588 Potter Park Drive, Suite 500
Sarasota, FL 34238

941-312-0400
800-926-4797
Fax: 941-312-0142
info@pwsausa.org
www.pwsausa.org

Fun and practical ways for parents and caregivers to help their child express their feelings, take medicine, get along with others, and make friends with their disability.

2003 2003 pages Ages 3-adult

John Heybach, Co-Chair
Ken Smith, Co-Chair
Dale Cooper, Interim Executive Directo

Newsletters

5879 Gathered View
Prader-Willi Syndrome Association
8588 Potter Park Drive, Suite 500
Sarasota, FL 34238

941-312-0400
800-926-4797
Fax: 941-312-0142
info@pwsausa.org
www.pwsausa.org

The official newsletter of PWSA USA. It offers current research findings, behavior and weight management techniques, educational news and more.

Bimonthly

Michelle˜ Torbert, Chair
James Koerber, Vice Chair
Ken Smith, Executive Director

Pamphlets

5880 Behavior Management - A Collection of Arti cles
Prader-Willi Syndrome Association
8588 Potter Park Drive, Suite 500
Sarasota, FL 34238

941-312-0400
800-926-4797
Fax: 941-312-0142
info@pwsausa.org
www.pwsausa.org

Includes general articles on behavior concerns, use of psychotropic medications, skin picking, and social skills teaching.

2003 49 pages softcover

Michelle˜ Torbert, Chair
James Koerber, Vice Chair
Ken Smith, Executive Director

5881 Child With Prader-Willi Syndrome: Birth to Three
Prader-Willi Syndrome Association
8588 Potter Park Drive, Suite 500
Sarasota, FL 34238

941-312-0400; 800-926-4797
Fax: 941-312-0142
info@pwsausa.org
www.pwsausa.org

Discusses the common concerns of the first three years and offers specific recommendations for early intervention strategies. A helpful and positive resource families, physicians, early intervention worker, and other care providers.

Revised 2004 34 pages Softcover

Michelle˜ Torbert, Chair
James Koerber, Vice Chair
Ken Smith, Executive Director

5882 Growing Up with Prader-Willi Syndrome - Pe rsonal Reflections of a Mother
Prader-Willi Syndrome Association
8588 Potter Park Drive, Suite 500
Sarasota, FL 34238

941-312-0400
800-926-4797
Fax: 941-312-0142
info@pwsausa.org
www.pwsausa.org

A collection of seventeen articles including tips for managing family life.

Revised 2003 37 pages Booklet

Michelle˜ Torbert, Chair
James Koerber, Vice Chair
Ken Smith, Executive Director

5883 Physical Therapy Intervention for Individu als With Prader-Willi Syndrome
Prader-Willi Syndrome Association
8588 Potter Park Drive, Suite 500
Sarasota, FL 34238   941-312-0400; 800-926-4797
Fax: 941-312-0142
info@pwsausa.org; www.pwsausa.org

Provides general information about physical therapy intervention. Includes copies of articles by Janice Agarwal, PT and mom of a son with PWS.

11 pages softcover

Michelle˜ Torbert, Chair
James Koerber, Vice Chair
Ken Smith, Executive Director

5884 Prader-Willi Syndrome: A Guide for Familie s & Professionals
Prader-Willi Syndrome Association
8588 Potter Park Drive, Suite 500
Sarasota, FL 34238   941-312-0400; 800-926-4797
Fax: 941-312-0142
info@pwsausa.org
www.pwsausa.org

Contains comprehensice information about PWS including description, evaluation, genetics, diagnostic testing, management.

Revised 2005 12 pages

Michelle˜ Torbert, Chair
James Koerber, Vice Chair
Ken Smith, Executive Director

5885 Prader-Willi Syndrome: Medical Alerts
Prader-Willi Syndrome Association
8588 Potter Park Drive, Suite 500
Sarasota, FL 34238   941-312-0400; 800-926-4797
Fax: 941-312-0142
info@pwsausa.org; www.pwsausa.org

Important resource for parents to give their child's doctor, Er staff, caregiver, etc.

2005

Michelle˜ Torbert, Chair
James Koerber, Vice Chair
Ken Smith, Executive Director

5886 Student with Prader-Willi Syndrome - Infor mation for Educators
Prader-Willi Syndrome Association
8588 Potter Park Drive, Suite 500
Sarasota, FL 34242   941-312-0400; 800-926-4797
Fax: 941-312-0142
info@pwsausa.org; www.pwsausa.org

An information packet for educators of children with PWS. It includes a handbook, worksheets and brochures. Applicable for Pre-k through high school.

Michelle Torbert, Chair
James Koerber, Vice Chair
Ken Smith, Executive Director

DESCRIPTION

5887 PRECOCIOUS PUBERTY

Synonym: Pubertas praecox

Covers these related disorders: Gonadotropin-dependent precocious puberty, Gonadotropin-independent precocious puberty

Involves the following Biologic System(s):

Endocrinologic Disorders

Precocious puberty refers to a condition in which the onset of sexual maturation occurs before the age of eight years in girls and nine years in boys. True precocious puberty refers to the premature sexual development of the sex glands (i.e., ovaries and testes) as well as the outward appearance of the child (secondary sexual characteristics). Precocious pseudopuberty refers to the early development of only the secondary sex characteristics with no involvement of the sex glands.

True precocious puberty results from the premature production and secretion by the pituitary gland of gonadotropin, a hormone that stimulates the ovaries and the testes. Because the release of hormones from the pituitary gland is controlled by another gland, the hypothalamus, functional abnormalities of or growth of a tumor in the pituitary or the hypothalamus may also result in premature sexual development. These abnormalities may include hormone-secreting tumors of the pituitary gland, brain lesions such as a hypothalamic hamartoma, and other lesions of the central nervous system that may activate the hypothalamus. True precocious puberty may also result from an underactive thyroid gland (hypothyroidism). However, for most children with precocious puberty, the exact cause is not known. More girls are affected by precocious puberty than boys. Although most cases appear sporadically, some patients have a family history of this condition. Sexual characteristics associated with true precocious puberty are always consistent with the sex of the affected child (isosexual characteristics). Such characteristics may include the early appearance of underarm and pubic hair, facial hair in boys, and breasts and menstrual cycles in girls. The penis, testes, and ovaries enlarge and acne may develop. Although height and weight may increase rapidly, advanced bone growth may result in premature closure of the growing ends of the bone (epiphyses) and, thus, slower linear growth leading to short stature.

Precocious pseudopuberty may be caused by a tumor of the ovary, testis, or adrenal gland. Such tumors may cause excessive production of sex hormones. This form of the disorder may also be inherited as an autosomal dominant trait. In addition, precocious pseudopuberty may be associated with other disorders such as McCune-Albright syndrome, which is a condition resulting from the overproduction of hormones of multiple glands. This syndrome is characterized by premature sexual development in girls, irregularities of skin color (pigmentation) and the skeletal system, and abnormalities of various glands. Physical characteristics associated with precocious pseudopuberty are similar to those of true precocious puberty, although the testes and ovaries are not usually involved. However, children affected with this form of the disorder may develop secondary sexual characteristics associated with those of the opposite sex (heterosexual characteristics). In addition, precocious pseudopuberty may prompt early maturation of the hormonal cycle that results in true precocious puberty.

Treatment for true precocious puberty may include the administration of gonadotropin-releasing hormones. These hormones work by diminishing the stimulatory response of the pituitary gland to the gonadotropin-releasing hormones produced naturally within the body until normal puberty begins. Treatment for precocious pseudopuberty may include the use of certain medications that reduce the levels of male and female sex hormones (i.e., testosterone and estrogen). In addition, surgery may be indicated in those patients who have precocious puberty as a result of certain types of tumors. Other treatment is symptomatic and supportive.

Government Agencies

5888 NIH/ Eunice Kennedy Shriver National Insti tute of Child Health & Human Development
31 Center Drive, Building 31
Bethesda, MD 20892

301-496-5113
800-370-2943
Fax: 866-760-5947
nichdpress@mail.nih.gov
www.nichd.nih.gov

Established in 1962 by congress, today the institute conducts and supports research on topics related to the health of children, adults, families and populations. Some of these topics include: developmental disabilities, growth and development, infant death, reproductive health and birth defects.

Diana W. Bianchi, Director
Paul Williams, Director, Communications

National Associations & Support Groups

5889 American Academy of Pediatrics
141 Northwest Point Boulevard
Elk Grove Village, IL 60007

847-434-4000
800-433-9016
Fax: 847-434-8000
www.aap.org

The American Academy of Pediatrics and its member pediatricians are committed to the attainment of optimal physical, mental and social health and well-being for all infants, children, adolescents, and young adults.

Fernando Stein, MD, FAAP, President
Karen Remley, MD, CEO/Executive VP

5890 Genetic Alliance
4301 Connecticut Avenue NW, Suite 404
Washington, DC 20008

202-966-5557
800-336-4363
Fax: 202-966-8553
info@geneticalliance.org
www.geneticalliance.org

A coalition of voluntary genetic support groups, consumers and professionals addressing the needs of individuals and families affected by genetic disorders from a national perspective.

Sharon Terry, President/CEO
Tetyana Murza, Managing Director
Natasha Bonhomme, VP, Strategic Development

5891 MAGIC Foundation: Major Aspects of Growth in Children
4200 Cantera Drive, #106
Warrenville, IL 60555

630-836-8200
800-362-4423
Fax: 630-836-8181
mary@magicfoundation.org
www.magicfoundation.org

A national nonprofit organization providing support and education regarding growth disorders in children and related adult disorders. Provides educational information, networking, a national conference, a kids' program and an extensive medical library.

Dianne Kremidas, Executive Director
Mary Andrews, CEO
Teresa Tucker, Patient Advocacy

5892 March of Dimes Foundation
1275 Mamaroneck Avenue
White Plains, NY 10605
914-997-4488
888-663-4637
Fax: 914-428-8203
answers@marchofdimes.com
www.marchofdimes.com

Partnership of volunteers and professionals dedicates to improving the health of babies by preventing birth defects and infant mortality. Over 100 chapters are located across the country and can be located through the National Office.

Stacey D. Stewart, President

Web Sites

5893 KidsHealth: Precocious Puberty
www.kidshealth.org/parents/

General overview of precocious puberty including signs, causes, diagnosis and treatment.

Neil Izenberg, MD, Editor-in-Chief & Founder

5894 Online Mendelian Inheritance in Man
National Library of Medicine, Building 38A
Bethesda, MD 20894
888-346-3656
info@ncbi.nlm.nih.gov
www.ncbi.nlm.nih.gov/entrez/dispomim.cgi?id=176400

This database contains textual information and references. It also contains copious links to MEDLINE and sequence records in the Entrez system, and links to additional related resources at NCBI and elsewhere.

5895 Society for Endocrinology
22 Apex Court, Woodlands
Bradley Stoke, BI BS32
145-464-2200
Fax: 145-464-2222
www.endocrinology.org

Aims to advance education and research in endocrinology for the benefit of the public. Lists resources such as journals, books, events, and training courses available.

5896 University of Michigan Health System
1500 E. Medical Center Drive
Ann Arbor, MI 48109
734-936-4000
kylaboys@umich.edu
www.med.umich.edu/yourchild/topics/puberty

Information on early puberty or precocious puberty.

Pamphlets

5897 Precocious Puberty
Human Growth Foundation
997 Glen Cove Avenue, Suite 5
Glen Head, NY 11545
800-451-6434
Fax: 516-671-4055
hgf1@hgfound.org
www.hgfound.org

Booklet

Pisit Pitukcheewanont, MD, President
Emily Germain-Lee, Vice President
Patricia D. Costa, Executive Director

DESCRIPTION

5898 PREMATURITY

Involves the following Biologic System(s):
Neonatal and Infant Disorders

Premature birth (also known as preterm birth) refers to the birth of an infant before the 37-week gestational period. Most pregnancies last for 40 weeks. About 12 percent of babies in the United States — or 1 in 8 — are born prematurely each year. Although at least 40 percent of premature births occur for unknown reasons, prematurity may result from many different factors including a condition in which the mother develops high blood pressure, large quantities of protein in the urine, and an abnormal accumulation of fluid in the body (preeclampsia); maternal heart disease, kidney disease, or diabetes; acute infection; trauma; uterine irregularities (e.g., bicornate uterus); and placental abnormalities (e.g., placenta previa). Other contributing factors may include multiple pregnancy, maternal drug use, and fetal distress. Poor nutrition and lack of appropriate prenatal care may also put the unborn child at risk for premature birth.

Premature infants usually have a characteristic appearance in addition to their small size. For example, their heads often appear too large for their bodies and their skin may be very pink, smooth, translucent, and covered with downy hair (lanugo). They may have sparse hair and very little subcutaneous fat. In girls, the genitals may be incompletely developed such that the labia majora do not cover the labia minora. In affected boys, the testes may not fully descend into the scrotum. Other findings may include the absence of the creases on the palms and soles, incomplete development of the ear, and other irregularities. In addition, the survival or health of a premature infant may be compromised as a result of the incomplete development of certain body systems. The earlier the delivery, the more immature the organs. Common irregularities associated with prematurity include inadequate development of the lungs and subsequent deficiency in the production of a substance that allows the air sacs in the lungs to remain open (surfactant). This condition may lead to respiratory distress syndrome (also called hyaline membrane disease) and associated life-threatening oxygen deficiency in the blood. Immature organ development may affect the brain, resulting in deficiencies in spontaneous breathing, inadequate sucking, and difficulty in swallowing. There is also an increased risk of bleeding in the brain (intraventricular hemorrhage). Premature infants are also particularly susceptible to serious infection resulting from incomplete placental transfer of maternal antibodies. Immature liver function may result in a temporary increase in blood levels of bilirubin causing yellowing of the eyes, skin, and mucous membranes (jaundice). Other complications of prematurity may include poor body temperature regulation, small stomach capacity, inadequacy of the intestinal tract that may result in injury or decreased blood flow to the intestines (necrotizing enterocolitis), immature kidney function, fluctuations in bloodsugar levels, reduced levels of calcium in the blood, and other irregularities related to underdevelopment of body systems. It has also been shown that premature babies are prone to developing depression as teenagers.

One of the most important steps to preventing prematurity is to receive prenatal care as early as possible in the pregnancy, and to continue such care until the baby is born. Statistics clearly show that early and good prenatal care reduces the chance of premature birth and related deaths. Two tactics are used to deal with a potential premature birth: delay the arrival of birth as much as possible, or prepare the premature fetus for arrival. Both of these tactics may be used simultaneously. Treatment for premature infants depends upon the maturity of the various organ systems at the time of birth. In many cases, these infants are cared for around the clock in a neonatal care unit where body temperature may be regulated in an incubator and respiration may be maintained through artificial ventilation, if necessary. Feeding may be accomplished through the use of intravenous feeding or through a feeding tube directly into the stomach. Nutritional supplementation may include the administration of iron and vitamins. In addition, liquids may be given to maintain fluid levels in the body. Antibiotics may be administered to help treat infection. Discharge from the hospital takes place once the infant has reached appropriate weight and certain functional criteria have been established. In addition, before discharge, parents or caregivers of these infants are given complete instructions in their proper care. Other treatment is symptomatic and supportive.

Government Agencies

5899 NIH/ Eunice Kennedy Shriver National Insti tute of Child Health & Human Development
31 Center Drive, Building 31
Bethesda, MD 20892

301-496-5113
800-370-2943
Fax: 866-760-5947
nichdpress@mail.nih.gov
www.nichd.nih.gov

Established in 1962 by congress, today the institute conducts and supports research on topics related to the health of children, adults, families and populations. Some of these topics include: developmental disabilities, growth and development, infant death, reproductive health and birth defects.

Diana W. Bianchi, Director
Paul Williams, Director, Communications

National Associations & Support Groups

5900 Alexis Foundation - Premature Infants and Children
PO Box 1126
Birmingham, MI 48012

248-543-4169
877-253-9470
thealexisfoundation@prodigy.net
www.home.vicnet.net.au/~garyh/mediarel.html

Their mission is to raise public and political awareness of the problems facing prematurely-born infants; education on the problems faced and how they can be foreseen and handled; make essential premature accessories readily available; and promote strong communication between doctors, nurses, and parents.

Elaine Sayers, Founder

5901 American Academy of Pediatrics
141 Northwest Point Boulevard
Elk Grove Village, IL 60007

847-434-4000
800-433-9016
Fax: 847-434-8000
www.aap.org

The American Academy of Pediatrics and its member pediatricians are committed to the attainment of optimal physical, mental and social health and well-being for all infants, children, adolescents, and young adults.

Fernando Stein, MD, FAAP, President
Karen Remley, MD, CEO/Executive VP

5902 March of Dimes Foundation
1275 Mamaroneck Avenue
White Plains, NY 10605   914-997-4488
                                          888-663-4637
                                     Fax: 914-428-8203
                            answers@marchofdimes.com
                                  www.marchofdimes.com

Partnership of volunteers and professionals dedicates to improving the health of babies by preventing birth defects and infant mortality. Over 100 chapters are located across the country and can be located through the National Office.

Stacey D. Stewart, President

5903 National Perinatal Association
457 State Street
Binghamton, NY 13901   607-772-0468
                                          888-971-3295
                                     Fax: 717-920-1390
                               ÿnpa@nationalperinatal.org
                                  www.nationalperinatal.org

The National Perinatal Association promotes the health and well being of mothers and infants enriching families, communities and the world.

Christine Lipoich, Manager
Mary Jo Crosby, VP Development

5904 Ropard: Association for Retinopathy of Pre maturity & Related Diseases
PO Box 250425
Franklin, MI 48025   800-788-2020
                                  ropard@yahoo.com
                                       www.ropard.org

Funds clinically relevant basic science and clinical research to eliminate retinopathy of prematurity and associated retinal diseases; innovative work leading directly to the development of new low vision devices and teaching techniques and services for children who are visually impaired and their families.

5905 Sidelines-National High Risk Pregnancy Sup port Network
PO Box 1808
Laguna Beach, CA 92652   888-447-4754
                                     Fax: 949-497-5598
                              sidelines@sidelines.org
                                    www.sidelines.org

Non profit organization that provides international support for women and their families experiencing premature births and complicated pregnancies.

Candace Hurley, Founder & Executive Director
Tracy Hoogenboom, Administrative Director
Nancy Veeneman, Volunteer Training Coordinator

State Agencies & Support Groups

Georgia

5906 Georgia Perinatal Association
c/o Terri Negron
5607 Walden Farm Drive
Powder Springs, GA 30127   www.georgiaperinatal.org

Works to promote perinatal health through education, collaboration and influence of state public policy. It collaborates with others to improve pregnancy and infant outcomes.

Bonnie Simmons, President
Diane Youmans, President
Margaret B. Hotz, Secretary

Texas

5907 Texas Perinatal Association
19 Cloister Parkway
Amarillo, TX 79121   lisaplat@aol.com
                                        www.txpa.org

Committed to achieving continuous improvement in the quality of health care to mothers and infants in the state of Texas.

Laura Street

Wisconsin

5908 Wisconsin Association for Perinatal Care
McConnell Hall
211 S. Paterson St.,ÿSuite 250
Madison, WI 53703   608-285-5858
                                     Fax: 608-285-5004
                               wapc@perinatalweb.org
                                  www.perinatalweb.org

Provides leadership and education for improved perinatal health outcomes of women, infants and their families through: increased public awareness; engaging the diverse community of perinatal health care advocates; and coordinating systems of perinatal care in Wisconsin.

Ann Conway, Executive Director
Kristine E Casto, Learning Coordinator

Libraries & Resource Centers

5909 National Center for Education in Maternal and Child Health
Georgetown University
2115 Wisconsin Ave NW, Suite 601
Washington, DC 20007   202-784-9770
                                     Fax: 202-784-9777
                               mchlibrary@ncemch.org
                                     www.ncemch.org

Information and advocacy resources for families and professionals. Includes listings of organizations providing general information and organizations focusing on more specific areas of concern to families and young adults who have disabilities.

Rochelle Mayer, Director

Research Centers

5910 NIH/ Eunice Kennedy Shriver National Insti tute of Child Health & Human Development
NICHD Clearinghouse
31 Center Drive, Building 31
Bethesda, MD 20892   301-496-5113
                                          800-370-2943
                                     Fax: 866-760-5947
                              nichdpress@mail.nih.gov
                                     www.nichd.nih.gov

The National Institute for Child Health and Human Development conducts and supports laboratory, clinical and epidemiological research on the reproductive, neurobiologic, developmental, and behavioral processes that determine and maintain the health of children, adults, families, and populations.

Diana W. Bianchi, Director
Paul Williams, Director, Communications

5911 NIH/National Institute of Mental Health Eating Disorders Program
6001 Executive Boulevard, Room 8184
Bethesda, MD 20892   301-443-4513
                                     Fax: 301-443-4279

Web Sites

5912 Children's Medical Ventures
3000 Minuteman Road
Andover, MA 01810   www.healthcare.philips.com/

The company offers high quality products which meet the unique needs of these special babies, including appropriately sized items, safety equipment and specialty feeding and skin care products.

5913 Newborns in Need
3323 Transou Road
Pfafftown, NC 27040   www.newbornsinneed.org

Charity organization for the care of sick and needy babies and
their families.

Sam Safrit, Chairman
Connie Edwards, President
Gayle McKeethan, Vice President

5914 PREBIC-International Preterm Birth Collabo rative
www.prebic.org

Supports and enhances international networking among researchers in preterm birth.

Craig Pennell, President
Hanns Helmer, Vice President
Melanie White, Treasurer

5915 Preemie Ring
hub.familynhome.org/hub/preemie

A collection of home pages about premature infants and premature infant care, etc.

5916 Preemie Twins
PO Box 12
Pierce, NE 68767   402-606-1820
                                    Fax: 402-606-1820
                                    www.preemietwins.com

Online resource for both parents of multiples and/or premature infants.

5917 Preemie World
preemie.info

A meeting place for family and friends of preemies.

5918 Premature Baby-Premature Child
www.prematurity.org

Preemie parent support for preemie special needs.

5919 Prematurely Yours
www.prematurelyyours.com

Special products for special babies.

Kim Bryant, RN, President
Becky Meloan, RN, VP
Curtis Bryant, Treasurer/Secretary

Book Publishers

5920 Prematurely Yours
6712 Townpoint Road
Suffolk, VA 23435   757-483-9879
                                    Fax: 757-484-8267
                                prematurely@PreMieProducts.com
                                    www.prematurelyyours.com

Designed exclusively to record milestones for the premature infant, from birth to six years of age. Such milestones as maintaining their body temperature, nippling their feedings, and breathing
without the aid of extra oxygen are, of course, taken for granted
with a full term infant.

40 pages Hardcover

Kim Bryant, RN, President
Becky Meloan, RN, VP
Curtis Bryant, Treasurer/Secretary

Magazines

5921 Left Side Lines
Sidelines
PO Box 1808
Laguna Beach, CA 92652   888-447-4754
                                    sidelines@sidelines.org
                                    www.sidelines.org

Offers articles, insights and tips related to the challange of coping with a high-risk pregnancy. Specific information is provided
on prematurity, NICU, multiples, and nutrition.

80 pages

Candace Hurley, Executive Director and Founder
Tracy Hoogenboom, Managing Director
Nancy Veeneman, Operations Director

5922 Preemie Magazine
6412 Brandon Avenue, Suite 274
Springfield, VA 22150   703-468-1005
                                    www.preemiemagazine.com

Started by five preemie parents, it provides free information and
an online community for preemeie parents and professionals.

Deborah A Discenza, Founder & Publisher
Nicole Hutzul, Sales & Marketing
Alicia Michaels, Director Operations/Development

Pamphlets

5923 March of Dimes-Preterm Birth Fact Sheets
March of Dimes Pregnancy & Newborn Health Edu Ctr
1275 Mamaroneck Avenue
White Plains, NY 10605   914-997-4488
                                    Fax: 914-997-4763
                                    answers@marchofdimes.com
                                    www.marchofdimes.org

Fact sheets discuss the possible causes of preterm birth, complications associated with, and current research.

DESCRIPTION

5924 PREVENTABLE CHILDHOOD INFECTIONS
Involves the following Biologic System(s):
Infectious Disorders

There are several infectious diseases that typically manifest in childhood, that are preventable with proper immunizations. This chapter will cover the following: Diphtheria; Tetanus; Pertussis; Rubella (German Measles); Measles; Mumps; Polio; Chickenpox; Influenza (flu); Meningococcal; Pneumococcal; Congenital Rubella; Genital Human Papillomavirus (HPV).

Diphtheria is an acute, contagious disease characterized at its onset by sore throat and painful swallowing. One to 4 days after exposure, infected individuals may also develop a low-grade fever, headache, nausea and vomiting, chills, and a rapid heart rate. Other symptoms may include signs associated with upper respiratory tract infection. Within a few days, a grayish-brown pseudomembrane may form over the tonsils, and the throat may swell. The lymph nodes in the neck may become swollen and enlarged. Damage to the heart or nervous system may occur. Diphtheria vaccine is usually combined with those for whooping cough (pertussis) and tetanus. This DPT combination is routinely given in a series in the first few months of life. Booster doses are required. In most cases, diphtheria is transmitted through coughed or exhaled droplets. Treatment is with antibiotics and an antitoxin.

Pertussis (whooping cough) is a highly contagious infectious disease in which inflammation of the respiratory tract results from a bacterial infection, transmitted through coughing or sneezing. Pertussis usually affects infants and children, but may occur at any age. Pertussis infection lasts about 6 weeks, occurring in 3 stages: moderate cold-like symptoms (catarrhal stage); severe coughing (paroxysmal stage); cessation of symptoms (convalescent stage). Treatment typically includes bed rest, proper nutrition and fluid intake. Erythromycin or other antibiotics may be given. Pertussis vaccine is usually combined with diptheria and tetanus.

Tetanus is an infectious disease of the central nervous system caused by a toxic bacteria that acts on nerves that control muscle activity. The bacterium typically enters puncture wounds caused by dirty objects such as nails, splinters or glass fragments, or via drug injection, surgical wounds, burns, animal bites or the umbilical cord stump. Symptoms usually appear from 2 to 14 days after infection, but could take months to appear. Tetanus may be classified into general or localized. Initial symptoms of generalized tetanus often include: prolonged spasms of the muscles of the jaw (trismus or lockjaw); difficulties in opening the mouth, chewing and swallowing (dysphagia); irritability, headaches and restlessness. Prolonged spasms of facial muscles, profuse sweating, a mild fever and rapid pulse may also occur. Progressed disease includes severe muscle contractions. Treatment includes human antibodies (tetanus immune globulin) and antibiotics, surgical cleaning of the wound site, and muscle relaxants. Children should receive the DPT (diptheria, pertussis, tetanus) vaccine and booster shots, which should also be given to anyone with wounds and unknown tetanus booster status.

German measles, or rubella, is a contagious viral disease characterized by swollen lymph nodes and a fine, reddish-pink rash that persists for 1 to 3 days. It is transmitted through inhalation of droplets coughed or exhaled by infected individuals. Early symptoms may include swollen lymph nodes, especially in the neck and back of the head; joint pain (arthralgia); low-grade fever; cold symptoms; and redness and discomfort of the throat. Within 1 or 2 days, a mildly itchy rash appears on the face, spreading to the trunk, arms and legs, accompanied by a spreading red flush. The rash usually subsides after 3 days. In some cases, enlargement of the spleen may occur. Measles symptoms range from slight to severe, the latter occuring primarily in older children and adults. Pregnant women with the disease are at risk of transmitting it to their newborn (congenital rubella, see below). Protection against infection is provided through rubella immunization, usually in combination with measles and mumps vaccine. Vaccines are recommended for women of child-bearing age who have not had German measles. Treatment for rubella is symptomatic.

Measles is a highly contagious infection caused by the measles virus. Infection is characterized by a spreading rash and other sypltoms. It typically infects the young, but may develop at any age. It is spread through airborne droplets from an infected individual. Infection usually results in life-long immunity. Early symptoms develop 1 to 2 weeks after exposure and include low-grade fever; inflammation of the nasal mucous membranes; runny nose; hacking cough; conjunctivitis; and increased sensitivity to light. These symptoms are followed 2 to 3 days later by tiny, grayish-white specks surrounded by an irregular red ring (Koplik's spots), that appear on the inside of the cheeks, usually near the back teeth. A rash, accompanied by a high fever, may develop within 3 to 5 days after the onset of symptoms, characterized by faint, reddish flat spots that first appear behind the ears, at the hairline and on the neck, and then spread over the entire body. Certain lymph nodes and the spleen may become enlarged. Immunization, usually in combination with mumps and rubella vaccines provides protection; a second vaccine is usually given upon entering school. Treatment includes fever-recuding medication, antibiotics, increased fluid intake, and bed rest in a warm humidified room. Other treatment is symptomatic and supportive.

Congenital rubella is a condition caused by the German measles virus that is passed from an infected mother to the fetus. Likelihood for transmission and the potential for miscarriage, stillbirth or severe developmental abnormalities (growth retardation, heart defects, eye problems, microcephaly, skin lesions) is highest during the first trimester. Many infants with congenital rubella have inner ear and/or hearing problems. Mental retardation and motor delays may also occur, along with a risk of hepatitis, anemia, lowered blood platelets, pneumonia and bone irregularities. Prevention is directed toward immunization of women of child-bearing age via the measles vaccine.

Mumps is an acute, infectious viral disease caused by a paramyxovirus. It is characterized by enlargement of the salivary glands, particularly those that lie below and in front of the ears (parotid glands). Mumps usually affects children from 5 through 15 years. It is spread through airborne droplets or direct contact with saliva, or possibly, urine, from an infected individual. Outbreaks most often occur in late winter or early spring. Infection usually results in lifelong immunity. Symptoms appear in 14 to 24 days after exposure and include fever, neck pain, weakness, discomfort and headache. One or both parotid glands may become enlarged or tender to the touch. Chewing and swallowing may become difficult, and fever and swelling of other salivary glands and the throat may occur. Swelling of the parotid glands usually lasts 7 to 10 days. Possible complications include meningitis, and joint swelling. A vaccine to prevent the disease is given to children 12 to 15 months, and again before entering school. Treatment is symptomatic and supportive.

Polio, or polimyelitis, is an acute infectious disease caused by one of three polio viruses transmitted through fecal contamination or, occasionally, through the air. It may produce no symptoms, but will grant immunity to those infected. In young children, it is usually accompanied by only mild symptoms that appear 3 to 5 days after infection — fever, headache, sore throat, vomiting, weakness and abdominal discomfort. Recovery often occurs in 1 to 3 days. In some cases, a brief recovery is followed by additional symptoms, including brain and spinal cord involvement with neck and back stiffness and skin sensitivity. This reappearance indicates major illness, and is more common in older children and adults, and may by paralytic or nonparalytic. Immunization to prevent polio is routinely administered. Treatment for the mild form includes bedrest and pain relievers. Paralysis requires physical therapy. Other treatment is symptomatic and supportive.

Chickenpox is a common, hightly contagious viral disease caused by the varicella zoster virus. Most cases occur before the age of 10. Those who do not contract the virus during childhood remain susceptible during adulthood, when symptoms are typically more severe. Chickenpox is spread by inhalation of airborne droplets or by direct contact with fluid from skin blisters. Older children particularly may experience fever,headache, mild abdominal pain, lack of appetite and malaise. A characteristic rash develops on the chest, abdomen, face or scalp, consisting of masses of small, red, extremely itchy spots that become fluid-filled blisters. As the first lesions dry, new ones form.Complication of chickenpox may include bacterial infection of the lesions, encephalitis, and impaired control of voluntary movements. Newborns may also experience a particularly severe, progressive form of chickenpox (neonatal chickenpox). Treatment of children with mild cases of chickenpox is symptomatic and supportive. In more severe cases, the antiviral drug acyclovir may be administered. A vaccine is available to help prevent chickenpox.

Influenza (flu) is a highly contagious viral infection of the nose, throat, and lungs. Spread easily through respiratory droplets of an infected person, influenza symptoms include sudden high fever, chills, dry cough, headache, runny nose, sore throat, muscle and joint pain, and extreme fatigue, which can last up to several weeks. Influenza can be prevented by the flu vaccine of thich there are two types: the flu shot is approved for children older than six months, inlcuding healthy children and those with chronic conditions. The nasal spray flu vaccine (LAIV) is approved for use in healthy individuals two to 49 years. Minor side effects of the flu shot include soreness, redness or swelling at the shot site, low-grade fever, and aches. These may occur soon after the shot and last one to two days. On rare occasions, flu vaccinations can cause severe allergic reactions. Side effects of the nasal spray can include runny nose, wheezing, headache, vomiting, muscle aches, and fever. A flu vaccine is needed every year to keep up with the changing flu virus. Also, studies show that the body's immunity to influenza viruses (either through infection or vaccination) declines over time.

Meningococcal disease is a leading cause of bacterial meningitis (infection of the covering of the brain and spinal cord) in children two to 18 years old, and can also cause blood infections. The bacteria that cause Meningococcal disease are spread through the exchange of nose and throat droplets through coughing, sneezing or kissing. Symptoms include nausea, vomiting, sensitivity to light, confusion and sleepiness. One of every 10 cases result in death. Meningococcal disease may leave patients limbless, with hearing and nervous system problems, developmental disabilities, and seizures or strokes. It is most common in infants less than one year, and in those 16 to 21 years. Children with certain medical conditions (i.e. no spleen), are at increased risk, as are college students living in dormitories. Meningococcal disease can be prevented by the MCV4 vaccine, which is recommended for those at risk, or who travel to countries where the disease is prevalant. The vaccine is given at age 11 to 12 years, and a booster dose at 16 years.

Genital human papillomavirus (HPV) is the most common sexually transmitted infection (STI) in the U.S. There are more than 40 types of HPV; some cause genital warts; some cause various cancers; some infect the mouth and throat. Aproximately 20 million Americans, including those 11-18 years, are currently infected with HPV, and about 6 million more are infected each year. The HPV virus can live for years in infected individuals, sometimes without symptoms. In rare cases, an infected pregnant woman can pass the HPV virus onto her newborn. HPV can be passed between straight and gay partners, even when the infected person has no symptoms. HPV can cause cervical cancer in women, and it is associated with other, less common cancers. HPV can be prevented by HPV vaccine which is given in three doses over six months. Children 11 to 12 years have the best protection from the vaccines. Two vaccines (Cervariz and Gardasil) are considered effective in protecting women against cancer and genital warts. Gardasil is considered effective in protecting men against genital warts and anal cancer; men at risk should receive the vaccine through 26 years. There is no cure for HPV.

Pneumococcal is an infection of the lungs that is caused by pneumococcus bacteria, which can also cause ear infections, sinus infections, meningitis, bacteremia and blood stream infection. In some cases pneumococcal disease can be fatal or result in brain damage, or hearing or limb loss. The bacteria is spread through infected respiratory droplets from the nose or mouth. It is common for children to carry the bacteria in their throats without becomming symptomatic. Children under two years, in group child care, or who have certain illnesses are at higher risk for pneumococcal disease, as are those with cochlear implants or cerebrospinal fluid (CSF) leaks. Pneumococcal disease is more common among certain ethnic groups, including Alaska Natives, American Indians, and African Americans. Meningitis is the most severe type of pneumococcal disease. Of children under five years with the disease, 5% will die from it, and others may have long-term effects, such as vision or hearing loss. Pneumococcal conjugate vaccine (PCV) prevents the infection. Treatment includes antibiotics which may slow or reverse emerging drug resistance found among pneumococcal infections. It is recommended that the vaccine be given to infants at two, four, and six months, followed by a booster dose at 12 to 15 months.

Hepatitis A and Hepatitis B also fall into the category of preventable childhood infections and are covered in depth in a separate chapter on Hepatitis.

Government Agencies

5925 Centers for Disease Control and Prevention
1600 Clifton Rd
Atlanta, GA 30333
800-232-4636
TTY: 888-232-6348
www.cdc.gov/vaccines

The CDC provides health and safety information. Many CDC publications are available to download, view online, or order at no cost.

5926 Department of Health
899 North Capitol St, NE
Washington, DC 20002
202-442-5955
Fax: 202-442-4795
doh@dc.gov
www.doh.dc.gov/page/vaccine-preventable-diseases

The DOH conducts investigations, tracking and reporting of vaccine preventable diseases.

Saul M. Levin, MD, MPA, Interim Director, DC Dept of Health

5927 NIH/National Institute of Allergy and Infectious Diseases
5601 Fishers Lane, MSC 9806
Bethesda, MD 20892
301-496-5717
866-284-4107
Fax: 301-402-3573
TDD: 800-877-8339
ocpostoffice@niaid.nih.gov
www.niaid.nih.gov

Conducts and supports basic and applied research to better understand, treat, and ultimately prevent infectious, immunologic, and allergic diseases.

Anthony S Fauci MD, Director

National Associations & Support Groups

5928 American Academy of Pediatrics
141 Northwest Point Boulevard
Elk Grove Village, IL 60007
847-434-4000
800-433-9016
Fax: 847-434-8000
www.aap.org

The American Academy of Pediatrics and its member pediatricians are committed to the attainment of optimal physical, mental and social health and well-being for all infants, children, adolescents, and young adults.

Fernando Stein, MD, FAAP, President
Karen Remley, MD, CEO/Executive VP

5929 American Association for Respiratory Care
9425 N. MacArthur Blvd. Suite 100
Irving, TX 75063
972-243-2272
info@aarc.org
www.aarc.org

The AARC encourages and promotes professional excellence, advances the science and practice of respiratory care, and serves as an advocate for patients and their families, the public, the profession and the respiratory therapist.

5930 American Association for Thoracic Surgery
500 Cummings Center, Suite 4550
Beverly, MA 1915
978-927-8330
Fax: 978-524-8890
aats.org

The American Association for Thoracic Surgery is an international organization of over 1,300 of the world's foremost cardiothoracic surgeons representing 41 countries.

Pedro J. del Nido, President
Thoralf M. Sundt, III, Vice President
Marc R. Moon, Secretary

5931 American Medical Association
AMA Plaza, 330 North Wabash Ave., Suite 39300
Chicago, IL 60611
800-262-3211
www.ama-assn.org/ama

AMA is dedicated to ensuring sustainable physician practices that result in better health outcomes for patients.

James L. Madara, MD, CEO/ EVP
Bernard L. Hengesbaugh, Chief Operating Officer
Kenneth J. Sharigian, SVP/ Chief Strategy Officer

5932 American Nurses Association
8515 Georgia Avenue, Suite 400
Silver Spring, MD 20910
800-274-4262
Fax: 301-628-5001
anf@ana.org
www.nursingworld.org

The American Nurses Association (ANA) is the only full-service professional organization representing the interests of the nation's 3.1 million registered nurses through its constituent and state nurses associations and its organizational affiliates.

Pamela F. Cipriano, PhD, President
Marla J. Weston, PhD, RN, FAAN, Chief Executive Officer
Cindy R. Balkstra, Vice President

5933 American Pregnancy Association
1425 Greenway Drive, Suite 440
Irving, TX 75038
info@americanpregnancy.org
americanpregnancy.org

The American Pregnancy Association is a 501(c)(3) nonprofit organization committed to promoting pregnancy wellness through education, advocacy and community awareness.

5934 American Public Health Association
800 I Street, NW
Washington, DC 20001
202-777-2742
Fax: 202-777-2534
TTY: 202-777-2500
www.apha.org

APHA champions the health of all people and all communities. They aim to strengthen the public health profession and speak out for public health issues and policies backed by science.

Georges C. Benjamin, MD, Executive Director
Kemi Oluwafemi, MBA, CPA, Chief Financial Officer
Susan Polan, PhD, Associate Executive Director

5935 American Society For Microbiology
1752 N Street, N.W.
Washington, DC 20036
202-737-3600
Fax: 202-942-9333
service@asmusa.org
www.asm.org

he American Society for Microbiology is a life science membership organization. Membership has grown from 59 scientists in 1899 to more than 39,000 members today, with more than one third located outside the United States. The members represent 26 disciplines of microbiological specialization plus a division for microbiology educators.

Nancy Sansalone, Interim Executive Director
Timothy Donohue, President
Joseph M. Campos, Secretary

5936 American Thoracic Society
25 Broadway
New York, NY 10004
212-315-8600
Fax: 212-315-6498
ATSInfo@Thoracic.org
www.Thoracic.org

The American Thoracic Society improves global health by advancing research, patient care, and public health in pulmonary disease, critical illness, and sleep disorders. Founded in 1905 to combat TB, the ATS has grown to tackle asthma, COPD, lung cancer, sepsis, acute respiratory distress, and sleep apnea, among other diseases.

Thomas W. Ferkol, MD, President
Atul Malhotra, MD, President-elect
Stephen C. Crane, PhD, MPH, Executive Director

5937 Association of Immunization Managers
620 Hungerford Dr. Suite 29
Rockville, MD 20850   301-424-6080
                                    Fax: 301-424-6081
                          www.immunizationmanagers.org

The Association of Immunization Managers (AIM) was created in
1999 to enable immunization managers to work together to effectively prevent and control vaccine-preventable diseases and improve immunization coverage in the United States and its
territories.

Pejman Talebian, Chair
Claire Hannan, Executive Director
Katelyn Wells, Research and Development Director

5938 Every Child By Two
1233 20th Street NW, Suite 403
Washington, DC 20036   202-783-7034
                                    Fax: 202-783-7042
                                        info@ecbt.org
                                        www.ecbt.org

Rosalynn Carter, President & Co-Founder
Betty Bumpers, Vice President & Co-Founder

5939 Immunization Action Coalition
2550 University Avenue West, Suite 415 North
Saint Paul, MN 55114   651-647-9009
                                    Fax: 651-647-9131
                                   admin@immunize.org
                                     www.immunize.org

The Immunization Action Coalition (IAC) works to increase immunization rates and prevent disease by creating and distributing
educational materials for health professionals and the public that
enhance the delivery of safe and effective immunization services.
The Coalition also facilitates communication about the safety, efficacy, and use of vaccines within the broad immunization community of patients, parents, health care organizations, and
government health agencies.

Deborah L. Wexler, MD, Executive Director
Litjen Tan, MS, PhD, Chief Strategy Officer
Robin VanOss, Operations Manager

5940 Infectious Diseases Society of America
1300 Wilson Blvd, Suite 300
Arlington, VA 22209   703-299-0200
                                    Fax: 703-299-0204
                                      www.idsociety.org

The Infectious Diseases Society of America (IDSA) represents
physicians, scientists and other health care professionals who specialize in infectious diseases. IDSA's purpose is to improve the
health of individuals, communities, and society by promoting excellence in patient care, education, research, public health, and
prevention relating to infectious diseases.

Stephen B. Calderwood, MD, FIDSA, President
Johan S. Bakken, MD, PhD, FIDSA, President-Elect
William G. Powderly, MD, FIDSA, Vice President

5941 National Association of Pediatric Nurse Practitioners
5 Hanover Square, Suite 1401
New York, NY 10004   917-746-8300
                                         877-662-7627
                                    Fax: 212-785-1713
                                        www.napnap.org

National Association of Pediatric Nurse Practitioners (NAPNAP)
is the professional association for pediatric nurse practitioners
(PNPs) and other advanced practice nurses who care for children.

Mary Chesney, PhD, President
Cate Brennan, Executive Director
Michele Stickel, Dir of Mrktng & Strategic Projects

5942 National Association of School Nurses
1100 Wayne Avenue Suite 925
Silver Spring, MD 20910   240-821-1130
                                         866-627-6767
                                    Fax: 301-585-1791
                                         www.nasn.org

The mission is to advance school nurse practice to keep students
healthy, safe and ready to learn.

Donna J. Mazyck, Executive Director
Nichole K. Bobo, Nursing Education Director
Margaret Cellucci, Director of Communications

5943 National Foundation for Infectious Diseases
7201 Wisconsin Avenue, Suite 750
Bethesda, MD 20814   301-656-0003
                                    Fax: 301-907-0878
                                         www.nfid.org

The National Foundation for Infectious Diseases (NFID) is a
non-profit, tax-exempt 501(c)(3) organization founded in 1973
dedicated to educating the public and healthcare professionals
about the causes, treatment, and prevention of infectious diseases
across the lifespan.

5944 National Healthy Mothers, Healthy Babies Coalition
Post Office Box 3360
Alexandria, VA 22302   703-837-4792
                                    Fax: 703-664-0485
                                        info@hmhb.org
                                         www.hmhb.org

The National Healthy Mothers, Healthy Babies Coalition
(HMHB) is a recognized leader and resource in maternal and
child health, reaching an estimated 10 million health care professionals, parents, and policymakers through its membership of
over 100 local, state and national organizations.

Janice Frey-Angel, CEO
Andrea Goodman, MCH Director
Jennifer Sharp, Deputy Director

5945 National Meningitis Association
P.O. Box 60143
Ft. Myers, FL 33906   866-366-3662
                                        www.nmaus.org

The National Meningitis Association (NMA) is a nonprofit organization founded by parents whose children have died or live
with permanent disabilities from meningococcal disease.

5946 National Tuberculosis Controllers Association
2452 Spring Rd, SE
Smyrna, GA 30080   678-503-0503
                                         877-503-0806
                                    Fax: 678-503-0805
                             dhwegener@tbcontrollers.org
                                    www.tbcontrollers.org

The NTCA was created in 1995 to bring together the leaders of
tuberculosis control programs in all states and territories, as well
as many counties and city health departments that organize their
own TB control activities.

Donna Hope Wegener, Executive Director
Jennifer Kanouse, Director of Comm. & Member Services
Eva Forest, Executive Assistant

5947 Pediatric Infectious Diseases Society
1300 Wilson Boulevard, Suite 300
Arlington, VA 22209   703-299-6764
                                    Fax: 703-299-0473
                                  cphillips@idsociety.org
                                         www.pids.org

PIDS is the world's largest organization of professionals dedicated to the treatment, control and eradication of infectious diseases affecting children. Membership is comprised of physicians,
doctoral-level scientists and others who have trained or are in
training in infectious diseases or its related disciplines, and who
are identified with the discipline of pediatric infectious diseases
or related disciplines through clinical practice, research, teaching
and/or administration activities.

David W. Kimberlin, MD, President
Terri Christene Phillips, Executive Director
Faith Ham, Membership and Comm. Assistant

5948 Polio Society
4200 Wisconsin Avenue NW, #106273
Washington, DC 20016   301-897-8180
                                    Fax: 202-994-3153
                                        jsh1@mhg.edu

A chartered nonprofit organization primarily for polio survivors and family members. It provides educational resources and support group services.

5949 Polio Survivors Association
12720 La Reina Avenue
Downey, CA 90242
562-862-4508
Fax: 562-862-5018
info@polioassociation.org
www.polioassociation.org

Nonprofit organization dedicated to education, advocacy, and support to promote the well being and improve the quality of life for severely disabled polio survivors.

Richard Dagget, President

5950 Post-Polio Health International
4207 Lindell Boulevard, Suite 110
Saint Louis, MO 63108
314-534-0475
Fax: 314-534-5070
info@post-polio.org
www.post-polio.org

Provides information to Polio survivors, their families and the health care community and promotes networking among the post-polio community.

Joan L Headley, Editor & Executive Director

5951 Shot At Life
www.shotatlife.org
202-862-6303
info@shotatlife.org
www.shotatlife.org

This organization aims to decrease vaccine-preventable childhood deaths and give every child a chance at a healthy life, by encouraging individuals to learn about, advocate for, and donate to vaccines to protect children worldwide.

5952 Shots For Tots
4747 Earhart Blvd - Ste 107
New Orleans, LA 70125
504-483-1900
800-251-2229
Fax: 504-483-1909
info@shotsfortots.com
www.shotsfortots.com

This organization provides up-to-date information for both parents and providers in order to ensure the highest level of immunizations for children.

Gina Deris, Coodinator

5953 World Health Organization
Avenue Appia 20
CH-1211 Geneva 27,
Switzerland
www.who.int

WHO is the directing and coordinating authority for health within the United Nations system.

Dr Margaret Chan, Director General

State Agencies & Support Groups

Arizona

5954 Maricopa Co Childhood Immunization Program
PO Box 44283
Phoenix, AZ 85064
602-262-2447
info@mcchip.org
www.mcchip.org

5955 The Arizona Partnership for Immunization
320 E. McDowell Rd
Phoenix, AZ 85004
602-253-0090
Fax: 602-262-2654
tapi@aachc.org
www.whyimmunize.org

Arkansas

5956 Arkansas Department of Health Div. of Comm Diseases/Immunizations
4815 West Markham St - Slot 48
Little Rock, AR 72205
501-661-2723
www.health.state.ar.us

California

5957 All Kids By Two Health Services Agency
1060 Emeline Ave - Bldg F
Santa Cruz, CA 95061
831-454-5477
Fax: 831-454-5049
katie.lebaron@health.co.santa-cruz.ca.us
www.santacruzhealth.org

5958 California Department of Health Services Immunization Branch
2151 Berkeley Way - Rm 712
Berkeley, CA 94704
510-540-2065
www.dhs.ca.gov

5959 Community Health Improvement Partners - Immunize San Diego (CHIP-ISD)
707 Broadway - Ste 905
San Diego, CA 92101
619-515-2858
Fax: 619-544-0888
tdanos@hasdic.org
www.sdchip.org

5960 Immunization Partnership of Alameda County
2000 Mowry Avenue
Fremont, CA 94538
510-494-7053
Fax: 510-791-3496
ruth_young@whhs.com
www.whhs.com

Colorado

5961 Colorado Dept. of Public Heand & Environme nt: Immunization Program, DCEED-IMM-A3
4300 Cherry Creek Drive South
Denver, CO 80222
303-692-2669
www.cdphe.state.co.us/health-h.asp

District of Columbia

5962 Commission of Public Health Immunization Program
1131 Spring Road, NW
Washington, DC 20010
202-576-7130

5963 Department of Health Division of Immunization
6323 Georgia Ave, NW - Ste 305
Washington, DC 20011
202-576-7130

Florida

5964 Florida Department of Health Immunization Program
2020 Capital Circle SE
Tallahassee, FL 32399
904-487-2755
www.doh.state.fl.us

Hawaii

5965 Hawaii Department of Health Immunization Program
1250 Punchbowl Street
Honolulu, HI 96813
808-586-4400
Fax: 808-586-4444
www.hawaii.gov/health

Idaho

5966 Idaho Dept. of Health & Welfare Immunizati on Program
PO Box 83720
Boise, ID 83720
208-334-5500
800-554-2922
Fax: 208-334-5942
idahovfc@idhw.state.id.us
www.healthandwelfare.idaho.gov

Indiana

5967 Indiana State Dept. of Health Immunization
2 North Meridian St
Indianapolis, IN 46204
317-233-1325
www.in.gov/isdh

Iowa

5968 Iowa Department of Public Health Bureau of Immunization
321 East 12th St - Lucas State Office Bldg
Des Moines, IA 50319
515-281-5787
www.idph.state.ia.us

Kansas

5969 Kansas Department of Health & Environment Immunization Program
109 SW 9th St - Ste 606
Topeka, KS 66612
785-296-5591
Fax: 785-296-6510
info@kdhe.state.ks.us
www.kdhe.state.ks.us/index.html

Maine

5970 Maine Dept. of Human Services: Bureau of Health Immunization Program
2 Bangor Street
Augusta, ME 04330 www.maine.gov/dhhs/boh/mip/index_home.htm

Maryland

5971 Dept. of Health & Mental Hygiene-Immunizat ion
201 West Preston St
Baltimore, MD 21201
410-767-6860
TDD: 800-735-2258
ww.dhmh.state.md.us

Mississippi

5972 Mississippi Dept. of Health Bureau of Preventative Health Immunization
2423 N State St - PO Box 1700
Jackson, MS 39215
601-576-7751
Fax: 601-576-7686
www.msdh.state.ms.us/msdhhome.htm

Nebraska

5973 Nebraska Dept. of Health Immunization Prog ram
PO Box 95044
Lincoln, NE 68509
402-471-3727
grey.borden@hhss.state.ne.us
www.hhs.state.ne.us

Nevada

5974 Nevada State Health Division Bureau of Com munity Health - Immunization Program
4150 Technology Way
Carson City, NV 89706
775-684-5900
http://health.nv.gov/immunization.htm

New Hampshire

5975 NH Dept. of Health & Human Services Immunization Program
28 Hazen Drive
Concord, NH 03301
603-271-4482
800-852-3345
www.dhhs.state.nh.us/dhhs/immunization/default.htm

New Jersey

5976 New Jersey Department of Health Immunizations Program
PO Box 369
Trenton, NJ 08625
609-588-7512
Fax: 609-588-7431
www.state.nj.us/health

New Mexico

5977 New Mexico Department of Health Immunization Program
1190 St. Francis Dr - S1260
Santa Fe, NM 87505
505-827-2463
ww.health.state.nm.us/immunize

New York

5978 New York State Department of Health Immunization Program
Corning Tower Building - Rm 649
Albany, NY 12237
518-473-4437
www.health.state.ny.us

Ohio

5979 Ohio Department of Health Immunization Program
246 N High St, PO Box 118
Columbus, OH 43216
614-466-0302
www.odh.state.oh.us

Oklahoma

5980 Oklahoma State Department of Health Immunization Division
1000 North East 10th St
Oklahoma City, OK 73117
405-271-5600
www.health.state.ok.us

Rhode Island

5981 Rhode Island Department of Health Immunization Program
3 Capitol Hill
Providence, RI 02908
401-222-2231
Fax: 401-222-6548
TTY: 800-745-5555
www.health.state.ri.us

South Carolina

5982 SC Dept. of Health & Environmental Control Immunization Division
1751 Calhoun St
Columbia, SC 29201
803-898-3432
www.scdhec.gov/health/disease/immunization

South Dakota

5983 South Dakota Department of Health Office of Disease Prevention
Health Building, 600 E. Capitol
Pierre, SD 57501   605-773-3737
doh.info@state.sd.us
www.state.sd.us/state/executive/doh/doh.html

Tennessee

5984 Tennessee Department of Health Immunization
Cordell Hull Building, 425 5th Ave, North - 3rd Fl
Nashville, TN 37247   615-741-3111
Fax: 615-741-3491
www.state.tn.us/health

Texas

5985 Texas Department oF Health Immunization Division
1100 West 49th Street
Austin, TX 78756   512-458-7284
ww.tdh.state.tx.us

Utah

5986 Utah Department of Health
PO Box 1010
Salt Lake City, UT 84114   801-538-6101
http://hlunix.ex.state.ut.us

Vermont

5987 Vermont Department oF Health State Immunication Program
108 Cherry Street
Burlington, VT 05402   800-464-4343
TDD: 802-863-7200
www.healthyvermonters.info

Virginia

5988 Virginia Department of Health Bureau of Immunization
1500 East Main Street
Richmond, VA 23219   804-786-6246
www.vdh.state.va.us

Washington

5989 Washington State Department of Health Immunization Program
1112 SE Quince St, PO Box 47890
Olympia, WA 98504   360-236-4010
www.doh.wa.gov

Web Sites

5990 Canadian Task Force on Preventive Health C are
3280 Hospital Drive Northwest
Calgary, AL T2N 4   info@canadiantaskforce.ca
canadiantaskforce.ca

This website is designed to serve as a practical guide to health care providers, planners and consumers for determining the inclusion or exclusion, content and frequency of a wide variety of preventive health interventions, using the evidence based recommendations of the Canadian Task Force on Preventice Health Care.

Marcello Tonelli, Chair
Richard Birtwhistle, Vice Chair
C. Maria Bacchus, Board Member

5991 Centers for Disease Control-Infection Cont rol
1600 Clifton Rd
Atlanta, GA 30333   800-232-4636
www.cdc.gov/hai/

Promotes health and quality of life by preventing and controlling disease, injury, and disability.

5992 Health Research Project (HaRP)
www.harpnet.org

A program by USAID, the project strives to improve the health status of infants, children, mothers and families through the development and research of new tools, technologies, policies and approaches.

5993 KidsHealth - Measles
kidshealth.org/parent/infections/lung/measles.html

KidsHealth provides doctor-approved health information about children from before birth through adolescence. KidsHealth provides families with accurate, up to date and jargon free health information they can use.

Neil Izenberg, MD, Editor-in-Chief & Founder

5994 KidsHealth - Rubella (German Measles)
kidshealth.org/parent/

KidsHealth provides doctor-approved health information about children from before birth through adolescence. KidsHealth provides families with accurate, up to date and jargon free health information they can use.

Neil Izenberg, MD, Editor-in-Chief & Founder

5995 KidsHealth - Tetanus
kidshealth.org/parent/

KidsHealth provides doctor-approved health information about children from before birth through adolescence. KidsHealth provides families with accurate, up to date and jargon free health information they can use.

Neil Izenberg, MD, Editor-in-Chief & Founder

5996 Pan American Health Organization (PAHO)
525 Twenty-third Street, N.W.
Washington, DC 20037   202-974-3000
Fax: 202-974-3663
www.paho.org

The mission is to strengthen national and local health systems and improve the health of the peoples of the Americas, in collaboraton with Ministries of Health, other government and international agencies, nongovernmental organizations, universities, social security agencies, community groups, and many others. Health topics include measles, mumps, rubella and diptheria.

5997 Polio Connection of America
www.geocities.com/w1066w/

For survivors of the Polio Survivors to chat and the site offers links to other polio sites.

5998 Polio Experience Network
825 Sherbrook Street
Winnipeg, MB R3A 1   204-975-3037
Fax: 204-975-3027
postpolionetwork@gmail.com
www.postpolionetwork.ca/pps

Offers information, inspiration, ideas and resources to help patients understand polio and post-poli syndrome, and to confidently manage life with it. Also helps loved ones cope with the effects of polio. Resources are also offered for students doing research on the disease as well as general resources available.

Cheryl Currie, President
Kathryn Harper, Vice President
Estelle Boissonneault, Secretary

5999 **Post Polio Awareness & Support Society of British Columbia**
#102-9775-4th Street
Sidney, BC V8L 2
250-665-8849
Fax: 250-665-8859
ppass@ppassbc.com
www.ppassbc.com

A non profit society formed as a network for polio survivors, those affected by polio, and any interested in polio.

Joan Toone, President

6000 **Slack Incorporated**
6900 Grove Road
Thorofare, NJ 8086
856-848-1000
Fax: 856-848-6091
email@slackinc.com
www.slackinc.com

A leading provider of healthcare information, educational programs, and meeting and exhibit management services worldwide.

6001 **Virtual Pediatric Hospital**
www.virtualpediatrichospital.org

A digital library of pediatric information including resources for patients and health care professionals.

Book Publishers

6002 **Everything You Need to Know About Measles and Rubella**

Trisha Hawkins, author

Rosen Publishing/PowerKids Press
29 E 21st Street
New York, NY 10010
212-777-3017
800-237-9932
Fax: 888-436-4643
rosenpub@tribeca.ios.com
www.rosenpublishing.com

Examines the continuing threat of these highly infectious respiratory diseases. Grades 7-12.

2001 64 pages
ISBN: 0-823933-22-9

Roger Rosen, President

6003 **IVUN Resource Directory**
4207 Lindell Boulevard, Suite 110
Saint Louis, MO 63108
314-534-0475
Fax: 314-534-5070
info@post-polio.org
www.post-polio.org

A networking tool for health professionals and both long-term and new ventilator users. Sections include health professionals, ventilator users, equipment and aids, manufacturers, service and repair, organizations, etc. Published annually in October.

34 pages Annually

Joan L Headley, Executive Director & Editor

6004 **Let's Talk About Having Chicken Pox**

Elizabeth Weitzman, author

Rosen Publishing/PowerKids Press
29 E 21st Street
New York, NY 10010
212-777-3017
800-237-9932
Fax: 888-436-4643
rosenpub@tribeca.ios.com
www.rosenpublishing.com

Highly contagious chicken pox is one of the childhood illnesses that few kids escape. This book tells kids how to handle the illness, where it comes from and how long it will take to recover. Grades K-5.

24 pages
ISBN: 0-823950-31-X

Roger Roger, President

6005 **Measles**

Maxine Rosaler, author

Rosen Publishing/PowerKids Press
29 E 21st Street
New York, NY 10010
212-777-3017
800-237-9932
Fax: 888-436-4643
rosenpub@tribeca.ios.com
www.rosenpublishing.com

An examination of the history of this once thought to be harmless disease, from its ancient origins to near eradication.

2005 64 pages
ISBN: 1-404202-56-0

Roger Roger, President

6006 **Post-Polio Directory**
4207 Lindell Boulevard, Suite 110
Saint Louis, MO 63108
314-534-0475
Fax: 314-534-5070
info@post-polio.org
www.post-polio.org

Over 32 pages of post polio clinics, health professionals, support groups, and other useful contacts. The directory includes international listings. Published annually in March.

Joan L Headley, Executive Director & Editor

Newsletters

6007 **Infectious Diseases in Children**
Slack Incorporated
6900 Grove Road
Thorofare, NJ 08086
856-848-1000
800-257-8290
editor@healio.com
www.healio.com/footer/healio-dot-com

Pediatric news source.

Monthly

Philip A Brunell MD, Chief Medical Editor

6008 **Post-Polio Health**
4207 Lindell Boulevard, Suite 110
Saint Louis, MO 63108
314-534-0475
Fax: 314-534-5070
info@post-polio.org
www.post-polio.org

Provides information to polio survivors, their families, and the health care community and promotes networking among the post-polio community.

12 pages Quarterly
ISSN: 1066-5331

William G. Stothers, President/Chairperson
Saul J. Morse, Vice President
Joan L Headley, Editor & Executive Director

Pamphlets

6009 **Tetanus and Diptheria Vaccine**
Centers for Disease Control & Prevention
1600 Clifton Road
Atlanta, GA 30333
404-639-3311
800-232-4636
www.cdc.gov/vaccines/pubs/vis/downloads/vis-td.pdf

Factsheet about the diseases and the vaccines.

DESCRIPTION

6010 PROTEIN C DEFICIENCY

Synonyms: PC deficiency, PROC deficiency

Covers these related disorders: Protein C deficiency Type I, Protein C deficiency Type II

Involves the following Biologic System(s):

Hematologic and Oncologic Disorders

Protein C deficiency is a blood clotting (thrombotic) disorder characterized by the recurrent formation of blood clots within the veins of the body (venous thrombosis). Protein C, which is formed in the liver, is a specialized protein that helps to prevent the formation of blood clots. When activated, protein C helps to dissolve fibrin, the semisolid portion of blood clots, thus inhibiting the formation of a clot. A deficiency of this protein, therefore, results in abnormal clot formation. Some signs of this disorder may become apparent during adolescence. Associated symptoms depend upon the organ or tissue affected by clot formation that leads to reduced or absent blood flow. Affected individuals may develop blood clots and inflammation in the veins of the legs (thrombophlebitis). This can occur when the blood moves slowly in the veins, such as from prolonged bed rest during an illness, surgery, or hospital stay. In some patients, these clots may dislodge from the vein and travel through the blood stream (embolus) to different parts of the body including the heart, lungs, or brain, potentially leading to life-threatening complications. However, not all patients with protein C deficiency experience all the signs associated with this disorder.

In the event of a blood clotting episode, the antithrombin factor heparin may be administered through injection into a vein (intravenous) or under the skin (subcutaneous). Other treatment may include continuing oral administration of the anti-coagulant drug warfarin to prevent a recurrence of thrombotic activity

Two types of protein C deficiency have been described in the general population. The more common form is Type I in which both protein C levels and activity are deficient. In the less common Type II, the amount of protein is normal but its activity or performance is impaired. The inherited form of protein C deficiency may be transmitted as an autosomal dominant trait. The gene for this disorder is located on the long arm of chromosome 2 (2q13-14). Protein C deficiency may also be acquired in connection with infection.

Government Agencies

6011 NIH/National Heart, Lung and Blood Institu te
National Institute of Health
31 Center Dr MSC 2486, Bldg 31, Room 5A52
Bethesda, MD 20892   301-592-8573
                                        Fax: 240-629-3246
                                        TTY: 240-629-3255
                                    NHLBIinfo@nhlbi.nih.gov
                                        www.nhlbi.nih.gov

Primary responsibility of this organization is the scientific investigation of heart, blood vessel, lung and blood disorders. Oversees research, demonstration, prevention, education, control and training activities in these fields and emphasizes the prevention and control of heart diseases.

Gary H Gibbons, MD, Director
Nakela Cook, MD, Chief of Staff

National Associations & Support Groups

6012 American Academy of Pediatrics
141 Northwest Point Boulevard
Elk Grove Village, IL 60007   847-434-4000
                                               800-433-9016
                                          Fax: 847-434-8000
                                               www.aap.org

The American Academy of Pediatrics and its member pediatricians are committed to the attainment of optimal physical, mental and social health and well-being for all infants, children, adolescents, and young adults.

Fernando Stein, MD, FAAP, President
Karen Remley, MD, CEO/Executive VP

6013 Genetic Alliance
4301 Connecticut Avenue NW, Suite 404
Washington, DC 20008   202-966-5557
                                               800-336-4363
                                          Fax: 202-966-8553
                                       info@geneticalliance.org
                                       www.geneticalliance.org

A coalition of voluntary genetic support groups, consumers and professionals addressing the needs of individuals and families affected by genetic disorders from a national perspective.

Sharon Terry, President/CEO
Tetyana Murza, Managing Director
Natasha Bonhomme, VP, Strategic Development

6014 March of Dimes Foundation
1275 Mamaroneck Avenue
White Plains, NY 10605   914-997-4488
                                               888-663-4637
                                          Fax: 914-428-8203
                                     answers@marchofdimes.com
                                        www.marchofdimes.com

Partnership of volunteers and professionals dedicates to improving the health of babies by preventing birth defects and infant mortality. Over 100 chapters are located across the country and can be located through the National Office.

Stacey D. Stewart, President

6015 Med Help International
6300 North Wickham Road, Suite 130
Melbourne, FL 32940   321-259-7505
                                          Fax: 321-751-0858
                                           office@medhelp.org
                                             www.medhelp.org

A not-for-profit organization dedicated to helping patients find the highest quality medical information in the world today. Patients are offered the tools necessary to make informed treatment decisions within the short time lines dictated by their illness or disease.

Cynthia ThompsonD, President & Co-Founder
Philip A Garfinkel, VP & Co-Founder

State Agencies & Support Groups

6016 Vitamin C Foundation
PO Box 130130
Spring, TX 77393   281-255-2679
                                               800-849-9025
                                          Fax: 630-416-1309
                                           ascorbade@aol.com
                                        www.vitamincfoundation.org

A Texas nonprofit organization devoted to preserving and distributing knowledge about ascorbic acid and its vital role in the life process.

Owen R Fonorow, Co-Founder
M S Till Sr, Co-Founder

Web Sites

6017 Factor V Leiden: Thrombophilia Support Pag e
www.fvleiden.org

Factor V Leiden is the most common hereditary blood coagulation disorder in the US. It is present in 3-7% of the population in Europe and America. It is associated with Venous thrombosis, DVT, unexplained miscarriage, blood clots in the lungs, gall bladder dysfunction, preeclampsia and/or eclapsia, stroke and/or heart attack.

6018 HealthCentral.com
750 Third Avenue, 6th Floor
New York, NY 10017   212-695-2223
                                        Fax: 212-695-2936
                                        www.healthcentral.com

Offering information on health issues for children, women, men and seniors. Information on Protein C Deficiency includes a description, causes, symptoms, diagnosis, treatment and questions that can be asked of the doctor.

Micheael Cunnion, Chief Executive Officer
Jim Curtis, Chief Revenue Officer
Rebecca Farwell, Chief Content Officer

6019 MedicineNet
www.medicinenet.com

An online, healthcare media publishing company. It provides easy to read, in-depth, authoritative medical information for consumers via an interactive web site.

6020 Merck
2000 Galloping Hill Road
Kenilworth, NJ 7033   908-740-4000
                                        www.merck.com

A site that offers research driven pharmaceutical products and services to improve human and animal health, directly and through its joint ventures.

Kenneth C.~ Frazier, Chairman & CEO
Robert M. Davis, EVP & CFO
Willie A. Deese, EVP & President

6021 Online Mendelian Inheritance in Man
National Library of Medicine, Building 38A
Bethesda, MD 20894   888-346-3656
                                        info@ncbi.nlm.nih.gov
                                        www.ncbi.nlm.nih.gov

This database is a catalog of human genes and genetic disorders.

Book Publishers

6022 Merck Manual of Diagnosis and Therapy
Merck Publishing Group
PO Box 2000 RY84-15
Rahway, NJ 07065   732-594-4600
                                        Fax: 732-388-3610
                                        www.merckbooks.com

Since it was first published in 1899, The Merck Manual has set the standard for excellence in the medical community for current, complete, and comprehensive information for all healthcare professionals. Written by more than 300 medical experts in all fields of medicine from around the world.

2006 18th Ed 2832 pages Hardcover
ISBN: 0-911910-18-2

Mark H Beers MD, Editor-in-Chief
Robert S Porter MD, Editor

6023 Protein Deficiency and Pesticide Toxicity
Eldon M Boyd, author

Charles C Thomas
2600 South First Street
Springfield, IL 62704   217-789-8980
                                            800-258-8980
                                        Fax: 217-789-9130
                                        books@ccthomas.com
                                        www.ccthomas.com

Discusses the approaches for analyzing Protein Deficiency and Pesticide Toxicity.

468 pages Hardcover
ISBN: 0-398024-76-6

DESCRIPTION

6024 PSORIASIS

Involves the following Biologic System(s):
Dermatologic Disorders

Psoriasis is a common, chronic skin disease characterized by red patches of skin that are covered by dry, thick, silvery scales. This disorder may occur at any age, but most commonly appears from the ages of 10 to 40 years. Although males and females are affected equally, females are more prone to development of this disorder when it appears during childhood. In addition, approximately half of those individuals who develop psoriasis in childhood have a family history of the disorder, but the pattern of transmission has not been determined. Individuals with psoriasis appear to produce new skin cells at a greatly accelerated rate while shedding their old cells at a normal rate. The subsequent buildup of new cells produces thickened areas of new skin that are covered by old skin, thus forming the characteristic dry, thickened, silvery patches associated with psoriasis.

Psoriatic lesions may appear anywhere on the body, but most commonly form on the scalp, elbows, knees, back, buttocks, navel area, and genitalia. In addition, relatively smaller lesions may appear on the face and pitting may develop on the nails. Peeling away a scale produces specks of bleeding from the capillaries (Auspitz's sign). Itching of the skin (pruritus) is common and scratching leads to more lesions (Koebner's phenomenon). On rare occasions, severe psoriasis may develop in newborns, accompanied by lesion formation in the diaper area.

There are different types of psoriasis. The most common form is called discoid psoriasis and is characterized by patches that form mainly on the elbows, knees, scalp, and other areas of the arms, legs, and trunk. Other findings may include nail irregul|arities such as pitting, thickening, and separation from the nail beds. In addition, psorasis is sometimes accompanied by painful swelling of the joints (arthritis). Guttate psoriasis occurs primarily in children and young adults and is characterized by the sudden appearance of small, oval, drop-like lesions on the trunk and upper portions of the arms and legs. Guttate psoriasis often develops following a streptococcal infection, viral infection, or sunburn. In addition, this form of the disorder sometimes follows the conclusion or withdrawal of corticosteroid treatment. Pustular psoriasis may be localized or generalized. In its localized form, eruptions of pustules develop over individual reddish patches that are present, usually, on the palms of the hands and the soles of the feet. Psoriasis is usually apparent on other parts of the body. Affected individuals may also experience localized discomfort. Generalized pustular psoriasis is an acute, severe, sometimes life-threatening form of the disorder that is characterized by the widespread eruption of small pustules in individuals with mild, moderate, or other types of psoriasis. Generalized pustular psoriasis is sometimes accompanied by high fever, pain in the joints, elevated levels of white blood cells (leukocytosis), low levels of blood calcium (hypocalcemia), and other irregularties.

Treatment of psoriasis is dependent upon age, area of involvement, and the type and severity of the disease. Many treatment protocols that are effective for adults may be too toxic for children; therefore, most treatment for children with psoriasis is conservative and mainly directed toward comfort and alleviation of pain. Such treatment may include the use of tar preparations in the form of gels, ointments, or bath emulsions. Additional topical treatments may include the cautious use of corticosteroid preparations, vitamin D analogs, and other ointments. Treatment for scalp lesions may include the use of a phenol and saline solution followed by tar shampoo and, when lesions are reduced, the application of a corticosteroid preparation. Severe psoriasis in children may indicate the use of various drugs such as methotrexate and certain oral retinoids; however, this therapy may be accompanied by severe side effects. Other treatment is symptomatic and supportive.

National Associations & Support Groups

6025 American Academy of Pediatrics
141 Northwest Point Boulevard
Elk Grove Village, IL 60007
847-434-4000
800-433-9016
Fax: 847-434-8000
www.aap.org

The American Academy of Pediatrics and its member pediatricians are committed to the attainment of optimal physical, mental and social health and well-being for all infants, children, adolescents, and young adults.

Fernando Stein, MD, FAAP, President
Karen Remley, MD, CEO/Executive VP

6026 National Psoriasis Foundation
6600 SW 92nd Avenue, Suite 300
Portland, OR 97223
503-244-7404
800-723-9166
Fax: 503-245-0626
getinfo@psoriasis.org
www.psoriasis.org

Promotes awareness and understanding of psoriasis and psoriatic arthritis through education and advocacy. The foundation also ensures access to treatment and supports research that leads to effective management of the condition.

Pam Field, CEO
Pam Field, VP Operations
Paula Fasano, Director Marketing/Communications

Research Centers

6027 University of California, San Francisco Dermatology Drug Research
515 Spruce Street
San Francisco, CA 94115
415-476-4701
Fax: 415-502-4126
ÿcommunications@cc.ucsf.edu
cc.ucsf.edu/people

Conducts clinical testing of new or existing pharmalogic agents used in the treatment of skin disorders.

John Koo, MD, Director

Audio Video

6028 National Library of Dermatologic Teaching Slides
American Academy Of Dermatology
PO Box 94020
Palatine, IL 60094
847-330-0230
Fax: 847-330-0050
www.aad.org/store/product/

A collection of dermatologic teaching slides offering the most comprehensive series ever assembled. Each set offers a realistic presentation of classic clinical skin conditions encountered by the dermatologist.

Brett M.~ Coldiron, President
Elise A. Olsen, MD, Vice President
Suzanne M.~ Olbricht, Secretary-Treasurer

Web Sites

6029 American Academy of Dermatology (AAD)
www.aad.org/aadpamphrework/Psoriasis.html

The American Academy of Dermatoloy is dedicated to achieving
the highest quality of dermatologic care for everyone.
Acheivement of this vision requires a dynamic organization
whose mission embodies: Excellence in patient care, education
and research, adherence to eithical conduct, respinsiveness to its
members and to the public unification and representation of the
specialty.

Brett M.~ Coldiron, President
Elise A. Olsen, MD, Vice President
Suzanne M.~ Olbricht, Secretary-Treasurer

6030 National Psoriasis Foundation
6600 SW 92nd Ave., Ste. 300
Portland, OR 97223
800-723-9166
getinfo@psoriasis.org
www.psoriasis.org

Promotes awareness and understanding of psoriasis and psoriatic
arthritis through education and advocacy. The foundation also ensures access to treatment and supports research that leads to effective management of the condition.

Krista Kellogg, Chair
Pete Redding, Vice Chair
Randy Beranek, President/ CEO

6031 Psoriasis Association
Dick Coles House, 2 Queensbridge
Northampton, NN4 7
845-676-0076
Fax: 160-425-1621
mail@psoriasis-association.org.uk
www.psoriasis-association.org.uk

Formed with these aims in view: to raise awareness of psoriasis;
support those who have psoriasis; and fund research into the
causes of and treatments for psoriasis.

4000 members

Ray Jobling, MBE, Chairman
Jonathan Swift, Vice Chairman
John Ford, MBE, Treasurer

6032 Psoriasis Connections
Thousand Oaks, CA 91320
www.psoriasisconnect.com

Connects people with medical experts on psoriasis, those affected
by the condition, family and friends, and other relevant resources.

6033 Skin Page
pinch.com/skin/

skinpage-0907-admin@pinch.com
pinch.com/skin/

Noncommercial site that provides shortcuts to search past messages in the skin diseases newsgroups and other databases. Includes a psoriasis information page and other resources.

6034 UnderstandingPsoriasis.org by Healthology
www.understandingpsoriasis.org

Current information on psoriasis gathered and presented by leaders in the field of dermatology.

Book Publishers

6035 Handbook of Psoriasis

Charles Camisa, author

Blackwell Publishing
Commerce Place, 350 Main Street
Malden, MA 02148
781-388-8200
800-216-2522
Fax: 781-388-8210
www.wiley.com

Reference for health care professionals, easy to read, yet detailed
information.

2005 2nd Ed Paperback
ISBN: 1-405109-27-7

Peter B. Wiley, Chairman
Stephen M. Smith, President & CEO
Ellis E. Cousens, Executive Vice President, Chief Fin

6036 Psychological Approaches to Dermatology

Linda Papadopoulos, author

Blackwell Publishing
Commerce Place, 350 Main Street
Malden, MA 02148
781-388-8200
800-216-2522
Fax: 781-388-8210
www.wiley.com

References all the main skin conditions - psoriasis, eczema,
vitiligo, dermatitis, alopecia, and others. The book blends theory
and practical experience, making it a highly recommended read.

1999 176 pages Paperback
ISBN: 1-854332-92-9

Peter B. Wiley, Chairman
Stephen M. Smith, President & CEO
Ellis E. Cousens, Executive Vice President, Chief Fin

6037 Textbook of Psoriasis

Peter Van de Kerkhof, author

Blackwell Publishing
Commerce Place, 350 Main Street
Malden, MA 02148
781-388-8200
800-216-2522
Fax: 781-388-8210
www.wiley.com

Written for dermatologists, it is a concise and clinical account of
psoriasis, divided into three sections: morphology of the skin, etiology and pathogenesis, and current treatments.

2003 2nd Ed Hardback
ISBN: 1-405107-17-4

Peter B. Wiley, Chairman
Stephen M. Smith, President & CEO
Ellis E. Cousens, Executive Vice President, Chief Fin

Magazines

6038 International Journal of Dermatology
International Society of Dermatology
2323 North State Street #30
Bunnell, FL 32110
386-437-4405
Fax: 386-437-4427
info@intsocderm.org
www.intsocderm.org

Focuses on information for dermatologists and the whole specialty of dermatology research and education.

10 times a year

Evangeline~ Handog, MD, President
Luca Borradori, Vice President
Paulo Rowilson Cunha, Vice President

6039   Journal of Dermatologic Surgery and Oncology
International Society for Dermatologic Surgery
930 N Meachan Road
Schaumburg, IL 60173   847-330-9830
                                              Fax: 847-330-1135

Focuses on medical updates and information on dermatology.
Monthly

6040   Psoriasis Advance
National Psoriasis Foundation
6600 SW 92nd Avenue, Suite 300
Portland, OR 97223   503-244-7404
                                                   800-723-9166
                                              Fax: 503-245-0626
                                            getinfo@psoriasis.org
                                              www.psoriasis.org

Member magazine that evolved from two formerly published
newsletters (Bulletin & Psoriasis Resource) connecting the psoriasis community.

36 pages Bi-monthly

Krista Kellogg, Chair
Pete Redding, Vice Chair
Randy Beranek, President/ CEO

Journals

6041   Psoriasis Forum
National Psoriasis Foundation
6600 SW 92nd Avenue, Suite 300
Portland, OR 97223   503-244-7404
                                                   800-723-9166
                                              Fax: 503-245-0626
                                            getinfo@psoriasis.org
                                              www.psoriasis.org

Journal for professional members of the foundation. It is dedicated to providing up-to-date, practical information to health care
providers on the front line of psoriasis treatment.

Krista Kellogg, Chair
Pete Redding, Vice Chair
Randy Beranek, President/ CEO

Newsletters

6042   Awareness
NAPVI
PO Box 317
Watertown, MA 2471   617-972-7441
                                                   800-562-6265
                                              Fax: 617-972-7444
                                           www.spedex.com/napvi

Newsletter offering regional news, sports and activities, conferences, camps, legislative updates, book reviews, audio reviews,
professional question and answer column and more for the visually impaired and their families.
Quarterly

6043   Bulletin
National Psoriasis Foundation
6600 SW 92nd Avenue, Suite 300
Portland, OR 97223   503-244-7404
                                                   800-723-9166
                                              Fax: 503-245-0626
                                            getinfo@psoriasis.org
                                              www.psoriasis.org

Published for 35 years by the National Psoriasis Foundation, past
issues are available online in pdf form. It covered both traditional
and alternative treatments, self-help techniques, research and a
wide variety of human-interest topics. Please refer to the foundation's magazine Psoriasis Advance for updated information and
resources.

Krista Kellogg, Chair
Pete Redding, Vice Chair
Randy Beranek, President/ CEO

6044   DVH Quarterly
University of Arkansas at Little Rock
2801 S University Avenue
Little Rock, AR 72204   Fax: 501-663-3536

Offers information on upcoming events, conferences and workshops on and for visual disabilities. Book reviews, information
on the newest resources and technology, educational programs,
want ads and more.
Quarterly
Bob Brasher, Editor

6045   Dermatology Focus
Dermatology Foundation
1560 Sherman Avenue, Suite 870
Evanston, IL 60201   847-328-2256
                                              Fax: 847-328-0509
                                    dfgen@dermatologyfoundation.org
                                        dermatologyfoundation.org

Includes membership activities, research articles and lists recipients of foundation awards.
Quarterly

Bruce U. Wintroub, Chairman
Michael D. Tharp, M.D., President
Staurt R. Lessin, M.D., Vice President

6046   Dermatology World
American Academy of Dermatology
PO Box 94020
Palatine, IL 60094   847-330-0230
                                              Fax: 847-330-0050
                                                   www.aad.org

Offers Academy members information outside the clinical realm.
It carries news of government actions, reports of socioeconomic
issues, societal trends and other events which impinge on the
practice of dermatology.
Monthly

Brett M.~ Coldiron, President
Elise A. Olsen, MD, Vice President
Suzanne M.~ Olbricht, Secretary-Treasurer

6047   Progress in Dermatology
Dermatology Foundation
1560 Sherman Avenue, Suite 870
Evanston, IL 60201   847-328-2256
                                              Fax: 847-328-0509
                                    dfgen@dermatologyfoundation.org
                                        dermatologyfoundation.org

Bulletin offering information on research reports and clinical
trials.
Quarterly

Bruce U. Wintroub, Chairman
Michael D. Tharp, M.D., President
Staurt R. Lessin, M.D., Vice President

6048   Psoriasis Resource
National Psoriasis Foundation
6600 SW 92nd Avenue, Suite 300
Portland, OR 97223   503-244-7404
                                                   800-723-9166
                                              Fax: 503-245-0626
                                            getinfo@psoriasis.org
                                              www.psoriasis.org

Published from 1999 to 2002, three times a year, by the National
Psoriasis Foundation, past issues are available online in pdf form.
It helped people make educated decisions about medication, therapy and product choices available for skin and joints. Please refer
to the foundation's magazine Psoriasis Advance for updated
information and resources.

Krista Kellogg, Chair
Pete Redding, Vice Chair
Randy Beranek, President/ CEO

Pamphlets

6049 Alternative Approaches
National Psoriasis Foundation
6600 SW 92nd Avenue, Suite 300
Portland, OR 97223

503-244-7404
800-723-9166
Fax: 503-245-0626
getinfo@psoriasis.org
www.psoriasis.org

Non-traditional therapies and treatments for both psoriasis and psoriatic arthritis including stress management, topical preparations and Chinese medicine.

2005 13 pages

Krista Kellogg, Chair
Pete Redding, Vice Chair
Randy Beranek, President/ CEO

6050 Conception, Pregnancy and Psoriasis
National Psoriasis Foundation
6600 SW 92nd Avenue, Suite 300
Portland, OR 97223

503-244-7404
800-723-9166
Fax: 503-245-0626
getinfo@psoriasis.org
www.psoriasis.org

Overview of the effect of pregnancy on psoriasis and treatment, risks and other considerations during conception.

2006 9 pages

Krista Kellogg, Chair
Pete Redding, Vice Chair
Randy Beranek, President/ CEO

6051 Phototherapy: Light Treatment for Psoriasi s
National Psoriasis Foundation
6600 SW 92nd Avenue, Suite 300
Portland, OR 97223

503-244-7404
800-723-9166
Fax: 503-245-0626
getinfo@psoriasis.org
www.psoriasis.org

Light treatment options: PUVA, lasers, broad-band UVB, and narrow-band UVB.

2006 13 pages

Krista Kellogg, Chair
Pete Redding, Vice Chair
Randy Beranek, President/ CEO

6052 Psoriasis 101: Learning to Live in the Ski n You're In
National Psoriasis Foundation
6600 SW 92nd Avenue, Suite 300
Portland, OR 97223

503-244-7404
800-723-9166
Fax: 503-245-0626
getinfo@psoriasis.org
www.psoriasis.org

Designed to educate young people, teens and college-age young adults about psoriasis. It is written from a young person's standpoint with bytes of information.

2006 12 pages

Krista Kellogg, Chair
Pete Redding, Vice Chair
Randy Beranek, President/ CEO

6053 Psoriasis Research: Progress & Promise
National Psoriasis Foundation
6600 SW 92nd Avenue, Suite 300
Portland, OR 97223

503-244-7404
800-723-9166
Fax: 503-245-0626
getinfo@psoriasis.org
www.psoriasis.org

Overview of present research and the foundation's role in supporting it. Includes new treatments and progress being made in genetics.

2004 11 pages

Krista Kellogg, Chair
Pete Redding, Vice Chair
Randy Beranek, President/ CEO

6054 Psoriasis on Specific Skin Sites
National Psoriasis Foundation
6600 SW 92nd Avenue, Suite 300
Portland, OR 97223

503-244-7404
800-723-9166
Fax: 503-245-0626
getinfo@psoriasis.org
www.psoriasis.org

Information on the disease affecting nails, ears, eyelids, face, mouth and lips, hands, feet and skin folds.

2005 9 pages

Krista Kellogg, Chair
Pete Redding, Vice Chair
Randy Beranek, President/ CEO

6055 Psoriasis: How it Makes You Feel
National Psoriasis Foundation
6600 SW 92nd Avenue, Suite 300
Portland, OR 97223

503-244-7404
800-723-9166
Fax: 503-245-0626
getinfo@psoriasis.org
www.psoriasis.org

Living with psoriasis and the emotional impact.

Krista Kellogg, Chair
Pete Redding, Vice Chair
Randy Beranek, President/ CEO

6056 Psoriatic Arthritis
National Psoriasis Foundation
6600 SW 92nd Avenue, Suite 300
Portland, OR 97223

503-244-7404
800-723-9166
Fax: 503-245-0626
getinfo@psoriasis.org
www.psoriasis.org

Overview of the joint disease that affects about 10-30% of psoriasis sufferers. Includes diagnosis and treatment details.

2005 11 pages

Krista Kellogg, Chair
Pete Redding, Vice Chair
Randy Beranek, President/ CEO

6057 Questions and Answers About Psoriasis
NAMSIC, National Institutes of Health
1 AMS Circle
Bethesda, MD 20892

301-495-4484
877-226-4267
Fax: 301-718-6366
TTY: 301-565-2966
NIAMSinfo@mail.nih.gov
www.niams.nih.gov

Offers various information for the psoriasis patient and their family regarding treatments, risks, nutrition and more.

2003 22 pages

Stephen I. Katz, M.D., Ph.D., Director

6058 Scalp Psoriasis
National Psoriasis Foundation
6600 SW 92nd Avenue, Suite 300
Portland, OR 97223

503-244-7404
800-723-9166
Fax: 503-245-0626
getinfo@psoriasis.org
www.psoriasis.org

Possible treatment, tips and regimens for psoriasis of the scalp.

2005 9 pages

Krista Kellogg, Chair
Pete Redding, Vice Chair
Randy Beranek, President/ CEO

6059   Specific Forms of Psoriasis
National Psoriasis Foundation
6600 SW 92nd Avenue, Suite 300
Portland, OR 97223   503-244-7404
                                                  800-723-9166
                                                  Fax: 503-245-0626
                                                  getinfo@psoriasis.org
                                                  www.psoriasis.org

Plaque, Pustular, guttate, inverse, and erythrodermic: overview
and treatment considerations for each type of the disease.

2006 7 pages

Krista Kellogg, Chair
Pete Redding, Vice Chair
Randy Beranek, President/ CEO

6060   Sun and Water Therapy
National Psoriasis Foundation
6600 SW 92nd Avenue, Suite 300
Portland, OR 97223   503-244-7404
                                                  800-723-9166
                                                  Fax: 503-245-0626
                                                  getinfo@psoriasis.org
                                                  www.psoriasis.org

Provides information on climatotherapy sites as well as an overview of natural sunlight and water treatment options.

2005 11 pages

Krista Kellogg, Chair
Pete Redding, Vice Chair
Randy Beranek, President/ CEO

6061   Things to Consider
National Psoriasis Foundation
6600 SW 92nd Avenue, Suite 300
Portland, OR 97223   503-244-7404
                                                  800-723-9166
                                                  Fax: 503-245-0626
                                                  getinfo@psoriasis.org
                                                  www.psoriasis.org

Discusses making treatment decisions, talking with your physician and knowing your rights.

Krista Kellogg, Chair
Pete Redding, Vice Chair
Randy Beranek, President/ CEO

6062   Your Diet & Psoriasis
National Psoriasis Foundation
6600 SW 92nd Avenue, Suite 300
Portland, OR 97223   503-244-7404
                                                  800-723-9166
                                                  Fax: 503-245-0626
                                                  getinfo@psoriasis.org
                                                  www.psoriasis.org

An overview of diet-related research and therapies.

2005 9 pages

Krista Kellogg, Chair
Pete Redding, Vice Chair
Randy Beranek, President/ CEO

Camps

6063   Camp Discovery
American Academy of Dermatology
930 E Woodfield Road
Schaumburg, IL 60173   847-240-1737
                                                  Fax: 847-330-8907
                                                  jmueller@aad.org
                                                  www.aad.org/dermatology-a-to-z/for-kids/camp-discove

A camp for young people with chronic skin conditions. There is
no fee and transportation is provided. Three locations: Camp Horizon in Millville, PA, Camp Knutson in Crosslake, MN, and
Camp Dermadillo in Burton, TX.

Brett M.˜ Coldiron, President
Elise A. Olsen, MD, Vice President
Suzanne M.˜ Olbricht, Secretary-Treasurer

DESCRIPTION

6064 PTOSIS

Synonym: Blepharoptosis

Covers these related disorders: Acquired ptosis, Congenital ptosis

Involves the following Biologic System(s):

Neurologic Disorders, Ophthalmologic Disorders

Ptosis, or blepharoptosis, refers to a condition in which one or both of the upper eyelids droop or sag as a result of an irregularity that is present at birth or an acquired weakness in the muscles of the upper eyelid that are responsible for movement. This condition may also be the result of irregularities of the nerve response for regulating muscle movements of the upper eyelids (third cranial nerve or oculomotor nerve). Congenital ptosis varies in severity; therefore, treatment depends upon the extent of the defect. If the eyelid droop is sufficient to cover the pupil, the ability to see is impaired. In some infants and children, the development of the affected eye may be slowed, resulting in reduced or lost vision (amblyopia) in that eye. In such cases, early intervention through surgery may aid in preventing the development of impaired vision. However, surgery to correct ptosis strictly for cosmetic reasons is often postponed until the affected child reaches the age of three or four years.

In some cases, ptosis is accompanied by an abnormality of certain eye muscles, resulting in irregular movements of the eyes. Other ocular irregularities often associated with congenital ptosis include misalignment of the eyes in relation to each other (strabismus) or an imbalance in the way each eye deflects light (anisometropia). Medical specialists recommended early treatment of any accompanying abnormalities to avert complications. Ptosis may also occur as a characteristic feature of several syndromes including congenital fibrosis syndrome, Horner syndrome, or Sturge-Weber syndrome. Congenital ptosis is transmitted as an autosomal dominant trait.

Acquired ptosis may develop secondary to several disorders or conditions including myasthenia gravis, a muscular disorder; botulism, a severe type of food poisoning; progressive lesions within the skull that impact on the third cranial nerve; inflammation or growths that impact the eye orbit or lid. Treatment for acquired ptosis depends upon and may be directed toward the underlying cause.

Government Agencies

6065 NIH/National Eye Institute
31 Center Drive MSC 2510
Bethesda, MD 20892

301-496-5248
2020@nei.nih.gov
www.nei.nih.gov

Conducts and supports research that helps prevent and treat eye diseases and other disorders of vision. This research leads to sight-saving treatments, reduces visual impairment and blindness, and improves the quality of life for people of all ages. NEI-supported research has advanced our knowledge of how the eye functions in health and disease.

Paul A Sieving M.D., Ph.D., Director

National Associations & Support Groups

6066 American Academy of Pediatrics
141 Northwest Point Boulevard
Elk Grove Village, IL 60007

847-434-4000
800-433-9016
Fax: 847-434-8000
www.aap.org

The American Academy of Pediatrics and its member pediatricians are committed to the attainment of optimal physical, mental and social health and well-being for all infants, children, adolescents, and young adults.

Fernando Stein, MD, FAAP, President
Karen Remley, MD, CEO/Executive VP

6067 Genetic Alliance
4301 Connecticut Avenue NW, Suite 404
Washington, DC 20008

202-966-5557
800-336-4363
Fax: 202-966-8553
info@geneticalliance.org
www.geneticalliance.org

A coalition of voluntary genetic support groups, consumers and professionals addressing the needs of individuals and families affected by genetic disorders from a national perspective.

Sharon Terry, President/CEO
Tetyana Murza, Managing Director
Natasha Bonhomme, VP, Strategic Development

6068 March of Dimes Foundation
1275 Mamaroneck Avenue
White Plains, NY 10605

914-997-4488
888-663-4637
Fax: 914-428-8203
answers@marchofdimes.com
www.marchofdimes.com

Partnership of volunteers and professionals dedicates to improving the health of babies by preventing birth defects and infant mortality. Over 100 chapters are located across the country and can be located through the National Office.

Stacey D. Stewart, President

6069 National Association for Visually Handicapped
111 E 59th St,ÿ
New York, NY 10022

212-889-3141
800-829-0500
Fax: 212-727-2931
navh@navh.org
www.navh.org

Serves as a clearinghouse for information about all services available to the partially-sighted from public and private sources. Conducts self-help groups. Provides information on large print books, textbooks and educational tools.

Lorianie Marchi, CEO

Web Sites

6070 National Association for Visually Handicapped
111 E 59th St
New York, NY 10022

800-284-4422
lighthouse.org/navh

Helps to cope with the difficulties of vision impairment.

6071 Online Mendelian Inheritance in Man
National Library of Medicine, Building 38A
Bethesda, MD 20894

888-346-3656
info@ncbi.nlm.nih.gov
www.ncbi.nlm.nih.gov

This database is a catalog of human genes and genetic disorders.

6072 **Royal National Institute of the Blind**
105 Judd Street
London, WC1H

303-123-9999
helpline@rnib.org.uk
www.rnib.org.uk

A leading UK charity offering information, support and advice to
over two million people with sight problems.

Lesley-Anne Alexander, Chief Executive
Wanda Hamilton, Group Director
Fazilet Hadi, Managing Director

DESCRIPTION

6073 PULMONARY HYPERTENSION

Covers these related disorders: Persistent fetal circulation (PFC)

Involves the following Biologic System(s):

Cardiovascular Disorders, Respiratory Disorders

Primary pulmonary hypertension is a condition in which the blood pressure within the pulmonary artery is abnormally high (hypertension). The pulmonary artery arises from the base of the lower right chamber of the heart (ventricle) and carries oxygen-poor blood to the lungs, where the exchange of oxygen and carbon dioxide occurs. When this occurs in newborn infants, it is known as persistent fetal circulation or more appropriately, persistent pulmonary hypertension in the newborn (PPHN).

PPHN is a condition in newborns in which blood continues to circulate through certain fetal openings or channels which usually close shortly after birth. These include the fetal opening between the left and right upper chambers of the heart (foramen ovale) and the fetal channel that joins the major artery of the body (aorta) and the pulmonary artery (ductus arteriosus). PPHN may occur in newborns for unknown reasons (idiopathic) or may result from a lack of oxygen during the birth process (birth asphyxia); certain abnormalities during pregnancy (e.g., amniotic fluid leak); certain birth defects (e.g., underdevelopment of the lungs seen in a diaphragmatic hernia); or other conditions, such as meconium aspiration, polycythemia (excess number of red blood cells, etc. PPHN affects approximately one in 500 t0 700 newborns.

Newborns with PPHN often experience symptoms immediately after birth or within the first 12 hours of life. Some may have bluish discoloration of the skin and mucous membranes (cyanosis) and increasing difficulties breathing (respiratory distress). Symptoms associated with respiratory distress may include rapid breathing (tachypnea), grunting upon exhalation, drawing in of the chest wall during inhalation, and a rapid heart rate (tachycardia).

In newborns with PPHN, immediate measures may be necessary to prevent or treat potentially life-threatening complications. Additional therapy is directed toward treating the underlying cause of the condition and providing ongoing supportive measures to increase the supply of oxygen to bodily tissues. Oxygen therapies may include the use of measures to mechanically assist breathing (mechanical ventilation), administration of certain medications (e.g., surfactant therapy; inhalation of nitric oxide to help widen pulmonary blood vessels), or use of a device known as an extracorporeal membrane oxygenator (ECMO). This device delivers oxygen to an infant's blood as it is circulated outside of the body and then returns the oxygenated blood to the body.

In contrast to PPHN, primary pulmonary hypertension is a progressive condition that often becomes apparent between the ages of 10 to 20 years. Females appear to be slightly more affected than males. Researchers suspect that th|e condition may be the result of the interactions of different genes, possibly in association with the involvement of certain environmental factors (multifactorial inheritance).

In patients with primary pulmonary hypertension, abnormal thickening and loss of elasticity of pulmonary arterial walls may cause abnormal obstruction and increased resistance of the blood flow from the right ventricle to the lungs. Consequently, the heart muscle must pump harder and at a higher pressure to adequately propel blood through the pulmonary artery, leading to enlargement of the right ventricle. Affected individuals may experience exercise intolerance (inability to do physical exercise at the level that would be expected of someone in his or her general physical condition), easy fatigability, and, in some cases, dizziness, fainting episodes (syncope), headaches, and chest pain. In addition, as the right ventricle begins to weaken in its ability to pump blood efficiently (right ventricular failure), patients may experience cyanosis, coldness of the affected limbs, enlargement of the liver (hepatomegaly), and an abnormal accumulation of fluid in body tissues (edema). Patients with severe pulmonary hypertension may experience sudden abnormalities in the rhythm or rate of the heartbeat (arrhythmias), resulting in life-threatening complications. Supportive therapies for the treatment of primary pulmonary hypertension may include intravenous administration of the medication prostacyclin to help widen pulmonary arteries (vasodilation) and increase blood flow. In addition, in some patients, the administration of calcium channel blocking agents by mouth may be beneficial. In many patients with severe primary pulmonary hypertension, heart-lung or lung transplantation may be required.

Government Agencies

6074 NIH/ Eunice Kennedy Shriver National Insti tute of Child Health & Human Development
31 Center Drive, Building 31
Bethesda, MD 20892

301-496-5113
800-370-2943
Fax: 866-760-5947
nichdpress@mail.nih.gov
www.nichd.nih.gov

Established in 1962 by congress, today the institute conducts and supports research on topics related to the health of children, adults, families and populations. Some of these topics include: developmental disabilities, growth and development, infant death, reproductive health and birth defects.

Diana W. Bianchi, Director
Paul Williams, Director, Communications

6075 NIH/National Heart, Lung and Blood Institu te
National Institute of Health
PO Box 30105
Bethesda, MD 20824

301-592-8573
Fax: 240-629-3246
TTY: 240-629-3255
nhlbiinfo@nhlbi.nih.gov
www.nhlbi.nih.gov

Primary responsibility of this organization is the scientific investigation of heart, blood vessel, lung and blood disorders. Oversees research, demonstration, prevention, education, control and training activities in these fields and emphasizes the prevention and control of heart diseases.

Gary H Gibbons, MD, Director
Nakela Cook, MD, Chief of Staff

National Associations & Support Groups

6076 American Academy of Pediatrics
141 Northwest Point Boulevard
Elk Grove Village, IL 60007

847-434-4000
800-433-9016
Fax: 847-434-8000
www.aap.org

The American Academy of Pediatrics and its member pediatricians are committed to the attainment of optimal physical, mental and social health and well-being for all infants, children, adolescents, and young adults.

Fernando Stein, MD, FAAP, President
Karen Remley, MD, CEO/Executive VP

6077 American Heart Association
7272 Greenville Avenue
Dallas, TX 75231
214-373-6300
800-242-8721
Fax: 214-706-1341
inquire@amhrt.org
www.heart.org/HEARTORG/

Supports research, education and community service programs with the objective of reducing premature death and disability from cardiovascular diseases and stroke; coordinates the efforts of health professionals, and others engaged in the fight against heart and circulatory disease.

Nancy Brown, CEO
Dr. Stephen Houser, President
Suzie Upton, Chief Operating Officer

6078 American Lung Association
55 W. Wacker Drive, Suite 1150
Chicago, IL 60601
312-801-7628
800-586-4872
info@lung.org
www.lung.org

The American Lung Association fights lung disease in all its forms, with special emphasis on asthma, tobacco control and environmental health. The American Lung Association is funded with contributions from the public, along with gifts and grants from corporations, foundations and government agencies. The association achieves its many successes through the work of thousands of committed volunteers and staff.

Harold P. Wimmer, National President & CEO
Susan Rappaport, National VP, Research/Scientific
Sue Swan, Chief Development Officer

6079 Genetic Alliance
4301 Connecticut Avenue NW, Suite 404
Washington, DC 20008
202-966-5557
800-336-4363
Fax: 202-966-8553
info@geneticalliance.org
www.geneticalliance.org

A coalition of voluntary genetic support groups, consumers and professionals addressing the needs of individuals and families affected by genetic disorders from a national perspective.

Sharon Terry, President/CEO
Tetyana Murza, Managing Director
Natasha Bonhomme, VP, Strategic Development

6080 March of Dimes Foundation
1275 Mamaroneck Avenue
White Plains, NY 10605
914-997-4488
888-663-4637
Fax: 914-428-8203
answers@marchofdimes.com
www.marchofdimes.com

Partnership of volunteers and professionals dedicates to improving the health of babies by preventing birth defects and infant mortality. Over 100 chapters are located across the country and can be located through the National Office.

Stacey D. Stewart, President

6081 Pulmonary Hypertension Association
801 Roeder Road, Ste 1000
Silver Spring, MD 20910
301-565-3004
800-748-7274
Fax: 301-565-3994
pha@phassociation.org
www.phassociation.org

PHA's mission is to seek a cure; provide hope, support and education; promote awareness, and advocate for the pulmonary hypertension community.

Rino Aldrighetti, Owner
Adrienne Dern, VP
Debbie Castro, Director Volunteer Services

Web Sites

6082 MayoClinic.com - Pulmonary Hypertension
13400 E. Shea Blvd.
Scottsdale, AZ 85259
480-301-8000
800-446-2279
mayoclinic.com/health/pulmonary-hypertension/DS00430

Introduction to the disorder, signs, symptoms, treatment, etc.

Samuel A. Di Piazza, Jr., Chairman
John H. Noseworthy, M.D., CEO and President
Jeffrey W.˜ Bolton, CAO and Vice President

DESCRIPTION

6083 PULMONARY VALVE STENOSIS

Covers these related disorders: Critical pulmonic stenosis
Involves the following Biologic System(s):
Cardiovascular Disorders

Pulmonary valve stenosis is a congenital heart defect characterized by abnormal narrowing (stenosis) of the valve between the lower right-sided, pumping chamber of the heart (right ventricle) and the pulmonary artery. Situated where the pulmonary artery arises from the base of the right ventricle, the pulmonary valve enables blood to flow from the right ventricle to the lungs while preventing the backward flow of blood. The pulmonary artery carries oxygen-depleted (deoxygenated) blood to the lungs, where the exchange of oxygen and carbon dioxide occurs. In infants and children with pulmonary valve stenosis, narrowing of the pulmonary valve opening increases resistance of the blood flow from the right ventricle to the pulmonary artery. As a result, the heart muscle must pump harder and at a higher pressure to propel blood to the pulmonary artery, potentially leading to thickening of the heart muscle (hypertrophy) of the right ventricle. Pulmonary valve stenosis affects approximately one in 1,250 individuals in the general population, comprising approximately 10 percent of all heart defects that are present at birth (congenital heart defects). Less commonly, pulmonary stenosis may be due to structural abnormalities other than a restricted valvular opening, such as narrowing within the upper region of the right ventricle or a portion of the pulmonary artery (e.g., isolated infundibular stenosis, branch pulmonary artery stenosis).

In infants and children with pulmonary valve stenosis, the severity of associated symptoms may vary, depending on the size of the restricted valvular opening and, in some patients, the presence of additional heart defects. For example, some affected children may also have relatively small septal defects, such as an abnormal opening in the fibrous partition (septum) that divides the ventricles or the two upper chambers (atria) of the heart (ventricular or atrial septal defects). Infants and children with mild pulmonary valve stenosis usually have no associated symptoms (asymptomatic), do not experience hypertrophy of heart muscle, and have normal growth and development. In such patients, the condition is usually initially suspected due to detection of characteristic, abnormal heart sounds (heart murmurs) during a physician's examination with a stethoscope. In patients with moderate pulmonary valve stenosis, the right ventricle may be of normal size or mildly thickened. Although such patients are usually asymptomatic, others may experience some symptoms, such as easy fatigability and exercise intolerance.

In newborns or young infants with severe pulmonary valve stenosis, the right ventricle may be unable to pump blood adequately (right ventricular failure) and become moderately or severely enlarged. Findings associated with right ventricular failure may include poor feeding, enlargement of the liver (hepatomegaly), an abnormal accumulation of fluid in body tissues (edema) or other abnormalities. In addition, blood may begin to circulate through a previously closed fetal opening in the heart (foramen ovale) between the left and right atria that closes shortly after birth. Abnormal opening of the foramen ovale in those with pulmonary valve stenosis may

cause oxygen-depleted blood to pass from the right to the left side of the atria (right-to-left shunting), into the left ventricle and into the aorta for transport to the body's tissues. Because this oxygen-depleted blood bypasses the lungs and instead recirculates throughout the body, bodily tissues receive less oxygenated blood (hypoxia). In such cases, affected newborns or infants are said to have critical pulmonic stenosis. In addition, in some infants, certain associated heart (cardiac) defects, such as atrial or ventricular septal defects, may also allow some mixing of oxygen-poor and oxygen-rich blood. Due to recirculation of oxygen-poor blood to the body's tissues, affected newborns or infants may experience mild to moderate bluish discoloration of the skin and mucous membranes (cyanosis), shortness of breath (dyspnea), and other serious symptoms and findings.

In these newborns or infants, emergency procedures are performed to widen the restricted valvular opening. Such procedures may include inflation of a balloon-tipped cathet|er (valvuloplasty) or surgical correction or resection of the valve (valvotomy). Although corrective measures may not be required in those with mild stenosis, such patients should receive regular follow-up evaluations. Such monitoring is necessary to ensure appropriate intervention for patients who may potentially experience increasing obstruction across the pulmonary valve or increasing hypertrophy of the right ventricle requiring surgical intervention. Other treatment is symptomatic and supportive.

Pulmonary valve stenosis may occur as a spontaneous, isolated finding; with other congenital heart defects; or in association with certain underlying disorders (e.g., Noonan syndrome). In some patients, the condition is thought to be determined by the interactions of several different genes, possibly in association with the involvement of certain environmental factors (multifactorial inheritance).

Government Agencies

6084 NIH/ Eunice Kennedy Shriver National Insti tute of Child Health & Human Development
31 Center Drive, Building 31
Bethesda, MD 20892
301-496-5113
800-370-2943
Fax: 866-760-5947
nichdpress@mail.nih.gov
www.nichd.nih.gov

Established in 1962 by congress, today the institute conducts and supports research on topics related to the health of children, adults, families and populations. Some of these topics include: developmental disabilities, growth and development, infant death, reproductive health and birth defects.

Diana W. Bianchi, Director
Paul Williams, Director, Communications

6085 NIH/National Heart, Lung and Blood Institu te
National Institute of Health
31 Center Dr MSC 2486, Bldg 31, Room 5A52
Bethesda, MD 20892
301-592-8573
Fax: 240-629-3246
TTY: 240-629-3255
NHLBIinfo@nhlbi.nih.gov
www.nhlbi.nih.gov

Primary responsibility of this organization is the scientific investigation of heart, blood vessel, lung and blood disorders. Oversees research, demonstration, prevention, education, control and training activities in these fields and emphasizes the prevention and control of heart diseases.

Gary H Gibbons, MD, Director
Nakela Cook, MD, Chief of Staff

National Associations & Support Groups

6086 American Academy of Pediatrics
141 Northwest Point Boulevard
Elk Grove Village, IL 60007
847-434-4000
800-433-9016
Fax: 847-434-8000
www.aap.org

The American Academy of Pediatrics and its member pediatricians are committed to the attainment of optimal physical, mental and social health and well-being for all infants, children, adolescents, and young adults.

Fernando Stein, MD, FAAP, President
Karen Remley, MD, CEO/Executive VP

6087 American Heart Association
7272 Greenville Avenue
Dallas, TX 75231
214-373-6300
800-242-8721
Fax: 214-706-1341
inquire@amhrt.org
www.heart.org/HEARTORG/

Supports research, education and community service programs with the objective of reducing premature death and disability from cardiovascular diseases and stroke; coordinates the efforts of health professionals, and others engaged in the fight against heart and circulatory disease.

Nancy Brown, CEO
Dr. Stephen Houser, President
Suzie Upton, Chief Operating Officer

6088 Division of Pediatric Pulmonology
New York Medical College
Pediatric Specialty Ctr, 19 Bradhurst Avenue
Hawthorne, NY 10532
914-372-3010
Fax: 914-594-4336
pedpulm@nymc.edu
www.nymc.edu

The division is dedicated to teaching and patient care.

6089 Genetic Alliance
4301 Connecticut Avenue NW, Suite 404
Washington, DC 20008
202-966-5557
800-336-4363
Fax: 202-966-8553
info@geneticalliance.org
www.geneticalliance.org

A coalition of voluntary genetic support groups, consumers and professionals addressing the needs of individuals and families affected by genetic disorders from a national perspective.

Sharon Terry, President/CEO
Tetyana Murza, Managing Director
Natasha Bonhomme, VP, Strategic Development

6090 March of Dimes Foundation
1275 Mamaroneck Avenue
White Plains, NY 10605
914-997-4488
888-663-4637
Fax: 914-428-8203
answers@marchofdimes.com
www.marchofdimes.com

Partnership of volunteers and professionals dedicates to improving the health of babies by preventing birth defects and infant mortality. Over 100 chapters are located across the country and can be located through the National Office.

Stacey D. Stewart, President

Web Sites

6091 Congenital Heart Information Network
www.tchin.org

An international organization that provides reliable information, support services and resources to families of children with congenital heart defects and acquired heart disease, adults with congenital heart defects, and the professionals who work with them.

6092 Southern Illinois University School of Medicine
PO Box 19658
Springfield, IL 62794
217-545-8000
800-342-5748
www.siumed.edu/peds/index.htm

The mission of SUI School of Medicine is to assist the people of central and southern Illinois in meeting their present and future health care needs through education, clinical service and research.

Book Publishers

6093 Congenital Disorders Sourcebook
Omnigraphics
PO Box 625
Holmes, PA 19043
800-234-1340
Fax: 800-875-1340
info@omnigraphics.com
www.omnigraphics.com

Basic consumer health information on disorders aquired during gestation, including spina bifida, hydrocephalus, cerebral palsy, heart defects, craniofacial abnormalities and fetal alcohol syndrome.

650 pages
ISBN: 0-780809-45-9

Peter Ruffner, Publisher

DESCRIPTION

6094 PYLORIC STENOSIS

Synonym: Infantile pyloric stenosis

Involves the following Biologic System(s):

Gastrointestinal Disorders

Pyloric stenosis refers to a condition in which the passageway (pyloric canal) that leads from the stomach to the first part of the small intestine known as the duodenum is narrowed or obstructed due to the thickening of the muscle that surrounds this opening (pyloric sphincter). Although the specific cause for this thickening is not known, many factors may be responsible, including breast-feeding, irregularities in nerve distribution to the muscle, and certain disorders such as Turner syndrome, Cornelia de Lange syndrome, trisomy 18 syndrome, and eosinophilic gastroenteritis. Pyloric stenosis is also commonly associated with certain birth defects of the gastrointestinal tract such as tracheoesophageal fistula.

Symptoms and findings associated with this disorder may develop as early as the first week of life; however, in some infants, this abnormality does not cause noticeable symptoms until the fourth or fifth month. At about the third week of life, episodes of forceful and explosive vomiting (projectile vomiting) may occur. After eating, rhythmic, wave-like movements (peristalsis) may be visible in the infant's abdominal area. Prolonged vomiting may result in excessive fluid loss (dehydration) and loss of essential elements known as electrolytes in the fluid portion of the blood (e.g., sodium, potassium, and calcium).

Treatment for infantile pyloric stenosis includes the administration of fluids to counteract the effects of dehydration. Once body fluids and electrolytes stabilize, a surgical procedure known as a pyloromyotomy may be performed. During this procedure, a lengthwise incision is made along the thickened pyloric muscle to correct the defect.

Pyloric stenosis affects approximately three in every 1,000 infants in the United States. Boys are more often affected than girls by a ratio of four to one. Children of parents who had pyloric stenosis are approximately 10 to 20 percent more likely to be affected. Infants with types B or O blood develop this defect more often than those with other blood types.

National Associations & Support Groups

6095 American Academy of Pediatrics

141 Northwest Point Boulevard
Elk Grove Village, IL 60007

847-434-4000
800-433-9016
Fax: 847-434-8000
www.aap.org

The American Academy of Pediatrics and its member pediatricians are committed to the attainment of optimal physical, mental and social health and well-being for all infants, children, adolescents, and young adults.

Fernando Stein, MD, FAAP, President
Karen Remley, MD, CEO/Executive VP

6096 American College of Gastroenterology

6400 Goldsboro Road, Suite 200
Bethesda, MD 20817

301-263-9000
info@acg.gi.org
www.gi.org

Founded to advance the scientific study and medical practice of diseases of the gastrointestinal (GI) tract.

13,000 members

Carol A. Burke, MD, FACG, President

6097 Cyclic Vomiting Syndrome Association

10520 W Bluemound Road, Suite #106
Milwaukee, WI 53226

414-342-7880
Fax: ÿ41- 34- 898
ÿcvsa@cvsaonline.org
www.cvsaonline.org

A volunteer organization serving the needs of CVS patients, their families around the world and the growing medical community studying CVS. The network has grown to over 37 medical advisors and over 90 volunteers in over 32 countries.

$75/year

Kathleen Adams, President/Research Liaison

6098 Digestive Disease National Coalition

507 Capitol Court NE, Suite 200
Washington, DC 20002

202-544-7497
Fax: 202-546-7105
hpayne@hmcw.org
www.ddnc.org

Advocacy organization comprised of over 30 voluntary and professional societies concerned with the many diseases of the digestive tract and liver.

Lynn Seim, Chairperson
Ralph McKibbin, President
Cathy Griffith, Vice Chairperson

6099 International Foundation for Functional Gastrointestinal Disorders

PO Box 170864
Milwaukee, WI 53217

414-964-1799
Fax: 414-964-7176
iffgd@iffgd.org
www.iffgd.org

Nonprofit education and research organization founded in 1991. IFFGD addresses the issues surrounding life with gastrointestinal (GI) functional and mobility disorders and increases the awareness about these disorders among the general public, researchers and the clinical care community.

Nancy J. Norton, President & Director
William Norton, Co-Founder

6100 March of Dimes Foundation

1275 Mamaroneck Avenue
White Plains, NY 10605

914-997-4488
888-663-4637
Fax: 914-428-8203
answers@marchofdimes.com
www.marchofdimes.com

Partnership of volunteers and professionals dedicates to improving the health of babies by preventing birth defects and infant mortality. Over 100 chapters are located across the country and can be located through the National Office.

Stacey D. Stewart, President

6101 North American Society for Pediatric Gastroenterology/Hepatology/Nutrition

714 N Bethlehem Pike, Suite 300
Ambler, PA 19002

215-641-9800
Fax: 215-641-1995
naspghan@naspghan.org
www.naspghan.org

Strives to improve the care of infants, children and adolescents with digestive disorders by promoting advances in clinical care of children with chronic abdominal pain, diarrhea, constipation, vomiting, bleeding from the GI tract, inflammatory bowel disease, liver diseases, diseases of the pancreas, poor weight gain and nutritional problems.

Margaret K Stallings, Executive Director
Kim Rose, Associate Director
Donna Murphy, Membership

6102 Pediatric/Adolescent Gastroesophageal Reflux Association (PAGER)
PO Box 7728
Silver Spring, MD 20907
301-601-9541
GERGROUP@aol.com
www.reflux.org

Non profit organization providing information and support to parents and children dealing with gastroesophageal reflux.

Beth Anderson, Director
Jan Gambino-Burns, Associate Director

Libraries & Resource Centers

6103 National Digestive Diseases Information Clearinghouse
9000 Rockville Pike
Bethesda, MD 20892
301-496-3583
800-860-8747
Fax: 703-738-4929
healthinfo@niddk.nih.gov
www.niddk.nih.govv

The National Institute of Diabetes and Digestive and Kidney Diseases conducts and supports research on many of the most serious diseases affecting public health. The Institute supports much of the clinical research on the diseases of internal medicine and related subspecialty fields as well as many basic science disciplines.

Dr. Griffin P. Rodgers, Director
Dr. Gregory G. Germino, Deputy Directortary
Camille M. Hoover, M.S.W., Executive Officer

Web Sites

6104 American Pediatric Surgical Association
111 Deer Lake Road, Suite 100
Deerfield, IL 60015
847-480-9576
Fax: 847-480-9282
eapsa@eapsa.org
www.eapsa.org/parents/pyloric.htm

For parents: an overview of Pyloric Stenosis including synptoms, treatment and complications.

Michael D. Klein, President
Mary L. Brandt, Secretary
Daniel von Almen, Treasurer

6105 Dr. Koop
750 Third Avenue, 6th Floor
New York, NY 10017
212-695-2223
Fax: 212-695-2936
www.healthcentral.com

Information on the condition, causes, symptoms, tests and treatment.

Micheael Cunnion, Chief Executive Officer
Jim Curtis, Chief Revenue Officer
Rebecca Farwell, Chief Content Officer

6106 KidsHealth-Pyloric Stenosis
www.kidshealth.org/parent/

Definition, causes, symptoms, treatment and complications.

Neil Izenberg, MD, Editor-in-Chief & Founder

6107 MEDLINEplus Medical Encyclopedia: Pyloric Stenosis
8600 Rockville Pike
Bethesda, MD 20894lm.nih.gov/medlineplus/ency/article/000970.htm

Definitions, causes, symptoms, treatment, prognosis and complications.

Donald A.B. Lindberg, Director

6108 National Digestive Diseases Information Clearinghouse
Bethesda, MD 20892
301-496-3583
www.digestive.niddk.nih.gov

The National Institute of Diabetes and Digestive and Kidney Diseases conducts and supports research on many of the most serious diseases affecting public health. The Institute supports much of the clinical research on the diseases of internal medicine and related subspecialty fields as well as many basic science disciplines.

Griffin P. Rodgers, M.D., M.A.C.P., Director

6109 Online Mendelian Inheritance in Man
National Library of Medicine, Building 38A
Bethesda, MD 20894
888-346-3656
info@ncbi.nlm.nih.gov
www.ncbi.nlm.nih.gov

This database is a catalog of human genes and genetic disorders.

6110 Southern Illinois University School of Medicine
PO Box 19658
Springfield, IL 62794
217-545-8000
800-342-5748
www.siumed.edu/peds/index.htm

The mission of SUI School of Medicine is to assist the people of central and southern Illinois in meeting their present and future health care needs through education, clinical service and research.

Journals

6111 Journal of Pediatric Gastroenterology and Nutrition
NASPGHAN, author

Lippincott Williams & Wilkins
530 Walnut Street
Philadelphia, PA 19106
215-521-8300
Fax: 215-521-8902
www.lww.com

Publication of the North American Society for Pediatric Gastroenterolgy, Hepatology and Nutrition, which strives to improve the care of infants, children and adolescents with digestive disorders by promoting advances in clinical care of children with chronic abdominal pain, diarrhea, constipation, vomiting, bleeding from the GI tract, inflammatory bowel disease, liver diseases, diseases of the pancreas, poor weight gain and nutritional problems.

Newsletters

6112 NASPGHAN News
714 N. Bethlehem Pike, Ste 300
Ambler, PA 19002
215-641-9800
Fax: 215-641-1995
naspghan@naspghan.org
www.naspgn.org

Publication of the North American Society for Pediatric Gastroenterolgy, Hepatology and Nutrition, which strives to improve the care of infants, children and adolescents with digestive disorders by promoting advances in clinical care of children with chronic abdominal pain, diarrhea, constipation, vomiting, bleeding from the GI tract, inflammatory bowel disease, liver diseases, diseases of the pancreas, poor weight gain and nutritional problems.

Margaret K Stallings, Executive Director
Kim Rose, Associate Director
Donna Murphy, Membership

DESCRIPTION

6113 REFRACTION DISTURBANCES

Synonym: Ametropia

Disorder Type: Vision

Covers these related disorders: Anisometropia, Astigmatism, Hyperopia (Farsightedness), Myopia (Nearsightedness)

Involves the following Biologic System(s):

Ophthalmologic Disorders

Refraction abnormalities are defects in the cornea and the lens of the eye to focus visual images appropriately on the nerve-rich membrane at the back of the eye (retina). The cornea is the convex, transparent area in front of the eye. The lens, which is located behind the pupil, is held in place by a circular muscle that changes the shape of the lens to make appropriate adjustments in focus (ciliary muscle). As light passes through the cornea and the lens, it is bent (refracted) so that it is properly focused on the retina, which contains millions of tiny nerve cells that respond to light (photoreceptors). However, in individuals with refraction defects, light rays are not properly focused on the retina (ametropia) due to abnormalities of the cornea, the lens, or the size of the eye. These refraction defects lead to visual abnormalities.

There are three primary types of refraction abnormalities: namely, farsightedness (hyperopia), nearsightedness (myopia), and astigmatism. In farsightedness, parallel light rays come to focus behind rather that on the retina. This may be due to shortness of the eyeball from front to back, abnormally reduced refractive power of the cornea or lens, or backward displacement of the lens. If farsightedness is mild or moderate, affected children may be able to clearly visualize near and far objects due to accommodation, a process by which the shape of the lens changes and brings the area of focus forward. The range and extent of accommodation is highest durign childhood and gradually decreases with age. With greater degrees of farsightedness, affected children may experience blurring of vision, eyestrain, fatigue, and recurrent headaches. They may also engage in repeated eye rubbing and squinting and appear uninterested in reading or schoolwork. Children with farsightedness may achieve clear vision with glasses or contact lenses with convex lenses.

In children with nearsightedness (myopia), parallel light rays come to focus in front of the retina due to increased length of the eyeball from front to back, abnormally increased refractive power of the cornea or lens, or forward displacement of the lens. Affected children experience blurring of vision when focusing on distant objects, tend to hold reading material and other objects close to their face, and often squint in an effort to improve clearness and clarity of vision. Nearsightedness usually becomes apparent during school age, particularly in the years prior to and up to adolescence. The degree of nearsightedness typically becomes more severe until early adulthood, when it tends to stabilize. Many affected children have a hereditary predisposition for nearsightedness; in addition, the condition may occur in association with other eye abnormalities (e.g., glaucoma, keratoconus) or other underlying disorders. Clear vision may be attained with glasses or contact lenses with concave lenses. Until the degree of nearsightedness stabilizes, prescriptions may need to be periodically increased in strength (e.g., varying from every few months to once every one or two years).

In children with astigmatism, parallel light rays are not clearly focused in a point on the retina due to unequal curvature of refractive surfaces of the eye. Astigmatism may result from irregularities in curvature of the cornea or, in some cases, abnormalities of the lens. Many individuals have minor degrees of astigmatism and have no associated symptoms. With more severe degrees of astigmatism, affected children may experience blurring and distortion of vision, fatigue, eyestrain, and recurrent headaches. In many cases, they may also engage in frequent eye rubbing, squint in an attempt to improve clearness and clarity of vision, hold reading materials and other objects close, and appear uninterested in schoolwork. In children with astigmatism, visual correction may be achieved with the part-time or ongoing use of glasses with cylindric or spherocylindric lenses. In some cases, contact lenses may be used to help correct vision.

Some children may also have a visual condition known as anisometropia in which the refractive or focusing ability of one eye significantly differs from the other. For example, one eye may have normal focusing ability, whereas the other may be affected by nearsightedness, farsightedness, and astigmatism. For proper vision to develop during infancy and early childhood, corresponding visual images mustform on both retinas to ensure the transmission of compatible nerve impulses (via the optic nerves) to the brain. If the images from one eye differ dramatically from the other, one may be suppressed, causing impaired visual development in one eye (amblyopia). Therefore, in infants and children with anisometropia, prompt detection and appropriate visual correction is essential to ensure proper visual development in both eyes.

Government Agencies

6114 NIH/National Eye Institute
31 Center Drive MSC 2510
Bethesda, MD 20892

301-496-5248
2020@nei.nih.gov
www.nei.nih.gov

Conducts and supports research that helps prevent and treat eye diseases and other disorders of vision. This research leads to sight-saving treatments, reduces visual impairment and blindness, and improves the quality of life for people of all ages. NEI-supported research has advanced our knowledge of how the eye functions in health and disease.

Paul A Sieving MD, PhD, Director

National Associations & Support Groups

6115 American Academy of Pediatrics
141 Northwest Point Boulevard
Elk Grove Village, IL 60007

847-434-4000
800-433-9016
Fax: 847-434-8000
www.aap.org

The American Academy of Pediatrics and its member pediatricians are committed to the attainment of optimal physical, mental and social health and well-being for all infants, children, adolescents, and young adults.

Fernando Stein, MD, FAAP, President
Karen Remley, MD, CEO/Executive VP

6116 Division on Visual Impairments
Council for Exceptional Children
1110 North Glebe Road, Suite 300
Arlington, VA 22201   800-224-6830
                                        Fax: 703-264-9494
                                        TTY: 866-915-5000
        www.ed.arizona.edu/dvi/welcome.htm; www.cec.sped.org

A division within the CEC, it handles concerns for Federal, state
and local issues and policies related to education of youths, children and infants with visual impairments.

Ellyn Ross, President
Shirley J Wilson, Secretary
Phyllis T Simmons, President Elect

6117 Lighthouse Guild
15 West 65th Street
New York, NY 10023   212-769-6200
                                             800-284-4422
                                      info@lighthouseguild.org
                                      www.lighthouseguild.org

Since 1905, Lighthouse International has led the charge in the
fight against vision loss through prevention, treatment and empowerment. In 2013, it merged with Jewish Guild Healthcare to
form a leading non profit vision and healthcare organization.

Alan R. Morse, President/CEO
Mark G. Ackermann, Executive VP/COO
Maura J. Sweeney, Senior VP, Programs & Services

6118 National Alliance of Blind Students
c/o Terry Pacheco
1155 15th Street NW, Suite 1004
Washington, DC 20005   202-467-5081
                                             800-424-8666
                                        Fax: 202-467-5085
                                      rj.hodson@verizon.net
                                        www.blindstudents.org

An advocacy and consumer organization for high school and college students who are blind or visually impaired. It works to facilitate progress toward full accessibility of college programs and
facilities, provides opportunities for discussion of issues important to students and assists with National Student Seminars.

Rebecca Hodson, President

**6119 National Association for Parents of Childr en with Visual
Impairments**
PO Box 317
Watertown, MA 02471   617-972-7441
                                             800-562-6265
                                        Fax: 617-972-7444
                                          napvi@perkins.org
                                        www.spedex.com/napvi/

Offers emotional support for parents of blind or visually impaired
children. Provides information, training and assistance, and help
in understanding and using available resources.

6120 National Association for Visually Handicapped
22 W 21st Street, 6th Floor
New York, NY 10010   212-889-3141
                                             888-205-5951
                                        Fax: 212-727-2931
                                          navh@navh.org
                                          www.navh.org

Serves as a clearinghouse for information about all services available to the partially-sighted from public and private sources. Conducts self-help groups. Provides information on large print books,
textbooks and educational tools.

Lorianie Marchi, CEO

State Agencies & Support Groups

Alabama

6121 Alabama Institute for the Deaf & Blind
PO Box 698
Talladega, AL 35161   256-761-3331
                                        Fax: 256-761-3344
                                             www.aidb.org

Services include central directory, representatives of agencies,
service providers, families, and coordinators of infant, toddler,
and preschool special education programs.

Terry Graham, President

Arizona

6122 National Association for Parents of the Visually Impaired
PO Box 317
Watertown, MA 02471   617-972-7441
                                             800-562-6265
                                        Fax: 617-972-7444
                                        www.spedex.com/napvi

Mary Ellen Simmons

California

6123 Blind Childrens Center
4120 Marathon Street
Los Angeles, CA 90029   323-664-2153
                                        Fax: 323-665-3828
                                   www.blindchildrenscenter.org

Family-centered agency that serves children with visual impairments from birth to school age. The center-based programs and
services help the children acquire skills and build their independence.

Midge Horton, Executive Director

Connecticut

**6124 Region 1 of the National Association for Parents of the Visually
Impaired**
252 Rye Street
Broad Brook, CT 06016   860-623-4129
Susan Ellsworth

Georgia

6125 Southeastern Region-Helen Keller National Center
1003 Virginia Avenue, Suite 104
Atlanta, GA 30354   404-766-9625
                                        Fax: 404-766-3447
                                        TTY: 404-766-2820

Susan Lascek, Supervisor of Reg Representatives

Illinois

6126 National Association for Parents of the Visually Impaired
PO Box 317
Watertown, MA 02471   617-972-7441
                                             800-562-6265
                                        Fax: 617-972-7444
                                        www.spedex.com/napvi

Mary Ellen Simmons

**6127 Region 3 of the National Association for Parents of the Visually
Impaired**
16 Thornfield Lane
Hawthorn Woods, IL 60047   847-438-0705
Kevin O'Connor

Kansas

6128 Great Plains Region-Helen Keller National Center
4330 Shawhee Mission Parkway, suite 108
Shawnee, KS 66205
913-677-4562
Fax: 913-677-1544
beth.jordan@hknc.org
www.helenkeller.org

Services are free and offer client advocacy, consultation and technical assistance to schools and agencies; assistance in developing local services information and referral; public education and awareness; maintenance of the National Registry.

Beth Jordan, Regional Representative

Maryland

6129 National Organization of Parents of Blind Children
350 Ignacio Blvd., Suite 200
Novato,, CA 94949
415-382-2530
Fax: 410-685-5653
nfb@iamdiyrx.net
www.nfh.org

Informational and emotional support to parents who have a child, adolescent, or adult family member with blindness or visual impairment.

Massachusetts

6130 New England Region-Helen Keller National Center
313 Washington Street
Newton, MA 02458
617-630-1580
Fax: 617-630-1579
hkncmeb@aol.com

New Mexico

6131 Region 5 of the National Association for Parents of the Visually Impaired
PO Box 1337
Alamogordo, NM 88311
505-682-2693

Ohio

6132 Region 2 of the National Association for Parents of the Visually Impaired
3910 Pocahontas Avenue
Cincinnati, OH 45227
513-561-8542
Victoria Gorman Miller

Pennsylvania

6133 East Central Region-Helen Keller National Center
4351 Garden City Drive
New Carrollton, MD 20785
301-459-5474
Fax: 301-459-5070
hkncreg3cl@aol.com
www.helenkeller.org

South Carolina

6134 Region 4 of the National Association for Parents of the Visually Impaired
1032 Trail Road
Belton, SC 29627
864-338-9593

Washington

6135 Northwestern Region-Helen Keller National Center
2366 Eastlake Avenue E
Seattle, WA 98102
206-324-9120
nwhknc@juno.com

Libraries & Resource Centers

Alabama

6136 Mobile Association for the Blind
2440 Gordon Smith Drive
Mobile, AL 36617
251-473-3585
Fax: 251-470-8622
www.mobileblind.org

Offers work adjustment training, activities of daily living, mobility, communication skills and sheltered employment for adults and children who are visually impaired.

Jim Bullock, Executive Director

Arizona

6137 Educational Services for the Visually Impaired
2402 Wildwood Avenue Suite 112
Sherwood, AR 72120
501-371-5448

Offers textbooks, Braille books and more to the visually impaired grades K-12 in the Arkansas area.

David Beavers, Director

Arkansas

6138 Arkansas Regional Library for the Blind and Physically Handicapped
1 Capitol Mall
Little Rock, AR 72201
501-682-1527
Fax: 501-682-1533
TDD: 501-682-1002
mindy@library.arkansas.gov
www.asl.lib.ar.us/ASL_LBPH.htm

Public library books in recorded or Braille format. Popular fiction and nonfiction books for all ages, books and players are on free loan, sent to patrons by mail and may be returned postage free. Anyone who cannot see well enough to read regular print with glasses on or who has a disability that makes it difficult to hold a book or turn the pages is eligible.

John D Hall, Director

California

6139 American Action Fund for Blind Children and Adults
18440 Oxnard Street
Tarzana, CA 91356
818-343-2022
Fax: 818-343-3219
lucyabba@aol.com
www.actinfund.org

A lending library for the visually impaired. We send out a weekly Braille newspaper for the deaf-blind (worldwide), we also send out pocket-sized Braille calendars. Our lending library is for pre-school thru high school. All of our services are free.

Lucille Abbazia, Manager

6140 Blind Children's Center
4120 Marathon Street
Los Angeles, CA 90029
323-664-2153
Fax: 323-665-3828
www.blindchildrenscenter.org

Offers support and informational groups.

Scott E. Schaldenbrand, President,Executive Committee
Danette M. Jones, Vice President
Lisa D. Hansen, Secretary

6141 Braille Institute Desert Center
70-251 Ramon Road
Rancho Mirage, CA 92270   760-321-1111
                                 Fax: 760-321-9715
                                 dc@brailleinstitute.org
                                 www.brailleinstitute.org

Dedicated to providing blind and visually impaired men, women
and children with the training, programs and services they need to
enjoy productive lives. Services offered include child development, youth programs, library services and adult education.

Lester M Sussman, Chairman
James B. Boyle Jr., Director
Thomas K. Callister, Director

6142 Braille Institute Sight Center
741 N Vermont Avenue
Los Angeles, CA 90029   323-663-1111
                                 Fax: 323-663-0867
                                 la@brailleinstitute.org
                                 www.brailleinstitute.org

Offers help, programs, services and information to the blind and
visually impaired children and adults.

Lester M Sussman, Chairman
James B. Boyle Jr., Director
Thomas K. Callister, Director

6143 Braille Institute Youth Center
741 N Vermont Avenue
Los Angeles, CA 90029   323-663-1111
                                 Fax: 323-663-0867
                                 la@brailleinstitute.org
                                 www.brailleinstitute.org

Offers various youth programs and services for the blind and visually impaired youngster.

Lester M Sussman, Chairman
James B. Boyle Jr., Director
Thomas K. Callister, Director

6144 New Beginnings - Blind Children's Center
4120 Marathon, Street
Los Angeles, CA 90029   323-664-2153
                                 800-222-3566
                                 Fax: 323-665-3828

Helps children and their families become independent by creating
a climate of safety and trust. Services include an infant stimulation program, educational preschool, interdisciplinary assessment
services, family services, correspondence program, toll-free national hotline and a publication and research service.

6145 San Francisco Public Library for the Blind and Print Disabled
100 Larkin Street
San Francisco, CA 94102   415-557-4400
                                 Fax: 415-557-4252
                                 lbphmgr@sfpl.lib.ca.us
                                 www.library.ca.us

Foreign-language books on cassette, children's books on cassettes
and more.

Luis Herrera, Manager

6146 Variety Audio
PO Box 5731
San Jose, CA 95150   408-277-4839

Summer reading programs, Braille writer, magnifiers, closed-circuit TV, large-print photocopier, cassette books and magazines,
children's books on cassette, home visits and other reference materials on blindness and other handicaps.

Louisa Griehshammer

6147 Council of Families with Visual Impairment
1155 15th Street NW
Washington, DC 20005   202-467-5081

Members are sighted parents of blind or visually impaired children. Offers a forum for support and outreach, sharing of experiences in parent-child relationships, and educational and cultural
information about child development. Monitors developments in
technical and legislative arenas.

Nola Webb, President

6148 Florida Bureau of Braille and Talking Book Library Services
1185 Dunn Avenue
Daytona Beach, FL 32114   386-254-3800
                                 Fax: 386-239-6069
                                 TDD: 800-226-6079
                                 mike_gunde@dbs.doe.state.fl.us
                                 www.state.fl.us/dbs/lswel.html

Discs, cassettes, closed-circuit TV, large-print photocopier, films,
children's books on cassettes and more.

Michael Gunde, Librarian

6149 Talking Book Library, Jacksonville Public Library
2233 Park Avenue, Suite 402
Orange Park, FL 32073   904-278-5620
                                 Fax: 904-278-5625
                                 TDD: 904-768-7822
                                 office@neflin.org
                                 www.neflin.org

Discs, cassettes and reference materials on blindness and other
disabilities.

Elizabeth Curry, President
Julie Sieg, Vice-President
Janet Loveless, Secretary

6150 Talking Book Service - Manatee County Central Library
6081 26th Street W
Bradenton, FL 34207   941-742-5914
                                 Fax: 941-751-7089
                                 TDD: 941-742-5951
                                 patricia.schubert@co.manatee.fl.us
                                 www.co.manatee.fl.us

Offers children's books on disc and cassette and more reference
materials for the blind and physically handicapped.

Patricia Schubert, Librarian

6151 Albany Library for the Blind and Physical Handicapped
300 Pine Avenue
Albany, GA 31701   229-420-3220
                                 Fax: 229-420-3215
                                 sinquefk@mail.dougherty.public.lib.ga.us
                                 www.docolib.org/LBPH/index.html

Offers discs, cassettes, reference materials on blindness and other
handicaps, large-print photocopiers, summer reading programs,
cassette books and more.

Katy Sinquefield, Manager

**6152 Bainbridge Subregional Library for the Blind and Physically
Handicapped**
301 S Monroe Street
Bainbridge, GA 39819   229-248-2665
                                 800-795-2680
                                 Fax: 229-248-2670
                                 TDD: 912-248-2665
                                 lbph@mail.deccatur.public.lib.ga.us
                                 www.swgrl.org

Discs, cassettes, summer reading programs, closed-circuit TV,
magnifiers and more.

Shelley Sudderth, Branch Manager
Susan Whittle, Director
Debbie Worthington, Administrative Secretary

6153 CEL Subregional Library for the Blind and Physically Handicapped
2708 Mechanics
Savannah, GA 31404   912-354-5864
                                          Fax: 912-354-5534
                                          TDD: 912-652-3635
                                          stokesl@cel.co.chatman.ga.us

Summer reading programs, Braille writer, magnifiers, closed-circuit TV, large-print photocopier, cassette books and magazines, children's books on cassette, home visits and other reference materials on blindness and other handicaps.

Linda Stokes, Librarian

Idaho

6154 Idaho State Talking Book Library
325 W State Street
Boise, ID 83702   208-334-2150
                                          Fax: 208-334-4016
                                          TDD: 800-377-1363
                                          tblbooks@isl.state.id.us
                                          www.lili.org/isl/tblinfo.htm

Summer reading programs, Braille writer, magnifiers, closed-circuit TV, large-print photocopier, cassette books and magazines, children's books on cassette, home visits and other reference materials on blindness and other handicaps.

Sue Walker, Manager

Illinois

6155 Chicago Library Service for the Blind
400 S State Street
Chicago, IL 60605   312-747-4300

Summer reading programs, Braille writer, magnifiers, closed-circuit TV, large-print photocopier, cassette books and magazines, children's books on cassette, home visits and other reference materials on blindness and other handicaps.

Carol Pellish, Librarian

6156 Illinois State Library, Talkng Book and Braille Service
213 State Capitol
Springfield, IL 62756   217-785-3000
                                          Fax: 217-558-4723
                                          TDD: 800-665-5576
                                          isltbbs@ilsos.net
                                          www.cyberdriveillinois.com

Summer reading programs, Braille writer, magnifiers, closed-circuit TV, large-print photocopier, cassette books and magazines, descriptive videos, children's books on cassette, home visits and other reference materials on blindness and other handicaps.

Anne Craig, Executive Director

6157 Mid Illinois Talking Book System
515 York Street
Quincy, IL 62301   217-224-6619
                                          Fax: 217-224-9818

Summer reading programs, Braille writer, magnifiers, closed-circuit TV, large-print photocopier, cassette books and magazines, children's books on cassette, home visits and other reference materials on blindness and other handicaps.

6158 Mid-Illinois Talking Book Center
600 High Point Lane #2
East Peoria, IL 61611   309-694-9200
                                          800-426-0709
                                          Fax: 309-799-7916
                                          hitbc@darkstar.rsa.lib.il.us
                                          www.mitbc.org

Summer reading programs, Braille writer, magnifiers, closed-circuit TV, large-print photocopier, cassette books and magazines, children's books on cassette, home visits and other reference materials on blindness and other handicaps.

Rose Chenoweth, Director
Valerie Brandon, Administrator

6159 Talking Book Center of Northwest Illinois
601 High Point Lane #2
East Peoria, IL 61612   309-694-9201
                                          800-426-0710
                                          Fax: 309-799-7917
                                          hitbc@darkstar.rsa.lib.il.us
                                          www.mitbc.org

Summer reading programs, Braille writer, magnifiers, closed-circuit TV, large-print photocopier, cassette books and magazines, children's books on cassette, home visits and other reference materials on blindness and other handicaps.

Rose Chenoweth, Director
Valerie Brandon, Administrator

Indiana

6160 Northwest Indiana Subregional Library for Blind and Physically Handicapped
1919 W 81st Street
Merrillville, IN 46410   219-769-3541
                                          Fax: 219-756-9358

Summer reading programs, Braille writer, magnifiers, closed-circuit TV, large-print photocopier, cassette books and magazines, children's books on cassette, home visits and other reference materials on blindness and other handicaps.

Renee Lewis

Iowa

6161 Iowa Library for the Blind and Physically Handicapped
Iowa Department for the Blind
524 4th Street
Des Moines, IA 50309   515-281-1333
                                          800-362-2587
                                          Fax: 515-281-1263
                                          TTY: 515-281-1355
                                          contact@idbonline.org
                                          www.blind.state.ia.us

Summer reading programs, magnifiers, closed-circuit TV, large-print photocopier, children's books on cassette, children's books in Braille and Print Braille, cassette magazines, home visits and reference materials on blindness and other handicaps.

Richard Sorey, Director
Bruce Snethen, Deputy Director

Kansas

6162 CKLS Headquarters
PO Box 515
Northampton, MA 01061   316-792-2393
                                          888-622-8527
                                          Fax: 316-792-5495
                                          cenks@ink.org
                                          www.macular.org

Summer reading programs, Braille writer, magnifiers, closed-circuit TV, large-print photocopier, cassette books and magazines, children's books on cassette, home visits and other reference materials on blindness and other handicaps.

Chip Goehring, President
Mark E. Torrey, Vice President
Paul F. Gariepy, Secretary

6163 Services for the Visually Disabled
629 Poyntz Avenue
Manhattan, KS 66502   785-776-4741
                                          Fax: 785-776-1545
                                          marionr@manhattan.lib.ks.us

Summer reading programs, Braille writer, magnifiers, closed-circuit TV, large-print photocopier, cassette books and magazines, children's books on cassette, home visits and other reference materials on blindness and other handicaps.

Marion Rice, Librarian

Kentucky

6164 Kentucky Library for the Blind and Physically Handicapped
PO Box 818
Frankfort, KY 40602

502-564-8300
800-372-2968
Fax: 502-564-5773
richard.feindel@kdla.net
www.kdla.net/libserv/ktbl.htm

Large-print photocopier, cassette books and magazines, children's books on cassette, and other reference materials on blindness and other handicaps.

5,200 members

Richard Feindel, Librarian

Maryland

6165 Maryland State Library for the Blind and Physically Handicapped
415 Park Avenue
Baltimore, MD 21201

410-230-2424
Fax: 410-333-2095
TTY: 800-934-2541
TDD: 410-333-8679
recept@lbta.lib.md.us
www.lbph.lib.md.us

Summer reading programs, Braille writer, magnifiers, large-print photocopier, cassette books and magazines, children's books on cassette, and other reference materials on blindness and other handicaps.

Jill Lewis, Manager

6166 Prince George's County Memorial Library Talking Book Center
6532 Adelphi Road
Hyattsville, MD 20782

301-699-3500

Summer reading programs, Braille writer, magnifiers, closed-circuit TV, large-print photocopier, cassette books and magazines, children's books on cassette, home visits and other reference materials on blindness and other handicaps.

Shirley Tuthill, Librarian

Massachusetts

6167 Braille and Talking Book Library Perkins School for the Blind
175 N Beacon Street
Watertown, MA 02472

617-924-3434
Fax: 617-972-7315
info@perkins.org
www.perkins.org

C. Richard Carlson, Chairman
Leslie Nordin, Vice Chairman
Michael Schnitman, Secretary

6168 Carroll Center for the Blind
770 Centre Street
Newton, MA 02458

617-969-6200
800-852-3131
Fax: 617-969-6204
www.carroll.org

Assists blind and visually impaired adults and adolescents to adjust to loss of vision. The goal of this dynamic program is to help the person become more independent, to restore self-confidence, prepare for employment and improve the quality of life. Programs of individual counseling are offered as part of the program.

Rachel Rosenbaum, President

Michigan

6169 Downtown Detroit Subregional Library for the Blind and Handicapped
5201 Woodward Avenue
Detroit, MI 48202

313-481-1300
Fax: 313-965-1977
TDD: 313-224-0584
deveans@cms.xx.wayne.edu
www.detroit.lib.mi.us

Summer reading programs, Braille writer, magnifiers, closed-circuit TV, large-print photocopier, cassette books and magazines, children's books on cassette, home visits and other reference materials on blindness and other handicaps.

Russell Bellant, President
Gregory Hicks, vice President
Jonathan C. Kinloch, Secretary

6170 Kent County Library for the Blind
775 Ball Avenue NE
Grand Rapids, MI 49503

616-336-3250
Fax: 616-336-3201
kdlem@lakeland.lib.mi.us

Summer reading programs, Braille writer, magnifiers, closed-circuit TV, large-print photocopier, cassette books and magazines, children's books on cassette, home visits and other reference materials on blindness and other handicaps.

Claudya Muller, Librarian

6171 Library of Michigan Service for the Blind
PO Box 30007
Lansing, MI 48909

517-373-5614
Fax: 517-373-5865
BTBL@michigan.gov

Summer reading programs, Braille writer, magnifiers, closed-circuit TV, large-print photocopier, cassette books and magazines, children's books on cassette, home visits and other reference materials on blindness and other handicaps.

Nancy Robertson, Manager

6172 Macomb Library for the Blind and Physically Handicapped
16480 Hall Road
Clinton Township, MI 48038

586-286-1580
Fax: 586-286-0634
TDD: 810-869-40
macbld@libcoop.net
www.macomb.lib.mi.us/macspe/

Summer reading programs, Braille writer, closed-circuit TV, cassette books and magazines, children's books on cassette, reference materials on blindness and other handicaps.

Beverlee Babcock, Executive Director

6173 Mideastern Michigan Library Co-op
503 S Saginaw Street Suite 711
Flint, MI 48502

810-232-7119
Fax: 810-232-6639
cnash@genesse.freeret.org
www.fakon.edu/gdl/talking.htm

Summer reading programs, Braille writer, magnifiers, closed-circuit TV, large-print photocopier, cassette books and magazines, children's books on cassette, home visits and other reference materials on blindness and other handicaps.

Carolyn Nash, Librarian

6174 Muskegon County Library for the Blind
4845 Airline Road
Muskegon, MI 49444

231-737-6310
Fax: 231-724-6675
TDD: 231-722-4103
www.muskcolib.org

Summer reading programs, Braille typewriter, magnifiers, closed-circuit TV, large-print photocopier, cassette books and magazines, children's books on cassette, home visits and other reference materials on blindness and other handicaps, The Reading Edge, Perkins Braille and large print books.

Linda Clapp, Librarian

6175 Upper Peninsula Library for the Blind Physically Handicapped
1615 Presque Isle Avenue
Marquette, MI 49855
906-228-7697
Fax: 906-228-5627
rruff@uproc.lib.mi.us
www.upesc.lib.mi.us/uplbph

Summer reading programs, Braille writer, magnifiers, closed-circuit TV, large-print photocopier, cassette books and magazines, children's books on cassette, home visits and other reference materials on blindness and other handicaps.

Suzanne Dees, Executive Director

6176 Washtenaw County Library
PO Box 8645
Ann Arbor, MI 48107
734-222-6850
Fax: 734-222-6715
mcdaniev@ewashtenaw.org
www.ewashtenaw.org

Summer reading programs, Braille writer, magnifiers, closed-circuit TV, large-print photocopier, cassette books and magazines, children's books on cassette, home visits and other reference materials on blindness and other handicaps.

Verna J. Mcdaniel, Administrator

6177 Washtenaw County Library for the Blind and Physically Disabled
PO Box 8645
Ann Arbor, MI 48107
734-222-6850
Fax: 734-222-6715
mcdaniev@ewashtenaw.org
www.ewashtenaw.org

Book lovers club. adaptive technology, cassette equipment, cassette books and magazines, described videos, low vision aids reference and referral services.

Verna J. Mcdaniel, Administrator

6178 Wayne County Regional Library for the Blind
30555 Michigan Avenue
Westland, MI 48186
734-727-7300
888-968-2737
Fax: 734-727-7333
TTY: 734-727-7330
werlbph@tln.lib.mi.us
www.wayneregional.lib.mi.us

Summer reading programs, Braille writer, magnifiers, closed-circuit TV, large-print photocopier, cassette books and magazines, children's books on cassette, home visits and other reference materials on blindness and other handicaps.

Reginald Williams, Wayne County Librarian

Minnesota

6179 Minnesota Library for the Blind & Physically Handicapped
Highway 298, PO Box 68
Fairbault, MN 55021
507-333-4828
800-722-0550
Fax: 507-333-4832
libblnd@state.mn.us

Summer reading programs, Braille writer, magnifiers, closed-circuit TV, large-print photocopier, cassette, large print, Braille books and magazines, children's books on cassette, and other reference materials on blindness and other handicaps.

Catherine A Durivage, Program Director

Missouri

6180 Adriene Resource Center for Blind Children
1445 Boonville Avenue
Springfield, MO 65802
417-831-8000
800-641-4310
Fax: 800-328-0294
blind@ag.org
www.gospelpublishing.com

Offers Braille and cassette lending library, Braille and cassette Sunday school materials for all ages, Braille and cassette periodicals and resource assistance, and resources for blind children and children of blind parents.

Paul Weingariner, Director

6181 Assemblies of God National Center for the Blind
1445 Boonville Avenue
Springfield, MO 65802
417-831-8001
800-641-4311
Fax: 800-328-0295
blind@ag.org
www.gospelpublishing.com

Offers Braille and cassette lending library, Braille and cassette Sunday school materials for all ages, Braille and cassette periodicals and resource assistance, and resources for blind children and children of blind parents.

Thomas Trask, Manager

6182 Wolfner Memorial Library for the Blind
PO Box 387
Jefferson City, MO 65102
573-751-8720
Fax: 573-526-2985
TDD: 800-347-1379
wolfner@sos.mo.gov

Summer reading programs, Braille writer, magnifiers, closed-circuit TV, large-print photocopier, cassette books and magazines, children's books on cassette, home visits and other reference materials on blindness and other handicaps.

Richard J Smith, Executive Director

Nebraska

6183 Nebraska Library Commission Talking Book & Braille Services
1200 N Street
Lincoln, NE 68508
402-471-2045
800-307-2665
Fax: 402-471-2083
TDD: 402-471-4038
doertli@nlc.state.ne.us
www.nlc.state.ne.us

Free loan of books and magazines on cassette and in Braille, including children's materials, along with specially designed playback equipment. Summer reading program for children, Braille embossing, closed circuit TV, large-print copier. Reference materials on blindness and other disabilities.

David Oerti, Librarian

New Jersey

6184 New Jersey State Library Talking Book and Braille Center
185 West State Street
Trenton, NJ 08625
609-278-2640
800-792-8322
Fax: 609-278-2647
TDD: 877-882-5593
njlbh@njstatelib.org
www.njstatelib.org

Free home delivery of large-print, audio, and Braille books and magazines, children's books on cassettes in Braille and other reference materials on blindness and other handicaps. Services are for New Jersey residents with print disabilities.

Adanrah Szczepaniak, Director
Anne McArthur, Head of Outreach and Audiovision

New Mexico

6185 New Mexico State Library for the Blind and Physically Handicapped
1209 Camino Carlos Ray
Santa Fe, NM 87507
505-476-9700
Fax: 505-476-9761
jbrewstr@stlib.state.nm.us
www.stlib.state.nm.us

Summer reading programs, Braille writer, magnifiers, closed-circuit TV, large-print photocopier, cassette books and magazines, children's books on cassette, home visits and other reference materials on blindness and other handicaps.

Susan Overland, Manager

New York

6186 New York State Talking Book & Braille Library
Empire State Plaza, CEC
Albany, NY 12230
518-474-5935
Fax: 518-486-1957
TDD: 518-474-7121
tbbl@mail.nysed.gov
www.suffolk.lib.ny.us

Books on audio cassette, cassette players, Braille books, summer reading programs, Braille writer, magnifiers, closed-circuit TV, large-print photocopier, cassette books and magazines, children's books on cassette, reference materials on blindness and other handicaps.

Jane Somers, Director

North Carolina

6187 North Carolina Library for the Blind
1841 Capital Boulevard
Raleigh, NC 27635
919-733-4376
Fax: 919-733-6910
TDD: 919-733-1462
nclbph@ncder.gov

Summer reading programs, Braille writer, magnifiers, closed-circuit TV, large-print photocopier, cassette books and magazines, children's books on cassette, home visits and other reference materials on blindness and other handicaps.

Francine Martin, Manager

Ohio

6188 American Council of Blind Parents
34400 Cedar Road, Apartment 108
University Heights, OH 44121
800-424-8666

Members are sighted parents of blind or visually impaired children. Offers a forum for support and outreach, sharing of experiences in parent-child relationships, and educational and cultural information about child development. Monitors developments in technical and legislative arenas.

Nola Webb, President

Oregon

6189 Oregon State Library, Talking Book and Braille Services
250 Winter Street NW
Salem, OR 97310
503-378-3849
Fax: 503-585-8059
TDD: 503-378-4276
tbabs@sparkie.osl.state.or.us
www.tbabs.org

Cassette books and magazines, children's books on cassette, home visits and other reference materials on blindness and other handicaps.

Susan Westin, Manager

Virginia

6190 Alexandria Library Talking Book Service
5005 Duke Street
Alexandria, VA 22304
703-746-1760
Fax: 703-519-5916
TDD: 703-838-4568
emccaffr@lea.eda
www.alexandria.lib.va.us

Summer reading programs, Braille writer, magnifiers, closed-circuit TV, large-print photocopier, cassette books and magazines, children's books on cassette, home visits and other reference materials on blindness and other handicaps.

Karen Russell, Manager

6191 Division for the Visually Handicapped
1920 Association Drive
Reston, VA 20191
703-620-3660

Members are teachers, college faculty members, administrators, supervisors and others concerned with the education and welfare of visually handicapped and blind children and youth. This is a division of the Council For Exceptional Children.

Dr. Kay Ferrell, President

6192 Division on Visual Impairments
Council for Exceptional Children
1110 North Glebe Road, Suite 300
Arlington, VA 22201
800-224-6830
Fax: 703-264-9494
TTY: 866-915-5000
www.ed.arizona.edu/dvi/welcome.htm; www.cec.sped.org

A division within the CEC, it handles concerns for Federal, state and local issues and policies related to education of youths, children and infants with visual impairments.

Ellyn Ross, President
Shirley J Wilson, Secretary
Phyllis T Simmons, President Elect

6193 Virginia State Library for the Visually and Physically Handicapped
1901 Roane Street
Richmond, VA 23222
804-367-0014

Summer reading programs, Braille writer, magnifiers, closed-circuit TV, large-print photocopier, cassette books and magazines, children's books on cassette, home visits and other reference materials on blindness and other handicaps.

Mary Ruth Halapatz, Librarian

Washington

6194 Washington Library for the Blind and Physically Handicapped
1000 Fourth Ave.
Seattle, WA 98104
206-386-4636
Fax: 206-386-4685
wtbbl@spl.lib.wa.us
www.spl.lib.wa.us

Summer reading programs, Braille writer, magnifiers, closed-circuit TV, large-print photocopier, cassette books and magazines, children's books on cassette, home visits and other reference materials on blindness and other handicaps.

Marcellus Turner, Librarian

West Virginia

6195 West Virginia School for the Blind
301 E Main Street
Romney, WV 26757
304-822-4801
Fax: 304-822-3370
cjohn@access.mountain.net

Summer reading programs, Braille writer, magnifiers, closed-circuit TV, large-print photocopier, cassette books and magazines, children's books on cassette, home visits and other reference materials on blindness and other handicaps.

Patsy Shank, Administrator

Research Centers

6196 Arlene R Gordon Research Institute
Lighthouse International
111 E 59th Street
New York, NY 10022

212-821-9525
800-829-0500
Fax: 212-821-9707
TTY: 212-821-9713
research@lighthouse.org
www.lighthouse.org

The institute is the only research institute within a vision rehabilitation agency. Trainees can come and acquire research skills in both laboratory and field settings. It is comprised on these major divisions: Evaluation research; Vision research; and Psychosocial research.

Amy Horowitz, Director
Joann P Reinhardt PhD, Director Psychosocial Research

6197 Center for the Partially Sighted
6101 W Centinela Ave, Suite 150
Los Angeles, CA 90230

310-988-1970
Fax: 310-988-1980
info@low-vision.org
www.low-vision.org

Provides professional, comprehensive vision rehabilitation services to visually impaired people of all ages. For those whose sight is severely limited due to macular degeneration, diabetic retinopathy, glaucoma, retinal detachment, stroke or other conditions not correctable medically or surgically.

La Donna Ringering, Executive Director
Herbert Ruderman, Psychiatrist
Marc Gerberick, IT Manager

6198 Mobile Association for the Blind
2440 Gordon Smith Drive
Mobile, AL 36617

251-473-3585
877-292-5463
Fax: 251-470-8622
sales@mobile.blind.com

Offers work adjustment training, activities of daily living, mobility, communication skills and sheltered employment for adults and children who are visually impaired.

Jim Bullock, Executive Director

6199 New Beginnings - The Blind Children's Center
4120 Marathon Street
Los Angeles, CA 90029

323-664-2153

The purpose of the Center is to turn initial fears into hope. Helps children and their families become independent by creating a climate of safety and trust. Children learn to develop self confidence and to master a wide range of skills. Services include an infant stimulation program, educational preschool, interdisciplinary assessment services, family services, correspondence program, toll free national hotline and a publication and research service.

6200 Research to Prevent Blindness
645 Madison Avenue
New York, NY 10022

212-752-4333
800-621-0026
Fax: 212-688-6231
www.rpbusa.org

Provides research grants to scientists interested in eye disease and vision disorders.

Diane Swift, President

Audio Video

6201 Heart to Heart
Blind Children's Center
4120 Marathon Street
Los Angeles, CA 90029

323-644-2153
Fax: 323-665-3828
www.blindcntr.org

Parents of blind and partially sighted children talk about their feelings.
Videotape

6202 Let's Eat
Blind Children's Center
4120 Marathon Street
Los Angeles, CA 90029

213-664-2153
Fax: 213-665-3828

Teaches competent feeding skills to children with visual impairments.
Videotape

6203 See What I Feel
Britannica Film Co.
345 4th Street
San Francisco, CA 94107

415-597-5555

A blind child tells her friends about her trip to the zoo. Each experience was explained as a blind child would experience it. A teacher's guide comes with this video.
Films

Web Sites

6204 Lighthouse Guild
15 West 65th Street
New York, NY 10023

212-769-6200
800-284-4422
info@lighthouseguild.org
www.lighthouseguild.org

Since 1905, Lighthouse International has led the charge in the fight against vision loss through prevention, treatment and empowerment. In 2013, it merged with Jewish Guild Healthcare to form a leading non profit vision and healthcare organization.

Alan R. Morse, President/CEO
Mark G. Ackermann, Executive VP/COO
Maura J. Sweeney, Senior VP, Programs & Services

6205 National Alliance of Blind Students
nabslink.org

The leading national advocacy and consumer organization for students in high school or college who are blind or visually impaired.

Sean Whalen, President
Karen Anderson, Vice President
Gabe Cazares, Vice President

6206 National Association for Visually Handicapped
111 E 59th St
New York, NY 10022

800-284-4422
lighthouse.org/navh

Helps to cope with the difficulties of vision impairment.

Book Publishers

6207 Children with Visual Impairments: A Parents' Guide
Peytral Publications
PO Box 1162
Minnetonka, MN 55345

952-949-8707
877-739-8725
Fax: 952-906-9777
help@peytral.com
www.peytral.com

Covers visual impairments ranging from low vision to total blindness. Offers authoritative information and empathy, parental insight on diagnosis and treatment, orientation and mobility, literacy, legal issues and more. Valuable to parents, educators and support staff.

395 pages

M Cay Holbrook PhD, Editor

6208 Mainstreaming the Visually Impaired Child: Blind & Partially Sighted Students
Michael D Oralnsky PhD, author

Nat'l Assn for Parents of Children with Visual
PO Box 317
Watertown, MA 02471

617-972-7441
800-562-6265
Fax: 617-972-7444
www.spedex.com/napvi

121 pages

6209 Ophthalmic Disorders Sourcebook
Omnigraphics
615 Griswold
Detroit, MI 48226

313-961-1340
800-234-1340
Fax: 800-875-1340
info@omnigraphics.com
www.omnigraphics.com

Basic consumer information about glaucoma, cataracts, macular degeneration, strabismus, refractive disorders and more.

1996 631 pages
ISBN: 0-780800-81-8

Magazines

6210 Journal of Visual Impairment and Blindness
American Foundation for the Blind
2 Penn Plaza, Suite 1102
New York, NY 10121

212-502-7600
Fax: 212-502-7777
afbinfo@afb.net
www.afb.org

Published in braille, regular print and on cassette this journal contains a wide variety of subjects including rehabilitation, psychology, education, legislation, medicine, technology, employment, sensory aids and childhood development as they relate to visual impairments.

10x Year

Carl R. Augusto, President & CEO
Kelly Bleach, Chief Administrative Officer
Rick Bozeman, Chief Financial Officer

6211 NAVH UPDATE
National Association for Visually Handicapped
111 E 59th St
New York, NY 10022

800-284-4422
Fax: 212-727-2931
navh@navh.org
lighthouse.org/navh

Free, large-print newsletter providing information about vision as well as general information to the partially sighted.
quarterly

6212 Reaching, Crawling, Walking - Let's Get Moving
Blind Children's Center
4120 Marathon Street
Los Angeles, CA 90029

323-664-2153
Fax: 323-665-3828
info@blindchildrenscenter.org
www.blindchildrenscenter.org

Orientation and mobility for visually impaired preschool children.
24 pages

6213 Tactic
Clovernook Home and School for the Blind
7000 Hamilton Avenue
Cincinnati, OH 45231

513-522-3860
Fax: 513-728-3950
clovernook@aol.com

Quarterly

Newsletters

6214 Awareness
Nat'l Assn for Parents of Children with Visual
PO Box 317
Watertown, MA 2471

617-972-7441
800-562-6265
Fax: 617-972-7444
www.spedex.com/napvi/awareness.html

Contains NAPVI regional news, commentary, letters to the editor, legislative updates, and information on conferences and events.
32 pages Quarterly

6215 National Library Service for the Blind & Physically Handicapped
Library of Congress Reference Section
1291 Taylor Street NW
Washington, DC 20542

202-707-5100
800-424-8567
Fax: 202-707-0712
TTY: 202-707-0744
TDD: 202-707-0744
nls@loc.gov
www.loc.gov/nls

Provides information and advocacy resources for families and professionals, including listings of organizations focusing on more specific areas of concern to families and young adults who have disabilities. Administers a natural library service that provides recorded and braille reading materials to eligible children and adults who cannot read standard print.

12 pages Quarterly
ISSN: 1046-1663

Vicki Fitzpatrick, Editor

6216 Talking Book Topics
National Library Services for the Blind
1291 Taylor Street NW
Washington, DC 20542

202-707-5100
Fax: 202-707-0712
nls@loc.gov
www.loc.gov/nls

Offers hundreds of listings of books, fiction and nonfiction, for adults and children on cassette. Also offers listings on foreign language books on cassette, talking magazines and reviews.
Bimonthly

Pamphlets

6217 Dancing Cheek to Cheek
Blind Children's Center
4120 Marathon Street
Los Angeles, CA 90029

213-664-2153
Fax: 213-665-3828
www.blindchildrenscenter.org

Discusses beginning social, play and language interactions.
33 pages

6218 Family Guide - Growth and Development of the Partially Seeing Child
National Association for Visually Handicapped
111 E 59th St
New York, NY 10022

800-284-4422
Fax: 888-305-9511
info@navh.org
lighthouse.org/navh

Offers information for parents and guidelines in raising a partially seeing child.

6219 Family Guide to Vision Care
American Optometric Association
243 N Lindbergh Boulevard
Saint Louis, MO 63141
314-991-4100
Fax: 314-991-4101
www.aoanet.org

Offers information on the early developmental years of your vision, finding a family optometrist and how to take care of your eyesight through the learning years, the working years and the mature years.

6220 Heart to Heart
Blind Children's Center
4120 Marathon Street
Los Angeles, CA 90029
213-664-2153
Fax: 213-665-3828
www.blindchildrenscenter.org

Parents of blind and partially sighted children talk about their feelings.
12 pages

6221 Learning to Play
Blind Children's Center
4120 Marathon Street
Los Angeles, CA 90029
213-664-2153
Fax: 213-665-3828
www.blindchildrenscenter.org

Discusses how to present play activities to the visually impaired preschool child.
12 pages

6222 Let's Eat
Blind Children's Center
4120 Marathon Street
Los Angeles, CA 90029
213-664-2153
Fax: 213-665-3828
www.blindchildrenscenter.org

Teaches competent feeding skills to children with visual impairments.
28 pages

6223 Move with Me
Blind Children's Center
4120 Marathon Street
Los Angeles, CA 90029
213-664-2153
Fax: 213-665-3828
www.blindchildrenscenter.org

A parent's guide to movement development for visually impaired babies.
12 pages

6224 Selecting a Program
Blind Children's Center
4120 Marathon Street
Los Angeles, CA 90029
213-664-2153
Fax: 213-665-3828
www.blindchildrenscenter.org

A guide for parents of infants and preschoolers with visual impairments.
28 pages

6225 Standing on My Own Two Feet
Blind Children's Center
4120 Marathon Street
Los Angeles, CA 90029
323-664-2153
Fax: 323-665-3828
info@blindchildrenscenter.org
www.blindchildrenscenter.org

A step-by-step guide to designing and constructing simple, individually tailored adaptive mobility devices for preschool-age children who are visually impaired.

36 pages

6226 Talk to Me
Blind Children's Center
4120 Marathon Street
Los Angeles, CA 90029
213-664-2153
Fax: 213-665-3828
www.blindchildrenscenter.org

A language guide for parents of deaf children.
11 pages

6227 Talk to Me II
Blind Children's Center
4120 Marathon Street
Los Angeles, CA 90029
213-664-2153
Fax: 213-665-3828
www.blindchildrenscenter.org

A sequel to Talk To Me, available in English and Spanish.
15 pages

Camps

6228 Bloomfield
5300 Angeles Vista Boulevard
Los Angeles, CA 90043
323-295-4555
800-352-2290
Fax: 323-296-0424
info@junoirblind.org
www.junoirblind.org

This camp is dedicated to serving blind and developmentally disabled children and adults.

6229 Florida School-Deaf and Blind Summer Camp
207 San Marco Avenue
Saint Augustine, FL 32084
904-827-2200
800-800-344
info@fsdb.k12.fl.us
www.fsdb.k12.fl.us

The Florida School for the Deaf and the Blind hosts summer campers from all over teh state of Florida for a week of fun and adventure. FSDB's 80 acre campus is where campers participate in a variety of activities including rock climbing, archery, swimming, kayaking, team games, arts and crafts, dance music, and much more.

L Daniel Hutto, President
Cindy Day, Executive Director of Parent Svcs
Terri Wiseman, Administrator of Business Services

6230 National Camps for Blind Children
Christian Record
4444 S 52nd Street
Lincoln, NE 68516
402-488-0981; Fax: 402-488-7582
info@christianrecord.org
www.christianrecord.org

Camps throughout the US and Canada are offered at no cost to the legally blind, ages 9-65. Activities include archery, beeper basketball, water sports, hiking and rock climbing and horseback riding.

Dan Jackson, Chair
Tom Lemon, Vice Chair
Larry Pitcher, Secretary

6231 VISIONS/Vacation Camp for the Blind
500 Greenwich Street, 3rd Floor
New York, NY 10013
212-625-1616
888-245-8333
Fax: 212-219-4078
info@visionsvcb.org
www.visionvcb.org

Family programs at Vacation Camp for the Blind in Rockland County, NY for children who are blind, severely visually impaired or multi-handicapped. Parent or guardian must attend winter weekends and summer session.

Nancy T. Jones, President
Richard P. Simon, Vice President
Burton M. Strauss, Treasurer

DESCRIPTION

6232   RESPIRATORY DISTRESS SYNDROME OF THE NEWBORN

Synonyms: Hyaline membrane disese (HMD), RDS

Covers these related disorders: Meconium aspiration syndrome

Involves the following Biologic System(s):

Neonatal and Infant Disorders, Respiratory Disorders

Respiratory distress syndrome of the newborn (RDS) is a breathing disorder characterized by insufficient production of surfactant, which consists of substances produced by certain cells in the lungs. Surfactant contributes to the elasticity of lung (pulmonary) tissue and enables the air sacs (alveoli) of the lungs to remain open between breaths. The exchange of oxygen and carbon dioxide takes place across the thin walls of the air sacs. Due to insufficient surfactant in newborns with RDS, greater pressure is required to expand the lungs' airways and air sacs. As a result, the air sacs may collapse and the lungs may become unable to properly provide oxygenated blood to the body.

Surfactant is produced as the lungs mature during fetal development. Sufficient levels of surfactant are often present after approximately 35 weeks of pregnancy (gestation). RDS primarily occurs in newborns who are born prior to 37 weeks of gestation (premature newborns), affecting up to 80 percent of those who are born before 28 weeks' gestation and up to 30 percent of infants born between 32 and 36 weeks' gestation. The condition also occurs with increased frequency in infants who are born to mothers with diabetes or those who are delivered by Cesarean section. In other newborns, RDS may occur in the absence of known predisposing factors or may be due to certain birth defects or other conditions, such as meconium aspiration syndrome.rome, or persistent fetal circulation. Respiratory distress syndrome of the newborn is sometimes referred to as hyaline membrane disease, because insufficient surfactant production may cause the formation of a fibrous membrane known as hyaline membrane lining the lungs' small airways (bronchioles), ducts (alveolar ducts), and air sacs (alveoli).

Symptoms associated with RDS usually occur within minutes of birth, although they may not be recognized for several hours. These symptoms may vary in severity, depending upon the degree of prematurity or other underlying causes responsible for the condition. Newborns may experience increasing difficulty breathing (dyspnea), characterized by rapid, labored, shallow breaths (tachypnea); grunting upon exhalation; drawing in of the chest wall during inhalation; and bluish discoloration of the skin and mucous membranes (cyanosis) due to lack of sufficient oxygen supply to bodily tissues (hypoxia). Air may leak into the chest cavity surrounding the lungs (pneumothorax), causing collapse of the lungs and further breathing difficulties. Without appropriate treatment, cyanosis and breathing difficulties may progressively worsen and body temperature and blood pressure may fall. As infants with severe RDS tire, grunting upon exhalation may subside, breathing becomes irregular, and life-threatening complications may result. Depending upon the severity of the condition, infants with RDS may begin to gradually improve in about three days or may experience life-threatening symptoms within approximately two to seven days after birth.

Meconium aspiration syndrome is characterized by blockage and irritation of the airways of the lungs due to passage of meconium before birth and inhalation of meconium before or during delivery. Meconium is the thick, sticky material that forms a newborn's first stools, and is typically passed during the first 24 to 48 hours after birth. In some cases, a fetus may pass meconium into the amniotic fluid before birth and then inhale this into the lungs before or right after birth. The skin of newborns with meconium aspiration is usually stained with meconium. In severe cases, symptoms include diminished muscle tone, an abnormally slow heartbeat, or absence of spontaneous respiration at birth.

In newborns with meconium aspiration syndrome, treatment may include immediate suctioning of an affected infant's mouth, throuat, and nose and placement of a tube into the windpipe to remove meconium from the airways. In most affected newborns, imporvement usually occurs in approximately three days.

If physicians suspect that a newborn may be born prematurely, steps may be taken to delay delivery in order to help decrease the risk of RDS. If delivery cannot be delayed, some women may be given certain corticosteroid medications (e.g., dexamethasone or betamethasone) approximately 48 to 72 hours before the delivery of premature newborns to help stimulate the production of surfactant before birth. In addition, an artificial surfactant may be administered into the windpipe of affected newborns immediately after birth or within 24 hours, to help reduce the severity of RDS and associated symptoms or complications. Additional treatment may include symptomatic and supportive measures, such as use of an oxygen hood or support with a ventilator.

Government Agencies

6233   NIH/ Eunice Kennedy Shriver National Insti tute of Child Health & Human Development
31 Center Drive, Building 31
Bethesda, MD 20892

301-496-5113
800-370-2943
Fax: 866-760-5947
nichdpress@mail.nih.gov
www.nichd.nih.gov

Established in 1962 by congress, today the institute conducts and supports research on topics related to the health of children, adults, families and populations. Some of these topics include: developmental disabilities, growth and development, infant death, reproductive health and birth defects.

Diana W. Bianchi, Director
Paul Williams, Director, Communications

6234   NIH/National Heart, Lung and Blood Institu te
National Institute of Health
31 Center Dr, Bldg 31 Rm 5A52
Bethesda, MD 20892

301-496-3245
Fax: 301-629-3246
TTY: 240-629-3255
NHLBIinfo@nhlbi.nih.gov
www.nhlbi.nih.gov

Primary responsibility of this organization is the scientific investigation of heart, blood vessel, lung and blood disorders. Oversees research, demonstration, prevention, education, control and training activities in these fields and emphasizes the prevention and control of heart diseases.

Gary H Gibbons, MD, Director
Nakela Cook, MD, Chief of Staff

National Associations & Support Groups

6235 American Academy of Pediatrics
141 Northwest Point Boulevard
Elk Grove Village, IL 60007
847-434-4000
800-433-9016
Fax: 847-434-8000
www.aap.org

The American Academy of Pediatrics and its member pediatricians are committed to the attainment of optimal physical, mental and social health and well-being for all infants, children, adolescents, and young adults.

Fernando Stein, MD, FAAP, President
Karen Remley, MD, CEO/Executive VP

6236 American Lung Association
55 W. Wacker Drive, Suite 1150
Chicago, IL 60601
312-801-7628
800-586-4872
info@lung.org
www.lung.org

The American Lung Association fights lung disease in all its forms, with special emphasis on asthma, tobacco control and environmental health. The American Lung Association is funded with contributions from the public, along with gifts and grants from corporations, foundations and government agencies. The association achieves its many successes through the work of thousands of committed volunteers and staff.

Harold P. Wimmer, National President & CEO
Susan Rappaport, National VP, Research/Scientific
Sue Swan, Chief Development Officer

6237 Genetic Alliance
4301 Connecticut Avenue NW, Suite 404
Washington, DC 20008
202-966-5557
800-336-4363
Fax: 202-966-8553
info@geneticalliance.org
www.geneticalliance.org

A coalition of voluntary genetic support groups, consumers and professionals addressing the needs of individuals and families affected by genetic disorders from a national perspective.

Sharon Terry, President/CEO
Tetyana Murza, Managing Director
Natasha Bonhomme, VP, Strategic Development

6238 March of Dimes Foundation
1275 Mamaroneck Avenue
White Plains, NY 10605
914-997-4488
888-663-4637
Fax: 914-428-8203
answers@marchofdimes.com
www.marchofdimes.com

Partnership of volunteers and professionals dedicates to improving the health of babies by preventing birth defects and infant mortality. Over 100 chapters are located across the country and can be located through the National Office.

Stacey D. Stewart, President

Web Sites

6239 American Lung Association
55 W. Wacker Drive, Suite 1150
Chicago, IL 60601
312-801-7628
info@lung.org
www.lung.org

The American Lung Association fights lung disease in all its forms, with special emphasis on asthma, tobacco control and environmental health.

Harold P. Wimmer, National President & CEO
Susan Rappaport, National VP, Research/Scientific
Sue Swan, Chief Development Officer

6240 KidsHealth
www.kidshealth.org

KidsHealth provides doctor-approved health information about children from before birth through adolescence.

Neil Izenberg, MD, Editor-in-Chief & Founder

6241 RSV Info Center
www.rsvinfo.com

A comprehensive overview about the most common cause of lower respiratory tract infections in children.

DESCRIPTION

6242 RESPIRATORY SYNCYTIAL VIRUS INFECTION
Synonym: RSV infection
Involves the following Biologic System(s):
Infectious Disorders, Respiratory Disorders

The respiratory syncytial virus (RSV) is the most common cause of lower respiratory tract infections in infants and young children. RSV is primarily spread by the inhalation of virus-containing airborne droplets. The virus is present worldwide and causes annual epidemics of RSV infection in late autumn, winter, or as late as May or June. Such outbreaks typically peak from January through March. Nearly every child is affected by RSV infection by age two, and many experience recurrent reinfection throughout childhood.

In older children and adults, RSV infection may cause no apparent symptoms (asymptomatic) or may result in mild to moderate lung infection and associated cold-like symptoms. However, RSV infection may be severe in others, particularly infants, young children, children with heart or lung disease, or individuals with compromised immune systems. In such patients, RSV infection may lead to inflammation of the lungs' small airways (bronchiolitis), inflammation of the airways and lung tissue (bronchopneumonia), or, in extremely severe cases, potentially life-threatening complications. RSV infection is known to be the leading cause of bronchiolitis or bronchopneumonia in children younger than one year of age.

In infants and young children with RSV infection, symptoms typically begin approximately four days after infection. Initial symptoms include a runny nose (rhinorrhea) and sore throat (pharyngitis). Patients may then develop a low fever, begin to cough and sneeze, and soon experience wheezing, which is the production of a whistling sound during breathing due to inflammation and associated narrowing of the airways. If RSV infection progresses, patients may develop additional symptoms, including increasing wheezing and coughing, an abnormally rapid rate of breathing (tachypnea), drawing in of the chest wall during inhalation, and bluish discoloration of the skin and mucous membranes (cyanosis). Patients with extremely severe disease progression may develop increasingly rapid breathing, temporary cessation of breathing (apnea), listlessness, and potentially life-threatening complications. In other infants or young children with RSV infection, initial running of the nose and coughing may be followed by poor feeding, listlessness, and difficulties breathing (dyspnea) with little or no wheezing.

As mentioned above, many children experience reinfection with RSV. Reinfection usually causes less severe symptoms than those associated with initial disease. However, depending upon the age of patients and other factors, secondary infections may also sometimes be associated with severe lower respiratory tract infections. Older children who experience reinfection with RSV generally have more mild symptoms.

In children with mild or moderate RSV infection without associated bronchiolitis or bronchopneumonia, treatment typically includes symptomatic and supportive measures. Affected infants, young children, children with heart or lung disease, or those with compromised immune systems may require hospitalization. Treatment may include providing respiratory therapy with humidified air to help supply adequate oxygen to bodily tissues; ensuring an adequate intake of fluids; or administering certain medications to relax the smooth muscles of the small airways (bronchodilators). Certain infants and children are at high risk for severe RSV disease, such as those with lung disease, congenital heart disease, or immunodeficiency. In these children, certain preventive or prophylactic therapies such as RSV-specific antibodies may be recommended to help reduce (or even prevent) the severity of RSV infection in these at-risk infants and young children.

Government Agencies

6243 NIH/ Eunice Kennedy Shriver National Insti tute of Child Health & Human Development
31 Center Drive, Building 31
Bethesda, MD 20892
301-496-5113
800-370-2943
Fax: 866-760-5947
nichdpress@mail.nih.gov
www.nichd.nih.gov

Established in 1962 by congress, today the institute conducts and supports research on topics related to the health of children, adults, families and populations. Some of these topics include: developmental disabilities, growth and development, infant death, reproductive health and birth defects.

Diana W. Bianchi, Director
Paul Williams, Director, Communications

6244 NIH/National Institute of Allergy and Infectious Diseases
5601 Fishers Lane, MSC 9806
Bethesda, MD 20892
301-496-5717
866-284-4107
Fax: 301-402-3573
TDD: 800-877-8339
ocpostoffice@niaid.nih.gov
www.niaid.nih.gov

Conducts and supports basic and applied research to better understand, treat, and ultimately prevent infectious, immunologic, and allergic diseases.

Anthony S Fauci MD, Director

National Associations & Support Groups

6245 American Academy of Pediatrics
141 Northwest Point Boulevard
Elk Grove Village, IL 60007
847-434-4000
800-433-9016
Fax: 847-434-8000
www.aap.org

The American Academy of Pediatrics and its member pediatricians are committed to the attainment of optimal physical, mental and social health and well-being for all infants, children, adolescents, and young adults.

Fernando Stein, MD, FAAP, President
Karen Remley, MD, CEO/Executive VP

6246 American Lung Association
55 W. Wacker Drive, Suite 1150
Chicago, IL 60601
312-801-7628
info@lung.org
www.lung.org

Founded in 1904 to fight tuberculosis, the American Lung Association today fights lung disease in all its forms, with special emphasis on asthma, tobacco control and environmental health.

Harold P. Wimmer, National President & CEO
Susan Rappaport, National VP, Research/Scientific
Sue Swan, Chief Development Officer

6247 World Health Organization
Avenue Appia 20
CH-1211 Geneva 27,
Switzerland
www.who.int

WHO is the directing and coordinating authority for health within the United Nations system.

Dr Margaret Chan, Director General

Web Sites

6248 American Lung Association
55 W. Wacker Drive, Suite 1150
Chicago, IL 60601
312-801-7628
info@lung.org
www.lung.org

Information regarding lung disease in all its forms, with special emphasis on asthma, tobacco control and environmental health.

Harold P. Wimmer, National President & CEO
Susan Rappaport, National VP, Research/Scientific
Sue Swan, Chief Development Officer

6249 KidsHealth
www.kidshealth.org/parent/infections/lung/rsv.html

Provides an explanation of the disorder as well as treatment and prevention.

Neil Izenberg, MD, Editor-in-Chief & Founder

6250 RSV Info Center
www.rsvinfo.com

An information center where anyone can find a comprehensive overview about the most common cause of lower respiratory tract infections in children.

DESCRIPTION

6251 RETINITIS PIGMENTOSA

Synonym: RP

Involves the following Biologic System(s):

Ophthalmologic Disorders

Retinitis pigmentosa (RP) refers to a group of inherited disorders in which changes occur in the light-sensitive, nerve-rich tissue membrane (retina) at the rear of the eye. This process is a slow, progressive degeneration leading to blindness. Changes in the retina include clumping (aggregation) or scattering (dispersion) of the retinal pigment, thinning or weakening of the vessels that supply the retina with oxygen-rich blood, and shrinking of the retina and the area where the optic nerve enters the retina (optic disk). Characteristic findings and symptoms of RP include difficulty in seeing at night or in dim light (night blindness; nyctalopia), a progressive reduction in the visual field with gradual loss of central vision, tunnel vision associated with loss of the peripheral visual field, and accompanying reduction of retinal function. Retinitis pigmentosa usually becomes apparent in childhood, progressing to blindness during middle age. However, the onset, severity, and rate of this progressive degeneration are widely variable.

Leber congenital retinal amaurosis (amaurosis congenita; congenital amaurosis) is a form of retinitis pigmentosa that occurs at birth or shortly thereafter and is characterized by shrinking of the optic disk (optic atrophy), thinning or weakening of the blood vessels of the retina, and widespread irregularities of retinal pigmentation. Leber congenital retinal amaurosis is transmitted as an autosomal recessive trait. In addition, retinitis pigmentosa-like degenerative changes may be associated with several metabolic, neurodegenerative, and multifold disorders.

Treatment for retinitis pigmentosa is supportive and may include the use of visual devices to enhance remaining vision. This disorder may appear as a sporadic occurrence or may be inherited, usually as an autosomal dominant disorder. There is also evidence of autosomal recessive and X-linked genetic transmission.

Government Agencies

6252 NIH/National Eye Institute
31 Center Drive MSC 2510
Bethesda, MD 20892
301-496-5248
2020@nei.nih.gov
www.nei.nih.gov

Conducts and supports research that helps prevent and treat eye diseases and other disorders of vision. This research leads to sight-saving treatments, reduces visual impairment and blindness, and improves the quality of life for people of all ages. NEI-supported research has advanced our knowledge of how the eye functions in health and disease.

Paul A Sieving M.D., Ph.D., Director

National Associations & Support Groups

6253 American Academy of Pediatrics
141 Northwest Point Boulevard
Elk Grove Village, IL 60007
847-434-4000
800-433-9016
Fax: 847-434-8000
www.aap.org

The American Academy of Pediatrics and its member pediatricians are committed to the attainment of optimal physical, mental and social health and well-being for all infants, children, adolescents, and young adults.

Fernando Stein, MD, FAAP, President
Karen Remley, MD, CEO/Executive VP

6254 National Association for Visually Handicapped
22 W 21st Street, 6th Floor
New York, NY 10010
212-889-3141
888-205-5951
Fax: 212-727-2931
navh@navh.org
www.navh.org

Serves as a clearinghouse for information about all services available to the partially-sighted from public and private sources. Conducts self-help groups. Provides information on large print books, textbooks and educational tools.

Lorianie Marchi, Ceo

6255 National Eye Health Education Program
National Eye Institute
31 Center Drive, MSC 2510
Bethesda, MD 20892
301-496-5248
Fax: 301-496-1065
www.nei.nih.gov/nehep

A program conducted by the National Eye Institute for large-scale professional and public education programs in partnership with national organizations.

Rosemary Janiszewski, Director
Karen Silver, Health Education Coordinator

6256 RP International
PO Box 900
Woodland Hills, CA 91365
818-992-0500
800-344-4877
Fax: 818-992-3265
info@rpinternational.org
www.rpinternational.org

Dedicated to promoting and supporting research to find effective treatments and cures for retinitis pigmentosa, macular degeneration, and other degenerative diseases. Provides referrals to genetic counselors and support groups and offers a variety of educational materials including a regular newsletter and brochures.

Helen Harris, President

Research Centers

6257 UIC Eye Center
Department of Ophthalmology & Visual Sciences
1855 W Taylor Street
Chicago, IL 60612
312-996-4356
Fax: 312-996-7770
eyeweb@uic.edu
www.uic.edu/com/eye/department

Offers help, support, information and research for persons with vision problems, including retinitis pigmentosa.

Gerald A Fishman

Web Sites

6258 British Retinitis Pigmentosa Society
PO Box 350
Buckingham, MK18
128-082-1334
Fax: 128-081-5900
info@rpfightingblindness.org.uk
www.rpfightingblindness.org.uk

Website aims to provide a better understanding of the inherited retinal disorders. The content of this website has been written by people who have many years experience of living with RP and by very knowledgeable professionals in the field of opththalmology.

David Head, Chief Executive Officer

6259 Foundation Fighting Blindness
7168 Columbia Gateway Drive, Suite 100
Columbia, MD 21046
410-423-0600
800-683-5555
TDD: 800-683-5551
info@FightBlindness.org
www.blindness.org

Searches for treatments and cures for macular degeneration, retinitis pigmentosa (RP), usher syndrome and the entire spectrum of retinal degenerative diseases.

William T. Schmidt, Chief Executive Officer
Stephen M. Rose, Ph.D., Chief Research Officer
Annette Hinkle, CPA, Chief Financial Officer

6260 National Association for Visually Handicapped
111 E 59th St
New York, NY 10022
800-284-4422
lighthouse.org/navh

Helps to cope with the difficulties of vision impairment.

6261 Retina South Africa - Fighting Blindness
www.rpsa.org.za/retinitis.htm

Represents retinitis pigmentosa, macular degeneration, usher syndrome and over 200 other rare conditions. Offers supports, education and counseling to affected people and their families. Self employment skills are also provided by unemployed sufferers to encourage financial independence and self esteem.

6262 Royal National Institute of the Blind
105 Judd Street
London, WC1H
303-123-9999
www.rnib.org.uk

A leading UK charity offering information, support and advice to over two million people with sight problems.

Lesley-Anne Alexander~, Chief Executive
Wanda~ Hamilton, Group Director~
Fazilet Hadi, Managing~Director~

6263 Texas Association of Retinitis Pigmentosa
www.geocities.com/HotSprings/7815/front.htm

Nonprofit organization based in Texas serving as a national information-sharing center to provide human services to persons with progressive vision loss from retinitis pigmentosa and other retinal degenerative disorders.

Book Publishers

6264 Children with Visual Impairments: A Parents' Guide
Peytral Publications
PO Box 1162
Minnetonka, MN 55345
952-949-8707
877-739-8725
Fax: 952-906-9777
help@peytral.com
www.peytral.com

Covers visual impairments ranging from low vision to total blindness. Offers authoritative information and empathy, parental insight on diagnosis and treatment, orientation and mobility, literacy, legal issues and more. Valuable to parents, educators and support staff.

395 pages

M Cay Holbrook PhD, Editor

Newsletters

6265 RP Messenger
Texas Association of Retinitis Pigmentosa
PO Box 8388
Corpus Christi, TX 78468
512-852-8515
Fax: 361-852-8515
www.jwen.com/rp

A biannual newsletter offering information on retinitis pigmentosa.

Biannual

DESCRIPTION

6266 RETINOBLASTOMA

Involves the following Biologic System(s):

Hematologic and Oncologic Disorders, Ophthalmologic Disorders

Retinoblastoma is a malignant tumor of the nerve-rich membrane at the back of the eye known as the retina. This membrane converts light waves into nerve impulses and transmits them to the brain via the optic nerve (the second cranial nerve), resulting in vision. Retinoblastoma occurs in approximately one in 18,000 live births. In most cases, one eye is affected (unilateral). However, both eyes may be involved (bilateral) in about 30 percent of affected children. In some severe cases, the tumor may spread to other parts of the body (metastasize), particularly when there is tumor invasion of the middle layer of the eye (choroid) or the optic nerve. If tumor growth occurs along the optic nerve, the brain may be affected. However, in most children with retinoblastoma, metastasis rarely occurs before the tumor is detected.

Unilateral retinoblastoma is usually detected at approximately 21 months to two years of age, whereas bilateral retinoblastoma is typically diagnosed at about 11 to 12 months. Rarely, the tumor may be detected at birth, during later childhood or adolescence, or adulthood. In most cases, the first sign associated with retinoblastoma is the appearance of a yellowish-white mass in the pupil area (leukokoria) due to the presence of the tumor behind the lens of the eye and reflection of light off the tumor. Additional symptoms and findings often include abnormal deviation of the affected eye in relation to the other (strabismus) and impaired or absent vision. In some cases, affected children experience secondary complications, such as detachment of the retina or abnormally increased pressure of the fluid of the eye (glaucoma). Children who have more advanced retinoblastoma may also experience bleeding (hemorrhaging) within the chamber of the eye in front of the iris (hyphema), irregularities of the pupil, pain, or other symptoms. In cases of severely advanced disease or metastasis, associated findings may include protusion of the eye ball (proptosis) and abnormally increased pressure within the skull (intracranial pressure).

A gene responsible for retinoblastoma (RB gene) has been located on the long arm chromosome 13 (13q14). Many cases of unilateral retinoblastoma are thought to be due to deletions or abnormal changes (mutations) of the gene that occur randomly, for unknown reasons (sporadic). In familial cases, the exact mechanisms of inheritance are not understood. However, bilateral retinoblastoma and some cases of unilateral disease are thought to result from deletion of the gene from one chromosome and inheritance of one mutated disease gene (hemizygous state) or inheritance of two mutated RB genes (homozygous state of RB gene). Individuals with familial retinoblastoma may also have an increased risk for other malignancies. About one percent of children treated for familial retinoblastoma eventually develop a malignant bone tumor (osteosarcoma) by 10 years of age. In addition, estimates in medical literature indicate that about 30 percent of those with familial retinoblastoma are affected by a second malignancy within 30 years after their initial diagnosis.

In some rare cases, affected children may have retinoblastoma in association with an underlying chromosomal deletion syndrome (chromosome 13, monosomy 13q syndrome) that is characterized by deletion (monosomy) of a portion of chromosome 13q including the RB gene at band 13q14. Although associated symptoms and findings may vary, affected children may have characteristic abnormalities of the head and facial (craniofacial) area including a high forehead, prominent eyebrows, a rounded (bulbous) tip of the nose and broad nasal bridge, prominent earlobes, a large mouth, and a thin upper lip.

The treatment of children with retinoblastoma is directed toward preserving vision. In children with unilateral retinoblastoma, treatment typically includes surgical removal of the affected eye and a portion of the optic nerve. However, if the tumor is very small, other measures may be indicated, such as the use of radiation or extremely cold temperatures (cryotherapy) to destroy the tumor. In children with bilateral retinoblastoma, treatment is directed toward preserving useful vision in at least one eye. Therefore, initial therapy may include cryotherapy or radiotherapy of one or both eyes. Bilateral therapy may be recommended since there have been cases in which the more severely affected eye has responded more dramatically to such measures. When one eye has no remaining vision or is affected by painful complications, removal of the eye may be advised. If tumor growth has begun to extend beyond the eye, radiation therapy may also be conducted. Therapy with anticancer drugs, such as cyclophosphamide and doxorubicin, may be considered with radiation therapy. Children and adults who have been affected by familial retinoblastoma should be carefully monitored for secondary malignancies. In addition, family members of affected children should be examined by an eye specialist to detect or help rule out the presence of retinoblastoma.

Government Agencies

6267 NIH/National Cancer Institute

BG 9609 / 9609 Medical Center Drive
Bethesda, MD 20892

800-422-6237
www.cancer.gov

The National Cancer Institute coordinates the National Cancer Program, which conducts and supports research, training, health information dissemination, and other programs with respect to the cause, diagnosis, prevention, and treatment of cancer, rehabilitation from cancer, and the continuing care of cancer patients and the families of cancer patients.

Douglas R. Lowy, MD, Acting Director
James Doroshow, MD, Deputy Director
Henry P. Ciolino, PhD, Acting Director, Cancer Centers

National Associations & Support Groups

6268 American Academy of Pediatrics

141 Northwest Point Boulevard
Elk Grove Village, IL 60007

847-434-4000
800-433-9016
Fax: 847-434-8000
www.aap.org

The American Academy of Pediatrics and its member pediatricians are committed to the attainment of optimal physical, mental and social health and well-being for all infants, children, adolescents, and young adults.

Fernando Stein, MD, FAAP, President
Karen Remley, MD, CEO/Executive VP

6269 American Childhood Cancer Organization (fo rmerly Candlelighters Childhood Cancer)
PO Box 498
Kensington, MD 20895
301-962-3520
800-366-2223
Fax: 310-962-3521
staff@acco.org
www.acco.org

The Candlelighters Childhood Cancer Foundation National Office was founded in 1970 by concerned parents of children with cancer. Today our membership of over 50,000 members of the national office and more than 100,000 members across the across the country, including Candlelighters affiliate groups, includes, parents of children who are being treated or have been treated for cancer.

Ruth I. Hoffman, MPH, Executive Director
Jessica DiBenedetto, Program Coordinator
Christy Perry, Director, Marketing/Communications

6270 Division on Visual Impairments
Council for Exceptional Children
1110 N Glebe Road, Suite 300
Arlington, VA 22201
800-224-6830
Fax: 703-264-9494
TTY: 866-915-5000
www.ed.arizona.edu/dvi/welcome.htm; www.cec.sped.org

A division within the CEC, it handles concerns for Federal, state and local issues and policies related to education of youths, children and infants with visual impairments.

Ellyn Ross, President
Shirley J Wilson, Secretary
Phyllis T Simmons, President Elect

6271 Genetic Alliance
4301 Connecticut Avenue NW, Suite 404
Washington, DC 20008
202-966-5557
800-336-4363
Fax: 202-966-8553
info@geneticalliance.org
www.geneticalliance.org

A coalition of voluntary genetic support groups, consumers and professionals addressing the needs of individuals and families affected by genetic disorders from a national perspective.

Sharon Terry, President/CEO
Tetyana Murza, Managing Director
Natasha Bonhomme, VP, Strategic Development

6272 Institute for Families
4650 Sunset Blvd, MS#111
Los Angeles, CA 90027
323-669-4649
Fax: 323-665-7869
info@instituteforfamilies.org
www.instituteforfamilies.org

A non-profit organization providing free of charge support and services to professionals and families of visually impaired children.

6273 Lighthouse Guild
15 West 65th Street
New York, NY 10023
212-769-6200
800-284-4422
info@lighthouseguild.org
www.lighthouseguild.org

Since 1905, Lighthouse International has led the charge in the fight against vision loss through prevention, treatment and empowerment. In 2013, it merged with Jewish Guild Healthcare to form a leading non profit vision and healthcare organization.

Alan R. Morse, President/CEO
Mark G. Ackermann, Executive VP/COO
Maura J. Sweeney, Senior VP, Programs & Services

6274 National Alliance of Blind Students
c/o Terry Pacheco
1155 15th Street NW, Suite 1004
Washington, DC 20005
202-467-5081
800-424-8666
Fax: 202-467-5085
rj.hodson@verizon.net
www.blindstudents.org

An advocacy and consumer organization for high school and college students who are blind or visually impaired. It works to facilitate progress toward full accessibility of college programs and facilities, provides opportunities for discussion of issues important to students and assists with National Student Seminars.

Rebecca Hodson, President

6275 National Association for Parents of Childr en with Visual Impairments
PO Box 317
Watertown, MA 02471
617-972-7441
800-562-6265
Fax: 617-972-7444
napvi@perkins.org
www.spedex.com/napvi/

Offers emotional support for parents of blind or visually impaired children. Provides information, training and assistance, and help in understanding and using available resources.

6276 National Childhood Cancer Foundation
4600 East West Highway, Suite 600
Bethesda, MD 20814
301-718-0042
800-458-6223
Fax: 301-718-0047
info@curesearch.org
www.curesearch.org

CureSearch unites the world's largest childhood cancer research organization, the Children's Oncology Group, and the National Childhood Cancer Foundation through our mission to cure childhood cancer. Research is the key to the cure.

Stacy Haller, Executive Director

6277 National Support & Information Network
NAPVI
PO Box 317
Watertown, MA 02471
617-972-7441
800-562-6265
www.spedex.com/napvi/network.html

Nationwide support group that provides direct support, information and referral services for parents of children with vision impairments and or multiple related disabilities.

6278 Retinoblastoma International
18030 Brookhurst Street, Box 408ÿ
Fountain Valley, CA 92708
323-669-2299
Fax: 323-660-8541
info@retinoblastoma.net
www.retinoblastoma.net

Retinoblastoma information for parents, family and friends of retinoblastoma patients, as well as online medical education and training for health care professionals.

Christina S Ashford, President
Robin Einstein, Treasurer

State Agencies & Support Groups

Connecticut

6279 Parents Association of Connecticut Childre n with Visual Impairments (PACVI)
PO Box 455
Newtown, CT 06470
203-364-1450
www.spedex.com/napvi/chapters.html

Sabeena Ali, Co-President
Jean Loberg,, President

Florida

6280 Florida Families of Children with Visual I mpairments
Ormond Beach, FL 32174
386-677-7760
ffcvi@yahoo.com

Sue Townsend, President

Massachusetts

6281 Massachusetts Association for Parents of t he Visually Impaired (MAPVI)
Maynard, MA 01754
978-897-3005
mapvi-info@viguide.com
www.mapvi.org

Anita Sullivan, President
Susan Rawlay, Regional Represenative
Chris Pine, Treasurer

New Hampshire

6282 New England Retinoblastoma Support Group (NERSG)
Salem, NH 03079
603-893-3908
Tom Gelinas, Treasurer

Web Sites

6283 A Parent's Guide to Understanding Retinobl astoma
1275 York Avenue
New York, NY 10065
212-639-2000
800-525-2225
www.mskcc.org

Craig B. Thompson, President
John Gunn, Chief Operating Officer
Kerry Bessey, Senior Vice President

6284 Children's Cancer Web
www.cancerindex.org/ccw

An independent nonprofit site, established to provide a directory of childhood cancer resources.

6285 Life With Retinoblastoma
www.mrmegabyte.net/rb/retino.html

A support site written by the parent of a child with retinoblastoma.

6286 Online Mendelian Inheritance in Man
National Library of Medicine, Building 38A
Bethesda, MD 20894
888-346-3656
info@ncbi.nlm.nih.gov
www.ncbi.nlm.nih.gov

This database is a catalog of human genes and genetic disorders.

6287 Retinoblastoma Solutions
1100 Bennett Road - Unit 4
Bowmanville, ON L1C 3
647-478-4902
877-624-9769
Fax: 905-697-9786
info@impactgenetics.com
impactgenetics.com

Dedicated to advancing retinoblastoma research and making available molecular diagnostic tests to families that cannot afford it.

Franny Jewett, CEO
David McDonald, CTO
Diane Rushlow, Scientific Director

Book Publishers

6288 Children with Visual Impairments: A Parents' Guide
Peytral Publications
PO Box 1162
Minnetonka, MN 55345
952-949-8707
877-739-8725
Fax: 952-906-9777
help@peytral.com
www.peytral.com

Covers visual impairments ranging from low vision to total blindness. Offers authoritative information and empathy, parental insight on diagnosis and treatment, orientation and mobility, literacy, legal issues and more. Valuable to parents, educators and support staff.

395 pages

M Cay Holbrook PhD, Editor

6289 Let's Talk About Going to the Hospital
Rosen Publishing Group's PowerKids Press
29 E 21st Street
New York, NY 10010
212-777-3017
800-237-9932
Fax: 888-436-4643
rosenpub@tribeca.ios.com
www.rosenpublishing.com

If a child has to check into the hospital, chances are he or she is already upset about being ill. Knowing how a hospital functions and what the procedures are, such as when family members can visit, will help in what is already a stressful situation. Grades K-5.

24 pages
ISBN: 0-823950-36-0

Roger Rosen, President

6290 Let's Talk About When Kids Have Cancer
Melanie Apel Gordon, author

Rosen Publishing Group's PowerKids Press
29 E 21st Street
New York, NY 10010
212-777-3017
800-237-9932
Fax: 888-436-4643
customerservice@rosenpub.com
www.rosenpublishing.com

In a straightforward yet comforting way, this book explains what cancer is, what kinds of treatments surround the disease and how to cope if a child or the friend of a child has cancer.

24 pages Paperback
ISBN: 0-823951-95-2

Roger Rosen, President

6291 My Fake Eye, The Story of My Prosthesis
Institute for Families
4650 Sunset Blvd, MS#111
Los Angeles, CA 90027
323-361-4649
Fax: 323-665-7869
info@instituteforfamilies.org
www.instituteforfamilies.org

A full color book and comforting tool for children, siblings and parents dealing with eye enucleation. Available in Spanish.

Peggy Yoshino, Chairman
Eric Dahl, CFO
Joni Dahl, Secretary

6292 My New Eye Patch
Institute for Families
4650 Sunset Blvd, MS#111
Los Angeles, CA 90027
323-361-4650
Fax: 323-665-7870
info@instituteforfamilies.org
www.instituteforfamilies.org

A book for describing the feelings and experiences surrounding wearing an eye patch, for children and parents. Available in Spanish.

Peggy Yoshino, Chairman
Eric Dahl, CFO
Joni Dahl, Secretary

6293 Surviving Childhood Cancer: A Guide for Families
New Harbinger Publications
5674 Shattuck Avenue
Oakland, CA 94609

510-652-0215
800-748-6273
Fax: 800-652-1613
customerservice@newharbinger.com
www.newharbinger.com

Cancer in a child is an overwhelming experience for a family. This book explains common medical procedures and offers readers practical advice about how to cope with emotions and stress during this time.
215 pages Paperback
ISBN: 1-572241-02-0

Newsletters

6294 Awareness
NAPVI
PO Box 317
Watertown, MA 2272

617-972-7441
800-562-6265
www.spedex.com/napvi/awareness.html

Contains regional NAPVI news and announcements, legislative updates, upcoming events and conferences and articles and letters to the editor.
32 pages Quarterly

6295 DVI Quarterly
Division on Visual Impairments (CEC)
2900 Crystal Drive, Suite 1000
Arlington, VA 22202

888-232-7733
TTY: 866-915-5000
www.cec.sped.org/mb/

News on the Division of Visual Impairments, articles and announcements having to do with the education of students with visual impairmnets.
1000+ Quarterly

James P. Heiden, President
Sharon Raimondi, Treasurer
Joni L. Baldwin, Associate Professor

6296 Retinoblastoma Support News
Institute for Families
4650 Sunset Blvd, MS#111
Los Angeles, CA 90027

323-669-4649
Fax: 323-665-7869
info@instituteforfamilies.org
www.instituteforfamilies.org

Newsletter for educational professionals and the families of children with retinoblastoma.
Quarterly

Peggy Yoshino, Chairman
Eric Dahl, Chief Financial Officer
Joni Dahl, Secretary

Pamphlets

6297 A Parent's Guide to Understanding Retinobl astoma
IRIS Medical Instruments/IRIDEX Corp
1275 York Avenue
New York, NY 10065

212-639-2000
800-525-2225
www.mskcc.org

Craig B. Thompson, President
John Gunn, Chief Operating Officer
Kerry Bessey, Senior Vice President

6298 Early Detection
Retinoblastoma International
18030 Brookhurst Street, Box 408
Fountain Valley, CA 92708

323-669-2299
Fax: 323-660-8541
info@retinoblastoma.net
www.retinoblastoma.net

A brochure promoting the early detection and treatment of retinoblastoma.
2 pages

DESCRIPTION

6299 RETINOPATHY OF PREMATURITY
Synonym: ROP
Involves the following Biologic System(s):
Neonatal and Infant Disorders, Ophthalmologic Disorders

Retinopathy of prematurity (ROP) is a condition characterized by improper development of blood vessels within the retinas of both eyes. The retinas are the nerve-rich membranes at the back of the eyes that contain specialized, light-sensitive nerve cells (rods and cones). The rods and cones convert visual images into nerve impulses that are transmitted to the brain via the optic nerve (second cranial nerve). ROP primarily occurs in newborns of low birth weight who are born at less than 37 weeks after conception (premature newborns). Premature infants who weigh less than approximately three pounds, are delivered before 33 weeks of pregnancy, and develop abnormally high levels of oxygen in the blood (hyperoxia) as a result of oxygen therapy for breathing difficulties are considered to be particularly at risk for retinopathy of prematurity. Less commonly, other factors may play some role in contributing to the condition, such as heart disease, infection, abnormally low levels of circulating red blood cells (anemia), or other conditions. Generally, the lower an infant's birthweight and the greater the degree of prematurity, the higher the risk for the development of ROP.

During fetal development, the blood vessels that will supply the retinas grow from the center of the retinas, gradually extending to their outer edges shortly after birth. However, in premature newborns, the retinal blood vessels are incompletely developed, potentially causing abnormalities in subsequent retinal growth and function. In infants with ROP, associated findings may range from mild or temporary changes of the outer edges of the retina to severe abnormalities affecting the entire retina. During the active or acute stage of ROP, which typically occurs within the first month or so of life, associated findings may include abnormal narrowing of certain retinal blood vessels and subsequent widening or abnormal twisting of other retinal vessels. In addition, there is an apparent lack of blood vessel growth in certain areas of the retina, particularly of the outer rim. There may also be a gradual development of new blood vessels outside the normal area of retinal blood vessel growth, such as over the surface of the retina or into the jelly-like fluid behind the lens of the eye (vitreous humor). These vessels may tend to bleed (hemorrhage) into the retina, and some patients may develop retinal scarring as well as the formation of retinal folds or breaks or detachment of the outer portion of the retina. In severe cases, patients may undergo chronic disease progression, leading to complete retinal detachment and progressive retinal degeneration. The retina may eventually appear as an abnormal whitish membrane behind the lens of the eye (leukokoria). As the condition continues to progress, infants may develop increased fluid pressure within the eye (glaucoma), gradual degeneration and shrinkage of the eye (phthisis bulbi), and associated visual impairment leading to blindness.

In many infants with ROP, the condition spontaneously subsides and regresses. Such children may have an increased risk of progressive nearsightedness (myopia) or other eye abnormalities. However, in fewer than 10 percent, there may be ongoing disease progression, potentially causing total retinal detachment and severe visual impairment or blindness. In fact, it is retinal detachment that is the main cause of visual impairment and blindness in ROP.

The prevention of ROP depends upon proper prenatal care and other measures to help prevent premature births. In addition, infants who are born prematurely are monitored closely to ensure prompt detection of ROP and appropriate treatment as required. In severe cases of ROP, a technique that freezes affected areas of the retina (cryotherapy) may help to reduce potentially severe complications. Laser therapy can "burn away" the periphery of the retina, which has no normal blood vessels. Both laser treatment and cryotherapy, only used in infants with advanced ROP, destroy the peripheral areas of the retina, slowing or reversing the abnormal growth of blood vessels. Unfortunately, the treatments also destroy some side vision but saves central vision.In some patients with total retinal detachment, surgical techniques may be used to help reattach the retina.

Government Agencies

6300 NIH/ Eunice Kennedy Shriver National Insti tute of Child Health & Human Development
31 Center Drive, Building 31
Bethesda, MD 20892

301-496-5113
800-370-2943
Fax: 866-760-5947
nichdpress@mail.nih.gov
www.nichd.nih.gov

Established in 1962 by congress, today the institute conducts and supports research on topics related to the health of children, adults, families and populations. Some of these topics include: developmental disabilities, growth and development, infant death, reproductive health and birth defects.

Diana W. Bianchi, Director
Paul Williams, Director, Communications

6301 NIH/National Eye Institute
31 Center Drive MSC 2510
Bethesda, MD 20892

301-496-5248
2020@nei.nih.gov
www.nei.nih.gov

Conducts and supports research that helps prevent and treat eye diseases and other disorders of vision. This research leads to sight-saving treatments, reduces visual impairment and blindness, and improves the quality of life for people of all ages. NEI-supported research has advanced our knowledge of how the eye functions in health and disease.

Paul A Sieving M.D., Ph.D., Director

National Associations & Support Groups

6302 American Academy of Pediatrics
141 Northwest Point Boulevard
Elk Grove Village, IL 60007

847-434-4000
800-433-9016
Fax: 847-434-8000
www.aap.org

The American Academy of Pediatrics and its member pediatricians are committed to the attainment of optimal physical, mental and social health and well-being for all infants, children, adolescents, and young adults.

Fernando Stein, MD, FAAP, President
Karen Remley, MD, CEO/Executive VP

6303 Association for Retinopathy of Prematurity and Related Diseases
PO Box 250425
Franklin, MI 48025

800-788-2020
ropard@yahoo.com
www.ropard.org

Funds clinically relevant basic science and clinical research to eliminate retinopathy of prematurity and associated retinal diseases.

Susan Campbell, Administrative Director
Paula Korelitz, Outreach Director

6304   Division on Visual Impairments
Council for Exceptional Children
1110 North Glebe Road, Suite 300
Arlington, VA 22201   800-224-6830
                                                     Fax: 703-264-9494
                                                     TTY: 866-915-5000
www.ed.arizona.edu/dvi/welcome.htm; www.cec.sped.org

A division within the CEC, it handles concerns for Federal, state and local issues and policies related to education of youths, children and infants with visual impairments.

Ellyn Ross, President
Shirley J Wilson, Secretary
Phyllis T Simmons, President Elect

6305   Lighthouse Guild
15 West 65th Street
New York, NY 10023   212-769-6200
                                                     800-284-4422
                                                     info@lighthouseguild.org
                                                     www.lighthouseguild.org

Since 1905, Lighthouse International has led the charge in the fight against vision loss through prevention, treatment and empowerment. In 2013, it merged with Jewish Guild Healthcare to form a leading non profit vision and healthcare organization.

Alan R. Morse, President/CEO
Mark G. Ackermann, Executive VP/COO
Maura J. Sweeney, Senior VP, Programs & Services

6306   National Alliance of Blind Students
c/o Terry Pacheco
1155 15th Street NW, Suite 1004
Washington, DC 20005   202-467-5081
                                                     800-424-8666
                                                     Fax: 202-467-5085
                                                     rj.hodson@verizon.net
                                                     www.blindstudents.org

An advocacy and consumer organization for high school and college students who are blind or visually impaired. It works to facilitate progress toward full accessibility of college programs and facilities, provides opportunities for discussion of issues important to students and assists with National Student Seminars.

Rebecca Hodson, President

6307   National Association for Parents of Childr en with Visual Impairments
PO Box 317
Watertown, MA 00247   617-972-7441
                                                     800-562-6265
                                                     Fax: 617-972-7444
                                                     napvi@perkins.org
                                                     www.spedex.com/napvi/

Offers emotional support for parents of blind or visually impaired children. Provides information, training and assistance, and help in understanding and using available resources.

6308   National Association for Visually Handicapped
111 E 59th St,
New York, NY 10022   212-889-3141
                                                     800-829-0500
                                                     Fax: 212-727-2931
                                                     navh@navh.org
                                                     www.navh.org

Serves as a clearinghouse for information about all services available to the partially-sighted from public and private sources. Conducts self-help groups. Provides information on large print books, textbooks and educational tools.

Lorianie Marchi, Ceo

Audio Video

6309   Management of Retinopathy of Prematurity V ideo
ROPARD
PO Box 250425
Franklin, MI 48025   800-788-2020
                                                     ropard@yahoo.com
                                                     www.ropard.org

Information on ROP related diseases including long term treatment considerations.

Web Sites

6310   National Association for Visually Handicapped
111 E 59th St
New York, NY 10022   800-284-4422
                                                     lighthouse.org/navh

Helps to cope with the difficulties of vision impairment.

Book Publishers

6311   Children with Visual Impairments: A Parents' Guide
Peytral Publications
PO Box 1162
Minnetonka, MN 55345   952-949-8707
                                                     877-739-8725
                                                     Fax: 952-906-9777
                                                     help@peytral.com
                                                     www.peytral.com

Covers visual impairments ranging from low vision to total blindness. Offers authoritative information and empathy, parental insight on diagnosis and treatment, orientation and mobility, literacy, legal issues and more. Valuable to parents, educators and support staff.

395 pages

M Cay Holbrook PhD, Editor

Newsletters

6312   Sight Lines
ROPARD
PO Box 250425
Franklin, MI 48025   800-788-2020
                                                     ropard@yahoo.com
                                                     www.ropard.org

Susan Campbell, Editor

Pamphlets

6313   Looking Ahead:A Parents Guide to the Devel opment Child w/ Retinopathy Prematurity
ROPARD
PO Box 250425
Franklin, MI 48025   800-788-2020
                                                     ropard@yahoo.com
                                                     www.ropard.org

Visual stimulation activity suggestions for the development of children up to five years of age with retinopathy of prematurity.

DESCRIPTION

6314 RHINITIS

Synonyms: Hay Fever, Allergic Rhinitis, Non-Allergic Rhinitis
Involves the following Biologic System(s):
Immunologic and Rheumatologic Disorders, Respiratory Disorders

Rhinitis is a condition in which plant pollens, chemicals, and certain other substances irritate the membranes that line the nose, throat, sinuses, and eyelids, causing them to become swollen and inflamed, with resulting nasal stuffiness and runniness (rhinorrhea), sneezing, burning and tearing of the eyes, and soreness of the throat. It falls into two categories — allergic and non-allergic rhinitis.

Allergic rhinitis is either seasonal (tending to recur in a particular season of every year), or perennial (likely to occur or persist regardless of season). It occurs when pollens, dust, animal dander, house dust mites, and other protein substances, known collectively as allergens, prompt the body cells named plasma cells to secrete an antibody named immunoglobulin E (IgE). The IgE secreted by these cells reacts with specialized structures known as IgE receptors, which exist both on the surfaces of the cells known as mast cells, in the mucous membranes of the nose, throat, and some other parts of the body, and also on the cells known as basophils, which circulate through the body in the blood and lymphatic fluid. The reaction between IgE and its receptors on mast cells and basophils causes these cells to release histamine, a substance that triggers inflammation and swelling in surrounding tissues. The reaction of IgE with its receptors also prompts mast cells and basophils to secrete other substances, known as inflammatory mediators, that promote inflammation in various ways. Allergic rhinitis often accompanies other disorders that affect the respiratory system, eyes, or ears, such as sinusitis, asthma, and inflammation of the ear (otitis), and its effects can interfere with sleep, alertness, and schoolwork. It typically begins from childhood through early adulthood, and in most cases develops by the age of 20 years.

Non-allergic rhinitis is typically caused by smoke, fumes, cold or heat, viral and other respiratory infections, and other sources of inflammation of the nose, throat, and eyes. Moreover, although the symptoms of non-allergic rhinitis often resemble those of allergic rhinitis, it is not triggered by IgE, as is allergic rhinitis, but rather by direct irritation of mucous membranes and other tissues, by effects of cold, heat, or other factors on the nervous system, and by other mechanisms. In the condition known as non-allergic rhinitis with eosinophilia syndrome (NARES), rhinitis and other symptoms of allergy recur without being traceable to any specific allergen, and nasal secretions contain the cells known as eosinophils, which are important members of the body's immune defense system.

Although it can be difficult to distinguish allergic from non-allergic rhinitis, the distinction can be important in terms of preventing and treating these conditions. The diagnosis of allergic rhinitis is based on symptoms that recur upon exposure to seasonal pollens and other specific substances, and by tests in which exposure of a small area of skin to various allergens results in reddening or swelling. A laboratory test known as the radioallergosorbent test (RAST), in which a small sample of blood is withdrawn and IgE in the blood serum is exposed to various allergens, can also show which specific allergens are responsible for a patient's rhinitis.

Because of its more generalized nature and lack of seasonality, non-allergic rhinitis can be difficult to diagnose. Its diagnosis is usually based on its particular symptoms and on linking its occurrence to a particular chemical or other causative agent.

A first step in controlling both allergic and non-allergic rhinitis is to prevent or avoid the allergens or other substances that cause these disorders. The medicines known as antihistamines, which block the inflammatory effects of histamine in the nose, eyes, and other parts of the body, are useful in preventing or easing the symptoms of allergic rhinitis, but are much less effective for non-allergic rhinitis. Although conventional antihistamines can cause drowsiness and other undesirable effects, such effects are often less severe with newer or second-generation antihistamines, which are in some cases also useful for non-allergic rhinitis. Nasal sprays containing corticosteroid drugs are sometimes prescribed for easing nasal swelling, stuffiness, rhinorrhea, and itching in rhinitis. Nasal decongestants, which reduces swelling in the mucous membranes of the nose, may also be effective.

National Associations & Support Groups

6315 American Academy of Allergy, Asthma & Immu nology
555 E. Wells Street, Suite 1100
Milwaukee, WI 53202

414-272-6071
Fax: 414-272-6070
mbrown@aaaai.org
www.aaaai.org

The American Academy of Allergy, Asthma & Immunology is the largest professional medical organization in the United States devoted to the allergy/immunology specialty.

Megan Brown, Communications Manager

6316 American Academy of Pediatrics
141 Northwest Point Boulevard
Elk Grove Village, IL 60007

847-434-4000
800-433-9016
Fax: 847-434-8000
www.aap.org

The American Academy of Pediatrics and its member pediatricians are committed to the attainment of optimal physical, mental and social health and well-being for all infants, children, adolescents, and young adults.

Fernando Stein, MD, FAAP, President
Karen Remley, MD, CEO/Executive VP

6317 American College of Allergy, Asthma & Immu nology
85 West Algonquin Road, Suite 550
Arlington Heights, IL 60005

847-427-1200
Fax: 847-427-9656
mail@acaai.org
www.acaai.org

The American College of Allergy, Asthma & Immunology is a professional association of 6,000 allergists/immunologists and allied health professionals. Established in 1942, the College is dedicated to improving the quality of patient care in allergy and immunology through research, advocacy and professional and public education.

Rick Slawny, Executive Director
Nancy Ryan, Associate Executive Director
Hollis Heavenrich-Jones, Public Relations Manager

6318 Asthma and Allergy Foundation of America
8201 Corporate Drive, Ste 1000
Landover, MD 20785

800-727-8462
www.aafa.org

AAFA provides practical information, community based services and support to people through a network of regional chapters, educational support groups and other local partners througout the United States.

6319   World Allergy Organization
555 East Wells Street, Ste 1100
Milwaukee, WI 53202   414-276-1791
Fax: 414-276-3349
info@worldallergy.org
www.worldallergy.org

A world-wide alliance of national and regional allergy and clinical immunology societies and organizations dedicated to raising awareness and advanceing excellence in clinical education, research and training in the field of allergy and pediatric allergy.

State Agencies & Support Groups

Colorado

6320   Parents of Asthmatic/Allergic Children, In c.
1024 S. Lemay Avenue
Fort Collins, CO 80524   970-495-8153
Fax: 970-495-7608
cmc@pvhs.org
www.coloradoallergy.com

Support group for parents and children ages 6 and older, focusing on asthma, and issues such as allergic and non-allergic rhinitis.

Cindy Coopersmith, Coordinator

Illinois

6321   Mothers of Children with Allergies (MOCHA)
Highland Park Hospital
777 Park Avenue West
Highland Park, IL 60035   847-735-8244
supportgroups@aafa.org
www.mochallergies.org

Support group serving Chicago & the Northern suburbs for parents and children having allergies associated with the environment, food, and Asthma.

Anne Thompson, Coordinator
Denise Bunning, Coordinator

New Jersey

6322   Allergy and Asthma Support Group of Centra l New Jersey
www.allergyfriendsnj.org

ainserro@allergyfriendsnj.org
www.allergyfriendsnj.org

The support group is for adults and parents of children with food allergies, environmental allergies, asthma, or a combination. The Allergy & Asthma Support Group of Central New Jersey supports families and friends afflicted by life threatening food allergies and other conditions such as environmental and non-environmental allergies.

Allison Inserro, Co-Facilitator

Libraries & Resource Centers

6323   The University of Iowa Libraries
100 Main Library (LIB)
Iowa City, IA 52242   319-335-5299
www.guides.lib.uiowa.edu/allergyimmunology

The libraries at the University of Iowa contain a collection of clinical resources on allergy and immunology.

6324   University of South Florida
12901 Bruce B. Downs Boulevard
Tampa, FL 33612   727-553-3533
Fax: 727-553-1295
sborst@health.usf.edu
www.health.usf.edu

Available libraries include ACH Medical Library, Bayfront Medical Center Library, and several libraries at USF such as: Hinks and Elaine Shimberg Health Sciences Library, Tampa Campus Library and many others. All libraries have access to MEDLINE.

Stacy Borst, Training Program Coordinator

Research Centers

6325   Allergy and Asthma Medical Group and Resea rch Center
9610 Granite Ridge Drive, Suite B
San Diego, CA 92123   858-268-2368
Fax: 858-268-5147
www.allergyandasthma.com

The Allergy and Asthma Medical Group and Research Center provide quality care given by a highly-trained team of physicians, nurse practitioners, nurses, medical assistants and office personnel with an understanding of the impact of these disorders on patients and their families.

6326   Children's National Health System
111 Michigan Avenue NW
Washington, DC 20010   202-476-5000
TTY: 800-855-1155
www.childrensnational.org

Children's National Medical Center's recognized staff of pediatric healthcare professionals deliver sophisticated care to thousands of families throughout the region and around the world.

George Zalzal, MD, Division Chief, Otolaryngology

6327   Duke University School of Medicine Pediatr ic and Allergy Immunology
T901/Children's Health Center
Durham, NC 27710   919-681-4080
Fax: 919-681-2714
http://pediatrics.duke.edu

Thd Division of Pediatric Allergy and Immunology and its faculty and staff ar committed to excellence in patient care, research, education and advocacy. Areas of expertise include all allergic diseases, anaphylaxis, primary immunodeficiency, asthma, rhinitis and others.

George Zalzal, MD, Division Chief, Otolaryngology

6328   Johns Hopkins Division of Allergy and Clin ical Immunology
5501 Hopkins Bayview Circle
Baltimore, MD 21224   410-550-2300
jhuallergy@jhmi.edu
www.hopkinsmedicine.org/allergy

The faculty and staff at the Johns Hopkins Division of Allergy and Clinical Immunology are working to meet the demand for advances in the treatment of allergies, asthma, and related disorders.

6329   The University of Chicago Comer Children's Hospital
5271 S. Maryland Avenue
Chicago, IL 60637   773-702-1000
888-824-0200
www.uchicagokidshospital.org/allergy

Doctors at Chicago Comer Children's Hospital are experts on a wide variety of childhood allergies, and specialize in diagnosing and treating the full range of allergic and immune disorders of infancy and childhood.

Web Sites

6330 American Academy of Pediatrics
141 Northwest Point Boulevard
Elk Grove Village, IL 60007   847-434-4000
                                               800-433-9016
                                               Fax: 847-434-8000
                                               www.aap.org

The American Academy of Pediatrics and its member pediatricians are committed to the attainment of optimal physical, mental and social health and well-being for all infants, children, adolescents, and young adults.

Fernando Stein, MD, FAAP, President
Karen Remley, MD, CEO/Executive VP

6331 http://children.webmd.com
WebMD
www.webmd.com/children

Includes comprehensive health information on pediatric allergic rhinitis, plus a variety of other pediatric health conditions. This site includes news, videos, FAQs, the opportunity to chat with other patients and parents, a glossary, and parenting topics. Users can search by condition, age, symptoms, and more.

Kristy Hammam, Senior Vice President
Denise Dym, Senior Director
Annic Jobin, Senior Director

6332 www.Nasal-Allergies.com
www.nasal-allergies.com/nasx

This web site offers education about pediatric and adult nasal allergies, inlcuding treatment and resources.

6333 www.aap.org
American Academy of Pediatrics
141 Northwest Point Boulevard
Elk Grove Village, IL 60007   847-434-4000
                                               800-433-9016
                                               Fax: 847-434-8000
                                               webeditor@aap.org
                                               www.aap.org

This site includes a variety of resources to help deal with allergic rhinitis, including a parenting corner, publications, advocacy, and recommendations on treatment.

Sandra Hassink, MD, FAAP, President
Benard P. Dreyer, MD, FAAP, President-Elect
Errol R. Alden, MD, FAAP, Executive Director/ CEO

6334 www.acaai.org
85 West Algonquin Road, Suite 550
Arlington Heights, IL 60005   847-427-1200
                                               Fax: 847-427-1294
                                               mail@acaai.org
                                               acaai.org

The American College of Allergy, Asthma & Immunology is a professional association of 5,500 allergists/immunologists and allied health professionals. Established in 1942, the College is dedicated to improving the quality of patient care in allergy and immunology through research, advocacy and professional and public education.

James L. Sublett, MD, President
Stephen A. Tilles, MD, Vice President
Bradley E. Chipps, MD, Treasurer

6335 www.pediatriccareonline.org
American Academy of Pediatrics
pediatriccare.solutions.aap.org/Pediatric-Care

This online publication includes definitions, clinical features, complications, laboratory findings, differential diagnosis, treatment, prognosis, tools, and references for a number of pediatric conditions, including allergic rhinitis. Users can also search for other relevant American Academy of Pediatrics publications.

6336 www.wrongdiagnosis.com
www.localhealth.com

WrongDiagnosis.com provides a free health information service to help people understand their health better. The site offers factual health information that is otherwise difficult to find. Topics include allergic rhinitis and the signs and symptoms associated with the allergy.

Richard G Grower, MD, President

6337 yourtotalhealth.ivillage.com

Contains information on numerous medical topics including pediatric allergies and asthma.

Richard G Grower, MD, President

Book Publishers

6338 Fast Facts: Rhinitis

Glenis K Scadding & Wytske J Fokkens, author

Health Press
30 Amberwood Parkway
Ashland, OH 44805   800-247-6553
                                               Fax: 419-281-6883
                                               info@atlasbooks.com
                                               www.fastfacts.com

This short and very practical book has been written for the individuals who are not seen by specialists for treatment of rhinitis, so treatment can be optimized and referral decisions are made easier.

6339 Immunology and Allergy Clinics of North Am erica
1600 John F Kennedy Boulevard, Suite 1800
Philadelphia, PA 19103   314-447-8871
                                               800-654-2452
                                               ElsevierClinics@elsevier.com
                                               www.immunology.theclinics.com

Comprehensive, state-of-the-art reviews by experts in the field of allergy and pediatric allergy provide current, practical information on the diagnosis and treatment of conditions affecting the respiratory system. Each issue focuses on a single topic.

Journals

6340 AAP News
American Academy of Pediatrics
141 Northwest Point Boulevard
Elk Grove Village, IL 60007   847-434-4000
                                               800-433-9016
                                               Fax: 847-434-8000
                                               webeditor@aap.org
                                               www.aap.org

A resource of product recall alerts, pediatric medication warnings, and key advancements in pediatric medicine, including allergies and related conditions.

Sandra Hassink, MD, FAAP, President
Benard P. Dreyer, MD, FAAP, President-Elect
Errol R. Alden, MD, FAAP, Executive Director/ CEO

6341 Ear, Nose and Throat Journal
www.entjournal.com

Monthly journal with articles on pediatric and adult conditions that affect the ear, nose and throat, including allergic rhinitis.

Robert T.ˇ Sataloff, MD, DMA, FACS, Editor-in-Chief
Linda Zinn, Managing Director
Mark C. Horn, Sales Manager

6342 Journal of Allergy and Clinical Immunology
www.elsevier.com

Includes articles written by experts in the fields of allergy, pediatric allergy and immunology that discuss current research, causes, diagnosis, treatments, and clinical studies relating to pediatric rhinitis and a varity of other allergic conditions. Also includes listings of new health products and medical equipment.

Youngsuk Chi, Chairman
Ron Mobed, Chief Executive Officer
Stuart Whayman, Chief Financial Officer

6343 Pediatrics
American Academy of Pediatrics
141 Northwest Point Boulevard
Elk Grove Village, IL 60007

847-434-4000
800-433-9016
Fax: 847-434-8000
webeditor@aap.org
www.aap.org

The flagship journal of the AAP, whose authoritative content has been recognized by medical experts for 60 years. Includes information on a variety of pediaric conditions, including allergic rhinitis.

Sandra Hassink, MD, FAAP, President
Benard P. Dreyer, MD, FAAP, President-Elect
Errol R. Alden, MD, FAAP, Executive Director/ CEO

6344 Pediatrics in Review
American Academy of Pediatrics
141 Northwest Point Boulevard
Elk Grove Village, IL 60007

847-434-4000
800-433-9016
Fax: 847-434-8000
webeditor@aap.org
www.aap.org

Features real-life cases, best practices, and review articles mapped to ABP content specifications for maintenance of certification-pediatrics. Conditions covered include pediatric allergy rhinitis and related conditions.

Sandra Hassink, MD, FAAP, President
Benard P. Dreyer, MD, FAAP, President-Elect
Errol R. Alden, MD, FAAP, Executive Director/ CEO

6345 World Allergy Organization Journal
236 Gray's Inn Road
London, WC1X

203-192-2009
Fax: 203-192-2010
waoj@worldallergy.org
www.waojournal.org

The official journal of the World Allergy Organization whose goals include to: be a premier journal of original scientific and clinically relevant information for practicing allergists/immunologists; to publish state-of-the-art review articles and editorials on translational and clincal medicine in the field of allergy, pediatric allergy and immunology; and to present a forum for scientific interaction between allergists, pediatric allergists and immunologists worldwide.

Alessandro Fiocchi, Editor-in-Chief
Johannes Ring, Executive Editor
Erika Jensen-Jarolim, Deputy Director

Newsletters

6346 AAP Grand Rounds
American Academy of Pediatrics
141 Northwest Point Boulevard
Elk Grove Village, IL 60007

847-434-4000
800-433-9016
Fax: 847-434-8000
webeditor@aap.org
www.aap.org

Features evidence-based summaries of clinical content from 100 journals. A key feature, 'Weighing the Evidence,' provides medical literature interpretation assistance.

Sandra Hassink, MD, FAAP, President
Benard P. Dreyer, MD, FAAP, President-Elect
Errol R. Alden, MD, FAAP, Executive Director/ CEO

6347 ACAAI eNews
85 West Algonquin Road, Suite 550
Arlington Heights, IL 60005

847-427-1200
Fax: 847-427-1294
enews@acaai.org
acaai.org

The ACAAI eNews is a monthly aggregated news service provided by the American College of Allergy, Asthma & Immunology.

Richard G Grower, MD, President

6348 Allergy & Asthma Issues
American Academy of Allergy Asthma & Immunology
555 E. Wells Street, Suite 1100
Milwaukee, WI 53202

414-272-6071
Fax: 414-272-6070
www.aaaai.org

A quarterly member publication produced by the AAAAI.

Megan Brown, Communications Manager

DESCRIPTION

6349 SARCOIDOSIS

Synonyms: Sarcoid of Boeck, Schaumann's disease

Involves the following Biologic System(s):

Connective Tissue Disorders

Sarcoidosis is a multisystem disorder that is characterized by the abnormal development of inflammatory growths or nodules (i.e., epithelioid granulomas) in various organs in the body. The cause of this inflammatory disorder is unknown; however, it is believed that granuloma formation associated with sarcoidosis may result from infection or an exaggerated immune response to specific agents (antigens). In addition, researchers believe that some people may be genetically predisposed to sarcoidosis and develop the disease only if triggered by environmental or other factors. Although this disorder most commonly occurs during young adulthood, it may occur in children and in the elderly. Symptoms and physical findings associated with sarcoidosis are dependent upon the organ(s) involved and, in children, the age of onset. Most affected children, however, share the common symptoms of fatigue, weight loss, cough, pain in the bones and joints, and abnormally low levels of circulating red blood cells (anemia).

The nodules or granulomas associated with sarcoidosis may develop in almost any organ of the body, but most commonly affect the lungs, upper respiratory tract, lymph nodes, skin, eyes, liver, bones, joints, bone marrow, skeletal muscles, heart, liver, spleen, or the central and peripheral nervous systems. In older children and adults, the lungs are most often affected (90 percent of patients), while younger children experience less lung involvement. Characteristic findings in older children may include swelling of the lymph nodes near the blood vessels that enter and exit the lungs (hilar lymphadenopathy) as well as the lymph nodes near the windpipe (paratracheal lymphadenopathy) and those under the skin (peripheral lymphadenopathy). In addition, nodule formation may cause inflammations in the eye (e.g., uveitis and iritis) and other eye lesions, skin lesions, and liver changes. Younger children may develop a reddish, combination-type rash consisting of waxy pimples and flat, discolored lesions (maculopapular erythematous rash) as well as inflammation of the joints (arthritis).

Diagnosis of sarcoidosis is usually a challenge as it is often difficult to distinguish from other disorders with similar symptoms and findings. Therefore, differential diagnosis often involves a physical examination, medical and environmental history, and the comprehensive evaluation of laboratory tests and chest x-rays, biopsy of tissue samples, and specialized testing. Laboratory findings may show excessive levels of calcium in the blood (hypercalcemia) and in the urine (hypercalciuria), abnormally high levels of protein in the blood (hyperproteinemia), excessive levels of certain granular white cells in the blood (eosinophilia), and other blood irregularities. For example, the cells of the nodules secrete a substance called angiotensin-converting enzyme, which, in some patients, is elevated to detectable levels in the blood. Testing for this enzyme may also be employed to measure disease activity. In addition, pulmonary function tests may be used to measure progress of the disease in those children with lung involvement, and repeat chest x-rays may also be indicated to monitor progress.

In some children, sarcoidosis may resolve spontaneously within a period of months or years; however, some children may have a more chronic form of the disease that may result in progressive lung involvement, eye disease that may cause blindness, and other prolonged symptoms and findings. Treatment for sarcoidosis may include the use of corticosteroid drops or ointments to alleviate eye inflammations and oral corticosteroids to alleviate acute symptoms such as resistant inflammatory lesions of the eyes, joint pain, fever, shortness of breath, and other symptoms. Approximately 90 percent of cases are responsive to corticosteroids and can be controlled with modest maintenance doses. If no symptoms are present, corticosteroid treatment is usually not advised. Other treatment is symptomatic and supportive.

National Associations & Support Groups

6350 American Academy of Pediatrics
141 Northwest Point Boulevard
Elk Grove Village, IL 60007
847-434-4000
800-433-9016
Fax: 847-434-8000
www.aap.org

The American Academy of Pediatrics and its member pediatricians are committed to the attainment of optimal physical, mental and social health and well-being for all infants, children, adolescents, and young adults.

Fernando Stein, MD, FAAP, President
Karen Remley, MD, CEO/Executive VP

6351 American Autoimmune Related Diseases Association
22100 Gratiot Avenue
Eastpointe, MI 48021
586-776-3900
800-598-4668
Fax: 586-776-3903
aarda@aarda.org
www.aarda.org

Dedicated to the eradication of autoimmune diseases and the alleviation of suffering and the socio-economic impact of autoimmunity through fostering and facilitating collaboration in the areas of education, public awareness, research and patient services in an effective, ethical and efficient manner.

Virginia T. Ladd, President/Executive Director
Patricia Barber, Assistant Director
Deb Patrick, Events Specialist

6352 National Sarcoidosis Resource Center and Networking Program
PO Box 1593
Piscataway, NJ 08855
732-463-0497
Fax: 732-463-0497
www.nsrc-global.net

Formed to heighten public awareness and to educate people about this often chronic and disabling disease; offers information and support. The center serves the United States, Canada, Europe.

Sandra Conroy, President

6353 Sarcoid Networking Association
12619 S. Wilderness Way
Molalla, OR 97308
541-905-2092
ÿsarcoidinformation@sarcoidosisnetwork.o
www.sarcoidosisnetwork.org

A nonprofit organization dedicated to improving the lives of those affected by sarcoidosis through providing support, eduation and other resources.

Kristi Anderson, Executive Director

6354 Sarcoid Registry
5239 SW Lance St
Roseburg, OR 97471
541-905-2092
admin@snaregistry.org
www.snaregistry.org

Operates under the laedership of SNA-Sarcoid Networking Association to bring the Sarcoidosis community together.

Kristi Anderson, Director

6355 Sarcoidosis Network Foundation
11428 E Artesia Blvd, Suite 10
Artesia, CA 90701
562-809-8500
Fax: 562-809-8182
www.sarcoid-network.org

A nonprofit organization that promotes awareness and education; supports research to find a cure; and supports those affected by sarcoidosis and their families.

Ruth Jacobs, President
Charles Walker, VP
Jean Johnson-Bell, Treasurer

6356 Sarcoidosis Research Institute
3475 Central Avenue
Memphis, TN 38111
901-219-6883
Fax: 901-774-7294
sarcoidosis@bellsouth.net
www.sarcoidosisresearch.org

Provides patient and professional education that will result in enhanced methods of diagnosis and treatment of the disease; information that will assist patients and their support network in the management of the disease; and engages in research initiatives that will result in a cure for the debilitating disease.

State Agencies & Support Groups

California

6357 REACH - Sarcoidosis Support
10843 Kenney St
Norwalk, CA 90650
714-739-4023
Ruth Jacobs

Colorado

6358 Denver Sarcoidosis Awareness Support Group
4351 Ireland St
Denver, CO 80249
303-375-9376
contacts@denversarcoidosisawareness.org
www.denversarcoidosisawareness.org

Provides support through sharing of experiences, discussing feeling and emotions, and sharing coping strategies.

Shirley R Holley, President

Georgia

6359 Sarcoidosis Support Group
St Joseph's/Chandler Health System
5353 Reynolds St
Savannah, GA 31405
912-819-8032
balkstra@sjchs.org

Cindy Balkstra RN

Indiana

6360 Central Indiana Sarcoidosis Support Group
Kindred Hospital
1700 W 10th St
Indianapolis, IN 46222
317-809-7011
cissg@usa.com
www.indysarcoid.org

The Central Indiana Sarcoidosis Support Group was started in 1998 to offer hope and support to those diagnosed with Sarcoidosis.

Gloria Hooks, President
Kelisa Walker, Vice President
Mary Wineglass, Secretary

Maryland

6361 Sarcoidosis Awareness Network
10313 Farrar Avenue
Cheltenham, MD 20623
301-372-2885
info@sarcoidosisawareness.org
www.sarcoidosisnetwork.net

The Sarcoidosis Awareness Network is a nonprofit organization established to increase and expand the public awareness of sarcoidosis; enhance the quality of life of sarcoidosis survivors; develop and implement a sarcoidosis registry; and to disseminate current literature on the disease so the general public is better informed about sarcoidosis and its impact on the lives of those afflicted with the disease.

Linda D. Lanier, Founder

Michigan

6362 Sarcoidosis Awareness Foundation
14540 Whitcomb St
Detroit, MI 48227
SarcoidAwareness@aol.com
Janie L Chuney

6363 Sarcoidosis Resource Support Group
PO Box 3231
Highland Park, MI 48203
315-575-4852
pmullins@detroitsworkplace.org
www.sarcoidosisnetwork.org/groups.htm
Pam Mullins
Dot Lawrence

6364 Sarcoidosis Support - Beaumont
William Beaumont Hospital
300 W 13 Mile Rd
Royal Oak, MI 48073
248-545-0320
lagalbrith@yahoo.com
www.sarcoidosisnetwork.org/groups.htm
Victoria Rice
Laura Galbraith, Contact
Sylvia Johnson, Contact

New Jersey

6365 Sarcoidosis Support Resource Central New Jersey
National Sarcoidosis Resource Center
PO Box 1593
Piscataway, NJ 08855
732-699-0733
Fax: 732-699-0882
www.sarcoidosisnetwork.org/groups.htm
Sandra Conroy

New York

6366 Long Island Sarcoidosis Support
1989 N Jerusalem Rd
E Meadow, NY 11554
516-483-2666
www.sarcoidosisnetwork.org/groups.htm
Robert Schoenfeld, Facilitator

North Carolina

6367 Sarcoidosis Support Group
1021 Fitzgerald Dr
Wilmington, NC 28405
910-395-0154
www.sarcoidosisnetwork.org/groups.htm

Uldridge Galloway

6368 University of North Carolina Sarcoidosis Support Group
Div. of Pulmonary Medicine
130 Mason Farm Rd, CB# 7020
Chapel Hill, NC 27599   919-966-5296
                                   juliem@med.unc.edu
                                   www.unceye.org

Ricky Bass, Manager

Pennsylvania

6369 Sarcoidosis Self-Help
2112 Highland Avenue
New Castle, PA 16105   412-652-6089
                                   www.sarcoidosisnetwork.org/groups.htm
Della Emmanuel

South Carolina

6370 Sarcoidosis Support
MUSC Medical Center
171 Ashley Ave
Charleston, SC 29425   803-792-0280
Kathy Lanza

Tennessee

6371 Middle Tennessee Sarcoidosis Support Group
PO Box 1342
Cookesville, TN 38503   931-528-7826
                                   www.sarcoidosisnetwork.org/groups.htm
Becky Robertson

6372 Sarcoidosis Patient Forum
Sarcoidosis Research Institute-SRI
3475 Central Avenue
Memphis, TN 38111   901-219-6883
                                   Fax: 901-774-7294
Paula Polite, President

Virginia

6373 Sarcoidosis Support Group
704 Woodnote Land
Newport News, VA 23608   804-988-3065
                                   www.sarcoidosisnetwork.org/groups.htm
Beverly Moses

Libraries & Resource Centers

6374 National Sarcoidosis Resource Center
PO Box 1593
Piscataway, NJ 08855   732-463-0497
                                   Fax: 732-463-0467
                                   www.nsrc-global.net

Provides general information about special services for
sarcoidosis patients; strives to increase public awareness about
this unknown disease, and to generate interest in sarcordosis and
support research, leading to easy diagnosis, better treatments and,
ultimately, a cure.
Sandra Conroy

6375 Sarcoidosis Center
Baptist Hospital East
6005 Park Avenue, Suite 501
Memphis, TN 38119   901-761-5877
                                   Fax: 901-761-2280
                                   sarcoid@sarcoidcenter.com
                                   www.sarcoidcenter.com

A nonprofit organization providing an exchange of information
regarding sarcoidosis for patients and professionals.
Norman T Soskel MD

Research Centers

6376 National Jewish Medical & Research Center
1400 Jackson St
Denver, CO 80206   303-388-4461
                                   800-222-5864
                                   www.nationaljewish.org/disease-info

Information on ongoing sarcoidosis research and available treatment programs at the center.
Russell P Bowler, Vice Chair/Associate Professor

6377 Sarcoidosis Research Institute
3475 Central Avenue
Memphis, TN 38111   901-219-6883
                                   Fax: 901-774-7294
                                   sarcoidosis@bellsouth.net
                                   www.sarcoidosisresearch.org

Provides patient and professional education that will result in enhanced methods of diagnosis and treatment of the disease; information that will assist patients and their support network in the
management of the disease; and engages in research initiatives
that will result in a cure for the debilitating disease.

Audio Video

6378 Dialogue with Doris
PC Publications
PO Box 1593
Piscataway, NJ 8855   732-699-0733
                                   Fax: 732-699-0882
                                   www.webmd.com

Kristy Hammam, Senior Vice President
Denise Dym, Senior Director
Annic Jobin, Senior Director

6379 Help with a Hidden Disease Update
PC Publications
PO Box 1593
Piscataway, NJ 8855   732-699-0733
                                   800-223-6429
                                   Fax: 732-699-0882
                                   www.webmd.com

Kristy Hammam, Senior Vice President
Denise Dym, Senior Director
Annic Jobin, Senior Director

**6380 International World Conference on Sarcoidosis-Patient
Symposium**
PC Publications
PO Box 1593
Piscataway, NJ 8855   732-699-0733
                                   Fax: 732-699-0882
                                   www.webmd.com

Cassette.
Kristy Hammam, Senior Vice President
Denise Dym, Senior Director
Annic Jobin, Senior Director

6381 Of Their Own-Person To Person Show
PC Publications
PO Box 1593
Piscataway, NJ 8855   732-699-0733
                                   Fax: 732-699-0882
                                   www.webmd.com

Kristy Hammam, Senior Vice President
Denise Dym, Senior Director
Annic Jobin, Senior Director

6382 Sarcoidosis Conference 2
PC Publications
PO Box 1593
Piscataway, NJ 8855   732-699-0733
                                   Fax: 732-699-0882
                                   www.webmd.com

Kristy Hammam, Senior Vice President
Denise Dym, Senior Director
Annic Jobin, Senior Director

6383 Sarcoidosis Conference 3
PC Publications
PO Box 1593
Piscataway, NJ 8855

732-699-0733
Fax: 732-699-0882
www.webmd.com

Kristy Hammam, Senior Vice President
Denise Dym, Senior Director
Annic Jobin, Senior Director

6384 Sarcoidosis and Lyme Disease
PC Publications
PO Box 1593
Piscataway, NJ 8855

732-699-0733
Fax: 732-699-0882
www.webmd.com

Kristy Hammam, Senior Vice President
Denise Dym, Senior Director
Annic Jobin, Senior Director

6385 Sarcoidosis-What's That?
PC Publications
PO Box 1593
Piscataway, NJ 8855

732-699-0733
Fax: 732-699-0882
www.webmd.com

Kristy Hammam, Senior Vice President
Denise Dym, Senior Director
Annic Jobin, Senior Director

Web Sites

6386 American Autoimmune Related Diseases Association
www.aarda.org

Dedicated to the eradiction of autoimmune diseases and the alleviation of suffering and the socio-economic impact of autoimmunity through fostering and facilitating collaboration in the areas of education, public awareness, research and patient services in an effective, ethical and efficient manner.

6387 Foundation for Sarcoidosis Research
1820 W. Webster Ave., Ste 304
Chicago, IL 60614

866-358-5477
www.stopsarcoidosis.org

Takes the lead as a nonprofit organization in funding research in finding a cure for sarcoidosis and improving patient care.

Andrea Wilson, Chairwoman
Anjan Chatterji, President
Reading Wilson, Treasurer

6388 Health Answers
410 Horsham Road
Horsham, PA 19044

215-442-9010
Michael.tague@healthanswers.com
www.healthanswers.com

HealthAnswers offers a breadth of services in medical education, sales force training, patient support solutions, professional promotion and consumer solutions.

Michael Tague, Managing Director

6389 NIH/National Heart, Lung and Blood Institu te
P.O. Box 30105
Bethesda, MD 20824

301-592-8573
nhlbiinfo@nhlbi.nih.gov
www.nhlbi.nih.gov/health/dci/Index/s.html

A part of the National Institutes of Health, this NHLBI site offers general information and answers to questions about Sarcoidosis.

Gary H. Gibbons, MD, Director

6390 National Sarcoidosis Resource Center
www.nsrc-global.net

The center provides information to people throughout the U.S., Canada, and Europe. They have an ongoing research study of the symptoms and demographics of Sarcoidosis patients.

6391 Online Mendelian Inheritance in Man
National Library of Medicine, Building 38A
Bethesda, MD 20894

888-346-3656
info@ncbi.nlm.nih.gov
www.ncbi.nlm.nih.gov

This database is a catalog of human genes and genetic disorders.

Christine E. Seidman, M.D., Chair
David J. Lipman, M.D., Executive Secretary

6392 Sarcoid Life
www.sarcoidlife.org

6393 Sarcoidosis
www.epler.com/wsarc.html

General information and answers to questions about Sarcoidosis.

6394 Sarcoidosis Center
www.sarcoidcenter.com

A nonprofit corporation designed to provide information for patients and physicians regarding sarcoidosis. The site includes a list of sarcoidosis experts by country.

6395 Sarcoidosis Research Institute
www.sarcoidosisresearch.org

Provides patient and professional education that will result in enhanced methods of diagnosis and treatment of the disease.

Book Publishers

6396 Sarcoidosis Resource Guide and Directory
PC Publications
PO Box 1593
Piscataway, NJ 08855

732-699-0733
Fax: 732-699-0882

1993 304 pages Paperback
ISBN: 0-963122-25-8

Newsletters

6397 Online Sarcoidosis Newsletter
National Sarcoidosis Resource Center
PO Box 1593
Piscataway, NJ 8855

732-699-0733
Fax: 732-699-0882

Offers information on the center's activities and events, medical and legislative updates for the patients and their families.

Quarterly

6398 Sarcoidosis Networking
Sarcoid Networking Association
6424 151st Avenue E
Sumner, WA 98390

253-891-6886
sarcoidosis_network@prodigy.net
www.sarcoidnetwork.org

Helps those affected by sarcoidosis network with one another and the medical community.

Quarterly

Dolores O'Leary, Executive Director

Pamphlets

6399 A Sarcoidosis Questionnaire: Demographics and Symptomatology-Patients Respond
PC Publications
PO Box 1593
Piscataway, NJ 8855
732-699-0733
800-223-6429
Fax: 732-699-0882

6400 Anemia of Sarcoidosis
PC Publications
PO Box 1593
Piscataway, NJ 8855
732-699-0733
Fax: 732-699-0882

6401 Bronchoalveolar Lymphocytes in Sarcoidosis
PC Publications
PO Box 1593
Piscataway, NJ 8855
732-699-0733
Fax: 732-699-0882

6402 Case Report-MR Imaging of Myocardial Sarcoidosis
PC Publications
PO Box 1593
Piscataway, NJ 8855
732-699-0733
Fax: 732-699-0882

6403 Case Report-Osseous Sarcoidosis and Chronic Polyarthritis
PC Publications
PO Box 1593
Piscataway, NJ 8855
732-699-0733
Fax: 732-699-0882

6404 Coping with Sarcoidosis
National Sarcoidosis Resource Center
PO Box 1593
Piscataway, NJ 8855
732-699-0733
Fax: 732-699-0882

A pamphlet offering information on how to manage and live with sarcoidosis.

6405 Drugs That Have Been Used for the Treatment of Sarcoidosis
PC Publications
PO Box 1593
Piscataway, NJ 8855
732-699-0733
Fax: 732-699-0882

6406 Effects of Sarcoid and Steroids on Angiotensin-Converting Enzyme
PC Publications
PO Box 1593
Piscataway, NJ 8855
732-699-0733
Fax: 732-699-0882

6407 Masqueraders of Sarcoidosis
PC Publications
PO Box 1593
Piscataway, NJ 8855
732-699-0733
Fax: 732-699-0882

6408 Multidisciplinary Clinico-Pathologic Conference
PC Publications
PO Box 1593
Piscataway, NJ 8855
732-699-0733
Fax: 732-699-0882

6409 National Sarcoidosis Resource Center
PC Publications
PO Box 1593
Piscataway, NJ 8855
732-699-0733
Fax: 732-699-0882
www.nsrc-global.net

A booklet offering a brief introduction to the illness and information on the role of the Center in finding a cure and educating the public on Sarcoidosis.

6410 Neurosarcoidosis
PC Publications
PO Box 1593
Piscataway, NJ 8855
732-699-0733
Fax: 732-699-0882

6411 Neurosarcoidosis or Multiple Sclerosis?
National Sarcoidosis Resource Center
PO Box 1593
Piscataway, NJ 8855
732-699-0733
Fax: 732-699-0882

6412 Paranoid Psychosis Due to Neurosarcoidosis
PC Publications
PO Box 1593
Piscataway, NJ 8855
732-699-0733
800-223-6429
Fax: 732-699-0882

6413 Patient Information Package
National Sarcoidosis Resource Center
PO Box 1593
Piscataway, NJ 8855
732-699-0733
Fax: 732-699-0882

Contains various brochures and pamphlets offering information about sarcoidosis.

6414 Presidential Proclamation-National Sarcoidosis Awareness Day
PC Publications
PO Box 1593
Piscataway, NJ 8855
732-699-0733
Fax: 732-699-0882

6415 Psychological Factors in Sarcoidosis
PC Publications
PO Box 1593
Piscataway, NJ 8855
732-699-0733
Fax: 732-699-0882

6416 Pulmonary Sarcoidosis: Evaluation with High Resolution
PC Publications
PO Box 1593
Piscataway, NJ 8855
732-699-0733
Fax: 732-699-0882

6417 Pulmonary Sarcoidosis: What We Are Learning
PC Publications
PO Box 1593
Piscataway, NJ 8855
732-699-0733
Fax: 732-699-0882

6418 Right & Left Ventricular Function At Rest In Patients with Sarcoidosis
PC Publications
PO Box 1593
Piscataway, NJ 8855
732-699-0733
Fax: 732-699-0882

6419 Sarcoidosis
PC Publications
PO Box 1593
Piscataway, NJ 8855
732-699-0733
Fax: 732-699-0882

Offers information on the illness, causes, symptoms and treatments.

6420 Sarcoidosis Questionnaire: Demographics and Symptomatology-The Patients Respond
PC Publications
PO Box 1593
Piscataway, NJ 8855
732-699-0733
Fax: 732-699-0882

6421 Sarcoidosis and Other Granulatomous
PC Publications
PO Box 1593
Piscataway, NJ 8855   732-699-0733
         800-223-6429
       Fax: 732-699-0882

6422 Sarcoidosis and You-A Listing of Possible Symptoms
PC Publications
PO Box 1593
Piscataway, NJ 8855   732-699-0733
       Fax: 732-699-0882

6423 Sarcoidosis-International Review
PC Publications
PO Box 1593
Piscataway, NJ 8855   732-699-0733
       Fax: 732-699-0882

6424 Sarcoidosis-Pleural Involvement Mimicking a Coin Lesson
PC Publications
PO Box 1593
Piscataway, NJ 8855   732-699-0733
       Fax: 732-699-0882

6425 Sarcoidosis: A Multisystem Disease
PC Publications
PO Box 1593
Piscataway, NJ 8855   732-699-0733
       Fax: 732-699-0882

Explains the effects of the illness on the lungs and joints.

6426 Sarcoidosis: Usual and Unusual Manifestations
PC Publications
PO Box 1593
Piscataway, NJ 8855   732-699-0733
       Fax: 732-699-0882

6427 Seasonal Clustering of Sarcoidosis
National Sarcoidosis Resource Center
PO Box 1593
Piscataway, NJ 8855   732-699-0733
       Fax: 732-699-0882

6428 Successful Treatment of Myocardial Sarcoidosis with Steriods
PC Publications
PO Box 1593
Piscataway, NJ 8855   732-699-0733
       Fax: 732-699-0882

6429 Support Group Listing
PC Publications
PO Box 1593
Piscataway, NJ 8855   732-699-0733
       Fax: 732-699-0882

6430 World Association Sarcoidosis Other Granulatomous
PC Publications
PO Box 1593
Piscataway, NJ 8855   732-699-0733
       Fax: 732-699-0882

DESCRIPTION

6431 SCLERODERMA

Covers these related disorders: Linear scleroderma, Morphea, Systemic sclerosis

Involves the following Biologic System(s):
Connective Tissue Disorders

Scleroderma is a connective tissue disease characterized by the build up of collagen (connective tissue) resulting in thickening and hardening of the skin and underlying tissues or, in some forms of scleroderma, other organs of the body. In patients with morphea, a form of the disease that primarily affects the skin and its underlying (subcutaneous) tissues, lesions appear as limited or localized patches. In linear scleroderma, lesions appear in a band-like pattern. In other patients, particularly in adults, scleroderma may occur as a generalized, systemic disease affecting the skin and subcutaneous tissues, blood vessels, and internal organs, such as the heart, lungs, kidneys, and certain parts of the digestive tract. Although the underlying cause of scleroderma is not known, some researchers speculate that it may be an autoimmune disease in which there is an abnormal immune response against the body's own tissues. During childhood, scleroderma is more common in girls than boys.

Children with scleroderma are primarily affected by morphea or linear scleroderma. Associated symptoms and findings usually become apparent at age two or older. Patients initially develop patchy skin lesions that are dry, red or violet, and shiny in appearance. These lesions may cause associated pain or unusual sensations, such as prickling feelings in affected areas. In some children, the lesions may have a linear distribution and develop primarily on one side of the body. The lesions gradually become hard (indurated) and develop waxy, pale centers and elevated borders. As the disease continues to progress, the lesions become larger and merge, potentially involving a large area, such as an entire arm or leg. Affected areas may eventually develop deep scar tissue and firmly bind to underlying tissues, potentially resulting in pain and permanent bending of affected joints in fixed postures (joint contractures). In children with morphea or linear scleroderma, active disease may spontaneously subside over months or years or may slowly progress over many years.

Rarely, children may develop generalized, systemic scleroderma (systemic sclerosis). In such cases, associated symptoms and findings usually become apparent at age four or older. Children with systemic sclerosis often initially experience Raynaud's phenomenon, a condition characterized by sudden contraction of blood vessels supplying the fingers or toes, causing an interruption of blood flow and a subsequent excess of blood in affected areas following the restoration of blood flow (reactive hyperemia). Such episodes are usually triggered by exposure to cold temperatures and are characterized by numbness, tingling, and bluish or whitish discoloration of the fingers or toes (cyanosis) due to lack of blood flow and subsequent reddening and pain.

Children with systemic sclerosis also often develop skin lesions on the hands and feet and, in some cases, the torso and facial area. These lesions may include groups of permanently widened (dilated) blood vessels (telangiectasias). As the disease progresses, skin lesions typically become hard, develop unusually light or dark pigmentation, and gradually bind to underlying tissues and structures. Children may also experience joint swelling, discomfort, and inflammation (arthritis) as well as degenerative changes of various organs, including those of the digestive tract, particularly the esophagus; the heart; the lungs and the kidneys. Associated symptoms may be extremely variable, depending upon the rate of disease progression and the specific bodily tissues and organs affected. In some patients, such abnormalities may include difficulty swallowing (dysphagia); chronic inflammation of the lungs due to unintended inhalation of foreign matter into the airways (aspiration pneumonia); high blood pressure (hypertension); or respiratory, heart, or kidney failure. Active disease may be gradually progressive or include periods during which symptoms temporarily subside (remit).

The treatment of children with scleroderma is symptomatic and supportive. Such measures may include the use of steroids, such as cortisone or prednisone, to decrease inflammation in muscles, joints or rarely in the skin itself. Non-steroidal anti-inflammatory drugs (NSAIDs) such as ibuprofen and naproxen are sometimes used for children who have arthritis to decrease joint inflammation early physical therapy to help prevent or minimize the development of joint contractures; systemic therapy with methotrexate or other medications (e.g., cytotoxic drugs), if appropriate; careful control of high blood pressure in those with systemic disease; and other measures as required. In addition, patients with Raynaud's phenomenon should avoid cold temperatures whenever possible and dress warmly before such exposure. Scleroderma is a chronic and slowly progressive disease, lasting for months or years. The outlook depends on the type of scleroderma, where and how much skin is involved and whether or not internal organs are affected.

Government Agencies

6432 NIH/National Institute of Arthritis and Musculoskeletal and Skin Diseases
1 AMS Circle
Bethesda, MD 20892

301-495-4484
877-226-4267
Fax: 301-718-6366
TDD: 301-565-2966
niamsinfo@mail.nih.gov
www.niams.nih.gov

The mission of the NIAMS, a part of the NIH, is to support research into the causes, treatment, and prevention of arthritis and musculoskeletal and skin diseases, the training of basic and clinical scientists to carry out this research, and the dissemination of information on research progress in these diseases.

Stephen I Katz MD PhD, Director
Robert H Carter MD, Deputy Director
Gahan Breithaupt, Assoc Dir for Management & Operatio

National Associations & Support Groups

6433 American Academy of Pediatrics
141 Northwest Point Boulevard
Elk Grove Village, IL 60007

847-434-4000
800-433-9016
Fax: 847-434-8000
www.aap.org

The American Academy of Pediatrics and its member pediatricians are committed to the attainment of optimal physical, mental and social health and well-being for all infants, children, adolescents, and young adults.

Fernando Stein, MD, FAAP, President
Karen Remley, MD, CEO/Executive VP

6434 American Autoimmune Related Diseases Association
22100 Gratiot Avenue
Eastpointe, MI 48021
586-776-3900
800-598-4668
Fax: 586-776-3903
aarda@aarda.org
www.aarda.org

Dedicated to the eradiction of autoimmune diseases and the alleviation of suffering and the socio-economic impact of autoimmunity through fostering and facilitating collaboration in the areas of education, public awareness, research and patient services in an effective, ethical and efficient manner.

Virginia T. Ladd, President/Executive Director
Patricia Barber, Assistant Director
Deb Patrick, Events Specialist

6435 International Scleroderma Network
7455 France Ave S, #266
Edina, MN 55435
952-831-3091
800-564-7099
isn@sclero.org
www.scerlo.org

Nonprofit organization for the research, education, support, and awareness for scleroderma and related illnesses. Website available in 20 languages.

Kevin Lenue Billups, Founder/President

6436 Juvenile Scleroderma Network
1204 W 13th Street
San Pedro, CA 90731
310-519-9511
866-338-5892
Fax: 800-369-8309
outreachJSDN@aol.com
www.jsdn.org

A nonprofit organization that provides support and friendship to children who have Juvenile Scleroderma.

Thomas J.A. Lehman, M.D., Chief, Pediatric Rheumatologist
Ronald Laxer, M.D., Chief, Pediatric Rheumatologist
Bernice Krafchik, M.D., Pediatric Dermatology

6437 Scleroderma Foundation
300 Rosewood Dr, Suite 105
Danvers, MA 01923
978-750-4950
800-722-4673
Fax: 978-463-5809
sfinfo@scleroderma.org
www.scleroderma.org

Nonprofit national organization for people with scleroderma and their family and friends. Provides support and promotes education and research.

Robert J. Riggs, Ceo
Kerri Connolly, Director of Programs and Services
Tracey O. Sperry, Director of Development and Researc

State Agencies & Support Groups

Florida

6438 Scleroderma Foundation Southeast Florida Chapter
3930 Oaks Clubhouse Drive, Suite 206
Pompano Beach, FL 33069
954-798-1854
sclerodermasefl@gmail.com
www.scleroderma.org/site/PageServer?pagename=sefl_ho
Ferne Robin, Executive Director
Jerry Lance, President
Ruth Greenspan, Vice President

Illinois

6439 Scleroderma Foundation Chicago Chapter
134 N. LaSalle St. Suite 1360
Chicago, IL 60602
312-660-1131
Fax: 312-660-1133
GCchapter@scleroderma.org
www.scleroderma.org/site/PageServer?pagename=gc_home

We provide assistance to patients with scleroderma adhering to our three-fold mission of support, education and research.

Ann Peterson, Executive Director
Mike Robbins, President
Julie L. Drewniak, Secretary

Nevada

6440 Scleroderma Foundation Nevada Chapter
Vegas TV Building, 6760 Surrey Street
Las Vegas, NV 89118
702-368-1572
Fax: 702-368-1582
NVchapter@scleroderma.org
http://www.scleroderma.org/site/PageServer?pagename=
Sheila Gray, President
Sheila Gray, VP, Support Group

New Jersey

6441 Scleroderma Foundation New Jersey Chapter
PO Box 285
Haddon Heights, NJ 08035
856-547-5010
866-675-5545
Fax: 856-547-5010
sfdv1@verizon.net

Liz Van Dzura, Executive Director

New York

6442 Scleroderma Foundation Tri-State, Inc (NY, NJ, CT)
59 Front St
Binghamton, NY 13905
607-723-2239
800-867-0885
Fax: 607-723-2039
sdtristate@aol.com
www.scleroderma.org/chapter/tristate

The mission of the Scleroderma Foundation/Tri State, Inc. Chapter is three fold: To provide educational and emotional support to people with scleroderma and their families; to stimulate and support research designed to identify the cause and cure of scleroderma as well as improve methods of treatment; and to enhance the public's awareness of this disease.

Jay Peak, Executive Director
Tom Knapp, Office Manager

Rhode Island

6443 Rhode Island Scleroderma Support Group
Roger Williams Medical Ctr
825 Chalkstone Ave
Providence, RI 02908
401-781-5013
scleroderma@hotmail.com
www.ri.sclerodermasupportgroup.net
Carole Cowell, Contact
Frank L. Fitzpatrick, Webmaster

Texas

6444 Scleroderma Foundation Texas Bluebonnet Ch apter
101 W. McDermott Dr. Suite 115
Allen, TX 75013
972-396-9400
866-532-7673
Fax: 972-649-7910
TXchapter@scleroderma.org
www.scleroderma.org/site/PageServer?pagename=tx_home
Emily Woods, President
Amber Paris, Vice President
Virginia Browne, Secretary

Virginia

6445 **Scleroderma Foundation Greater Washington DC Chapter**
2010 Corporate Ridge, 7th Fl, PMB 126
McLean, VA 22102
202-999-4562
888-233-4779
GWDCchapter@scleroderma.org
www.scleroderma.org/site/PageServer?pagename=dc_invo
Carol Sodetz, Contact

Washington

6446 **Scleroderma Foundation Evergreen Chapter**
PO Box 84506
Seattle, WA 98124
206-285-9822
WAchapter@scleroderma.org
www.scleroderma.org/site/PageServer?pagename=wa_home
Bunny Garthe, President
Nic Evans, Vice President
Gloria Blanco-Duque, Secretary

Research Centers

Alabama

6447 **University of Alabama - Birmingham Arthrit is Clinical Intervention Program**
1717 6th Avenue South SRC 076
Birmingham, AL 35249
205-934-7727
866-876-2247
Fax: 205-975-5554
rand1951@uab.edu
www.uab.edu/medicine/acip/

Since 1990, the Arthritis Clinical Intervention Program (ACIP) has conducted over 300 rheumatology trials (Phase I-IV). All our doctors are Board Certified Rheumatologists with many years of research experience. Dr. Jeffrey Curtis is our Medical Director.

Randall Parks, MBA, RN, Program Director
David J. Mackey, MPH, Regulatory Manager
Martha R. Sanderson, MSN, NP, Nurse Practitioner

Arizona

6448 **Mayo Clinic Scleroderma Service**
13400 E Shea Blvd
Scottsdale, AZ 85259
480-301-8000
Fax: 480-301-8673
www.mayoclinic.org/rheumatology-sct/
Heidi Garcia, Research Info

California

6449 **Scleroderma Research Foundation**
220 Montgomery St, Suite 1411
San Francisco, CA 94104
415-834-9444
800-441-2873
Fax: 415-834-9177
info@sclerodermaresearch.org
www.srfcure.org

The Scleroderma Research Foundation's mission is to find a cure for scleroderma, a life-threatening and degenerative illness, by funding and facilitating the most promising, highest quality research and placing the disease and its need for a cure in the public eye.

Luke Evnin, PhD, Chairman
Charles Spaulding, Vice President, Communications
Jill Wayne, Director, Cure Advocate Program

District of Columbia

6450 **Georgetown University**
Dept of Rheumatology
PHC Bldg, 3800 Reservoir Rd, 6th Fl
Washington, DC 20007
202-784-6671
Fax: 202-784-4332
memory@georgetown.edu
www.memory.georgetown.edu/

For adult and pediatric patients with localized and systemic scleroderma.

Raoul L Wientzen, President
R. Scott Turner, MD, PhD, Program Director
Carolyn Ward, MSPH, Program Coordinator

Pennsylvania

6451 **National Registry for Childhood Onset Scleroderma (NRCOS)**
University of Pittsburgh School of Medicine
M240 Scaife Hall, 3550 Terrace Street
Pittsburge, PA 15261
412-383-8674
800-603-8960
jablonj@msx.dept-med.pitt.edu
www.sctc-online.org/studies/nrcos.htm

This registry provides a unique opportunity for researchers to study a variety of aspects of scleroderma. The registry will include systemic sclerosis and various forms of localized scleroderma such as morphea, linear scleroderma, and eosinophilic fasciitis.

Jennifer Jablon, Research Coordinator
Thomas A Medsger Jr, MD, Principal Investigator

Web Sites

6452 **American Autoimmune Related Diseases Association**
22100 Gratiot Avenue
Eastpointe, MI 48021
586-776-3900
800-598-4668
Fax: 586-776-3903
aarda@aarda.org
www.aarda.org

Dedicated to the eradiction of autoimmune diseases and the alleviation of suffering and the socio-economic impact of autoimmunity through fostering and facilitating collaboration in the areas of education, public awareness, research and patient services in an effective, ethical and efficient manner.

Virginia T. Ladd, President/Executive Director
Patricia Barber, Assistant Director
Deb Patrick, Events Specialist

6453 **Health Answers**
410 Horsham Road
Horsham, PA 19044
215-442-9010
Michael.tague@healthanswers.com
www.healthanswers.com

HealthAnswers offers a breadth of services in medical education, sales force training, patient support solutions, professional promotion and consumer solutions.

Michael Tague, Managing Director

6454 **Online Mendelian Inheritance in Man**
www.omim.org

This database is a catalog of human genes and genetic disorders.

6455 **Scleroderma A to Z**
7455 France Ave So #266
Edina, MN 55435
952-831-3091
800-564-7099
isn@sclero.org
www.sclero.org

Presented by the International Scleroderma Network, it has over 1000 pages of scleroderma and scleroderma related information, resources, and links in over 20 languages.

Shelley Ensz, Founder and President
Sid Strong, Vice President
Gene Ensz, Treasurer

6456 Scleroderma Foundation
300 Rosewood Drive, Suite 105
Danvers, MA 1923

978-463-5843
800-722-4673
Fax: 978-463-5809
sfinfo@scleroderma.org
www.scleroderma.org

The national organziation for people with scleroderma and their families and friends.

Joseph Camerino, Ph.D., Chair
Carol Feghali-Bostwick, Ph.D., Vice Chair
Robert J. Riggs, Chief Executive Officer

6457 Scleroderma Message Board
disc.server.com/Indices/7571.html

An online message board about scleroderma and related conditions.

6458 Scleroderma Support
health.groups.yahoo.com/group/sclerodermasupport2/

A place where people who live with scleroderma can talk online.

Book Publishers

6459 Cooking Up A Storm for Scleroderma: Recipe s from the Scleroderma Foundation
Scleroderma Foundation
300 Rosewood Dr, Suite 105
Danvers, MA 01923

978-463-5843
800-722-4673
Fax: 978-463-5809
info@scleroderma.org
www.scleroderma.org

Over 480 recipes contributed by the foundations members, including patients, friends and family.

6460 It's Not Just Growing Pains
Thomas J.A. Lehman, PhD, author

Oxford University Press
198 Madison Ave
New York, NY 10016

212-726-6000
800-445-9714
Fax: 919-677-1303
custserv.us@oup.com
www.oup.com/usa

2004 Hardback
ISBN: 0-195157-28-1

6461 Let's Talk About Going to the Hospital
Rosen Publishing Group's PowerKids Press
29 E 21st Street
New York, NY 10010

212-777-3017
800-237-9932
Fax: 888-436-4643
rosenpub@tribeca.ios.com
www.rosenpublishing.com

If a child has to check into the hospital, chances are he or she is already upset about being ill. Knowing how a hospital functions and what the procedures are, such as when family members can visit, will help in what is already a stressful situation. Grades K-5.

24 pages
ISBN: 0-823950-36-0

Roger Rosen, President

6462 Medifocus Guidebook on Scleroderma
Medifocus.com, Inc
11529 Daffodil Lane, Suite 200
Silver Spring, MD 20902

301-649-9300
800-965-3002
Fax: 301-649-7809
info@medifocus.com
www.medifocus.com

This guidebook has four sections: an overview for patients; a guide to medical literature; research centers; and a resource and organization guide. Updates are available online for a year with purchase of the book. Also available in electronic format.

105 pages

Ovadia Abulafia, Board Member
William I. Bensinger, M.D., Board Member
Glenn D. Braunstein, M.D., Board Member

6463 Scleroderma Book (The)
Maureen Mayes, MD, author

Oxford University Press
198 Madison Ave
New York, NY 10016

212-726-6000
800-445-9714
Fax: 919-677-1303
custserv.us@oup.com
www.oup.com/usa

2005 Hardback
ISBN: 0-195169-40-9

Magazines

6464 Scleroderma Voice
Scleroderma Foundation
300 Rosewood Dr, Suite 105
Danvers, MA 1923

978-463-5843
800-722-4673
Fax: 978-463-5809
sfinfo@scleroderma.org
www.scleroderma.org

Includes articles and stories, answers to medical questions, updates on research and treatments, and advice on dealing with scleroderma.

Quarterly

Joseph Camerino, Ph.D., Chair
Carol Feghali-Bostwick, Ph.D., Vice Chair
Robert J. Riggs, Chief Executive Officer

Journals

6465 Scleroderma Care and Research
Scleroderma Clinical Trials Consortium
715 Albany St, E-5
Boston, MA 2118

617-638-4486
trials@blackmule.com
www.sclero.org/medical/journals/scar/a-to-z.html

Published by a group of international scleroderma researchers, it covers topics of interest to rheumatologists and others involved in scleroderma care, worldwide.

Pamphlets

6466 Handout on Health: Scleroderma
NIAMS, National Institutes of Health
31 Center Dr, Bldg 31, Rm 4C02
Bethesda, MD 20892

301-496-8190
Fax: 301-480-2814
www.niams.nih.gov/hi

Information including current research efforts for scleroderma.

Revised 7/2006
Stephen I. Katz, M.D., Ph.D., Director
Robert H Carter, Deputy Director
Gahan Breithaupt, Ass Dir for Management & Operations

Camps

6467 Camp Discovery
American Academy of Dermatology
930 E Woodfield Road
Schaumburg, IL 60173

847-240-1737
Fax: 847-330-8907
jmueller@aad.org
www.campdiscovery.org

A camp for young people with chronic skin conditions. There is no fee and transportation is provided. Three locations: Camp Horizon in Millville, PA, Camp Knutson in Crosslake, MN, and Camp Dermadillo in Burton, TX.

Brett M. Coldiron, MD, President
Janine Mueller, Program Coordinator
Elise A. Olsen, MD, Vice President

6468 Camp Wonder
Children's Skin Disease Foundation
712 Bancroft Rd, #511
Walnut Creek, CA 94598

925-947-3825
Fax: 866-236-6474
www.csdf.org

Established by the CSDF for young people who suffer from skin diseases. Medically staffed camps are free to children, ages 7-17 with skin diseases that are serious or life threatening.

Christine Tenconi, Vice-President
Christine Clakley, Executive Director

DESCRIPTION

6469 SCOLIOSIS

Synonym: Rachioscoliosis

Covers these related disorders: Compensatory scoliosis, Congenital scoliosis, Idiopathic kyphosis (Scheuermann's disease), Idiopathic scoliosis, Kyphosis, Neuromuscular scoliosis, Syndrome-associated scoliosis

Involves the following Biologic System(s):

Orthopedic and Muscle Disorders

The term scoliosis refers to a condition characterized by a sideward (lateral) curvature of the spine. Idiopathic scoliosis is the most common form of this disorder and occurs for no known reason in otherwise healthy individuals who range in age from infancy to adolescence. Adolescent scoliosis is the most common form and accounts for 80 percent of idiopathic scoliosis. Approximately 20 percent of people with scoliosis report at least one other affected family member. Therefore, in these cases, scoliosis is thought to have a genetic component. Idiopathic scoliosis that develops during infancy often corrects itself, but it may become progressive in older children. Treatment is dependent upon age and the degree of curvature progression. Mild curvatures may require little or no treatment, while more severe involvement may require surgery or the use of braces, etc. (orthotics). Although men and women are affected in about equal numbers, women are more at risk for more significant curvature progression. Girls between onset of puberty growth spurt and cessation of spinal growth are at the greatest risk for idiopathic scoliosis. Physical examination reveals asymmetry in the height of the shoulder and hip, with forward bending.

Congenital scoliosis, apparent at birth or soon thereafter, results from the improper or incomplete development of the vertebrae during the first trimester of pregnancy. This condition may appear singularly or in association with abnormalities of other systems of the body including the heart (i.e., congenital heart disease) and genitourinary tract (e.g., absence of one kidney, duplication of the tubes that carry urine, horseshoe kidney, and other malformations). Congenital scoliosis is often accompanied by other spinal cord defects (spinal dysraphism) that may range from mild to severe. In addition, children born with certain genetic disorders such as Klippel-Feil syndrome may experience associated scoliosis. The progression of the curvature is dependent upon the specific underlying vertebral malformation, its particular growth potential, and its location. About one quarter of affected children experience no progression of the curvature and, therefore, require no treatment. Approximately half of those remaining may require early treatment, such as spinal fusion of the affected area, to stop progression of the curvature.

Neuromuscular scoliosis is associated with certain childhood diseases (e.g., cerebral palsy, Duchenne muscular dystrophy, polio, and other disorders). This type of scoliosis tends to be progressive, with the degree of deformity dependent upon many factors. Those affected children who are unable to walk (nonambulatory) often develop additional skeletal irregularities involving the pelvis and spine. In severe cases, respiratory difficulties may develop. Early evaluation and intervention through surgery and other means help to alter the progression of the spinal deformity and its associated complications.

Kyphosis is characterized by an exaggerated backward curvature of the spine. Children with poor posture resulting in mild kyphosis who have no associated spinal irregularities may be treated by maintaining good posture. Congenital kyophosis, however, results from various malformations in the spinal column and may range from mild to severe deformity. Scoliosis also is present in one-third of patients with kyphosis. When several vertebrae are involved, there is a round back appearance; when only one vertebra is involved, there is an angular curve. As affected children grow, progression of the spinal abnormality may continue until growth is complete, possibly resulting in partial paralysis. Idiopathic kyphosis or Scheuermann's disease is common to both adolescent boys and girls; cause remains unknown. Examination and x-ray screening may determine whether kyphosis is postural or a result of a spinal malformation. Symptoms of Scheuermann's disease may include mild but chronic back pain and a round-shouldered appearance.

Children with mild kyphosis may be advised to refrain from strenuous activities, while those with more severe symptoms may benefit from sleeping on a very firm mattress, or using a brace or cast. Surgery is rarely indicated.

Certain syndromes (e.g., Marfan syndrome, neurofibromatosis) place affected children at risk for spinal irregularities such as scoliosis and kyphosis. Treatment for these children includes regular orthopedic examination and intervention to prevent progression of the irregularity.

Scoliosis sometimes results from unequal leg length resulting from an irregular tilt (obliquity) of the pelvis. Treatment for this compensatory scoliosis may include the use of special orthopedic shoes.

Government Agencies

6470 NIH/National Institute of Arthritis and Musculoskeletal and Skin Diseases
1 AMS Circle
Bethesda, MD 20892

301-495-4484
877-226-4267
Fax: 301-718-6366
TDD: 301-565-2966
niamsinfo@mail.nih.gov
www.niams.nih.gov

The mission of the NIAMS, a part of the NIH, is to support research into the causes, treatment, and prevention of arthritis and musculoskeletal and skin diseases, the training of basic and clinical scientists to carry out this research, and the dissemination of information on research progress in these diseases.

Stephen I Katz MD PhD, Director
Robert H Carter MD, Deputy Director
Gahan Breithaupt, Assoc Dir for Management & Operatio

National Associations & Support Groups

6471 American Academy of Pediatrics
141 Northwest Point Boulevard
Elk Grove Village, IL 60007

847-434-4000
800-433-9016
Fax: 847-434-8000
www.aap.org

The American Academy of Pediatrics and its member pediatricians are committed to the attainment of optimal physical, mental and social health and well-being for all infants, children, adolescents, and young adults.

Fernando Stein, MD, FAAP, President
Karen Remley, MD, CEO/Executive VP

6472 National Dissemination Center for Children with Disabilities
1825 Connecticut Ave NW
Washington, DC 20009   202-884-8200
                                        800-695-0285
                                        Fax: 202-884-8441
                                        nichcy@fhi360.org
                                        www.nichcy.org

A national information and referral center for families, educators
and other professionals on: disabilities in children and youth; programs and services; IDEA, the nation's special education law;
and research-based information on effective practices.

Suzanne Ripley, Executive Director

6473 National Scoliosis Foundation
5 Cabot Place
Stoughton, MA 02072   781-341-6333
                                        800-673-6922
                                        Fax: 781-341-8333
                                        nsf@scoliosis.org
                                        www.scoliosis.org

Promotes school screening, offers public awareness materials to
promote public education, maintains a resource center for professional information, conducts scoliosis conferences, and offers
support groups to people affected by the disease.

Joseph O'Brien, President/CEO
Dennis J. Fusco, CPA, Treasurer
Laura B. Gowen, LHD, Founder & President Emeritus

6474 Scoliosis Association
PO Box 811705
Boca Raton, FL 33481   561-994-4435
                                        800-800-0669
                                        Fax: 561-994-2455
                                        scolioassn2@aol.com
                                        www.scoliosis-assoc.org

Sponsors and encourages spinal screening programs. Disseminates information throughout the country, and raises funds for
scoliosis research. Membership fee of $20.00 includes subscrip-
tion to newsletter. Videos and printed information available.

Stanley Sacks, Ceo

Libraries & Resource Centers

6475 Johns Hopkins Department of Orthopaedics Surgery
601 N Caroline Street
Baltimore, MD 21287   410-955-5000
                                        Fax: 410-955-1719
                                        www.hopkinsinteractive.com

Scoliosis is a three-dimensional curvature of the spine, best ap-
preciated on an anteroposterior radiograph and physical examination. Many different causes have been identified. The most
common type is idiopathic scoliosis.

Claudia L Thomas

Research Centers

6476 Scoliosis Research Society
555 E Wells Street, Suite 1100
Milwaukee, WI 53202   414-289-9107
                                        Fax: 414-276-3349
                                        info@srs.org
                                        www.srs.org

An international society that is committed to research and education for health care professionals in the field of spinal deformities. It is recognized as one of the world's premier spine societies.
Current membership includes over 1000 of the world's leading
spine surgeons as well as researchers, physician assistants and
orthotists.

Tressa Goulding, Executive Director
Kamal N. Ibrahim, MD, FRCS(C), MA, President
John P. Dormans, MD, Vice President

6477 Shriners Hospital for Children
Headquarters
2900 Rocky Point Drive
Tampa, FL 33607   813-281-0300
                                        800-237-5055
                                        Fax: 813-281-8113
                                        patientreferrals@shrinenet.org
                                        www.shrinershospitalsforchildren.org/

Shrine's official philanthropy is Shriners Hospital for Children, a
network of 22 hospitals that provide expert, no-cost orthopaedic
and burn care to children under 18.

Alan W. Madsen, Chairman of the Board
John McCabe, Executive Vice President
Kenneth Guidera, M.D., Chief Medical Officer

Audio Video

6478 Cutting Edge Medical Report
National Scoliosis Foundation
5 Cabot Place
Stoughton, MA 2072   781-341-6333
                                        800-673-6922
                                        Fax: 781-341-8333
                                        nsf@scoliosis.org
                                        www.scoliosis.org

As seen on the Discovery Channel, this video is an in-depth examination of the latest developments in the diagnosis and treatment of scoliosis.

18 Minutes

**6479 Dealing with Scoliosis: A Patient Guide to Diagnosis and
Treatment**
National Scoliosis Foundation
5 Cabot Place
Stoughton, MA 2072   781-341-6333
                                        800-673-6922
                                        Fax: 781-341-8333
                                        nsf@scoliosis.org
                                        www.scoliosis.org

An upbeat video featuring Miss North Carolina Michelle Mauney
and that explains diagnosis and treatment of scoliosis through the
experience of several teenagers and young adults.

20 Minutes

6480 Ellie's Back
National Scoliosis Foundation
5 Cabot Place
Stoughton, MA 2072   781-341-6333
                                        800-673-6922
                                        Fax: 781-341-8333
                                        nsf@scoliosis.org
                                        www.scoliosis.org

An eight-year-old, and her mother team up together to produce a
film that portrays life with scoliosis through the eyes of a young
child.

15 Minutes

6481 Growing Straighter and Stronger
National Scoliosis Foundation
5 Cabot Place
Stoughton, MA 2072   781-341-6333
                                        800-673-6922
                                        Fax: 781-341-8333
                                        nsf@scoliosis.org
                                        www.scoliosis.org

Produced for the pre-screening education of students in grades
5-9. It emphasizes the importance of follow-up screening, encourages peer support and prescribed follow-up treatment. Video is
also available on loan for a refundable deposit plus shipping and
handling.

15 Minutes

6482 Preparing Yourself for Spinal Surgery (For Teenagers with Severe Scoliosis)
National Scoliosis Foundation
5 Cabot Place
Stoughton, MA 2072

781-341-6333
800-673-6922
Fax: 781-341-8333
nsf@scoliosis.org
www.scoliosis.org

Patient educational video helping to reduce the anxiety for teenagers facing surgery by giving a sense of what to expect before, during, and after surgery.

18 Minutes

6483 School Screening with Dr. Robert Keller
National Scoliosis Foundation
5 Cabot Place
Stoughton, MA 2072

781-341-6333
800-673-6922
Fax: 781-341-8333
nsf@scoliosis.org
www.scoliosis.org

A training video that teaches the proper technique for doing spinal screening. Defines scoliosis and kyphosis. Four teenagers, three with curves and one without, are examined and the findings explained.

60 Minutes

6484 Sharing Scoliosis: You're Not Alone
National Scoliosis Foundation
5 Cabot Place
Stoughton, MA 2072

781-341-6333
800-673-6922
Fax: 781-341-8333
nsf@scoliosis.org
www.scoliosis.org

The Missouri chapter of the NSF, shares their experience with scoliosis including diagnosis, wearing a brace, surgery, and recovery. It is a good source of support for patients of all ages and their families.

26 Minutes

6485 Taking the Mystery Out of Spinal Deformities
Children's Hospital of LA, Div. of Orthopaedics
4650 Sunset Boulevard
Los Angeles, CA 90027

323-660-2450
888-631-2452
www.childrenshospitalla.org

Answers questions most often asked by screeners, patients and parents.

Videotape

Richard D. Cordova, FACHE, President/ CEO
Rodney B. Hanners, SVP/ COO
Barry L. Mangels, MS, CPHRM, Chief Compliance & Privacy Officer

6486 Understanding Scoliosis
National Scoliosis Foundation
5 Cabot Place
Stoughton, MA 2072

781-341-6333
800-673-6922
Fax: 781-341-8333
nsf@scoliosis.org
www.scoliosis.org

A Kaiser Permanente educational video that clearly and positively addresses the patient community. In this video four teenagers at various stages of treatment talk about their life with scoliosis.

8 Minutes

6487 What's This Thing Called Scoliosis
Dr Charles Ray, author

National Scoliosis Foundation
5 Cabot Place
Stoughton, MA 2072

781-341-6333
800-673-6922
Fax: 781-341-8333
nsf@scoliosis.org
www.scoliosis.org

A comprehensive overview of scoliosis using the latest computer technology. The anatomical spine and animated model work together to truly show the 3D aspects of scoliosis and the corresponding impact on the patient.

17 Minutes

Web Sites

6488 American Academy of Orthopaedic Surgeons
9400 West Higgins Road
Rosemont, IL 60018

847-823-7186
Fax: 847-823-8125
custserv@aaos.org
www.aaos.org

Provides an informational fact sheet on scoliosis in children and adolescents.

Frederick M Azar, MD, President
Karen L. Hackett, FACHE, CAE, Chief Executive Officer
William Bruce, Chief Technology Officer

6489 Health Answers
410 Horsham Road
Horsham, PA 19044

215-442-9010
Michael.tague@healthanswers.com
www.healthanswers.com

HealthAnswers offers a breadth of services in medical education, sales force training, patient support solutions, professional promotion and consumer solutions.

Michael Tague, Managing Director

6490 John Hopkins Department of Orthopaedics Surgery
601 N. Caroline Street, JHOC #5215
Baltimore, MD 21287

443-997-2663
hopkinsortho@jhmi.edu
www.hopkinsmedicine.org/orthopedicsurgery/

The orthopaedics faculty works together as a team to provide optimum patient care, seeking out a role in patient care as both educators and treating physicians working together with you and your community health care providers to offer you the best possible medical and surgical care available.

6491 Natalie's Brace
www.nataliesbrace.com/scoliosis/

Personal website offering personal details and photos on scoliosis braces, general information and support.

6492 North Ameerican Spine Society
7075 Veterans Blvd.
Burr Ridge, IL 60527

630-230-3600
www.spine.org

Provides information on adolescent idiopathic scoliosis, including a description of, common problems associated with the curvature, and possible treatments.

Heidi Prather, DO, President
Christopher Bono, MD, First Vice President
Eric Muehlbauer, Executive Director

6493 Online Mendelian Inheritance in Man
www.omim.org

This database is a catalog of human genes and genetic disorders.

6494 Scoliosis Help
www.scoliosishelp.org

6495 Scoliosis Message Forum
www.scoliosis.org/forum/index.php

jpobrien@scoliosis.org
www.scoliosis.org/forum/index.php

An independent list maintained by people who have scoliosis.
You can find people with whom you can share your experiences
and ask questions.

6496 Scoliosis Research Society
555 East Wells Street, Suite 1100
Milwaukee, WI 53202

414-289-9107
Fax: 414-276-3349
info@srs.org
www.srs.org

An international society that is committed to research and education for health care professionals in the field of spinal deformities. It is recognized as one of the world's premier spine societies.
Current membership includes over 1000 of the world's leading
spine surgeons as well as researchers, physician assistants and
orthotists.

John P. Dormans, MD, President
Tressa Goulding, CAE, CMP, Executive Director
Ashtin Neuschaefer, Administrative Manager

6497 Wheeless' Textbook of Orthopaedics
www.wheelessonline.com

Derives from a variety of sources, including journals, articles, national meetings lectures and other textbooks.

Clifford R. Wheeless III, MD, Editor-in-Chief
James A. Nunley, II, MD, Managing Editor
James R. Urbaniak, MD, Managing Editor

Book Publishers

6498 Deenie
Simon & Schuster/Atheneum Books
100 Front Street
Riverside, NJ 08075

856-461-6500
800-488-4308
Fax: 800-943-9831
www.simonandschuster.com

Deenie, a beautiful thirteen-year-old girl, had a mother who was
pushing her to become a model. The agency representatives told
Deenie she had the looks but walked differently. Deenie's main
wish was to become a cheerleader. Her close friend, Janet, made
the cheerleading squad but Deenie didn't make the finalist list.
After this her gym teacher noticed her posture and called her family. After seeing therapists, the diagnosis of adolescent idiopathic
scoliosis was made.

159 pages Hardcover
ISBN: 0-689866-10-0

Carolyn Reidy, President/CEO
Liz Perl, Senior Vice President, Marketing
Dennis Eulau, Executive Vice President, Operation

6499 Getting Ready, Getting Well
Mary Knapp, author

National Scoliosis Foundation
5 Cabot Place
Stoughton, MA 02072

781-341-6333
800-673-6922
Fax: 781-341-8333
nsf@scoliosis.org
www.scoliosis.org

A guide for those anticipating surgery; divided into three sections: Making Up Your Mind, Taking Charge, and Home Again.

73 pages

Laura B. Gowen, Founder & President
W.Hugh M. Morton, Chairman
Joseph P. O'Brien, President & CEO

6500 Growing Up with Scoliosis: A Young Girl's Story
Michelle Spray, author

National Scoliosis Foundation
5 Cabot Place
Stoughton, MA 02072

781-341-6333
800-673-6922
Fax: 781-341-8333
nsf@scoliosis.org
www.scoliosis.org

A personal account of growing up with scoliosis and the different
stages of treatment, progression and surgery.

Laura B. Gowen, Founder & President
W.Hugh M. Morton, Chairman
Joseph P. O'Brien, President & CEO

6501 Handbook of Scoliosis
Scoliosis Research Society
555 East Wells Street, Suite 1100
Milwaukee, WI 53202

414-289-9107
Fax: 414-276-3349
info@srs.org
www.srs.org

Kamal N. Ibrahim, MD, President
John P. Dormans, MD, Vice President
Hubert Labelle, MD, Secretary

6502 Nothing Hurts But My Heart
Linda Barr, author

National Scoliosis Foundation
5 Cabot Place
Stoughton, MA 02072

781-341-6333
800-673-6922
Fax: 781-341-8333
nsf@scoliosis.org
www.scoliosis.org

For every boy, girl, and their parents who learn that bracing may
be needed to treat their scoliosis. The story is of a young gymnast
dealing with the issues of wearing a brace.

Laura B. Gowen, Founder & President
W.Hugh M. Morton, Chairman
Joseph P. O'Brien, President & CEO

**6503 Scoliosis Surgery, The Definitive Patient's Reference: Second
Edition**
Dave Wolpert, author

National Scoliosis Foundation
5 Cabot Place
Stoughton, MA 02072

781-341-6333
800-673-6922
Fax: 781-341-8333
nsf@scoliosis.org
www.scoliosis.org

For all those contemplating surgery or that know someone who
is; it explains in detail everything you need to know, written in
layman's terms by someone who has gone through it.

Laura B. Gowen, Founder & President
W.Hugh M. Morton, Chairman
Joseph P. O'Brien, President & CEO

6504 Scoliosis: What Young People and Parents N eed to Know
American Physical Therapy Association
1111 N Fairfax Street
Alexandria, VA 22314

703-684-2782
800-999-2782
Fax: 703-706-8556
TDD: 703-683-6748
www.apta.org

A physical therapist's perspective about what scoliosis is and
what parents and young people should look for to detect
scoliosis. Also available in Spanish.

12 pages Packet of 25

Paul Rocker, President
Sharon l. Dunn, Vice President
Laurita M. Hack, Secretary

6505 Stopping Scoliosis

Nancy Schommer, author

National Scoliosis Foundation
5 Cabot Place
Stoughton, MA 02072

781-341-6333
800-673-6922
Fax: 781-341-8333
nsf@scoliosis.org
www.scoliosis.org

Filled with accurate, currently researched information for adults concerned with their condition or that of a young person.

Laura B. Gowen, Founder & President
W.Hugh M. Morton, Chairman
Joseph P. O'Brien, President & CEO

6506 There's an S on My Back: S is for Scoliosi s

Mary Mahony, author

National Scoliosis Foundation
5 Cabot Place
Stoughton, MA 02072

781-341-6333
800-673-6922
Fax: 781-341-8333
nsf@scoliosis.org
www.scoliosis.org

The medical journey of a fifth grader diagnosed with idiopathic scoliosis at a school screening. A realistic fiction, the story gives us a day-by-day account of what a preadolescent experiences.

Laura B. Gowen, Founder & President
W.Hugh M. Morton, Chairman
Joseph P. O'Brien, President & CEO

6507 Twenty Years At Hull House

Jane Addams, author

New American Library/Penguin Group
375 Hudson Street
New York, NY 10014

212-366-2372
Fax: 212-366-2933
online@us.penguingroup.com
us.penguingroup.com

336 pages
ISBN: 0-451527-39-4

John Makinson, CHAIRMAN
Coram Williams, CFO
David Shanks, CEO

6508 What Can I Give You?

Mary Mahony, author

National Scoliosis Foundation
5 Cabot Place
Stoughton, MA 02072

781-341-6333
800-673-6922
Fax: 781-341-8333
nsf@scoliosis.org
www.scoliosis.org

A wounderful story of a loving mother's care for her daughter. The medical saga of Erin and Mary offers insight and inspiration to families living with congenital scoliosis and valuable guidance to the physicians who treat them.

Laura B. Gowen, Founder & President
W.Hugh M. Morton, Chairman
Joseph P. O'Brien, President & CEO

Newsletters

6509 Backtalk
Scoliosis Association
PO Box 811705
Boca Raton, FL 33481

561-994-4435
Fax: 561-994-2455
normlipin@aol.com
www.scoliosis-assoc.org

Information for families, patients and health care professionals. Includes a section for pen pals, an Ask the Doctor column, and a highlighted personal story.

3-4/yr

6510 Spinal Connection
National Scoliosis Foundation
5 Cabot Place
Stoughton, MA 2072

781-341-6333
800-673-6922
Fax: 781-341-8333
nsf@scoliosis.org
www.scoliosis.org

Offers updated information, the latest medical advances, and new research studies in the area of abnormal spinal curvatures.

8 pages Bi-annual

Pamphlets

6511 1 in Every 10 Persons Has Scoliosis
National Scoliosis Foundation
5 Cabot Place
Stoughton, MA 2072

781-341-6333
800-673-6922
Fax: 781-341-8333
nsf@scoliosis.org
www.scoliosis.org

Explains what scoliosis is and illustrates how to screen for it. It also contains facts about the Foundation.

6512 Adolescent Idiopathic Scoliosis-Prevalence ,Natural History, Treatments
National Scoliosis Foundation
5 Cabot Place
Stoughton, MA 2072

781-341-6333
800-673-6922
Fax: 781-341-8333
nsf@scoliosis.org
www.scoliosis.org

6513 Boston Bracing System for Idiopathic Scoli osis
National Scoliosis Foundation
5 Cabot Place
Stoughton, MA 2072

781-341-6333
800-673-6922
Fax: 781-341-8333
nsf@scoliosis.org
www.scoliosis.org

6514 Brace & Her Brace is No Handicap
National Scoliosis Foundation
5 Cabot Place
Stoughton, MA 2072

781-341-6333
800-673-6922
Fax: 781-341-8333
nsf@scoliosis.org
www.scoliosis.org

Contains two illustrated short stories, each about a teenage girl coping successfully with scoliosis.

6515 Getting a Second Opinion
National Scoliosis Foundation
5 Cabot Place
Stoughton, MA 2072

781-341-6333
800-673-6922
Fax: 781-341-8333
nsf@scoliosis.org
www.scoliosis.org

Reprinted from Health Tips.

6516 Medical Update Column
National Scoliosis Foundation
5 Cabot Place
Stoughton, MA 2072　　　　　　　781-341-6333
　　　　　　　　　　　　　　　　800-673-6922
　　　　　　　　　　　　Fax: 781-341-8333
　　　　　　　　　　　　nsf@scoliosis.org
　　　　　　　　　　　　www.scoliosis.org

Reprints from past issues of the Spinal Connections Medical Update Column available on various topics.

6517 NSF Packets
National Scoliosis Foundation
5 Cabot Place
Stoughton, MA 2072　　　　　　　781-341-6333
　　　　　　　　　　　　　　　　800-673-6922
　　　　　　　　　　　　Fax: 781-341-8333
　　　　　　　　　　　　nsf@scoliosis.org
　　　　　　　　　　　　www.scoliosis.org

Packet contains information for parents and young people, adults, and health care professionals.

6518 Postural Screening Program
National Scoliosis Foundation
5 Cabot Place
Stoughton, MA 2072　　　　　　　781-341-6333
　　　　　　　　　　　　　　　　800-673-6922
　　　　　　　　　　　　Fax: 781-341-8333
　　　　　　　　　　　　nsf@scoliosis.org
　　　　　　　　　　　　www.scoliosis.org

Guidelines for physicians and school nurses.

6519 Questions Most Often Asked the NSF
National Scoliosis Foundation
5 Cabot Place
Stoughton, MA 2072　　　　　　　781-341-6333
　　　　　　　　　　　　　　　　800-673-6922
　　　　　　　　　　　　Fax: 781-341-8333
　　　　　　　　　　　　nsf@scoliosis.org
　　　　　　　　　　　　www.scoliosis.org

Answers the most frequently asked questions about scoliosis and the foundation in general.

6520 Questions and Answers About Scoliosis
Federal Citizen Information Center
Pueblo, CO 81009　　　　　　　　719-295-2675
　　　　　　　　　　　　　　　　888-878-3256
　　　　　　　　　　　　pueblo@gpo.gov
　　　　　　　　　　publications.usa.gov/USAPubs.php

6521 Scoliosis and Kyphosis
Scoliosis Research Society
555 East Wells Street, Suite 1100
Milwaukee, WI 53202　　　　　　414-289-9107
　　　　　　　　　　　　Fax: 414-276-3349
　　　　　　　　　　　　info@srs.org
　　　　　　　　　　　　www.srs.org

Information and advice from parents.

John P. Dormans, MD, President
Tressa Goulding, CAE, CMP, Executive Director
Ashtin Neuschaefer, Administrative Manager

6522 Scoliosis: A Handbook for Patients
National Scoliosis Foundation
5 Cabot Place
Stoughton, MA 2072　　　　　　　781-341-6333
　　　　　　　　　　　　　　　　800-673-6922
　　　　　　　　　　　　Fax: 781-341-8333
　　　　　　　　　　　　nsf@scoliosis.org
　　　　　　　　　　　　www.scoliosis.org

Information on detection and treatment of adolescent scoliosis, kyphosis and lordosis and adult scoliosis.

6523 When the Spine Curves
National Scoliosis Foundation
5 Cabot Place
Stoughton, MA 2072　　　　　　　781-341-6333
　　　　　　　　　　　　　　　　800-673-6922
　　　　　　　　　　　　Fax: 781-341-8333
　　　　　　　　　　　　nsf@scoliosis.org
　　　　　　　　　　　　www.scoliosis.org

Camps

6524 Hemlocks Easter Seals Recreation
85 Jones Street
Hebron, CT 6248　　　　　　　　860-228-9496
　　　　　　　　　　　　　　　　800-832-4409
　　　　　　　　　　　　Fax: 860-228-2091
　　　　　　　　info@eastersealscamphemlocks.org
　　　　　　　　www.eastersealscamphemlocks.org

Accepts campers, ages 6 and under, whose major disability is orthopedic. First preference is given to Connecticut residents. A computer camp is also available.

Carl Larson

DESCRIPTION

6525 SEIZURES

Synonyms: Convulsions, Epilepsy

Covers these related disorders: Absence (petit mal) seizures, Complex partial seizures, Generalized (grand mal) tonic-clonic seizures, Simple partial seizures, Epilepsy

Involves the following Biologic System(s):

Neurologic Disorders

Seizures are a neurologic condition characterized by sudden episodes of uncontrolled electrical activity in the brain. These electrical disturbances may cause abnormal motor activities, lost or impaired consciousness, impaired control of certain involuntary functions (autonomic dysfunction), or sensory or behavioral abnormalities. Seizures are a common neurologic condition of childhood, affecting approximately six in 1,000 children. Approximately 70 percent of children who experience one seizure never experience another, whereas about 30 percent develop recurring seizures, which is referred to as epilepsy. Seizures may result from many different causes, including fever, head injury, infection or inflammation of the brain, insufficient oxygen supply to the brain, or certain metabolic imbalances. Seizures may also be caused by brain tumors, particular degenerative metabolic or neurological diseases, abnormal reactions to certain medications, or drug intoxication. There are also a number of syndromes and genetic disorders in which seizures are a primary feature. In many children, the exact underlying cause of recurrent seizures cannot be determined and the disorder is termed idiopathic epilepsy.

The specific form that a seizure takes and its associated symptoms may depend upon a number of factors, including the region of the brain in which the electrical disturbance arises and how widely it spreads from its point of origin. Epileptic seizures may be broadly classified into two groups: partial and generalized seizures. Partial seizures often result due to damage or impairment of a limited area of the brain, whereas generalized seizures may affect a wide area of the brain. In addition, some partial seizures may begin in a particular brain region but spread to affect most of the brain, ultimately becoming a generalized seizure. Because different seizure types may cause similar symptoms, specialized techniques that record brain wave activity (electroencephalography or EEG) and other neurologic imaging tests (such as MRI or CT scans) may play an important role in classifying certain seizure disorders.

Partial seizures, which may account for up to 40 percent of childhood seizures, may be subdivided into simple partial seizures, during which consciousness is retained, and complex partial seizures, during which consciousness is impaired. Simple partial seizures are characterized by abnormal, rhythmic muscle contractions and relaxations (clonic activity) and increased muscle tone and rigidity (tonic activity), particularly affecting muscles of the neck, face, arms, and legs. Simple partial seizures, which usually last about 10 to 20 seconds, are frequently associated with abnormal eye movements and head turning. In many children, simple partial seizures may be preceded by an aura consisting of headache, chest discomfort, and a feeling of anxiety, fear, or dread.

Complex partial seizures are characterized by a sudden pause in activity and a blank stare and may be preceded by an aura that consists of a vague feeling of fear or unpleasantness, headache, and chest discomfort. Most patients also perform certain involuntary actions following loss of consciousness. In infants, such actions may include lip smacking, swallowing, or chewing, whereas older children may conduct incoordinated, semipurposeful actions, such as rubbing objects or pulling at clothing. Such seizures may last approximately one to two minutes.

Generalized seizures may be subdivided into nonconvulsive (petit mal, absence) seizures and convulsive (grand mal or tonic-clonic) seizures. Absence seizures, which rarely occur before the age of five, usually last from a few seconds up to half a minute. During an episode, children experience a momentary loss of consciousness during which they cease speaking or performing other motor activities. They typically have a blank facial expression, their eyelids may flicker, and the head may fall forward. Patients typically have no awareness of the episode and resume the activity they were performing before the seizure.

Generalized tonic-clonic seizures may be preceded by an aura and occasionally begin with a shrill cry as patients lose consciousness. During an episode, the eyes roll back, muscles of the entire body stiffen, and all muscle groups begin to rhythmically contract and relax. If temporary cessation of breathing (apnea) occurs, patients may quickly develop an abnormal, bluish discoloration of the skin and mucous membranes (cyanosis). Bladder and bowel control may be temporarily lost. After an episode, patients are typically semiconscious and disoriented and may remain in a deep sleep for up to two hours (postictal state). During such a seizure episode, patients should be placed on one side, tight clothing around the neck should be loosened, and the jaw should be gently extended to enhance breathing. However, the mouth should not be forcibly opened nor should an object be placed between the teeth.

Generalized seizures also include a form of epilepsy known as infantile spasms, which typically begin between the ages of four and eight months and continue to approximately 18 months. Infantile spasms are characterized by sudden, brief, symmetric contractions of the arms and legs, neck, and torso. Spasms may occur for several minutes with brief intervals between each spasm. Episodes tend to occur when children are drowsy or immediately upon awakening. Depending upon the underlying cause, the condition may evolve into different forms of epilepsy later in life and may be associated with an increased risk of mental retardation.

Seizures that occur in association with a rapidly rising fever, known as febrile seizures, are the most common seizure disorder of childhood. Febrile seizures most commonly occur between nine months to five years of age and may affect up to four percent of all children. This type of seizure rarely develops into epilepsy. In many cases, there is a history of such seizures among siblings and parents, indicating that genetic factors may play some causative role. Febrile seizures often occur in association with certain upper respiratory infections and acute inflammation of the middle ear (otitis media). However, because convulsions may result from serious infections of the brain (e.g., meningitis), a thorough medical evaluation must be conducted to determine the cause of the fever. Febrile seizures are typically characterized by muscle rigidity followed by abnormal, rhythmic contractions and relaxations of muscle groups (generalized tonic-clonic seizures). The seizure may last from seconds up to about 10 minutes and is often followed by a brief period of drowsiness.

Generalized or partial seizures that continue for more than 30 minutes without a return to consciousness are known as status epilepticus. Such seizures may occur due to underlying metabolic abnormalities, neurologic disorders, congenital brain malformations, or inflammation of the brain. They may also represent prolonged febrile seizures, develop due to sudden withdrawal of antiseizure (anticonvulsant) medication, or result from unknown causes. Status epilepticus may result in life-threatening complications and is considered a medical emergency, requiring hospitalization. Treatment may include supplemental oxygen, intravenous fluids, physical and neurologic evaluations, intravenous medications including appropriate antiseizure drugs, and other measures as required. Children affected by the condition before one year of age are more likely to have mental retardation and other long-term effects, secondary to an underlying CNS disorder.

The treatment of seizures depends on the underlying cause, the type of seizure present, and other factors. If a treatable condition or disorder is identified, such as a fever, abnormal blood sugar levels, or certain tumors, measures are taken as required to treat the underlying cause. For example, in t|he case of febrile seizures, thorough evaluations are conducted to determine the fever's cause and measures are then taken as necessary to control the fever. If an underlying cause cannot be identified or adequately treated or controlled, treatment typically includes the administration of antiseizure (anticonvulsant) medications to help prevent, reduce, or control seizures. The specific anticonvulsant medication prescribed may depend on several factors, including the classification of the seizure, patient history, and possible side effects. Anticonvulsant drugs used to treat certain types of seizures may include carbamazepine, phenobarbital, primidone, phenytoin, gabapentin, or valproate. In addition, adrenocorticotropic hormone (ACTH) is often used to treat children with infantile spasms. If seizure control is not obtained with a particular medication, other anticonvulsants may be substituted. In some patients, combination drug therapy may be necessary to adequately control seizures. If seizure control is not obtained with anticonvulsant medications, surgery may be considered. Additional treatment is symptomatic and supportive.

National Associations & Support Groups

6526 American Academy of Pediatrics
141 Northwest Point Boulevard
Elk Grove Village, IL 60007
847-434-4000
800-433-9016
Fax: 847-434-8000
www.aap.org

The American Academy of Pediatrics and its member pediatricians are committed to the attainment of optimal physical, mental and social health and well-being for all infants, children, adolescents, and young adults.

Fernando Stein, MD, FAAP, President
Karen Remley, MD, CEO/Executive VP

6527 American Epilepsy Society
342 N Main Street
W Hartford, CT 06117
860-586-7505
Fax: 860-568-7550
www.aesnet.org

A society of clinicians, researchers, and health care professionals which promotes education and research of epilepsy.

M. Suzanne C. Berry, MBA, CAE, Executive Director
Jacqueline A. French, M.D., President
Elson So, M.D., Vice President

6528 Cleveland Clinic Children's Hospital & Epilepsy Center
9500 Euclid Avenue
Cleveland, OH 44195
216-445-8585
800-223-2273
Fax: 216-445-7792
TTY: 216-444-0261
cms.clevelandclinic.org/childrenshospital/

Provides innovative care for infants, children, and adolescents with complex medical problems. Includes medical, surgical, rehabilitation, psychiatric and intensive care, latest technology, including a computerized epilepsy monitoring unit, a consolidated pediatric intensive care unit and operating suites. Physicians are known for their expertise in treating major medical problems, such as cardiovascular disease, cancer, digestive disorders, musculoskeletal problems and neurosensory disorders.

Gene Altus, Executive Director
Prakash Kotagal MD, Pediatric Epilepsy Head

6529 Epilepsy Foundation
8301 Professional Place
Landover, MD 20785
301-459-3700
800-332-1000
Fax: 301-459-1569
ContactUs@efa.org
www.epilepsyfoundation.org

A national, charitable, nonprofit, volunteer agency dedicated to the welfare of people with epilepsy and their families. Its goals are the prevention and cure of seizure disorders, the alleviation of their effects, and the promotion of independence and optimal quality of life for people who have these disorders. The organization offers education, advocacy, service and research support groups, and has a network of local affiliates serving nearly 100 communities.

Phil Gattone, President/CEO
Ty Broadway, Director Web Design and Development
Dawn Leeks, Program Coordinator

6530 Epilepsy Institute
65 Broadway, Ste. 505
New York, NY 10006
212-677-8550
Fax: 212-677-5825
info@efmny.org
www.epilepsyinstitute.org

Program services are available to residents of NYC and Westchester County. The institute is a nonprofit social service organization with information available in Spanish, French, Chinese and Russian.

Pamela Conford, Executive Director

6531 FACES: Finding a Cure for Epilepsy & Seizures
223 East 34th Street
New York, NY 10016
646-558-0900
Fax: 646-385-7163
FACESinfo@nyumc.org
www.nyufaces.org

Nonprofit organization affiliated with NYU Medical Center and its Comprehensive Epilepsy Center. It strives to accomplish its mission through research, clinical programs, awareness, and community education and events.

Orrin Devinsky, MD, Founder
Orrin Devinsky, MD, Chair
Pamela B. Mohr, Executive Director

6532 Genetic Alliance
4301 Connecticut Avenue NW, Suite 404
Washington, DC 20008
202-966-5557
800-336-4363
Fax: 202-966-8553
info@geneticalliance.org
www.geneticalliance.org

A coalition of voluntary genetic support groups, consumers and professionals addressing the needs of individuals and families affected by genetic disorders from a national perspective.

Sharon Terry, President/CEO
Tetyana Murza, Managing Director
Natasha Bonhomme, VP, Strategic Development

6533 National Association of Epilepsy Centers
5775 Wayzata Blvd, Suite 200
Washington, DC 20024 202-484-1100
888-525-6232
Fax: 202-484-1244
info@naec-epilepsy.org
www.naecepilepsy.org

A nonprofit organization that encourages and supports professional and technical education in the treatment of epilepsy. Over 120 centers nationwide are members of the trade association, which will make referrals to its member centers.

Robert J Gumnit, MD, President
Gregory L Barkley MD, VP

6534 Parents Against Childhood Epilepsy (PACE)
7 E 85th St, Suite A3
New York, NY 10028 212-327-3070
Fax: 212-327-3075
pacenyemail@aol.com
www.paceusa.org

Research and education fund for severe seizure disorders and epilepsy.

Susan Fahey, Manager
Lauren Beck, President
Elizabeth Aquino, VP

State Agencies & Support Groups

Arkansas

6535 Epilepsy Education Association of Arkansas
2902 E Kiehl, Suite 1B
Sherwood, AR 72120 501-833-8680
sharon@epilepsyarkansas.com
www.epilepsyarkansas.com

A resource and provider of support and education in Arkansas for those with epilepsy.

Sharon Wingo McGinn, Director
Judy Hess RN, Co-Director

California

6536 Epilepsy Foundation of Northern California
155 Montgomery Street, Suite 309
San Francisco, CA 94104 415-677-4011
800-632-3532
Fax: 415-677-4190
tiffany@epilepsynorcal.org
www.epilepsynorcal.org

Nonprofit center serving families affected by epilepsy since 1953.

Katherine Keeney, President
Mary Cascino, Program Manager
Tiffany Manning, Events and Communications Manager

Florida

6537 Epilepsy Association of the Big Bend
1215 Lee Ave, Suite M-4
Tallahassee, FL 32303 850-222-1777
866-778-4583
Fax: 850-222-7440
epilepsyassoc@embarqmail.com
www.epilepsyassoc.org

Services include: case management, prevention education, counseling and advocacy, information and referral.

Scott Mehle, Executive Director

6538 Epilepsy Foundation of Florida
1200 NW 78 Ave, Suite 400
Miami, FL 33126 305-670-4949
877-553-7453
Fax: 305-670-0904
www.epilepsyfla.org

The Epilepesy Foundation of Florida (EFOF) leads the fight to stop seizures, find a cure, and overcome challenges created by epilepsy.

Karen Basha Egozi, CEO
Ivonne Anton, VP Director of Operations
Jesus Barraque, Director of Finance

6539 Florida Epilepsy Services Providers Associ ation
11200 NW 8th Avenue
Gainesville, FL 32601 352-392-6449
800-330-9746
Fax: 352-392-5792
fespa@floridaepilepsy.org
www.floridaepilepsy.org

A nonprofit membership organization of epilepsy services providers in the state of Florida, that serve the needs of those with epilepsy and their families. Local offices for services can be found for different regions and counties of Florida.

Jim Lyons, Program Director

New Jersey

6540 Epilepsy Foundation New Jersey
1 AAA Drive, Suite 203
Trenton, NJ 08691 609-392-4900
800-336-5843
Fax: 609-392-5621
TDD: 800-852-7899
aracioppi@efnj.com
www.efnj.com

A nonprofit organization providing support services for those with seizure disorders and their families.

Eric M Joice, Executive Director
Liza Grundell, Deputy Director
Jessica Goldsmith Barzilay, Assistant Director

New York

6541 Chrissy & Friends
930 Willowbrook Rd
Staten Island, NY 10302 718-698-1800
info@chrissyandfriends.org
www.chrissyandfriends.org

Offers children with epilepsy an opportunity to develop friendships through a variety of activities and tutoring programs.

RoseAnne DeRenzo, President
RoseAnne Zielechowski, VP
Joan DeRenzo, Secretary

6542 Epilepsy Foundation of Long Island
506 Stewart Avenue
Garden City, NY 11530 516-739-7733
888-672-7154
Fax: 516-739-1860
info@efli.org
www.efli.org

The Epilepsy Foundation of Long Island was founded in 1953 by a small group of parents who were determined to see their children lead productive and satisfying lives.

Jeffrey L. Nagel, President
Henry E. Klosowski, Vice President
Robert C. Creighton, Secretary

Pennsylvania

6543 Epilepsy Foundation Eastern Pennsylvania
919 Walnut Street, Suite 700
Philadelphia, PA 19107
215-629-5003
800-887-7165
Fax: 215-629-4997
efepa@efepa.org
www.efepa.org

The mission of the EPEA is to lead the fight to stop seizures, find a cure and overcome challenges created by epilepsy. They choose to fulfill the mission by meeting the non-medical needs for people affected by epilepsy/seizure disorder to enhance their lives and build supportive communities.

Frank Kotulka, Board President
Allison McCartin, Executive Director
Sue Livingston, Education Coordinator

6544 Epilepsy Foundation Western/Central Pennsylvania
1501 Reedsdale Street, Suite 3002
Pittsburgh, PA 15219
412-261-5880
800-316-5585
Fax: 412-322-7885
staff@efwp.org
www.efwp.org

The EFWCP is a private, non-profit service organization providing public education and supportive services to individuals and families affected by epilepsy/seizure disorders. The mission is to lead the fight to stop seizures, find a cure and overcome challenges created by epilepsy.

Judith K. Painter, Executive Director
Peggy Beem, Associate Director
Colleen K Fulkerson, Special Events Coordinator

Washington

6545 Epilepsy Foundation Northwest
2311 N. 45th St., #134
Seattle, WA 98103
206-547-4551
800-752-3509
Fax: 206-547-4557
mail@epilepsynw.org
www.epilepsynw.org

Serves all of Oregon & Washington.

Michael Reeves, Chair
Brent Herrmann, President/CEO
Rose Cain, Administrative Assistant

Libraries & Resource Centers

6546 EFWCP Resource Library
Epilepsy Foundation Western/Central Pennsylvania
1501 Reedsdale Street, Suite 3002
Pittsburgh, PA 15233
412-322-5880
800-361-5585
Fax: 412-322-7885
staff@efwp.org
www.efwp.org

For people with epilepsy and their families, comprehensive information on the disorder is often a valuable, yet hard-to-find asset. Living with epilepsy often requires special services to help better understand what epilepsy is and to learn how to deal with it. EFWCP can provide information beyond what is available in physician offices and in most cases the public library. The EFWCP maintains an Epilepsy Resource Library of brochures, books, reference manuals, videos and professional articles.

Judith Painter, Executive Director
Peggy Beem, Associate Director
Colleen K Fulkerson, Special Events Coordinator

Research Centers

California

6547 EpiCenter
University of California, Irvine
Irvine, CA 92697
949-824-5011
www.ucihs.uci.edu/epilepsyresearch/index.htm

Researchers, scientists and physicians studying the mechanisms and consequences of epilepsies through a variety of scientific approaches and research.

Tallie Z Baram, Chair

Illinois

6548 Citizens United for Research in Epilepsy (CURE)
223 W. Erie, Suite 2SW
Chicago, IL 60654
312-255-1801
800-765-7118
Fax: 312-255-1809
info@CUREepilepsy.org
www.cureepilepsy.org

Citizens United for Research in Epilepsy is a nonprofit organization dedicated to finding a cure for epilepsy by raising funds for research and by increasing awareness of the prevalence and devastation of this disease.

Susan Axelrod, Chair
Bogdan Ewendt, Executive Director
Samantha Kreindel, Director of Communications

Maryland

6549 Epilepsy Research Laboratory, Department of Neurology
Johns Hopkins University
Meyer 2-147, 600 N Wolfe St
Baltimore, MD 21287
410-276-8560
Fax: 410-563-0559
pfranasz@jhimi.edu
www.erl.neuro.jhmi.edu/

The Epilepsy Center evaluates and cares for seizure disorder patients from pediatric through adult.

Gregory K. Bergey, M.D., Professor/Director Epilepsy Center/
Christophe Jouny, Ph.D., Assistant Professor/Co-Director Epi
Joanne Barnett, Senior Medical Office Coordinator

Missouri

6550 Pediatric Epilepsy Center
St Louis Children's Hospital
One Children's Place, Suite 12E47
St Louis, MO 63110
314-454-6120
Fax: 314-454-4225
www.neuro.wustl.edu/

A comprehensive and one of the largest centers for epilepsy and seizure disorder care and research in the nation. It includes dedicated staff and an inpatient Epilepsy Monitoring Unit.

W. Edwin Dodson, M.D., Professor of Neurology & Pediatrics
Mary Bertrand, M.D., Associate Professor of Neurology
Christina Gurnett, M.D., Ph.D., Assistant Professor of Neurology an

New York

6551 Center for Neural Recovery & Rehabilitation Research
Helen Hayes Hospital
Route 9W
West Haverstraw, NY 10993
845-786-4225
888-707-3422
Fax: 845-947-3097
www.helenhayeshospital.org/research/
Helen E Scharfman PhD, Director

6552 Duke University Comprehensive Epilepsy Cen ter
200 Trent Drive, Room 4517, Busse Building
Durham, NC 27710
919-416-3853
Fax: 919-681-7973
koeni002@mc.duke.edu
neuro.surgery.duke.edu

Evaluation of potential surgical candidates by epilepsy specialists.
Roger L Cothran, Director
Allan H. Friedman, MD, Division Chief
Karen Koenig, Division Administrator

Tennessee

6553 Neuroscience Institute, University of Tenn essee Health Science Center
875 Monroe Ave, Suite 426
Memphis, TN 38163
901-448-5960
Fax: 901-448-4685
www.uthsc.edu/neuroscience

Epilepsy research and studies.
William E. Armstrong, Ph.D., Director
Anton J. Reiner, Ph.D., Co-Director
Shannon Guyot, Administrative Services Assistant

Texas

6554 Baylor Comprehensive Epilepsy Center
Baylor College of Medicine
Smith Tower, 18th Floor, 6550 Fannin, Suite 1801
Houston, TX 77030
713-798-8259
Fax: 713-798-7533
www.bcm.edu/neurology/epilepsy/

Individualized care for those with seizure disorders.
Richard A. Hrachovy, M.D., Director
David K. Chen, M.D., Epileptology and Neurophysiology
Alica M. Goldman, M.D., Ph.D., Epileptology and Neurophysiology

Wisconsin

6555 Regional Epilepsy Center
Aurora St. Luke's Medical Center
2801 W Kinnickic River Pkwy, Ste 570
Milwaukee, WI 53215
414-385-8780
www.aurorahealthcare.org/services/epilepsy/
Christopher Inglese, Director

Audio Video

6556 Because You Are My Friend
Epilepsy Foundation
8301 Professional Place East, Suite 200
Landover, MD 20785
866-330-2718
800-332-1000
Fax: 301-459-1569
ContactUs@efa.org
www.epilepsyfoundation.org

Video tape for children that provides a clear explanation of epilepsy, first aid and the importance of friendship. Cartoon slide presentation with child narration.
Warren Lammert, Chair
Phil Gattone, President/ CEO
Roger Heldman, Treasurer

6557 Epilepsy: The Untold Story
Fanflight Productions
32 Court Street, 21st Floor
Brooklyn, NY 11201
718-488-8900
800-876-1710
Fax: 718-488-8642
info@fanlight.com
www.fanlight.com

This video tells the story of six people with Temporal Lobe Epilepsy.
1993 Video - 27 mins
ISBN: 1-572951-37-0
Nicole Johnson, Publicity Coordinator

6558 How to Recognize and Classify Seizures
Epilepsy Foundation
8301 Professional Place East, Suite 200
Landover, MD 20785
866-330-2718
800-332-1000
Fax: 301-459-1569
ContactUs@efa.org
www.epilepsyfoundation.org

Discusses the classification of seizures and epileptic syndromes.
25 minutes
Warren Lammert, Chair
Phil Gattone, President/ CEO
Roger Heldman, Treasurer

6559 Just Like You and Me
WellMe/State of the Art
2201 Wisconsin Ave NW, Ste 350
Washington, DC 20008
202-537-0818
Fax: 202-537-0828
contact@wellme.com
wellme.stateart.com/productions/health/epilepsy/

A video/patient info guide package on successfully living with epilepsy.

6560 Rest of the Family
Epilepsy Foundation
8301 Professional Place East, Suite 200
Landover, MD 20785
866-330-2718
800-332-1000
Fax: 301-459-1569
ContactUs@efa.org
www.epilepsyfoundation.org

Presents the feelings and concerns of other family members, including siblings, of children with epilepsy.
Videocassette
Warren Lammert, Chair
Phil Gattone, President/ CEO
Roger Heldman, Treasurer

6561 Seizure First Aid
Epilepsy Foundation
8301 Professional Place East, Suite 200
Landover, MD 20785
866-330-2718
800-332-1000
Fax: 301-459-1569
ContactUs@efa.org
www.epilepsyfoundation.org

This video combines footage of real seizures with reenactments to demonstrate proper first aid procedures. In addition, people with epilepsy talk about how they feel when they have a seizure, and discuss how they would like friends, family and the general public to react when a seizure occurs. 10 minutes.
Video & DVD
Warren Lammert, Chair
Phil Gattone, President/ CEO
Roger Heldman, Treasurer

6562 Understanding Seizures & Epilepsy
Epilepsy Foundation
8301 Professional Place East, Suite 200
Landover, MD 20785

866-330-2718
800-332-1000
Fax: 301-459-1569
ContactUs@efa.org
www.epilepsyfoundation.org

Provides an explanation of seizure disorders in everyday language and dispels many misconceptions about epilepsy with medically accurate information.

Videocassette

Warren Lammert, Chair
Phil Gattone, President/ CEO
Roger Heldman, Treasurer

Web Sites

6563 American Epilepsy Society
www.aesnet.org

860-586-7505
emurray@aesnet.org
www.aesnet.org

The society promotes research and education of professionals in the field of epilepsy and related disorders. The site includes a comprehensive listing of postgraduate training opportunities in the fields related to epilepsy.

Amy Brooks-Kayal, M.D., President
Eileen M. Murray, MM, CAE, Executive Director
Jeffrey Melin, M.Ed., CMP, Director of Education

6564 Curing Epilepsy: Focus on the Future/Bench marks for Epilepsy Research
P.O. Box 5801
Bethesda, MD 20824

301-496-5751
800-352-9424
www.ninds.nih.gov/funding/research/epilepsyweb/

Summary of March 2000, White House-initiated conference.

Walter J. Koroshetz, M.D., Acting Director
Alan L. Willard, Ph.D., Acting Deputy Director
Caroline Lewis, Executive Officer

6565 Epilepsy Foundation of America
8301 Professional Place East, Suite 200
Landover, MD 20785

866-330-2718
800-332-1000
Fax: 301-459-1569
ContactUs@efa.org
www.epilepsyfoundation.org

Through its efforts the organization ensures that people with seizures are able to participate in all life experiences. Its goals are to eventually prevent, control and cure epilepsy through research, education, advocacy, and services.

Warren Lammert, Chair
Phil Gattone, President/ CEO
Roger Heldman, Treasurer

6566 Epilepsy.com
8301 Professional Place East, Suite 200
Landover, MD 20785

866-330-2718
800-332-1000
Fax: 301-459-1569
ContactUs@efa.org
www.epilepsy.com

Epilepsy resources made available through an initiative by the Epilepsy Therapy Development Project.

Warren Lammert, Chair
Phil Gattone, President/ CEO
Roger Heldman, Treasurer

6567 HealingWell.com
www.healingwell.com/epilepsy/

admin@healingwell.com
www.healingwell.com/epilepsy/

Offers information and resources including books, newsletters, and videos on a variety of diseases and chronic illnesses including epilepsy.

Peter Waite, Founder/ CEO

6568 NIH/National Institute of Neurological Dis orders and Stroke (NINDS)
PO Box 5801
Bethesda, MD 20824

301-496-5751
800-352-9424
www.ninds.nih.gov

The mission of NINDS is to reduce the burden of neurological disease - a burden borne by every age group, by every segment of society, by people all over the world.

Walter J. Koroshetz, MD, Director

6569 North Pacific Epilepsy Research
The Northrup Center, 2311 NW Northrup Street, Suit
Portland, OR 97210

503-291-5300
Fax: 503-291-5303
www.seizures.net/

Provides information to the public and health care professionals.

Dr. Mark Yerby, Founder

Book Publishers

6570 Brainstorms Companion: Epilepsy in Our Vie w
Steven C Schachter MD, author

Epilepsy Foundation
8301 Professional Place
Landover, MD 20785

301-459-3700
800-332-1000
Fax: 301-577-2684
www.epilepsyfoundation.org

Family members, friends and coworkers of those with seizure disorders describe their feelings and observations.

1994 160 pages Paperback
ISBN: 0-781702-30-5

Phil Gattone, President & CEO
Michele Dawson, Manager of Executive operations
Sandy Finucane, Senior Advisor

6571 Brainstorms: Epilepsy in Our Words
Steven C Schachter MD, author

Epilepsy Foundation
8301 Professional Place
Landover, MD 20785

301-459-3700
800-662-6922
Fax: 301-577-2684
www.epilepsyfoundation.org

Patients describe their experiences with seizures. Sixty-eight in-depth personal accounts of actual seizures are followed by a short section on how epilepsy affects the lives of the patients.

1993 197 pages Paperback
ISBN: 0-802774-65-2

Phil Gattone, President & CEO
Michele Dawson, Manager of Executive operations
Sandy Finucane, Senior Advisor

6572 Children with Seizures: A Guide For Parent s, Teachers and Other Professionals
Epilepsy Foundation
8301 Professional Place
Landover, MD 20785

301-459-3700
800-332-1000
Fax: 301-577-2684
www.epilepsyfoundation.org

Phil Gattone, President & CEO
Michele Dawson, Manager of Executive operations
Sandy Finucane, Senior Advisor

6573 Dotty the Dalmatian Has Epilepsy
Tim Peters & Company, Inc
87 Main St, PO Box 370
Peapack, NJ 07977

908-234-2050
800-543-2230
Fax: 908-234-1961
info@timpetersandcompany.com
www.timpetersandcompany.com

Part of the Dr. Wellbook® series, this is the story of Dotty the Dalmatian who discovers she has epilepsy.

16 pages Softcover
ISBN: 1-879874-35-0

6574 Embrace the Dawn

Andrea Davidson, author

Epilepsy Foundation
8301 Professional Place
Landover, MD 20785

301-459-3700
800-332-1000
Fax: 301-577-2684
www.epilepsyfoundation.org

A moving biographical account of one person's lifelong experience with epilepsy.

127 pages Softcover

Phil Gattone, President & CEO
Michele Dawson, Manager of Executive operations
Sandy Finucane, Senior Advisor

6575 Epilepsy A to Z
Demos Medical Publishing
11 West 42nd Street, 15th Floor
New York, NY 10036

212-683-0072
800-532-8663
Fax: 212-683-0118
orderdept@demosmedpub.com
www.demosmedpub.com

Easy reference in finding brief answers to questions regarding epilepsy terminology.

1995 322 pages Softcover
ISBN: 0-939957-75-0

Kathy Gonzalez, Order Dept/Fulfillment Coordinator
Paul Choi, Vice-President of Finance and Opera
Richard Winters, Executive Editor

6576 Epilepsy, A Guide to Balancing Your Life
Ilo E Leppik MD, author

Demos Medical Publishing
11 West 42nd Street, 15th Floor
New York, NY 10036

212-683-0072
800-532-8663
Fax: 212-683-0118
orderdept@demosmedpub.com
www.demosmedpub.com

Part of the Quality of Life Guide Series from the American Academy of Neurology Press. Provides reliable and practical information for those diagnosed with epilepsy and seizure disorders.

2006 192 pages Softcover
ISBN: 1-932603-20-0

Kathy Gonzalez, Order Dept/Fulfillment Coordinator
Paul Choi, Vice-President of Finance and Opera
Richard Winters, Executive Editor

6577 Epilepsy: 199 Answers

Andrew N Wilner MD, author

Demos Medical Publishing
11 West 42nd Street, 15th Floor
New York, NY 10036

212-683-0072
800-532-8663
Fax: 212-683-0118
orderdept@demosmedpub.com
www.demosmedpub.com

Helps to better understand conversations with the doctor and empowers the patient/caregiver to ask the right questions, resulting in optimal care.

2003 180 pages Softcover
ISBN: 1-888799-70-5

Kathy Gonzalez, Order Dept/Fulfillment Coordinator
Paul Choi, Vice-President of Finance and Opera
Richard Winters, Executive Editor

6578 Epilepsy: Frequency, Causes and Consequenc es
Epilepsy Foundation
8301 Professional Place
Landover, MD 20785

301-459-3700
800-332-1000
Fax: 301-577-2684
www.epilepsyfoundation.org

Statistical study that addresses the causes, natural history, prevalence and risk factors of epilepsy in certain populations and the impact on the community.

1990

Phil Gattone, President & CEO
Michele Dawson, Manager of Executive operations
Sandy Finucane, Senior Advisor

6579 Epilepsy: I Can Live with That

Sue Goss, author

Epilepsy Foundation
8301 Professional Place
Landover, MD 20785

301-459-3700
800-332-1000
Fax: 301-577-2684
www.epilepsyfoundation.org

The experience of epilepsy as recorded by a group of ordinary men and women living in Australia. Each story focuses on personal growth, triumph over disability and emphasizes individual courage and hope.

1995 Softcover

Phil Gattone, President & CEO
Michele Dawson, Manager of Executive operations
Sandy Finucane, Senior Advisor

6580 Growing Up With Epilepsy

Lynn Bennett Blackburn MD, author

Demos Medical Publishing
11 West 42nd Street, 15th Floor
New York, NY 10036

212-683-0072
800-532-8663
Fax: 212-683-0118
orderdept@demosmedpub.com
www.demosmedpub.com

Guidance in raising a child with epilepsy, including navigating the educational system, discipline, and social development.

2003 168 pages Softcover
ISBN: 1-888799-74-3

Kathy Gonzalez, Order Dept/Fulfillment Coordinator
Paul Choi, Vice-President of Finance and Opera
Richard Winters, Executive Editor

6581 Keto Kid, Helping Your Child to Succeed on the Ketogenic Diet

Deborah Ann Snyder DO, author

Demos Medical Publishing
11 West 42nd Street, 15th Floor
New York, NY 10036

212-683-0072
800-532-8663
Fax: 212-683-0118
orderdept@demosmedpub.com
www.demosmedpub.com

2006 176 pages Softcover
ISBN: 1-932603-29-3

Kathy Gonzalez, Order Dept/Fulfillment Coordinator
Paul Choi, Vice-President of Finance and Opera
Richard Winters, Executive Editor

6582 Lee the Rabbit with Epilepsy

Deborah M. Moss, author

Epilepsy Foundation
8301 Professional Place
Landover, MD 20785

301-459-3700
800-332-1000
Fax: 301-459-1569
www.epilepsyfoundation.org

Written for children ages three to six, this illustrated picture book follows the adventures of a small rabbit who has seizures. It follows her journey from the first seizure, the initial doctors visit through to treatment.

1989 21 pages Hardcover

Phil Gattone, President & CEO
Michele Dawson, Manager of Executive operations
Sandy Finucane, Senior Advisor

6583 Living Well with Epilepsy

Robert Gumnit MD, author

Demos Medical Publishing
11 West 42nd Street, 15th Floor
New York, NY 10036

212-683-0072
800-532-8663
Fax: 212-683-0118
orederdept@demosmedpub.com
www.demosmedpub.com

Designed to help both health-care professionals and patients to understand all aspects of diagnosis and management; to enable patients to participate more knowledgeably in interactions with their health care team and to help steer them toward a more normal, fulfilling life.

1997 249 pages Soft / 2nd Ed
ISBN: 1-888799-11-0

Kathy Gonzalez, Order Dept/Fulfillment Coordinator
Paul Choi, Vice-President of Finance and Opera
Richard Winters, Executive Editor

6584 Missing Michael - A Mother's Story of Love

Epilepsy Foundation
8301 Professional Place
Landover, MD 20785

301-459-3700
800-332-1000
Fax: 301-459-1569
www.epilepsyfoundation.org

A mother's story of her struggle with raising her son with epilepsy. Deatils in dealing with the health care system, the school system, and the complications of medication.

Paperback

Phil Gattone, President & CEO
Michele Dawson, Manager of Executive operations
Sandy Finucane, Senior Advisor

6585 Mom I Have a Staring Problem

Epilepsy Foundation
8301 Professional Place
Landover, MD 20785

301-459-3700
800-332-1000
Fax: 301-459-1570
www.epilepsyfoundation.org

Tiffany, a seven-year old, describes her experiences with petit mal seizures; her feelings, wishes and fears. Written to help adults recognize a hidden problem that could be occuring with a child who has learning problems.

1994 24 pages Softcover
ISBN: 0-802774-65-2

Phil Gattone, President & CEO
Michele Dawson, Manager of Executive operations
Sandy Finucane, Senior Advisor

6586 My Friend Matty: A Story About Living with Epilepsy

Epilepsy Foundation
8301 Professional Place
Landover, MD 20785

301-459-3700
800-332-1000
Fax: 301-459-1571
www.epilepsyfoundation.org

A comic-book style publication for educating children written by parents whose 5-year old boy passed away.

Paperback

Phil Gattone, President & CEO
Michele Dawson, Manager of Executive operations
Sandy Finucane, Senior Advisor

6587 Pediatric Epilepsy

Demos Medical Publishing
11 West 42nd Street, 15th Floor
New York, NY 10036

212-683-0072
800-532-8663
Fax: 212-683-0118
orderdept@demosmedpub.com
www.demosmedpub.com

Covers the diagnosis, treatment, classification and management of childhood epilepsies.

2001 666 pages Hardcover
ISBN: 1-888799-30-9

Kathy Gonzalez, Order Dept/Fulfillment Coordinator
Paul Choi, Vice-President of Finance and Opera
Richard Winters, Executive Editor

6588 Pediatric Epilepsy Resource Handbook

FACES/NYU Medical Center
223 East 34th Street
New York, NY 10016

646-558-0900
Fax: 646-385-7163
FACESinfo@nyumc.org
www.faces.med.nyu.edu

3rd Edition

Pamela Mohr, Executive Director
Nako Ishii, Project Co-ordinator
Luis L. Valero, Associate Director of Special Event

6589 School Planning

Epilepsy Foundation
8301 Professional Place
Landover, MD 20785

301-459-3700
800-332-1000
Fax: 301-577-2684
TDD: 800-332-2070
www.epilepsyfoundation.org

This guide describes some epilepsy-related problems that children and youth may face in the areas of academics, school achievement and social development. Suggests ways parents can take a proactive approach to ensure appropriate testing, placement and achievement of educational goals for their children.

125 pages Hardcover
ISBN: 0-802774-65-2

Phil Gattone, President & CEO
Michele Dawson, Manager of Executive operations
Sandy Finucane, Senior Advisor

6590 Seizures and Epilepsy In Childhood: A Guid e

Johns Hopkins University Press
2715 N Charles Street
Baltimore, MD 21218

410-516-6900
800-537-5487
Fax: 410-516-6968
www.press.jhu.edu

A standard resource for parents in need of comprehensive medical information about their child with epilepsy.

2002 432 pages 3rd Ed / Hard
ISBN: 0-801870-50-x

Kathleen Keane, Director
Timothy D. Fuller, Chief Information Officer
Erik A. Smist, Director, Finance and Administratio

6591 Your Child and Epilepsy
Roger J Gumnit MD, author

Demos Medical Publishing
11 West 42nd Street, 15th Floor
New York, NY 10036   212-683-0072
                                       800-532-8663
                                   Fax: 212-683-0118
                              orderdept@demospub.com
                                 www.demosmedpub.com

Provides information to help parents understand their child's epilepsy, suggestions on how to evaluate health care, to find better care if necessary and advice on how to help children with epilepsy to develop self-confidence and self-motivation.

1995 256 pages Softcover
ISBN: 0-939957-76-0

Kathy Gonzalez, Order Dept/Fulfillment Coordinator
Paul Choi, Vice-President of Finance and Opera
Richard Winters, Executive Editor

Magazines

6592 Epilepsy Foundation
Epilepsy Foundation
8301 Professional Place East, Suite 200
Landover, MD 20785   866-330-2718
                                       800-332-1000
                                   Fax: 301-459-1569
                                 ContactUs@efa.org
                            www.epilepsyfoundation.org

Catalog of epilepsy information materials, including pamphlets, books, manuals, videotapes and other items is available upon request.

Warren Lammert, Chair
Phil Gattone, President/ CEO
Roger Heldman, Treasurer

6593 EpilepsyUSA
Epilepsy Foundation
8301 Professional Place East, Suite 200
Landover, MD 20785   866-330-2718
                                       800-332-1000
                                   Fax: 301-459-1569
                                   TDD: 800-332-2070
                                 ContactUs@efa.org
                            www.epilepsyfoundation.org

Information on concerns about seizure disorders and epilepsy and new developments in treatment.

24 pages 6 issues/yr

Warren Lammert, Chair
Phil Gattone, President/ CEO
Roger Heldman, Treasurer

Journals

6594 Epilepsy & Behavior
Elsevier
Marquis One, 245 Peachtree Center Avenue, Suite 19
Atlanta, GA 30303   404-669-9400
                                       800-999-6274
                                   Fax: 404-669-9339
                               usjcs@elsevier.com
                www.journals.elsevier.com/epilepsy-and-behavior/

An international journal that offers current information on the behavioral aspects of seizures and epilepsy.

Bi-monthly
ISSN: 1525-5050

Ron Mobed, Chief Executive Officer
Stuart Whayman, Chief Financial Officer
Gavin Howe, EVP, Human Resources

Newsletters

6595 AES News
American Epilepsy Society
342 N Main Street
W Hartford, CT 6117   860-586-7505
                                   Fax: 860-568-7550
                                      www.aesnet.org

16 pages 3x/year
Deepak K Lachhwani, Editor
Amy Brooks-Kayal, M.D., President
Eileen M. Murray, MM, CAE, Executive Director

6596 Epilepsia: Journal of the International League Against Epilepsy
Blackwell Publishing
350 Main Street, Commerce Place
Malden, MA 2148   781-388-8200
                                       888-661-5800
                                   Fax: 781-388-8210
                            www.blackwellpublishing.com

A leading international journal on the epilepsies for more than 30 years, Epilepsia provides comprehensive coverage of current clinical and research results.

12 per year
ISSN: 0013-9580

Philip A Schwartzkroin, Co-Editor
Simon Shorvon, Co-Editor

6597 FACES: Finding a Cure for Epilepsy & Seizu res
223 East 34th Street (between 2nd and 3rd Avenues)
New York, NY 10016   646-558-0900
                                   Fax: 646-385-7163
                              FACESinfo@nyumc.org
                                  faces.med.nyu.edu

Covers new studies, research, events and special interest stories.

Quarterly
Orrin Devinsky, MD, Founder
Pamela B. Mohr, Executive Director
Luis L. Valero, Associate Director

Pamphlets

6598 Child with Epilepsy at Camp
Epilepsy Foundation
8301 Professional Place East, Suite 200
Landover, MD 20785   866-330-2718
                                       800-332-1000
                                   Fax: 301-459-1569
                                 ContactUs@efa.org
                            www.epilepsyfoundation.org

Written for camp counselors, it helps parents explain to them the specific needs of children with epilepsy at camp to ensure a safe camping experience.

14 pages Pamphlet

Warren Lammert, Chair
Phil Gattone, President/ CEO
Roger Heldman, Treasurer

6599 Child's Guide To Seizure Disorders
Epilepsy Foundation
8301 Professional Place East, Suite 200
Landover, MD 20785   866-330-2718
                                       800-332-1000
                                   Fax: 301-459-1569
                                 ContactUs@efa.org
                            www.epilepsyfoundation.org

A pamphlet for children, brightly-colored and explains seizures, why medication should be taken, etc.

Warren Lammert, Chair
Phil Gattone, President/ CEO
Roger Heldman, Treasurer

6600 Epilepsy in Children: The Teacher's Role
Epilepsy Foundation
8301 Professional Place East, Suite 200
Landover, MD 20785   866-330-2718
                                            800-332-1000
                                            Fax: 301-459-1569
                                            ContactUs@efa.org
                                            www.epilepsyfoundation.org

Provides an explanation for teachers on handling seizures in the classroom, the need for good communication between students and first aid procedures.

Warren Lammert, Chair
Phil Gattone, President/ CEO
Roger Heldman, Treasurer

6601 Epilepsy: You and Your Child
Epilepsy Foundation
8301 Professional Place East, Suite 200
Landover, MD 20785   866-330-2718
                                            800-332-1000
                                            Fax: 301-459-1569
                                            ContactUs@efa.org
                                            www.epilepsyfoundation.org

This instructional booklet offers information on emotional aspects of epilepsy, how to handle seizures, medication, diet and nutrition, and offers referral organizations for parents.

Warren Lammert, Chair
Phil Gattone, President/ CEO
Roger Heldman, Treasurer

6602 Febrile Seizures Fact Sheet
NINDS/NIH Neurological Institute
Office of Communications and Public Liaison, NINDS
Bethesda, MD 20892   301-496-5751
                                            800-352-9424
                                            TTY: 301-468-5981
                        www.ninds.nih.gov/disorders/febrile_seizures/

Also available in Spanish.

Walter J. Koroshetz, M.D., Acting Director
Alan L. Willard, Ph.D., Acting Deputy Director
Caroline Lewis, Executive Officer

6603 Finding Out About Seizures: A Guide to Medical Tests
Epilepsy Foundation
8301 Professional Place East, Suite 200
Landover, MD 20785   866-330-2718
                                            800-332-1000
                                            Fax: 301-459-1569
                                            ContactUs@efa.org
                                            www.epilepsyfoundation.org

Introduces adults and children with epilepsy to the types of tests they may have to undergo.

Warren Lammert, Chair
Phil Gattone, President/ CEO
Roger Heldman, Treasurer

6604 H.O.P.E. Series: Seizures in Childhood
Epilepsy Foundation
8301 Professional Place East, Suite 200
Landover, MD 20785   866-330-2718
                                            800-332-1000
                                            Fax: 301-459-1569
                                            ContactUs@efa.org
                                            www.epilepsyfoundation.org

Provides an overview of the challenges associated with living with epilepsy and other seizure disorders, including potential hazards, first aid procedures, and overall help in daily living.

Warren Lammert, Chair
Phil Gattone, President/ CEO
Roger Heldman, Treasurer

6605 H.O.P.E. Series: Seizures in the Teen Years
Epilepsy Foundation
8301 Professional Place East, Suite 200
Landover, MD 20785   866-330-2718
                                            800-332-1000
                                            Fax: 301-459-1569
                                            ContactUs@efa.org
                                            www.epilepsyfoundation.org

Provides general information specifically for teens with epilepsy and seizure disorders.

Warren Lammert, Chair
Phil Gattone, President/ CEO
Roger Heldman, Treasurer

6606 Infantile Spasms
NINDS/NIH Neurological Institute
Office of Communications and Public Liaison, NINDS
Bethesda, MD 20892   301-496-5751
                                            800-352-9424
                                            TTY: 301-468-5981
                        www.ninds.nih.gov/disorders/infantilespasms/

Information sheet on infantile spasms (West Syndrome).

Walter J. Koroshetz, M.D., Acting Director
Alan L. Willard, Ph.D., Acting Deputy Director
Caroline Lewis, Executive Officer

6607 Kids and Seizures: Know the Hidden Signs
Epilepsy Foundation
8301 Professional Place East, Suite 200
Landover, MD 20785   866-330-2718
                                            800-332-1000
                                            Fax: 301-459-1569
                                            ContactUs@efa.org
                                            www.epilepsyfoundation.org

Written for camp counselors, it helps parents explain to them the specific needs of children with epilepsy at camp to ensure a safe camping experience.

Warren Lammert, Chair
Phil Gattone, President/ CEO
Roger Heldman, Treasurer

6608 Managing Seizures, Information for Caregivers
Epilepsy Foundation
8301 Professional Place East, Suite 200
Landover, MD 20785   866-330-2718
                                            800-332-1000
                                            Fax: 301-459-1569
                                            ContactUs@efa.org
                                            www.epilepsyfoundation.org

Explains seizures, routine and special care, emergency aid and first aid for caregivers. Includes a poster size chart for medicines and general guidance in handling a seizure.

Warren Lammert, Chair
Phil Gattone, President/ CEO
Roger Heldman, Treasurer

6609 Me and My World Storybook
Epilepsy Foundation
8301 Professional Place East, Suite 200
Landover, MD 20785   866-330-2718
                                            800-332-1000
                                            Fax: 301-459-1569
                                            TDD: 800-332-2070
                                            ContactUs@efa.org
                                            www.epilepsyfoundation.org

An excellent pamphlet for explaining epilepsy to children and their friends. It also discusses various types of epilepsy and its effects on family members. Ages 4-8.

Warren Lammert, Chair
Phil Gattone, President/ CEO
Roger Heldman, Treasurer

6610 Medicines for Epilepsy
Epilepsy Foundation
8301 Professional Place East, Suite 200
Landover, MD 20785
866-330-2718
800-332-1000
Fax: 301-459-1569
ContactUs@efa.org
www.epilepsyfoundation.org

Offers information on medication and treatments, generic drugs, side effects, drug abuse and more. Contains a color chart with pictures of the most common medications for epilepsy.

Warren Lammert, Chair
Phil Gattone, President/ CEO
Roger Heldman, Treasurer

6611 Safety and Seizures
Epilepsy Foundation
8301 Professional Place East, Suite 200
Landover, MD 20785
866-330-2718
800-332-1000
Fax: 301-459-1569
ContactUs@efa.org
www.epilepsyfoundation.org

Warren Lammert, Chair
Phil Gattone, President/ CEO
Roger Heldman, Treasurer

6612 Seizures and Epilepsy: Hope Through Resear ch
NINDS/NIH Neurological Institute
Office of Communications and Public Liaison, NINDS
Bethesda, MD 20892
301-496-5751
800-352-9424
TTY: 301-468-5981
www.ninds.nih.gov/disorders/epilepsy/

Also available in Spanish.

Walter J. Koroshetz, M.D., Acting Director
Alan L. Willard, Ph.D., Acting Deputy Director
Caroline Lewis, Executive Officer

6613 Seizures, Epilepsy and Your Child
Epilepsy Foundation
8301 Professional Place East, Suite 200
Landover, MD 20785
866-330-2718
800-332-1000
Fax: 301-459-1569
ContactUs@efa.org
www.epilepsyfoundation.org

A pamphlet for parents, providing guidance on daily life, first aid and treatment for children with epilepsy.

Warren Lammert, Chair
Phil Gattone, President/ CEO
Roger Heldman, Treasurer

6614 Surgery for Epilepsy
Epilepsy Foundation
8301 Professional Place East, Suite 200
Landover, MD 20785
866-330-2718
800-332-1000
Fax: 301-459-1569
ContactUs@efa.org
www.epilepsyfoundation.org

Describes current surgical treatment and the testing that precedes it.
12 pages

Warren Lammert, Chair
Phil Gattone, President/ CEO
Roger Heldman, Treasurer

6615 Talking to Your Doctor About Seizure Disorders
Epilepsy Foundation
8301 Professional Place East, Suite 200
Landover, MD 20785
866-330-2718
800-332-1000
Fax: 301-459-1569
ContactUs@efa.org
www.epilepsyfoundation.org

Designed to help the patient talk with medical personnel about treatment of epilepsy.

Warren Lammert, Chair
Phil Gattone, President/ CEO
Roger Heldman, Treasurer

6616 The ADA: Questions and Answers
Epilepsy Foundation
8301 Professional Place East, Suite 200
Landover, MD 20785
866-330-2718
800-332-1000
Fax: 301-459-1569
ContactUs@efa.org
www.epilepsyfoundation.org

Offers a brief overview of the Americans with Disabilities Act and how it covers those with epilepsy.

Warren Lammert, Chair
Phil Gattone, President/ CEO
Roger Heldman, Treasurer

6617 What Everyone Should Know About Epilepsy
Epilepsy Foundation
8301 Professional Place East, Suite 200
Landover, MD 20785
866-330-2718
800-332-1000
Fax: 301-459-1569
ContactUs@efa.org
www.epilepsyfoundation.org

Warren Lammert, Chair
Phil Gattone, President/ CEO
Roger Heldman, Treasurer

6618 When Seizures Don't Look Like Seizures
Epilepsy Foundation
8301 Professional Place East, Suite 200
Landover, MD 20785
866-330-2718
800-332-1000
Fax: 301-459-1569
ContactUs@efa.org
www.epilepsyfoundation.org

Describes and helps with the subtle signs of a seizure for parents, child care providers and school personnel.
ISBN: 0-802774-65-2

Warren Lammert, Chair
Phil Gattone, President/ CEO
Roger Heldman, Treasurer

Camps

6619 Camp Achieve
Epilepsy Foundation Eastern Pennsylvania
919 Walnut Street, Suite 700
Philadelphia, PA 19107
215-629-5003
800-887-7165
Fax: 215-629-4997
camp@efepa.org
www.efepa.org/programs-and-resources/camp-achieve

Camp Achieve is a week long, overnight, summer camp for youth with a primary diagnosis of epilepsy/seizure disorder that is held every year in August. Camp Achieve is a unique opportunity for the children ages 8-17 to connect with other individuals coping with the same day to day challenges. Many individuals with epilepsy/seizure disorder face isolation, bullying, and discrimination from their classmates, their neighbors, and the general public.

Frank Kotulka, Board President
Allison McCartin, Executive Director
Sue Livingston, Education Coordinator

6620 Camp Frog
Epilepsy Foundation Western/Central Pennsylvania
1501 Reedsdale Street, Suite 3002
Pittsburgh, PA 15233
412-261-5880
800-316-5585
Fax: 412-322-7885
astein@efwp.org
www.efwp.org/programs/ProgramsCampFrog.xml

The EFWCP sponsors two-week long, overnight summer camping programs called Camp Frog. This nationally recognized activity allows kids with epilepsy/seizure disorders to be integrated into a typical camping experience with hundreds of other children. The overnight program is available to boys and girls with epilepsy/seizure disorders from grades 4 to 11. Campers enjoy a host of activities such as arts and crafts, campfire sing-alongs, swimming, team games, sailing, archery and horseback riding.

Peggy Beem, President/ CEO
Francine Reyher, Adult Services Coordinator
Colleen K Fulkerson, Special Events Coordinator

6621 Camp Ramah in New England Tikvah Program
39 Bennett Street
Palmer, MA 01609
413-283-9771
Fax: 413-283-6661
info@campramahne.org
www.campramahne.org

The Tikvah program is one of the first summer programs for Jewish children with special needs. It continues to grow and evolve as it strives to serve campers with a wide range of special needs including, but not limited to, congitive impairments, autism, cerebral palsy and seizure disorder.

Howard Blas, Tikvah Program Director
Talya Kalender, Director, Camper Care
Benjamin Greene, Director of Education

6622 Camp Roehr
140 Iowa Ave # A
Belleville, IL 62220
618-236-2181
866-848-0472
Fax: 618-236-3654
www.epilepsyfoundation.org/local/swillinois/camp.cfm

Seven day residential camp for children designed to meet the special needs of children diagnosed with epilepsy, providing a safe and fun camp experience.

Ellen Becker, Executive Director
Trudy Baxter, Director of Programs and Services
Jan Conder, Development Coordinator

6623 Crotched Mountain School & Rehabilitation Center
1 Verney Drive
Greenfield, NH 3047
603-547-3311
800-800-966
Fax: 603-547-3232
info@crotchedmountain.org
www.cmf.org

Currently serves children ages 6-22 with multiple-handicaps including: Cerebral Palsy, Spina Bifida, visual and hearing impairments and neurological disabilities, developmental disorders, mental retardation, autism, behavioral and emotional disorders, seizure disorders, spinal cord and head injuries. Member of the National Association of Independent Schools and accredited with the NE Association of Schools and Colleges, Independent Schools of Northern NE.

Donald L. Shumway, President/ CEO
Kathleen C. Brittan, VP, Development
Frederick R. Bruch, Jr., Medical Director

DESCRIPTION

6624 SICKLE CELL DISEASE

Synonyms: Homozygous Hb S, Sickle cell anemia

Involves the following Biologic System(s):

Hematologic and Oncologic Disorders

Sickle cell disease is an inherited blood disorder that primarily affects African Americans and is characterized by the presence of crescent or sickle-shaped red cells in the blood and the chronic premature destruction of red blood cells (hemolytic anemia). In this disorder, the red blood cells contain an abnormal form of the oxygen-carrying protein (hemoglobin) called hemoglobin S (Hgb S). This abnormality reduces the level of available oxygen (ischemia) in the blood cells and results in their characteristic sickle shape. These irregular cells tend to block the tiny blood vessels of various tissues and organs; they may cause restricted or obstructed blood flow resulting in tissue or organ damage (infarction). In addition, their unusual shape renders them fragile, leading to their premature destruction and thus anemia.

The symptoms of sickle cell disease tend to appear at or around six months of age and may include headaches; shortness of breath (dyspnea); paleness; fatigue; and a yellowish hue of the eyes, skin, and mucous membranes (jaundice). Any activity that would normally reduce the blood oxygen levels (e.g., exercise, exertion, illness, or high-altitude flying) may induce a sickle cell crisis or sudden worsening of the anemic condition accompanied by abdominal and bone pain, dyspnea, and vomiting. Infarction or a blocked blood vessel (vaso-occlusion) may also result in sickle cell crisis with the affected child experiencing chest pain and increased dyspnea. By adolescence most of those affected develop an|enlarged spleen (splenomegaly) that is no longer capable of assisting in fighting certain infections, leaving the body more vulnerable to certain types of infections (encapsulated organisms, notably pneumococcal pneumonia). Other symptoms may include skin changes resulting from poor circulation, stroke resulting from insufficient oxygen reaching the brain, or blood in the urine (hematuria) resulting from kidney damage. As the affected child grows to adulthood, the liver and heart may enlarge (hepatosplenomegaly) and a heart murmur may develop. The lungs, intestines, and gall bladder may also be affected. In addition, affected children may develop such distinct characteristics as a short torso with long extremities, fingers, and toes.

Because there is no known cure for sickle cell disease, treatment is geared toward prevention, control, and pain management. Such treatment may include the avoidance of activities that reduce blood oxygen levels, a full immunization regimen, and prompt medical intervention for any illness or viral infection. Other treatment may include folic acid supplementation, antibiotic medication for treatment and prevention of infection, oxygen therapy to improve the level of oxygen in the blood, and acetaminophen or other medication to relieve pain. To manage a sickle cell crisis, as well as the pain associated with it, affected children may be given intravenous fluids, pain-relieving drugs,and possibly blood transfusions. Other treatments being studied include certain drugs, gene therapy, and bone marrow transplantation.

Sickle cell dis|ease is inherited as an autosomal recessive trait. In this case, the defective gene for hemoglobin S is transmitted by both parents. If a child inherits this gene from only one parent (and one normal gene from the other parent, that child will usually be symptom-free, but will be a carrier of the sickle cell trait. The incidence of this disorder in the United States is approximately 150 African American children in 100,000; however, approximately one in 12 black children carries the sickle cell trait.

Government Agencies

6625 NIH/ Eunice Kennedy Shriver National Insti tute of Child Health & Human Development
31 Center Drive, Building 31
Bethesda, MD 20892

301-496-5113
800-370-2943
Fax: 866-760-5947
nichdpress@mail.nih.gov
www.nichd.nih.gov

Established in 1962 by congress, today the institute conducts and supports research on topics related to the health of children, adults, families and populations. Some of these topics include: developmental disabilities, growth and development, infant death, reproductive health and birth defects.

Diana W. Bianchi, Director
Paul Williams, Director, Communications

6626 NIH/National Heart, Lung and Blood Institu te
National Institute of Health
31 Center Dr MSC 2486, Bldg 31, Room 5A52
Bethesda, MD 20892

301-592-8573
Fax: 301-592-8563
TTY: 240-629-3255
NHLBIinfo@nhlbi.nih.gov
www.nhlbi.nih.gov

Primary responsibility of this organization is the scientific investigation of heart, blood vessel, lung and blood disorders. Oversees research, demonstration, prevention, education, control and training activities in these fields and emphasizes the prevention and control of heart diseases.

Gary H. Gibbons, M.D., Director
Nakela Cook, MD, Chief of Staff

National Associations & Support Groups

6627 American Academy of Pediatrics
141 Northwest Point Boulevard
Elk Grove Village, IL 60007

847-434-4000
800-433-9016
Fax: 847-434-8000
www.aap.org

The American Academy of Pediatrics and its member pediatricians are committed to the attainment of optimal physical, mental and social health and well-being for all infants, children, adolescents, and young adults.

Fernando Stein, MD, FAAP, President
Karen Remley, MD, CEO/Executive VP

6628 American Sickle Cell Anemia Association
10900 Carnegie Avenue
Cleveland, OH 44106

216-229-8600
Fax: 216-229-4500
irabragg@ascaa.org
www.ascaa.org

Provides education, testing, counseling, supportive services to the population at risk for sickle cell anemia and its hemoglobin variants. Bilingual educator on staff, educational materials and distribution of literature is provided by ASCAA. Referrals for children and families with special needs.

Ira Bragg-Grant, Executive Director

6629 Genetic Alliance
4301 Connecticut Avenue NW, Suite 404
Washington, DC 20008
202-966-5557
800-336-4363
Fax: 202-966-8553
info@geneticalliance.org
www.geneticalliance.org

A coalition of voluntary genetic support groups, consumers and professionals addressing the needs of individuals and families affected by genetic disorders from a national perspective.

Sharon Terry, President/CEO
Tetyana Murza, Managing Director
Natasha Bonhomme, VP, Strategic Development

6630 Sickle Cell Disease Association of America
231 E Baltimore St, Suite 800
Baltimore, MD 21202
410-528-1555
800-421-8453
Fax: 410-528-1495
scdaa@sicklecelldisease.org
www.sicklecelldisease.org

Promotes the finding of a universal cure for sickle cell disease while improving the quality of life for individuals and families where sickle cell related conditions exists. It also assists in the organization and development of local chapters.

Willarda Edwards, President
Sonya I Ross, VP Programs/Services
Asha Hamilton, Membership Services Coordinator

6631 Sickle Cell Information Center
Grady Memorial Hospital
80 Jesse Hill Jr Drive, PO Box 109
Atlanta, GA 30301
404-616-3572
Fax: 404-616-5998
aplatt@emory.edu
www.scinfo.org

Sickle cell resources, education, news and research updates for caregivers, patients and professionals.

State Agencies & Support Groups

Alabama

6632 Sickle Cell Foundation of Greater Montgomery
3180 US Highway 80 W
Montgomery, AL 36108
334-286-9122
800-742-5534
Fax: 334-286-4804
sickle2@aol.com
www.scfgm.org

Willie Owens, Executive Director

California

6633 Sickle Cell Disease Foundation of California
5777 W. Century Blvd. Suite 1230
Los Angeles, CA 90045
310-693-0247
877-288-2873
Fax: 310-216-0307
info@scdfc.org
www.scdfc.org

Educates, screens and offers counsel to those at risk for having children with sickle cell disease and other hemoglobin disorders.

Mary E Brown, President
Roger Brown, Director Development/Public Affairs

Connecticut

6634 Sickle Cell Disease Association of America - Connecticut Chapter
Hartford Regional Office
231 E Baltimore St, Suite 800
Baltimore, MD 21202
410-528-1555
800-421-8453
Fax: 410-528-1495
scdaa@sicklecelldisease.org
www.sicklecelldisease.org

Regional office loactions in Hartford, New Haven and New London.

Georgia

6635 Sickle Cell Foundation of Georgia
2391 Benjamin E Mays Drive
Atlanta, GA 30311
404-755-1641
800-326-5287
Fax: 404-755-7955
info@sicklecellga.org
www.sicklecellga.org/

Provides education, screening, and counseling programs for sickle cell and other abnormal hemoglobins. The Foundation has a deep-rooted commitment to making strides in monitoring the occurrence of sickle cell, improving the quality of life for those with the disease and cooperating with individuals conducting research.

Jean Brannan, Executive Director
Harold Dobbs, Outreach Coordinator
Nesby Gibson, Project Director

Louisiana

6636 NE Louisiana Sickle Cell Anemia Foundation
PO Box 1165
Monroe, LA 71210
318-322-0896
Fax: 318-387-4740
sickle@bayou.com
www.sicklecelldisease.org/index.cfm?page=chapter&id=

The Northeast Louisiana Sickle Cell Anemia Foundation is a community based tax exempt organization that assists victims with the inherited blood disease sickle cell anemia.

Christopher Hollins, Chair
Sonja L. Banks, President/Chief Operating Officer
Francis Aofolaju, Chief Financial Officer

Massachusetts

6637 Community Sickle Cell Support Group
1542 Tremont St
Roxbury, MA 02120
617-427-4100
cscsginc@aol.com
www.cscsginc.org

Jackie Rodriguez, Executive Director

New Mexico

6638 Sickle Cell Council of New Mexico, Inc.
1300 San Pedro NE
Albuquerque, NM 87108
505-254-9550
Fax: 505-254-9642
victoria@sicklecellnm.org
www.sicklecellnm.org

Blood screening, education, and genetic counseling.

Victoria A Jones, Executive Director

North Carolina

6639 Eastern North Carolina Chapter (SCDAA)
PO Box 5253
Jacksonville, NC 28540   910-346-2510
800-826-1314
Fax: 910-346-2614
sickle@bizec.rr.com
www.sicklecelleasternnc.org/index.php?pr=Home_Page

The North Carolina Sickle Cell Program was established in 1973. It provides services to persons with sickle cell disease, a lifelong red blood cell disorder that is passed from parents to children through genes. The program focuses on early detection and treatment, which can prevent many serious health prblems. It also offers education and genetic counseling for the general public.

Marcia M Wright, Executive Director

6640 Sickle Cell Disease Association of the Piedmont
231 E Baltimore St, Suite 800
Baltimore, MD 21202   410-528-1555
800-421-8453
Fax: 410-528-1495
scdaa@sicklecelldisease.org
www.sicklecelldisease.org/index.cfm?page=chapter&id=

Dedicated to educating the public and providing support to people affected by sickle cell disease. Serving the following counties: Alamance, Forsyth, Caswell, Guilford, Randolph, and Rockingham.

Gladys A Robinson, Executive Director

6641 Sickle Cell Regional Network
Ste 404
Charlotte, NC 28202   704-332-4184
800-435-6004
Fax: 704-332-2246
plambright@sc-cnc.org

Patricia Lambright, Executive Director

Pennsylvania

6642 Lehigh Valley Sickle Cell Support Group
PO Box 1711
Allentown, PA 18105   610-706-0636
SororW@aol.com
www.members.aol.com/SororW/index.html

For anyone affected/effected by Sickle Cell and all interested persons. Learn more about sickle cell disease and how you can help.

**6643 Sickle Cell Disease Association of America ,
Philadelphia/Delaware Valley Chapter**
5070 Parkside Avenue- Suite 1404
Philadelphia, PA 19139   215-471-8686
Fax: 215-471-7441
scdaa.pdvc@verizon.net
www.sicklecelldisorder.com

A support group for parents of a child or children with sickle cell disease.

Stanley A Simpkins, Executive Director

South Carolina

6644 James R Clark Memorial Sickle Cell Foundation
1420 Gregg Street
Columbia, SC 29201   803-765-9916
800-506-1273
Fax: 803-799-6471
office@jamesrclarksicklecell.org
www.jamesrclarksicklecell.org/?

The mission of the foundation is to optimize the social and psychological well being of residents with sickle cell disease within the fifteen county area of South Carolina. This mission is accomplished through the provision of comprehensive services to individuals, families, and communities and is further enhanced by collaboration with appropriate federal, state, and local resources and through the involvement of volunteers and contributors.

Melodie Helms-Desilet, Executive Director

Texas

6645 Sickle Cell Association of Austin - Marc Thomas Chapter
1 Highland Ctr, 314 E Highland Mall Blvd, Ste 108
Austin, TX 78752   512-458-9767
Fax: 512-458-9714
sicklecellaustin@sbcglobal.net
www.sicklecellaustin.org/

To raise awareness, resources and support for clients with sickle cell disease.

Linda Thomas, Manager
Nora Bouie-Burleson, Office Manager

6646 Sickle Cell Association of the Texas Gulf Coast
501 S. Main St.
Galena Park, TX 77547   713-921-1400
888-908-2355
Fax: 713-921-4525
mbruce@steelassociates.net
www.steelassociates.net

Michael Bruce
Zachary Kitchens
Jaime Lozano

Libraries & Resource Centers

6647 Children's Center for Cancer and Blood Disorders
University of South Carolina School of Medicine
5 Richland Memorial Park
Columbia, SC 29203   803-434-3533

Joint clinical and basic research of juvenile cancer and blood disorders.

Fauni Lowe, Manager

Research Centers

California

6648 Northern California Comprehensive Sickle Cell Center
Children's Hospital at Oakland
747 52nd St
Oakland, CA 94609   510-450-5647
evichinsky@mail.cho.org

Sickle cell disease research.

Elliott Vichinsky MD, Director

6649 University of Southern California Comprehensive Sickle Cell Center
2025 Zonal Avenue, Room 304
Los Angeles, CA 90033   323-442-1259
Fax: 323-442-1255
cagejohn@hsc.usc.edu

Cage S Johnson MD, Director

District of Columbia

6650 Howard University Center for Sickle Cell Disease
1840 7th Street NW
Washington, DC 20000   202-865-8292
Fax: 202-806-4517
sicklecell@howard.edu.
www.sicklecell.howard.edu

Okay H Odocha, Director

State-of-the-art patient care, clinical and basic lab research, education and advocacy programs.

Chen Shi, Director

Georgia

6651 Comprehensive Sickle Cell Center
Medical College of Georgia
1521 Pope Ave
Augusta, GA 30904
706-721-0174
Fax: 706-721-2643
www.mcg.edu/center/sicklecell/

New York

6652 Bronx Comprehensive Sickle Cell Center
Albert Einstein College of Medicine
Ullman Bldg, 1300 Morris Park Ave
Bronx, NY 10461
718-430-2088
Fax: 718-824-3153
nagel@aecom.yu.edu

Ronald L Nagel MD, Director

North Carolina

6653 Duke University Comprehensive Sickle Cell Center
Medical Center
Box 2615
Durham, NC 27710
919-684-5378
Fax: 919-681-7688
telen002@mc.duke.edu
www.sicklecell.mc.duke.edu

Research into sickle cell disease including molecular and organ studies.

Marilyn Telen MD, Director

Ohio

6654 Comprehensive Sickle Cell Center
Cincinnati Children's Hospital Medical Ctr
3333 Burnet Avenue, MLC 7015
Cincinnati, OH 45229
513-636-4200
800-344-2462
Fax: 513-636-5562
TTY: 513-636-4900
blood@cchmc.org
www.cincinnatichildrens.org

Offers research and statistical information in the area of sickle cell disease.

Russell E. Ware, MD, PhD, Director, Hematology Division
Cindi Tillman, RN, Center Contact

Texas

6655 Center for Cancer and Blood Disorders
Children Medical Center Dallas
1935 Medical District Dr.
Dallas, TX 75235
214-456-7000
Fax: 214-456-6133
ccbdinfo@childrens.com
www.childrens.com/ccbd/

A comprehensive program for diagnosis, patient/family education and management of sickle cell diseases in childhood and adolesance. Offers access to state-of-the art research projects and clinical management.

George R Buchanan, Medical Director
Zora R Rogers, MD, Associate Medical Director
Shirley Miller, Community Relations

6656 Southwestern Comprehensive Sickle Cell Cen ter
UT Southwestern Medical Ctr/Pediatrics Dept
5323 Harry Hines Blvd
Dallas, TX 75390
214-648-3111
Fax: 214-648-3122
George.Buchanan@UTsouthwestern.edu

Web Sites

6657 American Sickle Cell Anemia Association
DD Bldg. at the Cleveland Clinic, Suite DD1-201, 1
Cleveland, OH 44106
216-229-8600
Fax: 216-229-4500
irabragg@ascaa.org
www.ascaa.org

The mission of the American Sickle Cell Anemia Association is to ensure the availability and accessibility of quality, comprehensive sickle cell services, and promote the public professional awareness about sickle cell anemis an it's hemoglobin diseases ad trait variants.

Ira Bragg-Grant, Executive Director
Leslie Carter, Newborn Screening Coordinator
Charlotte Martin, Receptionist

6658 Information Center for Sickle Cell and Tha lassemic Disorders
sickle.bwh.harvard.edu

Free online information to the biomedical community, health care personnel and patients. The information can be of particular help to patients in enabling them to have a fuller and more knowledgeable role in their care.

6659 International Association of Sickle Cell Nurses and Physician Assistants
www.iascnapa.org

The association is made up of over 300 sickle cell nurses and physician assistants worldwide. It recognizes its responsibility to maintain high standards in the provision of quality and accessible health care services for individuals with sickle cell disease.

Coretta Jenerette, RN, PhD, President
Pat Corley, RN, Vice-President
Bonita Conley, MSN, RN, PNP-BC, Secretary

6660 Online Mendelian Inheritance in Man
www.omim.org

This database is a catalog of human genes and genetic disorders.

6661 Sickle Cell Disease Association of America
3700 Koppers Street, Suite 570
Baltimore, MD 21227
410-528-1555
800-421-8453
Fax: 410-528-1495
scdaa@sicklecelldisease.org
www.sicklecelldisease.org

Promotes the finding of a universal cure for sickle cell disease while improving the quality of life for individuals and families where sickle cell related conditions exists.

Sonja L. Banks, President/Chief Operating Officer
Francis Aofolaju, Vice President, Business & Finance
Natasha Thomas, Director, Planning & Development

6662 Sickle Cell Disease Forum
www.sicklecelldisease.org/forum/

Online forum for sickle cell disease discussion/chat sponsored by the Sickle Cell Disease Association of America.

6663 Sickle Cell Kids
www.sicklecellkids.org

Teaches children how to stay healthy and answers questions about sickle cell disease. A joint venture of the Georgia Comprehensive Sickle Cell Center at Grady Health System and Cynthia Gentry, artist.

787

Book Publishers

6664 Blood & Circulatory Disorders Sourcebook 4th Edition
Omnigraphics
615 Griswold, Ste 901
Detroit, MI 48226
610-461-3548
800-234-1340
Fax: 800-875-1340
info@omnigraphics.com
www.omnigraphics.com

Basic consumer health information on blood and its components, anemias, leukemias, bleeding disorders, and circulatory disorders, including sickle cell disease, aplastic anemia, thrombophilia, RH disease and hemophilia.

2005 600 pages 2nd Edition
ISBN: 0-780807-46-9

Peter Ruffner, Publisher

6665 Let's Talk About Going to the Hospital
Rosen Publishing Group's PowerKids Press
29 E 21st Street
New York, NY 10010
212-777-3017
800-237-9932
Fax: 888-436-4643
rosenpub@tribeca.ios.com
www.rosenpublishing.com

If a child has to check into the hospital, chances are he or she is already upset about being ill. Knowing how a hospital functions and what the procedures are, such as when family members can visit, will help in what is already a stressful situation. Grades K-5.

24 pages
ISBN: 0-823950-36-0

Roger Rosen, President

6666 Let's Talk About Sickle Cell Anemia
Melanie Apel Gordon, author

Rosen Publishing Group's PowerKids Press
29 E 21st Street
New York, NY 10010
212-777-3017
800-237-9932
Fax: 888-436-4643
rosenpub@tribeca.ios.com
www.rosenpublishing.com

Explains why sickle cell anemia is a disease that strikes more African Americans than any other people in the country. Describes symptoms and explains how a kid can help take care of himself during a pain crisis. Grades K-5.

24 pages
ISBN: 0-823954-17-X

Roger Rosen, President

6667 Understanding Sickle Cell Disease
Miriam Bloom PhD, author

University Press of Mississippi
3825 Ridgewood Road
Jackson, MS 39211
601-432-6205
800-737-7788
Fax: 601-432-6217
press@ihl.state.ms.us
www.upress.state.ms.us

Part of the Understanding Health and Sickness Series. For general readers, a guide to understanding a debilitating genetic disease that affects tens of thousands who are of African heritage.

128 pages Paperback
ISBN: 0-878057-45-5

Leila W. Salisbury, Director
Cynthia Foster, Administrative Assistant
Tracey Curtis, Assistant For Development

Pamphlets

6668 Sickle Cell Disease
March of Dimes Resource Center
1275 Mamaroneck Avenue
White Plains, NY 10605
914-997-4488
Fax: 914-997-4763
TTY: 914-977-4764
resourcecenter@modimes.org
www.marchofdimes.org/professionals/681_1221.asp

Fact Sheets: one to two page review written for the general public. Also available electronically from website www.modimes.org. Brochures: 3 panel color brochures written for the general public.

Camps

6669 Camp Crescent Moon
Sickle Cell Disease Foundation of California
6133 Bristol Parkway, Suite 240
Culver City, CA 90230
310-693-0247
877-288-2873
Fax: 310-693-0266
info@scdfc.org
www.campcrescentmoon.org

A specialized camp for children with sickle cell disease between the ages of 8 and 14 in southern & central California.

Mary E Brown, Camp Director
Deborah Green, Assistant Camp Director
Cage Johnson MD, Medical Director

6670 Camp Good Days & Special Times
1332 Pittsford-Mendon Rd, P.O. Box 665
Mendon, NY 14506
585-624-5555
800-785-2135
Fax: 585-624-5799
www.campgooddays.org

Camp for children ages 8 to 17 with sickle cell anemia. The camp is dedicated to improving the quality of life for children, adults and families whose lives have been touched by cancer and other life challenges.

Gary Mervis, Chairman/ Founder
Wendy Bleier-Mervis, Executive Director
Lisa Booz, Western New York Regional Director

6671 Camp Vacamas
256 Macopin Road
West Milford, NJ
973-838-1394
Fax: 973-838-7534
info@vacamas.org
www.vacamas.org

Disadvantaged children with asthma or sickle cell anemia, ages 8-16, are offered special programs in canoeing, backpacking, camping, music and leadership training. Sliding scale tuition. Year round programs for groups.

Michael Friedman, Executive Director
Philip Smith, Camp Director

DESCRIPTION

6672 SLEEP APNEA

Involves the following Biologic System(s):
Respiratory Disorders

Obstructive sleep apnea (OSA) is a breathing disorder that is commonly seen in the pediatric population. Specifically, it is when normal ventilation during sleep is disrupted because of upper airway obstruction. This process occurs intermittently throughout sleep and causes significant disruptions in normal sleep patterns. Although in adults this can result in excessive daytime sleepiness, children typically manifest changes in behavior or deficits in attention, thus affecting school performance.

Studies indicate that roughly 2% of children between the ages of 2-18 years are affected by this disorder. Girls and boys are equally likely to have OSA and African American children are more commonly affected than children of other ethnicities. OSA is also more common in children with obesity, craniofacial abnormalities and/or neurologic disorders. Children with Down syndrome are at especially increased risk.

The cause of obstructive sleep apnea is not well understood. Adenotonsillar (adenoids and tonsils) hypertrophy (increase in size) seems to be part of the process but even after tonsillectomy and adenoidectomy (removal of these tissues) many patients relapse, implying other processes involved.

The clinical features commonly seem with OSA include noisy breathing during sleep, prominent snoring often in a crescendo pattern that ends with a pause in respirations for performance, nocturnal enuresis (bed wetting) and frequent daytime napping. Complications of OSA can be failure to thrive or gain weight appropriately, pulmonary hypertension which cause stress on the right side of the heart and neurological sequelae.

Diagnosis should not be based solely on a history of snoring. Many children snore who do not suffer from OSA, however, a careful history focusing on some of the clinical features mentioned above should raise the suspicion of OSA and further evaluation can be considered. The physical exam of tonsillar hypertrophy may help support the diagnosis but often a polysomnography test, commonly called sleep study, is the most accurate way to diagnose OSA. The sleep study is a comprehensive diagnostic tool involving monitoring a patient during sleep using multiple parameters including the visual surveillance, monitoring of the heart rate and rhythm, monitoring of the respiratory rate, measurement of expired lung gases, oxygen saturation in the blood, chest wall rise with breathing and others. While the necessity of this study in children may be debated, it is considered a definitive way to establishthe diagnosis of OSA.

In general, nonsurgical therapy is very limited for the typical patient with OSA. Treatment of childhood OSA is primarily surgical. Removal of the tonsils and adenoids are often the first line of treatment as well as targeting weight reduction when relevant. Most children respond well to tonsillectomy and adenoidectomy, but for those who do not improve, nasal continued positive airway pressure (NCPAP) is another effective option which enhances the infant's respiratory function.

OSA is an important cause of health, emotional and behavioral problems in school aged children and effective and timely treatment can significantly improve school performance, and productivity and well-being of these children.

National Associations & Support Groups

6673 American Academy of Pediatrics
141 Northwest Point Boulevard
Elk Grove Village, IL 60007
847-434-4000
800-433-9016
Fax: 847-434-8000
www.aap.org

The American Academy of Pediatrics and its member pediatricians are committed to the attainment of optimal physical, mental and social health and well-being for all infants, children, adolescents, and young adults.

Fernando Stein, MD, FAAP, President
Karen Remley, MD, CEO/Executive VP

6674 American Academy of Sleep Medicine
2510 North Frontage Road
Darien, IL 60561
630-737-9700
Fax: 630-737-9790
www.aasmnet.org

National not-for-profit professional membership organization dedicated to the advancement of sleep medicine. The Academy's mission is to assure quality care for patients with sleep disorders, promote the advancement of sleep research and provide public and professional education. The AASM delivers programs, information and services to and through its members and advocates sleep medicine supportive policies in the medical community and the public sector.

Jerry Barrett, Executive Director
Jennifer Markkanen, Assistant Executive Director

6675 American Sleep Apnea Association
641 S Street NW, 3rd Floor
Washington, DC 20001
888-293-3650
Fax: 888-293-3650
asaa@sleepapnea.org
www.sleepapnea.org

Offers help and information to persons with sleep apnea and their families.

Will Headapohl, Chair (Emeritus)
Justine Amdur, Program Coordinator, AWAKE
Valerie Danielson, Program Coordinator, CPAP

6676 Center for Disabilities and Development
University of Iowa Stead Family Children's Hospita
100 Hawkins Drive
Iowa City, IA 52242
319-353-6900
877-686-0031
Fax: 319-356-7700
cdd-scheduling@uiowa.edu
www.uichildrens.org/cdd

A trusted resource for healthcare, training, research and information for people with disabilities that include: behavior disorders, brain injury, cerebral palsy, diabetes, down syndrome, learning disabilities, mental retardation, sleep disorders and spina bifida.

Dianne McBrien, MD, Medical Director

6677 National Sleep Foundation
1010 N Glebe Road
Arlington, VA 22201
703-243-1697
Fax: 202-347-3472
nsf@sleepfoundation.org
www.sleepfoundation.org

An independent, nonprofit organization dedicated to improving public health and safety by achieving public understanding of sleep and sleep disorders, and by supporting public education, sleep-related research, and advocacy. Actively collaborates with sleep centers and support groups for patients with sleep disorders and safety organizations.

789

David Cloud, CEO

Libraries & Resource Centers

6678 American Academy of Somnology
PO Box 27077
Las Vegas, NV 89126   702-371-0947
                                   somnology@aol.com
                          www.hopperinstitute.com/aas_intro.html

Covers about 75 physicians, dentists, nurses, psychologists, technicians, and students and sponsoring organizations, including associations, institutions, and corporations, with a special interest in sleep. Newsletter, published yearly.

David Hopper, Director

Research Centers

6679 Sleep Disorders Center
Beth Israel Deaconess Medical Ctr
330 Brookline Avenue
Boston, MA 02215   617-667-7000
                                   Fax: 617-975-5506
                                   www.bidmc.harvard.edu

Provides testing and treatment for those with sleep disorders and offers educational workshops, plus support for their families.

Jean K Matheson, MD, Division Chief

Web Sites

6680 About.com on Sleep Disorders
www.sleepdisorders.about.com

Well-organized information including new developments and a chat room.

6681 American Academy of Sleep Medicine
2510 North Frontage Road
Darien, IL 60561   630-737-9700
                                   Fax: 630-737-9790
                                   inquiries@aasmnet.org
                                   www.aasmnet.org

The mission is to assure quality care for patients with sleep disorders, promote the advancement of sleep research and provide public and professional education.

Timothy I. Morgenthaler, MD, President
Ronald D. Chervin, MD, MS, Secretary/Treasurer
Jerome A. Barrett, Executive Director

6682 American Sleep Apnea Association
641 S Street NW, 3rd Floor
Washington, DC 20001   888-293-3650
                                   Fax: 888-293-3650
                                   asaa@sleepapnea.org
                                   www.sleepapnea.org

Is dedicated to reducing injury, disbility, and death from sleep apnea and to enhancing the well being of those affected by this common disorder. The ASAA promotes education and awareness, the ASAA A.W.A.K.E. Network of voluntary mutual suport groups, research, and continuous improvement of care.

Will Headapohl, Chair (Emeritus)
Justine Amdur, AWAKE Program Coordinator
Valerie Danielson, CPAP Program Coordinator

6683 MEDLINEplus on Sleep Apnea
8600 Rockville Pike
Bethesda, MD 20894   custserv@nlm.nih.gov
                     www.nlm.nih.gov/medlineplus/sleepapnea.html

Offers information about Sleep Apnea.

Dr. Donald A.B. Lindberg, Director

6684 NIH/National Center on Sleep Disorders Research
www.nhlbi.nih.gov/about/org/ncsdr/

Coordinates sleep research, training and education supported by the government.

6685 National Sleep Foundation
1010 N. Glebe Road Suite 310
Arlington, VA 22201   703-243-1697
                                   nsf@sleepfoundation.org
                                   www.sleepfoundation.org

Is an independent nonprofit organization dedicated to improving public health and safety by achieving understanding of sleep and slepp disorders, and by supporting education, sleep-related research, and advocacy.

David Cloud, CEO

6686 Sleepdisorders.com
www.sleepdisorders.com

Provides a full range of internet communications and technology solutions from strategic consulting to concept design, content development, software engineering, and ongoing enhancements and maintenance. Our projects have encompassed direct-to-consumer marketing, direct-to-patient education, healthcare professional training, corporate intranets and database management systems, dynamic database-driven websites and hospital training.

John Douglas Hudson, M.D., Medical Director

6687 Sleepnet.com
www.sleepnet.com/sleepapnea2000.html

Categorizes sleep disorders for research, forums are up-dated frequently and posts are thoughtful and insightful.

Book Publishers

6688 Concise Guide to Evaluation and Management of Sleep Disorders
American Psychiatric Publishing
1000 Wilson Boulevard, Suite 1825
Arlington, VA 22209   703-907-7322
                                        800-368-5777
                                   Fax: 703-907-1091
                                        appi@psych.org
                                        www.appi.org

Overview of sleep disorders medicine, sleep physiology and pathology, insomnia complaints, excessive sleepiness disorders, parasomnias, medical and psychiatric disorders and sleep, medications with sedative - hypnotic properties, special problems and populations.

2002 296 pages Paper 3rd Ed
ISBN: 1-585620-45-6

Robert E. Hales, M.D., Editor-in-Chief
Rebecca D. Rinehart, Publisher
John McDuffie, Editorial Director

6689 Let's Talk About Going to the Hospital
Rosen Publishing Group's PowerKids Press
29 E 21st Street
New York, NY 10010   212-777-3017
                                        800-237-9932
                                   Fax: 888-436-4643
                                   rosenpub@tribeca.ios.com
                                   www.rosenpublishing.com

If a child has to check into the hospital, chances are he or she is already upset about being ill. Knowing how a hospital functions and what the procedures are, such as when family members can visit, will help in what is already a stressful situation. Grades K-5.

24 pages
ISBN: 0-823950-36-0

Roger Rosen, President

6690 Principles and Practice of Sleep Medicine
Elsevier Health Sciences Division
1600 John F Kennedy Blvd, Suite 1800
Philadelphia, PA 19103   215-239-3900
                                        800-523-1649
                                   Fax: 215-239-3990
                                   www.us.elsevierhealth.com

Covers the recent advances in basic sciences as well as sleep pathology in adults. Encompasses developments in this rapidly advancing field and also includes topics related to psychiatry, circadian rhythms, cardiovascualr diseases and sleep apnea diagnosis and treatment. Hardcover.

2005 1552 pages 4th Edition
ISBN: 0-721607-97-7

6691 Restless Nights
Yale University Press
PO Box 209040
New Haven, CT 06520

203-432-0960
800-405-1619
Fax: 203-432-0948
marketing@yale.edu.
yalepress.yale.edu/yupbooks

This book provides an explanation of sleep apnea symptoms, risk-factors, advice on diagnosis and consultation, and current available treatments.

2003 288 pages
ISBN: 0-300085-44-0

John Donatich, Director

6692 Sleep Disorders Sourcebook
Omnigraphics
PO Box 8002
Aston, PA 19014

800-234-1340
Fax: 800-875-1340
info@omnigraphics.com
omnigraphics.com

Basic consumer health information about sleep and its disorders, including sleep apnea, insomnia, sleepwalking, restless leg syndrome and narcolepsy.

567 pages 2nd Edition
ISBN: 0-780807-43-0

Peter Ruffner, Publisher

6693 Sleeping Like a Baby

Avi Sadeh, author

Yale University Press
PO Box 209040
New Haven, CT 06520

203-432-0960
800-405-1619
Fax: 203-432-0948
marketing@yale.edu.
yalepress.yale.edu/yupbooks

A practical and sensitive guide to solving your child's sleep problems.

2001 224 pages
ISBN: 0-300088-24-3

John Donatich, Director

6694 Snoring From A to Zzzz
Spencer Press
2525 NW Lovejoy Street, Suite 402
Portland, OR 97210

503-223-4959
Fax: 503-223-1608
dereklipman@aol.com

Covers organizations, associations, support groups, and manufactorers of sleep-related medical products relevant to sleep disorders. Discussess every aspect of snoring and sleep apnea from causes to cures.

256 pages Paperback
ISBN: 0-965070-81-6

Derek S Lipman, MD, Author/Editor

6695 Snoring and Sleep Apnea
Demos Medical Publishing
386 Park Avenue S
New York, NY 10016

212-683-0072
800-532-8663
Fax: 212-683-0118
orderdept@demosmedpub.com
www.demosmedpub.com

A straightforward, jargon-free approach to dealing with snoring and sleep problems.

286 pages 3rd Ed/Soft
ISBN: 1-888799-29-3

Kathy Gonzalez, Order Dept/Fulfillment Coordinator
Paul Choi, Vice-President of Finance and Opera
Richard Winters, Executive Editor

Pamphlets

6696 Get the Facts About Sleep Apnea
American Sleep Apnea Association
1717 Pennsylvania Avenue, NW Ste. 1025
Washington, DC 20006

202-293-3650
888-293-3650
Fax: 888-293-3650
asaa@sleepapnea.org
www.sleepapnea.org

Brochures are also available in bulk.

Will Headapohl, Chair
Tracy R. Nasca, Executive Director
Justine Amdur, AWAKE Program Coordinator

6697 Sleep Apnea
National Sleep Foundation
1010 N. Glebe Road Suite 310
Arlington, VA 22201

703-243-1697
Fax: 202-347-3472
nsf@sleepfoundation.org
www.sleepfoundation.org

A brochure about sleep apnea, a breathing disorder characterized by brief interruptions of breathing during sleep. Brochure explains what it is, who gets it, and how it is diagnosed and treated.

Charles A. Czeisler, PhD, MD, Chairman
Max Hirshkowitz, PhD, Vice Chairman
Joseph Ojile, MD, Secretary

DESCRIPTION

6698 SLEEPWALKING

Synonym: Somnambulism

Involves the following Biologic System(s):
Developmental/Behavioral/Psychiatric Disorders

Sleepwalking, also known as somnambulism, is a condition where the child engages in activities that are normally associated with wakefulness while asleep or in a sleeplike state. It occurs most commonly in children, particularly those from approximately four to six years of age. About 10 to 15 percent of children experience at least one episode of sleepwalking during childhood. In addition, approximately one in five children who sleepwalk has a family history of the condition. In many patients, sleepwalking occurs in association with bed-wetting (nocturnal enuresis) or night terrors (sleep disturbances that typically occur shortly after the onset of sleep). In some cases, a stressful event may lead to an episode of sleepwalking.

In children, sleepwalking occurs during stage four of NREM (nonrapid eye movement) sleep. NREM sleep consists of four progressively deeper stages of sleep that are typically characterized by slow, deep brain waves, muscle relaxation and slowed breathing rate, slowed heart rate, and lowered blood pressure. In contrast, REM (rapid eye movement) sleep, which is associated with dreaming, is characterized by increased levels of brain activity, rapid eye movements, and involuntary muscle jerks.

During an episode of sleepwalking, affected children may simply sit up in bed or move to the edge of the bed, without engaging in actual sleepwalking. In other cases, however, children may get out of bed and walk through their home. They may also perform certain routine acts, such as turning on a hallway light. Unless children are simultaneously experiencing night terrors, they usually do not have associated anxiety. During an episode, most children have their eyes open and are guided by their vision. Therefore, they typically move around familiar obstacles; however, some children may make no effort to avoid certain objects in their path, potentially resulting in injury. In addition, some children may mumble simple words or phrases or repeatedly perform certain acts, such as turning a doorknob back and forth. If children are urged to return to bed during such an episode, they may sometimes follow such instruction; however, they usually must be gently steered back to their beds. Sleepwalking episodes typically last only a few minutes, and children usually have little or no memory of the experience. In children, sleepwalking is rarely associated with psychologic abnormalities, and the number of episodes usually decreases by early adolescence. However, the persistence of sleepwalking episodes into adulthood is thought to be associated with a significant risk of psychiatric disease. Parents or caregivers of children who sleepwalk should take precautions to help protect them against injury. Possible obstacles or breakable objects should be removed from their paths. It may be advisable to block staircases and to have children sleep on the ground floor of the house, if possible.

Government Agencies

6699 NIH/National Institute of Mental Health
6001 Executive Boulevard, Room 6200, MSC 9663
Bethesda, MD 20892

301-443-4536
866-615-6464
Fax: 301-443-4279
TTY: 301-443-8431
nimhinfo@nih.gov
www.nimh.nih.gov

Conducts strategic planning for specific research areas as well as for the Institute as a whole.

Joshua Gordon, MD, PhD, Director
Shelli Avenevoli, MD, Deputy Director

National Associations & Support Groups

6700 American Academy of Pediatrics
141 Northwest Point Boulevard
Elk Grove Village, IL 60007

847-434-4000
800-433-9016
Fax: 847-434-8000
www.aap.org

The American Academy of Pediatrics and its member pediatricians are committed to the attainment of optimal physical, mental and social health and well-being for all infants, children, adolescents, and young adults.

Fernando Stein, MD, FAAP, President
Karen Remley, MD, CEO/Executive VP

6701 American Academy of Sleep Medicine
2510 North Frontage Road
Darien, IL 60561

630-737-9700
Fax: 630-737-9790
www.aasmnet.org

National not-for-profit professional membership organization dedicated to the advancement of sleep medicine. The Academy's mission is to assure quality care for patients with sleep disorders, promote the advancement of sleep research and provide public and professional education. The AASM delivers programs, information and services to and through its members and advocates sleep medicine supportive policies in the medical community and the public sector.

Jerry Barrett, Executive Director
Jennifer Markkanen, Assistant Executive Director

6702 Center for Disabilities and Development
University of Iowa Stead Family Children's Hospita
100 Hawkins Drive
Iowa City, IA 52242

319-353-6900
877-686-0031
Fax: 319-356-7700
cdd-scheduling@uiowa.edu
www.uichildrens.org/cdd

A trusted resource for healthcare, training, research and information for people with disabilities that include: behavior disorders, brain injury, cerebral palsy, diabetes, down syndrome, learning disabilities, mental retardation, sleep disorders and spina bifida.

Dianne McBrien, MD, Medical Director

6703 Federation of Families for Children's Mental Health
9605 Medical Center Drive, Suite 280
Rockville, MD 20850

240-403-1901
Fax: 240-403-1909
ffcmh@ffcmh.org
www.ffcmh.org

The National family run organization is dedicated exclusively to helping children with mental health needs and their families achieve a better quality of life.

Sandra Spencer, Executive Director

6704 National Mental Health Consumers' Self-Help Clearinghouse
1211 Chestnut Street, Suite 1207
Philadelphia, PA 19107 215-751-1810
800-553-4539
Fax: 215-636-6312
info@mhselfhelp.org
www.mhselfhelp.org

Offers information, support and appropriate referrals; and promotes public and professional education. Provides networking for those with special interests related to albinism. Promotes and supports research and funding that will improve diagnosis and management of albinism and hypopigmentation.

Joseph Rogers, Executive Director & Founder

6705 National Sleep Foundation
1010 N Glebe Road
Arlington, VA 22201 703-243-1697
Fax: 202-347-3472
nsf@sleepfoundation.org
www.sleepfoundation.org

An independent, nonprofit organization dedicated to improving public health and safety by achieving public understanding of sleep and sleep disorders, and by supporting public education, sleep-related research, and advocacy. Actively collaborates with sleep centers, support groups for patients with sleep disorders and safety organizations.

David Cloud, CEO

Libraries & Resource Centers

6706 American Academy of Somnology
PO Box 27077
Las Vegas, NV 89126 702-371-0947
somnology@aol.com
www.hopperinstitute.com/aas_intro.html

Covers about 75 physicians, dentists, nurses, psychologists, technicians, and students and sponsoring organizations, including associations, institutions, and corporations, with a special interest in sleep.

David Hopper, Director

Web Sites

6707 About.com on Sleep Disorders
www.sleepdisorders.about.com

Well-organized information including new developments and a chat room.

6708 National Sleep Foundation
1010 N. Glebe Road Suite 310
Arlington, VA 22201 703-243-1697
nsf@sleepfoundation.org
www.sleepfoundation.org

Is an independent nonprofit organization dedicated to improving public health and safety by achieving understnading of sleep and sleep disorders, and by supporting education, sleep-related research, and advocacy.

David Cloud, CEO

6709 Online Mendelian Inheritance in Man
www.omim.org

This database is a catalog of human genes and genetic disorders.

6710 Sleep Walking in Children
familydoctor.org/160.xml

Brief overview of possible parental concerns of sleep walking in children.

6711 SleepEducation.com
2510 North Frontage Road
Darien, IL 60561 630-737-9700
Fax: 630-737-9790
www.sleepeducation.com

Online resources on sleep related topics and sleep disorders including sleepwalking.

6712 Sleepdisorders.com
www.sleepdisorders.com

Provides a full range of internet communications and technology solutions from strategic consulting to concept design, content development, software engineering, and ongoing enhancements and maintenance. Our projects have encompassed direct-to-customer marketing, direct-to-patient education, healthcare professional training, corporate intranets and database management systems, dynamic database-driven web sites and hospital training.

John Douglas Hudson, M.D., Medical Director

Book Publishers

6713 Concise Guide to Evaluation and Management of Sleep Disorders
American Psychiatric Publishing
1000 Wilson Boulevard, Suite 1825
Arlington, VA 22209 703-907-7322
800-368-5777
Fax: 703-907-1091
appi@psych.org
www.appi.org

Over view of sleep disorders medicine, sleep physiology and pathology, insomnia complaints, excessive sleepiness disorders, parasomnias, medical and psychiatric disorders and sleep, medications with sedative-hypnotic properties, special problems and populations.

2002 296 pages Paper 3rd Ed
ISBN: 1-585620-45-6

Robert E. Hales, M.D., Editor-in-Chief
Rebecca D. Rinehart, Publisher
John McDuffie, Editorial Director

6714 Sleep Disorders Sourcebook
Omnigraphics
PO Box 8002
Aston, PA 19014 800-234-1340; Fax: 800-875-1340
info@omnigraphics.com; omnigraphics.com

Basic consumer health information about sleep and its disorders, including insomnia, sleepwalking, sleep apnea, restless leg syndrome and narcolepsy.

567 pages 2nd Edition
ISBN: 0-780807-43-0

Peter Ruffner, Publisher

6715 Sleep: The Brazelton Way

T Berry Brazelton; Joshua D Sparrow, author

Perseus Books Group-Da Capo Press
250 West 57th Street, 15th Floor
New York, NY 10107 617-252-5200
www.perseusbooksgroup.com

Pediatrician provide highly effective and affordable guides to lead parents through struggles of getting babies and toddlers to sleep.

2003 Paperback
ISBN: 0-738207-82-9

David Steinberger, President & CEO

6716 Snoring From A to Zzzz
Spencer Press
2525 NW Lovejoy Street, Suite 402
Portland, OR 97210 503-223-4959; Fax: 503-223-1608
dereklipman@aol.com

Covers organizations, associations, support groups, and manufactorers of sleep-related medical products relevant to sleep disorders. Discussess every aspect of snoring and sleep apnea from causes to cures.

256 pages Paperback
ISBN: 0-965070-81-6

Derek S Lipman, MD, Author/Editor

DESCRIPTION

6717 SOCIAL ANXIETY DISORDER
Synonym: Social phobia
Involves the following Biologic System(s):
Neurologic Disorders

Social Anxiety Disorder (also called social phobia) is diagnosed in individuals who are overwhelmingly anxious and excessively self-conscious in everyday social situations. Children with social anxiety disorder are usually diagnosed once they reach school age, but symptoms have been seen in children as young as two years. Symptoms include an intense, chronic fear of being watched and judged by others, and fear of doing things that will embarrass them. This fear causes anxiety for days or weeks before a dreaded situation, and may become so severe that it interferes with school and other ordinary activities, often making it difficult to make and keep friends.

Social anxiety disorder is a fear reaction to a danger that isn't actually dangerous—although the body and mind react as if the danger is real. The physical responses to fear—fast hearbeat, quick breathing actually occur as adrenaline and other chemicals prepare the body to either fight or flee the danger (fight-flight). This biological mechanism kicks in when we feel afraid, alerting us to danger so we can protect ourselves. Those with the disorder experience this response too frequently, too strongly, and in situations where it's not appropriate (dangerous). Because the physcial sensations are real, however, the danger seems real, too.

Indivduals with social anxiety disorder are often unable to do common things in front of other people, like signing a check in front of a cashier, eating or drinking in a resta urant, or using a public restroom. Most people with the disorder know they shouldn't be afraid, but can't control their fear. They usually interact easily only with their family and a few close friends. Physical symptoms often accompany the anxiety, including blushing, profuse sweating, trembling, nausea, and difficulty speaking. These symptoms increase the feeling of being watched, which intensifies the anxiety.

Like many other anxiety-based disorders, social anxiety disorder usually results from the combination of three factors: genetics; learned behaviors; and life experiences. Those who constantly receive criticism may grow to expect that reaction from everyone they meet. Children who are teased or bullied are more likely to retreat into themselves. They will be paranoid of making a mistake or disappointing someone, and be overly sensitive to criticism.

Social anxiety disorder can increase feelings of loneliness or disappointment over missed opportunities for friendship, getting the most out of school, sharing talents, and learning new skills. Some children and teens are so shy and fearful about talking to others that they exhibit selective mutism—not speaking at all to certain people (i.e. teachers or students they don't know) or in certain places (i.e. at someone else's house). These individuals have normal conversations with people and places they are comfortable with, and their selective silence is sometimes mistaken for a stuck-up attitude or rudeness. Instead, selective mutism stems from feeling uncomfortable and afraid.

Psychotherapy is a successful treatment for social anxiety disorder, and is used sometimes in combination with certain medications. A physical examination will rule out physical reasons for the symptoms being exhibited. Cognitive behavior therapy is especially useful for treating social anxiety. It teaches different ways of thinking, behaving, and reacting to situations that help reduce the feelings of anxiousness and fear. It can also help people learn and practice social skills. Sometimes anti-anxiety or anti-depressant medications are prescribed. Although safe and effective for many people, they may be risky for some, especially children, teens, and young adults. Those taking anti-depressants should be monitored closely, especially at the start of their treatment.

Family and other supportive adults are especially important to children with social anxiety disorder. It is often a supportive environment that gives those with the disorder the courage to go outside their comfort zone.

Government Agencies

6718 Center for Mental Health Services Knowledge Exchange Program
US Department of Health and Human Services
PO Box 42557
Washington, DC 20015
800-789-2647
Fax: 240-747-5470
TDD: 866-889-2647
http://mentalhealth.samhsa.gov

Supplies the public with expert responses to commonly asked questions about various mental health disorders, and directs the caller to appropriate resources.

6719 NIH/National Institute of Mental Health
6001 Executive Boulevard, Room 6200, MSC 9663
Bethesda, MD 20892
301-443-4536
866-615-6464
Fax: 301-443-4279
TTY: 301-443-8431
nimhinfo@nih.gov
www.nimh.nih.gov

Conducts strategic planning for specific research areas as well as for the Institute as a whole.

Joshua Gordon, MD, PhD, Director
Shelli Avenevoli, MD, Deputy Director

National Associations & Support Groups

6720 American Academy of Pediatrics
141 Northwest Point Boulevard
Elk Grove Village, IL 60007
847-434-4000
800-433-9016
Fax: 847-434-8000
www.aap.org

The American Academy of Pediatrics and its member pediatricians are committed to the attainment of optimal physical, mental and social health and well-being for all infants, children, adolescents, and young adults.

Fernando Stein, MD, FAAP, President
Karen Remley, MD, CEO/Executive VP

6721 American Counseling Association
6101 Stevenson Ave
Alexandria, VA 22304
703-823-9800
800-347-6647
Fax: 703-823-0252
webmaster@counseling.org
www.counseling.org

Represents professional counselors in various practice settings, and stands ready to serve more than 55,000 members with the resources they need to make a difference. From webinars, publications, and journals to Conference education sessions and legislative action alerts, ACA is where counseling professionals turn for powerful, credible content and support.

Robert L. Smith, President

6722 American Mental Health Foundation (AMHF)
PO Box 3
Riverdale, NY 10028
212-737-9027
elomke@americanmentalhealthfoundation.or
americanmentalhealthfoundation.org

Dedicated to the extensive and intensive research in the theories and techniques of treatment of emotional illness and to the implementation of reforms in the mental health system. Efforts have resulted in development of better and less expensive treatment methods. Findings are disseminated in English and other major languages.

Monroe W Spero, MD
Evander Lomke, Executive Director

6723 American Psychiatric Association
1000 Wilson Boulevard, Suite 1825
Arlington, VA 22209
703-907-7300
888-35 -7924
apa@psych.org
www.psychiatry.org

It is a medical specialty society representing growing membership of more than 36,000 psychiatrists.

6724 American Psychological Association
750 First St. NE
Washington, DC 20002
202-336-5500
800-374-2721
TTY: 202-336-6123
www.apa.org

The mission is to advance the creation, communication and application of psychological knowledge to benefit society and improve people's lives.

Norman B. Anderson, PhD, CEO/ EVP
L. Michael Honaker, PhD, Deputy Chief Executive Officer
Ellen G. Garrison, PhD, Senior Policy Advisor

6725 American School Counselor Association
1101 King Street, Suite 310
Alexandria, VA 22314
703-683-2722
800-306-4722
Fax: 703-997-7572
asca@schoolcounselor.org
www.schoolcounselor.org

The mission of ASCA is to represent professional school counselors and to promote professionalism and ethical practices.

Richard Wong, Executive Director
Jeff Broderson, Information Technology Admin.
Kathleen M Rakestraw, Director of Communications

6726 Anxiety Disorders Association of America
8730 Georgia Avenue, Suite 600
Silver Spring, MD 20910
240-485-1001
Fax: 240-485-1035
information@adaa.org
www.adaa.org

Offers resources and information for persons with anxiety and stress-related disorders.

Alies Muskin, Executive Director

6727 Anxiety Disorders Institute
1 Dunwoody Park Suite 112
Atlanta, GA 30338
770-395-6845

Provides support, training, and services for those suffering from anxiety disorders, and their families.

6728 Anxiety and Phobia Treatment Center
Whire Plains Hospital Center
Davis Avenue & East Post Road
White Plains, NY 10601
914-681-1038
Fax: 914-681-2284
jchessa@wphospital.org
phobia-anxiety.com

Treatment groups for individuals suffering from phobias. Deals with fears through contextual therapy, a treatment and study of the phobia in the actual setting in which the phobic reactions occur. Conducts Intensive Courses, Phobia Self-Help Groups, 8-week Phobia Clinics and individual treatment. Publications: PM Newsletter, bimonthly. Articles and papers. Annual conference.

Fredrick J Neumen, MD, Director

6729 Federation of Families for Children's Mental Health
9605 Medical Center Drive, Suite 280
Rockville, MD 20850
240-403-1901
Fax: 240-403-1909
ffcmh@ffcmh.org
www.ffcmh.org

The National family run organization is dedicated exclusively to helping children with mental health needs and their families achieve a better quality of life.

Sandra Spencer, Executive Director

6730 National Anxiety Foundation
3135 Custer Drive
Lexington, KY 40517
859-281-0003
www.lexington-on-line.com/naf.html

Nonprofit organization that provides education to the public and professionals about anxiety through printed and electronic media.

Stephen Cox MD, President & Medical Director

6731 Phobia Society of America
133 Rollins Avenue, Suite 4B
Rockville, MD 20852
301-231-9350
Fax: 301-231-7392
www.adaa.org

Offers support for those suffering from phobia and panic attacks.

6732 Phobics Anonymous
PO Box 1180
Palm Springs, CA 92263
706-327-2148

Twelve-step program for panic disorders and anxiety. Publications available.

Marily Gellis PhD, Contact

6733 Selective Mutism Foundation
PO Box 25972
Tamarac, FL 33320
305-748-7714
Fax: 305-748-7714
www.selectivemutismfoundation.org

Promotes awareness and understanding for individuals and families affected by selective mutism, an inherited anxiety disorder in which children with normal or deficient language skills are unable to speak in school or social situations. SM is often mistaken for normal shyness and may go undetected for as long as two years. Encourages research and treatment. Maintains speakers' bureau. Publications: Let's Talk, annual newsletter. Selective Mutism, A Silent Cry for Help, brochure.

Sue Newman, Co-Founder & Director

6734 Social Anxiety Association
socialphobia.org

The Social Anxiety Association is a non-profit organization founded in 1997 to meet the growing needs of people with social anxiety.

Thomas A. Richards, Ph.D., President

6735 Special Interest Group on Phobias and Related Anxiety Disorders (SIGPRAD)
245 E 87th Street
New York, NY 10128
212-860-5560
Fax: 212-744-5751
lindy@interport.net
www.cyberpsych.org

For psychologists, psychiatrists, social workers and other individuals interested in treatment of anxiety disorders. Objectives are to increase knowledge, facilitate communication, and support research and treatment of phobias and related anxiety disorders. Conducts programs at professional meetings. Affiliated with the Association for Advancement of Behavior Therapy. Periodic symposiums and workshops.

Carol Lindemann, PhD, CEO

Audio Video

6736 Acquiring Courage: Audio Cassette Program for the Rapid Treatment of Phobias
New Harbinger Publications
5674 Shattuck Avenue
Oakland, CA 94609
510-652-2002
800-748-6273
Fax: 800-652-1613
customerservice@newharbinger.com
newharbinger.com

ISBN: 1-879237-03-2

6737 Anxiety Disorders
American Counseling Association
6101 Stevenson Ave, Suite 600
Alexandria, VA 22304
703-823-9800
800-347-6647
Fax: 800-473-2329
webmaster@counseling.org
counseling.org

Increase your awareness of anxiety disorders, their symptoms, and effective treatments. Learn the effect these disorders can have on life and how treatment can change the quality of life for people presently suffering from these disorders. Includes 6 audiotapes and a study guide.

Robert L. Smith, President

Book Publishers

6738 Anxiety & Phobia Workbook
Edmund J Bourne, author

New Harbinger Publications
5674 Shattuck Avenue
Oakland, CA 94609
510-652-2002
800-748-6273
Fax: 510-652-5472
TTY: 800-652-1613
customerservice@newharbinger.com
www.newharbinger.com

This comprehensive guide is recommended to those struggling with anxiety disorders. Includes step-by-step instructions for the crucial cognitive-behavioral techniques that have given real help to hundreds of thousands of readers struggling with anxiety disorders.

448 pages 4th Edition
ISBN: 1-572244-13-5

6739 Anxiety Cure: An Eight-Step Program for Getting Well
John Wiley & Sons
10475 Crosspoint Boulevard
Indianapolis, IN 46256
877-762-2974
Fax: 800-597-3299
www.wiley.com

A practical guide, written by a father and his two daughters, featuring a step-by-step program for curing the six main kinds of anxiety.

272 pages 2nd Edition
ISBN: 0-471464-87-2

Peter B. Wiley, Chairman
Stephen M. Smith, President & CEO
Ellis E. Cousens, Executive Vice President, Chief Fin

6740 Anxiety Disorders
Cambridge University Press
40 W 20th Street
New York, NY 10011
212-924-3900
800-872-7423
Fax: 914-937-4712
marketing@cup.org
cup.org

This comprehensive text covers all the anxiety disorders found in the latest DSM and ICD classifications. Provides detailed information about seven principal disorders, including anxiety in the medically ill. For each disorder, the book covers diagnosis criteria, epidemiology, etiology and pathogenesis, clinical features, natural history and different diagnoses. Describes treatment approaches, both psychological and pharmacological.

354 pages

6741 Anxiety Disorders: Practioner's Guide
John Wiley & Sons
111 River Street
Hoboken, NJ 7030-
212-850-6000
Fax: 212-850-6008
info@wiley.com
wiley.com

210 pages
ISBN: 0-471931-12-8

Stephen M. Smith, President/ CEO
John Kritzmacher, EVP/ CFO
MJ O'Leary, EVO, Human Resources

6742 Encyclopedia of Phobias, Fears, and Anxieties
Facts on File
11 Penn Plaza, Room M274
New York, NY 10001
212-290-8090
800-322-8755

500 pages

6743 Helping Your Anxious Child
New Harbinger Publications
5674 Shattuck Avenue
Oakland, CA 94609
510-652-2002
800-748-6273
Fax: 510-652-5472
TTY: 800-652-1613
customerservice@newharbinger.com
www.newharbinger.com

Step-by-step guide for parents of anxious children to help them overcome their fears and anxieties. Detailed strategies and techniques.

168 pages Paperback
ISBN: 1-572241-91-8

6744 Psychological Trauma
American Psychiatric Press
1400 K Street, NW
Washington, DC 20005
202-682-6262
800-368-5777
Fax: 202-789-2648
order@appi.org
www.appi.org

Epidemiology of trauma and post-tramatic stress disorder. Evaluation, neuroimaging, neuroendocrinology and pharmacology.

1998 206 pages

Robert E. Hales M.D, Editor-in-Chief
Rebecca D. Rinehart, Publisher
John McDuffie, Editorial Director

6745 Shy Children, Phobic Adults: Nature and Treatment of Social Phobia
American Psychological Press
1400 K Street, NW
Washington, DC 20005

202-682-6262
800-368-5777
Fax: 202-789-2648
orders@appi.org
www.appi.org

Describes the simuliarities and differences in the syndrome across all ages. Draws from the clinical, social and developmental literatures, as well as from extensive clinical experience. Illustrates the impact of developmental stage on phenomenology, diagnosis and assessment and treatment of social phobia.

1998 321 pages

Robert E. Hales M.D, Editor-in-Chief
Rebecca D. Rinehart, Publisher
John McDuffie, Editorial Director

Pamphlets

6746 Anxiety Disorders
National Institute of Mental Health
6001 Executive Boulevard, Room 6200, MSC 9663
Bethesda, MD 20892

301-443-4536
866-615-6464
Fax: 301-443-4279
TTY: 301-443-8431
NIMHpress@mail.nih.gov
www.nimh.nih.gov

This brochure helps to identify the symptoms of anxiety disorders, explains the role of research in understanding the causes of these conditions, describes effective treatments, helps you learn how to obtain treatment and work with a doctor or therapist, and suggests ways to make treatment more effective.

6747 Anxiety Disorders Fact Sheet
Center for Mental Health Services
PO Box 42490
Washington, DC 20015

800-789-2647
Fax: 301-984-8796
ken@mentalhealth.org
mentalhealth.org

This fact sheet presents basic information on the symptoms, formal diagnosis, and treatment for generalized anxiety disorder, panic disorders, phobias, and post traumatic stress disorder.

3 pages

6748 Anxiety Disorders in Children and Adolescents
Center for Mental Health Services
PO Box 42490
Washington, DC 20015

800-789-2647
Fax: 301-984-8796
ken@mentalhealth.org
mentalhealth.org

This fact sheet defines anxiety disorders, identifies warning signs, discusses risk factors, describes types of help available, and suggests what parents or other caregivers can do.

3 pages

6749 Families Can Help Children Cope with Fear, Anxiety
Center for Mental Health Services
PO Box 42490
Washington, DC 20015

800-789-2647
Fax: 301-984-8796
ken@mentalhealth.org
mentalhealth.org

This fact sheet defines conduct disorder, identifies risk factors, discusses types of help available, and suggests what parents or other caregivers responses should be to common signs of fear and anxiety.

DESCRIPTION

6750 SPEECH IMPAIRMENT

Synonym: Speech dysfunction

Involves the following Biologic System(s):

Neurologic Disorders

Speech impairment refers to the decreased ability or inability to effectively communicate through vocalizations or uttered sounds. Difficulty speaking or more profound dysfunctions of speech may result from many different factors that include neurologic influences; muscular defects, injuries, or paralysis; structural irregularities of the vocal cords; psychologic influences; mental retardation; and other factors.

In some children, speech impairment may be classified as a dysfunction of articulation characterized by the inability to articulate or produce words properly (dysarthria) as a result of damage to the part of the brain responsible for regulation of the muscles that control the speech apparatus (e.g., mouth, lips, and voice box or larynx). Such damage may result from head or brain injuries, tumors, strokes, and certain diseases. Characteristic speech patterns of children with dysarthria are varied and may be described as unintelligible, slow, slurred, halting, tremulous, hoarse, or possessing a nasal quality. Additional causes of articulation dysfunction or delay include structural defects such as cleft lip or palate, hearing impairment or deafness, and other nervous system irregularities. In addition, speech impairment may result from irregularities directly related to the vocal cords that may affect the quality of the voice.

Impaired ability to communicate (aphasia or dysphasia) may also result from injury to the part of the brain responsible for language comprehension, resulting in the reduced ability or inability to express, write, or understand language. Such injury may be caused by head trauma, brain lesions, infection, or other factors. This type of impairment may be present in many different variations such as garbled sentences, extremely slow and difficult speech, absence of speech (mutism), and other irregularities. In addition, children with behavioral, emotional, or psychologic irregularities as well as those with hearing impairment may also experience delays in language comprehension and development.

It is important to identify the underlying cause of any dysfunction of speech or delay in speech development in order to allow for the most favorable educational and social outcome. Specialists in the diagnosis and treatment of these types of disorders (e.g., otolaryngologists and speech therapists) may base their treatment plans on the evaluation of family and medical histories, physical examination of essential speech structures, and specialized testing that may include speech, language, and hearing assessments. Treatment is directed toward the specific cause of impairment and may include exercises tailored to the specific patient's needs, as well as the cooperation of parents or caregivers, pediatricians, educators, and others to provide a supportive environment.

Government Agencies

6751 NIH/National Institute on Deafness and Other Communication Disorders (NIDCD)
31 Center Drive, MSC 2320
Bethesda, MD 20892

800-241-1044
TTY: 800-241-1055
nidcdinfo@nidcd.nih.gov
www.nidcd.nih.gov

A National Institute of Health, the NIDCD supports research and provides education and information on these following health topics: voice, speech, language, hearing, ear infections, deafness, balance, smell and taste.

Dr James F Battey Jr, MD, PhD, Director
Judith A Cooper PhD, Deputy Director
Timothy J Wheeles, Executive Officer

National Associations & Support Groups

6752 Advocure NF2
P.O. Box 4118
Clearwater, FL 33758

contact@advocurenf2.org
www.advocurenf2.org

Advocure NF2 Inc. is a working advocacy group, liaison, and 501(c)(3) public charity for the NF2 international community and NF2 Crew.

Barbara Franklin, Vice President, Interim President
Sheila Heal, Secretary
Cynthia Henrion, Treasurer

6753 American Academy of Pediatrics
141 Northwest Point Boulevard
Elk Grove Village, IL 60007

847-434-4000
800-433-9016
Fax: 847-434-8000
www.aap.org

The American Academy of Pediatrics and its member pediatricians are committed to the attainment of optimal physical, mental and social health and well-being for all infants, children, adolescents, and young adults.

Fernando Stein, MD, FAAP, President
Karen Remley, MD, CEO/Executive VP

6754 American Board of Fluency and Fluency Disorders
563 Carter Court, Suite B
Kimberly, WI 54136

920-750-7720
Fax: 920-882-3655
info@stutteringspecialists.org
www.stutteringspecialists.org

The mission is to promote among speech-language pathologists the highest standards for training and service delivery to impact positively the communication skills and thereby the lives of those who demonstrate fluency disorders.

Kristin Chmela, Co-Chair
Lynne Shields, Co-Chair
June Campbell, Treasurer

6755 American Laryngological Association
www.alahns.org

Founded in 1878, the ALA is a scholarly organization of physicians and scientists who have made significant contributions to the care of patients with disorders of the larynx and upper aerodigestive tract. The ALA recognizes the accomplishments of these individuals through membership, seeks to encourage research in laryngology and elevate the standards of the fundamental teaching of laryngology in medical schools and postgraduate medical education.

6756 American School Counselor Association
1101 King Street, Suite 310
Alexandria, VA 22314

703-683-2722
800-306-4722
Fax: 703-997-7572
asca@schoolcounselor.org
www.schoolcounselor.org

The mission of ASCA is to represent professional school counselors and to promote professionalism and ethical practices.

Richard Wong, Executive Director
Jeff Broderson, Information Technology Admin.
Kathleen M Rakestraw, Director of Communications

6757 American Speech Language Hearing Associati on (ASHA)
2200 Research Boulevard
Rockville, MD 20850   301-897-5700
                                             800-638-8255
                                        Fax: 301-571-0457
                                             pr@asha.org
                                             www.asha.org

A professional and credentialing association made up of more than 123,000 international pathologists, audiologists and scientists. The association promotes the interests of and provides services for those in the hearing, speech, and language field, and advocates for people with communication disorders.

Patricia A. Prelock, PhD, President
Elizabeth S. McCrea, PhD, CCC-SLP, President-Elect
Shelly S. Chabon, PhD, CCC-SLP, Immediate Past President

6758 Aphasia Hope Foundation
P.O. Box 79701
Houston, TX 77279   855-764-4673
                                sandycaudell@aphasiahope.org
                                        www.aphasiahope.org

Aphasia Hope Foundation is a public 501(c) 3 non-profit foundation that has a two-fold mission: (1) to promote research into the prevention and cure of aphasia and (2) to ensure all survivors of aphasia and their caregivers are aware of and have access to the best possible treatments available.

6759 Association for Research in Otolaryngology
19 Mantua Rd.
Mt Royal, NJ 8061   856-423-0041
                                        Fax: 856-423-3420
                                        headquarters@aro.org
                                             www.aro.org

ARO Midwinter Meetings bring together over 1500 investigators from around the world to present current results in hearing, vestibular function, and related fields, as well as representatives of funding agencies, publishers, and scientific vendors.

6760 Association of Academic Physiatrists
10461 Mill Run Circle, Suite 730
Owings Mills, MD 21117   410-654-1000
                                        Fax: 410-654-1001
                                        tknowlton@physiatry.org
                                             www.physiatry.org

The Association of Academic Physiatrists (AAP) is the only academic association dedicated to the specialty of physical medicine and rehabilitation (PM&R) in the world. AAP is a community of leading physicians, researchers, in-training physiatrists, and others involved or interested in leadership, mentorship, and discovery in PM&R.

Tiffany Knowlton, JD, MBA, Executive Director
Bernadette M. Rensing, Comm. & Marketing Manager
Amy Schnappinger, Member Services Manager

6761 Association of University Centers on Disabilities
1100 Wayne Ave., Suite 1000
Silver Spring, MD 20910   301-588-8252
                                        Fax: 301-588-2842
                                        aucdinfo@aucd.org
                                             www.aucd.org

The Association of University Centers on Disabilities (AUCD) is a membership organization that supports and promotes a national network of university-based interdisciplinary programs.

Andrew J. Imparato, JD, Executive Director
Abigail (Abbey) Alberico, MPH, Project Manager
Leon Barnett, MSEd, Program Specialist

6762 Auditory-Verbal Learning Institute
7205 North Habana Ave
Tampa, FL 33614   813-227-8766
                                        Fax: 813-932-9583
                                             info@avli.org
                                             www.avli.org

Promotes and teaches Auditory-Verbal Therapy.

Pamela Sullins, Director/CEO
Alisa Jenkins, Marketing/Product Consultant
Judith Marlowe PhD, Program Development Consultant

6763 CHERAB Foundation
P.O. Box 8524
Port St. Lucie, FL 34952   772-335-5135
                                             help@cherab.org
                                             www.cherab.org

Provides communication help, eductaion, research.

6764 Center for Parent Information and Resources
35 Halsey St., Fourth Floor
Newark, NJ 7102   malizo@spannj.org
                                        www.parentcenterhub.org

The Center for Parent Information and Resources (CPIR) serves as a central resource of information and products to the community of Parent Training Information (PTI) Centers and the Community Parent Resource Centers (CPRCs), so that they can focus their efforts on serving families of children with disabilities.

Myriam Alizo, Project Assistant
Debra Jennings, Project Director
Lisa K□pper, Product Development Coordinator

6765 Center for Speech and Language Disorders
310-D S. Main St.
Lombard, IL 60148   630-652-0200
                                             lynns@csld.org
                                             www.csld.org

Works with the mission to help children with communication disorders reach their full potential through family centered services.

Lynn Scheuer Kozak, Executive Director
Mary Catherine Brady, Operations Manager
Phyllis Kupperman, M.A., CCC-SLP, Founder

6766 Childhood Apraxia of Speech Association
416 Lincoln Avenue 2nd Fl.
Pittsburgh, PA 15209   www.apraxia-kids.org

The Childhood Apraxia of Speech Association is a 501(c)(3) non-profit publicly funded charity whose mission is to strengthen the support systems in the lives of children with apraxia so that each child is afforded their best opportunity to develop speech and communication.

Sue Freiburger, Board Secretary
Sharon Gretz, M.Ed, Executive Director
Kathy Hennessy, Education Director

6767 Council of Academic Programs in Communication
3000 South Jamaica Ct., Ste 390
Aurora, CO 80014   303-835-9089
                                        Fax: 800-805-5932
                                        mchavez@capcsd.org
                                             www.capcsd.org

CAPCSD is dedicated to promoting academic excellence, visionary leadership and collaboration among communication sciences and disorders academic programs.

Judith Vander Woude, Ph.D., President
Rich Folsom, VP for Student Development
Mary Chavez Rudolph, Ph.D., Executive Director

6768 Educational Audiology Association
700 McKnight Park Drive, Suite 708
Pittsburgh, PA 15237   800-460-7322
                                        Fax: 888-729-3489
                                             admin@edaud.org
                                             edaud.org

The Educational Audiology Association is an international organization of audiologists and related professionals who deliver a full spectrum of hearing services to all children, particularly those in educational settings.

Mike Sharp, AuD, CCC-A, President
Gary Pillow, President-Elect
Erin Schafer, PhD, Secretary

6769 National Aphasia Association
www.aphasia.org

The National Aphasia Association (NAA) is a non-profit organization founded in 1987 by Martha Taylor Sarno, MA, MD, (hon) as the 1st National organization dedicated to advocating for persons with aphasia and their families. Several of our board members, including the President, are people with Aphasia or family members.

Darlene S. Williamson, President
Daniel Martin, VP Strategic Planning
Barbara Kessler, VP, Community Outreach & Education

6770 National Black Association for Speech-Language and Hearing
700 McKnight Park Drive, Suite 708
Pittsburgh, PA 15237 855-727-2836
Fax: 888-729-3489
nbaslh@nbaslh.org
www.nbaslh.org

The Association was incorporated in Washington D.C., June 30, 1978. The committee wanted to establish a viable mechanism through which the professional needs of the Black professionals, students, and the communicatively handicapped community could be met.

Rachel M. Williams, PhD, CCC-SLP, Chair
Kellie E. Green, MA, CCC-SLP, Secretary, PR Co-Chair
Linda McCabe Smith, Treasurer, Membership Co-Chair

6771 National Spasmodic Dysphonia Association
300 Park Boulevard, Suite 335
Itasca, IL 60143 800-795-6732
Fax: 630-250-4505
NSDA@dysphonia.org
www.dysphonia.org

The National Spasmodic Dysphonia Association (NSDA) is a not-for-profit 501c(3) organization dedicated to advancing medical research into the causes of and treatments for SD, promoting physician and public awareness of the disorder, and providing support to those affected by SD through symposiums, support groups, and on-line resources.

Charlie Reavis, President
Marcia Sterling, Treasurer
Mary Bifaro, Support Services Director

6772 Voice Foundation (The)
219 N. Broad St. 10th Floor
Philadelphia, PA 19107 215-735-7999
Fax: 215-762-5572
voicefoundation.org

The Voice Foundation was founded in 1969 by the internationally celebrated voice specialist Wilbur James Gould, M.D.. At that time interdisciplinary care of the human voice was non-existent. Dr. Gould's groundbreaking foresight brought together physicians, scientists, speech-language pathologists, performers, and teachers to share their knowledge and expertise in the care of the professional voice user.

Robert Thayer Sataloff, Chairman
Stuart Orsher, MD, President
Michael S. Benninger, MD, Vice President

6773 Voice Health Institute
1 Bowdoin Square
Boston, MA 2114 617-720-5000
Fax: 617-720-5001
info@voicehealthinstitute.org
www.voicehealthinstitute.org

Since its inception and qualification as a federally-approved non-profit public charity (501-C-3), the VHI has funded educational and award-wining pioneering research programs.

Julie Andrews, Chairman
John L. Ward, Ph.D., President

State Agencies & Support Groups

New York

6774 Brooklyn College Speech and Hearing Center
2900 Bedford Ave, 4400 Boylan Hall
Brooklyn, NY 11210 718-951-5186
Fax: 718-951-4363
mbergen@brooklyn.cuny.edu
www.brooklyn.cuny.edu/bc/spotlite/news/110804.htm

Provides diagnostic and rehabilitative services to children and adults with speech, language, hearing and voice impairments.

Christopher Kimmich, President
Susan Bohne, Assistant Director

North Carolina

6775 North Carolina Speech, Hearing and Languag e Association
PO Box 28359
Raleigh, NC 27611 919-833-3984
Fax: 919-832-0445
info@ncshla.org
www.ncshla.org

Promotes the professional practice of speech, language and hearing sciences and works to enhance the lives of those who are communicatively impaired, through a variety of programs and opportunities.

Louise Raleigh, President
Tracie Rice, President-Elect
Kathleen Cox, Ph.D., CCC-SLP, Past President

Ohio

6776 Cleveland Hearing and Speech Center
11635 Euclid Avenue
Cleveland, OH 44106 216-231-0787
Fax: 216-795-2135
www.chsc.org

A nonprofit organization in Northeast Ohio dedicated to serving the needs of those with special communication needs.

Hilary Beatrez, Director of Finance and Administrat
Susan M. Bungard, CCDHH Program Director
Michelle L. Burnett, Director of Clinical Services

6777 Speech and Hearing Clinic
Kent State University
A104 Music & Speech Bldg, PO Box 5190
Kent, OH 44242 330-672-2672
Fax: 330-672-2643
www.kent.edu/spa

Services provided include: full-service clinic diagnoses, therapy, treatment and hearing aid repair.

Lynn Rowan, Executive Director

Oklahoma

6778 Oklahoma Speech Language Hearing Associati on
1741 S Cleveland Ave, Suite 301
Sioux Falls, SD 57103 405-802-1630
Fax: 405-271-3360
office@oslha.org
www.oslha.org

Deborah Earley, President
Sarah Baker, President Elect
Tracy Grammer, Past President

Oregon

6779 **Reading and Speech Clinic**
Unit 9
Bend, OR 97701
541-389-3302
800-283-0818
ellen@readingandspeechclinic.com
www.readingandspeechclinic.com

Provides alternate therapies for improving speech, language, spelling and reading difficulties.

Ellen Jacobs PhD, Director

Tennessee

6780 **Memphis State University, Center for the Communicatively Impaired**
807 Jefferson Avenue
Memphis, TN 38105
901-678-2009
Fax: 901-525-1282
www.memphis.edu/csd/crisci.htm

Offers research into hearing loss, deafness, and speech impairments.

Maurice I Mendel, Director

Texas

6781 **Callier Center for Communication Disorders**
University of Texas at Dallas
1966 Inwood Road
Dallas, TX 75235
214-905-3000
Fax: 214-905-3022
TDD: 214-905-3012
barbara.ember@utdallas.edu
www.callier.utdallas.edu

Multidisciplinary center serving infants through adults with all types of communcation disorders: diagnostic and treatment; hearing aid services; cochlear implant evalution and follow-up; N Texas Cochlear Implant Summer Listening Camp; aural rehabilitation services; assistive listening device program; tinnitus and hyperacusis clinic; speech-language pathology and psychological diagnostic and therapy services; research.

Thomas Campbell, Executive Director
Christine A Dollaghan, Child Language Development
Robert Stillman PhD, Communication Disorders

Washington

6782 **Scottish Rite Centers for Childhood Langua ge Disorders**
2800 16th Street, NW
Washington, DC 20009
202-232-8155
Fax: 202-483-8169
www.dcsr.org/clinic.php

Association offering speech-language evaluations and treatment, hearing screening and consultation and referrals to children ages birth to 18 years with hearing or speech disorders. Seven locations/clinincs are offered throughout the state of Washington.

Tommie L. Robinson, Jr., Ph.D, Director

6783 **University of Washington Department of Spe ech & Hearing Sciences**
1417 NE 42nd Street
Seattle, WA 98105
206-685-7400
Fax: 206-543-1093
sphscadv@u.washington.edu
www.depts.washington.edu/sphsc/

Committed to understanding the basic processes and mechanisms involved in human speech, hearing, language, their disorders and to improving the quality of life for individuals affected by communication disorders across the life span.

Stacy Betz, Child Language Disorders

Research Centers

Arizona

6784 **National Center for Neurogenic Communicati on Disorders**
University of Arizona
Speech & Hearing Sciences Bldg, Rm 500
Tucson, AZ 85721
520-621-1472
cnet.shs.arizona.edu

The center is supported by a grant from the NIDCD, a National Institute of Health, and is staffed by scientists, educators and students who are concerned with speech and language disorders caused by diseases of the nervous system.

Thomas J Hixon PhD, Director
Kathryn A Bayles PhD, Associate Director

Colorado

6785 **Speech, Language, and Hearing Center**
University of Colorado, Boulder
2501 Kittregde Loop Rd
Boulder, CO 80309
303-492-5375
slhs.colorado.edu/clinical-services?

Focuses on communication disorders including speech and hearing impairments.

Susan M Moore, Director

Michigan

6786 **University Center for the Development of L anguage & Literacy**
University of Michigan
1111 E Catherine Street
Ann Arbor, MI 48109
734-764-8440
Fax: 734-647-2489
www.languageexperts.org/research/

Focuses on communicative disorders including hearing impairments and speech disorders. Provides intensive language intervention for adults with aphasia as well as children with language disorders. Clinic offers residential program for adults and school liasion for children.

Carol C. Persad, PhD., ABPP, Director of the University Center f
Mimi Block, MS, CCC-SLP, Clinical Services Manager

Nebraska

6787 **Boys Town National Research Hospital**
555 N 30th Street
Omaha, NE 68131
402-498-6511
Fax: 402-498-6638
TTY: 402-498-6543
www.boystownhospital.org

An internationally recognized center for state-of-the-art research, diagnosis, treatment of patients with ear diseases, hearing and balance disorders, cleft lip and palate, and speech/language problems.

Patrick E Brookhouser, President

Nevada

6788 **University of Nevada - Department of Speec h-Language Pathology**
School of Medicine
Redfield Bldg, MS 152
Reno, NV 89557
775-784-4887
Fax: 775-784-4095
lgoldberg@medicine.nevada.edu
www.medicine.nevada.edu/spa/

The department includes an active clinic and nine faculty for research in language, speech and hearing.

Thomas Watterson, Chair
Leslie Goldberg, Clinical Director

New York

6789 Henry Youngerman Center for Communication Disorders
SUNY Fredonia/Dept of Comm Disorders/Sciences
Thompson Hall W123
Fredonia, NY 14063 716-673-3202
Fax: 716-673-3235

Studies communications disorders including hearing and speech.
It features a newly constructed research labs and an in-house
clinic that serves as a training ground for graduate clinicians. The
clinic provides speech/language and hearing services to members
of the college, student, and local community.

Melissa A Sidor MS, CCC/SLP Clinic Director
Dr Kim Tillery PhD, CCC/Aud-Chair, Professor

North Carolina

6790 Communications Disorders Clinic
Reich College of Education
400 University Hall Drive, PO Box 32041
Boone, NC 28608 828-262-2185
Fax: 828-262-6766
www.cdclinic.appstate.edu

The clinic provides prevention, assessment, and treatment of
speech, language and hearing disorders for all ages. It also provides several outreach programs.

Mary Ruth Sizer, Director

Washington

6791 University of Washington Speech and Hearin g Clinic
1417 N.E. 42nd St
Seattle, WA 98105 206-685-7400
Fax: 206-616-1185
shclinic@u.washington.edu
depts.washington.edu/sphsc/

A center for education and research serving speech, language, and
hearing needs within the university and the community. Serves as
a teaching facility in the fields of speech-language pathology and
audiology, with state of the art technology, innovative diagnostic
and treament methods, and internationally and nationally
recognized areas of research.

Nancy Alarcon MS, CCC-SLP, Director
Joan Hanson, Manager

Wisconsin

6792 Waisman Center - Auditory Physiology Resea rch Laboratory
University of Wisconsin, Madison
1500 Highland Ave
Madison, WI 53705 608-263-1656
www.physiology.wisc.edu/brugge/bruggelab.html?

The research laboratory is part of the Waisman Center which is
dedicated to advancing the knowledge about human development,
developmental disabilities, and neurodegenerative disorders.

James S Malter, Director

Web Sites

6793 Parent Pals
parentpals.com/gossamer/pages/Speech_and_Language

specialed@parentpals.co m
parentpals.com/gossamer/pages/Speech_and_Language

Their goal is to provide special education and gifted information,
continuing education, support, weekly tips, games, book resources, and news and views for parents and professionals.

Book Publishers

6794 Listen Little Star
Auditory-Verbal Learning Institute
7205 North Habana Ave
Tampa, FL 33614 813-227-8766
Fax: 813-932-9583
info@avli.org
www.avli.org

A family activity kit for parents designed to help their babies develop listening and speaking skills. It includes 12 activities, a
workbook, checklist, plush toy, and note-taking section.

**6795 Management of Motor Speech Disorders in Children and
Adults**
Pro-Ed
8700 Shoal Creek Boulevard
Austin, TX 78757 512-451-3246
800-897-3202
Fax: 800-397-7633
general@proedinc.com
www.proedinc.com

Second edition of this popular text incorporates information
about both dysarthria and apraxia of speech in children and adults
and reviews techniques for physical and motor speech examination and treatment techniques.

618 pages Hardcover
ISBN: 0-890797-84-6

6796 Preschool Motor Speech Evaluation & Interv ention
Pro-Ed
8700 Shoal Creek Boulevard
Austin, TX 78757 512-451-3246
800-897-3202
Fax: 800-397-7633
general@proedinc.com
www.proedinc.com

Comprehensive resource manual for evaluating and treating oral
motor and motor speech disorders in children 18 months to six
years of age.

Journals

6797 American Journal of Speech-Language Pathol ogy
American Speech Language Hearing Association
2200 Research Blvd
Rockville, MD 20850 301-296-5700
800-478-2071
Fax: 301-296-8580
TTY: 301-296-5650
TDD: 301-296-5650
www.asha.org

Pertains to all aspects of clinical practice in speech-language pathology.

Quarterly
Dr Laura Justice, Editor

6798 Communication Disorders Quarterly
Hammill Institute on Disabilities/Sage Publication
2455 Teller Road
Thousand Oaks, CA 91320 800-818-7243
Fax: 800-583-2665
journals@sagepub.com
www.sagepub.com

Presents cutting-edge information on typical and atypical communication disorders across the continuum-from oral language development to literacy. CDQ is the official journal of the Division
for Communicaative Disabilities and Deafness of the CEC. ISSN:
Print: 1525-722; Electronic: 1538-4837; Subscriptions available:
Institutional - Print Only $141, Insitutional - Print & E-access
$144, Personal $57.

Quarterly
ISSN: 1528-7401

Judy K Montgomery, PhD, Editor

6799 Journal of Speech, Language, and Hearing Research
American Speech Language Hearing Association
2200 Research Blvd
Rockville, MD 20850
301-296-5700
800-478-2071
Fax: 301-296-8580
TTY: 301-296-5650
TDD: 301-296-5650
www.asha.org

Pertains broadly to studies of the processes and disorders of hearing, language, and speech and to the diagnosis and treatment of such disorders.

Bi-monthly

Dr Anne Smith, Editor, Speech
Dr Karla McGregor, Editor, Language
Dr Robert Schlauch, Editor, Hearing

6800 Language, Speech, and Hearing in Schools
American Speech Language Hearing Association
2200 Research Blvd
Rockville, MD 20850
301-296-5700
800-478-2071
Fax: 301-296-8580
TTY: 301-296-5650
TDD: 301-296-5650
www.asha.org

An archival journal for research and practice in educational settings. Publishes studies and articles that pertain to speech, language, and hearing disorders and differences in children and adolescents, as well as to professional issues affecting service delivery in educational settings.

Quarterly

Dr Kenn Apel, Editor

Newsletters

6801 Callier Communications
Callier Center - University of Texas at Dallas
1966 Inwood Road
Dallas, TX 75235
214-905-3000
Fax: 214-905-3022
TDD: 214-905-3012
www.callier.utdallas.edu

W. Bennett Cullum, President
Jodelle Oakley, MS, Director, Education Division
Jan Lougeay, MA, CCC/SLP, Director of Clinical Education

6802 Communique
NCSHLA Publications
PO Box 28359
Raleigh, NC 27611
919-833-3984
Fax: 919-832-0445
info@ncshla.org
www.ncshla.org

The official newsletter of NCSHLA.

Quarterly

G Peyton Maynard, Executive VP
AJ Jacques, Executive Secretary
Cindy Davis Ling, President

Camps

6803 Central Michigan University Summer Clinics
444 Moore
Mount Pleasant, MI
517-774-3803

Designed for children, ages 6 and up, with speech, language and hearing disorders who can benefit from intensive clinical work. A wide range of recreational and social activities form part of the clinical program and promote the social use of skills learned in class.

6804 Meadowood Springs Speech and Hearing Camp
PO Box 1025
Pendleton, OR 97801
541-276-2752
Fax: 541-276-7227
info@meadowoodsprings.org
www.meadowoodsprings.org

On 143 acres in the Blue Mountains of Eastern Oregon, this camp is designed to help young people who have diagnosed clinical disorders of speech, hearing or language. A full range of activities in recreational and clinical areas is available. For cabin reservations 541-566-2191.

Rosemarie Atfield, Executive Director
Marie Story, Camp Manager
Cliff Story, Camp Manager

6805 University of Iowa - Wendell Johnson Speech and Hearing Clinic
Wendell Johnson Speech And Hearing Center
Iowa City, IA 52242
319-335-8718
Fax: 319-335-8851
speech-path-aud@uiowa.edu
clas.uiowa.edu/comsci/

The clinic offers assessment and remediation for disordered communication in adults and children. The clinic also offers an Intensive Summer Residential Clinic for school age children needing intervention services because of speech, language, hearing and/or reading problems.

Ruth Bentler, Professor / Department Chair
Dorothy Albright, Secretary
Vicki Jennings, Secretary

DESCRIPTION

6806 SPINA BIFIDA

Covers these related disorders: Encephalocele, Meningocele, Myelocele (Myelomeningocele, Meningomyelocele), Spina bifida occulta

Involves the following Biologic System(s):

Neurologic Disorders, Orthopedic and Muscle Disorders

Spina bifida, literally meaning "cleft spine," is a congenital abnormality, known as a neural tube defect, which is characterized by the failure during embryonic development of one or more of the developing vertebrae to develop completely or fuse. This frequently results in the exposure of part of the spinal cord. It is the most common neural tube defect in the United States—affecting 1,500 to 2,000 of the more than 4 million babies born in the country each year. Spina bifida occulta, the most common and least severe form of this defect, is characterized by a dimpling, dark tufts of hair, spider-like fine lines (telangiectasia), or a benign fatty tumor (lipoma) on the lower back or lumbosacral area. There is no protrusion or exposure of the spinal cord and it rarely involves problems with the nervous system. Some affected children, however, may experience weakness in the legs and feet and difficulty in bladder and bowel control resulting from an adhesion of the spinal cord to the area of the abnormality.

Meningocele occurs when the three membranes surrounding the spinal cord (meninges) protrude through the vertebral defect. Most meningoceles are covered by skin and contain cerebrospinal fluid. Although most affected children have no apparent neurologic involvement, some children may experience nerve dysfunction and associated irregularities (e.g., tethered spinal cord, diastematomyelia, and syringomyelia). If cerebrospinal fluid is leaking from the meningocele, immediate surgery is usually required to avoid infection or inflammation of the meninges (meningitis). Surgery to correct the meningocele may be performed at a later date in those children who are not at risk for such infection.

Myelocele is a severe form of spina bifida that affects one in 1,000 newborns. This form of the disorder is characterized by a protrusion of the spinal cord and meninges through the vertebral canal, covered by a raw swelling. Most myeloceles are located in the lumbosacral region. This abnormality may result in impaired function of the skeletal system, the skin, the genitourinary tract, and the peripheral and central nervous systems. Physical findings associated with myelocele are widely variable and depend upon the portion of the spinal cord affected and may include the inability to control the bladder and bowel functions, lack of muscle tone in the legs, and other irregularities of the lower extremities. Some children with myelocele develop an unusual accumulation of cerebrospinal fluid in the skull, resulting in enlargement of the head (hydrocephalus) and associated symptoms that may include choking and difficulty in feeding and breathing. The insertion of a tube or shunt is often indicated to relieve fluid buildup. Treatment of myelocele often involves a team of medical specialists working closely to manage care for the affected child. This care usually involves surgery to repair the myelocele. Other approaches to treatment are geared toward correction, alleviation, or management of symptoms. For example, training children or their parents how to empty the bladder through catheterization may help to avoid urinary tract infections and kidney disease. Also, laxatives or enemas may be used to relieve the constipation often associated with this abnormality. Other treatment may include the use of braces and canes or crutches and physical therapy to maintain joint mobility and to strengthen muscular function. Further treatment is supportive. The exact cause of myelocele is unknown; however, it is thought that environmental and nutritional influences may be contributing factors.

Encephalocele, a very severe and rare type of spina bifida, is characterized by the protrusion of the brain through a defect in the cranium. Affected children often experience visual difficulties, mental retardation, and seizures.

A common screening method used to look for spina bifida during pregnancy is a second trimester maternal serum alpha fetoprotein (MSAFP) screening. The MSAFP screen measures the level of a protein called alpha-fetoprotein (AFP), which is made naturally by the fetus and placenta. During pregnancy, a small amount of AFP normally crosses the placenta and enters the mother's bloodstream. But if abnormally high levels of this protein appear in the mother's bloodstream it may indicate that the fetus has a neural tube defect. Amniocentesis, an exam in which a sample of fluid is obtained from the amniotic sac that surrounds the fetus, may also be used to diagnose spina bifida. Research has shown that supplementation with folic acid, starting before pregnancy, reduces the risk of neural tube defects. It is recommended that all women of childbearing age consume 400 micrograms of folic acid daily.

Government Agencies

6807 NIH/National Institute of Arthritis and Musculoskeletal and Skin Diseases
1 AMS Circle
Bethesda, MD 20892

301-495-4484
877-226-4267
Fax: 301-718-6366
TDD: 301-565-2966
niamsinfo@mail.nih.gov
www.niams.nih.gov

The mission of the NIAMS, a part of the NIH, is to support research into the causes, treatment, and prevention of arthritis and musculoskeletal and skin diseases, the training of basic and clinical scientists to carry out this research, and the dissemination of information on research progress in these diseases.

Stephen I Katz MD PhD, Director
Robert H Carter MD, Deputy Director
Gahan Breithaupt, Assoc Dir for Management & Operatio

National Associations & Support Groups

6808 American Academy of Pediatrics
141 Northwest Point Boulevard
Elk Grove Village, IL 60007

847-434-4000
800-433-9016
Fax: 847-434-8000
www.aap.org

The American Academy of Pediatrics and its member pediatricians are committed to the attainment of optimal physical, mental and social health and well-being for all infants, children, adolescents, and young adults.

Fernando Stein, MD, FAAP, President
Karen Remley, MD, CEO/Executive VP

6809 Center for Disabilities and Development
University of Iowa Stead Family Children's Hospita
100 Hawkins Drive
Iowa City, IA 52242   319-353-6900
                            877-686-0031
                        Fax: 319-356-7700
                    cdd-scheduling@uiowa.edu
                    www.uichildrens.org/cdd

A trusted resource for healthcare, training, research and information for people with disabilities that include: behavior disorders, brain injury, cerebral palsy, diabetes, down syndrome, learning disabilities, mental retardation, sleep disorders and spina bifida.

Dianne McBrien, MD, Medical Director

6810 Easter Seals Disability Services Chicago, IL 60606
                            312-726-6200
                            800-221-6827
                        Fax: 312-726-1494
                        TDD: 312-726-4258
                    extranetinfo@easterseals.com
                    www.extraneteasterseals.com

Helps individuals with special needs and disabilities and their families to lead better lives through a variety of services including job training, development centers, rehabilitation, and education.

Lou Lowenkron, Chairman
James E Williams Jr, President/CEO

6811 Genetic Alliance
4301 Connecticut Avenue NW, Suite 404
Washington, DC 20008   202-966-5557
                            800-336-4363
                        Fax: 202-966-8553
                        info@geneticalliance.org
                        www.geneticalliance.org

A coalition of voluntary genetic support groups, consumers and professionals addressing the needs of individuals and families affected by genetic disorders from a national perspective.

Sharon Terry, President/CEO
Tetyana Murza, Managing Director
Natasha Bonhomme, VP, Strategic Development

6812 March of Dimes Foundation
1275 Mamaroneck Avenue
White Plains, NY 10605   914-997-4488
                            888-663-4637
                        Fax: 914-997-4763
                    answers@marchofdimes.com
                    www.marchofdimes.com

Partnership of volunteers and professionals dedicated to improving the health of babies by preventing birth defects and infant mortality. Over 100 chapters are located across the country and can be located through the national office.

Stacey D. Stewart, President

6813 National Center for Education in Maternal and Child Health
Georgetown University
2115 Wisconsin Ave NW, Suite 601
Washington, DC 20007   202-784-9770
                        Fax: 202-784-9777
                        mchlibrary@ncemch.org
                        www.ncemch.org

Provides leadership in disseminating information, program development, and education to individuals with an interest in maternal and child health (MCH), public health policy, and systems of care.

Rochelle Mayer, Director
Olivia Pickett, Director Library Services

6814 National Dissemination Center for Children with Disabilities
1825 Connecticut Ave NW
Washington, DC 20009   202-884-8200
                            800-695-0285
                        Fax: 202-884-8441
                        nichcy@fhi360.org
                        www.nichcy.org

A national information and referral center for families, educators and other professionals on: disabilities in children and youth; programs and services; IDEA, the nation's special education law; and research-based information on effective practices.

Suzanne Ripley, Executive Director

6815 National Rehabilitation Information Center
4200 Forbes Blvd, Suite 202
Lanham, MD 20706   301-459-5900
                            800-346-2742
                        Fax: 301-459-4263
                        TTY: 301-459-5984
                    naricinfo@heitechservices.com
                    www.naric.com

An online gateway to over 70,000 disability and rehabilitation related documents and journal articles, and other resources.

Mark Odum, Director

6816 Spina Bifida Association
4590 MacArthur Boulevard NW, Suite 250
Washington, DC 20007   202-944-3285
                            800-621-3141
                        Fax: 202-944-3295
                        sbaa@sbaa.org
                        www.spinabifidaassociation.org

Serves as the national office representing approximately 60 chapters of parents and other members of families having children born with spina bifida, individuals with spina bifida, and health professionals who work with them. Operates a national information and referral service, periodic public awareness campaigns, scholarships and an annual meeting.

Cindy Brownstein, Ceo
Caroline Alston, Director, Programs/Field Initiative
Mary E Johnson, Director Communications

State Agencies & Support Groups

Alabama

6817 Spina Bifida Association of Alabama
PO Box 13254
Birmingham, AL 35202   256-325-8600
                        info@sbaofal.org
                        www.sbaofal.org

Providing medical, social, and financial support to those afflicted with spina bifida.

Betsy Hopson, President
Angie Pate, Executive Director
Jamie Martin, Field Service Coordinator

Arizona

6818 Arizona Spina Bifida Association
1001 E Fairmount Avenue
Phoenix, AZ 85014   602-274-3323
                        Fax: 602-274-7632
                        office@sbaaz.org
                        www.sbaaz.org/?

Arlene Plouff, Manager

Arkansas

6819 Spina Bifida Association of Arkansas
4590 MacArthur Blvd., NW, Suite 250
Washington, DC 20007   202-944-3285
                        Fax: 202-944-3295
                        sbaa@sbaa.org
                        www.spinabifidaassociation.org

Providing medical, social, and financial support to those afflicted with spina bifida.

Vicki Rucker, Executive Director

California

6820 Spina Bifida Association of Greater Bay Ar ea
4590 MacArthur Blvd., NW, Suite 250
Washington, DC 20007   202-944-3285
                                    Fax: 202-944-3295
                                    sbaa@sbaa.org
                                    www.spinabifidaassociation.org

Providing medical, social, and financial support to those afflicted
with spina bifida.

Traci Whittemore, President

6821 Spina Bifida Association of Greater San Di ego
4590 MacArthur Blvd., NW, Suite 250
Washington, DC 20007   202-944-3285
                                    Fax: 202-944-3295
                                    sbaa@sbaa.org
                                    www.spinabifidaassociation.org

Providing medical, social, and financial support to those afflicted
with spina bifida.

Mary Robbins Wade, President

Colorado

6822 Spina Bifida Association of Colorado
PO Box 22994
Denver, CO 80222   303-797-7870
                                    sbacolorado@gmail.com
                                    www.coloradospinabifida.org

Providing medical, social, and financial support to those afflicted
with spina bifida.

Chris Mestas, Board Chair / SBACO Website
Rev. John Anderson, Immediate Past Chair
LaVon Birney, Executive Director

Connecticut

6823 Spina Bifida Association of Connecticut
370 Osgood Avenue Suite 106
New Britain, CT 06053   860-839-0115
                                         800-574-6274
                                    Fax: 860-832-6260
                                    sbac@sbac.org
                                    www.sbac.org

Providing medical, social, and financial support to those afflicted
with spina bifida.

Carol Toomey, Chair
Rebecca Hajosy, Treasurer/Secretary
Kiley J Carlson, Executive Director

Florida

6824 Spina Bifida Association of Central Florid a
100 W. Lucerne Circle, Suite 100-M
Orlando, FL 32801   407-248-9210
                                    Fax: 407-248-9227
                                    info@sbacfl.org
                                    sbacentralflorida.org

Providing medical, social, and financial support to those afflicted
with spina bifida.

Beccy Hosoda, President

**6825 Spina Bifida Association of Jacksonville N emours Childrens
Clinic**
807 Children's Way
Jacksonville, FL 32207   904-390-3686
                                         800-722-6355
                                    Fax: 904-390-3466
                                    Sbaj@sbaj.org
                                    www.sbaj.org

Providing medical, social, and financial support to those afflicted
with spina bifida.

Stephanie King, Executive Director
Margaret Quintana, Treasurer

6826 Spina Bifida Association of Southeast Florida
4590 MacArthur Blvd., NW, Suite 250
Washington, DC 20007   202-944-3285
                                    Fax: 202-944-3295
                                    sbaa@sbaa.org
                                    www.spinabifidaassociation.org

Providing medical, social, and financial support to those afflicted
with spina bifida.

Irene Ballart, President

6827 Spina Bifida Association of Tampa Bay
PO Box 16603
Tampa, FL 33687   813-933-4827
                                    sbatampabay@aol.com
                                    www.sbatampabay.org

Providing medical, social, and financial support to those afflicted
with spina bifida.

Dianne Gore, President

Georgia

6828 Spina Bifida Association of Georgia
5072 Bristol Industrial Way, Suite F
Buford, GA 30518   770-939-1044
                                    Fax: 770-939-1049
                                    sbag@spinabifidaga.org
                                    spinabifidaga.org

Jim Okula, Executive Director

Illinois

6829 Spina Bifida Association of Illinois
8765 W Higgins Rd, Suite 403
Chicago, IL 60631   773-444-0305
                                         800-969-4722
                                    Fax: 773-444-0327
                                    sbail@sbail.org
                                    www.sbail.org

The Illinois Spina Bifida Association is dedicated to improving
the quality of life of people with spina bifida through direct services, information and referral and public awareness. Direct services include family outreach, education advocacy and more.

Amy Maggio, Executive Director

Indiana

6830 Spina Bifida Association of Central Indian a
PO Box 19814
Indianapolis, IN 46219   317-592-1630
                                    membership@sbaci.org
                                    www.sbaci.org

Providing medical, social, and financial support to those afflicted
with spina bifida.

Lisa Jones, President

6831 Spina Bifida Association of Northern Indiana
4590 MacArthur Blvd., NW, Suite 250
Washington, DC 20007   202-944-3285
                                    Fax: 202-944-3295
                                    sbaa@sbaa.org
                                    www.spinabifidaassociation.org

Providing medical, social, and financial support to those afflicted
with spina bifida.

Tim Yoder, President

Iowa

6832 Spina Bifida Association of Iowa
8525 Douglas Avenue Suite 39
Urbandale, IA 50322   515-964-8810
                                      contact@sbaia.org
                                      www.sbaia.org

Providing support, a reimbursement program, quarterly newsletter
and public awareness campaigns.

Maryanne Lorenz, Manager

Kentucky

6833 Spina Bifida Association of Kentucky
982 Eastern Parkway, Box 18
Louisville, KY 40217   502-637-7363
                                      866-340-7225
                                      Fax: 502-637-1010
                                      sbak@sbak.org
                                      www.spinabifidakentucky.org

Providing support to those afflicted with spina bifida.

Joe O'Bryan, Board Chair/President
Eddie Brown Jr., Incoming Chair
Cris Miller, Secretary

Louisiana

6834 Spina Bifida Association of Greater New Orleans
PO Box 1346
Kenner, LA 70063   504-737-5181
                                      sbagno@sbagno.org
                                      www.sbagno.org

Providing support to those afflicted with spina bifida.

Julie Johnston, Coordinator

Maryland

6835 Spina Bifida Association of Chesapeake-Pot omac
PO Box 1750
Annapolis, MD 21404   888-733-0988
                                      Fax: 410-295-9744
                                      cpbs@kennedykrieger.org
                                      www.chesapeakespinabifida.org

Providing support to those afflicted with spina bifida.

Toni Shumate, Executive Director

Massachusetts

6836 Spina Bifida Association of Massachusetts
25 Birch Street, Building B
Milford, MA 01757   888-479-1900
                                      Fax: 504-482-5301
                                      edugan@sbamass.org
                                      www.sbamass.org

SBA Mass is a community of support for a large group of Massachusetts residents who sometimes need an empathetic ear or a
voice of advocacy. They are staffed entirely be volunteers dedicated to supporting their mission.

Ellen Heffernan-Dugan, LIOSOW, Operations Associate
Cara Packard, President
Matt Neal, Vice Chair and Treasurer

Michigan

6837 Spina Bifida Association of Upper Peninsula Michigan
1220 N 3rd Street
Ishpeming, MI 49849   906-485-5127
                                      cbengson@chartermi.net
                                      sba-up.8m.com

Providing support to those affected by spina bifida.

Lois Bengson, President

6838 Spina Bifida Association of West Michigan
235 Wealthy SE
Grand Rapids, MI 49503   616-949-3428
                                      wmisbo@gmail.com
                                      www.wmspinabifida.org/

Providing support to those afflicted with spina bifida.

Carol Carpenter, Interim President

Minnesota

6839 Spina Bifida Association of Minnesota
PO Box 29323
Brooklyn Center, MN 55429   651-222-6395
                                      Fax: 651-228-0914
                                      sbamn@hotmail.com
                                      www.sbamn.org

Providing support to those afflicted with spina bifida.

James Thayer, Executive Director

Mississippi

6840 Spina Bifida Association of Mississippi
PO Box 180594
Richland, MS 39218   601-420-0030
                                      Fax: 601-420-0300
                                      sbafms@yahoo.com
                                      www.spinabifidams.com

Providing support to those afflicted with spina bifida.

Amy Wilkinson, Executive Director

Missouri

6841 Spina Bifida Association of Greater Saint Louis
9201 Watson Road, Suite 125
Crestwood, MO 63126   314-843-2244
                                      800-784-0983
                                      Fax: 314-765-6246
                                      sbastl@charter.net
                                      www.sbstl.com

Providing support to those afflicted with spina bifida.

Mark Abbott, Chairman

Nebraska

6842 Spina Bifida Association of Nebraska
7612 Maple St
Omaha, NE 68134   402-572-3570
                                      Fax: 402-572-3002
                                      sbamom@cox.net
                                      www.spinabifidanebraska.org

Providing support to those afflicted with spina bifida.

Megan Sorensen, President

New Jersey

6843 Spina Bifida Association of the Tri-State Region
84 Park Avenue
Flemington, NJ 08822   908-782-7475
                                      Fax: 908-782-6102
                                      info@sbatsr.org
                                      www.sbatsr.org

Serves New Jersey, New York metro area and Southern Connecticut. Providing medical, social, and financial support to those afflicted with spina bifida.

Jane Horowitz, Executive Director
Haley Hopper, Director Development

New York

6844 Spina Bifida Association of Albany/Capital District
109 Spring Road
Scotia, NY 12302
518-399-9151
Sbaalbany102@aol.com
www.sbaalbany.org

Providing support to those afflicted with spina bifida.

Karen Wentworth, Director

6845 Spina Bifida Association of Greater Roches ter
PO Box 3
Fairport, NY 14450
585-388-7450
pritch50@yahoo.com
www.sbaa.com

Providing support to those afflicted with spina bifida.

Mary Pritchard, Manager

6846 Spina Bifida Association of Nassau County
12 Hampton Rd
South Beach, NY 11789
631-821-9028
kid3418@optonline.net
www.sbancny.org

Providing support to those afflicted with spina bifida.

Leslieann Sussman, President

6847 Spina Bifida Association of Western New York
137 Warner Ave
N Tonawanda, NY 14120
716-446-5595
Fax: 716-735-7561
pmorris@sbawny.org
www.sbawny.org

Providing support to those living with spina bifida.

Cynthia Carlson, President

North Carolina

6848 Spina Bifida Association of North Carolina
3915 Grace Court
Indian Trail, NC 28079
800-847-2262
Fax: 800-847-2262
sbanc@mindspring.com
sbanc.home.mindspring.com

Providing support to those afflicted with spina bifida. There are five regional support groups in the state.

Kim Gates, Charlotte/Piedmont Contact
Jolyne Wagner, Raleigh Area Contact

Ohio

6849 Spina Bifida Association of Canton
PO Box 9024
Canton, OH 44711
330-863-2531
cmgriffin@neo.rr.com
www.sbacanton.org

Providing support to those afflicted with spina bifida.

Connie Griffin, President

6850 Spina Bifida Association of Central Ohio
7574 Danbridge Way
Westerville, OH 43082
614-818-3840
lauriedvm@sbcglobal.net
www.sbaco.blogspot.com

Providing support to those afflicted with spina bifida.

Laurie Schulze, President

6851 Spina Bifida Association of Cincinnati
644 Linn Street, Suite 635
Cincinnati, OH 45203
513-923-1378
sbacincy@excel.com
www.sbacincy.org

Providing support to those afflicted with spina bifida.

Diane Burns, President

6852 Spina Bifida Association of Greater Dayton
4801 Springfield St
Dayton, OH 45431
937-236-1122
Fax: 937-434-4899
sbadayton@yahoo.com
www.sbadayton.org

Providing support to those afflicted with spina bifida.

David Skinner, President

6853 Spina Bifida Association of North West Ohio
302 Conant St., Suite C
Maumee, OH 43537
419-794-0561
jobrien@sbanwo.org
www.sbaofnorthwestohio.org

Providing support to those afflicted with spina bifida.

Mindy Gallant, Chair
Christina Fulton, Vice Chair
Jennifer O'Brien, Executive Director

6854 Spina Bifida Association of Tri-County Ohio
PO Box 8701
Warren, OH 44484
330-793-8544
jchappel@sbcglobal.net
www.spaa.org

Providing support to those living with spina bifida, from youth into adulthood. Also places an emphasis on parent support groups.

Julie Solomon, President

Pennsylvania

6855 Spina Bifida Association Pittsburgh
4590 MacArthur Blvd., NW, Suite 250
Washington, DC 20007
202-944-3285
Fax: 202-944-3295
sbaa@sbaa.org
www.spinabifidaassociation.org

Providing medical, social, and financial support to those afflicted with spina bifida.

Shannon Williams, President

6856 Spina Bifida Association of Delaware Valley
PO Box 1235
Havertown, PA 19803
610-584-5530
800-223-0222
info@sbadv.org
www.sbadv.org

Providing medical, social, and financial support to those living with spina bifida.

Keri Mascaro, President

6857 Spina Bifida Association of Greater Pennsy lvania
215 E State St, Suite D
Quarryville, PA 17566
717-786-9280
Fax: 717-786-8821
SBAofPA@aol.com
spinabifidaresource.weebly.com

Providing medical, social, and financial support to those afflicted with spina bifida.

Patricia Fulvio, Executive Director

Tennessee

6858 Spina Bifida Association of Tennessee
4590 MacArthur Blvd., NW, Suite 250
Washington, DC 20007
202-944-3285
Fax: 202-944-3295
sbaa@sbaa.org
www.spinabifidaassociation.org

Providing medical, social, and financial support to those living with spina bifida.

Lynn Hess, President

Texas

6859 Spina Bifida Association of Houston-Gulf Coast
440 Benmar Suite 3052
Houston, TX 77060
281-447-2707
Fax: 281-997-2378
president@sbahgc.org
www.sbahgc.org

Providing medical, social, and financial support to those afflicted with spina bifida.

Jennifer Franklin, Vice President
Joan Peck, Treasurer
Michelle Lockstedt, Secretary, Fundraising

6860 Spina Bifida Association of North Texas
705 Ave B, Suite 204
Garland, TX 75040
972-238-8755
Fax: 214-703-1981
sbnorthtexas@aol.com
www.spinabifidant.org/?

Providing medical, social, and financial support to those living with spina bifida.

Carol Barrett, Contact

6861 Spina Bifida Association of Texas
1550 NE Loop 410, Suite 224
San Antonio, TX 78209
210-826-7289
866-597-2289
sbinfo@sbatx.org
www.sbatx.org

Providing medical, social, and financial support to those afflicted with spina bifida.

Nora Oyler, Executive Director

Utah

6862 Spina Bifida Association of Utah
900 S 1500 East, Apt C124
Clearfield, UT 84015
801-214-8070
support@utahspinabifida.org
www.utahspinabifida.org/

Providing medical, social, and financial support to those living with spina bifida.

Ilene Hall, President

Virginia

6863 Spina Bifida Association of the Roanoke Valley
PO Box 7652
Roanoke, VA 24019
540-342-1231
Fax: 540-890-1244
sbaroanokevalley@yahoo.com
www.sbarv.org

Providing medical, social, and financial support to those living with spina bifida.

Millie Wilson, President

Washington

6864 Evergreen Spina Bifida Association
611 2nd street, Suite A
Snohomish, WA 98290
253-589-3700
sbaws@yahoo.com
www.sbaws.org/?

Providing medical, social, and financial support to those afflicted with spina bifida.

Ed Kennedy, President

Wisconsin

6865 Spina Bifida Association of Greater Fox Valley
4590 MacArthur Blvd., NW, Suite 250
Washington, DC 20007
202-944-3285
Fax: 202-944-3295
sbaa@sbaa.org
www.spinabifidaassociation.org

Providing support to those living with spina bifida.

Kelly Richard

6866 Spina Bifida Association of Northern Wisconsin
PO Box 421
Schofield, WI 54476
715-359-9674
dtackley@cheqnet.net

Providing medical, social, and financial support to those afflicted with spina bifida.

David Bouchard, President

6867 Spina Bifida Association of Wisconsin
830 N 109th Street, Suite 6
Wauwatosa, WI 53226
414-607-9061
Fax: 414-607-9602
sbawi@sbawi.org
www.sbawi.org

SBAWI is made up of those with spina bifida, as well as family, friends and health care providers. The association is dedicated to helping its membership emotionally, educationally, and financially.

Karen Drzewiecki, President
James B. Hanley, Secretary
Alexandria Sluis, Treasurer

Conferences

6868 SBA National Conference
Spina Bifida Association
4590 MacArthur Boulevard NW, Suite 250
Washington, DC 20007
202-944-3285
800-621-3141
Fax: 202-944-3295
sbaa@sbaa.org
www.spinabifidaassociation.org

Children and adults with Spina Bifida, their families, physicians, nurses, and other clinicians have the unique opportunity to gain information on the latest medical care and network on various issues which affect their lives and professions.

June

Cindy Brownstein, CEO

Audio Video

6869 Challenge
Spina Bifida Association
1600 Wilson Blvd., Suite 800
Arlington, VA 22209
202-944-3285
800-621-3141
Fax: 202-944-3295
sbaa@sbaa.org
www.spinabifidaassociation.org

A human look of how people come to grips with and overcome the challenges related to living with Spina Bifida.

1992 14 minutes

Sara Struwe, President/ CEO
Elizabeth Merck, Director of Development
Lisa Raman, Director

| **Web Sites** | **Book Publishers** |

6870 Association for Spina Bifida and Hydroceph alus
www.asbah.org

A UK charity that provides information and advice to those with spina bifida and their families.

6871 Children with Spina Bifida: A Resource Page for Parents
www.waisman.wisc.edu/~rowley/sb-kids/

rowley@waisman.wisc.edu
www.waisman.wisc.edu/~rowley/sb-kids/

A resource page for parents with children with Spina Bifida.

6872 International Federation for Spina Bifida and Hydrocephalus
Cellebroersstraat 16/Rue des Alexiens 16
Brussels, B-100   32 -0 2-502
info@ifglobal.org
www.ifglobal.org

The world-wide umbrella organization for spina bifida and hydracephalus organizations. It's primary goal is prevention through the dissemination of information and education.

Margo Whiteford, President
Jackie Bland, Treasurer
Lieven Bauwens, Secretary General

6873 LFSN: Lipomyelomeningecele Family Support Network
www.lfsn.org

A network of families providing support and information sharing to those affected by Occult Spinal Dysraphisms.

6874 March of Dimes Birth Defects Foundation
1275 Mamaroneck Avenue
White Plains, NY 10605   914-997-4488
www.marchofdimes.org

March of Dimes researchers, colunteers, educators, outreach workers and advocates work together to give all babies a fighting chance against the threats to their health: prematurity, birth defects, low birthweight.

6875 Online Mendelian Inheritance in Man
www.omim.org

This database is a catalog of human genes and genetic disorders.

6876 Spina Bifida Association of America
1600 Wilson Blvd., Suite 800
Arlington, VA 22209   202-944-3285
Fax: 202-944-3295
sbaa@sbaa.org
www.spinabifidaassociation.org

The mission is to promote the prevention os spina bifida and to enhance the lives of all affected. The association was founded to address the specific needs of the spina bifida community and serves as the national representative of almost 60 chapters. SBAA's efforts benefit thousands of infants, children, adults, parents and professionals each year.

Sara Struwe, President/ CEO
Elizabeth Merck, Director of Development
Lisa Raman, Director

6877 Wheeless' Textbook of Orthopaedics
www.wheelessonline.com

Derives from a variety of sources, imcluding journals, articles, national meetings lectures and other textbooks.

Clifford R. Wheeless, III, M.D., Author

6878 All Kinds of Friends, Even Green!

Ellen B Sensi, author

Spina Bifida Association
4590 MacArthur Boulevard NW, Suite 250
Washington, DC 20007   202-944-3285
800-621-3141
Fax: 202-944-3295
sbaa@sbaa.org
www.spinabifidaassociation.org

Moses has spina bifida and a lot of friends. Which one will he choose to write about for his school project?

Cindy Brownstein, President & CEO
Sara Struwe, Chief Operating Officer & Director
Christopher Vance, Director of Development

6879 Answering Your Questions About Spina Bifida
Spina Bifida Association
4590 MacArthur Boulevard NW, Suite 250
Washington, DC 20007   202-944-3285
800-621-3141
Fax: 202-944-3295
sbaa@sbaa.org
www.spinabifidaassociation.org

Provides information to help people understand the basic medical, educational and social issues which commonly affect people with Spina Bifida.

Cindy Brownstein, President & CEO
Sara Struwe, Chief Operating Officer & Director
Christopher Vance, Director of Development

6880 Bowel Continence and Spina Bifida
Spina Bifida Association
4590 MacArthur Boulevard NW, Suite 250
Washington, DC 20007   202-944-3285
800-621-3141
Fax: 202-944-3295
sbaa@sbaa.org
www.spinabifidaassociation.org

An excellent book aimed at anyone (infant or adult) trying to attain bowel continence. Focuses on continence programs, bowel management development and includes a chart and glossary of terms.

Cindy Brownstein, President & CEO
Sara Struwe, Chief Operating Officer & Director
Christopher Vance, Director of Development

6881 Children with Spina Bifida: A Parent's Gui de
Spina Bifida Association
4590 MacArthur Boulevard NW, Suite 250
Washington, DC 20007   202-944-3285
800-621-3141
Fax: 202-944-3295
sbaa@sbaa.org
www.spinabifidaassociation.org

Comprehensive publication provides easy-to-understand coverage of neurosurgery, physical therapy, emotional health, education, urological concerns, orthopedic concerns, childhood development and more. Valuable for parents, educators and libraries.

Cindy Brownstein, President & CEO
Sara Struwe, Chief Operating Officer & Director
Christopher Vance, Director of Development

6882 Complete IEP Guide: How to Advocate for Your Special Ed Child
Spina Bifida Association
4590 MacArthur Boulevard NW, Suite 250
Washington, DC 20007   202-944-3285
800-621-3141
Fax: 202-944-3295
sbaa@sbaa.org
www.spinabifidaassociation.org

This all-in-one guide will help you understand special education law, identify your child's needs, prepare for meetings, develop the IEP and resolve disputes.

Cindy Brownstein, President & CEO
Sara Struwe, Chief Operating Officer & Director
Christopher Vance, Director of Development

6883 Confronting the Challenges of Spina Bifida
Spina Bifida Association
4590 MacArthur Boulevard NW, Suite 250
Washington, DC 20007   202-944-3285
                                        800-621-3141
                                        Fax: 202-944-3295
                                        sbaa@sbaa.org
                                        www.spinabifidaassociation.org

A group curriculum addressing self-care, self-esteem, and social skills in eight to 13 year olds.

Cindy Brownstein, President & CEO
Sara Struwe, Chief Operating Officer & Director
Christopher Vance, Director of Development

6884 Congenital Disorders Sourcebook
Omnigraphics
PO Box 8002
Aston, PA 19014   800-234-1340
                                        Fax: 800-875-1340
                                        info@omnigraphics.com
                                        www.omnigraphics.com

Basic consumer health information on disorders aquired during gestation, including spina bifida, hydrocephalus, cerebral palsy, heart defects, craniofacial abnormalities and fetal alcohol syndrome.

650 pages
ISBN: 0-780809-45-9

Peter Ruffner, Publisher

6885 Featherless/Desplumado
Juan Felipe Herrera, author

Spina Bifida Association
4590 MacArthur Boulevard NW, Suite 250
Washington, DC 20007   202-944-3285
                                        800-621-3141
                                        Fax: 202-944-3295
                                        sbaa@sbaa.org
                                        www.spinabifidaassociation.org

Tomasito, although confined to a wheelchair, feels free when on the soccer field.

Cindy Brownstein, President & CEO
Sara Struwe, Chief Operating Officer & Director
Christopher Vance, Director of Development

6886 Friends No Matter What
Rose Blivins, author

Spina Bifida Association
4590 MacArthur Boulevard NW, Suite 250
Washington, DC 20007   202-944-3285
                                        800-621-3141
                                        Fax: 202-944-3295
                                        sbaa@sbaa.org
                                        www.spinabifidaassociation.org

The story of two boys, one in a wheelchair and one who loves to play basketball. How will it work out?

Cindy Brownstein, President & CEO
Sara Struwe, Chief Operating Officer & Director
Christopher Vance, Director of Development

6887 Guidelines for Spina Bifida and Health Car e Services Throughout Life
Spina Bifida Association
4590 MacArthur Boulevard NW, Suite 250
Washington, DC 20007   202-944-3285
                                        800-621-3141
                                        Fax: 202-944-3295
                                        sbaa@sbaa.org
                                        www.spinabifidaassociation.org

Guidelines designed to help spina bifida sufferers throughout their entire lives.

Cindy Brownstein, President & CEO
Sara Struwe, Chief Operating Officer & Director
Christopher Vance, Director of Development

6888 Introduction to Spina Bifida
Spina Bifida Association
4590 MacArthur Boulevard NW, Suite 250
Washington, DC 20007   202-944-3285
                                        800-621-3141
                                        Fax: 202-944-3295
                                        sbaa@sbaa.org
                                        www.spinabifidaassociation.org

An aid and guide for those who care for someone with spina bifida, written in non-medical terms and language.

Cindy Brownstein, President & CEO
Sara Struwe, Chief Operating Officer & Director
Christopher Vance, Director of Development

6889 Looking for Goodwill
Patt & Scott Price, author

Spina Bifida Association
4590 MacArthur Boulevard NW, Suite 250
Washington, DC 20007   202-944-3285
                                        800-621-3141
                                        Fax: 202-944-3295
                                        sbaa@sbaa.org
                                        www.spinabifidaassociation.org

An inspirational read, the result of a trek across the US and random interviews showing the heart and attitude of America.

Cindy Brownstein, President & CEO
Sara Struwe, Chief Operating Officer & Director
Christopher Vance, Director of Development

6890 Negotiating the Special Education Maze: A Guide for Parents and Teachers
Spina Bifida Association
4590 MacArthur Boulevard NW, Suite 250
Washington, DC 20007   202-944-3285
                                        800-621-3141
                                        Fax: 202-944-3295
                                        sbaa@sbaa.org
                                        www.spinabifidaassociation.org

An excellent aid for the development of an effective special education program.

Cindy Brownstein, President & CEO
Sara Struwe, Chief Operating Officer & Director
Christopher Vance, Director of Development

6891 New Language of Toys: Teaching Communicati on Skills to Children with Special Needs
Spina Bifida Association
4590 MacArthur Boulevard NW, Suite 250
Washington, DC 20007   202-944-3285
                                        800-621-3141
                                        Fax: 202-944-3295
                                        sbaa@sbaa.org
                                        www.spinabifidaassociation.org

A guide for parents and teachers, this reader-friendly resource guide provides a wealth of information on how play activities affect a child's language development (with a focus on special needs) and where to get the toys and materials to use in these activities.

Cindy Brownstein, President & CEO
Sara Struwe, Chief Operating Officer & Director
Christopher Vance, Director of Development

6892 Nick Joins In

Joe Lasker, author

Spina Bifida Association
4590 MacArthur Boulevard NW, Suite 250
Washington, DC 20007   202-944-3285
                                        800-621-3141
                                   Fax: 202-944-3295
                                        sbaa@sbaa.org
                         www.spinabifidaassociation.org

When Nick, who is in a wheelchair, enters a regular classroom, for the first time he realizes that he has much to contribute.

Cindy Brownstein, President & CEO
Sara Struwe, Chief Operating Officer & Director
Christopher Vance, Director of Development

6893 Rolling Along with Goldilocks and the Three Bears

Cindy Meyers, author

Spina Bifida Association
4590 MacArthur Boulevard NW, Suite 250
Washington, DC 20007   202-944-3285
                                        800-621-3141
                                   Fax: 202-944-3295
                                        sbaa@sbaa.org
                         www.spinabifidaassociation.org

The familiar folktale with a special-needs twist.

Cindy Brownstein, President & CEO
Sara Struwe, Chief Operating Officer & Director
Christopher Vance, Director of Development

6894 SPINAbilities: A Young Person's Guide to Spina Bifida

Spina Bifida Association
4590 MacArthur Boulevard NW, Suite 250
Washington, DC 20007   202-944-3285
                                        800-621-3141
                                   Fax: 202-944-3295
                                        sbaa@sbaa.org
                         www.spinabifidaassociation.org

Practical suggestions and tips for young people on becoming independent and managing their healthcare.

Cindy Brownstein, President & CEO
Sara Struwe, Chief Operating Officer & Director
Christopher Vance, Director of Development

6895 Sexuality and the Person with Spinabifida

Stephen Sloan PhD, author

Spina Bifida Association
4590 MacArthur Boulevard NW, Suite 250
Washington, DC 20007   202-944-3285
                                        800-621-3141
                                   Fax: 202-944-3295
                                        sbaa@sbaa.org
                         www.spinabifidaassociation.org

Focuses on sexuality, sexual development, sexual activity, and other important issues.

Cindy Brownstein, President & CEO
Sara Struwe, Chief Operating Officer & Director
Christopher Vance, Director of Development

6896 Steps to Independence: Teaching Everyday Skills to Children with Special Needs

Spina Bifida Association
4590 MacArthur Boulevard NW, Suite 250
Washington, DC 20007   202-944-3285
                                        800-621-3141
                                   Fax: 202-944-3295
                                        sbaa@sbaa.org
                         www.spinabifidaassociation.org

A guide to help parents teach life skills to their disabled child.

Cindy Brownstein, President & CEO
Sara Struwe, Chief Operating Officer & Director
Christopher Vance, Director of Development

6897 Teaching Students with Spina Bifida

BOSC Books-Books on Special Children
PO Box 3378
Amherst, MA 01004   413-256-8164
                                   Fax: 413-256-8896
                                        www.boscbooks.com

Explores the vital issues of concern to students with spina bifida including aspects of their social, personal and cognitive development. The book is sensitively written and abounds with useful tips covering such things as crutch storage, work space organization, etc.

460 pages Softcover

6898 Unlocking Potential: College and Other Choices for People with LD and AD/HD

Spina Bifida Association
4590 MacArthur Boulevard NW, Suite 250
Washington, DC 20007   202-944-3285
                                        800-621-3141
                                   Fax: 202-944-3295
                                        sbaa@sbaa.org
                         www.spinabifidaassociation.org

An indispensible tool for high school students with learning disabilities and AD/HD. Includes a comprehensive listing of resources.

Cindy Brownstein, President & CEO
Sara Struwe, Chief Operating Officer & Director
Christopher Vance, Director of Development

6899 Views from Our Shoes: Growing Up with a Brother or Sister with Special Needs

Spina Bifida Association
4590 MacArthur Boulevard NW, Suite 250
Washington, DC 20007   202-944-3285
                                        800-621-3141
                                   Fax: 202-944-3295
                                        sbaa@sbaa.org
                         www.spinabifidaassociation.org

A balanced view of the positives and negatives of living with a disabled sibling. Written for siblings ages nine and up.

Cindy Brownstein, President & CEO
Sara Struwe, Chief Operating Officer & Director
Christopher Vance, Director of Development

Newsletters

6900 Insights into Spina Bifida

Spina Bifida Association
1600 Wilson Blvd., Suite 800
Arlington, VA 22209   202-944-3285
                                        800-621-3141
                                   Fax: 202-944-3295
                                        sbaa@sbaa.org
                         www.spinabifidaassociation.org

Includes articles on the latest research, legislation, features, emotional aspects, educational information, and information on the Association's national conference.

Bimonthly

Sara Struwe, President/ CEO
Elizabeth Merck, Director of Development
Lisa Raman, Director

Pamphlets

6901 Educational Issues Among Children With Spina Bifida

Spina Bifida Association
1600 Wilson Blvd., Suite 800
Arlington, VA 22209   202-944-3285
                                        800-621-3141
                                   Fax: 202-944-3295
                                        sbaa@sbaa.org
                         www.spinabifidaassociation.org

Sara Struwe, President/ CEO
Elizabeth Merck, Director of Development
Lisa Raman, Director

6902 Learning Among Children with Spina Bifida
Spina Bifida Association
1600 Wilson Blvd., Suite 800
Arlington, VA 22209

202-944-3285
800-621-3141
Fax: 202-944-3295
sbaa@sbaa.org
www.spinabifidaassociation.org

Sara Struwe, President/ CEO
Elizabeth Merck, Director of Development
Lisa Raman, Director

6903 Monetary Allowance, Health Care and Vocational Training & Rehabilitation
National Veterans Services Fund
PO Box 2465
Darien, CT 06820

203-656-0003
800-521-0198
Fax: 203-656-1957
nvsf@NVSF.org
www.nvsf.org

Monetary allowance, health care, vocational training and rehabilitation for Vietnam Veterans' children with spine bifida.

Pamphlet

6904 SBAA General Information Brochure
Spina Bifida Association
1600 Wilson Blvd., Suite 800
Arlington, VA 22209

202-944-3285
800-621-3141
Fax: 202-944-3295
sbaa@sbaa.org
www.spinabifidaassociation.org

Sara Struwe, President/ CEO
Elizabeth Merck, Director of Development
Lisa Raman, Director

6905 SBAA General Information Packet
Spina Bifida Association
1600 Wilson Blvd., Suite 800
Arlington, VA 22209

202-944-3285
800-621-3141
Fax: 202-944-3295
sbaa@sbaa.org
www.spinabifidaassociation.org

Sara Struwe, President/ CEO
Elizabeth Merck, Director of Development
Lisa Raman, Director

6906 Social Development and the Person With Spina Bifida
Spina Bifida Association
1600 Wilson Blvd., Suite 800
Arlington, VA 22209

202-944-3285
800-621-3141
Fax: 202-944-3295
sbaa@sbaa.org
www.spinabifidaassociation.org

20 pages

Sara Struwe, President/ CEO
Elizabeth Merck, Director of Development
Lisa Raman, Director

6907 Urologic Care of the Child with Spina Bifida
David Joseph MD, author

Spina Bifida Association
1600 Wilson Blvd., Suite 800
Arlington, VA 22209

202-944-3285
800-621-3141
Fax: 202-944-3295
sbaa@sbaa.org
www.spinabifidaassociation.org

2001

Sara Struwe, President/ CEO
Elizabeth Merck, Director of Development
Lisa Raman, Director

Camps

6908 Camp Boggy Creek
30500 Brantley Branch Road
Eustis, FL 32736

352-483-4200
866-462-6449
Fax: 352-483-0589
info@campboggycreek.org
www.boggycreek.org

A year round camp serving seriously ill children throughout Florida. We offer week-long summer sessions for the children and family retreat weekends for the whole family.

June Clark, President/CEO
David Mann, Camp Director
Kimmy Lamborn, Assistant Camp Director

6909 Camp Oakhurst
111 Monmouth Road
Oakhurst, NJ 7755

732-531-0215
Fax: 732-531-0292
info@nysh.org
www.campoakhurst.com

A summer camp and year round respite program for children and adults with physical disabilities.

Robert Pacenza, Executive Director
Charles Sutherland, Camp Director

6910 Mountaineer Spina Bifida Camp
350 Capital Street
Charleston, WV 800-6

304-558-7098
800-800-642
Fax: 304-558-2866
www.kidscamps.com

The mission is to help children and teens to develop self-esteem, social skills, and self reliance while they participate in recreational and social activities.

DESCRIPTION

6911 SPINAL MUSCULAR ATROPHIES

Synonym: SMA

Covers these related disorders: Fazio-Londe disease (Progressive bulbar palsy of childhood), SMA type I (Werdnig-Hoffmann disease; Acute SMA), SMA type II (Intermediate SMA), SMA type III (Kugelberg-Welander disease)

Involves the following Biologic System(s):
Neurologic Disorders, Orthopedic and Muscle Disorders

The spinal muscular atrophies (SMAs) refer to a group of progressive, inherited neuromuscular disorders characterized by the progressive degeneration of motor neurons. Motor neurons are nerves that originate in the spinal cord and stimulate and control muscle movement (motor neurons). Spinal muscular atrophy type I, also called Werdnig-Hoffmann disease, usually becomes apparent between the second and fourth month of life; however, some infants may have symptoms at birth, including difficult breathing and the inability to feed. Other characteristic symptoms and findings include lack of muscle tone (hypotonia), muscle weakness, the inability to control head movements, absence of tendon stretch reflexes, and uncontrollable twitching or small movements (fasciculations) of the tongue and possibly other muscles. Within two to three years of age, continued breathing and feeding difficulties, along with other progressive problems, may lead to life-threatening complications. Treatment is symptomatic and supportive.

Children with SMA type II usually show signs of progressive muscle weakness of the legs and, to a lesser degree, the arms during the first or second year of life. As the disease progresses, many affected children develop side-to-side curvature of the spine (scoliosis), difficulty swallowing, and a nasal quality to their speech. Children with SMA type II may be severely physically handicapped and are usually of average or above average intelligence. Affected chidren are prone to repeated respiratory infections and breathing difficulties. Life-threatening complications may occur during adolescence or early adulthood.

SMA type III or chronic spinal muscular atrophy may become apparent between the ages of two to 17 years. This is the mildest form of SMA. Progressive weakness associated with chronic SMA is most apparent in the trunk area of the body, especially in the muscles of the shoulder girdle area. There is muscle weakness and loss of muscle mass (atrophy). In addition, deep tendon reflexes may be decreased or absent and muscle twitching (fasciculations) may be present. Some affected children may also have a tremor when the hands are outstretched. Repeated respiratory infections are common.

Fazio-Londe disease, also called progressive bulbar palsy of childhood, is a rare type of spinal muscular atrophy that results from degeneration of motor neurons located, for the most part, in the brain stem. This rare disorder is characterized by progressive palsy or paralysis of the nerves that emerge from the skull (cranial nerves). Symptoms and physical findings associated with Fazio-Londe disease include progressive loss of muscle mass (atrophy) and paralysis of the muscles of the tongue, mouth, lips, throat (pharynx), and voice box (larynx).

A team approach involving specialists such as neurologists, orthopedists, and physical therapists, in cooperation with parents or caregivers, may be helpful in providing care for children with spinal muscular atrophies. Other treatment is symptomatic and supportive.

SMA is usually inherited as an autosomal recessive trait, although some cases of autosomal dominant transmission have been reported. This disorder occurs in approximately one out of every 25,000 births. The genes for SMA types I, II, and III seem to be related and are located on the long arm of chromosome 5 (5q11-13).

National Associations & Support Groups

6912 American Academy of Pediatrics
141 Northwest Point Boulevard
Elk Grove Village, IL 60007
847-434-4000
800-433-9016
Fax: 847-434-8000
www.aap.org

The American Academy of Pediatrics and its member pediatricians are committed to the attainment of optimal physical, mental and social health and well-being for all infants, children, adolescents, and young adults.

Fernando Stein, MD, FAAP, President
Karen Remley, MD, CEO/Executive VP

6913 Families of Spinal Muscular Atrophy
925 Busse Road
Elk Grove Village, IL 60007
847-367-7620
800-886-1762
Fax: 847-357-7623
info@fsma.org
www.fsma.org

Families of SMA was founded for the purpose of encouraging support and raising funds to promote research into the causes and cure of spinal muscular atrophy. Funds are specifically directed to scientific, educational, or literary purposes in keeping with a charitable organization. It has more than 24 chapters worldwide and over 5000 member families.

Kenneth Hobby, President
Jill Jarecki, Research Director
Karen O'Brien, General Information

6914 Fight SMA / Andrew's Buddies
1807 Libbie Ave, Suite 104
Richmond, VA 23226
804-515-0080
Fax: 804-515-0081
heatherlennon@fightsma.com
www.fightsma.org/?

Corporation with 15 US chapters that works to raise awareness of SMA and accelerate treatment and a cure.

Martha Slay, President
Sarah Williams, Treasurer

6915 Genetic Alliance
4301 Connecticut Avenue NW, Suite 404
Washington, DC 20008
202-966-5557
800-336-4363
Fax: 202-966-8553
info@geneticalliance.org
www.geneticalliance.org

A coalition of voluntary genetic support groups, consumers and professionals addressing the needs of individuals and families affected by genetic disorders from a national perspective.

Sharon Terry, President/CEO
Tetyana Murza, Managing Director
Natasha Bonhomme, VP, Strategic Development

6916 March of Dimes Foundation
1275 Mamaroneck Avenue
White Plains, NY 10605 914-428-7100
888-663-4637
Fax: 914-428-8203
resourcecenter@marchofdimes.com
www.marchofdimes.com

Partnership of volunteers and professionals dedicated to improving the health of babies by preventing birth defects and infant mortality. Over 100 chapters are located across the country and can be located through the national office.

Stacey D. Stewart, President

6917 Muscular Dystrophy Association
3300 E Sunrise Drive
Tucson, AZ 85718 520-529-2000
800-572-1717
Fax: 520-529-5300
mda@mdausa.org
www.mda.org

The MDA is a voluntary health agency, and a partnership between scientists and concerned citizens, aimed at conquering neuromuscular diseases affecting more than 1 million Americans. MDA works worldwide with research, medical, and community programs, and supports more research on neuromuscular diseases than any other private-sector organization in the world.

Robert Ross, CEO

6918 Spinal Muscular Atrophy Coalition (SMA Coalition)
119 W 72nd Street, PO Box 187
New York, NY 10023 646-253-7100
Fax: 212-247-3079
info@smafoundation.org
www.smafoundation.org

A group of nonprofit organizations that stand together to raise awareness and advocate for progress towards the treatment and cure of SMA.

6919 Spinal Muscular Atrophy Foundation
119 W 72nd St, #187
New York, NY 10023 646-253-7100
Fax: 212-247-3079
info@smafoundation.org
www.smafoundation.org
Loren Eng, President
Cynthia Joyce, Executive Director
Yevgeniy Izrayelit, Operations Manager

State Agencies & Support Groups

Arizona

6920 Families of SMA - Arizona Chapter
P.O. Box 43861 Phoenix
Phoenix, AZ 85080 602-314-4902
arizona@fsma.org
www.fsma.org
Angel Wolff, President

California

6921 Families of SMA - Northern California Chapter
PO Box 9014
Santa Rosa, CA 95405 707-571-8990
ncalif@fsma.org
www.fsma.org

David Sereni, President

Connecticut

6922 Families of SMA - Connecticut Chapter
PO Box 124
Rowayton, CT 06853 203-288-1488
800-866-1762
conn@fsma.org
www.fsma.org

Jonathan Goldsberry, President

Indiana

6923 SMA Support Inc
PO Box 6301
Kokomo, IN 46904 765-688-0247
Fax: 801-460-2813
www.smasupport.com
Laura Stants, Contact

New York

6924 Families of SMA - Long Island NY Chapter
PO Box 322
Rockville Center, NY 11571 516-214-0348
greaterny@fsma.org
www.fsma.org
Debbie Cuevas, President

Tennessee

6925 Families of SMA - Tennessee Chapter
PO Box 7025
Knoxville, TN 37921 865-945-7636
tennessee@fsma.org
www.fsma.org
Sarah Boggess, President

Research Centers

6926 SMA Research Group
Stanford University School of Medicine
300 Pasteur Dr, Rm A343
Stanford, CA 94305 650-723-6469
Fax: 650-320-9443
mitzine@stanford.edu
neurology.stanford.edu

SMA clinical trials.

Mitzine Wright, Resident & Fellowship Coordinator
Chris Hopkins, Clerkship & Grand Rounds Coordinato
Diane Madsen, Administrative Associate to the Cha

6927 Spinal Muscular Atrophy Clinic
Columbia Pediatric Neuromuscular Disease Ctr
180 Ft Washington Ave, Harkness Pavilion, Ste 525
New York, NY 10032 212-342-0263
Fax: 212-342-2893
kidsmda@columbia.edu
www.columbiasma.org

Dr Darryl De Vivo, Director
Dr Petra Kaufmann, Associate Director
Leslie Disla, Clinic Coordinator

6928 Spinal Muscular Atrophy Project
NINDS
PO Box 5801
Bethesda, MD 20824 301-496-5751
800-352-9424
smaproject-fd@saic.com
www.smaproject.org

Research program established by NINDS (National Institute of Neurological Disorders and Stroke) as a model of developing a safe and effective treatment for SMA. The program adopts the methods used by the pharmaceutical industry to carry out drug discovery according to accepted standards.

Audio Video

6929 Living with SMA
Families of SMA
925 Busse Rd
Elk Grove Village, IL 60007
847-367-7620
800-886-1762
Fax: 847-357-7623
info@curesma.org
www.curesma.org

Tapes 3 and 4 are available and are part of the Living with SMA video series. Overview of Type II and Type III/Kennedy's.

18 pages

Kenneth Hobby, President
Jill Jarecki, PhD, Research Director
Colleen McCarthy O'Toole, Family Support Director

Web Sites

6930 Families of Spinal Muscular Atrophy
925 Busse Rd
Elk Grove Village, IL 60007
800-886-1762
info@curesma.org
www.curesma.org

Families of SMA was founded for the purpose of encouraging support and raising funds to promote research into the causes and cure of spinal muscular atrophy.

Kenneth Hobby, President
Jill Jarecki, PhD, Research Director
Colleen McCarthy O'Toole, Family Support Director

6931 Online Mendelian Inheritance in Man
www.omim.org

This database is a catalog of human genes and genetic disorders.

6932 Spinal Muscular Atrophy Information Page
Office of Communications and Public Liaison, NINDS
Bethesda, MD 20892
301-496-5751
800-352-9424
www.ninds.nih.gov/disorders/sma/
Walter J. Koroshetz, M.D., Acting Director
Alan L. Willard, Ph.D., Acting Deputy Director
Caroline Lewis, Executive Officer

6933 Spinal Muscular Atrophy Project
www.smaproject.org

Research program established by NINDS (National Institute of Neurological Disorders and Stroke) as a model of developing a safe and effective treatment for SMA. The program adopts the methods used by the pharmaceutical industry to carry out drug discovery according to accepted standards.

Newsletters

6934 Compass
Families of SMA
925 Busse Rd
Elk Grove Village, IL 60007
847-367-7620
800-886-1762
Fax: 847-357-7623
info@curesma.org
www.curesma.org

Newsletter dedicated solely to SMA research updates and information.

42 pages Quarterly

Kenneth Hobby, President
Jill Jarecki, PhD, Research Director
Colleen McCarthy O'Toole, Family Support Director

6935 Directions
Families of SMA
925 Busse Rd
Elk Grove Village, IL 60007
847-367-7620
800-886-1762
Fax: 847-357-7623
info@curesma.org
www.curesma.org

32 pages Quarterly

Kenneth Hobby, President
Jill Jarecki, PhD, Research Director
Colleen McCarthy O'Toole, Family Support Director

6936 SMA Newsletter
Columbia Pediatric Neuromuscular Disease Ctr
Harkness Pavilion, Floor 5, 180 Fort Washington Av
New York, NY 10032
212-342-0263
Fax: 212-342-2893
kidsmda@columbia.edu
www.columbiasma.org

Research updates, upcoming events and conferences, news, and a kids page.

Jessica Rascoll DPT, Newsletter Contact
Dr. Darryl C. De Vivo, Director

Pamphlets

6937 Facts About Spinal Muscular Atrophy
Muscular Dystrophy Association
222 S. Riverside Plaza, Suite 1500
Chicago, IL 60606
520-529-2000
800-572-1717
Fax: 520-529-5300
publications@mdausa.org
mda.org/publications/facts-about-spinal-muscular-atr

Covers the four forms of the disease and outlines the characteristics and genetic patterns of the SMAs. Research efforts aimed at finding the causes, treatments, and cures are also described. Online and in Spanish.

2003

Kristine Welker, Interim President/CEO
Valerie A. Cwik, MD, EVP, Chief Medical & Scientific
Julie Faber, EVP, CFO

6938 Understanding SMA
Families of SMA
925 Busse Rd
Elk Grove Village, IL 60007
847-367-7620
800-886-1762
Fax: 847-357-7623
info@curesma.org
www.curesma.org

This booklet is for the educaton and support of those with SMA.

18 pages

Kenneth Hobby, President
Jill Jarecki, PhD, Research Director
Colleen McCarthy O'Toole, Family Support Director

DESCRIPTION

6939 STRABISMUS

Synonyms: Heterotropia, Manifest deviation, Squint

Covers these related disorders: Accommodation strabismus, Nonparalytic strabismus, Paralytic strabismus

Involves the following Biologic System(s):

Neurologic Disorders, Ophthalmologic Disorders, Orthopedic and Muscle Disorders

Strabismus refers to a condition in which the eyes are not aligned properly in relation to each other and are focused on different objects simultaneously. Approximately four percent of all children under six years of age are affected by some form of strabismus. The eye deviations associated with this condition are classified according to the direction of the deviation. An eye that is turned inward is considered esotropic or convergent; an eye turned outward is exotropic or divergent; an eye turned upward is hypertropic; and an eye turned downward is hypotropic. In normal vision, both eyes focus as a unit to produce a single, three-dimensional image. In children with strabismus, the divergent images sent to the brain from the eyes may produce double vision (diplopia). In many cases, the brain will compensate for this error by blocking the image from the deviated eye, often resulting in poor vision or loss of vision in that eye (suppression amblyopia).

The most common type of strabismus is nonparalytic, in which this often-inherited ocular deviation is constant and results from a defect in the actual positioning of the eyes. Approximately 50 percent of individuals with nonparalytic strabismus have one eye turned inward. These inward-turned or esotropic deviations that appear before six months of age are classified as congenital or infantile esotropia. Outward-turned or exotropic deviations, the second most common type of strabismus, usually occur in children between six months and four years of age. Some outward deviations may result from neurologic disorders and craniofacial abnormalities.

Paralytic strabismus results from dysfunction of an eye muscle as the result of ocular muscle paralysis or a deficit of the nerves that supply the muscles. This resultant muscular imbalance causes the degree of deviation in the affected eye to vary as the eyes move.

Farsighted children are at particular risk for developing accommodative strabismus (accommodative esotropia), in which the lens of the eye tries to compensate for blurred images received by the brain by focusing the eyes inward (converging). If the compensation or accommodation demands are too great, some children may develop this additional eye abnormality.

Strabismus may result from many different factors; therefore, medical specialists make every effort to determine and treat the underlying cause as soon as possible after diagnosis. Such factors may include hereditary influences; trauma; neurologic abnormalities resulting from intracranial tumors or weaknesses in the walls of blood vessels in the brain (aneurysms); infection; systemic disorders; blood vessel malformations; structural abnormalities; and association with certain syndromes such as Duane syndrome.

Permanent loss of vision can occur if strabismus and its attendant amblyopia are not treated before age 4 to 6 years. Interventions may include wearing a patch over the normal eye in order to compel the brain to receive images from the affected eye. Patching often improves the vision in the deviating eye. Upon improvement, surgery may be performed to equalize the pull of the eye muscles. Children affected with paralytic strabismus may also benefit from wearing glasses with special lenses (prisms) that deflect light, thus altering positioning of objects seen through the lenses. In addition, children with paralytic strabismus with significant ocular deviation may benefit from eye muscle surgery to improve alignment. Farsighted children with accommodative strabismus may be treated with prescription glasses that lessen the need for ocular accommodation when focusing on objects that are far away. Certain medications in the form of eye drops may also aid in focusing on objects that are nearby. Other treatment is aimed toward the underlying cause of the ocular deviation.

Government Agencies

6940 NIH/National Eye Institute
31 Center Drive MSC 2510
Bethesda, MD 20892
301-496-5248
2020@nei.nih.gov
www.nei.nih.gov

Conducts and supports research that helps prevent and treat eye diseases and other disorders of vision. This research leads to sight-saving treatments, reduces visual impairment and blindness, and improves the quality of life for people of all ages. NEI-supported research has advanced our knowledge of how the eye functions in health and disease.

Paul A Sieving M.D., Ph.D, Director
Dr. Belinda Seto, Deputy Director

National Associations & Support Groups

6941 American Academy of Pediatrics
141 Northwest Point Boulevard
Elk Grove Village, IL 60007
847-434-4000
800-433-9016
Fax: 847-434-8000
www.aap.org

The American Academy of Pediatrics and its member pediatricians are committed to the attainment of optimal physical, mental and social health and well-being for all infants, children, adolescents, and young adults.

Fernando Stein, MD, FAAP, President
Karen Remley, MD, CEO/Executive VP

6942 Genetic Alliance
4301 Connecticut Avenue NW, Suite 404
Washington, DC 20008
202-966-5557
800-336-4363
Fax: 202-966-8553
info@geneticalliance.org
www.geneticalliance.org

A coalition of voluntary genetic support groups, consumers and professionals addressing the needs of individuals and families affected by genetic disorders from a national perspective.

Sharon Terry, President/CEO
Tetyana Murza, Managing Director
Natasha Bonhomme, VP, Strategic Development

6943 National Association for Visually Handicapped
111 E 59th St
New York, NY 10022
212-889-3141
800-829-0500
Fax: 212-727-2931
navh@navh.org
www.navh.org

Serves as a clearinghouse for information about all services available to the partially-sighted from public and private sources. Conducts self-help groups. Provides information on large print books, textbooks and educational tools.

Lorianie Marchi, Ceo

Research Centers

6944 Emory Eye Center - Strabismus Research
1365B Clinton Rd NE
Atlanta, GA 30322
404-778-2020
www.eyecenter.emory.edu/clinical_specialties/strabis

Clinical strabismus research.

Anastasios Costarides
Amy K Hutchinson MD

Web Sites

6945 National Association for Visually Handicapped
111 E 59th St
New York, NY 10022
212-821-9497
800-284-4422
kcampbell@lighthouse.org
lighthouse.org

Helps to cope with the difficulties of vision impairment.

6946 Online Mendelian Inheritance in Man
www.omim.org

This database is a catalog of human genes and genetic disorders.

6947 Royal National Institute of the Blind
105 Judd Street
London, WC1H
303-123-9999
www.rnib.org.uk

A leading UK charity offering information, support and advice to over two million people with sight problems.

Wanda Hamilton, Group Director
Fazilet Hadi, Managing Director
Sally Harvey, Managing Director

Book Publishers

6948 Ophthalmic Disorders Sourcebook
Omnigraphics
615 Griswold
Detroit, MI 48226
313-961-1340
800-234-1340
Fax: 313-961-1383
info@omnigraphics.com
www.omnigraphics.com

Basic consumer information about glaucoma, cataracts, macular degeneration, strabismus, refractive disorders and more.

1996 631 pages
ISBN: 0-780800-81-8

Journals

6949 Journal of AAPOS
Elsevier
P.O. Box 193832
San Francisco, CA 94119
415-561-8505
Fax: 415-561-8531
aapos@aao.org
www.jaapos.org

Covers pediatric ophthalmology and strabismus as it affects all groups. Presenting important clinical information on everything from the fundamentals to the finer points of diagnostic problem-solving, the Journal provides a comprehensive view of the field.

6 issues/yr
ISSN: 1091-8531

David G Hunter MD, PhD, Editor-in-Chief
T D Kozachek PhD, Managing Editor

DESCRIPTION

6950 STUTTERING

Involves the following Biologic System(s):

Developmental/Behavioral/Psychiatric Disorders, Neurologic Disorders

Stuttering refers to a type of speech dysfunction that interferes with the normal flow of speech (dysfluency). This dysfunction is characterized by difficulty in uttering certain sounds, letters, syllables, words, or phrases and is usually manifested by frequent hesitations, stumbling, or delay in enunciation, as well as prolongation of certain sounds. As young children develop language skills, they typically experience hesitations in speech as a result of still-developing muscle coordination and limited vocabulary. If excessive attention is given to these temporary speech deficiencies, some children may become self-conscious, anxious, and fearful of speaking. These types of emotional reactions may be manifested as persistent and compulsive movements of certain muscle groups that interfere with the normal flow of speech. Children who stutter may have difficulty with only particular letters, sounds, or words. In addition, the severity of the stutter is often related to the amount of stress evoked by the particular situation. Some affected children and adults may have associated tremors or tics. It is estimated that over three million Americans stutter. Stuttering affects individuals of all ages but occurs most frequently in young children between the ages of 2 and 6 who are developing language. Boys are three times more likely to stutter than girls.

Although most stuttering results from psychological causes, this speech dysfunction may sometimes occur as a result of certain disorders of the central nervous system, neuromuscular abnormalities, or injury to organs related to speech. Stuttering that results from behavioral influences is often self-limited and, in 80 percent of those affected, resolves during childhood.

There are a variety of treatments available for stuttering. Any of the methods may improve stuttering to some degree, but there is at present no cure for stuttering. Stuttering therapy, however, may help prevent developmental stuttering from becoming a life-long problem. In young children, treatment for stuttering is mainly supportive. Parents or caregivers are often counseled not to place undue emphasis on speech irregularities. Additional supportive care may include recognition of accomplishments and other gestures that will contribute to the development of self-worth. If stuttering persists beyond early childhood or into adulthood, speech therapy is usually indicated.

Government Agencies

6951 NIH/National Institute on Deafness and Oth er Communication Disorders (NIDCD)
31 Center Drive, MSC 2320
Bethesda, MD 20892
800-241-1044
TTY: 800-241-1055
nidcdinfo@nidcd.nih.gov
www.nidcd.nih.gov

Conducts and supports biomedical research and research training on normal mechanisms, as well as diseases and disorders of hearing, balance, smell, taste, voice, speech and language.

James F Battey Jr, MD, PhD, Director
Judith A Cooper PhD, Deputy Director
Timothy J Wheeles, Executive Officer

National Associations & Support Groups

6952 American Academy of Pediatrics
141 Northwest Point Boulevard
Elk Grove Village, IL 60007
847-434-4000
800-433-9016
Fax: 847-434-8000
www.aap.org

The American Academy of Pediatrics and its member pediatricians are committed to the attainment of optimal physical, mental and social health and well-being for all infants, children, adolescents, and young adults.

Fernando Stein, MD, FAAP, President
Karen Remley, MD, CEO/Executive VP

6953 American School Counselor Association
1101 King Street, Suite 310
Alexandria, VA 22314
703-683-2722
800-306-4722
Fax: 703-997-7572
asca@schoolcounselor.org
www.schoolcounselor.org

The mission of ASCA is to represent professional school counselors and to promote professionalism and ethical practices.

Richard Wong, Executive Director
Jeff Broderson, Information Technology Admin.
Kathleen M Rakestraw, Director of Communications

6954 American Speech Language Hearing Associati on (ASHA)
2200 Research Boulevard
Rockville, MD 20850
301-897-5700
800-638-8255
Fax: 301-571-0457
pr@asha.org
www.asha.org

A professional and credentialing association made up of more than 123,000 international pathologists, audiologists and scientists. The association promotes the interests of and provides services for those in the hearing, speech, and language field, and advocates for people with communication disorders.

Patricia A. Prelock, PhD, President
Elizabeth S. McCrea, PhD, CCC-SLP, President-Elect
Shelly S. Chabon, PhD, CCC-SLP, Immediate Past President

6955 Genetic Alliance
4301 Connecticut Avenue NW, Suite 404
Washington, DC 20008
202-966-5557
800-336-4363
Fax: 202-966-8553
info@geneticalliance.org
www.geneticalliance.org

A coalition of voluntary genetic support groups, consumers and professionals addressing the needs of individuals and families affected by genetic disorders from a national perspective.

Sharon Terry, President/CEO
Tetyana Murza, Managing Director
Natasha Bonhomme, VP, Strategic Development

6956 National Center for Stuttering
388 2nd Ave, Suite 136
New York, NY 10010
800-221-2483
Fax: 212-683-1372
executivedirector@stuttering.com
www.stuttering.com

Distributes information for parents of young children showing early signs of stuttering. For older children and adults, free information is available on treatment programs nationwide.

Martin F Schwartz, Executive Director

6957 National Stuttering Association
119 W 40th Street, 14th Fl
New York, NY 10018 212-944-4050
800-937-8888
Fax: 212-944-8244
info@westutter.org
www.westutter.org

A self-help support organization for people who stutter. It maintains a toll-free hotline on stuttering and a nationwide resource list for individuals seeking a speech-language pathologist who specializes in stuttering. Several publications are also directed toward medical professionals who serve the stuttering community.

Elaine Saitta, Executive Director
Katia Skowronska, Assistant Director

6958 Speak Easy International Foundation
233 Concord Drive
Paramus, NJ 07652 201-262-0895
Fax: 201-262-0895

A self-help support group for stutters.

Bob Gathman, Founder/President

6959 Stuttering Foundation of America
1805 Moriah Woods Blvd., Suite 3
Memphis, TN 38117 901-761-0343
800-992-9392
Fax: 901-761-0484
info@stutteringhelp.org
www.stutteringhelp.org

Provides free online resources, services and support to those who stutter and their families, as well as support for research into the causes of stuttering. Extensive educational programs on stuttering for professionals are also offered.

Jane H Fraser, President

State Agencies & Support Groups

6960 Speech, Language, & Hearing Center University of Colorado
2501 Kittredge Loop Rd., Campus Box 409
Boulder, CO 80309 303-492-5375
Fax: 303-492-3274
susan.moore@colorado.edu
slhs.colorado.edu/clinical-services?

Informational and emotional support to parents who have a child, adolescent, or adult family member with special needs.

Web Sites

6961 NIH/National Institute on Deafness and Other Communication Disorders (NIDCD)
www.nidcd.nih.gov/health/voice/stutter.asp

Fact sheet and information page on stuttering and other resources.

6962 Online Mendelian Inheritance in Man
www.omim.org

This database is a catalog of human genes and genetic disorders.

6963 Parent Pals
parentpals.com/gossamer/pages/Speech_and_Language
specialed@parentpals.com
parentpals.com/gossamer/pages/Speech_and_Language

Their goal is to provide special education and gifted information, continuing education, support, weekly tips, games, book resources, and news and views for parents and professionals.

Book Publishers

6964 Programmed Therapy for Stuttering in Child ren and Adults
Charles C Thomas Publisher
2600 S 1st Street
Springfield, IL 62704 217-789-8980
800-258-8980
Fax: 217-789-9130
books@ccthomas.com
www.ccthomas.com

This book highlights the systematic scientific approach to studying and treating stuttering by way of learning theory, single-subject research design and operant conditioning.

2001 360 pages 2nd Edition
ISBN: 0-398071-07-3

6965 Straight Talk on Stuttering: Information, Encouragement, and Counsel
Lloyd M Hulit, author

Charles C Thomas Publisher
2600 S 1st Street
Springfield, IL 62704 217-789-8980
800-258-8980
Fax: 217-789-9130
books@ccthomas.com
www.ccthomas.com

Written for stutterers and those who interact with stutterers, including parents, caregivers, teachers, and speech-language pathologists. The author dispels myths, corrects the misperceptions and creates a message of hope for all people who have this fascinating communication disorder.

338 pages 2nd Ed/ Hard
ISBN: 0-398075-19-4

6966 Stutter No More
Dr Martin F Schwartz, author

National Center for Stuttering
388 2nd Ave, Suite 136
New York, NY 10010 800-221-2483
Fax: 212-683-1372
executivedirector@stuttering.com
www.stuttering.com

The book covers a simple learning technique to stop stuttering in 9-12 months.

Martin F. Schwartz, Executive Director

Newsletters

6967 Stuttering Foundation of America Newslette r
Stuttering Foundation of America
1805 Moriah Woods Blvd., Suite 3
Memphis, TN 38117 901-761-0343
800-992-9392
Fax: 901-761-0484
info@stutteringhelp.org
www.stutteringhelp.org

Quarterly newsletter available online in pdf format.

Jane H Fraser, President

Camps

6968 Meadowood Springs Speech and Hearing Camp
PO Box 1025
Pendleton, OR 97801 541-276-2752
Fax: 541-276-7227
info@meadowoodsprings.org
www.meadowoodsprings.org

On 143 acres in the Blue Mountains of Eastern Oregon, this camp is designed to help young people who have diagnosed clinical disorders of speech, hearing or language. A full range of activities in recreational and clinical areas is available. For cabin reservations 541-566-2191.

Rosemarie Atfield, Executive Director
Marie Story, Camp Manager
Cliff Story, Camp Manager

6969 University of Iowa - Wendell Johnson Speech and Hearing Clinic

Wendell Johnson Speech And Hearing Center
Iowa City, IA 52242   319-335-8718
                                        Fax: 319-335-8851
                              speech-path-aud@uiowa.edu
                                    clas.uiowa.edu/comsci/

The clinic offers assessment and remediation for disordered communication in adults and children. The clinic also offers an Intensive Summer Residential Clinic for school age children needing intervention services because of speech, language, hearing and/or reading problems.

Ruth Bentler, Professor / Department Chair
Dorothy Albright, Secretary
Vicki Jennings, Secretary

DESCRIPTION

6970 SUBACUTE SCLEROSING PANENCEPHALITIS (SSPE)

Synonyms: Dawson's encephalitis, Van Bogaert's encephalitis

Involves the following Biologic System(s):

Immunologic and Rheumatologic Disorders, Neurologic Disorders

Subacute sclerosing panencephalitis (SSPE) is a rare, life-threatening, slow viral infection of the brain caused by a measles-like virus. SSPE appears months or years after a typical mild or severe measles infection and occurs most frequently in children and adolescents between the ages of five and 15 years. This disease occurs more often in children who develop measles before 18 months of age and is twice as prevalent in boys as it is in girls. Symptoms develop gradually and may commence with subtle behavorial changes such as forgetfulness or outbursts of temper, deterioration in school performance, sleeplessness, and hallucinations. These symptoms are often followed by more bizarre behavior, seizures, repetitive muscular jerks (myoclonic jerks) and other abnormal movements, eye irregularities, and mental deterioration (dementia). Late findings may include muscular rigidity or, in some patients, weak muscles, difficulty swallowing, blindness, or coma. In addition, due to generalized weakness and impaired muscle control associated with SSPE, life-threatening complications such as pneumonia may occur. Subacute sclerosing panencephalitis is incompatible with life; its usual duration is from one to three years.

The diagnosis of SSPE may be confirmed through laboratory tests that detect the presence of antibodies to the measles virus in the cerebrospinal fluid and the presence of large numbers of measles antibodies in the serum. In most cases, subacute sclerosing pnencephalitis may be prevented by immunization with attenuated measles virus vaccine.

Treatment of SSPE is geared toward chronic care. Over the last decade, however, stabilization of disease and in clinical progression has been observed with medications that alter the body's immune system response to this virus (immunomodulators), such as interferon and certain antiviral drugs including ribavirin and isoprinosine. Studies of other therapeutic programs are ongoing. Other treatment is symptomatic and supportive.

Government Agencies

6971 NIH/National Institute of Allergy and Infectious Diseases
5601 Fishers Lane, MSC 9806
Bethesda, MD 20892

301-496-5717
866-284-4107
Fax: 301-402-3573
TDD: 800-877-8339
ocpostoffice@niaid.nih.gov
www.niaid.nih.gov

Conducts and supports basic and applied research to better understand, treat, and ultimately prevent infectious, immunologic, and allergic diseases.

Anthony S Fauci MD, Director

6972 NIH/National Institute of Neurological Dis orders and Stroke (NINDS)
PO Box 5801
Bethesda, MD 20824

301-496-5751
800-352-9424
www.ninds.nih.gov/disorders/subacute_panencephalitis

Walter J. Koroshetz, MD, Director

National Associations & Support Groups

6973 American Academy of Pediatrics
141 Northwest Point Boulevard
Elk Grove Village, IL 60007

847-434-4000
800-433-9016
Fax: 847-434-8000
www.aap.org

The American Academy of Pediatrics and its member pediatricians are committed to the attainment of optimal physical, mental and social health and well-being for all infants, children, adolescents, and young adults.

Fernando Stein, MD, FAAP, President
Karen Remley, MD, CEO/Executive VP

6974 Genetic Alliance
4301 Connecticut Avenue NW, Suite 404
Washington, DC 20008

202-966-5557
800-336-4363
Fax: 202-966-8553
info@geneticalliance.org
www.geneticalliance.org

A coalition of voluntary genetic support groups, consumers and professionals addressing the needs of individuals and families affected by genetic disorders from a national perspective.

Sharon Terry, President/CEO
Tetyana Murza, Managing Director
Natasha Bonhomme, VP, Strategic Development

6975 World Health Organization
Avenue Appia 20
CH-1211 Geneva 27,
Switzerland

publications@who.int
www.who.int

WHO is the directing and coordinating authority for health within the United Nations system.

Dr Margaret Chan, Director General

Web Sites

6976 Encephalitis Information Resource
www.encepahlitis.info

Site is provided by the Encephalitis Society

6977 MedlinePlus
www.nlm.nih.gov/medlineplus/aboutmedlineplus.html

custserv@nlm.nih.gov
www.nlm.nih.gov/medlineplus/aboutmedlineplus.html

Information on the condition, causes, symptoms, tests, and treatment.

Dr. Donald A.B. Lindberg, Director

6978 NIH/National Institute of Neurological Dis orders and Stroke (NINDS)
Office of Communications and Public Liaison, NINDS
Bethesda, MD 20824

301-496-5751
800-352-9424
www.ninds.nih.gov/disorders/subacute_panencephalitis

Information fact sheet on the disorder.

Walter J. Koroshetz, MD, Director

6979 Let's Talk About Going to the Hospital
Rosen Publishing Group's PowerKids Press
29 E 21st Street
New York, NY 10010

212-777-3017
800-237-9932
Fax: 888-436-4643
rosenpub@tribeca.ios.com
www.rosenpublishing.com

If a child has to check into the hospital, chances are he or she is already upset about being ill. Knowing how a hospital functions and what the procedures are, such as when family members can visit, will help in what is already a stressful situation. Grades K-5.

24 pages
ISBN: 0-823950-36-0

Roger Rosen, President

DESCRIPTION

6980 SUDDEN INFANT DEATH SYNDROME

Synonyms: Cot death, Crib death, SIDS

Involves the following Biologic System(s):

Neonatal and Infant Disorders

Sudden infant death syndrome (SIDS) refers to the sudden, unexpected, and unexplained death of an apparently healthy infant. This syndrome may occur from the ages of two weeks to one year, but most commonly occurs between the ages of two to four months. Approximately 75 to 95 percent of all deaths related to SIDS occur by the age of six months. Sudden infant death syndrome is responsible for approximately half of all infant deaths that occur between the ages of 1 month and one year and, in the United States, affects approximately 1.3 of every 1,000 infants in that age group. SIDS is somewhat more common in boys and in infants born to individuals of African-American or Native American descent. In addition, sudden infant death syndrome occurs more often during the winter months.

Very little is sure about the exact cause of SIDS, but researchers believe that certain brain stem abnormalities may be a contributing factor to its occurrence. Such irregularities may affect the regulation of body temperature, cardiorespiratory function, and associated sleep and arousal mechanisms. Although the relationship is not fully understood, brain stem abnormalities, especially sleep and arousal deficit, may interact with certain other influencing factors (epidemiologic risk factors) to put infants at risk for SIDS. Such epidemiologic risk factors may include prematurity, low birth weight, bottle feeding, exposure to smoking, recent illness with fever and previous near death episodes requiring resuscitation. Also, mothers with abnormally low levels of circulating red blood cells (anemia) or those who smoke or use drugs during pregnancy may be at increased risk for having an infant with SIDS. Other factors may include insufficient prenatal care and low socioeconomic status. In addition, recent studies have shown that putting infants to sleep on their stomachs is a significant risk factor, as is the use of soft bedding or extra linens and toys (e.g., comforters, quilts, stuffed animals, etc.) in the crib.

To alleviate certain risk factors, appropriate prenatal care is essential in the possible prevention of SIDS. Also, after birth, parents are counseled to be alert to any respiratory changes or distress and to closely observe infants during and after any illness. In addition, new guidelines recommend that infants be placed in the crib on their backs, as statistics have shown declines in SIDS rates among those who have complied with this recommendation. Sleeping on the back has been recommended for some time to avoid SIDS, with the catchphrase "Back To Bed" and "Back to Sleep." Other guidelines include the advice that crib mattresses should be firm and should fit tightly within the crib frame; that comforters, quilts, pillows, toys, etc. should be removed from the crib; that, if possible, sleeper-type pajamas be used instead of blankets; that if a blanket must be used, it should be thin, should reach no further than the infant's chest, and shou ld be tucked around the infant's chest and mattress; and that the baby's head should be uncovered at all times during sleep. Infants who die from SIDS tend to have higher concentrations of nicotine and cotinine (a biological marker for secondhand smoke expo-

sure) in their lungs than those who die from other causes. Parents who smoke can significantly reduce their children's risk of SIDS by either quitting or smoking only outside and leaving their house completely smoke-free. In the event of the death of an infant from SIDS, counseling by trained specialists is strongly advised for parents and remaining siblings. In addition, support groups composed of families who have been affected by SIDS may be comforting and helpful.

Government Agencies

6981 National Center for Health Statistics

4770 Buford Hwy, NE

Atlanta, GA 30341

800-232-4636

800-311-3435

www.cdc.gov

National Associations & Support Groups

6982 American Academy of Pediatrics

141 Northwest Point Boulevard

Elk Grove Village, IL 60007

847-434-4000

800-433-9016

Fax: 847-434-8000

www.aap.org

The American Academy of Pediatrics and its member pediatricians are committed to the attainment of optimal physical, mental and social health and well-being for all infants, children, adolescents, and young adults.

Fernando Stein, MD, FAAP, President

Karen Remley, MD, CEO/Executive VP

6983 American SIDS Institute

528 Raven Way

Naples, FL 34110

239-431-5425

800-232-7437

Fax: 239-431-5536

prevent@sids.org

www.sids.org

A national nonprofit organization dedicated to the prevention of sudden infant death syndrome and the promotion of infant health.

Marc Peterzell, Chairman

Betty McEntire PhD, Executive Director

6984 Compassionate Friends

PO Box 3696

Oak Brook, IL 60522

630-990-0010

877-969-0010

Fax: 630-990-0246

nationaloffice@compassionatefriends.org

www.compassionatefriends.org

Compassionate Friends assists families toward the positive resolution of grief following the death of a child of any age and provides information to help others be supportive. A national nonprofit, self-help support organization that offers friendship, understanding, and hope to bereaved parents, grandparents and siblings.

Patricia Loder, Executive Director

Ronald Haynes, VP

Patricia Loder, Executive Director

6985 Council of Guilds for Infant Survival

PO Box 3586

Davenport, IA 52808

319-322-4870

Conducts research and provides information on SIDS.

Chris Elliott

6986 **First Candle/SIDS Alliance**
2105 Laurel Bush Road,, Suite 201
Bel Air, MD 21015 443-640-1049
800-221-7437
Fax: 410-653-8709
info@firstcandle.org
www.sidsalliance.org; www.firstcandle.org

First Candle started as the National SIDS Foundation focusing on supporting families that experienced SIDS. In 2002, it broadened its scope to include other areas of infant death, committing its resources in hopes of having an impact on all these areas. It's mission is to help babies survive and thrive.

Marian Sokol, President
Deborah M Boyd, Executive Director
Laura L Reno, Director Public Affairs/Marketing

6987 **National Center for Education in Maternal and Child Health**
Georgetown University
2115 Wisconsin Ave NW, Suite 601
Washington, DC 20007 202-784-9770
Fax: 202-784-9777
mchlibrary@ncemch.org
www.ncemch.org

6988 **National Center for the Prevention of SIDS**
4770 Buford Hwy, NE
Atlanta, GA 30341 800-232-4636
Fax: 410-653-8709
www.cdc.gov/sids/?

Offers medical updates and information on prevention of SIDS and other disorders to parents and professionals.

6989 **National SIDS/Infant Death Resource Center (Resource Center)**
2115 Wisconson Avenue, NW, Suite 601
Washington, DC 20007 202-687-7437
866-866-7437
Fax: 202-784-9777
info@sidscenter.org
www.sidscenter.org

NSIDRC (Resource Center) serves as a central source of information on sudden infant death and on promoting healthy outcomes for infants from birth through the first year of life and beyond.

Rochelle Mayer, Project Director

6990 **National Sudden Infant Death Syndrome Foundation**
31 Center Drive, Room 2A32
Bethesda, MD 20892 301-496-5133
Fax: 301-496-7101

6991 **Parents Helping Parents - A Family Resource Center**
1400 Parkmoor Avenue Suite 100
San Jose, CA 95126 408-727-5775
Fax: 408-727-0182
general@php.com
www.php.com

A group of parents and professionals committed to alleviating some of the problems, hardships and concerns of families with children having special needs.

Candy Smith, Director

6992 **Pregnancy and Infant Loss Center**
402 Jackson St
St. Charles, MO 63301 366-437-7014
800-821-6819
info@nationalshare.org
nationalshare.org

Offers support, resources, and education on miscarriage, stillbirth and newborn death. Nonprofit organization, membership and quarterly newsletter $20 per year.

6993 **SHARE National Headquarters**
Saint Elizabeth's Hospital
402 Jackson St
St. Charles, MO 63301 636-947-6164
800-821-6819
Fax: 636-947-7486
info@nationalshare.org
nationalshare.org

Serve those whose lives are touched by the tragic death of a baby through early pregnancy loss, stillbirth, or in the first few months of life.

Cathie Lamert, Executive Director
Rose Carlson, Program Director
Megan Nichols, Outreach &Public Relatons Director

6994 **SIDS Educational Services**
PO Box 2426
Hyattsville, MD 20784 301-322-2620
Fax: 301-322-9822
SIDSES@aol.com
www.sidssurvivalguide.org

Supports families grieving the loss of children to Sudden Infant Death Syndrome and other infant death causes. Information and support services are also provided to children grieving any type of death.

6995 **SIDS Information and Referral Hotline**
SIDS Alliance
1314 Bedord Avenue
Baltimore, MD 21208 410-653-8226
800-221-7437
Fax: 410-653-8709

24 hour information and referral line for parents who wish to discuss their concerns with a SIDS counselor, request additional information about SIDS and to receive referrals to the local SIDS affiliate in their area.

State Agencies & Support Groups

Alabama

6996 **Bureau of Family Health Services-Alabama Child Death Review**
Alabama Department of Public Health
43 Foundry Avenue
Waltham, MA 02453 617-618-2918
Fax: 334-206-2972
jallison@edc.org
www.childrenssafetynetwork.org
Jennifer Allison, CSN Assistant Director, State Partn

Alaska

6997 **SIDS Information & Counseling Program Alaska Department of Health**
1231 Gambell Street, Suite 302
Anchorage, AK 99501 907-272-1534
Fax: 907-274-1384
sid-network.org/map

Linda D Vlastuin, RN, MPH, Program Consultant

Arizona

6998 **Office of Women's & Children's Health**
Arizona Department of Health Services
150 N 18th Ave, Suite 320
Phoenix, AZ 85007 602-542-1025
Fax: 602-542-0883
newbers@azdhs.gov
www.azdhs.gov

The Unexplained Infant Death Council comes under the OWCH and assists the department to develop unexplained infant death training and educational programs.

Sheila Sjolander, Manager

Arkansas

6999 Arkansas Department of Health - SIDS Information & Counseling Program
4815 W Markham Street
Little Rock, AR 72205

501-661-2000
800-462-0599
Fax: 501-671-1450
www.healthy.arkansas.gov

Rosalind Abernathy, Project Coordinator

California

7000 California SIDS Program
11344 Coloma Road
Gold River, CA 95670

916-851-437
800-369-7437
Fax: 916-851-5937
info@californiasids.com
www.californiasids.com

Gwen Edelstein, Program Director
Susan More MA, Grief Counselor and Educator

7001 CorStone-Children & Loss Group
CorStone
250 Camino Alto
Mill Valley, CA 94941

415-331-6161
Fax: 415-388-6165
info@corstone.org
www.corstone.org

For children who have suffered the loss of a close loved one. Parent group meets separately at the same time.

Richard Cuadra MFT, Program Director
Melissa Mullin MFT, Program Coordinator

7002 Region IX Office Program Consultants for Maternal and Child Health
50 United Nations Plaza
San Francisco, CA 94102

415-437-8101
Fax: 415-437-8105
nrc.uchsc.edu

Lyn Headley, MD

Colorado

7003 Colorado SIDS Program
425 S Cherry Street, Suite 890
Denver, CO 80246

303-320-7771
888-285-7437
Fax: 303-320-7827
shelia@coloradosids.org
www.angeleyes.org

Donna Buss, President
Daniel Trujillo, Vice President
Luanne Chavez, Assisstant Vice President

7004 Region VIII Office Program Consultants for Maternal and Child Health
1961 Stout Street
Denver, CO 80294

303-844-7854
Fax: 303-844-2019
laurie.konsella@hhs.gov

Laurie Konsella, M.P.A

Delaware

7005 SIDS Information & Counseling - Division of Public Health
501 Ogletown Road
Newark, DE 19711

302-368-6840

Elaine Markell, LCSW, BCD, Program Coordinator

District of Columbia

7006 Division of Community Health Nursing
825 N Capitol Street, NE
Washington, DC 20002

202-698-0705
Fax: 202-645-7030

Mary Breach, RN, MSN, Nursing Coordinator

Florida

7007 Children's Medical Services Program Florida SIDS Program
Bin A-13 4025 Bald Cypress Way
Tallahassee, FL 32399

850-245-4444
Fax: 850-245-4047
susann-arbor@doh.state.fl.us
www.doh.state.fl.us

Georgia

7008 Georgia Department of Human Resources Children's Health Services
2 Peach Tree Street NW
Atlanta, GA 30303

404-656-6750
dhs.georgia.gov

Linette Jackson Hunt, MD, MPH, Chief

7009 Georgia Department of Human Resources - Center for Family Resource Planning
2 Peach Tree Street NW
Atlanta, GA 30303

404-656-7660
www.dhs.georgia.gov

Provides grief support for parents.
Lee Hackel

7010 Region IV Office Program Consultants For Maternal and Child Health
Atlanta Federal Center
61 Forsyth Street, SW, Suite 3M60
Atlanta, GA 30303

404-562-7980
Fax: 404-562-7974
kgonzalez@hrsa.gov
nrc.uchsc.edu

Dorothy Redfern, RN, MSPH

Hawaii

7011 Hawaii SIDS Information & Counseling Project
Kapiolani Children's Medical Center
1319 Punahou Street #1100
Honolulu, HI 96826

808-983-8368

Sharon Morton, RN, Nurse Consultant

Idaho

7012 Child Health Improvement Program Idaho Department of Health
211 Idaho CareLine, PO Box 83720
Boise, ID 83720

208-334-5945
800-926-2588
Fax: 208-334-5531
careline@dhw.idaho.gov
www.idahocareline.org

Simonne deGlee, MS, PNP, SIDS Coordinator

Illinois

7013 Region V Office Program Consultants for Maternal and Child Health
233 N Michigan Avenue
Chicago, IL 60601
312-353-4042
Fax: 312-886-3770
dparker@hrsa.gov

Kathryn Vedder, MD, MPH

7014 Statewide SIDS Program - Illinois Department of Public Health
535 W Jefferson Street
Springfield, IL 62761
217-785-4528
www.illinois.gov

Lori Bennett, Coordinator

Indiana

7015 Indiana State Board of Health - SIDS Project
2 N Meridian Street
Indianapolis, IN 46204
317-233-1325
Fax: 317-233-7394
opac@isdh.state.in.us
www.in.gov/isdh/

Judith Monroe, Manager

Iowa

7016 Iowa SIDS Program
Iowa Department of Public Health
406 SW School St
Ankeny, IA 50023
515-965-7655
866-480-4741
www.iowasids.org

Beverly Richardson, MA, MCH Consultant

Kansas

7017 Kansas Department of Health & Environment Bureau of Family Health
1000 SW Jackson Street, Suite 220
Topeka, KS 66612
785-296-1500
800-332-6262
Fax: 785-296-1562
www.kdheks.gov

Azzie N Young, PhD, Director

Kentucky

7018 Kentucky Department of Human Resources Bureau of Health Services
700 Capitol Avenue, Suite 100
Frankfort, KY 40601
502-564-2611
governor.ky.gov

Ida Lyons, RN, SIDS Coordinator

Louisiana

7019 Public Health Services of Louisiana
628 N 4th Street
Baton Rouge, LA 70802
225-342-9500
Fax: 225-342-5568
dhhwebinfo@la.gov
www.dhh.louisiana.gov/

Dorris Brown, Center Director
Myrra Lowe, Chief Financial Officer
Beth Scalso, Chief of Staff

Maine

7020 Department of Human Services
221 State Street
Augusta, ME 04333
207-287-3707
Fax: 207-287-3005
TTY: 800-606-0215
www.maine.gov/dhhs

Brenda Harvey, Manager
Mary Mayhew, Commisioner

Maryland

7021 Center for Infant & Child Loss
737 W. Lombard Street, Room 233
Baltimore, MD 21201
410-706-5062
800-808-7437
Fax: 410-328-4596
caring@infantandchildloss.org
www.infantandchildloss.org

Donna C Becker, RN, MSN, Director

7022 Maryland SIDS Information & Counseling Program
2905 64th Avenue
Cheverly, MD 20785
301-773-9671
sids-network.org

Daniel Timmel, MSW, Project Director
Jodi Shaefer, Director

Massachusetts

7023 Massachusetts Chapter of SIDS Alliance
Boston Medical Center
1 Boston Medical Place
Boston, MA 02118
617-638-8000
800-641-7437
Fax: 617-414-5555
www.bmc.org

State chapter offering educational resources and information on SIDS, parent groups, support networks, monthly meetings and workshops to the community.

Mary McClain, Manager
Mary McClain, RN, MS

7024 Region I Office Program Consultants For Maternal and Child Health
John F Kennedy Building
Room 1826
Boston, MA 02203
617-565-1433
Fax: 617-565-3044
btausey@hrsa.gov
www.mchb.hrsa.gob

Shirley A Smith, RN, MS

Michigan

7025 Apnea Identification Program
Children's Hospital of Michigan
3901 Beaubien Street
Detroit, MI 48201
313-745-5437
888-DMC-2500
www.chmkids.org

Karen Braniff, RN, MSW, Nurse Specialist

7026 Genesee County Health Department
630 S Saginaw Street
Flint, MI 48502
810-257-3612
Fax: 810-257-3147
gchd-info@gchd.us
www.gchd.us

Robert Pestronk, Manager
Mark Valck, Health Director
Gary Johnson, Medical Director

7027 Kent County Health Department
300 Monroe Avenue NW
Grand Rapids, MI 49503
616-632-7590
Fax: 616-632-7083
www.accesskent.com

Cathy Raevsky, Executive Director

7028 Oakland County Health Division - SIDS Project
1200 N Telegraph Road
Pontiac, MI 48341
248-858-1280
Fax: 248-858-0178
www.oakgov.com/health

Rosemary Rowney, Manager

7029 SIDS LEAD - Children's Special Health Care Services
Michigan Department of Public Health
3423 N Martin Luther King Jr Boulevard
Lansing, MI 48906
517-373-3500
arias@state.mi.us
www.mdmh.state.mi.us/

Cheryl Lauber, MSN

7030 SIDS Nursing Intervention Program
43525 Elizabeth Road
Mount Clemens, MI 48043
810-469-5520

Loretta Lindsay, RN, Coordinator

Minnesota

7031 Minnesota Sudden Infant Death Center
Minneapolis Children's Medical Center
2525 Chicago Avenue
Minneapolis, MN 55404
612-813-6285
TTY: 800-732-3812

Kathleen Farnbach, PHN, Project Coordinator

Mississippi

7032 Mississippi State Department of Health and Child Health Services
570 East Woodrow Wilson Drive
Jackson, MS 39216
601-576-7634
www.msdh.state.ms.us

Jenny Griffin, Manager

Missouri

7033 Region VII Office Program Consultants for Maternal and Child Health
Federal Building
601 E 12th Street
Kansas City, MO 64106
816-426-5291
Fax: 816-426-3633
bappelbaum@hrsa.gov

Bradley Appelbaum, MD, MPH

7034 SIDS Resources
1120 South Sixth Street, Suite 100
Saint Louis, MO 63104
314-822-2323
800-421-3511
Fax: 314-588-0850
www.sidsresources.org

Helen Fuller, MSW, Executive Director
Laura Hillman, President
Karl Barnickol, Secretary

Montana

7035 Montana Department of Health & Environmental Sciences
Family & Maternal & Child Health Bureau
Cogswell Building
Helena, MT 59620
406-444-4740
Maxine Ferguson, RN, MN, Bureau Chief

Nebraska

7036 Nebraska SIDS Foundation
University of Nebraska Medical Center
600 S 42nd Street
Omaha, NE 68198
402-559-4212
www.nebraskasidsfoundation.org
Valerie Ciciulla, Coordinator

Nevada

7037 Nevada State Division of Health, Maternal & Child Health
505 E King Street, Room 205
Carson City, NV 89701
702-687-4885
www.health.nv.gov/MCH.htm

Luana Ritch, Health Educator

New Hampshire

7038 New Hampshire SIDS Program
New Hampshire Division of Public Health Services
6 Hazen Drive
Concord, NH 03301
603-271-4533
800-852-3345
Fax: 603-271-3745

Audrey Knight, MSN, CPNP, SIDS Coordinator

New Jersey

7039 New Jersey Department of Health - Child Health Program
CN 364, 363 W State Street
Trenton, NJ 08625
609-292-5616
Judith Hall, BSN, RNC, Evaluator

7040 New Jersey SIDS Resource Center
254 Easton Avenue
New Brunswick, NJ 08901
732-249-2160

New York

7041 NYS Center for SIDS Office
Stony Brook University
School of Social Welfare Health Science Center
Stony Brook, NY 11794
631-632-6000
Fax: 631-444-6475
marie.chandick@stonybrook.edu
www.stonybrook.edu

Marie Chandrick, Director

7042 New York City Information & Counseling Program for SIDS
520 1st Avenue, Room 506
New York, NY 10016
212-757-1051
800-522-5006

Judith Gaines, CSW, PhD, SIDS Program Director

7043 Region II Office Program Consultants for Maternal and Child Health
26 Federal Plaza
New York, NY 10278
212-264-2571
Fax: 212-264-2673
ssmith@hrsa.gov

Margaret Lee, MD

7044 Western New York SIDS Center
200 Fairport Village Lane
Fairport, NY 14450
716-223-5110
Gabrielle Weiss, BPS, Director

North Carolina

7045 North Carolina SIDS Information and Counseling Program
North Carolina Department Of Environmental Health
2709 Water Ridge Parkway
Charlotte, NC 28217   704-644-4200
                                       800-868-8777
                                       Fax: 704-644-4210
                                       www.safetync.org

Dianne Tyson, BSW, Administrative Assistant

North Dakota

7046 North Dakota SIDS Management Program
600 E Boulevard Avenue
Bismarck, ND 58505   701-328-4464
                                       800-472-2286
                                       Fax: 701-328-1412
                                       www.ndhealth.gov/SIDS

Bertie Hagberg, RN, Coordinator
Katie Schimdt, North Dakota SIDS Management Progra
Peggy Stanton, Administrative Assistant

Ohio

7047 Perinatal and Infant Health Unit - SIDS Information and Counseling Program
Ohio Department Of Health
246 N High Street
Columbus, OH 43266   614-466-4716
                                       webmaster@ghodh.state.oh.us
                                       www.adh.state.oh.us/

Ben Chukwumah, MD, MPH, Project Director

Oklahoma

7048 Oklahoma State Department of Health - Maternal and Child Health Services
1000 NE 10th Street
Oklahoma City, OK 73117   405-271-5600
                                       Fax: 405-271-3431
                                       webmaster@health.ok.gov.
                                       www.ok.gov/health

Mike Crutcher, Manager

Oregon

7049 Oregon State Health Division - SIDS Information and Counseling Program
1400 SW 5th Avenue
Portland, OR 97201   503-229-6617
Sue Omel, RN, MPH, Child Coordinator

7050 SIDS Resource of Oregon
4035 NE Sandy Boulevard, Suite 209
Portland, OR 97212   503-287-8265
                                       800-221-7437
                                       Fax: 503-287-8693
                                       sidsor@teleport.com
                                       www.teleport.com/~sidsor

Todd Llinchliffer

Pennsylvania

7051 Pennsylvania SIDS Center
Suite 250 Riverfront Place
Pittsburgh, PA 15212   412-322-5680
                                       800-258-7437
                                       Fax: 215-923-2989
                                       www.sids-pa.org/

Rosanne English, RN, Executive Director

7052 Region III Office Program Consultants for Maternal and Child Health
Public Ledger Building
150 S Independence Mall West, Suite 1172
Philadelphia, PA 19106   215-861-4379
                                       Fax: 215-861-4338
                                       valos@hrsa.gov

Jane Coury, MSN, RN

Rhode Island

7053 Rhode Island Department of Health National SIDS Foundation
3 Capitol Hl
Providence, RI 02908   401-222-5960
                                       Fax: 401-444-3422
                                       www.health.ri.gov/

Anne M Roach, RN, SIDS Coordinator

South Carolina

7054 South Carolina Department of Health & Environmental Control - SIDS Information
2600 Bull Street
Columbia, SC 29201   803-898-3300
                 www.scdhec.gov/administration/hplhc/health.htm
Brenda Creswell, ACSW, LMSW, SIDS Coordinator

South Dakota

7055 South Dakota Department of Health
Health Building
500 East Capitol Avenue
Pierre, SD 57501   605-773-3361
                                       800-738-2301
                                       Fax: 605-773-5683
                                       dolt.info@state.sd.us
                                       www.doh.sd.gov

Doneen Hollingsworth, Manager

Tennessee

7056 Tennessee SIDS Program
Tennessee Department Of Health
425 5th Ave, N Cordell Hull Bldg, 3rd Fl
Nashville, TN 37243   615-741-7335
                                       Fax: 615-741-1063
                                       tn.health@tn.gov
                    health.state.tn.us/MCH/SIDS/SIDS_program.htm
Judith Womack, RN, Director Child Health

Texas

7057 Harris County Health Department
2223 West Loop South
Houston, TX 77027   713-439-6000
                                       publicinfo@hd.co.harris.tx.us
                                       www.hcphes.org

Kathleen Ingrando, RN, BSN, Program Coordinator

7058 North Texas SIDS Information And Counseling Program
5000 Harry Hines
Dallas, TX 75235   214-590-0135
                                       Fax: 214-590-0173

Leslie U Malone, SIDS Coordinator

7059 Region VI Office Program Consultants For Maternal and Child Health
1301 Young Street 10th Floor
Dallas, TX 75202   214-767-3003
                                       Fax: 214-767-3038
                                       twells@hrsa.gov

Marianne Davenport, CPNP, MPH

7060 Texas Department of Health - SIDS Information and Counseling Program
211 N. Florence, Suite 101
El Paso, TX 79901
915-532-1006
888-963-7111
Fax: 512-458-7750
bhc@borderhealth.org
www.borderhealth.org

Eduardo J Sanchez, Manager

Utah

7061 Utah Department of Health
Child Health Bureau
PO Box 141010
Salt Lake City, UT 84114
801-538-6003
health.utah.gov

Judith Ahrano, SIDS Director

Vermont

7062 Vermont Department of Health - SIDS Information and Counseling Program
108 Cherry Street
Burlington, VT 05401
802-863-7200
Fax: 802-865-7754
sshepar@udh.state.ut.us
www.healthvermont.gov

Wendy Davis, Manager

Virginia

7063 Virginia SIDS Program - Virginia Department of Health
Virginia Department of Health
P.O. Box 2448
Richmond, VA 23218
804-864-7001
Fax: 804-864-7001
schuettd@aol.com
www.vdh.state.va.us

Arlethia V Rogers, RN, Nurse Consultant

Washington

7064 Region X Office Program Consultants for Maternal and Child Health
2201 6th Avenue
Seattle, WA 98121
206-553-0215
Kay Girl, RNC, MN, Acting

7065 SIDS Northwest Regional Center
Washington Department of Health
4800 Sand Point Way NE
Olympia, WA 98504
360-236-3560
800-441-4392
www.doh.wa.gov

Lauren Valk Lawson, MN, Program Director

West Virginia

7066 West Virginia Department of Health and Human Services
One Davis Square, Suite 100, East
Charleston, WV 25301
304-558-0684
Fax: 304-558-1130
www.wvdhhr.org

Joan R Kenny, RN, SIDS Director

Wisconsin

7067 Counseling and Research Center for SIDS
2115 Wisconsin Avenue- NW Suite 601
Washington, DC 20007
202-687-7437
866-866-7437
Fax: 202-784-9777
info@sidscenter.org
www.sidscenter.org

Rochelle Mayer, Director

Wyoming

7068 Wyoming Department of Health
Division of Health and Medical Services
401 Hathaway Building
Cheyenne, WY 82002
307-777-7656
Fax: 307-777-7439
wdh@state.wy.us
www.health.wyo.gov

J Richard Hillman, MD, PhD, Administrator

Libraries & Resource Centers

7069 National Sudden Infant Death Syndrome Resource Center
Circle Solutions, Inc
8280 Greensboro Drive, Suite 300
McLean, VA 22102
703-893-6383
Fax: 703-821-2098
marketing@circlesolutions.com
www.circlesolutions.com

Resource Center provides information on keeping children safe through their first year and beyond, about SIDS, and about handling the grief of losing a child to SIDS, and so much more.

Kristina Lewis, Chairman, Executive Committee
Louis Cartwright, jr., Vice President-Finance
Michael Collins, Vice President-IT

7070 Sudden Infant Death Syndrome (SIDS) Network
PO Box 520
Ledyard, CT 06339
Fax: 860-887-7309
sids-network.org/

Research Centers

7071 American SIDS Institute
528 Raven Way
Naples, FL 34110
239-431-5425
800-232-7437
Fax: 239-431-5536
prevent@sids.org
www.sids.org

A national nonprofit organization dedicated to the promotion of infant health and the prevention of sudden infant death syndrome.

Marc Peterzell, Chairman
Betty McEntire PhD, Executive Director

7072 CJ Foundation for SIDS
Don Imus WFAN Pediatric Center
30 Prospect Ave
Hackensack, NJ 07601
201-996-5111
800-620-7832
Fax: 201-996-5326
info@cjsids.org
www.cjsids.org

Barry Bornstein, Executive Director

7073 Center for Research for Mothers & Children
National Institute of Child Health & Development
31 Center Drive, Building 31
Bethesda, MD 20892   301-496-5575
                                                       1 8-0 3-0 29
                                                 Fax: 866-760-5947
                              NICHDInformationResourceCenter@mail.nih.
                                                   www.nichd.nih.gov

This institute conducts and supports research on all stages of human development, from the preconception to adulthood, to better understand the health of children, adults, families, and communities.

7074 Massachusetts Sudden Infant Death Syndrome
Boston City Hospital
818 Harrison Avenue
Boston, MA 02118   617-638-8131

A joint program of Boston City Hospital and Children's Hospital. Services provided include around-the-clock availability for consultation to health professionals and families, counseling of families, parent group meetings and supportive home visits.

7075 National Sudden Infant Death Syndrome Research Center
Circle Solutions, Inc
8280 Greensboro Drive, Suite 300
McLean, VA 22102   703-821-8955
                                                 Fax: 703-821-2098
                                       marketing@circlesolutions.com
                                             www.circlesolutions.com

Provides information services and technical assistance concerning SIDS and related topics in order to promote understanding of SIDS and to comfort those affected by a SIDS loss. Offers its services to parents, family members, caregivers, counselors, medical and legal professionals, and the general public.

7076 Pathology Department SIDS/SUDC Research Project
Children's Hospital San Diego
3020 Children's Way, MC5007
San Diego, CA 92123   858-966-5944
Dr Henry Krous, Director
Amy Chadwick, Project Manager

7077 Pediatric Pulmonary Unit
Massachusetts General Hospital
55 Fruit Street
Boston, MA 02114   617-726-2000
                                                 www.massgeneral.org

Sudden infant death syndrome and childhood disorders research.

Douglas R Johnson, Associate Director

7078 Southwest SIDS Research Institute
Brazosport Memorial Hospital
100 Medical Drive
Lake Jackson, TX 77566   979-297-4411
                                                 Fax: 979-297-6682
                                 admin@brazosportmemorial.com
                                     www.brazosportmemorial.com

Mari Uranga, Manager

7079 Sudden Infant Death Syndrome Institute of The University of Maryland
2105 Laurel Bush Road,, Suite 201
Bel Air, MD 21015   443-640-1049
                                                 Fax: 410-653-8709
                                                  info@firstcandle.org
                                                 www.firstcandle.org

Debora Boyd, Executive Director

7080 USC - Neonatology Research Units
1240 Mission Road
Los Angeles, CA 90033   323-266-3813
                                                 Fax: 323-266-5049
                                                      www.usc.edu

Focuses on clinical problems of the newborn and premature infant.

Paul YK Wu, MD, Director

Conferences

7081 National Sudden Infant Death Syndrome Alliance Conference
www.healthyplace.com
                                                      210-225-4388
                                                      800-221-7437
                                                 www.healthyplace.com

Unites parents, caregivers, and researchers with government, business, and community service groups in a nationwide movement to advance the support of SIDS families and hasten the elimination of SIDS through medical research. Funds medical research and offers emotional support nationally and locally.

Gary Koplin, President
Harry Croft, M.D, Medical Director
Patricia Avila, Editor

Audio Video

7082 7 Steps to Reducing the Risk of SIDS
InJoy Productions
7107 La Vista Place
Longmont, CO 80503   303-447-2082
                                                      800-326-2082
                                                 Fax: 303-449-8788
                                          custserv@injoyvideos.com
                                                 www.injoyvideos.com

Shows how to dramatically lower infant's risk of using simple, important safety steps. Although SIDS is a frightening subject, this video's positive and compassionate tone will help ease parent's anxieties by showing them how to give their baby a healthy and happy first year.

14 minutes

Web Sites

7083 American SIDS Institute
528 Raven Way
Naples, FL 34110   239-431-5425
                                                 Fax: 239-431-5536
                                                      www.sids.org

A national nonprofit health care organization that is dedicated to the prevention of sudden infant death and the promotion of infant health through an aggresive, comprehensive nationwide program of: Research, Clinical Services, Education and Family Support.

Marc Peterzell, JD, Chairman
Betty McEntire, PhD, CEO/ Executive Director

7084 Center for Research for Mothers & Children
31 Center Drive, Building 31, Building 31, Room 2A
Bethesda, MD 20892   800-370-2943
                                                 Fax: 866-760-5947
                                                 TTY: 888-320-6942
                              NICHDInformationResourceCenter@mail.nih.
                                                   www.nichd.nih.gov

Composed of several branches the principle NIH source of support for research and research training in maternal and child health, through grants, contracts, and cooperative agreements. Through this research, CRMC-supported scientists are advancing fundamental and clinical knowledge concerning maternal health and child development problems such as low birth wieght, mental retardation and developmental disabilities, specific learning disabilities, congenital and genetic defects and others.

Alan E. Guttmacher, M.D., Director
Lisa Kaeser, Program Analyst
Lisa Williams Simons, Senior Research Assistant

7085 Compassionate Friends
www.compassionatefriends.org

Assists families toward the positive resolution of grief following the death of a child of any age and provides information to help others be supportive.

7086 Health Answers
410 Horsham Road
Horsham, PA 19044   215-442-9010
Michael.tague@healthanswers.com
www.healthanswers.com

HealthAnswers offers a breadth of services in medical education, sales force training, patient support solutions, professional promotion and consumer solutions.

Michael Tague, Managing Director

7087 National Center for Education in Maternal and Child Health
www.ncemch.org

202-784-9552
rmayer@ncemch.org
www.ncemch.org

The National Center for Education in Maternal and Child Health provides national leadership to the maternal and child health community in three key areas - program development, policy analysis and education, and knowledge to improve the health and well-being of the nation's children and families.

Rochelle Mayer, Ed.D., Director

7088 Online Mendelian Inheritance in Man
www.omim.org

This database is a catalog of human genes and genetic disorders.

7089 SID Network
PO Box 520
Ledyard, CT 6339   sidsnet1-at-sids-network-dot-org
sids-network.org/net.htm

Nonprofit voluntary agency that is dedicated to eliminate sudden infant death syndrome through the support of SIDS research projects, provide support for those who have been touched by the tragedy of sudden Infant Death Syndrome and to raise public awareness of sudden infant death syndrome through education.

Book Publishers

7090 Apparent Life - Threatening Event and Sudden Infant Death Syndrome
Circle Solutions, Inc
8280 Greensboro Drive, Suite 300
McLean, VA 22102   703-821-8955
866-866-7437
Fax: 703-821-2098
marketing@circlesolutions.com
www.circlesolution.com

Provides information about ALTE and its relationship to SIDS.

1992 29 pages

Kristina Lewis, Chairman, Executive Committee
Louis Cartwright, jr., Vice President-Finance
Michael Collins, Vice President-IT

7091 Crib Death: The Sudden Infant Death Syndrome
Futura Publishing Company
135 Bedford Road
Armonk, NY 10504   914-273-1014
Fax: 914-273-1015
www.growinghealthcare.com

A thorough book, that discusses the theories of SIDS and their implications. Athough it is aimed at the medical professional, lay people will also gain a clearer understanding of SIDS.

1995 456 pages Hardcover

7092 Death Investigations and Sudden Infant Death Syndrome
Circle Solutions, Inc
8280 Greensboro Drive, Suite 300
McLean, VA 22102   703-821-8955
Fax: 703-821-2098
marketing@circlesolutions.com
www.circlesolutions.com

Contains abstracts of articles on autopsies, death certification, and infant death scene investigation and SIDS.

1991 104 pages

Kristina Lewis, Chairman, Executive Committee
Louis Cartwright, jr., Vice President-Finance
Michael Collins, Vice President-IT

7093 Death of a Child, the Grief of the Parents A Lifetime Journey
Circle Solutions, Inc
8280 Greensboro Drive, Suite 300
McLean, VA 22102   703-821-8955
Fax: 703-821-2098
marketing@circlesolutions.com
www.circlesolutions.com

1997 38 pages

Kristina Lewis, Chairman, Executive Committee
Louis Cartwright, jr., Vice President-Finance
Michael Collins, Vice President-IT

7094 Grief, Bereavement and Sudden Infant Death Syndrome
Circle Solutions, Inc
8280 Greensboro Drive, Suite 300
McLean, VA 22102   703-821-8955
Fax: 703-821-2098
marketing@circlesolutions.com
www.circlesolutions.com

Contains abstracts of selected materials on the grief and bereavement process specific to the loss of a child to SIDS.

1991 28 pages

Kristina Lewis, Chairman, Executive Committee
Louis Cartwright, jr., Vice President-Finance
Michael Collins, Vice President-IT

7095 SIDS Research
Circle Solutions, Inc
8280 Greensboro Drive, Suite 300
McLean, VA 22102   703-821-8955
Fax: 703-821-2098
marketing@circlesolutions.com
www.circlesolutions.com

Contains abstracts of relevant articles published during 1993.

1995 146 pages

Kristina Lewis, Chairman, Executive Committee
Louis Cartwright, jr., Vice President-Finance
Michael Collins, Vice President-IT

7096 SIDS Survival Guide
Independent Publishers Group
814 N Franklin Street
Chicago, IL 60610   312-337-0747
800-888-4741
Fax: 312-337-5985
frontdesk@ipgbook.com
www.ipgbook.com

Offers information and comfort for grieving family, friends and professionals who seek to help them.

1994 290 pages Paperback
ISBN: 0-964121-87-5

Curt Matthews, CEO

7097 SIDS: A Parents Guide to Understanding & Preventing SIDS
Hachette Book Group USA
322 South Enterprise Blvd
Lebanon, IN 46052   800-759-0190
Fax: 800-286-9471
customer.service@hbgusa.com
www.hachettebookgroup.biz

1995
ISBN: 0-316779-12-1

David Young, Chairman
Evan Schnittman, Executive Vice President
Jamie Raab, President & Publisher

7098 Smoking and Sudden Infant Death Syndrome
Circle Solutions, Inc
8280 Breensboro Drive, Suite 300
McLean, VA 22102

703-821-8955
Fax: 703-821-2098
TTY: 703-556-4831
marketing@circlesolutions.com
www.circlesolutions.com

Contains abstracts of materials about tobacco use, its relationship to SIDS, and the dangers to the unborn and the newly born from passive and secondary smoking.

1992 34 pages

Kristina Lewis, Chairman, Executive Committee
Louis Cartwright, jr., Vice President-Finance
Michael Collins, Vice President-IT

7099 Sudden Death in Infancy, Childhood & Adolescence
Cambridge University Press
32 Avenue Of The Americas
New York, NY 10013

212-924-3900
Fax: 212-691-3239
newyork@cambridge.org
www.cambridge.org/us

1994 400 pages
ISBN: 0-521420-31-8

7100 Sudden Infant Death Syndrome Risk Factors
Circle Solutions, Inc
8280 Greensboro Drive, Suite 300
McLean, VA 22102

703-821-8955
Fax: 703-821-2098
TTY: 703-556-4831
marketing@circlesolutions.com
www.circlesolutions.com

Contains selected articles published between 1989 and 1993 on the risk factors for SIDS.

1994 131 pages

Kristina Lewis, Chairman, Executive Committee
Louis Cartwright, jr., Vice President-Finance
Michael Collins, Vice President-IT

Newsletters

7101 Illuminations
First Candle/SIDS Alliance
9 Newport Drive, Suite 200
Forest Hill, MD 21050

443-640-1049
800-221-7437
Fax: 410-653-8709
info@firstcandle.org
www.firstcandle.org

Quarterly

Christopher Blake, CEO
Barb Himes, IBCLC, Director of Education and Training
Shannon Carswell, Creative Director

7102 Network
Parent Care
9041 Colgate Street
Indianapolis, IN 46268

317-872-9913
Fax: 317-872-0795

Offers information on support groups, meetings, organizations and resources for parents and professionals dealing with the chronically ill child.

7103 Newsletter: SIDS
Massachusetts Center For SIDS
1 Boston Medical Center Place
Boston, MA 2118

617-638-8000
www.bmc.org/program/sids/

Offers information on SIDS, articles pertaining to the latest information available on the mystery condition, latest research and fund-raising news and professional resources available.

Monthly

Pamphlets

7104 After Sudden Infant Death Syndrome
Circle Solution, Inc
8280 Greensboro Drive, Suite 300
McLean, VA 22102

703-821-8955
Fax: 703-821-2098
marketing@circlesolutions.com
www.circlesolutions.com

1993 16 pages

Kristina Lewis, President/ Chair
Louis Cartwright, Jr., Vice President of Finance
Laura Scherzer, CMP, PMP, Vice President of Operations

7105 Bilingual Risk Reduction Brochure
First Candle/SIDS Alliance
9 Newport Drive, Suite 200
Forest Hill, MD 21050

443-640-1049
800-221-7437
Fax: 410-653-8709
info@firstcandle.org
www.firstcandle.org

Provides an understanding of the risk of SIDS and the steps that can be taken to help the baby survive and thrive.

2 pages

Christopher Blake, CEO
Barb Himes, IBCLC, Director of Education and Training
Shannon Carswell, Creative Director

7106 Facts About Apnea and Other Apparent Life-Threatening Events
Circle Solution, Inc
8280 Greensboro Drive, Suite 300
McLean, VA 22102

703-821-8955
Fax: 703-821-2098
marketing@circlesolutions.com
www.circlesolutions.com

Explains apparent life-threatening events in infants, their relationship to SIDS and current views on home monitoring.

1987 2 pages

Kristina Lewis, President/ Chair
Louis Cartwright, Jr., Vice President of Finance
Laura Scherzer, CMP, PMP, Vice President of Operations

7107 Facts About SIDS
Sudden Infant Death Syndrome Alliance
1314 Bedford Avenue
Baltimore, MD 21208

410-653-8226
Fax: 410-653-8709

Offers information on basic facts, answers to the most frequently asked questions about SIDS and information on numbers to call and referral centers for more help.

7108 Infant Positioning and Sudden Infant Death Syndrome
Circle Solutions, Inc
8280 Greensboro Drive, Suite 300
McLean, VA 22102

703-821-8955
Fax: 703-821-2098
marketing@circlesolutions.com
www.circlesolutions.com

Contains abstracts of selected articles on the topic of sleep position and SIDS.

1994

Kristina Lewis, President/ Chair
Louis Cartwright, Jr., Vice President of Finance
Laura Scherzer, CMP, PMP, Vice President of Operations

7109 National SIDS Resource Center Brochure
Circle Solutions, Inc
8280 Greensboro Drive, Suite 300
McLean, VA 22102
   703-821-8955
   Fax: 703-821-2098
   marketing@circlesolutions.com
   www.circlesolutions.com

1994

Kristina Lewis, President/ Chair
Louis Cartwright, Jr., Vice President of Finance
Laura Scherzer, CMP, PMP, Vice President of Operations

7110 Nationwide Survey of Sudden Infant Death Syndrome (SIDS) Service
Circle Solutions, Inc
8280 Greensboro Drive, Suite 300
McLean, VA 22102
   703-821-8955
   Fax: 703-821-2098
   marketing@circlesolutions.com
   www.circlesolutions.com

Analysis of availability of SIDS services.

1994

Kristina Lewis, President/ Chair
Louis Cartwright, Jr., Vice President of Finance
Laura Scherzer, CMP, PMP, Vice President of Operations

7111 Pacifiers and SIDS: Reducing the Risk
First Candle/SIDS Alliance
9 Newport Drive, Suite 200
Forest Hill, MD 21050
   443-640-1049
   800-221-7437
   Fax: 410-653-8709
   info@firstcandle.org
   www.firstcandle.org

A brochure for parents and caregivers.

Christopher Blake, CEO
Barb Himes, IBCLC, Director of Education and Training
Shannon Carswell, Creative Director

7112 SIDS Prevention
Corporate Office
100 Enterprise Way, Suite G300
Scotts Valley, CA 95066
   831-438-4060
   800-620-8884
   Fax: 831-438-4284
   support@etr.freshdesk.com
   www.etr.org

Gives overview, risk factors, prevention of Sudden Infant Death Syndrome.

50 pamphlets

Dan McCormick, MHA, Chief Executive Officer
David Kitchen, MBA, Chief Financial Officer
Erin Cassidy-Eagle, PhD, Director, Research

7113 SIDS: Toward Prevention and Improved Infant Health
American SIDS Institute
528 Raven Way
Naples, FL 34110
   239-431-5425
   800-232-sids
   Fax: 239-431-5536
   prevent@sids.org
   www.sids.org

Practical guide for those planning a pregnancy, for parents-to-be and for new parents.

Marc Peterzell, JD, Chairman
Betty McEntire, PhD, CEO/ Executive Director

7114 Surviving the Death of a Baby
First Candle/SIDS Alliance
9 Newport Drive, Suite 200
Forest Hill, MD 21050
   443-640-1049
   800-221-7437
   Fax: 410-653-8709
   info@firstcandle.org
   www.firstcandle.org

13 pages

Christopher Blake, CEO
Barb Himes, IBCLC, Director of Education and Training
Shannon Carswell, Creative Director

DESCRIPTION

7115 SYNCOPE

Synonyms: Swoon, Faint

Involves the following Biologic System(s):

Cardiovascular Disorders

Syncope is a medical term describing a phenomenon more commonly known as fainting. Specifically, syncope is a brief loss of consciousness that resolves without intervention. In the pediatric population most episodes of syncope are uncomplicated without neurologic or cardiac after effects (sequelae).

The true incidence of syncope is difficult to ascertain since many episodes are not reported to a medical provider. Roughly 15-25% of all children experience at least one episode of syncope or near-syncope, although adolescents are are the most common segment of the pediatric population to experience syncope and the most likely to have recurrent episodes.

The most common cause of fainting in pediatrics is neurocardiogenic (related to a problem of the nervous system and the heart) syncope, also known as vasovagal or vasodepressor syncope. The other cases of syncope can be divided into neurologic, cardiac, metabolic, toxin (drug abuse), and psychogenic. While greater than 95% of syncopal episodes have a benign etiology (cause), such as the simple vasovagal syncope, there are several rare causes that are fatal, accounting for 4-5 deaths per 100,000 pediatric patients. The possibility of a fatal etiology necessitates the need for a thorough investigation into any syncopal episode.

An appropriate evaluation begins with a thorough history and physical exam. The history should focus on details around the event, change in position (from sitting to standing, for instance), exercise, trauma, and past history of similar events. Family history is critical when evaluating unexplained sudden deaths, hearing loss, cardiac disease, recurrent fainting, seizure disorders or arrhythmias. The physical exam should include a careful neurologic exam as well as a thorough cardiac exam looking for murmurs, clicks or gallops (unusual heart sounds) and careful blood pressure measurements including orthostatic measurements (when the patient is sitting and then stands up. In individuals who have fainted, the blood pressure can drop significantly upon standing, indicating at least one possible cause of the syncopal episode.

The diagnostic evaluation continues with an electrocardiogram looking at abnormal rhythms as well as signs of cardiomyopathy (heart disease). If the physical examination and ECG are normal and the history is consistent with a simple 'faint', no further workup may be necessary. If the history is inconsistent with vasovagal syncope or if there are any abnormalities on the physical or ECG, referral to a specialist, usually a pediatric cardiologist or adult cardiologist, is appropriate. Further testing may include a tilt table test, 24-hour holter monitor, echocardiography, exercise stress testing or electrophysiology testing.

Treatment for syncope varies depending on the etiology. For simple vasodepressor syncope, management is often focused on increasing fluid and salt intake in an effort to improve blood volume and pressure. Often discovering the triggers for these patients enables them to avoid them or anticipate their response more effectively (i.e. lying on the ground with feet up before syncope occurs). Medication is an option if the syncopal episodes are frequent and impact on the patient's lifestyle. The most widely used and successfully used medication class has been beta-blockers. More serious cardiac causes of syncope may need to be treated with antiarrhythmics, pacemakers or defibrillators. These interventions can be life-saving and allow patients to lead full productive lives.

National Associations & Support Groups

7116 American Academy of Pediatrics
141 Northwest Point Boulevard
Elk Grove Village, IL 60007

847-434-4000
800-433-9016
Fax: 847-434-8000
www.aap.org

The American Academy of Pediatrics and its member pediatricians are committed to the attainment of optimal physical, mental and social health and well-being for all infants, children, adolescents, and young adults.

Fernando Stein, MD, FAAP, President
Karen Remley, MD, CEO/Executive VP

7117 NIH/National Heart, Lung and Blood Institu te
National Institute of Health
31 Center Dr MSC 2486, Bldg 31, Rm5A52
Bethesda, MD 20892

301-592-8573
Fax: 301-592-8563
TTY: 240-629-3255
NHLBIinfo@nhlbi.nih.gov
www.nhlbi.nih.gov

Primary responsibility of this organization is the scientific investigation of heart, blood vessel, lung and blood disorders. Oversees research, demonstration, prevention, education, control and training activities in these fields and emphasizes the prevention and control of heart diseases.

Gary H. Gibbons, M.D., Director
Nakela Cook, MD, Chief of Staff

7118 NIH/National Institute of Neurological Dis orders and Stroke (NINDS)
PO Box 5801
Bethesda, MD 20824

301-496-5751
800-352-9424
Fax: 301-496-0296
TTY: 301-468-5981
www.ninds.nih.gov

Information and advocacy resources for families and professionals. Includes listings of organizations providing general information and organizations focusing on more specific areas of concern to families and young adults who have disabilities.

Walter J. Koroshetz, MD, Director

Web Sites

7119 EMedicine Journal: Syncope
www.emedicine.com/med/topic3385.htm

Syncope information covering background, pathophysiology, frequency, mortality/morbidity, causes, lab studies and tests, diet, activity, drugs used in treatment, complications and patient education. Authored by Dr Jatin Dave and co-authored by Dr John Michael Gaziano.

7120 NINDS Syncope Information Page
Office of Communications and Public Liaison, NINDS
Bethesda, MD 20892

301-496-5751
800-352-9424
www.ninds.nih.gov/disorders/syncope/

Walter J. Koroshetz, M.D., Acting Director
Alan L. Willard, Ph.D., Acting Deputy Director
Caroline Lewis, Executive Officer

7121 Syncope Information Page
7272 Greenville Ave.
Dallas, TX 75231

800-242-8721
www.heart.org/HEARTORG/

American Heart Association information page about Syncope
such as what it is and what causes it.

Elliott Antman, President
Bernie Dennis, Chairman
Alvin Royse, Chairman-Elect

DESCRIPTION

7122 SYNDACTYLY

Synonyms: Syndactylia, Syndactylism

Involves the following Biologic System(s):

Orthopedic and Muscle Disorders

Syndactyly refers to an abnormality that is present at birth (congenital) and characterized by the joining together (fusing) of two or more fingers or toes. This relatively common abnormality seems to occur more frequently in boys than in girls. It is often inherited as an autosomal dominant trait. Syndactyly often results from incomplete or abnormal embryonic development of the fingers or toes. In some infants, it occurs spontaneously as the hands or feet of the developing fetus may be unnaturally constricted within the uterus. Classification of syndactyly is based on the severity of the clinical presentation. Defects associated with syndactyly may range from a simple or incomplete joining or webbing of the skin between two digits to fusion from the base to the tip of the digits, complete with fusion of the bones and nails.

Syndactyly of the foot may involve complete or incomplete webbing that usually affects the second and third toes. This simple condition is referred to as zygosyndactyly and often requires no treatment. Syndactyly may also involve webbing and bone fusion (synostosis) of the fourth and fifth toes with duplication of the fifth toe in a condition called syndactyly/polysyndactyly.

As in the foot, syndactyly of the hand may involve a simple webbing. However, in some cases, the fusion of certain fingers may be more complex and involve shared nerves and blood supply. Syndactyly of the fingers should be carefully evaluated to determine the best method of treatment, allowing for growth and dexterity of the fingers.

Syndactyly may also occur in association with several genetic disorders. Such disorders include acrocephalopolysyndactyly type II (Carpenter's syndrome), characterized by mental retardation and irregularities involving the head, hand, and genitalia; acrocephalosyndactyly type I (Apert's syndrome), characterized by craniofacial irregularities and syndactyly of the hands and feet; trisomy 18 syndrome, a chromosomal abnormality characterized by multiple craniofacial abnormalities, irregularities of the hands and feet, and severe mental retardation; and other inherited diseases. Treatment of syndactyly associated with these and other inherited disorders depends upon the nature of the underlying disorder. In itself, a minor incomplete syndactyly is not an indication for surgery if the only issue is its appearance. However, a syndactyly that prevents full range of motion in the involved fingers warrants surgical release to increase the fingers' ability to function. The timing of surgery is variable. However, as more fingers are involved and as the syndactyly becomes more complex, release should be performed earlier.

Government Agencies

7123 NIH/National Institute of Arthritis and Musculoskeletal and Skin Diseases
1 AMS Circle
Bethesda, MD 20892

301-495-4484
877-226-4267
Fax: 301-718-6366
TDD: 301-565-2966
niamsinfo@mail.nih.gov
www.niams.nih.gov

The mission of the NIAMS, a part of the NIH, is to support research into the causes, treatment, and prevention of arthritis and musculoskeletal and skin diseases, the training of basic and clinical scientists to carry out this research, and the dissemination of information on research progress in these diseases.

Stephen I Katz MD PhD, Director
Robert H Carter MD, Deputy Director
Gahan Breithaupt, Assoc Dir for Management & Operatio

National Associations & Support Groups

7124 American Academy of Pediatrics
141 Northwest Point Boulevard
Elk Grove Village, IL 60007

847-434-4000
800-433-9016
Fax: 847-434-8000
www.aap.org

The American Academy of Pediatrics and its member pediatricians are committed to the attainment of optimal physical, mental and social health and well-being for all infants, children, adolescents, and young adults.

Fernando Stein, MD, FAAP, President
Karen Remley, MD, CEO/Executive VP

7125 CHERUB-Association of Families and Friends of Children with Limb Disorders
Children's Hospital of Buffalo
936 Delaware Avenue
Buffalo, NY 14209

716-762-9997

Answers the questions and problems that families of juveniles diagnosed with a disorder may be experiencing.

Sandra Richenberg
Kathy Gura

7126 Genetic Alliance
4301 Connecticut Avenue NW, Suite 404
Washington, DC 20008

202-966-5557
800-336-4363
Fax: 202-966-8553
info@geneticalliance.org
www.geneticalliance.org

A coalition of voluntary genetic support groups, consumers and professionals addressing the needs of individuals and families affected by genetic disorders from a national perspective.

Sharon Terry, President/CEO
Tetyana Murza, Managing Director
Natasha Bonhomme, VP, Strategic Development

7127 March of Dimes Foundation
1275 Mamaroneck Avenue
White Plains, NY 10605

914-428-7100
888-663-4637
Fax: 914-428-8203
askus@marchofdimes.com
www.marchofdimes.com

Partnership of volunteers and professionals dedicated to improving the health of babies by preventing birth defects and infant mortality. Over 100 chapters are located across the country.

Stacey D. Stewart, President

7128 Shriners Hospitals for Children
Headquarters
2900 Rocky Point Drive
Tampa, FL 33607   813-281-0300
                             800-237-5055
                   Fax: 813-281-8113
          www.shrinershospitalsforchildren.org

Network of 22 hospitals that provide expert, no-cost orthopedic and burn care to children under 18.

Peter F Armstrong, VP

Web Sites

7129 A-to-Z Health & Disease Information
www.hmc.psu.edu/healthinfo/pq/poly.htm

Information page on polydactyly and syndactyly provided by Penn State Medical Center. Information includes a listing of physicians who treat the disorder, causes, symptoms, a general overview, diagnosis and treatment.

7130 Online Mendelian Inheritance in Man
www.omim.org

This database is a catalog of human genes and genetic disorders.

7131 Pediatric Plastic Surgery
One Hospital Drive, MC504
Columbia, MO 65212   573-882-4158
                   Fax: 573-884-4585
              mumedicine@missouri.edu
             medicine.missouri.edu/surgery/

Answers to questions about syndactyly and surgery provided by the University of Missouri Children's Hospital.

7132 Syndactyly
www.pncl.co.uk/~belcher/information/Syndactyly.pdf

Information sheet on syndactyly.

DESCRIPTION

7133 SYSTEMIC LUPUS ERYTHEMATOSUS

Synonyms: Lupus, SLE

Involves the following Biologic System(s):

Immunologic and Rheumatologic Disorders

Systemic lupus erythematosus (SLE) is a chronic, inflammatory, multisystem disorder of connective tissue that may affect many organ systems in the body including the skin, joints, membranes that line the walls of certain bodily cavities (serosal membranes), or kidneys. In children with the disorder, associated symptoms are often progressive and, without appropriate treatment, may result in life-threatening complications. However, in some patients, symptoms may spontaneously subside and periodically recur with varying levels of severity (relapsing-remitting). SLE usually becomes apparent during late adolescence or a patient's 20s or 30s. However, in up to 20 percent of patients, symptoms may begin during childhood, usually after the age of eight. Females are more commonly affected than males in all age groups.

The specific underlying cause of SLE is unknown. However, the disorder is thought to result from abnormalities in the regulating mechanisms of the immune system that normally prevent it from attacking the body's own cells and tissues. In addition, researchers speculate that certain microorganisms or other environmental factors may play some role in causing SLE. Familial cases have also been reported, suggesting potential genetic mechanisms. In some individuals, SLE-like symptoms may also occur after exposure to certain medications, such as particular antiseizure drugs or certain antibiotics known as sulfonamides. Drug-induced symptoms are usually relatively mild and subside when the responsible medication is removed.

The range and severity of associated symptoms and findings may vary. Although associated symptoms may begin suddenly or gradually, most children with SLE tend to have more acute, severe symptoms than adults. In some children, symptoms may tend to recur or worsen in association with certain infections. In addition, exposure to sunlight may worsen associated skin or other symptoms. Many children with SLE initially experience generalized symptoms, such as a fever, a general feeling of ill health (malaise), joint swelling and inflammation (arthritis) or pain (arthralgia), loss of appetite (anorexia), and weight loss. Most children also have associated skin abnormalities, including a scaly, reddish or bluish rash that is in a distinctive butterfly distribution across the cheeks and the bridge of the nose (butterfly rash). The affected area may be abnormally sensitive to sunlight (photosensitive), and the rash may gradually spread to other facial areas, the neck, scalp, chest, and arms. Additional skin symptoms may include flat, reddish, dot-like spots (punctate lesions) on the fingertips, palms, soles, arms, legs, and torso; abnormal changes of the tissues beneath t|he fingernails and toenails (nail beds); tender, reddish-purple swellings or nodules on the legs (erythema nodosum); and itchy, reddish, flat or raised lesions of the skin and mucous membranes (erythema multiforme). Patients may also develop painless sores of the mucous membranes of the mouth and nose. The hair may be abnormally coarse and dry, and some children may have patchy areas of baldness on the scalp (alopecia).

Many children with SLE may also experience joint stiffness; inflammation of muscles (myositis), causing muscle pain and weakness; abnormal changes and localized loss of bone in certain areas (aseptic necrosis), particularly the head of the thigh bone (femur); and Raynaud's phenomenon. This condition is characterized by sudden contraction of the relatively small blood vessels supplying the fingers and toes (digits), causing an interruption of blood flow to the digits and a subsequent excess of blood in affected areas following restoration of blood flow (reactive hyperemia). Such episodes are usually triggered by exposure to cold temperatures and are characterized by numbing, tingling, and bluish or whitish discoloration of the digits due to lack of blood flow and subsequent reddening and pain as blood flow is reestablished. Many children with SLE may also develop inflammation of the membranes that line the lungs and chest cavity (|pleurisy), surround the heart (pericarditis), and line the wall of the abdomen and cover the abdominal organs (peritonitis). Additional heart abnormalities may also be present, such as abnormal heart murmurs, inflammation of heart muscle (myocarditis), enlargement of the heart (cardiomegaly), a decreased ability of the heart to pump blood effectively to the lungs and the rest of the body (heart failure), and, in some severe cases, heart attacks (myocardial infarctions), potentially causing life-threatening complications.

Kidney involvement is common among children with SLE and may be the only disease manifestation. Associated inflammation of the filtering units of the kidneys (glomerulonephritis) may be mild, moderate, or severe. Symptoms and findings may range from small amounts of blood in the urine (hematuria) of mildly increased levels of protein in the urine (proteinuria) to kidney failure that causes potentially life-threatening complications. Some children with SLE may also experience symptoms due to involvement of the brain and spinal cord (central nervous system). Associated neurologic abnormalities may include personality changes, episodes of abnormally increased electrical activity in the brain (seizures), or other findings. In addition, in some children, disease progression may also affect other tissues and organs, causing additional symptoms and findings.

The treatment of SLE is individualized and based upon the severity of the disease and the specific organ systems affected. Episodes of active disease should be considered emergencies that require immediate evaluation and aggressive treatment to help prevent damage to affected tissues and organs. In addition, careful follow-up and ongoing monitoring is required to detect worsening disease and to ensure prompt, appropriate treatment as required. Therapy may include the use of nonsteroidal antiinflammatory drugs (NSAIDs)s or salicylates (aspirin) to help alleviate joint pain and antimalarial agents or topical corticosteroid creams to treat skin symptoms. In severe cases, immunosuppressive drugs may also be administered; however, such agents must be used with great caution in children. Treatment of kidney inflammation may also include the use of certain corticosteroids, such as prednisone, and in some patients, the addition of immunosuppressive agents, such as azathioprine. Children with severe kidney disease may require regular dialysis or kidney transplantation. Dialysis is a medical procedure that removes excess fluid from the body and waste products from the blood. Additional treatment is symptomatic and supportive.

National Associations & Support Groups

7134 American Academy of Pediatrics
141 Northwest Point Boulevard
Elk Grove Village, IL 60007 847-434-4000
800-433-9016
Fax: 847-434-8000
www.aap.org

The American Academy of Pediatrics and its member pediatricians are committed to the attainment of optimal physical, mental and social health and well-being for all infants, children, adolescents, and young adults.

Fernando Stein, MD, FAAP, President
Karen Remley, MD, CEO/Executive VP

7135 American Autoimmune Related Diseases Association
22100 Gratiot Avenue
Eastpointe, MI 48021 586-776-3900
800-598-4668
Fax: 586-776-3903
aarda@aarda.org
www.aarda.org

Dedicated to the eradiction of autoimmune diseases and the alleviation of suffering and the socio-economic impact of autoimmunity through fostering and facilitating collaboration in the areas of education, public awareness, research and patient services in an effective, ethical and efficient manner.

Virginia T. Ladd, President/Executive Director
Patricia Barber, Assistant Director
Deb Patrick, Events Specialist

7136 American Juvenile Arthritis Organization
1330 W. Peachtree Street., Suite 100
Atlanta, GA 30309 404-872-7100
800-283-7800
Fax: 404-237-8153
info.ga@arthritis.org
www.arthritis.org

Devoted to serving the special needs of children, teens, and young adults with childhood rheumatic diseases and their families. Offers both support and information through national and local programs that serve the needs of families, friends and health professionals. Serves as a clearinghouse of information, sponsors an annual national conference, monitors and promotes legislation, sponsors research, and offers training to both parents and health professionals.

Sage Rhodes, President

7137 Children's Hospital Boston
300 Longwood Avenue
Boston, MA 02115 617-355-6000
TTY: 617-730-0152
www.childrenshospital.org

Mission is to provide the highest quality care; be the leading source of research and discovery; educate the next generation of leaders in child health and enhance the health and well-being of the children and families in our local community.

Leslie M Higuchi, President & CEO
Sandra Fenwick, Chief Operating Officer

7138 Genetic Alliance
4301 Connecticut Avenue NW, Suite 404
Washington, DC 20008 202-966-5557
800-336-4363
Fax: 202-966-8553
info@geneticalliance.org
www.geneticalliance.org

A coalition of voluntary genetic support groups, consumers and professionals addressing the needs of individuals and families affected by genetic disorders from a national perspective.

Sharon Terry, President/CEO
Tetyana Murza, Managing Director
Natasha Bonhomme, VP, Strategic Development

7139 Lupus Foundation of America
2000 L Street NW, Suite 710
Washington, DC 20036 202-349-1155
800-558-0121
Fax: 202-349-1156
LupusInfo@aol.com
www.lupus.org/newsite/

The LFA mission is to educate and support those affected by lupus. It supports research into the cause and cure of lupus. Information resources are available on request, including free pamphlets, brochures (English/Spanish), and articles for people seeking an understanding of lupus. Books and materials on lupus are also available through the LFA. There are nearly 300 chapters, branches, and support groups in 32 states throughout the US.

Sandra Raymond, President
Cindy Coney, Board Secretary

Research Centers

7140 Lupus Research Institute
330 Seventh Ave, Suite 1701
New York, NY 10001 212-812-9881
Fax: 212-545-1843
lupus@LupusNY.org
www.lupusresearchinstitute.org

Established exclusively for lupus research. It has invested almost $20 million in new research and has funded 73 studies in 22 states.

Robert J Ravitz, Co-Chair
John A Luke, Treasurer

7141 SLE Lupus Foundation
330 Seventh Ave, Suite 1701
New York, NY 10001 212-685-4118
800-745-8787
Fax: 212-545-1843
lupus@LupusNY.org
www.lupusny.org

Purpose is to raise funds for research grants, provide information and services to lupus patients, and educate the public about lupus. Patient services include self-help groups, orientation meetings, referrals, publications, and counseling on personal and financial problems related to the disease.

Richard K DeScherer, President
Margaret G Dowd, Executive Director

Web Sites

7142 American Autoimmune Related Diseases Association
22100 Gratiot Avenue
Eastpointe, MI 48021 586-776-3900
800-598-4668
Fax: 586-776-3903
aarda@aarda.org
www.aarda.org

Dedicated to the eradiction of autoimmune diseases and the alleviation of suffering and the socio-economic impact of autoimmunity through fostering and facilitating collaboration in the areas of education, public awareness, research and patient services in an effective, ethical and efficient manner.

Virginia T. Ladd, President/Executive Director
Patricia Barber, Assistant Director
Deb Patrick, Events Specialist

7143 Children's Hospital Boston
300 Longwood Avenue
Boston, MA 2115 617-355-6000
800-355-7944
www.childrenshospital.org

Mission is to provide the highest quality care; be the leading source of reseach and discovery; educate the next generation of leaders in child health and enhance the health and well-being of the children and families in our local community.

Sandra L. Fenwick, President/ CEO
Kevin Churchwell, MD, EVP, Health Affairs & COO
Naomi Fried, PhD, Chief Innovation Officer

Book Publishers

7144 Are You Tired Again...I Understand

Marilyn Deutsch PhD, author

Lupus Foundation of America
PO Box 932615
Atlanta, GA 31193   866-484-3532
                                  Fax: 770-442-9742
                                    orders@lupus.org
                                       www.lupus.org

An activity workbook for children to help them understand and
what to expect when living with someone with lupus.

1996 42 pages Paperback

Sandra C. Raymond, President & CEO
Mary Schwarz, COO
Seung-Ae Chung, CFO

7145 Coping with Lupus

Robert Phillips PhD, author

Lupus Foundation of America
PO Box 932615
Atlanta, GA 31193   866-484-3532
                                  Fax: 770-442-9742
                                   LupusInfo@aol.com
                                       www.lupus.org

A practicing psychologist offers sound, meaningful and compassionate advice to individuals who must live with lupus.

2001 373 pages Softcover

Sandra C. Raymond, President & CEO
Mary Schwarz, COO
Seung-Ae Chung, CFO

7146 Disability Handbook for Social Security Applicants

Douglas Smith, author

Lupus Foundation of America
PO Box 932615
Atlanta, GA 31193   866-484-3532
                                   LupusInfo@aol.com
                                       www.lupus.org

The handbook also includes the Disability Evaluation Guide for
People with Systemic Lupus Erythematosus: Writing Medical Reports to the Social Security Administration. It helps people get
their disability benefits promptly, without unnecessary appeals.
Tells what you have to prove and how to prove it.

1995 137 pages Softcover

Sandra C. Raymond, President & CEO
Mary Schwarz, COO
Seung-Ae Chung, CFO

7147 Get to Sleep! How To Sleep Well...Despite Lupus

Robert Phillips PhD, author

Lupus Foundation of America
PO Box 932615
Atlanta, GA 31193   770-280-4177
                                      866-484-3532
                                  Fax: 770-442-9742
                                    orders@lupus.org
                                       www.lupus.org

Written in a simple, straightforward style, this easy to follow action guide teaches you the most effective strategies for enabling
you to get the sleep you want and need.

1995 14 pages
ISBN: 0-895294-75-3

Sandra C. Raymond, President & CEO
Mary Schwarz, COO
Seung-Ae Chung, CFO

7148 Immune System Disorders Sourcebook

Omnigraphics
PO Box 8002
Aston, PA 19014   800-234-1340
                                  Fax: 800-875-1340
                                  info@omnigraphics.com
                                   www.omnigraphics.com

Basic information about lupus, multiple sclerosis, guillain-barre
syndrome and other disorders of the immune system.

671 pages 2nd Edition
ISBN: 0-780807-48-0

Peter Ruffner, Publisher

7149 Let's Talk About Going to the Hospital

Rosen Publishing Group's PowerKids Press
29 E 21st Street
New York, NY 10010   212-777-3017
                                      800-237-9932
                                  Fax: 888-436-4643
                                  rosenpub@tribeca.ios.com
                                   www.rosenpublishing.com

If a child has to check into the hospital, chances are he or she is
already upset about being ill. Knowing how a hospital functions
and what the procedures are, such as when family members can
visit, will help in what is already a stressful situation. Grades
K-5.

24 pages
ISBN: 0-823950-36-0

Roger Rosen, President

7150 Loopy Lupus Helps Tell Scott's Story

Lupus Foundation of America
PO Box 932615
Atlanta, GA 31193   770-280-4177
                                      866-484-3532
                                  Fax: 770-442-9742
                                    orders@lupus.org
                                       www.lupus.org

Written by a boy named Scott and his 3rd grade class explaining
what it is like to live with lupus.

2002 34 pages Paperback

Sandra C. Raymond, President & CEO
Mary Schwarz, COO
Seung-Ae Chung, CFO

7151 Lupus Book

Daniel J Wallace MD, author

Lupus Foundation of America
PO Box 932615
Atlanta, GA 31193   770-280-4177
                                      866-484-3532
                                  Fax: 770-442-9742
                                    orders@lupus.org
                                       www.lupus.org

Packed with useful, easy to understand information and practical
guidance for people with lupus, their family members, friends
and physicians. This hardcover book explains virtually every aspect of the disease and will help people better manage their day
to day fight with lupus.

2005 271 pages 3rd Edition
ISBN: 0-195181-81-4

Sandra C. Raymond, President & CEO
Mary Schwarz, COO
Seung-Ae Chung, CFO

7152 Lupus Erythematosus: A Patient's Guide

Lupus Foundation of America
PO Box 932615
Atlanta, GA 31193   770-280-4177
                                      866-484-3532
                                  Fax: 770-442-9742
                                    orders@lupus.org
                                       www.lupus.org

A popular LFA publication, the handbook provides a brief but detailed overview of the disease and guide for living well with
lupus.

2000 27 pages

Sandra C. Raymond, President & CEO
Mary Schwarz, COO
Seung-Ae Chung, CFO

7153 Lupus Q&A: Everything You Need To Know
Lupus Foundation of America
PO Box 932615
Atlanta, GA 31193   770-280-4177
                                            866-484-3532
                                      Fax: 770-442-9742
                                       orders@lupus.org
                                         www.lupus.org

Resource written for patients that want to learn more about lupus
than what their doctors may or may not tell them.

2004 240 pages Paperback

Sandra C. Raymond, President & CEO
Mary Schwarz, COO
Seung-Ae Chung, CFO

7154 Sick and Tired of Feeling Sick and Tired
Lupus Foundation of America
PO Box 932615
Atlanta, GA 31193   770-280-4177
                                            866-484-3532
                                      Fax: 770-442-9742
                                       orders@lupus.org
                                         www.lupus.org

Written in simple terms, the author offers understanding and practical guidance to people who live with ICI's and those who care
for and about them.

2000 304 pages New Ed/ Paper
ISBN: 0-393320-65-0

Sandra C. Raymond, President & CEO
Mary Schwarz, COO
Seung-Ae Chung, CFO

7155 When Mom Gets Sick
Rebecca Samuels, author
Lupus Foundation of America
PO Box 932615
Atlanta, GA 31193   770-280-4177
                                            866-484-3532
                                      Fax: 770-442-9742
                                       orders@lupus.org
                                         www.lupus.org

Written and illustrated by a nine-year-old, this is a compelling
story based on the experiences of a sensitive and insightful young
girl who makes the best from what could be a devastating
situation.

27 pages

Sandra C. Raymond, President & CEO
Mary Schwarz, COO
Seung-Ae Chung, CFO

Magazines

7156 Lupus Now®
Lupus Foundation of America
2000 L Street NW, Suite 410
Washington, DC 20036   202-349-1155
                                            800-558-0121
                                      Fax: 202-349-1156
                                          info@lupus.org
                                    www.lupus.org/newsite/

National and official magazine of the LFA. It includes lifestyle
and wellness features and articles, research news, upcoming
events, and other timely information for people with lupus, their
families and health professionals.

48 pages 3x/year

Sandra C. Raymond, President/ CEO
Joan T. Merrill, MD, Medical Director
Seung-Ae Chung, CPA, Chief Financial Officer

DESCRIPTION

7157 TAY-SACHS DISEASE

Synonyms: GM2 gangliosidosis, type I, Hexa deficiency, Hexosaminidase A deficiency, Tay-Sachs disease, infantile type, TSD

Covers these related disorders: Tay-Sachs disease, juvenile type (GM2 gangliosidosis, type III)

Involves the following Biologic System(s):

Genetic/Chromosomal/Syndrome/Metabolic Disorders

Tay-Sachs disease, also known as GM2 gangliosidosis type I or infantile type, is a progressive degenerative metabolic disorder that occurs when two copies of the disease gene are inherited from the parents (autosomal recessive trait). The disorder, which belongs to a group of diseases known as lysosomal storage disorders, results from insufficient activity of the enzyme beta-hexosaminidase A. Enzymes within lysosomes, which are the major digestive units of cells, break down particles of nutrients such as certain fats and carbohydrates. In individuals with Tay-Sachs disease, insufficient activity of the enzyme hbeta-exosaminidase A causes an abnormal accumulation of particular fats (i.e., gangliosides) in certain tissues of the body, particularly nerve cells of the brain. Tay-Sachs disease affects approximately one in 3,500 to 4,000 newborns. The disease occurs predominantly in people of Ashkenazi Jewish (i.e., northeastern European Jewish) descent. About one in 30 individuals of Ashkenazi Jewish ancestry carries a single copy of the disease gene (heterozygous carrier).

Infants with Tay-Sachs disease appear to develop as expected until approximately four to six months of age, except for a marked startle reaction to sudden noises (hyperacusis) that may be apparent soon after birth. From four to six months of age, affected infants may begin to have decreased focusing and eye contact and appear listless and irritable. As the disease progresses, infants have delays in the acquisition of skills requiling the coordination of mental and physical activities (psychomotor delays) and lose previously acquired skills. By about one year of age, most affected children lose the ability to roll over, sit, stand, or vocalize sounds. In addition, muscle tone is severely diminished (hypotonia). With continuing disease progression, children experience increasing muscle rigidity and associated restrictions of movement (spasticity); uncontrolled electrical disturbances in the brain (seizures) that may be accompanied by prolonged contractions and relaxations of certain muscles (tonic-clonic convulsions); development of abnormal red circular areas of the middle layer of the eyes (cherry-red spots or Tay's sign); blindness; deafness; and loss of cognitive abilities (dementia). In many affected children, there is also enlargement of the brain (metabolic megalencephaly) due to abnormal accumulation of gangliosides in brain cells. Life-threatening complications often develop by approximately two to four years of age.

There are also variants of Tay-Sachs disease in which the onset of symptoms occurs later in life. For example, in children with the variant known as Tay-Sachs disease, juvenile type (GM2 gangliosidosis, type III), symptoms typically become apparent during mid-childhood although they may sometimes develop as early as the second year of life. This disease vari-

ant, which is characterized by varying levels of hexosaminidase deficiency, is also inherited as an autosomal recelssive trait. Associated symptoms may include progressive impairment of voluntary movements (ataxia); involuntary movements characterized by rapid, jerking or slow, repetitive, writhing movements (choreoathetosis); loss of speech; seizures; and visual loss. Patients may experience life-threatening complications by approximately 15 years of age.

The disease gene responsible for Tay-Sachs disease is located on the long arm of chromosome 15 (15q23-24). Several distinct changes (mutations) in this disease gene have been identified in individuals with Tay-Sachs disease. In addition, different mutations are responsible for the infantile and juvenile forms of the disorder. Tests have been developed to help confirm carrier status in individuals who may carry a single copy of the disease gene (e.g., serum or leukocyte hexosaminidase A testing). It is recommended that individuals of Askenazi Jewish descent obtain testing prior to starting a family. In addition, genetic counseling is provided for those individuals who are heterozygous carriers and desire to start a family or have additional children. Specialized testing is also available that may confirm a diagnosis of Tay-Sachs disease before birth (e.g., chorionic villus sampling). The treatment of infants and children with Tay-Sachs disease includes symptomatic and supportive measures. Even with the best of care, children with Tay-Sachs disease usually die by age 4, from recurring infection.

Government Agencies

7158 NIH/ Eunice Kennedy Shriver National Insti tute of Child Health & Human Development
31 Center Drive, Building 31
Bethesda, MD 20892
301-496-5113
800-370-2943
Fax: 866-760-5947
nichdpress@mail.nih.gov
www.nichd.nih.gov

Established in 1962 by congress, today the institute conducts and supports research on topics related to the health of children, adults, families and populations. Some of these topics include: developmental disabilities, growth and development, infant death, reproductive health and birth defects.

Diana W. Bianchi, Director
Paul Williams, Director, Communications

7159 NIH/National Institute of Neurological Dis orders and Stroke (NINDS)
PO Box 5801
Bethesda, MD 20824
301-496-5751
800-352-9424
Fax: 301-496-0296
TTY: 301-468-5981
www.ninds.nih.gov

Works to reduce the burden of neurological disease by conducting, fostering, coordinating and guiding research on the causes, prevention, diagnosis and treatment of neurological disorders and stroke, while supporting basic research in related scientific areas.

Walter J. Koroshetz, MD, Director

National Associations & Support Groups

7160 American Academy of Pediatrics
141 Northwest Point Boulevard
Elk Grove Village, IL 60007
847-434-4000
800-433-9016
Fax: 847-434-8000
www.aap.org

The American Academy of Pediatrics and its member pediatricians are committed to the attainment of optimal physical, mental and social health and well-being for all infants, children, adolescents, and young adults.

Fernando Stein, MD, FAAP, President
Karen Remley, MD, CEO/Executive VP

7161 Canadian Society for Mucopolysaccharid e & Related Diseases Inc
PO Box 30034, RPO Parkgate, North Vancouver
Britich Columbia,
Canada 604-924-5130
800-667-1846
Fax: 604-924-5131
www.mpssociety.ca

Committed to supporting families affected with MPS and related diseases, educating medical professionals and the general public about MPS and related diseases, and raising funds for research.

Kirsten Harkins, Executive Director

7162 Chicago Center for Jewish Genetic Disorder
Ben Gurion Way, 30 South Wells Street
Chicago, IL 60606 312-357-4718
jewishgeneticsctr@juf.org
www.jewishgeneticscenter.org

Provides public and professional education and to empower community members to seek out information and prevention strategies. Represents the blending of science with religious, cultural and historical sensitivity and awareness.

Karen Litwack, Director
Rachel Sacks, Community Outreach Coordinator

7163 Conner's Way Foundation for Tay-Sachs Dise ase
7746 Rockburn Drive
Ellicott City, MD 21043 410-379-0568
www.connersway.com

Provides support for parents and families with Tay-Sachs disease. Also, provides fundraising events.

Desiree Hopf, Co-Chair
Carl Hopf, Co-Chair

7164 Genetic Alliance
4301 Connecticut Avenue NW, Suite 404
Washington, DC 20008 202-966-5557
800-336-4363
Fax: 202-966-8553
info@geneticalliance.org
www.geneticalliance.org

A coalition of voluntary genetic support groups, consumers and professionals addressing the needs of individuals and families affected by genetic disorders from a national perspective.

Sharon Terry, President/CEO
Tetyana Murza, Managing Director
Natasha Bonhomme, VP, Strategic Development

7165 Genetic Alliance, Inc
4301 Connecticut Avenue NW, Suite 404
Washington, DC 20008 202-966-5557
Fax: 202-966-8553
info@geneticalliance.org
www.geneticalliance.org

Dedicated to improving the quality of life for everyone living with genetic conditions. Provide accuracy organizations results in measurable growth: increased funding for research, access to services, and support for emerging technologies.

Sharon Terry, President/CEO
Tetyana Murza, Managing Director
Natasha Bonhomme, VP, Strategic Development

7166 Jewish Genetic Disease Consortium
450 West End Avenue
New York, NY 10024 855-642-6900
866-370-4363
info@jewishgeneticdiseases.org
www.jewishgeneticdiseases.org

Created as a means by which a number of smaller, individual organizations could join together to heighten awareness of Jewish genetic diseases with a strong and unified voice.

Randy Yudenfriend-Glaser, Chair
Richard N. Gladstein, Co-Chair

7167 March of Dimes Foundation
1275 Mamaroneck Avenue
White Plains, NY 10605 914-428-7100
Fax: 914-428-8203
www.marchofdimes.com

Mission is to improve the health of babies by preventing birth defects, premature birth, and infant mortality. Provide research, community services, education and advocacy to save babies' lives, to give all babies a fighting chance against the threats to their health: prematurity, birth defects, low birth weight.

Stacey D. Stewart, President

7168 NIH/National Institute of Neurological Dis orders and Stroke (NINDS)
PO Box 5801
Bethesda, MD 20824 301-496-5751
800-352-9424
Fax: 301-496-0296
TTY: 301-468-5981
www.ninds.nih.gov

Mission is to reduce the burden of neurological disease - a burden borne by every age group, by every segment of society, by people all over the world.

Walter J. Koroshetz, MD, Director

7169 National Tay-Sachs and Allied Diseases Association
2001 Beacon Street, Suite 204
Boston, MA 2135 617-277-4463
800-906-8723
Fax: 617-277-0134
info@ntsad.org
www.ntsad.org

Direct, fund and promote research to develop treatments and cures; provide comprehensive support services to affected families and individuals; guide prevention, education, awareness and screening through effective grassroots collaborations with chapters and affiliates; lead advocacy efforts as the recognized authority for this family of genetic diseases.

Shari Ungerleider, President
Merle Adelman, Development
Sue Kahn, Executive Director

Web Sites

7170 Chicago Center for Jewish Genetic Disorder
www.jewishgeneticscenter.org

jewishgeneticsctr@juf.org
www.jewishgeneticscenter.org

Provides public and professional education and to empower community members to seek out information and prevention strategies.Represents the blending of science with religious, cultural and historical sensitivity and awareness.

7171 Genetic Alliance, Inc
4301 Connecticut Avenue NW, Suite 404
Washington, DC 20008 202-966-5557
Fax: 202-966-8553
info@geneticalliance.org
www.geneticalliance.org

Dedicated to improving the quality of life for everyone living with genetic conditions. Provide accuracy organizations results in measurable growth: increased funding for research, access to services, and support for emerging technologies.

Sharon Terry, President/CEO
Tetyana Murza, Managing Director
Natasha Bonhomme, VP, Strategic Development

7172 Health Answers
410 Horsham Road
Horsham, PA 19044
215-442-9010
Michael.tague@healthanswers.com
www.healthanswers.com

HealthAnswers offers a breadth of services in medical education, sales force training, patient support solutions, professional promotion and consumer solutions.

Michael Tague, Managing Director

7173 Healthfinder
1101 Wootton Parkway
Rockville, MD 20852
healthfinder@hhs.gov
www.healthfinder.gov

A key resource for finding the best government and nonprofit health and human services information on the internet. Links to carefully selected information and web sites from over 1,500 health-related organizations.

7174 Jewish Genetic Disease Consortium
450 West End Avenue
New York, NY 10024
855-642-6900
info@JewishGeneticDiseases.org
www.jewishgeneticdiseases.org

Created as a means by which a number of smaller, individual organizations could join together to heighten awareness of Jewish genetic diseases with a strong and unified voice.

Randy Yudenfriend-Glaser, Chair
Richard N. Gladstein, Co-Chair
Shari Ungerleider, Project Coordinator

7175 March of Dimes Birth Defects Foundation
1275 Mamaroneck Avenue
White Plains, NY 10605
914-997-4488
www.marchofdimes.org

Mission is to improve the health of babies by preventing birth defects, premature birth, and infant mortality. Provide research, community services, education and advocacy to save babies' lives, to give all babies a fighting chance against the threats to their health: prematurity, birth defects, low birthweight.

7176 NIH/National Institute of Neurological Dis orders and Stroke (NINDS)
PO Box 5801
Bethesda, MD 20824
301-496-5751
800-352-9424
www.ninds.nih.gov

Mission is to reduce the burden of neurological disease - a burden borne by every age group, by every segment of society, by people all over the world.

Walter J. Koroshetz, MD, Director

7177 National Tay-Sachs and Allied Disease Foundation
2001 Beacon Street, Suite 204
Boston, MA 2135
617-277-4463
800-906-8723
info@ntsad.org
www.ntsad.org

Dedicated to the treatment and prevention of Tay-Sachs and related diseases, and to provide information and support services to individuals and families affected by these diseases through education, research, genetic screening, family services and advocacy.

Shari Ungerleider, President
Merle Adelman, Development
Sue Kahn, Executive Director

7178 Online Mendelian Inheritance in Man
www.omim.org

This database is a catalog of human genes and genetic disorders.

7179 The Canadian Society for Mucopolysaccharid e & Related Diseases Inc
PO Box 30034, RPO Parkgate, North Vancouver
British Columbia, BC V7
604-924-5130
800-667-1846
Fax: 604-924-5131
info@mpssociety.ca
www.mpssociety.ca

Committed to supporting families affected with MPS and related diseases, educating medical professionals and the general public about MPS and related diseases, and raising funds for research.

Bernie Geiss, Chair
Jamie Myrah, Executive Director
Karen Saxvik, Executive Assistant

Book Publishers

7180 Home Care Book
National Tay-Sachs and Allied Diseases Association
2001 Beacon Street, Suite 204
Boston, MA 02135
617-277-4463
800-906-8723
Fax: 617-277-0134
info@ntsad.org
www.ntsad.org

Written by parents for parents and professionals, a guide to caring for children with progressive neuological disorders at home.

Kevin Romer, President
Stuart Altman, Vice President
Jayne Gershkowitz, Vice President-Finance

7181 International Quality for Adult Tay-Sachs Carrier Testing
National Tay-Sachs and Allied Diseases Association
2001 Beacon Street, Room 204
Boston, MA 02135
617-277-4463
800-906-8723
Fax: 617-277-0134
info@ntsad.org
www.ntsad.org

Kevin Romer, President
Stuart Altman, Vice President
Jayne Gershkowitz, Vice President-Finance

7182 Let's Talk About Going to the Hospital
Rosen Publishing Group's PowerKids Press
29 E 21st Street
New York, NY 10010
212-777-3017
800-237-9932
Fax: 888-436-4643
rosenpub@tribeca.ios.com
www.rosenpublishing.com

If a child has to check into the hospital, chances are he or she is already upset about being ill. Knowing how a hospital functions and what the procedures are, such as when family members can visit, will help in what is already a stressful situation. Grades K-5.

24 pages
ISBN: 0-823950-36-0

Roger Rosen, President

7183 Lifting of Canavan's Carrier Testing Facilities
National Tay-Sachs and Allied Diseases Association
2001 Beacon Street, Room 204
Boston, MA 02135
617-277-4463
800-906-8723
Fax: 617-277-0134
info@ntsad.org
www.ntsad.org

Kevin Romer, President
Stuart Altman, Vice President
Jayne Gershkowitz, Vice President-Finance

7184 Monograph on Canavan's Disease
National Tay-Sachs and Allied Diseases Association
2001 Beacon Street, Room 204
Boston, MA 02135
617-277-4463
800-906-8723
Fax: 617-277-0134
info@ntsad.org
www.ntsad.org

Kevin Romer, President
Stuart Altman, Vice President
Jayne Gershkowitz, Vice President-Finance

7185 Tay-Sachs Disease
Rosen Publishing
29 East 21st Street
New York, NY 10010
212-777-3017
800-237-9932
Fax: 888-436-4643
rosenpub@tribeca.ios.com
www.rosenpublishing.com

With colorful graphics and photographs, and a clear presentation of a tragic genetic disease, this title looks at gentic inheritance, dominant and recessive genes, and the carrier screening programs working to prevent Tay-Sachs.

6-12 64 pages 2007
ISBN: 1-404206-97-3

Roger Rosen, President

7186 Tay-Sachs Disease-A Bibliography, Medical Dictionary, & Annotated Research Guide
ICON Health Publications/ICON Group International
9606 Tierra Grande St., Suite 205
San Diego, CA 92126
Fax: 858-635-9414
orders@icongroupbooks.com
www.icongrouponline.com

A 3-in-1 reference book that provides a complete medical dictionary covering hundreds of terms and expressions relating to Tay-Sachs disease. Also gives extensive lists of bibliographic citations. Provides information to users on how to update their knowledge using various internet resources.

132 pages

7187 The Official Parent's Sourcebook on Tay-Sa chs Disease
ICON Health Publications/ICON Group International
9606 Tierra Grande St., Suite 205
San Diego, CA 92126
Fax: 858-635-9414
orders@icongroupbooks.com
www.icongrouponline.com

A comprehensive manual for anyone interested in self-directed research on tay-Sachs. Fully referenced with ample Internet listings and glossary.

128 pages

Newsletters

7188 Breakthrough
National Tay-Sachs and Allied Diseases Association
2001 Beacon Street, Room 204
Boston, MA 2135
617-277-4463
800-906-8723
Fax: 617-277-0134
info@ntsad.org
www.ntsad.org

Annual newsletter for friends and supporters that focuses on the latest advances in research, profiles of families and individuals helped by NTSAD and disease profiles.

Shari Ungerleider, President
Merle Adelman, Development
Sue Kahn, Executive Director

7189 The Connection
The Canadian MPS Society
PO Box 30034, RPO Parkgate, North Vancouver
British Columbia, BC V7
Canada
604-924-5130
800-667-1846
Fax: 604-924-5131
info@mpssociety.ca
www.mpssociety.ca

Members only quarterly newsletter, a valuable resource filled with information on MPS-related news, including updates on new treatments and care options, current research and clinical trials, MPS-related events, and family news.

Bernie Geiss, Chair
Jamie Myrah, Executive Director
Karen Saxvik, Executive Assistant

Pamphlets

7190 Late Onset Tay-Sachs Fact Sheet
National Tay-Sachs and Allied Diseases Association
2001 Beacon Street, Room 204
Boston, MA 2135
617-277-4463
800-906-8723
Fax: 617-277-0134
info@ntsad.org
www.ntsad.org

Quick reference information sheet on the chronic or late onset of Tay-Sachs is available for no charge.

Shari Ungerleider, President
Merle Adelman, Development
Sue Kahn, Executive Director

7191 Services to Families
National Tay-Sachs And Allied Diseases Association
2001 Beacon Street, Room 204
Boston, MA 2135
617-277-4463
800-906-8723
Fax: 617-277-0134
info@ntsad.org
www.ntsad.org

Offers information on the Association parent peer groups, referrals and advocacy services to families and patients.

Shari Ungerleider, President
Merle Adelman, Development
Sue Kahn, Executive Director

7192 Tay-Sachs & Sandhoff Disease
The Canadian MPS Society
PO Box 30034, RPO Parkgate, North Vancouver
British Columbia, BC V7
Canada
604-924-5130
800-667-1846
Fax: 604-924-5131
info@mpssociety.ca
www.mpssociety.ca

Bernie Geiss, Chair
Jamie Myrah, Executive Director
Karen Saxvik, Executive Assistant

7193 What Every Family Should Know
National Tay-Sachs & Allied Diseases Association
2001 Beacon Street, Room 204
Boston, MA 2135
617-277-4463
800-906-8723
Fax: 617-277-0134
info@ntsad.org
www.ntsad.org

50 page booklet detailing lysosomal storage and leukodystrophy disorders, with sections on Tay-Sachs, Sandhoff, Niemann-Pick, Gaucher, Canavan, Fabry, Pompe, therapeutic approaches and unique disease table.

Shari Ungerleider, President
Merle Adelman, Development
Sue Kahn, Executive Director

7194 What is Tay-Sachs?
National Tay-Sachs and Allied Diseases Association
2001 Beacon Street, Room 204
Boston, MA 2135

617-277-4463
800-906-8723
Fax: 617-277-0134
info@ntsad.org
www.ntsad.org

Informative educational pamphlet describing Infantile tay-Sachs, its inheritance and prevention is available for no charge.

Shari Ungerleider, President
Merle Adelman, Development
Sue Kahn, Executive Director

DESCRIPTION

7195 TELANGIECTASIA

Synonym: Telangiectasis

Covers these related disorders: Ataxia-telangiectasia (AT), Phlebectasia, Cutis marmorata, Hereditary hemorrhagic telangiectasia, Rendu-Osler-Weber disease, Spider Angioma

Involves the following Biologic System(s):

Dermatologic Disorders

Telangiectasia refers to the permanent widening or dilation of small blood vessels near the surface of the skin (superficial capillaries, arterioles, and venules). This results in the appearance of relatively small, red, well-defined skin lesions that have fine or coarse red lines or a spider-like network of red lesions that radiate from a central point (spider telangiectasia). Telangiectasias may develop as the result of an underlying disorder such as lupus erythematosus, dermatomyositis, rosacea, or psoriasis. These skin lesions may also result from exposure to sunlight, x-rays, or other forms of radiation.

Ataxia-telangiectasia (AT) is a rare, inherited, progressive disorder of the nervous system involving degenerative changes in the central nervous system along with defects in the immune system. AT is transmitted as an autosomal recessive trait and is characterized by the appearance during early childhood of telangiectasias involving the ears, face, the membranes that line the white outer coat of the eyes (bulbar conjunctiva), or other areas. Affected children are at risk for recurrent respiratory infections. Degeneration of the cerebellum, which is the part of the brain responsible for the regulation and coordination of voluntary movement and other vital functions, also occurs in children with AT.

Congenital generalized phlebectasia, sometimes called cutis marmorata telangiectatica congenita, is a benign telangiectasia that is apparent at birth and is characterized by red or purple-hued net-like lesions that may have a somewhat marbled appearance. These telangiectasias may be localized to an arm or leg or the trunk of the body; however, sometimes these skin lesions are more widely spread. In addition, the lesions may become more prominent with changes in outside temperature, crying, or exertion. This condition often resolves spontaneously by adolescence. Treatment is supportive.

Generalized essential telangiectasia is a rare condition that may affect children or adults and is characterized by the appearance of solitary or convergent patches of network-like telangiectasias. These lesions may appear on large but localized areas of the body such as the arms or legs or may sometimes involve or progress to the entire body. This disorder is limited to the skin with no health-associated irregularities. Treatment is supportive.

Hereditary benign telangiectasia is a rare, genetic disorder that is inherited as an autosomal dominant trait and is characterized by the appearance of telangiectasias on the skin of the face, arms, and upper portion of the trunk. This progressive disorder is limited to the skin.

Hereditary hemorrhagic telangiectasia, also called Rendu-Osler-Weber disease, is an inherited disorder that is transmitted as an autosomal dominant trait and is characterized by recurrent nosebleeds and the development of small telangiectasias of the skin and mucous membranes. These lesions range in color from red to purple and most often appear on the face, lips, and the membranes of the nose and mouth. In addition, the gastrointestinal tract, genitourinary tract, liver, brain, lungs, throat, voice box (larynx), and the membrane that lines the eyelids and whites of the eyes (conjunctiva) may be involved. Because the affected blood vessels may be fragile, they often break resulting in bleeding or hemorrhage from the gastrointestinal and genitourinary tracts, lungs, mouth, and nose.

Spider angioma, sometimes called spider nevus, is a telangiectasia characterized by the central, elevated, red lesion that is surrounded by a radiating, spider-like network of small blood vessels. Although these types of telangiectasias are often associated with conditions in which levels of circulating estrogen are elevated (e.g., pregnancy and liver disease), spider angiomas may also occur in preschool and school-age children. These lesions usually appear on the face, ears, forearms, and hands and often resolve on their own. Treatment is directed toward the removal of persistent angiomas and may include various methods such as freezing with liquid nitrogen (cryotherapy), the use of electric current to promote coagulation (electrocoagulation), or certain laser techniques such as intensed pulse light using a specially constructed flash lamp and focusing optics.

Telangiectasias can result in naevus flammeus (port-wine stain), which is a flat birthmark on the head or neck that spontaneously regresses. A port-wine stain, if present, will grow proportionately with the child. There is a high association with Sturge-Weber syndrome, a nevus formation in the skin and is associated with glaucoma, meningeal angiomas, and mental retardation. Unilateral nevoid telangiectasia refers to the appearance of telangiectasias on one side of the body in conjunction with an increase in the levels of circulating estrogen. These lesions sometimes develop in adolescent girls when they begin menstruation. Pregnancy may also prompt their development. When apparent in men, telangiectasias are the result of circulating estrogen secondary to liver disease. If this condition results from pregnancy, the lesions often fade or resolve during the postpartum period. Chronic treatment with corticosteroids may also lead to telangiectasias.

Government Agencies

7196 NIH/National Institute of Arthritis and Musculoskeletal and Skin Diseases
1 AMS Circle
Bethesda, MD 20892

301-495-4484
877-226-4267
Fax: 301-718-6366
TTY: 301-565-2966
niamsinfo@mail.nih.gov
www.niams.nih.gov

The mission of the NIAMS, a part of the NIH, is to support research into the causes, treatment, and prevention of arthritis and musculoskeletal and skin diseases, the training of basic and clinical scientists to carry out this research, and the dissemination of information on research progress in these diseases.

Stephen I Katz MD PhD, Director
Robert H Carter MD, Deputy Director
Gahan Breithaupt, Assoc Dir for Mngmnt & Operations

National Associations & Support Groups

7197 American Academy of Dermatology (AAD)
PO Box 4014
Schaumburg, IL 60168

847-240-1280
866-503-7546
Fax: 847-240-1859
mrc@aad.org
www.aad.org

Dedicated to achieving high quality dermatologic care for everyone which encompasses: responsiveness, unification and representation of the specialty, and excellence in patient care, education and research.

Brett M. Coldiron, MD, President
Elise A. Olsen, MD, VP
Suzanne M. Olbricht, MD, Secretary/Treasurer

7198 American Academy of Pediatrics
141 Northwest Point Boulevard
Elk Grove Village, IL 60007

847-434-4000
800-433-9016
Fax: 847-434-8000
www.aap.org

The American Academy of Pediatrics and its member pediatricians are committed to the attainment of optimal physical, mental and social health and well-being for all infants, children, adolescents, and young adults.

Fernando Stein, MD, FAAP, President
Karen Remley, MD, CEO/Executive VP

7199 American Skin Association
6 East 43rd Street, 28th Floor
New York, NY 10017

212-889-4858
800-499-7546
Fax: 212-889-4959
info@americanskin.org
www.americanskin.org

The American Skin Association is the only volunteer led health organization dedicated through research, education and advocacy to saving lives and alleviating human suffering caused by the full spectrum of skin disorders.

Philip G. Prioleau, MD, President
Kathleen Reichert, Executive Vice President
Ashley R. Jutchenko, Assistant Director

7200 Ataxia-Telangiectasia Children's Project
5300 W. Hillsboro Blvd., Suite 105
Coconut Creek, FL 33073

954-481-6611
800-543-5728
Fax: 954-725-1153
info@atcp.org
www.atcp.org

A non-profit organization that raises funds to support and coordinate biomedical research projects, scientific conferences and a clinical center aimed at finding a cure for ataxia-telagiectasia, a lethal genetic disease that attacks children, causing progressive loss of muscle control, cancer and immune system problems.

Brad Margus, Founder
Vicki Margus, Founder
Jennifer Thornton, Executive Director

7201 Children's Hospital Boston
300 Longwood Avenue
Boston, MA 2115

617-355-6000
800-355-7944
TTY: 617-355-0443
www.childrenshospital.org

Mission is to provide the highest quality care; be the leading source of research and discovery; educate the next generation of leaders in child health and enhance the health and well-being of the children and families in our local community.

Sandra L. Fenwick, President/ CEO
Kevin Churchwell, MD, EVP, Health Affairs & COO
Naomi Fried, PhD, Chief Innovation Officer

7202 Hereditary Hemorrhagic Telangiectasia (HHT) Foundation International
PO Box 329
Monkton, MD 21111

410-357-9932
800-448-6389
Fax: 410-357-0655
hhtinfo@curehht.org
curehht.org

Dedicated to increasing public and professional awareness and understanding of hereditary hemorrhagic telangiectasia (HHT). Supports ongoing medical research into the cause, prevention, and treatment of HHT; and offers a variety of materials including informational brochures and a quarterly newsletter.

Marianne Clancy, Executive Director

7203 NIH/National Institute of Neurological Dis orders and Stroke (NINDS)
PO Box 5801
Bethesda, MD 20824

301-496-5751
800-352-9424
Fax: 301-496-0296
TTY: 301-468-5981
www.ninds.nih.gov

Mission is to reduce the burden of neurological disease - a burden borne by every age group, by every segment of society, by people all over the world.

Walter J. Koroshetz, MD, Director

7204 National Ataxia Foundation
2600 Fernbrook Lane Suite 119
Minneapolis, MN 55447

763-553-0020
Fax: 763-553-0167
naf@ataxia.org
www.ataxia.org

Objectives of this organization are to make an early diagnosis of ataxia by locating all potential victims and encouraging them to have an examination, public information and professional education materials and basic research on the disease.

Charlene Danielson, President
Camille Daglio, Vice-President
Michael Parent, Executive Director

7205 Society for Pediatric Dermatology
8365 Keystone Crossing, Suite 107
Indianapolis, IN 46240

317-202-0224
Fax: 317-205-9481
info@pedsderm.net
www.pedsderm.net

Objective is to promote, develop and advance education, research and care of skin disease in all pediatric age groups.

Kent Lindeman, CMP, Executive Director
Stephanie Garwood, MTA, Meeting Manager
Barbara Case, Accounting Manager

Web Sites

7206 American Academy of Dermatology (AAD)
PO Box 4014
Schaumburg, IL 60168

847-240-1280
866-503-7546
Fax: 847-240-1859
mrc@aad.org
www.aad.org

Dedicated to achieving high quality dermatologic care for everyone which encompasses: responsiveness, unification and representation of the specialty, and excellence in pateint care, education and research.

Brett M. Coldiron, MD, President
Elise A. Olsen, MD, VP
Suzanne M. Olbricht, MD, Secretary/Treasurer

7207 American Skin Association
6 East 43rd Street, 28th Floor
New York, NY 10017
212-889-4858
800-499-7546
Fax: 212-889-4959
info@americanskin.org
www.americanskin.org

The American Skin Association is the only volunteer led health
organization dedicated through research, education and advocacy
to saving lives and alleviating human suffering caused by the full
spectrum of skin disorders.

Philip G. Prioleau, MD, President
Kathleen Reichert, Executive Vice President
Ashley R. Jutchenko, Assistant Director

7208 Ataxia-Telangiectasia Children's Project
5300 W. Hillsboro Blvd., Suite 105
Coconut Creek, FL 33073
954-481-6611
800-543-5728
Fax: 954-725-1153
info@atcp.org
www.atcp.org

A non-profit organization that raises funds to support and coordinate biomedical research projects, scientific conferences and a
clinical center aimed at finding a cure for ataxia-telagiectasia, a
lethal genetic disease that attacks childre, causing progressive
loss of muscle control, cancer and immune system problems.

Brad Margus, Founder
Vicki Margus, Founder
Jennifer Thornton, Executive Director

7209 Children's Hospital Boston
300 Longwood Avenue
Boston, MA 2115
617-355-6000
800-355-7944
www.childrenshospital.org

Mission is to provide the highest quality care; be the leading
source of reseach and discovery; educate the next generation of
leaders in child health and enhance the health and well-being of
the children and families in our local community.

Sandra L. Fenwick, President/ CEO
Kevin Churchwell, MD, EVP, Health Affairs & COO
Naomi Fried, PhD, Chief Innovation Officer

**7210 Hereditary Hemorrhagic Telangiectasia (HHT) Foundation
International**
PO Box 329
Monkton, MD 21111
410-357-9932
Fax: 410-357-0655
hhtinfo@curehht.org
curehht.org

Dedicated to increasing public and professional awareness and
understanding of hereditary hemorrhagic telangiectasia (HHT).
Supports ongoing medical research into the cause, prevention,
and treatment of HHT; and offers a variety of materials including
informational brochures and a quarterly newsletter.

**7211 NIH/National Institute of Neurological Dis orders and Stroke
(NINDS)**
PO Box 5801
Bethesda, MD 20824
301-496-5751
800-352-9424
www.ninds.nih.gov

Mission is to reduce the burden of neurological disease - a burden
borne by every age group, by every segment of society, by people
all over the world.

Walter J. Koroshetz, MD, Director

7212 National Ataxia Foundation
2600 Fernbrook Lane Suite 119
Minneapolis, MN 55447
763-553-0020
Fax: 763-553-0167
naf@ataxia.org
www.ataxia.org

Objectives of this organization are to make an early diagnosis of
ataxia by locating all potential victims and encouraging them to
have an examination, public information and professional education materials and basic research on the disease.

Charlene Danielson, President
Camille Daglio, Vice-President
Michael Parent, Executive Director

7213 Online Mendelian Inheritance in Man
www.omim.org

This database is a catalog of human genes and genetic disorders.

7214 Society for Pediatric Dermatology
8365 Keystone Crossing, Suite 107
Indianapolis, IN 46240
317-202-0224
Fax: 317-205-9481
info@pedsderm.net
www.pedsderm.net

Objective is to promote, develop and advance education, research
and care of skin disease in all pediatric age groups.

Kent Lindeman, CMP, Executive Director
Stephanie Garwood, MTA, Meeting Manager
Barbara Case, Accounting Manager

Journals

7215 Pediatric Dermatology Journal
Society for Pediatric Dermatology
8365 Keystone Crossing, Suite 107
Indianapolis, IN 46240
317-202-0224
Fax: 317-205-9481
info@pedsderm.net
www.pedsderm.net

6 issues/yr
Kent Lindeman, Executive Director

Newsletters

**7216 Hereditary Hemorrhagic Telangiectasia Foundation
International Newsletter**
PO Box 329
Monkton, MD 21111
410-357-9932
800-448-6389
Fax: 410-357-0655
hhtinfo@curehht.org
curehht.org

The Foundation is dedicated to increasing public and professional
awareness and understanding of hereditary hemorrhagic
telangiectasia (HHT). Supports ongoing medical research into the
cause, prevention, and treatment of HHT.

Quarterly

Pamphlets

7217 Ataxia-Telangiectasia and Cancer Risk
5300 W. Hillsboro Blvd., Suite 105
Coconut Creek, FL 33073
954-481-6611
800-543-5728
Fax: 954-725-1153
info@atcp.org
www.atcp.org

Brad Margus, Founder
Vicki Margus, Founder
Jennifer Thornton, Executive Director

7218 Ataxia-Telangiectasia and Estrogen Replace ment in Females
5300 W. Hillsboro Blvd., Suite 105
Coconut Creek, FL 33073
954-481-6611
800-543-5728
Fax: 954-725-1153
info@atcp.org
www.atcp.org

Brad Margus, Founder
Vicki Margus, Founder
Jennifer Thornton, Executive Director

7219 Ataxia-Telangiectasia and Immune Function
5300 W. Hillsboro Blvd., Suite 105
Coconut Creek, FL 33073
954-481-6611
800-543-5728
Fax: 954-725-1153
info@atcp.org
www.atcp.org

Brad Margus, Founder
Vicki Margus, Founder
Jennifer Thornton, Executive Director

7220 Ataxia-Telangiectasia and Swallowing Probl ems
5300 W. Hillsboro Blvd., Suite 105
Coconut Creek, FL 33073
954-481-6611
800-543-5728
Fax: 954-725-1153
info@atcp.org
www.atcp.org

Brad Margus, Founder
Vicki Margus, Founder
Jennifer Thornton, Executive Director

7221 Ataxia-Telangiectasia and X-Rays
5300 W. Hillsboro Blvd., Suite 105
Coconut Creek, FL 33073
954-481-6611
800-543-5728
Fax: 954-725-1153
info@atcp.org
www.atcp.org

Brad Margus, Founder
Vicki Margus, Founder
Jennifer Thornton, Executive Director

DESCRIPTION

7222 TETRALOGY OF FALLOT

Synonym: Fallot's syndrome

Involves the following Biologic System(s):

Cardiovascular Disorders

Tetralogy of Fallot is a combination of four specific heart malformations that are present at birth (congenital heart defects). Normally, oxygen-poor blood that returns from the body to the heart into the right upper chamber of the heart (right atrium), is pumped into the right lower chamber (right ventricle), and is then pumped into the pulmonary artery and on to the lungs, where the exchange of oxygen and carbon dioxide occurs. Oxygen-rich blood returns from the lungs to the heart via the left atrium, is pumped into the left ventricle, and is subsequently pumped into the major artery of the body (aorta) for circulation to the body's tissues. However, newborns with tetralogy of Fallot typically have four coexisting cardiac defects: i.e., (1) obstruction of the normal outflow of blood from the right ventricle due to abnormal narrowing (stenosis) of the opening between the right ventricle and the pulmonary artery (pulmonary stenosis); (2) an abnormal opening in the partition (septum) that separates the ventricles of the heart (ventricular septal defect or VSD); (3) displacement or override of the aorta, allowing oxygen-poor blood to flow directly from the right ventricle into the aorta; and (4) abnormal thickness of the right ventricle (right ventricular hypertrophy). Tetralogy of Fallot is thought to affect approximately one in 1,000 infants and children.

In patients with tetralogy of Fallot, the onset and severity of associated symptoms depend, in part, upon the degree of right ventricular outflow obstruction. Primary symptoms and findings in mild cases may be only a an unusual heart sound (murmur) heard through the stethoscope. In other cases, there may be a bluish discoloration of the skin and mucous membranes (cyanosis) due to decreased levels of oxygen in the blood; an insufficient supply of oxygen to bodily cells (hypoxia); and difficulties feeding. In infants with tetralogy of Fallot, cyanosis is typically most apparent in the nail beds of the fingers and toes and in the mucous membranes of the mouth and lips. In severe cases, cyanosis may be apparent soon after birth. In such newborns, pulmonary blood flow may primarily depend upon the fetal vascular channel that joins the pulmonary artery and the aorta (ductus arteriosus). Because this fetal vascular channel closes shortly after birth, severe cyanosis may develop within the first hours or days after birth. In other patients, cyanosis may not become apparent until later during the first year of life.

Some affected infants experience periodic attacks or spells during which cyanosis worsens (hypoxic or blue spells). During such hypoxic spells, patients may become restless and cyanotic; develop extreme shortness of breath; and potentially lose consciousness (syncope). Although the onset of these attacks is unpredictable, they may tend to occur after severe crying episodes or upon awakening (Tet spells). The duration of the spells may range from a few minutes to a few hours, and they should be considered life-threatening and an indication for surgical repair.

Tetralogy of Fallot may be diagnosed based upon a complete clinical examination and patient history, detection of distinctive heart murmurs, and various specialized tests (e.g., x-ray studies, echocardiogram, electrocardiogram, cardiac catheterization). Surgery is performed in the first year of life, and often in the first six months of life, depending upon the severity of right ventricular outflow obstruction. Corrective open-heart surgery patches the ventricular septal defect, and enlarges the opening between the pulmonary artery and right ventricle. In many cases, corrective open-heart surgery may be recommended during the neonatal or infant period to avoid the risk of cyanotic spells later in infancy. Before and after corrective open-heart surgery, patients may be susceptible to bacterial infection of certain areas of the heart (e.g., bacterial endocarditis). Therefore, patients should be provided with antibiotic medication (antibiotic prophylaxis) with dental visits and certain surgical procedures. Additional treatment is symptomatic and supportive.

Tetralogy of Fallot may occur as an isolated condition, with other congenital heart defects, or in some cases, in association with certain chromosomal abnormalities (e.g., DiGeorge syndrome — a partial gene deletion that results in heart defects, low calcium levels, and immune deficiency — and Down syndrome.) Prenatal factors associated with higher than normal risk for this condition include maternal rubella (German measles) or other viral illnesses during pregnancy, poor prenatal nutrition, maternal alcoholism, mother over 40 years old, and diabetes. Researchers indicate that, in some patients, tetralogy of Fallot may be due to the interaction of one or more genes v(22q11). As with patients that have undergone any heart surgery, antibiotic prophylaxis (prevention) is indicated during dental treatment in order to prevent infective endocarditis, inflammation of the heart's inner lining or the heart valves.

Government Agencies

7223 NIH/ Eunice Kennedy Shriver National Insti tute of Child Health & Human Development

31 Center Drive, Building 31

Bethesda, MD 20892

> 301-496-5113
> 800-370-2943
> Fax: 866-760-5947
> TTY: 888-320-6942
> nichdpress@mail.nih.gov
> www.nichd.nih.gov

Established in 1962 by congress, today the institute conducts and supports research on topics related to the health of children, adults, families and populations. Some of these topics include: developmental disabilities, growth and development, infant death, reproductive health and birth defects.

Diana W. Bianchi, Director

Paul Williams, Director, Communications

7224 NIH/National Heart, Lung and Blood Institu te

National Institute of Health

31 Center Dr MSC 2486, Bldg 31, Room 5A52

Bethesda, MD 20892

> 301-592-8573
> Fax: 240-629-3246
> TTY: 240-629-3255
> NHLBIinfo@nhlbi.nih.gov
> www.nhlbi.nih.gov

Primary responsibility of this organization is the scientific investigation of heart, blood vessel, lung and blood disorders. Oversees research, demonstration, prevention, education, control and training activities in these fields and emphasizes the prevention and control of heart diseases.

Gary H. Gibbons, M.D., Director

Nakela Cook, MD, MPH, Chief of Staff

Kathleen B. O'Sullivan, Executive Officer

National Associations & Support Groups

7225 American Academy of Pediatrics
141 Northwest Point Boulevard
Elk Grove Village, IL 60007   847-434-4000
                                                800-433-9016
                                                Fax: 847-434-8000
                                                www.aap.org

The American Academy of Pediatrics and its member pediatricians are committed to the attainment of optimal physical, mental and social health and well-being for all infants, children, adolescents, and young adults.

Fernando Stein, MD, FAAP, President
Karen Remley, MD, CEO/Executive VP

7226 American Heart Association
7272 Greenville Avenue
Dallas, TX 75231   214-373-6300
                                                800-242-8721
                                                Fax: 214-706-1341
                                                inquire@amhrt.org
                                                www.heart.org/HEARTORG/

Supports research, education and community service programs with the objective of reducing premature death and disability from cardiovascular diseases and stroke; coordinates the efforts of health professionals, and others engaged in the fight against heart and circulatory disease.

Nancy Brown, CEO
Dr. Stephen Houser, President
Suzie Upton, Chief Operating Officer

7227 Children's Hospital Boston
300 Longwood Avenue
Boston, MA 2115   617-355-6000
                                                800-355-7944
                                                TTY: 617-355-0443
                                                www.childrenshospital.org

Mission is to provide the highest quality care; be the leading source of research and discovery; educate the next generation of leaders in child health and enhance the health and well-being of the children and families in our local community.

Sandra L. Fenwick, President/ CEO
Kevin Churchwell, MD, EVP, Health Affairs & COO
Naomi Fried, PhD, Chief Innovation Officer

7228 Congenital Heart Anomalies, Support, Education & Resources (CHASER)
2112 N Wilkins Road
Swanton, OH 43558   419-825-5575
                                                Fax: 419-825-2880
                                                chaser@compuserve.com
                                                www.csun.edu/~hcmth011/chaser/

National organization for support, education and resources for families and patients who deal with children born with congenital heart malformations.

Anita Myers, Executive Director

7229 Genetic Alliance
4301 Connecticut Avenue NW, Suite 404
Washington, DC 20008   202-966-5557
                                                800-336-4363
                                                Fax: 202-966-8553
                                                info@geneticalliance.org
                                                www.geneticalliance.org

A coalition of voluntary genetic support groups, consumers and professionals addressing the needs of individuals and families affected by genetic disorders from a national perspective.

Sharon Terry, President/CEO
Tetyana Murza, Managing Director
Natasha Bonhomme, VP, Strategic Development

7230 Little Hearts
110 Court Street, Suite 3A, PO Box 171
Cromwell, CT 6416   860-635-0006
                                                866-435-4673
                                                info@littlehearts.org
                                                www.littlehearts.org

Provides support, resources, networking, and hope to families affected by congenital heart defects. Membership consists of families nationwide who have or are expecting a child with a congenital heart defect.

Lenore Cameron, Director

Web Sites

7231 American Heart Association
7272 Greenville Avenue
Dallas, TX 75231   800-242-8721
                                                www.heart.org/HEARTORG/

Supports research, education and community service programs with the objective of reducing premature death and disability from cardiovascular diseases and stroke; coordinates the efforts of health professionals, and others engaged in the fight against heart and circulatory disease.

Nancy Brown, CEO
Dr. Stephen Houser, President
Suzie Upton, Chief Operating Officer

7232 Children's Hospital Boston
300 Longwood Avenue
Boston, MA 2115   617-355-6000
                                                800-355-7944
                                                www.childrenshospital.org

Mission is to provide the highest quality care; be the leading source of reseach and discovery; educate the next generation of leaders in child health and enhance the health and well-being of the children and families in our local community.

Sandra L. Fenwick, President/ CEO
Kevin Churchwell, MD, EVP, Health Affairs & COO
Naomi Fried, PhD, Chief Innovation Officer

7233 Congenital Heart Anomalies, Support, Education & Resources (CHASER)
2112 N Wilkins Road
Swanton, OH 43558   419-825-5575
                                                Fax: 419-825-2880
                                                chaser@compuserve.com
                                                www.csun.edu/~hcmth011/chaser/

National organization for support, education and resources for families and patients who deal with children born with congenital heart malformations.

7234 Congenital Heart Information Network
www.tchin.org

An international organization that provides reliable information, support services and resources to families of children with congenital heart defects and acquired heart disease, adults with congenital heart defects, and the professionals who work with them.

7235 Little Hearts
P.O. BOX 171
Cromwell, CT 6416   860-635-0006
                                                866-435-4673
                                                www.littlehearts.org

Provides support, resources, networking, and hope to families affected by congenital heart defects. Membership consists of families nationwide who have or are expecting a child with a congenital heart defect.

7236 Southern Illinois University School of Medicine
PO Box 19639
Springfield, IL 62794   217-545-8000
                                                800-342-5748
                                                admin@siuhealthcare.org
                                                www.siumed.edu/peds/index.htm

The mission of SUI School of Medicine is to assist the people of central and southern Illinois in meeting their present and future health care needs through education, clinical service and research.

Book Publishers

7237 Congenital Disorders Sourcebook
Omnigraphics
PO Box 8002
Aston, PA 19014

800-234-1340
Fax: 800-875-1340
info@omnigraphics.com
www.omnigraphics.com

Basic consumer health information on disorders aquired during gestation, including spina bifida, hydrocephalus, cerebral palsy, heart defects, craniofacial abnormalities and fetal alcohol syndrome.

650 pages
ISBN: 0-780809-45-9

Peter Ruffner, Publisher

DESCRIPTION

7238 THALASSEMIAS

Covers these related disorders: Alpha-thalassemia, Beta-thalassemia, Beta-thalassemia minor, Beta-thalassemia major

Involves the following Biologic System(s):
Genetic/Chromosomal/Syndrome/Metabolic Disorders, Hematologic and Oncologic Disorders

The term thalassemia refers to a group of inherited blood disorders that includes the alpha-thalassemias and the more common beta-thalassemias. The thalassemias are characterized by the faulty production of hemoglobin, the protein that carries oxygen within the red blood cells. Hemoglobin is composed of two pairs of amino acid chains (globins), the alpha chains and the beta chains. The improper synthesis of hemoglobin is caused by a defect within the globin genes and results in abnormal, fragile red blood cells. Beta-thalassemia minor, a less severe form of the disease, is inherited when the defective gene is transmitted by one parent, while beta-thalassemia major is inherited through the defective genes of both parents.

A mild anemia is usually present in individuals with beta-thalassemia minor; however, it is not unusual for affected individuals to be symptom-free. Symptoms of beta-thalassemia major include fatigue; shortness of breath (dyspnea); and yellowing of the skin, eyes, and mucous membranes (jaundice). Other symptoms, usually associated with the premature destruction of red blood cells (hemolytic anemia) and subsequent release of iron, may include bronzed or freckled skin and enlargement of the spleen (splenomegaly). In severe cases, iron that gets deposited in the heart, liver, and pancreas may eventually lead to impaired function. In addition, extreme activity of the bone marrow may result in thickened and enlarged bones in the skull and face, while normal growth may be retarded.

Alpha-thalassemia, far less common than beta-thalassemia, ranges in severity from a carrier state with no symptoms to the most severe form that is incompatible with life. The severity of symptoms is dependent upon the level of alpha-chain involvement. The most severe form of alpha-thalassemia involves the complete absence of alpha-chain production.

Thalassemia patients vary a lot in their treatment needs depending on the severity of their anemia. Treatment for symptomatic thalassemias includes blood transfusion therapy to ensure normal growth. However, repeated blood transfusions may exacerbate iron deposition into the internal organs (hemosiderosis), necessitating treatment with iron-chelating drugs that increase iron excretion. Other treatment may include bone marrow transplantation.

Thalassemia is inherited as an autosomal recessive trait and is most prevalent among people living in or originating from the Mediterranean, the Middle East, and Southeast Asia. As with other genetically acquired disorders, aggressive birth screening and genetic counseling is recommended.

Government Agencies

7239 NIH/ Eunice Kennedy Shriver National Insti tute of Child Health & Human Development
31 Center Drive, Building 31
Bethesda, MD 20892
301-496-5113
800-370-2943
Fax: 866-760-5947
nichdpress@mail.nih.gov
www.nichd.nih.gov

Established in 1962 by congress, today the institute conducts and supports research on topics related to the health of children, adults, families and populations. Some of these topics include: developmental disabilities, growth and development, infant death, reproductive health and birth defects.

Diana W. Bianchi, Director
Paul Williams, Director, Communications

7240 NIH/National Heart, Lung and Blood Institu te
National Institute of Health
31 Center Dr MSC 2486, Bldg 31, Rm5A52
Bethesda, MD 20892
301-592-8573
Fax: 301-592-8563
TTY: 240-629-3255
NHLBIinfo@nhlbi.nih.gov
www.nhlbi.nih.gov

Primary responsibility of this organization is the scientific investigation of heart, blood vessel, lung and blood disorders. Oversees research, demonstration, prevention, education, control and training activities in these fields and emphasizes the prevention and control of heart diseases.

Gary H. Gibbons, M.D., Director

7241 NIH/National Institute of Arthritis and Musculoskeletal and Skin Diseases
1 AMS Circle
Bethesda, MD 20892
301-495-4484
877-226-4267
Fax: 301-718-6366
TDD: 301-565-2966
niamsinfo@mail.nih.gov
www.niams.nih.gov

The mission of the NIAMS, a part of the NIH, is to support research into the causes, treatment, and prevention of arthritis and musculoskeletal and skin diseases, the training of basic and clinical scientists to carry out this research, and the dissemination of information on research progress in these diseases.

Stephen I Katz MD PhD, Director
Robert H Carter MD, Deputy Director
Gahan Breithaupt, Assoc Dir for Management & Operatio

National Associations & Support Groups

7242 AHEPA Cooley's Anemia Foundation
1909 Q Street NW, Suite 500
Washington, DC 20009
202-232-6300
Fax: 202-232-2140
ahepa@ahepa.org
www.ahepa.org

Dedicated to advancing the treatment and cure of cooley's anemia, an inherited blood disorder. Provides information, referrals to local medical sources, medical supplies to people in need, and listings of informational materials available from the Foundation.

Basil Mossaidis, Executive Director
Patricia Farish, Controller
Phil Attey, Internet Strategist and Webmaster

7243 American Academy of Dermatology (AAD)
PO Box 4014
Schaumburg, IL 60168
847-240-1280
866-503-7546
Fax: 847-240-1859
mrc@aad.org
www.aad.org

Dedicated to achieving high quality dermatologic care for everyone which encompasses: responsiveness, unification and representation of the specialty, and excellence in patient care, education and research.

Stephen P Stone MD, President
William P Coleman III, MD, VP
David M Pariser MD, Secretary/Treasurer

7244 American Academy of Pediatrics
141 Northwest Point Boulevard
Elk Grove Village, IL 60007   847-434-4000
                                                     800-433-9016
                                                     Fax: 847-434-8000
                                                     www.aap.org

The American Academy of Pediatrics and its member pediatricians are committed to the attainment of optimal physical, mental and social health and well-being for all infants, children, adolescents, and young adults.

Fernando Stein, MD, FAAP, President
Karen Remley, MD, CEO/Executive VP

7245 American Heart Association
7272 Greenville Avenue
Dallas, TX 75231   214-373-6300
                                                     800-242-8721
                                                     Fax: 214-706-1341
                                                     inquire@amhrt.org
                                                     www.heart.org/HEARTORG/

Supports research, education and community service programs with the objective of reducing premature death and disability from cardiovascular diseases and stroke; coordinates the efforts of health professionals, and others engaged in the fight against heart and circulatory disease.

Nancy Brown, CEO
Dr. Stephen Houser, President
Suzie Upton, Chief Operating Officer

7246 American Skin Association
6 East 43rd Street, 28th Floor
New York, NY 10017   212-889-4858
                                                     800-499-7546
                                                     Fax: 212-889-4959
                                                     info@americanskin.org
                                                     www.americanskin.org

The American Skin Association is the only volunteer led health organization dedicated through research, education and advocacy to saving lives and alleviating human suffering caused by the full spectrum of skin disorders.

Joyce Weidler, Manager
George W Hambrick, Jr, President/Founder
David R Bickers, MD, Executive VP

7247 Ataxia-Telangiectasia Children's Project
5300 W. Hillsboro Blvd., Suite 105
Coconut Creek, FL 33073   954-481-6611
                                                     800-543-5728
                                                     Fax: 954-725-1153
                                                     info@atcp.org
                                                     www.atcp.org

A non-profit organization that raises funds to support and coordinate biomedical research projects, scientific conferences and a clinical center aimed at finding a cure for ataxia-telagiectasia, a lethal genetic disease that attacks children, causing progressive loss of muscle control, cancer and immune system problems.

Brad Margus, Founder
Vicki Margus, Founder

7248 Children's Cancer & Blood Foundation
333 East 38th Street, Suite 380
New York, NY 10016   212-297-4336
                                                     Fax: 212-297-4340
                                                     info@childrenscbf.org
                                                     www.childrenscbf.org

Mission is to support the comprehensive clinical care of children living with blood disorders; to foster research to help understand the causes of childhood blood disorders; and to sponsor the fellowship training of pediatricians of the subspecialty of pediatric hematology and oncology.

1952

Drew Phillips, President
Greg Karakashian, Operations Associate

7249 Children's Hospital Boston
300 Longwood Avenue
Boston, MA 02115   617-355-6000
                                                     617-355-6000
                                                     Fax: 800-355-7944
                                                     TTY: 617-730-0152
                                                     www.childrenshospital.org

Mission is to provide the highest quality care; be the leading source of research and discovery; educate the next generation of leaders in child health and enhance the health and well-being of the children and families in our local community.

Leslie M Higuchi, President & CEO
Sandra Fenwick, Chief Operating Officer

7250 Congenital Heart Anomalies, Support, Education & Resources (CHASER)
2112 N Wilkins Road
Swanton, OH 43558   419-825-5575
                                                     Fax: 419-825-2880
                                                     chaser@compuserve.com
                                                     www.csun.edu/~hcmth011/chaser/chaser-news.html?

National organization for support, education and resources for families and patients who deal with children born with congenital heart malformations.

Anita Myers, Executive Director

7251 Cooley's Anemia Foundation
330 Seventh Avenue, #900
New York, NY 10001   212-279-8090
                                                     800-522-7222
                                                     Fax: 212-279-5999
                                                     info@cooleysanemia.org
                                                     www.thalassemia.org

Advancing the treatment and cure for this fatal blood disease, enhancing the quality of life of patients and educating the medical profession, trait carriers and the public about Cooley's anemia/thalassemia major.

1954

Gina Cioffi Esq, National Executive Director

7252 Genetic Alliance
4301 Connecticut Avenue NW, Suite 404
Washington, DC 20008   202-966-5557
                                                     800-336-4363
                                                     Fax: 202-966-8553
                                                     info@geneticalliance.org
                                                     www.geneticalliance.org

A coalition of voluntary genetic support groups, consumers and professionals addressing the needs of individuals and families affected by genetic disorders from a national perspective.

Sharon Terry, President/CEO
Tetyana Murza, Managing Director
Natasha Bonhomme, VP, Strategic Development

7253 Hereditary Hemorrhagic Telangiectasia (HHT) Foundation International
PO Box 329
Monkton, MD 21111   410-357-9932
                                                     800-448-6389
                                                     Fax: 410-357-9931
                                                     hhtinfo@hht.org
                                                     www.hht.org

Dedicated to increasing public and professional awareness and understanding of hereditary hemorrhagic telangiectasia (HHT). Supports ongoing medical research into the cause, prevention, and treatment of HHT; and offers a variety of materials including informational brochures and a quarterly newsletter.

Marianne Clancy, Executive Director

7254 Little Hearts
110 Court Street, Suite 3A, PO Box 171
Cromwell, CT 06416
860-635-0006
866-435-4673
info@littlehearts.org
www.littlehearts.org

Provides support, resources, networking, and hope to families affected by congenital heart defects. Membership consists of families nationwide who have or are expecting a child with a congenital heart defect.

Lenore Cameron, Director

7255 March of Dimes Foundation
1275 Mamaroneck Avenue
White Plains, NY 10605
914-428-7100
Fax: 914-428-8203
www.marchofdimes.com

Mission is to improve the health of babies by preventing birth defects, premature birth, and infant mortality. Provide research, community services, education and advocacy to save babies' lives, to give all babies a fighting chance against the threats to their health: prematurity, birth defects, low birth weight.

Stacey D. Stewart, President

7256 NIH/National Institute of Neurological Dis orders and Stroke (NINDS)
PO Box 5801
Bethesda, MD 20824
301-496-5751
800-352-9424
Fax: 301-496-0296
TTY: 301-468-5981
www.ninds.nih.gov

Mission is to reduce the burden of neurological disease - a burden borne by every age group, by every segment of society, by people all over the world.

Walter J. Koroshetz, MD, Director

7257 National Ataxia Foundation
2600 Fernbrook Lane Suite 119
Minneapolis, MN 55447
763-553-0020
Fax: 763-553-0167
naf@ataxia.org
www.ataxia.org

Objectives of this organization are to make an early diagnosis of ataxia by locating all potential victims and encouraging them to have an examination, public information and professional education materials and basic research on the disease.

Mike Parent, Executive Director

7258 National Tay-Sachs and Allied Diseases Association
2001 Beacon Street, Suite 204
Boston, MA 02135
617-277-4463
800-906-8723
Fax: 617-277-0134
info@ntsad.org
www.ntsad.org

Direct, fund and promote research to develop treatments and cures; provide comprehensive support services to affected families and individuals; guide prevention, education, awareness and screening through effective grassroots collaborations with chapters and affiliates; lead advocacy efforts as the recognized authority for this family of genetic diseases.

Diana Pangonis, Executive Director

7259 Society for Pediatric Dermatology
8365 Keystone Crossing, Suite 107
Indianapolis, IN 46240
317-202-0224
Fax: 317-205-9481
info@pedsderm.net
www.pedsderm.net

Objective is to promote, develop and advance education, research and care of skin disease in all pediatric age groups.

Kent Lindeman, Executive Director

7260 Thalassemias Action Group (TAG)
330 Seventh Avenue, #900
New York, NY 10001
800-522-7222
tag@cooleysanmeia.org
www.studygroup.com

Started by a group of young adults who realized that by helping and sharing with each other, coping with the daily struggles of life with thalassemia was made a little easier.

1985

Jesal Kapasi, President

State Agencies & Support Groups

California

7261 Cooley's Anemia Foundation-California
2629 Foothill Boulevard, #319
La Crescenta, CA 91214
800-601-2821
ca_chapter@hotmail.com
www.thalassemia.org

Robert Yamashita, President
Christine Giannamore, Coordinator

Georgia

7262 Cooley's Anemia Foundation-Buffalo Chapter
781 Eagle Crossing Drive
Lawrenceville, GA 30044
678-357-4021
Fax: 678-969-0367
supermom2kids@earthlink.net
www.thalassemia.org

Tahseen Mahmood, President

Maryland

7263 Cooley's Anemia Foundation-Capital Area (DC, VA, MD)
15321 Peach Orchard Road
Silver Spring, MD 20905
301-989-8947
cvitaliti@aol.com
www.thalassemia.org/get-involved/chapters/capitol-ch

Carl C Vitaliti, President

Massachusetts

7264 Cooley's Anemia Foundation-Massachusetts Chapter
44 Joseph Road
Newton, MA 02460
617-332-5952
rvscomi@comcast.net
www.thalassemia.org/get-involved/chapters/massachuse

Rudi Viscomi, President

New York

7265 Cooley's Anemia Foundation - Staten Island
16 Dreyer Ave
Staten Island, NY 10314
718-761-5380
streganonaterri@aol.com
www.thalassemia.org/get-involved/chapters/staten-isl

Terri DiFilippo, President

7266 Cooley's Anemia Foundation-Buffalo
135 Wellington Road
Buffalo, NY 14216
716-832-3055
www.thalassemia.org

Dennis Locurto, President

7267 Cooley's Anemia Foundation-Long Island/Bro oklyn Chapter
PO Box 190
Franklin Square, NY 11010
516-697-5310
Fax: 516-358-9101
findacure.caf@gmail.com
www.thalassemia.org/get-involved/chapters/l-i-chapte

Thomas Rotolo, President

7268 Cooley's Anemia Foundation-Queens
157-26 9th Avenue
Beachurst, NY 11357
718-746-7677
Fax: 718-746-7678
JohnPoPs55@aol.com
www.thalassemia.org/get-involved/chapters/queens-cha
Paul Tucci, President
Abbey Chakalis, Events Manager
John Mancino, Contact

7269 Cooley's Anemia Foundation-Suffolk Chapter
740 Smithtown Bypass #201
Smithtown, NY 11787
631-863-0532
Fax: 631-863-0535
darlene@suffolkcaf.com
www.thalassemia.org/get-involved/chapters/suffolk-ch
Tony Laurino, Executive Director

7270 Cooley's Anemia Foundation-Westchester/Roc kland Chapter
3 Sammuel Purdy Lane
Katonah, NY 10536
914-232-1808
anemia@optonline.net
www.thalassemia.org/get-involved/chapters/westcheste
Peter Chieco, President
Janet Manning, Executive Director

Texas

7271 Cooley's Anemia Foundation - Texas
1004 Field Trail
Mesquite, TX 75150
214-324-6147
Fax: 214-324-0612
www.thalassemia.org
Mateen Shah, President

Conferences

7272 TAG Conference
Thalassemia Action Group
330 Seventh Avenue, #900
New York, NY 10001
800-522-7222
Fax: 212-279-5999
info@cooleysanemia.org
www.cooleysanemia.org

Held annually around March-April, look at website for more information.

Anthony J. Viola, President
Gina Cioffi, Executive Director
Amy Celento, Vice President

Web Sites

7273 Children's Cancer & Blood Foundation
www.childrenscbf.org

Mission is to support the comprehensve clinical care of children living with blood disorders; to foster research to help understand the causes of childhood blood disorders; and to sponsor the fellowship training of pediatricians of the subspecialty of pediatric hematology and oncology.

7274 Children's Hospital Boston
300 Longwood Avenue
Boston, MA 2115
617-355-6000
800-355-7944
www.childrenshospital.org

Mission is to provide the highest quality care; be the leading source of reseach and discovery; educate the next generation of leaders in child health and enhance the health and well-being of the children and families in our local community.

Sandra L. Fenwick, President/ CEO
Kevin Churchwell, MD, EVP, Health Affairs & COO
Naomi Fried, PhD, Chief Innovation Officer

7275 Cooley's Anemia Foundation
330 Seventh Avenue, #200
New York, NY 10001
800-522-7222
Fax: 212-279-5999
www.cooleysanemia.org

The only US-based voluntary health organization that aids in patient services, medical research, education and public information to fight thalassemia, a blood disease also known as Cooley's anemia. Members of CAF work alongside the Thalassemia Action Group (TAG) to provide national support, encouragement and friendship to other patients and families.

Anthony J. Viola, President
Gina Cioffi, Esq., National Executive Director
Eileen Scott, Patient Services Manager

7276 March of Dimes Birth Defects Foundation
1275 Mamaroneck Avenue
White Plains, NY 10605
914-997-4488
www.marchofdimes.org

Mission is to improve the health of babies by preventing birth defects, premature birth, and infant mortality. Provide research, community services, education and advocacy to save babies' lives, to give all babies a fighting chance against the threats to their health: prematurity, birth defects, low birthweight.

7277 NIH/National Heart, Lung and Blood Institu te
31 Center Dr MSC 2486, Bldg 31, Room 5A52
Bethesda, MD 20892
301-592-8573
NHLBIinfo@nhlbi.nih.gov
www.nhlbi.nih.gov

Primary responsibility of this organization is the scientific investigation of heart, blood vessel, lung and blood disorders. Oversees research, demonstration, prevention, education, control and training activities in these fields and emphasizes the prevention and control of heart diseases.

Gary H. Gibbons, M.D., Director
Nakela Cook, MD, MPH, Chief of Staff
Kathleen B. O'Sullivan, Executive Officer

7278 Online Mendelian Inheritance in Man
www.omim.org

This database is a catalog of human genes and genetic disorders.

7279 Thalassemias Action Group (TAG)
330 Seventh Avenue, #200
New York, NY 10001
800-522-7222
Fax: 212-279-5999
www.cooleysanemia.org

Promotes positive attidtude toward life; stresses the importance of compliance and chelation therapy; and provides patients with a channel of communication and information.

Anthony J. Viola, President
Gina Cioffi, Esq., National Executive Director
Eileen Scott, Patient Services Manager

Book Publishers

7280 Blood & Circulatory Disorders Sourcebook 4th Edition
Omnigraphics
615 Griswold, Ste 901
Detroit, MI 48226
800-234-1340
Fax: 800-875-1340
contact@omnigraphics.com
www.omnigraphics.com

Basic consumer health information on blood and its components, anemias, leukemias, bleeding disorders, and circulatory disorders, including aplastic anemia, thrombophilia, RH disease and hemophilia.

2005 600 pages
ISBN: 0-780807-46-9

Peter Ruffner, Publisher

7281 Coloring Book on Thalassemia
Cooley's Anemia Foundation
330 Seventh Avenue, #200
New York, NY 10001
212-279-8090
800-522-7222
Fax: 212-279-5999
info@cooleysanemia.org
www.cooleysanemia.org

Available in English, Italian, Greek and Chinese.

Anthony J. Viola, President
Gina Cioffi, Executive Director
Amy Celento, Vice President

7282 Cooley's Anemia 7th Annual Symposium
Cooley's Anemia Foundation
330 Seventh Avenue, #200
New York, NY 10001
800-522-7222
Fax: 212-279-5999
info@cooleysanemia.org
www.cooleysanemia.org

Published by the New York Academy of Sources.
1997

Anthony J. Viola, President
Gina Cioffi, Executive Director
Amy Celento, Vice President

7283 Genes, Blood & Courage
Cooley's Anemia Foundation
330 Seventh Avenue, #200
New York, NY 10001
800-522-7222
Fax: 212-279-5999
info@cooleysanemia.org
www.cooleysanemia.org

Anthony J. Viola, President
Gina Cioffi, Executive Director
Amy Celento, Vice President

7284 Let's Talk About Going to the Hospital
Rosen Publishing Group's PowerKids Press
29 E 21st Street
New York, NY 10010
212-777-3017
800-237-9932
Fax: 888-436-4643
rosenpub@tribeca.ios.com
www.rosenpublishing.com

If a child has to check into the hospital, chances are he or she is already upset about being ill. Knowing how a hospital functions and what the procedures are, such as when family members can visit, will help in what is already a stressful situation. Grades K-5.

24 pages
ISBN: 0-823950-36-0

Roger Rosen, President

Journals

7285 Pediatric Dermatology Journal
Society for Pediatric Dermatology
8365 Keystone Crossing, Suite 107
Indianapolis, IN 46240
317-202-0224
Fax: 317-205-9481
info@pedsderm.net
www.pedsderm.net

6 issues/yr
Kent Lindeman, Executive Director

Newsletters

7286 CAF Medical Update
Cooley's Anemia Foundation
330 Seventh Avenue, #200
New York, NY 10001
800-522-7222
Fax: 212-279-5999
info@cooleysanemia.org
www.cooleysanemia.org

Medical information.
Biannual

Anthony J. Viola, President
Gina Cioffi, Esq., National Executive Director
Eileen Scott, Patient Services Manager

7287 Lifeline
Cooley's Anemia Foundation
330 Seventh Avenue, #200
New York, NY 10001
800-522-7222
Fax: 212-279-5999
info@cooleysanemia.org
www.cooleysanemia.org

Cooley's Anemia Foundation
Biannual
Anthony J. Viola, President
Gina Cioffi, Esq., National Executive Director
Eileen Scott, Patient Services Manager

7288 TAG Newsletter
Cooley's Anemia Foundation
330 Seventh Avenue, #200
New York, NY 10001
800-522-7222
Fax: 212-279-5999
info@cooleysanemia.org
www.cooleysanemia.org

Anthony J. Viola, President
Gina Cioffi, Esq., National Executive Director
Eileen Scott, Patient Services Manager

Pamphlets

7289 Cooley's Anemia Fact Cards
Cooley's Anemia Foundation
330 Seventh Avenue, #200
New York, NY 10001
800-522-7222
Fax: 212-279-5999
info@cooleysanemia.org
www.cooleysanemia.org

Anthony J. Viola, President
Gina Cioffi, Esq., National Executive Director
Eileen Scott, Patient Services Manager

7290 Cooley's Anemia Foundation (CAF) Pamphlet
Cooley's Anemia Foundation
330 Seventh Avenue, #200
New York, NY 10001
800-522-7222
Fax: 212-279-5999
info@cooleysanemia.org
www.cooleysanemia.org

Anthony J. Viola, President
Gina Cioffi, Esq., National Executive Director
Eileen Scott, Patient Services Manager

7291 Desferal Q & A
Cooley's Anemia Foundation
330 Seventh Avenue, #200
New York, NY 10001
800-522-7222
Fax: 212-279-5999
info@cooleysanemia.org
www.cooleysanemia.org

Guidelines for home infusion.

Anthony J. Viola, President
Gina Cioffi, Esq., National Executive Director
Eileen Scott, Patient Services Manager

7292 Sibling Donor Cord Blood Program Pamphlet
Cooley's Anemia Foundation
330 Seventh Avenue, #200
New York, NY 10001
800-522-7222
Fax: 212-279-5999
info@cooleysanemia.org
www.cooleysanemia.org

Anthony J. Viola, President
Gina Cioffi, Esq., National Executive Director
Eileen Scott, Patient Services Manager

7293 Thalassemia Action Group (TAG) Patient Sup port Group Brochure
Cooley's Anemia Foundation
330 Seventh Avenue, #200
New York, NY 10001
800-522-7222
Fax: 212-279-5999
info@cooleysanemia.org
www.cooleysanemia.org

Anthony J. Viola, President
Gina Cioffi, Esq., National Executive Director
Eileen Scott, Patient Services Manager

7294 What is Thalassemia Trait?
Cooley's Anemia Foundation
330 Seventh Avenue, #200
New York, NY 10001
800-522-7222
Fax: 212-279-5999
info@cooleysanemia.org
www.cooleysanemia.org

This booklet offers information on the thalassemia trait.

Anthony J. Viola, President
Gina Cioffi, Esq., National Executive Director
Eileen Scott, Patient Services Manager

DESCRIPTION

7295 THROMBOCYTOPENIAS

Covers these related disorders: Idiopathic thrombocytopenia purpura (ITP)

Involves the following Biologic System(s):

Hematologic and Oncologic Disorders

Thrombocytopenia is a term that describes a condition in which the level of circulating platelets in the blood is reduced, resulting in a tendency to bleed. By changing shape and adhering to each other and the walls of broken blood vessels, platelets, also known as thrombocytes, play an essential role in the clotting process. Normal blood levels usually demonstrate 150,000 to 350,000 platelets per microliter. When the platelet count is reduced to 30,000 per microliter or lower, abnormal bleeding under the skin may occur and result in purple bruising or spots (purpura). Nosebleeds (epistaxis), bleeding of the gums , and blood in the urine (hematuria) are also common. Often, low platelet levels do not lead to clinical problems; rather, they are picked up on a routine full blood count.

Thrombocytopenia may result from a slowdown in platelet production or the rapid destruction of these cells. Certain diseases such as anemia, leukemia, lymphoma, bone marrow disorders, or autoimmune diseases may cause thrombocytopenia. Other causes include enlargement of the spleen (splenomegaly), cirrhosis, certain drugs, viral infection, and x-ray or radiation exposure.

The treatment of thrombocytopenia is based upon its underlying cause. For example, if the low platelet count is caused by a specific underlying disease, treatment is geared toward that disease. Low platelet counts caused by a specific drug necessitate the withdrawal of that drug. If bleeding is severe, platelet transfusions may be administered.

Idiopathic thrombocytopenia purpura (ITP) is a term used to describe thrombocytopenia of unknown origin. This condition often follows a viral infection and, in children, usually disappears within a month or so with no treatment. The duration of ITP in adolescents and adults is often more prolonged, and close medical follow up and avoidance of contact sports and activities is essential.

Government Agencies

7296 NIH/National Heart, Lung and Blood Institu te
National Institute of Health
31 Center Dr MSC 2486, Bldg 31, Room 5A52
Bethesda, MD 20892

301-592-8573
Fax: 301-592-8563
TTY: 240-629-3255
NHLBIinfo@nhlbi.nih.gov
www.nhlbi.nih.gov

Primary responsibility of this organization is the scientific investigation of heart, blood vessel, lung and blood disorders. Oversees research, demonstration, prevention, education, control and training activities in these fields and emphasizes the prevention and control of heart diseases.

Gary H. Gibbons, M.D., Director
Nakela Cook, MD, Chief of Staff

National Associations & Support Groups

7297 American Academy of Pediatrics
141 Northwest Point Boulevard
Elk Grove Village, IL 60007

847-434-4000
800-433-9016
Fax: 847-434-8000
www.aap.org

The American Academy of Pediatrics and its member pediatricians are committed to the attainment of optimal physical, mental and social health and well-being for all infants, children, adolescents, and young adults.

Fernando Stein, MD, FAAP, President
Karen Remley, MD, CEO/Executive VP

7298 American Heart Association
7272 Greenville Avenue
Dallas, TX 75231

214-373-6300
800-242-8721
Fax: 214-706-1341
inquire@amhrt.org
www.heart.org/HEARTORG/

Our mission is to reduce disability and death from cardiovascular diseases and stroke. Parents will find education and support to you better care for a child with arrhythmias.

Nancy Brown, CEO
Dr. Stephen Houser, President
Suzie Upton, Chief Operating Officer

7299 Children's Cancer & Blood Foundation
333 East 38th Street, Suite 380
New York, NY 10016

212-297-4336
Fax: 212-297-4340
info@childrenscbf.org
www.childrenscbf.org

Promotes the welfare of and addresses the issues that affect people with immune or idiopathic thrombocytopenic purpura. Goals are to provide patient support, ongoing medical research to advance the knowledge and treatment and educate the public and medical communities about the disorder. Provides educational and support materials including fact sheets, brochures, and a booklet entitled 'What's It Called Again?'

Drew Phillips, President
Greg Karakashian, Operations Associate

7300 Children's Hospital Boston
300 Longwood Avenue
Boston, MA 02115

617-355-6000
TTY: 617-730-0152
www.childrenshospital.org

Mission is to provide the highest quality care; be the leading source of research and discovery; educate the next generation of leaders in child health and enhance the health and well-being of the children and families in our local community.

Dr. James Mandell, CEO
Sandra Fenwick, President & COO
James Mandell, MD, Chief Executive Officer

7301 Genetic Alliance
4301 Connecticut Avenue NW, Suite 404
Washington, DC 20008

202-966-5557
800-336-4363
Fax: 202-966-8553
info@geneticalliance.org
www.geneticalliance.org

A coalition of voluntary genetic support groups, consumers and professionals addressing the needs of individuals and families affected by genetic disorders from a national perspective.

Sharon Terry, President/CEO
Tetyana Murza, Managing Director
Natasha Bonhomme, VP, Strategic Development

7302 Platelet Disorder Support Association
33 Rollins Avenue, #5
Rockville, MD 20852

301-770-6636
877-528-3538
Fax: 301-770-6638
pdsa@pdsa.org
www.itppeople.com

Our organization is devoted to bringing you the most timely, accurate and comprehensive information about ITP and assisting you in meeting others who share your interests.

Peter Pruitt, Board Chairman
Caroline Kruse, Executive Director
Marjorie Ligelis, Chief Financial Officer

Web Sites

7303 American Heart Association
7272 Greenville Avenue
Dallas, TX 75231

800-242-8721
www.heart.org/HEARTORG/

Our mission is to reduce disability and death from cardiovascular diseases and stroke. Parents will find education and support to you better care for a child with arrhythmias.

Nancy Brown, CEO
Dr. Stephen Houser, President
Suzie Upton, Chief Operating Officer

7304 Children's Cancer & Blood Foundation
www.childrenscbf.org

Promotes the welfare of and addresses the issues that affect people with immune or idiopathic thrombocytopenic purpura. Goals are to provide patient support, ongoing medical research to advance the knowledge and treatment and educate the public and medical communities about the disorder. Provides educational and support materials including fact sheets, brochures, and a booklet entitled 'What's It Called Again?'

7305 Children's Hospital Boston
300 Longwood Avenue
Boston, MA 2115

617-355-6000
800-355-7944
www.childrenshospital.org

Mission is to provide the highest quality care; be the leading source of reseach and discovery; educate the next generation of leaders in child health and enhance the health and well-being of the children and families in our local community.

Sandra L. Fenwick, President/ CEO
Kevin Churchwell, MD, EVP, Health Affairs & COO
Naomi Fried, PhD, Chief Innovation Officer

7306 Online Mendelian Inheritance in Man
www.omim.org

This database is a catalog of human genes and genetic disorders.

7307 Platelet Disorder Support Association
8751 Brecksville Road, Suite 150
Cleveland, OH 44141

440-746-9003
877-528-3538
Fax: 844-270-1277
pdsa@pdsa.org
www.pdsa.org

Our organization is devoted to bringing you the most timely, accurate and comprehensive information about ITP and assisting you in meeting others who share your interests.

Caroline Kruse, Executive Director
Marjorie Ligelis, Chief Financial Officer
Nancy Potthast, Director of Marketing

Book Publishers

7308 Harrison's Principles of Inernal Medicine 15th Edition
McGraw-Hill
PO Box 182605
Columbus, OH 43218

800-338-3987
Fax: 609-308-4480
customer.service@mheducation.com
www.mcgraw-hill.com

Raises the bar for internal medicine references. Features over 90 new chapters, Harrison's continues to provide authoritative record of internal medicine as practiced by the leading experts in the field.

Lloyd G. Waterhouse, President & CEO
Patrick Milano, CFO
David Stafford, Senior Vice President

7309 Let's Talk About Going to the Hospital
Rosen Publishing Group's PowerKids Press
29 E 21st Street
New York, NY 10010

212-777-3017
800-237-9932
Fax: 888-436-4643
rosenpub@tribeca.ios.com
www.rosenpublishing.com

If a child has to check into the hospital, chances are he or she is already upset about being ill. Knowing how a hospital functions and what the procedures are, such as when family members can visit, will help in what is already a stressful situation. Grades K-5.

24 pages
ISBN: 0-823950-36-0

Roger Rosen, President

DESCRIPTION

7310 THUMBSUCKING

Involves the following Biologic System(s):
Developmental/Behavioral/Psychiatric Disorders

Thumbsucking is a common habit that is prevalent among infants and young children. This behavior is usually used as a device for providing pleasure, amusement, comfort, oral gratification, and release of stress or tension. Sometimes a security object, such as a blanket, may become part of the thumbsucking habit. In most children, thumbsucking reaches a plateau between the ages of 18 months to two years and then slowly but steadily decreases until it disappears at about five to six years of age. One reason to encourage children to give up the habit before they enter school is to prevent the teasing they would otherwise receive. By adolescence, most normal children abandon thumbsucking because of peer pressure.

Although it is generally thought that thumbsucking does not cause any long-term developmental irregularities, thumbsucking that continues beyond age six may lead to acquired problems with the bones and tissues of the thumb and an abnormal bite or contact pattern between upper and lower teeth (malocclusion). The longer the habit persists, the more likely affected children are to develop these types of problems. Conversely, the earlier this habit comes to an end, the more likely that irregular positioning of the teeth will improve without intervention.

Many physicians agree that, as a general rule, the best treatment for thumbsucking is to ignore the behavior and wait patiently for the children to outgrow the habit or to discontinue the behavior on their own. Treatment is generally supportive as punishing or reprimanding often adds to stress levels, becomes a power struggle with the parent, and may actually worsen the problem. Other treatment may include the use of certain appliances that are fitted with small projections that alert children to their behavior when they attempt to suck their thumbs. Older children may require the use of orthodontic appliances to correct irregularities associated with malocclusion.

Government Agencies

7311 NIH/National Institute of Dental and Craniofacial Research (NIDCR)

National Institutes of Health
31 Center Drive, MSC 2290, Building 31
Bethesda, MD 20892

301-496-4261
Fax: 301-402-2185
nidcrinfo@mail.nih.gov
www.nidcr.nih.gov

The mission is to promote the general health of American people by improving their oral, dental and craniofacial health. Through the conduct and support of research and training of researchers, the NIDCR aims to promote health, prevent diseases and conditions, and develop new diagnostic and therapeutics.

Dr Martha J. Somerman, Director
John W Kusiak, PhD, Acting Deputy Director
Kathleen G Stephen, Executive Officer

7312 National Oral Health Information Clearinghouse

1 NOHIC Way
Bethesda, MD 20892

301-402-7364
866-232-4528
Fax: 301-480-4098
nidcrinfo@mail.nih.gov
www.nidcr.nih.gov

Produces and distributes patient and professional education materials including fact sheets, brochures, information packets and provides referrals to other organizations dealing with special care in oral health. Special care is an approach to oral health management that is tailored to the specific needs of persons with a variety of medical, disabling or mental conditions.

National Associations & Support Groups

7313 American Academy of Pediatrics

141 Northwest Point Boulevard
Elk Grove Village, IL 60007

847-434-4000
800-433-9016
Fax: 847-434-8000
www.aap.org

The American Academy of Pediatrics and its member pediatricians are committed to the attainment of optimal physical, mental and social health and well-being for all infants, children, adolescents, and young adults.

Fernando Stein, MD, FAAP, President
Karen Remley, MD, CEO/Executive VP

7314 American Dental Association

211 East Chicago Avenue
Chiacgo, IL 60611

312-266-7255
Fax: 312-266-9867
www.aae.org

Committed to the public's oral health, ethics, science and professional advancement; leading a unified profession through initiatives in advocacy, education, research and the development of standards.

James Drinan, Executive Director

7315 C.S. Mott Children's Hospital

1540 East Hospital Drive
Ann Arbor, MI 48109

734-936-4000
www.mottchildren.org

Provides information on how to handle a child's thumb sucking. Why they do it; how long it will last; how to help overcome the issue?

7316 Children's Hospital Boston

300 Longwood Avenue
Boston, MA 02115

617-355-6000
TTY: 617-730-0152
www.childrenshospital.org

Mission is to provide the highest quality care; be the leading source of research and discovery; educate the next generation of leaders in child health and enhance the health and well-being of the children and families in our local community.

Leslie M Higuchi, President & CEO
Sandra Fenwick, Chief Operating Officer

Web Sites

7317 American Dental Association

211 East Chicago Ave.
Chicago, IL 60611

312-440-2500
affiliates@ada.org
www.ada.org

Committed to the public's oral health, ethics, science and professional advancement; leading a unified profession through initiatives in advocacy, education, research and the development of standards.

Dr. Maxine Feinberg, President
Dr. Carol Gomez Summerhays, President-Elect
Dr. Kathleen T. O'Loughlin, Executive Director

7318 C.S. Mott Children's Hospital
1540 East Hospital Drive
Ann Arbor, MI 48109

734-936-6641
mottchildren@umich.edu
www.mottchildren.org

Provides information on how to handle a child's thumbsucking. Why they do it; how long it will last; how to help overcome the issue?

Paul King, Executive Director
John M. Park, M.D., Associate Professor
Chris Dickinson, Chief Medical Officer

7319 Children's Hospital Boston
300 Longwood Avenue
Boston, MA 2115

617-355-6000
800-355-7944
www.childrenshospital.org

Mission is to provide the highest quality care; be the leading source of reseach and discovery; educate the next generation of leaders in child health and enhance the health and well-being of the children and families in our local community.

Sandra L. Fenwick, President/ CEO
Kevin Churchwell, MD, EVP, Health Affairs & COO
Naomi Fried, PhD, Chief Innovation Officer

7320 NIH/National Institute of Dental and Crani ofacial Research (NIDCR)
Bethesda, MD 20892

301-496-4261
866-232-4528
Fax: 301-480-4098
nidcrinfo@mail.nih.gov
www.nidcr.nih.gov

The mission is to promote the general health of American people by improving their oral, dental and craniofacial health. Through the conduct and support of research and training of researchers, the NIDCR aims to promote health, prevent diseases and conditions, and develop new diagnostic and therapeutics.

Dr Martha J. Somerman, DDS, PhD, Director
John W Kusiak, PhD, Acting Deputy Director
Kathleen G Stephen, Executive Officer

7321 National Oral Health Information Clearinghouse
Bethesda, MD 20892

301-496-4261
866-232-4528
Fax: 301-480-4098
nidcrinfo@mail.nih.gov
www.nidcr.nih.gov

Produces and distributes patient and professional education materials including fact sheets, brochures, information packets and provides referrals to other organizations dealing with special care in oral health. Special care is an approach to oral health management that is tailored to the specific needs of persons with a variety of medical, disabling or mental conditions.

Martha J. Somerman, DDS, PhD, Director
Kathleen G. Stephan, Executive Officer
Michelle A. Culp, Director

Pamphlets

7322 A Healthy Mouth for Your Baby
National Oral Health Information Clearinghouse
1 NOHIC Way
Bethesda, MD 20892

301-496-4261
866-232-4528
Fax: 301-480-4098
nidcrinfo@mail.nih.gov
www.nidcr.nih.gov

Martha J. Somerman, DDS, PhD, Director
Kathleen G. Stephan, Executive Officer
Michelle A. Culp, Director

7323 Seal Out Tooth Decay
National Oral Health Information Clearinghouse
1 NOHIC Way
Bethesda, MD 20892

301-496-4261
866-232-4528
Fax: 301-480-4098
nidcrinfo@mail.nih.gov
www.nidcr.nih.gov

Martha J. Somerman, DDS, PhD, Director
Kathleen G. Stephan, Executive Officer
Michelle A. Culp, Director

DESCRIPTION

7324 TICS

Covers these related disorders: Chronic motor tic disorder, Tourette syndrome, Transient tics of childhood

Involves the following Biologic System(s):

Neurologic Disorders

Tics are repetitive or stereotypical, compulsive, abrupt (spasmodic) movements of a muscle or muscle groups. Although any muscle may be affected, tics most commonly involve muscles of the eyes, face, neck, or shoulders. Movements may include blinking, sniffing, facial grimacing, lip smacking, tongue thrusting, or shoulder shrugging. Tics may begin as intentional movements to relieve perceived tension. However, they may rapidly become unintentional or involuntary in nature. Although tics are extremely difficult to suppress, most patients are able to do so for short periods. Tics are often worsened by stress or any perceived attention to the condition; in contrast, they typically disappear during sleep.

In most patients, tics become apparent between approximately five to 10 years of age. According to some estimates, as many as 25 percent of children may be affected. Most children may experience a spontaneous disappearance of tics within a few weeks or less than one year after onset. In such patients, the condition is referred to as transient tics of childhood. Supportive measures that may be helpful in alleviating transient tics include providing children with a tranquil environment as well as additional rest.

Some children may experience chronic motor tics that persist throughout adult life. In such patients, the condition is known as chronic motor tic disorder. Chronic motor tics may simultaneously affect muscles in up to three different muscle groups.

In contrast to transient tics of childhood and chronic motor tics, which are considered relatively benign, restricted tic disorders, a genetic, neurologic disorder known as Tourette syndrome is characterized by multiple, chronic, complex tics. Tourette syndrome usually becomes apparent in children between the ages of two to 14 years. Initial symptoms typically include motor tics of the face, eyelids, shoulders, and neck. Movements may include grimacing, excessive eye blinking, or stretching of the neck. Vocal (phonic) tics, such as involuntary coughing, grunting, barking, or throat clearing, are also common. Additional symptoms may include involuntary repetition of obscene words (coprolalia) or words spoken by other individuals (echolalia); aggressive behaviors; the performance of repetitive actions or impulses in response to recurrent, persistent thoughts (obsessive-compulsive behaviors); and secondary learning, emotional, or social difficulties. Researchers suggest that variable expression of the disease gene responsible for Tourette syndrome may cause transient tics of childhood or chronic motor tics in other individuals, indicating possible overlap between the conditions. Several studies have demonstrated that immediate (first-degree) relatives of patients with Tourette syndrome have an increased frequency of such tic conditions.

In some patients with severe chronic motor tic disorder, treatment may include therapy with certain medications (e.g., certain benzodiazepines or haloperidol). The treatment of Tourette syndrome is symptomatic and supportive and may include therapy with certain medications, such as haloperidol, pimozide, clonidine, clonazepam, or carbamazepine. In addition, for those with learning, behavioral, and social difficulties, multidisciplinary management and the provision of special social, academic, and vocational services may be important in helping patients achieve their potential. (Please refer to the section entitled Tourette Syndrome for further information on this disorder.)

Government Agencies

7325 NIH/National Institute of Neurological Disorders and Stroke (NINDS)
PO Box 5801
Bethesda, MD 20824
301-496-5751
800-352-9424
Fax: 301-496-0296
TTY: 301-468-5981
www.ninds.nih.gov

Works to reduce the burden of neurological disease by conducting, fostering, coordinating and guiding research on the causes, prevention, diagnosis and treatment of neurological disorders and stroke, while supporting basic research in related scientific areas.

Walter J. Koroshetz, MD, Director

National Associations & Support Groups

7326 American Academy of Child & Adolescent Psychiatry
3615 Wisconsin Avenue NW
Washington, DC 20016
202-966-7300
Fax: 202-966-2891
clinical@aacap.org
www.aacap.org

Mission is to promote mentally healthy children, adolescents and families through research, training, advocacy, prevention, comprehensive diagnosis and treatment, peer support and collaboration.

Elizabeth Hughes, Asst. Director of Education & Recer
Quentin Bernhard III, CME Coordinator
Alan Ezagui, Deputy Director of Development

7327 American Academy of Pediatrics
141 Northwest Point Boulevard
Elk Grove Village, IL 60007
847-434-4000
800-433-9016
Fax: 847-434-8000
www.aap.org

The American Academy of Pediatrics and its member pediatricians are committed to the attainment of optimal physical, mental and social health and well-being for all infants, children, adolescents, and young adults.

Fernando Stein, MD, FAAP, President
Karen Remley, MD, CEO/Executive VP

7328 American School Counselor Association
1101 King Street, Suite 310
Alexandria, VA 22314
703-683-2722
800-306-4722
Fax: 703-997-7572
asca@schoolcounselor.org
www.schoolcounselor.org

The mission of ASCA is to represent professional school counselors and to promote professionalism and ethical practices.

Richard Wong, Executive Director
Jeff Broderson, Information Technology Admin.
Kathleen M Rakestraw, Director of Communications

7329 Genetic Alliance
4301 Connecticut Avenue NW, Suite 404
Washington, DC 20008
202-966-5557
800-336-4363
Fax: 202-966-8553
info@geneticalliance.org
www.geneticalliance.org

A coalition of voluntary genetic support groups, consumers and professionals addressing the needs of individuals and families affected by genetic disorders from a national perspective.

Sharon Terry, President/CEO
Tetyana Murza, Managing Director
Natasha Bonhomme, VP, Strategic Development

7330 NADD: National Association for the Dually Diagnosed
132 Fair Street
Kingston, NY 12401
845-331-4336
800-331-5362
Fax: 845-331-4569
info@thenadd.org
www.thenadd.org

Nonprofit organization designed to promote the interests of professional and parent development with resources for individuals who have the coexistence of mental illness and mental retardation. Provides conferences, educational services and training materials to professionals, parents, concerned citizens and service organizations.

Dr Robert Fletcher, CEO
Michelle Jordan, Office Manager
Edward Seliger, Project Coordinator

7331 WE MOVE (Worldwide Education and Advocacy for Movement Disorders)
5731 Mosholu Avenue
Bronx, NY 10024
212-875-8312
800-437-6682
Fax: 212-875-8389
wemove@wemove.org
www.wemove.org

Provides movement disorder information and education materials to physicians, patients, the media and the public via its comprehensive web sites, training courses, and more. It's goal is to make early diagnosis, up-to-date treatment and patient support a reality for all people living with movement disorders.

Susan Bressman, President
Mo Moadeli, Vice President
Wendy Borow-Johnson, Secretary

Audio Video

7332 Dakota
Tourette Syndrome Association
42-40 Bell Boulevard
Bayside, NY 11361
718-224-2999
888-486-8738
Fax: 718-279-9596
ts@tsa-usa.org
tsa-usa.org

A happy eleven year old baseball playing, video game whiz, Dakota is diagnosed with Tourette's Syndrome and ADHD.

7 minutes

7333 Family Life with Tourette Syndrome... Personal Stories
Tourette Syndrome Association
42-40 Bell Boulevard
Bayside, NY 11361
718-224-2999
888-486-8738
Fax: 718-279-9596
ts@tsa-usa.org
tsa-usa.org

In extended, in-depth interviews, all the people engagingly profiled in After the Diagnosis...The Next Steps, reveal the individual ways they developed to deal with TS. Each shows us that the key to leading a successful life in spite of having TS, is having a loving, supportive network of family and friends. Available in its entirety or as separate vignettes.

58 minutes

7334 Ryan
Tourette Syndrome Association
42-40 Bell Boulevard
Bayside, NY 11361
718-224-2999
888-486-8738
Fax: 718-279-9596
ts@tsa-usa.org
tsa-usa.org

Ryan's family first thought his behavior was a deliberate way to get attention, lateer educate themselves and others about Ryan's Tourette's Syndrome.

11 minutes

7335 The Turners
Tourette Syndrome Association
42-40 Bell Boulevard
Bayside, NY 11361
718-224-2999
888-486-8738
Fax: 718-279-9596
ts@tsa-usa.org
tsa-usa.org

Three of the four Turner daughters have Tourette's Syndrome in varying degress.

12 minutes

Web Sites

7336 American Academy of Child & Adolescent Psychiatry
3615 Wisconsin Avenue, N.W.
Washington, DC 20016
202-966-7300
Fax: 202-966-2891
communications@aacap.org
www.aacap.org

Mission is to promote mentally healthy children, adolescents and families through research, training, advocacy, prevention, comprehensive diagnosis and treatment, peer support and collaboration.

Paramjit T. Joshi, M.D., President
Gregory K. Fritz, M.D., President-Elect
Aradhana Sood, M.D., Secretary

7337 NADD: National Association for the Dually Diagnosed
132 Fair Street
Kingston, NY 12401
845-331-4336
800-331-5362
Fax: 845-331-4569
info@thenadd.org
www.thenadd.org

Nonprofit organization designed to promote the interests of professional and care providers for individuals who have the coexistence of mental illness and mental retardation. NADD provides conferences, educational services and training materials to professionals, parents, concerned citizens and service organizations.

Dr Robert Fletcher, CEO
Michelle Jordan, Office Manager
Edward Seliger, Project Coordinator

7338 NIH/National Institute of Neurological Dis orders and Stroke (NINDS)
PO Box 5801
Bethesda, MD 20824
301-496-5751
800-352-9424
www.ninds.nih.gov

Works to reduce the burden of neurological disease by conducting, fostering, coordinating and guiding research on the causes, prevention, diagnosis and treatment of neurological disorders and stroke, while supporting basic research in related scientific areas.

Walter J. Koroshetz, MD, Director

7339 Online Mendelian Inheritance in Man
www.omim.org

This database is a catalog of human genes and genetic disorders.

7340 Parents Helping Parents
Sobrato Center For Nonprofits-San Jose, 1400 Parkm
San Jose, CA 95126   408-727-5775
                                                  855-727-5775
                                         Fax: 408-286-1116
                                                    php.com

Mission is to help children with special needs revive the resources, love, hope, respect, health care, education, and other services they need to reach their full potential by providing them
with strong families, dedicated professionals and responsive systems to serve them.

Mary Ellen Peterson, M.A., Executive Director/CEO
Nancy O'Rourke, Chief Development Officer
Jane Floethe-Ford, Director of Education Services

7341 Tourette Syndrome Online
www.tourette-syndrome.com

Devoted to children and adults with Tourette syndrome disorder
and their families, friends, teachers and medical professionals.

**7342 WE MOVE (Worldwide Education and Advocacy for
Movement Disorders)**
www.wemove.org

Provides movement disorder information and education materials
to physicians, patients, the media and the public via its comprehensive web sites, training courses, and more. It's goal is to make
early diagnosis, up-to-date treatment and patient support a reality
for all people living with movement disorders.

Book Publishers

7343 Cognitive-Behavioral Management of Tic Dis orders
John Wiley & Sons
111 River Street
Hoboken, NJ 07030   201-748-6000
                                         Fax: 201-748-6088
                                              info@wiley.com
                                                www.wiley.com

Provides a comprehensive review of what is known about the
occurance and diagnosis of Tics.

2005 Paperback
ISBN: 0-470093-80-1

Peter B. Wiley, Chairman
Stephen M. Smith, President & CEO
Ellis E. Cousens, Executive Vice President, Chief Fin

7344 Hi, I'm Adam
Hope Press
PO Box 188
Duarte, CA 91009   800-321-4039
                                         Fax: 626-358-3520
                                       dcomings@earthlink.net
                                              www.hopepress.com

Adam Buehrens is ten years old and has Tourette syndrome.
Adam wrote and illustrated this book because he wants everyone
to know he and other children with Tourette syndrome are not
crazy. They just hava a common neurological disorder. If you
know a child that has tics, temper tantrums, unreasonable fears, or
problems dealing with school, you will find this a reassuring
story.

7345 Teaching the Tiger
Hope Press
PO Box 188
Duarte, CA 91009   800-321-4039
                                         Fax: 626-358-3520
                                       dcomings@earthlink.net
                                              www.hopepress.com

A handbook for individuals involved in the education of students
with Attention Deficit Disorder, Tourette Syndrome, or Obsessive
Compulsive Disorder.

ISBN: 1-878267-34-5

David E Comings MD, Presenter

**7346 Tourette's Syndrome - Tics, Obsession, Com pulsions:
Developmental Psychopathology**
John Wiley & Sons
111 River Street
Hoboken, NJ 07030   201-748-6000
                                         Fax: 201-748-6088
                                              info@wiley.com
                                                www.wiley.com

Once thought to be rare, Tourette's Syndrome is now seen as a
relatively common childhood disorder either in its complete or
partial incarnations. Drawing on the work of contributors hailing
from the prestigious Yale University Child Psychiatry Department, this edited volume explores the disorder from many perspectives, mapping out the diagnosis, genetics, phenomenology,
natural history, and treatment of Tourette's syndrome.

1998 600 pages Hardcover
ISBN: 0-471160-37-7

Peter B. Wiley, Chairman
Stephen M. Smith, President & CEO
Ellis E. Cousens, Executive Vice President, Chief Fin

7347 What Makes Ryan Tic?
Hope Press
PO Box 188
Duarte, CA 91009   800-321-4039
                                         Fax: 626-358-3520
                                       dcomings@earthlink.net
                                              www.hopepress.com

Covers Ryan's very difficult adolescent years-a period when his
symptoms were so severe he had to be placed in a residential
treatment facility-and the subsequent period of returning home
and pursuing a virtually normal life following his excellent response to the right combination of medication, family and school
support.

Susan Hughes, Author

Journals

7348 Movement Disorders
John Wiley & Sons
111 River Street
Hoboken, NJ 7030-   201-748-6000
                                         Fax: 201-748-6088
                                              info@wiley.com
                                                www.wiley.com

Publishes reviews, viewpoints, full length articles, historical reports, brief reports, clinical/scientific notes, videotape briefs, pa-
tient/imaging briefs, and letters. ISSN: 0885-3185

Vol 22 13 Issues

Stephen M. Smith, President/ CEO
John Kritzmacher, EVP/ CFO
MJ O'Leary, EVO, Human Resources

Pamphlets

7349 Matthew and Tics
Tourette Syndrome Association
42-40 Bell Boulevard
Bayside, NY 11361   718-224-2999
                                                  888-486-8738
                                         Fax: 718-279-9596
                                               ts@tsa-usa.org
                                                   tsa-usa.org

A story for young children with Tourette's Syndrome and their
peers; promotes acceptance and understanding.

7350 Tics and Tourette's Syndrome Fact Sheet
Movement Disorder Resource Center - WE MOVE
204 E 84th Street
New York, NY 10024   212-241-8567
                                                  800-437-6682
                                         Fax: 212-987-7363
                                          www.life-in-motion.org

Provides overviews of both diseases.

DESCRIPTION

7351 TOURETTE SYNDROME

Synonyms: Gilles de la Tourette syndrome, GTS

Involves the following Biologic System(s):

Neurologic Disorders

Tourette syndrome is a neurologic disorder that typically becomes apparent in children between the ages of two to 14 years, with approximately 50 percent of cases occurring before seven years of age. The disorder, which is thought to affect about one in 2,000 individuals, is approximately three times more prevalent in males than females and is more common among Caucasians than other populations. In children with Tourette syndrome, associated symptoms and findings vary greatly in range and severity. Initial symptoms may include involuntary, repetitive (stereotypical) muscle movements (motor tics) of the face, eyelids, shoulders, and neck, such as grimacing, abrupt head turning, excessive eye blinking, or stretching of the neck. In some patients with severe symptoms, motor tics may evolve to include self-mutilating behaviors, such as nail biting, lip biting, or facial punching. Children with Tourette syndrome may also develop vocal tics, such as involuntary coughing, grunting, barking, sniffling, or throat clearing. As the disease progresses, additional symptoms may develop including involuntary repetition of obscene words (coprolalia), words spoken by other individuals (echolalia), or one's own words (palilalia) or imitation of other individuals' behaviors (echokinesis or echopraxia). The symptoms associated with Tourette syndrome may periodically decrease or increase in intensity; may subside during high levels of concentration, such as when reading or studying; and may worsen with stress. Tourette syndrome is considered a life-long disorder; however, in approximately 50 to 66 percent of patients, symptoms significantly decrease about 10 to 15 years after initial diagnosis and treatment.

Children with Tourette syndrome may also experience associated behavioral abnormalities, such as aggressive behavior or the performance of repetitive actions or impulses in response to recurrent, persistent thoughts (obsessive-compulsive behaviors). Obsessive-compulsive behaviors are typically performed to help neutralize obsessive thoughts and relieve anxieties. Many affected children may also develop learning, emotional, or social difficulties. The treatment of Tourette syndrome is symptomatic and supportive and may include therapy with certain medications, such as haloperidol, pimozide, clonidine, clonazepam, or carbamazepine. In addition, for those with learning, behavioral, and social difficulties, multidisciplinary management and the provision of special social, academic, and vocational services may be important in helping patients achieve their potential.

Although the exact cause of Tourette syndrome is unknown, studies suggest that the disorder may result due to abnormalities of neurotransmitter (dopamine) activity within a certain area of the brain (basal ganglia). In most cases, Tourette syndrome is thought to be inherited as an autosomal dominant trait that occurs as the result of changes (mutations) in a gene located on the long arm (q) of chromosome 18 (18q22.1). Some children with mutations of this disease gene may not have symptoms associated with the disorder (incomplete penetrance). In addition, in those children with the defective gene who do have symptoms associated with Tourette syndrome, such symptoms may vary in range and severity from case to case (variable expressivity). Such variability of gene expression and penetrance may be suggested by the fact that immediate (first-degree) relatives of patients have an increased frequency of Tourette syndrome, tic conditions, and obsessive-compulsive disorder. In addition, some researchers suspect that Tourette syndrome may result from inheritance of a disease gene in combination with certain environmental factors that may trigger the gene's expression (multifactorial inheritance). Research suggests that individuals who have two copies of a disease gene for Tourette syndrome (homozygotes) typically express the disorder, whereas some who inherit one disease gene (heterozygotes) may not develop the disorder unless particular environmental factors (e.g., infection, such as due to exposure to Group A beta-hemolytic streptococcus) trigger its expression. Tourette syndrome is associated with a vary of misconceptions, for instance, that people with Tourette syndrome are mentally disturbed and that they always exhibit coprolalia. Tourette's is a neurological condition that (according to the most recent research) is primarily genetic in nature. Although there may be learning disabilities associated with Tourette's, the brain is wholly undamaged in respect to intellectual functioning. Statistically, coprolalia is present in less than 5% of TS patients.

Government Agencies

7352 Centers for Disease Control and Prevention Division: Tuberculosis Elimination
1600 Clifton Road NE, MS E-10
Atlanta, GA 30323

404-639-8813
800-232-4636
TTY: 888-232-6348
cdcinfo@cdc.gov
www.cdc.gov/nchstp/tb/contact.html

Raymond Strikas, Director
Tom Frieden, MD, MPH, Director, Centers for Disease Contr
Linda C. Degutis, DrPH, MSN, Director, National Center for Injur

7353 NIH/ Eunice Kennedy Shriver National Institute of Child Health & Human Development
31 Center Drive, Building 31
Bethesda, MD 20892

301-496-5113
800-370-2943
Fax: 866-760-5947
TTY: 888-320-6942
nichdpress@mail.nih.gov
www.nichd.nih.gov

Established in 1962 by congress, today the institute conducts and supports research on topics related to the health of children, adults, families and populations. Some of these topics include: developmental disabilities, growth and development, infant death, reproductive health and birth defects.

Diana W. Bianchi, Director
Paul Williams, Director, Communications

7354 NIH/National Heart, Lung and Blood Institute, g
31 Center Dr MSC 2486, Bldg 31, Room 5A52
Bethesda, MD 20892

301-592-8573
Fax: 301-629-3246
TTY: 240-629-3255
nhlbiinfo@nhlbi.nih.gov
www.nhlbi.nih.gov

Provides leadership for a national program in diseases of the heart, blood vessels, lungs, and blood; blood resources; and sleep disorders.

Gary H Gibbons, MD, Director
Nakela Cook, MD, Chief of Staff

7355 NIH/National Heart, Lung and Blood Institu te
31 Center Dr MSC 2486, Bldg 31, Room 5A52
Bethesda, MD 20892
301-592-8573
Fax: 240-629-3246
TTY: 240-629-3255
NHLBIinfo@nhlbi.nih.gov
www.nhlbi.nih.gov

Primary responsibility of this organization is the scientific investigation of heart, blood vessel, lung and blood disorders. Oversees research, demonstration, prevention, education, control and training activities in these fields and emphasizes the prevention and control of heart diseases.

Gary H Gibbons, MD, Director
Nakela Cook, MD, Chief of Staff

7356 NIH/National Institute of Allergy and Infectious Diseases
5601 Fishers Lane, MSC 9806
Bethesda, MD 20892
301-496-5717
866-284-4107
Fax: 301-402-3573
TDD: 800-877-8339
ocpostoffice@niaid.nih.gov
www.niaid.nih.gov

Conducts and supports basic and applied research to better understand, treat, and ultimately prevent infectious, immunologic, and allergic diseases.

Anthony S Fauci MD, Director
Hugh Auchincloss, M.D., Principal Deputy Director
John J. McGowan, Ph.D., Deputy Director for Science Managem

7357 NIH/National Institute of Allergy and Infe ctious Diseases
5601 Fishers Lane, MSC 9806
Bethesda, MD 20892
301-496-5717
866-284-4107
Fax: 301-402-3573
TDD: 800-877-8339
ocpostoffice@niaid.nih.gov
www.niaid.nih.gov

Conducts and supports basic and applied research to better understand, treat, and ultimately prevent infectious, immunologic, and allergic diseases.

Anthony S Fauci MD, Director
Hugh Auchincloss, M.D., Principal Deputy Director
John J. McGowan, Ph.D., Deputy Director for Science Managem

7358 New York City Department of Health Bureau of Tuberculosis Control
125 Worth Street
New York, NY 10013
212-346-7572
www.nyc.gov/html

Michael R Bloomberg, Mayor
Desiree Kim, Executive Director

National Associations & Support Groups

7359 American Academy of Child & Adolescent Psychiatry
3615 Wisconsin Avenue NW
Washington, DC 20016
202-966-7300
Fax: 202-966-2891
clinical@aacap.org
www.aacap.org

Mission is to promote mentally healthy children, adolescents and families through research, training, advocacy, prevention, comprehensive diagnosis and treatment, peer support and collaboration.

Elizabeth Hughes, Asst. Director of Education & Recer
Quentin Bernhard III, CME Coordinator
Alan Ezagui, Deputy Director of Development

7360 American Academy of Pediatrics
141 Northwest Point Boulevard
Elk Grove Village, IL 60007
847-434-4000
800-433-9016
Fax: 847-434-8000
www.aap.org

The American Academy of Pediatrics and its member pediatricians dedicate their efforts and resources to the health, safety and well-being of infants, children, adolescents and young adults.

Fernando Stein, MD, FAAP, President
Karen Remley, MD, CEO/Executive VP

7361 American Heart Association
7272 Greenville Avenue
Dallas, TX 75231
214-373-6300
800-242-8721
Fax: 214-706-1341
inquire@amhrt.org
www.heart.org/HEARTORG/

Supports research, education and community service programs with the objective of reducing premature death and disability from cardiovascular diseases and stroke; coordinates the efforts of health professionals, and others engaged in the fight against heart and circulatory disease.

Nancy Brown, CEO
Dr. Stephen Houser, President
Suzie Upton, Chief Operating Officer

7362 American Lung Association
55 W. Wacker Drive, Suite 1150
Chicago, IL 60601
312-801-7628
800-548-8252
info@lung.org
www.lung.org

The American Lung Association fights lung disease in all its forms, with special emphasis on asthma, tobacco control and environmental health. The American Lung Association is funded by contributions from the public, along with gifts and grants from corporations, foundations and government agencies. The association achieves its many successes through the work of thousands of committed volunteers and staff.

Harold P. Wimmer, National President & CEO
Susan Rappaport, National VP, Research/Scientific
Sue Swan, Chief Development Officer

7363 American School Counselor Association
1101 King Street, Suite 310
Alexandria, VA 22314
703-683-2722
800-306-4722
Fax: 703-997-7572
asca@schoolcounselor.org
www.schoolcounselor.org

The mission of ASCA is to represent professional school counselors and to promote professionalism and ethical practices.

Richard Wong, Executive Director
Jeff Broderson, Information Technology Admin.
Kathleen M Rakestraw, Director of Communications

7364 American Society for Reproductive Medicine
1209 Montgomery Highway
Birmingham, AL 35216
205-978-5000
Fax: 205-978-5005
asrm@asrm.org
www.asrm.org

The American Society for Reproductive Medicine is an organization devoted to advancing knowledge and expertise in infertility, reproductive medicine and biology. The ASRM is a voluntary nonprofit organization.

Linda C. Giudice, President
Rebecca Sokol, M.D., Vice President
Robert W. Rebar, M.D, Executive Director

7365 Arc of the United States
1660 L Street, NW, Suite 301
Washington, DC 20036
202-534-3700
800-433-5255
Fax: 202-534-3731
info@thearc.org
www.thearc.org

The Arc of the United States works to include all children and adults with cognitive, intellectual, developmental disabilities in every community. We are a national organization of and for the people with mental retardation and related developmental disabilities and their families. It is devoted to promoting and improving supports and services for people with mental retardation and their families. The ARC was founded by a small group of parents and other concerned individuals.

Peter V. Berns, CEO
Karen Wolf-Branigin, Senior Program Officer
Amy Goodman, Co-Director, Autism NOW

7366 Children's Hospital Boston
300 Longwood Avenue
Boston, MA 02115

617-355-6000
800-355-7944
TTY: 617-730-0152
www.childrenshospital.org

Mission is to provide the highest quality care; be the leading source of research and discovery; educate the next generation of leaders in child health and enhance the health and well-being of the children and families in our local community.

Sandra Fenwick, President/Chief Operating Officer
James Mandell, MD, Chief Executive Officer
Dick Argys, Senior Vice President and Chief Adm

7367 Chromosome 18 Registry & Research Society
7155 Oakridge Drive
San Antonio, TX 78229

210-657-4968
Fax: 210-657-4968
office@chromosome18.org
www.chromosome18.org

The purpose of the Chromosome 18 Registry & Research Society is to offer support to patients and families, to educate the public about different available treatments and to connect families and doctors to the research community.

Jannine Cody, President
Ben Flowe Jr, VP Public Relations
Claudia Traa, Executive Director

7368 Congenital Heart Anomalies, Support, Education & Resources (CHASER)
2112 N Wilkins Road
Swanton, OH 43558

419-825-5575
Fax: 419-825-2880
chaser@compuserve.com
www.csun.edu/~hcmth011/chaser/

National organization for support, education and resources for families, patients and professionals who deal with children born with congenital heart malformations. Information on hospitals, medical assistance, and schooling. Offers Chaser News, an international newsletter and Chaser's Pediatric Heart Surgeons Facility Directory.

Anita Myers, Executive Director

7369 Congenital Heart Information Network
PO Box 3397
Margate City, NJ 08402

609-823-4507
Fax: 215-627-4036
mb@tchin.org
www.tchin.org

CHIN is an international organization that provides reliable information, support services and resources to families of children with congenital heart defects and acquired heart disease.

Mona Barmash, President

7370 Epilepsy Foundation
8301 Professional Place
Landover, MD 20785

866-330-2718
800-332-1000
Fax: 301-459-1569
ContactUs@efa.org
www.epilepsyfoundation.org

An organization works to ensure that people with seizures are able to participate in all life experiences; and to prevent, control and cure epilepsy through research, education, advocacy and services.

Phil Gattone, President/CEO
Sandy Finucane, Senior Advisor
Priscilla Burton, Senior Advisor

7371 Family Support Network
7514 Big Bend Blvd.
Saint Louis, MO 63119

314-644-5055
800-255-6872
Fax: 314-644-5057
info@familysupport.org
www.familysupportnet.org/

The Support Network is an organized partnership of individuals whose lives have been affected by Tuberous Sclerosis. Across the nation, the Support Network is providing the latest medical information, education and support to those individuals who are seeking understanding about the genetic disease and offering them words of encouragement and empowerment.

Susan Didier, MSW, LCSW, Director of Family Services
Julia Pickup, MSW, LCSW, Lead Therapist
Ayriel Hadley, BA, Office Manager

7372 Genetic Alliance
4301 Connecticut Avenue NW, Suite 404
Washington, DC 20008

202-966-5557
800-336-4363
Fax: 202-966-8553
info@geneticalliance.org
www.geneticalliance.org

A coalition of voluntary genetic support groups, consumers and professionals addressing the needs of individuals and families affected by genetic disorders from a national perspective.

Sharon Terry, President/CEO
Tetyana Murza, Managing Director
Natasha Bonhomme, VP, Strategic Development

7373 MUMS: National Parent to Parent Network
150 Custer Street
Green Bay, WI 54301

920-336-5333
877-336-5333
Fax: 920-339-0995
mums@netnet.net
www.netnet.net/mums

A national parent-to-parent organization for parents or care providers of a child with any disability, rare or not so rare disorder, chromosomal abnormality or health condition.

Julie J Gordon, Director

7374 National Dissemination Center for Children with Disabilities
1825 Connecticut Ave NW
Washington, DC 20009

202-884-8200
800-695-0285
Fax: 202-884-8441
TTY: 800-695-0285
nichcy@aed.org
www.nichcy.org

A national information and referral center for families, educators and other professionals on: disabilities in children and youth; programs and services; IDEA, the nation's special education law; and research-based information on effective practices.

Suzanne Ripley, Executive Director

7375 National Tuberculosis Center at New Jersey Medical School
185 South Orange Avenue, MSB C-696
Newark, NJ 07107

973-972-4300
Fax: 973-972-3268
njmsadmiss@umdnj.edu
www.umdnj.edu

The National Tuberculosis Center was established in 1993 in response to the resurgence of tuberculosis in the United States. The center operates under the direction of Lee B. Reichmann, MD, MPH. The center operates a toll-free information line to provide state-of-the-art information to health care professionals and the public. Senior medical staff and nurses are available to respond to calls Monday-Friday from 9am-5pm.

Kevin M. Barry, M.D., MBA, Chairperson
Mary Ann Christopher, RN, MSN, Vice-Chairperson
Bradford W. Hildebrandt, Secretary

7376 National Tuberous Sclerosis Association
801 Roeder Road, Suite 750
Landover, MD 20785   301-562-9890
                                      800-225-6872
                                      Fax: 301-562-9870
                                      info@tsalliance.org
                                      www.tsalliance.org

Nonprofit organization.

Matt Bolger, Chair
Kari Luther Rosbeck, President/CEO
Keith Hall, Vice Chair

**7377 Support Organization for Trisomy 18, 13, and Related
Disorders (SOFT)**
2982 S Union Street
Rochester, NY 14624   585-594-4621
                                      800-716-7638
                                      barbsoft@rochester.rr.com
                                      www.trisomy.org

SOFT is a network of families and professional dedication to providing support and understanding to families involved in the issue
and decision surrounding the diagnosis and care in related chromosome disorders. Support is provided throughout pre-natal diagnosis, the child's life and after their passing. It is committed to
the support of families personal decision in alliance with a parent-professional partnership. Site includes a listing of local
chapters in 25 states.

Barb Vanherreweghe, President
Steve Wagner, Board Member
Raquel Wagner, Board Member

7378 Trisomy 18 Foundation
4491 Cheshire Station Plaza, Suite 157
Dale City, VA 22193   810-867-4211
                                      t18info@trisomy18.org
                                      www.trisomy18.org

The foundation's mission is to search for a cure and treatments;
to educate and support medical professionals; and to create a
worldwide caring community for those affected.

Victoria Miller, Executive Director
Sean Brown, Vice-President of Development
Kris Shaughnessy, M.A., Community Affairs Program Office

7379 Tuberous Sclerosis Alliance
801 Roeder Road, Suite 750
Silver Spring, MD 20910   301-562-9890
                                      800-225-6872
                                      Fax: 301-562-9870
                                      info@tsalliance.org
                                      www.tsalliance.org

The Tuberous Sclerosis Alliance is dedicated to finding a cure for
Tuberous Sclerosis complex while improving the lives of those
affected. TSC is a genetic disease causing tumors to grow
throughout the body and is the leading cause of epilepsy and
autism.

Matt Bolger, Chair
Kari Luther Rosbeck, President/CEO
Keith Hall, Vice Chair

7380 United Network for Organ Sharing
700 N 4th Street, PO Box 2484
Richmond, VA 23219   804-782-4800
                                      Fax: 804-782-4816
                                      www.unos.org

Our mission is to advance organ availability and transplantation
by uniting and supporting our communities for the benefit of patients through education, technology and policy development.

Walter K Graham, CEO
Vicki F Sauer, Executive VP/COO
Marcia D Manning, Director Community Affairs

**7381 WE MOVE (Worldwide Education and Advocacy for
Movement Disorders)**
5731 Mosholu Avenue
Bronx, NY 10024   212-875-8312
                                      800-437-6682
                                      Fax: 212-875-8389
                                      wemove@wemove.org
                                      www.wemove.org

A nonprofit organization dedicated to educating and informing
patients, professionals and the public about the latest clinical advances, management and treatment options for neurologic
movement disorders.

Susan Bressman, President
Mo Moadeli, Vice President
Wendy Borow-Johnson, Secretary

7382 World Health Organization
Avenue Appia 20
CH-1211 Geneva 27,   www.who.int

WHO is the directing and coordinating authority for health within
the United Nations system.

Dr Margaret Chan, Director General
Dr Anarfi Asamoa-Baah, Deputy Director-General
Bruce Aylward, Assistant Director General

State Agencies & Support Groups

Arizona

7383 Tourette Syndrome Association - Arizona Chapter
6501 E. Greenway Pkwy, PO Box 103-414
Scottsdale, AZ 85254   520-620-2288
                                      800-203-7490
                                      info@tsa-az.org
                                      www.tsa-az.org

The Arizona chapter of the Tourette Syndrome Association was
established to serve the community touched by Touretty
Syndrome.

Kelly Medlyn, President
Marci Frantz, Vice President
Teri Mendenhall, Secretary

California

**7384 Tourette Syndrome Association - Northern California/Hawaii
Chapter**
www.tsanorcal-hawaii.org

                                      925-548-3605
                                      gibsonohare@sbcglobal.net
                                      www.tsanorcal-hawaii.org

A voluntary organization dedicated to providing assistance and
support for individuals with Tourette Syndrome, their families,
friends & loved ones.

Sandy Gibson-O'Hare, Chair
Sandra Brackett, Vice Chair
Samantha Phillips, Secretary

7385 Tourette Syndrome Association - Southern California Chapter
PO Box 3778
Cerritos, CA 90703   866-478-1935
                                      bcourdy@ca.rr.com
                                      www.tourettesyndrome-sca.org

The TSA of Southern California is an all volunteer, non-profit organization whose missions is to support the needs of families affected by Tourette Syndrome. The goal is to advocate for
individuals with TS, educate the public and professionals about
TS, and promote awareness.

Colorado

7386 Tourette Syndrome Association - Rocky Mountain Region
992 S 4th Avenue, Suite 100, PMB 198
Brighton, CO 80601   720-212-7535
                                       support@tsa-rmr.org
                                       www.tsa-rmr.org

The TSARMR serves Colorado, Montana, Wyoming, and Nevada.

Sally Mescher Allen, Chair
Donna Davies, Vice Chair
Lorraine Alcott, Secretary

Connecticut

7387 Tourette Syndrome Association - Connecticut Chapter
PO Box 185883
Hamden, CT 06518   203-980-4215
                                       joytavo@tsact.org
                                       www.tsact.org

The mission of the Connecticut chapter of the Tourette Syndrome Association, Inc. is to educate the general public about Touretty Syndrome and further the acceptance of people with Tourette Syndrome in all settings.

Peter Tavolacci, Vice-Chairman
Paul Nazario, Treasurer
Jeanette Nazario, Board Member

Florida

7388 Tourette Syndrome Association of Florida
PO Box 411416
Melbourne, FL 32941   727-418-0240
                                       support@tsa-fl.org
                                       www.tsa-fl.org

The TSA of Florida is a voluntary organization dedicated to helping individuals with Tourette Syndrome and their families by gathering and distributing information, promoting local self-help and professional services, and providing local TS support groups and meetings.

Donna Sakuta, Executive Director

Hawaii

7389 Tourette Syndrome Association - Northern California/Hawaii Chapter
www.tsanorcal-hawaii.org

                                       925-548-3605
                                       gibsonohare@sbcglobal.net
                                       www.tsanorcal-hawaii.org

A voluntary organization dedicated to providing assistance and support for individuals with Tourette Syndrome, their families, friends & loved ones.

Sandy Gibson-O'Hare, Chair
Sandra Brackett, Vice Chair
Samantha Phillips, Secretary

Illinois

7390 Tourette Syndrome Association of Illinois
800 Roosevelt Road, Suite A-10
Glen Ellyn, IL 60137   630-790-8083
                                       877-TSA-IL55
                                       Fax: 630-790-8084
                                       tsaillinois@yahoo.com
                                       www.tsa-illinois.org

TSA of Illinois' mission is to serve and support those whose lives are affected by Tourette Syndrome. TSA-IL promotes awareness, advocates, and educates the public, health care providers, and educators about Tourette Syndrome. TSA-IL supports medical and scientific research about Tourette Syndrome.

Sande S Shamash, President
Jen Johnson, Vice President, Membership
Joan Lindauer, Vice President, Government Relation

Indiana

7391 Tourette Syndrome Association of Indiana
PO Box 3797
West Lafayette, IN 47996   765-714-9880
                                       tsaofindiana@gmail.com
                                       www.tsaindiana.org

One of TSA of Indiana's many priorities is to establish access to current information and easy communication for its members. The leaders are committed to serving and supporting those whose lives are affected by Tourette Syndrome.

Michele Lehman, President
Brenda Leopold, Youth Ambassador Program Coordin.
John Leopold, Youth Ambassador Program Coordin.

Maine

7392 Tourette Syndrome Association - Maine/New Hampshire Chapter
www.tsa-maine.org

                                       207-699-4258
                                       info@tsa-maine.org
                                       www.tsa-maine.org

The Tourette Syndrome Association is a non-profit organization aimed at identifying the cause of, finding the cure for, and controlling the effects of this disorder. TSA also seeks to broaden awareness of Tourette Syndrome and provide support for families and individuals who deal with it.

Maryland

7393 Tourette Syndrome Association of Greater Washington
5851 Deale Churchton Road, Suite 4
Deale, MD 20751   410-867-1151
                                       877-295-2148
                                       Fax: 301-576-4527
                                       info@tsagw.org
                                       www.tsagw.org

The TSA of Greater Washington is a non-profit organization comprised of an all volunteer Board of Directors, two paid Staff and numerous unaffiliated volunteers. The mission is to improve the quality of life in those affected by Tourette Syndrome through education, advocacy and awareness in Maryland, Virginia and Washington D.C.

Marla Shea Gabala, Chairman
Judy Krauthamer, Vice Chair/Treasurer
Mark Etzel, Secretary

Massachusetts

7394 Tourette Syndrome Association of Massachusetts
39 Godfrey Street
Taunton, MA 02780   617-277-7589
                                       info@tsa-ma.org
                                       www.tsa-ma.org

The Tourette Syndrome Association of Massachusets is an all volunteer, non-profit organization whose mission is to support the needs of families affected by Tourette Syndrome. The goal is to advocate for individuals with TS, educate the public and professionals about TS, and promote awareness.

Chrissy Joyal, President
Liliane Larsen, Vice President/Treasurer
Judy Storeygard, Education Specialist

7395 Tourette Syndrome Association - Minnesota Chapter
2233 University Avenue, Suite 338
St. Paul, MN 55114   651-646-0099
Fax: 952-918-0350
director@tsa-mn.org
www.tsa-mn.org

The mission is to assist Minnesotan's with Tourette syndrome in achieving their fullest potential through education, support and public awareness programs.

Lee Baker, Executive Director

7396 Tourette Syndrome Association - Greater Missouri Chapter
6526 Parkwood Place
St. Louis, MO 63116   314-984-9019
lmchd52@gmail.com
www.missouritsa.org

Serves individuals and families in the St. Louis and Kansas City metropolitan areas and beyond. In concert with the national TSA, they provide information about Tourette Syndrome (TS) and the resources available to help affected families throughout the service area.

Lynn Dunlap, Chair
Pete Abel, Co-Chair/ Government Liaison
Marty Guise, Secretary

7397 Tourette Syndrome Association - Rocky Mountain Region
992 S 4th Avenue, Suite 100, PMB 198
Brighton, CO 80601   720-212-7535
support@tsa-rmr.org
www.tsa-rmr.org

The TSARMR serves Colorado, Montana, Wyoming, and Nevada.

Sally Mescher Allen, Chair
Donna Davies, Vice Chair
Lorraine Alcott, Secretary

7398 Tourette Syndrome Association - Rocky Mountain Region
992 S 4th Avenue, Suite 100, PMB 198
Brighton, CO 80601   720-212-7535
support@tsa-rmr.org
www.tsa-rmr.org

The TSARMR serves Colorado, Montana, Wyoming, and Nevada.

Sally Mescher Allen, Chair
Donna Davies, Vice Chair
Lorraine Alcott, Secretary

7399 Tourette Syndrome Association of New Jersey
50 Division Street, Suite 205
Somerville, NJ 08876   732-972-4459
info@tsanj.org
www.tsanj.org

The Tourette Syndrome Association of New Jersey, Inc., a chapter of the national Tourette Syndrome Association, is a non-profit organization whos membership includes individuals with Tourette Syndrome, their families and friends, and interested professionals.

7400 Tourette Syndrome Association - New Mexico Chapter
42-40 Bell Boulevard
Bayside, NY 11361   718-224-2999
info@tsanm.org
www.tsanm.org

The purpose is to provide information, support, and assistance to adults, children, and families affected by Tourette Syndrome. The hope is to provide education and to encourage an understanding and acceptance of this disorder.

Jennifer Johns, President
Helen Gutierrez, Secretary
Tanya Mueller, Treasurer

7401 Tourette Syndrome Association - Greater Rochester and Finger Lakes Area
92 Windmere Road
Rochester, NY 14617   585-752-6190
info@rochestertourette.org
www.rochestertourette.org

The TSA of Greater Rochester and the Finger Lakes, Inc. is a non-profit organization whose mission is to provide support, information and advocacy to people with TS and their families in friends. The chapter serves the community at large with support groups, in-services, and public awareness programs to the local, educational, and medical communities.

Diana Pratt, Chair
Patrick Scanlon, Vice Chair
Bob Gleason, Treasurer

7402 Tourette Syndrome Association - Greater New York State Chapter
20 Thomas Jefferson Lane
Synder, NY 14226   716-839-4430
Fax: 716-839-1956
info@tsa-gnys.org
www.tsa-gnys.org

The Tourette Syndrome Association of Greater New York State is an affiliate chapter of the TSA, Inc. The chapter serves an area from Buffalo to the Pennsylvania border to the south. There is a Greater Rochester TSA chapter that serves greater Rochester, NY. TSA-GNYS then picks up from Rochester and continues east to serve Syracuse and all of the central NY area.

Susan Conners, President
Marge Henning, Co-Chair
John Silverwood, Co-Chair

7403 Tourette Syndrome Association - Hudson Valley Chapter
PO Box 517
Ardsley, NY 10502   914-378-5025
info@tsa-nyhv.org
www.tsa-nyhv.org

The mission of the Hudson Valley Chapter is; to provide service, information, and support to people with TS and their families; to educate medical and educational professionals in order to increase their understanding of TS; and to promote a greater understanding of TS in the community at large.

Shelly Cooler, President
Marilyn Trichon, Vice President
Richard Yannetti, Executive Director

7404 Tourette Syndrome Association - Long Island Chapter
PO Box 615
Jericho, NY 11753   516-876-6947
longisland.tsa@gmail.com
www.li-tsa.org

The Long Island TSA's mission is to provide help (at the community level) to families affected by Tourette Syndrome by providing services to its members in Nassau and Suffolk counties.

Lisa Filippi, Co Chair
Kate Callan, Co-Vice Chair
Jane Zwilling, 1st Vice Chair and Chair, Education

7405 Tourette Syndrome Association - New York City Chapter
www.tsa-nyc.org

646-395-0162
chapter@tsa-nyc.org
www.tsa-nyc.org

The New York city chapter offers a variety of services to people with Tourette Syndrome, their families, educators, and professionals.

Chelsea White, Chairperson
Linda McAndrew, Secretary
Jonathan Marks, Treasurer

Ohio

7406 Tourette Syndrome Association of Ohio
PO Box 40163
Cincinnatti, OH 45240

513-320-7161
800-543-2675
admin@tsaohio.org
www.tsaohio.org

The Tourette Syndrome Association of Ohio is a nonprofit organization whose membership includes individuals with Tourette Syndrome, their families, friends, and interested professionals.

Coreen Brown, Chair of the Board
Joleah Dean, Executive Director of the Board

Oregon

7407 Tourette Syndrome Association - Washington and Oregon Chapter
318 West Galer Street
Seattle, WA 98119

718-224-2999
tsawashingtonchapter@yahoo.com
www.tsa-waor.org

This chapter exists to offer information, support and resources regarding Tourette Syndrome and its related conditions. They work together with the medical community, the schools and families whose lives are touched by TS.

Todd Henry, Chair
Erin Farrar, Vice Chair
Bernadette Witty, Secretary

Pennsylvania

7408 PA Tourette Syndrome Alliance
PO Box 148
McSherrystown, PA 17344

717-337-1134
800-990-3300
Fax: 717-698-1420
info@patsainc.org
www.patsainc.org

The services provided by PA-TSA are focused on increasing understanding of the disorder and providing proven accommodations and strategies so the child or adult can succeed.

Melinda Bowling, President
Lesley Geye, Vice-President
Susan Lutz, Treasurer

Rhode Island

7409 Tourette Syndrome Association of Rhode Island
6946 Post Road, Suite 402
North Kingstown, RI 00285

401-886-0887
info@oshean.org
www.ri.net/tsari

TSARI tries to define the needs of Rhode Islanders with TS and their families and design services for them. They offer support and education to families with TS.

Susan Cerrone Abely, Chair
John Smithers, Vice-Chair
Michael Pickett, Treasurer

Utah

7410 Tourette Syndrome Association - Utah Chapter
PO Box 701312
West Valley City, UT 84170

801-967-2125
866-274-0700
chair@tsa-utah.org
www.tsa-utah.org

The local chapter of the national TSA organization, serving as a resource for individuals who have Tourette Syndrome and their families. Membership is open to anyone who is interested in Tourette Syndrome.

Kelsey Brown, Chairman
Adam Westwood, Treasurer
Gerri Harper, Secretary

Washington

7411 Tourette Syndrome Association - Washington and Oregon Chapter
318 West Galer Street
Seattle, WA 98119

718-224-2999
tsawashingtonchapter@yahoo.com
www.tsa-waor.org

This chapter exists to offer information, support and resources regarding Tourette Syndrome and its related conditions. They work together with the medical community, the schools and families whose lives are touched by TS.

Todd Henry, Chair
Erin Farrar, Vice Chair
Bernadette Witty, Secretary

Wyoming

7412 Tourette Syndrome Association - Rocky Mountain Region
992 S 4th Avenue, Suite 100, PMB 198
Brighton, CO 80601

720-212-7535
tsarmr@att.net
www.tsa-rmr.org

The TSARMR serves Colorado, Montana, Wyoming, and Nevada.

Sally Mescher Allen, Chair
Donna Davies, Vice Chair
Lorraine Alcott, Secretary

Research Centers

7413 Tourette Syndrome and Tic Disorder Clinic
Cincinnati Children's Hospital Medical Center
3333 Burnet Avenue
Cincinnati, OH 45229

513-636-4200
800-344-2462
TTY: 513-636-4900
tics@cchmc.org
www.cincinnatichildrens.org

Clinic that specializes in evaluating, diagnosing and treating kids, adolescents and adults with Tourette's Syndrome symptoms, including tics, hyperactivity, attention deficits, obsessive compulsive behaviors and other symptoms of Tourette Syndrome.

Donald L Gilbert, MD, MS, Director
Steve W. Wu, MD, Medical Director

7414 Trisomy 18 Foundation
4491 Cheshire Station Plaza, Suite 157
Dale City, VA 22193

810-867-4211
t18info@trisomy18.org
www.trisomy18.org

The foundation's mission is to search for a cure and treatments; to educate and support medical professionals; and to create a worldwide caring community for those affected.

Victoria Miller, Executive Director
Sean Brown, Vice-President of Development
Kris Shaughnessy, M.A., Community Affairs Program Office

7415 **University of Illinois at Chicago Institute for Tuberculosis Research**
904 W Adams Street
Chicago, IL 60607   202-318-2476
                                        www.uic.edu

Michael J Groves, PhD, Director
Paula Allen-Meares, Chancellor
Lon S. Kaufman, Vice Chancellor for Academic Affair

Audio Video

7416 **After the Diagnosis...The Next Steps**
Tourette Syndrome Association
42-40 Bell Boulevard, Suite 205
Bayside, NY 11361   718-224-2999
                                        888-486-8738
                                        Fax: 718-279-9596
                                        ts@tsa-usa.org
                                        www.tsa-usa.org

When the diagnosis is Tourette syndrome, what do you do first? How do you sort out the complexities of the disorder? Whose advice do you follow? What steps do you take to lead a normal life? Six people with TS—as different as any six people can be—relate the sometimes difficult, but finally triumphant path each took to lead the rich, fulfilling life they now enjoy. Narrated by Academy Award-winning actor, Richard Dreyfuss, the stories are refreshing blends of poignancy, fact and inspiration.

35 Minutes

7417 **Clinical Counseling: Toward a Better Understanding of TS**
Tourette Syndrome Association
42-40 Bell Boulevard, Suite 205
Bayside, NY 11361   718-224-2999
                                        888-486-8738
                                        Fax: 718-279-9596
                                        ts@tsa-usa.org
                                        www.tsa-usa.org

Certain key issues often surface during the counseling sessions of people with TS and their families. These important areas of concern are explored for counselors, social workers, educators, psychologists and other allied professionals. Expert clinical practitioners offer invaluable insights for those working with people affected by Tourette syndrome.

14 Minutes

7418 **Complexities of TS Treatment: A Physician's Roundtable**
Tourette Syndrome Association
42-40 Bell Boulevard, Suite 205
Bayside, NY 11361   718-224-2999
                                        888-486-8738
                                        Fax: 718-279-9596
                                        ts@tsa-usa.org
                                        www.tsa-usa.org

Three of the most highly regarded experts in the diagnosis and treatment of Tourette syndrome offer insight, advice and treatment strategies to fellow physicians and other healthcare professionals.

15 Minutes

7419 **Dakota**
Tourette Syndrome Association
42-40 Bell Boulevard
Bayside, NY 11361   718-224-2999
                                        888-486-8738
                                        Fax: 718-279-9596
                                        ts@tsa-usa.org
                                        www.tsa-usa.org

A happy eleven year old baseball playing, video game whiz, Dakota is diagnosed with Tourette's Syndrome and ADHD.

7 minutes

7420 **Echolalia**
Hope Press
PO Box 188
Duarte, CA 91009   800-321-4039
                                        Fax: 626-358-3520
                                        dcomings@earthlink.net
                                        www.hopepress.com

A story about a best selling writer who is diagnosed at age 35 with having Tourette syndrome.

David E Comings, MD, Presenter

7421 **Family Life with Tourette Syndrome**
Tourette Syndrome Association
42-40 Bell Boulevard, Suite 205
Bayside, NY 11361   718-224-2999
                                        888-486-8738
                                        Fax: 718-279-9596
                                        ts@tsa-usa.org
                                        www.tsa-usa.org

In extended, in-depth interviews, all the people engagingly profiled in After the Diagnosis...The Next Steps, reveal the individual ways they developed to deal with TS. Each show us that the key to leading a successful life in spite of having TS, is having a loving, supportive network of family and friends.

7422 **Family Life with Tourette Syndrome... Personal Stories**
Tourette Syndrome Association
42-40 Bell Boulevard
Bayside, NY 11361   718-224-2999
                                        888-486-8738
                                        Fax: 718-279-9596
                                        ts@tsa-usa.org
                                        tsa-usa.org

In extended, in-depth interviews, all the people engagingly profiled in After the Diagnosis...The Next Steps, reveal the individual ways they developed to deal with TS. Each shows us that the key to leading a successful life in spite of having TS, is having a loving, supportive network of family and friends. Available in its entirety or as separate vignettes.

58 minutes

7423 **Gift of Hope**
Tourette Syndrome Association
42-40 Bell Boulevard, Suite 205
Bayside, NY 11361   718-224-2999
                                        Fax: 718-279-9596
                                        www.tsa-usa.org

The cause of Tourette syndrome lies in the brain. This video offers five people who have TS explaining their reasons for agreeing to register with TSA's Brain Bank Program.

14 minutes

7424 **Kevin and Me**
Hope Press
PO Box 188
Duarte, CA 91009   800-321-4039
                                        Fax: 626-358-3520
                                        dcomings@earthlink.net
                                        www.hopepress.com

A memoir of a single moter who struggled with her son's Tourette syndrome and discovered music therapy as a magincal influence on him and their relationship.

David E Comings, MD, Presenter

7425 **Ryan**
Tourette Syndrome Association
42-40 Bell Boulevard
Bayside, NY 11361   718-224-2999
                                        888-486-8738
                                        Fax: 718-279-9596
                                        ts@tsa-usa.org
                                        tsa-usa.org

Ryan's family first thought his behavior was a deliberate way to get attention, lateer educate themselves and others about Ryan's Tourette's Syndrome.

11 minutes

7426 The Turners
Tourette Syndrome Association
42-40 Bell Boulevard
Bayside, NY 11361

718-224-2999
888-486-8738
Fax: 718-279-9596
ts@tsa-usa.org
tsa-usa.org

Three of the four Turner daughters have Tourette's Syndrome in varying degress.

12 minutes

Web Sites

7427 American Academy of Child & Adolescent Psychiatry
3615 Wisconsin Avenue, N.W.
Washington, DC 20016

202-966-7300
Fax: 202-966-2891
communications@aacap.org
www.aacap.org

Mission is to promote mentally healthy children, adolescents and families through research, training, advocacy, prevention, comprehensive diagnosis and treatment, peer support and collaboration.

Paramjit T. Joshi, M.D., President
Gregory K. Fritz, M.D., President-Elect
Aradhana Sood, M.D., Secretary

7428 American Academy of Neurology: Tourette Syndrome
201 Chicago Avenue
Minneapolis, MN 55415

612-928-6000
800-879-1960
Fax: 612-454-2746
memberservices@aan.com
www.aan.com

A specialty medical society established to advance the art and science of neurology and theryby promote the best possible care for patients with neurological disorders by: ensuring appropriate access to neurological care, supporting and advocating for an environment which ensures ethical, high quality neurological care, and providing excellence in professional education by offering a variety of programs in the clinical aspects of neurology and the basic neuroscience to healh professionals.

Timothy A. Pedley, MD, FAAN, President
Catherine M. Rydell, CAE, Executive Director/CEO
Lisa Larson, Executive Assistant

7429 Children's Hospital Boston
300 Longwood Avenue
Boston, MA 2115

617-355-6000
800-355-7944
www.childrenshospital.org

Mission is to provide the highest quality care; be the leading source of reseach and discovery; educate the next generation of leaders in child health and enhance the health and well-being of the children and families in our local community.

Sandra L. Fenwick, President/ CEO
Kevin Churchwell, MD, EVP, Health Affairs & COO
Naomi Fried, PhD, Chief Innovation Officer

7430 Health Answers
410 Horsham Road
Horsham, PA 19044

215-442-9010
Michael.tague@healthanswers.com
www.healthanswers.com

HealthAnswers offers a breadth of services in medical education, sales force training, patient support solutions, professional promotion and consumer solutions.

Michael Tague, Managing Director

7431 NIH/National Institute of Neurological Dis orders and Stroke (NINDS)
PO Box 5801
Bethesda, MD 20824

301-496-5751
800-352-9424
www.ninds.nih.gov

The mission of NINDS is to reduce the burden of neurological disease - a burden borne by every age group, by every segment of society, by people all over the world.

Walter J. Koroshetz, MD, Director

7432 Online Mendelian Inheritance in Man
www.omim.org

This database is a catalog of human genes and genetic disorders.

7433 Parents Helping Parents
Sobrato Center For Nonprofits-San Jose, 1400 Parkm
San Jose, CA 95126

408-727-5775
855-727-5775
Fax: 408-286-1116
www.php.com

Mission is to help children with special needs revive the resources, love, hope, respect, health care, education, and other services they need to reach their full potential by providing them with strong families, dedicated professionals, and responsive systems to serve them.

Mary Ellen Peterson, M.A., Executive Director/CEO
Nancy O'Rourke, Chief Development Officer
Jane Floethe-Ford, Director of Education Services

7434 Tourette Syndrome Association
42-40 Bell Boulevard
Bayside, NY 11361

718-224-2999
Fax: 718-279-9596
www.tsa-usa.org

Is the only voluntary nonprofit membership organization in this field. Its mission is to identify the cause of, find the cure for and control the effects of this disorder.

7435 Tourettes Syndrome Online
www.tourettes-syndrome.com

Devoted to children and adults with Tourette Syndrome disorder and their families, friends, teachers and medical professionals.

Book Publishers

7436 Adam and the Magic Marble
Hope Press
PO Box 188
Duarte, CA 91009

800-321-4039
Fax: 626-358-3520
dcomings@earthlink.net
www.hopepress.com

Constantly taunted by bullies, the boys find a marble full of magic powers that are nearly impossible to control. Humorous and delightful, this fantasy will take you from laughter to tears and happily back to laughter again every time you read it.

Adam Buehrens, Author
Carol Buehrens, Author

7437 Children with Tourette Syndrome: A Parent's Guide-2nd Edition
ADD WareHouse
300 NW 70th Avenue, Suite 102
Plantation, FL 33317

954-792-8100
800-233-9273
Fax: 954-792-8545
www.addwarehouse.com

The first guide written specifically for parents and other family members is a collaboration by a team of medical specialists, therapists, people with TS, and parents. It provides a complete introduction to TS and how it's diagnosed and treated. Also, chapters on family life, emotions, education and legal rights

2007 361 pages

7438 Don't Think About Monkeys: Extraordinary Stories Written by People with Tourette
Hope Press
PO Box 188
Duarte, CA 91009
800-321-4039
Fax: 626-358-3520
dcomings@earthlink.net
www.hopepress.com

A collection of stories written by fourteen people who live with Tourette syndrome. Ranging from three teenagers learning to come to grips with treatment to adults encountering discrimination, the collection represents the incredible diversity of a disorder as diverse as life itself.

200 pages
ISBN: 1-878267-33-7

Adam Seligman, Author
John Hilkevich, Author

7439 Hi! I'm Adam!
Hope Press
PO Box 188
Duarte, CA 91009
800-321-4039
Fax: 626-358-3520
www.hopepress.com

Adam Buehrens is ten years old and has Tourette syndrome. Adam wrote and illustrated this book because he wants everyone to know he and other children with Tourette syndrome are not crazy. They just have a common neurological disorder. If you know a child that has tics, temper tantrums, unreasonable fears, or problems dealing with school, you will find this a reassuring story.

Adam Buehrens, Author

7440 Matthew and the Tics
Tourette Syndrome Association
42-40 Bell Boulevard, Suite 205
Bayside, NY 11361
718-224-2999
Fax: 718-279-9596
ts@tsa-usa.org
www.tsa-usa.org

A story for young children with TS and their peers.

2 pages

7441 RYAN: A Mother's Story of Her Hyperactive/ Tourette Syndrome Child
Hope Press
PO Box 188
Duarte, CA 91009
800-321-4039
Fax: 626-358-3520
dcomings@earthlink.net
www.hopepress.com

Tells of the struggles with understanding Ryan's unusual behaviors, of getting a diagnosis, and of struggling with her own feelings of guilt. The message is written in the ultimately understandable language of parent to parent. It is written so others need not feel alone or struggle through so many years of uncertainty.

Susan Hughes, Author

7442 Raising Joshua
Hope Press
PO Box 188
Duarte, CA 91009
800-321-4039
Fax: 626-358-3520
dcomings@earthlink.net
www.hopepress.com

The harrowing and heartwarming story of Josh, a boy caught in Tourette Syndrome, and Attention Deficit Hyperactivity Disorder, as told by his mother. The true story of two souls caught in a modern jungle of medical ignorance, powerful drugs, and the ravaging behavior of a mysterious condition.

Sheryl Johnson Hamer RN, Author

7443 Teaching the Tiger
Hope Press
PO Box 188
Duarte, CA 91009
800-321-4039
Fax: 626-358-3520
dcomings@earthlink.net
www.hopepress.com

A handbook for individuals involved in the education of students with Attention Deficit Disorder, Tourette Syndrome, or Obsessive Compulsive Disorder.

ISBN: 1-878267-34-5

David E Comings MD, Presenter

7444 Tourette Syndrome and Human Behavior
Hope Press
PO Box 188
Duarte, CA 91009
800-321-4039
Fax: 626-358-3520
dcomings@earthlink.net
www.hopepress.com

Packed with information on all aspects of Tourette syndrome, the diagnosis; chapters on ADHD, obsessive-compulsive behaviors, conduct disorder, learning disorders and dyslexia, sexual problems, phobias, anxiety attacks, depression, mood swings, addictive behaviors, sleep and other problems; genetics; structure and chemistry of the brain, role of dopamine and serotonin in behvior; detailed chapters on all the medications used and their side effects; psychological treatment and school problems.

828 pages

David E Comings MD, Author

7445 Tourette Syndrome: The Facts
Oxford University Press
2001 Evans Road
Cary, NC 27513
212-726-6000
800-445-9714
Fax: 919-677-1303
custserv.us@oup.com
www.oup-usa.org

A guide for clinicians, general practitioners, school teachers, and anyone seeking an accsible introduction the disorder.

1998 122 pages
ISBN: 0-198523-98-X

7446 Tourette's Syndrome
ADD WareHouse
300 NW 70th Avenue, Suite 102
Plantation, FL 33317
954-792-8100
800-233-9273
Fax: 954-792-8545
www.addwarehouse.com

Provides any information needed on Torette's Syndrome.

2001 400 pages
ISBN: 0-596500-07-6

7447 What Makes Ryan Tic?
Hope Press
PO Box 188
Duarte, CA 91009
800-321-4039
Fax: 626-358-3520
dcomings@earthlink.net
www.hopepress.com

Covers Ryan's very difficult adolescent years-a period when his symptoms were so severe he had to be placed in a residential treatment facility-and the subsequent period of returning home and pursuing a virtually normal life following his excellent response to the right combination of medication, family and school support

Susan Hughes, Author

Pamphlets

7448 Coping with Tourette Syndrome, A Parent's Viewpoint
Tourette Syndrome Association
42-40 Bell Boulevard, Suite 205
Bayside, NY 11361
718-224-2999
Fax: 718-279-9596

An acclaimed medical writer and mother of three children with TS, the author sensitively addresses common concerns and feelings of parents.

7449 Development of Behavioral and Emotional Problems in Tourette Syndrome
Tourette Syndrome Association
National Library of Medicine, Building 38A
Bethesda, MD 20894
718-224-2999
888-346-3656
Fax: 718-279-9596
info@ncbi.nlm.nih.gov
www.ncbi.nlm.nih.gov/pubmed/

Using the Child Behavior Checklist, 78 male children were assessed for a variety of behavioral problems. Relation to tic severity covered.

Christine E. Seidman, M.D., Chair
David J. Lipman, M.D., Executive Secretary

7450 Discipline and the Child with Tourette Syndrome
Tourette Syndrome Association
42-40 Bell Boulevard, Suite 205
Bayside, NY 11361
718-224-2999
Fax: 718-279-9596

Helps children redirect impulses and compulsions through teaching cause and effect relationships.

7451 Georges Gilles de la Tourette-The Man and His Times
Tourette Syndrome Association
National Library of Medicine, Building 38A
Bethesda, MD 20894
718-224-2999
888-346-3656
Fax: 718-279-9596
info@ncbi.nlm.nih.gov
www.ncbi.nlm.nih.gov/pubmed/

Rare historical biography of the famous French neurologist G. Gilles De La Tourette.

Christine E. Seidman, M.D., Chair
David J. Lipman, M.D., Executive Secretary

7452 Getting Into College: Strategies for the Student with Tourette Syndrome
Tourette Syndrome Association
42-40 Bell Boulevard, Suite 205
Bayside, NY 11361
718-224-2999
Fax: 718-279-9596

7453 Guide to Diagnosis & Treatment
Tourette Syndrome Association
42-40 Bell Boulevard, Suite 205
Bayside, NY 11361
718-224-2999
Fax: 718-279-9596

Covers symptoms, pharmacology and clinical assessments.

7454 Health Insurance Issues and Solutions for People with Torette Syndrome
Tourette Syndrome Association
42-40 Bell Boulevard, Suite 205
Bayside, NY 11361
718-224-2999
Fax: 718-279-9596

Detailed, up-to-date packet of medical information for obtaining health insurance as well as information for submission to insurance carriers.

7455 Learning Problems & the Student with Tourette Syndrome
Tourette Syndrome Association
42-40 Bell Boulevard, Suite 205
Bayside, NY 11361
718-224-2999
Fax: 718-279-9596

Report on learning problems identified through a study of 200 children with TS.

7456 NINDS Seeks Patients with Tourette Syndrome
National Inst. of Neurological Disorders/Stroke
PO Box 5801
Bethesda, MD 20824
301-496-5751
800-352-9424
www.ninds.nih.gov

New program announcements and requests for applications.

Walter J. Koroshetz, M.D., Acting Director
Alan L. Willard, Ph.D., Acting Deputy Director
Caroline Lewis, Executive Officer

7457 Need to Know
Tourette Syndrome Association
42-40 Bell Boulevard, Suite 205
Bayside, NY 11361
718-224-2999
Fax: 718-279-9596

Recollections of a young woman who was diagnosed with TS in her 20s.

7458 Peer Problems in Tourette's Disorder
Tourette Syndrome Association
National Library of Medicine, Building 38A
Bethesda, MD 20894
718-224-2999
888-346-3656
Fax: 718-279-9596
info@ncbi.nlm.nih.gov
www.ncbi.nlm.nih.gov/pubmed/

Detailed research findings of peer problems in children with TS. Includes statistical results obtained from these studies.

Christine E. Seidman, M.D., Chair
David J. Lipman, M.D., Executive Secretary

7459 Problem Behaviors & Tourette Syndrome
Tourette Syndrome Association
42-40 Bell Boulevard, Suite 205
Bayside, NY 11361
718-224-2999
Fax: 718-279-9596

Describes recent research and what is now known about the relationship of a variety of behaviors and TS.

7460 Specific Classroom Strategies and Techniqu es for Students with TS-2nd Edition
Tourette Syndrome Association
42-40 Bell Boulevard, Suite 205
Bayside, NY 11361
718-224-2999
Fax: 718-279-9596

An educator with TS spells out concrete methods for managing students with TS. She outlines many valuable classroom interventions to help youngsters deal with tic symptons, ADHD, visual motor and fine motor integration, and behavioral difficulties.

7461 TS: A Look at the Interface Between Tourette Syndrome and the Law
Tourette Syndrome Association
42-40 Bell Boulevard, Suite 205
Bayside, NY 11361
718-224-2999
Fax: 718-279-9596

Summarizes important legislation protecting the rights of students with TS. Also covers resources and hints about how to prepare for dealing successfully with educators and school systems.

7462 Teens and Tourette Syndrome
Tourette Syndrome Association
42-40 Bell Boulevard, Suite 205
Bayside, NY 11361   718-224-2999
                              Fax: 718-279-9596
                              ts@tsa-usa.org
                              tsa-usa.org

Covers self esteem, friends, dating, drugs and alcohol, stress, depression, academic and vocational planning, sibling relationships and medication.

7463 Tourette Syndrome and the School Psychologist
Tourette Syndrome Association
42-40 Bell Boulevard, Suite 205
Bayside, NY 11361   718-224-2999
                              Fax: 718-279-9596

The role of the school psychologist is covered including testing procedures, counseling strategies and social implications.

7464 Tourette Syndrome and the School Nurse
Tourette Syndrome Association
42-40 Bell Boulevard, Suite 205
Bayside, NY 11361   718-224-2999
                              Fax: 718-279-9596

Comprehensive professional guide to educational, social and medical implications.

7465 What School Bus Drivers Need to Know About Students with Tourette Syndrome
Tourette Syndrome Association
42-40 Bell Boulevard, Suite 205
Bayside, NY 11361   718-224-2999
                              Fax: 718-279-9596
                              ts@tsa-usa.org
                              tsa-usa.org

Includes a description of the disorder, as well as related disorders and suggestions as to what school bus drivers can do for students with TS.

Camps

7466 Tourette Syndrome Camp Organization
6933 N Kedzie, #816
Chicago, IL 60640   773-465-7536
                              info@tourettecamp.com
                              www.tourettecamp.com

Dedicated to promoting camping opportunities for children with Tourette Syndrome and its associated disorders, Obsessive Compulsive Disorder (OCD) and Attention Deficit/Hyperactivity Disorder (ADD/ADHD).

Scott Loeff, President
Monica Newman, Camp Director

DESCRIPTION

7467 TOXOPLASMOSIS

Covers these related disorders: Congenital toxoplasmosis
Involves the following Biologic System(s):

Infectious Disorders

Toxoplasmosis is a common infection caused by the single-celled parasite Toxoplasma gondii. This parasite multiplies in the intestines of cats, and its eggs (oocysts) are shed in cat feces. Humans may acquire toxoplasmosis due to contact with cat feces (e.g., in litter boxes), from exposure to contaminated soil, or by eating undercooked or raw meat (lamb, pork, and beef) that contains a form of the parasite (tissue cysts). In addition, if a woman acquires toxoplasmosis during pregnancy, the developing fetus may be affected (congenital toxoplasmosis) due to transmission via the placenta.

Most children who acquire toxoplasmosis after birth and have normally functioning immune systems do not have any apparent symptoms (asymptomatic). However, some children may experience enlargement of one or more lymph nodes (lymphadenopathy). More rarely, such patients may also have other, variable symptoms and findings, such as fever; joint or muscle pain; enlargement of the liver (hepatomegaly); or inflammation of the lungs (pneumonia), the liver (hepatitis), or the middle layer of and the nerve-rich membrane at the back of the eyes (chorioretinitis). Most children with normal immune systems who acquire toxoplasmosis after birth recover spontaneously. However, others may require treatment with certain medications.

Toxoplasmosis is typically more severe in children who acquire the disease during fetal development or who have compromised immune systems. When the infection is transmitted via the placenta during pregnancy (or, in some cases, during vaginal delivery), patients are said to have congenital toxoplasmosis. The disease is typically more severe if the infection is acquired during early pregnancy (first trimester), but the risk of disease transmission is greatest during later pregnancy (third trimester). Approximately 50 percent of women who acquire toxoplasmosis during pregnancy and do not receive treatment transmit the infection to the developing fetus. In the United States, congenital toxoplasmosis affects approximately one in 1,000 newborns.

Without treatment, almost all patients demonstrate certain findings associated with toxoplasmosis by adolescence, particularly chorioretinitis. Chorioretinitis may cause blurred vision, abnormal sensitivity to light (photophobia), and possible visual impairment. In some affected infants, findings may include short height and low weight at birth (intrauterine growth retardation); persistent yellowish discoloration of the skin, whites of the eyes, and mucous membranes (jaundice); retinal scarring; skin rash; lymphadenopathy; decreased levels of circulating blood platelets (thrombocytopenia); hepatitis; hearing loss; or other findings. Severely affected infants may have an abnormally small head (microcephaly), an abnormal accumulation of cerebrospinal fluid around the brain (hydrocephalus), chorioretinitis, episodes of abnormally increased electrical activity in the brain (seizures), delays in the acquisition of skills requiring the coordination of physical and mental activities (psychomotor retardation), and calcium deposits in the brain. Life-threatening complications may occur shortly after birth.

In children who have compromised immune systems, such as those with acquired immunodeficiency syndrome (AIDS), toxoplasmosis often occurs suddenly and is extremely severe (fulminant). In such patients, infection may rapidly affect the lungs, heart, and brain. In fulminant toxoplasmosis, the most common symptoms are often neurological and may include headache, impaired cognition (thinking), seizures, and impaired control of voluntary movement (ataxia). Without treatment, life-threatening complications result.

The treatment of newborns with congenital toxoplasmosis, affected children with compromised immune systems, and other patients with acquired toxoplasmosis may include the use of combination drug therapies with such medications as pyrimethamine, folinic acid, sulfadiazine or triple sulfonamides, leukovorin, or spiramycin. Additional treatment is symptomatic and supportive. It is important to note that all newborns with congenital toxoplasmosis should receive appropriate drug therapy, regardless of whether they have severe, mild, or no associated symptoms. Appropriate drug therapy for women who contract toxoplasmosis any time during pregnancy may reduce the risk of congenital toxoplasmosis by approximately 60 percent. Such therapy may includeclindamycin and pyrimethamine combined trimethoprim-sulfamethoxasole or sulfadiazine. Pyrimethamine is not given during early pregnancy since it may increase the risk of birth defects during early fetal development. Treatment in AIDS patients is continued as long as the immune system is weak, to prevent reactivation of the disease.In addition, certain measures may be helpful in preventing toxoplasmosis, such as thoroughly cooking all meat, washing hands after handling raw meat, and avoiding direct contact with cat feces.

Government Agencies

7468 Centers for Disease Control and Prevention
1600 Clifton Road
Atlanta, GA 30329

404-639-8813
800-232-4636
TTY: 888-232-6348
www.cdc.gov

Mission is to promote health and quality of life by preventing and controlling disease, njury, and disability.

Dr. Tom Frieden, Director
Ileana Arias, PhD, Principal Deputy Director
John M. Auerbach, MBA, Associate Director of Policy

7469 NIH/National Institute of Allergy and Infectious Diseases
5601 Fishers Lane, MSC 9806
Bethesda, MD 20892

301-496-5717
866-284-4107
Fax: 301-402-3573
TDD: 800-877-8339
ocposfoffice@niaid.nih.gov
www.niaid.nih.gov

Conducts and supports basic and applied research to better understand, treat, and ultimately prevent infectious, immunologic, and allergic diseases.

Anthony S Fauci MD, Director
Hugh Auchincloss, M.D., Principal Deputy Director
John J. McGowan, Ph.D., Deputy Director for Science Mngmnt

7470 NIH/National Institute of Allergy and Infectious Diseases
5601 Fishers Lane, MSC 9806
Bethesda, MD 20892   301-496-5717
                                                866-284-4107
                                           Fax: 301-402-3573
                                           TDD: 800-877-8339
                                     ocposfoffice@niaid.nih.gov
                                                www.niaid.nih.gov

Conducts and supports basic and applied research to better understand, treat, and ultimately prevent infectious, immunologic, and allergic diseases.

Anthony Fauci MD, Director
Hugh Auchincloss, M.D., Principal Deputy Director
John J. McGowan, Ph.D., Deputy Director for Science Mngmnt

National Associations & Support Groups

7471 American Academy of Pediatrics
141 Northwest Point Boulevard
Elk Grove Village, IL 60007   847-434-4000
                                                800-433-9016
                                           Fax: 847-434-8000
                                                www.aap.org

The American Academy of Pediatrics and its member pediatricians are committed to the attainment of optimal physical, mental and social health and well-being for all infants, children, adolescents, and young adults.

Fernando Stein, MD, FAAP, President
Karen Remley, MD, CEO/Executive VP

7472 Arc of the United States
National Organization Mental Retardation
1825 K Street, NW, Suite 1200
Washington, DC 20006   202-534-3700
                                                800-433-5255
                                           Fax: 202-534-3731
                                                info@thearc.org
                                                www.thearc.org

The Arc of the United States works to include all children and adults with cognitive, intellectual, developmental disabilities in every community. We are a national organization of and for the people with mental retardation and related developmental disabilities and their families. It is devoted to promoting and improving supports and services for people with mental retardation and their families. The ARC was founded by a small group of parents and other concerned individuals.

Peter V. Berns, CEO
Ronald Brown, President
Elise McMillan, Vice President

7473 Children's Hospital Boston
300 Longwood Avenue
Boston, MA 2115   617-355-6000
                                                800-355-7944
                                           TTY: 617-355-0443
                                          www.childrenshospital.org

Mission is to provide the highest quality care; be the leading source of research and discovery; educate the next generation of leaders in child health and enhance the health and well-being of the children and families in our local community.

Sandra L. Fenwick, President/ CEO
Kevin Churchwell, MD, EVP, Health Affairs & COO
Naomi Fried, PhD, Chief Innovation Officer

7474 World Health Organization
Avenue Appia 20
CH-1211 Geneva 27,
Switzerland   www.who.int

WHO is the directing and coordinating authority for health within the United Nations system.

Dr Margaret Chan, Director General
Dr Anarfi Asamoa-Baah, Deputy Director-General
Bruce Aylward, Assistant Director-General

Web Sites

7475 Children's Hospital Boston
www.childrenshospital.org

Mission is to provide the highest quality care; be the leading source of reseach and discovery; educate the next generation of leaders in child health and enhance the health and well-being of the children and families in our local community.

Sandra L. Fenwick, President/ CEO
Kevin Churchwell, MD, EVP, Health Affairs & COO
Naomi Fried, PhD, Chief Innovation Officer

7476 Toxoplasmosis Fact Sheet
750 3rd Avenue, 6th Floor
New York, NY 10017   212-541-8500
                                      www.thebody.com/treat/toxo.html

Offers information about what the disease is, how to treat it, what treatments to use, and if it can be prevented.

Myles Helfand, Editorial Director
Julie Davids, Managing Editor
Mathew Rodriguez, Community Editor

Pamphlets

7477 Toxoplasmosis Fact Sheet
Division of Parasitic Diseases
1600 Clifton Road
Atlanta, GA 30329   404-639-3534
                                                800-232-4636
                                           TTY: 888-232-6348
                                                www.cdc.gov

Dr. Tom Frieden, Director
Ileana Arias, PhD, Principal Deputy Director
John M. Auerbach, MBA, Associate Director of Policy

881

DESCRIPTION

7478 TRANSPOSITION OF THE GREAT ARTERIES

Synonym: Transposition of the great vessels

Involves the following Biologic System(s):

Cardiovascular Disorders

Transposition of the great arteries is a heart defect that is present at birth (congenital) in which the major blood vessels that transport blood away from the heart (aorta and pulmonary artery) are switched (transposed) from their normal position. The pulmonary artery normally arises from the base of the lower right-sided pumping chamber (right ventricle) of the heart and carries oxygen-poor blood to the lungs, where the exchange of oxygen and carbon dioxide occurs. The aorta, the main artery of the body, normally arises from the base of the left ventricle and carries oxygen-rich (oxygenated) blood to the body's tissues. However, in infants with transposition of the great arteries, the aorta arises from the right ventricle and the pulmonary artery arises from the left ventricle. As a result, oxygenated blood recirculates to the lungs, while the oxygen-poor blood recirculates throughout the body, and bodily tissues receive insufficient levels of oxygenated blood (hypoxia).

Transpositon of the great arteries is not compatible with life unless there is some communication between the pulmonary and systemic circulation, thus allowing for some mixing of deoxygenated and oxygenated blood. Certain fetal shunts may provide such mixing. These include persistence of the fetal channel that joins the pulmonary artery and the aorta (ductus arteriosus), an opening in the fibrous partition (septum) between the upper chambers (atria) of the heart (patent foramen ovale). Some patients with transposition have mixing of blood through openings in the septum between the ventricles (ventricular septal defect, VSD) or atria (atrial septal defects, ASD)

In newborns with transposition of the great arteries, symptoms are primarily cyanosis (bluish discoloration of fingers and toes and mucous membranes). Shortly after birth, affected infants may experience abnormally rapid and deep breathing (tachypnea, hyperpnea) and cyanosis. Without treatment, life-threatening complications will result. Medical treatment includes a medication called prostaglandin E to open the ductus arteriosus and allow mixing. A cardiac catheterization to place a balloon catheter across the atrial septum (balloon septostomy) may be necessary to allow for mixing of blood. Permanent treatment of infants with transposition of the great arteries includes surgery to switch the aorta and coronary arteries and pulmonary artery back to their normal positions (arterial switch operation). This operation is done in the first weeks of life.

Transposition of the great arteries is more common in males than females and affects approximately one in 2,000 newborns. Infants are most often normal sized, full term, and otherwise healthy. The condition is thought to result from the interactions of several different genes, possibly in association with the involvement of environmental factors (multifactorial inheritance). Although the exact underlying cause of this heart defect is unknown, rese archers suggest that it may result from an error during the development of an embryonic structure that later divides the aorta and pulmonary artery.

Government Agencies

7479 NIH/ Eunice Kennedy Shriver National Insti tute of Child Health & Human Development

31 Center Drive, Building 31

Bethesda, MD 20892

301-496-5113
800-370-2943
Fax: 866-760-5947
TTY: 888-320-6942
nichdpress@mail.nih.gov
www.nichd.nih.gov

Established in 1962 by congress, today the institute conducts and supports research on topics related to the health of children, adults, families and populations. Some of these topics include: developmental disabilities, growth and development, infant death, reproductive health and birth defects.

Diana W. Bianchi, Director

Paul Williams, Director, Communications

7480 NIH/National Heart, Lung and Blood Institu te

National Institute of Health

31 Center Dr MSC 2486, Bldg 31, Room 5A52

Bethesda, MD 20892

301-592-8573
Fax: 240-629-3246
TTY: 240-629-3255
NHLBIinfo@nhlbi.nih.gov
www.nhlbi.nih.gov

Primary responsibility of this organization is the scientific investigation of heart, blood vessel, lung and blood disorders. Oversees research, demonstration, prevention, education, control and training activities in these fields and emphasizes the prevention and control of heart diseases.

Gary H. Gibbons, M.D., Director

Nakela Cook, MD, MPH, Chief of Staff

Kathleen B. O'Sullivan, Executive Officer

7481 NIH/National Heart, Lung, and Blood Instit ute

31 Center Dr MSC 2486, Bldg 31, Room 5A52

Bethesda, MD 20824

301-592-8573
Fax: 301-629-3246
TTY: 240-629-3255
nhlbiinfo@nhlbi.nih.gov
www.nhlbi.nih.gov

Provides leadership for a national program in diseases of the heart, blood vessels, lungs, and blood; blood resources; and sleep disorders.

Gary H. Gibbons, M.D., Director

Nakela Cook, MD, MPH, Chief of Staff

Kathleen B. O'Sullivan, Executive Officer

National Associations & Support Groups

7482 American Academy of Pediatrics

141 Northwest Point Boulevard

Elk Grove Village, IL 60007

847-434-4000
800-433-9016
Fax: 847-434-8000
www.aap.org

The American Academy of Pediatrics and its member pediatricians dedicate their efforts and resources to the health, safety and well-being of infants, children, adolescents and young adults.

Fernando Stein, MD, FAAP, President

Karen Remley, MD, CEO/Executive VP

7483 American Heart Association

7272 Greenville Avenue

Dallas, TX 75231

214-373-6300
800-242-8721
Fax: 214-706-1341
inquire@amhrt.org
www.heart.org/HEARTORG/

Supports research, education and community service programs with the objective of reducing premature death and disability from cardiovascular diseases and stroke; coordinates the efforts of health professionals, and others engaged in the fight against heart and circulatory disease.

Nancy Brown, CEO
Dr. Stephen Houser, President
Suzie Upton, Chief Operating Officer

7484 Congenital Heart Information Network
600 North 3rd Street, First Floor
Philadelphia, PA 19123
215-627-4034
Fax: 215-627-4036
mb@tchin.org
www.tchin.org

CHIN is an international organization that provides reliable information, support services and resources to families of children with congenital heart defects and acquired heart disease.

Mona Barmash, President

7485 Genetic Alliance
4301 Connecticut Avenue NW, Suite 404
Washington, DC 20008
202-966-5557
800-336-4363
Fax: 202-966-8553
info@geneticalliance.org
www.geneticalliance.org

A coalition of voluntary genetic support groups, consumers and professionals addressing the needs of individuals and families affected by genetic disorders from a national perspective.

Sharon Terry, President/CEO
Tetyana Murza, Managing Director
Natasha Bonhomme, VP, Strategic Development

7486 United Network for Organ Sharing
700 N 4th Street, PO Box 2484
Richmond, VA 23219
804-782-4800
Fax: 804-782-4817
webmaster@unos.org
www.unos.org

Our mission is to advance organ availability and transplantation by uniting and supporting our communities for the benefit of patients through education, technology and policy development.

Brian M. Shepard, CEO
Mary D. Ellison, Ph.D., MSHA, Chief External Relations Officer
Douglas E. Harvey, Chief Financial Officer

Web Sites

7487 American Academy of Pediatrics
141 Northwest Point Boulevard
Elk Grove Village, IL 60007
847-434-4000
800-433-9016
Fax: 847-434-8000
www.aap.org

The American Academy of Pediatrics and its member pediatricians are committed to the attainment of optimal physical, mental and social health and well-being for all infants, children, adolescents, and young adults.

Fernando Stein, MD, FAAP, President
Karen Remley, MD, CEO/Executive VP

7488 American Heart Association
7272 Greenville Avenue
Dallas, TX 75231
800-242-8721
www.heart.org/HEARTORG/

Supports research, education and community service programs with the objective of reducing premature death and disability from cardiovascular diseases and stroke; coordinates the efforts of health professionals, and others engaged in the fight against heart and circulatory disease.

Nancy Brown, CEO
Dr. Stephen Houser, President
Suzie Upton, Chief Operating Officer

7489 Congenital Heart Information Network
www.tchin.org

An international organization that provides reliable information, support services and resources to families of children with congenital heart defects and acquired heart disease and adults with congenital heart defects, and the professionals who work with them.

7490 NIH/National Heart, Lung and Blood Institute
31 Center Dr MSC 2486, Bldg 31, Room 5A52
Bethesda, MD 20892
301-592-8573
NHLBIinfo@nhlbi.nih.gov
www.nhlbi.nih.gov

Provides leadership for a national program in diseases of the heart, blood vessels, lungs, and blood; blood resources; and sleep disorders.

Gary H. Gibbons, M.D., Director
Nakela Cook, MD, MPH, Chief of Staff
Kathleen B. O'Sullivan, Executive Officer

7491 Southern Illinois University School of Medicine
PO Box 19639
Springfield, IL 62794
217-545-8000
800-342-5748
admin@siuhealthcare.org
www.siumed.edu/peds/index.htm

The mission of SUI School of Medicine is to assist the people if Central and Southern Illinois in meeting thier present and future health care needs through education, clinical service and research.

7492 United Network for Organ Sharing
700 North 4th Street
Richmond, VA 23219
804-782-4800
Fax: 804-782-4817
webmaster@unos.org
www.unos.org

Our mission is to advance organ availability and transplantation by uniting and supporting our communities for the benefit of patients through education, technology and policy development.

Brian M. Shepard, CEO
Mary D. Ellison, Ph.D., MSHA, Chief External Relations Officer
Douglas E. Harvey, Chief Financial Officer

7493 Yale University School of Medicine
333 Cedar Street
New Haven, CT 6510
203-432-4771
www.info.med.yale.edu/intmed/cardio/chd

A site that offers information on Transposition of the Great Arteries and other congenital heart conditions.

Peter Salovey, President of the University
Richard Belitsky M.D., Deputy Dean for Education
Benjamin Polak, B.A., M.A., Ph.D., Provost of the University

DESCRIPTION

7494 TRISOMY 18 SYNDROME

Synonyms: Chromosome 18, trisomy 18, Edwards syndrome

Covers these related disorders: Trisomy 18 mosaicism

Involves the following Biologic System(s):

Genetic/Chromosomal/Syndrome/Metabolic Disorders

Trisomy 18 syndrome is a chromosomal disorder that affects about one in 300 newborns. With the exception of reproductive cells, cells of the body normally have 23 pairs of chromosomes that are numbered from 1 to 22 (with a 23rd pair consisting of one X chromosome from the mother and an X or a Y chromosome from the father). However, in infants with trisomy 18 syndrome, all or a portion of chromosome 18 is present three times (trisomy) rather than twice in cells of the body. In some affected infants, only a percentage of cells may contain the trisomy 18 chromosomal abnormality (mosaicism).

The symptoms and physical findings associated with trisomy 18 syndrome are variable and depend upon the exact location, and percentage, of body cells containing the additional chromosomal material from chromosome 18. However, infants with trisomy 18 syndrome experience development delays, usually severe mental retardation, low birth weight, difficulties feeding and breathing, and a failure to gain weight and grow at the expected rate (failure to thrive). In addition, almost all infants with trisomy 18 have complex structural heart defects, failure of one or both testes to descend into the scrotum (cryptorchidism) in affected males, malformations of the hands and feet, additional skeletal abnormalities, and characteristic malformations of the head and facial (craniofacial) area.

In infants with trisomy 18 syndrome, defects of the hands and feet of ten include closed fists with overlapping, abnormally bent fingers; underdeveloped or absent thumbs; and webbing between certain fingers or toes (syndactyly). Affected infants also often have additional skeletal abnormalities, such as a small pelvis, narrow hips with limited movements, fusion of certain bones of the spinal column (vertebrae), or sideways curvature of the spine (scoliosis). Characteristic craniofacial abnormalities associated with trisomy 18 syndrome typically include an abnormally small head (microcephaly); a prominent back portion of the head (occiput); a small mouth (microstomia) and a small jaw (micrognathia); malformed, low-set ears; and short, narrow eyelid folds (palpebral fissures). Additional craniofacial malformations may be present, such as incomplete closure of the roof of the mouth (cleft palate), an abnormal groove in the upper lip (cleft lip), and drooping of the upper eyelids (ptosis). Some infants may have kidney defects . The abnormalities of trisomy 18 are generally not compatible with more than a few months of life. Fifty percent of the affected infants do not survive beyond the first week of life. Although the exact cause of trisomy 18 syndrome is unknown, it is thought to result from errors during division of a parent's reproductive cells (meiosis) and, in some cases of mosaicism, errors during cellular division after fertilization (e.g., postzygotic nondisjunction). Parents who have a child with translocational trisomy 18 and want additional children should have chromosome studies, because they are at increased risk to have another child with trisomy 18.

Government Agencies

7495 NIH/ Eunice Kennedy Shriver National Insti tute of Child Health & Human Development

31 Center Drive, Building 31
Bethesda, MD 20892

301-496-5113
800-370-2943
Fax: 866-760-5947
TTY: 888-320-6942
nichdpress@mail.nih.gov
www.nichd.nih.gov

Established in 1962 by congress, today the institute conducts and supports research on topics related to the health of children, adults, families and populations. Some of these topics include: developmental disabilities, growth and development, infant death, reproductive health and birth defects.

Diana W. Bianchi, Director
Paul Williams, Director, Communications

National Associations & Support Groups

7496 American Academy of Pediatrics

141 Northwest Point Boulevard
Elk Grove Village, IL 60007

847-434-4000
800-433-9016
Fax: 847-434-8000
www.aap.org

The American Academy of Pediatrics and its member pediatricians are committed to the attainment of optimal physical, mental and social health and well-being for all infants, children, adolescents, and young adults.

Fernando Stein, MD, FAAP, President
Karen Remley, MD, CEO/Executive VP

7497 Chromosome 18 Registry & Research Society

7155 Oakridge Drive
San Antonio, TX 78229

210-657-4968
Fax: 210-657-4968
office@chromosome18.org
www.chromosome18.org

The purpose of the Chromosome 18 Registry & Research Society is to offer support to patients and families, to educate the public about different available treatments and to connect families and doctors to the research community.

500 Members

Jannine DeMars Cody, PhD, President
Jason Fisher, CFRE, VP Public Relations
Kathy Borello, VP, Member Relations

7498 Congenital Heart Anomalies, Support, Education & Resources (CHASER)

2112 N Wilkins Road
Swanton, OH 43558

419-825-5575
Fax: 419-825-2880
chaser@compuserve.com
www.csun.edu/~hcmth011/chaser/

National organization for support, education and resources for families and patients who deal with children born with congenital heart malformations.

Anita Myers, Executive Director

7499 Genetic Alliance

4301 Connecticut Avenue NW, Suite 404
Washington, DC 20008

202-966-5557
Fax: 202-966-8553
info@geneticalliance.org
www.geneticalliance.org

The Genetic Alliance promotes healthy living by working to speed the translation of genetic advances into quality and affordable healthcare, public awareness and consumer-centered public policies.

Sharon Terry, President/CEO
Tetyana Murza, Managing Director
Natasha Bonhomme, VP, Strategic Development

7500 MUMS: National Parent to Parent Network
150 Custer Street
Green Bay, WI 54301   920-336-5333
                                              877-336-5333
                                         Fax: 920-339-0995
                                           mums@netnet.net
                                        www.netnet.net/mums

A national parent-to-parent organization for parents or care providers of a child with any disability, rare or not so rare disorder,
chromosomal abnormality or health condition.

Julie J Gordon, Director

**7501 Support Organization for Trisomy 18, 13, and Related
Disorders (SOFT)**
2982 S Union Street
Rochester, NY 14624   585-594-4621
                                              800-716-7638
                                     barbsoft@rochester.rr.com
                                             www.trisomy.org

SOFT is a network of families and professional dedication to provide support and understanding to families involved in the issue
and decision surrounding the diagnosis and care related to chromosome disorders. Support is provided throughout prenatal diagnosis, the child's life and after their passing. It is committed to
the support of families and personal decisions in alliance with a
parent-professional partnership. Includes listings of local chapters
in 25 states.

Barb Vanherreweghe, Co-President
Dave Vanherreweghe, Co-President
John C. Carey, MD, MPH, Medical Advisor

7502 Trisomy 18 Foundation
4491 Cheshire Station Plaza, Suite 157
Dale City, VA 22193   810-867-4211
                                        t18info@trisomy18.org
                                           www.trisomy18.org

The foundation's mission is to search for a cure and treatments;
to educate and support medical professionals; and to create a
worldwide caring community for those affected.

Victoria J. Miller, M.A., Executive Director/ President
Kris Shaughnessy, M.A., Community Affairs Program Office
Cathy Howard, Administration and Finance Office

Research Centers

7503 Trisomy 18 Foundation
4491 Cheshire Station Plaza, Suite 157
Dale City, VA 22193   t18info@trisomy18.org
                                           www.trisomy18.org

The foundation's mission is to search for a cure and treatments;
to educate and support medical professionals; and to create a
worldwide caring community for those affected.

Victoria J. Miller, M.A., Executive Director/ President
Kris Shaughnessy, M.A., Community Affairs Program Office
Cathy Howard, Administration and Finance Office

Book Publishers

7504 Introduction to Trisomy 18
SOFT
2982 S Union Street
Rochester, NY 14624   585-594-4621
                                              800-716-7638
                                     barbsoft@rochester.rr.com
                                             www.trisomy.org

Addresses parent question regarding the disorder as well as explains the chromosomes, diagnosis and characteristics.
Revised 1998

Barb Vanherreweghe, President
Jim Dye Holladay, Secretary
Kris & Hal Holladay Founders

DESCRIPTION

7505 TRISOMY 13 SYNDROME

Synonyms: Chromosome 13, trisomy 13, D1 trisomy syndrome, Patau syndrome

Covers these related disorders: Trisomy 13 mosaicism

Involves the following Biologic System(s):

Genetic/Chromosomal/Syndrome/Metabolic Disorders

Trisomy 13 syndrome is a chromosomal disorder that is thought to affect approximately one in 5,000 newborns. With the exception of reproductive cells, cells of the body normally have 23 pairs of chromosomes that are numbered from 1 to 22. The 23rd pair includes one X chromosome from the mother and an X or a Y chromosome from the father. In infants with trisomy 13 syndrome, all or a portion of chromosome 13 is present three times (trisomy) rather than twice. In some affected infants, a certain percentage of cells contain the extra chromosome 13, whereas other cells have the normal two. This finding is known as chromosomal mosaicism.

In infants with trisomy 13 syndrome, associated symptoms and physical findings are pronounced and depend upon the specific length and location of the duplicated portion of chromosome 13 as well as the percentage of the body cells containing the defect.

Abnormalities associated with trisomy 13 syndrome include severe developmental delays, profound mental retardation, incomplete closure of the roof of the mouth (cleft palate), an abnormal groove in the upper lip (cleft lip), and unusually small eyes (microphthalmia). Additional characteristic symptoms and findings include abnormal bending of the fingers, the presence of extra fingers and toes (polydactyly), failure of the testes to descend into the scrotum (cryptorchidis in affected males, and malformation of the uterus in affected females, i.e., bicornuate uterus). Many infants have severe feeding difficulties, abnormally diminished muscle tone (hypotonia), and episodes of temporary cessation of breathing (apnea).

Defects in the brain can result in seizure activity and deafness. Most infants with trisomy 13 syndrome also have additional physical malformations, including an abnormally small head (microcephaly) with a sloping forehead; widely set eyes (ocular hypertelorism); a broad, flat nose; low-set, malformed ears; and a small jaw (micrognthia). Reddish, purplish benign growths (hemangiomas) may be present on the forehead or other areas due to an abnormal distribution of minute blood vessels (capillaries). Many affected infants may also have additional skeletal abnormalities, heart defects, and brain malformations. More than 80% of children with trisomy 13 die in the first month.. Because of the severity of congenital defects, life-sustaining procedures are generally not attempted. Parents of infants with trisomy 13 caused by a translocation should have genetic testing and counseling, which may help them prevent recurrence. The exact cause of trisomy 13 syndrome is unknown.

Government Agencies

7506 NIH/ Eunice Kennedy Shriver National Insti tute of Child Health & Human Development

31 Center Drive, Building 31
Bethesda, MD 20892

301-496-5113
800-370-2943
Fax: 866-760-5947
TTY: 888-320-6942
nichdpress@mail.nih.gov
www.nichd.nih.gov

Established in 1962 by congress, today the institute conducts and supports research on topics related to the health of children, adults, families and populations. Some of these topics include: developmental disabilities, growth and development, infant death, reproductive health and birth defects.

Diana W. Bianchi, Director
Paul Williams, Director, Communications

National Associations & Support Groups

7507 American Academy of Pediatrics

141 Northwest Point Boulevard
Elk Grove Village, IL 60007

847-434-4000
800-433-9016
Fax: 847-434-8000
www.aap.org

The American Academy of Pediatrics and its member pediatricians are committed to the attainment of optimal physical, mental and social health and well-being for all infants, children, adolescents, and young adults.

Fernando Stein, MD, FAAP, President
Karen Remley, MD, CEO/Executive VP

7508 Congenital Heart Anomalies, Support, Education & Resources (CHASER)

2112 N Wilkins Road
Swanton, OH 43558

419-825-5575
Fax: 419-825-2880
chaser@compuserve.com
www.csun.edu/~hcmth011/chaser/

National organization for support, education and resources for families, patients and professionals who deal with children born with congenital heart malformations. Information on hospitals, medical assistance, and schooling. Offers Chaser News, an international newsletter and Chaser's Pediatric Heart Surgeons Facility Directory.

Anita Myers, Executive Director

7509 Genetic Alliance

4301 Connecticut Avenue NW, Suite 404
Washington, DC 20008

202-966-5557
800-336-4363
Fax: 202-966-8553
info@geneticalliance.org
www.geneticalliance.org

A coalition of voluntary genetic support groups, consumers and professionals addressing the needs of individuals and families affected by genetic disorders from a national perspective.

Sharon Terry, President/CEO
Tetyana Murza, Managing Director
Natasha Bonhomme, VP, Strategic Development

7510 National Dissemination Center for Children with Disabilities

PO Box 1492
Washington, DC 20013

202-884-8200
800-695-0285
Fax: 202-884-8441
nichcy@aed.org
www.nichcy.org

A national information and referral center for families, educators and other professionals on: disabilities in children and youth; programs and services; IDEA, the nation's special education law; and research-based information on effective practices.

Suzanne Ripley, Executive Director

7511 Support Organization for Trisomy 18, 13, and Related Disorders (SOFT)
2982 S Union Street
Rochester, NY 14624
585-594-4621
800-716-7638
barbsoft@rochester.rr.com
www.trisomy.org

SOFT is a network of families and professional dedication to providing support and understanding to families involved in the issue and decision surrounding the diagnosis and care in related chromosome disorders. Support is provided throughout pre-natal diagnosis, the child's life and after their passing. It is committed to the support of families personal decision in alliance with a parent-professional partnership. Site includes a listing of local chapters in 25 states.

Barb Vanherreweghe, Co-President
Dave Vanherreweghe, Co-President
John C. Carey, MD, MPH, Medical Advisor

Web Sites

7512 Living with Trisomy 13
www.livingwithtrisomy.org/trisomy-13-links.htm

fawna33@mindspring.com
www.livingwithtrisomy.org/trisomy-13-links.htm

Brings together families of children diagnosed with Trisomy 13 Syndrome through the use of photos and videos.

Book Publishers

7513 Introduction to Trisomy 13
SOFT
2982 S Union Street
Rochester, NY 14624
585-594-4621
800-716-7638
barbsoft@rochester.rr.com
www.trisomy.org

Addresses parent question regarding the disorder as well as explains the chromosomes, diagnosis and characteristics.

Revised 1998

Barb Vanherreweghe, President
Jim Dye Holladay, Secretary
Kris & Hal Holladay Founders

DESCRIPTION

7514 TUBERCULOSIS

Synonym: TB

Involves the following Biologic System(s):

Infectious Disorders, Respiratory Disorders

Tuberculosis (TB) is an infectious disease that is most often caused by the bacterium Mycobacterium tuberculosis, but may sometimes result from infection with Mycobacterium bovis or Mycobacterium africanum. As a result of improvements in living conditions, the number of people in the United States infected with this disease declined dramatically throughout most of the twentieth century. However, tuberculosis rates once again began to rise in the mid-1980s in association with such factors as immigration of individuals from countries that had high incidence rates of TB, poverty, poor access to health care among groups at high risk, the increase in AIDS infections, overcrowded and sometimes unsanitary conditions in certain institutional settings, and the development of antibiotic-resistant strains of tuberculosis bacteria. The neglect of TB control programs has also contributed to the resurgence of TB. This disease is most prevalent among the elderly, people with compromised immune systems, and those of low socioeconomic status.

Tuberculosis is usually transmitted through airborne droplets coughed or sneezed into the air by an infected person. The droplets are inhaled into the lungs where the bacteria multiply and travel to the lymph nodes that are responsible for draining the lungs; however, in the vast majority of cases, the immune system either destroys or seals off the bacteria. If this primary pulmonary tuberculosis infection is not completely resolved, the bacteria may become dormant within certain white blood cells called macrophages and be later reactivated. This reemergence of symptoms at a later date may be due to influences such as an impaired immune system, corticosteroid drug usage, or advancing age. In addition to the lungs, the tuberculosis bacteria may sometimes spread throughout the body via the bloodstream and affect other parts of the body (extrapulmonary tuberculosis). This type of disseminated disease may infect the lymph nodes, upper respiratory tract, skin, liver, spleen, kidneys, gastrointestinal tract, bones, joints, brain, spine, the sac surrounding the heart (pericardium), and other organs.

Symptoms and physical findings associated with primary pulmonary tuberculosis in children may include enlargement of the lymph nodes and the subsequent compression and obstruction of the large air passages of the lungs (bronchial tubes). This obstruction may result in lung collapse, cough, and less commonly wheezing, rapid breathing (tachypnea), and respiratory distress. Other symptoms may be absent or mild, but more pronounced in infants, and may include moderate difficulty in breathing (dyspnea), a nonproductive cough, and occasionally fever, loss of appetite (anorexia), and night sweats. In addition, some infants may have failure to thrive, a condition in which the current weight or rate of weight gain is significantly below that of other children of similar age and sex. Pneumonia may develop and, in rare instances, blister-type lesions may develop in the lungs that sometimes rupture, resulting in the presence of air between the lungs and the chest wall (pneumothorax) and possible associated lung collapse.

On rare occasions, tuberculosis may be transmitted from mother to fetus through a placental lesion or by the inhalation or swallowing of infected amniotic fluid by the baby before or during birth. Congenital tuberculosis is rare and more commonly occurs soon after birth, usually through inhalation of airborne droplets from an infected person. Symptoms and findings associated with congenital tuberculosis may not develop for two or three weeks and may include drowsiness, fever, difficulty in breathing, poor feeding, drainage from the ears, enlarged lymph glands, enlarged liver and spleen (hepatosplenomegaly), abdominal swelling, skin lesions, and failure to thrive.

Diagnosis of tuberculosis may be established through evaluation of family and medical history, physical examination, skin and sputum testing, chest x-ray, and sometimes testing of cerebrospinal and other fluids as well as microscopic examination of tissue samples (biopsy).

Treatment for tuberculosis includes the prolonged administration of at least two different types of antibiotics to assure that all bacteria are destroyed. The antibiotics most often used for children with this disease include combinations of isoniazid, rifampin, pyrazinamide as well as streptomycin, and ethionamide that are especially effective for drug-resistant disease. The primary difference between treatment of TB in adults and children is ethambutol since one of the side effects is impaired vision. Because this effect is difficult to monitor in young children, ethambutol is not routinely recommended for children less then five years old. Corticosteroids may also be administered, especially in children with associated inflammatory irregularities that adversely affect organ function. In addition, the medication isoniazid may sometimes be preventively administered to those at high risk of tuberculosis infection, such as other members of the household, or to those with positive skin test results but no symptomatic or x-ray evidence of disease. The best method to prevent cases of pediatric tuberculosis is to find, diagnose, and treat cases of active tuberculosis among adults. Routine testing for TB with a tuberculin skin test is now only recommended in children who are at high risk for having the illness.

Government Agencies

7515 Centers for Disease Control and Prevention Division:
Tuberculosis Elimination
National Center For Prevention Services
1600 Clifton Road
Atlanta, GA 30329

404-639-8813
800-232-4636
TTY: 888-232-6348
cdcinfo@cdc.gov
www.cdc.gov/nchstp/tb/contact.html

Dr. Tom Frieden, Director
Ileana Arias, PhD, Principal Deputy Director
John M. Auerbach, MBA, Associate Director of Policy

7516 NIH/National Institute of Allergy and Infectious Diseases
5601 Fishers Lane, MSC 9806
Bethesda, MD 20892

301-496-5717
866-284-4107
Fax: 301-402-3573
TDD: 800-877-8339
ocposfoffice@niaid.nih.gov
www.niaid.nih.gov

Conducts and supports basic and applied research to better understand, treat, and ultimately prevent infectious, immunologic, and allergic diseases.

Anthony S Fauci MD, Director
Hugh Auchincloss, M.D., Principal Deputy Director
John J. McGowan, Ph.D., Deputy Director for Science Mngmnt

7517 New York City Department of Health Bureau of Tuberculosis Control
125 Worth Street
New York, NY 10013   212-346-7572
Pressoffice@health.nyc.gov
www.nyc.gov/html/doh/html/diseases/tb.shtml
Mary Travis Bassett, M.D., MPH, Commissioner
Desiree Kim, Executive Director

National Associations & Support Groups

7518 American Academy of Pediatrics
141 Northwest Point Boulevard
Elk Grove Village, IL 60007   847-434-4000
800-433-9016
Fax: 847-434-8000
www.aap.org

The American Academy of Pediatrics and its member pediatricians are committed to the attainment of optimal physical, mental and social health and well-being for all infants, children, adolescents, and young adults.

Fernando Stein, MD, FAAP, President
Karen Remley, MD, CEO/Executive VP

7519 American Lung Association
55 W. Wacker Drive, Suite 1150
Chicago, IL 60601   312-801-7628
800-548-8252
info@lung.org
www.lung.org

The American Lung Association fights lung disease in all its forms, with special emphasis on asthma, tobacco control and environmental health. The American Lung Association is funded by contributions from the public, along with gifts and grants from corporations, foundations and government agencies. The association achieves its many successes through the work of thousands of committed volunteers and staff.

Harold P. Wimmer, National President & CEO
Susan Rappaport, National VP, Research/Scientific
Sue Swan, Chief Development Officer

7520 National Tuberculosis Center at New Jersey Medical School
University of Medicine and Dentistry of New Jersey
185 South Orange Avenue
Newark, NJ 7103   973-972-4300
Fax: 973-972-3268
douglawa@njms.rutgers.edu
www.umdnj.edu

The National Tuberculosis Center was established in 1993 in response to the resurgence of tuberculosis in the United States. The center operates under the direction of Lee B. Reichmann, MD, MPH. The center operates a toll-free information line to provide state-of-the-art information to health care professionals and the public. Senior medical staff and nurses are available to respond to calls Monday-Friday from 9am-5pm.

Robert L. Johnson, MD, FAAP, Dean
David Roe, Associate Dean/ CFO
Walter L. Douglas, Jr., Chief Operating Officer

7521 World Health Organization
Avenue Appia 20
CH-1211 Geneva 27,
Switzerland   www.who.int

WHO is the directing and coordinating authority for health within the United Nations system.

Dr Margaret Chan, Director General
Dr Anarfi Asamoa-Baah, Deputy Director-General
Bruce Aylward, Assistant Director-General

Research Centers

7522 Francis J. Curry National Tuberculosis Center
300 Frank H. Ogawa Plaza, Suite 520
Oakland, CA 94612   510-238-5100
877-390-6682
Fax: 415-861-7888
CurryTBcenter@ucsf.edu
www.currytbcenter.ucsf.edu

The Curry International Tuberculosis Center (CITC) creates, enhances and disseminates state-of-the-art resources and models of excellence and performs research to control and eliminate tuberculosis in the United States and internationally.

Francis Ho, President
Lisa Chen, MD, Medical Director, Principal Investi
James Sederberg, Deputy Director

7523 University of Illinois at Chicago Institute for Tuberculosis Research
904 W Adams Street
Chicago, IL 60607   202-318-2476
Michael J Groves, PhD, Director

Web Sites

7524 American Lung Association
55 W. Wacker Drive, Suite 1150
Chicago, IL 60601   312-801-7628
800-548-8252
info@lung.org
www.lung.org

Information regarding lung disease in all its forms, with special emphasis on asthma, tobacco control and environmental health.

Harold P. Wimmer, National President & CEO
Susan Rappaport, National VP, Research/Scientific
Sue Swan, Chief Development Officer

7525 Centers for Disease Control
1600 Clifton Road
Atlanta, GA 30329   800-232-4636
TTY: 888-232-6348
www.cdc.gov

Mission is to promote health and the quality of life by preventing and controlling disease, injury, and disability.

Dr. Tom Frieden, Director
Ileana Arias, PhD, Principal Deputy Director
John M. Auerbach, MBA, Associate Director of Policy

7526 Columbia University
630 West 168th St.
New York, NY 10032   212-305-CUMC
www.cpmc.columbia.edu

Provides what you need to know about tuberculosis, and what kind of treatment to prevent tuberculosis.

Joanne M. J. Quan, SVP/ CFO
Mark McDougle, MPH, SVP/ COO
Amelia J. Alverson, SVP, Development

7527 Health Answers
410 Horsham Road
Horsham, PA 19044   215-442-9010
Michael.tague@healthanswers.com
www.healthanswers.com

HealthAnswers offers a breadth of services in medical education, sales force training, patient support solutions, professional promotion and consumer solutions.

Michael Tague, Managing Director

7528 National Tuberculosis Center
www.nationaltbcenter.edu/

Creates, enhances and disseminiates state of the art resources and models of excellence to control and eliminate tuberculosis nationally and internationally. We are committed to the belief that everyone deserves the highest quality of care in a manner consistent with his or her culture, values and language. We develop and deliver highly versatile, culturally appropriate trainings and educational products, provide technical assistance and facilitate regional, state and national initiatives.

Book Publishers

7529 Forgotten Plague: How the Battle Against Tuberculosis Was Won & Lost
Hachette Book Group USA
1271 Avenue Of The Americas
New York, NY 10020   617-227-0730
                    Fax: 617-227-4633
              www.hachettebookgroupusa.com

1994 Paperback
ISBN: 0-316763-81-0

Alison Lindsay, Director Of Marketing

7530 Know About Tuberculosis
Walker & Company
1385 Broadway, 5 Floor
New York, NY 10018   212-419-5300
                    Fax: 212-727-0984
              marketingusa@bloomsbury.com
                   www.bloomsbury.com/us

1994 hardcover
ISBN: 0-802783-38-4

Jeremy Wilson, Chairman
Nigel Newton, Executive Director
Wendy Pallot, Executive Director

7531 Lung Disorders Sourcebook
Omnigraphics
PO Box 8002
Aston, PA 19014   800-234-1340
                    Fax: 800-875-1340
                 info@omnigraphics.com
                    omnigraphics.com

Basic consumer health information on lung disorders including tuberculosis, asthma and cystic fibrosis.

678 pages
ISBN: 0-780803-39-6

Peter Ruffner, Publisher

Pamphlets

7532 Classification of Tuberculosis and Other Mycrobacterial Diseases
American Lung Association
1740 Broadway
New York, NY 10019   212-315-8700

Chart listing different classes of tuberculosis and other mycrobacterial diseases.

7533 Facts About Tuberculosis
American Lung Association
1740 Broadway
New York, NY 10019   212-315-8700

Primary public information leaflet on TB as well as on its impact and treatment.
8 pages

7534 Global Epidemic Multi-Drug Resistant Tuberculosis
American Lung Association
55 W. Wacker Drive, Suite 1150
Chicago, IL 60601   312-801-7630
                         800-548-8252
                    Fax: 202-452-1805
                      www.lungusa.org

Kathryn A. Forbes, CPA, Chair
John F. Emanuel, JD, Vice Chair
Harold Wimmer, President/ CEO

7535 TB Skin Test
American Lung Association
1740 Broadway
New York, NY 10019   212-315-8700

Primary public information leaflet on the TB skin test.
8 pages

7536 TB: What You Should Know
American Lung Association
55 W. Wacker Drive, Suite 1150
Chicago, IL 60601   312-801-7630
                         800-548-8252
                    Fax: 202-452-1805
                      www.lungusa.org

Offers a brief overview of tuberculosis, how transmission is possible, and TB skin testing.

Kathryn A. Forbes, CPA, Chair
John F. Emanuel, JD, Vice Chair
Harold Wimmer, President/ CEO

7537 This Is Mr. TB Germ
American Lung Association
1740 Broadway
New York, NY 10019   212-315-8700

Lively booklet of drawings and very brief text giving a basic description of TB and its treatments.
20 pages

DESCRIPTION

7538 TUBEROUS SCLEROSIS

Synonyms: Epiloia, TS

Involves the following Biologic System(s):

Dermatologic Disorders, Neurologic Disorders

Tuberous sclerosis (TS) is a hereditary multisystem disorder that is one of a group of diseases described as neuro-cutaneous syndromes, because of large involvement of both the skin and the central nervous system (brain and/or spinal cord). It is characterized by multiple, wart-like, raised areas (papules) on the skin of the face (adenoma sebaceum); benign, tumor-like nodules (hamartomas) of the brain, the heart, the kidneys, the nerve-rich membrane at the back of the eyes (retinas), or other organs; episodes of abnormally increased, uncontrolled electrical activity in the brain (seizures); and mental retardation. Associated symptoms and findings may vary greatly from patient to patient, including among members of the same family. TS is caused by abnormal changes (mutations) in a gene or genes. These mutations may occur randomly for unknown reasons (sporadically) or may be inherited as an autosomal dominant trait. At least two genes have been identified that may cause TS. One disease gene, known as TSC1 gene, is located on the long arm (q) of chromosome 9 (9q34). A second gene, called the TSC2 gene, is on the short arm (p) of chromosome 16 (16p13.3). Tuberous sclerosis affects approximately one in 30,000 individuals.

TS is often apparent shortly after birth and presents as distinctive skin abnormalities and the development of either infantile spasms (hypsarrhythmia) or partial seizures characterized by sudden, repeated flexion or extension of the muscles of the neck, torso, arms, and legs. Seizures may later take the form of myoclonic epilepsy, in which there are sudden, shock-like contractions of a muscle or muscle groups. As many as 90 percent of infants with TS also have sharply defined areas of abnormally diminished skin coloration (hypopigmentation) on the torso, face, arms, or legs. These areas typically have an ashleaf-like appearance.

Seizures that begin during later childhood are often characterized by prolonged muscle contractions and alternating relaxation and contraction of muscles (generalized tonic-clonic seizures). Seizures tend to become progressively more severe and are often difficult to treat. In addition, approximately 60 to 70 percent of children with TS experience mental retardation, almost all of whom also have seizure disorders. However, seizures also occur in most of those without mental retardation. Generally, the younger a patient experiences symptoms associated with TS, the greater the risk for mental retardation.

Beginning at about age two to six, about 80 percent of children with TS also develop red, shiny nodules (lesions) over the cheeks and nose. These nodules gradually become larger and assume a wart-like, fleshy appearance (adenoma sebaceum). Similar nodules may also develop on the forehead. Many children have additional, distinctive skin lesions. These may include raised, knobby, skin-colored lesions with an orange-peel consistency (shagreen patches) primarily located onthe lower back; firm, skin-colored nodules that develop around the nails of the fingers and toes during puberty, and rarely, coffee-colored discolorations of the skin (cafe-au-lait spots).

In patients with TS, the characteristic tumor-like nodules that develop in the brain are known as tubers. These growths often become hardened due to an abnormal accumulation of calcium salts (calcification). In addition, depending upon their size and location, tubers may block the normal flow of cerebrospinal fluid (CSF), causing an abnormal accumulation of CSF in the brain (hydrocephalus). The severity of neurologic impairment typically increases with the number of tubers within the brain. Rarely, a tuber may differentiate into a malignant brain tumor (astrocytoma).

Approximately 50 percent of affected children also have benign tumors of the heart muscle (rhabdomyoma). Although rhabdomyomas may disrupt the normal rhythm or rate of the heartbeat (arrythmias), these tumors tend to gradually resolve on their own. Benign, tumor-like nodules or multiple cysts may also develop in the kidneys, causing blood in the urine (hematuria), pain, or, in severe cases, kidney failure. Hamartomas may also develop in other tissues and organs of the body, such as the retinas and the lungs. In patients with severe TS, life-threatening complications may occur by adulthood.

The management of patients with TS is symptomatic and supportive, including therapy with anticonvulsant medications to help control seizures. In addition, physicians may regularly monitor patients to detect certain serious conditions potentially associated with TS, such as abnormal accumulations of cerebrospinal fluid or malignant transformation of hamartomas in the brain. If such conditions are confirmed, immediate surgical intervention or other measures are performed as required. Medications are required for controlling seizures, which is often difficult. The need for special schooling or care is determined by the severity of mental retardation.

National Associations & Support Groups

7539 American Academy of Pediatrics

141 Northwest Point Boulevard

Elk Grove Village, IL 60007

847-434-4000
800-433-9016
Fax: 847-434-8000
www.aap.org

The American Academy of Pediatrics and its member pediatricians are committed to the attainment of optimal physical, mental and social health and well-being for all infants, children, adolescents, and young adults.

Fernando Stein, MD, FAAP, President
Karen Remley, MD, CEO/Executive VP

7540 Epilepsy Foundation

8301 Professional Place East, Suite 200

Landover, MD 20785

866-330-2718
800-332-1000
Fax: 301-459-1569
ContactUs@efa.org
www.epilepsyfoundation.org

An organization works to ensure that people with seizures are able to participate in all life experiences; and to prevent, control and cure epilepsy through research, education, advocacy and services.

Warren Lammert, Chair
Phil Gattone, President/ CEO
Roger Heldman, Treasurer

7541 Family Support Network
Tuberous Sclerosis Alliance
110 N. Elm Ave.
Saint Louis, MO 63119

314-961-5718
800-255-6872
Fax: 314-644-5057
info@familysupport.org
www.familysupportnet.org/

The Support Network is an organized partnership of individuals whose lives have been affected by Tuberous Sclerosis. Across the nation, the Support Network is providing the latest medical information, education and support to those individuals who are seeking understanding about the genetic disease and offering them words of encouragement and empowerment.

Kevin Drollinger, CEO
Rebecca Cornatzer, Chief Administrative Officer
Shannon Grass, Chief Development Officer

7542 Genetic Alliance
4301 Connecticut Avenue NW, Suite 404
Washington, DC 20008

202-966-5557
800-336-4363
Fax: 202-966-8553
info@geneticalliance.org
www.geneticalliance.org

A coalition of voluntary genetic support groups, consumers and professionals addressing the needs of individuals and families affected by genetic disorders from a national perspective.

Sharon Terry, President/CEO
Tetyana Murza, Managing Director
Natasha Bonhomme, VP, Strategic Development

7543 National Tuberous Sclerosis Association
801 Roeder Road, Suite 750
Silver Spring, MD 20910

301-562-9890
800-225-6872
Fax: 301-562-9870
info@tsalliance.org
www.ntsa.org

Nonprofit organization.

Carolyn Wilson, Contact

7544 Tuberous Sclerosis Alliance
801 Roeder Road, Suite 750
Silver Spring, MD 20910

301-562-9890
800-225-6872
Fax: 301-562-9870
info@tsalliance.org
www.tsalliance.org

The Tuberous Sclerosis Alliance is dedicated to finding a cure for Tuberous Sclerosis complex while improving the lives of those affected. TSC is a genetic disease causing tumors to grow throughout the body and is the leading cause of epilepsy and autism.

Kari Luther Rosbeck, President/ CEO
Mary Jane Perraut, Chief Financial Officer
Steven L. Roberds, PhD, Chief Scientific Officer

Web Sites

7545 Health Answers
410 Horsham Road
Horsham, PA 19044

215-442-9010
Michael.tague@healthanswers.com
www.healthanswers.com

HealthAnswers offers a breadth of services in medical education, sales force training, patient support solutions, professional promotion and ocnsumer solutions.

Michael Tague, Managing Director

7546 Online Mendelian Inheritance in Man
www.omim.org

This database is a catalog of human genes and genetic disorders.

7547 TS International
www.stsn.nl/tsi/tsi.htm

Goals and objectives are to increase the knowledge of TS throughout the world, to stimulate, co-ordinate and originate research on TS, to interest statutory international organizations in the welfare of TS sufferers, to support national TS associations in the work, to initiate the realistation of new TS associatons, to exchange information of mutual interest between TS associations.

Book Publishers

7548 Early Years Guide of the Life Stage Program
Tuberous Sclerosis Alliance
801 Roeder Road, Suite 750
Silver Spring, MD 20910

301-562-9890
800-225-6872
Fax: 301-562-9870
info@tsalliance.org
www.tsalliance.org

A resource guide for families of infants and young children with tuberous sclerosis.

Kari Luther Carlson, CEO

7549 School-Aged Guide of the Life Stages Program
Tuberous Sclerosis Alliance
801 Roeder Road, Suite 750
Silver Spring, MD 20910

301-562-9890
800-225-6872
Fax: 301-562-9870
info@tsalliance.org
www.tsalliance.org

A resource guide for parents of school-aged children with Tuberous Sclerosis.

Kari Luther Carlson, CEOsident/CEO
Becky Bull, VP Development/Communications
Kari Luther Carson, VP Community Outreach

7550 Tuberous Sclerosis: 3rd Edition
Oxford University Press
2001 Evans Road
Cary, NC 27513

Fax: 919-677-1303
www.oup-usa.org

A revision offering up-to-date medical information to families, researchers, and professionals on TS.
ISBN: 0-195122-10-0

Newsletters

7551 Perspective
National Tuberous Sclerosis Association
801 Roeder Road, Suite 750
Silver Spring, MD 20910

301-562-9890
800-225-6872
Fax: 301-562-9870
info@tsalliance.org
www.ntsa.org

Offers the latest research and medical information on tuberous sclerosis to physicians and health care professionals.
Bimonthly

Holly Knorr, Managing Editor

Pamphlets

7552 Living with Tuberous Sclerosis
National Tuberous Sclerosis Association
801 Roeder Road, Suite 750
Silver Spring, MD 20910

301-562-9890
800-225-6872
Fax: 301-562-9870
info@tsalliance.org
www.ntsa.org

True stories of people living with Tuberous Sclerosis.

Softcover

7553 Tuberous Sclerosis: Fact Sheet
National Inst. of Neurological Disorders/Stroke
P.O. Box 5801
Bethesda, MD 20824
                                                      301-496-5751
                                                      800-352-9424
                                            www.ninds.nih.gov

Walter J. Koroshetz, M.D., Acting Director
Alan L. Willard, Ph.D., Acting Deputy Director
Caroline Lewis, Executive Officer

DESCRIPTION

7554 TURNER SYNDROME

Synonyms: Chromosome 45,X syndrome, XO syndrome

Involves the following Biologic System(s):
Genetic/Chromosomal/Syndrome/Metabolic Disorders

Turner syndrome is a chromosomal disorder that affects only females. In most cases, females have two X chromosomes and males have one X and one Y chromosome in cells of the body. However, in females with Turner syndrome, one of the X chromosomes is deleted (missing) from cells or is functionally defective; some cells have the normal pair of X chromosomes whereas others do not (mosaicism). Although associated symptoms and findings may be variable, the most consistent abnormalities associated with the disorder include short stature and defective development of the ovaries (gonadal dysgenesis).

Many newborns with Turner syndrome have an abnormal accumulation of fluid in and associated swelling of the backs of the hands and the tops of the feet (peripheral lymphedema). Additional features that may be apparent at birth include an abnormally short, webbed neck (pterygium colli) with a low hairline; a narrow roof of the mouth (palate) or a small jaw (micrognathia); abnormal outward deviation of the elbows upon extension (cubitus valgus); a broad chest with widely spaced, underdeveloped, and/or inverted nipples; or deeply set, narrow, and/or outwardly curved (convex) nails. In most cases, females with Turner syndrome also have kidney (renal) malformations (e.g., horseshoe kidney and/or cleft or double renal pelvis). In addition, in some cases, heart (cardiac) defects may be present, such as abnormalities affecting the major artery (aorta) that arises from the lower left chamber (ventricle) of the heart (e.g., bicuspid aortic valve, coarctation of the aorta). In almost all affected females, there is also defective development of the ovaries (ovarian dysgenesis), i.e., the paired glands within which the female reproductive cells are produced (ova or eggs) and from which certain female hormones are secreted. Consequently, in most cases, female secondary sexual characteristics fail to develop (e.g., breast development, appearance of hair in the pubic area and under the arms, menstruation) and most affected females are infertile. In addition, although intelligence is typically normal, some females with Turner syndrome may experience learning disabilities (e.g., difficulty with visual-spatial relationships) and may have poor coordination. The treatment of children with Turner syndrome may include hormone replacement therapy (e.g., estrogen therapy, human growth hormone therapy); surgical intervention for congenital heart defects, renal malformations, webbing of the neck, or other abnormalities; special education for those with learning disabilities; and other treatment measures as required. Turner syndrome is thought to result from errors during the division of a parent's reproductive cells (meiosis). According to estimates in the medical literature, the disorder may affect from approximately one in 2,000 to one in 4,000 female newborns.

Government Agencies

7555 NIH/ Eunice Kennedy Shriver National Insti tute of Child Health & Human Development
31 Center Drive, Building 31
Bethesda, MD 20892

301-496-5113
800-370-2943
Fax: 866-760-5947
TTY: 888-320-6942
nichdpress@mail.nih.gov
www.nichd.nih.gov

Established in 1962 by congress, today the institute conducts and supports research on topics related to the health of children, adults, families and populations. Some of these topics include: developmental disabilities, growth and development, infant death, reproductive health and birth defects.

Diana W. Bianchi, Director
Paul Williams, Director, Communications

National Associations & Support Groups

7556 American Academy of Pediatrics
141 Northwest Point Boulevard
Elk Grove Village, IL 60007

847-434-4000
800-433-9016
Fax: 847-434-8000
www.aap.org

The American Academy of Pediatrics and its member pediatricians are committed to the attainment of optimal physical, mental and social health and well-being for all infants, children, adolescents, and young adults.

Fernando Stein, MD, FAAP, President
Karen Remley, MD, CEO/Executive VP

7557 American Society for Reproductive Medicine
1209 Montgomery Highway
Birmingham, AL 35216

205-978-5000
Fax: 205-978-5005
asrm@asrm.org
www.asrm.org

The American Society for Reproductive Medicine is an organization devoted to advancing knowledge and expertise in infertility, reproductive medicine and biology. The ASRM is a voluntary nonprofit organization.

Rebecca Sokol, M.D., M.P.H., President
Richard Paulson, M.D., Vice President
Richard H. Reindollar, M.D., Executive Director

7558 Genetic Alliance
4301 Connecticut Avenue NW, Suite 404
Washington, DC 20008

202-966-5557
800-336-4363
Fax: 202-966-8553
info@geneticalliance.org
www.geneticalliance.org

A coalition of voluntary genetic support groups, consumers and professionals addressing the needs of individuals and families affected by genetic disorders from a national perspective.

Sharon Terry, President/CEO
Tetyana Murza, Managing Director
Natasha Bonhomme, VP, Strategic Development

7559 Human Growth Foundation
997 Glen Cove Avenue, Suite 5
Glen Head, NY 11545

516-671-4041
800-451-6434
Fax: 516-671-4055
hgfl@hgfound.org
www.hgfound.org

A voluntary, nonprofit organization whose mission is to help children and adults with disorders of growth and growth hormones through research, education, support and advocacy. The foundation is dedicated to helping medical science to better understand the process of growth. It is composed of concerned parents and friends of children and adults with growth problems and interested health professionals.

Pisit Pitukcheewanon, MD, President
Emily Germain-Lee, Vice President
Patricia D Costa, Executive Director

7560 MAGIC Foundation: Major Aspects of Growth in Children: Turner's Syndrome Division
4200 Cantera Drive, #106
Warrenville, IL 60555   630-836-8200
                                               800-362-4423
                                          Fax: 630-836-8181
                        ContactUs@magicfoundation.org
                        www.magicfoundation.org

A national nonprofit organization providing support and education regarding growth disorders in children and related adult disorders. Provides educational information, networking, a national conference, a kids' program and an extensive medical library.

Dianne Kremidas, Executive Director
Mary Andrews, CEO
Teresa Tucker, Patient Advocacy

7561 Turner's Syndrome Society of the US
11250 West Road˜#G
Houston, TX 77065   832-912-6006
                                               800-365-9944
                                          Fax: 832-912-6446
                        tssus@turnersyndrome.org
                        www.turnersyndrome.org

More than 38 chapters across the country. Goals are to promote public awareness of the disease, support those affected by the condition and aid in continuing research. Membership dues for a single person are $40, a family, $60, and for professionals, $60.

2,500 members

Brenda Gruwell, President
Emily Havrilak, Secretary
Carol Crawford, Treasurer

State Agencies & Support Groups

Alaska

7562 Turner's Syndrome Society of Alaska
1334 N Street
Anchorage, AK 99501   907-279-3202
                        marytullius@hotmail.com
                        www.turnersyndrome.org
Mary Tullius

Arizona

7563 Turner's Syndrome Society of Arizona
2215 Wickenburg Road
Ponopah, AZ 85354   602-443-3805
                        www.turnersyndrome.org
Tracie Holley

California

7564 Turner's Syndrome Society Central And Northern
Bay Point, CA 94565   925-299-7729
                        rosie1038@attbi.com
                        www.turnersyndrome.org
Rosemary Morris

7565 Turner's Syndrome Society of Southern California
8902 Heil Avenue #24
Westminster, CA 92683   714-749-7313
                        colleencurby1@gmail.com
                        www.turnersyndrome.org
Colleen Curby, President

Colorado

7566 Turner's Syndrome Society of Rocky Mountain
4972 S Garland
Littleton, CO 80123   720-981-2632
                        www.turnersyndrome.org
Donna Landrum

Connecticut

7567 Turner's Syndrome Society of Connecticut
57 Cianci Drive
Southington, CT 06489   860-329-2990
                        dmj_lewis@sbcglobal.net
                        www.turnersyndrome.org
Jessica Fitzgibbon Lewis, Contact

Florida

7568 Turner's Syndrome Society - Tampa Support Group
3202 W Fair Oaks Avenue
Tampa, FL 33611   813-837-0582
                        heddyb@gateway.net
                        www.turnersyndrome.org
Heddy Brown

7569 Turner's Syndrome Society of Northern Florida
6447 Cooper Lane
Jacksonville, FL 32210   407-859-3131
                        elrcook3@bellsouth.net
                        www.turnersyndrome.org
Kim Brown
Randy Cook, Contact

7570 Turner's Syndrome Society of South Florida
235 NE 23rd Street #204
Ft. Lauderdale, FL 33305   407-859-3131
                        elrcook3@bellsouth.net
                        www.turnersyndrome.org
Rachel Nowak
Randy Cook, Contact

Iowa

7571 Turner's Syndrome Society of Iowa/New Found Friends
2615 Meadow Glen Road
Ames, IA 50014   515-321-6021
                        ashley.artzer@yahoo.com
                        www.turnersyndrome.org
Ashley Artzer, Contact

Kentucky

7572 Turner's Syndrome Society of Kentucky
380 Bob-O-Link Drive
Lexington, KY 40503   502-292-2742
                        timrhon@insightbb.com
                        www.turnersyndrome.org
Rhonda Curtis, Contact

Louisiana

7573 Turner's Syndrome Society of Gulf Coast
7731 Butterfield Road
New Orleans, LA 70126   334-476-7940
www.turnersyndrome.org

Donna Baudier

Maryland

7574 Turner's Syndrome Society of Maryland
2206 229th Street
Pasadena, MD 21122   410-360-5571
jmatts@erols.com
www.turnersyndrome.org

Kathy Mattson

Massachusetts

7575 Turner's Syndrome Society of New England
60 Joy Street, Apartment 303
Boston, MA 02114   617-557-4837
Fax: 617-636-6131
www.turnersyndrome.org

Geralyn Dwyer

Michigan

7576 Turner's Syndrome Society of Southeastern Michigan
7490 Drew Circle, Apartment 8
Westland, MI 48185   248-921-6298
hahoey@comcast.net
www.turnersyndrome.org

Heather Hoey, Contact

7577 Turner's Syndrome Society of West Michigan
1569 Sibley Street NW
Grand Rapids, MI 49504   517- 85- 959
maohler@att.net
www.turnersyndrome.org

Mary Ohler, Contact

Minnesota

7578 Turner's Syndrome Society of Minnesota
7109 Autumn Terrace
Eden Prairie, MN 55346   952-854-1224
jleon101@hotmail.com
www.tssminnesota.org

Julie Leon, Contact

Missouri

7579 Turner's Syndrome Society of St. Louis/ West Illinois
1514 Azalia Drive
Saint Louis, MO 63119   314-892-2635
www.turnersyndrome.org

Cheryl Jost

Nevada

7580 Turner's Syndrome Society of Nevada
1003 Mylert St
Jessup, PA 18434   702-731-3452
www.turnersyndrome.org

Joelle Barnes

New Hampshire

7581 Turner's Syndrome Society of Northern New England
1261 Old North Main Street
Laconia, NH 03246   603-528-3510
www.turnersyndrome.org

Lori Ann Pawlowski
Dawn And Matt Dragon

New Jersey

7582 Turner's Syndrome Society of New Jersey
238 Hempstead Drive
Somerset, NJ 08873   732-249-3727
www.turnersyndrome.org

Linda Kalb

New York

7583 Turner's Syndrome Society of Central New York
Apt 18
Owego, NY 13827   607-223-4124
tlkwwjd@gmail.com
www.turnersyndrome.org

Tammy Kozak, Contact

7584 Turner's Syndrome Society of Upstate New York
115 Union Avenue #205
Saratoga Springs, NY 12866   518-209-1793
saratogatif@aol.com
www.turnersyndrome.org

Tiffany Festo

North Carolina

7585 Turner's Syndrome Society of North Carolina
1223 Pine Springs Drive
Hendersonville, NC 28739   919-387-7974
denise.culin@gmail.com
www.turnersyndromenc.com

Denise Culin, Chapter President
Barbara Flink, Vice President
Megan Edwards, Secretary

Ohio

7586 Turner's Syndrome Society of Southwestern Ohio
8530 Gateview Court
Dayton, OH 45424   513-697-0941
lisa_lorigan@hotmail.com
www.swohioturnersyndrome.com

Lisa Lorigan, Chapter President

Oklahoma

7587 Turner's Syndrome Society of Oklahoma
5904 East Lattimer
Tulsa, OK 74115   405-271-6764
traci-schaeffer@ouhsu.edu
www.turnersyndrome.org

Traci Schaeffer, Contact

Pennsylvania

7588 Turner's Syndrome Society of Philadelphia
2322 Taggart Court
Wilmington, DE 19810   302-475-5780
jmkurze@aol.com
www.turnersyndrome.org

Joann Kurzeknabe

Rhode Island

7589 **Turner's Syndrome Society of Rhode Island**
24 Turner Street, Unit 3
Warwick, RI 02886
401-732-2136
deb_pomerantz@hotmail.com
www.turnersyndrome.org

South Carolina

7590 **Turner's Syndrome Society of South Carolina**
153 Gannet Point Road
Beaufort, SC 29907
843-522-8508
www.turnersyndrome.org

Robin Butler

Tennessee

7591 **Turner's Syndrome Society of Mid-South**
2541 Clydes Place Cove
Memphis, TN 38133
901-385-1720
hmschlmom3@yahoo.com
www.turnersyndrome.org

Penny Williams

7592 **Turner's Syndrome Society of Tennessee**
9202 Shady Bend Lane
Knoxville, TN 37922
423-539-2210
www.turnersyndrome.org

Kathy Blackbourne

Texas

7593 **Turner's Syndrome Society of Houston**
11602 Bexhil
Houston, TX 77065
832-689-3901
heatherandben@earthlink.net
www.turnersupport.org

Heather DeRousse, Contact

7594 **Turner's Syndrome Society of North Texas**
3211 W Division #28
Arlington, TX 76012
832-689-3901
smithar1@earthlink.org
www.turnersyndrome.org

Patricia Burton

7595 **Turner's Syndrome Society of San Antonio**
923 Escalon Avenue
San Antonio, TX 78221
210-647-8981
xpictinaki@hotmail.com
www.turnersyndrome.org

Christine Ashenfelter, Contact

Utah

7596 **Turner's Syndrome Society of Salt Lake City**
2337 Chateau Drive
Roy, UT 84067
801-825-4118
kristyne70@hotmail.com
www.turnersyndrome.org

Kristyne Rudolph

Virginia

7597 **Turner's Syndrome Society of National Capitol Area**
6200 Westchester Park Drive #406
College Park, MD 20740
301-345-3136
www.turnersyndrome.org

Deb Shoup

Washington

7598 **Turner's Syndrome Society of Inland Northwest**
5317 N Washington Street
Spokane, WA 99205
509-326-3703
www.turnersyndrome.org

Nancy Owen

Wisconsin

7599 **Turner's Syndrome Society of Southeastern Wisconsin**
10122 63rd Street
Kenosha, WI 53142
608-385-5910
thejohnsonact@earthlink.net
www.turnersyndrome.org

Melissa Caulum

Libraries & Resource Centers

7600 **Turner's Syndrome Society Resource Center**
Turner Syndrome Society of the United States
11250 West Road, Suite #G
Houston, TX 77065
832-912-6006
800-365-9944
Fax: 832-912-6446
tssus@turnersyndrome.org
www.turnersyndrome.org

Allows members to have access to the most recent articles being published in the area of Turner Syndrome, a listing of local chapters, physician referrals and booklets and videos offering guidance to families and physicians.

Brenda Gruwell, President
Cindy Scurlock, Executive Director
Emily Havrilak, Secretary

Web Sites

7601 **Endocrine Society**
2055 L Street NW, Suite 600
Washington, DC 20036
202-971-3636
888-363-6762
Fax: 202-736-9705
societyservices@endocrine.org
www.endocrine.org

Is the worlds largest and most active professional organization of endocrinologists in the world. The society is internationally known as the leading source of state of the art research and clinical advancements in endocrinology and metabolism. The society is dedicated to promoting excellence in research, education and clinical practice in the field of endocrinology.

Richard J. Santen, MD, President
Carol A. Lange, PhD, Vice President
Susan J. Mandel, MD, MPH, Vice President

7602 **Health Answers**
410 Horsham Road
Horsham, PA 19044
215-442-9010
Michael.tague@healthanswers.com
www.healthanswers.com

HealthAnswers offers a breadth of services in medical education, sales force training, patient support solutions, professional promotion and consumer solutions.

Michael Tague, Managing Director

7603 **Human Growth Foundation**
997 Glen Cove Avenue, Suite 5
Glen Head, NY 11545
800-451-6434
Fax: 516-671-4055
hgf1@hgfound.org
www.hgfound.org

A voluntary nonprofit organization whose mission is to help chidren, and adults with disorders of growth and growth hormones through research, education, support and advocacy.

Pisit Pitukcheewanont, MD, President
Emily Germain-Lee, MD, Vice President
Patricia D Costa, Executive Director

**7604 MAGIC Foundation: Major Aspects of Growth in Children:
Turner's Syndrome Division**
4200 Cantera Drive, #106
Warrenville, IL 60555   630-836-8200
                                               800-362-4423
                                          Fax: 630-836-8181
                            ContactUs@magicfoundation.org
                                    www.magicfoundation.org

Is a national nonprofit organization created to provide support
services for the families of children afflicted with a wide variety
of chronic and or critical disorders, syndromes and diseases that
affected a child's growth.

Dianne Kremidas, Executive Director
Mary Andrews, CEO
Teresa Tucker, Patient Advocacy

7605 Online Mendelian Inheritance in Man
www.omim.org

This database is a catalog of human genes and genetic disorders.

7606 Turner's Syndrome Society of the United States
11250 West Road, Suite G
Houston, TX 77065   832-912-6006
                                               800-365-9944
                                          Fax: 832-912-6446
                                    www.turnersyndrome.org

A nonprofit organization that provides assistance, support, and
education to girls and women with turner syndrome, their families, physicians, and the interested public.

Trudy McCarthy, President
Cindy Scurlock, Executive Director
Shawn Wier, Conference Coordinator

Newsletters

7607 Turner's Syndrome News
Turner's Syndrome Society of the United States
11250 West Road, Suite G
Houston, TX 77065   832-912-6006
                                               800-365-9944
                                          Fax: 832-912-6446
                                    www.turnersyndrome.org

Includes articles addressing current issues in turner syndrome,
updates on national and local activities and letters from girls and
women with Turner's syndrome and their families.

Quarterly

Trudy McCarthy, President
Cindy Scurlock, Executive Director
Shawn Wier, Conference Coordinator

Pamphlets

7608 Answers to Some Commonly Asked Questions
Turner Syndrome Society of the United States
11250 West Road, Suite G
Houston, TX 77065   832-912-6006
                                               800-365-9944
                                          Fax: 832-912-6446
                                    www.turnersyndrome.org

Offers information on the Society's activities and the role they
play in supporting people with Turner Syndrome.

Trudy McCarthy, President
Cindy Scurlock, Executive Director
Shawn Wier, Conference Coordinator

7609 Facing the Challenges of Turner Syndrome Together
Turner Syndrome Society of the United States
11250 West Road, Suite G
Houston, TX 77065   832-912-6006
                                               800-365-9944
                                          Fax: 832-912-6446
                                    www.turnersyndrome.org

Brochure offering information on Turner's syndrome, statistics
on how widespread the disease is and the Society's role in conquering this disease and supporting its members.

Trudy McCarthy, President
Cindy Scurlock, Executive Director
Shawn Wier, Conference Coordinator

7610 Facts About Turner Syndrome
Turner Syndrome Society of the United States
11250 West Road, Suite G
Houston, TX 77065   832-912-6006
                                               800-365-9944
                                          Fax: 832-912-6446
                                    www.turnersyndrome.org

Offers statistical and factual information on the disease of Turner
Syndrome, causes, symptoms, prevention and treatment.

Trudy McCarthy, President
Cindy Scurlock, Executive Director
Shawn Wier, Conference Coordinator

7611 How to Start a Turner Syndrome Support Group
Turner Syndrome Society of the United States
11250 West Road, Suite G
Houston, TX 77065   832-912-6006
                                               800-365-9944
                                          Fax: 832-912-6446
                                    www.turnersyndrome.org

Offers information to the lay person on how to obtain material
from medical professionals, and publicity aspects and funding aspects in pertaining to starting a support group.

Trudy McCarthy, President
Cindy Scurlock, Executive Director
Shawn Wier, Conference Coordinator

7612 Turner's Syndrome
Human Growth Foundation
11250 West Road, Suite G
Houston, TX 77065   832-912-6006
                                               800-365-9944
                                          Fax: 832-912-6446
                                    www.turnersyndrome.org

Background of a tremendous need for further information about
Turner's Syndrome.

Trudy McCarthy, President
Cindy Scurlock, Executive Director
Shawn Wier, Conference Coordinator

7613 Turner's Syndrome Society Resource Bibliographies
Turner's Syndrome Society of the United States
11250 West Road, Suite G
Houston, TX 77065   832-912-6006
                                               800-365-9944
                                          Fax: 832-912-6446
                                    www.turnersyndrome.org

These fact sheets offer information on books, videos and other resources available on Turner Syndrome.

Trudy McCarthy, President
Cindy Scurlock, Executive Director
Shawn Wier, Conference Coordinator

7614 Turner's Syndrome: A Personal Perspective
Turner's Syndrome Society of the United States
11250 West Road, Suite G
Houston, TX 77065   832-912-6006
                                               800-365-9944
                                          Fax: 832-912-6446
                                    www.turnersyndrome.org

A reprint from the Adolescent and Pediatric Gynecology Journal
offering a personal account of a woman with Turner Syndrome
and her experiences.

Trudy McCarthy, President
Cindy Scurlock, Executive Director
Shawn Wier, Conference Coordinator

7615 Turner's Syndrome: Guide for Families
Turner's Syndrome Society of the United States
11250 West Road, Suite G
Houston, TX 77065   832-912-6006
                                            800-365-9944
                                            Fax: 832-912-6446
                                            www.turnersyndrome.org

Offers information to parents on the causes, symptoms, diagnosis
and prognosis of Turner's syndrome, includes resources of where
to go for help and support.

Trudy McCarthy, President
Cindy Scurlock, Executive Director
Shawn Wier, Conference Coordinator

**7616 Turner's Syndrome: The Hows and Whys of the Missing X
Chromosome**
Human Growth Foundation
11250 West Road, Suite G
Houston, TX 77065   832-912-6006
                                            800-365-9944
                                            Fax: 832-912-6446
                                            www.turnersyndrome.org

Women with Turner's Syndrome lack one of the X chromosomes.
This carries genes for conditions relating to the development of
ovaries, sex hormone production, and physical development in
general.

Trudy McCarthy, President
Cindy Scurlock, Executive Director
Shawn Wier, Conference Coordinator

DESCRIPTION

7617 ULCERATIVE COLITIS

Involves the following Biologic System(s):

Gastrointestinal Disorders

Ulcerative colitis is an inflammatory bowel disease (IBD) characterized by chronic inflammation and ulceration of the lining of the colon, the major part of the large intestine. The disease initially affects the lowest region of the large intestine (rectum) and gradually progresses to involve varying lengths or all of the colon. The range and severity of associated symptoms is extremely variable and may depend in part on the amount of the colon that is affected. Ulcerative colitis usually becomes apparent during adolescence or young adulthood. However, in some patients, associated symptoms may occur as early as the first year of life. The frequency of the disorder varies greatly in different countries and is thought to be higher in urban areas. In the United States and northern Europe, ulcerative colitis affects approximately 100 to 200 per 100,000 individuals in the general population. In developed countries, inflammatory bowel disease, including ulcerative colitis, is the most common cause of chronic intestinal inflammation during mid-childhood. The exact cause of ulcerative colitis is unknown. However genetic, immune, and environmental factors are thought to be contributing factors.

In patients with ulcerative colitis, the onset of symptoms may be gradual (insidious) or sudden, rapid, and severe (fulminant). Most patients experience episodes of watery diarrhea with varying amounts of blood, mucus, or pus. Associated findings may include abdominal cramping and pain; persistant, inability or difficulty emptying the bowel at defecation (tenesmus); and an urgent, compelling urge to defecate. Fulminant colitis is characterized by over six daily bowel movements, a high fever, chills, abnormally low levels of iron or the protein albumin in the blood, an increase in certain circulating white blood cells (leukocytosis), and other findings. In some children, additional findings include failure to grow and gain weight at the expected rate and lack of appetite (anorexia). The frequency of episodes may vary greatly. Most patients experience periods of remission during which symptoms subside and eventual, periodic recurrences (exacerbations). However, some patients may have infrequent episodes and others may experience severe, ongoing symptoms.

Certain complications may occur in association with ulcerative colitis. For example, because of blood loss during episodes, there may be inadequate levels of iron and abnormally reduced levels of the oxygen-carrying protein of the blood (iron-deficiency anemia). Some individuals with ulcerative colitis may develop sudden massive enlargement of the colon (toxic megacolon). Without prompt, appropriate treatment, toxic megacolon may result in tearing or perforation of the colon, potentially causing life-threatening complications. In addition, patients who have ulcerative colitis for more than 10 years have an increased risk of colon cancer. Regular examination of the colon (colonoscopies) and biopsies are recommended beginning at eight to 10 years after disease onset to help ensure prompt detection and treatment. During a colonoscopy, tissue inside the colon is examined using a flexible viewing instrument. To obtain a biopsy, small samples of tissue are removed from the colon for examination under a microscope.

Many patients with ulcerative colitis may also eventually experience more generalized, systemic symptoms. By the third decade of life, some patients may develop ankylosing spondylitis (AS), a chronic, progressive, inflammatory disease that affects joints of the spine and results in pain, stiffness, and possible loss of spinal mobility. In patients with ulcerative colitis, AS most commonly affects joints of the back and the hips and may cause lower back pain and stiffness, particularly in the morning. Some patients with ulcerative colitis may also develop a chronic skin condition characterized by irregular, bluish-red skin sores (pyoderma gangrenosum); chronic inflammation of the liver (chronic active hepatitis); and inflammation of the bile ducts (primary sclerosing cholangitis).

Since ulcerative colitis cannot be cured, the goals of treatment with medication are to induce remissions, maintain remissions, minimize side effects of treatment, and improve the quality of life. In patients with mild colitis, treatment often includes administration of anti-inflammatory drugs, such as sulfasalazine, which may alleviate symptoms and potentially prevent recurrences. Patients with moderate to severe colitis who do not respond to such treatment may receive corticosteroid therapy, such as with the drug prednisone or immunomodulators that suppress the body's immune system, thus reducing inflammation. If affected individuals have fulminant colitis or colitis that is unresponsive to drug therapy, treatment may include surgical removal of the colon (colectomy). Additional treatment is symptomatic and supportive. An interesting new treatment uses nicotine. It has long been observed that the risk of ulcerative colitis appears to be higher in nonsmokers and in ex-smokers. In certain circumstances, patients improve when treated with nicotine where other medications have not been effective.

Government Agencies

7618 NIH/National Institute of Diabetes and Dig estive and Kidney Diseases
9000 Rockville Pike
9000 Rockville Pike
Bethesda, MD 20892

301-496-4000
TTY: 301-402-9612
niddkinquiries@nih.gov
www.niddk.nih.gov

Offers information and referrals to persons afflicted with ulcerative colitis.

Griffin P. Rodgers, MD, Director

National Associations & Support Groups

7619 American Academy of Pediatrics
141 Northwest Point Boulevard
Elk Grove Village, IL 60007

847-434-4000
800-433-9016
Fax: 847-434-8000
www.aap.org

The American Academy of Pediatrics and its member pediatricians are committed to the attainment of optimal physical, mental and social health and well-being for all infants, children, adolescents, and young adults.

Fernando Stein, MD, FAAP, President
Karen Remley, MD, CEO/Executive VP

7620 Crohn's & Colitis Foundation of America
386 Park Avenue South, 17th Floor
New York, NY 10016
212-685-8707
800-932-2423
Fax: 212-779-4098
info@ccfa.org
www.ccfa.org

Supports basic and clinical research into a cure and prevention for Crohn's disease and ulcerative colitis; conducts professional and patient education activities; produces public service programs and a wide variety of literature about inflammatory bowel disease for patients and their families, professionals and the public; and sponsors chapters nationwide.

Maura Breen, Chairman
Vance Gibbs, General Counsel
Paul Salerno, Treasurer

7621 Digestive Disease National Coalition
507 Capitol Court NE, Suite 200
Washington, DC 20002
202-544-7497
Fax: 202-546-7105
hpayne@hmcw.org
www.ddnc.org

Advocacy organization comprised of over 30 voluntary and professional societies concerned with the many diseases of the digestive tract and liver.

Lynn Seim, Chairperson
Ralph McKibbin, President
Cathy Griffith, Vice Chairperson

7622 Genetic Alliance
4301 Connecticut Avenue NW, Suite 404
Washington, DC 20008
202-966-5557
800-336-4363
Fax: 202-966-8553
info@geneticalliance.org
www.geneticalliance.org

A coalition of voluntary genetic support groups, consumers and professionals addressing the needs of individuals and families affected by genetic disorders from a national perspective.

Sharon Terry, President/CEO
Tetyana Murza, Managing Director
Natasha Bonhomme, VP, Strategic Development

7623 International Foundation for Functional Gastrointestinal Disorders
PO Box 170864
Milwaukee, WI 53217
414-964-1799
Fax: 414-964-7176
iffgd@iffgd.org
www.iffgd.org

Nonprofit education and research organization founded in 1991. IFFGD addresses the issues surrounding life with gastrointestinal (GI) functional and mobility disorders and increases the awareness about these disorders among the general public, researchers and the clinical care community.

Nancy J. Norton, President & Director
William Norton, Co-Founder
Eleanor Cautley, Vice Presidents and Directors

7624 Intestinal Disease Foundation
1323 Forbes avenue Suite 200
Pittsburgh, PA 15219
416-261-5888
877-587-9606
Fax: 412-471-2722
info@intestinalfoundation.org
www.intestinalfoundation.org

Nonprofit organization whose mission is to improve the quality of life of adults and children affected by chronic digestive illness through information, guidance and support. IDF offers a quarterly newsletter, Intestinal Fortitude, educational seminars, volunteer phone network, and Pittsburgh area support groups.

Linda Schurr, Executive Director

7625 Pediatric Crohn's & Colitis Association
PO Box 188
Newton, MA 02468
617-489-5854
questions@pcca.hypermart.net
www.pcca.hypermart.net

Focuses on all aspects of pediatric and adolescent Crohn's disease and ulcerative colitis, including medical, nutritional, psychological and social factors. Activities include information sharing, educational forums, newsletters and hospital outreach programs, as well as support of research.

7626 United Ostomy Association Hotline
PO Box 512
Northfield, MN 55057
949-660-8624
800-826-0826
Fax: 949-660-9262
info@ostomy.org
www.ostomy.org

An advocate for ostomy and alternative procedure patients answering questions from employment issues to insurability practices. Also publishes magazines, patient care guides, conducts conferences and youth rally summer camps. We sponsor networks and resources for children, teens young adults, and parents.

Ken Aukett, Chairman
Dave Illinois, President
Susan Burns, Vice President

Libraries & Resource Centers

7627 National Digestive Diseases Information Clearinghouse
9000 Rockville Pike
Bethesda, MD 20892
301-496-3583
800-860-8747
Fax: 301-907-8906
healthinfo@niddk.nih.gov
www.niddk.nih.govv

The National Institute of Diabetes and Digestive and Kidney Diseases conducts and supports research on many of the most serious diseases affecting public health. The Institute supports much of the clinical research on the diseases of internal medicine and related subspecialty fields as well as many basic science disciplines.

Dr. Griffin P. Rodgers, Director
Dr. Gregory G. Germino, Deputy Directortary
Camille M. Hoover, M.S.W., Executive Officer

Research Centers

7628 Center for Digestive Disorders
Central Dupage Hospital
One Boston Medical Center Place
Boston, MA 02118
617-638-8000
Fax: 617-638-7448
TTY: 800-439-2370
www.bmc.org/digestivedisorders

Kate Walsh, President/CEO

Web Sites

7629 Ask NOAH About: Stomach and Intestinal (Gastrointestinal) Disorders
noah-health.org/english/illness/gastro/gastro.html

Provides access to high quality full-text consumer health information in English and Spanish that is accurate, timely, relevant and unbiased.

7630 Colitis Cookbook
www.colitiscookbook.com/

A cookbook for people with colitis and other diseases.

Denise Weale, Co-Author
Ross Weale, Co-Author

7631 Crohn's & Colitis Foundation of America
733 Third Ave, Suite 510
New York, NY 10017 800-932-2423
info@ccfa.org
www.ccfa.org

Our mission is to prevent Crohn's disease and ulcerative colitis through research, and to improve the quality of life of children and adults affected by these digestive diseases through eduation and support.

Richard Geswell, President/ CEO
Judi Brown, Chief Development Officer
Aki Cipriani, MS, Human Resources Director

7632 Health Answers
410 Horsham Road
Horsham, PA 19044 215-442-9010
Michael.tague@healthanswers.com
www.healthanswers.com

HealthAnswers offers a breadth of services in medical education, sales force training, patient support solutions, professional promotion and consumer solutions.

Michael Tague, Managing Director

7633 IBS Self-help group
www.ibsgroup.org/

Works to educate those who are living with IBS and to increase awareness about his and other functional gastrointesinal disorders. The group was founded in support for those who suffer from IBS, those who are looking for support for someone who has IBS, and medical professionals who want to learn more about IBS.

Jeffrey D. Roberts, MSEd, B.Sc., Founder

7634 National Digestive Diseases Information Clearinghouse
Bethesda, MD 20892 301-496-3583
www.digestive.niddk.nih.gov

The National Institute of Diabetes and Digestive and Kidney Diseases conducts and supports research on many of the most serious diseases affecting public health. The Institute supports much of the clinical research on the diseases of internal medicine and related subspecialty fields as well as many basic science disciplines.

Griffin P. Rodgers, M.D., M.A.C.P., Director
Kevin Abbott, Program Director
Kristin Abraham, Program Director

7635 Online Mendelian Inheritance in Man
www.omim.org

This database is a catalog of human genes and genetic disorders.

7636 Pediatric Crohn's & Colitis Association
PO Box 188
Newton, MA 2468 617-489-5854
pcca.hypermart.net

We are committed to helping children with IBD and their families better understand the Crohn's disease and ulcerative colitis.

Book Publishers

7637 Angry Gut, The: Coping with Colitis and Crohn's Disease
Plenum Publishing Corporation
10 E 53 Street
New York, NY 10022 212-207-7600
Fax: 212-463-0742
onlineservice@springer.com
www.link.springer.com

Overview of the symptoms, diagnosis, complications, and treatment of IBD.

1993 364 pages
ISBN: 0-306444-70-4

7638 Ask Audrey
7466 Pebble Lane
West Bloomfield, MI 48322 248-626-6960

A compilation of material and the personal story of a medical psychotherapist who has inflammatory bowel disease. Includes practical tips on issues such as handling diarrhea, sexuality, relationships, traveling, coping with hospital stays, ostomies, and TPN.

7639 Digestive Diseases & Disorders Sourcebook
Omnigraphics
PO Box 625
Holmes, PA 19043 800-234-1340
Fax: 800-875-1340
info@omnigraphics.com
omnigraphics.com

Basic consumer health information including celiac disease, crohn's disease, diarrhea, hernias, irritable bowel syndrome and ulcers.

335 pages
ISBN: 0-780803-27-2

7640 IBD Nutrition Book
John Wiley & Sons
432 Elizabeth Avenue
Somerset, NJ 08875 800-225-5945
Fax: 732-302-2300
custserv@wiley.com
www.wiley.com

Clinical dietitian/nutritionist's overview of the role of diet in IBD, including recipes and meal plans.

Peter B. Wiley, Chairman
Stephen M. Smith, President & CEO
Ellis E. Cousens, Executive Vice President, Chief Fin

7641 Inflammatory Bowel Disease
Lippincott Williams & Wilkins
351 W Camden Street
Baltimore, MD 21201 410-528-4000
800-638-3030
www.lww.com

Detailed information on every aspect of IBD. Topics include medical and surgical management, epidemiology, fertility and pregnancy, psychosocial factors, and diagnostic techniques. Written for medical professionals and laypersons who are comfortable with medical terminology.

Edward B. Hutton Jr., Chief Executive Officer, President
E. Passano Jr., Vice Chairman of the Board and Secr

7642 Inflammatory Bowel Disease - From Bench to Bedside
Williams & Wilkins
351 W Camden Street
Baltimore, MD 21201 301-528-4000
www.lww.com

Offers in-depth information on the impact of basic research developments on the management of Crohn's disease and ulcerative colities. Written for medical professionals and laypersons who are comfortable with medical terminology.

Edward B. Hutton Jr., Chief Executive Officer, President
E. Passano Jr., Vice Chairman of the Board and Secr

7643 New People Not Patients: A Source Book for Living with IBD
Crohn's and Colitis Foundation of America
4930 Del Ray Avenue
Bethesda, MD 20814 301-654-2055
Fax: 301-654-5920
member@gastro.org
www.gastro.org/public/ibd.html

Anil K. Rustgi, President
Michael Camiller, Vice President
J. Sumner Bell III, Secretary/Treasurer

7644 Ostomy Book: Living Comfortably with Colostomies, Ileostomies and Urostomies
United Ostomy Association
P.O. Box 512
Northfield, MN 55057 949-660-8624
800-826-0826
Fax: 949-660-9262
info@ostomy.org
www.ostomy.org

An in-depth resource on how to adapt to an ostomy.

Dave Ruzdin, President
Diane Miterko, Advocacy Chair
Joan McGorry, Director of Administrative Services

7645 Treating IBD: A Patient's Guide to the Medical and Surgical Management
Crohn's and Colities Foundation of America
386 Park Avenue S
New York, NY 10016   212-685-3440
                           www.gastro.org/public/ibd.html

7646 You're Bigger than It
Hotel Dieu Hospital
Ontario, Canada,   613-544-3310

This cartoon book offers a lively, brief introduction to the basics of living with IBD. Contact can be reached at extension 2400.

Newsletters

7647 Inner Circle
Reach Out for Youth with Ileitis and Colitis
15 Chemung Place
Jericho, NY 11753   516-822-8010
            reachoutforyouth@reachoutforyouth.org
                     www.reachoutforyouth.org

Newsletter for youth with ileitis and colitis.

Pamphlets

7648 Bleeding in the Digestive Tract
Nat'l Digestive Diseases Information Clearinghouse
9000 Rockville Pike
Bethesda, MD 20892   301-496-3583
                           www.niddk.nih.gov

Informational fact sheet.

Griffin P. Rodgers, M.D., M.A.C.P., Director
Kevin Abbott, Program Director
Kristin Abraham, Program Director

7649 Crohn's Disease, Ulcerative Colitis, and Your Child
Crohn's and Colitis Foundation of America
733 Third Ave, Suite 510
New York, NY 10017   212-685-3440
                                   800-932-2423
                                   info@ccfa.org
                                   www.ccfa.org

Richard Geswell, President/ CEO
Judi Brown, Chief Development Officer
Aki Cipriani, MS, Human Resources Director

7650 Guide for Children & Teenagers
Crohn's and Colitis Foundation of America
733 Third Ave, Suite 510
New York, NY 10017   212-685-3440
                                   800-932-2423
                                   info@ccfa.org
                                   www.ccfa.org

Richard Geswell, President/ CEO
Judi Brown, Chief Development Officer
Aki Cipriani, MS, Human Resources Director

7651 Inside Story
Reach Out for Youth with Illeitis and Colitis
15 Chemung Place
Jericho, NY 11753   516-822-8010

Educational brochure for youth with illeitis and colitis.

7652 Living with IBD: A Guide for Teenagers
Crohn's and Colitis Foundation of America
733 Third Ave, Suite 510
New York, NY 10017   212-685-3440
                                   800-932-2423
                                   info@ccfa.org
                                   www.ccfa.org

Richard Geswell, President/ CEO
Judi Brown, Chief Development Officer
Aki Cipriani, MS, Human Resources Director

7653 Questions and Answers About Ulcerative Colitis
Crohn's and Colitis Foundation of America
733 Third Ave, Suite 510
New York, NY 10017   212-685-3440
                                   800-932-2423
                                   info@ccfa.org
                                   www.ccfa.org

Richard Geswell, President/ CEO
Judi Brown, Chief Development Officer
Aki Cipriani, MS, Human Resources Director

7654 Teacher's Guide to Crohn's Disease & Ulcerative Colitis
Crohn's & Colitis Foundation of America
733 Third Ave, Suite 510
New York, NY 10017   212-665-3440
                                   800-932-2423
                              Fax: 212-779-4098
                                   info@ccfa.org
                                   www.ccfa.org

Richard Geswell, President/ CEO
Judi Brown, Chief Development Officer
Aki Cipriani, MS, Human Resources Director

7655 Ulcerative Colitis
National Organization for Rare Disorders
55 Kenosia Avenue
Danbury, CT 6810   203-744-0100
                                   800-999-6673
                              Fax: 203-798-2291
                           orphan@rarediseases.org
                              www.rarediseases.org

Informational fact sheet.

Sheldon M. Schuster, Acting Chair
Peter L. Saltonstall, President & CEO
Pamela Gravin, COO

DESCRIPTION

7656 URTICARIA

Synonym: Hives

Involves the following Biologic System(s):

Dermatologic Disorders

Urticaria, more commonly known as hives, is a skin condition characterized by the development of raised, usually itchy (pruritic), white or reddish lesions (wheals). The wheals associated with urticaria vary in size and may sometimes blend together to form large, patchy skin lesions. Although individual lesions may disappear within minutes, hours, or days, new eruptions may continue to appear for weeks. Urticaria is considered to be a chronic skin disorder if wheals continue to appear for 6 weeks or longer.

Although the cause of urticaria is sometimes unknown, it is often the result of an immune or allergic response in which cells in the skin release various substances that create the effects of this condition. One of these substances is histamine, a protein produced by nerve cells and certain specialized blood and tissue cells. Released into the skin by these cells in response to an allergen or other triggering factor, histamine allows fluid to escape from small blood vessels into surrounding tissues to create the characteristic blister-like wheals associated with hives. The triggers for urticaria include allergic reactions caused by the ingestion of certain foods such as shellfish, strawberries, nuts, and eggs; drugs such as aspirin, penicillin, or codeine; and food dyes or other additives. Urticarial reactions may also be triggered by contact with pollens or other plant substances, insects, animals; chemicals or drugs that come into contact with the skin; certain drugs that are taken orally or by injection; blood transfusions; and insect bites or stings; well as by viral, bacterial, fungal, and parasitic infections; and by cold or heat, pressure on the skin, sunlight, and exercise.

Beyond this, hives may develop in conjunction with the swelling of certain areas of soft tissue (angioedema or angioneurotic edema) in deeper layers of the skin or in the upper respiratory tract, gastrointestinal tract, face and neck, hands and feet, and genitalia. A distinct disorder that may develop during early childhood is urticaria pigmentosa which is characterized by reddish-brown skin lesions occurring across the body, which change into hive-like lesions when stroked, rubbed, or scratched. Hives may also be associated with other systemic disorders and with certain inherited disorders such as amyloidosis; familial cold urticaria, a hereditary disorder characterized by urticaria occurring in response to coldness; and hereditary angioedema, a severe and potentially life-threatening form of angioedema.

The rash derived from poison ivy is commonly mistaken for urticaria, but is instead what is known as a contact dermatitis, caused by a toxin named urushiol that is present in this plant.

Hives often disappear rapidly and spontaneously, without treatment, but in some cases may be part of a more severe reaction known as an anaphylactic reaction, that may affect the heart and respiratory system as well as other organs and systems of the body. Consequently, children with acute, severe urticaria or those who experience difficulty in breathing or swallowing should be given immediate medical attention.

Other treatment for urticaria depends upon its underlying cause. In most instances, treatment of urticaria is directed at alleviating its symptoms. This may be accomplished with the drugs known as antihistamines, which block the effects of hitasmine; with oral steroids, which can be safely given over a short period to relieve inflammation and swelling; and by topical ointments or creams than relieve itching and swelling when applied directly to the skin. Avoidance to the agents or factors that trigger urticaria is often the best defense. Reducing or avoiding stress is often effective in preventing or limiting this condition. Other treatment is symptomatic and supportive.

Government Agencies

7657 NIH/ Eunice Kennedy Shriver National Insti tute of Child Health & Human Development

31 Center Drive, Building 31
Bethesda, MD 20892

301-496-5113
800-370-2943
Fax: 866-760-5947
TTY: 888-320-6942
nichdpress@mail.nih.gov
www.nichd.nih.gov

Established in 1962 by congress, today the institute conducts and supports research on topics related to the health of children, adults, families and populations. Some of these topics include: developmental disabilities, growth and development, infant death, reproductive health and birth defects.

Diana W. Bianchi, Director
Paul Williams, Director, Communications

7658 NIH/National Institute of Allergy and Infectious Diseases

5601 Fishers Lane, MSC 9806
Bethesda, MD 20892

301-496-5717
866-284-4107
Fax: 301-402-3573
TDD: 800-877-8339
ocpostoffice@niaid.nih.gov
www.niaid.nih.gov

Conducts and supports basic and applied research to better understand, treat, and ultimately prevent infectious, immunologic, and allergic diseases.

Anthony S Fauci MD, Director

7659 NIH/National Institute of Arthritis and Musculoskeletal and Skin Diseases

1 AMS Circle
Bethesda, MD 20892

301-495-4484
877-226-4267
Fax: 301-718-6366
TTY: 301-565-2966
TDD: 301-565-2966
niamsinfo@mail.nih.gov
www.niams.nih.gov

The mission of the NIAMS, a part of the NIH, is to support research into the causes, treatment, and prevention of arthritis and musculoskeletal and skin diseases, the training of basic and clinical scientists to carry out this research, and the dissemination of information on research progress in these diseases.

Stephen I Katz MD PhD, Director
Robert H Carter MD, Deputy Director

National Associations & Support Groups

7660 American Academy of Pediatrics

141 Northwest Point Boulevard
Elk Grove Village, IL 60007

847-434-4000
800-433-9016
Fax: 847-434-8000
www.aap.org

The American Academy of Pediatrics and its member pediatricians are committed to the attainment of optimal physical, mental and social health and well-being for all infants, children, adolescents, and young adults.

Fernando Stein, MD, FAAP, President
Karen Remley, MD, CEO/Executive VP

7661 Genetic Alliance
4301 Connecticut Avenue NW, Suite 404
Washington, DC 20008   202-966-5557
                                        800-336-4363
                                        Fax: 202-966-8553
                                        info@geneticalliance.org
                                        www.geneticalliance.org

A coalition of voluntary genetic support groups, consumers and professionals addressing the needs of individuals and families affected by genetic disorders from a national perspective.

Sharon Terry, President/CEO
Tetyana Murza, Managing Director
Natasha Bonhomme, VP, Strategic Development

7662 Society for Pediatric Dermatology
8365 Keystone Crossing, Suite 107
Indianapolis, IN 46240   317-202-0224
                                        Fax: 317-205-9481
                                        info@pedsderm.net
                                        www.pedsderm.net

Objective is to promote, develop and advance education, research and care of all skin disease in all pediatric age groups.

Karen Wiss, President
Andrea Zaenglen, President-Elect
Kent Lindeman, Executive Director

Web Sites

7663 Allergy Web
Asthma & Allergy Associates of Florida
7800 SW 87th Avenue, Suite C-340
Miami, FL 33173   305-595-0109
                                        Fax: 305-595-7092
                                        www.allergyweb.com

Provides information that may help you learn more about allergies and asthma.

Dr. Morris Beck, Founder
Mark Young, MD, Physician
Elena Ubals, MD, Physician

Journals

7664 Pediatric Dermatology Journal
Society for Pediatric Dermatology
8365 Keystone Crossing, Suite 107
Indianapolis, IN 46240   317-202-0224
                                        Fax: 317-205-9481
                                        info@pedsderm.net
                                        www.pedsderm.net

6 issues/yr

Kent Lindeman, Executive Director

DESCRIPTION

7665 VENTRICULAR SEPTAL DEFECTS
Synonym: VSDs
Involves the following Biologic System(s):
Cardiovascular Disorders

Ventricular septal defects (VSDs) are considered the most common structural heart malformations, comprising up to 20 percent of all heart defects that are present at birth (congenital). VSDs are characterized by the presence of an abnormal opening in the fibrous muscular partition (septum) that separates the two lower pumping chambers (ventricles) of the heart. The ventricles are the chambers that pump blood out of the heart via large blood vessels (arteries). The pulmonary artery arises from the base of the right ventricle and carries oxygen-poor (deoxygenated) blood to the lungs, where the exchange of oxygen and carbon dioxide occurs. The aorta, the main artery of the body, arises from the base of the left ventricle and carries oxygen-rich (oxygenated) blood to the body's tissues.

In infants with ventricular septal defects, the abnormal opening in the septum between the two ventricles allows oxygenated blood in the left ventricle to flow into the right ventricle and recirculate to the lungs rather than to the rest of the body's tissues. Symptoms and findings may vary, depending upon the size and location of the ventricular septal defect and the associated effects on pulmonary blood pressure and flow. If the VSD is large, it may result in significantly increased blood flow through the lungs' blood vessels.

Small VSDs usually cause no associated symptoms and, in up to 50 percent of patients, may close spontaneously before school age. Small ventricular septal defects may be detected during a routine physical examination based upon a characteristic heart sound (heart murmur) heard with a stethoscope. In infants with larger VSDs, too much blood is pumped to the lungs. This may result in persistent elevation of blood pressure in the pulmonary circulation (pulmonary hypertension), enlargement of the heart (cardiomegaly), and abnormally rapid breathing (tachypnea). Additional symptoms and findings may include difficulty with lower respiratory tract infections, increased sweating, difficulties feeding, and failure to grow and gain weight at the expected rate (failure to thrive). When these symptoms and findings occur, the infant is said to have congestive heart failure (CHF). Large VSDs may be diagnosed upon a complete clinical examinationand various specialized tests, such as x-ray studies, echocardiogram (ultrasound of the heart), electrocardiogram, or cardiac catheterization.

Children and adolescents with unclosed VSDs may be at an increased risk of bacterial infection of the lining of the heart (endocarditis). Such infection is rare before the age of two years. Due to the increased risk of bacterial endocarditis, affected individuals are cautioned to take antibiotic medication before dental visits and surgical procedures. After the VSD is successfully closed, preventive treatment is needed only during a six-month healing period. Closing small ventricular septal defects may not be needed. They often close on their own in childhood or adolescence. But if the opening is large, even in patients with few symptoms, closing the hole in the first two years of life is recommended to prevent serious problems later.

In some patients, VSDs may occur in association with certain underlying genetic syndromes, chromosomal abnormalities, or malformation syndromes that are caused by exposure to certain infectious agents, medications, or other environmental factors (teratogenic syndromes).

National Associations & Support Groups

7666 American Academy of Pediatrics
141 Northwest Point Boulevard
Elk Grove Village, IL 60007
847-434-4000
800-433-9016
Fax: 847-434-8000
www.aap.org

The American Academy of Pediatrics and its member pediatricians are committed to the attainment of optimal physical, mental and social health and well-being for all infants, children, adolescents, and young adults.

Fernando Stein, MD, FAAP, President
Karen Remley, MD, CEO/Executive VP

7667 American Heart Association
7272 Greenville Avenue
Dallas, TX 75231
214-373-6300
800-242-8721
Fax: 214-706-1341
inquire@amhrt.org
www.heart.org/HEARTORG/

Supports research, education and community service programs with the objective of reducing premature death and disability from cardiovascular diseases and stroke; coordinates the efforts of health professionals, and others engaged in the fight against heart and circulatory disease.

Nancy Brown, CEO
Dr. Stephen Houser, President
Suzie Upton, Chief Operating Officer

Web Sites

7668 Congenital Heart Information Network
3181 S.W. Sam Jackson Park Rd.
Portland, OR 97239
503-494-8311
www.ohsu.edu

An international organization that provides reliable information, support services and resources to families of children with congenital heart defects and acquired heart disease and adults with congenital heart defects, and the professionals who work with them.

7669 Southern Illinois University School of Medicine
PO Box 19639
Springfield, IL 62794
217-545-8000
800-342-5748
admin@siuhealthcare.org
www.siumed.edu

The mission of SUI School of Medicine is to assist the people of central and southern Illinois in meeting their present and future needs through education, clinical service and research.

7670 Yale University School of Medicine
www.info.med.yale.edu

A site that offers information on Ventricular Septal Defects and other congenital heart conditions.

DESCRIPTION

7671 VIOLENCE BY CHILDREN & TEENAGERS

Involves the following Biologic System(s):
Behavioral/Developmental/Psychiatric Disorders

Some children and teenagers prey on vulnerable people, exhibiting antisocial behavior, neurological dysfunctions, and mental illnesses. These youths may assault other children or adults for a variety of reasons, ranging from invoking fear as a form of entertainment to causing bodily harm as retribution for perceived wrongs such as social ostracism.

Criminal behavior by children and teenagers doubled during the late 1980s and early 1990s. Although homicide rates for teenage perpetrators began to decline in the United States by 1997, youth violence remained an urgent issue. By the beginning of the twenty-first century, violent youths were committing callous acts at increasingly younger ages. They also behaved more extremely with regard to weapons used or number of victims attacked during violent sprees. Crimes such as school shootings targeted individuals both known and unfamiliar to perpetrators. The fatal school shooting at Columbine High School in 1999 prompted many studies of why teenagers become violent.

Violent youths represent varying social classes and ethnicities, living in both rural and urban areas. Young males are twice as likely to act violently outside the home than are young females, but both genders are equally likely to be violent toward their families.

Violent tendencies sometimes emerge when children are toddlers. Aggressive children may fight with other youngsters, act up in class, challenge authority figures, or steal. Some sadistically abuse animals. Such aberrant behaviors can intensify during adolescence.

Researchers offer contrasting theories about why some youths become violent. Violent youths may suffer from severe mental illnesses, display disruptive behavior disorders or antisocial personalities, or have experienced brain damage. Some researchers suggest that brain circuits containing the neurotransmitter serotonin have malfunctioned in violent youths. A few researchers speculate that some infants have innate repressed violent characteristics that develop when the child encounters biological or psychological triggers, such as sexual or physical abuse, illegal substances, or peer pressure.

Authorities agree that many violent children and teenagers have been exposed to violence in their homes or communities. Inadequate or abusive parenting can prevent children from learning appropriate values of right and wrong. Neglected or abused children can feel emotionally abandoned and become self-centered. Egocentric youths are more likely to lack consciences and to be incapable of feeling empathy or compassion for others. Emotions such as depression, frustration, rage, and shame can intensify a child's perceived inadequacies. Many violent youths are alienated from emotional support systems and feel isolated and discriminated against. They may become desensitized to violence or emotionally numb and seek excitement through violence. Some are suicidal and resigned to accepting and participating in violence.

Youth violence can be categorized into four major types. **Situational violence**, one of the most common types of violence committed by children and teenagers, is sparked by an event that upsets or enrages the victimizer. For example, a student might assault a teacher who gave a failing grade. **Relational violence** occurs when a child or teenager is violent toward a relative or friend with whom he or she has a personal dispute. **Dating violence** is one of the most prevalent forms of this type of violence, as when a teenage boy attacks a girl who terminates their relationship. **Predatory violence** describes thefts and muggings involving violence or violent activities carried out to prove loyalty and ensure acceptance by a group. Violence connected to competition, drug dealing, riots, and gang fights and the use of concealed weapons with intent to maim or murder is considered predatory. Less than 1 percent of juvenile cases involve psychopathological violence, which involves perpetrators who probably are neurologically damaged or mentally ill and who commit extremely violent acts. These individuals require pharmaceutical and management therapy. Other violent acts that may be committed by youths include hate crimes, vandalism, bombings, or activism such as ecoterrorism. Some violent youths are attention seekers who believe that they will become celebrities through their acts.

While engaged in violent acts, youths may be dissociated from what they are doing and may feel as if they are experiencing a dreamlike or fantastical state instead of reality. Violent youths may verbally antagonize and ridicule their victims, who are often people whom the perpetrators view as weak, such as young children, the elderly, and handicapped individuals. Sometimes, groups of youths plan assaults to surround and attack one person. Preteens have raped or murdered children their own age or younger. Some children who commit violent acts are not sufficiently mature, intellectually and morally, to realize that their actions can hurt other people. In 2000, a six-year-old who shot a classmate at a Michigan school expressed confusion when she died.

Mental health professionals stress that children who display violent behaviors should be identified as young as possible so that intervention measures can be implemented to prevent them from harming other youths. Facilities that treat violent juvenile offenders include boot camps, detention centers, wilderness programs, and group or private psychotherapy sessions. Both public and private schools attempt to identify emotionally disturbed students who might interfere with the learning process of other students by disrupting classes and challenging faculty members.

Violent youths who are mentally ill should receive counseling and medication. Other options are available to those whose behavior has social and emotional roots. These youths may be enrolled in programs that promote self-esteem, emotional resilience, and self-control. Parents can teach their children appropriate coping techniques to prevent violence. Communities and churches can provide children with supervised recreational activities during afternoons, which are the hours when youths are most likely to act violently. Mentoring programs can demonstrate alternatives to destructive behavior. Peer counseling has been shown to be an effective deterrent to violence. Violence-prevention curricula can teach children to resolve conflicts creatively and help them develop skills to control emotional outbursts.

Government Agencies

7672 NIH/National Institute of Mental Health
6001 Executive Boulevard, Room 6200, MSC 9663
Bethesda, MD 20892
301-443-4536
866-615-6464
Fax: 301-443-4279
TTY: 301-443-8431
nimhinfo@nih.gov
www.nimh.nih.gov

The mission of NIMH is to transform the understanding and treatment of mental illnesses through basic and clinical research, paving the way for prevention, recovery, and cure.

Joshua Gordon, MD, PhD, Director
Shelli Avenevoli, MD, Deputy Director

National Associations & Support Groups

7673 American Academy of Child and Adolescent Psychiatry
3615 Wisconsin Avenue, N.W.
Washington, DC 20016
202-966-7300
Fax: 202-966-2891
clinical@aacap.org
www.aacap.org

The mission of AACAP is to promote the healthy development of children, adolescents, and families through advocacy, education, and research, and to meet the professional needs of child and adolescent psychiatrists throughout their careers.

Paramjit T. Joshi, MD, President
Aradhana Sood, MD, Secretary
David G. Fassler, MD, Treasurer

7674 American Academy of Family Physicians
11400 Tomahawk Creek Parkway
Leawood, KS 66211
913-906-6000
800-274-2237
Fax: 913-906-6075
www.aafp.org

The mission of the AAFP is to improve the health of patients, families, and communities by serving the needs of members with professionalism and creativity.

Reid B. Blackwelder, MD, FAAFP, Board Chair
Robert L. Wergin, MD, FAAFP, President
Douglas E. Henley, MD, FAAFP, EVP/ CEO

7675 American Academy of Pediatrics
141 Northwest Point Boulevard
Elk Grove Village, IL 60007
847-434-4000
800-433-9016
Fax: 847-434-8000
csc@aap.org
www.aap.org

The organization is committed to the optimal physical, mental, and social health and well-being for all infants, children, adolescents, and young adults.

Fernando Stein, MD, FAAP, President
Karen Remley, MD, CEO/Executive VP

7676 American College of Neuropsychopharmacology
5034-A Thoroughbred Lane
Brentwood, TN 37027
615-324-2360
Fax: 615-523-1715
acnp@acnp.org
www.acnp.org

The American College of Neuropsychopharmacology (ACNP), founded in 1961, is a professional society in brain, behavior, and psychopharmacology research. The field of neuropsychopharmacology involves the evaluation of the effects of natural and synthetic compounds upon the brain, mind, and human behavior.

Raquel E. Gur, M.D., Ph.D., President
Ronnie Wilkins, Ed.D., CAE, Executive Director
Sarah Timm, CAE, CMP, Deputy Director

7677 American Congress of Obstetricians and Gynecologists
409 12th Street SW
Washington, DC 20024
202-638-5577
800-673-8444
www.acog.org

Founded in 1951 in Chicago, Illinois, The College has over 58,000 members and is the nation's leading group of professionals providing health care for women. Based in Washington, DC, it is a private, voluntary, nonprofit membership organization.

Dr. Hal C. Lawrence III, EVP/ CEO
Richard C. Bailey, CPA, MBA, CFO/ VP, Finance
Dr. Sandra Ann Carson, MD, VP Education

7678 American Counseling Association
6101 Stevenson Ave
Alexandria, VA 22304
703-823-9800
800-347-6647
Fax: 703-823-0252
webmaster@counseling.org
www.counseling.org

Represents professional counselors in various practice settings, and stands ready to serve more than 55,000 members with the resources they need to make a difference. From webinars, publications, and journals to Conference education sessions and legislative action alerts, ACA is where counseling professionals turn for powerful, credible content and support.

Robert L. Smith, President

7679 American Medical Association
AMA Plaza, 330 North Wabash Ave., Suite 39300
Chicago, IL 60611
800-262-3211
www.ama-assn.org/ama

AMA is dedicated to ensuring sustainable physician practices that result in better health outcomes for patients.

James L. Madara, MD, CEO/ EVP
Bernard L. Hengesbaugh, Chief Operating Officer
Kenneth J. Sharigian, SVP/ Chief Strategy Officer

7680 American Mental Health Foundation (AMHF)
PO Box 3
Riverdale, NY 10471
USA
212-737-9027
elomke@americanmentalhealthfoundation.or
americanmentalhealthfoundation.org

Dedicated to the extensive and intensive research in the theories and techniques of treatment of emotional illness and to the implementation of reforms in the mental health system. Efforts have resulted in development of better and less expensive treatment methods. Findings are disseminated in English and other major languages.

Sister Joan Curtin. CND, Director
Evander Lomke, President/Executive Director
Eugene Gollogly, Vice President

7681 American Psychiatric Association
1000 Wilson Boulevard, Suite 1825
Arlington, VA 22209
703-907-7300
888-35 -7924
apa@psych.org
www.psychiatry.org

It is a medical specialty society representing growing membership of more than 36,000 psychiatrists.

7682 American Psychological Association
750 First St. NE
Washington, DC 20002
202-336-5500
800-374-2721
TTY: 202-336-6123
www.apa.org

The mission is to advance the creation, communication and application of psychological knowledge to benefit society and improve people's lives.

Norman B. Anderson, PhD, CEO/ EVP
L. Michael Honaker, PhD, Deputy Chief Executive Officer
Ellen G. Garrison, PhD, Senior Policy Advisor

7683 **American Public Health Association**
800 I Street, NW
Washington, DC 20001   202-777-2742
Fax: 202-777-2534
TTY: 202-777-2500
www.apha.org

APHA champions the health of all people and all communities.
They aim to strengthen the public health profession and speak out
for public health issues and policies backed by science.

Georges C. Benjamin, MD, Executive Director
Kemi Oluwafemi, MBA, CPA, Chief Financial Officer
Susan Polan, PhD, Associate Executive Director

7684 **American School Counselor Association**
1101 King Street, Suite 310
Alexandria, VA 22314   703-683-2722
800-306-4722
Fax: 703-997-7572
asca@schoolcounselor.org
www.schoolcounselor.org

The mission of ASCA is to represent professional school counselors and to promote professionalism and ethical practices.

Richard Wong, Executive Director
Jeff Broderson, Information Technology Admin.
Kathleen M Rakestraw, Director of Communications

7685 **Association for Behavioral and Cognitive Therapies**
305 7th Avenue, 16th Floor
New York, NY 10001   212-647-1890
Fax: 212-647-1865
membership@abct.org
www.abct.org/Home/

Formerly known as the Association for Advancement of Behavior
Therapy; this organization is concerned with the application of
behavioral and cognitive sciences to understanding human behavior, developing interventions to enhance the human condition,
and promoting the appropriate utilization of these interventions.

Stefan G. Hofmann, Ph.D., President
Dean McKay, Ph.D, President- Elect
Denise D. Davis, Ph.D., Secretary/Treasurer

7686 **Center for Disabilities and Development**
University of Iowa Stead Family Children's Hospita
100 Hawkins Drive
Iowa City, IA 52242   319-353-6900
877-686-0031
Fax: 319-356-7700
cdd-webmaster@uiowa.edu
www.uichildrens.org/cdd/

A trusted resource for healthcare, training, research and information for people with disabilities that include: behavior disorders,
brain injury, cerebral palsy, diabetes, down syndrome, learning
disabilities, mental retardation, sleep disorders and spina bifida.

Dianne McBrien, MD, Medical Director

7687 **Center for Mental Health Services Knowledge Exchange
Network**
US Department of Health and Human Services
PO Box 42557
Washington, DC 20015   800-662-4357
800-789-2647
Fax: 240-747-5470
TTY: 800-487-4889
TDD: 866-889-2647
samhsa.media@ees.hhs.gov
www.store.samhsa.gov/home

Develops national mental health policies that promote Fed-
eral/State coordination and benefit from input from consumers,
family members and providers. Ensures that high quality mental
health services programs are implemented to benefit seriously
mentally ill populations, disasters or those involved in the
criminal justice system.

Mirtha R. Beadle M.P.A., Deputy for Operations
Kana . Enomoto, M.A, Principal Deputy Administrator
Pamela S. Hyde, J.D., Administrator

7688 **Center on Media and Child Health**
CMBH BCH3186, 300 Longwood Avenue
Boston, MA 2115   617-355-5420
Fax: 617-730-0004
cmch@childrens.harvard.edu
cmch.tv

The Center on Media and Child Health (CMCH) at Boston Children's Hospital (BCH) is an academic research center whose mission is to educate and empower children and those who care for
them to create and consume media in ways that optimize children's health and development.

Michael Rich, MPH, Director, Founder
David S. Bickham, PhD, Research Scientist
Lauren Rubenzahl, EdM, Program Administrative Manager

7689 **Child Trends**
7315 Wisconsin Avenue, Suite 1200W
Bethesda, MD 20814   240-223-9200
Fax: 240-200-1238
agreen@childtrends.org
www.childtrends.org

Child Trends is a nonprofit, nonpartisan research center that provides valuable information and insights on the well-being of children and youth. - See more at:
http://www.childtrends.org/about-us/#sthash.M6MuEoBz.dpuf

The Hon. William A. Thorne, Chair
Carol Emig, President
Natalia E. Pane, SVP, Research and Operations

7690 **Family Online Safety Institute**
400 7th Street NW, Suite 506
Washington, DC 20004   202-775-0158
fosi@fosi.org
www.fosi.org

The Family Online Safety Institute brings a unique, international
perspective to the potential risks, harms as well as the rewards of
our online lives.

Stephen Balkam, Founder & CEO
Jennifer Hanley, Director, Legal & Policy
Emma Morris, International Policy Manager

7691 **Federation of Families for Children's Mental Health**
9605 Medical Center Drive, Suite 280
Rockville, MD 10205   240-403-1901
Fax: 240-403-1909
ffcmh@ffcmh.org
www.ffcmh.org

The National family run organization is dedicated exclusively to
helping children with mental health needs and their families
achieve a better quality of life.

Teka Dempson, President
Sherri Luthe, Vice President
Sheila Pires, Treasurer

7692 **Foundation for Child Development**
295 Madison Avenue, 40th Floor
New York, NY 10017   212-867-5777
Fax: 212-867-5844
info@fcd-us.org
fcd-us.org

There mission is to harness the power of research to ensure that
all children benefit from early learning experiences that affirm
their individual, family, and community assets, fortify them
against harmful consequences arising from economic instability
and social exclusion, and that strengthen their developmental
potential.

Jacqueline Jones, President and CEO
Jessica Chao, Chief Operating Officer
Annette Chin, Senior Program Officer

7693 **International Society for Research in Child and Adolescent
Psychopathology**
University of Washington, Child Health Institute,
Seattle, WA 98195   206-543-1538
Fax: 206-616-4623
annv@uw.edu
isrcap.org

909

The International Society for Research in Child and Adolescent Psychopathology (ISRCAP) was founded in 1988 by Herbert C. Quay, so that mental health professionals interested in child psychopathology would have a forum to exchange ideas concerning the nature and treatment of childhood mental disorders.

Joel Nigg, PhD, President
Ann Vander Stoep, PhD, Secretary/ Treasurer
Joan Luby, MD, President Elect

7694 Mental Health America
500 Montgomery Street, Ste 820
Alexandria, VA 22314
703-684-7722
800-969-6642
Fax: 703-684-5968
TTY: 800-433-5959
info@mentalhealthamerica.net
www.mentalhealthamerica.net

MHA, the leading advocacy organization addressing the full spectrum of mental and substance use conditions and their effects nationwide, works to inform, advocate and enable access to quality behavioral health services for all Americans.

Paul Gionfriddo, President/CEO
Shavonne Carpenter, Sr Assoc., Support & Services
Mallory Pernell, Assoc. Dir, Comments/Marketing

7695 NADD: National Association for the Dually Diagnosed
132 Fair Street
Kingston, NY 12401
845-331-4336
800-331-5362
Fax: 845-331-4569
info@thenadd.org
www.thenadd.org

Nonprofit organization designed to promote the interests of professional and care providers for individuals who have the coexistence of mental illness and mental retardation. NADD provides conferences, educational services and training materials to professionals, parents, concerned citizens and service organizations.

Dr Robert Fletcher, CEO
Michelle Jordan, Office Manager
Edward Seliger, Project Coordinator

7696 National Alliance for the Mentally Ill
3803 N. Fairfax Dr., Suite 100
Arlington, VA 22203
703-525-7600
800-950-6264
Fax: 703-524-9094
TDD: 703-516-7227
info@nami.org
www.nami.org

NAMI is a nonprofit, grassroots, self-help, support and advocacy organization of consumers, families and friends of people with severe mental illness, such as schizophrenia, bipolar disorder, major depressive disorder, obsessive compulsive disorder, anxiety disorders, autism and other severe and persistent mental illnesses that affect the brain.

Keris J,,n Myrick, President
Kevin B Sullivan, First Vice President
Jim Payne, Second Vice President

7697 National Association for the Education of Young Children
1313 L Street, NW, Suite 500
Washington, DC 20005
202-232-8777
800-424-2460
Fax: 202-328-1846
www.naeyc.org

NAEYC promotes high-quality early learning for all children, birth through age 8, by connecting practice, policy, and research. We advance a diverse, dynamic early childhood profession and support all who care for, educate, and work on behalf of young children.

Derry Koralek, Chief Publishing Officer
Rhian Evans Allvin, Executive Director
Stephanie A. Morris, Deputy Executive Director

7698 National Association of School Psychologists
4340 East West Highway, Suite 402
Bethesda, MD 20814
301-657-0270
866-331-NASP
Fax: 301-657-0275
www.nasponline.org

NASP empowers school psychologists by advancing effective practices to improve students' learning, behavior, and mental health.

Stephen E. Brock, President
Todd A. Savage, President-Elect
Sally Baas, Past President

7699 National Center for Injury Prevention and Control
4770 Buford Hwy, NE Mail Stop MS F-63
Atlanta, GA 30341
800-232-4636
TTY: 888-232-6348
www.cdc.gov/injury

CDC works to protect America from health, safety and security threats, both foreign and in the U.S. Whether diseases start at home or abroad, are chronic or acute, curable or preventable, human error or deliberate attack, CDC fights disease and supports communities and citizens to do the same.

Sue Binder, M.D., Director

7700 National Institute of Mental Health
6001 Executive Boulevard
Rockville, MD 20852
866-615-6464
Fax: 301-443-4279
TTY: 301-443-8431
NIMHinfo@mail.nih.gov
www.nimh.nih.gov

The mission of NIMH is to transform the understanding and treatment of mental illnesses through basic and clinical research, paving the way for prevention, recovery, and cure.

Tom Insel, MD, Director

7701 National Medical Association
8403 Colesville Road, Suite 920
Silver Spring, MD 20910
202-347-1895
Fax: 202-347-0722
www.nmanet.org

The National Medical Association (NMA) is the collective voice of African American physicians and the leading force for parity and justice in medicine and the elimination of disparities in health.

Garfield Clunie, M.D., Chairman of the Board
Lawrence Sanders, President
Martin Hamlette, J.D., M.H.A., Executive Director

7702 The Future of Children
267 Wallace Hall, Princeton University
Princeton, NJ 8544
609-258-5894
foc@princeton.edu
www.futureofchildren.org

The mission of the Future of Children is to translate the best social science research about children and youth into information that is useful to policymakers, practitioners, grant-makers, advocates, the media, and students of public policy.

Sara McLanahan, Editor-in-Chief
Janet Currie, Senior Editor
Ron Haskins, Senior Editor

Research Centers

7703 Menninger Child & Family Program
Menninger Clinic
2801 Gessner Drive, PO Box 809045
Houston, TX 77280
713-275-5000
800-351-9058
Fax: 713-275-5117
www.menninger.edu

Menninger's research strategies are developed through the Menninger Child & Family Program. Projects are designed to develop a better understanding of the mind in order to more effectively treat mental disorders.

Ian Aitken, Ceo

7704 National Technical Assistance Center for Children's Mental Health
Georgetown University
Center for Child and Human Development Georgetown
Washington, DC 20057   202-687-5000
Fax: 202-687-8899
TDD: 202-687-5503
gucdc@georgetown.edu
www.gucchd.georgetown.edu/67211.html

Devoted to helping states, tribes, territories, and communities discover, apply, and sustain innovative and collaborative solutions that improve the social, emotional, and behavioral well being of children and families.

James Wotring MSW, Director

7705 Research & Training Center for Children's Mental Health at University of South FL
Louis de la Parte Florida Mental Health Institute
13301 Bruce B. Downs Boulevard
Tampa, FL 33612   813-974-3154
Fax: 813-974-3078
friedman@fmhi.usf.edu
www.rtckids.fmhi.usf.edu/default.cfm

Working towards increasing the effectiveness of service systems by strengthening the empirical base for such systems through research and dissemination to key audiences. With its new, five-year research program, the Center expands its mission with an integrated research, training, and dissemination program targeted specifically at implementation issues for developing effective systems of care.

Robert M. Friedman, Ph.D, Center Director
Albert Duchnowski, Ph.D, Deputy Director
Krista Kutash, Ph.D, Deputy Director

7706 Research and Training Center on Family Support and Children's Mental Health
1600 SW 4th Avenue, Suite 900
Portland, OR 97201   503-725-4040
Fax: 503-725-4180
flemingd@pdx.edu
www.rtc.pdx.edu

Funded to pursue an integrated set of research, training, technical assistance, and dissemination activities. The center's work will focus on two related themes; community integration for children and adolescents with emotional and behavioral disorders and their families; and strengthening family and youth participation in child and adolescent mental health services.

Donna Flemming, Information Director

7707 Technical Assistance Partnership for Child and Family Mental Health
1000 Thomas Jefferson Street NW, Suite 400
Washington, DC 20007   202-403-6827
Fax: 202-342-5007
tapartnership@air.org
www.tapartnership.org

A staff of family members and professionals with extensive practice experience, grounded in an organization with vast research experience in children with serious emotional disturbance and their families.

Sharon Hunt, Deputy Director of Operations
Jeffrey Poirier, Continuous Quality Improvement
Regenia Hicks, Project Director Continuous Quality

Conferences

7708 FFCMH Annual Conference
Federation of Families for Childrens Mental Health
9605 Medical Center Drive, Suite 280
Rockville, MD 20850   240-403-1901
Fax: 240-403-1909
ffcmh@ffcmh.org
www.ffcmh.org

Address the complex issue of trauma; the impact it has on children and families; the promotion of healing and prevention strategies; knowledge about how to address trauma through resiliency-based interventions, utilizing a familydriven, youth guided approach; and examples of how family organizations and the partners they work with are raising awareness and improving trauma-focused services and supports.

November

Teka Dempson, President
Sherri Luthe, Vice President
Sheila Pires, Treausrer

7709 NADD Conference & Exhibit Show
National Association for the Dually Diagnosed
132 Fair Street
Kingston, NY 12401   845-331-4336
800-331-5362
Fax: 845-331-4569
info@thenadd.org
www.thenadd.org

Educating professionals, families and clients of services on standard and state-of-the-art information across many specialties; Enhancing specific skills required to provide maximum benefit to individuals with special or specific cognitive and/or developmental needs; Providing a forum for an exchange of ideas and information among professionals, families and those who may receive services.

November

Dr Robert Fletcher, CEO
Michelle Jordan, Office Manager
Edward Seliger, Project Coordinator

7710 NAMI Convention
National Alliance on Mental Illness
3803 N Fairfax Drive, Suite 100
Arlington, VA 22203   703-524-7600
888-999-6264
Fax: 703-524-9094
TDD: 703-516-7227
info@nami.org
www.nami.org

The NAMI Convention is packed with information, chances to network, leadership development opportunities, and lots more

July

Keris Jan Myrick, President
Kevin B Sullivan, Vice President
Clarence Jordan, Secretary

Audio Video

7711 Managing the Defiant Child
Courage To Change Publishing
PO Box 486
Wilkes-Barres, PA 18703   800-440-4003
Fax: 800-772-6499
www.couragetochange.com

An information-packed video brings to life a proven approach to behavior management. Shows clinicians, school practitioners, teachers, parents and students how enhanced parenting skills can dramatically improve the parent-child relationship.

Russell A Barkley, Editor

7712 Understanding and Treating the Hereditary Psychiatric Spectrum Disorders

Hope Press
PO Box 188
Duarte, CA 91009

818-303-0644
800-321-4039
Fax: 818-358-3520
hopepress.com

Learn with ten hours of audio tapes from a two day seminar given in May 1997 by David E Comings MD. Tapes cover: ADHD, Tourette syndrome, Obsessive-Compulsive Disorder, Conduct Disorder, Oppositional Defiant Disorder, Autism and other Hereditary Psychiatric Spectrum Disorders. Eight audio tapes.

David E Comings, MD, Presenter

7713 Understanding the Defiant Child

Courage To Change
PO Box 486
Wilkes-Barres, PA 18703

800-440-4003
Fax: 800-772-6499
www.couragetochange.com

Provides a vivid picture of what we know about Oppositional Defiant Disorder and presents real-life scenes of family interactions and commentary from parents. Illuminates the nature and causes of ODD, why it should be dealt with early, and what can be done. Ideal viewing for school practitioners, clinical child psychologists, counselors and parents coping with a defiant child.

Russell A Barkley, Editor

Web Sites

7714 ADDitude
www.additudemag.com

Founded in 1998 by Ellen Kingsley, an award-winning journalist with a unique ability to convey credible information with empathy and inspiration, ADDitude magazine has provided clear, accurate, user-friendly information and advice from the leading experts and practitioners in mental health and learning for almost 10 years.

Susan Caughman, Publisher
Wayne Kalyn, Editor

7715 BookRags
www.bookrags.com

BookRags was founded in 1999 by two recent college graduates interested in providing on-demand educational resources to students around the world. Launched with just 40 book notes, BookRags has expanded over the past seven years into one of the largest, most respected student education websites, with over 4 million unique pages of content.

7716 Child Welfare Information Gateway
www.childwelfare.gov

Child Welfare Information Gateway promotes the safety, permanency, and well-being of children, youth, and families by connecting child welfare, adoption, and related professionals as well as the public to information, resources, and tools covering topics on child welfare, child abuse and neglect, out-of-home care, adoption, and more.

7717 Circle of Parents
www.circleofparents.org

Circle of Parents provides a friendly, supportive environment led by parents and other caregivers. It's a place where anyone in a parenting role can openly discuss the successes and challenges of raising children. Where they can find and share support.

Julie Rivnak-McAdam, CEO

7718 Conductdisorders.com
www.conductdisorders.com

Site for parents, teachers, and family members who deal with a child with one of the defined behavioral disorders.

7719 Empowering Parents
www.empoweringparents.com

Empowering Parents has been giving the readers straight talk and real results since 2007. They are committed to providing parents and caregivers with sound advice using the same Cognitive Behavioral Therapy principles that The Total Transformation and there other programs are based upon.

Elisabeth Wilkins, Editor

7720 Enough Is Enough
www.enough.org

The Enough Is Enoughr mission is to Make the Internet Safer for Children and Families. EIE is dedicated to continuing to raise public awareness about online dangers, specifically the dangers of Internet pornography and sexual predators.

Dee Jepsen, President Emeritus
Donna Rice Hughes, President and CEO

7721 FRIENDS
friendsnrc.org

FRIENDS, the National Center for Community-Based Child Abuse Prevention (CBCAP), provides training and technical assistance to Federally funded CBCAP Programs. This site serves as a resource to those programs and to the rest of the Child Abuse Prevention community.

Linda Baker, Program Director
Dr. Valerie Spiva Collins, Training/ Technical Assis Sup.
Casandra Firman, Technical Assistance Coordinator

7722 Find Counseling.com
www.findcounseling.com

Since inception in 1996, the Find Counseling.com Network is a resource for those in need of mental health services. They enable users to find the therapist who is right for them.

7723 FindYouthInfo.gov
www.findyouthinfo.gov

FindYouthInfo.gov is the U.S. government Web site that helps you create, maintain, and strengthen effective youth programs.

7724 Guide to Psychology and its Practice (A)
www.guidetopsychology.com

This website provides freewill information about the practice of Clinical Psychology, especially in regard to psychotherapy, counseling, self-growth, and mental health in general.

Raymond Lloyd Richmond, Ph.D., Author

7725 Helpguide.org
www.helpguide.org

Guide for improving mental and emotional health.

Robert Segal, M.A., Publisher/ Managing Director
Jeanne Segal, Ph.D., Publisher/ Editorial Director
Melinda Smith, M.A., Senior Editor

7726 Internet Mental Health
www.mentalhealth.com

internetmentalhealth@shaw.ca
www.mentalhealth.com

Our goal is to improve understanding, diagnosis, and treatment of mental illness throughout the world.

Phillip W. Long, M.D., Psychiatrist

7727 NADD: National Association for the Dually Diagnosed

132 Fair Street
Kingston, NY 12401

845-331-4336
800-331-5362
Fax: 845-331-4569
info@thenadd.org
www.thenadd.org

Nonprofit organization designed to promote the interests of professional and care providers for individuals who have the coexistence of mental illness and mental retardation. NADD provides conferences, educational services and training materials to professionals, parents, concerned citizens and service organizations.

Dr Robert Fletcher, CEO
Michelle Jordan, Office Manager
Edward Seliger, Project Coordinator

7728 Online Mendelian Inheritance in Man
National Library of Medicine, Building 38A
Bethesda, MD 20894
888-346-3656
info@ncbi.nlm.nih.gov
www.ncbi.nlm.nih.gov

This database is a catalog of human genes and genetic disorders.

Christine E. Seidman, M.D., Chair
David J. Lipman, M.D., Executive Secretary

7729 Online Parenting Coach
www.onlineparentingcoach.com

A resource for children, parents, teachers, mental health professionals, and others who deal with the challenges of Oppositional Defiant Disorder, Conduct Disorder, ADHD and other childhood disorders.

7730 ParentsMedGuide.org
www.parentsmedguide.org

Resources for parents developed by the American Psychiatric Association and the American Academy of Child and Adolescent Psychiatry.

7731 Planetpsych
www.planetpsych.com

webmaster@PlanetPsych.com
www.planetpsych.com

Planetpsych is an online resource for mental health information.

7732 Psych Central
psychcentral.com

Since 1995, an award-winning website has been run by mental health professionals offering reliable, trusted information and over 200 support groups to consumers.

John M. Grohol, Psy.D., CEO/ Founder/ Editor-in-Chief
Rick Nauert, Ph.D., Senior News Editor
Bailey Apple, Associate Editor, Newsletters

7733 PsychAlive
www.psychalive.org

PsychAlive draws on the contribution of leading psychology experts who specialize in a broad spectrum of subjects related to our emotional well-being.

7734 StopBullying.gov
www.stopbullying.gov

StopBullying.gov provides information from various government agencies on what bullying is, what cyberbullying is, who is at risk, and how you can prevent and respond to bullying.

7735 The Successful Parent
www.thesuccessfulparent.com

The impetus for The Successful Parent comes from 60 years of combined experience in providing psychotherapy for parents, children, and families.

7736 Violence Prevention Works
www.violencepreventionworks.org

7737 Violentkids.com
www.violentkids.com

Dr. Helen Smith

7738 domesticshelters.org
www.domesticshelters.org

A searchable directory of domestic violence service providers in the United States providing users the ability to find services best suited to their needs and providing domestic violence providers with invaluable online resources.

Book Publishers

7739 Aggression and Violence Throughout the Life Span
Sage Publications
2455 Teller Road
Thousand Oaks, CA 91320
800-818-7243
Fax: 800-583-2665
info@sagepub.com
www.sagepub.com

A unique life span developmental perspective on some of society's most perplexing and pernicious problems, aggressive and violent behaviors. Examines issues in the development of aggressive behaviors in young children, the progression of these behaviors to older children and adolescents and cause, effect and treatment of aggressive and violent behaviors in adults. Integrates empirical research with clinical applications.

360 pages Softcover
ISBN: 0-803945-51-5

Sara Miller McCune, Founder/Chairman
Blaise R Simqu, President/CEO
Chris Hickok, Senior Vice President/CFO

7740 Antisocial Behavior by Young People
Cambridge University Press
32 Avenue of the Americas
New York, NY 10013
617-264-2300
Fax: 617-264-2323
info@cambridge.com
www.cambridge.org

Written by a child psychiatrist, a criminologist and a social psychologist, this book is a major international review of research evidence on anti-social behavior. Covers all aspects of the field, including descriptions of different types of delinquency and time trends, the state of knowledge on the individuals, social-psychological and cultural factors involved and recent advances in prevention and intervention.

490 pages Paperback
ISBN: 0-521646-08-1

Michael Rutter, Editor
Ann Hagell, Editor
Henri Giller, Editor

7741 Conduct Disorders in Childhood and Adolescence (Developmental Clinical)
Sage Publications
2455 Teller Road
Thousand Oaks, CA 91320
800-818-7243
800-818-7243
Fax: 800-583-2665
info@sagepub.com
www.sagepub.com

Conduct disorder is a clinical problem among children and adolescents that includes aggressive acts, theft, vandalism, firesetting, running away, truancy, defying authority and other antisocial behaviors. This book describes the nature of conduct disorder and what is currently known from research and clinical work. Topics include psychiatric diagnosis, parent psychopathology and child-rearing processes.

192 pages Hardcover
ISBN: 0-803971-81-8

Sara Miller McCune, Founder/Chairman
Blaise R Simqu, President/CEO
Chris Hickok, Senior Vice President/CFO

7742 Conduct Disorders in Children and Adolescents
American Psychiatric Publishing
1000 Wilson Boulevard, Suite 1825
Arlington, VA 22009
703-907-7322
800-368-5777
Fax: 703-907-1091
appi@psych.org
www.appi.org

Examines the phenomenology, etiology, and diagnosis of conduct disorders, and describes therapeutic and preventive interventions. Includes the range of treatments now available, including individual, family, group, and behavior therapy; hospitalization; and residential treatment.

1995 414 pages Hardcover
ISBN: 0-880485-17-5

G Pirooz Sholevar, MD, Editor

7743 Conduct Problem/Emotional Problem Interventions: A Holistic Perspective
Slosson Educational Publications
PO Box 544
East Aurora, NY 14052

716-625-0930
888-756-7766
Fax: 800-655-3840
slosson@slosson.com
www.slosson.com

This innovative book is broad in scope and addresses the now what sensation that many professionals get when charged with the education or treatment of individuals with conduct disorders or emotional disturbance. Distinct intervention and screening strategies and patient involvement strategies are offered in clear and practical terms.

Edward J Kelly, Editor

7744 Disruptive Behavior Disorders in Children and Adolescents
Robert L Hendren, DO, author

American Psychiatric Publishing
1000 Wilson Boulevard, Suite 1825
Arlington, VA 22209

703-907-7322
800-368-5777
Fax: 703-907-1091
appi@psych.org
www.appi.org

Discusses attention deficit hyperactivity disorder, conduct disorder, substance abuse and disruptive behavior disorders. Examines the relationship between violence and mental illness in adolescence.

1999 216 pages Paperback
ISBN: 0-880489-60-7

7745 Preventing Antisocial Behavior: Interventions
Guilford Press
72 Spring Street
New York, NY 10012

212-431-9800
800-365-7006
Fax: 212-966-6708
info@guilford.com
www.guilford.com

Establishes the crucial link between theory, measurement and intervention. Brings together a collection of studies that utilize experimental approaches for evaluating intervention programs, both the feasibility, and necessity of independent evaluation. Also shows how the information obtained in such studies can be used to test and refine prevailing theories about human behavior in general, and behavior changes in particular.

1992 391 pages
ISBN: 0-898628-82-1

Joan McCord, Editor
Richard Tremblay, Editor

7746 Skills Training for Children with Behavior Disorders
Courage To Change
PO Box 486
Wilkes-Barres, PA 18703

800-440-4003
Fax: 800-772-6499
www.couragetochange.com

Designed for use by both parents and therapists, provides background information, step-by-step instructions and many useful, reproducible worksheets. Techniques offered help children with anger management, compliance and following rules, academic success, emotional well-being and self-esteem and much more.

272 pages

Michael L Bloomquist, Editor

Journals

7747 Best Practices of Youth Violence Prevention
4770 Buford Hwy, NE Mail Stop MS F-63
Atlanta, GA 30341

800-232-4636
TTY: 888-232-6348
www.cdc.gov/injury

Timothy N. Thornton, M.P.A., Editor
Carole A. Craft, Editor
Linda L. Dahlberg, Ph.D., Editor

7748 Children, Adolescents, and Media Violence
2455 Teller Road
Thousand Oaks, CA 91320

800-818-7243
Fax: 800-583-2665
marketingservices@sagepub.com
www.sagepub.com

This revised text provides updates that reflect new findings in the field of media violence research during childhood and adolescence

Steven J. Kirsh, Author

7749 Disruptive Behavior Disorders in Children
1000 Wilson Boulevard, Suite 1825
Arlington, VA 22209

703-907-7322
800-368-5777
Fax: 703-907-1091
appi@psych.org
www.appi.org

The authors look at three subtypes of attention-deficit/hyperactivity disorder (ADHD), conduct disorder, and oppositional defiant disorder, all of which are common among youths and often share similar symptoms of impulse control problems.

John M. Oldham, M.D., M.S., Series Editor
Michelle B. Riba, M.D., M.S., Series Editor
Robert L. Hendren, D.O., Editor

7750 Electronic Media and Youth Violence - A CDC Issue Brief
4770 Buford Hwy, NE Mail Stop MS F-63
Atlanta, GA 30341

800-232-4636
TTY: 888-232-6348
www.cdc.gov/injury

Electronic Media and Youth Violence: A CDC Issue Brief for Educators and Caregivers focuses on the phenomena of electronic aggression.

Marci Feldman Hertz, M.S, Co-Author
Corinne David-Ferdon, Ph.D., Co-Author

7751 Facts for Families
3615 Wisconsin Avenue, N.W.
Washington, DC 20016

202-966-7300
Fax: 202-966-2891
clinical@aacap.org
www.aacap.org

AACAP's Facts for Families provide concise and up-to-date information on issues that affect children, teenagers, and their families.

7752 Handbook of Children and the Media
2455 Teller Road
Thousand Oaks, CA 91320

800-818-7243
Fax: 800-583-2665
marketingservices@sagepub.com
www.sagepub.com

Cyber-bullying, sexting, and the effects that violent video games have on children are widely discussed and debated.

Dorothy G. Singer, Co-Author
Jerome L. Singer, Co-Author

7753 Helping Kids in Crisis: Managing Emergencies in Children & Adolescents
1000 Wilson Boulevard, Suite 1825
Arlington, VA 22209   703-907-7322
                            800-368-5777
                        Fax: 703-907-1091
                          appi@psych.org
                           www.appi.org

7754 Journal of Abnormal Child Psychology
University of Washington, Child Health Institute,
Seattle, WA 98195   206-543-1538
                        Fax: 206-616-4623
                           annv@uw.edu
                            isrcap.org

The Journal of Abnormal Child Psychology brings together the latest research on psychopathology in childhood and adolescence, with an emphasis on empirical studies of the major childhood disorders.

7755 Measuring Bullying Victimization, Perpetration and Bystander Experiences
4770 Buford Hwy, NE Mail Stop MS F-63
Atlanta, GA 30341   800-232-4636
                        TTY: 888-232-6348
                         www.cdc.gov/injury

This compendium provides researchers, prevention specialists, and health educators with tools to measure a range of bullying experiences: bully perpetration, bully victimization, bully-victim experiences, and bystander experiences.

Merle E. Hamburger, PhD, Editor
Kathleen C. Basile, PhD, Editor
Alana M. Vivolo, MPH, CHES, Editor

7756 Measuring Violence-Related Attitudes, Behaviors and Influences
4770 Buford Hwy, NE Mail Stop MS F-63
Atlanta, GA 30341   800-232-4636
                        TTY: 888-232-6348
                         www.cdc.gov/injury

This compendium provides researchers and prevention specialists with a set of tools to assess violence-related beliefs, behaviors, and influences, as well as to evaluate programs to prevent youth violence.

Linda L. Dahlberg, PhD, Editor
Susan B. Toal, MPH, Editor
Monica H. Swahn, PhD, Editor

7757 Media Violence and Children: A Complete Guide
130 Cremona Drive
Santa Barbara, CA 93117   805-968-1911
                                800-368-6868
                            Fax: 866-270-3856
                    CustomerService@abc-clio.com
                           www.abc-clio.com

Stripping away the hype, this book describes how, when, and why media violence can influence children of different ages, giving parents and teachers the power to maximize the media's benefits and minimize its harm.

Douglas A. Gentile, Editor

7758 Media and Youth: A Developmental Perspective
111 River Street
Hoboken, NJ 07030   201-748-6000
                        Fax: 201-748-6088
                           info@wiley.com
                           www.wiley.com

Media & Youth: A Developmental Perspective provides a comprehensive review and critique of the research and theoretical literature related to media effects on infants, children, and adolescents, with a unique emphasis on development.

Steven J. Kirsh, Author

7759 Peer Violence Among Teenagers: Trends in Violence
295 Madison Avenue, 40th Floor
New York, NY 10017   212-867-5777
                        Fax: 212-867-5844
                          info@fcd-us.org
                            fcd-us.org

This report raises key questions and highlights an urgent need for further research to address current issues.

Kenneth C. Land, Author

7760 Technology and Youth - Protecting Your Child
4770 Buford Hwy, NE Mail Stop MS F-63
Atlanta, GA 30341   800-232-4636
                        TTY: 888-232-6348
                         www.cdc.gov/injury

This tipsheet provides an overview of electronic aggression, any type of harassment or bullying that occurs through e-mail, a chat room, instant messaging, a website (including blogs), or text messaging. It provides parents and caregivers with strategies for protecting children from this type of violence.

7761 Violence in the Media: A Reference Handbook
130 Cremona Drive
Santa Barbara, CA 93117   805-968-1911
                                800-368-6868
                            Fax: 866-270-3856
                    CustomerService@abc-clio.com
                           www.abc-clio.com

From the popular video game Mortal Kombat to reality TV, this book offers a candid compilation of the history, problems, impacts, and solutions relating to media violence.

Nancy Signorielli, PhD, Author

7762 Your Adolescent
3615 Wisconsin Avenue, N.W.
Washington, DC 20016   202-966-7300
                          Fax: 202-966-2891
                          clinical@aacap.org
                            www.aacap.org

David Pruitt M.D., Author

Pamphlets

7763 Conduct Disorder in Children and Adolescents
National Mental Health Information Center
PO Box 42557
Washington, DC 20015   800-789-2647
                          Fax: 240-747-5470
                           TDD: 866-889-2647
                        ken@mentalhealth.org
                      www.mentalhealth.samhsa.gov

This fact sheet defines conduct disorder, identifies risk factors, discusses types of help available, and suggests what parents or other caregivers can do.

1997 2 pages

7764 Mental, Emotional, and Behavior Disorders in Children and Adolescents
National Mental Health Information
PO Box 42557
Washington, DC 20015   240-747-5484
                              800-789-2647
                          Fax: 240-747-5470
                      mentalhealth.samhsa.gov

This fact sheet describes mental, emotional, and behavioral problems that can occur during childhood and adolescence and discusses related treatment, support services, and research.

4 pages

7765 Treatment of Children with Mental Disorder
National Institute of Mental Health
PO Box 5801
Bethesda, MD 20824

301-496-5751
800-352-9424
Fax: 301-443-4279
TTY: 301-443-8431
nimhinfo@nih.gov
www.nimh.nih.gov

A short booklet that contains questions and answers about therapy for children with mental disorders. Includes a chart of mental disorders and medications used.

Walter J. Koroshetz, M.D., Acting Director
Alan L. Willard, Ph.D., Acting Deputy Director
Caroline Lewis, Executive Officer

7766 Understanding Bullying - Fact Sheet
4770 Buford Hwy, NE Mail Stop MS F-63
Atlanta, GA 30341

800-232-4636
TTY: 888-232-6348
www.cdc.gov/injury

7767 Understanding School Violence Fact Sheet
4770 Buford Hwy, NE Mail Stop MS F-63
Atlanta, GA 30341

800-232-4636
TTY: 888-232-6348
www.cdc.gov/injury

This fact sheet provides an overview of school violence.

7768 Understanding Youth Violence: Fact Sheet
4770 Buford Hwy, NE Mail Stop MS F-63
Atlanta, GA 30341

800-232-4636
TTY: 888-232-6348
www.cdc.gov/injury

This 2-page fact sheet provides a basic overview of youth violence. It is intended for the general public.

Camps

7769 Adventure Learning Center Camp Programs
Eagle Village
4507 170th Avenue
Hersey, MI 49639

231-832-2234
800-748-0061
Fax: 231-832-1468
summercamp@eaglevillage.org
www.eaglevillage.org

Offers a variety of fun camp experiences for children, including those with emotional and/or behavioral impairments. A low staff-to-camper ratio and exciting, challenging activities make the camps rewarding experiences. As funding is available, we will offer camp scholarships to eligible participants.

Sara Kofal, Camp Director

7770 Life Adventure Center
Life Adventure Center of the Bluegrass
PO Box 447
Versailles, KY 40383

859-873-3271
Fax: 859-873-2410
www.lifeadventurecamp.org

A unique experience of discovery and development where life-long lessons are learned. Through purposeful play, using a combination of physical and mental problem-solving exercises, participants engage in opportunities to make positive choices, gain self-confidence, improve decision making, build on group strengths and much more.

7771 Talisman Summer Camps
Talisman Schools
64 Gap Creek Road
Zirconia, NC 28790

855-588-8254
Fax: 828-669-2521
summer@talismancamps.com
www.talismansummercamp.com/

Camps for children ages 6 to 17 and young adults 18-21 with LD, ADD and ADHD, Asperger's Syndrome, and high functioning autism. Talisman has been offering such experiences since 1980 and is ACA accredited. The unique summer camps specialize in creating camps that offer not only adventure, but learning experiences, for children and teenagers with learning disabilities, attention deficit hyperactivity disorder, Asperger's syndrome and high-functioning autism.

Linda Tatsapaugh, Director
Aaron McGinley, Base Camp Program Manager

DESCRIPTION

7772 WILLIAMS SYNDROME

Synonyms: WBS, Williams-Beuren syndrome, WMS, WS

Involves the following Biologic System(s):

Cardiovascular Disorders,

Genetic/Chromosomal/Syndrome/Metabolic Disorders

Williams syndrome is a genetic disorder characterized by mild growth delays before birth (prenatal growth retardation); growth delays after birth (postnatal growth retardation); mild short stature; characteristic abnormalities of the head and face (craniofacial area); and variable levels of mental deficiency. Unusual features of the head and face may result in a distinctive appearance that becomes more pronounced with advancing age. Characteristic features include a rounded face with full cheeks; full, thick lips and a large mouth that is typically in an open position, prominent ears; flared eyebrows; short eyelid folds (palpebral fissures); and a broad nasal bridge with a wide tip and nostrils that flare forward (anteverted). Dental abnormalities are often present, such as small teeth (hypodontia) with underdeveloped (hypoplastic) tooth enamel. Distinctive abnormalities of the eyes may also occur, including divergence of one eye in relation to the other (strabismus) and an unusual star-like (stellate) pattern in the colored portions of the eyes (irides).

Most children and adults with Williams syndrome also have mild to moderate mental retardation. Affected individuals may have an intelligence quotient (I.Q.) ranging from 80, which is considered the low end of average, to 40, which is considered moderate mental retardation. The average I.Q. is approximately 56, which is considered at the lower end of the range for mild mental retardation. Other findings associated with Williams syndrome may include a short attention span, easy distractibility, a poor relationship between visual stimuli and resultant movements (motor-visual integration skills), and strong general language skills as opposed to general cognitive abilities. Most affected children and adults have a friendly personality and a talkative, outgoing manner of speech.

Some infants and children with Williams syndrome may also have additional physical abnormalities, such as heart defects, musculoskeletal abnormalities, or unusually increased blood calcium levels during infancy (transient infantile hypercalcemia). For example, affected infants may develop narrowing (stenosis) in the area above the valve leading from the lower left-sided pumping chamber (ventricle) of the heart to the main artery (aorta) of the body (supravalvular aortic stenosis); obstruction of normal blood flow from the right ventricle of the heart to the lungs (branch pulmonary stenosis); high blood pressure (hypertension); or other cardiovascular abnormalities including narrowing of the blood vessels to the head and abdominal organs. Musculoskeletal defects may include limited movements of certain joints; abnormal curvature of the spine (e.g., scoliosis, kyphosis, lordosis); and an awkward gait. Some individuals with Williams syndrome also have abnormalities affecting the urinary tract, such as the return flow of urine from the urinary bladder back into a ureter (vesicoureteral reflux), recurrent urinary tract infections, and other findings (e.g., nephrocalcinosis, bladder diverticula). Digestive problems may also occur, including chronic constipation. Depending upon the specific abnormalities present, treatment may include limitation of calcium in and elimination of vitamin D from the diet in those with high levels of calcium in the blood; heart surgery for those with certain structural cardiac defects; and special educational and supportive services, such as physical therapy, individualized educational programs, speech therapy, and occupational therapy. Other treatment is symptomatic and supportive.

Most cases of Williams syndrome appear to occur randomly (sporadically) for unknown reasons; however, some familial cases have been reported. Sporadic and inherited cases of the disorder appear to occur due to missing genetic material (deletion) from genes located next to one another (contiguous genes) on the long arm (q) of chromosome 7 (7q11.23). The syndrome is thought to affect approximately one in 10,000 newborns.

Government Agencies

7773 NIH/ Eunice Kennedy Shriver National Institute of Child Health & Human Development

31 Center Drive, Building 31
Bethesda, MD 20892

301-496-5113
800-370-2943
Fax: 866-760-5947
TTY: 888-320-6942
nichdpress@mail.nih.gov
www.nichd.nih.gov

Established in 1962 by congress, today the institute conducts and supports research on topics related to the health of children, adults, families and populations. Some of these topics include: developmental disabilities, growth and development, infant death, reproductive health and birth defects.

Diana W. Bianchi, Director
Paul Williams, Director, Communications

National Associations & Support Groups

7774 American Academy of Pediatrics

141 Northwest Point Boulevard
Elk Grove Village, IL 60007

847-434-4000
800-433-9016
Fax: 847-434-8000
www.aap.org

The American Academy of Pediatrics and its member pediatricians are committed to the attainment of optimal physical, mental and social health and well-being for all infants, children, adolescents, and young adults.

Fernando Stein, MD, FAAP, President
Karen Remley, MD, CEO/Executive VP

7775 Cincinnati Center for Developmental & Behavioral Pediatrics

Cincinnati Children's Hospital Medical Center
3333 Burnet Avenue, MLC 4002
Cincinnati, OH 45229

513-636-4200
800-344-2462
Fax: 513-636-7361
TTY: 513-636-4900
tics@cchmc.org
www.cincinnatichildrens.org

Cincinnati Center for Developmental Disorders provides diagnosis, evaluation, treatment, training and education for infants, children and adolescents with a variety of developmental disorders.

Patricia M. Manning-Courtney, MD, Co-Director
Susan E. Wiley, MD, Co-Director

7776 Genetic Alliance

4301 Connecticut Avenue NW, Suite 404
Washington, DC 20008

202-966-5557
800-336-4363
Fax: 202-966-8553
info@geneticalliance.org
www.geneticalliance.org

A coalition of voluntary genetic support groups, consumers and professionals addressing the needs of individuals and families affected by genetic disorders from a national perspective.

Sharon Terry, President/CEO
Tetyana Murza, Managing Director
Natasha Bonhomme, VP, Strategic Development

7777 Williams Syndrome Association
570 Kirts Blvd, #223
Troy, MI 48084
284-244-2229
800-806-1871
Fax: 248-244-2230
info@williams-syndrome.org
www.williams-syndrome.org

Devoted to improving the lives of individuals with Williams Syndrome and their families. The WSA supports research into all facets of the syndrome, and the development of the most up to date educational materials regarding Williams Syndrome.

Deborah Payne, President
Anthony Vecchia, Vice President
Terry Monkaba, Executive Director

7778 Williams Syndrome Foundation
University of California
Irvine, CA 92697
949-240-1400
hlenhoff@uci.edu
www.wsf.org

The WSF offers support for those affected with the condition through opportunities in education, housing, employment and recreation.

William Lane, Treasurer/President
Patrick S Smith, Secretary

Research Centers

7779 Patient Recruitment & Public Liaison Office Clinical Center
10 Cloister Court, Building 61
Bethesda, MD 20892
800-411-1222
Fax: 301-480-9793
TTY: 866-411-1010
prpl@mail.cc.nih.gov
www.cc.nih.gov

The NIH Clinical Center is a federally funded biomedical research facility that supports clinical investigations conducted by the institutes of the National Institute of Health.

Martin Blaser, MD, Chair
Peter Markell, Vice Chair
Robert S. Balaban, PhD, Vice Chair

Web Sites

7780 Healthfinder
1101 Wootton Parkway
Rockville, MD 20852
healthfinder@hhs.gov
www.healthfinder.gov

A guide for health information.

Dr. Wright, Chief Medical Advisor

7781 Kansas University Medical Center
3901 Rainbow Boulevard
Kansas City, KS 66160
913-588-5000
dgirod@kumc.edu
www.kumc.edu

A nationally recognized biomedical research center, offers educational programs through its Schools of Allied Health, Medicine, Nursing, Pharmacy and Graduate Studies.

Doug Girod, MD, Executive Vice Chancellor
Richard J. Barohn, MD, Vice Chancellor for Research
Natalie Lutz, Communications Director

7782 Lili Claire Foundation
3540 West Sahara Ave., #182
Las Vegas, NV 89102
702-862-8141
Staff@LiliClaire.org
www.liliclairefoundation.org/

Helps to ease the challenges families face by providing a unique and comprehensive blend of programs and support services.

Leslie Litt, Founder
Keith Resnick, Co-Founder
Lydia Murphy, Board Member

7783 Online Mendelian Inheritance in Man
www.omim.org

This database is a catalog of human genes and genetic disorders.

7784 Rare Genetic Diseases in Children (NYU)
550 First Avenue
New York, NY 10016
212-263-7300
www.med.nyu.edu/rgdc/homenow.htm

We target issues arising from rare genetic diseases affecting children, and to assist in the endeavor to bring knowledge and hope to those for whom there is, at present, so little.

Kenneth G. Langone, Chair
Laurence D. Fink, Co-Chair
Robert I. Grossman, MD, Dean & CEO

7785 Williams Syndrome Foundation Home Page
www.williamssyndrome.org/

Seeks to create or enhance opportunities in education, housing, employment and recreation for people who have Willimas Syndrome and other related or similar conditions. The WSF identifies, initiates, funds and provides strategic guidance for major, long range development projects, either by itself, or by cooperating with other organizations.

7786 Williams Syndrome Monthly Medline Alert
www.geocities.com/HotSprings/8172/

Camps

7787 ACM Lifting Lives Music Camp
110 Magnolia Circle
Nashville, TN 37203
615-322-8240
www.acmliftinglives.org

A week-long residential camp designed for people with Williams syndrome and other developmental disabilities who are at least 16 years-old.

Bill Mayne, Chairman of the Board
Lori Badgett, President
Ed Warm, Vice President

7788 Eden Wood Center
Friendship Ventures
6350 Indian Chief Road
Eden Prairie, MN
952-852-0101
800-450-8376
Fax: 952-852-0123
fv@friendshipventures.org
truefriends.org

Offers resident camp programs for children, teenagers and adults with developmental, physical or multiple disabilities, Down Syndrome, special medical conditions, Williams Syndrome, autism and/or other conditions. Fishing, creative arts, golf, sports and other activities are available. Creative Options Respite Care offers weekend camps year round for children, teenagers and adults. Ventures Travel offers guided vacations for teens and adults with developmental disabilities or other unique needs.

Jon Salmon, Director of Programs and Services
Mel Kloek, Program Director
Dawn Brenner, Director of Health Care

DESCRIPTION

7789 WILMS TUMOR

Synonyms: Nephroblastoma, Renal Tumor, Kidney Tumor

Involves the following Biologic System(s):

Hematologic and Oncologic Disorders

Wilms tumor (also known as nephroblastoma) is a rare malignant tumor of the kidney that accounts for about 8% of childhood cancers. It typically develops at about the age of 3 years and rarely after age 8, and occurs with equal frequency among males and females. Wilms tumor may develop in any region of either kidney. In most cases the tumor develops in only one kidney (unilateral). However, both kidneys may be involved (bilateral) in about 5-10% of affected children. In some severe cases the tumor may spread from the kidney to other parts of the body (metastasize), particularly the lungs.

Wilms tumor typically becomes apparent by approximately 3 to 5 years of age. The most common sign of its presence is a smooth, firm mass in the abdominal area. About 50% of children with Wilms tumor experience associated abdominal pain or vomiting (emesis), and about 10-25% have blood in their urine (microscopic or gross hematuria). Up to 60% of children with Wilms tumor also have high blood pressure (hypertension) caused by pressure exerted by the tumor on the major artery that carries blood to the kidney (renal artery). In severe cases, long-term hypertension may impair the ability of the heart to pump blood effectively through the body (cardiac failure). Other indicators of Wilms tumor may be loss of appetite, weight loss, constipation, and blood in the urine

The exact cause of Wilms tumor is unknown but the tumor is thought to be caused by mutations in genes that normally prevent cells from becoming cancerous and multiplying. These mutations either occur in a seemingly random manner, for unknown reasons (sporadic) in children who develop Wilms tumor, or can be inherited in an autosomal dominant manner, which means from only one parent.. In most instances, Wilms tumor begins to develop before birth, in cells destined to develop into normal kidney tissue.

Treatment for Wilms tumor is based on the stage of this cancer, or degree to which it has progressed, and whether its histology (appearance of the tumor tissue under the microscope) indicates a likelihood of rapid tumor growth or less aggressive growth. Treatment typically begins with surgical removal of the affected kidney (nephrectomy). During surgery, the remaining kidney is examined to determine whether it too contains any tumor. Treatment after surgery for Wilms tumor may consist of chemotherapy, in which drugs are used to destroy any residual tumor that may not have been removed surgically, and radiation therapy, in which X-rays or other sources of radioactivity are used to destroy residual tumor.In children with Wilms tumor in both kidneys, chemotherapy and radiation therapy may be given before surgical removal of their tumors. Children in whom both kidneys must be removed to eliminate Wilms tumors will require periodic, intermittent kidney dialysis to rid their bodies of toxic wastes, a need that usually continues for life.

Government Agencies

7790 Cancer Information Service

National Cancer Institute
9609 Medical Center Drive
Bethesda, MD 20892

800-422-6237
Fax: 301-330-7968
TTY: 800-332-8615
www.cancer.gov

The Cancer Information Service provides the latest and most accurate cancer information to patients, their families, the public, and health professionals. Through its network of regional offices, the CIS serves the United States, Puerto Rico, the U.S. Virgin Islands, and the Pacific Islands.

Andrew C Von Eschenback, Director
Harold Varmus, M.D, Director

7791 NIH/National Cancer Institute

BG 9609 / 9609 Medical Center Drive
Bethesda, MD 20892

800-422-6237
www.cancer.gov

The National Cancer Institute coordinates the National Cancer Program, which conducts and supports research, training, health information dissemination, and other programs with respect to the cause, diagnosis, prevention, and treatment of cancer, rehabilitation from cancer, and the continuing care of cancer patients and the families of cancer patients.

Douglas R. Lowy, MD, Acting Director
James Doroshow, MD, Deputy Director
Henry P. Ciolino, PhD, Acting Director, Cancer Centers

National Associations & Support Groups

7792 American Academy of Pediatrics

141 Northwest Point Boulevard
Elk Grove Village, IL 60007

847-434-4000
800-433-9016
Fax: 847-434-8000
www.aap.org

The American Academy of Pediatrics and its member pediatricians are committed to the attainment of optimal physical, mental and social health and well-being for all infants, children, adolescents, and young adults.

Fernando Stein, MD, FAAP, President
Karen Remley, MD, CEO/Executive VP

7793 American Cancer Society

250 Williams Street NW
Atlanta, GA 30303

404-315-1123
800-227-2345
Fax: 404-315-9348
angelina.veal@cancer.org
www.cancer.org

The American Cancer Society is a nationwide, community-based voluntary health organization. Headquartered in Atlanta, Georgia, the ACS has state divisions and more than 3,400 local offices. For more than 80 years, ACS has led the way in cancer research. The goal is to prevent cancer, save lives, and diminish suffering from cancer.

Gary M. Reedy, Chair
Robert E. Youle, Vice Chair
Vincent T. DeVita, President

7794 American Childhood Cancer Organization (fo rmerly Candlelighters Childhood Cancer)

PO Box 498
Kensington, MD 20895

301-962-3520
800-366-2226
Fax: 310-962-3521
staff@acco.org
www.acco.org

The Candlelighters Childhood Cancer Foundation National Office was founded in 1970 by concerned parents of children with cancer. Today our membership of over 50,000 members of the national office and more than 100,000 members across the across the country, including Candlelighters affiliate groups, includes, parents of children who are being treated or have been treated for cancer.

Ruth I. Hoffman, MPH, Executive Director
Jessica DiBenedetto, Program Coordinator
Christy Perry, Director, Marketing/Communications

7795 CancerCare
275 7th Avenue, Floor 22
New York, NY 10001
212-712-8400
800-813-4673
Fax: 212-712-8495
info@cancercare.org
www.cancercare.org

CancerCare is a national nonprofit, 501(c)(3) organization that provides free, professional support services to anyone affected by cancer: people with cancer, caregivers, children, loved ones, and the bereaved. CancerCare programs - including counseling and support groups, education, financial assistance and practical help - are provided by professional oncology social workers and are completely free of charge.

Patricia J Goldsmith, CEO
John Rutigliano, Chief Operating Officer
Ahuva Morris, Children's Program Coordinator

7796 Children's Cancer Research Institute
University of Texas Health Science Ctr
8403 Floyd Curl Drive
San Antonio, TX 78229
210-562-9000
Fax: 210-562-9014
rodriguezdr@uthscsa.edu
www.ccri.uthscsa.edu

The Children's Cancer Research Institute was created by the State of Texas with $200 million from the State's tobacco settlement. Fulfilling its legislative mandate, it is CCRI's mission to advance scientific knowledge relevant to childhood cancer, to accelerate the translation of knowledge into novel therapies, and to eliminate cancer at all ages through discovery, development, and dissemination of scientific knowledge relevant to childhood cancer.

Sharon Murphy MD, Director
Gail Tomlinson, Division Chief of Hematology, Oncol

7797 Children's Hopes and Dreams
138 Cloudland Road
Dahlonega, GA 30533
706-482-2248
Fax: 706-482-2289
chdfdover@juno.com
www.helpingnow.org

Children's Hopes & Dreams has been serving children with serious childhood illnesses since 1983. We are one of the oldest wish fulfillment organizations in the world.

Mariann Oswald, Program Director

7798 Children's Hopes and Dreams Foundation
Wish Fulfillment Foundation
138 Cloudland Road
Dahlonega, GA 30533
706-482-2248
Fax: 706-482-2289
chdfdover@juno.com
www.helpingnow.org

Children's Hopes & Dreams Foundation has been serving children with serious childhood illnesses since 1983.

10,000 Members

Mariann Oswald, Program Director

7799 Children's Wish Foundation International
8615 Roswell Road
Atlanta, GA 30350
770-393-9474
800-323-9474
Fax: 770-393-0683
wish@childrenswish.org
www.childrenswish.org

A nonprofit organization that fulfills wishes for children with life threatening illnesses. The criteria for wish fulfillment are: the child must be under the age of eighteen, and have been diagnosed with a life threatening illness.

Arthur Stein, President
Linda Dozoretz, Founder/Executive Director

7800 National Childhood Cancer Foundation
4600 East West Highway, Suite 600
Bethesda, MD 20814
301-718-0042
800-458-6223
Fax: 301-718-0047
info@curesearch.org
www.curesearch.org

CureSearch unites the world's largest childhood cancer research organization, the Children's Oncology Group, and the National Childhood Cancer Foundation through our mission to cure childhood cancer. Research is the key to the cure.

Stuart Siegel, MD, Chairman
Timothy Harmon, Vice Chairman
Stacy Haller, Executive Director

Research Centers

7801 National Wilms Tumor Study
Fred Hutchinson Cancer Research Center
1100 Fairview Ave. N, M2-A876, PO Box 19024
Seattle, WA 98109
206-667-4842
800-553-4878
Fax: 206-667-6623
nwtsg@fhcrc.org
www.nwtsg.org

To improve the survival of children with Wilms tumor and other renal tumors, to study the long-term outcome of children with successfully treated by identifying adverse effects of treatment, to study the epidemiology and biology of Wilms tumor and to make information regarding successful treatment strategies for Wilms tumor available to physicians around the world.

Web Sites

7802 CancerCare
275 Seventh Avenue (between 25th & 26th Streets)
New York, NY 10001
800-813-4673
info@cancercare.org
www.cancercare.org

CancerCare is a national nonprofit, 501(c)(3) organization that provides free, professional support services to anyone affected by cancer: people with cancer, caregivers, children, loved ones, and the bereaved. CancerCare programs - including counseling and support groups, education, financial assistance and practical help - are provided by professional oncology social workers and are completely free of charge.

Patricia J Goldsmith, CEO
John Rutigliano, Chief Operating Officer
Ahuva Morris, Children's Program Coordinator

7803 Children's Cancer Web
www.cancerindex.org/ccw

An independent nonprofit site, established to provide a directory of childhood cancer resources.

7804 OncoLink: The University of Pennslyvania Cancer Center Resource
www.oncolink.upenn.edu/about/index

Mission to help cancer patients, families, health care professionals, and the general public get accurate cencer-related information at no charge.

7805 Online Mendelian Inheritance in Man
www.omim.org

This database is a catalog of human genes and genetic disorders.

Book Publishers

7806 Let's Talk About Going to the Hospital
Rosen Publishing Group's PowerKids Press
29 E 21st Street
New York, NY 10010   212-777-3017
                                   800-237-9932
                              Fax: 888-436-4643
                           senpub@tribeca.ios.com
                           www.powerkidspress.com

If a child has to check into the hospital, chances are he or she is already upset about being ill. Knowing how a hospital functions and what the procedures are, such as when family members can visit, will help in what is already a stressful situation. Grades K-5.

24 pages
ISBN: 0-823950-36-0

7807 Let's Talk About When Kids Have Cancer

Melanie Apel Gordon, author

Rosen Publishing Group's PowerKids Press
29 E 21st Street
New York, NY 10010   212-777-3017
                                   800-237-9932
                              Fax: 888-436-4643
                        customerservice@rosenpub.com
                           www.powerkidspress.com

In a straightforward yet comforting way, this book explains what cancer is, what kinds of treatments surround the disease and how to cope if a child or the friend of a child has cancer.

24 pages Paperback
ISBN: 0-823951-95-2

7808 Surviving Childhood Cancer: A Guide for Families
New Harbinger Publications
5674 Shattuck Avenue
Oakland, CA 94609   510-652-0215
                                   800-748-6273
                              Fax: 800-652-1613
                     customerservice@newharbinger.com
                           www.newharbinger.com

Cancer in a child is an overwhelming experience for a family. This book explains common medical procedures and offers readers practical advice about how to cope with emotions and stress during this time.

215 pages Paperback
ISBN: 1-572241-02-0

Camps

7809 Arizona Camp Sunrise & Sidekicks
PO Box 27872
Tempe, AZ 85285   480-382-8564
                                   928-478-4564
                         melissa@azcampsunrise.org
                           www.azcampsunrise.org

The camp is dedicated to provide an exciting, medically safe camp program for children whose families have been affected by cancer.

Melissa Lee, Camp Director

7810 Camp Catch-A-Rainbow
American Cancer Society
1205 E Saginaw Street
Lansing, MI 800-A   517-371-2920
                        kwilson@ymcastorercamps.org
                www.ymcastorercamps.org/ccar/camp-catch-a-rainbow/

Open to any child (age 7 thru 15) who has, or has had, cancer.

Becky Spencer, Vice President of Camping
Angela Hayner, Program Director
Katie Wilson, Coordinator

7811 Camp Sunshine Dreams
PO Box 28232
Fresno, CA 93729   contact@campsunshinedreams.com
                          www.campsunshinedreams.com

Summer camp for children with cancer.

Anthony Aiello, Board Member
Jeff Clem, Board Member
Pam Aiello, Board Member

7812 Okizu Foundation Camps
16 Digital Drive, Suite 130
Novato, CA 94949   415-382-9083
                              Fax: 415-382-8384
                                   info@okizu.org
                                   www.okizu.org

This foundation runs family camp programs for children who have cancer and their families, and for children who have or had a parent with cancer.

Lori Sparrow, Executive Director
Heather Ferrier, Camp Director of Operations

DESCRIPTION

7813 WILSON DISEASE

Synonyms: Hepatolenticular degeneration, WD, WND
Involves the following Biologic System(s):
Gastrointestinal Disorders

Wilson disease is a genetic disorder in which a defect in copper metabolism causes an abnormal accumulation of copper in the liver, brain, kidneys, corneas of the eyes, and other tissues of the body. The disorder is often characterized by progressive liver disease, degenerative changes in the brain, kidney failure, and characteristic grayish-green or reddish-gold rings (Kayser-Fleischer rings) at the outer margins of the corneas. Wilson disease is a progressive disorder, and if untreated can cause severe brain damage, liver failure, and death.

The age at which Wilson disease begins may vary from one patient to another. Symptoms and findings may not become apparent until 5 or 6 years of age and most commonly originate during mid-adolescence. In some patients, however, the disease may not become apparent until adulthood. Wilson disease is thought to occur in about 1 in 30,000 individuals worldwide. Wilson disease that results from alteration (mutation) in a gene that regulates the body's metabolism and handling of copper, with the result that copper accumulates excessively in the liver. Genetically, the disease is defined as an autosomal recessive disorder, meaning that it cannot occurunless the gene that causes it is inherited from both parents.

In Wilson disease, copper progressively collects in the liver and is released into other organs and tissues of the body, particularly the brain, corneas of the eyes, and kidneys. Associated symptoms and findings may be variable, but similar characteristics of the disease are typically observed in members of different generations of families within which the disease tends to occur with a greater than usual frequency.

In Wilson disease, the liver is typically enlarged (hepatomegaly) and may be acutely or chronically inflamed, and this may or may not be accompanied by enlargement of the spleen (splenomegaly). Internal scarring of the liver, as well as the condition known as cirrhosis and abnormalities in liver function, are uncommon in children under 10 years of age with Wilson disease, but do tend to occur in young adults with the disease.

Persons in whom Wilson disease causes cirrhosis may have yellowish discoloration of the skin, mucous membranes, and whites of the eyes (jaundice); unusually high blood pressure (hypertension) the veins that carry blood from the liver (portal hypertension); an abnormal accumulation of fluid in certain body tissues (edema) and in the abdominal cavity (ascites); and enlargement of blood vessels in the wall of the esophagus (esophageal varices), potentially causing them to rupture and bleed. In severe cases, affected individuals may develop fulminant hepatitis, a severe form of liver disease characterized by localized loss of liver tissue (necrosis), defects of blood clotting (coagulation), coma (hepatic encephalopathy), and other potentially life-threatening complications.

Neurologic symptoms associated with Wilson disease occur in about a third of all cases, and can develop suddenly or may occur gradually, but are rare in children under10 years of age. Many such symptoms are thought to result from progressive involvement of a region of the brain (basal ganglia) that assists in regulating muscular movements. Neurologic symptoms often initially include abnormalities of muscle tone (progressive dystonia), muscle stiffness, and rigidity. In addition, persons withWilson disease may experience involuntary, rhythmic, quivering movements of the extremities on one side of the body (unilateral) that may eventually become generalized. Other neurologic symptoms include difficulties in speech (dysphonia), drooling, a fixed smile caused by involuntary drawing back of the upper lip, and involuntary, rapid, jerky movements in association with slow, writhing movements of the limbs, head, and neck (choreoathetosis). Wilson disease may also result in the premature breakdown of red blood cells (hemolysis), which may progress to the chronic condition known as hemolytic anemia. In this type of anemia, premature destruction of red blood cells reduces these cells' transport of oxygen to all of the body's other cells. Wilson disease may also cause the condition known as progressive renal failure, by damaging the ability of the kidneys to maintain a proper balance between the body's water and salt contents, as well as their ability to filter waste products from the blood and excrete these wastes in urine, and to perform other vital functions. Inaddition to these effects, Wilson's disease can produce sudden changes in personality and behavior, which can interfere with a child's social development and performance in school, and are sometimes mistaken for other kinds of psychological problems.

The goal in treating Wilson disease is twofold: to remove excess copper and to prevent the mineral from building up again. This treatment often consists of giving penicillamine, a medication that binds with copper (chelation) and enables it to be excreted from the body. This is accompanied by vitamin B6 to supplement the quantity of this vitamin present in foods. For persons who cannot tolerate penicillamine, the medications trientine and zinc acetate may be appropriate substitutes. Physicians and other health care professionals may also recommend a diet that provides the body with only a small daily quantity of copper (less than 1 mg/day), and may recommend the avoidance of such foods that contain copper, such as chocolate, liver, and nuts. Liver transplantation may be considered for persons with Wilson disease who develop severe, fulminant hepatitis, since this can be life-threatening. Other treatment for Wilson disease is symptomatic and supportive.

National Associations & Support Groups

7814 American Academy of Pediatrics
141 Northwest Point Boulevard
Elk Grove Village, IL 60007

847-434-4000
800-433-9016
Fax: 847-434-8000
www.aap.org

The American Academy of Pediatrics and its member pediatricians are committed to the attainment of optimal physical, mental and social health and well-being for all infants, children, adolescents, and young adults.

Fernando Stein, MD, FAAP, President
Karen Remley, MD, CEO/Executive VP

7815 American Liver Foundation
39 Broadway, Suite 2700
New York, NY 10006
212-668-1000
800-465-4837
Fax: 212-483-8179
info@liverfoundation.org
www.liverfoundation.org

Nonprofit, national voluntary health organization dedicated to the prevention, treatment and cure of hepatitis and other liver diseases through research, education, and advocacy on behalf of those affected by or at risk of liver disease.

Thomas F. Nealon III, Chairman of the Board of Directors/
David Ticker, Chief Financial Officer
Cynthia Gardner, Vice President, Field Development

7816 Children's Liver Alliance
1500 E. Medical Center Drive, SPC 5391
Ann Arbor, MI 48109
734-232-1113
Fax: 734-232-1111
transweb@umich.edu
www.transweb.org

Aids in easing the physical and emotional strains that the child is experiencing, so they can better deal with the disorder through different media resources that are also available to family and friends.

Kathie DeLuca, Office Manager

7817 Children's Liver Association for Support Services
PO Box 15061
Monaca, PA 15061
724-888-2568
info@classkids.org
www.classkids.org

CLASS is an all volunteer, nonprofit organization dedicated to serving the emotional, educational and financial needs of families coping with childhood liver disease and transplantation. Our goal is to be both a service to families and a valuable resource for the medical community.

Diane Sumner, Co-Founder
Mark Sumner, Co-Founder
Aimee Seningen, MD, Treasurer

7818 Genetic Alliance
4301 Connecticut Avenue NW, Suite 404
Washington, DC 20008
202-966-5557
800-336-4363
Fax: 202-966-8553
info@geneticalliance.org
www.geneticalliance.org

A coalition of voluntary genetic support groups, consumers and professionals addressing the needs of individuals and families affected by genetic disorders from a national perspective.

Sharon Terry, President/CEO
Tetyana Murza, Managing Director
Natasha Bonhomme, VP, Strategic Development

7819 United Liver Foundation
5777 W Century Boulevard
Los Angeles, CA 90045
310-670-4624
Fax: 310-670-4672
pbrady@liver411.com
www.liver411.com

A national organization that promotes research and cures for hepatitis and other liver diseases.

Pam Brady, Contact Person
Donna Gracon, Chapter Director

7820 Wilson's Disease Association
5572 North Diversey Blvd
Milwaukee, WI 53217
414-961-0533
866-961-0533
Fax: 330-264-0974
info@wilsondisease.org
www.wilsonsdisease.org

Provides patients and their families with a membership list, e-mail correspondence, meetings for support and education, and a newsletter. Supports patients with financial assistance for medication and travel, and develops centers of excellence.

800 Members
Mary L. Graper, President
Stefanie F. Kaplan, Vice President
Jean P. Perog, Treasurer

Libraries & Resource Centers

7821 National Digestive Diseases Information Clearinghouse
9000 Rockville Pike
Bethesda, MD 20892
301-496-3583
800-860-8747
Fax: 703-738-4929
TTY: 866-569-1162
healthinfo@niddk.nih.gov
www.niddk.nih.govdk.nih.gov

The National Institute of Diabetes and Digestive and Kidney Diseases conducts and supports research on many of the most serious diseases affecting public health. The Institute supports much of the clinical research on the diseases of internal medicine and related subspecialty fields as well as many basic science disciplines.

Dr. Griffin P. Rodgers, Director
Dr. Gregory G. Germino, Deputy Director
Camille M. Hoover, M.S.W., Executive Officer

Research Centers

7822 National Center for the Study of Wilson's Disease
5572 North Diversey Blvd
Milwaukee, WI 53217
414-961-0533
866-961-0533
Fax: 330-264-0974
info@wilsondisease.org
www.wilsonsdisease.org

Mary L. Graper, President
Stefanie F. Kaplan, Vice President
Jean P. Perog, Treasurer

Web Sites

7823 Children's Liver Alliance
www.livertx.org

Offers a fact sheet on liver conditions.

7824 Children's Liver Association for Support Services
www.classkids.org

CLASS is an all volunteer, nonprofit organization dedicated to serving the emotional, educational and financial needs of families coping with childhood liver disease and transplantation. Our goal is to be both a service to families and a valuable resource for the medical community.

7825 Wilson's Disease Association International
5572 North Diversey Blvd.
Milwaukee, WI 53217
414-961-0533
866-961-0533
info@wilsonsdisease.org
www.wilsonsdisease.org

Funds research and facilitates and promotes the identification, education, treatment, and support of patients and other individuals affected by Wilson's Disease.

Mary L. Graper, President
Len Pytlak, Vice President
Carol Terry, Secretary & Founder

7826 Wilson's Disease Patient Information Exchange
www.gourmandizer.com/wilsons/indexx.html

Pages provide Wilson's Disease patients and their families a forum to share and compare their symptoms, treatments and to tell how the disease has affected thier lives.

Newsletters

7827 Children's Liver Alliance Newsletter
University of Michigan Transplant Center, 3868 Tau
Ann Arbor, MI 48109   734-232-1113
                                            Fax: 734-232-1111
                                         transweb@umich.edu
                                           www.transweb.org

Aids in easing the physical and emotional strains that the child is
experiencing, so they can better deal with the disorder through
different media resources that are also available to both friends
and family.

4-12 pages

Kathie DeLuca, Office Manager

Pamphlets

7828 Wilson's Disease
Nat'l Digestive Diseases Information Clearinghouse
9000 Rockville Pike
Bethesda, MD 20892   301-496-3583
                                            Fax: 301-907-8906
                                        nddic@info.niddk.nih.gov
                                           www.niddk.nih.gov

Griffin P. Rodgers, M.D., M.A.C.P., Director
Kevin Abbott, Program Director
Kristin Abraham, Program Director

Government Agencies

7829 Administration on Developmental Disabilities
Department of Health and Human Services
150 S. Independence
W. Philadelphia, PA 19106   215-861-4000
Fax: 215-861-4070
TTY: 202-690-6415
www.acf.hhs.gov

Information and advocacy resources for families and professionals. Includes listings of organizations providing general information and organizations focusing on more specific areas of concern to families and young adults who have disabilities.

Mary Riley, MPH, RN, CPH, Director, Office of Human Services

7830 Agency for Health Care Research
Department of Health and Human Services
540 Gaither Road
Rockville, MD 20850   301-427-1364
Fax: 301-427-1364
www.ahrq.gov

Healthcare information and advocacy resources for families and professionals.

Carolyn M. Clancy, M.D., Director

7831 Centers for Disease Control
Department of Health and Human Services
1600 Clifton Road
Atlanta, GA 30333   404-639-3311
800-232-4636
TTY: 888-232-6348
www.cdc.gov

Federal agency that protects America's health and safety, provides information to guide health decisions, and builds strong partnerships to promote health.

Raymond Strikas, Director
Tom Frieden, MD, MPH, Director, Centers for Disease Contr
Linda C. Degutis, DrPH, MSN, Director, National Center for Injur

7832 Educational Help for the Handicapped
Nat'l Info Center for Children and Youth
PO Box 1492
Washington, DC 20013   800-999-5599

Offers Federal assistance at many levels to enable children, youth and adults to receive education and training. Under the provisions of the Education for All Handicapped Children Act (EHA) of 1975, state and local school districts must provide an appropriate elementary and secondary education for disabled children from age 6 through 21. Presently, some states provide educational and related services for preschool age children.

7833 NIH/ Eunice Kennedy Shriver National Insti tute of Child Health & Human Development
Department of Health and Human Services
31 Center Drive, Building 31
Bethesda, MD 20892   301-496-5113
800-370-2943
Fax: 866-760-5947
TTY: 888-320-6942
nichdpress@mail.nih.gov
www.nichd.nih.gov

The National Institute for Child Health and Human Development conducts and supports laboratory, clinical and epidemiological research on the reproductive, neurobiologic, developmental, and behavioral processes that determine and maintain the health of children, adults, families, and populations.

Diana W. Bianchi, Director
Paul Williams, Director, Communications

7834 NIH/National Cancer Institute
BG 9609 / 9609 Medical Center Drive
Bethesda, MD 20892   800-422-6237
www.cancer.gov

Leads a national effort to reduce the burden of cancer morbidity and mortality and ultimately to prevent the disease. Through basic and clinical biomedical research and training, NCI conducts and supports programs to understand the causes of cancer; prevent, detect, diagnose, treat, and control cancer; and disseminate information to the practitioner, patient, and public.

Douglas R. Lowy, MD, Acting Director
James Doroshow, MD, Deputy Director
Henry P. Ciolino, PhD, Acting Director, Cancer Centers

7835 NIH/National Eye Institute
31 Center Drive MSC 2510
Bethesda, MD 20892   301-496-5248
2020@nei.nih.gov
www.nei.nih.gov

Conducts and supports research that helps prevent and treat eye diseases and other disorders of vision. This research leads to sight-saving treatments, reduces visual impairment and blindness, and improves the quality of life for people of all ages. NEI-supported research has advanced our knowledge of how the eye functions in health and disease.

Paul A Sieving M.D., Ph.D, Director

7836 NIH/National Genome Research Institute (NH GRI)
31 Center Drive, Building 31, Room 4B09
Bethesda, MD 20892   301-402-0911
Fax: 301-402-2218
www.genome.gov

Supports the NIH component of the Human Genome Project, a worldwie research effort designed to analyze the structure of human DNA and determine the location of the estimated 30,000 to 40,000 human genes. The NHGRI Intramural Research Program develops and implements understanding, diagnosing, and treating of genetic diseases.

Alan E. Guttmacher, Director
James. D. Watson, Ph.D., Director
Michael M. Gottesman, M.D., Director

7837 NIH/National Heart, Lung and Blood Institu te
Department of Health and Human Services
31 Center Drive, MSC 2480, Building 31, Room 5A52
Bethesda, MD 20892   301-594-1348
301-480-4907
TTY: 123-019-9912
nhlbiinfo@nhlbi.nih.gov
www.nhlbi.nih.gov

Provides leadership for a national research program in diseases of the heart, blood vessels, lungs, and blood and in transfusion medicine through support of innovative basic, clinical, population-based and health education research. NHLBI also maintains an information clearinghouse.

Gary H Gibbons, MD, Director
Nakela Cook, MD, Chief of Staff

7838 NIH/National Insitute of Allergy and Infectious Diseases
Department of Health and Human Services
6610 Rockledge Drive, MSC 6612
Bethesda, MD 20892   301-496-5717
866-284-4107
Fax: 301-402-3573
TDD: 800-877-8339
ocposfoffice@niaid.nih.gov
www.niaid.nih.gov

NIAID's research strives to understatnd, treat and ultimately prevent the many infectious, immunologic and allergic diseases that threaten millions of American lives.

Anthony S Fauci MD, Director
Hugh Auchincloss, M.D., Principal Deputy Director
John J. McGowan, Ph.D., Deputy Director for Science Managem

7839 NIH/National Institute of Arthritis and Musculoskeletal and Skin Diseases
1 AMS Circle
Bethesda, MD 20892   301-495-4484
                                       877-226-4267
                                  Fax: 301-718-6366
                                  TTY: 301-565-2966
                                  TDD: 301-565-2966
                            niamsinfo@mail.nih.gov
                                www.niams.nih.gov

The mission of the NIAMS, a part of the NIH, is to support research into the causes, treatment, and prevention of arthritis and musculoskeletal and skin diseases, the training of basic and clinical scientists to carry out this research, and the dissemination of information on research progress in these diseases. The Institute also maintains an information clearinghouse.

Stephen I Katz PhD, Director
Robert H Carter MD, Deputy Director

7840 NIH/National Institute of Dental and Crani ofacial Research (NIDCR)
National Institutes of Health
Bldg 31, Rm 9A06, 31 Center Drive, MSC 2560
Bethesda, MD 20892   301-496-4261
                                  Fax: 301-402-2185
                             nidcrinfo@mail.nih.gov
                                www.nidcr.nih.gov

The National Institute of Dental and Craniofacial Research promotes the general health of the American people by improving their oral, dental and craniofacial health. The NIDCR aims to promote health, to prevent diseases and conditions, and to develop new diagnostics and therapeutics.

Dr Martha J. Somerman, Director
John W Kusiak, PhD, Acting Deputy Director
Kathleen G Stephen, Executive Officer

7841 NIH/National Institute of Diabetes and Dig estive and Kidney Diseases
9000 Rockville Pike
Bethesda, MD 20892   301-654-3810
                                  Fax: 301-907-8906
                             niddkinquiries@nih.gov
                                www.niddk.nih.gov

Conducts and supports basic and applied research and provides leadership for a national program in diabetes, endrocrinology, and metabolic diseases; digestive diseases and nutrition and kidney, urologic and hemotologic diseases. Several of these diseases are among the leading causes of disability and death; all seriously affect the quality of life of those who have them. NIDDK also maintains an information clearinghouse.

Griffin P. Rodgers, Director

7842 NIH/National Institute of Mental Health
Department of Health and Human Services
6001 Executive Boulevard, Room 6200, MSC 9663
Bethesda, MD 20892   301-443-4536
                                       866-615-6464
                                  Fax: 301-443-4279
                                  TTY: 301-443-8431
                              nimhinfo@nih.govh.org
                                www.nimh.nih.gov

NIMH provides national leadership dedicated to understanding, treating, and preventing mental illnesses through basic research on the brain and through clinical, epidemiological, and services research.

Joshua Gordon, MD, PhD, Director
Shelli Avenevoli, MD, Deputy Director

7843 NIH/National Institute of Neurological Dis rs and Stroke (NINDS)
PO Box 5801
Bethesda, MD 20824   301-496-5751
                                       800-352-9424
                                  Fax: 301-496-0296
                                  TTY: 301-468-5981
                                www.ninds.nih.gov

Information and advocacy resources for families and professionals. Includes listings of organizations providing general information and organizations focusing on more specific areas of concern to families and young adults who have disabilities.

Walter J. Koroshetz, MD, Director

7844 NIH/National Institute on Alcohol Abuse an d Alcoholism (NIAAA)
5635 Fishers Lane
Bethesda, MD 20892   www.niaaa.nih.gov

NIAAA conducts research focused on improving the treatment and prevention of alcoholism and alcohol-related problems to reduce the enormous social and economic consequences of this disease.

George F. Koob, PhD, Director
Dr Patricia Powell, Acting Deputy Director

7845 NIH/National Institute on Deafness and Oth er Communication Disorders (NIDCD)
31 Center Drive, MSC 2320
Bethesda, MD 20892   301-496-7243
                                       800-241-1044
                                  Fax: 301-402-0018
                                  TTY: 800-241-1055
                              nidcdinfo@nidcd.nih.gov
                                www.nidcd.nih.gov

The National Institute on Deafness and Other Communication Disorders (NIDCD) is a national resource center for health information about hearing, balance, smell, taste, voice, speech, and language for health professionals, patients, industry, and the public.

James F Battey Jr, MD, PhD, Director
Judith A Cooper PhD, Deputy Director
Timothy J Wheeles, Executive Officer

7846 NIH/Office of Rare Diseases (ORD)
Department of Health and Human Services
31 Center Drive, MSC 2082. Room 1B03
Bethesda, MD 20892   301-402-4336
                                      sg18b@nih.gov
                            www.rarediseases.info.nih.gov

Information and advocacy resources for families and professionals. Includes listings of organizations providing general information and organizations focusing on more specific areas of concern to families and young adults who have disabilities.

Stephen Groft, Pharm.D., Director

7847 National Center for Education in Maternal and Child Health
Georgetown University
2115 Wisconsin Ave NW, Suite 601
Washington, DC 20007   202-784-9770
                                  Fax: 202-784-9777
                             mchlibrary@ncemch.org
                                www.ncemch.org

Information and advocacy resources for families and professionals. Includes listings of organizations providing general information and organizations focusing on more specific areas of concern to families and young adults who have disabilities.

Rochelle Mayor, Director

7848 National Center for Health Statistics
Department of Health and Human Services
3311 Toledo Rd, Room 5419
Hyattsville, MD 20782   301-458-4636
                                       800-232-4636
                                  TTY: 888-232-6348
                               nchsquery@cdc.gov
                                www.cdc.gov/nchs

Information and advocacy resources for families and professionals. Includes listings of organizations providing general information and organizations focusing on more specific areas of concern to families and young adults who have disabilities.

Edward J. Sondik, Ph.D., Director

7849 National Clearinghouse on Postsecondary Education: HEATH Resource Center
Department of Health and Human Services
1 Dupont Circle NW, Suite 800
Washington, DC 20036
Fax: 202-401-2608
TTY: 202-205-8241
www2.ed.gov

Provides information for individuals with disabilities and resources for families and professionals. Includes listings of organizations providing general information and organizations focusing
on more specific areas of concern to families and young adults
who have disabilities.

Arne Duncan, Secretary of Education
Tony Miller, Deputy Secretary
Martha Kanter, Under Secretary

7850 National Coalition of Title 1 Chapter 1 Parents
3609 Georgia Avenue
Washington, DC 20010
202-291-8100
Fax: 202-291-8200

Information and advocacy resources for parents and professionals. Includes listings of organizations providing general information and organizations focusing on more specific areas of concern
to families and young adults who have disabilities.

7851 National Council on Disability
Department of Health and Human Services
1331 F Street NW, Suite 850
Washington, DC 20004
202-272-2004
Fax: 202-272-2022
TTY: 202-272-2074
www.ncd.gov

Information and advocacy resources for families and professionals. Includes listings of organizations providing general information and organizations focusing on more specific areas of concern
to families and young adults who have disabilities.

7852 National Council on Patient Information and Education
200-A Monroe Street, Suite 212
Rockville, MD 20850
301-340-3940
Fax: 301-340-3944
ncpie@ncpie.info
www.talkaboutrx.org

N. Lee Rucker, Chair
W. Ray Bullman, M.A.M., Executive Vice President
Deborah E. Davidson, Membership Director

7853 National Health Council
410 Horsham Road
Horsham, PA 19044
215-442-9010
Fax: 202-785-5923
info@nhcouncil.org
www.healthanswers.com

Information and advocacy resources for families and professionals. Includes listings of organizations providing general information and organizations focusing on more specific areas of concern
to families and young adults who have disabilities.

Michael Tague, Managing Director

7854 National Health Information Center: Office of Disease Preventive/Health Promotion
US Dept of Health and Human Services
PO Box 1133
Washington, DC 20013
301-565-4167
800-336-4797
Fax: 301-984-4256
info@nhif.org
www.health.gov/nhic

The National Health Information Center is a health information
referral service that links consumers and health professionals who
have health questions to organizations best able to provide reiable
health information.

7855 National Library Service for the Blind and Physically Handicapped
Library of Congress Reference Section
1291 Taylor Street NW
Washington, DC 20011
202-707-5100
800-424-8567
Fax: 202-707-0712
TTY: 202-707-0744
TDD: 202-707-0744
nis@loc.gov
www.loc.gov/nls

Administers a national library service that provides recorded and
braille reading materials to eligible children and adults who cannot read standard print.

Karen Keninger, Director

7856 National Maternal & Child Health Clearinghouse
2070 Chain Bridge Road, Suite 450
Vienna, VA 22182
703-821-8955
Fax: 703-821-2098
nmchc@circsol.com
www.circsol.com

Information and advocacy resources for families and professionals. Includes listings of organizations providing general information and organizations focusing on more specific areas of concern
to families and young adults who have disabilities.

7857 National Mental Health: Knowledge Exchange Network
Department of Health and Human Services
1 Choke Cherry Road
Rockville, MD 20857
800-789-2647
Fax: 240-221-4292
TTY: 800-487-4889
ken@mentalhealth.com
www.store.samhsa.gov

Information and advocacy resources for families and professionals. Includes listings of organizations providing general information and organizations focusing on more specific areas of concern
to families and young adults who have disabilities.

7858 National Oral Health Information Clearinghouse
Institute of Dental and Craniofacial Research
31 Center Drive, MSC 2290, Building 31, Room 2C39
Bethesda, MD 20892
301-496-4261
866-232-4528
Fax: 301-480-4098
nidcrinfo@mail.nih.gov
www.nidcr.nih.gov

Produces and distributes patient and professional education materials including fact sheets, brochures, information packets and
provides referrals to other organizations dealing with special care
in oral health. Special Care is an approach to oral health management that is tailored to the specific needs of persons with a variety of medical, disabling, or mental conditions. Database includes
bibliographic citations, abstracts, and availability information for
a variety of printed materials.

Martha J. Somerman, D.D.S., Ph.D., Director

7859 National Prevention Information Network
Center for Disease Control
PO Box 6003
Rockville, MD 20849
301-562-1098
800-458-5231
Fax: 888-282-7681
TTY: 888-232-6348
info@cdcnpin.org
www.cdcnpin.org

Information and advocacy resources for families and professionals. Includes listings of organizations providing general information and organizations focusing on more specific areas of concern
to families and young adults who have disabilities.

7860 National Recreation and Park Association
22377 Belmont Ridge Road
Ashburn, VA 20148
703-858-0784
800-626-6772
info@nrpa.org
www.nrpa.org

Information on adaptive sports and recreation activities for people of many abilities. Includes local chapters, referrals, fun and social interaction and support groups.

Steven J. Thompson, Chair
Barbara Tulipane, CAE, President/Chief Executive Officer
Peter Camin, Treasurer

7861 National Rehabilitation Information Center
8400 Corporate Drive, Suite 500
Landover, MD 20785

301-459-5900
800-346-2742
Fax: 301-459-4263
TTY: 301-459-5984
naricinfo@heitechservices.com
www.naric.com

Resources for families and professionals dealing with the rehabilitation of people with disabilities.

Mark X. Odum, Program Director
Jessica H. Chaiken, Media and Information Services Mana
Natalie J. Collier, Library and Acquisitions Manager

7862 Office for Fair Housing & Equal Opportunity
U.S. Department of Housing & Urban Development
451 7th Street SW
Washington, DC 20410

202-708-1112
TTY: 202-708-1455
nis@loc.gov
www.portal.hud.gov

Information and advocacy resources for families and professionals. Includes listings of organizations providing general information and organizations focusing on more specific areas of concern to families and young adults who have disabilities.

David Sidari, Deputy Chief Finanical Officer
Shaun Donovan, Secretary, HUD
Maurice Jones, Deputy Secretary

7863 Office of Special Education and Rehabilitation Services
400 Maryland Avenue, SW
Washington, DC 20202

202-401-2000
800-872-5327
Fax: 202-401-2608
TTY: 202-205-8241
www.ed.gov

Information and advocacy resources for families and professionals. Includes listings of organizations providing general information and organizations focusing on more specific areas of concern to families and young adults who have disabilities.

Ruth E Ryder, Assistant Secretary
Paul Steenen, Director, Communications

7864 President's Committee on Employment of People with Disabilities
1331 F Street NW, 3rd Floor
Washington, DC 20004

202-376-6200
Fax: 202-376-6250
www.pcepd.gov

Information and advocacy resources for families and professionals. Includes listings of organizations providing general information and organizations focusing on more specific areas of concern to families and young adults who have disabilities.

John Lancaster, Executive Director

7865 President's Committee on Mental Retardation
370 L'Enfant Promenade SW, Suite 701
Washington, DC 20447

202-619-0634
Fax: 202-205-9519
prma@acp.dhhs.govprograms/pcmr
www.acf.dhhs.gov/

Information and advocacy resources for families and professionals. Includes listings of organizations providing general information and organizations focusing on more specific areas of concern to families and young adults who have disabilities. Serves in an advisory capacity to the President of the U.S. and the Secretary of the Dept. of Health and Human Services.

National Associations & Support Groups

7866 ABLEDATA
103 W. Broad Street, Suite 400
Falls Church, VA 22046

800-227-0216
Fax: 703-356-8314
TTY: 703-992-8313
abledata@neweditions.net
www.abledata.com

ABLEDATA provides objective information on assistive technology and rehabilitation equipment available from domestic and international source to consumers, organizations, professionals, and caregivers within the United States. We serve the nation's disability, and senior communities.

David Johnson, Publications Director
Katherine Belknap, Project Director
Steve Lowe, Associate Project Manager

7867 ADARA
1022 7th Street, NE
Washington, DC 20002

501-224-6678
Fax: 501-868-8812
TTY: 501-868-8850
ADARAorgn@aol.com
www.adara.org

Our mission is to facilitate excellence in human service delivery with individuals who are Deaf or Hard of Hearing. This mission is accomplished by enhancing the professional competencies of the membership, expanding opportunities for networking among ADARA colleagues and supporting positive public policies for individuals who are Deaf or Hard of Hearing.

Charlene Crump, President
Dr John Gournaris, President Elect

7868 AIM for the Handicapped Adventures in Movement
945 Danbury Road
Dayton, OH 45420

937-294-4611
800-332-8210
Fax: 937-294-3783
aimforthehandicapped@aimforthehandicappe
www.aimforthehandicapped.org

To help individuals achieve their highest potential through the AIM Method of Specialized Movement Education.

Jo Geiger, Founder & National Executive Direct
J. Voss, President
Nancy Lopez, National Ambassadors

7869 ARC of the United States
1825 K Street, NW, Suite 1200
Washington, DC 20006

301-565-3842
800-433-5255
Fax: 301-565-5342
info@thearc.org
www.thearc.org

The ARC is the national organization of and for people with mental retardation and related developmental disabilities and their families. Devoted to promoting and improving supports and services for people with mental retardation and their families. The association also fosters research and education regarding the prevention of mental retardation in infants and young children. The ARC was founded in 1950 by a small group of parents and other concerned individuals.

Peter V. Berns, Chief Executive Officer
Darcy Rosenbaum, Senior Exec. Officer, Operations
Marty Ford, Senior Exec. Offcr, Public Policy

7870 Academic Pediatric Association
6728 Old McLean Village Drive
McLean, VA 22101

703-556-9222
Fax: 703-556-8729
info@ambpeds.org
www.ambpeds.org

The Ambulstory Pediatric Association fosters the health of children, adolescents, and families by promoting generalism in academic pediatrics and academics in general pediatrics.

Jessica K. O'Hara, Executive Director
Stephanie Blyskal, Association Manager
Holly Tyrrell, Research/Network Coordinator

7871 Academy for Guided Imagery
30765 Pacific Coast Highway, Suite 355
Malibu, CA 90265
424-242-6369
800-726-2070
Fax: 310-589-9523
info@acadgi.com
www.acadgi.com

The Academy for Guided Imagery is dedicated to educating and supporting practicing clinicians in their uses of imagery and imagery related approaches to therapy and healing. The Academy is an accredited Post-graduate training provider for health professionals, and a source of self-care products and programs for those struggling with a chronic, difficult, or painful illness.

David E. Bresler PhD,LAc, President
Jeanne Achterberg, PhD, Conference Faculty
Mark Atkinson, MBBS, Conference Faculty

7872 Academy of Rehabilitative Audiology
P.O. Box 2323
Albany, NY 12220
952-920-0484
Fax: 952-920-6098
ara@audrehab.org
www.audrehab.org

The primary purpose of ARA is to promote excellence in hearing care through the provision of comprehensive rehabilitative and habilitative services.

350 Members

Claire Bernstein, PhD, President
Kristin Vasil-Dilaj, Ph.D., Secretary
Sherri Smith, Ph.D., Treasurer

7873 Access Board
1331 F Street NW, Suite 1000
Washington, DC 20004
202-272-0080
800-872-2253
Fax: 202-272-0081
TTY: 800-993-2822
info@access-board.gov
www.access-board.gov

The Access Board is an independent Federal agency devoted to accessibility for people with disabilities. Created in 1973 to ensure access to federally funded facilities, the Board is now a leading source of information on accessible design. The Board develops and maintains design criteria for the built environment, transit vehicles, telecommunications equipment, and for electronic and information technology.

Deborah A. Ryan, Chairman
David M. Capozzi, Executive Director
James J. Raggio, General Counsel

7874 Adoptive Families
108 West 39th Street, Suite 805
New York, NY 10018
646-366-0830
800-372-3300
Fax: 646-366-0842
letters@adoptivefamilies.com
www.adoptivefamilies.com

Information and advocacy resources for families and professionals interested in adoption.

Susan Caughman, Editor/Publisher
Eve Gilman, Editor

7875 Alexander Graham Bell Association for the Deaf and Hard of Hearing
3417 Volta Place NW
Washington, DC 20007
202-337-5220
800-432-7543
Fax: 202-337-8314
TTY: 202-337-5221
info@agbell.org
www.agbell.org

Gathers and disseminates information on pediatric hearing loss, and educational issues for hearing impaired children, promotes better public understanding of hearing loss in children and adults, provides scholarships and financial aid to families of children with hearing loss, and promotes early detection of hearing loss in infants. Publishes magazine for parents and professionals who work with children.

Emilio Alonso-Mendoza, Chief Executive Officer

7876 Alliance for Technology Access (ATA)
1119 Old Humboldt Road
Jackson, TN 38305
731-554-5282
800-914-3017
Fax: 731-554-5283
TTY: 731-554-5284
TDD: 707-778-3015
ATAinfo@ATAcess.org
www.ataccess.org

The mission of the Alliance for Technology Access (ATA) is to increase the use of technology be children and adults with disabilities and functional limitations.

James Allison, President
Bob Van der Linde, Vice President
Mike Hewitt, Secretary/Treasurer

7877 American Academy of Audiology
11480 Commerce Park Drive, Suite 220
Reston, VA 20191
703-790-8466
800-222-2336
Fax: 703-790-8631
info@audiology.org
www.audiology.org

A professional organization dedicated to providing high quality and balanced hearing care to the public. Provides professional development, education and research and provides increased public awareness of hearing disorders and audiologic services.

12,000 members

Deborah Carlson, PhD, President
Shilpi Banerjee, PhD, Members-at-Large
Thomas Littman, PhD, Members-at-Large

7878 American Academy of Child and Adolescent Psychiatry
3615 Wisconsin Avenue NW
Washington, DC 20016
202-966-7300
Fax: 202-464-0131
clinical@aacap.org
www.aacap.org

The AACAP (American Academy of Child and Adolescent Psychiatry) is the leading national professional medical association dedicated to treating and improving the quality of life for children, adolescents, and families affected by these disorders. The AACAP is a 501 (c)(3) nonprofit organization established in 1953.

Gregory K Fritz, MD, President
Heidi B. Fordi, Executive Director

7879 American Academy of Dermatology (AAD)
PO Box 4014
Schaumburg, IL 60168
847-240-1280
866-503-7546
Fax: 847-240-1859
MRC@aad.org
www.aad.org

Largest, most influential and most representative of all dermatologic associations. Committed to the highest quality standards in continuing medical education. Developed a platform to promote and advance the science and art of medicine and surgery related to the skin; promotes the highest possible standards in clinical practice, education and research in dermatology and related disciplines; and supports and enhances patient care and promotes the public interest relating to dermatology.

Henry W. Lim, President
Brian Berman, VP
Barbara M. Mathes, Secretary/Treasurer

7880   American Academy of Pediatrics
141 Northwest Point Boulevard
Elk Grove Village, IL 60007   847-434-4000
800-433-9016
Fax: 847-434-8000
www.aap.org

The American Academy of Pediatrics and its member pediatricians dedicate their efforts and resources to the health, safety and well-being of infants, children, adolescents and young adults.

Fernando Stein, MD, FAAP, President
Karen Remley, MD, CEO/Executive VP

7881   American Amputee Foundation
P.O. Box 94227
North Little Rock, AR 72190   501-835-9290
Fax: 501-835-9292
info@americanamputee.org
www.americanamputee.org

AAF empowers amputees, their families, and care providers to make informed decisions be providing them information, referral, peer counseling, literature, and education.

Catherine J. Walden, Executive Director
Shelly Soderlund, Executive Assistant

7882   American Association of Children's Residential Centers (AACRC)
11700 W. Lake Park Drive
Milwaukee, WI 53224   877-332-2272
877-332-2272
Fax: 877-332-2272
info@aacrc-dc.org
www.aacrc-dc.org

The American Association of Children's Residential Centers brings professionals together to advance the frontiers of knowledge pertaining to the spectrum of therapeutic living environments for children and adolescents with behavioral health disorders.

Richard Altman, MSW, ACSW, Chief Executive Officer
William Powers, Chief Executive Officer
Christopher Bellonci, President

7883   American Association of the Deaf-Blind
PO Box 24493
Federal Way, WA 98093   301-495-4403
Fax: 301-495-4404
TTY: 301-495-4402
aadb-info@aadb.org
www.aadb.org

The American Association of the Deaf-Blind is a national consumer organization of, by, and for deaf-blind Americans. Deaf-blind does not necessarily mean totally deaf and totally blind. It is a broad term that describes people who have varying degrees and types of both vision and hearing loss together. Our mission is to endeavor to enable deaf-blind persons to achieve their maximum potential through increased independence, productivity and integration into the community.

600 Members

Mark Gasaway, President
Adam Drake, Treasurer

7884   American Association on Intellectual and D evelopmental Disabilities
501 3rd Street, NW Suite 200
Washington, DC 20001   202-387-1968
800-424-3688
Fax: 202-387-2193
aamr@access.digex.net
www.aamr.org

American Association on Intellectual and Developmental Disabilities' mission is to promote progressive policies, sound research, effective practices, and universal human rights for people with intellectual disabilities.

Marc J. Tass,, PhD, President
Amy S. Hewitt, PhD, Vice President
Margaret Nygren, EdD, Executive Director

7885   American Auditory Society
PO Box 779
Pennsville, NJ 08070   877-746-8315
Fax: 650-763-9185
amaudsoc@comcast.net
www.amauditorysoc.org

The primary aims of the Society are to increase knowledge and understanding of the ear, hearing and balance; disorders of the ear, hearing and balance, and preventions of these disorders; and habilitation and rehabilitation of individuals with hearing and balance dysfunction.

Linda Hood, President
Wayne J Staab, PhD, Executive Director
Harvey Abrams, Board of Director

7886   American Autoimmune Related Diseases Association
22100 Gratiot Avenue
Eastpointe, MI 48021   586-776-3900
800-598-4668
Fax: 586-776-3903
aarda@aarda.org
www.aarda.org

Dedicated to the eradication of autoimmune diseases and the alleviation of suffering and the socio-economic impact of autoimmunity through fostering and facilitating collaboration in the areas of education, public awareness, research and patient services in an effective, ethical and efficient manner.

Virginia T. Ladd, President/Executive Director
Patricia Barber, Assistant Director
Deb Patrick, Events Specialist

7887   American Blind Bowling Association
7232 South Ridgeland
Chicago, IL 60649   773-255-3121
Fax: ica-go -
president@abba1951.org
www.abba1951.org

Information on adaptive bowling activities for people who are blind.

Robert McDonald, President
Rozella Campbell, Secretary/Treasurer
Wilbert Turner, Public Relations Committee Chair

7888   American Blind Skiing Foundation
609 Crandell Lane
Schaumburg, IL 60193   312-409-1605
ABSF@absf.org
www.absf.org

ABSF is committed to serving visually impaired children and adults, giving them the opportunities and experiences that build confidence and independence.

Michelle Hulscher, President
Beth Zange, Vice President
William Kopp, Treasurer

7889   American Board of Dermatology
2 Wells Avenue
Newton, MA 02459   617-910-6400
abderm@hfhs.org
www.abderm.org

Sole mission is to ensure competence for patients with cutaneous diseases through board representation.

Stanley J. Miller, President
Karen E. Warschaw, Vice President
Thomas D. Horn, Executive Director

7890   American Board of Pediatrics
111 Silver Cedar Court
Chapel Hill, NC 27514   919-929-0461
Fax: 919-929-9255
abpeds@abpeds.org
www.abp.org

The American Board is Pediatrics certifies general pediatricians and pediatric subspecialists based on standards of excellence that lead to high quality health care for infants, children and adolescents.

Dr. David G. Nichols, President/CEO

7891   American Camping Association
5000 State Road, 67 N
Martinsville, IN 46151
765-342-8456
800-428-2267
Fax: 765-342-2065
Wo.turner5@sbcglobal.net
www.acacamps.org

The American Camping Association is a community of camp professionals who, for nearly 100 years, have joined together to share our knowledge and experience and to ensure the quality of camp program.

Wilbert Turner, Chair
Peg Smith, CEO
Tisha Bolger, President

7892   American Cancer Society
250 Williams Street NW
Atlanta, GA 30303
800-227-2345
Fax: 404-315-9348
angelina.veal@cancer.org
www.cancer.org

The American Cancer Society is a nationwide, community-based voluntary health organization. Headquartered in Atlanta, Georgia, the ACS has state divisions and more than 3,400 local offices. For more than 80 years, ACS has led the way in cancer research. The goal is to prevent cancer, save lives, and diminish suffering from cancer.

Gary M. Reedy, Chair
Robert E. Youle, Vice Chair
Vincent T. DeVita, President

7893   American Canoe Association
108 Hanover St
Fredricksburg, VA 22401
540-907-4460
Fax: 888-229-3792
aca@americancanoe.org
www.americancanoe.org

The mission of the American Canoe Association is to promote the health, social and personal benefits of canoeing, kayaking and rafting and to serve the needs off all paddlers for safe, enjoyable and quality paddling opportunities.

Wade Blackwood, Executive Director
Cireena Katto, Office Manager
Kelsey Bracewell, Safety Education, Instruction, & Ou

7894   American Childhood Cancer Organization (fo rmerly Candlelighters Childhood Cancer)
PO Box 498
Kensington, MD 20895
301-962-3520
800-366-2226
Fax: 301-962-3521
staff@acco.org
www.acco.org

The Candlelighters Childhood Cancer Foundation was founded by concerned parents of children with cancer. The foundation is a national nonprofit membership organization whose mission is to educate, support, serve, and advocate for families of children with cancer, survivors of childhood cancer, and the professionals who care for them.

Ruth I. Hoffman, MPH, Executive Director
Jessica DiBenedetto, Program Coordinator
Christy Perry, Director, Marketing/Communications

7895   American Dermatological Association
PO Box 551301
Davie, FL 33355
954-452-1113
Fax: 305-945-7063
info@amer-derm-assn.org
www.amer-derm-assn.org

Professional society of physicians specializing in dermatology. Promotes teaching, practice, public education and research into dermatology.

Rex Amonette, President
John Wolf, Vice President
Julie Odessky, Executive Manager

7896   American Epilepsy Society
342 N Main Street
W Hartford, CT 06117
860-586-7505
800-332-1000
Fax: 860-568-7550
www.aesnet.org

A society of clinicians, researchers, and health care professionals which promotes education and research of epilepsy.

Suzanne C Berry, Executive Director
Cheryl-Ann Tubby, Assistant Executive Director
Elizabeth Kunsey, Senior Meeting Planner

7897   American Hearing Research Foundation
8 South Michigan Avenue, Suite #1205
Chicago, IL 60603
312-726-9670
Fax: 312-726-9695
ahrf@american-hearing.org
www.american-hearing.org

A nonprofit foundation serving two vital roles — funding significant research in hearing and balance disorders and helping educate the public.

Richard G. Muench, Chair
Alan G. Micco, M.D, President
Mark R. Muench, Vice President

7898   American Heart Association
7272 Greenville Avenue
Dallas, TX 75231
214-373-6300
800-242-8721
Fax: 214-706-1341
inquire@amhrt.org
www.heart.org/HEARTORG/

Supports research, education and community service programs with the objective of reducing premature death and disability from cardiovascular diseases and stroke; coordinates the efforts of health professionals, and others engaged in the fight against heart and circulatory disease.

Nancy Brown, CEO
Dr. Stephen Houser, President
Suzie Upton, Chief Operating Officer

7899   American Juvenile Arthritis Organization
1330 W. Peachtree Street., Suite 100
Atlanta, GA 30309
404-872-7100
800-933-7023
Fax: 404-237-8153
info.ga@arthritis.org
www.arthritis.org

Devoted to serving the special needs of children, teens, and young adults with childhood rheumatic diseases and their families. Offers both support and information through national and local programs that serve the needs of families, friends and health professionals. Serves as a clearinghouse of information, sponsors an annual national conference, monitors and promotes legislation, sponsors research, and offers training to both parents and health professionals.

Daniel T. McGowan, Chair
John H. Klippel, President
Michael V. Ortman, Secretary

7900   American Liver Foundation
39 Broadway, Suite 2700
New York, NY 10006
212-668-1000
800-465-4837
Fax: 212-483-8179
info@liverfoundation.org
www.liverfoundation.org

National, voluntary, nonprofit organization dedicated to the prevention, treatment and cure of liver diseases. The foundation offers support groups, advocacy, medical research support and education.

Thomas F. Nealon III, Chair
David Ticker, Chief Financial Officer
Cynthia Gardner, Vice President, Field Development

7901 American Lung Association
55 W. Wacker Drive, Suite 1150
Chicago, IL 60601   312-801-7628
                                     800-586-4872
                                     info@lung.org
                                     www.lung.org

The American Lung Association fights lung disease in all its forms, with special emphasis on asthma, tobacco control and environmental health. The American Lung Association is funded with contributions from the public, along with gifts and grants from corporations, foundations and government agencies. The association achieves its many successes through the work of thousands of committed volunteers and staff.

Harold P. Wimmer, National President & CEO
Susan Rappaport, National VP, Research/Scientific
Sue Swan, Chief Development Officer

7902 American Pediatrics Society
3400 Research Forest Drive, Suite B-7
The Woodlands, TX 77381   281-419-0052
                                Fax: 281-419-0082
                                     info@aps-spr.org
                                     www.aps-spr.org

The objects of the Society shall be to bring together men and women for the advancement of the study of children and their diseases, for the prevention of illness and the promotion of health in childhood, for the promotion of pediatric education and research, and to honor those who, by their contributions to pediatrics, have aided in its advancement.

Debbie Anagnostelis, Executive Director
Kathy Cannon, Associate Executive Director
Kate Culliton, Accounting Manager

7903 American Red Cross
2025 E Street NW
Washington, DC 20006   202-303-4498
                                     800-733-2767
                                Fax: 202-303-0044
                                     info@usa.redcross.org
                                     www.redcross.org

The American Red Cross has been the nation's premier emergency response organization. As part of a worldwide movement that offers neutral humanitarian care to the victims of war, the American Red Cross distinguished itself by also aiding victims of devastating natural disasters.

Bonnie McElveen-Hunter, Chair
Gail J. McGovern, President and CEO
Brian J. Rhoa, Chief Financial Officer

7904 American Skin Association
6 East 43rd Street, 28th Floor
New York, NY 10017   212-889-4858
                                     800-499-7546
                                Fax: 212-889-4959
                                     info@americanskin.org
                                     www.americanskin.org

The American Skin Association is the only volunteer led health organization dedicated through research, education and advocacy to saving lives and alleviating human suffering caused by the full spectrum of skin disorders.

Howard P. Milstein, Chair
George W Hambrick, Jr, President/Founder
David R Bickers, MD, Executive VP

7905 American Society for Deaf Children
800 Florida Ave NE, #2047
Washington, DC 20002   800-942-2732
                                Fax: 410-795-0965
                                     asdc@deafchildren.org
                                     www.deafchildren.org

A nonprofit, parent-helping-parent organization promoting a positive attitude toward signing and deaf culture. Also provides support, encouragement, and current information about deafness to families with deaf and hard of hearing children.

Jodee Crace, President
Avonne Brooker-Rutowski, Vice President
Timothy G. Frelich, Treasurer

7906 American Speech Language Hearing Associati on (ASHA)
2200 Research Boulevard
Rockville, MD 20850   301-296-5700
                                      800-498-2071
                                 Fax: 301-296-8580
                                 TTY: 301-296-5650
                                      actioncenter@asha.org
                                      www.asha.org

A professional organization made up of over 123,000 hearing, speech and language professionals. It is a credentialing organization as well promotes the interests of provides services and information for those with communication disorders.

Arlene A. Pietranton, PhD, CAE, Chief Executive Officer
Patricia A. Prelock, President
Neil T. Shepard, PhD, CCC-A (Bio, Vice President for Academic Affairs

7907 American Wheelchair Table Tennis Association
P.O. Box 5266
Kendall Park, NJ 08824   732-266-2634
                                Fax: 732-355-6500
                                     johnsonjennifer@yahoo.com
                                     www.wsusa.org

AWTTA is the National Governing Body of Wheelchair Sports, U.S.A., for table tennis. Information on adaptive table tennis activities for people of many abilities. Includes local chapters, referrals, fun and social interaction and support groups.

Barbara Chambers, Chairperson
Jessica Galli, Secretary
Mike Burns, Treasurer

7908 Association for Children's Mental Health
6017 W. St. Joseph Hwy., Suite #200
Lansing, MI 48917   517- 37- 401
                                     888-226-4543
                                Fax: 517-372-4032
                                     www.acmh-mi.org

ACMH is a family organization with statewide staff and membership who support activities to enhance the system or services which address the needs of children with serious emotional disorders and their families. ACMH is a statewide chapter of the national Federation of families for Children's Mental Health and our membership of over 1200 individuals is comprised of family members, professionals and concerned.

Malisa Pearson, Executive Director
Mary Porter, Business Manager
Terri Henrizi, Training Coordinator and Family Sup

7909 Association for Education & Rehabilitation of the Blind & Visually Impaired
1703 N Beauregard Street, Suite 440
Alexandria, VA 22311   703-671-4500
                                     877-492-2708
                                Fax: 703-671-6391
                                     markr@aerbvi.org
                                     www.aerbvi.org

This association is the only international membership organization dedicated to rendering all possible support and assistance to the professionals who work in all phases of education and rehabilitation of blind and visually impaired children and adults.

Jim Adams, President
Susan Jay Spungin, Secretary
Lou Tutt, Executive Director

7910 Association for Persons with Severe Handicaps (TASH)
1001 Connecticut Avenue, NW, Suite 235
Washington, DC 20036   202-540-9020
                                Fax: 202-540-9019
                                     info@tash.org
                                     www.tash.org

An international association of people with disabilities, their family members, other advocates, and professionals fighting for a society in which inclusion of all people in all aspects of society is the norm.

David Westling, President
Jean Trainor, Vice President
Barbara Trader, Executive Director

7911 Association for the Gifted Child
Council for Exceptional Children
2900 Crystal Drive, Suite 1000
Arlington, VA 22202

703-620-3660
888-232-7733
Fax: 703-264-9494
TTY: 866-915-5000
service@cec.sped.org
www.cec.sped.org

Focuses on the delivery of information to both professionals and parents about gifted and talented children and their needs.

Lynda Van Kuren, Contact

7912 Association for the Handicapped
350 5th Avenue, Suite 3304
New York, NY 10118

212-868-1217
Fax: 212-868-1219

Information on adaptive sports and recreation activities for people of many abilities. Includes local chapters, referrals, fun and social interaction and support groups.

7913 Association for the Help of Retarded Children
83 Maiden Lane
New York, NY 10038

212-780-2690
800-662-1220
Fax: 212-777-5893
ahrcnyc@dti.net
www.ahrcnyc.org

Developmentally disabled children and adults, their families, and interested individuals. Provides support services, training programs, clinics, schools and residential facilities to the developmentally disabled. Publications: The Chronicle, quarterly newsletter.

Amy West, Chief Financial Officer
Laura J. Kennedy, President
Gary Lind, Executive Director

7914 Association of Blind Athletes
1 Olympic Plaza
Colorado Springs, CO 80909

719-630-0422
Fax: 719-630-0616
usaba@usa.net
www.usaba.org

The mission of the United States Association of Blind Athletes is to increase the number and quality of grassroots through competitive, world-class athletic opportunities for Americans who are blind or visually impaired. We value the life enhancing aspects of sports and the opportunity to demonstrate the abilities of people who are blind and visually impaired.

Dave Bushland, President
Tracie Foster, Vice President
Mark A. Lucas, MS, Executive Director

7915 Association of Children's Prosthetic/ Orthotic Clinics
6300 N River Road, Suite 727
Rosemont, IL 60018

847-698-1637
Fax: 847-823-0536
acpoc@aaos.org
www.acpoc.org

An association of professionals who are involved in clinics which provide prosthetic-orthotic care for children with limb loss or orthopedic disabilities.

J Ivan Krajbich, MD, President
David B Rotter, CPO, Vice President
Jorge Amelio Fabregas, MD, Secretary-Treasurer

7916 Association of University Centers on Disabilities
1100 Wayne Ave., Suite 1000
Silver Spring, MD 20910

301-588-8252
800-424-3410
Fax: 301-588-2842
TTY: 301-588-3319
aucdinfo@aucd.org
www.aucd.org

The Association of University Centers on Disabilities (formerly the American Association of University Affiliated Programs) is a nonprofit organization that promotes and supports the national network of university centers on disabilities, which includes University Centers for Excellence in Developmental Disabilities Education, Research, and Service Leadership Education in Neurodevelopment and Related Disabilities Programs and Developmental Disabilities Research Centers.

Julie Fodor, PhD, President
George S. Jesien, PhD, Executive Director
Laura Martin, MA, Director of Operations

7917 Barbara DeBoer Foundation
79 Fifth Avenue/16th Street
New York, NY 10003

212-620-4230
800-424-9836
Fax: 212-807-3677
order@foundationcenter.org
www.foundationcenter.org

Offers a variety of programs that include advocacy services, donor awareness, referral information, medication and medical center information.

Bradford K. Smith, President
Lisa Philp, Vice President for Strategic Philan
Lawrence T. McGill, Vice President for Research

7918 Beneficial Designs
2240 Meridian Boulevard, Suite C
Minden, NV 89423

425-373-5787
Fax: 775-783-8823
hello@beneficialdesign.com
www.beneficialdesign.com

Beneficial Designs works towards universal access through research, design, and education. We believe all individuals should have access to the physical, intellectual, and spiritual aspects of life. We seek to enhance the quality of life for people of all abilities, and work to achieve this aim by developing and marketing technology for daily living, vocational, and leisure activities.

Peter Axelson, Founder/Research Director
Denise Yamada Axelson, Research Coordinator

7919 Benetech
480 S California Avenue, Suite 201
Palo Alto, CA 94306

650-644-3400
Fax: 650-475-1066
info@benetech.org
www.benetech.org

Benetech (formerly Arkenstone) is a nonprofit venture that combines the impact of technological solutions with the social entrepreneurship business model to help disadvantaged communities in our society and across the world.

Jim Fruchterman, President/CEO
Marc Levine, Senior Project Manager
Jane Simchuk, Administration Manager

7920 Birth Defect Research for Children
976 Lake Baldwin Lane, Suite 104
Orlando, FL 32814

407-895-0802
Fax: 407-895-0824
staff@birthdefects.org
www.birthdefects.org

A nonprofit organization that provides information about birth defects of all kinds to parents and professionals. Offers a library of medical books and files of information on less common categories of birth defects and is involved in research to discover possible links between environmental exposures and birth defects.

Betty Mekdeci, Executive Director

7921 Boundless Playgrounds
401 Chestnut St, Suite 410
Chattanooga, TN 37402

423-648-5619
877-268-6353
Fax: 860-243-5854
info@boundlessplaygrounds.org
www.boundlessplaygrounds.org

Boundless Playgrounds helps communities create extraordinary playgrounds where all children, with and without disabilities, can develop essential skills for life as they learn together through play.

Frederick Leone, Chief Executive Officer
Monique Farias, Technical Services Manager
Antonio Mulkusack, Director of Technical Services

7922 Boy Scouts of America National Council
9190 Rockville Pike
Bethseda, MD 20814
301-530-9360
Fax: 301-564-9513
www.boyscouts-ncac.org

The mission of the Boy Scouts of America is to prepare young people to make ethical and moral choices over their lifetimes by instilling in them the values of the values of the Scouts Oath and Law.

Hugh Redd, Council President
Ed Yarbrough, Council Commissioner
Les Baron, Scout Executive

7923 Braille Revival League
American Council of the Blind
1155 15th Street NW, Suite 1004
Washington, DC 20005
202-467-5081
800-424-8666
Fax: 202-467-5085
info@acb.org
www.acb.org

Encourages blind people to read and write in Braille, advocates for mandatory Braille instruction in educational facilities for the blind, strives to make available a supply of Braille materials from libraries and printing houses and more.

7924 Brass Ring Society
500 Macaw Lane, #5
Fern Park, FL 32730
407-339-6188
800-666-9474
Fax: 407-339-6369
www.brassring.org

Society that seeks to fulfill the dreams of children with life-threatening illnesses.

Ray Esposito, Director

7925 Breckenridge Outdoor Education Center
PO Box 697
Breckenridge, CO 80424
970-453-6422
800-383-2632
Fax: 970-453-4676
boec@boec.org
www.boec.org

The Breckenridge outdoor Education Center is a non-profit organization whose mission is to expand the potential of people with disabilities and special needs through meaningful, educational, and inspiring outdoor experiences.

Tim Casey, Chairman
John Ebright, Vice-Chairman
Bruce Fitch, Executive Director

7926 CANDU Parent Group
Riverwalk Community Center
2100 Manchester Rd., Bldg. B, Suite. 925
Wheaton, IL 60187
630-752-0066
Fax: 630-752-1064
il@namidupage.org
www.namidupage.org

Support and advocacy group for parents of children with serious emotional disturbance, behavioral disorders, or mental illness.

Tony Davis, President
Cora Corley, Secretary
Bob Barger, Treasurer

7927 CHERUB-Association of Families and Friends of Children with Limb Disorders
Children's Hospital of Buffalo
936 Delaware Avenue
Buffalo, NY 14209
716-762-9997

Answers the questions and problems that families of juveniles diagnosed with a disorder may be experiencing.

Sandra Richenberg
Kathy Compliance Officer

7928 Cancer Information Service
National Cancer Institute
6116 Executive Boulevard, Suite 3036A
Bethesda, MD 20892
800-422-6237
Fax: 301-330-7968
TTY: 800-332-8615
www.cis.nic.nih.gov

The Cancer Information Service provides the latest and most accurate cancer information to patients, their families, the public, and health professionals. Through its network of regional offices, the CIS serves the United States, Puerto Rico, the U.S. Virgin Islands, and the Pacific Islands.

Andrew C Von Eschenback, Director

7929 Center for Best Practices in Early Childhood
College of Education and Human Services
1 University Circle
Macomb, IL 61455
309-298-1634
Fax: 309-298-2305
jk-johanson@wiu.edu
www.wiu.edu/thecenter

Operates the following: Early Childhood Interactive Technology Literacy Curriculum Project; Disseminating and Replicating an Effective Early Childhood Comprehensive Technology System; Expressive Arts Outreach; ECCSPLOR-IT; LiTECH Interactive Outreach; STARNET Regions I and III; and Provider Connections.

Joyce Johanson, Associate Director
Linda Robinson, Assistant Director
Patricia Hutinger, Director

7930 Center for Literacy and Disability Studies
321 South Columbia Street Suite 1100 Bondurant Hal
Chaple Hill, NC 27599
919-966-8566
Fax: 919-843-3250
clds@unc.edu
www.med.unc.edu

The Center for Literacy and Disability Studies is a unit within the Department of Allies Health Sciences, school of Medicine, at the University of North Carolina at Chapel Hill.

Karen Erickson

7931 Center for Mental Health Services Knowledge Exchange Network
US Department of Health and Human Services
PO Box 42557
Washington, DC 20015
800-789-2647
Fax: 240-747-5470
TDD: 866-889-2647
www.mentalhealth.samhsa.gov

Supplies the public with responses to their commonly asked questions about mental health issues and services.

7932 Chai Lifeline/Camp Simcha National Office
151 W 30th Street
New York, NY 10001
212-465-1300
800-242-4543
Fax: 212-465-0949
info@chailifeline.org
www.chailifeline.org

Chai Life is a not for profit organization dedicated to helping children suffering from serous illness as well as their family members. We offer a comprehensive range is services to address the multiple needs of patients, parents, and siblings.

Esther Schwartz, Director of Hospital Services

7933 Child Abuse Prevention Association
503 E 23rd Street
Independence, MO 64055
816-252-8388
Fax: 816-252-1337
capa@childabuseprevention.org
www.childabuseprevention.org

Mission is to prevent and treat all forms of child abuse by creating changes in individuals, families and society which strengthen relationships and promote healing.

Shelly Hall, Chairman
Jeanetta Issa, CEO
Karen Costa, Clinical Director

7934 Child Care Plus+
Univ. of Montana Rural Institute on Disabilities
634 Eddy Avenue
Missoula, MT 59812   406-243-6355
                                      800-235-4122
                                 Fax: 406-243-4730
                                 TDD: 406-243-5467
                                 ccplus@selway.umt.edu
                                 www.ccplus.org

Provides inclusion information and resources for child care providers and other professionals: written materials (newsletter, curriculum, articles), training, workshops, technical assistance and various other resources.

Sandra L. Morris, Center Co-Director
Susan Harper-Whalen, Consultant
Karen Martin, Inclusion I and II Instructor

7935 Children's Defense Fund
25 E Street NW
Washington, DC 20001   202-628-8787
                                      800-233-1200
                                 Fax: 202-662-3510
                                 cdfinfo@childrensdefense.org
                                 www.childrensdefense.org

Information and advocacy resources for families and professionals. Includes listings of organizations providing general information and organizations focusing on more specific areas of concern to families and young adults who have disabilities.

Geoffrey Canada, Chairman
Kenneth Troshinsky, Chief Financial Officer
Marian Wright Edelman, President

7936 Children's Hopes and Dreams
138 Cloudland Road
Dahlonega, GA 30533   706-482-2248
                                 Fax: 706-482-2289
                                 chdfdover@juno.com
                                 www.helpingnow.org

Three programs: Dream fulfillment program is for children age four through seventeen with life threatening illness who have not received a dream before; Pen Pal Program matches children five through seventeen with chronic or life threatening illnesses, conditions, disabilities or major trauma to other ill children by their age, sex and illness category; Kid's Kare Package program supplies new donated items to children through Pen Pal Program and/or health care professionals.

Luke Oswald, Program Director

7937 Children's Hopes and Dreams Foundation
Wish Fulfillment Foundation
138 Cloudland Road
Dahlonega, GA 30533   706-482-2248
                                 Fax: 706-482-2289
                                 chdfdover@juno.com
                                 www.helpingnow.org

Children's Hopes & Dreams Foundation has been serving children with serious childhood illnesses since 1983.

10,000 Members

Luke Oswald, Program Director

7938 Children's Hospice International
1101 King Street Suite 360
Alexandria, VA 22314   703-684-0330
                                      800-242-4453
                                 Fax: 703-684-0330
                                 info@chionline.org
                                 www.chionline.org

This nonprofit organization works to improve hospice care for children. Free services include information and referral service for child care, counseling, support groups, pain management, professional education, and research. This is a membership group, with a membership fee for other services.

Ann Armstrong-Dailey, Founding Director/CEO
Richard Larkin, Secretary/Treasurer
Rebecca Brant, Directors

7939 Children's Hospital Boston
300 Longwood Avenue
Boston, MA 02115   617-355-6000
                                 Fax: 617-277-4832
                                 TTY: 617-730-0152
                                 webteam@tch.harvard.edu
                                 www.childrenshospital.org

Children's Hospital Boston is a 325 bed comprehensive center for pediatric health care. As the largest pediatric medical center in the United States, Children's offers a complete range of health care services for children from 15 weeks gestation through 21 years of age (and older in some cases).

James Mandell, MD, Chief Executive Officer
Sandra Fenwick, President and Chief Operating Offic
Naomi Fried, PhD, Chief Innovation Officer

7940 Children's Organ Transplant Association
2501 Cota Drive
Bloomington, IN 47403   800-366-2682
                                 Fax: 812-336-8885
                                 cota@cota.org
                                 www.cota.org

The association provides fundraising assistance for children needing life-saving transplants and promotes organ, marrow and tissue donation.

Rick Lofgren, President/CEO
Lisa Fulkerson, VP/CFO
Judy Sutton, Administrative Assisstant

7941 Children's Wish Foundation International
8615 Roswell Road
Atlanta, GA 30350   770-393-9474
                                      800-323-9474
                                 Fax: 770-393-0683
                                 wish@childrenswish.org
                                 www.childrenswish.org

A nonprofit organization that fulfills wishes for children with life threatening illnesses. The criteria for wish fulfillment are: The child must be under the age of eighteen, and have been diagnosed with a life threatening illness.

Arthur Stein, President
Linda Dozoretz, Founder/Executive Director

7942 Chill: Straight Talk About Stress
Childs Work/Childs Play
303 Crossways Park Drive
Woodbury, NY 11797   516-349-5520
                                      800-962-1141
                                 Fax: 800-262-1886
                                 info@Childswork.com
                                 www.Childswork.com

Childswork/Childsplay uses a prevention and intervention model when creating its high-quality products. These programs focus on the behavioral, social, and emotional issues children deal with at home and at school. Through the use of games, print materials and visual media, counselors and educators have a superior array of counseling tools at their disposal.

7943 Christian Horizons
25 Sportsworld Crossing Road
Kitchener, ON N2P 0   519-650-0966
                                      866-362-6810
                                 Fax: 519-650-8984
                                 info@christian-horizons.org
                                 www.christian-horizons.org

Devoted to assisting individuals, with developmental disabilities, on a day-to-day basis.

Nigel Wilford, Chair
Janet Nolan, CEO
Claire Lebold, Vice Chair

7944 Compassionate Friends
PO Box 3696
Oak Brook, IL 60522
630-990-0010
877-969-0010
Fax: 630-990-0246
nationaloffice@compassionatefriends.org
www.compassionatefriends.org

Compassionate Friends assists families toward the positive resolution of grief following the death of a child of any age and provides information to help others be supportive. A national nonprofit, self-help support organization that offers friendship, understanding, and hope to bereaved parents, grandparents and siblings.

Rick Yotti, President
Ronald Haynes, VP
Patricia Loder, Executive Director

7945 Cooperative Wilderness Handicapped Outdoor Group
Idaho State University
921 South 8th Avenue
Pocatello, ID 83209
208-282-3912
Fax: 208-282-2127
krindavi@isu.edu
www.isu.edu

A regional self-help group to provide recreational opportunities for people of all disabilities. The program is part of the Idaho State University.

Dr. Michael McCurry, Professor Of Geosciences
Dr. Leslie Devaud, Associate Professor Of Ph Sciences

7946 Council for Educational Diagnostic Services (CEDS)
Council for Exceptional Children
1664 N. Virginia Street
Reno, NV 89557
775-784-1110
888-232-7733
Fax: 775-784-6429
TTY: 703-264-9446
www.unr.edu

Promotes the highest quality of diagnostic and prescriptive procedures involved in the education of individuals with disabilities and/or who are gifted. Members include educational diagnosticians, psychologists, social workers, speech and language specialists, physicians, and other professionals and related service professionals.

Dr. Marc Johnson, President
Patricia Richard, Assistant Vice President for Consti
Janet Sanderson, Executive Assistant to the Presiden

7947 Council for Exceptional Children
2900 Crystal Drive, Suite 1000
Arlington, VA 22202
703-620-3660
888-232-7733
Fax: 703-264-9494
TTY: 866-915-5000
service@cec.sped.org
www.cec.sped.org

Advocates appropriate policies, standards and development for students with special needs.

Lynda Van Kuren, Contact

7948 Council of Administrators of Special Education
Council for Exceptional Children
101 Katelyn Circle, Suite E
Warner Robins, GA 31088
478-333-6892
888-232-7733
Fax: 478-333-2453
TTY: 703-264-9446
lpurcell@casecec.org
www.casecec.org

A international professional educational organization which is affiliated with the Council for Exceptional Children (CEC) whose members are dedicated to the enhancement of the worth, dignity, potential, and uniqueness of each individual in society. The mission is to provide leadership and support to members by shaping policies and practices which impact the quality of education.

Laurie VanderPloeg, President
Tom Adams, Finance Committee Chairman
Dr. Luann Purcell, Executive Director

7949 Council of Families with Visual Impairments
American Council of the Blind
6686 Capricorn Lane N.E.
Bremerton, WA 98311
360-698-0827
800-424-8666
Fax: 202-467-5085
cindybur@comcast.net
www.cfvi.info/keep.html

A network of parents with blind or visually impaired children that offers support and outreach, shares experiences in parent/child relationships, exchanges educational, cultural and medical information about child development and more.

7950 Courage Center
3915 Golden Valley Road
Minneapolis, MN 55422
763-588-0811
888-846-8253
Fax: 612-520-0577
TTY: 763-520-0245
Information@CourageCenter.org
www.couragecenter.org

The mission of Courage Center is to empower people with physical disabilities to reach for their full potential in every aspect of life. We are guided by the vision that one day, all people will live, work, learn and play in a community based on abilities, not disabilities.

John Church, Chair
Kathy Connors, Treasurer
Jan Malcolm, Secretary

7951 CureSearch: The National Childhood Cancer Foundation
4600 East West Highway, Suite 600
Bethseda, MD 20814
800-458-6223
Fax: 301-718-0047
info@curesearch.org
www.curesearch.org

Cure Search unites the Children's Oncology Group (COG) and the National Childhood Center Foundation (NCCF) through a shared mission to cure and prevent childhood and adolescent cancer through scientific discovery and compassionate care.

Stuart Siegel, Chair
Laura Thrall, President and CEO
Christine Bor, Chief Development Officer

7952 Deafness Research Foundation
363 Seventh Avenue, 10th Floor
New York, NY 10001
212-257-6140
866-454-3924
info@hearinghealthfoundation.org
www.hearinghealthfoundation.org

The nation's largest voluntary health organization entirely committed to public awareness and support for basic and clinical research into deafness and hearing disabilities. Sponsors a broad program of innovative research and education into the causes, treatments and prevention of nerve deafness, increases the number of young scientists entering and engaged in otologic studies, increases the nation's awareness and creates an understanding of serious hearing dysfunctions.

Shari Eberts, Chairman
Mark Angelo, President
Andrea Boidman, Executive Director

7953 Developmental Delay Resources
5801 Beacon St.
Pittsburgh, PA 15217
800-497-0944
Fax: 412-422-1374
www.devdelay.org

A nonprofit organization dedicated to meeting the needs of those working with children who have developmental delays in sensory motor, language, social, and emotional areas. DDR provides a network for parents and professionals and current information after the diagnosis to support children with special needs.

Patricia S. Lemer, Executive Director
Teresa Badillo, Executive Board
Margaret Britt, Executive Board

7954 Developmental Disabilities Nurses Association
Po Box 536489
Orlando, FL 32853
407-835-0642
800-888-6733
Fax: 407-426-7440
ddnahq@aol.com
www.ddna.org

A nonprofit professional nursing organization founded to meet the professional needs of nurses serving individuals with developmental disabilities.

Kathleen Brown, President
Wendy Herbers, Vice President
Richanne Cunningham, Secretary

7955 Disability Rights Education & Defense Fund
2212 6th Street
Berkeley, CA 94710
510-644-2555
Fax: 510-841-8645
dredf@dredf.org
www.dredf.org

Nonprofit law and public policy center that specializes in laws affecting more than 45 million Americans with disabilities. DREDF was founded 16 years ago to challenge the barriers that exclude people with disabilities from participating in all aspects of society.

Jenny Kern, President/Chair
Susan Henderson, Executive Director
Arlene B. Mayerson, Directing Attorney

7956 Disabled Shooting Services
National Rifle Association of America
11250 Waples Mill Road
Fairfax, VA 22030
703-267-1495
800-672-3888
info@nrpa.org
www.compete.nra.org

Information on adaptive shooting activities for people of many abilities. Includes local chapters, referrals, fun and social interaction and support groups.

Dave Baskin, Department Head

7957 Disabled Sports USA
451 Hungerford Drive, Suite 100
Rockville, MD 20850
301-217-0960
Fax: 301-217-0968
info@dsusa.org
www.dsusa.org

A national nonprofit, organization established in 1967 by disabled Vietnam veterans to serve the war injured. DS/USA now offers nationwide sports rehabilitation programs to anyone with a permanent disability.

Kirk Bauer, Executive Director
Cheryl Collins, Administrative Services Manager
Orlando Gill, Field Representative

7958 Division for Early Childhood
27 Fort Missoula Road, Suite 2
Missoula, MT 59804
406-543-0872
Fax: 406-543-0887
TTY: 703-264-9446
dec@dec-sped.org
www.dec-sped.org

This division is one of seventeen divisions of the Council for Exceptional Children, the largest international professional organization dedicated to improving educational outcomes for individuals with exceptionalities, students with disabilities, and/or the gifted.

Leah Weiner, Executive Director
Cynthia Wood, Associate Executive Director

7959 Division for Physical and Health Disablities
Council for Exceptional Children
1110 N Glebe Road, Suite 300
Arlington, VA 22201
703-620-3660
888-232-7733
Fax: 703-264-9474
TTY: 703-264-9446
www.education.gsu.edu

Advocates for quality education for individuals with physical disabilities and special health care needs in schools, hospitals, or home settings.

Pam DeLoach, President
Blanche Jackson Glimps, Vice President
Peggy Allgood, Interim Secretary

7960 Division of Birth Defects & Developmental Disabilities
National Center for Environmental Health
4770 Buford Highway NE
Atlanta, GA 30341
770-488-7150
888-232-6789
Fax: 770-488-7156
www.cdc.gov

Information and advocacy resources for families and professionals dealing with children with birth defects and developmental disabilities.

Raymond Strikas, Director
Tom Frieden, MD, MPH, Director, Centers for Disease Contr
Linda C. Degutis, DrPH, MSN, Director, National Center for Injur

7961 Division on Career Development and Transition
Council for Exceptional Children
1110 N Glebe Road, Suite 300
Arlington, VA 22201
703-620-3660
888-232-7733
Fax: 703-264-9474
TTY: 866-915-5000
www.dcdt.org

Focuses on the career development of individuals with disabilities and their transition from school to adult life.

Audrey Trainor, President
Joseph W. Madaus, Vice President
Darlene Unger, Treasurer

7962 ERIC Clearinghouse on Disabilities & Gifted Children
Council for Exceptional Children
1110 N Glebe Road Suite 300
Arlington, VA 22201
703-620-3660
888-232-7733
Fax: 703-264-9494
TTY: 866-915-5000
ericec@cec.sped.org
www.cec.sped.org/ericec.htm

Information and advocacy resources for families and professionals. Includes listings of organizations providing general information and organizations focusing on more specific areas of concern to families and young adults who have disabilities.

7963 Easter Seals Disability Services
233 South Wacker Drive, Suite 2400
Chicago, IL 60606
205-759-1211
800-221-6827
Fax: 312-726-1494
TDD: 312-726-4258
info@easterseals.com
www.easterseals.com

Easter Seals mission is to create solutions that change lives for children and adults with disabilities and to provide appropriate developmental and rehabilitation services. Services provided include early intervention, after-school programs, preschool, tutoring, medical rehabilitation, vocational services, adult and senior day services, respite and in home care, camping and recreation, residential housing, support services, support groups, transportation and referrals.

Stephen F. Rossman, Chairman
Richard W. Davidson, 1st Vice Chairman
James E Williams Jr, President/CEO

7964 Endocrine Society
8401 Connecticut Avenue, Suite 900
Chevy Chase, MD 20815
301-941-0200
Fax: 301-941-0259
endostaff@endo-society.org
www.endo-society.org/

To advance excellence in endocrinology and promote its essential role as an integrative force in scientific research and medical practice.

William F. Young, Jr., M.D., M.Sc., President
Ursula Kaiser, M.D., Vice President (Basic Scientist)
Margaret E. W ierman, M.D., Vice President (Clinical Scientist)

7965 Family Caregiver Alliance
180 Montgomery Street Suite 900
San Francisco, CA 94104   415-434-3388
                                                 800-445-8016
                                           Fax: 415-434-3508
                                             info@caregiver.org
                                              www.caregiver.org

Good information with resources and hotline numbers.

Ping Hao, MBA, President
Jacquelyn Kung, Vice President
Kathleen Kelly, MPA, Executive Director

7966 Family Voices
3701 San Mateo Blvd NE, Suite 200
Albuguerque, NM 87110   505-872-4774
                                                 888-835-5669
                                           Fax: 505-872-4780
                                     kidshealth@familyvoices.org
                                            www.familyvoices.org

Family Voices, a national grassroots network of families and
friends, advocates for health care services that are famliy-cen-
tered, community-based, comprehensive. coordinated and culturally competent for all children and youth with special health care
needs; promotes the inclusion of all families as decision makers
at all levels of health care; and supports essential partnerships
between families and professionals.

Molly Cole, President
Marcia O'Malley, Vice-President
Lynn Pedraza, Executive Director

7967 Federation for Children with Special Needs Center
529 Main Street, Suite 1102
Boston, MA 02129   617-236-7210
                                                 800-331-0688
                                           Fax: 617-241-0330
                                               fcsninfo@fcsn.org
                                                   www.fcsn.org

The Federation is a center for parents and parent organizations to
work together on behalf of children (up to age 22) with special
needs and their families. The Federation operates a Parent Center
in Massachusetts that offers a variety of services to parents, parent groups and others who are concerned with children with
special needs.

James F. Whalen, President
Michael Weiner, Treasurer
Kate Brewe, Information Specialist

7968 Federation of Families for Children's Mental Health
9605 Medical Center Drive, Suite 280
Rockville, MD 20850   240-403-1901
                                           Fax: 240-403-1909
                                               ffcmh@ffcmh.org
                                                  www.ffcmh.org

The National family run organization is dedicated exclusively to
helping children with mental health needs and their families
achieve a better quality of life.

Teka Dempson, President
Sherri Luthe, Vice President
Sandra Spencer, Executive Director

7969 Foundation for Exceptional Children
16 Lake Shore Road
Grosse Poimte Farm, MI 48236   313-885-8660

To improve the well-being of children and families by providing
theapeutic, social and educational services.

7970 Friends' Health Connection
PO Box 114
New Brunswick, NJ 08903   732-418-1811
                                                 800-483-7436
                                           Fax: 732-249-9897
                                  info@friendshealthconnection.org
                                    www.friendshealthconnection.org

Organization Mission Friends' Health Connection is a nonprofit
organization that connects people who are currently experiencing
or who have overcome the same disease, illness, handicap or injury in order to communicate for mutual support.

1989

Roxanne Black-Weisheit, FHC Founder and Executive Director

7971 Genetic Alliance
4301 Connecticut Avenue NW, Suite 404
Washington, DC 20008   202-966-5557
                                                 800-336-4363
                                           Fax: 202-966-8553
                                        info@geneticalliance.org
                                          www.geneticalliance.org

A nonprofit tax exempt organization founded in 1986 as a national coalition of consumers, professionals and genetic support
groups to voice the common concerns of children and adults and
families living with, and at risk of, genetic conditions. The Alliance builds partnerships among consumers and professionals and
the private and public sectors to promote optimum healthcare and
enhanced quality of life for individuals identified with genetic
conditions.

Sharon Terry, President/CEO
Tetyana Murza, Managing Director
Natasha Bonhomme, VP, Strategic Development

7972 Girl Scouts of the USA
Membership and Program Group
420 5th Avenue
New York, NY 10018   212-852-8000
                                                 800-478-7248
                                           Fax: 212-852-6515
                                                www.girlscouts.org

Girl Scout of the USA is the world's preeminent organization
dedicated solely to girls-all girls-where, in an accepting and nurturing environment, girls build character and skills for success in
the real world.

Anna Maria Ch vez, CEO
Nhadine Leung, Chief of Staff
Connie L. Lindsey, Chairman

7973 Handicapped Scuba Association
1104 El Prado
San Clemente, CA 92672   949-498-4540
                                                 800-673-5084
                                           Fax: 949-498-6128
                                              hsa@hsascuba.com
                                               www.hsascuba.com

Information on adaptive scuba diving activities for people of
many abilities. Includes local chapters, referrals, fun and social
interaction and support groups.

7974 Handle with Care
184 McKinstry Road
Gardnier, NY 12525   845-255-4031
                                                 888-590-5049
                                           Fax: 845-256-0094
                                         info@handlewithcare.com
                                           www.handlewithcare.com

Information and advocacy resources for families and professionals. Includes listings of organizations providing general information and organizations focusing on more specific areas of concern
to families and young adults who have disabilities.

Bruce Chapman, Founder/President
Hilary Adler, Vice President
Jeanette Smith, Accounting Dept. & Office Manager

7975 Heriditary Disease Foundation
3960 Broadway, 6th Floor
New York, NY 10032   212-928-2121
                                           Fax: 212-928-2172
                                           cures@hdfoundation.org
                                             www.hdfoundation.org

Conducts interdisciplinary workshop program that recruits scientists to develop and apply new technologies, supports basic research on genetic illness through grant and postdoctoral
fellowship programs at major universities, and provides research
tissue to medical investigators.

Nancy Wexler, President
Frank O. Gehry, Vice President
Alice Wexler, Secretary

7976 Houston Challengers TIRR Sports
1475 W Gray
Houston, TX 77019   713-521-3737

Information on adaptive sports and recreation activities for people of many abilities. Includes local chapters, referrals, fun and social interaction and support groups.

7977 Human Growth Foundation
997 Glen Cove Avenue, Suite 5
Glen Head, NY 11545   516-671-4041
                                      800-451-6434
                                      Fax: 516-671-4055
                                      hgfl@hgfound.org
                                      www.hgfound.org

Provides referrals to support groups, services, and genetic counseling on its toll-free telephone line. Encourages communication among support groups and continuing education.

Pisit Pitukcheewanon, MD, President
Emily Germain-Lee, Vice President
Patti D Costa, Executive Director

7978 Independent Living Research Utilization Program
2323 S Shepard, Suite 1000
Houston, TX 77019   713-520-0232
                                      Fax: 713-520-5785
                                      TTY: 713-520-5136
                                      ilru@ilru.org
                                      www.ilru.org

Information and advocacy resources for families and professionals on independent living for people with disabilities.

Lex Frieden, Director, ILRU
Linda CoVan, Grant Coordinator
Maria Del Bosque, Project Associate

7979 Indian Health Service
Mental Health/Social Service Programs Branch
801 Thompson Avenue, Suite 400
Rockville, MD 20852   301-443-1083

Includes listings of organizations providing general information and organizations focusing on more specific areas of concern to Native American families and young adults who have disabilities.

7980 Institute for Families of Blind Children
4650 Sunset Blvd, Mail Stop 111
Los Angeles, CA 90027   213-669-4649
                                      800-669-4549
                                      Fax: 323-665-7869
                                      info@instituteforfamilies.org
                                      www.instituteforfamilies.org

Offers support and information to families of blind children. Provides direct counseling and nation-wide telephone counseling.

Peggy Yoshino, Chairman
Eric Dahl, Chief Financial Officer
Joni Dahl, Secretary

7981 International Braille and Technology Center for the Blind
National Federation of the Blind
1800 Johnson Street
Baltimore, MD 21230   410-659-9314
                                      Fax: 410-685-5653
                                      nfb@nfb.org
                                      www.nfb.org

World's largest and most complete evaluation and demonstration center of all assistive technology used by the blind from around the world. Includes all Braille, synthetic speech, print-to-speech scanning, internet and portable devices and programs. Available for tours by appointment to blind persons, employers, technology manufacturers, teachers, parents and those working in the assistive technology field.

Curtis Chong, President, Computer Science

7982 International Society of Dermatology
2323 North State Street #30
Bunnell, FL 32110   386-437-4405
                                      Fax: 386-437-4427
                                      info@IntSocDermatol.org
                                      www.intsocderm.org

Promotes interest, education and research in dermatology.

Francisco Kerdel, President
Mark D P Davis, MD, Vice President
Martin Kassir, MD, Vice President

7983 International Wheelchair Aviators
82 Corral Drive
Keller, TX 76244   817-229-4634
                                      wheelchairaviators@yahoo.com
                                      www.wheelchairaviators.org

Provides information for pilots or future pilots who have a disability.

Mike Smith, President

7984 Iron Overload Diseases Assocation
525 Mayflower Rd.
West Palm Beach, FL 33405   561-586-8246
                                      Fax: 561-842-9881
                                      iod@ironoverload.org
                                      www.ironoverload.org

Committed to providing information and support to affected individuals and their families, educating the general public, promoting and supporting research, and pressing for earlier diagnosis and more effective treatment. Acts as a clearinghouse for affected individuals and family members, provides telephone consultations, offers referrals to genetic counseling and support groups. Provides a variety of educational and support materials including books, newsletters, pamphlets, and fact sheets.

7985 Jewish Children's Adoption Network
PO Box 147016
Denver, CO 80214   303-573-8113
                                      Fax: 303-893-1447
                                      jcan@qwest.net
                                      www.jcan.qwestoffice.net

Information and advocacy resources for families and professionals. Includes listings of organizations providing general information.

Stephen Krausz, PhD, President

7986 Job Opportunities for the Blind
1800 Johnson Street
Baltimore, MD 21230   410-659-9314
                                      Fax: 410-685-5653
                                      nfb@nfb.org
                                      www.nfb.org

Information and resources for those with visual impairments.

Curtis Chong, President, Computer Science

7987 Just One Break
570 Seventh Avenue, 6th Floor
New York, NY 10018   212-785-7300
                                      Fax: 212-785-4513
                                      TTY: 212-785-4515
                                      justonebreak@interactive.net
                                      www.justonebreak.com

Information and advocacy resources for families and professionals dealing with families and young adults who have disabilities.

C. Jeffrey Knittel, Chairman
Russ Cusick, Chief People Officer
John D. Kemp, President

7988 Learning Disabilities Association of Ameri ca
4156 Library Road
Pittsburgh, PA 15234   412-341-1515
                                      888-300-6710
                                      Fax: 412-344-0224
                                      info@LDAAmerica.org
                                      www.ldaamerica.org

Helps families of the affected individual through information and referral to professionals in their area. A membership organization with affiliates across the country.

Sheila Buckley, Executive Director

7989 Lifespire (A.C.R.M.D.)
1 Whitehall Street, 9th Floor
New York, NY 10004
212-741-0100
Fax: 212-320-0407
info@lifespire.org
www.lifespire.org

Life is committees to the principle that all individuals with a development disability are able to become contributing members of their family and community. It is Lifespire's aim to provide these individuals with the assistance and support necessary so that they can attain the skills necessary to maintain themselves in their community in the most integrated and independent manner possible.

Mark Van Voorst, CEO/President
Tom Lydon, COO
Keith Lee, CFO

7990 MUMS: National Parent to Parent Network
150 Custer Street
Green Bay, WI 54301
920-336-5333
877-336-5333
Fax: 920-339-0995
mums@netnet.net
www.netnet.net/mums/

Matches parents of children with rare disorders. Provides information and advocacy resources for families and professionals. Includes listings of organizations providing general information and organizations focusing on more specific areas of concern to families and young adults who have disabilities.

Julie Gordon, Director

7991 Make Today Count
101 1/2 S Union Street
Alexandria, VA 22314
703-548-9674

An organization that helps patients and their families cope with cancer and other serious diseases and improve their quality of life.

7992 March of Dimes Foundation
1275 Mamaroneck Avenue
White Plains, NY 10605
914-997-4488
888-663-4637
Fax: 914-428-8203
resourcecenter@marchofdimes.com
www.marchofdimes.com

Partnership of volunteers and professionals dedicated to the mission of the March of Dimes to improve the health of babies by preventing birth defects and infant mortality. Chapters are situated across the country and can be located through the web site, National Office, or telephone book. The Resource Center answers questions relating to preconception health, pregnancy, childbirth and birth defects.

Stacey D. Stewart, President

7993 March of Dimes Nursing Modules
1275 Mamaroneck Avenue
White Plains, NY 10605
914-997-4488
888-663-4637
Fax: 914-428-8203
productquestions@marchofdimes.com
www.marchofdimes.com/catalog

Nursing modules are self-directed learning monographs designed for registered nurses and nurse-midwives. Created to help nurses meet the challenges posed by a rapidly changing world of technological advances, evolving demographics and greater cultural diversity, they focus on effective care delivery during the pre-conceptional, prenatal, intrapartum, postpartum and inter-conceptional periods.

Dr Jennifer Howse, President

7994 NADD: National Association for the Dually Diagnosed
132 Fair Street
Kingston, NY 12401
845-331-4336
800-331-5362
Fax: 845-331-4569
info@thenadd.org
www.thenadd.org

Nonprofit organization designed to promote the interests of professional and parent development with resources for individuals who have the coexistence of mental illness and mental retardation. Provides conferences, educational services and training materials to professionals, parents, concerned citizens, and service organizations.

Dr Robert Fletcher, CEO
Michelle Jordan, Office Manager
Edward Seliger, Project Coordinator

7995 NAEYC: National Association for the Education of Young Children
1313 L Street, NW, Suite 500
Washington, DC 20005
202-232-8777
800-424-2460
Fax: 202-328-1846
pubaff@aeyc.org
www.naeyc.org

Information and advocacy resources for families and professionals. Includes listings of organizations providing general information and organizations focusing on more specific areas of concern to families and young adults who have disabilities.

Gera Jacobs, President
Roberta Schomburg, Vice President
Jerlean E. Daniel, Executive Director

7996 National Ability Center
PO Box 682799, 1000 Ability Way
Park City, UT 84068
435-649-3991
Fax: 435-658-3992
TDD: 435-649-3991
info@DiscoverNAC.org
www.discovernac.org

Information on adaptive sports and recreation activities for people of many abilities. Includes local chapters, referrals, fun and social interaction and support groups.

Gail Loveland, Executive Director
Ellen Hall Adams, Program Director
Kristi Brangle, Executive Assistant - Resource Deve

7997 National Academy for Child Development (NACD)
549 25th Street
Ogden, UT 84401
801-621-8606
Fax: 801-621-8389
info@nacd.org
www.nacd.org

International organization of parents and professionals dedicated to helping children and adults reach their full potential.

Julian Neil, Director of Health

7998 National Adoption Center
1500 Walnut Street, Suite 701
Philadelphia, PA 19102
215-735-9988
800-862-3678
Fax: 215-735-9410
nac@nationaladoptioncenter.org
www.adopt.org

Information and advocacy resources for families and professionals interested in or dealing with adoption. Includes listings of organizations providing general information and organizations focusing on specific areas of concern.

Ken Mullner, Executive Director
Gloria Hochman, Director of Communications
Christine Jacobs, Program Director

7999 National Alliance for the Mentally Ill
3803 N. Fairfax Dr., Ste. 100
Arlington, VA 22203
703-524-7600
800-950-6264
Fax: 703-524-9094
TDD: 703-516-7227
info@nami.org
www.nami.org

NAMI is a nonprofit, grassroots, self-help, support and advocacy organization of consumers, families and friends of people with severe mental illness, such as schizophrenia, bipolar disorder, major depressive disorder, obsessive compulsive disorder, anxiety disorders, autism and other severe and persistent mental illnesses that affect the brain.

David Levy, Chief Financial Officer
Lynn Borton, Chief Operating Officer
Jean-Michel Texier, Chief Information Officer

8000 National Amputee Golf Association
11 Walnut Hill Road
Amherst, NH 03031
603-672-6444
800-633-6242
Fax: 603-672-2987
webmaster@nagagolf.org
www.nagagolf.org

Information on adaptive golf activities for people of many abilities. Includes local chapters, referrals, fun and social interaction and support groups.

Kenny Greene, Executive Director
Virgil Price, Treasurer
Bob Wilson, Consultant

8001 National Archery Association
4065 Sinton Road, Suite 110
Colorado Springs, CO 80907
719-578-4576
Fax: 719-632-4733
dparker@usarchery.org
www.usarchery.org

Information on adaptive archery activities for people of many abilities. Includes local chapters, referrals, fun and social interaction and support groups.

Denise Parker, Chief Executive Officer
Cindy Clark, Office/Finance Manager
Amber Hildebrand, Accounting Assistant

8002 National Arts and Disability Center
760 Westwood Plaza
Los Angeles, CA 90095
310-794-1141
800-UCL-MD1
Fax: 310-794-1143
TTY: 310-267-2356
oraynor@mednet.ucla.edu
www.semel.ucla.edu

Information and advocacy resources for families and professionals. Includes listings of organizations providing general information on art and disabilities.

Olivia Raynor, Director
Beth Stoffmacher, Technical Assisstance Coordinator
Peter Whybrow, Director

8003 National Association for Parents of Childr en with Visual Impairments
PO Box 317
Watertown, MA 02471
617-972-7441
800-562-6265
Fax: 617-972-7444
napvi@perkins.org
www.spedex.com/napvi/

Julie Urban, President
Venetia Hayden, Vice President
Susan LaVenture, Executive Director

8004 National Association of Blind Students
National Federation of the Blind
1800 Johnson Street
Baltimore, MD 21230
410-659-9314
Fax: 410-685-5653
www.nabslink.org

Provides support, information and encouragement to blind college and university students. Leads the way in offering resources for national testing, accessible textbooks and materials, overcoming negative attitudes about blindness from school personnel, developing new techniques of accomplishing laboratory or field assignments and many other college experiences. Offers strong advocacy and motivational support.

Sean Whalen, President
Shelby Ball, Treasurer
Cindy Bennett, Secretary

8005 National Association of Protection and Advocacy Systems
900 2nd Street NE, Suite 211
Washington, DC 20002
202-408-9514
Fax: 202-408-9520
TTY: 202-408-9521
NAPAS@earthlink.net
www.napas.org

Information and advocacy resources for families and professionals. Includes listings of organizations providing general information and organizations focusing on more specific areas of concern to families and young adults who have disabilities.

Curtis L Decker, Executive Director

8006 National Association of the Dually Diagnosed
132 Fair Street
Kingston, NY 12401
845-331-4336
800-331-5362
Fax: 845-331-4569
info@thenadd.org
www.thenadd.org

Seeks to stimulate the public and professional awareness regarding the dually diagnosed population, and to encourage the exchange of pertinent information, promoting educational and training programs, advocating for appropriate governmental policies, supporting research focusing on identification, diagnosis, and treatment.

Robert J. Fletcher DSW, Chief Executive Officer
Michelle Jordan, Office Manager
Lisa Christie, Conference Planner

8007 National Center for Learning Disabilities
381 Park Avenue S, Suite 1401
New York, NY 10016
212-545-7510
888-575-7373
Fax: 212-545-9665
www.ncld.org

Works to ensure that the nation's 15 million children, adolescents and adults with learning disabilities have every opportunity to succeed in school, work and life. NCLD provides essential information to parents, professionals and individuals with learning disabilities, promotes research and programs to foster effective learning and advocates for policies to protect and strengthen educational rights and opportunities.

Sheldon Horowitz MD, LD Resources/Essential Information
James H Wendorf, Executive Director
Alan Bendich, Director, Finance & Operations

8008 National Center for Sight
National Society To Prevent Blindness
500 Remington Road
Schaumburg, IL 60173
847-843-2020
Fax: 847-843-8458

A toll-free line offering information on a broad range of vision, eye health and safety topics including sports eye safety, lazy eye, diabetic retinopathy, glaucoma, cataracts, children's eye disorders, and more.

8009 National Center for Vision and Child Development
Lighthouse
111 E 59th Street
New York, NY 10022
212-821-9200
800-829-0500
Fax: 212-821-9707
TTY: 212-821-9713
info@lighthouse.org
www.lighthouse.org

The mission is to overcome vision impairment for people of all ages through worldwide leadership in rehabilitation services, education, research, prevention and advocacy.

Joseph A. Ripp, Chairman
Mark G. Ackermann, President/Chief Executive Officer
Robert P. Hoak Jr., Chief Development Officer

8010 National Center on Accessbility
University of Indiana
501 North Morton Street, Suite 109
Bloomington, IN 47404   812-856-4422
                                          800-424-1877
                                          Fax: 812-856-4480
                                          TTY: 812-856-4421
                                          nca@indiana.edu
                                          www.ncaonline.org

Information on adaptive activities for people of many abilities. Includes local chapters, referrals, fun and social interaction and support groups.

Sherril York, Director
Ray Bloomer, Director of Education & Technical A
Jennifer Skulski, Director of Marketing and Special P

8011 National Children's Cancer Society
One South Memorial Drive, Suite 800
Saint Louis, MO 63102   314-241-1600
                                          800-532-6459
                                          Fax: 314-241-6949
                                          nccs@children-cancer.com
                                          nationalchildrenscancersociety.com

NCCS offers a multifaceted outreach program, which includes financial assistance, education, information, and emotional support. They provide financial assistance for bone marrow transplantation, donor harvest, donor search, donor recruitment, and family emergency expenses (such as travel, hotel, food). They also have an active advocacy program to help families with insurance companies and hospitals.

Mark Stolze, President
Julie Komanetsky, Director Patient/Family Services

8012 National Christian Resource Center
Bethesda Lutheran Homes
300 N. Kanawha Street, Suite 100
Beckley, WV 25801   304-252-9494
                                          800-369-4636
                                          Fax: 304-252-9004
                                          ernie@CRCbeckley.com
                                          www.crcbeckley.com

Information and advocacy resources for families and professionals. Includes listings of organizations providing general information and organizations focusing on more specific areas of concern to families and young adults who have disabilities.

Ernie Drumheller, CRC Director
Mike Carter, WOAY Operations Manager
Jim Hale, CRC Director of Communications

8013 National Disability Sports Alliance
4101 W. Green Oaks, Suite 305, #149
Arlington, TX 76016   401-792-7130
                                          Fax: 401-792-7132
                                          info@ndsaonline.org
                                          www.chasa.org

Nonprofit organization. Coordinates sports, recreation and fitness activities for individuals with physical disabilities. Main focus is on cerebral palsy, traumatic brain injury and stroke.

Nancy Atwood, Executive Director
Jana Smoot White, Board Director
Julie Ring, Board Director

8014 National Dissemination Center for Children with Disabilities
1825 Connecticut Ave NW
Washington, DC 20009   202-884-8200
                                          800-695-0285
                                          Fax: 202-884-8441
                                          TTY: 800-695-0285
                                          nichcy@aed.org
                                          www.nichcy.org

A national information and referral center that provides information on disabilities and disability-related issues for families, educators and other professionals.

Suzanne Ripley, Executive Director

8015 National Early Childhood Technical Assistance System
500 NationsBank Plaza, 137 East Franklin Street
Chapel Hill, NC 27514   919-962-2001
                                          Fax: 919-966-7463
                                          TDD: 919-966-4041
                                          nectas@unc.edu
                                          www.unc.edu

Assists states and other designated governing jurisdictions as they develop multidisciplinary, coordinated and comprehensive services for children with special needs.

8016 National Family Caregivers Association
10400 Connecticut Avenue, Suite 500
Kensington, MD 20895   301-942-6430
                                          800-896-3650
                                          Fax: 301-942-2302
                                          info@caregiveraction.org
                                          www.caregiveraction.org

The only not-for-profit organization dedicated to making life better for all of America's family caregivers. Services include information support and validation, public awareness and advocacy; NFCA strives to minimize the disparity between a caregivers quality of life and that of mainstream Americans.

Jon Shanfield, Chair
John Schall, CEO
Lisa Winstel, Chief Operating Officer

8017 National Father's Network
Kindering Center
16120 NE 8th Street
Bellevue, WA 98008   425-653-4286
                                          800-224-6827
                                          Fax: 425-747-1069
                                          jmay@fathersnetwork.org
                                          www.fathersnetwork.org

Information and advocacy resources for fathers. Includes listings of organizations providing general information and organizations focusing on more specific areas of concern to fathers and young adults who have disabilities.

Greg Schell, Director

8018 National Foundation for Facial Reconstruction
333 East 30th Street, Lobby Unit
New York, NY 10016   212-263-6656
                                          Fax: 212-263-7534
                                          info@nffr.org
                                          www.nffr.org

The National Foundation for Facial Reconstruction, founded in 1951 by the late Dr. John Marquis Converse, to enable patients with facial deformities to lead productive fulfilling lives. NFFR lends its support to the multidisciplinary craniofacial team at the Institute of Reconstructive Plastic Surgery at NYU Medical Center. An assembly of world-renowned surgeons, mental health professionals, research specialists and staff, give their time and expertise, using the latest reconstructive techniques

Whitney Burnett, Executive Director
Kelly Strantz, Director of Development and Events
Deborah Malkoff, Pediatric Dietitian

8019 National Foundation for Transplants
5350 Poplar Avenue, Suite 430
Memphis, TN 38119   901-684-1697
                                          800-489-3863
                                          Fax: 901-684-1128
                                          info@transplants.org
                                          www.transplants.org

Nonprofit organization that assists transplant candidates and recipients nationwide when public or private insurance does not cover all their transplant-related costs. Offers a fund raising program for patients who need to raise $10,000 or more, and grant program that helps patients with smaller, one-time needs.

Jackie D. Hancock, Jr., President/CEO
Kristin Clay, Database Coordinator
Annalisa Daughety, Online Marketing and Database Manag

8020 National Foundation of Wheelchair Tennis
70 West Red Oak Lane
White Plains, NY 10604　　　　　　　914-696-7000
　　　　　　　　　　　　　　　　　　Fax: 714-361-6603
　　　　　　　　　　　　　　　　　　nfwt@aol.com
　　　　　　　　　　　　　　　　　　www.usta.com

Information on adaptive tennis for people of many abilities. Includes local chapters, referrals, fun and social interaction and support groups.

Jon Vegosen, Chairman of the Board/President
Geoffrey Russell, Manager, Talent ID and Development
Joe Ceriello, Manager, USTA Training Center

8021 National Handicapped Sports
451 Hungerford Drive, Suite 100
Rockville, MD 20850　　　　　　　　301-217-0960
　　　　　　　　　　　　　　　　　　Fax: 301-217-0968
　　　　　　　　　　　　　　　　　　dsusa@dsusa.org
　　　　　　　　　　　　　　　　　　www.disabledsportsusa.org

Information on adaptive sports and recreation activities for people of many abilities, including local chapters, referrals, fun and social interaction and support groups.

Kirk Bauer, Executive Director
Cheryl Collins, Administrative Services Manager
Orlando Gill, Field Representative

8022 National Hospice Organization
1731 King Street, Suite 100
Alexandria, VA 22314　　　　　　　　703-837-1500
　　　　　　　　　　　　　　　　　　800-338-8898
　　　　　　　　　　　　　　　　　　Fax: 703-837-1233
　　　　　　　　　　　　　　　　　　nhpco_info@nhpco.org
　　　　　　　　　　　　　　　　　　www.nhpco.org

The nation's only advocate for terminally ill children, patients and their families. Provides member programs, represents hospice care interests in Congress, regulatory agencies and the public.

Ronald Fried, Chair
J. Donald Schumacher, PsyD, President/CEO
Galen Miller, PhD, Executive Vice President

8023 National Industries for the Blind
1310 Braddock Place
Alexandria, VA 22314　　　　　　　　703-310-0500
　　　　　　　　　　　　　　　　　　Fax: 703-998-8268
　　　　　　　　　　　　　　　　　　communications@nib.org
　　　　　　　　　　　　　　　　　　www.nib.org

A nonprofit organization that represents over 100 associated industries serving people who are blind in thirty-six states. These agencies serve people who are blind or visually impaired and help them to reach their full potential. Services include job and family counseling, job skills training, instruction in Braille and other communication skills, children's programs and more.

Gary J. Krump, Chairperson
Kevin A. Lynch, President and Chief Executive Offic
Claudia Knott, Chief Operating Officer

8024 National Industries for the Severely Handicapped
2235 Cedar Lane
Vienna, VA 22182　　　　　　　　　703-560-6800
　　　　　　　　　　　　　　　　　　Fax: 703-849-8916
　　　　　　　　　　　　　　　　　　info@nish.org
　　　　　　　　　　　　　　　　　　www.nish.org

Information and advocacy resources for families and professionals. Includes listings of organizations providing general information and organizations focusing on more specific areas of concern to families and young adults who have disabilities.

8025 National Mental Health Consumers' Self-Help Clearinghouse
1211 Chestnut Street, Suite 1207
Philadelphia, PA 19107　　　　　　　267-507-3810
　　　　　　　　　　　　　　　　　　800-553-4539
　　　　　　　　　　　　　　　　　　Fax: 215-636-6312
　　　　　　　　　　　　　　　　　　info@mhselfhelp.org
　　　　　　　　　　　　　　　　　　www.mhselfhelp.org

Offers information, support, and appropriate referrals and promotes public and professional education. Provides networking for those with special interest related to albinism and management of albinism and hypopigmentation.

Joseph Rogers, Executive Director
Susan Rogers, Director
Christa Burkett, Technical Assistance Coordinator

8026 National Organization for Rare Disorders
55 Kenosia Avenue, PO Box 1968
Danbury, CT 06810　　　　　　　　　203-744-0100
　　　　　　　　　　　　　　　　　　800-999-6673
　　　　　　　　　　　　　　　　　　Fax: 203-798-2291
　　　　　　　　　　　　　　　　　　TDD: 203-797-9590
　　　　　　　　　　　　　　　　　　orphan@rarediseases.org
　　　　　　　　　　　　　　　　　　www.rarediseases.org

The National Organization for Rare Disorders (NORD), a 501(c)(3) organization, is a unique federation of voluntary health organization dedicated to helping with rare 'orphan' diseases and assisting the organization that serve them. NORD is committed to the identification, treatment, and cure of rare disorders through programs of education, advocacy, research, and service.

Peter L Saltonstall, President & CEO
Pamela Gavin, Chief Operating Officer
Mary Cobb, SVP Membership & Organiz. Strategy

8027 National Organization on Disability
77 Water Street, Suite 204
New York, NY 10005　　　　　　　　646-505-1191
　　　　　　　　　　　　　　　　　　Fax: 646-505-1184
　　　　　　　　　　　　　　　　　　TDD: 202-293-5968
　　　　　　　　　　　　　　　　　　info@nod.org
　　　　　　　　　　　　　　　　　　www.nod.org

The mission of the National Organization on Disability (N.O.D.) is to expand the participation and contribution of America's 54 million men, women and children with disabilities in all aspects of life, by raising awareness through programs and information.

Thomas J. Ridge, Chairman
Cory Olicker Henkel, Chief Operating Officer
Miranda Pax, Chief of Staff

8028 National Parent Network on Disabilities
1130 17th Street NW, Suite 400
Washington, DC 20036　　　　　　　202-463-2299
　　　　　　　　　　　　　　　　　　Fax: 202-463-9403
　　　　　　　　　　　　　　　　　　www.npnd.org

Information and advocacy resources for families and professionals. Includes listings of organizations providing general information and organizations focusing on more specific areas of concern to families and young adults who have disabilities.

8029 National Parent Resource Center
Federation for Children with Special Needs
95 Berkeley Street, Suite 104
Boston, MA 02116　　　　　　　　　617-482-2915
　　　　　　　　　　　　　　　　　　800-695-2939
　　　　　　　　　　　　　　　　　　Fax: 617-572-2094
　　　　　　　　　　　　　　　　　　fcsninfo@fcsn.org
　　　　　　　　　　　　　　　　　　www.fcsn.org

A parent-run resource system designed to further the needs and goals of family-centered, community-based coordinated care for children with special health needs and their families. Offers written materials, training packages, workshops and presentations for parents and professionals on special education, health care financing and other topics.

8030 National Parent to Parent Support and Information System
457 State Street
Binghamton, NY 13901　　　　　　　706-632-8822
　　　　　　　　　　　　　　　　　　888-971-3295
　　　　　　　　　　　　　　　　　　Fax: 607-772-0468
　　　　　　　　　　　　　　　　　　npa@nationalperinatal.org
　　　　　　　　　　　　　　　　　　www.nationalperinatal.org

NPPSIS is a nonprofit organization established to support, strengthen, and empower families through one-on-one parent contacts. Links families nationally whose children have special health care needs and rare disorders, and provides parents with heath care information, resources and referrals to allow them to identify appropriate services.

Bernadette Hoppe, MA, JD, MPH, President
Karen D'Apolito, PH.D., APN, N, VP of Programs
Mona Liza Hamlin, BSN, RN, IB, VP of Development

8031 National Perinatal Association (NPA)
457 State Street
Binghamton, NY 13901
    813-971-1008
    888-971-3295
    Fax: 607-772-0468
    npa@nationalperinatal.org
    www.nationalperinatal.org

Information and advocacy resources for families and professionals. Includes listings of organizations providing general information and organizations focusing on more specific areas of concern to families and young adults who have disabilities.

Bernadette Hoppe, MA, JD, MPH, President
Karen D'Apolito, PH.D., APN, N, VP of Programs
Mona Liza Hamlin, BSN, RN, IB, VP of Development

8032 National Rehabilitation Information Center
8400 Corporate Drive, Suite 500
Landover, MD 20785
    301-459-5900
    800-346-2742
    Fax: 301-459-4263
    TTY: 301-459-5984
    naricinfo@heitechservices.com
    www.naric.com

NARIC is a library and information center focusing in disability and rehabilitation research. Information specialists provide quick information and referrals free of charge. Other services include customized searches of REHABDATA, the premier database of disability and rehabilitation literature, and documents from NARIC's collection of more than 70,000 documents are available for nominal fee.

Mark X. Odum, Project Director
Jessica H. Chaiken, Media and Information Services Mana
Natalie J. Collier, Library and Acquisitions Manager

8033 National Respite Locator Service
800 Eastowne Drive, Suite 105
Chapel Hill, NC 27514
    919-490-5577
    800-773-5433
    Fax: 919-490-4905
    mmathers@chtop.org
    www.chtop.org

Information for families and professionals interested in repite care. Includes listings of organizations that provide respite services to families.

Patricia Parker, Board Chair
Angela Poole, Treasurer
Mike Mathers, Executive Director

8034 National Self-Help Clearinghouse
365 5th Avenue, Suite 3300
New York, NY 10016
    212-817-1822
    info@selfhelpweb.org
    www.selfhelpweb.org

Information and advocacy resources for families and professionals. Includes listings of organizations providing general information and organizations focusing on more specific areas of concern to families and young adults who have disabilities.

Frank Riessman, Executive Director

8035 National Skeet & Sporting Clay Headquarters
5931 Roft Road
San Antonio, TX 78253
    210-688-3371
    800-877-5338
    Fax: 210-688-3014

Information on adaptive skeet and sporting clay activities for people of many abilities.

8036 National Sleep Foundation
1010 N. Glebe Road, Suite 310
Arlington, VA 22201
    703-243-1697
    Fax: 202-347-3472
    nsf@sleepfoundation.org
    www.sleepfoundation.org

Works to improve the quality of life for millions of Americans who suffer from sleep disorders, and to prevent the catastrophic accidents that are related to poor or disordered sleep through research, education and the dissemination of information towards the cause of Narcolepsy Project. Seeks patients to aid new research project targeting the cause of the disorder.

David Cloud, CEO

8037 National Technical Assistance Center for Children's Mental Health
Georgetown University Child Development Center
PO Box 571485
Washington, DC 20007
    202-687-5000
    Fax: 202-687-8899
    gucdc@georgetown.edu
    www.gucchd.georgetown.edu

Provides services to children experiencing emotional and mental problems.

Phyllis R. Magrab, Ph.D., Principal Investigator
James R. Wotring, M.S.W., A.C.S.W, Director of the National TA Center
Bruno Anthony, Ph.D., Senior Policy Associate

8038 National Vaccines Information Center
407 Church Street, Suite H
Vienna, VA 22180
    703-938-0342
    Fax: 703-938-5768
    contactNVIC@gmail.com
    www.nvic.org

Information and advocacy resources for families and professionals. Includes listings of organizations providing general information and organizations focusing on more specific areas of concern to families and young adults who have disabilities.

Barbara Loe Fisher, Co-Founder and President
Kathi Williams, Co-Founder and Vice President
Paul Arhtur, Director of Operations

8039 National Wheelchair Racquetball Association
2380 McGinley Road
Monroeville, PA 15146
    412-856-2400
    Fax: 412-856-2437

Information on adaptive racquetball activities for people of many abilities.

8040 National Wheelchair Shooting Federation
102 Park Avenue
Rockledge, PA 19111
    215-379-2359
    Fax: 215-663-9662

Information on adaptive shooting activities for people of many abilities.

8041 National Wheelchair Softball Association
13414 Paul Street
Omaha, NE 68145
    402-305-5020
    Fax: 612-437-3889
    bfroendt@cox.net
    www.wheelchairsoftball.org

Information on adaptive softball activities for people of many abilities.

Brian Chavez, President
Bruce Froendt, Commissioner
Thomas Dodd, 1st Director at Large

8042 National Youth Crisis Hotline
5331 Mount Alifan Drive
San Diego, CA 92111
    800-448-4663

Information and referral for runaways; also youth and parents with problems.

8043 New England Center for Children
33 Turnpike Road
Southborough, MA 01772
    508-481-1015
    Fax: 508-485-3421
    info@necc.org
    www.necc.org

Serving students between the ages of 3 and 22 diagnosed with autism, learning disabilities, language delays, mental retardation, behavior disorders and related disabilities; educational curriculum encompasses both the teaching of functional life skills and traditional academics; communication skills are taught throughout all activities in the school, residence, and community. Tuition and fees are set by the state. Consulting services also available.

Lisel Macenka, Chair
Vincent Strully, Chief Executive Officer & Founder
Katherine E. Foster, MEd., Chief Operating Officer

8044 NineLine
460 W 41st Street
New York, NY 10036 212-613-0300
 800-999-9999
 www.covenanthouse.org

Nationwide crisis/suicide hotline.

Andrew P. Bustillo, Board Chair
Kevin Ryan, President/CEO
Daniel C. McCarthy, Senior Vice President/Chief Financi

8045 North American Riding for the Handicapped
7475 Dakin Street, Suite 600
Denver, CO 80223 303-452-1212
 800-369-7433
 Fax: 303-252-4610
 narha.org
 www.pathintl.org

Information on adaptive riding activities for people of many abilities. Includes local chapters, referrals, fun and social interaction and support groups. NARHA is a membership organization that promotes and supports equine activities for the disabled. Membership dues are $50 - $150.

Kay Green, Chief Executive Officer
Carolyn Malcheski, Director of Human Resource and Fina
Kaye Marks, Director of Marketing and Communica

8046 Oak-Leyden Developmental Services
411 Chicago Avenue
Oak Park, IL 60302 708-524-1050
 Fax: 708-524-2469
 vplomin@oak-leyden.org
 www.oak-leyden.org

The mission of Oak-Leyden Developmental Services is to help people with developmental disabilities meet life's challenges and reach their highest potential.

Bob Atkinson, President & CEO
Valerie Plomin, Director of Development
Darlene Ehling, Director of Development

8047 Pan American Health Organization (PAHO)
525 23rd Street NW
Washington, DC 20037 202-974-3000
 Fax: 202-974-3663
 postmaster@paho.org
 www.paho.org

Acts as the directing and co-ordinating authority on international health work; aids in the prevention and control of epidemic, endemic and other diseases; promotes the improvement of nutrition, housing, sanitation, recreation, economic or working conditions; promotes improved standards of teaching and training in the health, medical and related professions; and fosters activities in the field of mental health.

Mirta Roses Periago, Director

8048 Parents Information Network FFCMH
1926 1700th Avenue
Lincoln, IL 62656 217-735-1662
 ffcmh.org/local.htm

Bridget Schneider

8049 Pathways Awareness Foundation
150 N Michigan Avenue, Suite 2100
Chicago, IL 60601 800-955-2445
 Fax: 888-795-8154
 TTY: 800-326-8154
 friends@pathwaysawareness.org
 www.pathwaysawareness.org

Established in 1988, Pathways Awareness Foundation is a national, nonprofit organization dedicated to raising awareness about the gift of early detection and early therapy for infants and children with physical movement differences. PAF provides informational materials to raise awareness of subtle indicators of physical development problems in infants and young children. We also have a parent answered toll-free phone. Our activities are based upon the expertise of our Medical Round Table.

Shirley W. Ryan, President
Sarah Kerndt, Education Director
Kathy O'Brien, Resource Director

8050 Pharmaceutical Manufacturers Association
1100 15th Street NW
Washington, DC 20005 800-762-4636
 www.pharmindex.com

Many drug companies have programs to provide free medicines (including chemotherapy) to needy patients. Eligibility requirements vary, but most are available to those not covered by private or public insurance programs. Ask your physician to request, on letterhead, a free copy of the Directory of Pharmaceutical Indigent Programs.

8051 Pike Institute on Law and Disability
Boston University School of Law
765 Commonwealth Avenue
Boston, MA 02115 Fax: 617-353-2906
 TTY: 617-353-2904
 pikeinst@bu.edu
 www.sph.bu.edu

Information and advocacy resources for families and professionals. Includes listings of organizations providing general information and organizations focusing on more specific areas of concern to families and young adults who have disabilities.

Edi Ablavs, Communications Specialist
Meg Comeau, Project Director
Cara Frigand, Project Director

8052 Pilot Parents (PP)
1941 S 42nd Street, Suite 122
Omaha, NE 68105 402-346-5220
 Fax: 402-346-5253
 aadamson@olliewebb.org
 www.olliewebb.org

Parents, professionals and others concerned with providing emotional and peer support to new parents of children with special needs. Sponsors a parent-matching program which allows parents who have had sufficient experience and training in the care of their own children to share their knowledge and expertise with parents of children recently diagnosed as disabled. Publications: The Gazette, newsletter, published 6 times a year.

Laurie Ackermann, Executive Director
Jennifer Varner, Coordinator

8053 Pioneers Division of CEC
Council for Exceptional Children
2900 Crystal Drive, Suite 1000
Arlington, VA 22202 703-620-3660
 888-232-7733
 Fax: 703-264-9474
 TTY: 866-915-5000
 www.cec.sped.org

Promotes activities and programs to increase awareness of the educational needs of children with disabilities and/or who are gifted, and the services that are available to them.

Lynda Van Kuren, Contact

8054 Planetree Health Information Service
2040 Webster Street
San Francisco, CA 94115 415-923-3680

A nonprofit consumer-oriented resource for health information, including relaxation and visualization techniques. Write or call for a catalog and price list.

8055 Prevent Blindness America
211 W Wacker Drive #1700
Chicago, IL 60606   800-331-2020
                                      Fax: 312-363-6001
                                      info@preventblindness.org
                                      www.preventblindness.org

A volunteer eye health and safety organization dedicated to fighting blindness and saving sight. Focused on promoting a continuum of vision care, Prevent Blindness America touches the lives of millions of people each year through public and professional education, advocacy, certified vision screening training, community and patient service programs and research.

Hugh R Parry, President/CEO
Jeff Todd, COO
Arzu Bilazer, Creative Director

8056 Rainbows
1111 Tower Road
Schaumburg, IL 60173   708-310-1880

Peer support groups for adults and children who are grieving.

8057 Resources for Children with Special Needs
116 E 16th Street, 5th Floor
New York, NY 10003   212-677-4650
                                      Fax: 212-254-4070
                                      info@resourcesnyc.org
                                      www.resourcesnyc.org

A not for profit agency providing information, referrals, advocacy, training and support for New York City parents of children with learning, developmental, emotional and physical disabilities and special needs and the professionals who serve them. Publishers of The Comprehensive Directory: Programs and Services for Children and Youth with Disabilities and their Families in the Metro New York Area, Camps 2004, Schools and services for Children with Autism Spectrum Disorders.

Rachel Howard, Executive Director
Stephen Stern, Director of Finance and Administrat
Todd Dorman, Director of Communications and Outr

8058 Roeher Institute
York University
Kinsmen Building, 4700 Keele Street
North York, ON, M3J
Canada   416-661-9611
                                      Fax: 416-661-5701
                                      TDD: 416-661-2023
                                      info@roeher.ca
                                      www.indie.ca/roeher

Conducts research for various pediatric disabilities.

8059 Ronald McDonald Houses
One Kroc Drive
Oak Brook, IL 60523   603-623-7048
                                      Fax: 630-623-7488
                                      info@rmhc.org
                                      www.rmhc.org

Provides national programs, funding and other support to network of 150 local Ronald McDonald Houses, homes-away-from-homes for families of seriously ill children

Martin J Coyne Jr, President and CEO
Aggie Dentice, Friends of Ronald McDonals House Ch
Linda Dunham, Ronald McDonald House Charities Boa

8060 Rural Institute on Disabilities
University of Montana
52 Corbin Hall
Missoula, MT 59812   406-243-5467
                                      800-732-0323
                                      Fax: 406-243-4730
                                      TTY: 403-243-5467
                                      rural@ruralinstitute.umt.edu
                                      www.ruralinstitute.umt.edu

Information and advocacy resources for families and professionals. Includes listings of organizations providing general information and organizations focusing on more specific areas of concern to families and young adults who have disabilities.

8061 SHAPE America: Society of Health and Physical Educators
1900 Association Drive
Reston, VA 20191   703-476-3400
                                      800-213-7193
                                      Fax: 703-476-9527
                                      aair@aahperd.org
                                      www.shapeamerica.org

Formerly the American Association for Leisure and Recreation, it serves recreation professionals practitioners, educators, and students who advance the profession and enhance the quality of life of all Americans through creative and meaningful leisure and recreation experiences.

Judith Young, Interim CEO

8062 Sexuality Information and Education Council of the US (SIECUS)
90 John Street, Suite 402
New York, NY 10038   212-819-9770
                                      Fax: 212-819-9776
                                      siecus@siecus.org
                                      www.siecus.org/

Information and advocacy resources for families and professionals. Includes listings of organizations providing general information and organizations focusing on more specific areas of concern to families and young adults who have disabilities.

Monica Rodriguez, President/CEO
Jason I. Osher, Chief Operating Officer
Kurt Conklin, MPH, MCHES, Program Director

8063 Sibling Support Project
Children's Hospital and Regional Medical Center
4800 Sand Point Way NE
Seattle, WA 98105   206-987-2000
                                      Fax: 206-527-5705
                                      TTY: 206-987-2280
                                      dmeyer@chmc.org
                                      www.seattlechildrens.org

Information and advocacy resources for families and professionals. Includes listings of organizations providing general information and organizations focusing on more specific areas of concern to families and young adults who have disabilities.

8064 Ski for Light
1455 West Lake Street
Minneapolis, MN 55408   612-827-3232
                                      info@sfl.org
                                      www.sfl.org

Nonprofit organization founded in 1975 to promote the physical fitness of visually and mobility impaired adults.

8065 Society for Pediatric Dermatology
8365 Keystone Crossing, Suite 107
Indianapolis, IN 46240   317-202-0224
                                      Fax: 317-205-9481
                                      info@pedsderm.net
                                      www.pedsderm.net

Objective is to promote, develop and advance education, research and care of skin disease in all pediatric age groups.

Karen Wiss, President
Andrea Zaenglen, President-Elect
Kent Lindeman, Executive Director

8066 Sparrow Foundation
1110 East Michigan Avenue
Seattle, WA 48912   517-364-5680
                                      Fax: 517-364-5698
                                      foundation@sparrow.org
                                      www.sparrow-fdn.org

This nonprofit charitable and educational organization was started by the family of a child who needed a bone marrow transplant, for which their insurance carrier refused to pay. The foundation provides seed money to schools, youth organizations, service clubs, and churches which help persons with medical needs.

John Pirich, Chair
Ron Simon, Vice Chair
Charles Blockett, Secretary/Treasurer

8067 Spaulding for Children
16250 Northland Drive, Suite 100
Southfield, MI 48075   248-443-7080
                                      Fax: 248-443-7099
                                      sfc@spaulding.org
                                      www.spaulding.org

Information and advocacy resources for families and professionals. Includes listings of organizations providing general information and organizations focusing on more specific areas of concern to families and young adults who have disabilities.

8068 Special Needs Advocate for Parents (SNAP)
1801 Avenue of the Stars #401
Century City, CA 90067   310-452-3759
                                           888-310-9889
                                      Fax: 310-450-5769
                                      TTY: 310-201-9889
                                      info@spapinfo.org
                                      www.icdri.org

Nonprofit organization with advisors nationwide and information and advocacy resources for families and professionals. Includes listings of organizations providing general information and organizations focusing on more specific areas of concern to families and young adults who have disabilities, support groups, educational advocates and medical insurance problem solving. Quarterly newsletter with articles of interest.

Marla Kraus, Executive Director

8069 Special Olympics
1133 19th Street, NW
Washington, DC 20036   202-628-3630
                                           800-700-8585
                                      Fax: 202-824-0200
                                      info@specialolympics.org
                                      www.specialolympics.org

Information on adaptive sports and recreation activities and related health issues for people of many abilities. Including local chapters, referrals, fun and social interaction and support groups.

Timothy P. Shriver, Ph.D., Chairman/Board of Directors/Chief E
J. Brady Lum, President & Chief Operating Officer
Peter Wheeler, Chief Strategic Properties

8070 Specialized Training of Military Parents (STOMP)
Washington PAVE
6316 S 12th Street
Tacoma, WA 98465   253-565-2266
                                           800-572-7368
                                      Fax: 253-566-8052
                                      TTY: 253-565-2266
                                      stomp@washingtonpave.com
                                      www.stompproject.org

Information and advocacy resources for military families who have children with special education or health needs. Includes listings of organizations providing general information and organizations focusing on more specific areas of concern and family to family connections.

Heather Hedbon, Founder & Director
Luz Adriana Martinez, Parent Education Coordinator
Valerie Patterson, Parent Education Coordinator

8071 Starbright
5757 Wilshire Boulevard, Suite M100
Los Angeles, CA 90036   310-479-1212
                                           800-315-2580
                                      Fax: 310-479-1235

The Foundation is dedicated to the development of projects that empower seriously ill children to combat the medical and emotional challenges they face on a daily basis. STARBRIGHT projects do more then educate and entertain, address the core issues that accompany illness, the pain, fear and loneliness and depression that can be as damaging as the sickness itself.

8072 Tech Connection
Family Resource Associates
1421 Park Ave., Ste. 100
Chico, CA 95928   732-747-5310
                                      Fax: 732-747-1896
                                      techhorin@aol.com
                                      www.techconnection.us

Tech Connection is a resource center to help children and adults who have disabilities gain access to the benefits of technology. Includes nationwide network of community-based assistive technology, resource centers, hands on consultants and product demonstrations and evaluations.

8073 Technology Assistance for Special Consumers
1856 Keats Drive
Huntsville, AL 35810   256-859-8300
                                      Fax: 256-859-4332
                                      TDD: 256-532-5996
                                      tasc@ucphuntsville.org
                                      www.ucptasc.org

Technology group of parents, consumers and professionals; provides resources to help children and adults who have disabilities gain access to the benefits of technology. Includes nationwide network of community-based assistive technology, resource centers, hands on consultants and product demonstrations.

Laura Parks, M.Ed., Assistive Technology Specialist
Julie Yockel, M.S., CCC-SLP, AAC Specialist
Mark Pepper, STAR Reutilization Specialist

8074 US Paralympics
U.S. Olympic Committee
1 Olympic Plaza, 30 Cimino Drive
Colorado Springs, CO 80903   719-866-2030
                                      Fax: 719-866-2029
                                      alison.nicholas@usoc.org
                                      www.teamusa.org

A division of the United States Olympic Committee, we focus our efforts on enhancing programs, funding and opportunities for persons with physical disabilities to participate in Paralympic sport. The Paralympic Games are the second largest sporting event in the world, conceding top honors only to the Olympics. The multi-sport competition showcases the talents and abilities of the world's most elite athletes with physical disabilities.

Alison Nicholas, Program Coordinator
Beth Bason, Communications Coordinator
Joe Walsh, Director

8075 Vision of Children Foundation
11975 El Camino Real, Suite 104
San Diego, CA 92130   858-314-7917
                                      Fax: 858-314-7920
                                      info@visionofchildren.org
                                      www.visionofchildren.org

Provides information, promotes research and assists the families of blind and visually impaired children in locating organizations and service providers who can give support.

Samuel A Hardage, Chairman
Elizabeth Dole, Senator, Honorary Co-Chair
Andria Kinnear, Executive Director

8076 WE MOVE (Worldwide Education and Advocacy for Movement Disorders)
Mt. Siani Medical Center
5731 Mosholu Avenue
Bronx, NY 10471   212-241-8567
                                           800-437-6682
                                      Fax: 212-875-8389
                                      wemove@wemove.org
                                      www.wemove.org

WE MOVE provides movement disorder information and educational materials to physicians, patients, the media, and the public via its comprehensive web site, training courses, patient support group and more. Its goal is to make early diagnosis, up-to-date treatment and patient support a reality for all people living with movement disorders.

Mark Stacy, MD, Chair, Education Committee
Susan Bressman, President
Mo Moadeli, Vice President

947

8077 World Institute on Disability
3075 Adeline Street, Suite 280
Berkeley, CA 94703

510-225-6400
Fax: 510-225-0477
TTY: 510-225-0478
wid@wid.org
www.wid.org

Information and advocacy resources for families and professionals. Includes listings of organizations providing general information and organizations focusing on more specific areas of concern to families and young adults who have disabilities.

Stanley K Yarnell MD, Chairman
Martin B Schulter, Vice Chair

8078 World Research Foundation
41 Bell Rock Plaza
Sedona, AZ 86351

928-284-3300
Fax: 928-248-3530
info@wrf.org
www.wrf.org

Nonprofit organization. Your global source of information on illnesses and therapies used around the world.

LaVerne Ross, Co-Founder
Steven Ross

8079 Young Adult Institute
460 West 34th St.
New York, NY 2382

212-273-6100
TDD: 212-290-2787
www.yai.org

A nonprofit professional organizations serving developmentally disabled children and adults in many programs throughout the New York metropolitan area. Provides over 50 program sites for thousands of participants.

Stephen E. Freeman, L.C.S.W., Chief Executive Officer
Thomas A. Dern, L.C.S.W., Chief Operating Officer
Sanjay Dutt, Chief Financial Officer

8080 Zero to Three
1255 23rd Street, NW, Suite 350
Washington, DC 20037

202-638-1144
800-899-4301
Fax: 202-638-0851
webhelp@zerotothree.org
zerotothree.org

The mission is to promote the healthy development of our nation's infants and toddlers by supporting and strengthening families, communities and those who work on their behalf. We are dedicated to advancing current knowledge , promoting beneficial policies and practices and providing training, technical assistance, and leadership development. A nonprofit organization.

Janice Im, Chief Program Officer
Laura Shiflett, Chief Financial/Administrative Offi
Matthew E Melmed, Executive Director

State Agencies & Support Groups

Alabama

8081 ARC of Morgan County
401 14th Street, Suite 4-E
Decatur, AL 35601

205-355-6192
Fax: 256-350-4502
arc@hiwaay.net
www.arcofmorgancounty.org

Informational and emotional support to parents who have a child, adolescent, or adult family member with special needs.

Lisa English, President
Sherry Stephenson, Vice President
Ireta Hogan, Secretary

8082 Early Intervention Program
2129 East South Blvd
Montgomery, AL 36111

334-281-8780
800-441-7607
Fax: 334-281-1973
oholder@rehab.state.al.us
www.rehab.state.al.us

Services include central directory, representatives of agencies, service providers, families, and coordinators of infant, toddler, and preschool special education programs.

Stephen G. Kayes, Board of Director
Jimmie Varnado, Board of Director

8083 Friends for Life Auburn United Methodist Church
99 South Street
Auburn, NY 13021

315-253-6295
www.auburnunitedmethodist.org

Informational and emotional support to parents who have a child, adolescent, or adult family member with special needs.

Richelle Duchaner, Pastor
Geri Jackson, Administrative Assisstant
Mary Howard, Coordinator of Congregational Life

8084 Special Education Action Committee Huntsville Outreach Office
3322 S Memorial Parkway, Suite 25
Huntsville, AL 35801

256-882-3911
Fax: 256-882-3974
seach@traveler.com
www.hsv.tis.net/~seachsv

Informational and emotional support to parents who have a child, adolescent, or adult family member with special needs.

8085 Special Education Services
Department of Education
PO Box 302101
Montgomery, AL 36130

334-242-8114
800-392-8020
Fax: 334-242-9192
jwaid@sdenet.alsde.edu
www.alsde.edu

Services include central directory, representatives of agencies, service providers, families, and coordinators of infant, toddler, and preschool special education programs.

Robert J. Bentley, President
Thomas R. Bice, Ed.D., Secretary/Executive Officer
Stephanie Bell, Vice President

8086 Statewide Technology Access & Response System for Alabamians with Disabilities
2125 E South Boulevard, PO Box 20752
Montgomery, AL 36120

334-613-3480
800-782-7656
Fax: 334-613-3485
TDD: 334-613-3519
tgannaway@rehab.state.al.us
www.mindspring.com/alstar/

State assisted programs and support group information for people of many abilities. Includes local chapters, referrals, fun and social interaction and support groups.

Alaska

8087 Alaska Department of Education
801 W 10th Street, Suite 200, PO Box 110500
Juneau, AK 99811

907-465-2800
Fax: 907-465-4156
TTY: 907-465-2815
eed.webmaster@alaska.gov
www.eed.state.ak.us

Individuals with Disabilities Education Act requires early intervention and preschool special education for children with disabilities and special health care needs. Services include central directory, representatives of agencies, service providers, families, and coordinators of infant, toddler, and preschool special education programs.

Steven J. Hostetter, President

8088 Assistive Technologies of Alaska
3330 Arctic Blvd., Suite 101
Anchorage, AK 99503
907-563-2599
800-723-2852
Fax: 907-563-0699
TTY: 907-561-2592
TDD: 907-269-3569
mystie@atlaak.org
www.atlaak.org

State assisted programs and support group information for people of many abilities. Includes local chapters, referrals, fun and social interaction and support groups.

8089 Leukemia & Lymphoma Society - Washington/ Alaska Chapter
Leukemia & Lymphoma Society
5601 6th Avenue, Ste 182
Seattle, WA 98108
206-628-0777
anne.gillingham@lls.org
www.lls.org/washingtonalaska

Dedicated to finding cures for leukemia and related cancers and to improving the quality of life for patients and their families.

Anne Gillingham, Executive Director
Courtney Hale, Operations Director
Victoria Wenick, Senior Campaign Director

8090 Maternal, Child & Family Health, Early Intervention/Infant Learning Program
State of Alaska Department of Health
1231 Gambell Street
Anchorage, AK 99501
907-269-3419
Fax: 907-269-3465
jbatuk@health.state.ak.us

Early intervention and preschool special education for children with disabilities and special health care needs. Services include administration of statewide early intervention programs for infants and toddlers with developmental delays or disabilities and their families.

Jane Atuk, Part C Coordinator
Karen Martinek, Special Needs Services Unit

8091 PARENTS
4743 E Northern Lights Boulevard
Anchorage, AK 99508
907-337-7678
800-478-7678
Fax: 907-337-7671
TDD: 907-337-7678
parentsss@alaska.com
www.parentsinc.org

Parent Training and Information (PTI) programs help parents to understand their children's specific needs, communicate more effectively with professionals, participate in the educational planning process, and obtain information about relevant programs, services and resources.

Arizona

8092 Arizona Early Intervention Program/ Department of Economic Security
3839 N. 3rd St, Suite 304 Site Code No. 801 A-6
Phoenix, AZ 85012
602-532-9960
888-439-5609
Fax: 602-200-9820
allazeip2@azdes.gov
www.azdes.gov/azeip

Early intervention and preschool special education for children with disabilities and special health care needs. Services include central directory, representatives of agencies, service providers, families, and coordinators of infant, toddler, and preschool special education programs.

8093 Arizona Technology Access Program Institute for Human Development
2400 N. Central Avenue, Suite 300
Pheonix, AZ 85004
602-728-9534
800-477-9921
Fax: 602-728-9353
TTY: 602-728-9536
Daniel.Davidson@nau.edu
www.nau.edu/ihd/aztap

State assisted programs and support group information for people of many abilities. Includes local chapters, referrals, fun and social interaction and support groups.

8094 Blake Foundation Children's Achievement Center
3825 E 2nd Street
Tucson, AZ 85716
520-325-0611
Fax: 520-327-5414
www.nectas.unc.edu

Services include central directory, representatives of agencies, service providers, families, and coordinators of infant, toddler, and preschool special education programs.

Annabell Rose, Interagency Coordinating Council

8095 Division of Special Education State Department of Education
1535 W Jefferson
Phoenix, AZ 85007
602-542-3852
Fax: 602-542-5404
lbusenb@mail1.ade.state.az.us
www.nectas.unc.edu

Individuals with Disabilities Education Act requires all states and territories to provide early intervention and preschool special education for children with disabilities and special health care needs. Services include central directory, representatives of agencies, service providers, families, and coordinators of infant, toddler, and preschool special education programs.

Lynn Busenbark, Preschool Special Ed. Coordinator

8096 Pilot Parents of Southern Arizona
2600 N Wyatt Drive
Tucson, AZ 85712
520-324-3150
877-365-7220
Fax: 520-324-3152
ppsa@pilotparents.org
www.pilotparents.org

Parent Training and Information (PTI) programs help parents to understand their children's specific needs, communicate more effectively with professionals, participate in the educational planning process, and obtain information about relevant programs, services and resources.

Lynn Kallis, Executive Director
Robert Snyder, Director of Education & Training
Cheryl McKenzie, Administrative Assistant

8097 Raising Special Kids
5025 E Washington Street, Suite 204
Phoenix, AZ 85034
602-242-4366
800-237-3007
Fax: 602-242-4306
info@specialkids.org
www.raisingspecialkids.org

Provides support and training to families of children who have disabilities and special health needs, helps parents communicate more effectively with professionals, participate in the educational planning process and obtain information about programs and resources available to them. Offers training to professionals in health, education and social services.

Paula Banahan, President
Joyce Millard-Hoie, Executive Director
Janna Murrell, Director of Family Support and Educ

8098 Southwest Human Development
PO BOX 28487
Austin, TX 78755
512-467-7916
800-369-9082
Fax: 512-467-1453
TTY: 888-467-1455
info@swhuman.org
www.swhuman.org

Services include central directory, representatives of agencies, service providers, families, and coordinators of infant, toddler, and preschool special education programs.

Blake Stanford, President/CEO

Arkansas

8099 Arkansas Disability Coalition
1501 N. University Avenue, Suite 268
Little Rock, AR 72207

501-614-7020
800-223-1330
Fax: 501-614-9082
TDD: 501-614-7020
adc@alltel.net
www.adcpti.org

Parent Training and Information (PTI) programs help parents to understand their children's specific needs, communicate more effectively with professionals, participate in the educational planning process, and obtain information about relevant programs, services and resources.

Wanda Horton, Executive Director
Karen Lutrick, Parent Educator
Bryan Cozart, Project Director

8100 Arkansas Disability Coalition Parent Train ing and Information Center
1501 N. University Avenue, Suite 268
Little Rock, AR 72207

501-614-7020
800-223-1330
Fax: 501-614-9082
TDD: 501-614-7020
adc@alltel.net
www.adcpti.org

The Arkansas Parent Training and Information Center (PTI) is a project of the Arkansas Disability Coalition. It is funded through a federal grant from the US Department of Education that serves families of children ages birth through 26 years of age who have a disability, but not yet diagnosed.

Wanda Horton, Executive Director
Karen Lutrick, Parent Educator
Bryan Cozart, Project Director

8101 DD Services, Department of Human Services
PO Box 1437, Slot 2520
Little Rock, AR 72203

501-682-8699
Fax: 501-682-8890
dds1@aristotle.net
www.chasa.org

Individuals with Disabilities Education Act requires all states and territories to provide early intervention and preschool special education for children with disabilities and special health care needs. Services include central directory, representatives of agencies, service providers, families, and coordinators of infant, toddler, and preschool special education programs.

Sherrill Archer, Coordinator

8102 FOCUS
305 W Jefferson Avenue
Jonesboro, AR 72401

870-935-2750
Fax: 870-931-3755
focusinc@ipa.net
www.taalliance.org

Parent Training and Information (PTI) programs help parents to understand their children's specific needs, communicate more effectively with professionals, participate in the educational planning process, and obtain information about relevant programs, services and resources.

8103 Family-2-Family Health Information Center of Arkansas
1501 N. University Avenue, Suite 268
Little Rock, AR 72207

501-614-7020
800-223-1330
Fax: 501-614-9082
TDD: 501-614-7020
adc@alltel.net
www.adcpti.org

The Family-2-Family Health Information Center of Arkansas (F2F HIC) is a nonprofit family-run organization that assists families of children and youth with special health care needs and the professionals who serve them. They provide health-related support, information, resources and training.

Bryan Cozart, Project Director
Karen Lutrick, Parent Educator
Wanda Horton, Executive Director

8104 Increasing Capabilities Access Network
Dept of Education/Arkansas Rehabilitation Services
525 W. Capitol
Little Rock, AR 72201

501-666-8868
800-828-2799
Fax: 501-666-5319
TTY: 501-666-8868
TDD: 800-828-2799
Barbara.Gullett@arkansas.gov
www.ar-ican.org

State assisted programs and support group information for people of many abilities. Includes local chapters, referrals, fun and social interaction and support groups.

Barry Vuletich, Program Administrator

8105 Parent to Parent Arc of Arkansas
2004 South Main Street
Little Rock, AR 72206

501-375-7770
Fax: 501-372-4621

Informational and emotional support to parents who have a child, adolescent, or adult family member with special needs.

8106 Special Education Section State Department of Education
4 Capitol Mall, Room 105-C
Little Rock, AR 72201

501-682-4225
Fax: 501-682-4313
sreifeiss@arkedu.k12.ar.us
www.unc.edu

Individuals with Disabilities Education Act requires all states and territories to provide early intervention and preschool special education for children with disabilities and special health care needs. Services include central directory, representatives of agencies, service providers, families, and coordinators of infant, toddler, and preschool special education programs.

Sandra Reifeissk, Preschool Special Ed. Coordinator

California

8107 ARC Family Resource Project
2421 Lomitas Avenue, PO Box 219
Santa Rosa, CA 95402

877-694-4335
Fax: 707-578-8601
arcsoco@sonic.net

Parent Training and Information (PTI) programs help parents to understand their children's specific needs, communicate more effectively with professionals, participate in the educational planning process, and obtain information about relevant programs, services and resources.

Traci N Turner, Program Coordinator
Elvis Bozarth, President

8108 CARE Family Resource Center
1350 Arnold Drive, Suite 203
Martinez, CA 94553

925-313-0999
800-281-3023
Fax: 925-370-8651

Informational and emotional support to parents who have a child, adolescent, or adult family member with special needs.

8109 Carolyn Kordich Family Resource Center
1135 W. 257th Street
Harbor City, CA 90710

310-325-7288
Fax: 310-325-7288
ckfrc@worldnet.att.net

Informational and emotional support to parents who have a child, adolescent, or adult family member with special needs.

8110 Challenged Family Resource Center
827 West 20th Street
Merced, CA 95340

209-385-5314
Fax: 209-385-5317
dkuneck@aol.com
www.challengedfrc.org

Informational and emotional support to parents who have a child, adolescent, or adult family member with special needs.

8111 Children Living with Illness
The Center for Attitudinal Healing
33 Buchanan Drive
Sausalito, CA 94965

415-331-6161
Fax: 415-331-4545

For children who are ill, have an ill sibling, or an ill. Parent group meets separately at the same time.

Jimmy Pete

8112 Comfort Connection Family Resource Center
12361 Lewis Street, Suite 101
Garden Grove, CA 92840

714-748-7491
Fax: 714-748-8149

Informational and emotional support to parents who have a child, adolescent, or adult family member with special needs.

8113 Department of Developmental Services of Early Start Program
1600 9th Street, PO Box 944202
Sacramento, CA 94244

916-654-1690
800-515-2229
Fax: 916-654-2054
TTY: 916-654-2054
TDD: 916-654-2054
earlystart@dds.ca.gov
www.dds.ca.gov

Individuals with Disabilities Education Act requires all states and territories to provide early intervention and preschool special education for children with disabilities and special health care needs. Services include central directory, representatives of agencies, service providers, families, and coordinators of infant, toddler, and preschool special education programs.

Mark Hutchinson, Chief Deputy Director
Terri Delgadillo, Director
Rick Ingraham, Quality Management/Development Bran

8114 Early Start Family Resource Network
1425 S. Waterman Ave.
San Bernadino, CA 92408

909-890-4794
800-974-5553
Fax: 909-890-4709
www.esfrn.org

Informational and emotional support to parents who have a child, adolescent, or adult family member with special needs.

8115 Exceptional Family Resource Center
9245 Sky Park Court, Suite 130
San Diego, CA 92123

619-594-7416
800-281-8252
Fax: 858-268-4275
efro@cybergate.com
www.efrconline.org

Informational and emotional support to parents who have a child, adolescent, or adult family member with special needs.

Sherry Torok, Executive Director
Susan Carlton-Bahm, Manager
Joyce Clark, Manager

8116 Exceptional Family Support, Education and Advocacy Center
6402 Skyway
Paradise, CA 95969

530-876-8321
Fax: 530-876-0346
sea@sunset.net
www.taalliance.org

Parent Training and Information (PTI) programs help parents to understand their children's specific needs, communicate more effectively with professionals, participate in the educational planning process, and obtain information about relevant programs, services and resources.

8117 Exceptional Parents
Family Resource Center
4440 N 1st Street
Fresno, CA 93726

559-229-2000
Fax: 559-229-2956
TTY: 559-225-6059
epu1@cybergate.com
www.exceptionalparents.org

Informational and emotional support to parents who have a child, adolescent, or adult family member with special needs.

Suzanne Ellis, Chief Financial Officer
Kyle Loreto, President
Marion Karian, Executive Director

8118 Families Caring for Families
Family Resource Center
113 W Pillsbury Street, Suite A1
Lancaster, CA 93534

661-949-1746
Fax: 661-948-7266

Informational and emotional support to parents who have a child, adolescent, or adult family member with special needs.

8119 Family First Program Alpha Resource Center
4501 Cathedral Oaks Road, Suite A1
Santa Barbara, CA 93110

805-683-2145
Fax: 805-967-3647
arcofsb@slcom.com

Informational and emotional support to parents who have a child, adolescent, or adult family member with special needs.

8120 Family Focus Resource Center
18111 Nordhoff Street
Northridge, CA 91330

818-677-6854
Fax: 818-677-5574
family.focus@csun.edu
www.familyfocusresourcecenter.org

Informational and emotional support to parents who have a child, adolescent, or adult family member with special needs.

Ivor Weiner, Principal Investigator
Victoria Berrey, Program Manager
Stacie Anderle, PRRS, Coordinator

8121 Family Resource Center
5828 North Clark Street
Chicago, IL 60660

773-334-2300
800-676-2229
Fax: 773-334-8228
www.f-r-c.org

Informational and emotional support to parents who have a child, adolescent, or adult family member with special needs.

Debbie Frisch, Board President
Richard Pearlman, Executive Director
Jane Turner, Associate Director

8122 H.E.A.R.T.S. Connection Family Resource Center
3101 N Sillect Avenue, Suite 115
Bakersfield, CA 93308

661-328-9055
800-210-7633
Fax: 661-328-9940
heartsfrc@igalaxy
www.heartsfrc.org

Informational and emotional support to parents who have a child, adolescent, or adult family member with special needs.

Susan Graham, Director
Ana Gomez, Family Resource Specialist
Ana Gomez, Family Resource Specialist

8123 Harbor Regional Center Family and Professional Resource Center
21231 Hawthorne Boulevard
Torrance, CA 90503

310-543-0691
Fax: 310-316-8843
familyresourcecntr@hddf.com
www.harborrc.org

Informational and emotional support to parents who have a child, adolescent, or adult family member with special needs.

8124 MATRIX: Parent Network and Family Resource Center
94 Galli Drive, Suite C
Novato, CA 94949
415-884-3535
800-578-2592
Fax: 415-884-3555
info@matrixparents.org
www.matrixparents.org

Informational and emotional support to parents who have a child, adolescent, or adult family member with special needs.

Lee Cox, Chief Financial Officer
Rhanda Dunn, Board President
Nora Thompson, Executive Director

8125 Matrix Parents Network and Resource Center
94 Galli Drive, Suite C
Novato, CA 94949
415-884-3535
800-578-2592
Fax: 415-884-3555
info@matrixparents.org
www.matrixparents.org

Matrix is a nonprofit agency that serves families of children with special needs and disabilities. Provides information and referral, individual support, technical assistance, support groups, training about special education and services, and direction to appropriate early start services.

Lee Cox, Chief Financial Officer
Rhanda Dunn, Board President
Nora Thompson, Executive Director

8126 Parents Helping Parents of San Francisco
4752 Mission St Ste 100
San Francisco, CA 94112
415-841-8820
Fax: 415-841-8824
www.parentcenternetwork.org

Parent Training and Information (PTI) programs help parents to understand their children's specific needs, communicate more effectively with professionals, participate in the educational planning process, and obtain information about relevant programs, services and resources.

Paula Goldberg, National ALLIANCE PTAC Co-Director
Sue Folger, National ALLIANCE PTAC Co-Director
Debbie Andrews, Communications Coordinator

8127 Parents Helping Parents of Santa Clara
3041 Olcott Street
Santa Clara, CA 95054
408-727-5775
Fax: 408-727-0182
info@php.com
www.php.com

Informational and emotional support to parents who have a child, adolescent, or adult family member with special needs.

Mary Ellen Peterson, M.A., Executive Director/CEO
Nancy O'Rourke, Chief Development Officer
Paul Schutz, Chief Financial Officer

8128 Peaks and Valleys Family Resource Center
20 Sherwood Place No. 4
Salinas, CA 93906
831-755-1450
800-400-2937
Fax: 831-755-1470
peaks@montereyk12.ca.us

Informational and emotional support to parents who have a child, adolescent, or adult family member with special needs.

8129 San Gabriel/Pomona Parents' Place
1500 S Hyacinth Avenue # B
West Covina, CA 91791
626-919-1091
800-422-2022
Fax: 626-337-2736
empower@gte.net
www.parentsplacefrc.com

Family Resource Center committed to supporting, promoting and enhancing family focused services in a parent driven atmosphere for families who have children with special needs. Family Resource Centers are part of the California Early Start Program which addresses the unique and individual needs of families raising a child with a disability. The Parent's Place is dedicated to empowering families through information/education, referrals and parent to parent support.

Sona Baghdassarian, Director
Judy Kyne, Administrative Secretary
Elena Sanchez, Parent Resource Specialist

8130 South Central Los Angeles Regional Center for Devlopmentally Disabled Persons
6500 W Adams Boulevard
Los Angeles, CA 90007
213-744-7000
Fax: 213-744-8494
TTY: 213-763-5634

Informational and emotional support to parents who have a child, adolescent, or adult family member with special needs.

8131 Special Connections Family Resource Center
400 Encinal Street
Santa Cruz, CA 95060
831-464-0669
Fax: 831-465-9177
frcedp@aol.com

Informational and emotional support to parents who have an infant or toddler (birth to 36 months) with special needs.

Leslie Burnham, Program Supervisor

8132 Special Education Division State Department of Education
PO Box 944272
Sacramento, CA 94244
916-327-3696
Fax: 916-327-8878
cbourne@mail515a.cde.ca.gov
www.nectas.unc.edu

Individuals with Disabilities Education Act requires all states and territories to provide early intervention and preschool special education for children with disabilities and special health care needs. Services include central directory, representatives of agencies, service providers, families, and coordinators of infant, toddler, and preschool special education programs.

Constance J Bourne, Preschool Special Ed. Coordinator

8133 Starlight Children's Foundation
2049 Century Park East. Suite 4320
Los Angeles, CA 90067
310-479-1212
800-274-7827
Fax: 323-634-0090
Jenny@starlight.org
www.starlight.org

International nonprofit organization dedicated to improving the quality of life for seriously ill children and their families. Working with more than 850 hospitals worldwide, the Foundation provides an impressive menu of both in-hospital and outpatient programs and services. A leader in delivering distractive entertainment therapies, over 85,000 children benefit from Starlight's programs each month.

Jacqueline Hart-Ibrahim, Chief Executive Officer
Clifford R. Ball, CFO/CTO
Denise Muniz, Development Director

8134 Support for Families of Children with Disabilities
1663 Mission Street, 7th Floor
San Francisco, CA 94103
415-282-7494
Fax: 415-282-1226
TTY: 415-920-5040
info@supportforfamilies.org
www.supportforfamilies.org

Parent Training and Information (PTI) programs help parents to understand their children's specific needs, communicate more effectively with professionals, participate in the educational planning process, and obtain information about relevant programs, services and resources.

Christian Dauer, SFCD, Board President
Laura Lanzone, SFCD, Vice President
Juno Duenas, SFCD, Executive Director

8135   Team Advocates for Special Kids, Anaheim
100 W. Cerritos Ave
Anaheim, CA 92805   714-533-8275
                                                    866-828-8275
                                              Fax: 714-533-2533
                                              taskca@yahoo.com
                                              www.taskca.org

Programs help parents to understand their children's specific
needs, communicate more effectively with professionals, participate in the educational planning process, and obtain information
about relevant programs, services and resources.

Marta Anchondo, Executive Director/CEO

8136   Team Advocates for Special Kids, San Diego
4550 Kearney Villa Road, #102
San Diego, CA 92123   858-874-2386
                                              Fax: 858-874-2375

Programs help parents to understand their children's specific
needs, communicate more effectively with professionals, participate in the educational planning process, and obtain information
about relevant programs, services and resources.

8137   Warmline Family Resource Center
6960 Destiny Dr., Suite 106
Rocklin, CA 95677   916-632-2100
                                                    800-660-7995
                                              Fax: 916-632-2103
                                              warmlinefrc@warmlinefrc.com
                                              www.warmlinefrc.org

Informational and emotional support to parents who have a child,
adolescent, or adult family member with special needs.

Heather Green, Contact
Amber Johnson, Contact

Colorado

8138   Assistive Technology Partners
601 E 18th Avenue, Suite 130
Denver, CO 80203   303-315-1280
                                                    800-255-3477
                                              Fax: 303-837-1208
                                              TTY: 303-837-8964
                                              GeneralInfo@AT-Partners.org
                                              www.ucdenver.edu

State assisted programs and support group information for people
of many abilities. Focuses on assistive technology devices and
services for persons with disabilities, training and technical assistance available.

**8139   Colorado Consortium of Intensive Care Nurseries United
         Parents (UP)**
1056 E 19th Avenue, B535
Denver, CO 80218   303-861-6557
                                              Fax: 303-764-8092
                                              McGinley.Pandora@ex.tchden.org

Informational and emotional support to parents who have a child,
adolescent, or adult family member with special needs.

8140   Delta/Montrose Parent to Parent
2091 E Locust Road
Montrose, CO 81401   970-249-2878
                                              Fax: 970-252-0544
                                              children@gi.net

Informational and emotional support to parents who have a child,
adolescent, or adult family member with special needs.

8141   Denver Early Childhood Connections
2727 W 92nd Avenue
Denver, CO 80204   303-458-0852
                                              Fax: 303-744-9502

Provides resource coordination for children eligible for Part C
services and referrals to other agencies for children with needs
outside of the Part C realm. Parent to parent support, parent education and community playgroups are some of the services that
are conducted. Forums are hosted on varied topics relevant to
parents of young children as well as in-service and pre-service
workshops on child development. IFSP development, parent's
rights under IDEA, and other resource packets are available

Newsletter

Judith Persoff, Executive Director

**8142   Disability Connection and RAFT, Larimer County's Early
         Childhood Connection**
PO Box 270714
Fort Collins, CO 80527   970-229-0224
                                              Fax: 970-229-0242
                                              bstuts@fornet.org

Informational and emotional support to parents who have a child,
adolescent, or adult family member with special needs.

8143   Effective Parent Project
255 Main Street
Grand Junction, CO 81501   970-241-4068
                                              Fax: 970-241-3725

Informational and emotional support to parents who have a child,
adolescent, or adult family member with special needs.

8144   El Groupo Vida
P.O. Box 11096
Denver, CO 80211   303-904-6073
                                              Fax: 303-296-4105
                                              info@elgrupovida.org
                                              www.elgrupovida.org

Informational and emotional support to parents who have a child,
adolescent, or adult family member with special needs.

Gabriela Perez, Board President
Italia Cortes-Santillan, Vice President
Gabriela Perez, Interim (Volunteer) Executive Direc

**8145   Help Parent Support Group Hope & Education for Loving
         Parents**
378 S Falcon
Pueblo West, CO 81007   719-545-2282
                                              Fax: 719-547-1282
                                              fastgram@aol.com

Informational and emotional support to parents who have a child,
adolescent, or adult family member with special needs.

8146   Oasis
1120 N Circle Drive, Suite 19
Colorado Springs, CO 80909   719-635-8722
                                              Fax: 719-577-9482
                                              oasis@juno.com

Informational and emotional support to parents who have a child,
adolescent, or adult family member with special needs.

8147   PEAK Parent Center
611 N Weber, Suite 200
Colorado Springs, CO 80903   719-531-9400
                                                    800-284-0251
                                              Fax: 719-531-9452
                                              TDD: 719-531-9403
                                              info@peakparent.org
                                              www.peakparent.org

Parent Training and Information (PTI) programs help parents to
understand their children's specific needs, communicate more effectively with professionals, participate in the educational planning process, and obtain information about relevant programs,
services and resources.

Kent Willis, President
Sarah Billerbeck, Vice President
Barbara Buswell, Executive Director

8148   Parent Support Group of Littleton & Auora
7600 E Arapahoe, Suite 219
Englewood, CO 80112   303-773-0044
                                              Fax: 303-773-8780

953

Informational and emotional support to parents who have a child, adolescent, or adult family member with special needs.

8149 Parents Supporting Parents of Eagle County
PO Box 2656
Vail, CO 81658　　　　　　　　　　970-926-6015
　　　　　　　　　　　　　　　Fax: 970-926-6015

Informational and emotional support to parents who have a child, adolescent, or adult family member with special needs.

8150 Parents Supporting Parents of Garfield and Pitkin County
PO Box 784
Silt, CO 81652　　　　　　　　　　970-876-5768
　　　　　　　　　　　　　　　Fax: 970-876-5204

Informational and emotional support to parents who have a child, adolescent, or adult family member with special needs.

8151 Prevention Initiatives State Department of Education
210 E Colfax, Room 301
Denver, CO 80203　　　　　　　　303-866-6600
　　　　　　　　　　　　　　　Fax: 303-866-0793
　　　　　　　　　　　　　smith_s@cde.state.co.us
　　　　　　　　　　　　　　www.cde.state.co.us

Provides early intervention and preschool special education for children with disabilities and special health care needs. Services include central directory, representatives of agencies, service providers, families, and coordinators of infant, toddler, and preschool special education programs.

Susan Smith, Infant/Toddler Program Coordinator
Marie Huchton, Senior Consultant
Dan Jorgensen, Principal Consultant

8152 Resources for Young Children and Families
1120 N Circle Drive, Suite 19
Colorado Springs, CO 80909　　　　719-577-9190
　　　　　　　　　　　　　　　Fax: 719-577-9482
　　　　　　　　　　　　　　　partc@rycf.org

Informational and emotional support to parents who have a child, adolescent, or adult family member with special needs.

8153 Wilderness on Wheels Foundation
PO Box 1007
Wheat Ridge, CO 80034　　　　　　303-403-1110
　　　　　　　　　　　　　www.wildernessonwheels.org

State assisted programs and support group information for people of many abilities. Includes local chapters, referrals, fun and social interaction and support groups.

Connecticut

8154 A.J. Pappanikou Center for Developmental D isabilities
263 Farmington Avenue, MC 6222
Farmington, CT 06030　　　　　　860-679-1500
　　　　　　　　　　　　　　　866-623-1315
　　　　　　　　　　　　　　Fax: 860-679-1571
　　　　　　　　　　　　　TTY: 860-679-1502
　　　　　　　　　　　contact.us.ucedd@uchc.edu
　　　　　　　　　　　　www.uconnucedd.org

Individuals with Disabilities Education Act requires all states and territories to provide early intervention and preschool special education for children with disabilities and special health care needs. Services include central directory, representatives of agencies, service providers, families, and coordinators of infant, toddler, and preschool special education programs.

Mary Beth Bruder, Director
Tierney Giannotti, Associate Director
Linda Procko, Program Coordinator

8155 Assistive Technology Project
Department of Social Services, BRS
25 Sigourney Street, 11th Floor
Hartford, CT 06106　　　　　　　860-424-4881
　　　　　　　　　　　　　　　800-537-2549
　　　　　　　　　　　　　　Fax: 860-424-4850
　　　　　　　　　　　　　TDD: 860-424-4850
　　　　　　　　　　　　　cttap@aol./com
　　　　　　　　　　　　www.tachact.uconn.edu

State assisted programs and support group information for people of many abilities. Includes local chapters, referrals, fun and social interaction and support groups.

8156 CPAC
338 Main Street
Niantic, CT 06357　　　　　　　　860-739-3089
　　　　　　　　　　　　　　　Fax: 860-739-7460
　　　　　　　　　　　　　　cpac@cpacinc.org
　　　　　　　　　　　　　　www.cpacinc.org

Programs help parents to understand their children's specific needs, communicate more effectively with professionals, participate in the educational planning process, and obtain information about relevant programs, services and resources.

8157 Department of Mental Retardation
460 Capital Avenue
Hartford, CT 06106　　　　　　　860-418-6134
　　　　　　　　　　　　　　　Fax: 860-418-6003
　　　　　　　　　　　　　　lbgood993@aol.com
　　　　　　　　　　　　　　www.birth23.org

Individuals with Disabilities Education Act requires all states and territories to provide early intervention and preschool special education for children with disabilities and special health care needs. Services include central directory, representatives of agencies, service providers, families, and coordinators of infant, toddler, and preschool special education programs.

Linda Goodman, Part C Director
Lynn.S Johnson, Assistant Director
Karyn Pitt, Administrative Assistant

8158 Parent to Parent Network of Connecticut the Family Center
Dept. of Connecticut Children's Medical Center
282 Washington
Hartford, CT 06106　　　　　　　860-545-9021
　　　　　　　　　　　　　　　Fax: 860-545-9201
　　　　　　　　　　　　　TTY: 860-545-9002
　　　　　　　　　　　　　mcole@ccmckids.org
　　　　　　　　　　　　　www.ccmckids.org

Informational and emotional support to parents who have a child, adolescent, or adult family member with special needs.

8159 State Department of Education
25 Industrial Park Road
Middletown, CT 06457　　　　　　860-632-1485
　　　　　　　　　　　　　　　Fax: 860-807-2062
　　　　　　　　　　　　　　　www.unc.edu

Individuals with Disabilities Education Act requires all states and territories to provide early intervention and preschool special education for children with disabilities and special health care needs. Services include central directory, representatives of agencies, service providers, families, and coordinators of infant, toddler, and preschool special education programs.

Leslie Averna, Acting Bureau Chief

Delaware

8160 Delaware Assisstive Technology Initiative (DATI)
University of Delaware
461 Wyoming Road
Newark, DE 19716　　　　　　　302-831-0354
　　　　　　　　　　　　　　　800-870-3284
　　　　　　　　　　　　　　Fax: 302-831-4690
　　　　　　　　　　　　　TDD: 302-651-6794
　　　　　　　　　　　　　dati@asel.udel.edu
　　　　　　　　　　　　　www.dati.org

The Delaware Assistive Technology Initiative (DATI) connects Delawareans who have disabilities with the tools they need in order to learn, work, play and participate in community life safely and independently. DATI services include: Equipment demonstration center in each county; no-cost, short-term equipment loans that let you try before you buy; Equipment Exchange Program; AT workshops and other training sessions; advocacy for improved AT access policies and funding and several more.

Beth Mineo, Director
Bob Piech, Project Coordinator
Ron Sibert, Funding Specialist

8161 Department of Public Instruction
PO Box 1402
Dover, DE 19903   302-739-5471
                                    Fax: 302-739-2388
                                    mbrooks@state.de.us
                                    www.unc.edu

Individuals with Disabilities Education Act requires all states and
territories to provide early intervention and preschool special education for children with disabilities and special health care
needs. Services include central directory, representatives of agencies, service providers, families, and coordinators of infant, toddler, and preschool special education programs.

Martha Brooks, Director

8162 Parent Information Center of Delaware
6 Larch Avenue, Suite 404, Larch Corporate Center
Wilmington, DE 19804   302-999-7394
                                         888-547-4412
                                    Fax: 302-999-7637
                                    PEP700@aol.com
                                    www.picofdel.org

Programs help parents to understand their children's specific
needs, communicate more effectively with professionals, participate in the educational planning process, and obtain information
about relevant programs, services and resources.

Verna Hensley, President
Marie-Anne Aghazadian, Executive Director
Mindy Cox, Office Manager

District of Columbia

8163 Advocates for Justice and Education
1012 Pennsylvania Ave SE
Washington, DC 20020   202-678-8060
                                         888-327-8060
                                    Fax: 202-678-8062
                                    aje.qpg.com
                                    www.aje-dc.org

Programs help parents to understand their children's specific
needs, communicate more effectively with professionals, participate in the educational planning process, and obtain information
about relevant programs, services and resources.

Tracey Davis, Board Chair
Kim Y. Jones, Executive Director & Member
Antoinette C. Bush, Board Secretary

8164 DC Arc
900 Vamum Street, NE
Washington, DC 20017   202-636-2950
                                    Fax: 202-636-2996
                                    www.taalliance.org

Programs help parents to understand their children's specific
needs, communicate more effectively with professionals, participate in the educational planning process, and obtain information
about relevant programs, services and resources.

8165 DC-EIP Services
717 14th Street, NW, Suite 730
Washington, DC 20002   202-727-1839
                                    Fax: 202-727-8166
                                    TDD: 202-727-2114
                                    www.chasa.org

Provides early intervention and preschool special education for
children with disabilities and special health care needs. Services
include central directory, representatives of agencies, service providers, families, and coordinators of infant, toddler, and preschool special education programs.

Joan Christopher, Infant/Toddler Program Coordinator

8166 Georgetown University Child Development Center
National Early Childhood Technical Assistance Ctr
3700 O St., N.W.
Washington, DC 20057   202-687-0100
                                    Fax: 202-687-8899
                                    www.georgetown.edu

Individuals with Disabilities Education Act requires all states and
territories to provide early intervention and preschool special education for children with disabilities and special health care
needs. Services include central directory, representatives of agencies, service providers, families, and coordinators of infant, toddler, and preschool special education programs.

Paul Tagliabue, Chair
Chris Augostini, Senior Vice President and Chief Ope
John J. DeGioia, Ph.D., President

8167 Giddings School Special Education Division
National Early Childhood Technical Assistance Ctr
Campus Box 8040 Unc-Ch
Chapel Hill, NC 27599   919-962-2001
                                    Fax: 919-966-7463
                                    TDD: 919-843-3269
                                    www.nectas.unc.edu

Services include central directory, representatives of agencies,
service providers, families, and coordinators of infant, toddler,
and preschool special education programs.

Ann Palmore, Preschool Special Ed. Coordinator

8168 Partnership for Assistive Technology
220 I Street NE, Suite 202
Washington, DC 20002   202-547-0198
                                    Fax: 202-547-2662
                                    TDD: 202-547-2657

State assisted programs and support group information for people
of many abilities. Includes local chapters, referrals, fun and social interaction and support groups.

Florida

8169 Alliance for Assistive Service and Technology (FAAST)
325 John Knox Road, Building 400, Suite 402
Tallahassee, FL 32301   850-487-3278
                                         888-788-9216
                                    Fax: 850-487-2805
                                    TDD: 850-922-5951
                                    faast@faast.org
                                    www.faast.org

State assisted programs and support group information for people
of many abilities. Includes local chapters, referrals, fun and social interaction and support groups.

2-8 pages Newsletter

Gayle Miller, Esq., Chair
Karen M. Clay, Chair-Elect
Lisa Taylor, Treasurer

8170 Early Intervention Unit, Division of Children's Medical Services
1309 Winewood Boulevard
Tallahassee, FL 32399   850-488-6005
                                    Fax: 850-921-5241
                                    Fran_L_Wilber@dcf.state.fl.us
                                    www.nectas.unc.edu

Individuals with Disabilities Education Act requires all states and
territories to provide early intervention and preschool special education for children with disabilities and special health care
needs. Services include central directory, representatives of agencies, service providers, families, and coordinators of infant, toddler, and preschool special education programs.

Fran Wilber, Infant/Toddler Program Coordinator

8171 Family Network on Disabilities
2735 Whitney Road
Clearwater, FL 33760   727-523-1130
                                         800-825-5736
                                    Fax: 727-523-8687
                                    TDD: 727-523-1130
                                    fnd@gate.net
                                    www.fndfl.org

Parent Training and Information (PTI) programs help parents to
understand their children's specific needs, communicate more effectively with professionals, participate in the educational planning process, and obtain information about relevant programs,
services and resources.

Richard La Belle, Executive Director
Christine Goulbourne, Director of Programs
Joseph Hecker, Director of Finance

8172 Florida Department of Education
325 W Gaines Street
Tallahassee, FL 32399

850-245-0505
Fax: 850-245-9667
westc@mail.doe.state.fl.us
www.fldoe.org

Individuals with Disabilities Education Act requires all states and territories to provide early intervention and preschool special education for children with disabilities and special health care needs. Services include central directory, representatives of agencies, service providers, families, and coordinators of infant, toddler, and preschool special education programs.

Carale Chu, Chief of Staff
Will Krebs, Deputy Chief of Staff
Dr. Tony Bennett, Commissioner, Florida Department of

8173 Florida's Collaboration for Young Children and their Families Head State
1310 Cross Creek Circle, Suite A
Tallahassee, FL 32301

850-487-8871
Fax: 850-487-0045
kkamiya@com1.med.usf.edu
www.nectas.unc.edu

Provides early intervention and preschool special education for children with disabilities and special health care needs. Services include central directory, representatives of agencies, service providers, families, and coordinators of infant, toddler, and preschool special education programs.

Katherine Kamiya, Interagency Coordinator

8174 US Blind Golfers Association
3093 Shamrock Street N
Tallahassee, FL 32308

904-893-4511
Fax: 904-893-4511
nightgolf@concentric.net
www.usblindgolf.com

State assisted programs and support group information for people of many abilities. Includes local chapters, referrals, fun and social interaction and support groups.

David Meador, President
Phil Hubbard, Vice President
Bill McMahon, Board Members

Georgia

8175 DHR/Division of Public Health - Babies Can t Wait Program
2 Peachtree Street NE, Room 7-315
Atlanta, GA 30303

404-657-2700
888-651-8224
Fax: 404-657-2763
skmoss@dhr.state.ga.us
www.health.state.ga.us/programs/bcw

Babies Can't Wait (BCW) Program is Georgia's Part C Early Intervention Program under Part C of the federal Individuals with Disabilities Education Improvement Act (IDEA). Services include a comprehensive, coordinated, multidisciplinary, interagency system of early intervention supports for infants and toddlers with disabilities from birth to age 3 and their families.

Janie Brodnax, Chief Operating Officer DHP
Brenda Fitzgerald, M.D., Commissioner, Georgia Department of
Russell Crutchfield, Deputy Chief of Staff

8176 Department for Exceptional Students Georgia Department of Education
205 Jessie Hill Jr. Drive, SE, Suite 1870
Atlanta, GA 30334

404-657-9965
Fax: 404-651-6457
tbowen@doe.k12.ga.us
www.nectas.unc.edu

Provides early intervention and preschool special education for children with disabilities and special health care needs. Services include central directory, representatives of agencies, service providers, families, and coordinators of infant, toddler, and preschool special education programs.

Toni Waylor Bowen, Preschool Special Ed. Coordinator

8177 Department of Counseling and Educational Leadership-Columbus State University
4225 University Avenue, Suite 754
Columbus, GA 31907

706-568-2222
Fax: 706-569-3134
www.nectas.unc.edu

Individuals with Disabilities Education Act requires all states and territories to provide early intervention and preschool special education for children with disabilities and special health care needs. Services include central directory, representatives of agencies, service providers, families, and coordinators of infant, toddler, and preschool special education programs.

Katherine McCormick, Interagency Coordinating Council

8178 Parent to Parent of Georgia
3070 Presidential Parkway, Suite 130
Atlanta, GA 30340

770-451-5484
800-229-2038
Fax: 770-458-4091
parenttoparent@fga.org
www.p2pga.org

Statewide informational and emotional support to families and individuals affected by disability.

8179 Parents Educating Parents and Professional for All Children (PEPPAC)
8318 Durelee Lane, Suite 101
Douglasville, GA 30134

770-577-7771
Fax: 770-577-7774
peppac@bellsouth.net
www.taalliance.org

Parent Training and Information (PTI) programs help parents to understand their children's specific needs, communicate more effectively with professionals, participate in the educational planning process, and obtain information about relevant programs, services and resources.

8180 Tools for Life Division of Rehabilitation Services
1700 Century Circle B-4
Atlanta, GA 30345

404-894-4960
800-578-8665
Fax: 404-894-9320
TDD: 404-657-3085
102476.1737@compuserve.com
www.gatfl.org

State assisted programs and support group information for people of many abilities. Includes local chapters, referrals, fun and social interaction and support groups.

Hawaii

8181 AWARE
200 N Vineyard Boulevard, Suite 310
Honolulu, HI 96817

808-536-9684
Fax: 808-537-6780
LDAH@gte.net
www.taalliance.org

Parent Training and Information (PTI) programs help parents to understand their children's specific needs, communicate more effectively with professionals, participate in the educational planning process, and obtain information about relevant programs services, and resources.

8182 Assistive Technology Resource Centers of H awaii (ATRC)
414 Kuiwii Street, Suite 104
Honolulu, HI 96817

808-532-7110
800-645-3007
Fax: 808-532-7120
atrc-info@atrc.org
www.atrc.org

State assisted programs and support group information for people of many abilities. Includes local chapters, referrals, fun and social interaction and support groups.

8183 Parents and Children Together (PACT) Honolulu, HI 96819

808-847-3285
Fax: 808-841-1485
admin@pacthawaii.org
www.pacthawaii.org

Individuals with Disabilities Education Act requires all states and territories to provide early intervention and preschool special education for children with disabilities and special health care needs. Services include central directory, representatives of agencies, service providers, families, and coordinators of infant, toddler, and preschool special education programs.

David Shibata, Chair
Dana Ann Takushi, Vice Chair
Lowell Kalapa, Treasurer

8184 Special Needs Branch Department of Education
637 18th Avenue, Building C, Room 101
Honolulu, HI 96816   808-733-4900
Fax: 808-733-4841
michael_fahley@notes.k12.hi.us
www.unc.edu

Individuals with Disabilities Education Act requires all states and territories to provide early intervention and preschool special education for children with disabilities and special health care needs. Services include central directory, representatives of agencies, service providers, families, and coordinators of infant, toddler, and preschool special education programs.

Michael Fahey, Preschool Special Ed. Coordinator

8185 Zero-To-3 Hawaii Project
1600 Kapiolani Boulevard, Suite 1401
Honolulu, HI 96814   808-957-0066
Fax: 808-946-5222
jeanj@hawaii.edu
www.chasa.org

Services include central directory, representatives of agencies, service providers, families, and coordinators of infant, toddler, and preschool special education programs.

Jean Johnson, Infant/Toddler Program Coordinator

Idaho

8186 Assistive Technology Project
1 West Old State Capitol Plaza, Suite 100
Springfield, ID 62701   217-522-7985
800-852-5110
Fax: 217-522-8067
TTY: 217-522-9966
TDD: 208-855-3559
seile861@uidaho.edu
www.iltech.org

State assisted programs and support group information for people of many abilities. Includes local chapters, referrals, fun and social interaction and support groups.

8187 Department of Education
PO Box 83720
Boise, ID 83720   208-332-6917
Fax: 208-334-4664
jkbrenn@sde.state.id.us
www.unc.edu

Individuals with Disabilities Education Act requires all states and territories to provide early intervention and preschool special education for children with disabilities and special health care needs. Services include central directory, representatives of agencies, service providers, families, and coordinators of infant, toddler, and preschool special education programs.

Nolene Weaver, Supervisor

8188 Idaho Parents Unlimited
500 S 8th Street
Boise, ID 83702   208-342-5884
800-242-4785
Fax: 208-342-1408
TDD: 208-342-5884
parents@ipulidaho.org
www.ipulidaho.org

Parent Training and Information (PTI) programs help parents to understand their children's specific needs, communicate more effectively with professionals, participate in the educational planning process, and obtain information about relevant programs services, and resources.

Angela Lindig, Executive Director

8189 Infant/Toddler Program
PO Box 83720
Boise, ID 83720   208-334-5523
Fax: 208-334-6664
jonesm@dhw.state.id.us
www.idahochild.org

Services include central directory, representatives of agencies, service providers, families, and coordinators of infant, toddler, and preschool special education programs.

Mary Jones, Infant/Toddler Program Coordinator

8190 Palouse Area Parent To Parent
317 17th Avenue
Lewiston, ID 83501   208-746-8599
TTY: 208-746-8599
irel102w@wonder.em.cdc.gov

Informational and emotional support to parents who have a child, adolescent, or adult family member with special needs.

8191 Parent Reaching Out to Parents
2195 Ironwood Court
Coeur d'Alene, ID 83814   208-769-1409
Fax: 208-769-1430
parentsreachingout.com

Informational and emotional support to parents who have a child, adolescent, or adult family member with special needs.

Lorena Freund, Coordinator
Kathy Dalberg, Secretary/Treasurer

Illinois

8192 Archway
PO Box 1180, 2751 W Main
Carbondale, IL 62903   618-549-4442
Fax: 618-549-0231

Informational and emotional support to parents who have a child, adolescent, or adult family member with special needs.

8193 Assistive Technology Project
1 W Old State Capitol Plaza, Suite 100
Springfield, IL 62701   217-522-7985
800-852-5110
Fax: 217-522-8067
TTY: 217-522-9966
TDD: 217-522-9966
iatp@iltech.org
www.ittech.org

State assisted programs and support group information for people of many abilities. Includes local chapters, referrals, fun and social interaction and support groups.

Wilhelmina Gunther, Executive Director
Shelly Lowe, Finance/Personnel Manager
Theresa Ganci, Finance/Personnel Assistant

8194 Child and Family Connections
PO Box 741280
Boynton Beach, FL 33474   773-233-1799
800-554-1802
Fax: 773-233-2011
www.cfcpbc.org

Informational and emotional support to parents who have a child, adolescent, or adult family member with special needs.

8195 Developmental Services Center
1304 W Bradley
Champaign, IL 61821
217-356-9176
Fax: 217-356-9851
jmcateer@dsc-illinois.org
www.dsc-illinois.org

Informational and emotional support to parents who have a child, adolescent, or adult family member with special needs.

Dale Morrissey, Chief Executive Officer
Danielle Matthews, Executive Vice President of Support
Patty Walters, Executive Vice President of Consume

8196 Family Resource Center on Disabilities
11 E. Adams St. Suite 1002
Chicago, IL 60603
312-939-3513
800-952-4199
Fax: 312-854-8980
TTY: 312-939-3519
TDD: 312-939-3519
info@frcd.org
www.frcd.org

Parent Training and Information (PTI) programs help parents to understand their children's specific needs, communicate more effectively with professionals, participate in the educational planning process, and obtain information about relevant programs, services and resources.

Karen Aguilar, Coalition Director
Melody Musgrove, Director, Special Education Program

8197 Family T.I.E.S. Network
830 S Spring Street
Springfield, IL 62704
217-544-5809
800-865-7842
Fax: 217-544-6018
FTIESN@aol.com
www.taalliance.org

Parent Training and Information (PTI) programs help parents to understand their children's specific needs, communicate more effectively with professionals, participate in the educational planning process, and obtain information about relevant programs, services and resources.

8198 Greater Interagency Council Parent to Parent Support Network
925 W 175th Street
Homewood, IL 60430
708-799-2718
Fax: 708-799-7974

Informational and emotional support to parents who have a child, adolescent, or adult family member with special needs.

8199 Leukemia Research Foundation
3520 Lake Avenue, Suite #202
Wilmette, IL 60091
847-424-0600
888-558-5385
Fax: 847-424-0606
info@lrfmail.org
www.allbloodcancers.org

Founded to conquer leukemia by funding research into the causes and cures of the disease and to enrich the quality of life by those touched by leukemia.

Kevin Radelet, Executive Director
Cindy Kane, Senior Director of Development
Carl Alston, Director of Communications

8200 National Center for Latinos with Disabilities
1921 S Blue Island Avenue
Chicago, IL 60608
312-666-3393
800-532-3393
Fax: 312-666-1787
TTY: 312-666-1788
ncld@ncld.com
homepage.interaccess.com/~ncld/

Parent Training and Information (PTI) programs help parents to understand their children's specific needs, communicate more effectively with professionals, participate in the educational planning process, and obtain information about relevant programs, services and resources.

Everardo Franco, Executive Director
Nancy Perez, Coordinator Info and Referral

8201 Next Steps - Parents Reaching Parents
100 W Randolph, Suite 8-100
Chicago, IL 60601
312-814-4042
Fax: 708-799-7974
TTY: 312-814-4042
caroldors@aol.com

Informational and emotional support to parents who have a child, adolescent, or adult family member with special needs.

8202 Office of Community Health and Prevention Bureau of Early Intervention, DHR
222 South College, 2nd Floor
Springfield, IL 62704
217-782-9260
Fax: 217-782-7849
www.dhs.state.il.us/ei

Provides early intervention and preschool special education for children with disabilities and special health care needs. Services include central directory, representatives of agencies, service providers, families, and coordinators of infant, toddler, and preschool special education programs.

Mary Miller, Infant/Toddler Program Coordinator
Brian Bond, Contact

8203 Parent to Parent Network
1530 Lincoln Avenue
Charleston, IL 61920
217-348-0127
Fax: 217-348-0740

Informational and emotional support to parents who have a child, adolescent, or adult family member with special needs.

8204 Southern IL Child and Family Connections
2751 W Main Street
Carbondale, IL 62903
888-340-6702
Fax: 618-549-8137

Informational and emotional support to parents who have a child, adolescent, or adult family member with special needs.

8205 State Board of Education Department of Special Education
National Early Childhood Technical Assistance Ctr
100 N 1st Street, Suite 233
Springfield, IL 62777
217-782-5589
Fax: 217-782-7849
preising@smtp.isbe.state.il.us
www.unc.edu

Individuals with Disabilities Education Act requires all states and territories to provide early intervention and preschool special education for children with disabilities and special health care needs. Services include central directory, representatives of agencies, service providers, families, and coordinators of infant, toddler, and preschool special education programs.

Jack Shook, Division Administrator

Indiana

8206 ATTAIN: Assistive Technology Through Action in Indiana
32 E Washington Street, Suite 1400
Indianapolis, IN 46204
317-486-8808
800-527-8246
Fax: 317-486-8809
TDD: 800-743-3333
attaininfo@attaininc.org
www.attaninc.org

State assisted programs and support group information for people of many abilities. Includes local chapters, referrals, fun and social interaction and support groups.

8207 About Special Kids (ASK)
7172 Graham Road, Suite 100
Indianapolis, IN 46250   317-257-8683
      800-964-4746
Fax: 317-251-7488
familynetw@aboutspecialkids.org
www.aboutspecialkids.org

Helping children with special needs live better lives by education, empowering and connecting their families.

Cindy Robinson, Director of Education and Informati
Jane Scott, Director of Family Support
Joe Brubaker, Executive Director

8208 Assistive Technology Training and Information Center
3354 Pine Hill Drive, PO Box 2441
Vincennes, IN 47591   812-886-0575
      800-962-8842
Fax: 812-886-1128
inattic1@aol.com
www.theattic.org

Technology group of parents, consumers and professionals that provides resources to help children and adults who have disabilities gain access to the benefits of technology. Includes nationwide network of community-based assistive technology, resource centers, hands on consultants and product demonstrations.

8209 Division of Exceptional Learners Indiana Department of Education
State House, Room 229
Indianapolis, IN 46204   317-232-0570
Fax: 317-232-0589
scochran@doe.state.in.us
www.doe.state.in.us/exceptional

Individuals with Disabilities Education Act requires all states and territories to provide preschool special education for children with disabilities. Special Education and related services are provided through the public schools.

Sheron Cochran, Preschool Special Ed Coordinator

8210 Down Syndrome Association of Central Indiana
10792 Downing Street
Carmel, IN 46033   317-574-9757
Fax: 317-574-9757
MKaye62801@aol.com

Provides informational and emotional support to parents who have a child, adolescent, or adult family member with special needs. Program offers an important connection for a parent who is seeking support for a special disability issue, by matching him or her with a trained veteran parent.

8211 Family Resource Center of Southeast Indiana
4101 Timberview Road
West Harrison, IN 47060   812-637-1445

Informational and emotional support to parents who have a child, adolescent, or adult family member with special needs.

8212 First Direction
PO Box 4234
Lafayette, IN 47903   765-423-1460

Informational and emotional support to parents who have a child, adolescent, or adult family member with special needs.

8213 First Steps
402 W Washington Street, Suite W-386
Indianapolis, IN 46204   317-233-9229
Fax: 317-232-7948
mgreer@fssa.state.in.us
www.chasa.org

Individuals with Disabilities Education Act requires all states and territories to provide early intervention and preschool special education for children with disabilities and special health care needs. Services include central directory, representatives of agencies, service providers, families, and coordinators of infant, toddler, and preschool special education programs.

Maureen Greer, Part C Director

8214 First Steps for Families
500 8th Avenue
Terre Haute, IN 47804   812-231-8419
Fax: 812-231-8208
famnetwork@aol.com

Informational and emotional support to parents who have a child, adolescent, or adult family member with special needs.

8215 First Steps, Early Interventions, New Horizons Rehabilitation
PO Box 98
Batesville, IN 47006   812-934-4528
Fax: 812-934-2522
TTY: 812-934-4528

Informational and emotional support to parents who have a child, adolescent, or adult family member with special needs.

8216 Future Choices
309 N High Street
Muncie, IN 47305   765-741-3494
Fax: 765-741-8333
futurechoicesinc@aol.com

Informational and emotional support to parents who have a child, adolescent, or adult family member with special needs.

8217 Knox County Advocates
1805 Indiana Avenue
Vincennes, IN 47591   812-882-0375
Fax: 812-886-1128
INATTIC1@aol.com

Informational and emotional support to parents who have a child, adolescent, or adult family member with special needs.

8218 NEO Fight
PO Box 17715
Indianapolis, IN 46217   317-446-3013
info@neofight.org
www.neofight.org

Informational and emotional support to parents who have a child, adolescent, or adult family member with special needs.

Michie Sebree, R.N., President
Kathleen Smith, Secretary
Amanda Blann, Board Member

8219 Project Special Care
4755 Kinsway Drive, Suite 105
Indianapolis, IN 46205   317-257-8683
Fax: 317-251-7488
www.ipin.org

Informational and emotional support to parents who have a child, adolescent, or adult family member with special needs.

8220 US Rowing Assocation
2 Wall Street
Princeton, NJ 08540   609-751-0700
      800-314-4769
Fax: 609-924-1578
members@usrowing.org
www.usrowing.org

State assisted programs and support group information for people of many abilities. Includes local chapters, referrals, fun and social interaction and support groups.

Brian Klausner, Chief Financial Officer
Glenn Merry, Chief Executive Officer
Beth Kohl, Chief Marketing Officer

Iowa

8221 ARC of East Central Iowa Pilot Parents
680 2nd Street SE, Suite 200
Cedar Rapids, IA 52404   319-365-0487
      800-843-0272
Fax: 319-365-9938

Informational and emotional support to parents who have a child, adolescent, or adult family member with special needs.

8222 Bureau of Children, Family, and Community Services
Grimes State Office Building, 3rd Floor
Des Moines, IA 50319
515-281-7145
Fax: 515-242-6019
dee.gethman@ed.state.ia.us
www.chasa.org

Individuals with Disabilities Education Act requires all states and territories to provide early intervention and preschool special education for children with disabilities and special health care needs. Services include central directory, representatives of agencies, service providers, families, and coordinators of infant, toddler, and preschool special education programs.

Lynda Pletcher, Preschool Special Ed. Coordinator

8223 Family & Educator Connection - Cedar Falls /Waterloo Region
3706 Cedar Heights Drive
Cedar Falls, IA 50613
219-273-8265
800-542-8375
Fax: 319-273-8275
TTY: 319-273-8291
dpaton@aea267.k12.ia.us
www.aea267.k12.ia.us

The Family & Educator Connection is part of the Parent & Educator Connection, a statewide network of families and educators working together to serve children and young adults with special needs. They work together in positive ways to improve educational programs for children and youth with disabilities.

Rod Ball, Administrator
Edie Penno, Special Education Coordinator and T
Sandy Lichty, Consultant for Challenging Behavior

8224 Family & Educator Connection - Clear Lake/ Mason City Region
Mason City Airport Grounds, 9184 B 265th Street
Clear Lake, IA 50428
641-357-6125
800-392-6640
skraschel@aea27.k12.ia.us
www.aea267.k12.ia.us

The Family & Educator Connection is part of the Parent & Educator Connection, a statewide network of families and educators working together to serve children and young adults with special needs. They work together in positive ways to improve educational programs for children and youth with disabilities.

Roberta Kraft-Abrahamson, Director District 1 - Vice Presiden
Sandy Kraschel, Administrator

8225 Family & Educator Connection - Marshalltow n Region
909 South 12th Street
Marshalltown, IA 50158
641-844-2469
800-735-1539
Fax: 641-752-0075
alawler@aea267.k12.ia.us
www.aea267.k12.ia.us

The Family & Educator Connection is part of the Parent & Educator Connection, a statewide network of families and educators working together to serve children and young adults with special needs. They work together in positive ways to improve educational programs for children and youth with disabilities.

Andy Lawler, Administrator
David Giese, Director District 5

8226 Iowa Program for Assistive Technology
University Hospital School
303A CDD, 100 Hawkins Drive
Iowa City, IA 52242
319-353-6108
800-331-3027
Fax: 319-356-8284
TDD: 800-331-3027
jane_gay@uiowa.edu
www.uiowa.edu

State assisted programs and support group information for people of many abilities. Includeslocal chapters, referrals, fun and social interaction and support groups.

Linda Monroe, Contact

8227 Iowa's System of EI Services
Grimes State Office Building, 3rd Floor
Des Moines, IA 50319
515-281-7145
Fax: 515-242-6019
lynda.pletcher@ed.state.ia.us
www.chasa.org

Individuals with Disabilities Education Act requires all states and territories to provide early intervention and preschool special education for children with disabilities and special health care needs. Services include central directory, representatives of agencies, service providers, families, and coordinators of infant, toddler, and preschool special education programs.

Lynda Pletcher, Infant/Toddler Program Coordinator

8228 Parent Educator Connection
Grimews State Office Bldg
Des Moines, IA 50318
515-242-5295
800-572-5073
Fax: 712-722-1643
bjones@aea5.k12.ia.uss

Informational and emotional support to parents who have a child, adolescent, or adult family member with special needs.

8229 Parent Educator Connection Program
Heartland AEA 11, 6500 Corporate Drive
Johnston, IA 50131
515-270-9030
800-362-2720
Fax: 515-270-5383
www.aea11.k12.ia.us/parents/PEC/

Provides informational and emotional support to parents who have a child, adolescent, or adult family member with special needs. Program offers an important connection for a parent who is seeking support for special disability issue, by matching him or her with a trained veteran parent.

Paula Vincent, Chief Administrator
David King, Chief Financial Officer
Kevin Fangman, Director of District Services

Kansas

8230 Assistive Technology for Kansas Project
2601 Gabriel, PO Box 738
Parsons, KS 67357
316-421-8367
800-526-3648
Fax: 620-421-8367
TDD: 316-421-0954
ssack@parsons.lsi.ukans.edu
www.atk.ku.edu/kansas/

State assisted programs and support group information for people of many abilities. Includes local chapters, referrals, fun and social interaction and support groups.

Sara Sack, ATK Director
Sheila Simmons, ATK Coordinator
Sarah Walters, Kansas Infant Toddler Services

8231 Department of Health & Environment
1000 Sw Jackson
Topeka, KS 66612
785-296-1500
Fax: 785-368-6368
info@kdheks.gov
www.kdheks.gov

Individuals with Disabilities Education Act requires all states and territories to provide early intervention and preschool special education for children with disabilities and special health care needs. Services include central directory, representatives of agencies, service providers, families, and coordinators of infant, toddler, and preschool special education programs.

Nathan Bainbridge, Senior Executive Policy Analyst
Tim Keck, Deputy Chief Counsel
Glen Yancey, Information Technology Director

8232 Families Together
3033 West 2nd, Suite 106
Wichita, KS 67203
316-945-7747
888-815-6364
Fax: 316-945-7795
wichita@familiestogetherinc.org
www.familiestogetherinc.org

Parent Training and Information (PTI) programs help parents to understand their children's specific needs, communicate more effectively with professionals, participate in the educational planning process, and obtain information about relevant programs, services and resources.

Linda Peterson, President
Eric Morrison, Vice President
Jill Elkins, Secretary

8233 Families Together/Parent to Parent of KS
501 Jackson, Suite 400
Topeka, KS 66603
785-233-4777
800-264-6343
Fax: 756-233-4787
TTY: 785-233-4777
family@inlandnet.net

Informational and emotional support to parents who have a child, adolescent, or adult family member with special needs.

8234 Special Education Administration Kansas St ate Department of Education
120 E 10th Avenue
Topeka, KS 66612
785-296-3201
Fax: 785-296-7933
tsmith@ksde.org
www.ksde.org/Default.aspx?tabid=4745

Individuals with Disabilities Education Act requires all states and territories to provide early intervention and preschool special education for children with disabilities and special health care needs. Services include central directory, representatives of agencies, service providers, families, and coordinators of infant, toddler, and preschool special education programs.

Tiffany Smith, Consultant
Colleen Riley, Team Director
Gayle Stuber, Early Learning & Preschool Coord.

Kentucky

8235 Assistive Technology Services Network
8412 Westport Road
Louisville, KY 40242
502-429-4484
800-327-5287
Fax: 502-429-7114
TDD: 502-327-9855
www.katsnet.org

State assisted programs and support group information for people of many abilities. Includes local chapters, referrals, fun and social interaction and support groups.

Stephen M. Johnson, Executive Director

8236 College of Education - Western Kentucky University
Interdisciplinary Early Childhood Education
#1 Big Red Way, Western Kentucky University
Bowling Green, KY 42101
270-745-5414
Fax: 270-745-6474
vicki.stayton@wku.edu
www.nectas.unc.edu

Individuals with Disabilities Education Act requires all states and territories to provide early intervention and preschool special education for children with disabilities and special health care needs. Services include central directory, representatives of agencies, service providers, families, and coordinators of infant, toddler, and preschool special education programs.

Vicki Stayton, Interagency Coordinating Council

8237 Division of Preschool Services
1711 Capotol Plaza Tower
Frankfort, KY 40601
502-564-7056
Fax: 502-564-6771
bsinglet@kde.state.ky.us
www.nectas.unc.edu

Provides early intervention and preschool special education for children with disabilities and special health care needs. Services include central directory, representatives of agencies, service providers, families, and coordinators of infant, toddler, and preschool special education programs.

Barbara Singleton, Preschool Special Ed. Coordinator

8238 Infant-Toddler Program, Division of Mental Retardation
275 E Main Street
Frankfort, KY 40621
502-564-7722
Fax: 502-564-0438
jhenson@mail.state.ky.us
www.nectas.unc.edu

Individuals with Disabilities Education Act requires all states and territories to provide early intervention and preschool special education for children with disabilities and special health care needs. Services include central directory, representatives of agencies, service providers, families, and coordinators of infant, toddler, and preschool special education programs.

Jim Henson, Infant/Toddler Program Coordinator

8239 Special Parent Involvement Network
10301-B Deering Road
Louisville, KY 40272
502-937-6894
800-525-7746
Fax: 502-937-6464
spininc@kyspin.com
www.kyspin.com

Parent Training and Information (PTI) programs help parents to understand their children's specific needs, communicate more effectively with professionals, participate in the educational planning process, and obtain information about relevant programs, services and resources.

Crump Caroline, Director

Louisiana

8240 Division of Special Populations
PO Box 94064
Baton Rouge, LA 70804
225-342-3633
800-737-2958
Fax: 225-342-5880
Vberidon@mail.doe.state.la.us
www.doe.state.la.us

Individuals with Disabilities Education Act requires all states and territories to provide early intervention and preschool special education for children with disabilities and special health care needs. Services include central directory, representatives of agencies, service providers, families, and coordinators of infant, toddler, and preschool special education programs.

Evelyn Johnson, Infant/Toddler Program Coordinator
Virginia C. Beridon, Director

8241 Families Helping Families of Greater New Orleans
1323 Division Street, Suite 110
Metairie, LA 70002
504-888-9111
800-766-7736
Fax: 504-888-0246
fhfgno@ix.netcom.com
www.fhfgno.org

Informational and emotional support to parents who have a child, adolescent, or adult family member with special needs.

8242 Louisiana Assistive Technology Access Network
3042 Old Forge Drive, Suite D
Baton Rouge, LA 70898
225-925-9500
800-270-6185
Fax: 225-925-9560
TDD: 225-925-9500
latanstate@aol.com
www.latan.org

961

State assisted programs and support group information for people of many abilities. Includes local chapters, referrals, fun and social interaction and support groups.

Charles Tate, Board Chair
Jim Parks, Vice Chair
Julie Nesbit, ATP, President/CEO

8243 Preschool Programs - Division of Special Populations
PO Box 94064
Baton Rouge, LA 70804   225-342-3633
                                        800-737-2958
                              Fax: 225-342-5880
                         Vberidon@mail.doe.state.la.us
                              www.doe.state.la.us

Individuals with Disabilities Education Act requires all states and territories to provide early intervention and preschool special education for children with disabilities and special health care needs. Services include central directory, representatives of agencies, service providers, families, and coordinators of infant, toddler, and preschool special education programs.

Evelyn Johnson, Infant/Toddler Program Coordinator
Virginia C. Beridon, Director

8244 Project PROMPT
4323 Division Street, Suite 110
Metairie, LA 70002   504-888-9111
                                        800-766-7736
                              Fax: 504-888-0246
                              thsgno@ix.netcom.com
                              www.taalliance.org

Parent Training and Information (PTI) programs help parents to understand their children's specific needs, communicate more effectively with professionals, participate in the educational planning process, and obtain information about relevant programs, services and resources.

Maine

8245 CDC Lincoln County
PO Box 1114
Damariscotta, ME 04543   207-563-1411
                              Fax: 207-563-6312
                              www.nectas.unc.edu

Individuals with Disabilities Education Act requires all states and territories to provide early intervention and preschool special education for children with disabilities and special health care needs. Services include central directory, representatives of agencies, service providers, families, and coordinators of infant, toddler, and preschool special education programs.

Jean Eaton, Interagency Coordinating Council

8246 Child Department Services
146 State House Station
Augusta, ME 04333   207-287-3272
                              Fax: 207-287-5900
                              jaci.holmes@state.me.us

Provides early intervention and preschool special education for children with disabilities and special health care needs. Services include central directory, representatives of agencies, service providers, families, and coordinators of infant, toddler, and preschool special education programs.

Joanne C Holmes, Infant/Toddler Program Coordinator

8247 Child Department Services, Department of Education
23 State House Station
Augusta, ME 04333   207-287-5950
                              Fax: 207-287-2550
                         Debbie.Violette@state.me.us
                              www.unc.edu

Provides early intervention and preschool special education for children with disabilities and special health care needs. Services include central directory, representatives of agencies, service providers, families, and coordinators of infant, toddler, and preschool special education programs.

Joanne C Holmes, Preschool Special Ed. Coordiantor

8248 Consumer Information and Technology Training Exchange (Maine CITE)
46 University Drive
Augusta, ME 04330   207-621-3195
                              Fax: 207-629-5429
                              TDD: 207-621-3195
                              powers@maine.maine.edu
                              www.mainecite.org

State assisted programs and support group information for people of many abilities. Includes local chapters, referrals, fun and social interaction and support groups.

Kathleen Powers, Program Director
Kathy Adams, OTR/L, ATP, Training Coordinator
Darcy York, Administrative Assistant

8249 Special Needs Parent Info Network
PO Box 2067
Augusta, ME 04338   207-623-2144
                                        800-870-7746
                              Fax: 207-623-2148
                              parentconnect@mpf.org
                              www.startingpointsforme.org

Parent Training and Information (PTI) programs help parents to understand their children's specific needs, communicate more effectively with professionals, participate in the educational planning process, and obtain information about relevant programs, services and resources.

Lorraine Christensen, President
Steve Ocean, Vice President/Treasurer
Janice LaChance, Executive Director

8250 York County Parent Awareness
150 Main Street, Midtown Mall
Sanford, ME 04027   207-324-2337
                              Fax: 207-324-5621
                              ycpa@mmp.org

Informational and emotional support to parents who have a child, adolescent, or adult family member with special needs.

Maryland

8251 ARC Family Connection Parent to Parent Program
11600 Nebel Street
Rockville, MD 20852   301-984-5777
                              Fax: 301-816-2429

Informational and emotional support to parents who have a child, adolescent, or adult family member with special needs.

8252 Developmental Pediatrics School of Medicine, University of Maryland
630 W Fayette Street, Room 5686
Baltimore, MD 21201   410-706-3542
                              Fax: 410-706-0835
                              www.nectas.unc.edu

Individuals with Disabilities Education Act requires all states and territories to provide early intervention and preschool special education for children with disabilities and special health care needs. Services include central directory, representatives of agencies, service providers, families, and coordinators of infant, toddler, and preschool special education programs.

Renee Wachtel, Interagency Coordinating Council

8253 MD Infant/Toddler/Preschool Services Division
200 W Baltimore Street
Baltimore, MD 21201   410-767-0238
                                        800-535-0182
                              Fax: 410-333-2661
                              TDD: 410-333-0781
                              cbaglin@msde.state.md.us
                              www.msde.state.md.us

Individuals with Disabilities Education Act requires all states and territories to provide early intervention and preschool special education for children with disabilities and special health care needs. Services include central directory, representatives of agencies, service providers, families, and coordinators of infant, toddler, and preschool special education programs.

Carol Ann Baglin, Assstant State Superintendent

8254 Maryland Infant and Toddlers Program Family Support Network
200 W Baltimore, 4th Floor
Baltimore, MD 21201 410-767-0652
Fax: 410-333-8165

Informational and emotional support to parents who have a child, adolescent, or adult family member with special needs.

8255 Parents Place of Maryland
801 Cromwell Park Drive, Suite 103
Glen Burnie, MD 21061 410-768-9100
Fax: 410-768-0830
TDD: 410-768-9100
info@ppmd.org
www.ppmd.org

Parent Training and Information (PTI) programs help parents to understand their children's specific needs, communicate more effectively with professionals, participate in the educational planning process, and obtain information about relevant programs, services and resources.

Josie Thomas, Executive Director
Suzie Shannon, Administration
Mary Baskar, Health Projects Coordinator

8256 Partners in Intensive Care
PO Box 41043
Bethesda, MD 20824 301-681-2708
Fax: 301-681-2707

Informational and emotional support to parents who have a child, adolescent, or adult family member with special needs.

8257 Technology Assistance Program Maryland Rehabilitation Center
2301 Argonne Drive, Room T-17
Baltimore, MD 21218 410-554-9230
800-832-4827
Fax: 410-554-9237
TTY: 866-881-7488
mdtap.org
www.mdtap.org

State assisted programs and support group information for people of many abilities. Includes local chapters, referrals, fun and social interaction and support groups.

Tony Rice, Loan Program Director
Tanya Goodman, Loan Program Assistant Director
Lori Markland, Director of Communications, Outreac

Massachusetts

8258 Bureau of Early Childhood Programs
350 Main Street
Malden, MA 02148 781-388-3300
Fax: 781-388-3394
eschaefer@doe.mass.edu
www.doe.mass.edu

Individuals with Disabilities Education Act requires all states and territories to provide early intervention and preschool special education for children with disabilities and special health care needs. Services include central directory, representatives of agencies, service providers, families, and coordinators of infant, toddler, and preschool special education programs.

David P. Driscoll, Commissioner

8259 Children's Happiness Foundation
PO Box 266
Marshfield, MA 02050 781-837-9609
Fax: 781-837-5229
rsvpmktg@aol.com

Serves New England children ages three to eighteen with life-threatening or chronic degenerative diseases.

8260 Early Intervention Services
250 Washington Street
Boston, MA 02108 617-624-5969
Fax: 617-624-5990
Ron.Benham@state.ma.us

Individuals with Disabilities Education Act requires all states and territories to provide early intervention and preschool special education for children with disabilities and special health care needs. Services include central directory, representatives of agencies, service providers, families, and coordinators of infant, toddler, and preschool special education programs.

Ron Benham, Infant/Toddler Program Coordinator

8261 Education Development Center - EDC
43 Foundry Avenue
Waltham, MA 02453 617-969-7100
800-225-4276
Fax: 617-969-5979
TTY: 617-964-5448
pprintz@edc.org
www.edc.org

One of the largest nonprofit education and health organizations. With programs for children and families combining research and practice, promoting professional development and systematic change, forging community links, and influencing the policies and legislation that affect the lives of children. The New England RAP incorporates proven strategies to enhance the efforts of organizations servicing children with disabilities and their families.

Luther Luedtke, President and Chief Executive Offic
Cheryl Hoffman-Bray, Vice President/Chief Financial Offi
Robert Spielvogel, Vice President/Chief Technology Off

8262 Family Ties at Massachusetts Department of Public Health
5 Randolph Street
Canton, MA 02021 781-774-6736
Fax: 781-774-6618
TTY: 781-774-6619
TDD: 508-947-0977
mcsummers@fcsn.org
www.massfamilyties.org

Informational and emotional support to parents who have a child, adolescent, or adult family member with special needs.

Mary Castro Summers, Program Director

8263 Federation for Children with Special Needs
1135 Tremont Street Suite 420
Boston, MA 02120 617-236-7210
800-331-0688
Fax: 617-572-2094
TDD: 617-482-2915
fcsninfo@fcsn.org
www.fcsn.org/

Parent Training and Information (PTI) programs help parents to understand their children's specific needs, communicate more effectively with professionals, participate in the educational planning process, and obtain information about relevant programs, services and resources.

James F. Whalen, President
Maureen Jerz, Director of Development
Tom Hamel, Director of Finance

8264 Greater Boston Arc Parent Support
1505 Commonwealth Avenue
Boston, MA 02135 617-783-3900
Fax: 617-783-9190
bostonarc@aol.com
gbarc.org

Informational and emotional support to parents who have a child, adolescent, or adult family member with special needs.

8265 Massachusetts Assistive Technology Partnership
1295 Boylston Street, Suite 310
Boston, MA 02215 617-355-7153
Fax: 617-355-6345
TDD: 617-355-7301
matp@matp.net
www.matp.org

State assisted programs and support group information for people of many abilities. Includes local chapters, referrals, fun and social interaction and support groups.

8266 National Birth Defects Center
40 2nd Avenue, Suite 520
Waltham, MA 02451   781-466-9555
                                    Fax: 781-487-2361

Treats patients with birth defects, mental retardation and genetic diseases.

Michigan

8267 CAUSE
2365 Woodlake Frive, Suite 100
Okemos, MI 48864   517-347-2283
                                      800-221-9105
                                   Fax: 517-886-9366
                                   TTY: 517-347-2283
                                   TDD: 517-886-9167
                                   www.causeonline.org

Parent Training and Information (PTI) programs help parents to understand their children's specific needs, communicate more effectively with professionals, participate in the educational planning process, and obtain information about relevant programs, services and resources.

8268 Early on Michigan
PO Box 30008
Lansing, MI 48909   517-335-4865
                                   Fax: 517-373-7504
                                 banfieldj@state.mi.us
                                  www.1800earlyon.org

Provides early intervention and preschool special education for children with disabilities and special health care needs. Services include central directory, representatives of agencies, service providers, families, and coordinators of infant, toddler, and preschool special education programs.

Julie Banfield, Infant/Toddler Program Coordinator

8269 Family Support Network of Michigan Parent Participation Program-MDCH
200 6th Street, 3rd Fl., S Tower, Suite 315
Detroit, MI 48226   517-373-3740
                                   Fax: 313-256-2605
                                   TDD: 517-373-3573

Informational and emotional support to parents who have a child, adolescent, or adult family member with special needs.

8270 Livingston County CMH Services
2280 East Grand River
Howell, MI 48843   517-546-4126
                                   Fax: 517-546-1300
                                   www.nectas.unc.edu

Provides early intervention and preschool special education for children with disabilities and special health care needs. Services include central directory, representatives of agencies, service providers, families, and coordinators of infant, toddler, and preschool special education programs.

Mac Miller, Interagency Coordinating Council

8271 Office of Special Education
608 W. Allegan Street, PO Box 30008
Lansing, MI 48909   517-373-9433
                                   Fax: 517-373-7504
                              webmaster@oses.mde.state.mi.us
                                   www.michigan.gov

Individuals with Disabilities Education Act requires all states and territories to provide early intervention and preschool special education for children with disabilities and special health care needs. Services include central directory, representatives of agencies, service providers, families, and coordinators of infant, toddler, and preschool special education programs.

Sally Vaughn, Deputy Superintendent, Chief Academ
Jacqueline Thompson, Director
Mike P. Flanagan, Superintendent of Public Instructio

8272 Parents are Experts
23077 Greenfield Road, Suite 205
Southfield, MI 48075   248-557-5070
                                      800-827-4843
                                   Fax: 248-557-4456
                                   TDD: 248-557-5070
                                   ucp@ameritech.net
                                   www.taalliance.org

Parent Training and Information (PTI) programs help parents to understand their children's specific needs, communicate more effectively with professionals, participate in the educational planning process, and obtain information about relevant programs, services and resources.

8273 TECH 2000 Project-Michigan Disability Rights Coalition
740 W Lake Lansing Road, Suite 400
East Lansing, MI 48823   517-333-2477
                                      800-760-4600
                                   Fax: 517-333-2677
                                   TDD: 517-333-2477
                                   roanne@match.org
                                   www.discoalition.org

State assisted programs and support group information for people of many abilities. Includes local chapters, referrals, fun and social interaction and support groups.

Minnesota

8274 ARC Suburban
1526 E 122nd Street
Burnsville, MN 56337   612-890-3057
                                   Fax: 612-890-3527

Informational and emotional support to parents who have a child, adolescent, or adult family member with special needs.

8275 Department of Children, Family, & Learning
1500 Highway 36 W
Roseville, MN 55113   651-582-8200
                                   Fax: 651-582-8872
                              michael.eastman@state.mn.us

Individuals with Disabilities Education Act requires all states and territories to provide early intervention and preschool special education for children with disabilities and special health care needs. Services include central directory, representatives of agencies, service providers, families, and coordinators of infant, toddler, and preschool special education programs.

Michael Eastman, Preschool Special Ed. Coordinator

8276 Family to Family Network ARC of Hennepin County
4301 Highway 7, Suite 104
Minneapolis, MN 55416   612-920-0855
                                   Fax: 612-920-1480

Informational and emotional support to parents who have a child, adolescent, or adult family member with special needs.

8277 Interagency Early Intervention Project
550 Cedar Street
Saint Paul, MN 55101   612-296-7032
                                   Fax: 612-296-5076
                              jan.rubenstein@state.mn.us
                                  www.pediatricservices.com

Individuals with Disabilities Education Act requires all states and territories to provide early intervention and preschool special education for children with disabilities and special health care needs. Services include central directory, representatives of agencies, service providers, families, and coordinators of infant, toddler, and preschool special education programs.

Jan Rubenstein, Infant/Toddler Program Coordinator

8278 Parents for Parents
345 N Smith Avenue, MS 70-403
Saint Paul, MN 55102   651-220-6731
                                   Fax: 651-220-6125
                              pat.schaffner@childrenshc.org

Informational and emotional one-to-one support to parents who have a child or adolescent with special needs.

Pat Schaffner, Parent to Parent Specialist

8279 Pilot Parents in Anoka and Ramsey Counties
1201 89th Avenue NE, Suite 305
Blaine, MN 55434 612-783-4958
Fax: 612-783-4900

Informational and emotional support to parents who have a child, adolescent, or adult family member with special needs.

8280 Pilot Parents of Northeast Minnesota
201 Ordean Building
Duluth, MN 55802 218-726-4725
Fax: 218-726-4722

Informational and emotional support to parents who have a child, adolescent, or adult family member with special needs.

8281 Vinland Center
PO Box 308
Loretto, MN 55357 763-479-3555
Fax: 763-479-2605
vinland@vinlandcenter.org
www.vinlandcenter.org

State assisted programs and support group information for people of many abilities. Includes local chapters, referrals, fun and social interaction and support groups.

Gerald Seck, President
Mary Roehl, Executive Director
Duane Reynolds, Associate Director

8282 Voyageur Outward Bound School
101 E Chapman, Suite 120
St. Ely, MN 55731 218-365-7790
800-321-4453
Fax: 218-365-7079
www.vobs.com

State assisted programs and support group information for people of many abilities. Includes local chapters, referrals, fun and social interaction and support groups.

Jack Lee, Executive Director
Suellen Sack, Program Director
Poppy Potter, Director of Operations

8283 Wilderness Inquiry
808 14th Avenue SE
Minneapolis, MN 55414 612-676-9400
800-728-0719
Fax: 612-676-9475
TTY: 800-728-0719
info@wildernessinquiry.org
www.wildernessinquiry.org

State assisted programs and support group information for people of many abilities. Includes local chapters, referrals, fun and social interaction and support groups.

Tom Nelson, Chair
Greg Lais, Executive Director
Beth Dooley, Communications Director

Mississippi

8284 First Steps Program
570 East Woodrow Wilson
Jackson, MS 39215 601-576-7816
Fax: 601-576-7540
www.nectas.unc.edu

Individuals with Disabilities Education Act requires all states and territories to provide early intervention and preschool special education for children with disabilities and special health care needs. Services include central directory, representatives of agencies, service providers, families, and coordinators of infant, toddler, and preschool special education programs.

Roy Hart, Infant/Toddler Program Coordinator

8285 Office of Special Education
359 NW Street, Suite 337, PO Box 771
Jackson, MS 39205 601-359-3498
Fax: 601-359-2078
dbowman@mdek12.state.ms.us
www.nectas.unc.edu

Individuals with Disabilities Education Act requires all states and territories to provide early intervention and preschool special education for children with disabilities and special health care needs. Services include central directory, representatives of agencies, service providers, families, and coordinators of infant, toddler, and preschool special education programs.

Dot Bowman, Preschool Special Ed. Coordinator

8286 Parent Partners
5 Old River Place, Suite 101
Jackson, MS 39202 601-354-3302
800-366-5707
Fax: 601-354-2426
ptiofms@misnet.com
www.parentpartners.org

Parent Training and Information (PTI) programs help parents to understand their children's specific needs, communicate more effectively with professionals, participate in the educational planning process, and obtain information about relevant programs, services and resources.

8287 Project Start
PO Box 1698
Jackson, MS 39215 601-987-4872
800-852-8328
Fax: 601-364-2349
dyoung@mdrs.ms.gov
www.msprojectstart.org

State assisted programs and support group information for people of many abilities. Includes local chapters, referrals, fun and social interaction and support groups.

Dorothy Young, Project Director
Kacee Mott, Administrative Assistant

Missouri

8288 Assistance Technology Project
4731 S Cochise, Suite 114
Independence, MO 64055 816-373-5193
Fax: 816-373-9314
TTY: 816-373-9315
matpmo@gni.com
www.doir.state.mo.us/matp/

State assisted programs and support group information for people of many abilities. Includes local chapters, referrals, fun and social interaction and support groups.

8289 Children's Therapy Center
600 E 14th Street
Sedalia, MO 65301 660-826-4400
Fax: 660-826-4420
www.nectas.unc.edu

Services include central directory, representatives of agencies, service providers, families, and coordinators of infant, toddler, and preschool special education programs.

Roger Garlich, Interagency Coordinating Council

8290 Department of Elementary and Secondary Education
PO Box 480
Jefferson City, MO 65102 573-751-2965
Fax: 573-526-4404
pgoff@mail.dese.state.mo.us
www.unc.edu

Individuals with Disabilities Education Act requires all states and territories to provide early intervention and preschool special education for children with disabilities and special health care needs. Services include central directory, representatives of agencies, service providers, families, and coordinators of infant, toddler, and preschool special education programs.

Melodie Friedebach, Coordinator

8291 Disabilities Advocacy & Support Network
PO Box 4067
Parker, CO 80134   417-895-7464
                                    Fax: 417-895-7412
                                    TTY: 417-895-7430
                                    sdasn@aol.com
                                    www.invisibledisabilities.org

Informational and emotional support to parents who have a child, adolescent, or adult family member with special needs.

Wayne Connell, Founder & President
Steve Tonkin, Vice-President
Rob Germundson, Treasurer

8292 Family Resource Network
Park A Plaza
601 Business Loop 70 W, Suite 2161
Columbia, MO 65203   573-449-8663
                                    betty@ece.missouri.edu

Informational and emotional support to parents who have a child, adolescent, or adult family member with special needs.

8293 Missouri Parents Act
8301 State Line Road, Suite 204
Kansas City, MO 64114   816-531-7070
                                    800-743-7634
                                    Fax: 816-531-4777
                                    info@ptimpact.org
                                    www.ptimpact.org

Parent Training and Information (PTI) programs help parents to understand their children's specific needs, communicate more effectively with professionals, participate in the educational planning process, and obtain information about relevant programs, services and resources.

Mary Kay Savage, Executive Director
Diana Biere, Associate Director

8294 Parent Act
1 W Armour Boulevard, Suite 301
Kansas City, MO 64111   816-531-7070
                                    Fax: 816-531-4777
                                    impactcs@coop.cm.org
                                    www.taalliance.org

Parent Training and Information (PTI) programs help parents to understand their children's specific needs, communicate more effectively with professionals, participate in the educational planning process, and obtain information about relevant programs, services and resources.

8295 Positive Solutions for Life Challenges
Route 3, Box 441
Warswaw, MO 65355   660-438-6990

Informational and emotional support to parents who have a child, adolescent, or adult family member with special needs.

8296 United Services
4140 Old Mill Parkway
Saint Peters, MO 63376   636-926-2700
                                    Fax: 636-447-4919
                                    ssalmo@unitedsrvcs.org
                                    www.unitedsrvcs.org

Provides services to children ages infant to five-years-old with special needs. Preschool and daycare onsite. We also offer support groups for siblings and family members, parent library available.

Denise Liebel, President/CEO
Windy Spalding, Chief Operating Officer
Dick Frizzell, CFO

Montana

8297 CO-TEACH/Division of Educational Research and Service
School of Education
University of Montana
Missoula, MT 59812   406-243-5344
                                    Fax: 406-243-2797
                                    coteach@selway.umt.edu

Informational and emotional support to parents who have a child, adolescent, or adult family member with special needs.

8298 Developmental Disabilities Program
PO Box 4210
Helena, MT 59604   406-444-5647
                                    Fax: 406-444-0230
                                    jspiegle@mt.gov
                                    www.nectas.unc.edu

Individuals with Disabilities Education Act requires all states and territories to provide early intervention and preschool special education for children with disabilities and special health care needs. Services include central directory, representatives of agencies, service providers, families, and coordinators of infant, toddler, and preschool special education programs.

Jan Spiegle, Infant/Toddler Program Coordinator

8299 Division of Special Education
PO Box 202501
Helena, MT 59620   406-444-4429
                                    Fax: 406-444-3924
                                    dmccarthy@opi.mt.gov
                                    www.unc.edu

Individuals with Disabilities Education Act requires all states and territories to provide early intervention and preschool special education for children with disabilities and special health care needs. Services include central directory, representatives of agencies, service providers, families, and coordinators of infant, toddler, and preschool special education programs.

Robert Runkel, Director

8300 MonTECH
634 Eddy Avenue, Rural Inst on Disab
Missoula, MT 59812   406-243-5676
                                    800-732-0323
                                    Fax: 406-243-4730
                                    TDD: 800-732-0323
                                    montech@selway.umt.edu
                                    www.rudi.montech.umt.edu/

State assisted programs and support group information for people of many abilities. Includes local chapters, referrals, fun and social interaction and support groups.

8301 Parents Let's Unite for Kids
516 N 32nd Street
Billings, MT 59101   406-255-0540
                                    800-222-7585
                                    Fax: 406-255-0523
                                    info@pluk.org
                                    www.pluk.org

Parent Training and Information (PTI) programs help parents to understand their children's specific needs, communicate more effectively with professionals, participate in the educational planning process, and obtain information about relevant programs, services and resources.

8302 Quality Life Concepts
215 Smelter Ave. N.E. PO Box 250
Great Falls, MT 59403   406-452-9531
                                    800-761-2680
                                    Fax: 406-453-5930
                                    www.qlc-gtf.org

Informational and emotional support to parents who have a child, adolescent, or adult family member with special needs.

Priscilla Halcro, Chief Executive Officer
Tracy Lane, Business Services Director
Lynn Morley, Community Support Services Director

Nebraska

8303 Assistive Technology Partnership
3901 N 27th Street, Suite 5
Lincoln, NE 68521   402-471-0734
                                    888-806-6287
                                    Fax: 402-471-6052
                                    TDD: 402-471-0734
                                    atp@nebraska.gov
                                    www.atp.ne.gov

State assisted programs and support group information for people of many abilities. Includes local chapters, referrals, fun and social interaction and support groups.

David Altman, Technology Specialist
Lauren Rock, Program Director
Leslie Novacek, Director

8304 Individual and Family Support Arc of Lincoln & Lancaster County
645 M Street, Suite 19
Lincoln, NE 68508 402-477-6925
Fax: 402-477-6927

Informational and emotional support to parents who have a child, adolescent, or adult family member with special needs.

8305 Nebraska Parents Center
1941 S 42nd Street, Suite 122
Omaha, NE 68105 402-346-0525
800-284-8520
Fax: 402-346-5253
TDD: 402-346-0525
npe@uswest.ne.net
www.neparentcenter.org

Parent Training and Information (PTI) programs help parents to understand their children's specific needs, communicate more effectively with professionals, participate in the educational planning process, and obtain information about relevant programs, services and resources. The Nebrask Parent Center services families statewide. There is no fee for services. Call for additional information.

Glenda Davis, Project Director

8306 Parent Assistance Network
310 W 24th
Kearney, NE 68847 308-237-6025
Fax: 308-237-6014

Informational and emotional support to parents who have a child, adolescent, or adult family member with special needs.

8307 Parent Support Group
123 S Webb Road
Grand Island, NE 68802 308-385-5925
Fax: 308-385-5797
msheen@genie.esu10.k12.ne.us

Informational and emotional support to parents who have a child, adolescent, or adult family member with special needs.

8308 Parents Encouraging Parents
NE Department of Education
301 Centennial Mall Street, PO Box 94987
Lincoln, NE 68509 402-471-2471
Fax: 402-471-0117
TTY: 402-471-2471
ginny_w@nde4.nde.state.ne.us

Informational and emotional support to parents who have a child, adolescent, or adult family member with special needs.

8309 Special Education Office State Department of Education
301 Centennial Mall South
Lincoln, NE 68509 402-471-9329
Fax: 402-471-6252
jan_t@nde4.nde.state.ne.us
www.chasa.org

Individuals with Disabilities Education Act requires all states and territories to provide early intervention and preschool special education for children with disabilities and special health care needs. Services include central directory, representatives of agencies, service providers, families, and coordinators of infant, toddler, and preschool special education programs.

Charlotte Lewis, Part C Co-Coordinator

Nevada

8310 Assistive Technology Collaborative
711 S Stewart Street, Rehab Division
Carson City, NV 89701 775-687-4452
Fax: 775-687-3292
TTY: 702-687-3388
pgowins@govmail.state.nv.us
www.state.nv.us.80

State assisted programs and support group information for people of many abilities. Includes local chapters, referrals, fun and social interaction and support groups.

8311 Early Intervention Services Division of Child & Family Services
3987 S McCarren Boulevard
Reno, NV 89502 775-688-2284
Fax: 775-688-2558
mkwalter@govmail.state.nv.us
www.nectas.unc.edu

Provides early intervention and preschool special education for children with disabilities and special health care needs. Services include central directory, representatives of agencies, service providers, families, and coordinators of infant, toddler, and preschool special education programs.

Marilyn K Walter, Infant/Toddler Program Coordinator

8312 Educational Equity, Special Education Branch
700 E 5th Street, Suite 113
Carson City, NV 89701 775-687-9171
800-992-0900
Fax: 775-687-9123
gdopf@nsn.scs.unr.edu
www.unc.edu

Individuals with Disabilities Education Act requires all states and territories to provide early intervention and preschool special education for children with disabilities and special health care needs. Services include central directory, representatives of agencies, service providers, families, and coordinators of infant, toddler, and preschool special education programs.

Gloria Dopf, Preschool Special Ed. Coordinator

8313 Nevada Parent Network
University of Nevada-Reno
COE, REPC/285
Reno, NV 89557 702-784-4921
800-216-7988
Fax: 702-702-4997
cdinnell@scs.unr.edu
www.iser.com/npn-NV.html

Informational and emotional support to parents who have a child, adolescent, or adult family member with special needs.

Cheryl Dinnell, Program Coordinator

8314 Nevada Parents Encouraging Parents (PEP)
2101 S. Jones Blvd., Suite 120
Las Vegas, NV 89146 702-388-8899
800-216-5188
Fax: 702-388-2966
pepinfo@nvpep.org
www.nvpep.org

Parent Training and Information (PTI) programs help parents to understand their children's specific needs, communicate more effectively with professionals, participate in the educational planning process, and obtain information about relevant programs, services and resources.

Karen Taycher, Executive Director
Stephanie Vrsnik, Community Development Director
Natalie Filipic, Director of Operations

8315 Parents Encouraging Parents
2101 S. Jones Blvd., Suite 120
Las Vegas, NV 89146

702-388-8899
800-216-5188
Fax: 702-388-2966
pepinfo@nvpep.org
www.nvpep.org

Informational and emotional support to parents who have a child, adolescent, or adult family member with special needs.

Karen Taycher, Executive Director
Stephanie Vrsnik, Community Development Director
Natalie Filipic, Director of Operations

New Hampshire

8316 Bureau of Early Learning
101 Pleasant Street
Concord, NH 03301

603-271-3791
Fax: 603-271-1953
rlittlefield@ed.state.nh.us
www.education.nh.gov

Individuals with Disabilities Education Act requires all states and territories to provide early intervention and preschool special education for children with disabilities and special health care needs. Services include central directory, representatives of agencies, service providers, families, and coordinators of infant, toddler, and preschool special education programs.

Ruth Littlefield, Preschool Special Ed. Coordinator

8317 Dartmouth-Hitchcock Sleep Disorders Center Dartmouth Medical Center
One Medical Center Drive
Lebanon, NH 03756

603-650-7534
Fax: 603-650-7820
www.dartmouth-hitchcock.org

Rocco R Addante, Director
Glen Greenough MD, Fellowship Director
Joanne MacQuarrie, BS,RPSGT,RRT, Administrator

8318 Division of Special Education
101 Pleasant Street
Concord, NH 03301

603-271-3791
Fax: 603-271-1953
www.education.nh.gov

Individuals with Disabilities Education Act requires all states and territories to provide early intervention and preschool special education for children with disabilities and special health care needs. Services include central directory, representatives of agencies, service providers, families, and coordinators of infant, toddler, and preschool special education programs.

Ruth Littlefield, Preschool Special Ed. Coordinator

8319 Family Center Early Supports & Services
105 Pleasant Street
Concord, NH 03301

603-271-5122
Fax: 603-271-5166
cohara@dhhs.state.nh.us
www.familyvoices.org

Services include central directory, representatives of agencies, service providers, families, and coordinators of infant, toddler, and preschool special education programs.

Molly Cole, President
Marcia O'Malley, Vice-President
Lynn Pedraza, Executive Director

8320 High Hopes Foundation of New Hampshire
301 Daniel Webster Hwy., Suite 6
Merrimack, NH 03054

603-529-1010
800-639-6804
Fax: 603-529-0037
HighHopeNH@aol.com
www.highhopesfoundation.org

Volunteer organization dedicated to granting wishes of seriously ill New Hampshire children from three through 18 years old.

60+ members
Shaunae Nolet, President
Tom Perkins, Vice President
Dana Wallace, Treasurer

8321 Parent Information Center
PO Box 2405
Concord, NH 03302

603-224-7005
Fax: 603-224-4365
TDD: 603-224-7005
mlewis@picnh.org
www.picnh.org

Parent Training and Information (PTI) programs help parents to understand their children's specific needs, communicate more effectively with professionals, participate in the educational planning process, and obtain information about relevant programs, services and resources.

Michelle Lewis, Executive Director
Sylvia Abbott, Administrative Supervisor
Jennifer Cunha, Project Staff

8322 Parent to Parent of New Hampshire
12 Flynn Street
Lebanon, NH 03766

603-448-6393
800-698-5465
Fax: 603-448-6311
www.p2pnh.org

Informational and emotional support to parents who have a child, adolescent, or adult family member with special needs.

Richard Cohen, Executive Director
Judith Iaconianni, Director/Co-founder

8323 Technology Partnership Project Institute on Disability/UAP
The Concord Center
10 West Edge Drive , Suite 101
Durham, NH 03824

603-862-4320
Fax: 603-862-0555
TDD: 603-224-0630
institute.disability@unh.edu
iod.unh.edu

State assistive programs funded by the National Institute on Disability and Rehabilitation Research. Includes directories, support group information, training and project information.

New Jersey

8324 Division of Student Services
Riverview Executive Plaza, Building 100
Trenton, NJ 08625

609-633-6833
Fax: 609-984-8422
btkach@doh.state.nj.us
www.unc.edu

Individuals with Disabilities Education Act requires all states and territories to provide early intervention and preschool special education for children with disabilities and special health care needs. Services include central directory, representatives of agencies, service providers, families, and coordinators of infant, toddler, and preschool special education programs.

Barbara Tkach, Preschool Special Ed. Coordinator

8325 Early Intervention System
PO Box 364
Trenton, NJ 08625

609-777-7734
Fax: 609-292-3580
Terry.Harrison@dob.state.nj.us
www.state.nj-us/health/8hs/eiphome.htm

Individuals with Disabilities Education Act requires all states and territories to provide early intervention and preschool special education for children with disabilities and special health care needs. Services include central directory, representatives of agencies, service providers, families, and coordinators of infant, toddler, and preschool special education programs.

Charles E. Drum, Director & Professor
Jennifer Donahue, Director of Finance
Matthew Gianino, Director of Communications

8326 Family Support Center of New Jersey
Lion's Head Office Park
1 AAA Drive, Suite 203
Trenton, NJ 08691   732-262-8020
                                      800-336-5843
                                  Fax: 609-392-5621
                                     FSCNJ@aol.com
                                        www.efnj.com

Informational and emotional support to parents who have a child,
adolescent, or adult family member with special needs.

Michael P. Rinaldo, Chairman
Robert L. D'Avanzo, President
Eric B. Geller, M.D., Vice President

8327 New Jersey Self-Help Clearinghouse
375 East McFarlan Street
Dover, NJ 07801   973-989-1122
                                      800-367-6274
                                  Fax: 973-989-1159
                                  TTY: 973-625-9053
                                info@selfhelpgroups.org
                                      www.njgroups.org

The NJ Self-Help Group Clearinghouse provides contacts for over
4,500 New Jersey support groups and over 1,100 national support
networks for most illnesses, addictions, disabilities, bereavement,
parenting and other stressful life situations. The organization also
helps individuals wanting to start a group.

8328 New Jersey Statewide Parent to Parent
2150 Highway 35, Suite 207C
Sea Girt, NJ 08750   800-372-6510
                                  Fax: 973-642-8080
                                      www.spannj.org

Informational and emotional support to parents who have a child,
adolescent, or adult family member with special needs.

Malia Corde, Program Coordinator|
Malia Corde, Coordinator
Jeannette Mejias, Bilingual (Spanish) Associate

8329 Statewide Parent Advocacy Network
35 Halsey Street, 4th Floor
Newark, NJ 07102   973-642-8100
                                     800-654-SPAN
                                  Fax: 973-642-8080
                                diana.autin@spannj.org
                                   www.spanadvocacy.org

Parent Training and Information (PTI) programs help parents to
understand their children's specific needs, communicate more effectively with professionals, participate in the educational planning process, and obtain information about relevant programs,
services and resources.

Diana Autin, Co-Director
Maria Docherty, Co-Director
Carolyn Hayer, Co-Director

New Mexico

8330 EPICS Project-SW Communication Resources
PO Box 788, 2000 Camino del Pueblo
Bernalilo, NM 87004   505-867-3396
                                      800-765-7320
                                  Fax: 505-867-3398
                                  TDD: 505-867-3396
                                  www.disabilityrights.org

Parent Training and Information (PTI) programs help parents to
understand their children's specific needs, communicate more effectively with professionals, participate in the educational planning process, and obtain information about relevant programs,
services and resources.

8331 Long Term Services Division
PO Box 26110
Santa Fe, NM 87502   505-827-0103
                                  Fax: 505-827-2455
                                   www.nectas.unc.edu

Individuals with Disabilities Education Act requires all states and
territories to provide early intervention and preschool special education for children with disabilities and special health care
needs. Services include central directory, representatives of agencies, service providers, families, and coordinators of infant, toddler, and preschool special education programs.

Cathy Stevenson, Infant/Toddler Program Coordinator

8332 Parents Reaching Out
1920 B Columbia Drive SE
Albuquerque, NM 87106   505-247-0192
                                      800-524-5176
                                  Fax: 505-247-1345
                                  TDD: 505-865-3700
                                info@parentsreachingout.org
                                   www.parentsreachingout.org

Provides peer support, technical assistance and information statewide to families in New Mexico who have family member with
unique or special needs and professionals who care for them.

Renata Witte, President
Johnny Wilson, Executive Director
Leon Emplit, Director of Operations

8333 Special Education Unit
300 Don Gaspar Avenue
Santa Fe, NM 87501   505-827-6541
                                  Fax: 505-827-6791
                                bpasternack@sde.state.mn.us
                                        www.unc.edu

Individuals with Disabilities Education Act requires all states and
territories to provide early intervention and preschool special education for children with disabilities and special health care
needs. Services include central directory, representatives of agencies, service providers, families, and coordinators of infant, toddler, and preschool special education programs.

Maria Landazuri, Preschool Special Ed. Coordinator

8334 Technology Assistance Program
435 St Michael's Drive, Building D
Santa Fe, NM 87505   505-954-8539
                                      800-866-2253
                                  Fax: 505-954-8562
                                  TDD: 800-866-2253
                                    nmdvrtap@aol.com
                                   www.tap.gcd.state.nm.us

State assisted programs for people of many abilities. Includes local chapters, referrals, fun and social interaction and support
groups.

New York

8335 Advocacy Center
590 South Avenue
Rochester, NY 14620   716-546-1700
                                      800-650-4967
                                  Fax: 716-546-7069
                                advocacy@frontiernet.net
                                   www.advocacycenter.com

Parent Training and Information (PTI) programs help parents to
understand their children's specific needs, communicate more effectively with professionals, participate in the educational planning process, and obtain information about relevant programs,
services and resources.

Stephen G. Schwarz, President
Adam Anolik, Vice President
Paul Visca, Treasurer

8336 Advocates for Children of New York
151 W 30th Street, 5th Floor
New York, NY 10001   212-947-9779
                                  Fax: 212-947-9790
                                info@advocatesforchildren.org
                                   www.advocatesforchildren.org

Parent Training and Information (PTI) programs help parents to
understand their children's specific needs, communicate more effectively with professionals, participate in the educational planning process, and obtain information about relevant programs,
services and resources.

Jamie A. Levitt, President
Kim Sweet, Executive Director
Matthew Lenaghan, Deputy Director

8337 Aurora of Central New York
518 James Street, Suite 100
Syracuse, NY 13203   315-422-7263
                                 Fax: 315-422-4792
                                 TTY: 315-422-9746
                                 TDD: 315-422-9746
                              auroracny@auroraofcny.org
                              www.auroraofcny.org

Professional counseling services to assist individuals and their families deal with the trauma of hearing or vision loss.

John McCormick, President
Scott Gucciardi, 1st Vice President
Robert C. Haege, Assistant Treasurer

8338 Early Intervention Program
Corning Tower Room 208, Empire Street Plaza
Albany, NY 12237   518-473-7016
                                 Fax: 518-473-8673
                              dmn02@health.state.ny.us
                              www.nectas.unc.edu

Individuals with Disabilities Education Act requires all states and territories to provide early intervention and preschool special education for children with disabilities and special health care needs. Services include a central directory, representatives of agencies, service providers, families, and coordinators of infant, toddler, and preschool special education programs.

Donna Noyes, Infant/Toddler Program Coordinator

8339 Friends of Karen
118 Titicus Road, PO Box 190
Purdys, NY 10560   845-277-4547
                                    800-637-2774
                              www.friendsofkaren.org

Dedicated to helping terminally and catastrophically ill children and their families in the New York metropolitan area only. They provide assistance with payments for physicians, hospitals and medications, help with extra expenses beyond medical bills, provide home nursing services and equipment, supplies for loans, and offers emotional support.

Pam Hervey, President
Bob Goldberg, Vice President
David Rosenberg, Vice President

8340 Marty Lyons Foundation
326 W 48th Street
New York, NY 10036   212-977-9474
                                    877-560-9474
                                 Fax: 212-977-1752
                          mlf_hq@martylyonsfoundation.org
                          www.martylyonsfoundation.org

Chapters in New Jersey, New York, Massachussets, Connecticut, Maryland, North Carolina, South Carolina, Georgia, Texas, Pennsylvania and Florida provide a special wish to children ages three to seventeen who are terminally ill or have a life-threatening disease.

300 volunteers

Marty Lyons, Chairman
Ken Schroy, Vice Chairman
Richard A. Miller, President

8341 New York Department of Education
1 Commerce Plaza
Albany, NY 12234   518-473-4823
                                 Fax: 518-486-4154
                              mplotzke@mail.nysed.gov

Individuals with Disabilities Education Act requires all states and territories to provide early intervention and preschool special education for children with disabilities and special health care needs. Services include central directory, representatives of agencies, service providers, families, and coordinators of infant, toddler, and preschool special education programs.

Michael Plotzker Vesid, Preschool Special Ed. Coordinator

8342 Parent Network Center
250 Delaware Avenue, Suite 3
Buffalo, NY 14202   716-853-1570
                                    800-724-7408
                                 Fax: 716-853-1574
                                 TDD: 716-853-1573
                              www.taalliance.org

Parent Training and Information (PTI) programs help parents to understand their children's specific needs, communicate more effectively with professionals, participate in the educational planning process, and obtain information about relevant programs, services and resources.

8343 Parent to Parent of New York State
500 Balltown Road
Schenectady, NY 12304   518-381-4350
                                    800-305-8817
                                 Fax: 518-382-1959
                              parent2par@aol.com
                              www.parenttoparentnys.org

Informational and emotional support to parents who have a child, adolescent, or adult family member with special needs.

1500 Members

Linda Coull, Vice President
Holly Bartczak, Coordinator
Tina Beauparlant, Parent Advocate

8344 Resources for Children with Special Needs
116 East 16th Street, 5th Floor
New York City, NY 10003   212-667-4650
                                 Fax: 212-254-4070
                              info@resourcesnyc.org
                              www.resourcesnyc.org

Parent Training and Information (PTI) programs help parents to understand their children's specific needs, communicate more effectively with professionals, participate in the educational planning process, and obtain information about relevant programs, services and resources.

Ellen Miller-Wachtel, Chair
Shon E. Glusky, President
Stephen Stern, Director of Finance and Administrat

8345 Saint Mary's Healthcare System for Children
One Penn Plaza Suite 2420
New York, NY 10119   212-586-8723
                                 Fax: 212-586-5170
                              www.nycharities.org

Information and advocacy resources for families and professionals. Includes listings of organizations providing general information and organizations focusing on more specific areas of concern to families and young adults who have disabilities.

8346 Sinergia/Metropolitan Parent Center
15 W 65th Street, 6th Floor
New York, NY 10023   212-496-1300
                                 Fax: 212-496-5608
                              Sinergia@panix.com
                              www.panic.com/~sinergia

Parent Training and Information (PTI) programs help parents to understand their children's specific needs, communicate more effectively with professionals, participate in the educational planning process, and obtain information about relevant programs, services and resources.

8347 TRIAD Project-Advocates for Persons with Disabilities
One Empire State Plaza, Suite 1001
Albany, NY 12223   518-474-2825
                                    800-522-4369
                                 Fax: 518-473-6005
                                 TTY: 518-473-4231
                              leffingw@emi.com

State assisted programs and support group information for people of many abilities. Includes local chapters, referrals, fun and social interaction and support groups.

8348 Ulster County Social Services
1061 Development Court
Kingston, NY 12401   845-334-5000
                                              Fax: 845-255-3202
                                              www.co.ulster.ny.us

Individuals with Disabilities Education Act requires all states and territories to provide early intervention and preschool special education for children with disabilities and special health care needs. Services include central directory, representatives of agencies, service providers, families, and coordinators of infant, toddler, and preschool special education programs.

Thomas Roach, Interagency Coordinating Council
Michael Iapoce, Commissioner

North Carolina

8349 Assistive Technology Project, Human Resources, Voc. and Rehab. Services
1110 Navaho Drive, Suite 101
Raleigh, NC 27609   919-850-2787
                                                 800-852-0042
                                              Fax: 919-850-2792
                                              TTY: 919-850-2787
                                              rickic@mindspring.com
                                              www.ncatp.org

State assisted programs and support group information for people of many abilities. Includes local chapters, referrals, fun and social interaction and support groups.

8350 ECAC
907 Barra Row, Suites 102/103
Davidson, NC 28036   704-892-1321
                                              Fax: 704-892-5028
                                              TDD: 704-892-1321
                                              ecac@ecac.org
                                              www.ecac-parentcenter.org

Parent Training and Information (PTI) programs help parents to understand their children's specific needs, communicate more effectively with professionals, participate in the educational planning process, and obtain information about relevant programs, services and resources.

Connie Hawkins, Executive Director
Mary Watson, Director of Exceptional Children Di

8351 Exceptional Children Division
301 N Wilmington Street
Raleigh, NC 27601   919-807-3300
                                              Fax: 919-807-3482
                                              kbaars@state.nc.us
                                              www.mcpublicschools.org

Individuals with Disabilities Education Act requires all states and territories to provide early intervention and preschool special education for children with disabilities and special health care needs. Services include central directory, representatives of agencies, service providers, families, and coordinators of infant, toddler, and preschool special education programs.

Kathy Baars, Preschool Special Ed. Coordinator

8352 Family Support Network of North Carolina
University of North carolina
200 N Greensboro St, Carr Mill Mall, 2nd Fl Ste D9
Carrboro, NC 27510   919-966-2841
                                                 800-852-0042
                                              Fax: 919-966-2916
                                              cdr@med.unc.edu
                                              www.fsnnc.org

Family Support Network of North Carolina promotes and provides support for families with children who have special needs. Families are in a unique position to offer information and support to other families. An experienced family member can share the most practical advice and help a parent navigate the complex service systems. Having support can make it easier for families to experience the joy and satisfaction that can come from parenting a child with special needs.

Laura Curtis, Education & Outreach Coordinator
Irene Nathan Zipper, Director

8353 Partnerships for Inclusion
2415 W Vernon Avenue
Kingston, NC 28501   919-559-5156
                                              msteele@greenvillenc.com
                                              www.nectas.unc.edu

Individuals with Disabilities Education Act requires all states and territories to provide early intervention and preschool special education for children with disabilities and special health care needs. Services include central directory, representatives of agencies, service providers, families, and coordinators of infant, toddler, and preschool special education programs.

Sandy Steele, Interagency Coordinating Council

8354 Rockingham County Schools
511 Harrington Highway
Eden, NC 27288   336-627-2615
                                              Fax: 336-627-2660
                                              speele@greenvillenc.com
                                              www.ncpublicschools.org/success/regionalcontacts

Individuals with Disabilities Education Act requires all states and territories to provide early intervention and preschool special education for children with disabilities and special health care needs. Services include central directory, representatives of agencies, service providers, families, and coordinators of infant, toddler, and preschool special education programs.

Susan Peele, Interagency Coordinating Council

North Dakota

8355 Developmental Disabilities Unit
1237 W Divide Avenue, Suite 1A
Bismarck, ND 58501   701-328-8936
                                                 800-755-8529
                                              Fax: 701-328-8969
                                              sobald@nd.gov
                                              www.nectas.unc.edu

Individuals with Disabilities Education Act requires all states and territories to provide early intervention and preschool special education for children with disabilities and special health care needs. Services include central directory, representatives of agencies, service providers, families, and coordinators of infant, toddler, and preschool special education programs.

Debra Balsdon, Infant/Toddler Program Coordinator

8356 Interagency Program Assistive Technology
3240-15th Street South, Suite B
Fargo, ND 58104   701-365-4728
                                                 800-895-4728
                                              Fax: 701-365-6242
                                              TDD: 701-265-4807
                                              lee@pioneer.state.nd.us
                                              www.ndipat.org

State assisted programs and support group information for people of many abilities. Includes local chapters, referrals, fun and social interaction and support groups.

8357 Special Education Division
600 E Boulevard
Bismarck, ND 58505   701-328-2277
                                              Fax: 701-328-4149
                                              TTY: 701-328-4920
                                              dpi@nd.gov
                                              www.dpi.state.nd.us

Individuals with Disabilities Education Act requires all states and territories to provide early intervention and preschool special education for children with disabilities and special health care needs. Services include central directory, representatives of agencies, service providers, families, and coordinators of infant, toddler, and preschool special education programs.

Ann Chase, Child Nutrition, Grant Manager
Jerry Coleman, School Finance, Director
Jim Bosch, Maintenance/Clerk

Ohio

8358 Bureau of EI Services
246 N High Strees, PO Box 118
Columbus, OH 43215

614-644-8389
Fax: 614-728-9163
coser@gw.odh.state.oh.us
www.ohiohelpmegrow.org

Individuals with Disabilities Education Act requires all states and territories to provide early intervention and preschool special education for children with disabilities and special health care needs. Services include central directory, representatives of agencies, service providers, families, and coordinators of infant, toddler, and preschool special education programs.

Cindy Oser, Infant/Toddler Program Coordinator

8359 Celebrating Families of Children & Adults with Special Needs
16 Vassar Drive
Dayton, OH 45406

937-275-0990
800-432-2199
Fax: 937-275-0277
families@erinet.com
www.eparent.com

Informational and emotional support to parents who have a child, adolescent, or adult family member with special needs.

Joseph M Valenzano, Jr., President, CEO & Publisher
James P. McGinnis, VP of Operations/CFO
Rick Rader, MD, Editor-in-Chief

8360 Division of Early Childhood Education
65 S Front Street, Room 309
Columbus, OH 43215

614-466-0224
Fax: 614-728-2338
www.dec-sped.org

Individuals with Disabilities Education Act requires all states and territories to provide early intervention and preschool special education for children with disabilities and special health care needs. Services include central directory, representatives of agencies, service providers, families, and coordinators of infant, toddler, and preschool special education programs.

Jane Wiechel, Preschool Special Ed. Coordinator

8361 East Central Regional Office
170 W High Avenue
New Philadelphia, OH 44663

330-364-5567
Fax: 330-343-3038
ECE_Greer@ode.ohio.gov@inet
www.nectas.unc.edu

Individuals with Disabilities Education Act requires all states and territories to provide early intervention and preschool special education for children with disabilities and special health care needs. Services include central directory, representatives of agencies, service providers, families, and coordinators of infant, toddler, and preschool special education programs.

Edith Greer, Preschool Special Ed. Coordinator

8362 Family Information Network
143 NW Avenue, Building A
Tallmadge, OH 44278

330-633-2055
Fax: 330-633-2658

Informational and emotional support to parents who have a child, adolescent, or adult family member with special needs.

8363 National Child Advocacy Center
210 Pratt Avenue
Huntaville, AL 35801

256-533-0531
Fax: 256-534-6883
TDD: 513-821-2400
CADCCenter@aol.com
www.nationalcac.org

Parent Training and Information (PTI) programs help parents to understand their children's specific needs, communicate more effectively with professionals, participate in the educational planning process, and obtain information about relevant programs, services and resources.

Tim Kauffman, President
Duz Packett, Vice President
Chris Kuffner, Secretary

8364 OCECD
165 W Center Street, Suite 302
Marion, OH 43302

614-382-5452
800-374-2806
Fax: 614-383-6421
ocecd@edu.gte.net
www.ocecd.org

Parent Training and Information (PTI) programs help parents to understand their children's specific needs, communicate more effectively with professionals, participate in the educational planning process, and obtain information about relevant programs, services and resources.

Margaret M. Burley, Director

8365 Ohio Protection and Advocacy Organization
5350 Brookpark Avenue
Cleveland, OH 44134

216-398-5501
800-672-1220
Fax: 216-398-5505

Informational and emotional support to parents who have a child, adolescent, or adult family member with special needs.

8366 Operation Liftoff of Ohio
PO Box 1094
Canti polise, OH 45663

Fulfills a dream for children in Ohio and surrounding states who have a life-threatening illness.

8367 Society for Rehabilitation
9521 Lake Shore Boulevard
Mentor, OH 44060

440-352-8993
Fax: 440-352-6632
info@societyhelps.org
www.societyhelps.org

Individuals with Disabilities Education Act requires all states and territories to provide early intervention and preschool special education for children with disabilities and special health care needs. Disability therapy is provided for children and adults.

Richard J Kessler, Executive Director

8368 Train-Ohio Super Computer Center
1224 Kinnear Road
Columbus, OH 43212

614-292-9248
Fax: 614-292-7168
TDD: 614-292-2426
www.osc.edu

State assisted programs and support group information for people of many abilities. Includes local chapters, referrals, fun and social interaction and support groups.

Pankaj Shah, Executive Director
Kevin Wohlever, Director of Supercomputing Operatio
Brian Guilfoos, Client and Technology Support Manag

Oklahoma

8369 Oklahoma ABLE Tech-Wellness Center
1514 W Hall of Fame
Stillwater, OK 74078

405-744-9748
800-257-1705
Fax: 405-744-7670
TTY: 800-257-1705
mljwell@okway.okstate.edu
www.okabletech.okstate.edu

State assisted programs and support group information for people of many abilities. Includes local chapters, referrals, fun and social interaction and support groups.

Linda Jaco, Director of Sponsored Programs
Milissa Gofourth, Program Manager
Diana Sargent, Staff Assistant

8370 Parents Reaching Out in Oklahoma
1917 S Harvard Avenue
Oklahoma City, OK 73128
405-681-9710
Fax: 405-685-4006
TDD: 405-681-9710
prook@aol.com
www.ucp.org/probase.htm

Parent Training and Information (PTI) programs help parents to understand their children's specific needs, communicate more effectively with professionals, participate in the educational planning process, and obtain information about relevant programs, services and resources.

8371 Special Education Office
2500 N Lincoln Boulevard
Oklahoma City, OK 73105
405-521-3351
Fax: 405-522-2066
TDD: 405-521-4875
mark_sharp@mail.sde.state.ok.us
www.ok.gov

Individuals with Disabilities Education Act requires all states and territories to provide early intervention and preschool special education for children with disabilities and special health care needs. Services include central directory, representatives of agencies, service providers, families, and coordinators of infant, toddler, and preschool special education programs.

Joel Robison, Chief of Staff
Mark Sharp, Associate Director
Janet Barresi, State Superintendent of Public Inst

Oregon

8372 Early Childhood CARES Program
1895 E 15th Avenue
Eugene, OR 97403
541-346-2639
Fax: 541-343-5650
Judy_Newman@ccmail.uoregon.edu

Individuals with Disabilities Education Act requires all states and territories to provide early intervention and preschool special education for children with disabilities and special health care needs. Services include central directory, representatives of agencies, service providers, families, and coordinators of infant, toddler, and preschool special education programs.

Judy Newman, Interagency Coordinating Council

8373 Early Intervention Programs
255 Capitol Street NE
Salem, OR 97301
503-378-3598
Fax: 503-373-7968
TDD: 503-378-2892
steve.johnson@state.or.us
www.unc.edu

Individuals with Disabilities Education Act requires all states and territories to provide early intervention and preschool special education for children with disabilities and special health care needs. Services include central directory, representatives of agencies, service providers, families, and coordinators of infant, toddler, and preschool special education programs.

Steven B. Johnson, Associate Superintendent

8374 Oregon Department of Education
255 Capitol Street NE
Salem, OR 97301
503-947-5747
Fax: 503-378-5156
nancy.johnson-dorn@state.or.us
www.ode.state.or.us

Provides early intervention and preschool special education for children with disabilities. Services include central directory, representatives of agencies, service providers, families, and coordinators of infant, toddler, and preschool special education programs.

Nancy Johnson-Dorn, Early Childhood Director
Susan Castillo, State Superintendent of Public Inst

8375 Oregon Parent Training and Information Center
2295 Liberty Street NE
Salem, OR 97303
503-581-8156
888-505-2673
Fax: 503-391-0429
orpti@orpti.org
www.orpti.org

Informational and emotional support to parents who have a child, adolescent, or adult family member with special needs.

8376 Technology Access for Life Needs Project
1257 Ferry Street, Se
Salem, OR 97310
503-361-1201
Fax: 503-370-4530
TDD: 503-361-1201
ati@orednet.org

State assisted programs and support group information for people of many abilities. Includes local chapters, referrals, fun and social interaction and support groups.

Pennsylvania

8377 Bureau of Special Education
333 Market Street, 7th Floor
Harrisburg, PA 17126
717-783-6788
800-874-2301
Fax: 717-783-6139
TTY: 717-783-8445
TDD: 717-787-7367
ebeck@state.pa.us
www.portal.state.pa.us

Services include central directory, representatives of agencies, service providers, families, and coordinators of infant, toddler, and preschool special education programs.

Esther Beck, Educational Supervisor
Rick Price, Division Chief
Patti Skunta, Preschool Spcl.Education Supervisor

8378 Division of Early Intervention Services
PO Box 2675
Harrisburg, PA 17105
717-783-7213
Fax: 717-772-0012
jackiee@dpw.state.pa.us
www.unc.edu

Individuals with Disabilities Education Act requires all states and territories to provide early intervention and preschool special education for children with disabilities and special health care needs. Services include central directory, representatives of agencies, service providers, families, and coordinators of infant, toddler, and preschool special education programs.

Jacqueline Epstein, Infant/Toddler Program Coordinator

8379 Montgomery County Intermediate Unit #23
1605 B W Main Street
Norristown, PA 19403
610-539-8550
Fax: 610-539-5973
www.mciu.org

Services include a central directory, representatives of agencies, service providers, families, and coordinators of infant, toddler, and preschool special education programs.

Burunda Prince-Jones, President
Louis A. Polaneczky, Vice President
Nancy Landes, Secretary

8380 Parent Education Network
2107 Industrial Highway
York, PA 17402
717-600-0100
800-441-5028
Fax: 717-600-8101
TTY: 717-600-0100
TDD: 717-600-0100
pen@parentednet.org
www.parentednet.org

Parent Training and Information (PTI) programs help parents to understand their children's specific needs, communicate more effectively with professionals, participate in the educational planning process, and obtain information about relevant programs, services and resources.

Kay Lipsitz, PEN Director
Jane Erdo, Parent Support Coordinator
Jackie Hines, Technology & Parent Support Coordin

8381 Parent to Parent ARC Allegheny
711 Bingham Street
Pittsburgh, PA 15203 412-995-5001
ptparc@arcallegheny.org
www.arcallegheny.org

Informational and emotional support to parents who have a child, adolescent, or adult family member with special needs.

8382 Parent to Parent of Pennsylvania
150 S Progress Avenue
Harrisburg, PA 17109 717-540-4722
Fax: 717-540-7603
bril1134@cdc.gov
www.parenttoparent.org

Informational and emotional support to parents who have a child, adolescent, or adult family member with special needs.

Fiona Patrick, Program Director
Janice Forosisky, Statewide Supervisor
Kim Huff, Database Coordinator

8383 Parents Union for Public Schools
1315 Walnut Street, Suite 1124
Philadelphia, PA 19107 215-546-1166
Fax: 215-731-1688
Parents@aol.com
www.nyfac.org

Parent Training and Information (PTI) programs help parents to understand their children's specific needs, communicate more effectively with professionals, participate in the educational planning process, and obtain information about relevant programs, services and resources.

8384 Pennsylvania's Initiative on Assistive Technology, Institute on Disabilities
University Affliated Program
423 Ritter Annex, Temple University
Philadelphia, PA 19122 215-204-5966
800-204-7428
Fax: 215-204-9371
TTY: 800-750-7428
piat@astro.temple.edu
www.temple.edu/inst_disabilities

Most of PAIT's activities are free to Pennsylvania residents, and are focused on the provision of public awareness of the benefit and scope of assistive technology (AT), information and referral, advocacy and funding, and training. PAIT is the state's contractor for the implementation of Pennsylvania's Assistive Technology Lending library.

8385 US Wheelchair Weightlifting Association
39 Michael Place
Levittown, PA 19057 215-945-1964

State assisted programs and support group information for people of many abilities. Includes local chapters, referrals, fun and social interaction and support groups.

Rhode Island

8386 Assistive Technology Access Partnership
40 Fountain Street
Providence, RI 02903 401-421-7005
Fax: 401-222-3574
TTY: 401-421-7016
reginac@ors.state.ri.us
www.atap.state.ri.us

State assisted programs and support group information for people of many abilities. Includes local chapters, referrals, fun and social interaction and support groups.

8387 Central Region Early Intervention Program
J Arthur Trudeau Memorial Center
250 Commonwealth Avenue
Warwick, RI 02886 401-823-1731
Fax: 401-823-1849

Informational and emotional support to parents who have a child, adolescent, or adult family member with special needs.

8388 Office Integrated Social Services
255 Westminister Road
Providence, RI 02903 401-222-4600
Fax: 401-222-6030
ride0032@ride.ri.net
www.unc.edu

Individuals with Disabilities Education Act requires all states and territories to provide early intervention and preschool special education for children with disabilities and special health care needs. Services include central directory, representatives of agencies, service providers, families, and coordinators of infant, toddler, and preschool special education programs.

Robert M. Pryhoda, Director

8389 Rhode Island Arc
99 Bald Hill Road
Cranston, RI 02920 401-463-9191
Fax: 401-463-9244
www.nectas.unc.edu

Individuals with Disabilities Education Act requires all states and territories to provide early intervention and preschool special education for children with disabilities and special health care needs. Services include central directory, representatives of agencies, service providers, families, and coordinators of infant, toddler, and preschool special education programs.

James Healey, Interagency Coordinating Council

8390 Rhode Island Department of Health
600 New London Avenue
Cranston, RI 02920 401-462-0318
Fax: 401-462-6253
www.nectas.unc.edu

Individuals with Disabilities Education Act requires all states and territories to provide early intervention and preschool special education for children with disabilities and special health care needs. Services include central directory, representatives of agencies, service providers, families, and coordinators of infant, toddler, and preschool special education programs.

Ron Caldarone, Infant/Toddler Program Coordinator

8391 Rhode Island Parent Information Network
1210 Pontiac Avenue
Cranston, RI 02920 401-270-0101
800-464-3399
Fax: 401-270-7049
info@ripin.org
www.ripin.org

Nonprofit organization providing information, training, support and advocacy to parents.

Kathleen DiChiara, Chair
Rebecca Kislak, Esq., Vice Chair
Louis J. Simon, CPA, MST, Treasurer

South Carolina

8392 Assistive Technology Project
Center for Developmental Disabilities
USC School of Medicine
Columbia, SC 29208 Fax: 803-935-5342
TDD: 803-935-5263
scatp@scsn.net
www.scsn.net/users/scatp

State assisted programs and support group information for people of many abilities. Includes local chapters, referrals, fun and social interaction and support groups.

8393 BabyNet
1751 Calhoun Street
Columbia, SC 29201
803-898-0784
Fax: 803-898-0613
strickll@dhec.sc.gov
www.scdhec.net/babynet

Individuals with Disabilities Education Act requires all states and territories to provide early intervention and preschool special education for children with disabilities and special health care needs. Services include central directory, representatives of agencies, service providers, families, and coordinators of infant, toddler, and preschool special education programs.

Kathy Hart, Infant/Toddler Program Coordinator

8394 Office of Exceptional Children South Carolina Department of Education
1429 Senate Street, Room 808
Columbia, SC 29201
803-734-8811
Fax: 803-734-4824
njenkins@sde.state.sc.us
www.myschools.com/offices/ec

Individuals with Disabilities Education Act requires all states and territories to provide early intervention and preschool special education for children with disabilities and special health care needs. Services include central directory, representatives of agencies, service providers, families, and coordinators of infant, toddler, and preschool special education programs.

Norma Donaldson-Jenkins, Preschool Special Ed. Coordinator
Susan Duranti, Director

8395 PRO-Parents
652 Bush River Road
Columbia, SC 29210
803-772-5688
800-759-4776
Fax: 803-772-5341
proparents@proparents.org
www.proparents.org

Parent Training and Information (PTI) programs help parents to understand their children's specific needs, communicate more effectively with professionals, participate in the educational planning process, and obtain information about relevant programs, services and resources.

3500 Members

Dana C. Reed, President
Melina Lee, Vice President
Erik Norton, Treasurer

South Dakota

8396 DakotaLink
P.O. Box 218
Sturgis, SD 57785
605-347-4476
605-394-1876
Fax: 605-394-5315
TTY: 800-645-0673
rreed@sdtie.sdserv.org
www.dakotalink.tie.net

State assisted programs and support group information for people of many abilities. Includes local chapters, referrals, fun and social interaction and support groups.

8397 Office of Special Education
700 Governors Drive
Pierre, SD 57501
605-773-3678
Fax: 605-773-6846
TTY: 605-773-6302
barbh@deca.state.sd.us
www.sd.gov

Individuals with Disabilities Education Act requires all states and territories to provide early intervention and preschool special education for children with disabilities and special health care needs. Services include central directory, representatives of agencies, service providers, families, and coordinators of infant, toddler, and preschool special education programs.

Barb Hemmelman, Education Program Assistant Manager

8398 South Dakota Parent Connection
3701 W 49th, Suite 102
Souix Falls, SD 57106
605-361-3171
Fax: 605-361-2928
bschreck@dakota.net
www.sdparent.org

Parent Training and Information (PTI) programs help parents to understand their children's specific needs, communicate more effectively with professionals, participate in the educational planning process, and obtain information about relevant programs, services and resources.

Elaine Roberts, Executive Director
Mary Pat Jones, Finance Director
Nykki Sutton, Office Coordinator

8399 University Affiliated Program, School of Medicine
414 E Clark Street
Vermillion, SD 57069
605-677-5311
Fax: 605-677-6274
jwounded@used.edu
www.nectas.unc.edu

Individuals with Disabilities Education Act requires all states and territories to provide early intervention and preschool special education for children with disabilities and special health care needs. Services include central directory, representatives of agencies, service providers, families, and coordinators of infant, toddler, and preschool special education programs.

Joanne Wounded Head, Interagency Coordinating Council

Tennessee

8400 Center for Early Childhood
E Tennessee State University, Box 70434
Johnson City, TN 37614
423-439-7555
Fax: 423-439-7561
doylel@etsu.edu
child.etsu.edu

Individuals with Disabilities Education Act requires all states and territories to provide early intervention and preschool special education for children with disabilities and special health care needs. Services include central directory, representatives of agencies, service providers, families, and coordinators of infant, toddler, and preschool special education programs.

Wesley Brown, Interagency Coordinating Council

8401 Office of Special Education, State Department of Education
710 James Robertson Parkway
Nashville, TN 37243
615-741-2851
Fax: 615-532-9412
dmattraw@mail.state.tn.us
www.state.tn.us

Individuals with Disabilities Education Act requires all states and territories to provide early intervention and preschool special education for children with disabilities and special health care needs. Services include central directory, representatives of agencies, service providers, families, and coordinators of infant, toddler, and preschool special education programs.

Joseph Fisher, Executive Director

8402 STEP (Support & Training for Exceptional Parents)
712 Professional Plaza
Greenvilles, TN 37745
800-975-2919
800-280-7837
Fax: 423-636-8217
TTY: 423-639-8802
TDD: 423-639-8802
information@tnstep.org
www.tnstep.org

STEP is the Parent Training and Information Center (PTI) for TN. The purpose of STEP is to support families by providing free information, advocacy training, and support services to parents of children in special education or that might need special education. STEP serves parents of children eligible to receive special education services under the Individuals with Disabilities Education Act (IDEA) who reside in Tennessee (birth through age 22).

Sally Ottinger, Information Coordinator
Karen Harrison, Executive Director
Donna Jennings, Business and Personnel Manager

8403 Technology Access Center of Middle Tennessee
2222 Metrocenter Boulevard, Suite 126
Nashville, TN 37228   615-248-6733
                                   800-368-4651
                             Fax: 615-259-2536
                             tactn@nashville.com
                             tac.ataccess.org

Technology group of parents, consumers and professionals; provides resources to help children and adults who have disabilities gain access to the benefits of technology. Includes nationwide network of community-based assistive technology, resource centers, hands on consultants and product demonstrations.

Texas

8404 Department of Assistive and Rehabilitation Services
4900 N Lamar Boulevard
Austin, TX 78751   512-424-6754
                                  800-250-2246
                            Fax: 512-424-6749
                            marytbetho'hanlon@dars.state.tx.us
                            www.eci.state.tx.us

Individuals with Disabilities Education Act part C requires all states and territories to provide early intervention to infants and toddlers with disabilities. Services include a full array of infant intervention fields and disciplines.

MaryBeth O'Hanlon, Assistant Commissioner

8405 Office of the Dean, University of Texas at Austin
College of Education, EBB 210
Austin, TX 78712   512-471-7255
                            Fax: 512-471-0846
                            www.nectas.unc.edu

Individuals with Disabilities Education Act requires all states and territories to provide early intervention and preschool special education for children with disabilities and special health care needs. Services include central directory, representatives of agencies, service providers, families, and coordinators of infant, toddler, and preschool special education programs.

Alba Ortiz, Interagency Coordinating Council

8406 Parent Case Management
4601 Hartford
Abilene, TX 79605   915-691-7232
                            Fax: 915-793-3549

Support network for parents of children with disabilities and/or chronic illness. Veteran parents offer support to parents who are just learning of their child's diagnosis. Offers support and insight into parenting a child with special needs, as well as referrals to trained veteran parents.

8407 Partners Resource Network
1090 Longfellow Drive, Suite B
Beaumont, TX 77706   409-898-4684
                                  800-866-4726
                            Fax: 409-898-4869
                            TTY: 409-898-4816
                            partnersresource@sbcglobal.net
                            www.partnerstx.org

Support network for parents of children with disabilities and/or chronic illness. Veteran parents offer support to parents who are just learning of their child's diagnosis. Offers support and insight into parenting a child with special needs, as well as referrals to trained veteran parents.

Janice Meyer, M. Ed., Executive Director
Alva Adkins, Business Manager
Shene St. Simone, Administrative Assistant

8408 Project PODER
1017 N Main Avenue, Suite 207
San Antonio, TX 78212   210-222-2637
                            Fax: 210-475-9283
                            TDD: 800-682-9747
                            poder@world-net.com
                            www.tfepoder.org/poder

Parent Training and Information (PTI) programs help parents to understand their children's specific needs, communicate more effectively with professionals, participate in the educational planning process, and obtain information about relevant programs, services and resources.

8409 South Central Region-Helen Keller National Center
4230 Lyndon B Johnson
Dallas, TX 75244   972-490-9677
                            Fax: 972-490-6042
                            ccfutbol@aol.com

8410 Special Education Programs - U.S. Dept. of Education Office of Special Ed Programs
400 Maryland Avenue SW
Washington, DC 20202   202-401-2000
                                  800-872-5327
                            Fax: 202-401-0689
                            TTY: 800-473-0833
                            education@custhelp.com
                            www.ed.gov

Early intervention and preschool special education for children with disabilities and special health care needs. Services include central directory, representatives of agencies, service providers, families, and coordinators of infant, toddler, and preschool special education programs.

Joanne Weiss, Chief of Staff
Thomas Skelly, Chief Financial Officer/Chief Finan
James W. Runcie, Chief Operating Officer, Federal St

8411 Texas Assistive Technology Partnership
Texas University Affiliated Program
10100 Burnet Road
Austin, TX 78758   512-232-0740
                                  800-828-7839
                            Fax: 512-232-0761
                            TTY: 512-232-0762
                            txcds@uttcds.org
                            www.tcds.edb.utexas.edu

State assisted programs and support group information for people of many abilities. Includes local chapters, referrals, fun and social interaction and support groups.

Penny Seay, Ph.D., Executive Director
Laura Buckner, M.Ed., L.P.C., Community Education Specialist, TCD
Karen Fonken, Office Manager, TCDS

Utah

8412 Baby Watch Early Intervention Program
288 North 1460 West
Salt Lake City, UT 84116   801-538-6003
                            Fax: 801-584-8496
                            sord@doh.state.ut.us
                            www.utahbabywatch.org

Individuals with Disabilities Education Act requires all states and territories to provide early intervention and preschool special education for children with disabilities and special health care needs. Services include central directory, representatives of agencies, service providers, families, and coordinators of infant, toddler, and preschool special education programs.

W. David Patton, Ph.D., Executive Director
Michael Hales, Director, Medicaid and Health Finan
Barry Nangle, Ph.D, Director, Center for Health Data

8413 Computer Center for Citizens with Disabilities
UT Center for Assistive Technology
1595 W 500 Street
Salt Lake City, UT 84104

801-887-9533
888-866-5550
Fax: 801-887-9382
cboogaar@usoe.k12.ut.us
www.usor.utah.gov/ucat/computers

Technology group of parents, consumers and professionals; provides resources to help children and adults who have disabilities gain access to the benefits of technology. Includes nationwide network of community-based assistive technology, resource centers, hands on consultants and product demonstrations.

8414 Special Education Services Unit
250 E 500 S
Salt Lake City, UT 84111

801-538-7706
Fax: 801-538-7991
TTY: 801-538-7876
mtaylor@usoe.k12.ut.us
www.unc.edu

Individuals with Disabilities Education Act requires all states and territories to provide early intervention and preschool special education for children with disabilities and special health care needs. Services include central directory, representatives of agencies, service providers, families, and coordinators of infant, toddler, and preschool special education programs.

Mae Taylor, Director

8415 US Disabled Ski Team
Box 100
Park City, UT 84060

435-649-9090
Fax: 435-649-3613
info@usaa.org

State assisted programs and support group information for people of many abilities. Includes local chapters, referrals, fun and social interaction and support groups.

8416 Utah Center for Assistive Technology
Center for Persons with Disabilities
Judy Ann Buffmire Building, 1595 West 500 South
Salt Lake City, UT 84104

801-887-9380
Fax: 801-887-9382
TDD: 801-797-2096
sharon@cpo2.usu.edu
www.ucat.usor.utah.gov

State assisted programs and support group information for people of many abilities. Includes local chapters, referrals, fun and social interaction and support groups.

Kent Remund, Director
Lynn Marcoux, Executive Secretary
Michael Offutt, Assistive Technology Specialist

8417 Utah Parent Center
230 West 200 South, Suite 1101
Salt Lake City, UT 84101

801-272-1051
800-468-1160
Fax: 801-272-8907
upc@inconnect.com
www.utahparentcenter.org

Parent Training and Information (PTI) programs help parents to understand their children's specific needs, communicate more effectively with professionals, participate in the educational planning process, and obtain information about relevant programs, services and resources. Offers free written materials, workshops, individual consultations, newsletter, statewide volunteer network, parent to parent support.

Helen Post, Director
Jennie Gibson, Associate Director, Programs and Se
Sherrie Wignall, Fiscal Manager

8418 Assistive Technology Project
103 S Main Street, Weeks Building, 1st Floor
Waterbury, VT 05671

Fax: 802-241-2174
TTY: 802-241-2620
TDD: 801-797-2096
lynnec@dad.state.vt.us
www.uvm.edu/uapvt/cats.html

State assisted programs and support group information for people of many abilities. Includes local chapters, referrals, fun and social interaction and support groups.

8419 Center on Disabilities and Community Inclusion
101 Cherry Street, Suite 450
Burlington, VT 05401

802-656-4031
Fax: 802-656-1357
TDD: 802-656-4031
ccloning@zoo.uvm.edu
www.uvm.edu/~cdci

In collaboration with individuals with disabilities, their families and communities, will promote the independence, inclusion, participation and personal choice of individuals with disabilities of all ages in all environments through the development and enhancement of culturally sensitive, responsive services and supports, interdisiplinary training, technical assistance, exemplary service models, research, dissemination of information and advocacy for the legal and civil rights of the disabled.

Rachel Cronin, Human Resources, CDCI Core Project
Michael Coleman, CDCI Alliliated Faculty Researcher:
Michaella Collins, Dissemination Coordinato

8420 Family, Infant, and Toddler Project
208 Colchester Avenue
Burlington, VT 05405

802-656-8112
Fax: 802-656-1357
bmccar@vdh.state.vt.us
www.nectas.unc.edu

Individuals with Disabilities Education Act requires all states and territories to provide early intervention and preschool special education for children with disabilities and special health care needs. Services include central directory, representatives of agencies, service providers, families, and coordinators of infant, toddler, and preschool special education programs.

Beverly MacCarty, Infant/Toddler Program Coordinator

8421 Special Education Unit
120 State Street
Montpelier, VT 05620

802-828-2755
Fax: 802-828-3140
kandrews@doe.state.vt.us
www.vermont.gov

Individuals with Disabilities Education Act requires all states and territories to provide early intervention and preschool special education for children with disabilities and special health care needs. Services include central directory, representatives of agencies, service providers, families, and coordinators of infant, toddler, and preschool special education programs.

Dennis Kane, Director

8422 Vermont Parent Information Center
1 Mill Street, Suite 310
Burlington, VT 05401

802-658-5315
800-639-7170
Fax: 802-658-5395
TDD: 802-658-5315
vpic@vtpic.com
www.allthebuzzmarketing.com/Vermont

Dedicated to increasing and expanding educational and developmental opportunities that improve the quality of life for children with special needs and their families. We believe that we can achieve this goal only when we provide families with the chance to build on their own strengths, and to feel respected for their values and beliefs.

Connie Curtain, Executive Director

8423 Infant & Toddler Program
PO Box 1797
Richmond, VA 23218

804-371-6592
Fax: 804-371-7959
alucas@dmhmrsas.state.va.us
www.nectas.unc.edu

Provides early intervention and preschool special education for children with disabilities and special health care needs. Services include central directory, representatives of agencies, service providers, families, and coordinators of infant, toddler, and preschool special education programs.

Anne Lucas, Infant/Toddler Program Coordinator

8424 Office of Special Education, Virginia
101 N 14th Street
Richmond, VA 23219

804-225-2675
Fax: 804-371-8796
prnondak@mail.vak12ed.edu
www.doe.virginia.gov

Individuals with Disabilities Education Act requires all states and territories to provide early intervention and preschool special education for children with disabilities and special health care needs. Services include central directory, representatives of agencies and coordinators preschool special education programs.

Thomas Broyles, Director, Business & Risk Managemen
Marie G. Williams, Director, Office of Accounting
June F. Eanes, Director, Office of Support Service

8425 Parent Educational Advocacy Training Cente r
100 N Washington Street, Suite 234
Falls Church, VA 22046

703-923-0010
800-869-6782
Fax: 800-693-3514
TTY: 703-923-0010
TDD: 703-923-0010
partners@peatc.org
www.peatc.org

Parent Training and Information (PTI) programs help parents to understand their children's specific needs, communicate more effectively with professionals, participate in the educational planning process, and obtain information about relevant programs, services and resources.

Cathy Healy, Chief Executive Officer
Francisco R. Ramirez, President
Suzanne Bowers, Executive Director

8426 Tidewater Center for Technology Access
1413 Laskin Road
Virginia Beach, VA 23451

757-437-6524
Fax: 757-474-6540
tcta@aol.com.vi
www.tcta.ataccess.org

Technology group of parents, consumers and professionals; provides resources to help children and adults who have disabilities gain access to the benefits of technology. Includes nationwide network of community-based assistive technology, resource centers, hands on consultants and product demonstrations.

8427 Virginia Assistive Technology System
8004 Franklin Farms Drive
8004 Franklin Farms Drive
Richmond, VA 23229

804-662-9990
800-552-5019
Fax: 804-662-9478
TTY: 757-662-9990
vatskhk@aol.com
www.vats.org

State assisted programs and support group information for people of many abilities. Includes local chapters, referrals, fun and social interaction and support groups.

Barclay Shepard, Manager, VATS
Robert W. Krollman, AT Specialist-Aging Coordinator
Elin Glass, Administrative Office Specialist, V

8428 Infant Toddler Early Intervention Program
640 Woodland Square Loop, SE
Olympia, WA 98504

360-725-3516
Fax: 360-725-3523
LoercSK@dshs.wa.govt
www.nectas.unc.edu

Early intervention and preschool special education for children with disabilities and special health care needs. Services include central directory, representatives of agencies, service providers, families, and coordinators of infant, toddler, and preschool special education programs.

Sandy Loerch, Infant/Toddler Program Coordinator

8429 Leukemia & Lymphoma Society - Washington/ Alaska Chapter
Leukemia & Lymphoma Society
5601 6th Avenue, Ste 182
Seattle, WA 98108

206-628-0777
anne.gillingham@lls.org
www.lls.org/washingtonalaska

Dedicated to finding cures for leukemia and related cancers and to improving the quality of life for patients and their families.

Anne Gillingham, Executive Director
Courtney Hale, Operations Director
Victoria Wenick, Senior Campaign Director

8430 Office of the Superintendent of Public Instruction
PO Box 47200
Olympia, WA 98504

360-753-6733
Fax: 360-586-0247
TTY: 360-586-0126
ashureen@inspire.ospi.wednet.edu
www.unc.edu

Services include central directory, representatives of agencies, service providers, families, and coordinators of infant, toddler, and preschool special education programs.

Anne Shureen, Preschool Special Ed. Coordinator

8431 Washington PAVE
6316 S 12th Street
Tacoma, WA 98465

253-565-2266
800-572-7368
Fax: 253-566-8052
TTY: 800-572-7368
pave@wapave.org
www.washingtonpave.org

Parent Training and Information (PTI) programs help parents to understand their children's specific needs, communicate more effectively with professionals, participate in the educational planning process, and obtain information about relevant programs, services and resources.

Joanna S Butts, Executive Director

8432 Early Intervention Program
350 Capitol Street, Room 427
Charleston, WV 25301

304-558-6311
Fax: 304-558-4984
www.unc.edu

Individuals with Disabilities Education Act requires all states and territories to provide early intervention and preschool special education for children with disabilities and special health care needs. Services include central directory, representatives of agencies, service providers, families, and coordinators of infant, toddler, and preschool special education programs.

Pam Roush, Part C Coordinator

8433 Office of Special Education Administration
1900 Kawanha Boulevard E
Charleston, WV 25305 304-558-2696
  800-642-8541
Fax: 304-558-3741
pcarte@access.k12.wv.us
www.unc.edu

Individuals with Disabilities Education Act requires all states and territories to provide early intervention and preschool special education for children with disabilities and special health care needs. Services include central directory, representatives of agencies, service providers, families, and coordinators of infant, toddler, and preschool special education programs.

Liza Cordeiro, Executive Director, Office of Commu
Dee Bodkins, Director
Allison Barker, Coordinator

8434 West Virginia Assistive Technology System
Airport Research and Office Park
959 Hartman Run Road
Morgantown, WV 26505 304-293-4692
  888-829-9426
Fax: 304-293-7294
TTY: 800-518-1448
TDD: 304-293-4692
stewiat@wvnvm.wvnet.edu
www.wvats.cedwvu.org

State assisted programs and support group information for people of many abilities. Includes local chapters, referrals, fun and social interaction and support groups.

Martha Ankney, Accountant
Donna J. Brewer, Database Manager
Lashanna Brunson, Research Coordinator

8435 West Virginia Parent Training and Information
1701 Hamill Ave.
Clarksburg, WV 26301 304-624-1436
  800-281-1436
Fax: 304-624-1438
WVPTI@aol.com
www.wvpti.org

Parent Training and Information (PTI) programs help parents to understand their children's specific needs, communicate more effectively with professionals, participate in the educational planning process, and obtain information about relevant programs, services and resources.

Wisconsin

8436 Birth to 3 Program
1 West Wilson St, Room 418, PO Box 7851
Madisonton, WI 53370 608-267-3270
Fax: 608-261-6752
kremema@dhfs.state.wi.us
www.nectas.unc.edu

Early intervention and preschool special education for children with disabilities and special health care needs. Services include central directory, representatives of agencies, service providers, families, and coordinators of infant, toddler, and preschool special education programs.

Mitchell Kremer, Infant/Toddler Program Coordinator

8437 Development and Training Center
2125 3rd Street
Eau Circle, WI 54703 715-833-7755
Fax: 715-833-7757
www.nectas.unc.edu

Individuals with Disabilities Education Act requires all states and territories to provide early intervention and preschool special education for children with disabilities and special health care needs. Services include central directory, representatives of agencies, service providers, families, and coordinators of infant, toddler, and preschool special education programs.

Stacy H Wigfield, Interagency Coordinating Council

8438 Division of Community Services
1 Wilson Street, Room 418, PO Box 7851
Madison, WI 53707 608-267-3270
Fax: 608-267-6752
dhfs.wisconsin.gov/bdds/birthto3

Individuals with Disabilities Education Act requires all states and territories to provide early intervention and preschool special education for children with disabilities and special health care needs. Services include central directory, representatives of agencies, service providers, families, and coordinators of infant, toddler, and preschool special education programs.

Beth Wroblewski, Preschool Special Ed. Coordinator

8439 Early Childhood Handicapped Prgrams
125 S. Webster St., PO Box 7841
Madison, WI 53707 608-266-1649
  800-441-4563
Fax: 608-267-3746
langejr@mail.state.wi.us
www.dpi.state.wi.us

Services include central directory, representatives of agencies, service providers, families, and coordinators of infant, toddler, and preschool special education programs.

Juanita S. Pawlisch, Ph. D.,, Assistant State Superintendent

8440 Parent Education Project of Wisconsin
2192 S 60th Street
West Allis, WI 53219 414-328-5520
Fax: 414-328-5530
TDD: 414-328-5520
pmcolletti@aol.com
www.members.aol.com/pepofwi

Parent Training and Information (PTI) programs help parents to understand their children's specific needs, communicate more effectively with professionals, participate in the educational planning process, and obtain information about relevant programs, services and resources.

8441 WisTech
1 W. Wilson Street, Room 527
Madison, WI 53703 608-266-7974
Fax: 608-266-3386
TTY: 608-267-9880
sarah.lincoln@DHS.wisconsin.gov
www.dhs.wisconsin.gov/disabilities/wistech/

State assisted programs and support group information for people of many abilities. Includes local chapters, referrals, fun and social interaction and support groups.

Sarah Lincoln, Contact

Wyoming

8442 Division of Developmental Disabilities
6101 Yellowstone Road
Cheyenne, WY 82002 307-777-7115
Fax: 307-777-3337
www.nectas.unc.edu

Provides early intervention and preschool special education for children with disabilities and special health care needs. Services include central directory, representatives of agencies, service providers, families, and coordinators of infant, toddler, and preschool special education programs.

Mitch Brauchie, Interagency Coordinating Council

8443 Parent Information Center
500 W. Lott St Suite A
Buffalo, WY 82834 307-684-2277
Fax: 307-684-5314
TDD: 307-684-2277
tdawson@wpic.org
www.wpic.org

Parent Training and Information (PTI) programs help parents to understand their children's specific needs, communicate more effectively with professionals, participate in the educational planning process, and obtain information about relevant programs, services and resources.

Terri Dawson, Executive Director
Betty Carmon, Outreach Parent Liaison
Janet Kinstetter, Outreach Parent Liaison

8444 Special Education Unit
2300 Cheyenne Avenue, 2nd Floor
Cheyenne, WY 82002
307-777-7414
Fax: 307-777-6234
smofie@educ.state.wy.uss
www.edu.wyoming.gov

Individuals with Disabilities Education Act requires all states and
territories to provide early intervention and preschool special education for children with disabilities and special health care
needs. Services include central directory, representatives of agencies, service providers, families, and coordinators of infant, toddler, and preschool special education programs.

Ron Micheli, Chairman

8445 Wyoming's New Options in Technology (WYNOT)
University of Wyoming
1000 East University Avenue
Laramie, WY 82072
307-766-2084
Fax: 307-721-2084
TTY: 800-861-4312
wynot.uw@uwyo.edu
www.uwyo.edu/wynot

State assisted programs and support group information for people
of many abilities. Includes local chapters, referrals, fun and social
interaction and support groups.

Libraries & Resource Centers

Arizona

8446 Special Needs Center/Phoenix Public Library
12 E McDowell Road
Phoenix, AZ 85004
602-261-8690
choh@lib.ci.phoenix.az.us
www.ci.phonix.az.us

Offers talking books and records, braille books and magazines,
large print books, video print enlarger, video magnifier and
VersaBraille software with synthetic speech for the blind, visually handicapped, physically/mentally handicapped and speech
and hearing impaired children and adults.

Mary Roatch, Supervisor

8447 Technology Access Center of Tucson
PO Box 13178
Tucson, AZ 85732
520-638-2733
Fax: 520-519-7954
tact1@qwestoffice.net
www.uacoe.arizona.edu/tact/

Technology group of parents, consumers and professionals; provides resources to help children and adults who have disabilities
gain access to the benefits of technology. Includes nationwide
network of community-based assistive technology, resource centers, hands on consultants and product demonstrations.

Arkansas

8448 Arkansas Easter Seals Technology Resource Center
3920 Woodland Heights Road
Little Rock, AR 72212
501-227-3602
Fax: 501-227-3601
atrce@aol.com
www.arkeasterseals.org

Technology group of parents, consumers and professionals; provides resources to help children and adults who have disabilities
gain access to the benefits of technology. Includes nationwide
network of community-based assistive technology, resource centers, hands on consultants and product demonstrations.

8449 Crowley Ridge Regional Library
315 W Oak
Jonesboro, AR 72401
870-935-5133
reference@libraryinjonesboro.org
www.libraryinjonesboro.org

Offers a children's summer reading program, large print and
books on cassette.

James Dunivan, Chairman
Mary Norris, Vice-Chairman

8450 Educational Services for the Visually Impaired
2402 Wildwood Avenue, Suite 112
Sherwood, AR 72120
501-835-5448
Fax: 501-835-6840
ayoung@esvi.org
www.esvi.org

Offers textbooks, braille books and more to the visually impaired
grades K-12 in the Arizona area.

Angyln Young, State Coordinator
Cindy Lester, Data Management Specialist/Preschoo
Cynthia Kelly, ESVI Office Manager

8451 Library for the Blind and Handicapped, Southwest
PO Box 668
Magnolia, AR 71754
870-234-0399
Fax: 870-234-5077
lbph@hotmail.com

Offers a children's summer reading program and a book collection featuring discs and casettes.

Susan Walker, Librarian

California

8452 Alliance for Technology Access (ATA)
1119 Old Humboldt Road
Jackson, TN 38305
731-554-5282
800-914-3017
Fax: 731-554-5283
TDD: 731-554-5284
atainfo@ataccess.org
www.ataccess.org

Technology group of parents, consumers and professionals; provides resources to help children and adults who have disabilities
gain access to the benefits of technology. Includes nationwide
network of community-based assistive technology, resource centers, hands on consultants and product demonstrations.

Margaret Doumitt, Executive Director
James Allison, President
Mike Hewitt, Secretary/Treasurer

8453 Assistive Technology Center Simi Valley Hospital
Rehabilatation Unit North
PO Box 1325
Simi Valley, CA 93062
805-582-1881
Fax: 805-582-2855
dssacca@aol.com

Technology group of parents, consumers and professionals; provides resources to help children and adults who have disabilities
gain access to the benefits of technology. Includes nationwide
network of community-based assistive technology, resource centers, hands on consultants and product demonstrations.

8454 Center for Accessible Technology
3075 Adeline Street, Suite 220
Berkeley, CA 94703
510-841-3224
Fax: 510-841-7956
TDD: 510-841-5621
info@cforat.org
www.cforat.org

Provides resources to help children and adults who have disabilities gain access to the benefits of technology. Clients are seen by
appointment only.

Guy Thomas, Board President
Sara Armstrong Ph.D., Board Treasure
Carol Cody, Executive Director

8455 Clearinghouse for Specialized Media and Technology (CSMT)
California Department of Education
1430 N Street, Suite 3207
Sacramento, CA 95814
916-445-5103
Fax: 916-323-9732
rbrawley@cde.ca.gov
http://csmt.cde.ca.gov

Assists California schools and students in the identification and acquisition of textbooks, reference books and study materials in aural media, braille, large print and electronic media access technology.

Rod Brawley, Manager

8456 Sacramento Center for Assistive Technology
701 Howe Avenue, Suite E-5
Sacramento, CA 95825
916-927-7228
scatca@quicknet.com
www.quicknet.com/~scat

Technology group of parents, consumers and professionals; provides resources to help children and adults who have disabilities gain access to the benefits of technology. Includes nationwide network of community-based assistive technology, resource centers, hands on consultants and product demonstrations.

District of Columbia

8457 Georgetown University Child Development Center
3300 Whitehaven Street, NW, Suite 3300
Washington, DC 20007
202-687-5000
Fax: 202-687-8899
gucdc@georgetown.edu
www.gucchd.georgetown.edu

8458 HEATH Resource Center
1 DuPont Circle, Suite 800
Washington, DC 20036
920-939-9320
800-544-3284
Fax: 202-833-5696
TTY: 202-939-9320
heath@ace.nche.edu
www.heath.gwu.edu/

Dan Gardner, Information Specialist

Florida

8459 Center for Independence Technology and Education, (CITE)
215 E New Hampshire Street
Orlando, FL 32804
407-898-2483
Fax: 407-895-5255
comcite@aol.com

Technology group of parents, consumers and professionals; provides resources to help children and adults who have disabilities gain access to the benefits of technology. Includes nationwide network of community-based assistive technology, resource centers, hands on consultants and product demonstrations.

8460 University of Miami, Mailman Center for Child Development
1601 NW 12th Avenue
Miami, FL 33136
305-243-6631
Fax: 305-284-4911
pediatrics.med.miani.edu/mccd1

Focuses on birth defects and children's illnesses.

Dr. Robert Stempfel, Jr, Director

8461 West Florida Regional Library
239 North Spring Street
Pensacola, FL 32502
850-436-5060
Fax: 850-436-5039
TDD: 850-435-1763
tlambert@ci.pensacola.fl.us
www.mywfpl.com/

Offers children's print/braille books.

Tamatha Lambert, Librarian

Georgia

8462 Augusta-Richmond County Public Library
425 9th Street
Augusta, GA 30901
706-821-2625
Fax: 706-724-5403
talkbook@mail.richmond.public.lib.ga.us
www.scescape.net/~ecgrl/lbph.htm

Discs, cassettes, braille writer, films, large print books, summer reading program, magnifiers and reference materials on blindness and other handicaps.

Gary Swint, Librarian

8463 Gainesville Subregional LBPH Hall County Public Library
2434 Old Cornelia Highway
Gainesville, GA 30507
770-531-2500
Fax: 770-531-2502
TDD: 770-531-2530
kevans@mail.hall.public.lib.ga.us
www.hall.public.lib.ga.us/ehmap.htm#program

Summer reading programs, braille writer, magnifiers, closed-circuit TV, large-print photocopier, cassette books and magazines, children's books on cassette, home visits and other reference materials on blindness and other handicaps.

Kathy Evans, Librarian

8464 La Fayette Subregional Library for the Blind and Physically Disabled
305 S Duke Street
La Fayette, GA 30728
706-638-2992
Fax: 706-638-4028
chelseak@chrl.org
www.chrl.org/

Summer reading programs, braille writer, magnifiers, closed-circuit TV, large-print photocopier, cassette books and magazines, children's books on cassette, home visits and other reference materials on blindness and other handicaps.

Chelsea Kovalevskiy, Youth Education Coordinator
Marilyn Southerland, Library Assistant
Carol Smith, Genealogy Librarian

8465 Macon Subregional Library for the Blind and Handicapped, Washington Memorial
1180 Washington Avenue
Macon, GA 31201
912-744-0877
800-805-7613
Fax: 912-742-3161
TDD: 912-744-0877
mgrltbc2@bibblib.org

Summer reading programs, braille writer, magnifiers, closed-circuit TV, large-print photocopier, cassette books and magazines, children's books on cassette, home visits and other reference materials on blindness and other handicaps.

Rebecca Sherrill, Librarian

8466 Oconee Regional Library, Library for the Blind and Physically Handicapped
801 Bellevue Avenue, PO Box 100
Dublin, GA 31040
478-272-5710
Fax: 478-275-5381
TDD: 478-275-3821
heritage@ocrl.org
www.ocrl.org/

Summer reading programs, braille writer, magnifiers, closed-circuit TV, large-print photocopier, cassette books and magazines, children's books on cassette, home visits and other reference materials on blindness and other handicaps.

Betty Schlid, Librarian

8467 Rome Subregional Library for the Blind and Physically Handicapped
205 Riverside Parkway NE
Rome, GA 30161 706-236-4618
Fax: 706-236-4631
TDD: 706-236-4618
dianam@mail.floyd.public.lib.ga.us
www.rome-lpd.org/romsub.htm

Summer reading programs, braille writer, magnifiers, closed-circuit TV, large-print photocopier, cassette books and magazines, children's books on cassette, home visits and other reference materials on blindness and other handicaps.

Diana Mills, Librarian

8468 Special Needs Library of NE Georgia Athens-Clarke County Regional Library
2025 Baxter Street
Athens, GA 30606 706-613-3655
Fax: 706-613-3660
TDD: 706-613-3655
burnsp@mail.clarke.public.lib.ga.us
www.clarke.public.lib.ga.us/tbc.htm

Discs, cassettes, large print books, reference materials on blindness, films, closed-circuit TV, magnifiers, braille writer, summer reading programs, cassette books and magazines and more.

Paige Burns, Librarian

8469 Subregional Library for the Blind and Physically Handicapped
1120 Bradley Drive
Columbus, GA 31906 706-649-0780
Fax: 706-649-1914
TDD: 706-649-0974
barness@mail.muscogee.public.lib.ga.us

Braille writer, magnifiers, closed-circuit TV, large-print photocopier, cassette books and magazines, children's books on cassette, home visits and other reference materials on blindness and other handicaps.

Suzanne Barnes, Librarian

8470 Tech-Able
1112A Brett Drive
Conyers, GA 30094 770-922-6768
Fax: 770-922-6769
techable@america.net
www.gatfl.org

Technology group of parents, consumers and professionals; provides resources to help children and adults who have disabilities gain access to the benefits of technology. Includes nationwide network of community-based assistive technology, resource centers, hands on consultants and product demonstrations.

Hawaii

8471 Aloha Special Technology Access Center
710 Green Street
Honolulu, HI 96813 808-523-5547
Fax: 808-536-3765
gstachi@yahoo.com
www.geocities.com/astachi/index.html

Technology group of parents, consumers and professionals; provides resources to help children and adults who have disabilities gain access to the benefits of technology. Member of nationwide network of community-based assistive technology, resource centers, hands on consultants and product demonstrations.

8472 Library for the Blind and Physically Handicapped, Hawaii State Library
402 Kapahulu Avenue
Honolulu, HI 96815 808-733-8444
Fax: 808-733-8449
TDD: 808-733-8444
olbcirc@state.lib.hi.us
www.hcc.hawaii.edu/hspls/oahu/lbph.html

Summer reading programs, braille writer, magnifiers, closed-circuit TV, large-print photocopier, cassette books and magazines, children's books on cassette, home visits and other reference materials on blindness and other handicaps.

Fusako Miyashiro, Librarian

Illinois

8473 Northern Illinois Center for Adaptive Technology
3615 Louisiana Road
Rockford, IL 61108 815-229-2163
Fax: 815-229-2135
davegrass@earthlink.net
www.nicat.ataccess.org

Technology group of parents, consumers and professionals; provides resources to help children and adults who have disabilities gain access to the benefits of technology. Includes nationwide network of community based assistive technology, resource centers, hands on consultants and product demonstrations.

Dave Grass, Director

8474 Parents Alliance Employment Project
Illinois Employment and Training Center
2525 Cabot Drive, Suite 302
Lisle, IL 60532 630-955-2075
Fax: 630-955-2080
TTY: 630-955-2098
TDD: 630-495-6055
ktribe@parents-alliance.org
www.parents-alliance.org

Information and advocacy resources for families and professionals. Includes listings of organizations providing general information and organizations focusing on more specific areas of concern to families and young adults who have disabilities.

Kristen Tribe, M.A., CRC, Executive Director
Roger Joseph B. Cave, Employment Coordinator
Paul Engman, Employment Specialist II

8475 Professional Assistance Center for Education (PACE)
National-Louis University
2840 Sheridan Road
Evanston, IL 60201 847-475-1100
Fax: 847-256-5190
cbur@evan1.nl.edu

A two-year, noncredit certification program servicing students with learning disabilities. The program provides a rare opportunity for students from all parts of the country to continue their education in an age appropriate environment. Committed to an instructional approach that integrates both group and individual teaching for career preparation, academics, life skills, and socialization. Transitional program offered to qualified graduates.

Carol Burns, Director

8476 Shawnee Library System
607 S Greenbriar Road
Carterville, IL 62918 618-985-3711
800-445-2665
Fax: 618-985-4211
dbrawley@shawls.lib.il.us
www.shawls.lib.il.us

Lends recorded books and magazines, descriptive videos, and braille to adults and children unable to read standard print due to blindness, visual impairment, physical disablity and reading disability. Information on blindness and disabilities. Public presentations.

Karen Bounds, President
Thomas Turner, Vice-President
Sarah Doerner, Secretary

8477 Suburban Audio Visual Service
920 Barnsdale Road
La Grange Park, IL 60526 630-352-7671

Summer reading programs, braille writer, magnifiers, closed-circuit TV, large-print photocopier, cassette books and magazines, children's books on cassette, home visits and other reference materials on blindness and other handicaps.

Leon Drolet, Jr, Librarian

Indiana

8478 Allen County Public Library
900 Library Plaza
Fort Wayne, IN 46802   260-421-1200
                                    Fax: 260-421-1386
                                    webmaster@acpl.lib.in.us
                                    www.acpl.lib.in.us

Summer reading programs, braille writer, magnifiers, closed-circuit TV, large-print photocopier, cassette books and magazines, children's books on cassette, home visits and other reference materials on blindness and other handicaps.

Gloria Shamanof, President
Martin E. Seifert, Vice-President
John Gerni, Secretary

8479 Assistive Technology Training and Information Center
3354 Pine Hill Drive
Vincennes, IN 47591   812-886-0575
                                        800-962-8842
                                    Fax: 812-886-1128
                                    TTY: 800-962-8842
                                    inattic2@aol.com

Informational and emotional support to parents who have a child, adolescent, or adult family member with special needs.

8480 Bartholomew County Public Library
536 Fifth Street
Columbus, IN 47201   812-379-1255
                                    Fax: 812-379-1275
                                    library@barth.lib.in.us
                                    www.barth.lib.in.us

Summer reading programs, braille writer, magnifiers, closed-circuit TV, large-print photocopier, cassette books and magazines, children's books on cassette, home visits and other reference materials on blindness and other handicaps.

Wilma Perry, Librarian

8481 Elkhart Public Library
300 S 2nd Street
Elkhart, IN 46516   574-522-5669
                                    www.myepl.org

Summer reading programs, braille writer, magnifiers, closed-circuit TV, large-print photocopier, cassette books and magazines, children's books on cassette, home visits and other reference materials on blindness and other handicaps.

Barbara G. Anderson, President
Janice E. Dean, Vice-President
Krystal Anderson, Secretary

8482 Special Services Division - Indiana State Library
140 N Senate Avenue
Indianapolis, IN 46204   317-232-3684
                                        800-622-4970
                                    Fax: 317-232-3728
                                    bph@statelib.lib.in.us

Summer reading programs, braille writer, magnifiers, closed-circuit TV, braille and large print books and magazines, children's books on cassette and in braiile, and other reference materials on blindness and other handicaps.

Lissa Shanahan, Librarian
Carole Rose, Childrens/Braille Services

Kansas

8483 Kansas State Library
State Capitol Building
Topeka, KS 66612   785-296-3296
                                        800-432-3919
                                    Fax: 785-296-6650
                                    TDD: 785-256-0733
                                    infodesk@library.ks.gov
                                    www.kslib.info/

Summer reading programs, braille writer, magnifiers, closed-circuit TV, large-print photocopier, cassette books and magazines, children's books on cassette, home visits and other reference materials on blindness and other handicaps.

Jo Budler, State Librarian
Daniel Eells, Production/Network/Technical Assist
Lianne Flax, Online Services and Programming Lib

8484 Manhattan Public Library
629 Poyntz Avenue
Manhattan, KS 66502   785-776-4741
                                    Fax: 785-776-1545
                                    refstaff@manhattan.lib.ks.us
                                    www.manhattan.lib.ks.us/

Summer reading programs, braille writer, magnifiers, closed-circuit TV, large-print photocopier, cassette books and magazines, children's books on cassette, home visits and other reference materials on blindness and other handicaps.

Linda Knupp, Director
John Pecoraro, Assistant Director
Teri Belin, Admistrative Assistant

8485 Prenatal Diagnostic and Genetic Center
HCA Wesley Medical Center
550 N Hillside
Wichita, KS 67214   316-688-2362
Sechin Cho, MD

8486 Solution Outreach Center at OCCK, Inc.
2941 Centennial
Salina, KS 67401   785-827-9383
                                        800-526-9731
                                    Fax: 785-452-9374
                                    TTY: 785-827-7051
                                    TDD: 785-827-9383
                                    kreed@occk.com
                                    www.occk.com

Technology group of parents, customers and professionals; provides resources to help children and adults who have disabilities gain access to the benefits of technology. Includes nationwide network of community-based assistive technology, resource centers, hands on consultants and product demonstrations.

Kathy Reed, Director
Sidney Gray, Coordinator

8487 South Central Kansas Library System
321 North Main Street
South Hutchinson, KS 67505   620-336-5441
                                        800-234-0529
                                    Fax: 620-663-9797
                                    sharon@sckls.info
                                    skyways.lib.ks.us/sckls/

Summer reading programs, braille writer, magnifiers, closed-circuit TV, large-print photocopier, cassette books and magazines, children's books on cassette, home visits and other reference materials on blindness and other handicaps.

Paul Hawkins, Director
Katherine Goodenberger, Library Support Specialist
Sharon Barnes, Technology Consultant

8488 Wesley Medical Research Institutes
3306 E Central
Wichita, KS 67208   316-686-7172
                                    Fax: 316-687-0033
                                    tjones@wichitamedicalresearch.org
                                    www.wichitamedicalresearch.org/

Respiratory and birth defects disorders research.

Peggy L Johnson, Executive Director/COO
William Hendry, PhD, President
Thomas R Kluzak, MD, MMM, President Elect

8489 Wichita Public Library
223 S Main Street
Wichita, KS 67202   316-261-8500
                                    Fax: 316-262-4540
                                    admin@wichita.lib.ks.us
                                    www.wichita.lib.ks.us/

Summer reading programs, braille writer, magnifiers, closed-circuit TV, large-print photocopier, cassette books and magazines, children's books on cassette, home visits and other reference materials on blindness and other handicaps.

Brad Reha, Librarian

Kentucky

8490 Bluegrass Technology Center
409 Southland Drive
Lexington, KY 40505
859-294-4343
800-209-7767
Fax: 866-576-9625
office@bluegrass.org
www.bluegrass-tech.org

Technology group of parents, consumers and professionals; provides resources to help children and adults who have disabilities gain access to the benefits of technology. Includes nationwide network of community-based assistive technology, resource centers, hands on consultants and product demonstrations.

Vicki Cooper, President
Bruce W. Turley, Treasurer
Jeanna Richardson, Secretary

8491 EnTech: Enabling Technologies of Kentuckiana
301 York Street
Louisville, KY 40203
502-574-1637
entech@iglou.org

Technology group of parents, consumers and professionals; provides resources to help children and adults who have disabilities gain access to the benefits of technology. Includes nationwide network of community-based assistive technology, resource centers, hands on consultants and product demonstrations.

8492 Louisville Talking Book Library
301 York Street
Louisville, KY 40203
502-574-1611
Fax: 502-574-1657
denning@lfpl.org
www.lfpl.org/

Summer reading programs, braille writer, magnifiers, closed-circuit TV, large-print photocopier, cassette books and magazines, children's books on cassette, home visits and other reference materials on blindness and other handicaps.

Tad Thomas, Chair
Deborah Williams, Vice-chair

8493 Northern Kentucky Talking Book Library
502 Scott Boulevard
Covington, KY 41011
859-962-4095
Fax: 859-962-4096
www.kenton.lib.ky.us/information/talking

Summer reading programs, braille writer, magnifiers, closed-circuit TV, large-print photocopier, cassette books and magazines, children's books on cassette, home visits and other reference materials on blindness and other handicaps.

Jama Rooney, Librarian

8494 Western Kentucky Assistive Technology Consortium
607 Poplar Street, Suite 211, PO Box 266
Murray, KY 42071
270-759-4233
Fax: 270-759-4208
wkatc@cablecomm-ky.net

Technology group of parents, consumers and professionals; provides resources to help children and adults who have disabilities gain access to the benefits of technology. Includes nationwide network of community-based assistive technology, resource centers, hands on consultants and product demonstrations.

Louisiana

8495 Louisiana State Library
701 N 4th Street
Baton Rouge, LA 70802
225-342-4923
Fax: 225-219-8404
admin@state.lib.la.us
www.state.lib.la.us/

Summer reading programs, braille writer, magnifiers, closed-circuit TV, large-print photocopier, cassette books and magazines, children's books on cassette, home visits and other reference materials on blindness and other handicaps.

Rebecca Hamilton, State Librarian
Beverly Dugas, Business Manager
Tabitha Tabitha Pimlott, Executive Assistant

8496 Louisiana State University Genetics Section of Pediatrics
1501 Kings Highway
Shreveport, LA 71130
318-675-5681
TF Thurman, MD, Director

Maine

8497 Bangor Public Library
145 Harlow Street
Bangor, ME 04401
207-947-8336
Fax: 207-945-6694
bplill@bpl.lib.me.us
www.bpl.lib.me.us/

Summer reading programs, braille writer, magnifiers, closed-circuit TV, large-print photocopier, cassette books and magazines, children's books on cassette, home visits and other reference materials on blindness and other handicaps.

Barbara McDade, Director
Matt Brown, Network Administrator
Caroline Hammond, Business Manager

8498 Cary Library
107 Main Street
Houlton, ME 04730
207-532-1302
Fax: 207-532-4350
faucherl@cary.lib.me.us
www.cary.lib.me.us

Summer reading programs, braille writer, magnifiers, closed-circuit TV, large-print photocopier, cassette books and magazines, children's books on cassette, home visits and other reference materials on blindness and other handicaps.

Leigh Cummings Jr., President
Forrest Barnes, Treasurer
Gary Hagan, Secretary

8499 Lewiston Public Library
200 Lisbon Street
Lewiston, ME 04240
207-513-3004
Fax: 207-784-3011
rspeer@LewistonMaine.gov
www.lplonline.org/

Summer reading programs, braille writer, magnifiers, closed-circuit TV, large-print photocopier, cassette books and magazines, children's books on cassette, home visits and other reference materials on blindness and other handicaps.

Rick Speer, Director
Beth Martel, Circulation Supervisor
David Moorhead, Children's Librarian

8500 Maine State Library
64 State House Station
Augusta, ME 04333
207-287-5650
Fax: 207-287-5615
TTY: 888-577-6690
reference.desk@maine.gov
www.state.me.us/

Summer reading programs, braille writer, magnifiers, closed-circuit TV, large-print photocopier, cassette books and magazines, children's books on cassette, home visits and other reference materials on blindness and other handicaps.

Linda H. Lord, State Librarian
Janet McKenney, Director of Library Development
James Ritter, Director of Reader & Information S

8501 New England Regional Genetics Group
PO Box 920288
Needham, MA 02492   781-444-0126
                                     Fax: 781-444-0127
                                  mfgnergg@verizon.net
                                        www.nergg.org

Human genetic services and educational planning pertaining to birth defects.

Mary-Frances Garber, Executive Director
Lisa Demers, MS, CGC, President
Marinell Newton, MSW, President Elect

8502 Portland Public Library
5 Monument Square
Portland, ME 04101   207-871-1700
                                     Fax: 207-871-1703
                             reference@portland.lib.me.us
                               www.portlandlibrary.com/

Summer reading programs, braille writer, magnifiers, closed-circuit TV, large-print photocopier, cassette books and magazines, children's books on cassette, home visits and other reference materials on blindness and other handicaps.

Janice Littlefield, Librarian
Steve Podgajny, Executive Director

8503 Waterville Public Library
73 Elm Street
Waterville, ME 04901   207-872-5433
                                     Fax: 207-873-4779
                                         wpl@borg.com
                               www.watervillelibrary.org/

Summer reading programs, braille writer, magnifiers, closed-circuit TV, large-print photocopier, cassette books and magazines, children's books on cassette, home visits and other reference materials on blindness and other handicaps.

Meta Vigue, Librarian

Maryland

8504 Learning Independence Through Computers
1001 Eastern Avenue, 3rd Floor
Baltimore, MD 21202   410-659-5462
                                     Fax: 410-659-5472
                                       lincmd@aol.com

Technology group of parents, consumers and professionals; provides resources to help children and adults who have disabilities gain access to the benefits of technology. Includes nationwide network of community-based assistive technology, resource centers, hands on consultants and product demonstrations.

Massachusetts

8505 Resources for Rehabilitation
22 Bonad Road
Winchester, MA 01890   781-368-9080
                                           800-621-0026
                                     Fax: 781-368-9096
                                          info@rfr.org
                                          www.rfr.org/

Provides training and information to professionals who serve individuals with vision loss and other disabilities. Publishes a variety of resource guides on coping with visual impairment.

8506 Talking Book Library at Worcester Public Library
3 Salem Square
Worcester, MA 01608   508-799-1730
                                           800-762-0085
                                     Fax: 508-799-1656
                                     TDD: 508-799-1731
                                   talkbook@cwmars.org
                             www.worcpublib.org/talkingbook

Massachusetts subregional library within the Library of Congress National Library Service for the Blind and Physically Handicapped network. Provides audiocassette books, large print books, described videos and print/braille books to registered partons. Has adapted computers and other assistive technology for on-site use. Offers reference and referral service.

James L Izatt, Librarian

8507 Worcester Public Library
3 Salem Square
Worcester, MA 01608   508-799-1655
                                     Fax: 508-799-1652
                                    jizatt@site.cwmars.org
                                   www.worcpublib.org/

Summer reading programs, braille writer, magnifiers, closed-circuit TV, large-print photocopier, cassette books and magazines, children's books on cassette, home visits and other reference materials on blindness and other handicaps.

Susan Gately, President
James Kersten, Vice-President
Jyoti Datta, Secretary

Michigan

8508 Frederick Douglas Branch for Specialized Services and Physically Handicapped
3666 Grand River/Trumbull
Detroit, MI 48226   313-883-9414
                                     Fax: 313-833-9717
                                     TDD: 313-833-5492
                                   www.detroit.lib.mi.us

Summer reading programs, braille writer, magnifiers, closed-circuit TV, large-print photocopier, cassette books and magazines, children's books on cassette, home visits and other reference materials on blindness and other handicaps.

Deborah Evans, Librarian

Minnesota

8509 PACER Center
8161 Normandale Blvd.
Minneapolis, MN 55437   952-838-9000
                                           888-248-0822
                                     Fax: 952-838-0199
                                     TTY: 952-838-0190
                                       pacer@pacer.org
                                        www.pacer.org

Parent Training and Information (PTI) programs help parents to understand their children's specific needs, communicate more effectively with professionals, participate in the educational planning process, and obtain information about relevant programs, services and resources.

Paula F. Goldberg, Executive Director
Mary Schrock, Chief Operating and Development Off
Alicia Kunin-Batson, Board Vice-President

8510 Star Center for Family Health
University of Minnesota Gateway
200 Oak Street SE, Suite 160
Minneapolis, MN 55455   612-626-4260
                                     Fax: 612-626-2134
                               www.peds.umn.edu/peds-adol/

Helps children, youth, and families develop new and enhanced ways of coping with stress, learn strategies for adjusting to living with a chronic illness, and discover new ways of finding health, balance and well-being.

Elizabeth Latts, MSW, Resource Coordinator

985

8511 Technology Access Center
475 Metroplex Drive, Suite 301
Nashville, TN 37211

615-248-6733
800-368-4651
Fax: 615-259-2536
TTY: 314-569-8446
TDD: 615-248-6733
techaccess@tacnashville.org
www.tacnashville.org/

Technology group of parents, consumers and professionals; provides resources to help children and adults who have disabilities gain access to the benefits of technology. Includes nationwide network of community-based assistive technology, resource centers, hands on consultants and product demonstrations.

Kenyatta Lovett, President
J P Williams, Vice President
Jeffery A. Betzler, Treasurer

8512 Whitney Library for the Blind
1445 Boonville Avenue
Springfield, MO 65802

417-862-2781
Fax: 417-862-7566
blind@ag.org
www.gospelpublishing.com

Offers braille and cassette lending library, braille and cassette Sunday school materials for all ages, braille and cassette periodicals and resource assistance, and resources for blind children and children of blind parents.

Paul Weingariner, Director

8513 Montana State Library
1515 E 6th Avenue, PO Box 201800
Helena, MT 59601

406-444-3009
Fax: 406-444-0266
TDD: 406-444-4799
jstapp2@mt.gov
www.apps.msl.mt.gov/

Summer reading programs, braille writer, magnifiers, closed-circuit TV, large-print photocopier, cassette books and magazines, children's books on cassette, home visits and other reference materials on blindness and other handicaps.

Jennie Stapp, State Librarian
Sarah McHugh, Director of Statewide Library Resou
Cara Orban, Statewide Projects Librarian

8514 North Platte Public Library
120 W 4th Street
North Platte, NE 69101

308-535-8036
Fax: 308-535-8296
library@ci.north-platte.ne.us
www.ci.north-platte.ne.us/library/

Summer reading programs, braille writer, magnifiers, closed-circuit TV, large-print photocopier, cassette books and magazines, children's books on cassette, home visits and other reference materials on blindness and other handicaps.

Brenda Behsman, Librarian
Cecelia Lawrence, Library Director

8515 Las Vegas-Clark County Library District
7060 W. Windmill Lane
Las Vegas, NV 89113

702-507-3400
Fax: 702-507-3482
www.lvccld.org/

Summer reading programs, braille writer, magnifiers, closed-circuit TV, large-print photocopier, cassette books and magazines, children's books on cassette, home visits and other reference materials on blindness and other handicaps.

Jeanne Goodrich, Executive Director

8516 Nevada State Library and Archives
100 N Stewart Street
Carson City, NV 89701

775-684-3360
800-922-2880
Fax: 775-684-3330
TDD: 775-687-8338
www.nsla.nevadaculture.org/

Summer reading programs, braille writer, magnifiers, closed-circuit TV, large-print photocopier, cassette books and magazines, children's books on cassette, home visits and other reference materials on blindness and other handicaps.

Kevin E Putnam, Librarian

8517 New Hampshire State Library
117 Pleasant Street
Concord, NH 03301

603-271-3429
800-491-4200
michael.york@dcr.nh.gov
www.nh.gov/nhsl/about/index.html

Summer reading programs, braille writer, magnifiers, closed-circuit TV, large-print photocopier, cassette books and magazines, children's books on cassette, home visits and other reference materials on blindness and other handicaps.

Michael Yorks, State Librarian
Janet Eklund, Administrator of Library Operations
Donna Gilbreth, Supervisor

8518 Center for Enabling Technology
622 Route 10 W, Suite 22B
Whippany, NJ 07981

973-428-1455
Fax: 973-560-9751
TTY: 973-428-1450
cetnj@aol.com

Technology group of parents, consumers and professionals; provides resources to help children and adults who have disabilities gain access to the benefits of technology. Includes nationwide network of community-based assistive technology, resource centers, hands on consultants and product demonstrations.

8519 Institute for Basic Research in Developmental Disabilities
1050 Forest Hill Road
Staten Island, NY 10314

718-494-0600
Fax: 718-494-0837
ibr@opwdd.ny.gov
www.opwdd.ny.gov/

Conducts research into neurodegenerative diseases, Alzheimer's disease, developmental disabilities, fragile X syndrome, Down syndrome, autism, epilepsy and basic science issues underlying all developmental disabilities.

Dr. Krystyna Wisniewski

8520 JGB Cassette Library International
Jewish Guild for the Blind
15 W 65th Street
New York, NY 10023

212-769-6331

Summer reading programs, braille writer, magnifiers, closed-circuit TV, large-print photocopier, cassette books and magazines, children's books on cassette, home visits and other reference materials on blindness and other handicaps.

Bruce Massis

8521 Keren-Or Jerusalem Center for Multi- Handicapped Blind Children
350 7th Avenue, Suite 200
New York, NY 10010
212-279-4070
Fax: 212-279-4043
info@keren-or.org
www.keren-or.org

Center houses and cares for over 85 resident and day students who in addition to blindness or very low vision suffer from other severe physical and or mental disabilities. Provides training in daily living skills, as well as therapy, rehabilitation and education. Funds aquired through government stipends, contributions, bequests and legacies. Keren-OR is an IRS 501(C)(3) tax exempt organization.

Dr. Edward L Steinburg, Chairman
Dr. Albert Hornblass, President
Madelyn Cohen, Executive Director

8522 Nassau Library System
900 Jerusalem Avenue
Uniondale, NY 11553
516-292-8920
Fax: 516-565-0950
nls@lilrc.org
www.nassaulibrary.org/

Summer reading programs, braille writer, magnifiers, closed-circuit TV, large-print photocopier, cassette books and magazines, children's books on cassette, home visits and other reference materials on blindness and other handicaps.

Dorothy Pruyear, Librarian

8523 Techspress Resource Center for Independent Living
401-409 Columbia Street, PO Box 210
Utica, NY 13503
315-797-4642
Fax: 315-797-4747
lana.gossin@rcil.com

Technology group of parents, consumers and professionals; provides resources to help children and adults who have disabilities gain access to the benefits of technology. Includes nationwide network of community-based assistive technology, resource centers, hands on consultants and product demonstrations.

North Carolina

8524 Carolina Computer Access Center
401 E 9th Street
Charlotte, NC 28202
704-342-3004
Fax: 704-342-1513
ccacnc@aol.com
ccac.ataccess.org

Enabling individuals with disabilities to control and direct their own lives by providing information about demonstrations of, and access to assistive technology tools.

Linda Schilling, Executive Director

Ohio

8525 Blick Clinic for Developmental Disabilities
640 W Market Street
Akron, OH 44303
330-762-5425
Fax: 330-762-4019
blickclinic@blickclinic.com
www.blickclinic.org/

Blick Clinic began providing services in 1969 during the philosophical era when warehousing individuals with mental retardation in state institutions were commonplace and considered appropriate treatment.

Karin Lopper, Executive Director
Tami Mastrojohn, Kevin
Kelly Director of Finance

8526 Cleveland Public Library
325 Superior Avenue N.E.
Cleveland, OH 44114
216-623-2800
Fax: 216-623-7015
lbphmgr1@library.cpl.org
www.cpl.org

Summer reading programs, braille writer, magnifiers, closed-circuit TV, large-print photocopier, cassette books and magazines, children's books on cassette, home visits and other reference materials on blindness and other handicaps.

Barbara Mates, Librarian

8527 Ohio Regional Library for the Blind and Physically Handicapped
800 Vine Street, Library Square
Cincinnati, OH 45202
513-369-6999
Fax: 513-369-3111
TDD: 513-369-6072

Summer reading programs, braille writer, magnifiers, closed-circuit TV, large-print photocopier, cassette books and magazines, children's books on cassette, home visits and other reference materials on blindness and other handicaps.

Donna Foust, Librarian

8528 Technology Resource Center
1133 Edwin C. Moses Boulevard, #370
Dayton, OH 45408
937-461-3305
Fax: 937-461-6304
TDD: 937-236-6110
trcdoh@aol.com
www.trcd.org

Technology group of parents, consumers and professionals; provides resources to help children and adults who have disabilities gain access to the benefits of technology. Includes nationwide network of community-based assistive technology, resource centers, hands on consultants and product demonstrations.

Kevin Leonard, Coordinator
Judy Havens, Community Based Rehab Technologist

Oklahoma

8529 Oklahoma Library for the Blind & Physically Handicapped
300 NE 18th Street
Oklahoma City, OK 73105
405-521-3514
800-523-0288
Fax: 405-521-4582
TTY: 405-521-4672
olbph@oltn.odl.state.ok.us
www.library.state.ok.us/

Summer reading programs, braille writer, magnifiers, closed-circuit TV, large-print photocopier, cassette books and magazines, children's books on cassette, home visits and other reference materials on blindness and other handicaps.

Geraldine Adams, Director

8530 Tulsa City-County Library System
400 Civic Center
Tulsa, OK 74103
918-549-7323
www.tulsalibrary.org

Summer reading programs, braille writer, magnifiers, closed-circuit TV, large-print photocopier, cassette books and magazines, children's books on cassette, home visits and other reference materials on blindness and other handicaps.

Ellen Ontko, Librarian

Oregon

8531 Oregon State Library
250 Winter Street NW
Salem, OR 97310
503-378-4243
Fax: 503-585-8059
TDD: 503-378-4276
library.help@state.or.us

987

Summer reading programs, braille writer, magnifiers, closed-circuit TV, large-print photocopier, cassette books and magazines, children's books on cassette, home visits and other reference materials on blindness and other handicaps.

Mary Mohr, Librarian

Pennsylvania

8532 Free Library of Philadelphia
1901 Vine Street
Philadelphia, PA 215-686-5322
flpblind@library.phila.gov
www.library.phila.gov

Summer reading programs, braille writer, magnifiers, closed-circuit TV, large-print photocopier, cassette books and magazines, children's books on cassette, home visits and other reference materials on blindness and other handicaps.

Tobey Gordon Dichter, Chair
Leslie Anne Miller, First Vice Chair
Siobhan A. Reardon, President/Director

8533 Library for the Blind & Physically Handicapped, Leonard C Staisey Building
Carnegie Library of Pittsburgh
4724 Baum Boulevard
Pittsburgh, PA 15213 412-687-2440
800-242-0586
Fax: 412-687-2442
lbph@carnegielibrary.org
www.clpgh.org/clp/lbph

Provides on loan recorded books and magazines, large print books, and described videos to Western Pennsylvania residents unable to use standard printed materials due to visual, physically-based reading disabilities. Also loans special cassette and disc machines; does not loan equipment to play described videos. Information about disabilities and related agencies is also available.

Lou Testoni, Chair, Carnegie Library of Pittsbur
Mary Frances Cooper, President/Director
Susan Banks, Deputy Director

Rhode Island

8534 TechACCESS of Rhode Island
100 Jefferson Boulevard
Warwick, RI 02888 401-463-0202
800-916-8324
Fax: 401-463-3433
TTY: 401-273-0202
techaccess@techaccess-ri.org
www.techaccess-ri.org/

Technology group of parents, consumers and professionals; provides resources to help children and adults who have disabilities gain access to the benefits of technology. Includes nationwide network of community-based assistive technology, resource centers, hands on consultants and product demonstrations.

Judith Hammerlind Carlson, M.S., Executive Director
Kelly Charlebois, ATP, Clinical Manager/AT Consultant
Matthew Provost, M.S., CCC-SLP, Augmentative Communication Consulta

South Carolina

8535 Family Connection of South Carolina
2712 Middleburg Dr., Suite 103
Columbia, SC 29204 803-252-0914
800-578-8750
Fax: 866-420-4082
info@FamilyConnectionSC.org
www.familyconnectionsc.org/

Support network for parents of children with disabilities and/or chronic illness. Veteran parents offer support to parents who are just learning of their child's diagnosis. Offers support and insight into parenting a child with special needs, as well as referrals to trained veteran parents.

Esther Dennis, President
McIver Williamson, Vice President
Jackie Richards, Executive Director

8536 South Carolina State Library
P.O. Box 11469
Columbia, SC 29211 803-734-8666
888-221-4643
Fax: 803-734-8676
TDD: 803-734-7298
reference@statelibrary.sc.gov
www.statelibrary.sc.gov/

Summer reading programs, braille writer, magnifiers, closed-circuit TV, large-print photocopier, cassette books and magazines, children's books on cassette, home visits and other reference materials on blindness and other handicaps.

Deborah P. Anderson, Administrative Coordinator
Leesa Benggio, Deputy Director
Paula James, Finance Director

South Dakota

8537 South Dakota State Library
800 Governors Drive
Pierre, SD 57501 605-773-3131
800-423-6665
Fax: 605-773-6962
TDD: 605-773-4950
lturchen@dakotablue.net?subject=SDSL%20B
www.library.sd.gov/

Summer reading programs, braille writer, magnifiers, closed-circuit TV, large-print photocopier, cassette books and magazines, children's books on cassette, home visits and other reference materials on blindness and other handicaps.

Lesta Turchen, President
Monte Loos, Vice President
Daria Bossman, State Librarian

Tennessee

8538 East Tennessee Technology Access Center
116 Childress Street
Knoxville, TN 37920 865-219-0130
Fax: 865-219-0137
ettacmain@gmail.com
www.ettac.org/

Assistive technology group of parents, consumers and professionals; provides resources to help children and adults who have disabilities gain access to the benefits of technology. Includes nationwide network of community-based assistive technology, resource centers, hands on consultants and product demonstrations.

Lois M. Symington, Executive Director
Bedros Bozdogan, President/Board of Directors
Mat Jones, Coordinator, Technology Support Ser

8539 Saint Jude Children's Research Hospital
262 Danny Thomas Place
Memphis, TN 38105 901-495-3300
www.stjude.org

Mike Canarios, SVP/Chief Financial Officer
Camille Sarrouf, Jr., Chair / President
Pam Dotson, SVP Patient Care Services/Chief Nur

Texas

8540 Baylor College of Medicine Birth Defects Center
One Baylor Plaza
Houston, TX 77030 713-798-4951
president@bcm.edu
www.bcm.tmc.edu

Baylor College of Medicine in Houston, the only private medical school in the Greater Southwest, is recognized as a premier academic health science center and is known for excellence in education, research and patient care.

Paul Klotman, M.D., President/CEO
Claire M. Bassett, Vice President, Communications and
Kristi Cooper, Vice President, Development

8541 Texas State Library
1201 Brazos St.
Austin, TX 78701   512-463-5455
                                           Fax: 512-463-5436
                                           TDD: 512-463-5449
                                           info@tsl.state.tx.us
                                           www.tsl.state.tx.us

Summer reading programs, braille writer, magnifiers, closed-circuit TV, large-print photocopier, cassette books and magazines, children's books on cassette, home visits and other reference materials on blindness and other handicaps.

Edward Seidenberg, Interim Director and Librarian
Donna Osborne, Administrative Services
Jelain Chubb, Archives & Information Services

Utah

8542 Utah State Library Commission
2150 S 300 W
Salt Lake City, UT 84115   801-468-6789

Summer reading programs, braille writer, magnifiers, closed-circuit TV, large-print photocopier, cassette books and magazines, children's books on cassette, home visits and other reference materials on blindness and other handicaps.

Gerald Buttars, Librarian

Vermont

8543 Vermont Department of Libraries Special Service Unit
109 State Street, Pavilion Office Building
Montpelier, VT 05609   802-828-3261
                                                 800-479-1711
                                           Fax: 802-828-2199
                                           ssu@dol.state.vt.us
                                           libraries.vermont.gov

Summer reading programs, braille writer, magnifiers, closed-circuit TV, large-print photocopier, cassette books and magazines, children's books on cassette, home visits and other reference materials on blindness and other handicaps.

Martha Reid, State Librarian
Christine Friese, Assistant State Librarian
Brittney Wilson, Executive Asst. to the State Librar

Virginia

8544 Arlington County Department of Libraries
1015 N Quincy Street
Arlington, VA 22201   703-228-5990
                                           Fax: 703-228-5962
                                           TDD: 703-358-6320
                                           www.co.arlington.va.us/lib/

Summer reading programs, braille writer, magnifiers, closed-circuit TV, large-print photocopier, cassette books and magazines, children's books on cassette, home visits and other reference materials on blindness and other handicaps.

Roxanne Barnes, Librarian

8545 ERIC Clearinghouse on Disabilities and Gifted Education
1110 N Glebe Road
Arlington, VA 22201   703-264-9474
                                                 800-328-0272
                                           Fax: 703-620-2521
                                           TTY: 703-264-9449
                                           ericec@cec.speed.org
                                           ericec.org

Offers educational materials and bibliographic information on topics such as ADD, gifted, behavior disorders, early childhood, inclusion and learning.

Susan Elting

8546 Fairfax County Public Library
12000 Government Center Parkway
Fairfax, VA 22035   703-324-3100
                                           Fax: 703-222-5921
                                           TDD: 703-660-8524
                                           sjapikse@leo.vsla.edu
                                           www.co.fairfax.va.us/library/defaylt

Summer reading programs, braille writer, magnifiers, closed-circuit TV, large-print photocopier, cassette books and magazines, children's books on cassette, home visits and other reference materials on blindness and other handicaps.

Jeanette Studley, Librarian

8547 Newport News Public Library System
110 Main Street
Newport News, VA 23601   757-597-2917
                                           Fax: 757-591-7425
                                           shalswin@leo.vsla.edu
                                           www.nnpls.libguides.com/

Summer reading programs, braille writer, magnifiers, closed-circuit TV, large-print photocopier, cassette books and magazines, children's books on cassette, home visits and other reference materials on blindness and other handicaps.

Sue Balswin, Librarian

8548 Roanoke City Public Library System
2607 Salem Turnpike NW
Roanoke, VA 24017   540-853-2648
                                           Fax: 540-853-1030

Summer reading programs, braille writer, magnifiers, closed-circuit TV, large-print photocopier, cassette books and magazines, children's books on cassette, home visits and other reference materials on blindness and other handicaps.

Rebecca Cooper, Librarian

8549 Virginia Beach Public Library
930 Independence Boulevard
Virginia Beach, VA 23455   757-385-0150
                                           Fax: 757-523-9452
                                           library@vbgov.com

Summer reading programs, braille writer, magnifiers, closed-circuit TV, large-print photocopier, cassette books and magazines, children's books on cassette, home visits and other reference materials on blindness and other handicaps.

Susan Head, Librarian

West Virginia

8550 Cabell County Public Library
455 Ninth Street Plaza
Huntington, WV 25701   304-528-5700
                                           Fax: 304-528-5701
                                           cabelllibrary@cabell.lib.wv.us.
                                           www.cabell.lib.wv.us/

Summer reading programs, braille writer, magnifiers, Arkenstone reader/scanner, cassette books and magazines, children's books on cassette, home visits and other reference materials on blindness and other handicaps.

Judy K. Rule, Director
Angela Strait, Assistant Director
Mary Lou Pratt, Adult Services Coordinator

8551 Kanawha County Public Library
123 Capitol Street
Charleston, WV 25301   304-343-4646
                                           Fax: 304-348-6530
                                           www.kanawhalibrary.org/

Summer reading programs, braille writer, magnifiers, closed-circuit TV, large-print photocopier, cassette books and magazines, children's books on cassette, home visits and other reference materials on blindness and other handicaps.

Michael Albert, President
Elizabeth O. Lord, First Vice President
Cheryl Morgan, Second Vice President

8552 West Virginia Library Commission
1900 Kanawha Boulevard E
Charleston, WV 25305
304-340-2041
800-642-9021
Fax: 304-558-2044
karen.e.goff@wv.gov
www.librarycommission.wv.gov/

Summer reading programs, braille writer, magnifiers, closed-circuit TV, large-print photocopier, cassette books and magazines, children's books on cassette, home visits and other reference materials on blindness and other handicaps.

Karen Goff, Secretary
Denise Seabolt, Library Administrative Services Dir
Deborah McNeal, Personnel Officer

Wisconsin

8553 Brown County Library
515 Pine Street
Green Bay, WI 54301
920-448-4400
Fax: 920-448-4376
www.co.brown.wi.us

Summer reading programs, braille writer, magnifiers, closed-circuit TV, large-print photocopier, cassette books and magazines, children's books on cassette, home visits and other reference materials on blindness and other handicaps.

Angela Basten, Librarian

Research Centers

8554 Association for Research of Childhood Cancer
PO Box 251
Buffalo, NY 14225
716-681-4433
www.arocc.org

A nonprofit organization staffed by volunteers and formed in 1971 by parents who had lost children to pediatric cancer. Chapter members raise funds by various projects in order to provide seed money to various pediatric research centers in order to find a cure and, ultimately, prevent the types of cancers that attack children.

Anne O'Donnell, President
Larry Lorenz, 1st Vice President
Phyllis Winkle, Treasurer

8555 Baylor College of Medicine Birth Defects Center
6621 Fannin Street
Houston, TX 77030
713-770-3013
Fax: 713-770-4294

Frank Greenberg, MD, Director

8556 Children's Cancer Research Institute
University of Texas Health Science Ctr
8403 Floyd Curl Drive
San Antonio, TX 78229
210-562-9000
Fax: 210-562-9014
chessher@uthscsa.edu
www.ccri.uthscsa.edu

A specialized cancer research center established by the largest single oncology endowment of $200 million from Texas' tobacco settlement. Through discovery, development and dissemination of scientific knowledge relevant to childhood cancer, the overall aim of the CCRI is to impact cancer at all ages.

Sharon Murphy MD, Director
Danette Besancon, Administrative Assistant Senior
Gail Tomlinson, MD, PhD, Interim Director

8557 Computer Access Center
PO Box 12464
Albuquerque, NM 87195
505-242-9588
Fax: 310-338-9318
cac@cac.org
www.cac.org

Includes nationwide network of community-based assistive technology, resource centers, hands on consultants and product demonstrations.

8558 Division for Research (CEC-DR)
Council for Exceptional Children
1920 Association Drive
Reston, VA 20191
703-620-3660
Fax: 703-264-9474
TTY: 703-264-9446
www.cecdr.org

Devoted to the advancement of research related to the education of individuals with disabilities and/or who are gifted. Members include university, public, and private school teachers, researchers, administrators, psychologists, speech/language clinicians, parents of children with special learning needs.

Kathleen Lane, President
David Houchins, Vice President
Tanya Santangelo, Treasurer

8559 Division of Birth Defects and Genetic Diseases
4770 Buford Highway
Chamblee, GA 30341
770-488-7150
Fax: 770-488-7156

Muin J Khoury, MD

8560 Early Intervention Research Institute, Developmental Center
Utah State University
9510 Old Main Hill
Logan, UT 84322
435-750-1172

8561 Georgetown University Child Development Center
3307 Main Street, NW
Washington, DC 20007
202-687-8899
Fax: 202-687-5000
gucdc@georgetown.edu
gucdc.georgetown.edu

8562 Institute for Basic Research in Developmental Disabilities
1050 Forest Hill Road
Staten Island, NY 10314
718-494-0600
Fax: 718-494-0837

Conducts research into neurodegenerative diseases, Alzheimer's disease, developmental disabilities, fragile X syndrome, Down's syndrome, autism, epilepsy and basic science issues underlying all developmental disabilities.

8563 Keren-Or Jerusalem Center for Multi- Handicapped Blind Children
350 7th Avenue, Suite 200
New York, NY 10001
212-279-4070
Fax: 212-279-4043
info@keren-or.org
www.karen-or.org

Center houses and cares for over 85 resident and day students who in addition to blindness or very low vision, suffer from other severe physical and or mental disabilities. Provides training in daily living skills, as well as therapy, rehabilitation and education. Funds aquired through government stipends, government contributions, grants, bequests and legacies. Keren-Or is an IRS 501 (C)(3) tax exempt organization.

Dr. Edward L Steinburg, Chairman
Dr. Albert Hornblass, President
Madelyn Cohen, Executive Director

8564 Louisiana State University Genetics Section of Pediatrics
1501 Kings Highway
Shreveport, LA 71103
318-675-5681
TF Thurman, MD, Director

8565 New England Regional Genetics Group
PO Box 920288
Needham, MA 02492
781-444-0126
Fax: 781-444-0127
mfgnergg@verizon.net
www.nergg.org

Human genetic services and educational planning pertaining to birth defects.

Lisa Demers, MS, CGC, President
Mary-Frances Garber, Coordinator
Lisa Demers, MS, CGC, Officer

8566 Parent and Information Center
5 N Lobban
Buffalo, WY 82834   307-684-2277
                                     800-660-9742
                                 Fax: 307-684-5314
                              tdawsonpic@vcn.com

Support network for parents of children with disabilities and/or chronic illness. Veteran parents offer support to parents who are just learning of their child's diagnosis. Offers support and insight into parenting a child with special needs, as well as referrals to trained veteran parents.

8567 Prenatal Diagnostic and Genetic Center
HCA Wesley Medical Center
550 N Hillside Street
Wichita, KS 67214   316-962-2000
                                 Fax: 316-962-7076
                                 www.wesleymc.com
Sechin Cho, MD

8568 Primary Children's Medical Center
Graduate Parents
100 North Mario Capecchi Drive
Salt Lake City, UT 84113   801-662-1000
                                 Fax: 801-588-3869
                               PCSWAR2@jhc.com
                          www.intermountainhealthcare.org

8569 Research and Training Center for Children' Mental Health
University of South Florida
13303 Bruce B Downs Boulevard
Tampa, FL 33612   813-974-4661
                                 Fax: 813-974-6257
                            www.rtckids.fmhi.usf.edu

Dedicated to promoting effective community based culturally competent family centered services for familes and thier children who are affeed by mental, emotional or behavoiral disorders.

Bob Frieman, PhD, Center Director
Albert Duchnowski, Ph.D., Deputy Director
Krista Kutash, Ph.D., Deputy Director

8570 Research and Training Center on Family Support and Children's Mental Health
Portland State University/Regional Research Instit
PO Box 751
Portland, OR 97207   503-725-4040
                                 Fax: 503-725-4180
                               rtcinfo@rri.pdx.edu
                                     rtc.pdx.edu

Dedicated to promoting effective community based, culturally competent, family centered services for families and their children who are or may be affected by mental, emotional or behavioral disorders. This goal is accomplished through collaborative research partnerships with family members, service providers, policy makers, and other concerned persons. Major efforts in dissemination and training include an annual conference and comprehensive web site.

Rachel Elizabeth, Public Information/Outreach

8571 Rusk Institute of Rehabilitation Medicine
NYU Langone Medical Center
301 East 17th Street, at Second Avenue
New York, NY 10003   212-263-7300
                                 Fax: 212-263-5499
                              Rusk.Info@nyumc.org.
                              www.rusk.med.nyu.edu

The world's first university-affiliated facility devoted entirely to rehabilitation medicine, Rusk is among the most renowned center of its kind for the treatment of adults and children with disabilities-home to innovations and advances that have set the standard in rehabilitation care for every stage of life and for every stage of recovery.

Dr. Steven Flanagan, Professor & Chairman
Marilyn Shoo, Pediatrics Director

8572 TIES, The Children's Hospital
1056 E 19th Avenue
Denver, CO 80218   303-861-6395
                                     800-332-2082
                                 Fax: 303-861-3992
Karen Prescott, MS

8573 Team of Advocates for Special Kids
100 W Cerritos Avenue
Anaheim, CA 92805   714-533-8275
                                     866-828-8275
                                 Fax: 714-533-2533
                                   taskca@aol.com
                                    www.taskca.org

Technology group of parents, consumers and professionals; provides resources to help children and adults who have disabilities gain access to the benefits of technology. Includes nationwide network of community-based assistive technology, resource centers, hands on consultants and product demonstrations.

Marta Anchondo, Executive Director/CEO

8574 Teratogen and Birth Defects Information Project
University of South Dakota
414 E Clark Street
Vermillion, SD 57069   605-677-5011
                                     www.usd.edu

8575 UC Berkeley School of Social Welfare
Mental Health & Social Welfare Research Group
303 Haviland Hall
Berkeley, CA 94720   510-642-3949
                               spsegal@berkeley.edu
                          www.socialwelfare.berkeley.edu
Steven P Segal, Director

8576 University of Alaska, Fairbanks
College of Rural Alaska
PO Box 7565000
Fairbanks, AK   907-474-7143
                                 www.uaf.edu/rural/
Bernice Joseph, Vice Chancellor/Executive Dean
Pete Pinney, Associate Executive Dean
Cecelia Chamberlain, CRCD Executive Officer

8577 University of Iowa Birth Defects and Genetic Disorders Unit
2614 JCP
Iowa City, IA 52242   319-335-9901
                              val-sheffield@uiowa.edu
                                    www.uiowa.edu
James M Smith, Director

8578 University of Miami, Mailman Center for Child Development
PO Box 16820
Miami, FL 33101   305-585-2703
                                 Fax: 305-547-6309
                www.pediatrics.med.miami.edu/mailman-center/
Focuses on birth defects and children's illnesses.
Dr. Robert Stempfel Jr, Director

8579 Wesley Medical Research Institutes
3306 E Central Avenue
Wichita, KS 67208   316-686-7172
                                 www.wesleymc.com
Respiratory and birth defects disorders research.
Dr. Sechin Cho, MD, Director

Conferences

8580 AACAP & CACAP Joint Annual Meeting
American Academy of Child & Adolescent Psychiatry
3615 Wisconsin Avenue NW
Washington, DC 20016   202-966-7300
                                 Fax: 202-966-2891
                                 clinical@aacap.org
                                    www.aacap.org

The world's largest gathering place for leaders in the field of child and adolescent psychiatry, children's mental health, and other allied disciplines.

Martin J. Drell, M.D., President
David R. DeMaso, M.D., Secretary
David R. DeMaso, M.D., Secretary

8581 ACLP Annual Conference
Association of Child Life Professionals
1820 N Fort Myer Drive, Ste 520
Arlington, MD 22209
501-483-4500
800-252-4515
Fax: 501-483-4482
aclpadmin@childlife.org
www.childlife.org

The premier educational experience for child life professionals. The largest gathering of child life specialists of the year, offers ample opportunities for both formal and informal networking with peers.

1,000 May

Jennifer Lipsey, Interim CEO
Yvonne Kassimatis, Marketing & Communications
Ramona Spencer, Manager, Conferences & Events

8582 ADAA Annual Conference
Anxiety Disorders Association of America
8701 Georgia Ave. #412
Silver Spring, MD 20910
240-485-1001
Fax: 240-485-1035
information@adaa.org
www.adaa.org

April

Alies Muskin, Executive Director
Terence M. Keane, PhD, President
Karen Cassiday, PhD, Secretary

8583 ARC Annual National Convention
The ARC
1825 K Street NW, Suite 1200
Washington, DC 20006
202-534-3700
800-433-5255
Fax: 202-534-3731
info@thearc.org
www.thearc.org

held in cities throughout the U.S. each fall which attracts nearly 1000 people for educational sessions, business meetings and social events.

Peter V. Berns, Chief Executive Officer
Trudy R. Jacobson, Chief Development & Marketing Offic
Elise McMillan, Secretary

8584 CEC Convention & Expo
Council for Exceptional Children
2900 Crystal Drive, Suite 1000
Arlington, VA 22201
703-243-0446
888-232-7733
Fax: 703-264-9494
TTY: 866-915-5000
service@cec.sped.org
www.cec.sped.org

April

Bruce Ramirez, Executive Director
Krista Barnes, Assistant Executive Director
Karen Niles, Assistant Executive Director

8585 FFCMH Annual Conference
Federation of Families for Childrens Mental Health
9605 Medical Center Drive, Suite 280
Rockville, MD 20850
240-403-1901
Fax: 240-403-1909
ffcmh@ffcmh.org
www.ffcmh.org

Address the complex issue of trauma; the impact it has on children and families; the promotion of healing and prevention strategies; knowledge about how to address trauma through resiliency-based interventions, utilizing a familydriven, youth guided approach; and examples of how family organizations and the partners they work with are raising awareness and improving trauma-focused services and supports.

November

Teka Dempson, President
Sherri Luthe, Vice President
Josh Ross, Secretary

8586 Genetic Alliance Annual Conference
Genetic Alliance
4301 Connecticut Avenue NW, Suite 404
Washington, DC 20008
202-966-5557
800-336-4363
Fax: 202-966-8553
info@geneticalliance.org
www.geneticalliance.org

Consistently inspirational and enables partnership among all stakeholders: advocates and community leaders, health and industry professionals, policymakers, and academicians.

July

Sharon Terry, President/CEO
Tetyana Murza, Managing Director
Natasha Bonhomme, VP, Strategic Development

8587 International Conference On Young Children With Special Needs & Their Familiies
Division for Early Childhood
27 Fort Missoula Road, Suite 2
Missoula, MT 59804
406-543-0872
Fax: 406-543-0887
TTY: 703-264-9446
dec@dec-sped.org
www.dec-sped.org

Attendees from around the world explore the evidence, present practical strategies, and engage in discussions that will change the way one thinks about early childhood special education. Topics include: policy, autism, recommended practices, tiered interventions, challenging behavior, personnel development, research, assessment, cultural diversity and more.

Dr. Leah Weiner, President
Cynthia Wood, Associate Executive Director
Sharon Walsh, Governmental Relations Consultant

8588 Long Term Survivor Conference
Childhood Brain Tumor Foundation
20312 Watkins Meadow Drive
Germantown, MD 20876
301-515-2900
877-217-4166
Fax: 301-540-8367
cbtf@childhoodbraintumor.org
www.childhoodbraintumor.org

In collaboration with the Children's National Medical Center, includes excellent topics and speakers from the region who shared their expertise.

Jeanne P. Young, President
Carol Cornman, Vice President
Kiren Day, Vice Pres./ Secretary

8589 NADD Conference & Exhibit Show
National Association for the Dually Diagnosed
132 Fair Street
Kingston, NY 12401
845-331-4336
800-331-5362
Fax: 845-331-4569
info@thenadd.org
www.thenadd.org

November

Dr Robert Fletcher, CEO
Michelle Jordan, Office Manager
Edward Seliger, Project Coordinator

8590 NAMI Convention
National Alliance on Mental Illness
3803 N. Fairfax Dr., Ste. 100
Arlington, VA 22203   703-524-7600
                                   800-950-6264
                                   Fax: 703-524-9094
                                   TDD: 703-516-7227
                                   info@nami.org
                                   www.nami.org

The NAMI Convention is packed with information, chances to
network, leadership development opportunities, and lots more

July

Keris J,,n Myrick, M.B.A., M.S., Ph, President
Kevin B. Sullivan, First Vice President
Jim Payne, J.D., Second Vice President

Audio Video

8591 A Mind of Your Own
Fanlight Productions
32 Court Street, 21st Floor
Brooklyn, NY 11201   718-488-8900
                                  800-876-1710
                                  Fax: 718-488-8642
                                  info@fanlight.com
                                  www.fanlight.com

Learning disabilities can make children feel lonely, confused,
hopeless and worthless, even if they know they are smart, but it
doesn't have to feel that way. Meet Henry, Matthew, Max and
Stephanie, four incredible kids who don't let learning differences
hold them back or get them down.

38 minutes DVD or VHS

Nicole Johnson, Publicity Coordinator

8592 Assisting Parents Through the Mourning Process
Hope
55 E 100 N
Logan, UT 84321   435-752-9533
                                  Fax: 435-752-9533

Describes the mourning process experienced by some parents of
children with disabilities and ways in which the professional can
help them through the process.

20 minutes

8593 CANCER
Rosen Publishing Group
29 E 21st Street
New York, NY 10010   800-237-9932
                                  Fax: 888-436-4643
                                  rosenpub@tribeca.ios.com
                                  www.rosenpublishing.com

Interviews with experts and cancer patients reveal the many
types, causes, and treatments for cancer. Recommended for
grades seven-twelve.

30 Minutes
ISBN: 0-823921-76-0

8594 Disability Awareness
Active Parenting Publishers
1220 Kennestone Circle, Suite 130
Marietta, GA 30066   770-429-0565
                                  Fax: 770-429-0334
                                  cservice@activeparenting.com
                                  www.activeparenting.com

Helps viewers think about how they feel when confronted by people with disabilities. Close-captioned with study guide.

19 minutes

Michael H. Popkin, PhD, Founder & President
Virginia Murray, Marketing Manager
Melody Popkin, Manager of Christian Resources

8595 It's Just Part of My Life
National Kidney Foundation
30 E 33rd Street
New York, NY 10016   212-889-2210
                                  800-622-9010
                                  Fax: 212-689-9261
                 info@kidney.org, membership@kidney.org
                                  www.kidney.org

A 15-minute program for adolescent dialysis patients and their
families.

Gregory W. Scott, Chairman
Jeffery S. Berns, President
Bruce Skyer, CEO

**8596 Kid's Health: TV Late Breaking News Video About Broken
Bones and Cast Care**
Aquarius Health Care Videos
5 Powderhouse Lane, PO Box 1159
Sherborn, MA 1770   508-651-2963
                                  888-440-2963
                                  Fax: 508-650-4216
                                  info@aquariusproductions.com
                                  www.aquariusproductions.com

You probably have lots of questions. How do doctors know if a
bone is really broken? What are casts and what do they do? What
are some ways to take good care of your cast so you won't need a
new one? The Kids Health TV News Tem answer these questions
and more in an entertaining format.

Donna Kaufman

8597 Laughter Therapy
PO Box 827
Monterey, CA 93942   408-625-3788

These people can supply tapes of old Candid Camera movies to
patients. Maintains a library of 50 topics.

8598 Meeting the Challenge: Parenting Children with Disabilities
Active Parenting Publishers
1220 Kennestone Circle, Suite 130
Marietta, GA 30066   770-429-0565
                                  800-825-0060

Award-winning video for parents of special-needs children. Other
parents share their stories.

94 minutes

8599 My Body Is Not Who I Am
Aquarius Health Care Videos
5 Powderhouse Lane, PO Box 1159
Sherborn, MA 1770   508-651-2963
                                  888-440-2963
                                  Fax: 508-650-4216
                                  info@aquariusproductions.com
                                  www.aquariusproductions.com

Children host this video and educate themselves and the viewer
about disabilities. While profiling adults and children who talk
candidly about their disabilites, they learn that people are more
alike than different. This video is crafted to foster senitivity toward others and acceptance of people with disabilities. It provides general disability etiquette guidelines that both children
and adults can benefit from. The video is fast paced and designed
to keep children's attention. Closed caption.

K - 12 25 Minutes

Donna Kaufman

8600 No Fears, No Tears
Fanlight Productions
32 Court Street, 21st Floor
Brooklyn, NY 11201   718-488-8900
                                  800-876-1710
                                  Fax: 718-488-8642
                                  info@fanlight.com
                                  www.fanlight.com

Dr. Leora Kuttner explores the pioneer pain management project
for children with cancer. The film proves the strenth of the human spirit and mind's ability to ease away excrutiating pain. See
No Fears, No Tears - 13 Years Later.

28 minutes DVD
ISBN: 1-572958-73-1

8601 No Fears, No Tears - 13 Years Later
Fanlight Productions
32 Court Street, 21st Floor
Brooklyn, NY 11201
718-488-8900
800-876-1710
Fax: 718-488-8642
info@fanlight.com
www.fanlight.com

Dr. Leora Kuttner explore the effects of children's pain management therapies 13 years after use. See original No Fears, No Tears. ISBN: DVD: 1-57295-874-X; VHS: 1-572952-77-6

47 minutes DVD or VHS

8602 Not Just a Cancer Patient
Fanlight Productions
32 Court Street, 21st Floor
Brooklyn, NY 11201
718-488-8900
800-876-1710
Fax: 718-488-8642
info@fanlight.com
www.fanlight.com

Focuses on several articulate teenagers who are undergoing cancer treatment to help caregivers understand the needs and feelings of this very special population.

23 minutes VHS
ISBN: 1-572950-86-2

Nicole Johnson, Publicity Coordinator

8603 Operation Sneek-a-Peek
Aquarius Health Care Videos
5 Powderhouse Lane, PO Box 1159
Sherborn, MA 1770
508-651-2963
888-440-2963
Fax: 508-650-4216
info@aquariusproductions.com
www.aquariusproductions.com

Helps children feel more comfortable and safe in a hospital environment. The puppets in the video take the children on an educational, comforting and at times, humorous tour of the hospital operating and recovery rooms. This video eases children's concerns and fears with factual information and truthful demonstrations. Closed captioned.

20 Minutes

Donna Kaufman

8604 Recognizing Children with Special Needs
Aquarius Health Care Videos
5 Powderhouse Lane, PO Box 1159
Sherborn, MA 1770
508-651-2963
888-440-2963
Fax: 508-650-4216
info@aquariusproductions.com
www.aquariusproductions.com

A great overview for caregivers of children on how to recognize special needs. Often times it is the little things children do everyday to compensate for, or express, a disability that can be observed by their caregiver. All types of disabilities are addressed, emotional, physical, psychological, and chonic illness. A wonderful tool for teachers, childcare staff, and students who play a vital role in our children's development. Closed captioned.

18 Minutes

Donna Kaufman

8605 Stress Reduction Tapes, Stress Reduction Clinic
University Massachusetts Medical
PO Box 547
Lexington, MA 2420
508-856-2656
mindfulness@umassmed.edu
www.mindfulnesstapes.com

There are two tapes sold separately that are appropriate for preteens or adolescents. Tapes may be ordered from the website.

Jon Kabat-Zinn, PhD, Author

8606 They're Just Kids
Aquarius Health Care Videos
5 Powderhouse Lane, PO Box 1159
Sherborn, MA 1770
508-651-2963
888-440-2963
Fax: 508-650-4216
info@aquariusproductions.com
www.aquariusproductions.com

This documentary explores the advantages of the inclusion of disabled children in the classroom, Cub Scouts and other extracurricular activities. Unfortunately, there is a great deal of fear, apprehension and concern regarding mainstreaming. This film is an excellent tool to expedite and ease that integration of children and adults into the community as well as into recreational, social and educational programs. Closed captioned, for schools, parents and those working with disabled children.

27 Minutes

Donna Kaufman

8607 When Parents Can't Fix It
Fanlight Productions
32 Court Street, 21st Floor
Brooklyn, NY 11201
718-488-8900
800-876-1710
Fax: 718-488-8642
info@fanlight.com
www.fanlight.com

Looks at the stresses and rewards in the lives of five families who are raising children with diabilities. Offers a realistic look and different family strengths and coping styles. ISBN: DVD: 1-57295-876-6; VHS: 1-572952-55-5

58 minutes DVD or VHS

Nicole Johnson, Publicity Coordinator

Web Sites

8608 Adolescent Health On-Line
AMA Plaza, 330 N. Wabash Ave.
Chicago, IL 60611
312-464-4430
800-621-8335
www.ama-assn.org

Includes state-to-state guide to poison control centers, database of pediatrician and hospitals, basic home care instructions and immunizations.

Barbara L. McAneny, MD, Chair
Robert M. Wah, MD, President
Andrew W. Gurman, MD, Speaker

8609 Adoptive Families
108 West 39th Street, Suite 805
New York, NY 10018
646-366-0830
800-372-3300
Fax: 646-366-0842
letters@adoptivefamilies.com
www.adoptivefamilies.com

Information and advocacy resources for families and professionals interested in adoption.

Susan Caughman, Editor/Publisher
Eve Gilman, Editor

8610 American Academy of Pediatrics
141 Northwest Point Boulevard
Elk Grove Village, IL 60007
847-434-4000
800-433-9016
Fax: 847-434-8000
www.aap.org

The American Academy of Pediatrics and its member pediatricians are committed to the attainment of optimal physical, mental and social health and well-being for all infants, children, adolescents, and young adults.

Fernando Stein, MD, FAAP, President
Karen Remley, MD, CEO/Executive VP

8611 American Autoimmune Related Diseases Association
22100 Gratiot Avenue
Eastpointe, MI 48021   586-776-3900
                                                       800-598-4668
                                                  Fax: 586-776-3903
                                                   aarda@aarda.org
                                                   www.aarda.org

Dedicated to the eradication of autoimmune diseases and the alleviation of suffering and the socio-economic impact of autoimmunity through fostering and facilitating collaboration in the areas of education, public awareness, research and patient services in an effective, ethical and efficient manner.

Virginia T. Ladd, President/Executive Director
Patricia Barber, Assistant Director
Deb Patrick, Events Specialist

8612 American Board of Pediatrics
111 Silver Cedar Court
Chapel Hill, NC 27514   919-929-0461
                                                  Fax: 919-929-9255
                                        abpeds@abpeds.org, ite@abpeds.org

Is an independent, nonprofit organization whose certificate is recognized throughout the world signifying a high level of physician competence. It consists of distinguished pediatricians in education, research, and clinical practice, as well as one or more nonphysicians who have a professional interest in the health and welfare of children and adolescents.

8613 American College of Medical Genetics
7220 Wisconsin Avenue, Suite 300
Bethesda, MD 20814   301-718-9603
                                                  Fax: 301-718-9604
                                                   acmg@acmg.net
                                                   www.acmg.net

Provides education, resources and a voice for the medical genetics profession. To make genetic services available to and improve the health of the public, the ACMG promoted the development and implementation of methods to diagnose, treat and prevent genetic disease.

8614 American Society of Pediatric Neurosurgeons
www.aspn.org

                                                   aspnhelp@aspn.org
                                                   www.aspn.org

The society is dedicated to the advancement of the subspecialty of Pediatric Neurosugery and to assure superlative care for children with neurosurgical disorders. It holds an annual meeting where recent advances in clinical and basic research into pediatric neurosurgical disorders are presented and discussed, and sponsors a journal, Pediatric Neurosurgery.

Alan R. St. Geme III, MD, President
James M. Drake, Secretary
John Ragheb, MD, Treasurer

8615 Archives of Pediatric and Adolescent Medicine
333 Seventh Avenue, 20th Floor
New York, NY 10001   646-674-6300
                                                       800-950-2035
                                                  Fax: 646-674-6301
                                                   sales@ovid.com
                                        www.ovid.com/site/cataloge/journal

It provides a forum for dialogue on a range of scientific, clinical, and humanistic issues relevant to the care of pediatric patients, from infancy to young adulthood. The journal's core articles are original clinical studies and reviews by experts.

8616 Association for Children with Hand or Arm Deficiency (REACH)
Provides a means by which patients and professionals share experiences, information, and support.

8617 Birth Defect Research for Children
976 Lake Baldwin Lane, Suite 104
Orlando, FL 32814   407-895-0802
                                                   staff@birthdefects.org
                                                   www.birthdefects.org

Nonprofit organization that provides parents and expectant parents with information about birth defects and support services for their children, including the National Birth Defect Registry.

8618 Cedars-Sinai Medical Center
8700 Beverly Road
Los Angeles, CA 90048   310-423-3277
                                                       800-233-2771
                                                   cedars-sinai.edu

Focused on providing the finest healthcare available, resulting in advances in all areas of healthcare for both children and adult disorders.

Vera S. Guerin, Chair
Marc H. Rapaport, Vice Chair
Thomas M. Priselac, President & CEO

8619 CenterWatch Clinical Trials Listings
10 Winthrop Square, Fifth Floor
Boston, MA 2110   617-948-5100
                                                       866-219-3440
                                                  Fax: 617-948-5101
                                        customerservice@centerwatch.com
                                                   www.centerwatch.com

CenterWatch is a Boston-based publishing and information services company. We provide information services used by patients, pharmaceutical, biotechnology and medical device companies, CRO's and research centers involved in clinical research around the world.

Kenneth A. Getz, Founder & Owner
Joan A. Chambers, COO
Cheryl Appel Rosenfeld, Editor-in-Chief

8620 Council for Exceptional Children
2900 Crystal Drive, Suite 1000
Arlington, VA 22202   888-232-7733
                                                   TTY: 866-915-5000
                                                   heidenj@cudahysd.org
                                                   www.cec.sped.org

The worldwide mission of The Council for Exceptional Children is to improve education outcomes for individuals with exceptionalities. CEC, a nonprofit association, accomplishes its mission in support of special education professionals and others working on behalf of individuals with exceptionalities, by advocating for appropriate governmental policies, by setting professional standards, and by providing continuing professional development.

James P. Heiden, President
Antonis Katsiyannis, President Elect
Sharon Raimondi, Treasurer

8621 CyberPsych
www.cyberpsych.org

CyberPsych presents information about psychoanalysis, psychotherapy, and special topics such as anxiety disorder, the problematic use of alcohol, homophobia, and the traumatic effects of racism. CyberPsych is a nonprofit network which offers free web hosting and technical support for internet communication, to nonprofit groups and individuals.

Carol Lindemann, PHD, Webmaster

8622 Dermatology Foundation
1560 Sherman Ave., Suite 870
Evanston, IL 60201   847-328-2256
                                                  Fax: 847-328-0509
                                                   dermatologyfoundation.org

Committed to advancing dermatologic through research and education. The foundation is a charitable organization that has the primary service to fund research in skin cancer and other diseases of the skin, hair, and nails.

Bruce U. Wintroub, MD, Chair
Michael D. Tharp, MD, President
Stuart R. Lessin, MD, Vice President

8623 Easter Seals Disability Services
233 South Wacker Drive, Suite 2400
Chicago, IL 60606   800-221-6827
                                                   www.easterseals.com

For more than 80 years, Easter Seals has helped people with disabilities in communities nationwide, from creating the first national voluntary act for children with disabilities in the 1920's to leading the creation and implementation of the Americans with Disabilities Act in the 1990's. Easter Seals child development services build strong foundations for children of all abilities.

Rick Davidson, Chair
Eileen Howard Boone, 1st Vice Chair
Ralph F. Boyd, Jr., 2nd Vice Chair

8624 European Society for Pediatric Urology
www.espu.org

Is a nonprofit society whose main purpose is to promote pediatric urology, appropriate practice, education as well as exchanges between practitioners involved in the treatment of genitourinary disorders in children.

Gianantonio Manzoni, President
Guy Bogaert, President-Elect
Serdar Tekgul, Secretary

8625 Federation for Children with Special Needs
529 Main Street, Suite 1M3
Boston, MA 2129   617-236-7210
                                         800-331-0688
                                     Fax: 617-241-0330
                                     fcsninfo@fcsn.org
                                              fcsn.org

Mission is to provide information, support, and assistance to parents of children with disabilites, their professional partners, and their communities. We are committed to listening to and learning from families and encouraging full participation in community life by all people, especially those with disabilities.

James F. Whalen, President
Rich Robison, Executive Director
Michael Weiner, Treasurer

8626 GeneTest
481B Edward H. Ross Drive
Elmwood Park, NJ 7407   888-729-1204
                                     Fax: 202-212-6457
                                 genetests@genetests.org
                                   www.geneclinics.org

By providing current, authoritative information on genetic testing and its use in diagnosis, management, and genetic couseling, GeneTests promotes the appropriate use of genetic services in patient care and personal decision making.

Roberta A. Pagon, MD, Founder & Medical Director
Amar Kamath, Commercial Director
Deb Eunpu, MS, CGC, Program Manager

8627 ICAN (International Child Amputee Network)
PO Box 13812
Tuscon, AZ 85732   child-amputee.net

Is an internet mailing list to provide information and support contacts to children with absent or underdeveloped limbs and their parents.

Sami Madden, President
Mike Holmes, Vice President
Joyce Baughn, Director

8628 International Foundation for Functional Gastrointestinal Disorders
PO Box 170864
Milwaukee, WI 53217   414-964-1799
                                     Fax: 414-964-7176
                                       iffgd@iffgd.org
                                         www.iffgd.org

Is a nonprofit education and research organization whoes mission is to inform, assist and support people affected by gastrointestinal disorders.

Nancy J. Norton, President & Director
William Norton, Co-Founder
Eleanor Cautley, Vice President & Director

8629 KidsHealth at the AMA
AMA Plaza, 330 N. Wabash Ave.
Chicago, IL 60611   312-464-4430
                                          800-621-8335
                                         www.ama-assn.org

Includes state-to-state guide to poison control centers, database of pediatricians and hospitals, basic home-care instructions and immunizations.

Barbara L. McAneny, MD, Chair
Robert M. Wah, MD, President
Andrew W. Gurman, MD, Speaker

8630 LSUMC Family Medicine Patient Education
lib-sh.lsumc.edu

Offers databases, E-journals, E-books, and a library catalog.

8631 Learning Disabilities Association of Ameri ca
www.ldaamerica.org

Helps families of the affected individual through information and referral to professionals in their area. A membership organization with affiliates across the country.

8632 Low Vision Gateway
www.lowvision.org

Devoted to issues of vision loss, low vision aids, vision rehabilitation and the role of the doctor.

8633 MUMS: National Parent to Parent Network
www.netnet.net/mums

A national parent-to-parent organization for parents or care providers of a child with any disability, rare or not so rare disorder, chromosomal abnormality or health condition. MUM's main purpose is to provide support to parents in the form of a networking system that matches them with other parents whose children have the same or similar condition.

8634 March of Dimes Birth Defects Foundation
1275 Mamaroneck Avenue
White Plains, NY 10605   914-997-4488
                                     www.marchofdimes.org

March of Dimes researchers, volunteers, educators, outreach workers and advocated work together to give all babies a fighting chance against the threats to their health: prematurity, birth defects, low birthweight.

8635 Medical Economics Company
24950 Country Club Drive, Suite 200
North Olmsted, OH 44070   www.medec.com

Full text for non-prescription drugs and the PDR Guide to Drug Interactions.

Georgiann DeCenzo, Executive Vice President
Ken Sylvia, Vice President
Don Berman, Director, Business Development

8636 Medical Matrix: Pediatrics
medmatrix.org/_SPages/Pediatrics.asp

Christoph U. Lehman, MD, Assoc. Professor
Andy Spooner, MD, Pediatrics Dept.

8637 Mental Help Net
P.O. Box 20709
Columbus, OH 43220   614-448-4055
                                          800-232-TALK
                            info@centersite.net, editor@centersite.n
                                          mentalhelp.net

Seeks to advance the state of online mental health communications. We wish to provide the following: to discuss, develop and debate in an open forum the future of the mental health field in America and throughout the world, to help coordinate various componests of the mental health field.

8638 NADD: National Association for the Dually Diagnosed
132 Fair Street
Kingston, NY 12401

845-331-4336
800-331-5362
Fax: 845-331-4569
info@thenadd.org
www.thenadd.org

Nonprofit organization designed to promote the interests of professional and care providers for individuals who have the coexistence of mental illness and mental retardation. NADD provides conferences, educational services and training materials to professionals, parents, concerned citizens and service organizations.

Dr Robert Fletcher, CEO
Michelle Jordan, Office Manager
Edward Seliger, Project Coordinator

8639 National Arthritis and Musculoskeletal & Skin Disease Info. Clearinghouse
NIAMS Information Clearinghouse
1 AMS Circle
Bethesda, MD 20892

301-495-4484
877-226-4267
Fax: 301-718-6366
TTY: 301-565-2966
NIAMSinfo@mail.nih.gov
www.niams.nih.gov

Supports and provides clinical and public information and research to increase understanding of the many skin diseases and related disorders. Also provides lists and order forms for their resources and materials.

Stephen I. Katz, Director
Robert H. Carter, Deputy Director
Gahan Breithaupt, Assoc. Dir. For Management

8640 National Association for Visually Handicapped
111 E 59th St
New York, NY 10022

212-821-9497
800-284-4422
kcampbell@lighthouse.org
lighthouse.org

Helps to cope with the difficulties of vision impairment.

8641 National Dissemination Center for Children with Disabilities
Two Sites under Parent Act the any the two disabilities in children and youth; programs and services for infants, children, and youth with disabilities; IDEA, the nation's special education law; No Child Left Behind, the nation's general education law; and research-based information on effective practices for children with disabilities.

8642 National Institute on Disability, Indepen dent Living & Rehabilitation Research
U.S. DHHS
330 C Street SW, Room 1304
Washington, DC 20201

202-795-7398
Fax: 202-205-0392
nidilrr-mailbox@acl.hhs.gov
acl.gov/Programs/NIDILRR/

Is committed to improving results and outcomes for people with dsiabilities of all ages. It supports programs that serve millions of children, youth and adults with disablities.

Kristi Hill, Acting Deputy Director
Ruth Brannon, Director, Research Sciences

8643 National Library Service for the Blind and Physically Handicapped
1291 Taylor Street, NW
Washington, DC 20542

202-707-5100
Fax: 202-707-0712
TDD: 202-707-0744
nls@loc.gov
www.loc.gov/nls

A free library program of braille and audio materials circulated to eligible borrowers in the United States by postage-free mail.

Karen Keninger, Director
Erica Vaughns, Executive Asst. to the Director
Isabella Marques de Castilla, Deputy Director

8644 National Newborn Screening and Genetic Resources Center
3907 Galacia Drive
Austin, TX 78759

512-345-5685
therrell@uthscsa.edu
genes-r-us.uthscsa.edu

The mission is to provide a forum for interaction between consumers, health care professionals, researchers, organizations, and policy-makers in-refining and developing public health, newborn screening and geneting programs, and to serve as a national resource center for information and education in the areas of newborn screening and genetics.

Bradford L. Therrell, Jr., Ph.D., Director
Celia Kaye, MD, PhD, Professor & Senior Associate Dean
Louis Bartoshesky, MD, MPH, Pediatrician & Clinical Geneticist

8645 National Organization of Parents of Blind Children
200 East Wells Street at Jernigan Place

a membership organization of parents and friends of blind chilren reaching out to each other to give support, encouragement and information. We believe the real problem of blindness is not the loss of eyesight, but the misunderstanding and lack of information which exists. With proper training opportunity, blindness can be reduced to a physical nuisance.

8646 National Resource Library on Youth With Disabilities
3 Morrill Hall, 100 Church St. SE
Minneapolis, MN 55455

www.cyfc.umn.edu/NRL/

Brings together comprehensive sources of information related to youth with chrionic or disabling conditions and their families. Topics include psychosocial issues, disability awareness, developmental processes, family, sexuality, education, employment, independent living, cultural issues, gender issues, service delivery, professional issues, advocacy and legal issues, and health issues.

Eric W. Kaler, President
Karen Hanson, Provost
Scott Studham, VP & CIO

8647 Nuclear Medicine at Children's Hospital, Boston
www.jpnm.org/contentch.html

8648 Office of Special Education and Rehabilitative Services
www2.ed.gov/about/offices/list/osers/

Mission is to strengthen the federal commitment to assuring access to equal opportunity for every individual; to supplement and complement the efforts of states, the local school systems and other instrumentalities of the states, the private nonprofit educational research institutions, community-based organizations, parents, and students to improve the quality of education; and to encourage the increased involvement of the public, parents, and students in federal education programs.

8649 Online Mendelian Inheritance in Man
www.omim.org

Conducts research on fundamental biomedical problems at the molecular level using mathematical and computational methods, maintains collaborations with several NIH institutes, academia, industry, and other governmental agencies, fosters scientific communication by sponsoring meetings, workshops, and lecture series, and supports training on basic and applied research in computational biology for postdoctoral fellows through the NIH Intramural Research Program.

8650 PDR - Physicians' Desk Reference
5 Paragon Drive
Montvale, NJ 7645

888-227-6469
PDRnet@pdr.net
www.pdr.net

Robert Carmignani, Sales & Marketing
Kim Marich, Sr. Director, Marketing

8651 PEDINFO: An index of the Pediatric Internet
www.pedinfo.org

Collection of links to pediatric information.

8652 Pediatric Behavior and Development
www.dbpeds.org

997

Is an independent web site created to promote better care and outcomes for children and families affected by developmental, learning, and behavioral problems by providing access to clinically relevant information and educational materials for physicians, fellows, resident physicians, and students. The site may also be of interest to psychologists, nurses, nurse practitioners, social workers, therapists, educators, and parents.

8653 Pediatric Points of Interest
www.pslgroup.com/dg/20112

Are a collection of updated links for pediatricians, parents and children to medical sources on the internet.

8654 Planetpsych
www.planetpsych.com

webmaster@PlanetPsych.com
www.planetpsych.com

Planetpsych is an online resource for mental health information.

8655 Pregnancy and Child Health Resource Center from Mayo Health Oasis
13400 E. Shea Blvd.
Scottsdale, AZ 85259

480-301-8000
800-446-2279
www.mayohealth.org

Our mission is to empower people to manage their health. We accomplish this by providing useful and up-to-date information and tools that reflect the expertise and standard of excellence of Mayo Clinic.

Roger W. Harms, MD, Medical Director, Content
Brooks S. Edwards, MD, Founding Medical Director
Philip T. Hagen, Senior Medical Editor

8656 Psych Central
55 Pleasant St., Suite 207
Newburyport, MA 1950

sales at psychcentral.com
www.psychcentral.com

Offers free informational and educational articles and resources on psychological support and mental health online.

John M. Grohol, Psy.D., CEO & Founder
Gilbert Levin, Ph.D., Member, Advisory Board
Holly R. Counts, Psy.D., Member, Advisory Board

8657 PubMed
National Library of Medicine, Building 38A
Bethesda, MD 20894

888-346-3656
info@ncbi.nlm.nih.gov
www.ncbi.nlm.nih.gov/pubmed/

Creates public databases, conducts research in computational biology, develops software tools for analyzing genome data, and disseminates biomedical information - all for better understanding molecular processes affecting human health and disease.

Christine E. Seidman, M.D., Chair
David J. Lipman, M.D., Executive Secretary

8658 Rare Genetic Diseases in Children (NYU)
550 First Avenue
New York, NY 10016

212-263-7300
www.med.nyu.edu/rgdc/homenow.htm

We target issues arising from rare genetic diseases affecting children, and to assist in the endeavor to bring knowledge and hope to those for whom there is, at present, so little.

Kenneth G. Langone, Chair
Laurence D. Fink, Co-Chair
Robert I. Grossman, MD, Dean & CEO

8659 Save Babies Through Screening Foundation
PO Box 42197
Cincinnati, OH 45242

888-454-3383
email@savebabies.org
www.savebabies.org

Is a national nonprofit public charity run by volunteers. Its mission is to improve the lives of babies by working to prevent disabilities and early death resulting from disorders detectable through newborn screening.

Jill Levy-Fisch, President
micki Gartzke, Vice President
Anne Rugari, Treasurer

8660 Society for Adolescent Medicine
111 Deer Lake Road, Suite 100
Deerfield, IL 60015

847-753-5226
Fax: 847-480-9282
info@adolescenthealth.org
www.adolescenthealth.org

A multidisciplinary organization of professionals committed to improving the physical and psychosocial health and well-being of all adolescents.

Carol Ford, President
Paula Braverman, Secretary-Treasurer
Michael Resnick, President Elect

8661 Southern Illinois University School of Medicine
PO Box 19639
Springfield, IL 62794

217-545-8000
800-342-5748
admin@siuhealthcare.org
www.siumed.edu/peds/index.htm

The mission of SUI School of Medicine is to assist the people of central and southern Illinois in meeting their present and future health care needs through education, clinical service and research.

Paul Castillo, CPA, CFO
Denise A. Gray-Felder, APR, Chief Communication Officer
Quinta Vreede, Chief Administrative Officer

8662 TRIP Database
www.tripdatabase.com

734-615-0863
800-211-8181
contact@tripdatabase.com
www.tripdatabase.com

The TRIP Database allows users to rapidly and easily identify high quality medical literature from a wide range of sources.

8663 TransWeb
www.transweb.org

Mission is to provide information about donation and transplantation to the general public in order to improve organ and tissue procurement efforts worldwide, to provide transplant patients and families world wide with information specifically dealing with transplant-related issues and concerns and to provide and index sources for transplant-related information available through the internet and otherwise.

8664 Virtual Childrens Hosptial
www.virtualpediatrichospital.org

Is dedicated to helping patients find the highest quality medical information in the world today. We offer patients the tools necessary to make informed treatment decisions within the short timlines dictated by their illness or disease.

8665 WebMD Community Services
my.webmd.com

Provides valuable health information, tools for managing youth health, and support to those who seek information.

Michael Smith, MD, MBA, CPT, Chief Medical Officer
Brunilda Nazario, MD, BC-ADM, Lead Medical Editor
Hansa Bhargava, MD, Medical Editor

Book Publishers

8666 Parental Alienation, DSM-5, and ICD-11
William Bernet, author

Charles C Thomas Publisher
2600 S 1st Street
Springfield, IL 62704   217-789-8980
                                          800-258-8980
                                     Fax: 217-789-9130
                                   books@ccthomas.com
                                     www.ccthomas.com

264 pages
ISBN: 0-398079-44-4
Sue F V Rakow, Co-Author
Carol B Carpenter, Co-Author

Magazines

8667 Adoptive Families
108 West 39th Street, Suite 805
New York, NY 10018   646-366-0830
                                          800-372-3300
                                     Fax: 646-366-0842
                              letters@adoptivefamilies.com
                                 www.adoptivefamilies.com

Information and advocacy resources for families and professionals interested in adoption.

Susan Caughman, Editor/Publisher
Eve Gilman, Editor

8668 Childswork Childsplay
135 Dupont Street, PO Box 760
Plainview, NY 11803   800-962-1141
                                     Fax: 888-803-3908
                                    www.childswork.com

Full of training tools for children of all ages.

63 pages

8669 Exceptional Parent
209 Harvard Street, Suite 303
Brookline, MA 2146   617-730-5800
                                     Fax: 617-730-8742
                                      www.eparent.com

Provides information and support for families, parents, physicians and professionals in the special needs community. Published 11 times monthly plus a special January issue.

Monthly
ISSN: 0046-9157
Joseph M. Valenzano, Jr., President, CEO & Publisher
Rick Rader MD, Editor-in-Chief
Vanessa B. Ira, Contributing Writer / Editor

8670 Future Reflections
National Federation of the Blind
200 East Wadsworth Street respectively for parents and educators
of blind children. Each issue addresses various topics important
to blind children, their families and to school personnel.

Quarterly

8671 Journal of the Academy of Dermatology
American Academy of Dermatology
PO Box 94020
Palatine, IL 60094   847-330-0230
                                     Fax: 847-330-0050

A scientific publication serving the clinical needs of the specialty and providing a wide selection of articles on various topics important to continuing medical education of Academy members and the international dermatologic community.

Monthly

8672 The Deaf-Blind American
American Association of the Deaf-Blind
PO Box 8064
Silver Spring, MD 20907   301-495-4403
                                     Fax: 301-495-4404
                                     TTY: 301-495-4402
                                   aadb-info@aadb.org
                                        www.aadb.org

The Deaf-Blind American (DBA), the official quarterly magazine of the AADB, is available only to its members. It contains articles of interest to deaf-blind individuals, their families, and service providers who work with people who are deaf-blind. The DBA is available in large print, Braille, disk and email.

Timothy Jackson, President
Jill Gaus, Vice President
Debby Lieberman, Secretary

Journals

**8673 International Journal of Nursing in Intell ectual &
Developmental Disabilities**
Developmental Disabilities Nurses Association
1501 South Loop 288, Suite 104-PMB 381
Denton, TX 76205   800-888-6733
                                     Fax: 844-336-2329
                                    ddnahq@aol.com
                                        www.ddna.org

Electronic journal for nurses, individuals, families and others interested in promoting health and nursing supports for individuals with intellectual and developmental disabilities. Provides information and resources, educational strategies and policy development on a variety of clinical topics.

Karen Green McGowan, RN, CDDN, President
Wendy Herbers, RN, CDDN, QDDP, Vice President
Linda Coley, RN, CDDN, Secretary

8674 Pediatric Dermatology Journal
Society for Pediatric Dermatology
8365 Keystone Crossing, Suite 107
Indianapolis, IN 46240   317-202-0224
                                     Fax: 317-205-9481
                                    info@pedsderm.net
                                     www.pedsderm.net

6 issues/yr
Kent Lindeman, Executive Director

Newsletters

8675 AADB E-News
American Association of the Deaf-Blind
PO Box 8064
Silver Spring, MD 20907   301-495-4403
                                     Fax: 301-495-4404
                                     TTY: 301-495-4402
                                   aadb-info@aadb.org
                                        www.aadb.org

A free newsletter, the AADB E-News is available to anyone during the months when the DBA is not being published. It contains information about the latest events occurring within AADB and in the deaf-blind community. One does not need to be an AADB member to receive the free AADB E-News newsletter.

Timothy Jackson, President
Jill Gaus, Vice President
Debby Lieberman, Secretary

8676 ABDC Newsletter
Association of Birth Defect Children
976 Lake Baldwin Lane, Suite 104
Orlando, FL 32814   407-895-0802
                                     Fax: 407-566-8341
                                  staff@birthdefects.org
                                    www.birthdefects.org

Offers updated information on the association activities, events and medical updates. Back issues available.

8 pages Quarterly

8677   ACLP Bulletin Newsletter
Association of Child Life Professionals
1820 N Fort Myer Drive, Ste 520
Arlington, MD 22209

501-483-4500
800-252-4515
Fax: 501-483-4482
aclpadmin@childlife.org
www.childlife.org

The Association of Child Life Professionals (formerly Child Life Council) newsletter provides information to promote the well-being of children and families in health care settings. Newsletter is provided to members only.

12 pages Quarterly

Jennifer Lipsey, Interim CEO
Yvonne Kassimatis, Marketing & Communications
Ramona Spencer, Manager, Conferences & Events

8678   BDRC Newsletter
Association of Birth Defect Children
976 Lake Baldwin Lane, Suite 104
Orlando, FL 32814

407-895-0802
Fax: 407-566-8341
staff@birthdefects.org
www.birthdefects.org

Offers updated information on the association activities, events and medical updates.

8 pages Quarterly

8679   Children's Hopes and Dreams
Wish Fulfillment Foundation
280 Route 46
Dover, NJ 7801

973-361-7366
Fax: 973-361-6627
chdfdover@juno.com
childrenscharities.org/childrens_wisheso

Dream Newsletter (describes dreams recently fulfilled, events, request and info about programs) available upon request; at no cost. 4 times per year.

10,000 Members

8680   Connecting
5025 E Washington Street, Suite 204
Phoenix, AZ 85034

602-242-4366
800-237-3007
Fax: 602-242-4306
TDD: 602-242-4366
info@raisingspecialkids.org
www.raisingspecialkids.org

Presenting informational and personal articles, calendar of events and news relevant to Arizona families of children with special needs. Subscription is free to families.

Bimonthly

Paula Banahan, President
Blanca Esparza-Pap, Vice President
Joyce Millard Hoie, Executive Director

8681   For Siblings Only
Family Resource Associates
35 Haddon Avenue
Shrewsbury, NJ 7702

732-747-5310
Fax: 732-747-1896

Quarterly newsletter for siblings of children with disabilities, aged four through 10.

S Levine, Editor

8682   Matchmaker
MUMS: National Parent to Parent Network
150 Custer Street
Green Bay, WI 54301

920-336-5333
877-336-5333
Fax: 920-339-0995
mums@netnet.net
www.netnet.net/mums/

Matches parents of children with rare disorders. Provides information and advocacy resources for families and professionals. Includes listings of organizations providing general information and organizations focusing on more specific areas of concern to families and young adults who have disabilities.

Quarterly

Julie Gordon, Director

8683   Newsline
Federation for Children with Special Needs
529 Main Street, Suite 1M3
Boston, MA 2129

617-236-7210
800-331-0688
Fax: 617-241-0330
TDD: 800-331-0688
fcsninfo@fcsn.org
www.fcsn.org

Carolyn Romano, Editor
Janet Vohs, Editor
Rich Robison, Executive Director

8684   Orphan Disease Update
National Organization for Rare Disorders
55 Kenosia Avenue
Danbry, CT 6810

203-744-0100
800-999-6673
Fax: 203-798-2291
orphan@rarediseases.org
www.rarediseases.org

It provides updates on research, advocacy, and special events, as well as advice and sources of help for caregivers, Web sites of interest, current clinical trials, and funding opportunities.

16 pages 3/year

Sheldon M. Schuster, Chair
Peter L Saltonstall, President & CEO
Pamela Gavin, COO

8685   PAL News
Parent Professional Advocacy League
529 Main Street, Suite 1M3
Boston, MA 2129

617-236-7210
800-331-0688
Fax: 617-241-0330
fcsninfo@fcsn.org
www.fcsn.org

Offers information on medical and technological updates in the area of research on birth defects, support groups and family resources for persons with disabled children.

Quarterly

Rich Robison, Executive Director
Sara Miranda, Associate Executive Director
John Sullivan, Associate Executive Director

8686   Sibling Forum
Family Resource Associates
35 Haddon Avenue
Shrewsbury, NJ 7702

732-747-5310
Fax: 732-747-1896
info@frainc.org
www.frainc.org

Quarterly newsletter for siblings of children with disabilities, aged 10 and up.

Allan Proske, President
Bill Sheeser, Vice President
Sue Levine, Editor

Pamphlets

8687   AAP Education Resource Guide
American Academy of Pediatrics
141 NW Point Boulevard
Elk Grove Village, IL 60007

847-434-4000
800-433-9016
Fax: 847-434-8000
cme@aap.org
www.aap.org

Sandra Hassink, MD, FAAP, President
Benard P. Dreyer, MD, FAAP, President-Elect
?Errol R. Alden, MD, FAAP, Executive Director/CEO

8688 About Children's Eyes
National Association for Visually Handicapped
111 E 59th St
New York, NY 10022
212-821-9497
800-284-4422
Fax: 212-727-2931
kcampbell@lighthouse.org
lighthouse.org

How to identify the child with a visual problem.

8689 About Children's Vision: A Guide for Parents
National Association for Visually Handicapped
111 E 59th St
New York, NY 10022
212-821-9497
800-284-4422
Fax: 212-727-2931
kcampbell@lighthouse.org
lighthouse.org

Offers a better understanding of the normal and possible abnormal development of a child's eyesight.

Eva Cohen, Assistant to the Director

8690 Advanced Cancer: Coping with Advanced Canc er
National Cancer Institute
6116 Executive Blvd, Room 3036A
Bethesda, MD 20892
800-422-6237
800-422-6237
TTY: 800-332-8615

Booklet delving into all aspects of everyday living with cancer. Offers information on coping, how children react, facing the unknown, living wills, additional resources and making treatment decisions.

30 pages

8691 Amyloidosis and Kidney Disease
Information Claringhouse
9000 Rockville Pike
Bethesda, MD 20892
301-496-3583
Fax: 301-907-8906
nddic@info.niddk.nih.gov
www.niddk.nih.gov

Griffin P. Rodgers, M.D., M.A.C.P., Director
Kevin Abbott, Program Director
Kristin Abraham, Program Director

8692 Birth Defects: A Brighter Future
March of Dimes Resource Center
1275 Mamaroneck Avenue
White Plains, NY 10605
914-997-4488
Fax: 914-997-4763
www.marchofdimes.org

8693 Heart Disease, High Blood Pressure, Stroke and Diabetes
Information Clearinghouse
9000 Rockville Pike
Bethesda, MD 20892
301-496-3583
Fax: 301-907-8906
nddic@info.niddk.nih.gov
www.niddk.nih.gov

Griffin P. Rodgers, M.D., M.A.C.P., Director
Kevin Abbott, Program Director
Kristin Abraham, Program Director

8694 How to Find Out More About Your Child's Bi rth Defect or Disability
Association of Birth Defect Children
976 Lake Baldwin Lane, Suite 104
Orlando, FL 32814
407-895-0802
Fax: 407-895-0824
staff@birthdefects.org
www.birthdefects.org

An informational fact sheet that encourages parents who have a child with a birth defect or disability to become the expert on the child's disability with some suggestions on how to educate themselves.

8695 Interstitial Cyctitis
Information Clearinghouse
9000 Rockville Pike
Bethesda, MD 20892
301-496-3583
Fax: 301-907-8906
ndoc@info.niddk.nih.gov
www.niddk.nih.gov

Griffin P. Rodgers, M.D., M.A.C.P., Director
Kevin Abbott, Program Director
Kristin Abraham, Program Director

8696 Liver Transplantation
American Liver Foundation
1425 Pompton Avenue
Cedar Grove, NJ 7009
973-857-2626
800-223-0179

8697 NPF Benefits of Membership Pamphlets
National Psoriasis Foundation
6600 SW 92nd Avenue, Ste. 300
Portland, OR 97223
503-244-7404
800-723-9166
Fax: 503-245-0626
getinfo@psoriasis.org
www.psoriasis.org

Offers all the pamphlets that are published through the foundation for members. Includes NPF 800 number and reply tear-off card.

Krista Kellog, Chair
Pete Redding, Vice Chair
Randy Beranek, President & CEO

8698 New Challenge: Responding to Families
Federation for Children with Special Needs
529 Main Street, Suite 1M3
Boston, MA 2129
617-236-7210
800-331-0688
Fax: 617-241-0330
fcsninfo@fcsn.org
www.fcsn.org

Addresses the needs of children with emotional, behavioral and mental disorders and their families.

Rich Robison, Executive Director
Sara Miranda, Associate Executive Director
John Sullivan, Associate Executive Director

8699 Nutrition for Early Chronic Kidney Disease
Information Clearing House
9000 Rockville Pike
Bethesda, MD 20892
301-496-3583
Fax: 301-907-8906
nddic@info.niddk.nih.gov
www.niddk.nih.gov

Griffin P. Rodgers, M.D., M.A.C.P., Director
Kevin Abbott, Program Director
Kristin Abraham, Program Director

8700 Nutrition for Later Chronic Disease
Information Clearinghouse
9000 Rockville Pike
Bethesda, MD 20892
301-496-3583
Fax: 301-907-8906
nddic@info.niddk.nih.gov
www.niddk.nih.gov

Griffin P. Rodgers, M.D., M.A.C.P., Director
Kevin Abbott, Program Director
Kristin Abraham, Program Director

8701 Pain, Pain Go Away: Helping Children with Pain
Association for the Care of Children's Health
7910 Woodmont Avenue, Suite 300
Bethesda, MD 20814
301-654-6549
800-808-2224
Fax: 301-986-4553

This booklet teaches parents about pain in children.

1993

8702 Proteinuria
Information Clearinghouse
9000 Rockville Pike
Bethesda, MD 20892

301-496-3583
Fax: 301-907-8906
nddic@info.niddk.nih.gov
www.niddk.nih.gov

Griffin P. Rodgers, M.D., M.A.C.P., Director
Kevin Abbott, Program Director
Kristin Abraham, Program Director

8703 Renal Tubular Acidosis
Information Clearinghouse
9000 Rockville Pike
Bethesda, MD 20892

301-496-3583
Fax: 301-907-8906
nddic@info.niddk.nih.gov
www.niddk.nih.gov

Griffin P. Rodgers, M.D., M.A.C.P., Director
Kevin Abbott, Program Director
Kristin Abraham, Program Director

8704 When Your Child Has a Life-Threatening Illness
Association for the Care of Children's Health
7910 Woodmont Avenue
Bethesda, MD 20814

301-654-6549
Fax: 301-986-4553

A concise, supportive booklet for parents. Sections include initial reactions, hope, communication, other children, impact on marriage, and single parent families.

1983

8705 Wish Fulfillment Organizations
Candlelighters' Childhood Cancer Foundation
7910 Woodmont Avenue, Suite 460
Bethesda, MD 20814

301-657-8401
800-366-2223

A list of groups granting wishes of children with life-threatening, chronic or terminal illnesses, with criteria and contacts.

8706 Young People with Cancer: A Handbook for Parents
National Cancer Institute
BG 9609 MSC 9760, 9609 Medical Center Drive
Bethesda, MD 20892

800-422-6237
TTY: 800-332-8615
www.cancer.gov

Discusses the most common types of childhood cancer, treatments, and side effects and issues that may arise when a child is diagnosed with cancer.

86 pages

Harold Varmus, M.D., Director

8707 Your Kidneys and How They Work
Information Clearinghouse
9000 Rockville Pike
Bethesda, MD 20892

301-496-3583
Fax: 301-907-8906
ndoc@info.niddk.nih.gov
www.niddk.nih.gov

Griffin P. Rodgers, M.D., M.A.C.P., Director
Kevin Abbott, Program Director
Kristin Abraham, Program Director

Camps

8708 Camp Brave Eagle
8326 Nabb Rd.
Indianapolis, IN 46260

317-871-0000
www.campbraveeagle.org

Summer camp for children with bleeding disorders and their siblings.

Angel Couch, Program Director
Jennifer Maahs, Pediatric Nurse Practitioner

8709 Camp Horizon
930 E Woodfield Road
Schaumburg, IL 60173

847-240-1280
866-503-7546
Fax: 847-240-1859
president@aad.org
www.campdiscovery.org

Camp for children with chronic dermatologic conditions. The camp offers the opportunity to experience summer camp and support each other in a setting of acceptance, love and fun.

Brett M. Coldiron, MD, President
Elise A. Olsen, MD, Vice President
Suzanne M. Olbricht, MD, Secretary-Treasurer

8710 Crotched Mountain School & Rehabilitation Center
One Verney Drive
Greenfield, NH 03047

603-547-3311
Fax: 603-547-3232
info@cmf.org
www.cmf.org

Crotched Mountain is a charitable organization with a mission to serve individuals with disabilities and their families, embracing personal choice and development and building communities of mutual support.

William Cossaboon, MS, Director of Education
Jerry Hunter, VP Information Services
Lorrie Rudis, Director of Human Resources

Alabama

8711 Camp ASCCA/Easter Seals
PO Box 21, 5278 Camp Ascca Dr
Jackson's Gap, AL 36861

256-825-9226
800-THE-CAMP
Fax: 256-825-8332
info@campascca.org
www.campascca.org

Camp for children and adults with disabilities, ages 6+.

Matt Rickman, Camp Director
John Stephenson, Administrator
Jocelyn Jones, Secretary

8712 Camp Merrimack
3320 Triana Boulevard
Huntsville, AL 35805

256-534-6455
ksimari@merrimackhall.com
www.merrimackhall.com

A unique arts half-day camp for children ages 3 through 12; open to children with special needs including Cerebral Palsy, Down Syndrome, autism and others.

Debra Jenkins, Executive Director, Founder
Melissa Reynolds, Program & Operations Dir.
Claire Lindsay, Marketing Manager

8713 Camp Rap A Hope
2701 Airport Blvd
Mobile, AL 36606

251-476-9880
Fax: 251-476-9495
info@camprapahope.org
www.camprapahope.org

A week-long summer camp in Alabama that is open to children between the ages of 7 and 17 who have and have ever had cancer.

Sandy Blount, President
Melissa McNichol, Executive Director
Roz Dorsett, Asst. Director

8714 Camp Smile-A-Mile
PO Box 550155
Birmingham, AL 35255

205-323-8427
888-500-7920
jennifer.amundsen@campsam.org
www.campsam.org

Camp for children who have or have had cancer. Year round programs are provided for the campers and their family at no cost.

Sam Heide, President
Ryan M. Weiss, Vice President
Fred Elliott, Vice President

Arizona

8715 Camp Abilities Tucson
PO Box 86838
Tucson, AZ 85754　　　　　　520-770-3204
campabilitiestucson@gmail.com
www.campabilitiestucson.org

Comprehensive developmental sports camp for children in middle
and high school who are blind, deaf-blind or multiply disabled.

Murry Everson, Camp Director

8716 Camp Civitan
12635 North 42nd Street
Phoenix, AZ 85032　　　　　　602-953-2944
Fax: 602-953-2946
info@campcivitan.org
www.campcivitan.org

A 501c3 non-profit organization, that has been providing multiple
ever-changing programs to meet the needs of children and adults
who are developmentally disabled.

Jane Armstrong, Director
Rob Adams, Camp Director
Mary Kellogg, Operations

Arkansas

8717 Camp Aldersgate
Med Camps Coordinator
2000 Aldersgate Road
Little Rock, AR 72205　　　　　　501-225-1444
Fax: 501-225-2019
info@campaldersgate.net
www.campaldersgate.net

The camps allow children and youth, ages 6-16, who have various
medical conditions and physical disabilities to enjoy traditional
camping experiences adapted to their abilities.

Sarah C. Wacaster, CEO
Bill Faggard, COO
Kerri Daniels, Dir. Of Development

California

8718 Ability First
1300 E Green Street
Pasadena, CA 91106　　　　　　626-396-1010
877-768-4600
Fax: 626-396-1021
info@abilityfirst.org
www.abilityfirst.org

Services include residential camping programs, aquatics, lifespan
programs and housing.

Steve Brockmeyer, Chair
John Kelly, Vice Chair
Lori Gangemi, President & CEO

8719 Ability First, Camp Paivika
600 Playground Drive
Cedarpines Park, CA 92332　　　　　　909-338-1102
Fax: 909-338-2502
jane.garcia@abilityfirst.org
camppaivika.org

Nonprofit camp owned and operated by Ability First to provide
outdoor, recreational camping services for children and adults
with physical and/or developmental disabilities. Located in the
San Bernadino mountains, the camp has a dining lodge and rec
room, four cabins, infirmary, program building and pool that are
all fully accessible. Camp is available to rent during winter/spring
for up to 80 people.

Kelly Kunsek, Camp Director
Ievgeniia (Jade) Garcia, Camper Services Coordinator
Sonia Ramirez, Marketing Manager

8720 All Nations Camp
1908 Grand Avenue
Nashville, TN 37212　　　　　　760-249-3822
877-899-2780
Fax: 760-249-4492
info@gbod.org
www.gbod.org

Camp for children with disabilities, ages 8 to 18.

Bishop Elaine Stanovsky, President
Eric Park, Vice President
Tim Bias, General Secretary

8721 Camp Alex A. Krem
Camping Unlimited
102 Brook Lane
Boulder Creek, CA 95006　　　　　　510-222-6662
Fax: 510-223-3046
campkrem@campingunlimited.com
www.campingunlimited.com

Camp serves people of all ages and all disabilities. Summer Program: six one- and two-week sessions of residential or outdoor
adventure camps. Year-round: weekend outings throughout the
year. Vendorized by the California Regional Centers;
camperships are available. Member of the American Camping
Association.

Mary Farfaglia, Executive Director
Leon Wong, Program Director

8722 Camp Joan Mier
Ability First
11677 E Pacific Coast Highway
Malibu, CA　　　　　　310-457-9863
Fax: 310-457-6374
www.kidscamps.com

8723 Camp Ronald McDonald at Eagle Lake
1250 Lyman Place~
Los Angeles, CA 90029　　　　　　310-268-8488
Fax: 310-473-3338
rmhcsc.org/camp/

Camp dedicated to creating a positive long-lasting impact on children with cancer and their families by providing, fun-filled, medically supervised year-round camp program.

Edward Lodgen, President
Jodie Lesh, Vice President
Martin Breidsprecher, Chief Executive Officer

8724 Camp Rubber Soul
325A East Redwood Avenue
Fort Bragg, CA 95437　　　　　　707-962-0906
camp@camprubbersoul.org
www.camprubbersoul.org

Summer camp for children and young adults with special needs
that is not affiliated with any church, School District or state program.

Rachel Miller, Director
Sayre Statham, Director

8725 Camp-A-Lot
3030 Market Street
San Diego, CA 92102　　　　　　619-685-1175
800-800-748
Fax: 619-234-3759
info@arc-sd.com
www.arc-sd.com

Residential camping program for children and adults, ages 7 and
up. San Diego locals offered transportation.

David W. Schneider, President/ CEO
Anthony J. DeSalis, Esq., EVP & COO
Rich Coppa, VP of Infra & Facilities/ CIO

8726 Christian Berets
1317 Oakdale Road, Suite 340
Modesto, CA 95355　　　　　　209-524-7993
Fax: 209-524-7979
www.christianberets.org

A community-based program for children and adults with developmental disabilities.

James Woodhead, President
Carletta Evans Steele, Treasurer
Kelly Luth, Secretary

8727 Dream Street Foundation
324 South Beverly Drive, Suite 500
Beverly Hills, CA 90212   424-333-1371
                                        Fax: 310-388-0302
                                     dreamstreatca@gmail.com
                                   www.dreamstreetfoundation.org

A customized camping program for children with terminal, chronic, and life threatening infirmities. Over 600 children with cancer, AIDS, cystic fibrosis, leukemia, blood disorders and other serious diseases are given the opportunity to enjoy activities.

Patty Grubman, Director

8728 Easter Seal Summer Camp Programs
2645 Pleasant Hill Road
Pleasant Hill, CA   925-689-1777

Offers education, adventure and the experience and enjoyment of living-out-of-doors in a striking and challenging wilderness environment. Serves ages 6 to 60, male and female.

Beverly Mayhall

8729 Gloriana Opera Company
210 N. Corry Street, PO Box 273
Fort Bragg, CA 95437   707-964-7469
                                        Fax: 707-965-9653
                                          info@gloriana.org
                                           www.gloriana.org

Since 1977 superlative music theater productions all year long, plus concerts, childrens workshops and classes.

Diane Larson, President
Ana Lucas, Artistic Director

8730 Junior Wheelchair Sports Camp
Santa Barbara Parks and Recreation Department
1819 Farnam St Suite 701
Omaha, NE 68183   402-444-5900
                                        Fax: 402-444-4921
                                     www.ci.omaha.ne.us/parks

This five-day camp is for children 5-19 years old that are physically disabled. Sports instruction in aquatics, tennis, track and field, basketball, archery and new sports activities introduced each year. The camp counselors and instructors are also physically disabled to provide the children with a role model. Fee based on fundraising efforts.

Colorado

8731 Magic of Music and Dance
PO Box M
Aspen, CO 800-5   970-923-0578
                                        Fax: 970-923-7338
                                         www.kidscamps.com

8732 Rocky Mountain Village
Easter Seals Colorado
PO Box 115
Empire, CO 80438   303-569-2333
                                        Fax: 303-569-3857
                                   kkoev@eastersealscolorado.org
              www.easterseals.com/co/our-programs/camping-recreati

Sessions are conducted for both developmentally and physically disabled children and adults. Activities include swimming, horseback riding, outdoor education, zigline challenge course elements.

Krasimir Koev, Camp Director

Connecticut

8733 Mansfield's Holiday Hill
41 Chaffeeville Road
Mansfield Center, CT 6250   860-423-1375
                                        Fax: 860-456-2444
                                    info@holidayrecreation.com
                                 www.holidayrecreation.com/camp

A home not far from home where beautiful fields, forests, facilities and a caring staff support the activities and relationships of our camp families. The camp offers many programs such as: Outdoor Adventure; Tumbling; Dance; Adventure Ropes Course; Swimming; Arts & Crafts; Archery; Tennis and more to thirty boys and girls.

Dudley Hamlin

Florida

8734 Camp Thunderbird
500 E. Colonial Drive
Orlando, FL 32803   407-218-4300
                                        Fax: 407-218-4301
                                    campthunderbird@questinc.org
                                           www.questinc.org

Residential summer camping program for children and adults with a developmental disability. Campers enjoy swimming, sports, nature hikes, canoeing, etc. In short, a real summer camp experience provided by people who understand the physical, and behavioral challenges associated with Down syndrome, autism, Cerebral Palsy, and other developmental disabilities. Camp provides the chance to try new things, learn new skills, and focus on can-do with new friends. 6- & 12-day overnights.

Rosa Figueroa, Camp Coordinator

8735 Easter Seals Camp Challenge
31600 Camp Challenge Road
Sorrento, FL   352-383-4711
                                        Fax: 352-383-0744
                                    camp@fl.easter-seals.org
                                         www.kidscamps.com

Micheal Currence, Director Camping/Recreation
Melissa Guinta, Summer Camp Director

Hawaii

8736 Camp Erdman YMCA
69-385 Farrington Highway
Waialua, HI   808-637-4615
                                        Fax: 808-637-8874
                                         www.camperdman.net

A specialized youth camp serving the needs of the disabled.

Lance Wihelm, Chair
Steven C. Ai, Vice Chair
Michael A. Pietsch, President & CEO

Illinois

8737 Camp Discovery
American Academy of Dermatology
930 E Woodfield Road
Schaumburg, IL 60173   847-240-1280
                                             866-503-7546
                                        Fax: 847-240-1859
                                           jmueller@aad.org
              www.aad.org/dermatology-a-to-z/for-kids/camp-discove

A camp for young people with chronic skin conditions. There is no fee and transportation is provided. Three locations: Camp Horizon in Millville, PA, Camp Knutson in Crosslake, MN, and Camp Dermadillo in Burton, TX.

David M Pariser, MD, President
Janine Mueller, Program Coordinator

8738 Easter Seals - Timber Pointe Outdoor Center
507 East Armstrong Avenue
Peoria, IL 61603   309-686-1177
                              Fax: 309-687-2035
                              www.easterseals.com/ci/

Handicapable camping for kids.

Brad Halverson, Chair
Don Young, 1st Vice Chair
Wes Blumenshine, 2nd Vice Chair

8739 Jewish Council for Youth Services
JCYS Camp Red Leaf
180 W. Washington Street, Suite 1100
Chicago, IL 60602   312-726-8891
                              Fax: 312-726-7920
                              jthomason@jcys.org
                                      jcys.org

Overnight summer camp for youth and adults with developmental
disabilites. Family Camps, respite weekends, trips, and other special events are offered throughout the year.

Jeffery Heftman, President
Adam Tarantur, President Elect
Jennifer Gartenberg, VP, Programming

8740 Olympia
Southern Illinois University
Mail Code 6519
Carbondale, IL   618-453-1423
                              Fax: 618-453-1445

Located on 6,500 acres of forests and meadows on the shores of
Little Grassy Lake, Olympia Camp is for mentally and physically
handicapped children and adults. Among the activities offered are
arts and crafts, hay wagon rides, canoeing and swimming.

Craig Dittmar

8741 Summer Wheelchair Sports Camp
University of Illinois
1207 S Oak Street, Division of Rehab Education
Champaign, IL   217-333-4606
                              Fax: 217-333-0248
                              TTY: 217-333-1970
                              www.kidscamps.com

8742 Touch of Nature Environmental Center
Southern Illinois University
Carbondale, IL 62901   618-453-6793
                              Fax: 618-453-1188
                              webdev@pso.siu.edu
                              www.pso.siu.edu

Providing a traditional camping experience for non-traditional
campers, including recreational and outdoor programs for adults
and children with various developmental, mental and physical
disabilities as well as learning and behavioral disorders.

Phil Gatton, Director
Dawn Wilson, Administrative Assistant
Tammy Baumharte, Customer Service Specialist

Indiana

8743 Camp Isanogel
7601 W Isanogel Road
Muncie, IN   765-288-1073
                              Fax: 765-288-3103
                              isanogel@iquest.net
                              www.isanogelcenter.og

Thirty-two years of programs for special needs of children
through adults.

Karen Kovacn, Executive Director
Monica Sauter, Recreation Director

8744 Camp Millhouse
25600 Kelly Road
South Bend, IN   219-287-9833
                              Fax: 812-358-4381
                              www.kidscamps.com

8745 Easter Seal Society
4251 S 600 E
Columbus, IN   812-342-0134
                              www.kidscamps.com

8746 Happiness Bag Incorporated
3833 Union Road
Terre Haute, IN 47802   812-234-8867
                              Fax: 812-238-0728
                              www.happinessbag.org

Serves developmentally disabled age 5-adult; day and residential
camp program; after school program; scouting; Special Olympic
anticipation (basketball, athletics, bowling, softball and aquatics); and a bowling league.

Trudy Rupska, President
Caren Elrod, Vice President
Jodi Moan, Executive Director

8747 Happy Hollow Children's Camp
3049 Happy Hollow Road
Nashville, IN   812-988-4900
                              Fax: 812-988-7505
                              hhcdir@aol.com
                              www.happyhollowcamp.net

Accepts disabled campers.

Bernard Schrader, Executive Director

8748 Kiwanis Twin Lakes Camp
15543 12th Road
Plymouth, IN   219-941-2750

Serving the orthopedically handicapped children and young
adults.

Iowa

8749 Camp Courageous
PO Box 418
Monticello, IA 52310   319-465-5916
                              info@campcourageous.org
                              www.campcourageous.org

Over 3,500 disabled campers have attended this recreational and
respite care facility. The camp is open 24 hours a day, 365 days a
year and operates entirely on donations.

Aly Jonson, Dietary Director
Amanda Brenneman, Assistant Nursing
Amatullah Richard, Communications Director

8750 Camp Courageous of Iowa
PO Box 418
Monticello, IA 52310   319-465-5916
                              Fax: 319-465-5919
                              info@campcourageous.org
                              www.campcourageous.com

A year round residential and respite care facility for individuals
with special needs. Campers range in age from 3-80 years old.
Activities include traditional activities like canoeing, hiking,
swimming, nature and crafts plus adventure activities like caving,
rock climbing, etc. Campers with disabilities have opportunities
to succeed at challenging activities. This feeling of self-worth
can transfer to home, work or school environments.

Aly Jonson, Dietary Director
Amanda Brenneman, Assistant Nursing
Amatullah Richard, Communications Director

8751 Camp Tanager
1614 W Mount Vernon Road
Mount Vernon, IA 52314   319-363-0681
                              Fax: 319-365-6411
                              www.camptanager.org

Nonprofit camp for children with disabilities.

Robin Butler

8752 Easter Seals Camp Sunnyside
Easter Seals Iowa
233 South Wacker Drive, Suite 2400
Chicago, IL 60606   515-289-1933
                                     800-221-6827
                                Fax: 515-289-1281
                                essia@netins.net
                                www.easterseals.com

Each summer from June through August, campers with disabilities ages five and up, take part in one week camping sessions, gaining skills and independence by participating in activities like swimming, horseback riding, canoeing, fishing, camping and more. Financial assistance available.

Brad Halverson, Chair
Don Young, 1st Vice Chair
Wes Blumenshine, 2nd Vice Chair

Kentucky

8753 Bethel Mennonite Camp
2773 Bethel Church Road
Clayhole, KY 41317   606-666-4911
                                Fax: 606-666-4911
                                grow@bethelcamp.org
                                www.bethelcamp.org

Roger Voth, Camp Director

8754 Easter Seal Kysoc
2050 Versailles Road~
Lexington, KY 40504   859-254-5701
                                     800-233-3260
                                Fax: 502-732-0783
                                ek1@cardinalhill.org
                                www.cardinalhill.org

Designed for the fullest camping experience for children or adults with physical disabilities, blind, deaf, behavior disorders, mental retardation, diabetes and multiple handicaps, ages 7 and up.

Gary Payne, President/ CEO
Heide Miller, CCD, CTRS, Director

Louisiana

8755 Camp Bon Coeur
405 W. Main St.~
Lafeyette, LA 70501   337-233-8437
                                Fax: 337-233-4160
                                www.heartcamp.com

8756 Louisiana Lions Camp for Crippled Children
292 L. Beauford Dr.
Anacoco, LA 71403   337-239-0782
                                     800-348-6567
                                Fax: 337-239-9975
                                lalions@lionscamp.org
                                www.lionscamp.org

Camp for disabled children.
Raymond Cecil III

8757 Med-Camps of Louisiana
102 Thomas Road Suite 615
West Monroe, LA 71291   318-329-8405
                                Fax: 318-329-8407
                                info@medcamps.com
                                www.medcamps.com

Maine

8758 Camp Waban
Waban Projects, Inc.
5 Dunaway Drive
Sanford, ME   207-324-7955
                                Fax: 207-324-6050
                                www.kidscamps.com

8759 Pine Tree Camp Children - Adults
149 Front Street
Bath, ME 4530   207-443-3341
                                Fax: 207-443-1070
                                ptcamp@pinetreesociety.org
                                www.pinetreesociety.org

Paul Jacques, Chair
Dean Paterson, 1st Vice Chair
Penny Plourde, 2nd Vice Chair

Maryland

8760 Easter Seals Camp Fairlee Manor
22242 Bay Shore Road
Chestertown, MD   410-778-0566
                                Fax: 410-778-0567
                                www.kidscamps.com

8761 Kamp-A-Kom-Plish
9035 Ironsides Road
Nanjemoy, MD 20662   301-870-3226
                                Fax: 301-870-2620
                                www.kampakomplish.org

8762 The League at Camp Greentop and The Therapeutic Recreation
League: Serving People with Disabilities
1111 E Cold Spring Lane
Baltimore, MD 21239   410-323-0500
                                Fax: 410-323-3298
                                TTY: 410-435-4298
                                jrondeau@leagueforpeople.org
                                www.campgreentop.org

Summer residential camp located in the Catoctin Mountain National Park. Since 1937, Greentop has been serving children and adults with physical, cognitive, emotional and multiple disabilities in a completely accessible camp setting. Campers enjoy a traditional camping program. Medical facilities, staffed with registered nurses 24 hours a day. ACA/MD Youth Camp. Year round travel programs also offered.

Jonathon Rondeau, Director
Katrina Johnson, Executive Director

Massachusetts

8763 Camp Ramah in New England Tikvah Program
39 Bennett Street
Palmer, MA 01609   413-283-9771
                                Fax: 413-283-6661
                                info@campramahne.org
                                www.campramahne.org

The Tikvah program is one of the first summer programs for Jewish children with special needs. It continues to grow and evolve as it strives to serve campers with a wide range of special needs including, but not limited to, congitive impairments, autism, cerebral palsy and seizure disorder.

Howard Blas, Tikvah Program Director
Talya Kalender, Director, Camper Care
Benjamin Greene, Director of Education

8764 Camp Ramah in New England (Summer)
39 Bennett Street
Palmer, MA 1069   413-283-9771
                                Fax: 413-283-6661
                                www.campramahane.org

8 week sleep-away camp for Jewish adolescents with developmental disabilities. Full camping program includes swimming, Hebrew singing and dancing, sports, arts and crafts, daily services, Kosher food, and Jewish studies classes.

Howard Blas, Director

8765 Camp Ramah in New England (Winter)
35 Highland Circle
Needham Heights, MA   701-449-7090
                                Fax: 413-283-6661
                                www.campramahane.org

8 week sleep-away camp for Jewish adolescents with developmental disabilities. Full camping program includes swimming, Hebrew singing and dancing, sports, arts and crafts, daily services, Kosher food, and Jewish studies classes.

Howard Blas, Director

8766 Carroll School Summer Programs
25 Baker Bridge Road
Lincoln, MA 1773
989-879-5199
Fax: 781-259-8852
admissions@carrollschool.org
www.carrollschool.org

Academic and recreational programs designed to improve learning skills and build self-confidence. The school is a tutorial program for students not achieving their potential due to poor skills in reading, writing and math. The summer camp complements the summer school offering outdoor activities in a supportive, non-competitive environment.

Sam Foster, Chair
Josh Levy, Co-Vice Chair
Laura Rehnert, Co-Vice Chair

8767 Handi-Kids/King Solomon Foundation
470 Pine Street
Bridgewater, MA
508-697-7557
Fax: 508-697-1529
handi7557@aol.com
www.handikids.com

A therapeutic recreational facility in Bridgewater, Massachusetts offering after-school programs, special events, school vacation full-week and summer day camp programs. Every individual is welcome regardless of the severity of a child's disability.

Mary L Gallant, Program Director

8768 Massachusetts Easter Seals Camping Program
484 Main Street
Worcester, MA 1608
800-922-8290
Fax: 508-831-9768
TTY: 800-564-9700
www.kidscamps.com

Michigan

8769 Camp Barakel
PO Box 159
Fairview, MI 48621
989-848-2279
Fax: 979-848-2280
info@CampBarakel.org
www.campbarakel.org

Five-day Christian camp experience in mid-August for campers ages 13-55 who are physically disabled, visually impaired, upper trainable mentally impaired or educable mentally impaired, bus transportation provided from locations in Lansing, Flint, Bay City, and Marshall, Michigan.

Lee Brown, Program Director
Mike Alchin, Resident Missionary Staff
Teresa Alchin, Resident Missionary Staff

8770 Camp Fish Tales
2177 Erickson Road
Pinconning, MI 48650
989-879-5199
www.campfishtales.org

Larry Hammond, Chair
Lara Beth Sullivan, Executive Director
Brad Sullivan, Assistant Director

8771 Eric RicStar Winter Music Therapy Summer Camp
4930 S. Hagadorn Rd.
East Lansing, MI 48823
517-353-7661
Fax: 517-355-3292
commusic@msu.edu
www.cms.msu.edu

The purpose of this camp is to provide opportunities for musical expression, enjoyment and interaction for all people with special needs and their siblings.

Cindy Edgerton, Director
Judy Winter, Co-Chair

8772 Indian Trails Camp
0-1859 Lake Michigan Drive NW
Grand Rapids, MI
616-677-5251
Fax: 616-677-2955
www.indiantrails-camp.org

Year round residential camping program for children and adults with physical disabilities.

Lynn Gust, Executive Director

Minnesota

8773 Camp Friendship
Friendship Ventures
10509 108th Street NW
Annandale, MN 55302
952-852-0101
800-450-8376
Fax: 952-852-0123
fv@friendshipventures.org
truefriends.org

Camp Friendship offers kids, teens, and adults the chance to have the time of their lives. The program focuses on building self-esteem and independence, and practicing social skills; and we nurture each person's strengths and abilities and encourage participation in activies at their own pace. Specially designed for persons with developmental, physical or multiple disabilities, special medical conditions, Down syndrome, autism or other conditions. Weekend camps and longer available.

Jon Salmon, Director of Programs and Services
Mel Kloek, Program Director
Dawn Brenner, Director of Health Care

8774 Camp New Hope
Friendship Ventures
53035 Lake Avenue
McGregor, MN 55760
952-852-0101
800-450-8376
Fax: 952-852-0123
fv@friendshipventures.org
truefriends.org

Camp New Hope is a great place for children, teens, and adults to have the time of their lives. The program provides a unique opportunity for having fun, learning skills, boosting confidence, and making friends. Services are specifically designed for persons with developmental, phyisical or multiple disabilities, special medical needs, Down syndrome, autism, or other conditions. Weekend camps and longer available. Other services available throughout the year.

Jon Salmon, Director of Programs and Services
Mel Kloek, Program Director
Dawn Brenner, Director of Health Care

8775 Camp Winnebago
19708 Camp Winnebago Road
Caledonia, MN 55921
507-724-2351
Fax: 507-724-3786
director@campwinnebago.org
www.campwinnebago.org

We offer one week summer sessions for children and adults with developmental disabilities. We also do integrated youth sessions to allow friends and siblings to attend with our traditional campers. Respite week-ends are offered monthly throughout the year. Travel vacations are also offered as an option. We also have a campground open to the public.

8-12 pages

Terry Chiglo, President
Eileen Loken, Vice President
Jane Palen, Secretary

8776 Courage Camps
Courage Center
3915 Golden Valley Road
Golden Valley, MN 55422
952-852-0101
800-450-8376
Fax: 952-852-0123
camping@mtn.org
truefriends.org

Summer resident camp serving children and adults who have physical or sensory disabilities. Also for children who need the help of a speech clinician. Special sessions include those for children who have been burned, children who have cancer and their siblings, and children who have hemophilia or sickle cell anemia. Offers special outdoor education or leadership sessions for deaf, or physically disabled teens and a sports camp for physically disabled and blind teens.

Jon Salmon, Director of Programs and Services
Mel Kloek, Program Director
Dawn Brenner, Director of Health Care

8777   Courage North
PO Box 1626
Lake George, MN 56458   952-852-0101
                                             800-450-8376
                                          Fax: 952-852-0123
                                             truefriends.org

Jon Salmon, Director of Programs and Services
Mel Kloek, Program Director
Dawn Brenner, Director of Health Care

8778   Eden Wood Center
Friendship Ventures
6350 Indian Chief Road
Eden Prairie, MN   952-852-0101
                                             800-450-8376
                                          Fax: 952-852-0123
                                        fv@friendshipventures.org
                                             truefriends.org

Offers resident camp programs for children, teenagers and adults with developmental, physical or multiple disabilities, Down Syndrome, special medical conditions, Williams Syndrome, autism and/or other conditions. Fishing, creative arts, golf, sports and other activities are available. Creative Options Respite Care offers weekend camps year round for children, teenagers and adults. Ventures Travel offers guided vacations for teens and adults with developmental disabilities or other unique needs.

Jon Salmon, Director of Programs and Services
Mel Kloek, Program Director
Dawn Brenner, Director of Health Care

8779   Knutson
523 N 3rd Street
Brainerd, MN   218-828-7610

Provides a camping program for mentally and physically disabled and emotionally disturbed children and adults. Campers must come with an established group that brings its own counselors. Swimming, sailing, archery, nature study and hiking are among the non-competitive activities.

Robert Larson

8780   Search Beyond Adventures
400 S Cedar Lake Road
Minneapolis, MN 800-8   612-374-4845
                                             800-800-800
                                          www.kidscamps.com

Mississippi

8781   Tik-A-Witha
PO Box 126
Van Vleet, MS   662-844-7577
                                          Fax: 662-680-3164
                                          www.kidscamps.com

Missouri

8782   Sidney R. Baer Day Camp
2 Millstone Drive serving campers ages 5-12 years old.
Saint Louis, MO
Astrid Balzer, Special Needs
Andy Brown, Camp Director

Nebraska

8783   Camp Easter Seals
609 N 60th Road
Nebraska City, NE 800-6   402-578-3992
                                             800-800-650
                                          www.kidscamps.com

New Hampshire

8784   Camp Allen
56 Camp Allen Road
Bedford, NH 03110   603-622-8471
                                          Fax: 603-626-4295
                                        mary@campallennh.org
                                        www.campallennh.org

A summer camp for individuals with disabilities.

Sebastian Grasso, Chair
Bret Cote, Vice Chair
Mary Constance, Executive Director

8785   Camp Dartmouth-Hitchcock
1 Medical Center Drive
Lebanon, NH   603-650-5597
                                          Fax: 603-650-8980
                                          www.kidscamps.com

8786   Crotched Mountain School & Rehabilitation Center
1 Verney Drive
Greenfield, NH 3047   603-547-3311
                                             800-800-966
                                          Fax: 603-547-3232
                                        info@crotchedmountain.org
                                             www.cmf.org

Currently serves children ages 6-22 with multiple-handicaps including: Cerebral Palsy, Spina Bifida, visual and hearing impairments and neurological disabilities, developmental disorders, mental retardation, autism, behavioral and emotional disorders, seizure disorders, spinal cord and head injuries. Member of the National Association of Independent Schools and accredited with the NE Association of Schools and Colleges, Independent Schools of Northern NE.

James W. Varnum, Chair
Donald L. Shumway, President & CEO
Tom Zubricki, CFO

New Jersey

8787   Bancroft Camp
1255 Caldwell Road
Cherry Hill, NJ 8034   856-429-0010
                                             800-774-5516
                                          Fax: 207-729-1603
                                          TTY: 856-428-2697
                                        lynn.tomaio@bancroft.org
                                             www.bancroft.org

Has served as a summer camp for children and adults enrolled in Bancroft programs. The camp recognizes the need for individuals with developmental disabilities to vacation with their families. The camp offers a resort program for people wishing to explore the fascinating coast of Maine or to relax in the clean New England air. Accommodations include accessible rustic cabins and bayfront cottages.

Toni Pergolin, MA, CPA, President & CEO
Charles McLister, COO
Thomas J. Burke, MBA, CFO

8788   Camp Chatterbox
200 Portland Rd A-20
Highlands, NJ 7732   908-301-5451
                                        campchatterbox@gmail.com
                                        www.campchatterbox.org

Joan Bruno, Ph.D., Director

8789 Camp Oakhurst
111 Monmouth Road
Oakhurst, NJ 908-531-0215
www.kidscamps.com

8790 Cross Roads Outdoor Ministries
29 Pleasant Grove Road
Port Murray, NJ 7865 908-832-7264
Fax: 908-832-6593
officemanager@crossroadsretreat.com
www.crossroadsretreat.com

Program for ages 6-15 offers Bible study, worship, swimming, crafts, hiking, canoeing and campfires. Special education program for those with developmental disabilities.

Anthony P. Briggs, Executive Director
Kathy Felch, Office Manager
Kathryn Schaefer, Program Director

New Mexico

8791 Santa Fe Mountain Center
PO Box 449
Tesuque, NM 505-983-6158
Fax: 505-983-0460
sky@santafemc.org
www.sf-mc.com

Camp sessions offered to disabled campers from the ages of 1-20.

Juanita Thorne-Connerty, Vice Chair
Seth R. Fullerton, President
Skye Gray, MS, Executive Director

New York

8792 Advocates for Children of New York
151 W 30th Street, 5th Floor
New York, NY 10001 212-947-9779
Fax: 212-947-9790
info@advocatesforchildren.org
www.advocatesforchildren.org

Mental Health

Eric F. Grossman, President
Jamie A. Levitt, Vice President
Kim Sweet, Executive Director

8793 Camp Sun 'N Fun
Routes 322 & 555
Williamstown, NJ 856-629-4502
Fax: 856-875-1499
www.kidscamps.com

8794 Freedom Camp
Carr Bldg, 188 Genesee St, Suite 109
Auburn, NY 13021 315-253-5465

A summer day camp for youths with disabilities sponsored by Freedom Recreational Services. Freedom Camp is offered in two-week sessions at Casey Park in Auburn, New York.

Mary Ellen Perry, Executive Director

8795 Gow School Summer Programs
2491 Emery Road, PO Box 85
South Wales, NY 14139 716-652-3450
Fax: 716-652-3457
summer@gow.org
www.gow.org

Co-ed summer programs for ages 8-16, offer a balanced blend of morning academics, afternoon/evening traditional camp activities and weekend overnight trips (teen-tours). The primary purpose of these programs is to provide a positive experience while balancing these three elements. Committed to the creation of a positive and enjoyable experience for each participant, by defining and merging the goals of the camp and the school, with those of camper students, their families and educators.

M. Bradley Rogers, Jr., Headmaster
Bekah D Atkinson, Admissions Director

8796 Marist Brothers Mid-Hudson Valley Camp Marist Brothers
1455 Broadway, 9W
Esopus, NY 12429 845-384-6620
Fax: 845-384-6479
kids2@esopuscamps.com
www.esopuscamps.com

Individual camps serve different special people: Special Children Camps 1 & 2; Deaf Camp; Young Adult Camp; Sacred Heart Camp; Sr. Pat's Camp; Camp Hope; Molloy Freshman Camp; and Adult Vacation. Cost varies.

Brother Don Nugent, President
Frances Rurley, Coordinator

8797 Oakhurst
853 Broadway
New York, NY 212-253-8680

Accepts children and young adults who are physically handicapped, ages 8-18. The program includes physical therapy, recreational activities and a work program for teenagers.

Marvin Raps

8798 Programs for Children with Special Health Care Needs
Tower Building
Albany, NY 518-474-2084
cx104@health.state.ny.us

Claudia Lee, Acting Director

8799 Programs for Infants and Toddlers with Disabilities: Ages Birth Through 2
Box 2000
Albany, NY 12220 518-473-7016
800-698-4543
TTY: 877-898-5849
dmn02@health.state.ny.us
www.autismgateway.com/resources_NY.html

Donna M Noyes, PhD, Director

8800 Ramapo Anchorage Camp
PO Box 266
Rhinebeck, NY 12572 Residential program for children, ages 4-16, with a wide range of emotional, behavoral, and learning problems. A one-to-one ratio of counselors-to-campers enables children to build healthy relationships, increase self-esteem and improve learning skills. Character values such as honesty, concern for others, responsibility, and the courage to do one's best are encouraged. Campers demonstrate significant gains in their ability to maintain relationships, control impulses and adjust.

8801 Wagon Road
Children's Aid Society
431 Quaker Road
Chappaqua, NY 10514 914-238-4761
Fax: 914-238-0714
www.childrensaidsociety.org

Provides residential respite services to developmentally disabled children ages 7-18. At its 50 acre campus which is entirely wheelchair accessible, 24 hour RN and MD services are provided.

Phoebe Boyer, President & CEO
William D. Weisberg, PhD, EVP & COO
Dan Lehman, VP & CFO

North Carolina

8802 Camp Winding Gap
Rural Route 1, Box 56
Lake Toxaway, NC 828-966-4520
Fax: 828-883-8720
www.campwindinggap.com

For boys and girls ages 8-16, with facilities for up to 75 campers. A high staff-camper ratio (less than 1 to 3) of carefully selected counselors provides a nurturing family atmosphere. A few children with disabilities are mainstreamed each session. Must be able to handle horseback riding and rugged terrain, this is a ranch type camp in a farm setting with many animals. Program includes regular camp activities.

Ann Hertzberg, Director

8803 Talisman Programs
64 Gap Creek Road
Zirconia, NC 28790   828-669-8639
                                       888-458-8226
                                       Fax: 828-669-2521
                            summer@stonemountainschool.com
                            www.talismansummercamp.com

Talisman Programs offers summer programs for kids ages 8-17
with ADHD, learning disabilities, high functioning autism, or
Aspergers Syndrome. Our high-adventure programs include paddling, hiking, rock climbing, an Alpine Tower, swimming, arts
and crafts, and many other activities designed to promote communication and cooperation skills. We focus on building social skills
and self esteem in 2 and 3 week programs. One session of
academics.

Linda Tatsapaugh, Director

Ohio

8804 Camp Allyn
1414 Lake Allyn Road
Batavia, OH   513-732-0240
                                       Fax: 513-735-1461
                                       ssc@one.net
                            www.steppingstonecenter.org

A camp for children and adults with disabilities.

Dennis Carter, Associated Director

8805 Highbrook Lodge Camp
12412 Aquilla Road
Chardon, OH   216-791-8118
                                       Fax: 216-791-1101
                            mmullin@clevelandsightcenter.org
                            www.clevelandsightcenter.org

A summer residential camp for blind and disabled children, adults
and families.

Mike Mullin, Director

Oregon

8806 Easter Seals Oregon Camping Program
5757 SW Macadam Avenue
Portland, OR 800-5   503-228-5108
                                       Fax: 503-228-1352
                                       camp@oregonseals.org
                            www.kidscamps.com

8807 Mt Hood Kiwanis Camp
9320 SW Barbur Blvd, Suite 165
Portland, OR 97219   503-272-3288
                                       Fax: 503-452-0062
                            www.kidscamps.com

Pennsylvania

8808 Briarwood Day Camp
1380 Creek Road
Furlong, PA 18925   215-598-7143
                                       Fax: 215-598-9813
                                       info@briarwood-camp.com
                            www.briarwood-camp.com

A comprehensive day camp providing lunch and transportation
for children with disabilities.

Ted Levin

8809 Camp Lee Mar
450 Route 590
Lackawaxen, PA   570-685-7188
                                       Fax: 570-685-7590
                                       gtour400@aol.com
                            www.leemar.com

A camp for children with developmental challenges, ages 5-21.
Offers a program of academics, speech therapy, vocational training and recreation. The academic program is designed to help
each child develop skills in the areas of communication, reading
and math. Activities include swimming, boating, team sports, tennis and perceptual motor training.

Ari Segal, MSW, Director
Lynsey Trohoske, BA, Asst. Dir./ Admissions Director
Laura Leibowitz, BA, M.Ed, Asst. Dir./ Academic Coordinator

8810 Camp Yomeca Upper Perkiomen Valley YMCA
476 Pottstown Avenue
Pennsburg, PA 18073   215-679-9622
                                       drothenberger@fvymca.org
                            www.fvymca.org/youth/

The YMCA day camp for children ages 4-18. Small group and
camp-wide activities are offered. Streams, woods and trails to explore. Children ages 10-12 also have several overnights offered
to them during the summer. Children continue to build upon established skills from earlier years, take on more leadership, challenge and responsibility and strengthen past friendships.

Debbie Rothensberger, Camp Contact; School Age Care Dir

8811 Keystone Community Resources
100 Abington Executive Park
Carks Summit, PA 18411   570-702-8000
                                       Fax: 570-702-8093
                            LCunningham@keycommres.com
                            www.keycommres.com

Keystone serves both children and adults with developmental disabilities in a variety of residential settings. Support services include 24 hour supervision, on site nursing services, special and
therapeutic recreation programs and psychological and
psychiatric services.

Robert Fleese, President
Lisa Cunningham, Director Admissions
Ignatz Deutsch, Founder

8812 Variety Club Camp & Development Center
Variety Club
A Bound campthe Poratioe Road
Feasterville, PA 19053

A camp and recreation facility for children with special needs and their families. Includes summer camping, aquatics,
weekend retreats and other specialty programs.

South Carolina

8813 Burnt Gin Camp
SC Department of Health and Environmental Control
Box 101106
Columbia, SC   803-898-0455
                                       Fax: 803-898-0613
                            aimonemi@columb60.dhec.state.sc.us
                            www.scdhec.net/hs/mch/burntgin/hsbgin5.htm

A residential camp for children who have physical disabilities
and/or chronic illnesses. Camper/staff ratio is 2:1. Four
seven-day sessions for 7-15 year olds and two six-day sesssions
for 16-19 year olds. Limited to residents of South Carolina.

Marie I Aimone, Camp Director

Tennessee

8814 Camp Easter Seal
750 Old Hickory Blvd, #2-260
Brentwood, TN 37027   615-292-6640
                                       Fax: 615-251-0994
                            www.tn.easter-seals.org

John Pfeiffer, Chair
Chuck Mataya, Vice Chair
Rita Baumgartner, President & CEO

Texas

8815 Children's Association for Maxiumum Potential CAMP
PO Box 27086
San Antonio, TX 78227   210-671-5411
                                          Fax: 210-671-5225
                                      campmail@campcamp.org
                                          www.campcamp.org

Overnight camping, day-care, respite and rehabilitation to children with severe medical, physical or mental disabilities. Large medical staff enables nationwide acceptance of children with severe problems.

Mike Zerda, Chair
Susan Osborne, Executive Director
Ben Elble, Camp Director

8816 Hughen Center
2849 9th Avenue
Port Arthur, TX 77642   409-983-6659
                                          Fax: 409-983-6408
                                  www.hughencenter.org/contact_us

The Center provides a therapeutic, educational, and recreational program for children with physical disabilities. Physical and occupational therapy are featured. Day and residential.

Jeff Kuchar, Executive Director

8817 Texas Lions Camp
Lions Clubs of Texas
PO Box 290247
Kerrville, TX 78029   830-896-8500
                                               830-896-8500
                                          Fax: 830-896-3666
                                              tlc@ktc.com
                                          www.lionscamp.com

The primary purpose of Texas Lions camp is to provide, without charge, a camp for physically disabled, hearing/vision impaired and diabetic children from the State of Texas, regardless of race, religion, or national origin. Our goal is to create an atmosphere wherein campers will learn the can do philosophy and be allowed to achieve maximum personal growth and self esteem. The camp welcomes boys and girls ages 7-16.

Stephen Mabry, Executive Director
Doug Parker, Business Manager
Steven King, Program/Client Service Director

Utah

8818 Camp Kostopulos
4180 Emigration Canyon Road
Salt Lake City, UT 84108   801-582-0700
                                          Fax: 801-583-5176
                                              www.campk.org

One of only a few camps in the Intermountain region that provides recreational opportunities for individuals of all ages with mental or physical disabilities. Activities include fifteen days of swimming, fishing, fieldtrips, nature study, arts and crafts and traditional outdoor adventure games. Five year-round programs offered.

John Miller, Chairman
Rick Lifferth, Vice Chairman
Layne Smith, Vice Chairman

Vermont

8819 Farm and Wilderness Camps
HCR 70, Box 27
Plymouth, VT   802-422-3761
                                               802-422-3761
                                          Fax: 802-422-8660
                                          www.kidscamps.com

Virginia

8820 Camp Baker Services
7600 Beach Road
Chesterfield, VA   804-748-4789
                                          Fax: 804-796-6889
                          www.veryspecialcamps.com/summer-camps/Camp-Baker-Ser

Year round support services for children and adults with disabilities. Operated by the Richmond Area ARC, programs include: an 8-week summer camp program; weekend congregate respite services; summer day camp (8 wks); spring fling (spring break).

Melissa Wahers, Director
Jolene Loving, Assistant Director
Heather Elliot, Administrative Assistant

8821 Camp Easter Seal East, Camp Easter Seal We st
201 E Main Street
Salem, VA 800-3   540-362-1656
                                          Fax: 540-563-8928
                                      www.campeasterseal-va.org

Six and 12 day summer camp sessions for children and adults ages 5 and older with physical disabilities, cognitive disabilities, sensory impairments. Therapeutic recreation activities including swimming, fishing, sports, horseback riding, rock climbing, and more. 26 speech therapy camp children with disabilities ages 8-16. 12 day Spina Bifida Self Help Skills Camp.

Deborah Duerk, Director
Devin Brown, Director

8822 Camp Holiday Trails
400 Holiday Trails Lane
Charlottesville, VA 22903   434-977-3781
                                          Fax: 434-977-8814
                      info@campholidaytrails.org, campisgood@c
                                      www.campholidaytrails.org

A nonprofit camp for children with special health needs, various chronic illnesses. Residential, 1 and 2 week sessions are open June - August; camperships are available. Coed 5-17, nationwide and international. Canoeing, swimming, horseback riding, arts and crafts, drama, ropes course, etc. 24-hr. medical supervision by doctor and nursing staff. Air conditioned cabins.

Tina LaRoche, Executive Director

8823 Makemie Woods Camp Conference Center
PO Box 39
Barhamsville, VA 23011   757-566-1496
                                               800-566-1496
                                          Fax: 757-566-8803
                                          mike@makwoods.org
                                          www.makwoods.org

Counselors serve as teachers, friends and activity leaders. The individual is important within the small group. No camper is lost in the crowd, but is an integral partner in the group process. Residential Christian Camp and conference center. Summer camp for children 8-18 special camp for children with diabetes.

Michelle Burcher, Director
Beth Martin, Office Assistant

8824 Overlook
RR 1, Box 203
Keezletown, VA   540-269-2267

A Christian life experience for youth and children, located at the base of the scenic Massanutten Mountains.

Ronald Robey

8825 Triangle D Camp for Children
1701 North Beauregard Street
Alexandria, VA 22311   414-248-1330
                                               800-342-2383

Disabled campers.

Marilyn Caras

8826 Mountain Milestones Stepping Stones
15 Cottage Street
Morgantown, WV 800-9
304-296-0150
800-800-982
Fax: 304-296-0194
stepping@westco.net
www.kidscamps.com

A nonprofit organization.

Missy Weimex, Recreation Coordinator

8827 Camp Joy
W7725 Kettle Moraine Drive
Whitewater, WI 53190
262-473-3132
Fax: 262-473-0941
www.campjoy.org

A year round residential camping program for children and adults with mental retardation and physical disabilities. Brochure, video, and application available upon request.

Charlie Hatchett, Camp Director
Todd Hatchett, Program & Promotion
Dannett Smith, JBCF Secretary & Promotion

8828 Timbertop Nature Adventure Camp
Stevens Point Area YMCA-Glacier Hollow
1000 Division Street
Stevens Point, WI 54481
715-342-2980
Fax: 715-342-2987
pmatthai@spymca.org
www.glacierhollow.com/timbertop-camp/

For children who can benefit from an individualized program of learning in a non-competitive outdoor setting under the skilled leadership of people who understand the environment and the unique potential of these children.

Pete Matthai, Camp Director

Grant a Wish Foundations

8829 Children's Dream Factory of Maine
400 US Route 1, ATTN: Doris Simard
Falmouth, ME 04105
207-781-3406
800-639-1492

Grants wishes for chronically or seriously ill children from Maine.

8830 Children's Wish Foundation
8615 Roswell Rd
Atlanta, GA 30350
770-393-WISH
800-323-WISH
Fax: 770-393-0683
www.childrenswish.org

Atlanta-based organization that grants wishes for children with life-threatening illnesses who have not yet reached their 18th birthday. Focuses primarily on children who reside in Florida, but has also granted wishes to children from other parts of the US, Canada, England, and Russia.

8831 Dream Factory
120 W Broadway, Suite 300
Louisville, KY 40202
502-561-3001
800-456-7556
Fax: 502-561-3004
dfinfo@dreamfactoryinc.org
www.dreamfactoryinc.org

The Dream Factory grants dreams to children disagnosed with critical or chronic illnesses who are 3 through 18 years of age.

David Zukowski, Director of Program Services
Janice Harris, President
Ralph Coldiron, Vice President

8832 Famous Fone Friends
9101 Sawyer Street
Los Angeles, CA 90035
310-204-5683
fonefriends@aol.com
www.famousfonefriends.org

Offers the ability for a sick child's doctor or nurse to arrange for a well-known actor, athlete or other celebrity to call the child.

8833 Freedom's Wings International
324 Charles Street
Coopersberg, PA 18036
800-382-1197
rrfucci@earthlink.net
www.freedomswings.org

Freedom's Wings International (FWI) is a non-profit organization run by and for people with physical disabilities. We provide the opportunity for those who are physically challenged to fly in specially adapted sailplanes, either as a passenger or as a member of the flight training program.

8834 Give Kids the World
210 S Bass Road
Kissimmee, FL 34746
407-396-1114
800-995-5437
Fax: 407-396-1207
dream@gktw.org
www.gktw.org

Makes dreams come true for children with life-threatening illnesses and their families with a week-long, cost-free fantasy vacation to our 'story book' village located near central Florida's most beloved attractions.

Sarah Jones, Communications Manager

8835 Magic Moments- Children's Hospital of Alabama
2112 11th Aves., Ste 219
Birmingham, AL 35205
205-939-9372
Fax: 205-939-6717
info@magicmoments.org
www.magicmoments.org

Grants wishes to children four to nineteen living or being treated in Alabama, who have chronic, life-threatening diseases, or who have severe trauma (burns, spinal cord, head trauma).

8836 Make A Wish Foundation of America
4742 N 24th St, Ste 400
Pheonix, AZ 85016
602-279-9474
800-722-9474
Fax: 602-279-0855
www.wish.org

Information and advocacy resources for families and professionals. Includes listings of organizations providing general information and organizations focusing on more specific areas of concern to families and young adults who have disabilities.

8837 Sunshine Foundation
1041 Mill Creek Drive
Feasterville, PA 19053
215-396-4770
800-767-1976
Fax: 215-396-4774
philly@sunshinefoundation.org
www.sunshinefoundation.org

Grants dreams of seriously ill, physically challenged and abused children ages 3-18 whose parents cannot fulfill their request due to the financial strain caused by the child's illness.

Diane Mazzeo, Admin Assistant

8838 Teddi Project
Camp Good Days and Special Times
356 North Midler Avenue
Syracuse, NY 13206
315-434-9477
Fax: 315-434-9590
www.campgooddays.org

Priority given to children from Central Florida and the upstate New York area, especially Buffalo, Rochester, Syracuse, Albany, and Binghamton. Services chronically or terminally ill children ages seven to seventeen.

8839 Thursday's Child
PO Box 95
Mt. Hope, WI 53816   608-988-4234
dorothyf@chorus.net

Grants wishes to seriously ill children who live in or are being
treated in southwest and south central Wisconsin.

8840 Wish Upon a Star
California Law Enforcement
PO Box 4000
Visalia, CA 93278   559-733-7753
Fax: 559-733-0962
info@wishuponastar.org
www.wishuponastar.org

Serves children in the state of California. Nonprofit, law enforcement effort designed to grant wishes of children afflicted with
high-risk and terminal illnesses.

Carmen Perez, Executive Director

8841 Wish with Wings
3817 Alamo Ave
Ft. Worth, TX 76107   817-469-9474
Fax: 817-275-6005
wish@awishwithwings.org
www.awishwithwings.org

Founded in 1982, grants wishes for children ages three-eighteen
years of age who have life threatening diseases. The organization
serves children who reside in or are receiving treatment in the
state of Texas.

Kim Christian, Executive Director

8842 Wishing Star Foundation
139 S Sherman
Spokane, WA 99202   509-744-3411
Fax: 509-744-3414
info@wishingstar.org
www.wishingstar.org

Serves Idaho, eastern and western Washington. Grants wishes to
children ages three to twenty-one with life-threatening diseases.

Paula Nordgaarden, Executive Director

8843 Wishing Well Foundation
3000 West Esplanade Ave, Ste 100
Metaine, LA 70002   888-663-9474
www.wishingwellusa.org

Grants wishes to children in the St. Louis area only who are
chronically or terminally ill.

Description

Cardiovascular

The cardiovascular system, also known as the circulatory system, consists of the heart and the blood vessels. The functions of the cardiovascular system include the following:

- To maintain the continual flow of blood throughout the body to provide cells with oxygen and vital nutrients

- To assist in the removal of carbon dioxide and other waste products from cells

The Heart

Anatomy

The heart, a hollow, muscular organ the approximate size and shape of a clenched fist, is an efficient pump that maintains the continuous flow of blood through the vessels to all areas of the body. It is located between the lungs in approximately the center of the chest, with its right margin located under the right side of the breastbone (sternum) and the remaining areas pointing toward the left. The "tip" or the lowest point of the heart, known as the apex, rests on the diaphragm and is situated beneath the left nipple.

The heart consists of four chambers and is divided into left and right sides by a thick, fibrous, central partition known as the septum. The upper chambers of the heart are known as atria, and the lower chambers are called ventricles. Each chamber is referred to by its location: i.e., the left and right atria and the left and right ventricles. The atria are smaller and have thinner walls than the ventricles. The walls of the chambers of the heart are composed of specialized cardiac muscle known as the myocardium, and their internal surfaces are lined with a thin layer of smooth membrane tissue called the endocardium.

The heart and the roots of its major blood vessels are surrounded by a membrane (pericardium) that consists of two fibrous layers. The pericardium has a tough outer layer (fibrous pericardium) that surrounds the heart like a loose-fitting bag, providing space for the heart to beat. The inner layer (serous pericardium) consists of an innermost "sheet" (visceral layer) that is attached to the heart and an outermost layer (parietal layer) that lines the inside of the fibrous pericardium. A space between the inner layers contains a thin film of fluid that lubricates the opposing surfaces of the inner membranes, enabling the heart to beat without friction.

Cardiac Function

Contraction of the heart muscle is termed systole, whereas relaxation is known as diastole. The atria and ventricles beat in a precise rhythmic pattern. One cycle of this pattern is known as a heartbeat. As the atria contract, they force blood into the ventricles. Once the ventricles fill with blood, they contract, pumping blood either to the lungs or out to the rest of the body.

The pumping action of the heart also involves the heart valves at the entrance to and exit from the ventricles. These valves control and direct the flow of blood through the heart. Two heart valves separate the atria from the ventricles (atrioventricular valves), preventing the backward flow of blood into the atria during ventricular contraction. The valves include the mitral or bicuspid valve, situated between the left atrium and left ventricle, and the tricuspid valve, located between the right atrium and right ventricle. In addition, two heart valves (semilunar valves) are situated between the two ventricles and the large blood vessels that transport blood away from the heart during ventricular contractions. The aortic semilunar valve, located where the major artery of the body (aorta) arises from the base of the left ventricle, enables blood to flow from the left ventricle into the aorta while preventing the backward flow of blood into the ventricle. The pulmonary semilunar valve, situated where the pulmonary artery arises from the base of the right ventricle, enables blood to flow from the right ventricle to the lungs while preventing the backward flow of blood.

"Oxygen-poor" or deoxygenated blood that has circulated through the body enters the right side of the heart into the right atrium through two large veins (the superior and inferior vena cava). The blood is then pumped through the tricuspid valve into the right ventricle. When the ventricle contracts, blood is pumped through the pulmonary semilunar valve into the pulmonary artery and on to the lungs, where the exchange of oxygen and carbon dioxide occurs. Oxygen-rich blood is returned to the left atrium by way of four pulmonary veins and is pumped through the bicuspid valve into the left ventricle. When the ventricle contracts, blood is pumped through the aortic semilunar valve into the aorta for circulation to the body's tissues.

The heart muscle or myocardium requires an ongoing supply of oxygen and other nutrients to function efficiently; thus, the coronary circulation transports vital oxygen-rich (oxygenated) and nutrient-rich arterial blood to the heart muscle and returns deoxygenated, nutrient-poor blood back to the venous system. Blood is transported to the myocardium by way of the left and right coronary arteries, which are the first branches of the aorta. Once blood is circulated to the myocardium, supplying the heart with oxygen and other nutrients, it passes into the cardiac veins, which then empty into the coronary sinus and into the right atrium.

Each heartbeat, also known as a cardiac cycle, consists of the contraction (systole) and relaxation (diastole) of the atria and ventricles. In order for the heart to pump efficiently, the different areas of the heart and the cardiac muscle fibers must work together in an exact sequence. Precise coordination is achieved through the transmission of electrical impulses originating from the heart's "pacemaker" (the sinoatrial node at the apex of the right atrium). These signals are then relayed to the various areas of the heart via a complex system of fibers (atrioventricular node, bundle of His, and Purkinje fibers). The electrical transmissions are delivered with precision timing to various areas of the heart, resulting in a rhythmic beat.

The Blood Vessels

Blood vessels are like a system of complex tubing of different sizes through which blood flows to various parts of the body. Different types of blood vessels have different purposes. For example:

- Some vessels ensure the movement of blood from one part of the body to another.

- Other much smaller vessels (i.e., the capillaries) facilitate the exchange of certain nutrients and waste products between the blood and the fluid surrounding cells within bodily tissues.

Function

There are several types of blood vessels including arteries, arterioles, capillaries, venules, and veins. The arteries, which carry blood away from the heart, progressively subdivide into smaller and smaller vessels known as arterioles, which control blood flow into the minute vessels known as capillaries. The arterioles help to regulate proper arterial blood distribution and pressure by constricting or expanding as necessary. The thin walls of microscopic capillaries facilitate the exchange of nutrients and waste products between the blood and tissue fluid surrounding the cells. For example, oxygen and glucose move from the blood in the capillaries to the fluid surrounding cells and then into the cells themselves; in contrast, carbon dioxide and other waste products move from the cells into the blood within the capillaries. The oxygen-poor blood then flows from the capillaries into the small blood vessels known as venules. The venules join with other venules and progressively increase in size, becoming larger veins that transport the blood toward the heart.

The systemic circulation also includes a specialized group of vessels known as the hepatic portal circulation, within which blood flow follows a somewhat different route. Veins from certain organs, such as the stomach, intestines, spleen, pancreas, and gallbladder, do not transport blood directly into the inferior vena cava but, rather, into the hepatic portal vein, which carries blood to veins, venules, and capillaries within the liver. Nutrients pass from the blood in the capillaries into liver cells where various toxic substances are filtered from the blood. Hepatic veins carry blood from the liver and rejoin the systemic circulation via the inferior vena cava.

Structure

Arteries and veins consist of three layers including an outermost layer (tunica adventitia), a middle layer of smooth muscle (involuntary muscle) tissue (tunica media), and an inner lining (tunica intima or endothelium). The middle layer of arteries is thicker than that of veins, enabling the arteries to withstand the pressure of ventricular contractions. In contrast, blood returning to the heart via the veins remains at a relatively low pressure. The passage of blood through the veins is assisted by involuntary muscle that compresses the walls of the veins; in addition, veins have one-way valves that prevent the backward flow of blood.

Capillaries have extremely thin walls and cannot be seen by the naked eye. They consist of only one layer (tunica intima), enabling oxygen and certain wastes to easily pass through them.

Fetal Blood Circulation

Because the developing fetus must obtain nutrients and oxygen from the mother's blood, the fetal circulation differs somewhat from the circulation after birth. During pregnancy, blood vessels carry fetal blood to the placenta, where oxygen and nutrients are exchanged between the fetal and maternal blood supply, and then return blood to the fetus. Two relatively small umbilical arteries carry deoxygenated blood, whereas a larger umbilical vein carries oxygen-rich blood. The fetal circulation also includes vascular channels or openings (e.g., ductus venosus, ductus arteriosus, foramen ovale), enabling most blood to bypass the developing liver and lungs. In most cases, once an infant is born and the pulmonary circulation is established, such vascular channels close and the umbilical blood vessels collapse soon after birth.

Description

Cells

The human body consists of literally trillions of atoms, molecules, and cells that are organized in several "structural levels."

Atoms and molecules. Atoms of oxygen, sodium, nitrogen, and carbon, for example, are the infinitesimal components of the most basic level of living matter of the body. Atoms link to one another to form molecules.

Cells. These are the smallest structural units that are able to live independently. The human body has billions of cells that are functionally integrated to perform the complex, vital tasks necessary for sustaining life. Cells are organized in the following ways:

- Tissues. Bodily tissues are organizations of structurally similar, specialized cells that carry out a common function.

- Organs. The organs of the body are groupings of two or more different types of tissues incorporated into a functional, structural unit to perform certain, specialized functions.

- Bodily systems. These comprise the final level of structural organization within the body. Bodily systems consist of several, interdependent organs that work together to perform integrated functions.

Certain mechanisms enable cells of the body to conduct activities that are vital for ongoing growth and survival. These include the processes of metabolism and homeostasis.

Metabolism

Metabolism refers to all the physical and chemical processes occurring within the body's tissues and includes catabolism and anabolism. Catabolism refers to the breakdown of large, complex substances into simpler, smaller substances, usually resulting in the release of energy. During anabolism, complex substances are built up from simpler substances, usually resulting in consumption of energy. The processes of respiration, circulation, digestion, and excretion, for example, collectively enable the body to provide those substances required for metabolism and remove the byproducts or waste products of metabolism. Abnormal changes in genetic material (mutations) or inherited defective genes may cause inborn errors of metabolism, affecting the body's ability to function properly.

Homeostasis

Homeostasis refers to the processes by which the body maintains a balanced internal environment (equilibrium). In order to maintain homeostasis, the body requires oxygen, water, other nutrients, and regulated atmospheric pressure and body temperature, for example. Because disturbances from the external environment as well as cellular activity continually challenge internal equilibrium, the body has ongoing self-regulating systems (feedback systems) that induce the responses necessary to maintain or restore homeostasis. For example, abnormally decreased levels of oxygen in the blood are counteracted by increased breathing rates that restore normal blood oxygen levels.

Cells

Cells are extremely complex, containing several subcellular structures vital to life. Human cells vary greatly in size and shape and are adapted for their specific functions. However, most cells are similar in structure. They contain fluid material known as cytoplasm surrounded by a thin, outer membrane (plasma membrane). The plasma membrane separates the fluid and specialized structures (organelles) within each cell from the fluid that surrounds and bathes the cells of the body. The cytoplasm of most human cells contains a circular, membrane-bound structure known as the nucleus.

Plasma Membrane

The plasma membrane serves to keep cells intact. In addition, it regulates the entry of oxygen and certain vital nutrients into cells and enables the passage of carbon dioxide and other waste materials out of cells. Certain protein molecules on the surface of the plasma membrane also bind with other protein molecules, activating particular cellular functions.

Cytoplasm

The cytoplasm is essentially the "living matter" of the cell, containing the fluid that comprises the cell's inner environment and the specialized parts known as organelles. The organelles include the following:

- Ribosomes are relatively tiny particles that function as "protein factories." They produce proteins, which are large molecules consisting of combinations of certain chemical "building blocks" (amino acids). Proteins play an essential role in the body. Particular proteins serve as the source of "building materials" for certain tissues and organs of the body (e.g., muscle, skin, blood, etc.). Other protein compounds known as enzymes accelerate the rate of chemical reactions in the body. Proteins also play an essential role in the elimination of waste materials and have many other functions.

- Endoplasmic reticulum (ER) is a complex network of small tubular membranes arranged in complex folds. This network winds throughout the cytoplasm of a cell. Passageways within the endoplasmic reticulum transport proteins and other substances to different areas within a cell. Rough ER has a rough texture due to the presence of ribosomes attached to its outer surface. Carbohydrates, fats, and certain types of proteins are manufactured within smooth ER.

- The Golgi apparatus, which is located near the nucleus, is a system of microscopic, stacked membranous sacs and spaces. Small "bubbles" or sacs (vesicles) from the smooth ER transport newly produced proteins to the Golgi apparatus, where they fuse with the Golgi sacs. The Golgi apparatus then processes and modifies the proteins and packages them into small vesicles. These vesicles break away and eventually fuse with the plasma membrane, at which point they break open and release their contents outside of the cell for transport to other cells.

- Centrioles are typically paired rod-like structures that participate in cell division.

- Mitochondria are tiny organelles that have double membranes and sacs with inner, folded partitions. Known as the "power plants" of the cells, the mitochondria serve as the major source of cellular energy production due to their complex, ongoing chemical reactions.

- Lysosomes are the major digestive units of cells. Enzymes within lysosomes break down (digest) particles of nutrients as well as certain invading particles such as bacteria.

- Cilia are hair-like projections on the surfaces of certain cells that move together in a wave-like manner. For example, cilia within the mucous membranes of the respiratory tract (respiratory mucosa) propel mucus upward and out of the tract.

Nucleus
The nucleus regulates cellular activities by controlling the functions of the organelles and cell reproduction. It is surrounded by a nuclear envelope that encloses a cellular material within the nucleus known as nucleoplasm. Pores within the nuclear envelope's membranes enable the interior of the nucleus to "communicate" with the cell's cytoplasm. The nucleoplasm of the nucleus contains several structures including the nucleolus and chromatin.

The nucleolus regulates the formation of ribosomes within the nucleus. Ribosomes then move through the nuclear envelope to the cell's cytoplasm where they engage in protein production.

Chromatin, the material within the nucleus from which chromosomes are created, consists of thread-like structures comprised of protein and deoxyribonucleic acid (DNA). DNA is the carrier of the genetic code and is described as a "double helix" because of its relatively long, spiraling, lad-

der-like structure. It consists of strands of certain chemical groups that are linked by pairs of substances known as "bases." There are four types of bases including adenine, which always pairs with thymine, and the base cytosine, which always pairs with guanine. Therefore, the sequence of bases on one strand of the helix coincides with the sequence on the other strand, enabling DNA molecules to duplicate before cell division.

Chromosomes
During the division and reproduction of cells, DNA condenses and gradually forms into the rod-like structures known as chromosomes. The DNA of the chromosomes carries the genetic information that controls the ultimate growth, development, and functioning of the body and determines the expression of certain inherited traits, such as blood groups, various physical characteristics (e.g., hair color, eye color, height), etc.

The cell that is produced when an egg (ovum) is fertilized by a sperm is known as a zygote. With the first and each subsequent division of the zygote, chromosomes within the zygote's nucleus are duplicated. Therefore, in most cases, all cells in the human body contain the same chromosomal material. In rare cases, some individuals may have some cells that contain differences in certain genetic material (mosaicism) due to an error in cellular division.

The nuclei of cells (except for ova and sperm) normally contain 46 individual chromosomes, one of each pair from the mother and the other from the father. Chromosome pairs are numbered from 1 to 22 with a 23rd pair consisting of one X chromosome from the mother and an X or a Y chromosome from the father. Males have an X and a Y chromosome and females have two X chromosomes within the 23rd pair. Each chromosome has a long arm designated "q" and a short arm designated "p." Both arms are further divided into numbered bands. Every individual chromosome contains thousands of genes, which are the hereditary units that contain segments of DNA. Genes function within cells by regulating the production of proteins. The 46 human chromosomes collectively contain approximately 100,000 genes that, together, are referred to as the "human genome."

Chromosomal Disorders
In some cases, due to certain abnormalities during cellular division (meiosis or mitosis), individuals may have abnormalities in the structure or number of chromosomes in the nuclei of cells of the body. There may be extra or missing whole chromosomes or chromosomal material within all or some of the body's cells. Because chromosomes contain many genes, the range and severity of associated symptoms and physical findings may vary greatly, depending upon the exact nature and location of the chromosomal abnormality.

RNA

Genes, which are sections of DNA, regulate the production of certain proteins. Ribonucleic acid or RNA is essential in "decoding" the inherited instructions within genes. RNA is similar in structure to one strand of DNA, with some differences-e.g., replacement of the base thymine with uracil. During the formation of RNA, a strand of DNA "unwinds" and a duplicate copy of a gene sequence is created. This copy is known as messenger RNA or mRNA. The mRNA migrates from the nucleus to the cytoplasm, promoting protein production in the ribosomes and endoplasmic reticulum. The ribosomes use information within the mRNA molecule to translate chemical "building blocks" known as amino acids into a properly sequenced protein strand.

Cellular Reproduction: Mitosis

Most cells of the body are replicated or reproduced during a complex process known as mitosis. During mitosis, a single cell divides in order to form two "daughter cells" with chromosomes identical to those within the original cell. The process of mitosis enables the body to produce new cells, to replace cells that have been damaged or lost due to injury or disease, and to replace cells that have aged and no longer function efficiently.

Sometimes mitosis may become uncontrolled, resulting in the development of an abnormal mass of replicating cells known as a neoplasm. Such growths may be noncancerous (benign tumors) or cancerous (malignant).

Cellular Reproduction: Meiosis

Reproductive cells in the male and female sex glands (gonads, including the testes and ovaries) carry out a different form of cell division known as meiosis. During mitosis, one cell division occurs, creating two daughter cells-each of which contains 46 chromosomes. Unlike mitosis, two cellular divisions occur during meiosis, resulting in four daughter cells-each of which contains half of the chromosomes (i.e., 23 chromosomes).

Genetic Mutations

During the processes of mitosis and meiosis, the chromosomes within an original cell and thus its genetic material (DNA) are replicated and passed along to its daughter cells. Sometimes, errors may occur during this replication process, resulting in small changes or mutations in genetic composition. Such genetic mutations are passed along with every subsequent division of the daughter cell. For example, a genetic mutation may occur during the production of a reproductive cell (ovum or sperm). If that cell is eventually involved in fertilization, the resultant zygote and all of its reproduced cells will contain the same genetic error. Thus, every cell of the developing embryo and fetus will contain the identical mutant gene.

Genes function within cells by directing the manufacture of a particular protein. Therefore, mutations of a particular gene may impair the appropriate production of its protein. The effects of a particular gene mutation depend upon the function of its protein within the body. Disorders that result due to such mutations are termed genetic disorders.

Genetic Disorders

Human traits are the result of the interaction of two genes, one received from the mother and one received from the father. There are typically two genes engaged in the regulation of a particular protein. If one such gene changes or mutates and "overrides" the instructions of the normal gene on the other chromosome, the abnormal gene is said to be dominant. If the mutated gene is not expressed and is "masked" by the normal gene on the other chromosome, the mutated gene is termed recessive. In such cases, two copies of the mutated gene are required for possible expression of the disease trait.

Genetic disorders may be classified into unifactorial and multifactorial defects. Unifactorial genetic disorders result due to abnormalities of a single gene or gene pair. Such disorders may be autosomal or X-linked.

In autosomal dominant disorders, the presence of a single copy of the disease gene results in the disorder. The mutated gene "overrides" or dominates the other normal gene. An affected individual may have inherited the disease gene from one of his or her parents, or the disease may arise as a result of an abnormal change (mutation) that occurred randomly, for unknown reasons (sporadically). If an individual with an autosomal dominant disorder has children, all offspring have a 50 percent risk of inheriting the defective gene.

In autosomal recessive disorders, two copies of the same disease gene are necessary for an individual to potentially develop the disorder. If both parents carry a single copy of the disease gene, all offspring have a 25 percent risk of inheriting both disease genes and expressing the disorder. Fifty percent of their children risk being carriers, and 25 percent may receive both normal genes for that trait.

In X-linked disorders, the disease gene is located on the X chromosome. As discussed earlier, females have two X chromosomes, whereas males have one X chromosome from the mother and one Y chromosome from the father. In females, certain disease traits on the X chromosome may be "masked" by the presence of a normal gene on the other X chromosome. In other cases, certain disease traits may not be fully masked by the normal gene; as a result, some females who carry a single copy of such a disease gene (heterozygous carriers) may express some of the symptoms associated with the disorder. In such cases, heterozygous females often have more variable, less severe symptoms than affected males. Because males have only one X chromosome, if they inherit such a disease gene, they generally express the physical characteristics or other findings associated with the disease and are typically more severely affected than females. Males with X-linked disorders transmit the disease gene to their daughters but not to their sons. Females with one copy of such a disease gene have a 50 percent risk of transmitting the gene to their daughters and their sons.

In multifactorial disorders, susceptibility to a disorder is determined by the interaction of several different genes, possibly in association with the involvement of certain environmental factors.

Tissues

As mentioned above, tissues are groups of structurally similar cells that perform a common function. Different tissues within the human body may vary greatly in terms of the size, shape, and specific functioning of their cells.

There are four main types of tissue in the human body including epithelial tissue, connective tissue, muscle tissue, and nervous tissue.

Epithelial tissue or epithelium covers the surfaces of the body, lines most of its hollow structures or cavities, and serves to provide protection and support. In addition, some epithelial tissues permit the absorption of certain nutrients (e.g., oxygen into the blood); help to protect the body against invading microorganisms; or produce and release certain secretions. The cells within epithelial tissue are tightly packed together and contain no blood vessels; however, blood vessels within underlying connective tissue provide epithelial cells with nutrients. Different types of epithelial tissue are categorized based upon cellular shape and thickness.

Connective Tissue

Connective Tissue

The purpose of connective tissue, the most widely distributed tissue of the body, is to bind together and, along with the skeleton, provide a supporting framework to bodily tissues and organs. The shape and arrangement of connective tissue cells and the intercellular substance between such cells differ depending upon the type of connective tissue. There are several major forms of connective tissue in the body including the following:

- Areolar tissue, which consists of cells embedded in webs of loosely arranged fibers, supports and provides form to most internal organs of the body.

- Adipose tissue, which consists of fat cells within a mesh of areolar tissue, serves to insulate the body against heat loss, protect and cushion certain areas of the body, and store fat as a future energy source.

- Fibrous connective tissue, which consists primarily of parallel rows of white collagen fibers, are the cords of strong, dense, flexible tissue that connect muscle to bone (tendons). Collagen is the major structural protein of the body.

- Bone, the hardest connective tissue of the body, provides a supportive framework, assists in movement, and houses bone marrow.

- Cartilage, which has the consistency of firm or gel-like plastic, helps to absorb shock and provides flexibility.

- Blood, interestingly, is considered to be a type of connective tissue. Even though it has a different function in comparison to other connective tissues, it does have an extracellular liquid matrix (plasma). Plasma has several functions including providing a defense against invading microorganisms, repairing damage to blood vessels and tissues through blood clotting, and transporting oxygen, vital nutrients, and waste products.

The purpose of the body's muscle tissue is to enable movement through muscle contraction and relaxation. The nervous tissue of the body includes specialized cells that ensure ongoing, rapid communication between structures of the body and the control of bodily functions necessary to maintain life.

Description

Dermatologic

The dermatologic system includes the skin, the largest organ of the body, and its derivatives, such as the skin glands, the hair, and the nails. The skin, the sheet-like, outermost covering of body tissue, has several vital functions:

- To serve as a sensory organ. The skin's millions of sensory nerve endings (receptors) serve as somatic sense organs, enabling the body to respond to pain, variations in temperature, pressure or touch sensations, and other important changes in the surrounding environment.

- To help protect the human body from the harmful effects of the sun, chemicals, invading microorganisms, injuries, fluid loss, and other hazards.

- To assist in normalizing the body's temperature through the regulation of blood flow close to the body's surface and sweat secretion. For example, when the body is too cold, blood vessels within the skin constrict to help conserve body heat. When the body is too hot, blood vessels within the inner layer of the skin (dermis) widen (dilate) and the sweat glands secrete perspiration to cool the body.

The skin comprises several tissue layers including a thin, outermost layer (epidermis); a thicker, inner layer (dermis); and a thick underlying layer of subcutaneous tissue, which is a loose layer of connective tissue and fat. The subcutaneous tissue helps to insulate the body from extremes in temperature, protects underlying tissues from injury, and serves as a stored energy source.

Epidermis
The epidermis, which serves as the protective outer layer of skin, is made up of tightly packed cells (epithelial cells) that are arranged in layers. The thickness of the epidermis is variable, depending on its function; for example, it is relatively thick on the palms of the hands, yet comparatively thin on the eyelids.

The outermost layer of the epidermis (stratum corneum epidermidis) consists of dead cells that create a tough, protective covering. As the dead cells are sloughed off, they are replaced by new cells that are produced by rapidly dividing cells within the innermost layer of the epidermis (stratum germinativum). As new cells rise upward though cellular layers (strata) and approach the surface, their cytoplasm-i.e., the inner substance of cells other than the nucleus-is replaced by the tough protein keratin. In addition, specialized cells (melanocytes) within the deepest layer of the epidermis produce melanin, a pigment that gives coloration to the skin.

Dermis
The dermis, the innermost layer of skin, consists of connective tissue; lymph vessels, blood vessels, sensory nerve endings (skin receptors), and muscle fibers; as well as other specialized structures, including sweat glands, sebaceous glands, and hair follicles.

The uppermost portion of the dermis contains rows of peg-like projections (dermal papillae) that help bind together the dermal and epidermal layers (dermal-epidermal junction) and form the characteristic grooves and ridges (dermatoglyphic patterns) on the skin of the palms and tips of the fingers. Such ridges, which are unique to each individual, develop before birth.

The deeper portion of the dermis contains a network of fibers including those that provide the skin with the necessary toughness (collagen fibers) as well as elasticity and the ability to stretch (elastic fibers). The number of elastic fibers decreases with advancing age and the level of fat stored within the subcutaneous tissue is also reduced. Consequently, the skin loses its elasticity.

Skin Glands
The sweat glands within the dermis are classified according to their location and type of secretion. These glands include the eccrine and apocrine glands.

The eccrine glands are the most widespread sweat glands in the body. Their function is to produce sweat or perspiration, which helps to eliminate certain waste products (e.g., uric acid, etc.) and to maintain a constant body temperature.

The apocrine glands, larger glands that produce a thicker secretion than that of the eccrine glands, are primarily located under the arms (axilla) and around the genitals. Such glands begin to function during puberty.

The dermis also contains sebaceous glands, tiny glands that open into hair follicles. They produce an oily secretion known as sebum that helps to lubricate the hair and skin and protect the skin from drying. Sebum secretion increases during adolescence (due to increased levels of certain sex hormones); however, it decreases during later adulthood, contributing to skin wrinkling and cracking.

Hair
When epidermal cells grow into the dermis, a small tube called a hair follicle may be formed. The growth of a hair begins from a tiny cluster of cells (hair papilla) at the base of the follicle. New hair replaces any that has been cut or plucked, for example, as long as the hair papilla is alive. The hair itself is a threadlike structure consisting of dead cells filled with keratin. The root is that portion of the hair that remains hidden within the follicle, whereas the shaft is the visible portion of the hair. A particular hair color results

from the amount and specific form of the pigment melanin that has been produced by melanocytes at the base of the hair follicle. The straightness or curliness of the hair depends upon the shape of the hair follicle.

A few areas of the body are hairless, including the palms of the hands, the soles of the feet, and the lips. Most hair on the body is fine and barely visible, with the most visible hair typically including that on the scalp, the eyebrows, and the eyelashes. Coarse hair also typically develops under the arms and in the pubic area during puberty (i.e., in response to the secretion of certain hormones). In addition, most males also develop coarser hair in the facial area, on the trunk, and on the arms and legs.

Skin Receptors

The dermis also has sensory nerve endings (skin receptors) that function as sense organs (i.e., somatic sense organs), transmitting messages to the brain concerning temperature, touch, pressure, and pain. For example, Pacini's corpuscle receptors, which are located deep within the dermis, detect pressure on the surface of the skin. Meissner's corpuscle receptors, which are usually close to the skin's surface, detect light touch sensations. Other skin receptors include those that detect other touch sensations, cold, heat, vibration, or pain.

Nails

The nails are produced when epidermal cells on the ends of the fingers and toes fill with the tough protein keratin. The nail body is the visible portion of the nail, whereas the remainder of the nail, known as the nail root, is hidden by a fold of skin (cuticle). A portion of the nail body that is closest to the root has a white, crescent-shaped area called the lunula. Tissue underneath the nail, known as the nail bed, contains many blood vessels, causing it to appear pinkish in color.

Description

Digestive

The digestive system consists of organs that break down food into small chemical components that ultimately may be used by cells of the body for energy (metabolism), growth, and repair. It includes the alimentary canal or gastrointestinal (GI) tract, which is the long, hollow passageway through which food passes, as well as associated organs, such as glands whose secreted juices help to break down (digest) food. Organs that comprise the GI tract include the mouth, pharynx, esophagus, stomach, small intestine, large intestine, and anus. Associated organs include the tongue, teeth, gallbladder, and digestive glands, such as the salivary glands, pancreas, and liver.

Nutrients
The foods of an individual's diet primarily include water as well as other nutrients necessary for growth and development. These include proteins, which play an essential role in cell repair and replacement; vitamins; carbohydrates, which serve as the primary energy source and assist in the breakdown and metabolism of other nutrients; fats; and minerals. Most minerals and vitamins may be absorbed into the blood circulation from the digestive system with no change in structure. However, other nutrients must be broken down into smaller, simpler (less complex) food molecules. Food is broken down (digested) through physical and chemical processes. Physical breakdown of food materials is performed by the chewing and grinding actions of the teeth, for example. The actions of certain digestive enzymes (i.e., substances that act as catalysts in the breakdown of proteins and other nutrients) as well as other substances (e.g., acids) chemically break down food as it travels through the GI tract. Thus, the nutrients are reduced into smaller molecules that may be absorbed through the lining of the intestinal wall for distribution to body cells.

Layers of the GI Tract
The hollow internal space within the alimentary canal or GI tract is known as the lumen. The walls of the GI tract consist of four layers of tissue, including an outermost covering (serosa); the mucous membrane (mucosa), which produces the mucus that lines the canal; the submucosa, a layer of connective tissue beneath the mucosa; and underlying layers of muscle tissue (muscularis). Regular, rhythmic contractions of involuntary (smooth) muscle within these layers of underlying muscle tissue propel food through the GI tract in a process known as peristalsis.

Mouth
Digestion begins in the mouth. The roof of the mouth, known as the palate, has a hard, bony, front portion (hard palate) and a soft, fleshy area (soft palate) that consists primarily of muscle. The tongue, which forms most of the floor of the mouth, is a flexible, muscular organ that helps manipulate food during chewing. It also contains the microscopic chemical receptors (taste receptors) that produce the nerve impulses necessary for taste (taste buds).

The teeth, which assist in the chewing and grinding of food, are firmly attached to the upper and lower jaws. The gums (gingiva), which consist of a mucous membrane and supporting fibrous tissues, surround the teeth, serving as "shock absorbers" and keeping the teeth tightly set into the jaws. Enclosing the oral cavity are the cheeks and the upper and lower lip. In addition, as with all of the GI tract, the mouth is lined by a mucous membrane. Saliva, a thin, watery fluid that is secreted by the salivary glands and the mucosa of the mouth, assists in the process of swallowing by moistening the oral mucosa; lubricating food; initiating the breakdown of certain food products through its digestive enzymes; and promoting the sense of taste.

Teeth
The teeth are essential for the chewing, tearing, and grinding of food (mastication) as it mixes with saliva. Humans typically have two sets of teeth including the primary (deciduous) teeth and the permanent (secondary) teeth. There are usually 20 primary teeth that erupt between the ages of six months and two to three years. The primary teeth are gradually replaced by the permanent teeth beginning at about six years of age. Adults typically have 32 permanent teeth.

There are four major types of teeth that are classified based upon their shape and location:

- Incisors are chisel shaped and have sharp edges for cutting during mastication. The incisors are the eight front teeth (i.e., four in the upper jaw and four in the lower jaw).

- Canines or cuspids are sharp, pointed teeth that tear or pierce food. The four canines (i.e., two in the upper jaw and two in the lower jaw) are situated next to the incisors.

- Premolars or bicuspids have large, flat surfaces with two grinding "cusps" to assist in the breakdown of food during mastication. The eight premolars are situated next to and in back of the canines. The primary teeth include no premolars.

- Molars or tricuspids also have large, flat surfaces, yet have three grinding "cusps." The 12 molars are located in back of the premolars. The primary teeth typically include only four molars in the upper jaw and four in the lower jaw. Wisdom teeth are typically known as third molars. They usually erupt in the late teens and early twenties.

The interior of each tooth contains living pulp, which includes connective tissue, sensory nerves, and blood and lymphatic vessels. The pulp is surrounded by the dental tissue known as dentin. In addition, each tooth is divided into a crown, neck, and root. The crown, the exposed portion of a tooth, is covered by enamel, the hardest tissue in the human body. The neck, which is the narrow portion of the tooth surrounded by the gums, and the root, which fits into the bony socket of the lower or upper jaw, are covered by the sensitive dental tissue cementum. A fibrous membrane (periodontal membrane) connects the cementum to the jaw and gums.

Salivary Glands

The salivary glands are the three pairs of glands that secrete saliva. Their secretions are released into ducts that empty into the mouth. Because the salivary glands release their secretions into ducts, they are exocrine glands. The salivary glands include the parotid, submandibular, and sublinqual. The parotid glands, the largest of the salivary glands, are located below and in front of the ears at the angle of the jaws. Their ducts open inside the cheeks. The submandibular glands are located toward the back of the mouth, and their ducts open under the tongue. The ducts of the sublingual glands secrete saliva onto the floor of the mouth. Saliva contains digestive enzymes (salivary amylase) that initiate the chemical digestion of certain foods (e.g. carbohydrates).

Pharynx

The pharynx, also known as the throat, is a muscular tube lined with mucous membranes and is part of the digestive and respiratory systems. Food and fluids enter the throat from the mouth and exit via the esophagus. However, air normally enters the pharynx from the nasal cavities and exits via the larynx. (For more information, please see the section entitled The Respiratory System.)

Esophagus

The esophagus is a muscular tube that transports food from the pharynx to the stomach. It is also lined with mucous membrane. The upper portion of the esophagus is encircled by a ring-shaped muscle (sphincter) that opens to allow the passage of food products. A similar muscle (cardiac sphincter) is located where the esophagus joins the stomach. The walls of the esophagus contain strong smooth muscles fibers, and rhythmic wavelike contractions of these involuntary muscles (peristalsis) propel food toward the stomach.

Stomach

The stomach is a hollow, pouch-like organ located in the upper portion of the abdominal cavity. It continues the breakdown of food that began in the mouth. Once food passes through the cardiac sphincter from the esophagus, it is contained in the stomach by contraction of the ring-shaped muscle at the end of the stomach (pyloric sphincter).

The walls of the stomach consist of three layers of smooth muscle and are lined with mucous membrane containing specialized cells that secrete gastric juices. These juices contain hydrochloric acid and digestive enzymes (e.g., rennin, pepsin) that are necessary for the breakdown of proteins. Rhythmic contractions of the stomach's smooth muscle layers mix digesting food with gastric juices, forming a semiliquid mixture known as chyme. Once partially digested food has been mixed into the chyme, relaxation of the pyloric sphincter and contractions of the stomach propel the chyme into the duodenum of the small intestine.

Small Intestine

The small intestine has three sections: the duodenum, jejunum, and the ileum. The function of the small intestine is to continue the breakdown of food products as they travel through the GI tract and to promote the absorption of nutrients into the bloodstream.

As rhythmic contractions of smooth muscles (peristalsis) propel food through the small intestine, digestive juices from the pancreas and bile from the liver are added to partially digested food within the duodenum. In addition, the mucus lining of the small intestine contains tiny glands that secrete intestinal digestive juice. Mucus, the enzymes within the intestinal digestive juice (e.g., maltase, sucrase, lactase, peptidase), and the secretions from the pancreas and liver serve to further break down food into smaller food molecules that may be more easily absorbed.

The mucosa of the small intestine is organized into several circular folds (plicae) covered with minute projections known as villi. Each villus contains finger-like lymphatic vessels (lacteals that absorb fat soluble nutrients (lipids) from the small intestine for transport to the blood circulation. Such fats are absorbed in the form of chyle, a cloudy milky substance containing products of digestion. The villi also contain blood capillaries that absorb certain products of digestion (e.g., amino acids, sugars).

Pancreas

The pancreas, an elongated gland located across the back of the abdomen, functions as both an exocrine and endocrine gland. It primarily consists of exocrine tissues that secrete pancreatic juice into ducts entering the duodenum. Pancreatic juice is an essential digestive juice that contains enzymes (e.g., trypsin, lipase, amylase) necessary for the breakdown of proteins, fats, carbohydrates, and certain acids. The pancreas also contains tiny clumps of endocrine cells (pancreatic islets) that secrete certain hormones, directly into the bloodstream.

The exocrine cells of the pancreas secrete their enzymes into several ducts that combine to form the main pancreatic duct. This duct joins with the common bile duct, which conveys bile from the gallbladder, and then opens into the duodenum. Most of the digestive enzymes secreted by the exocrine cells are activated by enzymes within the duodenum. In addition, exocrine cells of the pancreas secrete sodium bicarbonate, a substance that neutralizes the hydrochloric acid within the stomach's gastric juice as it enters the duodenum.

Liver, Bile Ducts, and Gallbladder

The liver, one of the largest organs of the body, is located within the upper right abdominal cavity. As part of the digestive system, the liver functions as an exocrine gland whose cells secrete the substance known as bile into a network of ducts (bile ducts). Bile, a liquid that consists of waste products, cholesterol, and bile salts, carries waste products from the liver and assists in the digestion and absorption of fats within the small intestine. The bile ducts transport bile from the liver to the gallbladder and on to the uppermost region of the small intestine (duodenum). The gallbladder, a small, muscular sac located under the liver, stores and concentrates bile from the liver. When chyme that contains fats (lipids) enters the duodenum from the stomach, the fats stimulate the secretion of a hormone (cholecystokinin) from the mucous membrane of the duodenum; in turn, the hormone stimulates contraction of the gallbladder, forcing bile into the small intestine.

The liver also has several additional essential functions in the body. These include regulating the blood levels of amino acids, the building blocks of proteins; helping to filter toxic substances from the blood; and producing certain proteins within the fluid portion of the blood (plasma). Such proteins include certain components that play a role in blood clotting (coagulation factors); particular blood proteins (complement system) that, when activated, destroy invading microorganisms; and the protein albumin, which helps to regulate the exchange of water between the bloodstream and bodily tissues. In addition, the liver produces cholesterol and certain proteins that transport fats in the bloodstream to cells throughout the body and processes hemoglobin for use of its iron content. Hemoglobin is the protein that enables red blood cells to transport large amounts of oxygen to cells.

Large Intestine

The large intestine is the organ that forms the lower portion of the GI tract. This organ, which has a larger diameter than the small intestine, consists of several areas. These include a pouch-like area (cecum); the ascending, transverse, descending, and sigmoid colons, the latter of which descends into the pelvic area and terminates in the rectum; and the end of the rectum known as the anal canal, which terminates at the external opening known as the anus. In addition, the appendix, a small, tubular structure, hangs from the cecum. Because the appendix contains lymphatic tissue, it may play a small role in helping to protect the body

against infection; however, it has no known role in the body's digestive system.

As food matter that has not been broken down or absorbed moves through the lower region of the small intestine (ileum), it passes into the large intestine through the ileocecal valve. Bacteria within the large intestine act upon the undigested material, potentially resulting in the release and absorption of additional nutrients. Water, vitamins, fats and minerals are absorbed into the bloodstream through the lining of the large intestine. Remaining undigested material is expelled through the rectum, anal canal, and anus as feces. Swelling (distension) of the rectum typically stimulates the desire to defecate, i.e., empty feces from the rectum. Two ring-shaped muscles (sphincters) usually remain contracted to keep the anus closed except during the process of defecation. The inner anal sphincter consists of involuntary (smooth) muscle, where the outer anal sphincter is composed of voluntary muscle.

Description

Endocrine

The term "endocrine system" is used to describe a group of specialized tissues, glands, and other structures that have the ability to produce and secrete certain complex chemical substances (hormones) into the bloodstream or lymphatic circulation for transport to particular tissues or ogans. These hormones have specific effects on certain bodily functions. Hormones assist in regulating the body's growth; controlling the rate of chemical processes in the body (metabolism); promoting the maturation and function of reproductive organs and the development of secondary sexual characteristics (puberty); and regulating many other bodily activities. Each hormone molecule may eventually combine with (or bind to) a specific area (receptor) on the surface of a cell within its "target organ," triggering the appropriate response. In contrast, exocrine glands are "outwardly secreting glands"-i.e., they secrete certain substances into ducts for emptying into a particular cavity or onto a bodily surface. (For example, the salivary glands of the digestive system secrete saliva via ducts that empty into the mouth.)

The endocrine glands include the pituitary gland, gonads (ovaries and testes), thyroid gland, parathyroid glands, adrenal glands, pancreatic islets, thymus, pineal gland, and placenta.

Pituitary Gland

The pituitary gland, also known as the "master gland," is a relatively small structure located deep in a saddle-shaped cavity in the skull (sella turcica). The gland is connected to a region of the brain known as the hypothalamus by a stalk of nerve fibers (pituitary stalk). The hypothalamus controls the functioning of the pituitary gland through direct nerve stimulation as well as through the actions of certain nerve cells that secrete hormones (hormone-releasing and hormone-inhibiting factors) into the bloodstream for transport directly to the pituitary. Hormone-releasing factors cause the secretion of certain hormones by the pituitary gland, whereas hormone-inhibiting factors inhibit the production and release of such hormones.

The pituitary gland is divided into two main regions: i.e., the anterior pituitary gland (adenohypophysis) and the posterior pituitary gland (neurohypophysis). Each region is responsible for producing different hormones. The anterior lobe of the pituitary gland produces the following hormones, most of which are considered tropic hormones, i.e., hormones that stimulate the growth of another endocrine gland and the secretion of its hormones.

- Prolactin stimulates the growth of the female breasts (mammary glands) during pregnancy and the secretion of milk by the mammary glands after birth.

- Growth hormone serves to stimulate body development.

- Melanocyte-stimulating hormone (MSH) controls the amount of dark brown or black pigment (melanin) produced by certain specialized skin cells (melanocytes).

- Thyroid-stimulating hormone (TSH) stimulates the production of thyroid hormones.

- Adrenocorticotropic hormone (ACTH) stimulates the growth of the outer regions of the adrenal glands (adrenal cortex) and their production of hormones.

- Follicle-stimulating hormone (FSH) and luteinizing hormone (LH), which are known as gonadotropins, stimulate the gonads, i.e., the sex glands (ovaries and testes) within which the reproductive cells (ova and sperm) are produced.

In addition, the posterior region of the pituitary gland releases two hormones:

- Antidiuretic hormone (ADH) decreases urine production by increasing the reabsorption of water from urine into the blood.

- Oxytocin stimulates powerful contractions of involuntary (smooth) muscle within the uterus during labor. This hormone also stimulates the secretion of milk (lactation) by the female mammary glands during breast-feeding.

Gonads

In females, the paired glands, known as the ovaries, produce the female sex cells (ova or eggs), and, in males, the paired structures, called the testes, produce the male sex cells (spermatozoa or sperm). Follicle-stimulating hormone produced by the pituitary gland promotes the growth and maturation of the cavities in the ovaries (follicles) within which the ova develop and mature; in addition, it stimulates the ovarian follicles' production of the female hormone estrogen. In males, FSH promotes the growth and maturation of and production of sperm by the long, coiled tubules (seminiferous tubules) that form the bulk of the testes. In addition, in females, luteinizing hormone produced by the pituitary gland stimulates the maturation of ovarian follicles and their eggs, the follicles' secretion of estrogen, and the monthly release of ova from the follicles (ovulation). LH stimulates the formation of glandular structures (corpus luteum) within the ruptured follicles that secrete the female hormones progesterone and estrogen. In males, LH stimulates the cells located between the seminiferous tubules in the testes to produce and secrete the male sex hormone testosterone.

Thyroid Gland

The horseshoe-shaped thyroid gland consists of two lobes on either side of the windpipe (trachea) that are joined by a narrow region of tissue (isthmus). Tissue within the thyroid gland consists of follicular cells and parafollicular cells. The follicular cells, which comprise most of the thyroid gland, secrete the thyroid hormones thyroxine (T4) and triiodothyronine (T3). Certain amounts of the thyroid hormones are stored as a semifluid material within the follicular cells, from which they are released into the bloodstream as required. The parafollicular cells secrete the hormone calcitonin.

Secretion of the thyroid hormones T4 and T3 is controlled by the pituitary gland. These hormones assist in regulation of the metabolic rate, i.e., chemical activities within cells that release energy from nutrients or consume energy to create certain substances. The thyroid hormones also play a vital role in the normal mental and physical development and growth of infants and children.

Release of the hormone calcitonin occurs independently of the pituitary gland and hypothalamus. This hormone-in coordination with parathyroid hormone released by the parathyroid glands-helps to regulate the concentrations of calcium in the body. Calcium is a mineral that is important for proper functioning of the cells, blood clotting, muscle contraction, nerve impulse transmission, and other vital functions. Most calcium in the body is stored in bones of the skeleton. Calcitonin has the ability to decrease blood levels of calcium. It suppresses resorption of bone by inhibiting the activity of cells that "digests" bone matrix (osteoclasts), releasing calcium and phosphorus into blood.

Parathyroid Glands

The parathyroid glands are the two pairs of small, oval glands on the back of both lobes of the thyroid gland. These glands produce parathyroid hormone, which serves to increase levels of calcium in the blood by stimulating osteoclasts to reabsorb bone mineral, thus liberating calcium into blood.

Adrenal Glands

The adrenal glands are small, triangular organs that curve over the top of each kidney. The outer region (adrenal cortex) and inner region (adrenal medulla) of the glands have different functions.

The secretion of hormones by the adrenal cortex is regulated by hormones produced by the pituitary gland (e.g., adrenocorticotropic hormone [ACTH]). The adrenal cortex consists of three distinct zones of cells. The outer zone secretes hormones known as mineralocorticoids that help to regulate the levels of certain mineral salts (e.g., sodium) in the blood. The main mineralocorticoid, known as aldosterone, assists in maintaining the delicate balance between sodium and potassium-ultimately helping to regulate blood pressure and blood volume.

The middle and inner zones of the adrenal cortex together secrete hormones known as glucocorticoids, such as hydrocortisone. Glucocorticoids help to regulate the body's use of carbohydrates, fats, and proteins; maintain normal blood pressure; produce certain anti-inflammatory effects; and decrease the production of certain white blood cells that produce antibodies (anti-allergic effect). The middle and inner zones of the adrenal cortex also secrete small amounts of sex hormones (androgens) that stimulate the development of male secondary sexual characteristics and the female sexual drive.

The adrenal medulla or inner region of the adrenal glands releases the hormones epinephrine and norepinephrine in response to nerve impulses from sympathetic nerve fibers. The release of such hormones into the bloodstream serves to increase the heart rate, widen the air passages of the lungs, and dilate blood vessels that supply the skeletal muscles of the body.

Pancreatic Islets

The pancreas, an elongated gland that is located across the back of the abdomen, is divided into a head, body, and tail. It primarily consists of exocrine tissue that secretes digestive enzymes necessary for the breakdown of proteins, fats, carbohydrates, and certain acids.

The endocrine tissue of the pancreas, known as pancreatic islets or islets of Langerhans, consists of tiny clumps of cells among the exocrine cells. The alpha cells of the pancreatic islets secrete glucagon, whereas the beta cells secrete insulin. Glucagon promotes a chemical process (glycogenolysis) during which glycogen, a carbohydrate that is stored in the liver, is broken down into glucose and released into the bloodstream. Insulin serves to regulate and stabilize blood glucose levels by promoting the movement of energy-rich glucose into the cells of the body. The secretion of glucagon increases blood glucose levels. In contrast, secretion of insulin decreases levels of glucose in the blood.

Thymus

The thymus, a small lymphoid organ located behind the breastbone (sternum) in the upper portion of the chest, consists of two lobes that join in front of the windpipe (trachea). This organ functions as an essential part of the immune system, beginning its functions at approximately the twelfth week of fetal development until puberty. The thymus serves as a source of certain white blood cells (lymphocytes) before birth. In addition, the organ secretes hormones (e.g., thymosin) that promote the development of specialized lymphocytes, known as T lymphocytes, which defend the body against certain microorganisms (i.e., during cell-mediated immunity.)

Pineal Gland

The pineal gland is a small, cone-shaped gland that is located deep in the brain. It secretes the hormone melatonin, which is thought to play a role in regulating puberty, ovarian cycles, mood, sleep, and the body's "internal clock" (e.g., 24-hour circadian cycle).

Placenta

The placenta, the organ that develops in the uterus during pregnancy, serves to connect the blood supplies of the mother and the developing fetus. It develops from the chorion, i.e., the outermost layer of cells from the fertilized egg (zygote). The placenta produces chorionic gonadotropin hormone, which stimulates the ovaries to produce the female sex hormones estrogen and progesterone. Both of these hormones are necessary for the functioning of the placenta during pregnancy.

Description

Growth and Development

Human growth and development may be encompassed in two broad categories: namely, prenatal growth and postnatal growth.

Prenatal Growth

The prenatal period, which means the "period before birth," begins when the male reproductive cell (sperm) fertilizes the female reproductive cell (egg or ovum). The fertilized egg (zygote) is a single cell containing all the genetic information (DNA) necessary for the growth and development of a human being. Half of the genetic information (in the form of 23 chromosomes) comes from the egg and half is from the sperm (for a total of 46 chromosomes).

As the zygote begins to travel down the mother's fallopian tube, its single cell immediately begins to divide (in the process called mitosis). (Please see the section entitled Cells for more information.) In approximately three days, the zygote has become a solid mass of cells known as a morula. About a week to 10 days after fertilization, what has become a hollow cellular "ball" (blastocyst) becomes implanted in the lining of the mother's uterus. During the zygote's journey to the uterus for implantation, the ovum supplies nutrients necessary for development of the embryo. The "embryonic phase" of development extends from fertilization until the end of the eighth week of pregnancy (gestation).

As the blastocyst continues to develop, its walls form an outer layer of membranes (chorion) that surround and protect the embryo. In addition, an inner layer of membranes (amnion) forms the amniotic sac, the fluid-filled sac within which the embryo grows and develops, protecting it from injury.

The chorion develops into the placenta, the organ attached to the lining of the uterus that serves to connect the blood supplies of the mother and the developing embryo, enabling the exchange of vital nutrients (including oxygen) and waste products. Blood from the embryo flows through a cord-like structure (umbilical cord) to the placenta and passes into tiny, finger-like blood vessels (chorionic villi) surrounded by maternal blood. The umbilical cord contains three blood vessels: two umbilical arteries that carry oxygen-poor (deoxygenated) blood and a larger umbilical vein that carries oxygen-rich (oxygenated) blood.

Teratogens and Birth Defects

A thin layer of tissue separates the developing embryo's blood and the mother's blood, thus providing protection from certain harmful substances that may circulate in the mother's bloodstream. However, in some cases, particular substances, such as certain infectious agents or drugs (teratogens), may cross this barrier, potentially interfering with prenatal growth and causing developmental abnormalities. The specific abnormalities that may result depend upon a number of factors, including the stage of development during which such exposure occurred, certain genetic influences, the specific teratogen in question, and other environmental factors. Birth defects are abnormalities that are apparent at birth (congenital) or early infancy. Such malformations may occur due to prenatal exposure to teratogens, genetic factors, or a combination of both (multifactorial).

As mentioned above, the embryonic stage of development takes place from fertilization until the end of the eighth week of gestation. The fetal stage of development extends from the ninth week of gestation until birth. Pregnancy is usually approximately 39 weeks in duration and is divided into three phases known as trimesters, each of which is about three months in length.

By approximately the third week of gestation, the head of the developing embryo begins to form and the region that will later become the brain and spinal cord (neural crest) starts to develop. At about four weeks, "buds" of tissue have begun to form that will later develop into certain organs (e.g., liver, lungs, pancreas, etc.) and into the arms, hands, legs, and feet (limb buds); the neural tube continues to develop; and rudimentary eyes form. By approximately five weeks, all internal organs have begun to develop, the jaws form, and the limb buds continue to grow. And by six weeks, the nose, mouth, and ears are beginning to develop and fingers and toes are becoming apparent.

Early during the first trimester, the growing embryo develops three layers of cells known as primary germ layers: an inner layer (endoderm), a middle layer (mesoderm), and an outer layer (ectoderm). Specific tissues and organs develop from each of these layers. For example, the lining of the lungs, gastrointestinal tract, and thyroid arise from the endoderm; the dermis of the skin, the muscles, most bones, the kidneys, and the circulatory system arise from the mesoderm; and the facial bones, the brain and spinal cord, the sensory organs such as the eyes and ears, and the epidermis of the skin arise from the ectoderm. By approximately the fourth month of gestation, the internal organs and organ systems are formed and almost mature. Growth and development continues until approximately nine months' gestation, when birth typically occurs.

Labor and Birth

Birth is the process during which the fetus moves from the uterus down through the cervix and passes out through the vagina. During the end of pregnancy, the uterus begins to contract in preparation for birth. The process known as labor begins when contractions become regular and occur at progressively shorter intervals. In addition, strong uterine muscular contractions cause the cervix to open and widen (dilate), and the membranes surrounding the amniotic fluid rupture, resulting in the release of the amniotic fluid through the vagina ("breaking of the waters"). The process of labor includes the following stages:

- First stage, which begins with the onset of contractions and ends with full dilation of the cervix

- Second stage, during which the baby exits through the vagina

- Third stage, during which the placenta is expelled through the vagina

Postnatal Growth and Development

The postnatal period, which means "the period after birth," begins at birth and extends until death. The most rapid rate of growth during one's development occurs prenatally ing embryonic and fetal development. Although the rate of growth decreases after birth, it remains high during childdhood, particularly during the first year of life. Individuals also experience a "growth spurt" at the onset of puberty that progresses until their adult height is obtained.

During the first five months of life, infants grow approximately 30 percent in height and their weight usually doubles. By the age of one year, their height has increased by about 50 percent from birth and their weight has typically tripled. Height and weight are carefully measured and recorded during regular visits to pediatricians to ensure that growth is progressing at a predictable, steady rate. Physiicians use measurements known as percentiles to compare the height and weight of infants who are of the same age. If an infant is said to be at the "fiftieth percentile" for weight, 50% of infants weigh more and 50% weigh less. If an infant is at the "tenth percentile" for height, 90% of infants have a higher height and 10% have a lower height. When assessing growth and development, physicians consider the actual percentile as well as changes in percentiles between visits.

Between birth and adolescence, the relative proportions of the head, limbs, and trunk change dramatically. For exammple, an infant's head tends to be about one quarter of the height of the body; however, an adult's head is approxiimately one eighth that of the height of the body. In addition, from childhood to adulthood, the trunk tends to become proportionally shorter and the legs proportionally longer.

Different organs have varying rates of growth. For example, the human brain is about one quarter of its adult size at birth. The brain grows primarily during the first year of life and is typically three quarters of its adult size by the age of one year. In contrast, the small lymphoid organ known as the thymus gradually enlarges until puberty, at which time it begins to decrease in size (involution).

Developmental Milestones

Infants and children develop mental, physical, and behavvioral skills in certain stages known as developmental mileestones. Although the particular rate of development may vary from child to child, most children typically acquire such skills at certain ages. The development of these skills depends upon a number of factors including the following:

Genetic factors-e.g., certain developmental patterns, such as developing the ability to speak earlier than otherwise exxpected, may be present in particular families.

Physical factors-e.g., visual or hearing impairment may innterfere with the ability to learn certain skills, potentially neecessitating the use of special supportive techniques or services to ensure that children have the best chance to reach their developmental potential.

Environmental factors-e.g., appropriate levels of stimulaation are important in helping children to develop certain skills, such as receiving regular verbal stimulation to proomote language development.

When infants are born, they primarily communicate any needs (e.g., hunger, thirst, etc.) by crying. In addition, cerrtain essential reflex reactions are typically present at birth. For example, when any objects touch newborns' lips, they usually respond by sucking (sucking reflex). When a side of the mouth is touched, newborns typically move their head toward that side, enabling them to locate the mother's nipple for breast-feeding (rooting reflex). And when newwborns are startled, they stretch their arms and legs forward and out and extend their fingers (startle or Moro's reflex). These reflex reactions gradually fade as infants develop muscle strength and the ability to conduct and coordinate certain voluntary movements. For example, hand-eye coorrdination skills include watching objects, developing the ability to focus, tracking moving objects, and forming an association between seeing and performing certain actions by focusing on hand movements.

Development is typically assessed by evaluating the acquiisition of skills in the areas of vision and fine movement, hearing and speech, locomotion, and social behavior. The following is a description of developmental milestones that are generally acquired during the first year of life:

By approximately one month of age, infants are usually able to:

- Focus on faces

- Bring their hands toward the face (e.g., mouth, eyes)

- Look at objects directly in front of them
- Turn toward familiar voices and respond to other sounds
- Move their head from side to side while lying on their stomach

At about three months, infants are usually able to:

- Track objects that move approximately 180 degrees
- Grasp objects placed in their hands
- Smile at familiar voices (e.g., mother's or father's)
- Make sounds that begin to resemble speech
- Raise their head 45 degrees when lying on their stomach

At approximately five months, infants are usually able to:

- Reach for objects
- Listen carefully to certain voices
- Hold their head steady while upright
- Roll from the stomach to the back
- Spontaneously smile

At about six months, infants are usually able to:

- Reach out for an move objects from one hand to another
- Turn their head to locate sounds
- Laugh, make certain vowel sounds, and babble to toys
- Roll from back to front and vice versa
- Sit with support
- Bear weight on their legs with support

At the age of nine months, infants are usually able to:

- Look for toys that have been hidden
- Grasp for toys that are out of reach
- Manipulate objects with both hands
- Listen to and comprehend certain sounds
- Occasionally utter strings of syllables (e.g., "mama" or "dada")
- Attempt to crawl, sit without support, and pull themselves to a sitting or standing position
- Step on alternative feet with support

By 12 months of age, infants are usually able to:

- Grasp and release objects
- Say several words
- Respond when they hear their names
- Wave good-bye
- Move from their stomach to a sitting position
- Crawl on their hands and knees
- Walk by holding furniture
- Walk without support for a few steps or with one hand held

Description

Hematologic

The blood is a circulating tissue composed of fluid and other formed elements such as red blood cells, white cells, and platelets. The study of the blood, its components, and blood-forming tissues is known as hematology. Blood is pumped by the heart through the body's arteries, veins, and capillaries. The noncellular, fluid portion of the blood is a pale, yellowish liquid known as plasma. The blood has several functions including:

- To serve as a transport system, carrying oxygen and other vital nutrients to body tissues and promoting the exchange and removal of carbon dioxide and other waste products from cells

- To help provide a defense against invading microorganisms, foreign tissue cells, and certain abnormal cells

- To help repair damage to blood vessels and tissues through the process of blood clotting

Blood Plasma

Approximately half of the blood's volume consists of plasma. This liquid, noncellular portion of the blood is approximately 95 percent water. In addition, the blood plasma also contains dissolved sugars (e.g., glucose, etc.), fats, salts, vitamins and minerals, amino acids necessary for the production of cellular proteins, and chemical messengers (such as hormones) that regulate specific cellular activities. Plasma also contains certain plasma proteins including globulins (e.g., antibodies, which are produced in response to a particular foreign protein [antigen]); albumin, which plays an important role in maintaining the balance of pressure from inside and outside the cell, ; and fibrinogen, a protein that is essential for blood clotting. In addition, certain waste products are dissolved in plasma and transported to the kidneys for excretion.

Formed Elements

The formed elements of the blood include red blood cells (erythrocytes), white blood cells (leukocytes), and platelets (thrombocytes). Red blood cells, platelets, and some white blood cells are produced in the bone marrow. However, most white blood cells are produced by lymphatic tissue (e.g., lymph nodes, spleen, thymus).

Red Blood Cells

The red blood cells (RBCs) are mostly rounded, double concave cells with thin centers and thicker edges. A cubic millimeter of blood contains approximately five million red blood cells. The relatively large surface area of the red blood cells because they are concave allows them to absorb and release oxygen molecules, and their shape facilitates

their movement through narrow blood vessels. As mentioned above, red blood cells are produced in the bone marrow, where the rate of their formation is regulated by erythropoietin, a hormone produced by the kidneys. They typically circulate in the blood for approximately four months, at which time they break apart and are removed from the blood by the liver.

The red blood cells perform several essential functions. For example, RBCs transport carbon dioxide from the body's cells to the lungs for release into the environment. Carbon dioxide is a harmful waste product that is generated by normal cellular activities. The red blood cells also carry hemoglobin, an essential protein that contains iron. This red pigmented protein chemically combines (binds) with oxygen, producing oxyhemoglobin, which enables the red blood cells to transport oxygen to cells.

The various blood groups, such as blood types A, B, AB, and O, are classified based upon the presence or absence of certain antigens (or "marker proteins"). Antigens are proteins that stimulate the body to produce antibodies. The red blood cells may have two types of antigens: namely, A and/or B. The different A or B blood types are classified according to whether the red blood cells have both, one or the other, or neither antigen. In individuals with type B blood, for example, the body does not produce antibodies to inactivate or destroy the type B antigen; however, the blood plasma contains anti-A antibodies. In individuals with type A blood, the red blood cells contain type A antigen and the blood plasma has anti-B antibodies. In type O blood, the red blood cells contain neither type A nor type B antigens, whereas the blood plasma has both anti-A and anti-B antibodies. In contrast, in individuals with type AB blood, the red blood cells have both type A and type B antigens, and the blood plasma contains neither anti-A nor anti-B antibodies.

In approximately 85 percent of individuals, red blood cells also contain an antigen called Rh factor. Those with this antigen are said to have Rh-positive blood, whereas those without the antigen have Rh-negative blood.

White Blood Cells

White blood cells (WBCs) are larger than red blood cells; however, they are present in the blood in lower quantities. A cubic millimeter of blood contains approximately 7,500 white blood cells.

The white blood cells include two major categories: granular leukocytes, which have granules in the substance of the cell outside the nucleus (cytoplasm), and nongranular leukocytes. Granular leukocytes include neutrophils, eosinophils, and basophils, and nongranular leukocytes include lymphocytes and monocytes.

Neutrophils and monocytes, which are also known as phagocytes, are responsible for isolating, engulfing, and destroying microorganisms that have invaded the bloodstream. These cells engulf the microorganisms and digest them in a process known as phagocytosis.

Lymphocytes originate in the bone marrow and mature in lymphatic tissue. They become active immune cells in response to the presence of invading microorganisms. Lymphocytes known as B lymphocytes produce specific antibodies to inhibit certain microorganisms, whereas those known as T lymphocytes may actively destroy microorganisms or assist in the functions of the B lymphocytes.

Eosinophils help protect the body from various irritants that may cause allergies and are able to participate in phagocytosis. In addition, white blood cells known as basophils also play a role in allergic reactions and secrete certain chemicals such as heparin, which assists in the prevention of clotting as the blood circulates through the blood vessels (intravascular clotting).

Although granular leukocytes may have a lifespan of only a few days, nongranular leukocytes may survive for over six months. In fact, in some cases, certain individual lymphocytes may remain in the bloodstream for years.

Platelets

Platelets, which are the smallest blood cells, are produced in the bone marrow by specialized cells known as megakaryocytes and typically survive for approximately nine days. A cubic millimeter of blood contains approximately 250,000 platelets.

Platelets usually circulate in the bloodstream in an inactive state. However, when a blood vessel wall is injured, platelets respond through a complex process by clumping at the injury site and sticking to one another. The platelets and damaged tissue cells also release certain chemicals that stimulate blood clotting (coagulation) factors in the blood plasma. Due to a series of complex reactions, known as a cascade, long filaments of fibrin, a fibrous gel, are produced that capture circulating platelets, red blood cells, and white blood cells. Once the damaged blood vessel is "plugged," the filaments contract, forming a solid blood clot.

In some cases, blood clots may form in undamaged blood vessels, potentially blocking vital blood supply to certain tissues and organs. A stationary blood clot is called a thrombus. If a portion of such a clot dislodges and circulates in the bloodstream, it is known as an embolus. Healthy blood vessel walls secrete the chemical prostacyclin, which helps to prevent the unnecessary activation of platelets and clot formation. However, under certain circumstances, emboli travel from their origin to other parts of the body, notably the lungs, heart, and brain.

Measurement of Blood Components

The complete blood count (CBC) is a calculation of the cellular (formed elements) of blood. These calculations are generally determined by specially designed machines that analyze the different components of blood in less than a minute. A major portion of the complete blood count is the measure of the concentration of white blood cells, red blood cells, and platelets in the blood. The complete blood count (also called CBC) is generated by testing a simple blood sample.

White Blood Count (WBC), also called leukocyte count. Normal range varies slightly between laboratories but is generally between 4,300 and 10,800 cells per cubic millimeter (cmm).

Automated white cell differential. A machine generated percentage of the different types of white blood cells, usually split into granulocytes, lymphocytes, monocytes, eosinophils, and basophils.

Red cell count (RBC), also called erythrocyte count. Normal range varies slightly between laboratories but is generally between 4.2 - 5.9 million cells/cmm.

Hemoglobin (Hb). Hemoglobin is the protein molecule within red blood cells that carries oxygen and gives blood its red color. Normal range for hemoglobin is different between the sexes and is approximately 13 - 18 grams per deciliter (g/dl) for men and 12 - 16 g/dl for women.

Platelet count, also called thrombocyte count. Normal range varies slightly between laboratories but is in the range of 150,000 - 400,000 per cubic millimeter.

Immune System

Description

Immune System

The body's immune system consists of specialized proteins, cells, and tissues that function to protect the body against...

- Invading microorganisms (e.g., bacteria, viruses, etc.) that may cause disease

- Foreign tissue cells (such as those that may have been transplanted from a donor)

- Toxins (such as harmful chemicals)

- Cells that have become cancerous

Nonspecific Immunity
Certain mechanisms provide the body with general protection from invading cells and toxins, maintaining "nonspecific immunity." For example, nonspecific immunity is provided by the presence of certain physical barriers that may prevent the entry of invading cells or toxins or expel them-as well as chemical barriers that may destroy invading cells or toxins. Such barriers include certain enzymes within the saliva of the mouth, tears, and sweat; the protective barrier of the skin; the cough reflex; hairs within the nose and the sneeze reflex; the presence of harmless bacteria within the intestines that help to control harmful microorganisms; and secretion of mucus by cells lining certain organs of the respiratory tract.

In addition, tissue injury results in an inflammatory response, which consists of a series of nonspecific immune reactions. During an inflammatory response-which produces characteristic swelling, discomfort, and redness-the blood vessels widen (dilate), increasing the blood supply and enabling certain white blood cells to move from the vessels to the site of injury. For example, invading microorganisms typically encounter white blood cells known as phagocytes, which contain the infection by engulfing and destroying the microbes (phagocytosis). Invading microorganisms may also encounter certain naturally produced substances, such as a group of blood proteins (complement system) that, when activated, serve to destroy such microbes, or interferon, proteins that are produced in response to viral infection.

Specific Immunity
Specific immunity consists of particular defenses against certain invading microorganisms or toxins and includes inborn and acquired immunity. From birth, individuals are immune to certain diseases that affect other animals (inborn immunity). Acquired immunity is obtained when certain protective proteins known as antibodies are passed to a developing fetus via the mother's placenta or to an infant via the mother's breast milk. Acquired immunity also results from casual exposure to certain disease-causing agents and

immunization (stimulation of the immune system to provide protection against a particular disease, such as through vaccination).

Humoral or Cellular Immune Responses
Specific immunity, which relies on the actions of the white blood cells known as lymphocytes, includes the humoral- and cell-mediated immune responses.

Humoral Response
A humoral-mediated immune response, also known as an antibody-mediated response, primarily consists of the production of antibodies by cells called B lymphocytes or B cells. B lymphocytes initially arise from primitive cells in the bone marrow known as stem cells. Shortly before and after birth, certain stem cells develop into immature B cells.

When immature B cells recognize a disease-causing agent as foreign (antigen), they develop into activated B cells. Activated B cells rapidly divide into two lines of cells (clones): plasma cells, which secrete large amounts of antibodies into the blood, and memory cells, which are stored within the lymph nodes until they are stimulated by the same antigen that prompted their formation. They then also develop into plasma cells, secreting antibodies into the blood in response to the recognized antigen.

When antibodies are secreted into the blood, they bind to their specific antigens (antibody-antigen complex), making the antigens or the cells on which they are located harmless. Phagocytes then engulf and destroy large numbers of such antibody-antigen complexes. The binding of antibodies and antigens may stimulate the complement system, thereby improving the efficiency of phagocytosis.

Cellular Response
Cell-mediated immunity defends the body against certain microorganisms and possibly cancerous cells through the actions of particular white blood cells known as T lymphocytes or T cells. These cells initially develop within the thymus before birth. They arise from stem cells that migrate from the bone marrow to the thymus, where their development is facilitated by certain hormones. Newly formed T cells then migrate from the thymus to other lymphatic tissues, primarily the lymph nodes.

There are two main types of T lymphocytes involved in cell-mediated immunity including the helper cells and killer cells. Helper cells assist in the recognition of certain antigens and help to activate killer cells. The killer cells bind to cells invaded by viruses or other microbes and destroy them. It is thought that killer cells may function similarly against cancerous cells or foreign tissue cells.

Allergies and Autoimmune Disease

In some cases, humoral- or cell-mediated immune responses may inappropriately occur against the body's own tissues. Such "autoimmunity" may result in hypersensitivity or autoimmune diseases. A hypersensitivity reaction is characterized by an excessive immune response to a substance that the body perceives as foreign (sensitizing antigen). For example, an allergic reaction is a hypersensitive response that occurs upon exposure to previously encountered, usually environmental substances (allergens), such as pollen, dust, or certain foods. Autoimmune diseases may be caused by the production of antibodies against the body's own cells (autoantibodies) and inappropriate cell-mediated immune responses against self antigens (autoantigens). One proposed theory suggests that certain viruses or bacteria may play some role in provoking an abnormal autoimmune reaction. For example, when a foreign protein from an invading bacterium or virus is very similar to one of the body's proteins, the immune system may be unable to distinguish between the invading and the "self" protein, potentially triggering an autoimmune response. It is not known what role genetic, hormonal, or other environmental factors may play in contributing to such a response. Autoimmune diseases may be localized, affecting a particular tissue, or may involve many tissues and organs of the body (systemic).

Infectious Diseases and Vaccination

The purpose of immunization is to induce immunity to provide protection against a certain disease. In response to a vaccine, the body's immune system produces certain immune defenses, such as antibodies or particular white blood cells that should protect against infection upon exposure to the disease-causing organism.

There are two major types of vaccination. In passive vaccination, antibodies obtained from a donor who was previously exposed to the microorganism are introduced into the body, thereby providing short-term protection against the disease-causing organism. In active vaccination, noninfectious portions of bacteria or viruses are introduced into the body, stimulating the production of antibodies against the foreign protein, resulting in longer-term immunity.

Some vaccines are intended for the general population, particularly infants and young children, such as immunization against the infectious diseases diphtheria, pertussis (whooping cough), and tetanus (DPT); measles, mumps, and rubella (German measles); hepatitis B; and polio. The recommended ages for immunization may vary from case to case. A child's pediatrician can recommend an appropriate immunization schedule.

Other vaccines are available for individuals who are at risk for certain infectious diseases due to their work situations (e.g., health care workers); their living situations or age groups (e.g., students living in dormitories, elderly individuals in nursing homes); local outbreaks of dangerous infectious diseases; or travel in certain countries.

Some individuals should not receive certain vaccinations, such as people with deficient immune systems. In individuals who have a fever or a preexisting infection, immunizations should be delayed. In addition, particular vaccines should not be given to young children or pregnant women.

Musculoskeletal

Neuromuscular Activities

The muscles of the body, collectively referred to as the muscular system, consist of bundles of specialized cells that, unlike other cells, have the ability to contract and re-lax, resulting in movement of body parts and organs. There are two main types of muscles: namely, skeletal muscle and smooth muscle. In addition, the cardiac muscle is a highly specialized muscle that is sometimes referred to as a third muscle type.

Skeletal Muscle

The skeletal muscles, so named because they attach to bones of the skeleton, are the most prominent muscles in the body and typically contribute to approximately 40 to 45 percent of an individual's body weight. These muscles may also be referred to as striated ("cross striped") muscles or called voluntary muscles because their movements are under voluntary control.

Each skeletal muscle consists of groups of threadlike mus-cle cells, known as muscle fibers, in a highly organized ar-rangement. Each muscle fiber is made up of slender, striated strands called myofibrils that, in turn, are com-posed of bunches of microscopic, threadlike structures known as myofilaments. The myofilaments contain minute fibers or threads of proteins known as myosin and actin. The interactions of these proteins are essential for muscle contraction. During voluntary movement, skeletal muscle contracts and the bone to which it is attached (via tendons) moves in response to the contraction.

Neuromuscular Activities and Voluntary Movement:

The brain regulates voluntary movements of skeletal mus-cles by sending impulses to the nerve fibers that supply the muscle fibers (motor neurons). The area where nerve end-ings and muscle fibers join is known as the neuromuscular junction. When the brain sends such impulses, nerve end-ings release a specialized chemical (the neurotransmitter acetylcholine) that serves to stimulate the muscle fibers. A complex series of electrical and chemical processes is initiated resulting in muscle contraction.

When voluntary movements occur, there are coordinated contractions and simultaneous relaxations of several mus-cles. In other words, as several muscles contract, one mus-cle is primarily responsible for producing the particular movement (prime mover or agonist) and the others (syner-gists) contract in order to assist the prime mover in making the movement in question. While such muscles contract, other muscles known as antagonists simultaneously relax, producing movements that oppose those of the prime mover and synergists. Such coordination of skeletal muscle

movements helps to ensure smooth rather than jerky motions.

In addition to producing movement, the skeletal muscles also function to maintain posture and to produce body heat. For example, skeletal muscles are typically maintained at a level of slight, continuous contraction (muscle tone). Such muscle tone helps the body to maintain proper posture-i.e., the specific positioning of body parts to support their opti-mum function, place the least strain on different areas of the body, and maintain proper weight distribution. In addi-tion, muscle fiber contraction creates most of the heat that the body needs to maintain its proper temperature.

Smooth Muscle

Smooth muscle cells have a smooth appearance when viewed under a microscope, lacking the striations of skele-tal muscle cells. Rather, they consist of elongated, "spin-dle-shaped" cells that are typically organized parallel to one another. Also known as involuntary muscles since their movements are not under voluntary control, the smooth muscles help to regulate certain functional movements of internal organs. For example, in the process known as peristalsis, the rhythmic contractions of smooth muscle propel food forward through the digestive tract. Smooth muscle is also located within the blood vessel walls and several other areas of the body.

The actions of the smooth muscles are regulated by the au-tonomic nervous system, the portion of the nervous system that controls involuntary activities of blood vessels, organs, and other tissues and organ systems. Neurotransmitters re-leased at nerve endings contribute to the series of events that lead to contraction of smooth muscles. As with the skeletal muscles, smooth muscle contractions rely upon the interactions between the myosin and actin filaments. In ad-dition, smooth muscle cell activities may be affected by changes in the chemical composition of the fluid surround-ing the cells as well as the release of certain hormones.

Cardiac Muscle

Cardiac muscle, also known as the myocardium, is a spe-cial type of striated muscle that is located only in the heart. Like the cells within the skeletal muscles, cardiac muscle cells also have cross striations. In addition, there are dark bands or disks (intercalated disks) at the junctures of adja-cent cardiac fibers. These disks enable the fibers to contract as a unit, thereby ensuring the heart's efficiency in pump-ing blood throughout the circulatory system.

As with the smooth muscles, contraction of cardiac muscle is regulated by the autonomic nervous system. Cardiac muscle activities may also be affected by the release of specific hormones. Electrical impulses that stimulate a reg-ulated, coordinated sequence of contractions originate from the heart's "pacemaker" (sinoatrial node), an area within the upper right chamber of the heart (right atrium).

Description

Nervous System

The nervous system is a complex network of structures that function to...

- obtain information about the body's internal environment and the external environment

- relay and analyze such "data"

- initiate, integrate, and control appropriate responses to this information

The nervous system includes the brain and spinal cord, known as the central nervous system; nerves that extend from the brain and spinal cord to all areas of the body, referred to as the peripheral nervous system; somatic sense organs, which are distributed in almost every area of the body but concentrated primarily in the skin; and special sensory organs, such as the eyes. In addition, the peripheral nervous system is further subdivided into the autonomic nervous system, which includes structures that regulate involuntary functions of the body.

Nervous System Cells

Cells of the nervous system ensure ongoing, rapid communications between different structures of the body and the control of bodily functions necessary to maintain life. There are two main types of cells within the nervous system:

- Nerve cells, also known as neurons, which conduct (transmit) impulses

- Glia, which are the connective tissue cells of the nervous system

Neurons contain a cell body, one or more slender, branching projections (dendrites) that transmit impulses toward the cell body, and a slender extension (axon or nerve fiber) that carries nerve impulses away from the cell body. A whitish, fatty substance known as myelin forms a protective "wrapping" or insulating sheath around certain axons, serving as an electrical insulator and ensuring the efficient conduction of nerve impulses.

There are three types of neurons:

- Sensory neurons (afferent ["toward"] neurons) carry impulses to the brain and spinal cord from all areas of the body.

- Motor neurons (efferent ["away from"] neurons) transmit impulses away from the brain and spinal cord to certain tissues (e.g., muscle or glandular tissues).

- Interneurons (connecting or central neurons) carry impulses from sensory neurons to motor neurons.

Glia hold together and protect neurons. The different types of glia include the following:

- Astrocytes are relatively large cells with thread-like projections. These "branches" connect with blood capillaries and neurons, holding them in proximity to one another. The walls of the capillaries and the projections of the astrocytes are said to form the "blood-brain barrier," which functions to separate systemic blood circulation from the central nervous system. This barrier prevents or slows the passage of certain toxic substances or infectious agents from the blood to the central nervous system.

- Oligodendroglia produce myelin and hold together nerve fibers.

- Microglia are relatively small cells with slender projections. When brain tissue becomes inflamed, these cells migrate toward the affected tissue, surround invading microorganisms or waste products, and digest them (phagocytosis).

Nerves and Nerve Impulses

Nerves consist of one or more bundles of impulse-carrying fibers known as axons that extend from the brain and spinal cord to all areas of the body. Certain nerves transmit impulses from particular receptor organs to the brain and spinal cord (afferent impulses) or from the CNS to certain specialized tissues (efferent impulses). White matter within the central nervous system and peripheral nervous system consists of bundles of axons that are myelinated; in contrast, gray matter of the nervous system primarily includes neuron cell bodies, dendrites, and unmyelinated axons.

The pathways by which nerve impulses are transmitted by neurons are known as neuron pathways. Nerve signals are electrical impulses or waves of electrical disturbances that result due to complex electrochemical changes in a neuron's environment. Such nerve impulses travel from the axon of one neuron (presynaptic neuron) to the dendrite of another neuron (postsynaptic neuron). The junction between two neurons is known as a synapse. As an electrical impulse reaches a synapse, the presynaptic neuron's axon releases small amounts of chemical substances known as neurotransmitters, which bind to certain areas (receptors) of the postsynaptic neuron. Consequently, the electrical impulse is conducted across the synapse to the postsynaptic neuron's dendrite. Thus, neurotransmitters are the chemical substances that enable neurons to communicate with one another.

Central Nervous System

The central nervous system includes the brain and the spinal cord. Bones of the skull enclose the brain, and bones of the spinal column (vertebrae) surround the spinal cord. In addition, a three-layered membrane (meninges) provides additional protection for the brain and spinal cord. The tough, fibrous outermost layer is known as the dura mater. The delicate middle layer, called the arachnoid mater, is separated from the elastic innermost layer (pia mater) by a space (subarachnoid space) that contains cerebrospinal fluid (CSF). This fluid, which acts as a protective "shock absorber," flows through the cavity within the vertebrae containing the spinal cord (spinal canal), the four cavities of the brain (ventricles), and the subarachnoid space.

Brain

The brain controls and regulates the many functions of the central nervous system including muscle control and coordination, sensory reception and response, and speech production as well as elaboration of thought and emotions. It consists of several major regions including the brain stem, diencephalon, cerebellum, and cerebrum.

Brain Stem

The brain stem consists of three structures: the medulla oblongata, pons, and midbrain. All regions of the brain stem serve as "two-lane" conduction "highways," with motor fibers relaying impulses from the brain to the spinal cord, and sensory fibers conducting messages from the spinal cord to other areas of the brain.

The medulla oblongata, a thick extension of the spinal cord, is located above the large opening (foramen magnum) in the bone that forms the back of the skull (occipital bone). It primarily consists of white matter mixed with bits of gray matter (reticular formation). The medulla contains groups of nerve cells (nuclei) of the ninth, eleventh, and twelfth cranial nerves (see below), thereby receiving and sending impulses involved in the sensation of taste and sending messages to muscles involved in swallowing, speech, and movements of the neck, shoulders, and tongue, for example. This region of the brain stem also contains nuclei of the tenth cranial nerve (vagus nerve) and thus receives and relays information concerning the regulation of blood vessel diameter (thus affecting blood pressure), beating of the heart, breathing, and digestion.

The pons and the midbrain both also contain white matter mixed with bits of gray matter. The pons has bundles of nerve fibers that connect with the region of the brain known as the cerebellum. In addition, it contains nuclei of the fifth, sixth, seventh, and eighth cranial nerves, thus relaying messages involved in movement of the eyes, jaws, and muscles of facial expression as well as receiving and transmitting sensory impulses from the face and ears. The midbrain contains nuclei of the third and fourth cranial nerves and there-fore relays messages to muscles involved in controlling the reactions of the pupils of the eyes as well as five of the six muscles that move the eyes.

Diencephalon

The diencephalon is the region of the brain located between the midbrain and the cerebrum. It includes the hypothalamus and the thalamus.

The hypothalamus, a relatively small area of the brain, is situated under the thalamus and above the pituitary gland. One of its functions is to regulate the sympathetic nervous system, a division of the autonomic nervous system. The sympathetic nervous system controls certain involuntary activities during times of stress, such as raising blood pressure, increasing the heart rate and the breathing rate, and widening (dilating) the pupils. The hypothalamus is also involved in regulating body temperature, appetite, moods and emotions (such as anger, fear, etc.), and the sleep cycle.

Sleep and the Brain

Sleep is a natural state characterized by reduced consciousness and metabolic activity. During sleep, the brain typically engages in two main cycles, known as REM (rapid eye movement) and NREM (nonrapid eye movement) sleep. NREM sleep, which makes up approximately 80 percent of sleep in adults (and about 50 percent of sleep in infants), consists of four progressively deeper stages of sleep characterized by slow, deep brain waves; muscle relaxation; and regular, reduced autonomic activities (e.g., slowed breathing and heart rate; lowered blood pressure; etc.). Episodes of REM sleep periodically alternate with NREM sleep. REM sleep, which is associated with dreaming, includes increased levels of brain activity, irregular autonomic activities, rapid eye movements, and involuntary muscle jerks. A complete sleep cycle is usually approximately 90 minutes. Most individuals experience approximately four or five sleep cycles each night. It is not completely understood why sleep is a necessity, although most scientists agree that the brain requires regular rest to ensure optimum functioning-and that dreaming may help the brain to sort, manipulate, and store information obtained during waking activities. Many different areas of the brain, including the hypothalamus, are thought to play a role in regulating sleep.

The hypothalamus also controls the functions of the pituitary gland, an endocrine gland also known as the "master gland." The hypothalamus is attached to the pituitary gland by a stalk of nerve fibers known as the pituitary stalk. It regulates the gland's activities through direct nerve stimulation as well as through the actions of certain nerve cells whose axons secrete chemicals (hormone-releasing and hormone-inhibiting factors) into the bloodstream for transport directly to the pituitary. Hormone-releasing factors cause the secretion of certain hormones by the pituitary gland, whereas hormone-inhibiting factors halt the production and release of such hormones. The balance of these factors, via a feedback mechanism, is crucial in maintaining effective function of many of the body's activities.

The thalamus consists of two masses of gray matter located above the hypothalamus. The neurons within the thalamus relay impulses from sense organs of the body to the outer region of the cerebrum (cerebral cortex); transmit motor impulses from the cerebral cortex toward the spinal cord; associate certain sensations with emotions (e.g., unpleasant or pleasant feelings); and play a role in the body's state of responsiveness to sensory stimulation (arousal or alerting mechanisms).

Cerebellum

The cerebellum, a two-lobed, rounded region of the brain, has a "wrinkled" surface and is located under the back portion of the cerebrum and behind the brain stem. The surface (cortex) of the cerebellum contains parallel ridges that are separated by deep fissures. Three stalks of nerve fibers (peduncles) that arise from the inner side of each cerebellar hemisphere link to different areas of the brain stem. Messages between the cerebellum and other regions of the brain travel along these nerve stalks. Through messages transmitted via the brain stem, the cerebellum receives information concerning muscle contraction and relaxation and posture. The cerebellum works in conjunction with the basal ganglia and the thalamus, adjusting messages relayed to muscle groups from a certain area of the cerebrum (motor cortex) in order to maintain normal postures, sustain balance, and produce smooth and coordinated movements.

Cerebrum

The cerebrum is the largest area of the brain and is responsible for voluntary movements, sensory perception, emotions, memory, and comprehensive thought. The cerebrum contains several ridges (gyri) and grooves (sulci or fissures) and one deep groove known as the longitudinal fissure that divides the cerebrum into two halves (cerebral hemispheres). The left cerebral hemisphere controls the right side of the body, whereas the right hemisphere controls the left side of the body due to crossing of nerve fibers in the medulla of the brain stem. A thick band of myelinated nerve fibers known as the corpus callosum joins the lower midportions of and carries messages between the cerebral hemispheres. In addition, each hemisphere contains a fluid-filled cavity known as a ventricle (first and second or lateral ventricles). These ventricles communicate with a third ventricle in the center of the brain, and a fourth ventricle is located between the brain stem and the cerebellum.

Two sulci divide each hemisphere into four lobes that are designated by the bones over them: i.e., frontal, temporal, parietal, and occipital lobes. The surface of the cerebrum, called the cerebral cortex, consists of a thin layer of gray matter, whereas most of the interior of the cerebrum con-

tains bundles of myelinated nerve fibers (white matter) known as tracts. In addition, deep within the white matter of the cerebrum are paired nerve cell clusters of gray matter known as the basal ganglia. Their function includes assisting in the regulation of muscular actions as well as initiating and ceasing movements.

The cerebrum has various areas that are responsible for particular complex functions. These areas include the following:

- Sensory areas, which receive sensory information from somatic sense organs (e.g., in the skin, muscles, internal organs) and special sense organs (e.g., ears, eyes, etc.) and analyze and sort such information

- Motor areas, which transmit messages that control muscles, resulting in movement

- Association areas, which link sensory and motor areas, integrate information received from the various sense organs, and engage in memory storage, recall, recognition, decision making, judgment, comprehensive thought, and the experience of emotions.

Spinal Cord

The spinal cord is housed inside a central canal within the spinal column and extends from the foramen magnum at the base of the skull to the bottom of the first vertebra of the lower back. It is a long, cylindrical structure of nerve tissue and is an extension of the medulla oblongata of the brain stem. As mentioned above, the spinal cord is enclosed and protected by a three-layered membrane (meninges) and is bathed by cerebrospinal fluid.

The inner core of the spinal cord consists of gray matter (i.e., primarily containing nerve cell bodies and dendrites). Its outer portion is composed of columns of white matter that contain bundles of myelinated nerve fibers (spinal tracts). These pathways transmit sensory impulses from the spinal cord to the brain (ascending tracts) and motor impulses from the brain to the spinal cord (descending tracts). Certain ascending tracts transmit impulses that produce sensations of temperature and pain, and certain descending tracts convey impulses that control specific voluntary movements.

Peripheral Nervous System

The peripheral nervous system refers to those nerves outside the central nervous system. This part of the nervous system establishes communications between the brain and spinal cord and outlying (peripheral) parts of the body, such as muscles, glands, and internal organs. Nerves of the peripheral nervous system include the cranial nerves and the spinal nerves.

The cranial nerves are the 12 nerve pairs that arise directly from the brain and emerge through various openings in the skull (foramen). The cranial nerve pairs...

- Carry sensory impulses to the brain that are analyzed, sorted, and integrated, resulting in vision, smell, taste, hearing, and/or balance.

- Transmit motor and/or sensory information to particular areas of the head and neck.

- Convey impulses to glands and organs, resulting in certain involuntary (autonomic) activities.

The cranial nerve pairs include the...
- First cranial nerves or olfactory nerves
- Second cranial nerves or optic nerves
- Third cranial nerves or oculomotor nerves
- Fourth cranial nerves or trochlear nerves
- Fifth cranial nerves or trigeminal nerves
- Sixth cranial nerve or abducens nerves
- Seventh cranial nerves or facial nerves
- Eighth cranial nerves or vestibulocochlear nerves
- Ninth cranial nerves or glossopharyngeal nerves
- Tenth cranial nerves or vagus nerves
- Eleventh cranial nerves or accessory nerves
- Twelfth cranial nerves or hypoglossal nerves

The spinal nerves are the 31 pairs of nerves that emerge from either side of the spinal cord through gaps between adjacent bones (vertebrae) in the spinal column. The nerves are assigned a specific letter and number based upon the level of the spinal column from which they emerge. Eight pairs of spinal nerves are attached to the cervical segments; 12 pairs to the thoracic segments; five pairs to the lumber segments; five pairs to the sacrospinal segments; and one pair to the coccygeal segment. The designation "C2," for example, refers to the pair of spinal nerves attached to the second segment of the cervical region of the spinal cord. The spinal nerves that emerge from the spinal cord branch to form many of the nerves supplying the trunk and limbs. The function of the spinal nerves is to transmit sensory and motor impulses between the spinal cord to those areas of the body that are not supplied (innervated) by the cranial nerve pairs. More specifically, the sensory nerve fibers of the spinal nerves transmit impulses from sensory receptors in muscles, internal organs, and the skin to the spinal cord, whereas the motor nerve fibers convey motor impulses from the spinal cord to glands and muscles.

Autonomic Nervous System

The autonomic nervous system (ANS) is that portion of the peripheral nervous system responsible for regulation of the involuntary functioning of certain tissues and organs. The ANS includes specialized motor neurons that transmit impulses from the brain stem or the spinal cord to involuntary muscle tissue, cardiac muscle tissue, and specialized glandular cells that produce and secrete certain chemical substances (e.g., hormones, enzymes).

The autonomic nervous system includes two groups of motor neurons (preganglionic and postganglionic neurons) and a group of nerve cell bodies (ganglia) located between them. The cell bodies and dendrites of preganglionic neurons are located in gray matter of the brain stem or spinal cord, and their axons extend to a set of ganglia in the peripheral nervous system. Within the ganglia, the endings of preganglionic neuron axons join with cell bodies or dendrites of postganglionic neurons, which, in turn, convey nerve impulses from ganglia to smooth muscle, cardiac muscle, or glandular tissue. The tissues to which postganglionic neurons transmit impulses are known as visceral effectors.

Autonomic Nervous System Neurotransmitters

There are four distinct types of nerve fibers (axons) in the autonomic nervous system that release certain neurotransmitters (i.e., acetylcholine or norepinephrine). The sympathetic and parasympathetic nervous systems work somewhat, although not completely, in opposition to each other (antagonistic), since each division may inhibit certain visceral effectors and activate others.

The autonomic nervous system is further subdivided into the sympathetic and the parasympathetic nervous systems.

Sympathetic Nervous System

The sympathetic nervous system functions to prepare the body for an emergency. When the body is affected by stress, such as occurs during strong emotions (fear, anger) or exercise, sympathetic nerve impulses increase to many of the body's visceral effectors, resulting in what is sometimes called the "fright-or-flight response." During this response, the heart and breathing rates increase; the pupils of the eyes widen (dilate); and secretions of certain glands increase, while those of other glands decrease. In addition, most blood vessels constrict, resulting in raised blood pressure; blood vessels that supply skeletal muscle widen, supplying additional blood; and the digestive process slows due to a reduction in the rate of the wave-like contractions of smooth muscle within the GI tract.

Parasympathetic Nervous System

The parasympathetic nervous system controls most visceral nerve transmission under normal circumstances, thus slowing and steadying certain bodily activities. For example, impulses conducted by parasympathetic neurons tend to increase peristalsis, speeding the digestive process; slow the heart and breathing rates; contract the pupils; and stimulate the salivary glands.

Description

Reproductive

The female reproductive system includes those organs that enable females to produce the specialized reproductive or sex cells (gametes) known as eggs (ova); engage in reproductive activity; provide nourishment to a fertilized ovum (zygote) during embryonic and fetal development; and give birth. The male reproductive system consists of those organs that enable males to produce and store the reproductive cells (gametes) known as sperm, engage in reproductive activity, and fertilize ova with sperm. The production and secretion of certain chemical substances (hormones) by glands of the endocrine system promote the maturation and normal functioning of reproductive organs and the development of secondary sexual characteristics (puberty) in males and females.

Female Reproductive System

The female reproductive system includes several organs, including the ovaries, fallopian tubes, uterus, vagina, and vulva. With the exception of the vulva (external genitalia), the female reproductive organs are located within the pelvic cavity. In addition, the female breasts (mammary glands) are supportive glands of the female reproductive system.

Ovaries

The female reproductive cells are produced in the paired structures known as the ovaries. These small, egg-shaped glands contain cavities known as follicles in which the female sex cells develop and mature (oogenesis). As females reach puberty (i.e., which typically has an onset between approximately nine to 13 years of age), the follicles begin to release eggs (ovulation) on a regular monthly cycle. This cycle is regulated by female sex hormones (estrogen and progesterone) that are also secreted by the ovaries.

The hormone estrogen promotes the development of female secondary sexual characteristics and normal functioning of reproductive organs (i.e., puberty). It promotes the development and maturation of female reproductive organs; development of the breasts; development of female body contours caused by fat deposition in the breasts and hip area, for example; and initiation (menarche) and regulation of the menstrual cycle. The menstrual cycle is the recurring monthly cycle during which the mucous membrane lining of the uterus (endometrium) is shed; begins to regrow, becoming thick and supplied with blood; is maintained in the uterus, and is again shed. The thickening of the endometrium is stimulated by the hormone progesterone in preparation for implantation of a fertilized egg (zygote). If such fertilization does not occur, progesterone and estrogen production decrease, causing the uterine lining and the unfertilized egg to be shed (menstruation). Progesterone also plays an essential role in the normal functioning of the placenta, the organ that nourishes the developing embryo and fetus during pregnancy.

Fallopian Tubes

A funnel-shaped duct, known as a fallopian tube, uterine tube, or oviduct, extends from each ovary to the uterus. Each tube ends in a structure shaped like a funnel whose edge has finger-like projections. When an egg is released from an ovary, it enters the fallopian tube with the assistance of the beating motions of these projections and microscopic hairs (cilia) on their surfaces. These motions help to propel the egg toward the uterus. In addition, the fallopian tubes serve as the passageways within which the male sex cells (sperm) move toward the ovaries.

Uterus

The uterus, a hollow, pear-shaped organ composed almost entirely of muscle (myometrium), is the organ within which a fertilized egg (zygote) becomes implanted and the developing embryo and fetus is nourished and grows during pregnancy. The organ consists of a lower narrow section known as the cervix and an upper portion called the body. The uterus usually lies in the pelvic cavity behind the bladder. However, during pregnancy, the uterus expands in size as the developing fetus grows and may eventually extend to the top of the abdominal cavity. During the end of pregnancy, strong uterine muscular contractions cause the cervix to open and widen (dilate) and expel the fetus through the vagina.

Other Components of the Female Reproductive System

The vagina is the muscular passage that connects the cervix and the external genitalia and is the portion of the female reproductive tract that opens to the exterior of the body. The vulva is the external, visible portion of the external genitalia.

Breasts

The female breasts, which are supportive glands of the female reproductive system, produce milk to nourish infants after birth (lactation). The female breast consists of approximately 15 to 20 divisions or lobes embedded within fatty tissue. Each lobe is comprised of smaller lobules of milk-secreting glandular cells that are organized in grape-like clusters (alveoli). The small ducts that drain the alveoli have their outlet within the nipple. The circular, colored (pigmented) area of skin surrounding the nipple is known as the areola. Due to secretion of the hormones progesterone and estrogen by the placenta and the ovaries during pregnancy, the milk-secreting glandular cells become active, causing the nipple to become enlarged. Before and after birth, the glands initially produce a thin, watery fluid (colostrum) containing antibodies and proteins that help to protect the newborn from certain infections. Another hormone known as prolactin is responsible for the secretion of milk.

Male Reproductive System

The male reproductive system also includes several organs, including the testes, reproductive ducts, seminal vesicles, bulbourethral glands, prostate gland, and penis.

Testes

In males, the gonads, i.e., the sex glands within which the reproductive cells are produced, are the paired oval-shaped structures known as the testes. The male sex cells produced by the testes, known as spermatozoa or sperm, are responsible for fertilizing the female ova. The testes are located in pouch-like structures called the scrotum.

Each testis is surrounded by a tough, fibrous membrane (tunica albuginea) and contains a long, narrow, coiled structure known as a seminiferous tubule. Sperm develop within the walls of the tubules in a process known as spermatogenesis. In addition, cells located between the tubules produce the male sex hormone testosterone. This male hormone and certain hormones produced in the pituitary gland (gonadotropin hormones) are responsible for the development and production of sperm.

As males reach puberty (i.e., which typically has an onset between approximately 12 to 14 years of age), increased secretion of testosterone promotes muscle and bone growth, stimulates the development of male secondary sexual characteristics, and promotes the normal functioning of the reproductive organs. More specifically, it stimulates sperm production; the development and maturation of male reproductive organs (e.g., seminal vesicles, prostate gland); and the development of male characteristics (e.g. deepening of the voice due to enlargement of the larynx and the vocal cords, growth of facial and body hair, etc.).

Reproductive Ducts

Sperm develop within the walls of the seminiferous tubules of the testes and pass through several reproductive ducts: i.e., the epididymis, ductus (vas) deferens, ejaculatory duct, and urethra. The first of these is the epididymis, a tightly coiled tube that runs along the top and behind the testes. The ductus or vas deferens is the muscular, movable tube that enables sperm to pass from the testes and the epididymis. The ductus deferens joins the duct from the seminal vesicles to form the ejaculatory duct. This duct enables sperm to empty into the urethra, the tube that passes along the length of the penis and carries sperm to the exterior of the body. In males, the urethra also serves as the passageway through which urine is excreted from the body.

Other Components of the Male Reproductive System

Semen (seminal fluid) is a fluid consisting of sperm as well as the secretions of certain supportive sex glands of the male reproductive tract. Such glands include the seminal vesicles, the prostate gland, and the bulbourethral glands.

Semen serves to protect sperm from the acidic environment within the female reproductive tract.

The seminal vesicles, a pair of pouch-like glands, produce the largest portion of the semen's volume. The secretions of the seminal vesicles contain the sugar fructose, which provides a source of energy promoting the mobility of the sperm. The prostate gland, the chestnut-shaped organ under the bladder and in front of the rectum, secretes a thin fluid that forms a portion of the semen's volume and helps sperm to maintain their mobility. The bulbourethral glands, also known as Cowper's glands, are two relatively small, pea-shaped organs located below the prostate gland. The glands produce mucus-like fluids that form a small portion of the semen's volume. In addition, such secretions help to lubricate the end of the urethra. The penis is the portion of the male genitalia through which semen and urine pass.

Description

Respiratory

The respiratory system, comprising the air passages from the nose, throat, bronchial tubes, and lungs, is responsible for filtering the air that enters the body, supplying oxygen to the body, and removing carbon dioxide from the blood. This process is known as respiration. Certain organs of the respiratory (pulmonary) system also influence speech and help to produce the sense of smell (olfaction).

The organs of the respiratory system are often classified into the upper and lower respiratory tract. The upper respiratory tract, which consists of organs that are located outside the actual chest cavity (thorax), includes the nose, pharynx, and larynx. The organs within the lower respiratory tract are located primarily within the thorax and include the trachea, the bronchial tree, and the lungs.

Nose
The nose functions as the uppermost portion of the respiratory tract. This hollow passage, which connects the naval cavities and the upper portion of the throat (nasopharynx), serves to filter, warm, and moisten the air entering the respiratory tract. Mucous membranes (respiratory mucosa) covered by microscopic hairs (cilia) line the entire nasal passage-as well as most passageways of the respiratory tract. Located within the nasal mucosa are specialized nerve receptors necessary for the sense of smell.

During inspiration, air enters the respiratory tract through the nostrils (external nares). Small hairs within the nostrils trap foreign particles, such as dust, pollen, or microorganisms, thus protecting against infection and allergic responses. Filtered air passes into the nasal cavities, which have moist surfaces due to mucus production. The nasal cavities are divided by a structure made of cartilage (nasal septum). Bones surrounding the nose contain hollow, air-filled cavities (paranasal sinuses) that affect the resonance of sound (e.g., during speech). In addition, these mucous-membrane lined cavities, which drain into the nasal cavities, assist in producing mucus for the respiratory tract.

As air passes through the nasal cavities, it is warmed, humidified, and filtered by three thin, mucosa-covered structures (conchae). Mucus on the surface of the conchae and other organs of the respiratory tract flows toward the nasopharynx due to the beating action of the cilia, thereby helping to move trapped foreign particles out of the respiratory tract.

Pharynx
The pharyx, also known as the throat, is a muscular tube lined with mucous membranes. The throat is part of both the respiratory and digestive systems and is divided into three regions: an uppermost portion (nasopharynx) that serves as an air passage; an area of the throat behind the mouth (oropharynx) that is a passage for food and air; and a lower segment (laryngopharynx) that functions as a passage for food only. Air normally enters the pharynx from the nasal cavities (although it may sometimes enter through the mouth) and exits via the larynx. However, food enters the pharynx from the mouth and continues through the digestive system via the esophagus.

The eustachian or auditory tubes also open into the nasopharynx, connecting the middle ears and the throat. In addition, the masses of lymphoid tissue that serve as the "front line" against invading microorganisms (tonsils) are located under the mucous membranes at the back of the pharynx.

Larynx
The larynx, also known as the voice box, connects the pharynx with the trachea. It consists of several areas of fibrous, flexible connective tissue (cartilage) and is also lined with mucous membranes. The larynx is responsible for producing the voice and preventing food from entering the airway during swallowing.

The opening of the larynx is partially covered by a "lid-like" flap of cartilage known as the epiglottis. This structure normally remains open, maintaining the larynx as part of the airway. However, when swallowing occurs, the epiglottis closes, sealing off the opening of the larynx and preventing food from passing into the larynx and the trachea. In addition, two strong, fibrous sheets of tissue known as the vocal cords stretch across the interior of the larynx. Passage of air over the vocal cords results in vibrations that help to create speech.

Trachea
The trachea, also known as the windpipe, extends from the larynx to an area behind the upper breastbone (sternum), where it then divides to form the two bronchi. The windpipe is a tube-like structure composed of elastic and fibrous tissues, smooth (involuntary) muscle, and rings of cartilage that help to keep the trachea open (patent). As with other organs of the respiratory tract, the trachea is also lined with mucous membranes (respiratory mucosa) covered by cilia. The secreted mucus helps to trap tiny foreign particles remaining in the inhaled air of the trachea, and the beating action of the cilia propels the mucus upward toward the pharynx and out of the respiratory tract.

Bronchial Tree
Because the numerous air passages of the lungs resemble an upside-down, tree-like structure, the bronchi and their branching airways are known as the bronchial tree. The trachea branches to form the main bronchi (primary bronchi) of the left and right lungs. Both of the primary bronchi then branch into smaller bronchi (secondary bronchi). The bron-

chi walls consist of three layers including an outer layer of fibrous, dense tissue; a middle layer of smooth muscle; and an inner layer of mucous membranes. In addition, the walls of the primary and secondary bronchi, like the trachea, are kept open by rings of cartilage, allowing the passage of air.

The bronchi divide into progressively smaller airways that eventually branch into tiny passages known as bronchioles. The walls of the bronchioles include only smooth muscle. The bronchioles then branch into microscopic tubes known as alveolar ducts that lead to the alveolar sacs. The walls of the alveolar sacs consist of many microscopic, grape-like structures called alveoli. The alveoli lie in contact with microscopic blood vessels (capillaries). The exchange of oxygen and carbon dioxide takes place across the thin walls of the alveoli, i.e., oxygen moves from the alveoli to the blood while carbon dioxide moves from the blood to the alveoli.

Lungs

The lungs, which are spongy, elastic organs located in the chest cavity, are divided into lobes: the left lung has two lobes, whereas the right lung has three. The narrow, rounded, upper area of each lung is known as the apex, and the broad, concave, lower portion of each lung that rests on the diaphragm is referred to as the base. In addition, a thin, moist, two-layered membrane known as the pleura lines the outside of the lungs and the inside of the chest cavity. A small amount of fluid separates the two layers of the pleura, serving as a lubricant as the lungs contract and expand during respiration.

The act of breathing (pulmonary ventilation) consists of two phases: inspiration and expiration. During inspiration, the chest and lungs expand, and air is drawn into the lungs. During expiration, the chest and lungs contract and air is forced out of the lungs.

Pulmonary Circulation

Pulmonary circulation refers to the movement of blood through vessels between the heart and the lungs for the removal of carbon dioxide and the addition of oxygen (oxygenation) to the blood. When the right lower chamber of the heart (ventricle) contracts, "oxygen-poor" (deoxygenated) blood is pumped to the lungs via the pulmonary artery. From there, the blood flows through the capillaries that lie in contact with the air-filled alveoli. Oxygen moves across the thin walls of the alveoli into the blood, whereas carbon dioxide is transported by the blood to the alveoli. Carbon dioxide exits the lungs during expiration. Oxygenated blood is returned to the left upper chamber of the heart (atrium) via four pulmonary veins and is propelled into the left ventricle. When the left ventricle contracts, the blood is pumped into the major artery of the body (aorta) for circulation to the body's tissues. In addition, the blood that nourishes the lungs themselves is supplied by the bronchial arteries.

Description

Sensory Organs

Certain specialized components of the nervous system, known as sense organs, are able to recognize specific stimuli in the external environment that affect the body, such as light, sound, temperature, or pressure. When the specialized microscopic structures that comprise the sensory organs (sensory receptors) recognize certain stimuli, they produce nervous impulses that are sent to the brain, the spinal cord, or both. The sense organs may be classified into two general categories: the somatic sense organs and the special sense organs.

Special Sense Organs

Sensory receptors for the special senses of hearing, vision, smell, and taste, are collected in the special sense organs, including the eyes (i.e., in the retinas), the ears (within the hearing apparatus), the nose (smell receptors), and the tongue (taste receptors). Sensory information received by these special sense organs travels to the brain via the cranial nerves, the 12 nerve pairs that arise from the brain and emerge through various openings in the skull. Most sensory information is transmitted to the sensory cortex of the brain.

Ears, Hearing, and Balance

The ear is the special sensory organ involved in hearing and balance. It consists of three major parts including
- external ear
- middle ear
- inner ear

The External Ear

The external ear includes the visible portion of the ear (pinna or auricle) and the external auditory canal. The pinna consists of folds of cartilage and skin surrounding the opening of the auditory canal, which is the tube that extends into the lower cranium bone (temporal bone) and ends at the partition between the external and middle ear (eardrum or tympanic membrane). The skin of the auditory canal contains specialized glands (ceruminous glands) that produce cerumen, a waxy substance that traps dust and other foreign bodies. Sound waves pass through the auditory canal and strike the eardrum, causing it to vibrate.

The Middle Ear

The middle ear, a tiny cavity between the eardrum and the inner ear, contains three minute, movable bones (ossicles) that conduct sound to the inner ear. The names of the bones essentially describe their shapes: i.e., the malleus (hammer), incus (anvil), and stapes (stirrup). When the eardrum vibrates in response to sound waves, the vibrations are transmitted and amplified by the three ear bones. The stapes' movement against a membrane-covered opening to the inner ear results in movement of the fluid within the inner ear.

The eustachian or auditory tube connects the middle ear to the uppermost region of the throat (nasopharynx). Although the eustachian tube is usually closed at rest, it opens due to muscle contractions associated with swallowing or yawning. The eustachian tube is shorter in infants and young children than in older children and adults. As a result, when an upper respiratory tract infection occurs, infants and young children have an increased likelihood of experiencing the backward flow of secretions from the nasopharynx into the middle ear space and associated infection of the middle ear (otitis media).

The Inner Ear

The inner ear contains a maze of complex, winding passages (known as the labyrinth) deep within the temporal bone. The major parts of the inner ear include the organ of hearing, known as the cochlea, and the organ of balance, the semicircular canals.

The cochlea, a hollow, coiled passage that resembles a snail's shell, contains the organ of Corti and thick fluid. The organ of Corti has tiny cells with hair-like extensions projecting into the fluid. Vibrations transmitted to the inner ear cause the fluid and the hair-like extensions to vibrate. As a result, the hair cells are stimulated to generate nerve impulses that are transmitted by the vestibulocochlear nerve (acoustic nerve or eighth cranial nerve) to the brain.

The three semicircular canals are fluid-filled tubes containing specialized hair cells that respond to movement of the fluid. When movements of the head cause fluid movement within a canal, the cells initiate nerve impulses to the brain via the vestibulocochlear nerve, resulting in necessary adjustments to maintain balance.

The Eyes and Vision

The eye is a specialized sensory organ that is actually part of the central nervous system. It focuses light waves to create an image on the nerve-rich membrane at the back of the eye (retina). The retina, in turn, converts the image into nerve impulses that are transmitted to the brain via the optic nerve (second cranial nerve).

Anatomy and Function of the Eye

The eye is embedded in pads of fat within the bony socket in the skull. Movements of the eye are regulated by a network of six muscles, each of which moves the eye in a particular direction or directions.

The outermost layer of the eye, known as the sclera, is a tough, fibrous tissue that includes the "white" of the eye and the cornea, which is the front, circular, transparent area that serves as the eye's primary lens. A flexible mucous membrane, the conjunctiva, covers the sclera and lines the eyelid; in addition, the conjunctiva contains several glands that secrete tears and mucus. The eyelid consists of a thin layer of skin over muscle that covers a thin plate of connective tissue (tarsal plate). The edge of the eyelid contains a row of strong protective hairs known as eyelashes as well as several glands (meibomian glands) that produce an oily secretion known as sebum. The combined actions of the tear-secreting and mucus-producing glands of the conjunctiva and the meibomian glands of the eyelid produce an essential tear film that protects the conjunctiva and cornea from damage due to drying. The eyelid spreads the tear film over the cornea during the blink reflex, helping to ensure clear vision. Moreover, the eyelid further protects the eye by closing quickly as an involuntary reaction (reflex action) to the approach of any foreign object.

The middle layer of the eye, known as the choroid, includes two involuntary muscles: the iris and the ciliary muscle. The iris, the pigmented area visible through the cornea, is a circular muscle with a hole in its center known as the pupil, which controls the amount of light entering the eye. When certain fibers in the iris contract, the pupil widens, allowing in additional light; in contrast, when other iris fibers contract, the pupil constricts, allowing in less light. The lens of the eye, which is behind the pupil, is held in place by the ciliary muscle, a circular muscle that changes the shape of the lens to make appropriate adjustments in focus. For example, the ciliary muscle contracts when the eye focuses on near objects and relaxes when the eye views distant objects.

The hollow main cavity of the eye is filled with fluids that help to ensure the proper shape of the eyeball and assist in bending light rays that fall on the retina. The fluids include the thin, watery fluid in front of the lens (aqueous humor) and the jelly-like fluid behind the lens (vitreous humor).

The retina, the innermost layer of the eye, is a complex nerve-rich membrane upon which images created by the cornea and the lens fall. More specifically, as light passes through the cornea, the pupil, the aqueous humor, the lens, and the vitreous humor, it is bent (refracted) so that it is properly focused on the retina, which contains millions of tiny nerve cells that respond to light (photoreceptors). Such nerve cells are named based upon their shapes: i.e., rods and cones. Rods are stimulated by dim light and are necessary for night vision. Cones are stimulated by brighter light and are the receptors for daytime vision. Three different types of cones respond to the colors red, blue, or green. The rods and cones convert images formed on the retina into nerve impulses that are transmitted by the optic nerve (second cranial nerve) to the brain.

The Nose and the Smell Receptors

In addition to serving as the uppermost region of the respiratory tract, the nose also functions as the special sensory organ involved in the sense of smell (olfaction). The chemical receptors necessary for olfaction are specialized nerve cell endings located in a small area of mucous membrane (nasal mucosa) lining the nasal cavities. The olfactory cells have specialized, microscopic hairs (cilia) that are stimulated by different chemicals. In response to such chemicals, the cilia generate nerve impulses that pass through the olfactory nerve (first cranial nerve) to the smell centers of the brain.

The Tongue and the Taste Receptors

The tongue is the muscular, flexible organ in the floor of the mouth. This organ-which also plays an essential role in producing speech, breaking down food during chewing (mastication), and swallowing - functions as a specialized sensory organ involved in taste.

There are approximately 10,000 microscopic chemical receptors known as taste buds that produce the nerve impulses required for taste. Although most are located on the tongue, there are also some taste buds on the roof of the mouth (palate) and the back of the throat. The taste buds surround the bases of nipple-shaped elevations (papillae) that cover the surface of the tone and other tissues. Specialized cells within the taste buds (gustatory cells) generate nerve impulses in response to dissolved chemicals within saliva. Most of these impulses pass through the facial nerve (seventh cranial nerve) and the glossopharyngeal nerve (ninth cranial nerve) to the taste center of the brain. Stimulation of the taste buds results in four types of taste sensations including sour, sweet, bitter, and salty. Other taste sensations or "flavors" result due to the combined stimulation of taste and olfactory receptors.

Description

Urologic

The urinary system, which consists of the two kidneys, the ureters, the bladder, and the urethra, filters waste products from the blood, returns essential nutrients back into the blood, and produces and excretes urine.

The Kidneys

The kidneys, which are located at the back of the abdominal cavity, are situated on either side of the spinal column above the waistline. The right kidney lies beneath the liver. The left kidney, which is usually slightly higher than the right, is located below the spleen.

The primary functions of the kidneys are to regulate the delicate balance of electrolytes including sodium and potassium; control the acid-base balance of the body (i.e., ensuring that the blood and other bodily fluids are neither too acidic nor alkaline); and filter soluble wastes from the blood and eliminate these waste products. More specifically, the purpose of the kidneys includes the following:

- To filter certain waste products (e.g., urea, ammonia) and excessive sodium and water from the blood

- To reabsorb particular substances and return them to the blood

- To regulate the levels of certain substances in the blood and maintain the appropriate balance between water and salt content in the body (i.e., by filtration, reabsorption, and secretion)

- To regulate blood pressure and the production and release of red blood cells. For example, cells of the juxtaglomerular apparatus of the kidneys secrete a hormone (renin) that results in the constriction of blood vessels, thereby raising blood pressure. In addition, the kidneys produce erythropoietin, a hormone that assists in stimulating and regulating the production and release of red blood cells (erythrocytes) from the bone marrow. An increase in the number of circulating red blood cells boosts the body's capacity to carry oxygen to its tissues and organs.

Urine Production and Excretion

The kidneys each contain approximately one million nephrons, the filtering units of the kidneys. Each nephron consists of two primary components, the renal corpuscle and the renal tubule, both of which are further divided into additional regions.

The top of each nephron consists of a cup-shaped structure known as Bowman's capsule. Within Bowman's capsule is a network of tiny capillaries known as a glomerulus. Together, the two structures are known as the renal corpuscle.

As blood flows through the kidneys, the fluid portion of the blood is filtered by minute pores in the blood vessels of the glomerulus and the inner layer of Bowman's capsule. The fluid then moves into the region between the inner and outer layers of Bowman's capsule and enters into the first portion of the renal tubule (proximal convoluted tubule), where most filtered substances (e.g., most of the water, glucose, and sodium) are reabsorbed into the blood via capillaries around the tubules (peritubular capillaries). Next, as fluid moves into the loop of Henle, sodium and other electrolytes are pumped out. As the fluid passes through the next portion of the renal tubule (distal convoluted tubule), additional sodium is removed in exchange for potassium. Diluted fluid from distal convoluted tubules then passes into a collecting tubule, where fluid may continue to pass through the urinary tract as dilute urine or be returned to the blood to ensure appropriate water content in the body.

Urine then drains from the collecting tubules into central collecting areas (renal pelvis) of each kidney, which are the upper portions of the ureters. The ureters are narrow muscular tubes lined by mucous membranes. Contractions of the ureters' muscular walls move small quantities of urine into the bladder, a hollow organ that gradually expands as the volume of urine increases. As the bladder nears its capacity, nerve signals are transmitted to the brain to signal that urination is necessary. When urination occurs, the circular muscle (sphincter) between the bladder and the urethra opens, allowing urine to pass out of the body. Contractions of the bladder create pressure that forces urine into the urethra and out its external opening (urinary meatus).

A

A&K Associates, 4438

A-TMRF Newsletter, 570

A-to-Z Health & Disease Information, 7129

A.J. Pappanikou Center for Developmental Disabilities, 8154

AAAAI Annual Meeting, 454

AABA Newsletter, 2970

AACAP, 2492

AACAP & CACAP Joint Annual Meeting, 1674, 8580

AACAP News, 5429

AACE Annual Meeting and Clinical Congress, 2231

AADB E-News, 3864, 8675

AADB National Symposium, 1895, 2046, 3579

AAP Education Resource Guide, 8687

AAP Grand Rounds, 6346

AAP News, 6340

AASCEND, 342

ABA Program Companion, 906

Abbott Northwestern Brain Tumor SupportGroup at Abbott Northwestern Hospital, 1201

ABC Stories DVD, 3592

ABC's of Finger Spelling, 3722

ABCs of AVT: Analyzing Auditory-Verbal Therapy, 3723

ABCs of AVT: Analyzing Auditory-VerbalTherapy, 3593

ABDC Newsletter, 8676

Ability First, 8718

Ability First, Camp Paivika, 8719

ABLEDATA, 7866

AbleData, 3545

About Children's Eyes, 8688

About Children's Vision: A Guide forParents, 8689

About Down Syndrome, 2756

About Ependymoma, 1274

About Glioblastoma Multiforme and Anaplastic Astrocytoma, 1275

About Headaches, 4768

About Hydrocephalus - Book for Families, 4265

About Medulloblastoma/PNET(Medulloblastoma), 1276

About Meningioma, 1277

About Metastatic Tumors to the Brain and Spine, 1278

About NDSS, 2754

About Neurofibromatosis 1, 5053

About Oligodendroglioma and Mixed Glioma, 1279

About Pituitary Tumors, 1280

About Special Kids (ASK), 8207

About the American Brain Tumor Association, 1281

About.com on Sleep Disorders, 5137, 6680, 6707

AboutFace USA, 1692

ACAAI Annual Meeting, 455

ACAAI eNews, 6347

Academic Pediatric Association, 7870

Academy for Eating Disorders (AED), 2887

Academy for Guided Imagery, 7871

Academy for Sports Dentistry, 2391

Academy of General Dentistry, 2392

Academy of Nutrition and Dietetics, 2835

Academy of Operative Dentistry, 2393

Academy of Osseointegration, 2394

Academy of Rehabilitative Audiology, 3477, 7872

Accelerate Brain Cancer Cure, 1079

Access Board, 7873

Accidents of Nature, 1499

Achieve Beyond, 715

Achieving in Spite of...A Booklet on Learning Disabilities, 5054

Achondroplasia, 2, 20

Achondroplasia UK, 13

ACLP Annual Conference, 97, 8581

ACLP Bulletin Newsletter, 8677

ACM Lifting Lives Music Camp, 7787

Acoustic Neuroma Association, 3353

Acoustical Society of America, 3478

Acoustics, Audition and Speech Reception, 3597

ACPOC Annual Meeting, 3172

Acquiring Courage: Audio Cassette Programfor the Rapid Treatment of Phobias, 5588, 6736

Action for Healthy Kids, 5304

Activity Schedules for Children withAutism, 907

Acute Gastrointestinal Infections, 21

Acute Lymphoblastic Leukemia, 61

Acute Lymphocytic Leukemia, 165

Acute Myeloid Leukemia, 121

AD-IN: Attention Deficit InformationNetwork, 600

ADA Technical Assistance Program, 1378

The ADA: Questions and Answers, 6616

ADAA Annual Conference, 2482, 8582

Adam and the Magic Marble, 7436

ADARA, 7867

ADD & Learning Disabilities, 641

ADD From A To Z-Understanding The Diagnosis & Treatment of ADD in Children & Adult, 621

ADD: Helping Your Child, 642

ADDitude, 7714

ADHD, 691

The ADHD Book of Lists, 684

ADHD Challenge, 601

ADHD in Schools: Assessment andIntervention Strategies, 645

ADHD in the Young Child, 646

ADHD Parenting Handbook: Practical Advicefor Parents from Parents, 643

ADHD Report, 688

ADHD Survival Guide for Parents andTeachers, 644

ADHD: Handbook for Diagnosis & Treatment, 647

ADHD: What Can We Do?, 622

ADHD: What Do We Know?, 623

Administration for Children & Families-Child Abuse and Neglect Prevention, 5646

Administration on DevelopmentalDisabilities, 7829

Adolescent Health On-Line, 8608

Adolescent Idiopathic Scoliosis-Prevalence ,Natural History, Treatments, 6512

Adolescents with Down Syndrome, 2728

Adoptive Families, 7874, 8609, 8667

Adriene Resource Center for Blind Children, 1873, 2020, 5252, 6180

Adult Brain Tumor Support Group, 1251

Adult Down Syndrome Center of LutheranGeneral Hospital, 2681

Adult Endocrine Disorders/GHDEducational Convention, 11, 333, 1810

Advanced Cancer: Coping with Advanced Cancer, 8690

Adventure Learning Center Camp Programs, 1801, 7769

Adventures of Maxx, 4056

Advocacy Center, 8335

Advocate Lutheran General Children'sHospital, Pediatric Research, 2682

Advocates for Children of New York, 8336, 8792

Advocates for Justice and Education, 8163

Advocure NF2, 6752

AEGIS, 3321

AER Regional Conference, 1896

AES News, 6595

African American Collaborative Obesity Research Network, 5305

After Sudden Infant Death Syndrome, 7104

After the Diagnosis...The Next Steps, 7416

After the Tears: Parents Talk AboutRaising a Child with a Disability, 1513

AG Bell Biennial Convention, 3580

Agency for Health Care Research, 7830

Agency for Healthcare Research and Quality, 2437

Aggression and Violence Throughout theLife Span, 1789, 7739

Aging with Autism, 716

Agoraphobics in Motion, 5562

AHA Association [Asperger Syndrome and High Functioning Autism Association, 343

AHEPA Cooley's Anemia Foundation, 7242

AIDS and the Education of Our Children, 3336

AIDS Awareness Library, 3335

AIDS Healthcare Foundation, 3281

AIDS Knowledge Base, 3322

AIDS Research Alliance, 3282

AIDS United, 3283

AIM for the Handicapped Adventures inMovement, 7868

Air Support America, 404

AJAO Newsletter, 4402

Al Capone Does My Shirts: A Novel, 908

Alabama Department of RehabilitationServices, 3988

Alabama Head Injury Foundation, 3364

Alabama Institute for the Deaf & Blind, 1824, 1969, 3551, 5202, 6121

Alabama/Northwest Florida Chapter of Crohns Colitis Foundation of America, 2144

Alandra's Lilacs, 3727

Alaska Chapter of Asthma and Allergy Foundation of America, 429

Alaska Department of Education, 8087

Albany Library for the Blind and PhysicalHandicapped, 1844, 1990, 5223, 6151

Albany Medical College Pediatric Pulmonary& Cystic Fibrosis Center, 2306

Albany New York Regional ComprehensiveHemophilia Treatment Center, 3991

Albinism, 172

Alcohol, Tobacco and Other Drugs May Harmthe Unborn, 3156

Aleh Foundation, 2635, 2719

Alert, 571

Alex's Journey: The Story of a Child witha Brain Tumor, 1266

Alex: The Life of a ChildRutledge Press, 2359

Alexander Graham Bell Association for theDeaf and Hard of Hearing, 3479, 7875

Alexandria Library Talking Book Service, 1883, 2030, 5262, 6190

Alexis Foundation - Premature Infants andChildren, 5900

All About Amblyopia (Lazy Eye), 4473

All About Vision, 4474

All About Vision.Com, 4475

All Ages Support Group, 1163

All Children Have Different Eyes, 4486

ALL Kids, 100

All Kids By TwoHealth Services Agency, 5957

All Kinds of Friends, Even Green!, 6878

All Kinds of Minds, 648

All Nations Camp, 8720

All of Us Together, 3728

Alleghenies United Cerebral Palsy, 1472

Allen County Public Library, 8478

Allergy & Asthma Issues, 458, 6348

Allergy & Asthma Network Mothers of Asthmatics, 405, 467

Allergy & Asthma Today, 485

Allergy and Asthma Medical Group and Research Center, 6325

Allergy and Asthma Support Group of Central New Jersey, 6322

Allergy and Pulmonary Medicine, 435

Allergy Control Begins at Home: House Dust Allergy, 459

Allergy Web, 7663

Alliance Brochure, 576

Alliance for a Healthier Generation, 5306

Alliance for Assistive Service andTechnology (FAAST), 8169

Alliance for Eating Disorder Awarenes, 2836

Alliance for Eating Disorders Awareness, 2903

Alliance for Technology Access (ATA), 7876, 8452

Alliance of Genetic Support Groups, 3253

Aloha Special Technology Access Center, 8471

Alone in the Mainstream: A Deaf Women Remembers Public School, 3729

Alopecia Areata, 197

Alpha Omega International Dental Fraternity, 2395

Alpha-1-Antitrypsin Deficiency, 210

Alphabet of Animal Signs, 3730

Alphabet Soup: A Recipe for Understanding& Treating ADD, 649

AlphaNet, Inc., 211

Alternative Approaches, 6049

Amblyopia, 4494

America's Special Kidz, 345

American Academy for Cerebral Palsy andDevelopmental Medicine, 1379, 1498, 1501

American Academy of Allergy, Asthma & Immunology, 6315

American Academy of Allergy, Asthma &Immunology, 406

American Academy of Allergy, Asthma and Immunology, 468

American Academy of Audiology, 3480, 5473, 7877

American Academy of Child & AdolescentPsychiatry, 7326, 7336, 7359, 7427

American Academy of Child and AdolescentPsychiatry, 1668, 5419, 5422, 7673, 7878

American Academy of Cosmetic Dentistry, 2396

American Academy of Dental Hygiene, 2397

American Academy of Dental Practice Administration, 2398

American Academy of Dermatology, 198

American Academy of Dermatology (AAD), 3917, 4417, 5740, 6029, 7197, 7206, 7243, 7879

American Academy of Esthetic Dentistry, 2399

American Academy of Family Physicians, 2095, 7674

American Academy of HIV Medicine, 3284

American Academy of Neurology, 4748, 4754

American Academy of Neurology: TouretteSyndrome, 7428

American Academy of Orthopaedic Surgeons, 6488

American Academy of Otolaryngology Head and Neck Surgery, 1008

American Academy of Otolaryngology-Headand Neck Surgery, 1002

American Academy of Pediatric DentistryFoundation, 2400, 2431

American Academy of Pediatrics, 6, 23, 64, 124, 174, 199, 212, 224, 235, 249, 259, 284, 295, 302, 312, 328, 346, 407, 501, 589, 603

American Academy of Periodontology, 2402

American Academy of Sleep Medicine, 4881, 5096, 5126, 6674, 6681, 6701

American Academy of Somnology, 5112, 5135, 6678, 6706

American Action Fund for Blind Childrenand Adults, 1832, 1978, 3553, 5211, 6139

American Amputee Foundation, 7881

American Annals of the Deaf, 3860

American Anorexia Bulimia Association of Philadelphia, 5337

American Asperger's Association, 347

American Association for Cancer Research, 1081

American Association for Dental Research, 2403

American Association for Marriage and Family Therapy, 348

American Association for Pediatric Opthalmology, 1889, 1901, 2637, 3141

American Association for Respiratory Care, 408, 5929

American Association for the Study ofLiver Diseases, 1014

American Association for Thoracic Surgery, 5930

American Association of Children'sResidential Centers (AACRC), 7882

American Association of ClinicalEndocrinologists, 2226, 4346, 4353

American Association of Diabetes Educators, 2551

American Association of Endodontists, 2404

American Association of Neurological Surgeons, 1082

American Association of Oral and Maxillofacial Surgeons, 2405

American Association of Orthodontics, 2406

American Association of Orthodontists, 2407

American Association of People with Disabilities, 4678

American Association of Public Health Dentistry, 2408

American Association of Sleep Technologists, 5097

American Association of Suicidology, 2439

American Association of the Deaf-Blind, 3482, 7883

American Association on Health and Disabilities, 4679

American Association on Intellectual and Developmental Disabilities, 4712, 7884

American Asthma Foundation, 409

American Auditory Society, 7885

American Autoimmune Related Diseases Association, 200, 250, 255, 1335, 1570, 1586, 2137, 2552, 3273, 3275, 3933, 3934, 5084, 5088, 5524, 5538, 6351, 6386, 6434, 6452, 7135

American Beverage Association, 5308

American Blind Bowling Association, 7887

American Blind Skiing Foundation, 7888

American Board of Dermatology, 7889

American Board of Fluency and Fluency Disorders, 6754

American Board of Pediatrics, 7890, 8612

American Board of Sleep Medicine, 5098

American Brain Tumor Association, 1083, 1260

American Brain Tumor Association MessageLine, 3463

American Brain Tumor Association PatientLine, 1084

American Camp Association, 4602

American Camping Association, 7891

American Cancer Society, 1085, 3105, 7793, 7892

American Canoe Association, 7893

American Celiac Disease Alliance, 1336

American Celiac Society, 1337, 1368

American Celiac Society Dietary Support, 1338

American Childhood Cancer Organization (formerly Candlelighters Childhood Cancer), 65, 125, 1086, 3106, 4188, 5065, 5079, 5166, 6269, 7794, 7894

American Cleft Palate-Craniofacial Association, 2409

American Cochlear Implant Alliance, 3483

American College Counseling Association, 2440

American College Health Association, 2441

American College of Allergy, Asthma & Immunology, 6317

American College of Allergy, Asthma andImmunology, 410

American College of Cardiology, 313

American College of Dentists, 2410

American College of Gastroenterology, 24, 260, 1745, 3091, 4126, 4133, 4976, 5408, 6096

American College of Medical Genetics, 3189, 8613

American College of Preventive Medicine, 3286

American College ofNeuropsychopharmacology, 7676

American Congress of Obstetricians andGynecologists, 7677

American Council of Blind Parents, 1881, 2028, 5260, 6188

American Council of the Blind, 175, 1819

American Counseling Association, 1032, 5564, 5781, 6721, 7678

American Deaf Culture: An Anthology, 3731

American Deafness and Rehabilitation Association (ADARA), 3484

American Dental Assistants Association, 2411

American Dental Association, 2412, 2980, 2990, 4742, 4743, 7314, 7317

American Dental Education Association, 2413

American Dental Hygienists Association, 2414

American Dental Society of Anesthesiology, 2415

American Dermatological Association, 7895
American Diabetes Association, 2553, 2602
American Dietetic Association, 1339
American Epilepsy Society, 6527, 6563, 7896
American Foundation for AIDS Research, 3317
American Foundation for Children with AIDS, 3287
American Foundation for Suicide Prevention, 2442
American Foundation for the Blind, 176, 4461
American Gastroenterological Association, 25, 36
American Group Psychotherapy Association, 1033
American Hair Loss Association, 201
American Headache Society, 4750
American Hearing Impaired Hockey Association, 3485
American Hearing Research Foundation, 3486, 5475, 7897
American Heart Association, 285, 314, 590, 1734, 4292, 4296, 5513, 6077,
    6087, 7226, 7231, 7245, 7298, 7303, 7361, 7483, 7488, 7667, 7898
American Institute for Preventive Medicine, 2093
American Journal of Gastroenterology, 44
American Journal of Speech-Language Pathology, 6797
American Journal on Mental Retardation, 4718
American Juvenile Arthritis Organization, 251, 4388, 7136, 7899
American Kidney Fund, 4992, 4995
American Laryngological Association, 6755
American Liver Foundation, 213, 3199, 3205, 4097, 4104, 4114, 4426,
    4977, 4984, 7815, 7900
American Lung Association, 214, 411, 469, 1305, 1309, 2239, 5752, 6078,
    6236, 6239, 6246, 6248, 7362, 7519, 7524, 7901
American Lung Association of the City of New York, 2353
American Lyme Disease Foundation, 4603, 4615
American Medical Association, 412, 1746, 5309, 5931, 7679
American Mental Health Counselors Association, 1034
American Mental Health Foundation (AMHF), 1610, 1764, 4680, 5099,
    5127, 5488, 5565, 6722, 7680
American Network of Community Options & Resources, 4681
American Nurses Association, 3288, 5932
American Nystagmus Network, 5198, 5275
American Obesity Treatment Association, 5310
American Occupational Therapy Association, 4682
American Osteopathic College of Dermatology, 1571, 1587, 4419
American Pediatric Surgical Association, 6104
American Pediatrics Society, 7902
American Porphyria Foundation, 5771
American Pregnancy Association, 1747, 3142, 5933
American Professional Society on the Abuse of Children, 5649, 5687
American Pseudo-Obstruction and Hirschsprung's Disease Society, 4157
American Psychiatric Association, 1035, 2443, 2838, 3289, 5566, 6723,
    7681
American Psychiatric Nurses Association, 1036
The American Psychiatric Publishing Textbook of Schizophrenia, 1657
American Psychoanalytic Association, 1037
American Psychological Association, 718, 1038, 2444, 2839, 3290, 5311,
    5567, 5782, 6724, 7682
American Public Health Association, 2445, 2840, 3291, 4683, 5934, 7683
American Red Cross, 7903
American School Counselor Association, 177, 349, 413, 719, 1381, 2446,
    2638, 2772, 2841, 4505, 5312, 5568, 6725, 6756, 6953, 7328, 7363, 7684
American Sickle Cell Anemia Association, 6628, 6657
American SIDS Institute, 6983, 7071, 7083
American Sign Language Dictionary Third Edition, 3732
American Sign Language Handshape Dictionary DVD, 3598
American Sign Language Teachers Association, 3487
American Sign Language V2.0, 3687
American Sign Language Video Series, 3599
American Sign Language Vocabulary, 3688
American Sign Language: A Student Text; Units 10-18, 3733
American Sign Language: A Student Text; Units 19-27, 3735
American Sign Language: A Student Text; Units 1-9, 3734
American Sign Language: Green Books Text and Tapes, 3600
American Skin Association, 3919, 4420, 7199, 7207, 7246, 7904
American Sleep Apnea Association, 296, 6675, 6682
American Sleep Association, 5100
American Sleep Medicine Foundation, 5101
American Social Health Association, 3292, 3323, 4143, 4147, 4962, 4965
American Society for Deaf Children, 3488, 7905
American Society for Dental Aesthetics, 2416
American Society for Gastrointestinal Endoscopy, 1340
American Society for Metabolic and Bariatric Surgery, 5313
American Society For Microbiology, 5935
American Society for Microbiology, 3293
American Society for Nutrition, 5314

American Society for Reproductive Medicine, 7364, 7557
American Society of Bariatric Physicians, 5315
American Society of Clinical Oncology, 3294, 5316
American Society of Clinical Psychopharmacology, 2447
American Society of Forensic Odontology, 2417
American Society of Pediatric Neurosurgeons, 8614
American Speech Language Hearing Association (ASHA), 2787, 2805,
    2817, 3489, 4506, 6757, 6954, 7906
American Speech Language Hearing Association (ASHA), 2773
American Speech-Language-Hearing Foundation, 3490
American Student Dental Association, 2418
American Thoracic Society, 414, 5317, 5936
American Tinnitus Association, 3491
American Urological Association, 1748
American Urological Association Foundation, 5152, 5158
American Wheelchair Table Tennis Association, 7907
AmeriFace, 1681, 2113, 3032, 4579
AmeriFace Newsletter, 1700, 3048
AMOR - A Cancer Support Group for Patients & Their Families, 1207
AMT Children of Hope Foundation, 5647
Amyloidosis and Kidney Disease, 8691
An End to Panic: Breakthrough Techniques for Overcoming Panic Disorder,
    5604
An Introduction to Cystic Fibrosis for Patients and Families, 2370
An Introduction to Pemphigus, 5542
An Introduction to Your Child Who Has Cerebral Palsy, 1514
ANA National Symposium Acoustic Neuroma Association, 3581
ANA Symposium, 3441
Analgesic Rebound Headaches-Fact Sheet, 4769
Anchor Point Camp, 392, 975, 4533
Ancient Greece, 3601
Anemia of Sarcoidosis, 6400
Anencephaly, 222
Anencephaly Support Foundation, 225
anfAR, 3316
Angels in the Sun Brain Tumor Support Group, 1155
Angels of Hope, 1213
Angry Gut, The: Coping with Colitis and Crohn's Disease, 7637
Animal Signs: A First Book of Sign Language, 3736
Animals, Insects, School, Colors Spanish/English Videos, 3602
Aniridia, 233
Aniridia Network, 241
Aniridia Web Site, 242
Ankylosing Spondylitis, 247, 257
Ann Whitehill Down Syndrome Program, 2684
Annual Education Conference & Food Faire, 1355
Annual International Conference on ADHD, 616
Annual Meeting & OTO Expo, 1007
Annual New York State Child Abuse Prevention Conference, 5684
Annual TEACCH Conference, 867
Annual World Symposium on Ocular Albinism, 186
Anorectal Malformations, 258
Anorectal Malformations- A Parent's Guide, 280
Anorexia Nervosa & Recovery: A Hunger for Meaning, 2929
Anorexia Nervosa & Related Eating Disorders, 2842
Anorexia Nervosa and Related Eating Disorders, 2920
Answering Your Questions About Spina Bifida, 6879
Answers to Some Commonly Asked Questions, 7608
Answers to Your Questions about Panic Disorder, 5593
Antisocial Behavior by Young People, 1790, 7740
Anxiety & Depression In Adults & Children, 2502
Anxiety & Phobia Workbook, 5605, 6738
Anxiety and Depression Association of America, 1039, 2449, 5571
Anxiety and Phobia Treatment Center, 5572, 6728
Anxiety Cure: An Eight-Step Program for Getting Well, 5606, 6739
Anxiety Disorders, 5589, 5607, 5616, 6737, 6740, 6746
Anxiety Disorders Association of America, 2448, 2493, 5360, 5378, 5569,
    5594, 5783, 6726
Anxiety Disorders Fact Sheet, 5617, 6747
Anxiety Disorders in Children and Adolescents, 5618, 6748
Anxiety Disorders Institute, 5570, 6727
Anxiety Disorders: Practitioner's Guide, 5608, 6741
Anxiety Panic Internet Resource, 5595
AOCD Annual Meeting, 1583
Aortic Stenosis, 281
APF Newsletter, 5776
Aphasia Hope Foundation, 6758
Apnea Identification Program, 7025
Apnea of Prematurity, 292, 298

Apparent Life - Threatening Event andSudden Infant Death Syndrome, 7090

Applying New Attitudes & Directions, 2974

Approaching Equality, 3737

APSAC Advisor, 5716

The Arc, 3154

Arc (The), 4684

ARC Annual National Convention, 2706, 3186, 4204, 8583

ARC Family Connection Parent to ParentProgram, 8251

ARC Family Resource Project, 8107

ARC National Convention, 3155

ARC of East Central Iowa Pilot Parents, 8221

Arc of Montgomery County, 2639

ARC of Morgan County, 8081

ARC of the United States, 602, 2634, 2718, 3139, 3178, 3188, 3213, 3218, 4200, 4206, 4627, 4634, 4676, 4730, 7869

Arc of the United States, 7365, 7472

ARC Suburban, 8274

Arc's National Convention, 617

Archives of Pediatric and AdolescentMedicine, 8615

Archway, 8192

Are You Tired Again...I Understand, 7144

Arizona Ataxia Support Group, 504

Arizona Camp Sunrise & Sidekicks, 114, 166, 1294, 3121, 5180, 7809

Arizona Chapter of Crohn's & ColitisFoundation of America, 2145

Arizona Early Intervention Program/Department of Economic Security, 8092

Arizona HeartLight, 4309

The Arizona Partnership for Immunization, 5955

Arizona Sleep Disorders Center, 4889

Arizona Spina Bifida Association, 6818

Arizona Technology Access ProgramInstitute for Human Development, 8093

Arkansas Department of Health - SIDSInformation & Counseling Program, 6999

Arkansas Department of Health Div. of CommDiseases/Immunizations, 5956

Arkansas Disability Coalition, 8099

Arkansas Disability Coalition Parent Training and Information Center, 8100

Arkansas Easter Seals Technology ResourceCenter, 8448

Arkansas Regional Library for the Blindand Physically Handicapped, 1831, 1977, 5210, 6138

Arkansas Rehabilitation Research andTraining Center for Deaf Persons, 3567

Arlene R Gordon Research Institute, 6196

Arlington County Department of Libraries, 8544

Armond V. Mascia CF Center, 2307

Arnold-Chiari Malformation, 300

Arrhythmias, 311

Art Projects for the Mentally RetardedChild, 4714

Art Show, 3603

Artery, 4070

Arthritis, 4394

Arthritis Foundation, 252, 1572, 1588, 4389

Arthritis in Children, 1603

Arthritis in Children and La ArtritisInfantojuvenil, 4404

Arthritis in Children: Resources forChildren, Parents and Teachers, 4405

Arthritis Information: Children, 4403

Arthritis Sourcebook, 4395

Arthrogryposis Multiplex Congenita, 326

Articles on Legg-Calve-Perthes, 4561

As You Get Older, 1701

ASCD Biennial Conference, 3582

ASHA Annual Convention, 3583

ASHA Convention, 2782, 2814

Ask Audrey, 7638

Ask NOAH About: Stomach and Intestinal(Gastrointestinal) Disorders, 7629

Ask the Doctor: Depression, 2503

ASL Babies: First Signs, 3724

ASL Babies: Let's Eat, 3725

ASL Clip and Create Version 3, 3681

ASL Songs for Kids, 3682

ASL Stories: Christmas Stories, 3594

ASL Stories: Fairy Tales I, 3595

ASL Stories: Fairy Tales II, 3596

ASL Tales and Games for Kids, 3683

ASL Tales and Games for Kids 2, 3684

ASL Tales and Songs for Kids CD-1, 3685

ASL Tales and Songs for Kids CD-2, 3686

Aspects of Lyme Borreliosis, 4618

ASPEN (Asperger Autism SPectrum Education Network), 344

ASPEN Annual Fall Conference, 370

Asperger Autism Spectrum Education Network (ASPEN), 350, 893

Asperger Syndrome, 338, 380, 390

Asperger Syndrome and Your Child: AParent's Guide, 381

Asperger Syndrome: A Practical Guide forTeachers, 382

Asperger Syndrome: Guide for Educatorsand Parents, Second Edition, 383

Asperger's Association of New England, 375

Asperger's Network Support for Well-being Education and Research, 351

Asperger's Syndrome: A Guide for Parentsand Professionals, 384

Asperger's Syndrome: Autism and Obsessive Behavior, 373

Asperger/Autism Network, 352, 720

Aspergers Women's Association, 353

Aspire of WNY, 1459

Assemblies of God National Center for theBlind, 1874, 2021, 5253, 6181

Assistance Technology Project, 8288

Assisting Parents Through the MourningProcess, 8592

Assistive Media, 192

Assistive Technologies of Alaska, 8088

Assistive Technology Access Partnership, 8386

Assistive Technology CenterSimi Valley Hospital, 8453

Assistive Technology Collaborative, 8310

Assistive Technology for Kansas Project, 8230

Assistive Technology Partners, 8138

Assistive Technology Partnership, 8303

Assistive Technology Project, 8155, 8186, 8193, 8392, 8418

Assistive Technology Project, HumanResources, Voc. and Rehab. Services, 8349

Assistive Technology Resource Centers of Hawaii (ATRC), 8182

Assistive Technology Services Network, 8235

Assistive Technology Training andInformation Center, 8208, 8479

Association for Behavioral and Cognitive Therapies, 1765, 7685

Association for Children with DownSyndrome, 2640, 2720

Association for Children with Hand or ArmDeficiency (REACH), 8616

Association for Children's Mental Health, 7908

Association for Education & Rehabilitationof the Blind & Visually Impaired, 1820, 7909

Association for Neuro-Metabolic Disorders, 4636, 4810

Association for Neurologically ImpairedBrain Injured Children, 1087, 3355

Association for Persons with SevereHandicaps (TASH), 7910

Association for Psychological Science, 1040

Association for Research in Otolaryngology, 6759

Association for Research of ChildhoodCancer, 8554

Association for Retinopathy ofPrematurity and Related Diseases, 6303

Association for Science in Autism Treatment, 721

Association for Size Diversity and Health, 2843

Association for Spina Bifida and Hydrocephalus, 6870

Association for the Bladder ExstrophyCommunity, 5153

Association for the Gifted Child, 7911

Association for the Handicapped, 7912

Association for the Help of RetardedChildren, 4720, 7913

Association of Academic Physiatrists, 6760

Association of Asthma Educators, 415

Association of Blind Athletes, 7914

Association of Child Life Professionals, 66, 126

Association of Children's Prosthetic/Orthotic Clinics, 3169, 3173, 7915

Association of Developmental Disabilities, 4685

Association of Gastrointestinal MotilityDisorders, 1341, 2904

Association of Immunization Managers, 5937

Association of Nurses in AIDS Care, 3295

Association of Professional Developmental Disabilities Administrators, 4686

Association of Professional SleepSocieties, 4882

Association of Professionals Treating Eating Disorders, 2844

Association of Reproductive Health Professionals, 3143

Association of State and Territorial Health Officials, 3296

Association of Traumatic Stress Specialists, 5784, 5793

Association of University Centers onDisabilities, 4687, 6761, 7916

Asthma, 400, 476

Asthma & Allergy Foundation of America, 433, 1342

Asthma - Understanding and Control, 460

Asthma and Allergy Answers: Patient Education Library, 489

Asthma and Allergy FAQs, 470

Asthma and Allergy Foundation of America, 416, 436, 471, 6318

Asthma and Allergy Foundation of America -North Texas Chapter, 437, 438, 440

Asthma Self Help Book, 477

Ataxia, 499

Ataxia Fact Sheet, 577

Ataxia Telangiectasia Children's Project, 553

Ataxia Telangiectasia Medical Research Foundation, 554

Ataxia Telangiectasia Project, 555
Ataxia-Telangiectasia and Cancer Risk, 7217
Ataxia-Telangiectasia and Estrogen Replacement in Females, 7218
Ataxia-Telangiectasia and Immune Function, 7219
Ataxia-Telangiectasia and Swallowing Problems, 7220
Ataxia-Telangiectasia and X-Rays, 7221
Ataxia-Telangiectasia Children's Project, 7200, 7208, 7247
Atrial Septal Defects, 586
ATTAIN: Assistive Technology ThroughAction in Indiana, 8206
Attention, 687
Attention Deficit Disorder and LearningDisabilities, 650
Attention Deficit Disorder and Parenting Site, 633
Attention Deficit Disorder Association, 604, 632
Attention Deficit Disorder: ConciseSource of Information for Parents, 651
Attention Deficit Disorders and Hyperactivity, 692
Attention Deficit Hyperactivity Disorder, 597
Attention Deficit Hyperactivity Disorder:What Every Parent Wants to
    Know, 652
Attention Deficit Information Network, 634
Attention Deficit-Hyperactivity Disorder: Is it a Learning Disability?, 693
Attention Disorders and Eyesight, 4476
Auditory - Verbal International, 3492, 3853
Auditory-Verbal Learning Institute, 6762
Auditory-Verbal Therapy and Practice, 3738
Augusta-Richmond County Public Library, 8462
Aurora of Central New York, 8337
AUSPLAN Auditory Speech and Language, 3726
Autism, 874
Autism Acceptance Book: Being A Friend toSomeone With Autism, 909
Autism Action Network, 722
Autism Advocate, 965
Autism and Asperger Syndrome, 385
Autism and Learning, 911
Autism and the Family: Problems, Prospectsand Coping with the Disorder,
    912
Autism as an Executive Director, 913
Autism Consortium, 723
Autism Fact Sheet, 391, 972
Autism Inclusion Resources, 724
Autism Is a World, 875
Autism National Committee, 725
Autism National Committee Conference, 868
Autism Network for Dietary Intervention, 895
Autism Network for Hearing and VisuallyImpaired Persons, 727
Autism Network International, 354, 726, 894
Autism New Jersey, 355
Autism Research Foundation, 728, 859
Autism Research Institute, 729, 860, 896
Autism Research Institute Conference, 730
Autism Research Review International, 970
Autism Resources, 376, 897
Autism Science Foundation, 731
Autism Services Center, 732, 857
Autism Society National Conference & Expo, 869
Autism Society National Conference andExposition, 371
Autism Society of Alabama, 777
Autism Society of America, 356, 733, 898
Autism Society of America BaltimoreChesapeake Chapter, 819
Autism Society of America BluegrassChapter, 816
Autism Society of America Broward Chapter, 801
Autism Society of America Coachella Valley, 781
Autism Society of America ConnecticutChapter, 798
Autism Society of America District ofColumbia Chapter, 800
Autism Society of America East TennesseeChapter, 842
Autism Society of America Emerald CoastChapter, 802
Autism Society of America Florida Chapter, 803
Autism Society of America Gateway Chapter, 825
Autism Society of America Greater AustinChapter, 843
Autism Society of America Greater GeorgiaChapter, 808
Autism Society of America Greater LongBeach/San Gabriel Valley, 782
Autism Society of America Greater PhoenixChapter, 779
Autism Society of America GreaterHarrisburg Area Chapter, 838
Autism Society of America Inland EmpireChapter, 783
Autism Society of America JacksonvilleChapter, 804
Autism Society of America Larimer CountyChapter, 794
Autism Society of America Los AngelesChapter, 784
Autism Society of America Manasota Chapter, 805
Autism Society of America MassachusettsChapter, 820
Autism Society of America North San DiegoCounty Chapter, 785
Autism Society of America NorthernVirginia Chapter, 845

Autism Society of America Orange CountyChapter, 786
Autism Society of America PanhandleChapter, 806
Autism Society of America Pikes PeakChapter, 795
Autism Society of America San DiegoChapter, 787
Autism Society of America San FranciscoBay Chapter, 788
Autism Society of America San GabrielValley Chapter, 789
Autism Society of America Santa Barbara Chapter, 790
Autism Society of America Southern ArizonaChapter, 780
Autism Society of America Treasure ValleyChapter, 810
Autism Society of America Tulare CountyChapter, 791
Autism Society of America: ColoradoChapter, 796
Autism Society of American Boulder CountyChapter, 797
Autism Society of California, 792
Autism Society of Delaware, 799
Autism Society of Greater Cincinatti, 834
Autism Society of Greater Orlando, 807
Autism Society of Hawaii, 809
Autism Society of Illinois, 811
Autism Society of Indiana, 812
Autism Society of Iowa, 813
Autism Society of Louisiana, 817
Autism Society of Maine, 818
Autism Society of Michigan, 822
Autism Society of Minnesota, 823
Autism Society of Mississippi, 824
Autism Society of Nebraska, 826
Autism Society of New Hampshire, 828
Autism Society of North Alabama, 778
Autism Society of North Carolina, 833, 856
Autism Society of Northern Nevada Chapter, 827
Autism Society of Ohio Tri-County Chapter, 835
Autism Society of Oklahoma, 836
Autism Society of Oregon, 837
Autism Society of Rhode Island, 839
Autism Society of South Carolina, 840
Autism Society of South DakotaBlack Hills Chapter, 841
Autism Society of the Heartland, 815
Autism Society of Vermont, 844
Autism Society of Washington, 846
Autism Society of West Virginia, 847
Autism Society of Wisconsin, 848
Autism Solution Center, 734
Autism Speaks, 735, 861, 899
Autism Spectrum Disorders: The CompleteGuide, 910
Autism Training Center, 858
Autism Treatment Center of America, 736
Autism, Strabismus & Amblyopia (Lazy Eye), 4462
Autism: A Strange, Silent World, 876
Autism: A World Apart, 877
Autism: Being Friends, 878
Autism: Effective Biomedical Treatments, 914
Autism: From Tragedy to Triumph, 915
Autism: Mind and Brain, 916
Autism: The Child Who Couldn't Play, 879
Autism: The Facts, 917
Autism: The Unfolding Mystery, 880
Autistic Disorder, 712
Autistic Services, 737
Autreat, 372, 738
AVKO Dyslexia Research Foundation, 4503
AWARE, 8181
Awareness, 1596, 3012, 4493, 5639, 6042, 6214, 6294
Awareness Foundation for OCD and Related Disorders, 5361

B

B.A.S.E. Camp Children's Cancer Foundation, 67, 127, 3107
Babies with Down Syndrome, 2729
Baby Breath, 461
Baby Center, 37, 274
Baby See 'n Sign, 3604
Baby See 'n Sign II, 3605
Baby Sign Language Basics, 3739
Baby Signing Time, 3606
Baby Signing Time DVD 2, 3607
Baby Watch Early Intervention Program, 8412
Baby's First Book of Signs: An ASL Word Book (Volume 1-3), 3689
Baby's First Book of Signs: Volumes I-III, 3690
Baby's First Signs, 3740

BabyNet, 8393
Bachelor Father, 3608
Backtalk, 6509
Bainbridge Subregional Library for theBlind and Physically Handicapped, 1845, 1991, 5224, 6152
A Balancing Act: Living with SpinalCerebellar Ataxia, 565
Bancroft Camp, 8787
Bangor Public Library, 8497
Barbara DeBoer Foundation, 7917
Bartholomew County Public Library, 8480
BASH Magazine, 2967
Basic Course in American Sign LanguageVideotape Package, 3609
A Basic Course in American Sign Lanuage,Second Edition, 3718
Basic Guided Relaxation: AdvancedTechnique, 5596
A Basic Vocabulary: American Sign Languagefor Parents and Children, 3719
Basics for the Gluten-free Diet, 1369
Baxter Healthcare Hyland Division, 3939
Baylor College of Medicine, 4833
Baylor College of Medicine Birth DefectsCenter, 8540, 8555
Baylor College of Medicine-Pathology & Pathogenesis of Otitis Media, 5478
Baylor Comprehensive Epilepsy Center, 6554
Baylor Sleep Wellness Center, 4944
Baystate Medical Center, 2285
BDRC Newsletter, 8678
Be Careful, 3741
Be Happy Not Sad, 3742
Because You Are My Friend, 6556
Bedwetting Online, 5159
Beech Brook, 976, 4534
Beez Foundation (The), 1088
Beginning Level Curriculum Tapes CompleteSet, 3610
Beginning Reading and Sign Language Video, 3611
BEGINNINGS for Parents of Children Who AreDeaf or Hard of Hearing, 3493
Behavior Management - A Collection of Articles, 5880
Behavioral and Developmental PediatricsDivision, University of Maryland, 2685
Believe In Tomorrow - National Children'sFoundation, 68
Believe In Tomorrow Children's Foundation, 128
Believe In Tomorrow National Children's Foundation, 3108
Bell's Palsy, 1000
Bell's Palsy Network, 1009
Bell's Palsy Research Foundation, 1006, 1010
Belonging, 3743
Ben and Catherine Ivy Foundation, 1089
Bend Support Group, 1235
Beneficial Designs, 7918
Benetech, 7919
Benign Brain Tumor Support Group, 1174
Benign Essential Blepharospasm ResearchFoundation Newsletter, 2812, 2824
Berkshire Center, 4517
Best of Superstuff Activity Booklet, 478
Best Practices of Youth ViolencePrevention, 7747
Beth Israel Medical Center-Hydrocephalus, 4245
Bethel Mennonite Camp, 8753
Bethesda Oak Hospital, Sleep DisordersCenter, 4917
Bethpage Mission, 4688
Bethphage, 4689
Better Hearing Institute, 3494
Beyond Ritalin: Facts About Medication andOther Strategies for Helping Children, 653
Beyond the Autism Diagnosis: A Professional's Guide to Helping Families, 918
BeyondHunger, 2845
Big Crystal Camp, 977
Big Hearts for Little Hearts, 4323
Big Red Factor, 4071
Big Sky Kids Cancer Camp, 115
The Big Test, 3669
Bikers Against Child Abuse, 5688
Biliary Atresia, 1012, 1026
Bilingual Risk Reduction Brochure, 7105
Bill Wilkerson Center, 3577
Billy's Story, 2930
Binge Eating Disorder Association, 2846
Bioengineering Center of Wayne StateUniversity, 3429
Biology of Schizophrenia and AffectiveDisease, 1641
Biomedical Concerns in Persons with Down'sSyndrome, 2730

Bipolar Disorder, 1028, 1072
Bipolar Disorders: A Guide to HelpingChildren & Adolescents, 1067
Bipolar Puzzle Solutions, 1068
Bipolar World, 1062
Birmingham Support Group, 503
Birth Defect Research for Children, 226, 3034, 4217, 4246, 4581, 4629, 4733, 7920, 8617
Birth Defects Research for Children, 2641, 2721
Birth Defects: A Brighter Future, 8692
Birth to 3 Program, 8436
Black AIDS Institute, 3297
Blake Foundation Children's AchievementCenter, 8094
Blank Children's Hospital: Department of Pulmonology, 2275
Bleeding Disorders Association of Northeastern New York, 3965
Bleeding Disorders Foundation ofWashington, 3985
Bleeding in the Digestive Tract, 47, 7648
Blick Clinic for DevelopmentalDisabilities, 8525
Blind Children's Center, 1833, 1979, 5212, 6140
Blind Childrens Center, 6123
Blood, 8845
Blood & Circulatory Disorders Sourcebook4th Edition, 104, 160, 6664, 7280
Blood Research Institute of SaintMichael's Medical Center, 3992
Bloodlines, 4072
Bloodstone Magazine, 4067
Bloomfield, 1927, 2080, 5299, 6228
Blue's Clues: All Kinds of Signs, 3612
Blueberry Eyes, 4487
Bluegrass Technology Center, 8490
Body Betrayed, 2931
Body Image, 2975
Body Language of the Abused Child, 5708
The Body Positive, 2882
Bold as Brianna, 3613
Bonnie Tapes, 1625
The Book of Choice, 3837
A Book of Colors: Baby's First Sign Book, 3720
BookRags, 7715
Books for Parents of Deaf and Hard-of-Hearing Children, 3875
Borderline Personality Disorder Sanctuary, 5496
Boston Bracing System for Idiopathic Scoliosis, 6513
Boston Children's HospitalDept. of Otolaryngology & Communication, 3566
Boston Hemophilia Center, 3993
Boundless Playgrounds, 7921
Bowel Continence and Spina Bifida, 6880
Boy in the World, 2712
The Boy Inside, 374
Boy Scouts of America National Council, 7922
Boy Who Couldn't Stop Washing: TheExperience and Treatment of OCD, 5388
Boys Town National Research Hospital, 6787
Brace & Her Brace is No Handicap, 6514
Brachial Plexus Palsy Foundation, 3074
Brady Institute for Traumatic BrainInjury, 3431
Braille and Talking Book LibraryPerkins School for the Blind, 1861, 2007, 5239, 6167
Braille Institute Desert Center, 1834, 1980, 5213, 6141
Braille Institute Sight Center, 1835, 1981, 5214, 6142
Braille Institute Youth Center, 1836, 1982, 5215, 6143
Braille Revival League, 7923
Brain & Behavior Research Foundation, 1041
Brain and Spinal Injury Center (BASIC)Research at University of California, 3426
Brain Cancer Support Group at Mid-AmericaCancer Center, 1208
Brain Center Brain Tumor Support Group, 1189
Brain Imaging Center at the University ofCalifornia, Irvine, 3424
Brain Injury Alliance of South Carolina, 3410
Brain Injury Association, 3444
Brain Injury Association of America Helpline, 3356
Brain Injury Association of America National Office, 3357
Brain Injury Association of Arizona, 3365
Brain Injury Association of Arkansas, 3366
Brain Injury Association of Colorado, 3369
Brain Injury Association of Connecticut, 3370
Brain Injury Association of Delaware, 3372
Brain Injury Association of Florida, 3374
Brain Injury Association of Hawaii, 3378
Brain Injury Association of Idaho, 3380
Brain Injury Association of Illinois, 3381
Brain Injury Association of Indiana, 3382

Brain Injury Association of Iowa, 3383
Brain Injury Association of Kansas &Greater Kansas City, 3384
Brain Injury Association of Kentucky, 3385
Brain Injury Association of Louisiana, 3386
Brain Injury Association of Maine, 3387
Brain Injury Association of Maryland, 3388
Brain Injury Association of Massachusetts, 3389
Brain Injury Association of Michigan, 3358, 3390, 3422
Brain Injury Association of Minnesota, 3392
Brain Injury Association of Mississippi, 3393
Brain Injury Association of Missouri, 3394
Brain Injury Association of Montana, 3395
Brain Injury Association of New Hampshire, 3396
Brain Injury Association of New Jersey, 3397
Brain Injury Association of New Mexico, 3398
Brain Injury Association of New York State, 3399
Brain Injury Association of North Carolina, 3402
Brain Injury Association of North Dakota, 3403
Brain Injury Association of Ohio, 3404
Brain Injury Association of Oklahoma, 3405
Brain Injury Association of Oregon, 3406
Brain Injury Association of Rhode Island, 3409
Brain Injury Association of South Carolina, 3411
Brain Injury Association of Tennessee, 3412
Brain Injury Association of Texas, 3413
Brain Injury Association of Utah, 3414
Brain Injury Association of Vermont, 3415
Brain Injury Association of Virginia, 3416
Brain Injury Association of Washington, 3417
Brain Injury Association of Washington DC, 3373
Brain Injury Association of West Virginia, 3419
Brain Injury Association of Wisconsin, 3420
Brain Injury Association of Wyoming, 3421
Brain Injury Glossary, 3468
Brain Injury Research Center of theInstitute for Rehabilitation & Research, 3439
Brain Injury Resource Foundation, 3377
Brain Injury Source, 3461
Brain Injury Support And Education Group, 1182
Brain Injury Support Group, 1181, 1183
Brain Injury Support Group at AbbottNorthwestern Hospital, 1202
Brain Injury Update, 3469
Brain Lock: Free Yourself from ObsessiveCompulsive Behavior, 5389
Brain Research Center, 1257
Brain Research Foundation, 1258
Brain Research Institute, 3425
Brain Research Institute (BRI) School ofMedicine University of California LA, 3445
Brain Trauma Foundation, 3359
Brain Tumor Education & Support Group, 1236
Brain Tumor Foundation - National, 1090
Brain Tumor Foundation for Children, 1091, 1164
Brain Tumor Networking Club, 1195
Brain Tumor Networking Group, 1187
Brain Tumor Patient & Family Support Group, 1124, 1148
Brain Tumor Patient/Family Group, 1149
Brain Tumor Resource & Support Group, 1169
Brain Tumor Support Group, 1150, 1151, 1156, 1165, 1167, 1170, 1175, 1178, 1190, 1196, 1209, 1214, 1218, 1230, 1250, 1252, 1253
Brain Tumor Support Group at Ann Arbor, 1197
Brain Tumor Support Group at Burlington, 1191
Brain Tumor Support Group at Dallas, 1245
Brain Tumor Support Group at Duluth, 1203
Brain Tumor Support Group at Indianapolis, 1176
Brain Tumor Support Group at Miami, 1157
Brain Tumor Support Group at Milwaukee, 1254
Brain Tumor Support Group at Newport Beach, 1125
Brain Tumor Support Group at NorthwesternMemorial Hospital, 1171
Brain Tumor Support Group at NovaCareRehabilitation Institute of Tucson, 1122
Brain Tumor Support Group at Park Ridge, 1172
Brain Tumor Support Group at Philadelphia, 1238
Brain Tumor Support Group at Phoenix, 1123
Brain Tumor Support Group at Pittsburgh, 1239
Brain Tumor Support Group at PlainfieldMuhlenberg Medical Center, Neuroscience, 1215
Brain Tumor Support Group at Plano, 1246
Brain Tumor Support Group at Providence, 1242
Brain Tumor Support Group at Robbinside, 1204
Brain Tumor Support Group at San Diego, 1126

Brain Tumor Support Group at San LuisObispo, 1127
Brain Tumor Support Group at Santa Monica, 1128
Brain Tumor Support Group at South NassauCommunity Hospital, 1219
Brain Tumor Support Group at St.Petersburg, 1158
Brain Tumor Support Group at Tampa, 1159
Brain Tumor Support Group at the NebraskaMedical Center, 1211
Brain Tumor Support Group at UnitedHospital, 1205
Brain Tumor Support Group at WauwatosaFroederdt Memorial Lutheran Hospital, 1255
Brain Tumor Support Group at Worcester, 1192
Brain Tumor Support Group for Patients & Families: University of Michigan Med Ctr, 1198
Brain Tumor Support Group of Greater StLouis, 1210
Brain Tumor Support Group of Maine, 1185
Brain Tumor Support Group of the Carolinasand Virginia Cancer Services, 1226
Brain Tumor Support Group of the LehighValley, 1240
Brain Tumor Support Program Cedars-SinaiNeurosurgical Inst. & Wellness Communit, 1129
Brain Tumor Survivor Support Group, 1193
Brain Tumor Trials Collaborative, 1092
Brain Tumors, 1075
Brain Tumors: Understanding Your Care, 1282
Brainstorms Companion: Epilepsy in Our View, 6570
Brainstorms: Epilepsy in Our Words, 6571
Brass Ring Society, 7924
Break the Silence: Kids Against ChildAbuse, 5685
Breaking Ground: Ten Families BuildingOpportunities Through Integration, 1515
Breakthrough, 5467, 7188
Breathe Easy: Respiratory Care in Neuromuscular Disorders, 4852
Breathing Association (The), 417
Breckenridge Outdoor Education Center, 1928, 7925
Brian Wesley Ray Cystic Fibrosis Center, 2247
Briarwood Day Camp, 8808
Bridges4Kids, 357
Brief Strategic Solution-Oriented Therapyof Phobic and Obsessive Disorders, 5390
Brigham and Women's Hospital, Asthma andAllergic Disease Research Center, 443
British Dyslexia Association, 2788
British Retinitis Pigmentosa Society, 6258
Bronchoalveolar Lymphocytes in Sarcoidosis, 6401
Bronchopulmonary Dysplasia, 1301
Bronx Comprehensive Sickle Cell Center, 6652
Brooklyn College Speech and Hearing Center, 6774
Broward County Support Group, 514
Brown County Library, 8553
Building Cue Reading, 3614
Bulimia, 2916
Bulimia Nervosa & Binge Eating: A Guide toRecovery, 2932
Bulimia: A Guide to Recovery, 2933
Bulletin, 6043
Bureau of Children, Family, and CommunityServices, 8222
Bureau of Early Childhood Programs, 8258
Bureau of Early Learning, 8316
Bureau of EI Services, 8358
Bureau of Family Health Services-AlabamaChild Death Review, 6996
Bureau of Special Education, 8377
Burger School for the Autistic, 851
Burn Injuries, 1311
Burn Institute, 1313, 1321
Burn Prevention Foundation, 1314, 1322
Burn Survivors Throughout the World, 1315, 1323
Burns Sourcebook, 1330
Burnt Gin Camp, 8813
Butterworth Hospital, Cystic FibrosisCenter, 2289

C

C.S. Mott Children's Hospital, 7315, 7318
Cabell County Public Library, 8550
CAF Medical Update, 7286
California Brain Injury Association, 3367
California Department of Health ServicesImmunization Branch, 5958
California SIDS Program, 7000
Callier Center for Communication Disorders, 6781
Callier Communications, 6801
Camelot For Children, 1241

Camp Abilities Tucson, 8715
Camp About Face, 2134
Camp Achieve, 6619
Camp Akeela, 393
Camp Aldersgate, 8717
Camp Alex A. Krem, 8721
Camp Allen, 8784
Camp Allyn, 8804
Camp ASCCA/Easter Seals, 8711
Camp Baker Services, 8820
Camp Barakel, 8769
Camp Barefoot, 3470
Camp Boggy Creek, 6908
Camp Bon Coeur, 8755
Camp Brave Eagle, 8708
Camp Buckskin, 701, 978, 4535
Camp Catch-A-Rainbow, 116, 167, 1295, 3122, 5181, 7810
Camp Chatterbox, 8788
Camp Civitan, 1929, 2081, 3897, 8716
Camp Courageous, 8749
Camp Courageous of Iowa, 8750
Camp Crescent Moon, 6669
Camp Dartmouth-Hitchcock, 8785
Camp de los Ninos - Diabetes Society, 2608
Camp Discovery, 196, 1605, 3019, 5644, 6063, 6467, 8737
Camp Discovery American Diabetes Association, 2603
Camp Dunnabeck at Kildonan, 2799
Camp Easter Seal, 8814
Camp Easter Seal East, Camp Easter Seal West, 8821
Camp Easter Seals, 8783
Camp Emanuel, 3898
Camp Erdman YMCA, 8736
Camp Fantastic, 117, 168, 1296
Camp Fish Tales, 8770
Camp Friendship, 979, 2762, 8773
Camp Frog, 6620
Camp Funshine, 2377
Camp Good Days & Special Times, 6670
Camp Grizzly, 3899
Camp Hawkins, 2763
Camp Heartland, 3347
Camp Hickory Wood, 3471
Camp Hodia, 2604
Camp Holiday Trails, 8822
Camp Horizon, 8709
Camp Huntington, 2764, 4536, 4722
Camp Isanogel, 8743
Camp Joan Mier, 8722
Camp Joslin, 2605
Camp Joy, 8827
Camp Juliena, 3900
Camp Kindle, 3348
Camp Kindle- Project Kindle, 3349
Camp Kostopulos, 8818
Camp Krem, 980
Camp Kudzu, 2606
Camp Kushtaka, 2607
Camp Lee Mar, 8809
Camp Lotsafun, 981
Camp Merrimack, 982, 1538, 2765, 8712
Camp Merry Heart/Easter Seals Easter Seal Society, 1297, 1539
Camp Millhouse, 8744
Camp New Friends, 5060
Camp New Hope, 983, 2766, 8774
Camp Northwood, 394
Camp Nuhop, 702, 984, 4537
Camp O' Fair Winds, 4538
Camp Oakhurst, 6909, 8789
Camp PALS, 2767
Camp Ramah in New England (Summer), 8764
Camp Ramah in New England (Winter), 8765
Camp Ramah in New EnglandTikvah Program, 985, 1540, 6621, 8763
Camp Rap A Hope, 8713
Camp Roehr, 6622
Camp Ronald McDonald at Eagle Lake, 8723
Camp Rubber Soul, 8724
Camp Shane, 5349
Camp Shane Arizona, 5350
Camp Shane California, 5351
Camp Shining Stars, 5352
Camp Shocco for the Deaf, 3901

Camp Smile-A-Mile, 8714
Camp Sun 'N Fun, 8793
Camp Sunshine Dreams, 118, 169, 1298, 3123, 5182, 7811
Camp Tanager, 8751
Camp Thunderbird, 8734
Camp Tushmehata, 1930
Camp Vacamas, 496, 6671
Camp Waban, 8758
Camp Winding Gap, 8802
Camp Winnebago, 8775
Camp Wonder, 6468
Camp Yomeca Upper Perkiomen Valley YMCA, 8810
Camp-A-Lot, 8725
The Campaign to End Obesity, 5331
Can I Tell You About Asperger Syndrome?:A Guide for Friends and Family, 386
Can Your Baby Hear?, 3876
Can't You be Still?, 1516
The Canadian Society for Mucopolysaccharide & Related Diseases Inc, 7179
Canadian Society for Mucopolysaccharide & Related Diseases Inc, 7161
Canadian Society for Mucopolysaccharide &Related Diseases, 4813
Canadian Task Force on Preventive Health Care, 5990
CANCER, 8593
Cancer & Blood Diseases Institute, 3994
Cancer Information Service, 7790, 7928
Cancer Support Group for Children, 1160
CancerCare, 69, 101, 129, 156, 1094, 1261, 3109, 3114, 5066, 5071, 5167, 5172, 7795, 7802
CANDU Parent Group, 7926
Capital Regional Sleep-Wake DisordersCenter, 4906
Cara: Growing with a Retarded Child, 2731
Cardeza Foundation Hemophilia Center, 3995
Cardiac Kids, 4324
Cardiac Kids/Association of Volunteers, 4310
Cardiovascular Research Foundation, 318
Cardiovascular System, 8846
CARE Family Resource Center, 8108
Care of the Ears and Hearing for Health, 3877
Caregiver Brain Tumor Support Group, 1265
CARES Foundation, 1806, 1811
CARES Foundation Newsletter, 1814
Caring for Infants and Children with Osteogenesis Imperfecta, 5468
Caring For Your Child With Hemophilia, 4082
Carolina Computer Access Center, 8524
Carolinas Chapter of Crohn's &Colitis Foundation of America, 2176
Carolinas Support Group, 548
Carolyn Kordich Family Resource Center, 8109
Carroll Center for the Blind, 2008, 4518, 5240, 6168
Carroll School Summer Programs, 8766
Cary Library, 8498
Case Report-MR Imaging of MyocardialSarcoidosis, 6402
Case Report-Osseous Sarcoidosis andChronic Polyarthritis, 6403
Case Western Research University, BoltonBrush Growth Study Center, 3247
Case Western Reserve UniversityCystic Fibrosis Center, 2319
Catholic Celiac Society, 1343
CAUSE, 8267
Causes of Anxiety and Panic Attacks, 5597
CCFA: A Case for Support, 2205
CDC Lincoln County, 8245
CdLS Biennial Conference, 2107
CEA-HOW Annual Global Convention, 2911
CEC Convention & Expo, 618, 8584
CEDAR Associates, 2847, 5785
Cedars-Sinai Medical Center, 8618
CEL Subregional Library for the Blind andPhysically Handicapped, 1846, 1992, 5225, 6153
Celebrating Families of Children & Adultswith Special Needs, 8359
Celiac Disease, 1333
Celiac Disease Foundation, 1344, 1358
Celiac Sprue Association/USA, 1345
Celiac Support Association, 1346
Celiac Support Page, 1359
Cells and Tissues, 8844
Center for Accessible Technology, 8454
Center for Auditory and SpeechSciences-Gallaudet University, 3555
Center for Autism and Related Disorders, 358, 739
Center for Best Practices in EarlyChildhood, 7929
Center for Cancer and Blood Disorders, 6655

Center for Cancer and Blood Disorders atChildren's Medical Center in Dallas, 3996
Center for Digestive Disorders, 7628
Center for Disabilities and Development, 1382, 1766, 2554, 2642, 2774, 3360, 4690, 5128, 6676, 6702, 6809, 7686
Center for Early Childhood, 8400
Center for Early Intervention of Deafness(CEID), 3495
Center for Eating Disorders, 2888
Center for Enabling Technology, 8518
Center for Family Support, 831, 1055, 1619, 2672, 4710, 5111, 5134, 5372, 5495, 5586
Center for Hearing and Communication, 3546
Center for Independence Technology andEducation, (CITE), 8459
Center for Infant & Child Loss, 7021
Center for Interdisciplinary Research onImmunologic Diseases, 444
Center for Literacy and Disability Studies, 7930
Center for Mental Health ServicesKnowledge Exchange Network, 1029, 1607, 1767, 5093, 5123, 5357, 5560, 6718, 7687, 7931
Center for Narcolepsy Research at theUniversity of Illinois at Chicago, 4939
Center for Neural Recovery & Rehabilitation Research, 6551
Center for Parent Information and Resources, 6764
Center for Pediatric Orthopaedic Surgery, 1716
Center for Peripheral Neuropathy, 4604
Center for Psychiatric Rehabilitation, 1042
Center for Research for Mothers &Children, 7073, 7084
Center for Sleep & Wake Disorders, MiamiValley Hospital, 4918
Center for Sleep Diagnostics, 4902
Center for Sleep Medicine of the MountSinai Medical Center, 4907
Center for Sleep Science at University ofMichigan, 4901
Center for Speech and Language Disorders, 6765
Center for the Disabled, 1460
Center for the Partially Sighted, 1890, 2036, 2558, 5268, 6197
Center for the Research and Treatment ofAnorexia Nervosa, 2907
Center for the Study of Anorexia andBulimia, 2908
Center for the Study of Autism, 900
Center for the Study of Bioethics, 2705
Center on Disabilities and CommunityInclusion, 8419
Center on Media and Child Health, 7688
Centers for Disease Control, 4105, 7525, 7831
Centers for Disease Control and PreventionDivision: Tuberculosis Elimination, 5925, 7352, 7468, 7515
Centers for Disease Control-Infection Control, 5991
CenterWatch Clinical Trials Listings, 8619
Central Brain Tumor Registry of the United States, 1095
Central California Chapter of the NationalHemophilia Foundation, 3944
Central Connecticut Chapter of Crohn's &Colitis Foundation of America, 2150
Central DuPage Hospital Center forDigestive Disorders, 1755
Central Indiana Sarcoidosis Support Group, 6360
Central Indiana Support Group, 523
Central Institute for the Deaf, 3570
Central Maine Medical Center, 2281
Central Michigan University Summer Clinics, 3902, 6803
Central Missouri Area Support Group, 534
Central New York Chapter of Crohn's &Colitis Foundation of America, 2169
Central Ohio Brain Tumor Support Group, 1231
Central Ohio Chapter of Crohn's & ColitisFoundation of America, 2177
Central Ohio Chapter of the NationalHemophilia Foundation, 3969
Central Pennsylvania Area Support Group, 545
Central Region Early Intervention Program, 8387
Central Texas Brain Tumor Support Group, 1247
Centre for Neuro Skills, 3446
Cephalic Disorders Fact Sheet, 4266
Cerebral Palsy, 1375
Cerebral Palsy Associations of NewYork State, 1461
Cerebral Palsy Center Summer Program, 1541
Cerebral Palsy-Facts & Figures, 1537
Cerebral Palsy: What Every Parent ShouldKnow, 1500
Cerebrospinal Fluid Shunt Systems for theManagement of Hydrocephalus, 4218, 4267
CERN Foundation, 1093
CF & Pediatric Pulmonary Care Center, 2308
CF & Pediatric Pulmonary Disease Center, 2262
CF Center at The Children's Hospital ofPhiladelphia, 2326
CF Center, Pulmonary Section, 2335
CF Center/Medical University of SouthCarolina, 2331
CF Index of Online Resources, 2354
CF Web, 2355

CF, Pediatric Pulmonary & GI Center, 2309
CHADD: Children and Adults with Attention Deficit Disorders, 605, 635
Chadder, 689
Chai Lifeline/Camp Simcha National Office, 7932
Challenge, 6869
Challenged Family Resource Center, 8110
Challenging Behaviour, 5506
Change for Good Coaching, 2848
Charcot-Marie-Tooth Association, 1552
Charcot-Marie-Tooth Disease, 1546
Charcot-Marie-Tooth Disorders: A Guide about Genetics for Patients, 1565
Charcot-Marie-Tooth Disorders: A Handbookfor Primary Care Physicians, 1555
CHARGE Syndrome Conference, 1020
CHARGE Syndrome Foundation, 1015
Charis Hills, 395
Charles Campbell Children's Camp, 1542
CHEF - Comprehensive Health Education Foundation, 5318
Chemotherapy of Brain Tumors, 1283
CHERAB Foundation, 6763
CHERUB-Association of Families andFriends of Children with Limb Disorders, 5762, 7125, 7927
CHERUBS: Association of CongenitalDiaphragmatic Hernia Research & Advocacy, 1941
Chesapeake Chapter, 529
Chicago Center for Jewish Genetic Disorder, 7162, 7170
Chicago Library Service for the Blind, 1848, 1994, 5227, 6155
Chicago, IL Area Ataxia Support Group, 522
Child Abuse Legislation, 5689
Child Abuse Prevention Association, 5650, 7933
Child Abuse Prevention Network, 5690
Child Abuse Prevention Project: Be'adHaYeled (For the Sake of the Child), 5678
Child Abuse Quilts: Revealing and Healingthe Pain of Child Abuse, 5691
Child Abuse.com, 5692
Child and Adolescent Bipolar Disorder, 1073
Child and Family Connections, 8194
A Child Called It: One Child's Courageto Survive, 5707
Child Care Aware of America, 5319
Child Care Plus+, 7934
Child Department Services, 8246
Child Department Services, Department ofEducation, 8247
Child Development Clinical Services, 2692
Child Development Institute, 5160
Child Health Improvement ProgramIdaho Department of Health, 7012
Child Sexual Abuse Treatment Program (Giarretto), 5673
Child Trauma Academy, 5693
Child Trends, 7689
Child Welfare Information Gateway, 5682, 7716
Child Welfare League of America, 5651
Child With A Bleeding Disorder GuidelinesFor Finding Childcare, 4083
Child With A Bleeding Disorder: First AidFor School Personnel, 4084
Child with Epilepsy at Camp, 6598
The Child with NF1, 5059
Child With Prader-Willi Syndrome: Birth to Three, 5881
Child's Guide To Seizure Disorders, 6599
Childhelp, 5652
Childhelp Children's Center of Virginia, 5681
Childhelp National Child Abuse Hotline, 5653
Childhood Apraxia of Speech Association, 6766
Childhood Asthma, 462
Childhood Asthma: A Matter of Control, 490
Childhood Brain Tumor Foundation (The), 1097
Childhood Brain Tumor Foundation Newsletter, 1096, 1270
Childhood Cancer Canada Foundation, 70
Childhood Dermatomyositis, 1568
Childhood Glaucoma: A Reference Guide forFamilies, 2058
Childhood Leukemia: A Guide for Families,Friends & Caregivers, 105
Childhood Nephrotic Syndrome, 5001
Childhood Obsessive Compulsive Disorder, 5391
Childhood Schizophrenia, 1606
Children and Adolescents, 5401
Children and Autism: Time is Brain, 881
Children and Kidney Disease, 5002
Children Living with Illness, 8111
Children of the Stars, 882
Children Special Needs-Pediatric Eye Care, 4477
Children with ADD: A Shared Responsibility, 695
Children with AIDS Project, 3324

Children with Autism and Asperger SyndromeA Guide for Practitioners and Carers, 921
Children with Autism: A DevelopmentalPerspective, 922
Children With Autism: A Parents Guide, 919
Children With Cerebral Palsy: A ParentsGuide, 1517
Children with Diabetes, 2588
Children With Fragile X Syndrome, 3192
Children with Hearing Difficulties, 3744
Children with Mental Retardation, 4715
Children with Osteogenesis Imperfecta: Strategies to Enhance Performance, 5460
Children with Seizures: A Guide For Parents, Teachers and Other Professionals, 6572
Children with Spina Bifida: A Parent's Guide, 6881
Children with Spina Bifida: A ResourcePage for Parents, 6871
Children wIth Starving Brains, 920
Children with Talipes (Clubfoot), 1721
Children with Tourette Syndrome: AParent's Guide-2nd Edition, 7437
Children with Traumatic Brain Injury, 3452
Children with Visual Impairments: AParents' Guide, 245, 1907, 2059, 6207, 6264, 6288, 6311
Children's Alopecia Project, 202, 206
Children's Association for Maximum Potential CAMP, 8815
Children's Beach House, 3903
Children's Brain Tumor Foundation, 1098
Children's Bureau, 5694
Children's Cancer & Blood Foundation, 71, 130, 3940, 7248, 7273, 7299, 7304
Children's Cancer Research Institute, 5070, 7796, 8556
Children's Cancer Web, 102, 157, 3115, 4193, 5072, 5173, 6284, 7803
Children's Center for Cancer and BloodDisorders, 3924, 3997, 6647
Children's Center for NeurodevelopmentalStudies, 862
Children's Clinical Research Center, 3318
Children's Craniofacial Association, 2102, 2115, 3035, 4582
Children's Defense Fund, 5654, 7935
Children's Dream Factory of Maine, 8829
Children's Gaucher Research Fund, 3219
Children's Glaucoma Foundation, 1964
Children's Happiness Foundation, 8259
Children's Heart Society, 4337
Children's Hopes and Dreams, 7797, 7936, 8679
Children's Hopes and Dreams Foundation, 7798, 7937
Children's Hospice International, 7938
Children's Hospital & Research Center ofOakland, 2678
Children's Hospital Association, 5320
Children's Hospital at Montefiore, 4376, 4380
Children's Hospital Boston, 2286, 7137, 7143, 7201, 7209, 7227, 7232, 7249, 7274, 7300, 7305, 7316, 7319, 7366, 7429, 7473, 7475, 7939
Children's Hospital Merit Care DownSyndrome Service, 2694
Children's Hospital of Los Angeles, 2248
Children's Hospital of Michigan CysticFibrosis Care, Teaching & Resource, 2290
Children's Hospital of New York Presbyterian, 4377, 4381, 4521
Children's Hospital of Orange County: Department of Pulmonology - Cystic Fibrosis, 2249
Children's Hospital of PhiladelphiaHemophilia Program, 3998
Children's Hospital of Pittsburgh GeneralClinical Research Center, 2698
Children's Hospital: Academic PediatricSurgery Department, 1737
Children's Hospital: Pediatric PulmonaryCenter, 2250
Children's House, 5695
Children's Legal Advocacy Program (CLA), 3496
Children's Leukemia Association, 72, 131
Children's Liver Alliance, 7816, 7823
Children's Liver Alliance Newsletter, 7827
Children's Liver Association for Support Services, 215, 219, 1016, 1023, 7817, 7824
Children's Lung and Cystic FibrosisCenter, 2310
Children's Lung Specialists, 2301
Children's Lyme Disease Network, 4605
Children's Medical Services ProgramFlorida SIDS Program, 7007
Children's Medical Ventures, 5912
Children's Mercy Hospital, Down SyndromeClinic, 2689
Children's Mercy Hospital, University ofMissouri, 2296
Children's National Health System, 95, 154, 1347, 6326
Children's Neurobiological SolutionsFoundation, 1383, 1502
Children's Neurodevelopment Center atHasbro Children's Hospital, 2702
Children's Organ Transplant Association, 7940
Children's PKU Network, 5546
Children's Seashore House, 2699
Children's Therapy Center, 8289
Children's Tumor Foundation, 5007, 5045

Children's Tumor Foundation - Colorado Chapter, 5017
Children's Tumor Foundation - Florida Chapter, 5018
Children's Tumor Foundation - Georgia, 5019
Children's Tumor Foundation - Illinois, 5020
Children's Tumor Foundation - Illinois Chapter, 5021
Children's Tumor Foundation - Indiana Affiliate, 5024
Children's Tumor Foundation - Iowa Chapter, 5025
Children's Tumor Foundation - Michigan Chapter, 5030
Children's Tumor Foundation - MidAtlanticRegion Chapter, 5039
Children's Tumor Foundation - Missouri Chapter, 5031
Children's Tumor Foundation - Nevada, 5032
Children's Tumor Foundation - Northern NewEngland, 5028
Children's Tumor Foundation - Ohio, 5033
Children's Tumor Foundation - Oregon Support Group, 5034
Children's Tumor Foundation - South Carolina Chapter, 5036
Children's Tumor Foundation - Tennessee Affiliate, 5037
Children's Tumor Foundation - Utah Chapter, 5038
Children's Tumor Foundation - Washington Chapter, 5040
Children's Tumor Foundation - Wisconsin Chapter, 5041
Children's Tumor Foundation-Arkansas Chapter, 5014
Children's Tumor Foundation-Arkansas Inforwww.php.com, 5015
Children's Wish Foundation, 8830
Children's Wish Foundation International, 5067, 7799, 7941
Children, Adolescents, and Media Violence, 7748
Childswork Childsplay, 8668
Chill: Straight Talk About Stress, 7942
Chilren's Heart Services, 4314
Chorea, 1666
Chris Gets Ear Tubes, 3745
Chris Gets Ear Tubes: Spanish Edition, 3746
Chrissy & Friends, 6541
Christian Berets, 8726
Christian Dental Society, 2419
Christian Horizons, 5102, 5129, 5489, 7943
Christian Medical & Dental Associations, 2420
Chromosome 18 Registry & Research Society, 7367, 7497
Chronic Viral Hepatitis Backgrounder, 4116
Cincinnati Center for Developmental &Behavioral Pediatrics, 7775
Cincinnati Children's Hospital Medical Center, 4338
Cincinnati Digestive Health Center, 1756
Circle of Parents, 7717
Citizens United for Research in Epilepsy(CURE), 6548
CJ Foundation for SIDS, 7072
CKLS Headquarters, 1856, 2002, 5234, 6162
Clara Barton Camp, 2609
Classification of Tuberculosis and OtherMycobacterial Diseases, 7532
Classroom GOALS, 3747
Classroom Notetaker, 3748
Clearinghouse for Specialized Media andTechnology (CSMT), 8455
Clearwater, FL Support Group, 515
Cleft Lip & Palate, 1703
Cleft Lip and Cleft Palate, 1680
Cleft Palate Foundation, 1683
Cleft Palate/Craniofacial Birth Defects:Cleft Palate Foundation, 1693
Cleft Surgery, 1704
Cleveland Brain Tumor Patient Network -Adult and Pediatric, 1232
Cleveland Clinic, 4236
Cleveland Clinic Children's Hospital & Epilepsy Center, 6528
Cleveland Clinic Foundation, SleepDisorders Center, 4919
Cleveland Hearing and Speech Center, 6776
Cleveland Public Library, 8526
CLIMB: Children Living with InheritedMetabolic Disorders, 4207
Clinical Assessment and Management ofSevere Personality Disorders, 5507
Clinical Counseling: Toward a BetterUnderstanding of TS, 7417
Clinical Diabetes, 2583
Clinical Research Center, Pediatrics, 1018
Clinical Trial for Brain Tumors, 1284
CLIPS: Clubfoot Information and ParentalSupport, 1720
Club Foot & Other Physical Deformities, 1727
Club Foot and Other Foot Deformities, 1728
Clubfoot, 1713
Cluster Headache-Fact Sheet, 4770
CMT Brochure, 1559
CMT Facts I, 1560
CMT Facts II, 1561
CMT Facts III, 1562
CMT Facts IV, 1563
CMT Facts V, 1564
CMT Net, 1551
CMTA Chapter - New York (Greater), 1548
CMTA Chapter - Ohio, 1549

CMTA Chapter - Pennsylvania, 1550
CMTA Report, 1558
CO-TEACH/Division of Educational Researchand Service, 8297
Coalition for Global Hearing Health, 3497
Coarctation of the Aorta, 1730
Cochlear Impant Auditory Training Guide, 3691
Cochlear Implant Assocciation, 3498
Cochlear Implant Auditory TrainingGuidebook, 3749
Cochlear Implant Awareness Foundation, 3499
Cochlear Implants for Kids, 3750
Cochlear Implants in Children, 3751
Cochlear Implants in Children: Ethics andChoices, 3752
Coconut Creek Eating Disorders SupportGroup, 2885
Cognition, Eduction, and Deafness: Directions for Research and Instruction, 3753
Cognitive Effects of Early Brain Injury, 3453
Cognitive Rehabilitation for Persons withTraumatic Brain Injury, 3454
Cognitive-Behavioral Management of Tic Disorders, 7343
COGREHAB, 694
Colic, 1743
Colitis Cookbook, 7630
College of Education - Western KentuckyUniversity, 8236
College of Psychiatric and Neurologic Pharmacists, 1043
Colorado Consortium of Intensive CareNurseries United Parents (UP), 8139
Colorado Dept. of Public Heand & Environment: Immunization Program, DCEED-IMM-A3, 5961
Colorado SIDS Program, 7003
Colorado Support Group, 512
Coloring Book on Thalassemia, 7281
Colors, 3754
Columbia Presbyterian Medical Center, 4829
Columbia Presbyterian Medical Center SleepDisorders Center, 4908
Columbia University, 7526
Columbus Children's Hospital, CysticFibrosis Center, 2320
Coma Recovery Association, 3361
Come Sign With Us: Sign Language Activities for Children, 3755
Come Sign with UsSign Language Activities for Children, 3756
Comfort Connection Family Resource Center, 8112
Commission of Public HealthImmunization Program, 5962
Commitment, 2369
Communicating Together, 2755
Communicating with People who Have aHearing Loss, 3878
Communication Disorders Quarterly, 6798
Communication Rules for Hard-of-HearingPeople, 3615
Communication Service for the Deaf, Inc., 3547
Communication Skills in Children withDown Syndrome: A Guide for Parents, 2732
Communications Disorders Clinic, 6790
Communique, 6802
Community Health Improvement Partners -Immunize San Diego (CHIP-ISD), 5959
Community Medical Center, Sleep DisordersClinic, 4925
Community Outreach for Prevention of Eating Disorders, 2849
Community Services for Autistic Adults & Children (CSAAC), 740, 901
Community Sickle Cell Support Group, 6637
Compass, 6934
Compassionate Friends, 6984, 7085, 7944
Complementary and Alternative Therapiesfor Diabetes Treatment, 2589
The Complete Family Guide to Schizophrenia, 1658
Complete IEP Guide: How to Advocate forYour Special Ed Child, 6882
Complex PTSD in Children, 5790
Complexities of TS Treatment: APhysician's Roundtable, 7418
Comprehensive Bleeding Disorder Center, 3999
Comprehensive Pediatric HemophiliaTreatment Center, 4000
Comprehensive Sickle Cell Center, 6651, 6654
Compulsive Eaters Anonymous, 2850, 5321
Computer Access Center, 8557
Computer Center for Citizens withDisabilities, 8413
Concentration Video, 624
Conception, Pregnancy and Psoriasis, 6050
Concise Guide to Evaluation and Managementof Sleep Disorders, 5144, 6688
Concise Guide to Evaluation andManagement of Sleep Disorders, 5119, 6713
Conduct Disorder, 1761
Conduct Disorder in Children andAdolescents, 1798, 7763
Conduct Disorders in Childhood andAdolescence (Developmental Clinical), 1791, 7741
Conduct Disorders in Children andAdolescents, 1792, 7742

Conduct Problem/Emotional ProblemInterventions: A Holistic Perspective, 1793, 7743
Conductdisorders.com, 1784, 7718
Conference on the Cause and Treatment ofFacioscapulohumeral Muscular Dystrophy, 4853
Confronting the Challenges of SpinaBifida, 6883
Congenital & Acquired Hypothyroidism, 4358
Congenital Adrenal Hyperplasia, 1804
Congenital Cataracts, 1816
Congenital Diaphragmatic Hernia, 1938
Congenital Disorders Sourcebook, 291, 596, 1518, 1742, 2132, 3047, 3157, 4256, 5519, 6093, 6884, 7237
Congenital Disorders Sourcebook 2nd Edit., 4597
Congenital Dysplasia of the Hip, 1950
Congenital Glaucoma, 1961
Congenital Heart Anomalies, Support,Education & Resources (CHASER), 7228, 7233, 7250, 7368, 7498, 7508
Congenital Heart Information Network, 1739, 4307, 4339, 4343, 5516, 6091, 7234, 7369, 7484, 7489, 7668
Congratulations? An Introduction to DownSyndrome for Parents/Family/Friends, 2713
Congressional Testimony on MuscularDystrophy, 4854
Conjunctivitis, 2089
Connect for Kids, 5696
Connecticut Brain Tumor Support Group(Adult), 1152
Connecticut Down Syndrome Congress, 2662
Connecticut Lead Poisoning PreventionProgram, 4498
Connecting, 8680
Connecting Students: A Guide to ThoughtfulFriendship Facilitation, 1519
The Connection, 7189
Connections Conference, 1690
Conner's Way Foundation for Tay-Sachs Disease, 7163
Constipation, 3058
Constipation in Children, 3059
Consumer Fact Sheet, 2371
Consumer Indicators of Quality Genetic Services, 578
Consumer Information and TechnologyTraining Exchange (Maine CITE), 8248
Consumer Product Safety Commission Hotline, 4499
Consumer Products Safety Commission, 1324
Contemporary Issues in the Treatment ofSchizophrenia, 1642
Controlling Asthma, 486
Conventional Radiation Therapy, 1285
Convergence Insufficiency, 4478
Conversation with Anorexics: ACompassionate & Hopeful Journey, 2934
Cook-Ft. Worth Medical Center, CF Center, 2336
Cookbook for the PWS Diet, 5870
Cooking Up A Storm for Scleroderma: Recipes from the Scleroderma Foundation, 6459
Cool the Burn, 1325
Cooley's Anemia 7th Annual Symposium, 7282
Cooley's Anemia Fact Cards, 7289
Cooley's Anemia Foundation, 7251, 7275
Cooley's Anemia Foundation (CAF) Pamphlet, 7290
Cooley's Anemia Foundation - Staten Island, 7265
Cooley's Anemia Foundation - Texas, 7271
Cooley's Anemia Foundation-Buffalo, 7266
Cooley's Anemia Foundation-Buffalo Chapter, 7262
Cooley's Anemia Foundation-California, 7261
Cooley's Anemia Foundation-Capital Area(DC, VA, MD), 7263
Cooley's Anemia Foundation-Long Island/Brooklyn Chapter, 7267
Cooley's Anemia Foundation-MassachusettsChapter, 7264
Cooley's Anemia Foundation-Queens, 7268
Cooley's Anemia Foundation-Suffolk Chapter, 7269
Cooley's Anemia Foundation-Westchester/Rockland Chapter, 7270
Cooperative Wilderness HandicappedOutdoor Group, 7945
Coping with Allergies and Asthma, 487
Coping with Cancer Magazine, 112
Coping with Childhood Cancer, 98, 155
Coping with Crohn's and Colitis is Tough, 2206
Coping with Depression, 2487, 2504
Coping with Eating Disorders, 2935
Coping with Lupus, 7145
Coping with Post-Traumatic Stress Disorder, 5801
Coping with Sarcoidosis, 6404
Coping with Tourette Syndrome, A Parent'sViewpoint, 7448
Coping with Your Inattentive Child, 696
Coping with Your Loved One's Brain Tumor, 1286
Cornelia de Lange Syndrome, 2100
Cornelia de Lange Syndrome Foundation, 2103

CorStone-Children & Loss Group, 7001
Cosmo Gets An Ear, 3757
COTT Washington Update, 4073
Council for Educational DiagnosticServices (CEDS), 7946
Council for Exception Children - Division on Autism and Development Disabilities, 4691
Council for Exceptional Children, 7947, 8620
The Council For Exceptional Children, 615
Council for Extended Care of Mentally Retarded Citizens, 4723
Council for Learning Disabilities, 4507
Council of Academic Programs in Communication, 6767
Council of Administrators of SpecialEducation, 7948
Council of Families with Visual Impairment, 1840, 1986, 5219, 6147
Council of Families with VisualImpairments, 7949
Council of Guilds for Infant Survival, 6985
Council of the American Instructors of the Deaf, 3500
Council on Education of the Deaf, 3501
Council on Quality and Leadership (The), 4692
Council on Size and Weight Discrimination(CSWD), 2851
Counseling and Research Center for SIDS, 7067
Count Us In: Growing up with Down Syndrome, 2733
Countdown, 2577
Courage Camps, 8776
Courage Center, 7950
Courage North, 8777
Covert Modeling and Reinforcement, 1069
Cowden Preautism Observation Inventory, 923
CPAC, 8156
CPF Teddy Bears, 1702
Craniofacial Center at University of Illinois, Chicago, 2128
Craniofacial Foundation of America, 1684, 1694
Craniosynostosis, 2112
Craniosynostosis and PositionalPlagiocephaly Support, 2116
CRI Worldwide Pediatric Center forExcellence, 1754
Crib Death: The Sudden Infant DeathSyndrome, 7091
Crisis Nursery, 5672
Crohn's & Colitis Foundation of America, 2138, 2155, 2190, 2194, 7620, 7631
Crohn's Disease, 2135
Crohn's Disease and Ulcerative ColitisFact Book, 2196
Crohn's Disease, Ulcerative Colitis, andYour Child, 2207, 7649
Cross Roads Outdoor Ministries, 8790
Crotched Mountain School & Rehabilitation Center, 986, 1543, 3472, 4724, 6623, 8710, 8786
Crowley Ridge Regional Library, 8449
Crozer-Chester Medical Center, 4926
Cry for Help - How to Help a Friend Who isDepressed or Suicidal, 2488
Cryptorchidism, 2214
CSA Annual Conference, 1356
Cued Speech Conference, 3584
Cued Speech Resource Book, 3758
Cult of Thinness, 2936
CureSearch: The National Childhood CancerFoundation, 7951
Curing Epilepsy: Focus on the Future/Benchmarks for Epilepsy Research, 6564
Current Approaches to Down's Syndrome, 2734
Cushing's Support & Research Foundation, 2227
Cushing's Support and Research Foundation, 1099, 2232
Cushing's Syndrome, 2224
Cutting Edge Medical Report, 6478
CyberPsych, 1063, 1629, 5113, 5138, 5379, 5497, 5598, 8621
Cyclic Vomiting Syndrome, 48
Cyclic Vomiting Syndrome Association, 6097
Cystic Fibrosis, 2237, 2360
Cystic Fibrosis and Chronic PulmonaryDisease Clinic, 2273
Cystic Fibrosis and Pediatric RespiratoryDiseases Center, 2254
Cystic Fibrosis Care, Teaching andResearch Center, 2337
Cystic Fibrosis Center - All Children'sHospital, 2263
Cystic Fibrosis Center at PolyclinicMedical Center, 2327
Cystic Fibrosis Center/Pediatric Pulmonaryand Sleep Medicine, 2291
Cystic Fibrosis Center/University ofVirginia Health System, 2342
Cystic Fibrosis Center: Cedars-SinaiMedical Center, 2251
Cystic Fibrosis Center: Children's Memorial Hospital, 2268
Cystic Fibrosis Center: Phoenix Children'sHospital, 2246
Cystic Fibrosis Center: University ofCalifornia at San Francisco, 2252
Cystic Fibrosis Foundation, 2240
Cystic Fibrosis Program of the MedicalCollege of Virginia, 2343
Cystic Fibrosis Research, Inc., 2241, 2253
Cystic Fibrosis, Pediatric Pulmonary andPediatric Gastrointestinal Center, 2297
Cystic Fibrosis-Lung Disease CenterSanta Rosa Children's Hospital, 2338

Cystic Fibrosis: A Guide for Patient andFamily, 2361
Cystic Fibrosis: Guide for Parents, 2372
Cystic Fibrosis: The Facts, 2362
Cytomegalovirus, 2380

D

Dad and Me in the Morning, 3759
Daddy's Girl, 2714
Dakota, 7332, 7419
DakotaLink, 8396
Dallas Academy, 703, 987, 4539
Dana Alliance for Brain Initiatives, 3432, 3447
Dancing Cheek to Cheek, 1916, 2067, 5288, 6217
Dangerous DecibelsOregon Health & Science University, 3548
The Daniel Jordan Fiddle Foundation, 769
Dartmouth-Hitchcock Sleep Disorders CenterDartmouth Medical Center, 4903, 8317
David Baldwin's Trauma InformationPages, 5794
Davis Dyslexia Association InternationalDyslexia: The Gift, 2775, 2789
Day for Night: Recognizing TeenageDepression, 2489
DBSA National Conference, 1058
DC Arc, 8164
DC-EIP Services, 8165
DD Services, Department of Human Services, 8101
Deadly Diet: Recovering From Anorexia andBulimia, 2937
A Deadly Hunger, 5860
Deaf Children in China, 3760
Deaf Children in Public Schools: Placement, Context, and Consequences, 3761
Deaf Children Signers, 3616
Deaf Counseling, Advocacy & Referral Agency, 3502
Deaf Daughter, Hearing Fahter, 3762
Deaf Life, 3854
Deaf REACH, 3503
Deaf Side Story: Deaf Sharks, Hearing Jets, and a Classic American Musical, 3763
Deaf Students Can Be Great Readers, 3764
Deaf USA, 3855
The Deaf-Blind American, 3858, 8672
Deafness Research Foundation, 7952
Deafness: A Fact Sheet, 3879
Dealing with Depression: Five Ways to Help, 2505
Dealing with Scoliosis: A Patient Guide toDiagnosis and Treatment, 6479
Death Investigations and Sudden InfantDeath Syndrome, 7092
Death of a Child, the Grief of the ParentsA Lifetime Journey, 7093
DebRA Currents, 3071
DebRA: Dystrophic Epidermolysis BullosaResearch Association of America, 3064
Deenie, 6498
Delaware Assisstive Technology Initiative(DATI), 8160
Delaware Division of Libraries for theBlind and Physically Handicapped, 1577, 3001, 5630
Delaware Valley Chapter of the NationalHemophilia Foundation, 3976
Delightful as Derek, 3617
Delta/Montrose Parent to Parent, 8140
Dental Conditions, 2388
Dental Consumer Advisory, 2432, 4744
Dental Problems with Growth HormoneDeficiency, 3266
Dental Resources on the Web, 2433, 2991, 4745
Denver Children's Hospital, 2259
Denver Early Childhood Connections, 8141
Denver Sarcoidosis Awareness Support Group, 6358
Department for Exceptional StudentsGeorgia Department of Education, 8176
Department of Assistive and RehabilitationServices, 8404
Department of Children, Family, & Learning, 8275
Department of Counseling and EducationalLeadership-Columbus State University, 8177
Department of Developmental Services ofEarly Start Program, 8113
Department of Education, 8187
Department of Elementary and SecondaryEducation, 8290
Department of Health & Environment, 8231
Department of Health and Human Services, 5753
Department of HealthDivision of Immunization, 5926, 5963
Department of Human Services, 7020
Department of Mental Retardation, 8157
Department of Pediatrics, Medical Collegeof Georgia, 2266
Department of Public Instruction, 8161
Depression, 2435

Depression & Related Affective DisordersAssociation, 2450
Depression and Bipolar Support Alliance, 1044, 2451
Depression and Its Treatment, 2506
Depression in Children and Adolescents: AFact Sheet for Physicians, 2538
Depression Is a Treatable Illness: APatients Guide, 2537
Depression, the Mood Disease, 2507
Depressive and Manic-DepressiveAssocation of Mount Sinai, 1056, 2476
Depressive Illnesses: Treatments Bring NewHope, 2508
Depressives Anonymous: Recovery fromDepression, 2452
Dept. of Health & Mental Hygiene-Immunization, 5971
Dermatologic System, 8847
Dermatology Focus, 1598, 3014, 5641, 6045
Dermatology Foundation, 8622
Dermatology Information Network(DERMINFONET), 1578, 3002, 5631
Dermatology World, 1599, 3015, 5642, 6046
DermNet NZ: The Dermatology Resource, 5743
Des Moines YMCA Camp, 119, 170, 497, 1299, 2378, 2610, 3904
Described and Captioned Media Program, 3565
Desferal Q & A, 7291
Detroit Michigian Ataxia Support Group, 531
Developing and Writing IEPs Under the New IDEA, 884
Developing Cognition in Young Children Whoare Deaf, 3880
Developing Friendships: Wonderful People to Get to Know, 883
Developing Good Speech, 1705
Development and Training Center, 8437
Development of Behavioral and EmotionalProblems in Tourette Syndrome, 7449
The Development of Deaf Children: AcademicAchievement Levels and Social Processes, 3838
Developmental Center, 704, 988, 4540
Developmental Delay Resources, 7953
Developmental Delay Resources (DDR), 741
Developmental Disabilities NursesAssociation, 4693, 7954
Developmental Disabilities Program, 8298
Developmental Disabilities Unit, 8355
Developmental Medicine Center, 3319
Developmental Pediatrics School ofMedicine, University of Maryland, 8252
Developmental Services Center, 8195
DevelopMentor, 5430
DHR/Division of Public Health - Babies Cant Wait Program, 8175
Diabetes, 2580
Diabetes 101, 2563
Diabetes Advisor, 2584
Diabetes Care, 2581
Diabetes Dateline, 2585
Diabetes Dictionary, 2564
Diabetes Educator, 2586
Diabetes Forecast, 2578
Diabetes in African Americans, 2592
Diabetes in Hispanic Americans, 2593
Diabetes Insipidus, 2590
Diabetes Medical Nutition Therapy, 2565
Diabetes Mellitus, 2549
Diabetes Overview, 2591
Diabetes Spectrum: From Research toPractice, 2582
Diabetes Teaching Guide for People Who UseInsulin, 2566
Diabetic Neuropathy: the Nerve Damageof Diabetes, 2594
Diabetics Control and Complications Trial, 2595
Diagnosis Autism: Now What? 10 Steps toImprove Treatment Outcomes, 924
Diagnosis Schizophrenia: A ComprehensiveResource, 1643
Diagnostic and Statistical Manual ofMental Disorders, 1676
Diagnostic Approach to the Dysmorphic Patient, 557
Diagnostic Tests, 49
Dial-a-Hearing Screening Test, 3504
Dialogue with Doris, 6378
Diarrhea, 50
Dictionary for Brain Tumor Patients, 1287
Diet and Headache-Fact Sheet, 4771
Diet Instruction, 1370
A Diet Management, 1366
Differences in Common: Straight Talk onMental Retardation/Down Syndrome & Life, 2735
Different Like Me: My Book of Autism Heroes, 925
Difficult Child, 1794
DiGeorge Syndrome, 2619
Digestive Disease National Coalition, 26, 261, 1749, 1942, 2139, 3092, 4978, 6098, 7621
Digestive Diseases & Disorders Sourcebook, 1362, 1949, 2197, 7639

Digestive Diseases Dictionary, 43
Digestive Diseases Self-Education Program (DDSEP 5.0), 35
Digestive System, 8848
Directions, 6935
Directory of National Genetic VoluntaryOrganizations, 566
Directory of Pediatric Neurosurgeons, 4268
Disabilities Advocacy & Support Network, 8291
Disability Awareness, 8594
Disability Connection and RAFT, LarimerCounty's Early Childhood Connection, 8142
Disability Handbook for Social SecurityApplicants, 7146
Disability Information and Resource Center, 3206
Disability Rights Education & Defense Fund, 7955
Disabled Shooting Services, 7956
Disabled Sports USA, 7957
Discipline and the Child with TouretteSyndrome, 7450
Discovering Cued Speech, 3618
Discovery Book, 1520
Disruptive Behavior Disorders in Children, 1795, 5423, 7744, 7749
Distant Drums, Different Drummers: A Guidefor Young People with ADHD, 654
District of Columbia Public Library/Librarian for the Deaf Community, 3556
Diverticular Disease, 51
Division for Early Childhood, 7958
Division for Learning Disabilities, 4508, 4522
Division for Physical and HealthDisablities, 7959
Division for Research (CEC-DR), 8558
Division for the Visually Handicapped, 1884, 2031, 5263, 6191
Division of Birth Defects & DevelopmentalDisabilities, 7960
Division of Birth Defects &Developmental Disabilities, 5406
Division of Birth Defects and GeneticDiseases, 8559
Division of Community Health Nursing, 7006
Division of Community Services, 8438
Division of Developmental Disabilities, 8442
Division of Early Childhood Education, 8360
Division of Early Intervention Services, 8378
Division of Exceptional LearnersIndiana Department of Education, 8209
Division of Pediatric Pulmonology, 6088
Division of Preschool Services, 8237
Division of Special Education, 8299, 8318
Division of Special Education StateDepartment of Education, 8095
Division of Special Populations, 8240
Division of Student Services, 8324
Division on Career Development andTransition, 7961
Division on Visual Impairments, 1885, 2032, 5264, 6116, 6192, 6270, 6304
DMRF/NINDS Dystonia Workshop: From Geneto Function in Dystonia, 2826
Do I Look Fat in This?: Life Doesn't BeginFive Pounds From Now, 2938
Does My Child Have Autism?, 926
Dogs for the Deaf, Inc., 3505
domesticshelters.org, 7738
Don't Give Up Kid, 655
Don't Think About Monkeys: ExtraordinaryStories Written by People with Tourette, 7438
Dotty the Dalmatian Has Epilepsy, 6573
The Doug Flutie, Jr. Foundation for Autism, 770
Down Sydrome: Living and Learning in theCommunity, 2736
Down Syndrome, 2632, 2757
Down Syndrome Affiliates in Action, 2643
Down Syndrome Association of Atlanta, 2665
Down Syndrome Association of CentralIndiana, 8210
Down Syndrome Association of Los Angeles, 2660
Down Syndrome Association of MiddleTennessee, 2674
Down Syndrome Association of Minnesota, 2671
Down Syndrome Association of NWI, 2667
Down Syndrome Clinic of MinneapolisChildren's Medical Center, 2688
Down Syndrome Clinic, Children's Hospitalof Alabama, 2677
Down Syndrome Clinic, Rainbow Babies andChildren's Hospital, 2695
Down Syndrome Community, 2644
Down Syndrome Guild, 2645, 2722
Down Syndrome Guild of Dallas, 2675
Down Syndrome Information Alliance, 2646
Down Syndrome News, 2752
Down Syndrome Program, Children's HospitalBoston, 2687
Down Syndrome Specialty Clinic, 2703
Down Syndrome Support Association ofSouthern Indiana (DSSASI), 2668
Down Syndrome: Birth to Adulthood: GivingFamilies an Edge, 2737
Down Syndrome: The Facts, 2738
Down's Syndrome Medical Clinic, 2690

Downtown Detroit Subregional Library forthe Blind and Handicapped, 1862, 2009, 5241, 6169
Dr. Gertrude A. Barber National Institute, 2700
Dr. Ivan's Depression Central, 2494
Dr. Koop, 1959, 2096, 5161, 6105
Draw Me a Picture, 106
Dream Factory, 8831
Dream Street Foundation, 8727
Dreams Come True Emery Clinic-Peds, 73, 132
The Driving Test, 3670
Drugs and Pregnancy: It's Not Worth TheRisk, 3158
Drugs That Have Been Used for theTreatment of Sarcoidosis, 6405
DSBA National Conference, 2483
Dual Diagnosis, 5498
Duchenne Parent Project Muscular Dystrophy, 4822
Duke Brain Tumor Support Group, 1227
Duke Pediatric Brain Tumor Family SupportProgram, 1228
Duke University Comprehensive Epilepsy Center, 6552
Duke University Comprehensive Sickle CellCenter, 6653
Duke University Medical Center/ CF Center, 2316
Duke University School of Medicine Pediatric and Allergy Immunology, 6327
Durable Power of Attorney for Health CareDecisions, 4269
DVH Quarterly, 1597, 3013, 5640, 6044
DVI Quarterly, 6295
Dwarf Athletic Association of America, 3230, 3254
Dysautonomia Foundation, 3127
Dyslexia, 2769, 2786
Dyslexia Research Institute, 2781, 4509
Dystonia, 2802
Dystonia Dialogue, 2825
Dystonia Medical Research Foundation, 2806, 2813, 2818
Dytonias: Fact Sheet, 2827

E

EA Message, 2533
Each of Us Remembers: Parents of ChildrenWith Cerebral Palsy, 1521
Eagle Eyes A Child's View od AttentionDeficit Disorder, 656
Eagle Eyes: A Child's View of AttentionDeficit Disorder, 657
Eagle Hill School - Summer Program, 705, 989, 4541
EAR Foundation, 3506
Ear, Nose and Throat Journal, 6341
Early Childhood CARES Program, 8372
Early Childhood Handicapped Prgrams, 8439
Early Detection, 6298
Early Intervention Program, 8082, 8338, 8432
Early Intervention Programs, 8373
Early Intervention Research Institute,Developmental Center, 8560
Early Intervention Services, 8260
Early Intervention Services Division ofChild & Family Services, 8311
Early Intervention System, 8325
Early Intervention Unit, Division ofChildren's Medical Services, 8170
Early on Michigan, 8268
The Early Stages of Schizophrenia, 1659
Early Start Family Resource Network, 8114
Early Years Guide of the Life StageProgram, 7548
East Central Region–Helen Keller NationalCenter, 1827, 1972, 5205, 6133
East Central Regional Office, 8361
East Tennessee Comprehensive HemophiliaCenter, 4001
East Tennessee Technology Access Center, 8538
Easter Seal Kysoc, 2612, 3905, 4725, 8754
Easter Seal Society, 8745
Easter Seal Summer Camp Programs, 8728
Easter Seals, 1384
Easter Seals - Timber Pointe Outdoor Center, 8738
Easter Seals Camp Challenge, 8735
Easter Seals Camp Fairlee Manor, 8760
Easter Seals Camp Sunnyside, 8752
Easter Seals Disability Services, 1385, 1503, 6810, 7963, 8623
Easter Seals Oregon Camping Program, 8806
Easter Seals WisconsinCamp Respite, 1544
Eastern Maine Medical Center: CysticFibrosis Center, 2282
Eastern Michigan Hemophilia Center, 4002
Eastern North Carolina Chapter (SCDAA), 6639
Eastern Virginia Medical Center, 2344
Eating Disorder AnonymousEDA, Inc., 2852
Eating Disorder Hope, 2853
Eating Disorder Recovery Support, 2854
Eating Disorder Referrals, 5727

Eating Disorder Sourcebook, 2939
Eating Disorder Video, 2917
Eating Disorders, 2830, 2940
Eating Disorders & Obesity, 2nd Ed., 2941
Eating Disorders and Education Network, 2859
Eating Disorders Association of New Jersey, 2890
Eating Disorders Coalition, 2855
Eating Disorders Group, 2856
Eating Disorders Information Network, 2857
Eating Disorders Online.com: 15 Styles ofDistorted Thinking, 2921
Eating Disorders Research and TreatmentProgram, 2909
Eating Disorders Research Society, 2858
Eating Disorders Resource Catalogue, 2942
Eating Disorders Review, 2971
Eating Disorders: When Food Turns AgainstYou, 2943
Eaton-Peabody Laboratory of AuditoryPhysiology, 3561
EB Medical Research Foundation, 3068
ECAC, 8350
Echolalia, 7420
Ecology and Enviromental Management ofLyme Disease, 4619
Economic Glitch, 3619
Ectodermal Dysplasias, 2976
Eczema, 2994
Eczema/Atopic Dermatitis, 3017
Eden Wood Center, 2768, 7788, 8778
EDI, 2611
Educating Boys with Fragile X Syndrome, 3193
Educating Deaf Children: An Introduction, 3881
Educating Deaf Students: Global Perspectives, 3765
Educating Inattentive Children, 625
Educating Peter, 2715
Educating Students with Autism: Implementation of Applied Bahavior Analysis, 885
Education and Care for Adolescents andAdults with Autism, 927
Education Development Center - EDC, 8261
Educational and Development Aspects ofDeafness, 3768
Educational and Developmental Aspects of Deafness, 3769
Educational Audiology Association, 3507, 6768
Educational Audiology for the Limited-Hearing Infant and Preschooler, 3766
Educational Equity, Special EducationBranch, 8312
Educational Help for the Handicapped, 7832
Educational Interpreting: How It Can Succeed, 3767
Educational Issues Among Children WithSpina Bifida, 6901
Educational Rights for Children WithArthritis: Parents Manual, 4396
Educational Services for the VisuallyImpaired, 1830, 1976, 5209, 6137, 8450
Effective Parent Project, 8143
Effective Treatments for PTSD, 2nd Ed, 5802
Effects of Alcohol on Pregnancy NationalClearinghouse for Alcohol Information, 3161
Effects of Sarcoid and Steroids onAngiotensin-Converting Enzyme, 6406
EFWCP Resource Library, 6546
Egleston Cystic Fibrosis Center: Department of Pediatrics, 2267
EHealth, 5427
Ehlers-Danlos National Foundation, 3023
Ehlers-Danlos National Foundation LearningConference, 3026
Ehlers-Danlos Syndrome, 3020, 3029
El Groupo Vida, 8144
El Rolphe Center, 5499
Electronic Media and Youth Violence - ACDC Issue Brief, 7750
Elf on a Shelf for Minimal Pairs: Giant CD Print Program, 3692
Elizabeth Glazer Pediatric AIDS Foundation, 3298, 3325
Elkhart Public Library, 8481
Ellie's Back, 6480
Embrace the Dawn, 6574
EMedicine Journal: Syncope, 7119
Emory Autism Resource Center, 849
Emory Eye Center - Strabismus Research, 6944
Empowering Parents, 7719
Encephalitis Information Resource, 6976
Encephalocele, 3030
Enchanted Hills Camp, 1931, 2082, 3906
Encopresis, 3050
Encyclopedia of Depression, 2509
Encyclopedia of Obesity and EatingDisorders, 2944
Encyclopedia of Phobias, Fears, andAnxieties, 5609, 6742
Encyclopedia of Schizophrenia and thePsychotic Disorders, 1644
Endeavor, 3865
Endocrine & Metabolic Disorders Sourcebook, 2233, 2567, 3261, 4356
Endocrine Practice, 2235

Endocrine Society, 7601, 7964
Endocrine System, 8849
Endorphins: Eating Disorders & OtherAddictive Behavior, 2945
Endoscopic Third Ventriculoscopy, 4270
Enough Is Enough, 7720
EnTech: Enabling Technologies ofKentuckiana, 8491
Environmental Protection Agency, 418
EpiCenter, 6547
EPICS Project-SW Communication Resources, 8330
Epidermoid Brain Tumor Society, 1100
Epidermolysis Bullosa, 3061
Epilepsia: Journal of the InternationalLeague Against Epilepsy, 6596
Epilepsy & Behavior, 6594
Epilepsy A to Z, 6575
Epilepsy Association of the Big Bend, 6537
Epilepsy Education Association of Arkansas, 6535
Epilepsy Foundation, 1386, 6529, 6592, 7370, 7540
Epilepsy Foundation Eastern Pennsylvania, 6543
Epilepsy Foundation New Jersey, 6540
Epilepsy Foundation Northwest, 6545
Epilepsy Foundation of America, 6565
Epilepsy Foundation of Florida, 6538
Epilepsy Foundation of Long Island, 6542
Epilepsy Foundation of Northern California, 6536
Epilepsy Foundation Western/Central Pennsylvania, 6544
Epilepsy in Children: The Teacher's Role, 6600
Epilepsy Institute, 6530
Epilepsy Research Laboratory, Department of Neurology, 6549
Epilepsy, A Guide to Balancing Your Life, 6576
Epilepsy.com, 6566
Epilepsy: 199 Answers, 6577
Epilepsy: Frequency, Causes and Consequences, 6578
Epilepsy: I Can Live with That, 6579
Epilepsy: The Untold Story, 6557
Epilepsy: You and Your Child, 6601
EpilepsyUSA, 6593
Episcopal Conference of the Deaf, 3508
Erb's Palsy, 3072
ERIC Clearinghouse on Disabilities &Gifted Children, 7962
ERIC Clearinghouse on Disabilities andGifted Education, 8545
Eric RicStar Winter Music Therapy Summer Camp, 1545, 8771
Erythema Infectiosum, 3081
Erythropoietic Protoporphyria Research &Education Fund, 5772
Esophageal Atresia, 3089
Essential Guide to Psychiatric Drugs, 2510
Eukee the Jumpy, Jumpy Elephant, 658
European Society for Pediatric Urology, 2221, 8624
Even Exchange Newsletter, 4446
Even Little Kids Get Diabetes, 2568
Evergreen Spina Bifida Association, 6864
Every Child By Two, 5938
Everybody is Different: A Book for Young People, 928
Everybody's Different, Nobody's Perfect, 4855
Everyday Solutions: A Practical Guide forFamilies of Children with Autism, 929
Everyone Likes to Eat, 2569
Everything You Need to Know About Measlesand Rubella, 6002
Everything You Need To Know AboutDepression, 2511
Ewing's Sarcoma, 3102
Ewing's Sarcoma Support Group ResourcesPage, 3116
Exceptional Children Division, 8351
Exceptional Family Resource Center, 8115
Exceptional Family Support, Education andAdvocacy Center, 8116
Exceptional Parent, 8669
Exceptional Parents, 8117
Explosive Child, 5421, 5424
Eye on NEI, 4490
Eye Patch Club, 4463
Eye Problems Associated with Hydrocephalusin Children, 4271
EyeCare America, 4464
EyeWorld, 4491

F

FAA World Convention, 2912
Face First, 2130, 2430, 3442
FACES: Finding a Cure for Epilepsy & Seizures, 6531, 6597
FACES: National Association for theCraniofacially Handicapped, 1685, 1695, 2117, 4583

FACES: National Craniofacial Foundation, 2118
FACES: The National CraniofacialAssociation, 2104
Facilitated Communication Institute atSyracuse University, 742, 863
Facing Neurofibromatosis: A Guide for Teens, 5055
Facing the Challenges, 2110
Facing the Challenges of Turner SyndromeTogether, 7609
Facioscapulohumeral Dystrophy Society, 4823
Fact Sheet: Guillain-Barre Syndrome, 3278
Fact Sheet: Hydrocephalus, 4272
Fact Sheet: Syringomyelia, 4273
Factor Nine News, 4074
Factor V Leiden: Thrombophilia Support Page, 6017
Facts & Fallacies About Digestive Diseases, 52
Facts About Apnea and Other ApparentLife-Threatening Events, 7106
Facts About Autism, 973
Facts About Charcot-Marie-Tooth Disease and Dejerine-Sottas, 1566
Facts About Duchenne and Becker MuscularDystrophies, 4856
Facts About Facioscapulohumeral MuscularDystrophy, 4857
Facts About Friedreich's Ataxia, 579
Facts About Inflammatory Myopathies-DM, PM and IBM, 4858
Facts About Limb-Girdle Muscular Dystrophy, 4859
Facts About Metabolic Diseases of Muscle, 4860
Facts About Mitochondrial Myopathies, 4861
Facts About Muscular Dystrophy, 4862
Facts About Myasthenia Gravis (MG, LEMS, &CMS), 4863
Facts About Myopathies, 4864
Facts About Myotonic Muscular Dystrophy, 4865
Facts About Plasmapheresis, 4866
Facts About Rare Muscular Dystrophies, 4867
Facts About SIDS, 7107
Facts About Spinal Muscular Atrophy, 6937
Facts About Tuberculosis, 7533
Facts About Turner Syndrome, 7610
Facts for Families, 7751
Facts for Health: PTSD, 5795
Facts on Liver Transplantation, 1027
Fairfax County Public Library, 8546
Fairfield/Westchester Chapter of Crohn's &Colitis Foundation of America, 2151, 2170
Familial Dysautonomia, 3125
Familial Dysautonomia Hope Foundation, 3128
Families Affected by Fetal Alcohol Spectrum Disorder, 3144
Families at Heart, 4318
Families Can Help Children Cope with Fear,Anxiety, 5619, 6749
Families Caring for Families, 8118
Families Coping with Mental Illness, 1061, 1626
Families Empowered and Supporting Treatment of Eating Disorders, 2905
Families for Depression Awareness, 1045, 2453
Families for Early Autism Treatment, 743, 902
Families Helping Families of Greater NewOrleans, 8241
Families of Adults Afflicted with Asperger's Syndrome, 359, 744
Families of SMA - Arizona Chapter, 6920
Families of SMA - Connecticut Chapter, 6922
Families of SMA - Long Island NY Chapter, 6924
Families of SMA - Northern California Chapter, 6921
Families of SMA - Tennessee Chapter, 6925
Families of Spinal Muscular Atrophy, 6913, 6930
Families Together, 8232
Families Together/Parent to Parent of KS, 8233
Families with Heart, 4321
Family & Educator Connection - Cedar Falls/Waterloo Region, 8223
Family & Educator Connection - Clear Lake/Mason City Region, 8224
Family & Educator Connection - Marshalltown Region, 8225
Family Caregiver Alliance, 7965
Family Center Early Supports & Services, 8319
Family Connection of South Carolina, 8535
Family Empowerment Network: SupportingFamilies Affected by FAS/FAE, 3145
Family First Program Alpha Resource Center, 8119
Family Focus Resource Center, 8120
Family Guide - Growth and Development ofthe Partially Seeing Child, 1917, 2068, 5289, 6218
Family Guide to Vision Care, 1918, 2069, 5290, 6219
Family Information Network, 8362
Family Life with Tourette Syndrome, 7421
Family Life with Tourette Syndrome...Personal Stories, 7333, 7422
Family Network on Disabilities, 8171
Family Online Safety Institute, 7690
Family Resource Center, 8121
Family Resource Center at Lucile PackardChildren's Hospital, 1752

Family Resource Center of SoutheastIndiana, 8211
Family Resource Center on Disabilities, 8196
Family Resource Network, 8292
Family Service Association, 2454
Family Support Bulletin, 1532
Family Support Center of New Jersey, 8326
Family Support Network, 1387, 1504, 7371, 7541
Family Support Network of MichiganParent Participation Program-MDCH, 8269
Family Support Network of North Carolina, 8352
Family T.I.E.S. Network, 8197
Family Ties at Massachusetts Departmentof Public Health, 8262
Family to Family Network ARC of HennepinCounty, 8276
Family Traditions, 3620
Family Village, 377, 1948, 3069, 3132, 4369, 4641, 5191
Family Voices, 7966
Family, Infant, and Toddler Project, 8420
Family-2-Family Health Information Centerof Arkansas, 8103
Family/Community Support Group of theBrain Injury Association of Florida, 3375
FamilyConnect, 4479
Famous Fone Friends, 8832
Fantastic Videos: Colonial Times, Chocolate, and Cars, 3621
Fantastic Videos: Dogs at Work and Play, 3622
Fantastic Videos: Exciting People, Placesand Things!, 3623
Fantastic Videos: From Post Offices to Dairy Goats!, 3624
Fantastic Videos: Imagination, Actors, and 'Deaf Way!', 3625
Fantastic Videos: Roller Coasters, Maps, and Ice Cream!, 3626
Fantastic Videos: Skiing, Factories, and Race Horses, 3627
Fantastic Videos: The Wonderful Worlds ofSports and Travel, 3628
Farm and Wilderness Camps, 8819
Fast Facts: Rhinitis, 6338
Fear of Being Fat, 2946
Fear of Illness, 5590
Featherless/Desplumado, 6885
Febrile Seizures Fact Sheet, 6602
Fecal Incontinence, 3060
Federal Hemophilia Treatment Center ofHawaii, 4004
Federal Hemophilia Treatment CenterProgram of Los Angeles, 4003
Federation for Children with Special Needs, 4510, 7967, 8263, 8625
Federation of Families for Children'sMental Health, 745, 1046, 1611, 1768, 2455, 5103, 5130, 5154, 5362, 5490, 5573, 6703, 6729, 7691, 7968
Feed Your Kids Well: How to Help YourChild Lose Weight and Get Healthy, 5340
Feeding Your Baby, 1706
Feingold Association of the US, 606, 636
Fetal Alcohol Education Program, 3146
Fetal Alcohol Syndrome, 3135, 3162
Fetal Alcohol Syndrome Family ResourceInstitute, 3147
Fetal Retinoid Syndrome, 3166
A Few Errands, 3588
FFCMH Annual Conference, 870, 1059, 1623, 1778, 2484, 7708, 8585
Fight Drug Abuse at Home, Work, School andin the Community, 3163
Fight SMA / Andrew's Buddies, 6914
Fighters for Encephalocele Support Group, 3036
Fighters for Encephaly Support Group, 4584
Financial Assistance and Insurance forPeople with Kidney Disease, 5003
Financial Help for Diabetics Care, 2596
Find Counseling.com, 7722
Finding Out About Seizures: A Guide toMedical Tests, 6603
FindYouthInfo.gov, 7723
Fingerspelling: Expressive and ReceptiveFluency, 3629
Fire Fighter Brown, 3770
Firefighters Kids Camp Camp Concord, 1332
First Candle/SIDS Alliance, 6986
First Direction, 8212
First Regional Hemophilia Center, 4005
First Signs at Home, 3771
First Signs at Play, 3772
First Steps, 8213
First Steps for Families, 8214
First Steps Program, 8284
First Steps, Early Interventions, NewHorizons Rehabilitation, 8215
The First Year, 1710
FIRST: Foundation for Ichthyosis andRelated Skin Types, 4364
5 Smart Steps to Less Stress, 5615
50 Freqently Asked Questions About Auditory-Verbal Therapy, 3717
50th Anniversary Collection, 3587
52 Proven Stress Reducers, 4767
Florida Bureau of Braille and Talking BookLibrary Services, 1841, 1987, 5220, 6148

Florida Camp for Children and Youth, 2613
Florida Chapter of Crohn's & Colitis Foundation of America, 2153
Florida Department of Education, 8172
Florida Department of Health ImmunizationProgram, 5964
Florida Epilepsy Services Providers Association, 6539
Florida Families of Children with Visual Impairments, 6280
Florida Hemophilia Association, 3949
Florida Narcolepsy Association, 4883
Florida Ophthalmic Institute, 2037
Florida School-Deaf and Blind Summer Camp, 1932, 2083, 3907, 5300, 6229
Florida's Collaboration for Young Childrenand their Families Head State, 8173
Floyd Rogers, 2614
Flying, 5591
FOCUS, 8102
Focus on Autism and Other Developmental Disabilities, 967
Focus On Recovery-United, 2860
Fontan Friends, 4327
Food Addicts Anonymous, 2861
Food Allergy Network, 2922
Food Allergy News, 2972
Food Allergy Research & Education, 1348
Food and Drug Administration, 3326
Food for Recovery, 2947
Food Research and Action Center, 5322
Food, Behavior and Beyond, 5862
For Siblings Only, 8681
Forgotten Plague: How the Battle AgainstTuberculosis Was Won & Lost, 7529
Forward Face, 2119, 3037
Forward Face: The Charity for Childrenwith Craniofacial Conditions, 4585
Foundation Fighting Blindness, 6259
Foundation for Child Development, 7692
Foundation for Exceptional Children, 7969
Foundation for Glaucoma Research, 2038
Foundation for Prader-Willi Research, 5816, 5859
Foundation for Sarcoidosis Research, 6387
Foundations of Spoken Language for Hearing-Impaired Children, 3773
Four for You! Fables and Fairy Tales Series, 3630
49 XXY Syndrome Association, 4437
Fox Valley Hydrocephalus Support Group, 4240
Fragile X - A to Z: Guide for Families byFamilies, 3194
Fragile X Alliance of Ohio, 3185
Fragile X Association of SouthernCalifornia, 3183
Fragile X Center of San Diego, 3184
Fragile X Syndrome, 3176
Francis J. CurryNational Tuberculosis Center, 7522
FRAXA Research Foundation, 3180, 3190
FRAXA Research Foundation Newsletter, 3196
Frederick Douglas Branch for SpecializedServices and Physically Handicapped, 8508
Free Hand: Enfranchising the Education ofDeaf Children, 3774
Free Library of Philadelphia, 8532
Freedom Camp, 8794
Freedom From Fear, 5574
Freedom From Headaches, 4757
Freedom's Wings International, 8833
Freeing Your Child from Obsessive-Compulsive Disorder, 5392
Fresno Brain Tumor Support Group, 1130
Friedrich's Ataxia, 580
FRIENDS, 7721
Friends for Life Auburn United MethodistChurch, 8083
Friends No Matter What, 6886
Friends of Karen, 8339
Friends of Libraries for Deaf Action, 3509
Friends' Health Connection, 7970
From Gesture to Language in Hearing and Deaf Children, 3775
From Mime to Sign, 3631
From the Ashes, 3455
Frontier Travel Camp, 396
Functional Behavior Assessment for Peoplewith Autism, 930
Future Choices, 8216
The Future of Children, 7702
Future Reflections, 8670

G

G. Advocacy, 4259
Gainesville Subregional LBPHHall County Public Library, 8463

Galactosemia, 3197
Galactosemia Resources and Information, 3207, 4789
Gallaudet Today, 3866
Gallstones, 53
Gas in the Digestive Tract, 54
Gastoparesis in Diabetes, 2597
Gastroesophageal Reflux Disease in Children, 55
Gateway Hemophilia Association of Missouri, 3963
Gathered View, 5879
Gaucher Disease Fact Sheet, 3225
Gaucher Disease Newsletter, 3224
Gaucher Registry, 3220
Gaucher's Disease, 3212
Gaylord Hospital Sleep Medicine, 4892
Gazoontite, 472
GBS Support Group of the UK, 3276
GBS/CIDP Foundation International, 3274
Geisinger Wyoming Valley Medical Center,Sleep Disorders Center, 4927
Gemma B Publishing, 1522
Gene Clinics, 561
Gene Testing for Ataxia, 581
Generating Business, 3632
Generation Rescue, 746
Generations, 572
Genes, Blood & Courage, 7283
Genesee County Health Department, 7026
GeneTest, 8626
Genetic Alliance, 178, 216, 227, 236, 286, 303, 329, 419, 591, 607, 747,
    1017, 1306, 1670, 1686, 1717, 1735, 1821, 1943, 1954, 1965
Genetic Alliance Annual Conference, 187, 218, 230, 240, 288, 306, 334,
    456, 593, 619, 871, 1021, 1308, 1691, 1719, 1738, 1897, 1947, 1958,
    2047, 2108
Genetic Alliance, Inc, 7165, 7171
Genetic Network of the Empire State, 537
Genetics and Neuromuscular Diseases, 4868
Genetics and You, 1707
Genetics Coloring Book, 4057
Genetics, Disability and Deafness, 3776
Georges Gilles de la Tourette-The Man andHis Times, 7451
Georgetown University, 6450
Georgetown University Child DevelopmentCenter, 8166, 8457, 8561
Georgetown University Sleep DisordersCenter, 4893
Georgia Ataxia Support Group, 518
Georgia Chapter of Crohn's & ColitisFoundation of America, 2154
Georgia Department of Human Resources -Center for Family Resource
    Planning, 7009
Georgia Department of Human ResourcesChildren's Health Services, 7008
Georgia Perinatal Association, 5906
Get a Grip on Asthma Programs, 420
Get Ready to Read!, 4527
Get the Facts About Sleep Apnea, 6696
Get to Sleep! How To Sleep Well...DespiteLupus, 7147
Getting a Grip on ADD: A Kid's Guide toUnderstanding & Coping with
    ADD, 659
Getting a Second Opinion, 6515
Getting Better Bit(e) by Bit(e), 2948
Getting Into College: Strategies for theStudent with Tourette Syndrome,
    7452
Getting Ready for the Big Date, 3633
Getting Ready, Getting Well, 6499
Getting Started with Facilitated Communication, 886
Getting Your Life Back Together When YouHave Schizophrenia, 1645
Ghost Investigation, 3634
Giddings School Special Education Division, 8167
Gift of Hope, 7423
GIG Quarterly, 1363
Girl Scouts of the USA, 7972
Give Kids the World, 8834
Give Me One Wish, 2363
Give Your ADD Teen a Chance: A Guide forParents of Teenagers with
    ADD, 660
Glaucoma, 2070
Glaucoma Associates, 2051
Glaucoma Laser Trabeculoplasty Study, 2039
Glaucoma Research Foundation, 1966, 2040, 2052
Glaucoma: The Sneak Thief of Sight, 2071
GLC Annual Education Conference, 1349
Gleams, 1912
Glenn Garcelon Foundation, 1101
Global and Regional Asperger Syndrome Partnership, 360, 748

Global Down Syndrome Foundation, 2648
Global EpidemicMulti-Drug Resistant Tuberculosis, 7534
Gloriana Opera Company, 8729
Gluten Intolerance Group of North America(GIG), 1350
Gluten-free Commercial Products, 1371
Gluten-Free Page, 1360
Go Togethers, 3777
Gold Coast Down Syndrome Organization, 2663
The Golden Fund for Autism, 771
Goldilocks and the Three Bears Told in Signed English, 3778
Good Morning Me!Hand and Voices, 3779
Goodwill Industries-Suncoast, 2664
Goodwill Industries-Suncoast: Choices forWork Program, 3376
The Gossip, 3671
Governor's Campaign, 3635
Gow School Summer Programs, 8795
Graduate School, 3636
Grandfather Moose!, 3780
Great Lakes Hemophilia Foundation, 3987
Great Plains Region-Helen Keller NationalCenter, 6128
Greater Atlanta Area Support Group, 519
Greater Boston Arc Parent Support, 8264
Greater Interagency Council Parent toParent Support Network, 8198
Greater Los Angeles Chapter, 4979
Greater Los Angeles/Orange County Chapterof Chron's & Colitis
    Foundation, 2146
Greater New York Chapter of Crohn's &Colitis Foundation of America,
    2171
Greater North Valley California SupportGroup, 505
Greater San Diego/Desert Chapter of Crohn's & Colitis Foundation of
    America, 2147
Gregory Fleming James Cystic Fibrosis Center, 2245
Grief, Bereavement and Sudden InfantDeath Syndrome, 7094
Grilled Cheese, 2570
The Grocer and the Cook, 3672
Group Psychotherapy for Eating Disorders, 2949
Groupworks West, 749
Groves Academy, 706, 990, 4542
Growing Children: A Parent's Guide, 3262
Growing Straighter and Stronger, 6481
Growing Up With Epilepsy, 6580
Growing Up with OI: Guide for Children, 5461
Growing Up with OI: Guide for Familiesand Caregivers, 5462
Growing Up with Prader-Willi Syndrome - Personal Reflections of a
    Mother, 5882
Growing Up with Scoliosis: A Young Girl'sStory, 6500
Growth Hormone and Prader-Willi Syndrome, 5871
Growth Hormone Deficiency, 3227, 3267
Growth Hormone Testing, 3268
Guardians of Hydrocephalus ResearchFoundation, 2121, 3038, 4220, 4247
Guide for Children & Teenagers, 7650
Guide for Children and Teenagers toCrohn's Disease/Ulcerative Colitis,
    2208
Guide to Diagnosis & Treatment, 7453
A Guide to Hydrocephalus, 4255
Guide to Insurance Coverage for PeopleWith Hemophilia, 4058
Guide to Psychology and its Practice (A), 7724
Guidelines for Families Coping with OCD, 5380
Guidelines for Spina Bifida and Health Care Services Throughout Life,
    6887
Guillain-Barre Syndrome, 3271
Gurze Books, 5338
Gurze Bookstore, 2923

H

H.E.A.R.T.S. Connection Family ResourceCenter, 8122
H.O.P.E. Series: Seizures in Childhood, 6604
H.O.P.E. Series: Seizures in the Teen Years, 6605
H.O.P.E.: Helping Other People Eat, 2862
Hair Club for Kids: Hair Club for Men, 74, 133, 3110
Hand Eczema, 3018
Handbook of Autism and Pervasive Developmental Disorders, 931
Handbook of Children and the Media, 7752
Handbook of Head Truma: Acute Care toRecovery, 3456
Handbook of Headache, 4758
The Handbook of Pediatric Audiology, 3839
Handbook of Psoriasis, 6035
Handbook of School-Based Interventions, 2512

Handbook of Scoliosis, 6501
Handi-Kids/King Solomon Foundation, 8767
Handicapped Scuba Association, 7973
Handle with Care, 7974
Handling the Young Cerebral Palsied Childat Home, 1523
Handout on Health: Scleroderma, 6466
Hands & Voices National, 3510
Hands Organization, 3511
Happiness Bag Incorporated, 8746
Happy Hollow Children's Camp, 8747
Harbor Regional Center Family andProfessional Resource Center, 8123
Hard of Hearing Advocates, 3549
Harold Goodglass Aphasia Research Center, 3428
Harold Talks About How He InheritedHemophilia, 4059
Harold's Secret: A Boy with Hemophilia, 4060
Harris County Health Department, 7057
Harrison's Principles of Inernal Medicine15th Edition, 7308
Having Leukemia Isn't So Bad, of Course,It Wouldn't Be My First Choice, 107
Hawaii Department of Health ImmunizationProgram, 5965
Hawaii Down Syndrome Congress, 2666
Hawaii SIDS Information & CounselingProject, 7011
HCMA - Heart Link Online, 4304
Head Injuries, 3351
Head Injury Hotline, 3362, 3418
Head Injury in Children and Adolescents: AResource and Review for School, 3457
Head Trauma Sourcebook, 3458
Headache, 4765
Headache Book: Prevention & Treatmentfor All Types of Headaches, 4759
Headache Facts-What Everyone Should Know, 4772
Headache Handbook, 4773
Headache in Children-Fact Sheet, 4775
Headache Q & A, 4774
Headaches and Hydrocephalus, 4274
Headline News, 4075
The Headliner, 3467
Headlines, 3464
Heads Up Brain Tumor Support Group, 1102
Headstrong Brain Tumor Support Group, 1180
Headway, 3465
Healing Exchange Brain Trust, 1103
Healing Hearts, 4326
Healing Well, 2356
HealingWell.com, 6567
Health Answers, 562, 637, 1361, 1505, 1553, 2195, 2723, 2924, 3221, 3255, 4053, 6388, 6453, 6489, 7086, 7172, 7430, 7527, 7545, 7602, 7632
Health Insurance Issues and Solutions forPeople with Torette Syndrome, 7454
Health Research Project (HaRP), 38, 275, 4148, 4966, 5992
Healthcare for Children on the AutismSpectrum, 932
HealthCentral.com, 6018
Healthfinder, 4803, 4814, 7173, 7780
A Healthy Mouth for Your Baby, 7322
Hear, 3867
Hear & Listen! Talk & Sing!, 3693
Hear Center, 3554
Hear Now, 3512
The Hearing Aid Handbook: Clinician's Guide to Client Orientation, 3840
Hearing Alert Informational Brochures, 3882
Hearing Education & Awareness for Rockers, 3550
Hearing Health, 3856
Hearing Health Foundation, 3513
Hearing Impairment/Deafness, 3474
Hearing ImpairmentsBetter Hearing Institute, 3514
Hearing is Believing, Volume One, 3694
Hearing is Believing, Volume Three, 3695
Hearing is Believing, Volume Two, 3696
Hearing Loss Association of America, 3515
Hearing Loss Magazine, 3861
HearingPlanet, 3516
Heart and Down Syndrome, 2758
Heart Burn, Hiatal Hernia, and Gastroesophageal Reflux Disease, 56
Heart Center Online, 320
Heart Disease, High Blood Pressure, Strokeand Diabetes, 8693
Heart Failure Society Newsletter, 325
Heart Failure Society of America, 315
The Heart Institute, 4308
Heart of the Matter, 4315
Heart to Heart, 1898, 1919, 2048, 2072, 4312, 4330, 4332, 4334, 5272, 5291, 6201, 6220

Heart to Heart - St. Louis, 4320
Heart to Heart Fund, 4317
Hearts and Homes For Youth, 3517
HEATH Resource Center, 8458
Heights, 5592
The Help Group, 772
Help Me, I'm Sad, 2513
Help Parent Support Group Hope & Educationfor Loving Parents, 8145
Help with a Hidden Disease Update, 6379
Helpguide.org, 7725
Helping Children & Youth with RSD/CRPSSucceed in School, 4849
Helping Children and Adolescents Cope withViolence and Disasters, 5809
Helping Children with Autism Learn, 933
Helping Hearts, 4325
Helping Kids Cope With a New Threat, 5796
Helping Kids Heal - 75 Activities to HelpChildren Recover from Trauma & Loss, 5803
Helping Kids in Crisis: ManagingEmergencies in Children & Adolescents, 7753
Helping the Noncompliant Child, 5425
Helping with Hearing, 1708
Helping Your Anxious Child, 5610, 6743
Helping Your Child Cope with Depressionand Suicidal Thoughts, 2514
Helping Your Depressed Child, 2515
Helping Your Hard-of-Hearing ChildSucceed, 3883
HEMALOG, 4068
Hemangioma Support System, 3920
Hemangiomas and Lymphangiomas, 3915
HemAware, 4069
Hemlocks Easter Seals Recreation, 1729, 6524
Hemochromatosis, 57
Hemolytic Disease of the Newborn, 3929
Hemophila Foundation of North Carolina, 3968
Hemophilia, 3937
Hemophilia and Coagulation Programs, 4012
Hemophilia and Mild Hemophilia What ToExpect, 4085
Hemophilia and Thrombosis Center at theUniversity of Minnesota Medical Center, 4013
Hemophilia and Thrombosis Center ofNevada, 4014
Hemophilia Association of San Diego County, 3945
Hemophilia Association of South Carolina, 3978
Hemophilia Association of the Capital Area, 3983
Hemophilia Camp Directory, 4061
Hemophilia Center of Arkansas, 3943, 4006
Hemophilia Center of the New EnglandMedical Center, 4009
Hemophilia Center of Western New York, 3966, 4007
Hemophilia Center of Western Pennsylvania, 4008
Hemophilia Diseases and People, 4062
Hemophilia Federation of America, 3300
Hemophilia Foundation of Georgia, 3951
Hemophilia Foundation of Greater Florida, 3950
Hemophilia Foundation of Hawaii, 3952
Hemophilia Foundation of Idaho, 3953
Hemophilia Foundation of Illinois, 3954
Hemophilia Foundation of Indiana, 3955
Hemophilia Foundation of Maryland, 3958
Hemophilia Foundation of Michigan, 3960
Hemophilia Foundation of Minnesota and theDakotas, 3961
Hemophilia Foundation of NorthernCalifornia, 3946
Hemophilia Foundation of Oregon, 3975
Hemophilia Foundation of SouthernCalifornia, 3947
Hemophilia Foundation of Washington, 3986
Hemophilia Handbook, 4063
Hemophilia Headlines, 4076
Hemophilia Health Services, 3941
Hemophilia Nursing Handbook, 4064
Hemophilia Outreach Center, 3990
Hemophilia Program at Children's NationalMedical Center, 4010
Hemophilia Society of Colorado, 3948
Hemophilia Treatment Center at theUniversity of Iowa, 4011
Hemophilia, Sports, and Exercise, 4086
Hemophilia: Current Medical Management, 4087
Henry Youngerman Center for CommunicationDisorders, 6789
Hepatitis, 4094, 4117
Hepatitis A, 39
Hepatitis B, 40
Hepatitis B Coalition, 4098, 4106
Hepatitis B Coalition News, 4115
Hepatitis B Foundation, 4099, 4107
Hepatitis B Prevention: A Resource Guide, 4110
Hepatitis B: Your Child at Risk, 4118

Hepatitis C, 41
Hepatitis C: An Information Resource, 4111
Hepatitis Education Project, 4100, 4108
Hepatitis Fact Sheet, 4119
Hepatitis International Foundation, 4101, 4109
Here's Everything You'll Need to SaveMoney with the CFF Health Services, 2373
Here's Everything You'll Need to StartSaving Money with the CFF Pharmacy, 2374
Here's What I Mean to Say, 1524
Hereditary Ataxia: A Guidebook forManaging Speech & Swallowing, 567
Hereditary Ataxia: The Facts, 582
Hereditary Fructose Intolerance, 4124
Hereditary Hemorrhagic Telangiectasia(HHT) Foundation International, 7202, 7210, 7216, 7253
Heriditary Disease Foundation, 7975
Hermansky-Pudlak Syndrome Network AnnualFamily Conference, 188
Hermansky-Pudlak Syndrome Network Newsletter, 179, 195
Heroes Against AIDS, 3337
Herpes Resource Center, 4146, 4964
Herpes Simplex, 4140
Herpes.com, 4150, 4968
HerpeSite, 4149, 4967
Hey! I'm Here, Too!, 4869
HFSA Annual Scientific Meeting, 319
Hi! I'm Adam!, 7439
Hi, I'm Adam, 7344
Hickory Hill, 2615
High Five! Fables and Fairy Tales, 3637
High Hopes Foundation of New Hampshire, 8320
Highbrook Lodge Camp, 1933, 2084, 8805
Hill School of Fort Worth, 707, 991, 4543
Hirschsprung Disease, 4155, 4173
Hispanic Dental Association, 2421
Histiocytosis, 4174
Histiocytosis Association of America, 4178
HIV Infection, 3279
HIV Medicine Association, 3299
Hodgkin's Disease, 4185
Hodgkin's Disease and Non-Hodgkin'sLymphomas, 4198
Hole in the Wall Gang Camp, 3350, 4092
Holidays CD-ROM, 3697
Holidays: An ASL Word Book, 3698
Holistic Dental Association, 2422
Home Care Book, 7180
Home Line, 2375
Homocystinuria, 4199
HOPE (Helping Oncology Parents Endure)Brain Tumor Foundation of the Southwest, 1248
Hope and Recovery: A Mother-Daughter StoryAbout Anorexia Nervosa & Bulimia, 2950
Hope and Solutions for OCD, 5375
Hope for Children with AIDS, 3346
Hope for Hypothalamic Hamartomas, 1104
Hospitalization Tips, 4275
House Ear Institute, 3518
House Guests, 3638
Houston Area Brain Tumor Network, 1249
Houston Challengers TIRR Sports, 7976
Houston Ear Research Foundation, 3578
Houston Support Group, 549
Houston-Gulf Coast/South Texas Chapter ofCrohn's & Colitis Foundation of America, 2185
How Children Learn Language, 3781
How Does Your Child Hear and Talk?, 3884
How I Am (Wie Ich Bin), 887
How Many Times a Day Do You Risk BeingInfected with Hepatitis B?, 4120
How to be an Assertive Member of theTreatment Team, 4276
How to Find Out More About Your Child's Birth Defect or Disability, 8694
How to get Your Kid to Eat..., 2951
How to Help Your Child Succeed in School, 626, 4520
How to Recognize and Classify Seizures, 6558
How to Start a Turner Syndrome SupportGroup, 7611
How to Take Care of Your Baby Before Birth, 3164
How to Talk to Your Doctor About Headaches, 4776
Howard University Center for Sickle CellDisease, 6650
http://children.webmd.com, 6331
Hughen Center, 8816

Human Growth Foundation, 7, 14, 330, 2228, 3232, 3256, 4662, 5187, 7559, 7603, 7977
Hungry Caterpillar and Goodnight Moon, 3639
Hy Feinstein Clubhouse, 3400
HYCEPH-L, 4248
Hydrocephalus, 4215
Hydrocephalus Association, 3039, 4221, 4249
Hydrocephalus Association Newsletter, 4260
Hydrocephalus Association of N Texas, 4238
Hydrocephalus Association of Rhode Island, 4237
Hydrocephalus Family Support Group ofCentral Florida, 4229
Hydrocephalus Foundation, 4222
Hydrocephalus Group - Children's Hospitalof New Jersey, 4233
Hydrocephalus Parent Support Group, 2122
Hydrocephalus Support Group, 3040, 4230, 4232
Hydrocephalus Support Group Newsletter, 4261
Hydrocephalus Support Group of Seattle, 4239
Hydrocephalus Support Group of SouthernCalifornia, 4228
Hydrocephalus, a Neglected Disease, 4244
Hydrocephalus: A Guide for Patients,Families, and Friends, 4257
Hydrocephalus: Fact Sheet, 4277
Hydrohaven Chat Room, 4250
Hyperactive Child, Adolescent, and Adult:ADD Through the Lifespan, 661
Hyperactivity: Why Won't My Child PayAttention?, 662
Hypertrophic Cardiomyopathy, 4290
Hypertrophic Cardiomyopathy Association, 4293, 4297
Hypertrophic Cardiomyopathy Program atSt. Luke's-Roosevelt Hospital Center, 4295
Hypertrophic Cardiomyopathy: Heart CenterOnline for Patients, 4298
Hypoplastic Left Heart Syndrome, 4305
Hypothyroidism, 4344

I

I Am the Boss of My Body: PreventingChild Sexual Abuse, 5686
I Can Sign my ABCs, 3782
I Can't Hear You in the Dark: How to Learnand Teach Lipreading, 3783
I Cue, U Cue, 3699
I Have Diabetes: How Much Should I Eat?, 2598
I Have Diabetes: What Should I Eat?, 2599
I Have Diabetes: When Should I Eat?, 2600
I Love You Story, 3784
I Remember it Well, 3640
I Want My Little Boy Back, 888
I Was a Fifteen-Year-Old Blimp, 2952
I'M Deaf and It's Okay, 3785
I.D. Weeks Library, 5500
IAEDP Symposium, 2913
Ian's Walk: A Story About Autism, 934
IBD Nutrition Book, 7640
IBS Self-help group, 7633
ICAN (International Child Amputee Network), 8627
iCanShine, 775
ICARE, 134
Ichthyosis, 4359
Ichthyosis Information, 4370
Ichthyosis: An Overview, 4372
Ichthyosis: The Genetics of ItsInheritance, 4373
ID Card for Third VentriculostomyPatients, 4278
Idaho Dept. of Health & Welfare Immunization Program, 5966
Idaho Parents Unlimited, 8188
Idaho State Talking Book Library, 1847, 1993, 5226, 6154
Identification and Treatment of Attention Deficit Disorders, 697
If Your Child Has Diabetes: An Answer Bookfor Parents, 2571
IFFGD Professional Symposia, 32, 270, 2193, 3055, 3096
IHS Annual Convention & Expo, 3585
Illinois State Library, Talkng Book andBraille Service, 1849, 1995, 5228, 6156
Illuminations, 7101
Illustrated Dictionary - 3D ASL, 3700
Immune Deficiency Foundation, 2623, 3301, 3327
Immune Deficiency Foundation NationalConference, 2626, 3320
Immune System, 8850
Immune System Disorders Sourcebook, 3277, 7148
Immunization Action Coalition, 5939
Immunization Partnership of Alameda County, 5960
Immunology and Allergy Clinics of North America, 6339
Impact of Migraine-A Disabling and CostlyCondition, 4777
Implantable Defibrillators in PreventingSudden Death, 4299

In Control: Guide for Teens with Diabetes, 2572
In Our House, 3786
In Silence: Growing Up Hearing in a Deaf World, 3787
Incorporating Consumers into Regional Genetics Networks, 583
Increasing Capabilities Access Network, 8104
Incredible 5-Point Scale, 935
Independent Holoprosencephaly SupportSite, 4593
Independent Living Research UtilizationProgram, 7978
Indian Health Service, 7979
Indian Trails Camp, 8772
Indiana Chapter of Crohn's & Colitis Foundation of America, 2156
Indiana Deaf Camp, 3908
Indiana Hemophilia and Thrombosis Center, 4015
Indiana Resource Center for Autism, 850
Indiana State Board of Health - SIDSProject, 7015
Indiana State Dept. of Health Immunization, 5967
Indiana State University School of Medicine, 5479
Individual and Family SupportArc of Lincoln & Lancaster County, 8304
Individualized Education Program (IEP) -Communication Skills for Parents, 4279
Infant & Toddler Program, 8423
Infant Behavior, Cry and Sleep Clinic, 1757
Infant Motor Development: A Look at thePhases, 2716
Infant Positioning and Sudden Infant DeathSyndrome, 7108
Infant Toddler Early Intervention Program, 8428
Infant-Toddler Program, Division of MentalRetardation, 8238
Infant/Toddler Program, 8189
Infantile Spasms, 6606
Infectious Diseases in Children, 4969, 6007
Infectious Diseases Society of America, 3302, 5940
Infinitec, 1506
Inflammatory Bowel Disease, 7641
Inflammatory Bowel Disease - From Bench toBedside, 7642
Infocus Newsletter, 208
Information Center for Sickle Cell and Thalassemic Disorders, 6658
Information for Adults, 1709
Informed Consent: Participation in Genetic Research Studies, 584
Infusions, 4077
Inheritance of Hemophilia, 4088
Initiatives, 4078
Injury Control Research Center for Suicide Prevention, 2456
Injury Prevention Center, 4227
Inland Empire Brain Tumor Support Group, 1131
Inner Circle, 7647
Inner Lives of Deaf Children: Interviews and Analysis, 3788
Inside Out: Stories of Bulimia, 2918
Inside Story, 7651
Insights in the Dynamic Psychotherapy ofAnorexia And Bulimia, 2953
Insights into Spina Bifida, 6900
Inspire - Cerebral Palsy Center, 1462
Institute for Basic Research inDevelopmental Disabilities, 854, 2693, 8519, 8562
Institute for Families, 6272
Institute for Families of Blind Children, 7980
Institute on Communication and Inclusion, 750, 864, 903
Institutes for Achievement of HumanPotential, 3436
Interagency Early Intervention Project, 8277
Interagency Program Assistive Technology, 8356
Internal Journal of Eating Disorders, 2968
International Albinism Center, 193
International Antiviral Society-USA, 3303
International Association for Orthodontics, 2423
International Association of Dental Research, 2424
International Association of EatingDisorders Professionals Foundation, 2863, 5721
International Association of Providers of AIDS Care, 3304
International Association of Sickle CellNurses and Physician Assistants, 6659
International Bone Marrow TransplantRegistry, 96
International Braille and TechnologyCenter for the Blind, 7981
International CDH Conference, 1944
International Center for SkeletalDysplasia Registry, 2986
International CHARGE Syndrome Conference, 1022
International Chiropractic Pediatric Assoc, 1750
International Conference On Young ChildrenWith Special Needs & Their Famililies, 872, 8587
International Critical Incident StressFoundation, 5786, 5797
International Deaf Education Association, 3519
International Dyslexia Association, 2777, 2784, 2790, 4511
International Federation for Spina Bifidaand Hydrocephalus, 6872
International Foundation for BowelDysfunction, 2141

International Foundation for FunctionalGastrointestinal Disorders, 27, 262, 2142, 3053, 3093, 4786, 4790, 4980, 6099, 7623, 8628
International Foundation for GeneticResearch/Michael Fund, 2701
International Hearing Society, 3520
International Herpes Alliance, 4970
International Herpes Management Forum, 4151
International Journal of Dermatology, 1592, 3009, 5636, 6038
International Journal of Nursing in Intellectual & Developmental Disabilities, 8673
International Mosaic Down Syndrome Association, 2649
International Network of Ataxia Friends, 563
International NF Summer Camp, 5061
International Patient Organization forPrimary Immunodeficiencies, 2627
International Pemphigus Foundation, 5526, 5534
International Pemphigus Foundation DallasSupport Group, 5535
International Pemphigus Foundation Promotional Video, 5537
International Pemphigus Foundation: Baltimore Support Group, 5530
International Pemphigus Foundation: Houston Support Group, 5536
International Pemphigus Foundation: Massachusetts Support Group, 5531
International Pemphigus Foundation: New York Support Group, 5532
International Pemphigus Foundation: SouthCarolina Support Group, 5533
International Pemphigus Foundation: Southern California Support Group, 5529
International Prader-Willi Syndrome Organization (IPWSO), 5866
International Quality for Adult Tay-SachsCarrier Testing, 7181
International Scleroderma Network, 6435
International Skeletal Dysplasia Registry, 4659
International Society for Burn Injuries, 1316, 1326
International Society for Research inChild and Adolescent Psychopathology, 7693
International Society for TraumaticStress Studies, 5789
International Society of Dermatology, 7982
International Wheelchair Aviators, 7983
International World Conference onSarcoidosis-Patient Symposium, 6380
Internet Mental Health, 1064, 1630, 1785, 2495, 7726
Interstitial Cyctitis, 8695
Intestinal Disease Foundation, 263, 7624
Intestinal Pseudoobstruction (IP) SupportNetwork, 4159
Intrafamilial (Incest) Abuse Resources, 5697
Intrauterine Growth Retardation, 3269
Intraventricular Hemorrhage, 4374
Introduction to Spina Bifida, 6888
Introduction to Trisomy 13, 7513
Introduction to Trisomy 18, 7504
Introductory Packet Brochure, 1372
Iowa Chapter of Crohn's Colitis Foundationof America, 2157
Iowa Department of Public HealthBureau of Immunization, 5968
Iowa Library for the Blind and PhysicallyHandicapped, 1854, 2000, 5233, 6161
Iowa Program for Assistive Technology, 8226
Iowa SIDS Program, 7016
Iowa's System of EI Services, 8227
IPF Quarterly, 5541
Iron Overload Diseases Assocation, 7984
Irritable Bowel Syndrome, 58
A is for Access: Creating Full & Interactive Access for Students, 3591
It Only Takes One Bite: Food Allergy andAnaphylaxis, 2919
It's Just Part of My Life, 8595
It's My Body, 5709
It's Nobody's Fault-New Hope and Help forDifficult Children and Their Parents, 5393
It's Nobody's Fault: New Hope and Help forDifficult Children and Their Parents, 5611
It's Not Just Growing Pains, 6460
It's Not Me...It's My OCD: A Look at Behavioral Therapy, 5376
It's So Much Work to Be Your Friend, 663
IVAT: Institute on Violence, Abuse and Trauma, 5655
IVH Parents, 4378, 4382
IVUN Resource Directory, 6003

J

Jackson Laboratory, 3248
Jake's Ride for Dystonia Research, 2816
James R Clark Memorial Sickle CellFoundation, 6644
James S. McDonnell Foundation, 1105
Jane and Richard Thomas Center for DownSyndrome, 2696
Jason's First Day!, 5463
The Jed Foundation, 1053
Jeffrey Modell Foundation, 2628

Jewish Children's Adoption Network, 7985
Jewish Council for Youth Services, 8739
Jewish Genetic Disease Consortium, 7166, 7174
JGB Cassette Library International, 8520
JM Companion, 1593
Job Opportunities for the Blind, 7986
Jodi House, 3368
John Hopkins Arthritis Center, 445
John Hopkins Children's Hospital, 2284
John Hopkins Department of OrthopaedicsSurgery, 6490
John Sierzant Brain Tumor Support Group, 1256
John Tracy Clinic, 3521
John Warvel, 2616
Johnny Rock's Christmas, 3701
Johns Hopkins Arthritis Center, 446
Johns Hopkins Brain Tumor Education Group, 1188
Johns Hopkins Department of OrthopaedicsSurgery, 6475
Johns Hopkins Department of OrthopaedicSurgery, 1722
Johns Hopkins Division of Allergy and Clinical Immunology, 6328
Johns Hopkins University Sleep DisordersCenter, 4899
Joslin Diabetes Center, 2559
Journal of AAPOS, 6949
Journal of Abnormal Child Psychology, 7754
Journal of Allergy and Clinical Immunology, 6342
Journal of Cardiac Failure, 323
Journal of Clinical Endocrinology, 4357
Journal of Dermatologic Surgery andOncology, 1594, 3010, 5637, 6039
Journal of Head Trauma Rehabilitation, 3462
Journal of Learning Disabilities, 4531
Journal of Pediatric Gastroenterologyand Nutrition, 45, 277, 1759, 3099, 4138, 4988, 5416, 6111
Journal of Pediatric Health Care, 4492
The Journal of Positive Behavior Interventions, 968
The Journal of Special Education, 969
Journal of Speech, Language, and Hearing Research, 3862, 6799
Journal of Spirochetal and Tick-borne Diseases, 4623
Journal of the Academy of Dermatology, 8671
Journal of the American Dietetic AssociatiOn, 2969
Journal of the American Medical Association, 4624
Journal of Visual Impairment andBlindness, 1909, 2061, 5282, 6210
Journey of Love: Parent's Guide toDuchenne Muscular Dystrophy, 4839
The Joy of Signing Second Edition, 3841
JRA and Me, 4397
Judevine Center for Autism, 852
Judge David L. Bazelon Center for Mental Health, 4694
Jumpin' Johnny Get Back to Work! A Child'sGuide to ADHD/Hyperactivity, 664
Junior National Association of the Deaf, 3522
Junior Wheelchair Sports Camp, 8730
Just In Time, 75, 135, 3111
Just Like You and Me, 6559
Just One Break, 7987
Just Take a Bite: Easy, Effective Answersto Food Aversions and Eating Challenges, 936
Juvenile Bipolar Research Foundation, 1047
Juvenile Dermatomyositis, 1573, 1604
Juvenile Diabetes Foundation International, 2555
Juvenile Rheumatoid Arthritis, 4384
Juvenile Scleroderma Network, 6436

K

Kaiser Permanente Medical Center, 2255
Kalamazoo Center for Medical Studies, 2292
Kalamazoo Comprehensive HemophiliaTreatment Center, 4016
Kamp-A-Kom-Plish, 8761
Kanawha County Public Library, 8551
Kansas City, Missouri Support Group, 535
Kansas Department of Health & EnvironmentBureau of Family Health, 5969, 7017
Kansas State Library, 8483
Kansas University Medical Center, 2629, 7781
Kansas University Medical Center: Department of Pulmonology, 2277
Kardiac Kids, 4313
Kathy's Hats: A Story of Hope, 108
Kawasaki Disease, 4408
Kawasaki Disease Foundation, 4413
Kawasaki Families' Network, 4414
Keep In Touch (KIT) Forum, 1600

Keloids, 4415
The Kempe Center: For the Prevention & Treatment of Child Abuse and Neglect, 5669
KenCrest Services, 4711
Kennedy Krieger Institute, 4753
Kennedy Krieger Institute, Down SyndromeClinic, 2686
Kent County Health Department, 7027
Kent County Library for the Blind, 1863, 2010, 5242, 6170
Kentucky Chapter of Crohn's & ColitisFoundation of America, 2159
Kentucky Department of Human ResourcesBureau of Health Services, 7018
Kentucky Hemophilia Foundation, 3956
Kentucky Library for the Blind andPhysically Handicapped, 1858, 2004, 5236, 6164
Keren-Or Jerusalem Center for Multi-Handicapped Blind Children, 8521, 8563
Kern Autism Network, 793
Kernicterus, 4423
Keto Kid, Helping Your Child to Succeed onthe Ketogenic Diet, 6581
Kettering Medical Center, Sleep DisordersCenter, 4920
Kevin and Me, 7424
Key Update, 5399
Keystone Community Resources, 8811
Kid Power Tactics for Dealing withDepression & Parent's Survival Guide, 2516
Kid's Corner, 2587
Kid's Health, 2386, 3086, 5754
Kid's Health: TV Late Breaking News VideoAbout Broken Bones and Cast Care, 8596
Kid-Friendly Parenting with Deaf and Hardof Hearing Children, 3789
Kidney Disease of Diabetes, 2601, 5004
Kids and Seizures: Know the Hidden Signs, 6607
Kids In the Syndrome Mix, 937
Kids on the Block Arthritis Programs, 4391
Kids with AIDS, 3338
Kids with Food Allergies, 1351
Kids With Heart, 4335
Kids with Incredible Potential Leader'sGuide, 666
Kids With Incredible Potential Parent'sGuide, 665
A Kids' Brain Tumor Cure Foundation, 1078
KidsHealth, 6240, 6249
KidsHealth - Measles, 5993
KidsHealth - Rubella (German Measles), 5994
KidsHealth - Tetanus, 5995
KidsHealth at the AMA, 8629
KidsHealth for Parents, 5728, 5735
KidsHealth-Pyloric Stenosis, 6106
KidsHealth: Precocious Puberty, 5893
KidsPeace, 5698
KidsPeace National Centers/Hospital, 5656
King Midas, 3790
Kingsmont, 5353
Kiss the Candy Days Good-Bye, 2573
Kiwanis Twin Lakes Camp, 8748
KlaasKids Foundation for Children, 5657
Klaman Eating Disorders Center at McLean Hospital, 2864
Klamath Falls Support Group, 1237
Klinefelter Syndrome, 4435
Klinefelter Syndrome and Associates, 4441
Klinefelter Syndrome Newsletter, 4447
Klinefelter Syndrome Support Group, 4444
Klinefelter's Syndrome Association, 4442
Klippel-Feil Syndrome, 4448
Klippel-Feil Syndrome Support Group, 4453
Know About Tuberculosis, 7530
Knox County Advocates, 8217
Knutson, 8779
Krancer Center for Inflammatory BowelDisease Research, 2191
Kris' Camp, 992
Kristin Brooks Hope Center, 1048
Kudos to Kuualoha, 3641

L

La Fayette Subregional Library for theBlind and Physically Disabled, 8464
LA Lions Camp Pelican, 2379
Lab School of Washington Summer Program, 708, 993, 4544
Laboratory of Dermatology Research, 1580, 3004, 5633
Lactose Intolerance, 4797
Landmark School, 2800

Language, Speech, and Hearing in Schools, 3863, 6800
Lankenau Hospital, Sleep Disorders Center, 4928
LaRabida Children's Hospital, DownSyndrome Clinic, 2683
Largesse, The Network for Size Esteem, 2865
Las Vegas-Clark County Library District, 8515
Late Onset Tay-Sachs Fact Sheet, 7190
Laughter Therapy, 8597
Laurent Clerc National Deaf EducationCenter-Gallaudet Universty, 3557
Lawson Wilkins Pediatric EndocrineSociety, 2229, 3233, 4348
Lazy Eye, 4458
Lazy Eye Discussion Group, 4480
LD Advocate, 4528
The LD Child and the ADHD Child: WaysParents and Professionals Can Help, 685
LD News, 4529
LDA Annual Conference, 2785
Lead Poisoning, 4495
Leading National Publications of and forDeaf People, 3885
The League at Camp Greentop and The Therapeutic Recreation, 8762
Learning Among Children with Spina Bifida, 6902
Learning Disabilities and Challenging Behaviors, 4526
Learning Disabilities Association of America, 608, 638, 2778, 2791, 4512, 4523, 7988, 8631
Learning Disabilities in Children withHydrocephalus, 4281
Learning Disability/Reading Dyslexia, 4502
Learning Independence Through Computers, 8504
Learning Ladder: Assessing and Teaching Text Comprehension, 3791
Learning Problems & the Student withTourette Syndrome, 7455
Learning to Live with NeuromuscularDisease: A Message for Parents, 4870
Learning to Play, 1920, 2073, 5292, 6221
Learning to See: American Sign Languageas a Second Language, 3792
Learning To Slow Down and Pay Attention, 667
Lee the Rabbit with Epilepsy, 6582
Left Hearts, 4336
Left Side Lines, 5921
Legacy Good Samaritan Hospital & Medical Center, 5035
Legal Rights for the Deaf and Hard of Hearing, 3793
Legal Rights: The Guide for Deaf andHard of Hearing People - Fifth Edition, 3794
Legg-Calve-Perthes Disease, 4554
Lehigh Valley Sickle Cell Support Group, 6642
A Lesson With Heart, 3589
Let's Eat, 1899, 1921, 2049, 2074, 3642, 5273, 5293, 6202, 6222
Let's Face It, 2123
Let's Talk About Being Overweight, 5341
Let's Talk About Depression, 2539
Let's Talk About Diabetes, 2574
Let's Talk About Down Syndrome, 2739
Let's Talk About Dyslexia, 2795
Let's Talk About Going to the Hospital, 109, 161, 221, 246, 310, 337, 479, 1267, 1556, 1591, 1960, 2198, 2234, 2364, 2387, 2631, 3118, 3339, 3459, 4065, 4112
Let's Talk About Having Asthma, 480
Let's Talk About Having Chicken Pox, 6004
Let's Talk About Having Lyme Disease, 4620
Let's Talk About Sickle Cell Anemia, 6666
Let's Talk About When Kids Have Cancer, 5075, 5177, 6290, 7807
Let's Talk About when Kids Have Cancer, 162, 1268, 3119, 4195
Let's Talk Facts About Childhood Disorders, 2540
Leukemia & Lymphoma Society - North Texas Chapter, 89
Leukemia & Lymphoma Society, 76, 103, 136, 158, 4189, 5168, 5174
Leukemia & Lymphoma Society - Central OhioChapter, 82, 142
Leukemia & Lymphoma Society - NationalCapital Area Chapter, 92, 152
Leukemia & Lymphoma Society - North TexasChapter, 149
Leukemia & Lymphoma Society - NorthCarolina Chapter, 81, 141
Leukemia & Lymphoma Society - NorthernOhio Chapter, 83, 143
Leukemia & Lymphoma Society - OklahomaChapter, 85, 145
Leukemia & Lymphoma Society - OregonChapter, 86, 146
Leukemia & Lymphoma Society - SouthCentral Texas - San Antonio Chapter, 90, 150
Leukemia & Lymphoma Society - Texas GulfCoast Chapter, 91, 151
Leukemia & Lymphoma Society - Tri-StateSouthern Ohio Chapter, 84, 144
Leukemia & Lymphoma Society - Washington/Alaska Chapter, 80, 93, 8089, 8429
Leukemia & Lymphoma Society - Westchester/Connecticut/Hudson Valley Chapter, 139
Leukemia & Lymphoma Society - Western &Central New York Chapter, 140
Leukemia & Lymphoma Society - WesternPennsylvania/West Virginia Chapter, 87, 147
Leukemia & Lymphoma Society - WisconsinChapter, 94, 153

Leukemia & Lymphoma Society, TennesseeChapter, 88, 148
Leukemia Research Foundation, 8199
Leukodystrophies, 4564
Lewis H. Walker, MD, Cystic FibrosisCenter, 2321
Lewiston Public Library, 8499
LFSN: Lipomyelomeningecele Family SupportNetwork, 6873
Library for the Blind & PhysicallyHandicapped, Leonard C Staisey Building, 8533
Library for the Blind and Handicapped,Southwest, 8451
Library for the Blind and PhysicallyHandicapped, Hawaii State Library, 8472
Library of Michigan Service for the Blind, 1864, 2011, 5243, 6171
Lied Learning and Technology Center for Childhood Deafness and Vision Disorders, 3571
Life Adventure Center, 1802, 7770
Life Beyond Your Eating Disorder, 2954
Life in the Country, 3643
Life Planning and Down Syndrome, 2759
Life with Diabetes: A Series of TeachingOutlines, 2575
Life With Retinoblastoma, 6285
Lifeline, 1364, 7287
Lifespire (A.C.R.M.D.), 7989
Lifting of Canavan's Carrier TestingFacilities, 7183
Lighthouse Guild, 237, 1902, 2053, 4465, 5276, 6117, 6204, 6273, 6305
Lili Claire Foundation, 7782
Ling Series, 3702
LINK, 4262
The Link, 814
LINK Directory Information, 4280
Linking Factor, 4079
Lions Club International, 4466
Lipomyelomeningocele Family Support, 4235
Lissencephaly, 4577
Lissencephaly Network, 4586
Listen - Hear for Parents of HearingImpaired Children, 3886
Listen Learn and Talk, 3644
Listen Little Star, 3795, 6794
Listen to This, Volume One, 3645
Listen to This, Volume Two, 3646
Listen with the Heart: Relationships and Hearing Loss, 3796
The Listener, 3842
Literacy and Your Deaf Child: What Every Parent Should Know, 3797
Literacy, Classroom Amplification and the Brain, 3648
Literacy, Classroom Amplification and the Brain DVD, 3647
Little Hearts, 7230, 7235, 7254
Little People of America, 8, 15, 3234, 3257, 5436, 5454
Little People of America - District 2, 3242, 3243, 3245, 5445, 5446, 5448
Little People of America - District 7, 3237, 3240, 3241, 3244, 5440, 5443, 5444, 5447
Little People of America - Front RangeChapter, 3239, 5442
Little People of America - San FranciscoBay Area Chapter, 3238, 5441
Little People of America - Utah Seagulls, 3246, 5449
Little Read Riding Hood: Told in Signed Enlish, 3798
Liver 411, 4985
Liver Disease in Children, 1025, 4113
Liver Transplantation, 8696
Living a Full Life with Celiac Sprue, 1373
Living in a World with AIDS, 3340
Living Well with Epilepsy, 6583
Living with Arthritis, 4398
Living with Asthma, 481
Living with Asthma and Allergies Brochure Series, 491
Living with Ataxia, 568
Living with Childhood Cancer: A PracticalGuide to Help Families Cope, 4196
Living with Cystic Fibrosis, 2352
Living with Depression and ManicDepression, 2490
Living with Gaucher Disease, 3226
Living with Hearing Loss, 3799, 5483
Living with HIV: Talking With Your Child, 4089
Living with IBD: A Guide for Teenagers, 7652
Living with Narcolepsy, 4957
Living with Schizophrenia, 1627
Living with SMA, 6929
Living with Trisomy 13, 7512
Living with Tuberous Sclerosis, 7552
Living Without Depression & ManicDepression: A Workbook, 2541
Livingston County CMH Services, 8270
Loma Linda University Sleep Disorders Center, 4890
Lone Star Chapter of the NationalHemophilia Foundation, 3980
Long Island Adult Brain Tumor SupportGroup, 1220

Long Island Chapter of Crohn's & ColitisFoundation of America, 2172
Long Island College Hospital, 2311
Long Island Sarcoidosis Support, 6366
Long Term Services Division, 8331
Long Term Survivor Conference, 1259, 8588
Lookin' Up, 5717
Looking After Louis, 938
Looking Ahead:A Parents Guide to the Development Child w/ Retinopathy Prematurity, 6313
Looking for Goodwill, 6889
Loopy Lupus Helps Tell Scott's Story, 7150
Los Angeles Ataxia Support Group, 506
Loss & FoundHands & Voices, 3649
Louisiana Assistive Technology AccessNetwork, 8242
Louisiana Chapter, 525
Louisiana Comprehensive Hemophilia CareCenter, 4017
Louisiana Hemophilia Foundation, 3957
Louisiana Lions Camp for Crippled Children, 8756
Louisiana State Library, 8495
Louisiana State University GeneticsSection of Pediatrics, 8496, 8564
Louisiana State University Health SciencesCenter, 2280
Louisiana Support Group, 526
Louisiana/Mississippi Chapter of Crohn's &Colitis Foundation of America, 2160
Louisiana/Mississippi Chapter of Crohn's& Colitis Foundation of America, 2165
Louisville Talking Book Library, 8492
Lovaas Institute, 751
Low Vision Gateway, 8632
Loyola University Medical Center/Department of Pediatrics, 2269
Loyola University of Children, ParmlyHearing Institute, 3559
LPA National Conference, 12, 3252, 5451
LSU Health Sciences Center, 2097
LSUMC Family Medicine Patient Education, 8630
Lucile Packard Children's Hospital, 4379
Lucky Lou Gets Game, 1525
Lung Disorders Sourcebook, 482, 2365, 7531
Lupus Book, 7151
Lupus Erythematosus: A Patient's Guide, 7152
Lupus Foundation of America, 7139
Lupus Now®, 7156
Lupus Q&A: Everything You Need To Know, 7153
Lupus Research Institute, 7140
Lydia's Lessons, 3650
Lyme Disease, 4600, 4621
Lyme Disease (Deadly Diseases andEpidemics), 4622
Lyme Disease Association, Inc. (LDA), 4606, 4616
Lyme Disease Foundation, 4607, 4617
Lyme Disease Research Foundation, 4608
Lyme Induced Autism Foundation, 4609
Lyme Research Alliance, 4610
Lymphatic System, 8851
Lymphoma Innovations, 5175
Lymphoma Research Foundation, 5169
Lymphoma Research Foundation of America, 4190

M

MA Report, 488
MAAP Newsletter, 971
Macomb Library for the Blind andPhysically Handicapped, 1865, 2012, 5244, 6172
Macon Subregional Library for the Blindand Handicapped, Washington Memorial, 8465
Macon Support Group, 520
Macrocephaly, 4625
Madison Institute of Medicine, 5798
Madisons Foundation, 4611
MAGIC Foundation: Major Aspects of Growthin Children: Turner's Syndrome Division, 9, 16, 331, 1807, 1812, 3235, 3264, 4660, 5188, 5891, 7560, 7604
Magic Moments- Children's Hospital of Alabama, 8835
Magic of Music and Dance, 8731
Maine Dept. of Human Services:Bureau of Health Immunization Program, 5970
Maine Hemophilia and Thrombosis Center, 4018
Maine State Library, 8500
Maine Support, 527

Mainstreaming the Visually Impaired Child:Blind & Partially Sighted Students, 6208
Major Depression in Children andAdolescents, 2542
Make A Wish Foundation of America, 8836
Make Today Count, 7991
Makemie Woods Camp Conference Center, 2617, 8823
Making Daughters Safe Again, 5699
Making Headway Foundation-Family SupportProgram, 1221
Making Peace with Food, 2955, 5342
Management of Eating Disorders and Obesity, 2956
Management of Headache & HeadacheMedications, 4760
Management of Motor Speech Disordersin Children and Adults, 6795
Management of Prader-Willi Syndrome, 5872
Management of Retinopathy of Prematurity Video, 6309
Managing Attention Deficit HyperactivityDisorder in Children, 668
Managing Childhood Asthma, 463
Managing Food Allergy and Intolerance, 4795
Managing Osteogenesis Imperfecta: aMedical Manual, 5465
Managing Seizures, Information for Caregivers, 6608
Managing the Defiant Child, 1781, 7711
Managing Your Child's Crohn's Disease orUlcerative Colitis, 2199
Mandy, 3800
Manhattan Public Library, 8484
Mansfield's Holiday Hill, 8733
Maple Syrup Urine Disease, 4633
Maplebrook School, 709, 994, 4545
March of Dimes Birth Defects Foundation, 1696, 3174, 4209, 4301, 6874, 7175, 7276, 8634
March of Dimes Foundation, 217, 228, 238, 253, 264, 287, 304, 332, 592, 609, 752, 1004, 1307, 1388, 1671, 1687, 1718, 1736, 1955, 2106, 2124
March of Dimes Nursing Modules, 7993
March of Dimes-Preterm Birth Fact Sheets, 5923
Marfan Syndrome, 4644, 4653
Maribel, 5863
Maricopa Co Childhood Immunization Program, 5954
Marist Brothers Mid-Hudson Valley Camp Marist Brothers, 8796
Marty Lyons Foundation, 8340
Marvelwood Summer, 2801
Marvin Teaches Fingerspelling, 3703
Mary M Gooley Hemophilia Center of theNational Hemophilia Foundation, 3967
Maryland Department of Health, 4210, 4671
Maryland Infant and Toddlers ProgramFamily Support Network, 8254
Maryland SIDS Information & CounselingProgram, 7022
Maryland State Library for the Blindand Physically Handicapped, 1859, 2005, 5237, 6165
Maryland-Greater Washington, DC Chapter Asthma and Allergy Foundation of America, 432
Maryland/South Delaware Chapter of Crohn's& Colitis Foundation of America, 2161
Masqueraders of Sarcoidosis, 6407
Massachusetts Assistive TechnologyPartnership, 8265
Massachusetts Association for Parents of the Visually Impaired (MAPVI), 6281
Massachusetts Chapter of SIDS Alliance, 7023
Massachusetts Down Syndrome Congress(MDSC), 2670
Massachusetts Easter Seals Camping Program, 8768
Massachusetts Eating Disorder Association(MEDA), 2889
Massachusetts General Hospital, 2287
Massachusetts Sudden Infant Death Syndrome, 7074
Massachusetts, New England HemophiliaAssociation, 3959
Mastering Asthma, 464
Matchmaker, 8682
Maternal, Child & Family Health, EarlyIntervention/Infant Learning Program, 8090
Matrix Parents Network and Resource Center, 8125
MATRIX: Parent Network and Family ResourceCenter, 8124
Matthew and the Tics, 7440
Matthew and Tics, 7349
Maudsley Parents, 2866
Maybe You Know My Kid: A Parent's Guide toIdentifying ADHD, 669
Mayo Clinic, 5755
Mayo Clinic and Foundation, 4828
Mayo Clinic Scleroderma Service, 6448
Mayo Comprehensive Hemophilia Center, 4019
MayoClinic.com, 5736
MayoClinic.com - Pulmonary Hypertension, 6082
McCallum Place, 2867
McCune-Albright Syndrome, 4654
MD Infant/Toddler/Preschool ServicesDivision, 8253

MDA Fact Sheet, 1567, 4871
MDA Services for the Individual, Familyand Community, 4872
MDA Summer Camp, 4877
MDA Summer Camp Brochure, 4873
MDA/ALS Newsmagazine, 4847
Me and My World Storybook, 6609
Meadowood Springs Speech and Hearing Camp, 3909, 6804, 6968
Meals Without Squeals Sense, 2957
Measles, 6005
Measuring Bullying Victimization,Perpetration and Bystander Experiences, 7755
Measuring Violence-Related Attitudes,Behaviors and Influences, 7756
Med Help International, 3087, 6015
Med-Camps of Louisiana, 8757
Media and Youth: A DevelopmentalPerspective, 7758
Media Violence and Children: A CompleteGuide, 7757
Media-Smart Youth: Eat, Think, and Be Active Fact Sheet, 5348
Medical and Surgical Care for Childrenwith Down Syndrome, 2740
Medical Center Hospital of Vermont, 2341
Medical College of Pennsylvania, SleepDisorders Center, 4929
Medical College of Wisconsin, 17, 4571
Medical College of Wisconsin CysticFibrosis Center, 2348
Medical Economics Company, 8635
Medical Genetics Clinic, 2691
Medical Illness and Schizophrenia, 1646
Medical Matrix: Pediatrics, 8636
Medical Sign Language: Easily Understood Definitions of Commonly Used Medical Term, 3801
Medical Update Column, 6516
Medication for ADHD, 627
MedicineNet, 6019
MedicineNet.com, 2098
Medicines for Epilepsy, 6610
Mediconsult, 159, 2561
Medifocus Guidebook On Reflex SympatheticDystrophy, 4841
Medifocus Guidebook on Scleroderma, 6462
MEDLINEplus, 4300
MedlinePlus, 6977
MEDLINEplus Medical Encyclopedia:Pyloric Stenosis, 6107
MEDLINEplus on Sleep Apnea, 6683
Meeting the Challenge: Parenting Childrenwith Disabilities, 8598
The Memo, 3673
Memorial Miller Children's HospitalCystic Fibrosis Center, 2256
Memphis Cystic Frosis Center, 2333
Memphis Regional Brain Tumor SurvivorsGroup, 1244
Memphis State University, Center for theCommunicatively Impaired, 6780
Meningitis, 4665
Meningitis Foundation of America, 4669, 4672
Menninger Child & Family Program, 1773, 7703
Mental Fitness, Inc., 2868
Mental Health America, 610, 753, 1049, 1612, 1769, 3149, 5104, 5155, 5364, 5491, 5575, 5722, 7694
Mental Health Net, 1065, 1631, 2496, 2792
Mental Help Net, 3056, 8637
Mental Help Net- Eating Disorders, 2925
Mental Retardation, 4675, 4719
Mental Wellness, 1632
Mental, Emotional, and Behavior Disorders in Children and Adolescents, 1799, 7764
Mercer Mayer Frog Stories, 3651
Merck, 6020
Merck Manual of Diagnosis and Therapy, 1677, 6022
Mercy Hospital of Johnstown, SleepDisorders Center, 4930
Mercy Sleep Laboratory, 4940
Message Line, 1271
Messy Monsters Jungle Joggers and Bubble Baths, 3802
Methodist Hospital Sleep Disorders Center, 4894
Metro Intergroup of Overeaters Anonymous, 2892
MGH Neurology Web Forums, 6670
Miami Children's Hospital, Division ofPulmonology, 2264
Miami Comprehensive Hemophilia Center, 4020
Miami Valley Downs Syndrome Association, 2673
Michigan Chapter of Allergy and AsthmaFoundation of America, 434
Michigan Chapter of Crohn's & ColitisFoundation of America, 2163
Michigan State University ComprehensiveCenter for Bleeding Disorders, 4021
Microcephaly, 4729
Microdontia, 4738
Mid Illinois Talking Book System, 1850, 1996, 5229, 6157
Mid-America Chapter of Crohn's & Colitis Foundation of America, 2158
Mid-Atlantic Regional Human GeneticsNetwork, 546

Mid-Illinois Talking Book Center, 1851, 1997, 5230, 6158
Middle Tennessee Sarcoidosis Support Group, 6371
Mideastern Michigan Library Co-op, 1866, 2013, 5245, 6173
MidWest Medical Center - Sleep DisordersCenter, 4895
Migraine and Coexisting Conditions-OtherIllnesses That May Affect Migraine, 4778
Migraine and Other Headaches: VascularMechanisms, 4761
Migraine Awareness Group: A NationalUnderstanding for Migraineurs, 4755
Migraine Awareness Group: NationalUnderstanding for Migraineurs (MAGNUM), 4751
Migraine Headaches, 4746
Migraine-Fact Sheet, 4779
Mile High Down Syndrome Association, 2661
Milk Protein Allergy/Lactose Intolerance, 4784
A Mind of Your Own, 8591
Mindblindness: An Essay on Autism & Theoryof Mind, 939
Minneapolis, MN Support Group, 532
Minnesota Cystic Fibrosis Center, 2294
Minnesota Library for the Blind &Physically Handicapped, 1872, 2019, 5251, 6179
Minnesota Sudden Infant Death Center, 7031
Minnesota/Dakotas Chapter of Crohn's &Colitis Foundation of America, 2164
Miracle to Believe In, 940
Mirror, Mirror, 2926
Missing Michael - A Mother's Story of Love, 6584
Mississippi Chapter, 533
Mississippi Dept. of Health Bureau ofPreventative Health Immunization, 5972
Mississippi Hemophilia Foundation, 3962
Mississippi State Department of Health andChild Health Services, 7032
Missouri Parents Act, 8293
Misunderstood Child, 2796
Mobile Association for the Blind, 1891, 1975, 2041, 5208, 5269, 6136, 6198
Mom I Have a Staring Problem, 6585
Monetary Allowance, Health Care andVocational Training & Rehabilitation, 6903
Monmouth Medical Center, Cystic Fibrosis& Pediatric Pulmonary Center, 2303
Monograph on Canavan's Disease, 7184
Montana Department of Health &Environmental Sciences, 7035
Montana State Library, 8513
MonTECH, 8300
Montgomery County Intermediate Unit #23, 8379
Montifiore Medical Center, 3572
Mood Apart, 2517
Mood Disorders, 1074
Mosaic, 4695
Most Frequently Asked Questions withGrowth Hormone Deficiency, 3270
A Mother's Persepctive on the IEP Process, 3590
A Mother's Touch: The Tiffany Callo Story, 1512
Mothers of Children with Allergies (MOCHA), 6321
Mothers of Omphaloceles, 5412
Mount Sinai Traumatic Brain Injury, 3401
Mountain Milestones Stepping Stones, 8826
Mountain States Regional Genetics ServicesNetwork, 513
Mountaineer Spina Bifida Camp, 6910
Move with Me, 1922, 2075, 5294, 6223
Movement Disorders, 7348
MSRGSN Newsletter, 573
MSUD Newsletter, 4643
MSUD:(Maple Syrup Urine Disease) FamilySupport Group, 4638
Mt Hood Kiwanis Camp, 8807
Mucolipidoses, 4798
Mucolipidosis IV Foundation, 4801, 4804
Mucopolysaccharidoses & Related Diseases, 4815
Mucopolysaccharidoses, 4808
Multidisciplinary Clinico-PathologicConference, 6408
MUMS: National Parent to Parent Network, 7373, 7500, 7990, 8633
Muscular Dystrophies, 4820
Muscular Dystrophy, 4835
Muscular Dystrophy and Allied Diseases: Impacts on Patients, Family, and Staff, 4842
Muscular Dystrophy and OtherNeuromuscular Diseases, 4843
Muscular Dystrophy Association, 1554, 1672, 2809, 2819, 4824, 4836, 6917
Muscular Dystrophy Family Foundation, 4825, 4837
Muscular System, 8852
Musella Foundation for Brain Tumor Research and Information, 1106

Music Curriculum Guidelines for ModeratelyRetarded Adolescents, 4716
Muskegon County Library for the Blind, 1867, 2014, 5246, 6174
My Baby Can Talk: First Signs, 3652
My Body is Mine, My Feelings are Mine, 5710
My Body Is Not Who I Am, 8599
My Brother has Fragile X, 3195
My Brother Sammy, 941
My Brother's a World Class Pain: ASibling's Guide To
　ADHD/Hyperactivity, 670
My Child Without Limits, 1507
My Child Without Limits Newsletter, 1533
My Fake Eye, The Story of My Prosthesis, 6291
My Friend Matty: A Story About Living withEpilepsy, 6586
My Friend With Autism, 942
My Hair's Falling Out...Am I Still Pretty?, 99
My Life-Melinda's Story, 4844
My New Eye Patch, 6292
My Social Stories Book, 943
My Surprise, 3653
My Travelin' Eye, 4488
Myositis Association of America, 1574, 1589
Myths and Facts About AIDS, 3341
MyTTY for Windows 95, 98, ME, 2000, XP, 3705
MyTTY Phone Messenger Software for Windows, 3704

N

NAAFA Annual Convention, 2914
NAD Biennial Conference, 3586
NAD Youth Leadership Camp, 3910
NADD Bulletin, 1662, 4721
NADD Conference & Exhibit Show, 1779, 2485, 7709, 8589
NADD: National Association for the Dually Diagnosed, 1613, 1633, 1770,
　1786, 2457, 2497, 4696, 4713, 5105, 5114, 5131, 5139, 5365, 5381,
　5492, 5501, 7330, 7337, 7695, 7727, 7994
NADezine, 3868
NADF News, 1815, 2236
NAEYC: National Association for theEducation of Young Children, 7995
NAMI Convention, 620, 1060, 1624, 1780, 2486, 7710, 8590
Narcolepsy, 4878, 4946, 4949, 4958
Narcolepsy Institute, 4886
Narcolepsy Network, 4887
Narcolepsy Primer, 4953
Narcolepsy: A Guide for Understanding, Diagnosing & Treating
　Narcolepsy, 4947
Narcolepsy: Evaluation and Treatment, 4948
NASPGHAN, 4791
NASPGHAN Annual Meeting and PostgraduateCourse, 33, 271, 1758,
　3097, 4132
NASPGHAN News, 46, 278, 1760, 3100, 4139, 4796, 4989, 5417, 6112
Nassau Library System, 8522
Natalie's Brace, 6491
Natalie's Way Foundation, 180
National Abandoned Infants AssistanceResource Center, 3306
National Ability Center, 7996
National Academy for Child Development(NACD), 7997
National Adoption Center, 7998
National Adrenal Diseases Foundation, 1808, 1813, 2230
National Advisory Allergic and Infectious Disease Council, 403
National AIDS Hotline, 3305
National Alliance for Research onSchizophrenia and Depression, 1057,
　1614, 1620, 1621, 2458, 2477, 5374
National Alliance for the Mentally Ill, 611, 1050, 1615, 1771, 2459, 5106,
　5366, 5493, 5576, 5724, 7696, 7999
National Alliance of Black Interpreters, 3523
National Alliance of Blind Students, 1903, 2054, 5277, 6118, 6205, 6274,
　6306
National Alliance of State & Territorial AIDS Directors, 3307
National Alliance on Mental Illness, 362, 2460, 3150, 4698, 5577
National Alopecia Areata Foundation AnnualConference, 205
National Alopecia Areata Foundation Newsletter, 203, 209
National Amputee Golf Association, 8000
National Anxiety Foundation, 2461, 5367, 5382, 5502, 5578, 5599, 6730
National Aphasia Association, 6769
National Archery Association, 8001
National Arthritis and Musculoskeletal &Skin Disease Info. Clearinghouse,
　8639
National Arts and Disability Center, 8002

National Association for Anorexia Nervosaand Associated Disorders
　(ANAD), 2927
National Association for Child Development, 2651
National Association for Down Syndrome(NADS), 2652, 2724
National Association for Dually Diagnosed, 4699
National Association for Hearing andSpeech Action, 3524
National Association for Males with Eating Disorders (The), 2869
National Association for Parents of Children with Visual Impairments,
　6119, 6275, 6307, 8003
National Association for Parents of theVisually Impaired, 1825, 1970,
　5203, 6122, 6126
National Association for Parents ofChildren with Visual Impairments, 1822,
　4467
National Association for Proton Therapy, 1107
National Association for the Education ofYoung Children, 7697
National Association for VisuallyHandicapped, 243, 1823, 1904, 1967,
　2055, 5201, 5278, 6069, 6070, 6120, 6206, 6254, 6260, 6308, 6310,
　6943, 6945, 8640
National Association of Addiction Treatmemt Professionals, 2870
National Association of Anorexia Nervosaand Associated Disorders
　(ANAD), 2871
National Association of Blind Students, 8004
National Association of Community Health Centers, 3308
National Association of Councils on Developmental Disabilities, 4700
National Association of Epilepsy Centers, 6533
National Association of Parents with Children in Special Education, 3525
National Association of Pediatric Nurse Practitioners, 5941
National Association of People with AIDS, 3309, 3328
National Association of Protection andAdvocacy Systems, 8005
National Association of QDDPs, 4701
National Association of Residential Providers for Adults with Autism, 754
National Association of School Nurses, 421, 5942
National Association of SchoolPsychologists, 3526, 7698
National Association of Special Education Teachers, 363, 755
National Association of State Agencies of the Deaf and Hard of Hearing,
　3527
National Association of State Directors of Developmental Disabilities
　Services, 4702
National Association of State Mental Health Program Directors, 1051, 4703
National Association of the Deaf (NAD), 3528
National Association of the DuallyDiagnosed, 8006
National Association to Advance FatAcceptance (NAAFA), 2872
National Asthma Educator Certification Board, 422
National Ataxia Foundation, 502, 564, 7204, 7212, 7257
National Ataxia Foundation Annual Membership Meeting, 556
National Autism Association, 364, 756
National Autism Hotline - Autism ServicesCenter, 757
National Birth Defects Center, 8266
National Black Association for Speech-Language and Hearing, 6770
National Black Deaf Advocates, 3529
National Black Leadership Commission on AIDS, Inc., 3310
National Bone Marrow Transplant Link, 77, 137
National Brachial Plexus/Erb's PalsyAssociation, 3076
National Brain Research Association, 1108
National Brain Tumor Foundation, 1109, 5010
National Brain Tumor Foundation Fact Sheets, 1288
National Brain Tumor Society, 1110
National Burn Victim Foundation, 1317, 1327
National Camps for Blind Children, 1934, 2085, 5301, 6230
National Capital Lyme Disease Association, 4613
National Captioning Institute, 3530
National Catholic Office for the Deaf, 3531
National Celiac Disease Society, 1352
National Center for BiotechnologyInformation, 2222, 4211
National Center for Education in Maternaland Child Health, 5909, 6813,
　6987, 7087, 7847
National Center for Environmental Health, 1714
National Center for Health Statistics, 6981, 7848
National Center for Hearing Assessment & Management, 3533
National Center for Injury Prevention andControl, 7699
National Center for Latinos withDisabilities, 8200
National Center for Learning Disabilities, 612, 639, 8007
National Center For Learning DisabilitiesWith Disabilities, 4513
National Center for Missing & ExploitedChildren, 5658
National Center for Missing and ExploitedChildren: 24-hour Hotline, 5659
National Center for Neurogenic Communication Disorders, 6784
National Center for Overcoming Overeating, 2873
National Center for PTSD, 5779
National Center for Sight, 8008
National Center for Stuttering, 6956

National Center for the Prevention of SIDS, 6988
National Center for the Study of Wilson'sDisease, 7822
National Center for Vision and ChildDevelopment, 8009
National Center for Voice and Speech, 3534
National Center on Accessbility, 8010
National Center on Child Abuse PreventionResearch, 5683
National Center On Deaf-Blindness, 3532
National Centers for Facial Paralysis, 1005
National Child Advocacy Center, 8363
National Child Pornography Tiplineand Cyber Tipline, 5660
National Child Traumatic Stress NetworkNCCTS - University of California, LA, 5787
National Childhood Cancer Foundation, 78, 1111, 3112, 4191, 5170, 6276, 7800
National Children's Advocacy Center, 5661
National Children's Alliance, 5662
National Children's Cancer Society, 1112, 8011
National Christian Resource Center, 8012
National Clearinghouse on PostsecondaryEducation: HEATH Resource Center, 7849
National Coalition for Cancer Survivorship, 79, 138, 3113
National Coalition of Title 1Chapter 1 Parents, 7850
National Collaborative on Childhood Obesity Research, 5323
National Comprehensive Cancer Network, 1113
National Conference of State Legislatures, 4500
National Conference on Hydrocephalus, 4224
National Conference on OI, 5452
National Congenital CMV Disease Registry, 2385
National Council for Behavioral Health, 1052
National Council of Hispano Deaf and Hard of Hearing, 3535
National Council on Child Abuse & FamilyViolence, 5700
National Council on Disability, 7851
National Council on Patient Informationand Education, 7852
National Craniofacial Foundation, 3042, 4588
National Cued Speech Association, 3536
National Cystic Fibrosis Family EducationConference, 2351
National Dental Association, 2425
National Diabetes Action Network for theBlind, 2556
National Diabetes InformationClearinghouse, 2557, 2562
National Digestive Diseases InformationClearinghouse, 31, 42, 269, 276, 1753, 1945, 2189, 2244, 3095, 3098, 3203, 4130, 4134, 4163, 4352, 4430, 4640, 4983, 4986, 5333, 5411
National Directory of HydrocephalusSupport Groups, 4282
National Disability Rights Network, 4704
National Disability Sports Alliance, 1389, 8013
National Dissemination Center for Children with Disabilities, 229, 265, 758, 1390, 1508, 1956, 2653, 4514, 4524, 4589, 4631, 4736, 5438, 6472, 6814, 7374, 7510, 8014, 8641
National Down Syndrome Adoption Network, 2654
National Down Syndrome Coalition, 2655
National Down Syndrome Congress, 2656, 2725
National Down Syndrome Society, 2657, 2726
National Down Syndrome Society AnnualNational Conference, 2709
National Down Syndrome Society Hotline, 2658
National Early Childhood TechnicalAssistance System, 2659, 8015
National Eating Disorder Association of Long Island (NEDA-LI), 2906
National Eating Disorders Association (NEDA), 2874, 5324, 5725
National Eating Disorders Association-LongIsland (NEDA-LI), 2893
National Eczema Association, 2998
National Eczema Association for Science and Education, 474
National Education Alliance for Borderline Personality Disorder, 2462
National Environmental Education Foundation, 423
National Exchange Club Foundation, 5663
National Eye Health Education Program, 6255
National Eye Research Foundation, 239, 2042
National Family Association for Deaf-Blind, 3537
National Family Caregivers Association, 8016
National Father's Network, 8017
National Federation of Families for Children's Mental Health, 2463
National Fire Protection Association, 1318, 1328
National Foundation for Cancer Research, 4192
National Foundation for Celiac Awareness, 1353
National Foundation for Depression, 2464
National Foundation for Depressive Illness, 2465, 2534
National Foundation for EctodermalDysplasias Annual Conference, 2983, 2985, 2988
National Foundation for FacialReconstruction, 2125, 4225, 8018
National Foundation for Infectious Diseases, 5943
National Foundation for Transplants, 8019
National Foundation of Wheelchair Tennis, 8020
National Fragile X Foundation, 3182, 3191

National Gaucher Foundation, 3215, 3222
National Handicapped Sports, 8021
National Headache Foundation, 4752, 4756
National Health Council, 7853
National Health Information Center: Officeof Disease Preventive/Health Promotion, 4963, 7854
National Healthy Mothers, Healthy Babies Coalition, 5944
National Hemophilia Foundation, 3942, 4054
National Hemophilia Foundation Annual Meeting, 4051
National Histicytosis Organizations, 4181
National Hospice Organization, 8022
National Human Genome Research Institute, 5549
National Hydrocephalus FoundationNewsletter, 2126, 2131, 2133, 3043, 3045, 3049, 4226, 4251, 4263, 4590, 4594, 4599
National Industries for the Blind, 8023
National Industries for the SeverelyHandicapped, 8024
National Information Center on Deafness, 3538, 3887, 4560
National Institute of Diabetes and Digestive and Kiney Diseases, 2832
National Institute of Environmental Health Sciences, 424
National Institute of Environmental Sciences, 365
National Institute of Health NINDSInformation Page, 307
National Institute of Mental Health, 7700
National Institute on Disability, Independent Living & Rehabilitation Research, 8642
National Jewish Center for Immunology andRespiratory Medicine, 447
National Jewish Health, 441
National Jewish Medical & Research Center, 448, 5751, 5756, 6376
National Kidney and Urologic DiseasesInformation Clearinghouse, 5150
National Kidney Foundation, 4993, 4996, 5162
National Lead Information Center, 4497
National Library of Dermatologic TeachingSlides, 1579, 3003, 3008, 5632, 6028
National Library Service for the Blind &Physically Handicapped, 1914, 2065, 5286, 6215
National Library Service for the Blind andPhysically Handicapped, 7855, 8643
National Marfan Foundation, 4649, 4650
National Maternal & Child HealthClearinghouse, 7856
National Medical Association, 425, 3311, 7701
National Meningitis Association, 5945
National Mental Health Consumers'Self-Help Clearinghouse, 181, 366, 613, 759, 1616, 1772, 3151, 5107, 5132, 5156, 5368, 5383, 5494, 5579, 5726, 6704, 8025
National Mental Health:Knowledge Exchange Network, 7857
National Minority AIDS Council, 3312
National MPS Society, 4802, 4805, 4812, 4816
National Multiple Sclerosis Society, 2466
National Network of Depression Centers, 2467
National Neutropenia Network, 5089
National Newborn Screening and GeneticResources Center, 8644
National Obesity Foundation, 5325
National Ophthalmic Research Institute, 2043
National Oral Health InformationClearinghouse, 7312, 7321, 7858
National Organization for Albinism andHypopigmentation Bi-Annual Conference, 182, 190
National Organization for People of Color Against Suicide, 2468
National Organization for Rare Disorders, 8026
National Organization for SeasonalAffective Disorder (SAD), 2469
National Organization of Parents of BlindChildren, 6129, 8645
National Organization on Disability, 8027
National Organization on Fetal AlcoholSyndrome, 3152
National Panic/Anxiety Disorder Newsletter, 5600
National Parent Network on Disabilities, 8028
National Parent Resource Center, 8029
National Parent to Parent Support andInformation System, 8030
National Pediatric & Family HIV ResourceCenter, 3329
National Pediatric AIDS Network, 3330
National Perinatal Association, 5903
National Perinatal Association (NPA), 8031
National PKU News, 5556
National Prevention Information Network, 7859
National Psoriasis Foundation, 6026, 6030
National Recreation and Park Association, 7860
National Registry for Childhood OnsetScleroderma (NRCOS), 6451
National Registry for Ichthyosis andRelated Disorders, 4367
National Rehabilitation Information Center, 1495, 3078, 3171, 3175, 3539, 6815, 7861, 8032
National Resource Center for Health & Safety in Child Care & Early Education, 5326
National Resource Center for Preventionof Perinatal Abuse of Alcohol, 3153

National Resource Library on Youth With Disabilities, 8646
National Respite Locator Service, 8033
National Sarcoidosis Resource Center, 6374, 6390, 6409
National Sarcoidosis Resource Center andNetworking Program, 6352
National Scoliosis Foundation, 6473
National Self-Help Clearinghouse, 8034
National SIDS Resource Center Brochure, 7109
National SIDS/Infant Death Resource Center(Resource Center), 6989
National Skeet & Sporting ClayHeadquarters, 8035
National Sleep Foundation, 297, 4888, 5108, 5133, 5157, 6677, 6685, 6705, 6708, 8036
National Society for Phenylketonuria (UK), 5550
National Spasmodic Dysphonia Association, 6771
National Spasmodic Torticollis Association, 2821
National Spasmodic TorticollisAssociation, 2810
National Stuttering Association, 6957
National Sudden Infant Death SyndromeAlliance Conference, 6990, 7069, 7075, 7081
National Support & Information Network, 6277
National Tay-Sachs and Allied DiseaseFoundation, 7177
National Tay-Sachs and Allied DiseasesAssociation, 3216, 4568, 7169, 7258
National Technical Assistance Center forChildren's Mental Health, 1774, 7704, 8037
National Technical Institute for the Deaf, 3540
National Temporal Bone, Hearing and Balance Pathology Resource Registry, 3568
National Tuberculosis Center, 7528
National Tuberculosis Center at New JerseyMedical School, 7375, 7520
National Tuberculosis Controllers Association, 5946
National Tuberous Sclerosis Association, 7376, 7543
National Vaccines Information Center, 8038
National Wheelchair RacquetballAssociation, 8039
National Wheelchair Shooting Federation, 8040
National Wheelchair Softball Association, 8041
National Wilms Tumor Study, 7801
The National Women's Health Information Center, 2834
National Youth Crisis Hotline, 8042
Nationwide Survey of Sudden Infant DeathSyndrome (SIDS) Service, 7110
The Natural History of Mania, Depression,and Schizophrenia, 1660
Natural Supports in School/Work/Communityfor the Severely Disabled, 1526
NAVH UPDATE, 6211
NAVH Update, 1913, 2064, 5283
NDSC Annual Convention, 2708
NE Florida Support Group, 516
NE Indiana Support Group, 524
NE Louisiana Sickle Cell Anemia Foundation, 6636
Nebraska Chapter of the NationalHemophilia Foundation, 3964
Nebraska Dept. of Health Immunization Program, 5973
Nebraska Library Commission Talking Book& Braille Services, 1876, 2023, 5255, 6183
Nebraska Parents Center, 8305
Nebraska Regional Hemophilia Center, 4022
Nebraska SIDS Foundation, 7036
NEDA Annual Conference, 2915
Need to Know, 7457
Negative Symptom and Cognitive Deficit Treatment Response in Schizophrenia, 1647
Negotiating the Special Education Maze: AGuide for Parents and Teachers, 6890
NEHA News, 4080
NEO Fight, 8218
Neonatal Herpes Simplex, 4959
Neonatal Jaundice, 4973
NephCure Foundation, 4994, 4997
NephCure Now, 4999
Nephrotic Syndrome, 4990
NERG News, 574
Nervous System, 8853
Network, 7102
Networker, 1534
Neuroanatomy: Text and Atlas3rd Edition, 1678
Neurobiology of Autism, 944
Neuroblastoma, 5062
Neuroblastoma Children's Cancer Society, 5069
Neurofibromatosis, 5005
Neurofibromatosis Center at North BrowardMedical Center, 5043
Neurofibromatosis Ink, 5051
Neurofibromatosis News, 5052

Neurofibromatosis Support & Information Group, 5011
Neurofibromatosis Type 1: A Guide for Educators, 5056
Neurofibromatosis Type 2: Information forPatients and Families, 5057
Neurofibromatosis, Inc, 5012, 5046
Neurofibromatosis, Inc - Arizona Chapter, 5013
Neurofibromatosis, Inc - California Chapter, 5016
Neurofibromatosis, Inc - Illinois, 5022
Neurofibromatosis, Inc - Illinois/Midwest, 5023
Neurofibromatosis, Inc - Kansas & CentralPlains, 5026
Neurofibromatosis, Inc - MidAtlantic, 5027
Neurofibromatosis, Inc - New England/Northeast, 5029
Neurofibromatosis: A Handbook for Patients, Families and Health Care Professionals, 5049
Neurofibromatosis: Questions and Answers, 5058
The Neurology of Autism, 959
Neurology of Down Syndrome, 2760
Neuromuscular Disease Guidebooks & Pamphlets, 4874
Neuropathy Association, 4569, 4573
Neurosarcoidosis, 6410
Neurosarcoidosis or Multiple Sclerosis?, 6411
Neuroscience Institute at Mercy Hospital, 5044
Neuroscience Institute Brain TumorSupport Group, 1132
Neuroscience Institute, University of Tennessee Health Science Center, 6553
Neutropenia, 5080
Nevada Parent Network, 8313
Nevada Parents Encouraging Parents (PEP), 8314
Nevada State Division of Health, Maternal& Child Health, 7037
Nevada State Health Division Bureau of Community Health - Immunization Program, 5974
Nevada State Library and Archives, 8516
Nevus Outreach, 1114
New Beginnings - Blind Children's Center, 1837, 1983, 5216, 6144
New Beginnings - The Blind Children'sCenter, 1892, 2044, 5270, 6199
New Challenge: Responding to Families, 8698
New England Center for Children, 760, 4515, 8043
New England Chapter of Crohn's & ColitisFoundation of America, 2162
New England Region-Helen Keller NationalCenter, 6130
New England Regional Genetics Group, 528, 8501, 8565
New England Retinoblastoma Support Group (NERSG), 6282
New England Support Group, 530
New Expectations, 2717
New Hampshire Cystic Fibrosis Care andTeaching Center, 2302
New Hampshire SIDS Program, 7038
New Hampshire State Library, 8517
New Heights (formerly Cerebral Palsy of Northeast Florida), 1420
New Image Camps, 5354
New Jersey Camp Jaycee, 4726
New Jersey Center for Outreach & Servicesfor the Autism Community (COSAC), 776, 829
New Jersey Center for Outreach and Services for the Autism Community (COSAC), 853
New Jersey Chapter of Crohn's & ColitisFoundation of America, 2167
New Jersey Department of Health - ChildHealth Program, 7039
New Jersey Department of HealthImmunizations Program, 5976
New Jersey Institute of Technology Centerfor Biomedical Engineering, 3249
New Jersey Medical School, 2304
New Jersey Self-Help Clearinghouse, 8327
New Jersey SIDS Resource Center, 7040
New Jersey State Library Talking Book andBraille Center, 1877, 2024, 5256, 6184
New Jersey Statewide Parent to Parent, 8328
New Language of Toys: Teaching Communication Skills to Children with Special Needs, 6891
New Mexico Autism Society, 830
New Mexico Department of HealthImmunization Program, 5977
New Mexico State Library for the Blind andPhysically Handicapped, 1878, 2025, 5257, 6185
New Neighbors, 3654
New Parents, 2761
New People Not Patients: A Source Book forLiving with IBD, 7643
New People...Not Patients: a Source Bookfor Living with Bowel Disease, 2200
New Pharmacotherapy of Schizophrenia, 1648
New Strong-Willed Child, 5426
New York Autism Network, 832
New York Brain Tumor Support Group, 1222
New York City Area Support Group, 538

New York City Department of Health Bureauof Tuberculosis Control, 7358, 7517
New York City Information & CounselingProgram for SIDS, 7042
New York Department of Education, 8341
New York Obesity Research Center, 2910, 5334
New York Online Access to Health, 5503
New York State Department of HealthImmunization Program, 3088, 5978
New York State Talking Book & BrailleLibrary, 1879, 2026, 5258, 6186
New York Support Group, 539
New York University Medical CenterAuxillary of Tisch Hospital, 4234, 4241
Newark Sleep Disorders Center, 4905
Newberry County Memorial HospitalBrain Tumor Support Group, 1243
Newborns in Need, 5913
Newport News Public Library System, 8547
Newsletter of American Hearing Research, 3869
Newsletter: SIDS, 7103
Newsline, 3870, 8683
Newsline Eight & Nine, 4081
Newslink, 966
Next Steps - Parents Reaching Parents, 8201
NF Clinic - University of PittsburghChildren's Hospital, 5042
NFB National Convention, 189
NH Dept. of Health & Human ServicesImmunization Program, 5975
NHF Camp Directory, 4093
NHF Head Lines, 4766
Nick Joins In, 6892
The Night Before Christmas told in Signedenglish, 3843
Night Terrors, 5122
Nightmares, 5092
NIH News Advisory, 4166
NIH/ Eunice Kennedy Shriver National Institute of Child Health & Human Development, 173, 223, 282, 293, 301, 361, 587, 1302, 1376, 1731, 1939, 1951, 2215, 2381, 2389, 2633, 2770, 2793, 3031,

3051, 3136

NIH/National Cancer Institute, 62, 122, 1076, 3103, 4175, 4186, 5063, 5164, 6267, 7791, 7834
NIH/National Center on Sleep DisordersResearch, 6684
NIH/National Eye Institute, 234, 1817, 1962, 2090, 4459, 4747, 5196, 5623, 6065, 6114, 6252, 6301, 6940, 7835
NIH/National Genome Research Institute (NHGRI), 7836
NIH/National Heart, Lung and Blood Institute, 7354
NIH/National Heart, Lung and Blood Institute, 283, 588, 1303, 1732, 3931, 4410, 5082, 5511, 6011, 6075, 6085, 6234, 6389, 6626, 7117, 7224, 7240, 7277, 7296, 7355, 7480
NIH/National Heart, Lung and BloodInstitute Information Center, 63, 123, 401
NIH/National Heart, Lung, and Blood Institute, 7481
NIH/National Insitute of Allergy andInfectious Diseases, 473, 7838
NIH/National Institute of Allergy and Infectious Diseases, 7357, 7470
NIH/National Institute of Allergy andInfectious Diseases, 22, 402, 2091, 2382, 2995, 3082, 3280, 4095, 4141, 4361, 4411, 4666, 4960, 5472, 5732, 5747, 5927, 6244, 6971, 7356, 7469
NIH/National Institute of Arthritis &Musculoskeletal & Skin Diseases, 1952, 4385, 4450, 4556
NIH/National Institute of Arthritis and Musculoskeletal and Skin Diseases, 3, 248, 327, 2977, 2996, 3021, 3062, 3916, 4362, 4386, 4416, 4557, 4612, 4645, 4656, 5522, 5624, 5739, 5760, 6432,

6470

NIH/National Institute of Dental and Craniofacial Research (NIDCR), 2390, 2978, 4740, 7311, 7320, 7840
NIH/National Institute of Diabetes and Digestive and Kidney Diseases, 7618, 7841
NIH/National Institute of EnvironmentalHealth Sciences (NIEHS), 4
NIH/National Institute of Mental Health, 339, 598, 1030, 1608, 1762, 2219, 2436, 2831, 3137, 4445, 5094, 5124, 5149, 5358, 5486, 5561, 5723, 5911, 6699, 6719, 7672
NIH/National Institute of Neurological Disrs and Stroke (NINDS), 294, 340, 500, 599, 713, 1001, 1011, 1077, 1377, 1667, 2803, 2820, 3352, 3448, 4879, 4885, 6568, 6972, 6978, 7118, 7159
NIH/National Institute on Alcohol Abuse and Alcoholism (NIAAA), 3138, 7844

NIH/National Institute on Deafness and Other Communication Disorders (NIDCD), 6961
NIH/National Institute on Deafness and Other Communication Disorders (NIDCD), 341, 714, 3475, 6751, 6951, 7845
NIH/National Institute on Drug Abuse(NIDA), 5
NIH/National Institutes of Health-Genetic and Rare Diseases Information Center, 3935
NIH/National Library of Medicine (NLM), 10
NIH/Office of Rare Diseases (ORD), 7846
NIH/Osteoporosis and Related Bone DiseasesNational Resource Center, 4451, 5433, 5450
NINDS Seeks Patients with GeneralizedDystonia, 2828
NINDS Seeks Patients with TouretteSyndrome, 7456
NINDS Syncope Information Page, 7120
NineLine, 8044
NM Alliance for the NeurologicallyImpaired, 1216
No Fears, No Tears, 8600
No Fears, No Tears - 13 Years Later, 8601
No Time for Jello: One Family's Experience, 1527
Nobody Knows, 1528
Nocturnal Enuresis, 5148
Non-Hodgkin's Lymphoma, 5163
Non-Malignant Brain Tumor Support Group, 1206
Nonverbal Learning Disorder Syndrome, 4283
Noonan Connection, 5194
Noonan Syndrome, 5184
Noonan Syndrome Support Group, 5190
North Ameerican Spine Society, 6492
North American Craniofacial Family Conference, 3044
North American Riding for the Handicapped, 8045
North American Society for Childhood OnsetSchizophrenia - NACOS, 1617
North American Society for PediatricGastroenterology/Hepatology/Nutrition, 28, 266, 1751, 3094, 4129, 4135, 4787, 4982, 5410, 6101
North American Society for the Study of Ce, 1354
North Carolina Library for the Blind, 1880, 2027, 5259, 6187
North Carolina SIDS Information andCounseling Program, 7045
North Carolina Speech, Hearing and Language Association, 6775
North Central Oklahoma Support Group, 542
North Dakota Comprehensive Hemophilia andThrombosis Treatment Center, 4023
North Dakota SIDS Management Program, 7046
North Pacific Epilepsy Research, 6569
North Platte Public Library, 8514
North Texas Chapter of Crohn's &Colitis Foundation of America, 2186
North Texas SIDS Information AndCounseling Program, 7058
North Texas Support Group, 550
Northeast Ohio Chapter of Crohn's &Colitis Foundation of America, 2178
Northeast Rehabilitation Health Network, 3449
Northern California Chapter of Asthma andAllergy Foundation of America, 430
Northern California Chapter of Crohn's andColitis Foundation, 2148
Northern California Comprehensive Sickle Cell Center, 6648
Northern California Support Group, 507
Northern Connecticut Affiliate Chapter ofCrohn's & Colitis Foundation of America, 2152
Northern Illinois Center for AdaptiveTechnology, 8473
Northern Kentucky Talking Book Library, 8493
Northern Ohio Chapter of the NationalHemophilia Foundation, 3970
Northern Regional Bleeding Disorder Center, 4024
Northridge Hospital: Leavey Cancer Center, 1133
Northwest Indiana Subregional Library forBlind and Physically Handicapped, 1853, 1999, 5232, 6160
Northwest Ohio Hemophilia Foundation, 3971
Northwest Ohio Hemophilia TreatmentCenter, 4025
Northwestern Region-Helen Keller NationalCenter, 1829, 1974, 5207, 6135
Northwestern University Asthma and AllergyDisease Center, 449
Not Just a Cancer Patient, 8602
Not So Sweet: Living With Diabetes, 2560
Nothing Hurts But My Heart, 6502
Now We Can Successfully Treat the IllnessCalled Depression, 2543
NPF Benefits of Membership Pamphlets, 8697
NSF Packets, 6517
Nuclear Medicine at Children's Hospital,Boston, 8647
Number Signs for Everyone: Numbering in American Sign Language, 3655
Nursery Rhymes from Mother Goose: Told inSigned English, 3803
Nutitional Care for Children with PWS, Infants and Toddlers, 5873
Nutrition for Early Chronic Kidney Disease, 8699
Nutrition for Later Chronic Disease, 8700
NW Ohio Sleep Disorders Center, 4921

NYS Center for SIDSOffice, 7041
NYSARC, 4697
Nystagmus, 5195
Nystagmus Network, 5279
NYU, 3133, 4572
NYU Rusk Institute, 4830

O

Oak-Leyden Developmental Services, 761, 8046
Oakhurst, 8797
Oakland County Health Division - SIDSProject, 7028
Oakland School & Camp, 4546
Oasis, 8146
Oasis at MAAP, 367, 762
Oasis Guide to Asperger Syndrome, 387
Obesity, 5303
Obesity Action Coalition, 5327
Obesity Online, 5339
The Obesity Society, 5332
Obesity Sourcebook, 5343
Obsessive Compulsive Anonymous, 5369
Obsessive Compulsive Disorder (OCD), 5384
Obsessive Compulsive Disorder General Packet, 5402
Obsessive Compulsive Disorder: HelpingChildren and Adolescents, 5394
Obsessive Compulsive Foundation, 5370, 5385
Obsessive Compulsive Foundation of Metropolitan Chicago, 5373
Obsessive-Compulsive Disorder, 5356
Obsessive-Compulsive Disorder in Childrenand Adolescents, 5395
Obsessive-Compulsive Disorder, A Real Illness, 5403
OCD Newsletter, 5400
OCECD, 8364
Oconee Regional Library, Library for theBlind and Physically Handicapped, 8466
Of Their Own-Person To Person Show, 6381
Office for Fair Housing & EqualOpportunity, 7862
Office Integrated Social Services, 8388
Office of Community Health and PreventionBureau of Early Intervention, DHR, 8202
Office of Exceptional ChildrenSouth Carolina Department of Education, 8394
Office of Special Education, 8271, 8285, 8397
Office of Special Education Administration, 8433
Office of Special Education and Rehabilitation Services, 3476
Office of Special Education andRehabilitative Services, 7863, 8648
Office of Special Education, StateDepartment of Education, 8401
Office of Special Education, Virginia, 8424
Office of the Dean, University of Texas atAustin, 8405
Office of the Superintendent of PublicInstruction, 8430
Office of Women's & Children's Health, 6998
Official Journal of the American Academyof Child and Adolescent Psychiatry, 5428
The Official Parent's Sourcebook on Tay-Sachs Disease, 7187
The Official Parent's Sourcebook onChildhood Nephrotic Syndrome, 4998
Ohio Department of HealthImmunization Program, 5979
Ohio Protection and Advocacy Organization, 8365
Ohio Regional Library for the Blind andPhysically Handicapped, 8527
Ohio Sleep Medicine Institute, 4922
Ohio State University Hospitals, SleepDisorders Center, 4923
Ohio State University Laboratory ofPsychobiology, 3435
Ohio Support Group, 541
OHSU Homepage Search, 3258
Okizu Foundation Camps, 120, 171, 1300, 3124, 5183, 7812
Oklahoma ABLE Tech-Wellness Center, 8369
Oklahoma Brain Injury Camp, 3473
Oklahoma Chapter of Crohn's & ColitisFoundation of America, 2180
Oklahoma Chapter of the NationalHemophilia Foundation, 3974
Oklahoma Library for the Blind &Physically Handicapped, 8529
Oklahoma Speech Language Hearing Association, 6778
Oklahoma State Department of Health -Maternal and Child Health Services, 7048
Oklahoma State Department of HealthImmunization Division, 5980
Oley Foundation, 29, 267
Oley Foundation Annual Conference, 34, 272
Olympia, 8740
Omphalocele, 5405
On The Other Hand, 5766
On the Threshold of a Cure...You Can Makethe Difference!, 2376

OncoLink: The University of PennslyvaniaCancer Center Resource, 3117, 7804
1 in Every 10 Persons Has Scoliosis, 6511
Onhealth, 2357
Online Asperger Syndrome Information and Support, 378
Online Mendelian Inheritance in Man, 18, 220, 231, 244, 256, 308, 335, 475, 904, 1024, 1262, 1634, 1675, 1697, 1787, 1905, 2056, 2109, 2223, 2358, 2498
Online Parenting Coach, 7729
Online Pediatric Surgery Handbook, 4170
Online Sarcoidosis Newsletter, 6397
Online Support Group, 4562
Open Support Group-All Kinds of CancerCare of Maine, 1186
Opening Doors: Strategies for IncludingAll Students in Regular Education, 1529
Operation Liftoff of Ohio, 8366
Operation SHHH, 3804
Operation Sneek-a-Peek, 8603
Ophthalmic Disorders Sourcebook, 1908, 2060, 6209, 6948
Opinion Section, 3656
Opposites, 3805
Oppositional Defiant Disorder, 5418
Option Institute, 2794
Option Institute: Son Rise Program, 614, 640, 763, 821, 2780
Optometrists Network, 4481
Oral Cancer Foundation, 2426
Orange County Support Group, 508
Oregon Brain Injury Resource Network, 3407
Oregon Department of Education, 8374
Oregon Health Sciences Unit, 2325
Oregon Health Sciences UniversityResearch Center, 3575
Oregon Parent Training and InformationCenter, 8375
Oregon State Health Division - SIDSInformation and Counseling Program, 7049
Oregon State Library, 8531
Oregon State Library, Talking Book andBraille Services, 1882, 2029, 5261, 6189
Organization for Autism Research, 764
Organizing and Facilitating a Support Group, 1289
Orphan Disease Update, 3265, 8684
Orthopaedic Biomechanics Laboratory, 1496
Orthopaedic Hospital's HemophiliaTreatment Center, 4026
Orthoseek, 1723
Osteogenesis Imperfecta, 5431
Osteogenesis Imperfecta Foundation, 5439, 5456
Osteogenesis Imperfecta: A Guide for Medical Professionals, Ind. & Families, 5469
Osteogenesis Imperfecta: A Guide for Nurses, 5466
Osteoporosis and Related Bone Diseases -National Resource Center, 5457
Ostomy Book: Living Comfortably withColostomies, Ileostomies and Urostomies, 7644
Otitis Media, 5471
Otto Learns About His Medicine A Story About Medication for Hyperative Children, 671
Our Brother Has Down's Syndrome: AnIntroduction for Children, 2741
Our Hearts, 4316
Our World, 4530
Out for a Walk: Baby's First Sign Book, 3806
Out of Darkness, 698
Out of Harm's Way: A Parent's Guide to Protecting Young Children from Sexual Abuse, 5711
Out-of-Sync Child: Recognizing and Copingwith Sensory Processing Disorder, 388
The OutLook, 1602
Outreach, 1071, 2535, 3080
Overcoming Depression, 2518
Overcoming Dyslexia in Children,Adolescents, and Adults, 2797
Overcoming Headaches & Migraines, 4762
Overeaters Anonymous, 2958
Overeaters Anonymous Lifeline Sampler, 5344
Overeaters Anonymous Support Group, 2894
Overeaters Anonymous, World Service Office, 2875
Overlook, 8824
Overview of the Prader-Willi Syndrome, 5874

P

PA Tourette Syndrome Alliance, 7408
PACER Center, 8509

Pacific Northwest Regional Genetics Group, 543
Pacific Southwest Regional Genetics Group, 509
Pacifiers and SIDS: Reducing the Risk, 7111
Pain, Pain Go Away: Helping Childrenwith Pain, 8701
PAL News, 8685
Palo Alto Brain Tumor Support Group, 1134
Palouse Area Parent To Parent, 8190
Pan American Health Organization (PAHO), 5996, 8047
Pandora's Box, 5701
Panic Attacks, 5620
Panic Disorder, 2544
Panic Disorder in the Medical Setting, 2519
Panic Disorder, Separation, AnxietyDisorder, 5601
Paranoid Psychosis Due to Neurosarcoidosis, 6412
Parent Act, 8294
Parent and Information Center, 8566
Parent Assistance Network, 8306
Parent Case Management, 8406
Parent Education Network, 8380
Parent Education Project of Wisconsin, 8440
Parent Education/Support Group, 1194
Parent Educational Advocacy Training Center, 8425
The Parent Educational Advocacy Training Center, 4525
Parent Educator Connection, 8228
Parent Educator Connection Program, 8229
Parent Information Center, 8321, 8443
Parent Information Center of Delaware, 8162
Parent Network Center, 8342
Parent Packets, 3888
Parent Pals, 6793, 6963
Parent Partners, 8286
Parent Project for Muscular DystrophyResearch, 4831
Parent Project Muscular Dystrophy, 4838
Parent Reaching Out to Parents, 8191
Parent Sign Series, 3657
Parent Support Group, 8307
Parent Support Group of Littleton & Auora, 8148
Parent to Parent ARC Allegheny, 8381
Parent to Parent Arc of Arkansas, 8105
Parent to Parent Network, 8203
Parent to Parent Network of Connecticutthe Family Center, 8158
Parent to Parent of Georgia, 8178
Parent to Parent of New Hampshire, 8322
Parent to Parent of New York State, 8343
Parent to Parent of Pennsylvania, 8382
Parent's Guide to Children's CongenitalHeart Defects, 4341
Parent's Guide to Chochlear Implants, 3807
Parent's Guide to Down Syndrome: Towarda Brighter Future, 2742
A Parent's Guide to Understanding Retinoblastoma, 6283, 6297
Parental Alienation, DSM-5, and ICD-11, 8666
Parenting Across the Autism Spectrum, 945
Parenting Attention Deficit Disordered Teens, 699
Parenting Children with ADHD: LessonsThat Medicine Cannot Teach, 672
PARENTS, 8091
Parents Against Childhood Epilepsy (PACE), 6534
Parents Alliance Employment Project, 8474
Parents and Children Together (PACT), 8183
Parents and Their Deaf Children: The Early Years, 3808
Parents are Experts, 8272
Parents Association of Connecticut Children with Visual Impairments (PACVI), 6279
Parents Educating Parents and Professionalfor All Children (PEPPAC), 8179
Parents Encouraging Parents, 8308, 8315
Parents For Heart of Minnesota, 4319
Parents for Parents, 8278
Parents Helping Parents, 3331, 7340, 7433
Parents Helping Parents - A FamilyResource Center, 6991
Parents Helping Parents of San Francisco, 8126
Parents Helping Parents of Santa Clara, 8127
Parents Helping Parents: A Directory ofSupport Groups for ADD, 673
Parents Helping Parents: Family Resourcesfor Children with Special Needs, 4516
Parents Information Network FFCMH, 8048
Parents Let's Unite for Kids, 8301
Parents of Asthmatic/Allergic Children, Inc., 431, 6320
Parents of Children with Brain Tumors(PCBT), 1173
Parents of Children with Down SyndromeArc of Montgomery County, 2669
Parents of Galactosemic Children, 3202, 3209, 4788, 4792
Parents of Infants and Children withKernicterus, 4432

Parents Place of Maryland, 8255
Parents Reaching Out, 8332
Parents Reaching Out in Oklahoma, 8370
Parents Supporting Parents of Eagle County, 8149
Parents Supporting Parents of Garfield andPitkin County, 8150
Parents Union for Public Schools, 8383
Parents' Hyperactivity Handbook: Helpingthe Fidgety Child, 674
ParentsMedGuide.org, 7730
Park Ridge, Cystic Fibrosis Center, 2270
Partners in Intensive Care, 8256
Partners Resource Network, 8407
Partnership for a Healthier America, 5328
Partnership for Assistive Technology, 8168
Partnerships for Inclusion, 8353
Passive-Aggressive Behavior, 5485
Passport: Global Treatment CentreDirectory, 4066
The Patch, 4489
Patent Ductus Arteriosus, 5509
Pathology Department SIDS/SUDC ResearchProject, 7076
Pathways Awareness Foundation, 8049
Patient Information Package, 6413
Patient Packets For Celiac Disease, 1374
Patient Recruitment & Public LiaisonOffice Clinical Center, 7779
Patients with Cervical or Focal HandDystonia Sought, 2829
Paws Sign Stories, 3706
PDR - Physicians' Desk Reference, 8650
PDR.net, 5480
PEAK Parent Center, 8147
Peaks and Valleys Family Resource Center, 8128
Pearls of Dysmorphology, 558
Pediatric AIDS Clinical Trials Group, 3332
Pediatric Behavior and Development, 8652
Pediatric Brain Tumor Foundation of the United States, 1263
Pediatric Brain Tumor Support Group, 1121, 1153
Pediatric Cancer Sourcebook, 110, 163, 1269, 3120, 5076, 5178
Pediatric Clinical Trials International, 2697
Pediatric Crohn's & Colitis Association, 7625, 7636
Pediatric Cystic Fibrosis Center, 2283
Pediatric Dermatology Journal, 194, 207, 1331, 1595, 2993, 3011, 3928, 4371, 4422, 5540, 5638, 5744, 7215, 7285, 7664, 8674
Pediatric Disabilities Clinic, DownSyndrome Clinic, 2679
Pediatric Epilepsy, 6587
Pediatric Epilepsy Center, 6550
Pediatric Epilepsy Resource Handbook, 6588
Pediatric Heart Foundation, 4311
Pediatric Hemophilia Program ofPennsylvania, 4027
Pediatric Infectious Diseases Society, 5947
Pediatric Neurodevelopmental Center atMarcus Institute, 2680
Pediatric Neurosurgery-Hydrocephalus, 4253
Pediatric Ophathalmology and Adult Strabismus Service Research, 1893
Pediatric Plastic Surgery, 7131
Pediatric Points of Interest, 8653
Pediatric Pulmonary and Cystic FibrosisCenter, 2328
Pediatric Pulmonary Center, 2312, 2322
Pediatric Pulmonary Medicine, 2334
Pediatric Pulmonary Unit, 7077
Pediatric Rheumatoid Clinic, 4392
Pediatric Surgery Update, 4171, 5415
Pediatric/Adolescent GastroesophagealReflux Association (PAGER), 6102
Pediatrics, 6343
Pediatrics CRPS Tri-Fold Brochure, 4850
Pediatrics in Review, 6344
PEDINFO: An index of the PediatricInternet, 8651
Peer Problems in Tourette's Disorder, 7458
Peer Violence Among Teenagers: Trends inViolence, 7759
Pemphigus, 5520
Pemphigus and Pemphigoid At a Glance, 5543
Pemphigus FAQ, 5539
Pen-Pal Directory, 585
Peninsula Support & Education Group forParents of Children with Brain Tumors, 1135
Penn Center for Sleep Disorders, Hospitalof the University of Pennsylvania, 4931
Penn Neurological Institute, 4832
Pennsylvania Chapter of the AmericanAnorexia Bulimia Association, 2898
Pennsylvania Educational Network forEating Disorders (PENED), 2899
Pennsylvania SIDS Center, 7051
Pennsylvania's Initiative on AssistiveTechnology, Institute on Disabilities, 8384
Pennsylvania/Delaware Valley Chapter ofCrohn's & Colitis Foundation of America, 2181

People First International, 4705
People Living Through Cancer, 1217
People Treated for Brain Tumors and TheirCaregivers, 1223
Perceptual-Motor Behavior in DownSyndrome, 2743
Perfectionism: What's Bad About Being TooGood, 5612
Perinatal and Infant Health Unit - SIDSInformation and Counseling
    Program, 7047
Personality and Psychopathology, 5508
Perspective, 7551
Perspectives Folio: Parent-Child, 3889
Perspectives in Education and Deafness, 3857
Perspectives Network, 3363, 3450
Perspectives on Language and Literacy, 4532
Pervasive Developmental Disorders, 974
The Pet Show, 3674
Pharmaceutical Manufacturers Association, 8050
Pharmacologic Therapy of Pediatric Asthma, 465
Pharmacotherapy of Schizophrenia, 1628
Phelps School, 4547
Phenylketonuria (PKU), 5544
Phenylketonuria (PKU) Information Sheet, 5558
Phobia Society of America, 5580, 6731
Phobias, 5559
Phobics Anonymous, 5581, 6732
Phoenix Center for Cancer and BloodDisorders, 4028
Photosensitivity, 5621
Phototherapy: Light Treatment for Psoriasis, 6051
Physical & Sexual Abuse, 5645
Physical Therapy Intervention for Individuals With Prader-Willi Syndrome,
    5883
Physician Referral and Information Line, 442
Physician's Research Network, 3313
PICA, 5719
Pica Information Page, 5729
Pike Institute on Law and Disability, 8051
Pilot Parents (PP), 8052
Pilot Parents in Anoka and Ramsey Counties, 8279
Pilot Parents of Northeast Minnesota, 8280
Pilot Parents of Southern Arizona, 8096
Pine Tree Camp Children - Adults, 8759
Pinworm (Enterobius Vermicularis), 5730
Pinworm Infection, 5737
Pioneers Division of CEC, 8053
Pittsburgh Area Brain Injury Alliance, 3408
Pituitary Network Association, 1115
Pityriasis Rosea, 5738, 5745
PKU Kid Zone, 5552
PKU Mailing List, 5553
PKU Organization of Illinois, 5548, 5554
PKU Press, 5557
Plain Talk About Depression, 2545
Plan for Success: Educator's Guide to Students with Osteogenesis
    Imperfecta, 5453
Planetpsych, 1066, 1635, 1788, 5115, 5140, 5386, 5504, 5602, 7731, 8654
Planetree Health Information Service, 8054
Plasma Homovanillic Asid in Schhizophrenia, 1649
Platelet Disorder Support Association, 7302, 7307
Pneumonia, 5746
Police Officer Jones, 3809
Polio Connection of America, 5997
Polio Experience Network, 5998
Polio Society, 5948
Polio Survivors Association, 5949
Polydactyly, 5758, 5767
Porphyria, 5768
Porphyria Fact Sheet, 5777
Portland Public Library, 8502
Positive Behavioral Strategies to SupportChildren & Young People with
    Autism, 946
Positive Exposure, 183
Positive Solutions for Life Challenges, 8295
Post Polio Awareness & Support Society ofBritish Columbia, 5999
Post Traumatic Stress Disorder Sourcebook, 5805
Post Traumatic Stress Disorder: A Guide, 5810
Post-Polio Directory, 6006
Post-Polio Health, 6008
Post-Polio Health International, 5950
Post-Traumatic Stress Disorder, 5778
Post-Traumatic Stress Disorder, A Real Illness, 5811
Postpartum Progress, 2470

Postpartum Support International, 2471
Posttraumatic Stress Disorder in Childrenand Adolescents, 5806
Postural Screening Program, 6518
Practice Guidelines for Eating Disorders, 2959
Prader-Willi Alliance of New York, 5846, 5868
Prader-Willi Association of New England(Maine, Mass, RI, NH, VT),
    5835, 5837
Prader-Willi California Foundation, 5822
Prader-Willi Colorado Association, 5823
Prader-Willi Connecticut Association, 5824
Prader-Willi Delaware Association, 5825
Prader-Willi Families of Ohio, 5849
Prader-Willi Northwest Association, 5820, 5828, 5841
Prader-Willi Northwest Association-Idaho, 5829
Prader-Willi Syndrome, 5813
Prader-Willi Syndrome - An Overview for Health Professionals, 5865
Prader-Willi Syndrome Advocates, 5833
Prader-Willi Syndrome Arizona Association, 5821
Prader-Willi Syndrome Association, 5819, 5869
Prader-Willi Syndrome is What I Have Not Who I Am!, 5875
Prader-Willi Syndrome: A Guide for Families & Professionals, 5884
Prader-Willi Syndrome: Medical Alerts, 5885
Prader-Willi Utah Association, 5856
PREBIC-International Preterm Birth Collaborative, 5914
Precious Hearts, 4333
Precocious Puberty, 5887, 5897
Preemie Magazine, 5922
Preemie Ring, 5915
Preemie Twins, 5916
Preemie World, 5917
Pregnancy and Child Health Resource Centerfrom Mayo Health Oasis, 8655
Pregnancy and Exposure to Alcohol andOther Drug Use, 3159
Pregnancy and Infant Loss Center, 6992
Premature Baby-Premature Child, 5918
Prematurely Yours, 5919, 5920
Prematurity, 5898
Prenatal and Postnatal Growth and Development, 8859
Prenatal Diagnostic and Genetic Center, 8485, 8567
Prenatal Exposures in Schizophrenia, 1650
Prenatal Hydrocephalus-Book for Parents, 4284
Preparing Yourself for Spinal Surgery (For Teenagers with Severe
    Scoliosis), 6482
Presbyterian-University Hospital,Pulmonary Sleep Evaluation Center, 4932
Preschool Issues in Autism, 947
Preschool Motor Speech Evaluation & Intervention, 6796
Preschool Programs - Division of SpecialPopulations, 8243
Prescription for Success, 948
Prescription Parents, 1688, 1698
President's Committee on Employmentof People with Disabilities, 7864
President's Committee on MentalRetardation, 7865
Presidential Proclamation-NationalSarcoidosis Awareness Day, 6414
Preuss Foundation, 1116
Prevent Blindness America, 1968, 8055
Prevent Blindness America Affiliates &Divisions, 4482
Prevent Child Abuse America, 5664, 5702
Prevent Child Abuse California, 5703
Prevent Child Abuse Georgia, 5674
Prevent Child Abuse Illinois, 5675
Prevent Child Abuse Indiana, 5676
Prevent Child Abuse Iowa, 5677
Prevent Child Abuse New York, 5679
Prevent Child Abuse North Carolina, 5680
Preventable Childhood Infections, 5924
Preventing Antisocial Behavior:Interventions, 1796, 7745
Prevention Initiatives State Department ofEducation, 8151
Prevention Resource Guide: Pregnant,Postpartum Women and Their
    Infants, 3160
Primary Brain Cancer Support Group, 1177
Primary Care Needs of Children withHydrocephalus, 4285
Primary Children's Medical Center, 8568
A Primer of Brain Tumors, 1273
Prince George's County Memorial LibraryTalking Book Center, 1860,
    2006, 5238, 6166
Principles and Practice of Sleep Medicine, 5145, 6690
PRO-Parents, 8395
Problem Behaviors & Tourette Syndrome, 7459
Professional Assistance Center forEducation (PACE), 8475
Programmed Therapy for Stuttering in Children and Adults, 6964
Programs for Children with Special Health Care Needs, 8798

Programs for Infants and Toddlers with Disabilities: Ages Birth Through 2, 8799
Progress in Dermatology, 1601, 3016, 5643, 6047
Project Cuddle, 5665
Project PODER, 8408
Project PROMPT, 8244
Project Special Care, 8219
Project Start, 8287
A Promising Future Together, 2710
Protein C Deficiency, 6010
Protein Deficiency and Pesticide Toxicity, 6023
Proteinuria, 8702
Prozac Nation: Young & Depressed inAmerica, A Memoir, 2520
Psoriasis, 6024
Psoriasis 101: Learning to Live in the Skin You're In, 6052
Psoriasis Advance, 6040
Psoriasis Association, 6031
Psoriasis Connections, 6032
Psoriasis Forum, 6041
Psoriasis on Specific Skin Sites, 6054
Psoriasis Research: Progress & Promise, 6053
Psoriasis Resource, 6048
Psoriasis: How it Makes You Feel, 6055
Psoriatic Arthritis, 6056
Psych Central, 1636, 5116, 5141, 5387, 5505, 7732, 8656
PsychAlive, 7733
Psychological Approaches to Dermatology, 6036
Psychological Factors in Sarcoidosis, 6415
Psychological Trauma, 5613, 6744
Psychosocial Aspects of Narcolepsy, 4954
Psychotherapy of Severe and MildDepression, 2521
PTN National Conference, 273
PTN News, 279
Ptosis, 6064
PTSD Alliance, 5799
PTSD in Children: Move in the Rhythm of the Child, 5791
PTSD Workbook, 5804
Public Health Services of Louisiana, 7019
Publications From the National InformationCenter on Deafness, 3890
PubMed, 8657
Puget Sound Blood Center, 4029
Pull-Thru Network, 268, 4161, 4168
Pull-Thru Network News, 4172
Pulmonary Care and Cystic Fibrosis Center, 2257
Pulmonary Hypertension, 6073
Pulmonary Hypertension Association, 6081
Pulmonary Sarcoidosis: Evaluation withHigh Resolution, 6416
Pulmonary Sarcoidosis: What We AreLearning, 6417
Pulmonary Valve Stenosis, 6083
Pulmonary Wellness Program, 2265
Pure Facts, 690
Putting on the Brakes, 676
Putting On The Brakes - Young People's Guide To Understanding ADHD, 675
The 'Putting On The Brakes' Activity BookFor Young People With ADHD, 683
PWS - The Early Years, 5864
PWS Project for New Mexico, 5845
PWSA - New Jersey Chapter, 5844
PWSA - South Carolina, 5853
PWSA - Tennessee, 5854
PWSA Chapter - Minnesota, 5839
PWSA Florida Chapter, 5826
PWSA Las Vegas/Nevada Support Group, 5843
PWSA Missouri Chapter, 5840
PWSA of Georgia, 5827
PWSA of Illinois, 5830
PWSA of Indiana, 5831
PWSA of Iowa, 5832
PWSA of Kentucky, 5834
PWSA of Maryland, Virginia & DC, 5836, 5857
PWSA of Michigan, 5838
PWSA of Nebraska, 5842
PWSA of North Carolina, 5847
PWSA of Ohio, 5848
PWSA of Oklahoma, 5850
PWSA of Oregon, 5851
PWSA of Pennsylvania, 5852
PWSA of Wisconsin, 5858
Pyloric Stenosis, 6094

Q

Q and A: Hepatitis B Prevention, 4121
Quad Cities Brain Tumor Support Group, 1179
Quality Life Concepts, 8302
Quest Magazine, 1557, 4848
Questions & Answers About Diet and Nutrition, 2209
Questions and Answers About Complications, 2210
Questions and Answers About Crohn's Disease & Ulcerative Colitis, 2211
Questions and Answers About Emotional Factors In Ileitis and Colitis, 2212
Questions and Answers About Psoriasis, 6057
Questions and Answers About Scoliosis, 6520
Questions and Answers About UlcerativeColitis, 7653
Questions and Answers on Hearing Loss, 3891
Questions Most Often Asked the NSF, 6519

T

The Race, 3675
Rainbow's End, 3658
Rainbows, 8056
Rainrock Treatment Center, 2897
Raising a Child with Diabetes: A Guide forParents, 2576
Raising Joshua, 7442
Raising Special Kids, 8097
Raising Your Child Without Milk:Reassuring Advice and Recipes For Parent, 4793
Raleigh TEACCH Center, 765
Ramapo Anchorage Camp, 4548, 8800
Rape, Abuse and Incest National Network(RAINN), 5666, 5704
Rare Genetic Diseases in Children (NYU), 232, 309, 3046, 3210, 3223, 4137, 4213, 4254, 4433, 4456, 4596, 7784, 8658
Rather Strange Stories, 3659
Raven Rock Lutheran Camp, 4727
REACH - Sarcoidosis Support, 6357
Reaching Out, 2111
Reaching the Autistic Child: A ParentTraining Program, 949
Reaching, Crawling, Walking - Let's GetMoving, 1910, 2062, 5284, 6212
Reading and Speech Clinic, 6779
Ready! Set! Sign!, 3707
Realities in Coping with ProgressiveNeuromuscular Diseases, 4845
Reality Matters - Obesity & Nutrition, 5336
Recognizing Children with Special Needs, 8604
Recovery, 2472
Recovery Panic Anxiety, 5603
Reflex Sympathetic Dystrophy SyndromeAssociation, 4826
Refraction Disturbances, 6113
Region 1 of the National Association forParents of the Visually Impaired, 6124
Region 2 of the National Association forParents of the Visually Impaired, 1826, 1971, 5204, 6132
Region 3 of the National Association forParents of the Visually Impaired, 6127
Region 4 of the National Association forParents of the Visually Impaired, 1828, 1973, 5206, 6134
Region 5 of the National Association forParents of the Visually Impaired, 6131
Region I Office Program Consultants ForMaternal and Child Health, 7024
Region II Office Program Consultants forMaternal and Child Health, 7043
Region III Office Program Consultants forMaternal and Child Health, 7052
Region IV Office Program Consultants ForMaternal and Child Health, 7010
Region IX Office Program Consultants forMaternal and Child Health, 7002
Region V Office Program Consultants forMaternal and Child Health, 7013
Region VI Office Program Consultants ForMaternal and Child Health, 7059
Region VII Office Program Consultants forMaternal and Child Health, 7033
Region VIII Office Program Consultants forMaternal and Child Health, 7004
Region X Office Program Consultants forMaternal and Child Health, 7064
Regional Epilepsy Center, 6555
Regional Hemophilia Program, 4030
Regional Resource Center on Deafness, 3564
A Regular Kid, 457
Rehabilitation Institute of Michigan, 3391, 3430
Rehabilitation Research and TrainingCenter on Traumatic Brain Injury, 3433
Rehabilitation Research Training Center on Developmental Disabilities and Health, 4706
Religious Signing: A Comprehensive Guide for All Faiths, 3810

Renal Tubular Acidosis, 8703
Renalink, 5000
Renfrew Center of Bryn Mawr, 2900
Renfrew Center of Connecticut, 2884
Renfrew Center of Miami, 2886
Renfrew Center of New York City, 2895
Renfrew Center of Northern New Jersey, 2891
Renfrew Center of Philadelphia, 2901
Report of the Secretary's Task Force onYouth Suicide, 2522
Reproductive Systems, 8854
Research & Training Center for Children'sMental Health at University of
    South FL, 1775, 7705
Research and Training Center for Children'Mental Health, 8569
Research and Training Center on Community Living, 4707
Research and Training Center on FamilySupport and Children's Mental
    Health, 1776, 7706, 8570
Research at BloodCenter of Wisconsin, 4031
Research to Prevent Blindness, 1894, 2045, 5271, 6200
Residential Eating Disorders Consortium, 2876
Resource Center for the American Alliance of Cancer - Pain Initiatives, 113
Resource Guide, 4286
Resource Survival Handbook, 5077
Resources for Children with Special Needs, 8057, 8344
Resources for Rehabilitation, 8505
Resources for Young Children and Families, 8152
Respiratory Distress Syndrome of the Newborn, 6232
Respiratory Health Association, 426
Respiratory Syncytial Virus Infection, 6242
Respiratory System, 8855
Rest of the Family, 6560
Restless Nights, 6691
Restricted Growth Association, 19
Retarded Isn't Stupid, Mom!, 4717
Rethink autism, 766
Rethinking Attention Deficit Disorders, 677
Retina South Africa - Fighting Blindness, 6261
Retinitis Pigmentosa, 6251
Retinoblastoma, 6266
Retinoblastoma International, 6278
Retinoblastoma Solutions, 6287
Retinoblastoma Support News, 6296
Retinopathy of Prematurity, 6299
Rewrite Beautiful, 2877
Rheumatoid Arthritis, 4406
Rhinitis, 6314
Rhode Island Arc, 8389
Rhode Island Department of Health, 5981, 7053, 8390
Rhode Island Hemostasis and ThrombosisCenter, 4032
Rhode Island Hospital, Cystic FibrosisCenter, 2330
Rhode Island Parent Information Network, 8391
Rhode Island Scleroderma Support Group, 6443
Rhode Island Test of Language StructureRITLS, 3811
Rid Alaska of Child Abuse, 5671
Riddle of Autism: A Psychological Analysis, 950
Right & Left Ventricular Function At RestIn Patients with Sarcoidosis,
    6418
Riley Cystic Fibrosis Center, 2274
Riley Hemophilia and Thrombophilia Center, 3989
The Rising of Lotus Flowers: Self-Educating Deaf Children in Thai
    Boarding Schools, 3844
Ritalin is Not the Answer, 678
River Centre Foundation, 2878
Roanoke City Public Library System, 8548
Robyn's Book: A True Diary, 2366
Rochester Chapter of Crohn's & ColitisFoundation of America, 2173
Rockefeller University Laboratory forInvestigative Dermatology, 1581,
    3005, 5634
Rockingham County Schools, 8354
Rocky Mountain Chapter of Crohn's &Colitis Foundation of America, 2149
Rocky Mountain Village, 8732
Roeher Institute, 8058
Rolling Along with Goldilocks and theThree Bears, 6893
Rome Subregional Library for the Blindand Physically Handicapped, 8467
Ronald McDonald Houses, 8059
Ropard: Association for Retinopathy of Prematurity & Related Diseases,
    5904
Round Lake Camp, 710, 995, 4549
Royal National Institute of the Blind, 1906, 2057, 5281, 6072, 6262, 6947
RP International, 6256
RP Messenger, 6265

RSDA Review, 4851
RSV Info Center, 6241, 6250
Rudd Center for Food Policy & Obesity, 5329
Rural Institute on Disabilities, 8060
Rush Children's Heart Center, 316, 321
Rusk Institute of Rehabilitation Medicine, 4827, 8571
Russian Soldier, 3660
Ryan, 7334, 7425
The Ryan Licht Sang Bipolar Foundation, 1054
RYAN: A Mother's Story of Her Hyperactive/Tourette Syndrome Child,
    7441

S

Sacramento Area Brain Tumor Support GroupLawrence J Ellison
    Ambulatory Care Ctr, 1136
Sacramento Center for Assistive Technology, 8456
Sad Days, Glad Days, 2523
Safe Drinking Water Hotline, 4501
Safe Place for Newborns, 5667
Safety and Seizures, 6611
Saint Alexius Medical Center/CF Center, 2318
Saint Francis Medical Center SpecialtyClinics, CF Center, 2271
Saint Joseph's Hospital Health CenterSleep Laboratory, 4909
Saint Jude Children's Research Hospital, 8539
Saint Louis Chapter of Crohn's & ColitisFoundation of America, 2166
Saint Mary's Healthcare System forChildren, 8345
Saint Vincent Medical Center, SleepDisorders Center, 4924
San Diego Support Group, 510
San Fernando Valley Support Group, 511
San Francisco Brain Tumor Support Group, 1137
San Francisco Public Library for the Blindand Print Disabled, 1838, 1984,
    5217, 6145
San Gabriel/Pomona Parents' Place, 8129
Santa Barbara Brain Tumor Support Group, 1138
Santa Cruz County Brain Tumor SupportGroup, 1139
Santa Fe Mountain Center, 8791
Santa Rosa Brain Tumor Support Group, 1140
Sarcoid Life, 6392
Sarcoid Networking Association, 6353
Sarcoid Registry, 6354
Sarcoidosis, 6349, 6393, 6419
Sarcoidosis and Lyme Disease, 6384
Sarcoidosis and Other Granulatomous, 6421
Sarcoidosis and You-A Listing ofPossible Symptoms, 6422
Sarcoidosis Awareness Foundation, 6362
Sarcoidosis Awareness Network, 6361
Sarcoidosis Center, 6375, 6394
Sarcoidosis Conference 2, 6382
Sarcoidosis Conference 3, 6383
Sarcoidosis Network Foundation, 6355
Sarcoidosis Networking, 6398
Sarcoidosis Patient Forum, 6372
A Sarcoidosis Questionnaire: Demographicsand Symptomatology-Patients
    Respond, 6399
Sarcoidosis Questionnaire: Demographicsand Symptomatology-The
    Patients Respond, 6420
Sarcoidosis Research Institute, 6356, 6377, 6395
Sarcoidosis Resource Guide and Directory, 6396
Sarcoidosis Resource Support Group, 6363
Sarcoidosis Self-Help, 6369
Sarcoidosis Support, 6370
Sarcoidosis Support - Beaumont, 6364
Sarcoidosis Support Group, 6359, 6367, 6373
Sarcoidosis Support Resource Central New Jersey, 6365
Sarcoidosis-International Review, 6423
Sarcoidosis-Pleural InvolvementMimicking a Coin Lesson, 6424
Sarcoidosis-What's That?, 6385
Sarcoidosis: A Multisystem Disease, 6425
Sarcoidosis: Usual and UnusualManifestations, 6426
Save Babies Through Screening Foundation, 3211, 4214, 4434, 8659
SBA National Conference, 6868
SBAA General Information Brochure, 6904
SBAA General Information Packet, 6905
SC Dept. of Health & Environmental ControlImmunization Division, 5982
Scalp Psoriasis, 6058
Schedules of Development for HearingImpaired Infants and Their Parents,
    3812
Schizophrenia, 1651, 1663

Schizophrenia and Comorbid ConditionsDiagnosis and Treatment, 1654
Schizophrenia Fact Sheet, 1664
Schizophrenia Into Later Life: Treatment,Research, and Policy, 1652
Schizophrenia Revealed: From Neurons toSocial Interactions, 1653
Schizophrenia Support Organizations, 1637
Schizophrenia.com, 1638
Schizophrenia.com Home Page, 1639
Schizophrenia: Handbook for Families, 1640
Schizophrenics Anonymous Forum, 1618
Schneider Children's Hospital of LongIsland, 2313
School Based Assessment of Attention Deficit Disorders, 700
School Days, 3708
School Days: An ASL Word Book, 3709
School Personnel: A Critical Link in theIdentification and Management of OCD, 5396
School Planning, 6589
School Screening with Dr. Robert Keller, 6483
The School-Aged Child, 1711
School-Aged Guide of the Life StagesProgram, 7549
Science, Math, 3661
Scizophrenia in a Molecular Age, 1655
Scleroderma, 6431
Scleroderma A to Z, 6455
Scleroderma Book (The), 6463
Scleroderma Care and Research, 6465
Scleroderma Foundation, 6437, 6456
Scleroderma Foundation Chicago Chapter, 6439
Scleroderma Foundation Evergreen Chapter, 6446
Scleroderma Foundation Greater WashingtonDC Chapter, 6445
Scleroderma Foundation Nevada Chapter, 6440
Scleroderma Foundation New Jersey Chapter, 6441
Scleroderma Foundation Southeast FloridaChapter, 6438
Scleroderma Foundation Texas Bluebonnet Chapter, 6444
Scleroderma Foundation Tri-State, Inc (NY, NJ, CT), 6442
Scleroderma Message Board, 6457
Scleroderma Research Foundation, 6449
Scleroderma Support, 6458
Scleroderma Voice, 6464
Scoliosis, 6469
Scoliosis and Kyphosis, 6521
Scoliosis Association, 6474
Scoliosis Help, 6494
Scoliosis Message Forum, 6495
Scoliosis Research Society, 6476, 6496
Scoliosis Surgery, The Definitive Patient's Reference: Second Edition, 6503
Scoliosis: A Handbook for Patients, 6522
Scoliosis: What Young People and Parents Need to Know, 6504
Scope (UK), 1509
Scottish Rite Centers for Childhood Language Disorders, 6782
Screening for Down Syndrome, 2744
Screening for Hearing Loss and Other Otitis Media, 5484
Screening for Hearing Loss and Otitis Media in Children, 3813
Screening for Mental Health, 2879
SE Pennsylvania Chapter of Asthma andAllergy Foundation of America, 439
Seal Out Tooth Decay, 7323
SEARCH, 1272
Search Beyond Adventures, 8780
A Season of Change, 3721
Seasonal Affective Disorder, 2499
Seasonal Clustering of Sarcoidosis, 6427
Seattle Area Support Group, 552
SEE Center for the Advancement of Deaf Children, 3541
See What I Feel, 1900, 2050, 5274, 6203
Seeking Techniques Advancing Research inShunts (STARS), 4242
Seizure First Aid, 6561
Seizures, 6525
Seizures and Epilepsy In Childhood: A Guide, 6590
Seizures and Epilepsy: Hope Through Research, 6612
Seizures, Epilepsy and Your Child, 6613
Selecting a Program, 1923, 2076, 5295, 6224
Selective Mutism Foundation, 5582, 6733
Self Help for Hard of Hearing PeopleHearing Loss Association of America, 3542
Self-Control Games & Workbook, 679
Self-Starvation: from Individual to FamilyTherapy in the Treatment of Anorexia Ne, 2960
A Sense of Belonging: Including Students with Autism in their School Community, 873

Sense of Belonging: Including Students with Autism in Their School Community, 889
Sensory Organs, 8856
SERGG Regional News, 575
Services for the Visually Disabled, 1857, 2003, 5235, 6163
Services to Families, 7191
7 Steps to Reducing the Risk of SIDS, 7082
Severe Chronic Neutropenia InternationalRegistry (SCNIR), 5087
Sexuality and the Person with Spinabifida, 6895
Sexuality Information and EducationCouncil of the US (SIECUS), 8062
SHAPE America: Society of Health andPhysical Educators, 8061
Shape Up America, 5330
SHARE National Headquarters, 6993
Sharing Scoliosis: You're Not Alone, 6484
Shattered Dreams - Lonely Choices: BirthParents of Babies with Disabilities, 2745
Shawnee Library System, 8476
Shelley The Hyperactive Turtle, 680
Short and OK, 3263
Shot At Life, 5951
Shots For Tots, 5952
Show Me No Mercy: Compelling Story ofRemarkable Courage, 2746
Shriner's Hospital Research Study Report, 5458
Shriners Hospital for Children, 6477
Shriners Hospitals for Children, 5765, 7128
Shy Children, Phobic Adults: Nature andTreatment of Social Phobia, 5614, 6745
Sibling Abuse Survivors' Information & Advocacy Network, 5705
Sibling Donor Cord Blood Program Pamphlet, 7292
Sibling Forum, 8686
Sibling Support Project, 8063
Sick and Tired of Feeling Sick and Tired, 7154
Sickle Cell Association of Austin - MarcThomas Chapter, 6645
Sickle Cell Association of the Texas GulfCoast, 6646
Sickle Cell Council of New Mexico, Inc., 6638
Sickle Cell Disease, 6624, 6668
Sickle Cell Disease Association of America, 6630, 6634, 6643, 6661
Sickle Cell Disease Association of thePiedmont, 6640
Sickle Cell Disease Forum, 6662
Sickle Cell Disease Foundation ofCalifornia, 6633
Sickle Cell Foundation of Georgia, 6635
Sickle Cell Foundation of GreaterMontgomery, 6632
Sickle Cell Information Center, 6631
Sickle Cell Kids, 6663
Sickle Cell Regional Network, 6641
SID Network, 7089
Sidelines-National High Risk Pregnancy Support Network, 5905
Sidney R. Baer Day Camp, 8782
Sidran Institute - Traumatic Stress Education & Advocacy, 5800
SIDS Educational Services, 6994
SIDS Information & Counseling - Divisionof Public Health, 7005
SIDS Information & Counseling ProgramAlaska Department of Health, 6997
SIDS Information and Referral Hotline, 6995
SIDS LEAD - Children's Special Health CareServices, 7029
SIDS Northwest Regional Center, 7065
SIDS Nursing Intervention Program, 7030
SIDS Prevention, 7112
SIDS Research, 7095
SIDS Resource of Oregon, 7050
SIDS Resources, 7034
SIDS Survival Guide, 7096
SIDS: A Parents Guide to Understanding &Preventing SIDS, 7097
SIDS: Toward Prevention and ImprovedInfant Health, 7113
Sight for Students - Vision Service Plan, 4468
Sight Lines, 6312
Sign Fine - Vacations, 3710
Sign Language for Babies, 3814
Sign Numbers, 3815
Sign Songs: Fun Songs to Sign and Sing, 3662
Sign With Kids Supplement, 3816
Sign With Your Baby-Complete Learning Kit, 3663
Sign-Me-Fine, 3817
Significant Event Childhood Trauma, 5792
Signing Exact English Using Affixes, 3818
Signing Family: What Every Parent Should Know About Sign Communication, 3819
Signing Fun: American Sign Language Vocabulary, Phrases, Games and Activities, 3820
Signing Naturally, 3664
Signing: How to Speak With Your Hands, Second Edition, 3821

Signs for Me, 3822

Signs for Me: Basic Sign Vocabulary for Children, Parents and Teachers, 3823

Signs for Me: Basic Sign Vocabulary forChildren, Parents, & Teachers, 3871, 3892

Signs of Sharing: An Elementary SignLanguage and Deaf Awareness Curriculum, 3824

Silent Garden, 3825

Silent Observer, 3826

Simple Signs, 3827

Simser Series, 3711

Since Owen, 2747

Sinergia/Metropolitan Parent Center, 8346

Sioux Valley Hospital, South DakotaCystic Fibrosis Center, 2332

Six-Sound Song, 3828

Skeletal System, 8857

Ski for Light, 8064

Skills Training for Children with BehaviorDisorders, 1797, 7746

Skin Page, 6033

Slack, 4152

Slack Incorporated, 6000

SLE Lupus Foundation, 7141

Sleep Apnea, 6672, 6697

Sleep Center, Community General Hospital, 4910

Sleep Disorder Center, St Elizabeth Medical Center, 4896

Sleep Disorders, 4951, 5117, 5142

Sleep Disorders and Psychiatry, 4956, 5120, 5146

Sleep Disorders Center, 6679

Sleep Disorders Center for Children, 4936

Sleep Disorders Center of Lifespan Hospitals, 4935

Sleep Disorders Center of Western New YorkMillard Fillmore Hospital, 4911

Sleep Disorders Center, UniversityHospital, 4912

Sleep Disorders Center-Good SamaritanHospital, 4897

Sleep Disorders Sourcebook, 4955, 6692, 6714

Sleep Disorders Unit, Beth Israel Hospital, 4900

Sleep Laboratory, Maine Medical Center, 4941

Sleep Medicine Associates of Texas, 4937

Sleep Research Society, 5109

Sleep Walking in Children, 6710

Sleep-Wake Disorders Center, MontefioreSleep Disorders Center, 4913

Sleep-Wake Disorders Center, New YorkPresbyterian Hospital, 4914

Sleep/Wake Disorders Center, HampsteadHospital, 4904

Sleep/Wake Disorders Center-Community Health Network, 4898

Sleep: The Brazelton Way, 6715

Sleepdisorders.com, 5118, 5143, 6686, 6712

SleepEducation.com, 6711

Sleeping Beauty, 3665

Sleeping Like a Baby, 6693

Sleepnet.com, 6687

Sleepwalking, 6698

SMA Newsletter, 6936

SMA Research Group, 6926

SMA Support Inc, 6923

Smile, 3712

Smoking and Sudden Infant Death Syndrome, 7098

Smooth Sailing, 2536

Snap! Kids American Sign Language, 3713

Snoring and Sleep Apnea, 6695

Snoring From A to Zzzz, 5121, 5147, 6694, 6716

The Snowman, 3676

So You Have Had An Ear Operation...WhatNext?, 3893

Social Anxiety Association, 5583, 6734

Social Anxiety Disorder, 6717

Social Development and the Person WithSpina Bifida, 6906

Social Skills Development in Children withHydrocephalus, 4287

Social Skills Picture Book, 951

Society for Adolescent Medicine, 8660

Society for Autistic Children, 767

Society for Endocrinology, 3260, 5895

Society for Mucopolysaccharide Diseases, 4818

Society for NeuroOncology, 1117

Society for Pediatric Dermatology, 184, 204, 1319, 1329, 1575, 1590, 2984, 2999, 3921, 4368, 4421, 5528, 5628, 5742, 7205, 7214, 7259, 7662, 8065

Society for Pediatric Dermatology Annual Meeting, 2989, 3007

Society for Pediatric Dermatology AnnualMeeting, 191, 1320, 1584, 3922

Society for Rehabilitation, 8367

Society for the Rehabilitation of theFacially Disfigured Inc., 4591

Society of Behavioral Sleep Medicine, 5110

Solution Outreach Center at OCCK, Inc., 8486

Solving Behavior Problems in Autism, 952

Something Fishy, 2928

Something Happened and I'm Scared to Tell, 5712

Sometimes I'm Mad, Sometimes I'm Glad - ASibling Booklet, 5876

Son-Rise: The Miracle Continues, 953

Song of Superman, 4052

Songs for Listening! Songs for Life!, 3714

Songs in Sign, 3829

Sontag Foundation, 1118

Soul Murder Revisited, 5713

Sound & Fury, 3666

Sound and Fury: Six Years Later, 3667

South Bay Brain Tumor Support Group, 1141

South Carolina Chapter of Crohn's &Colitis Foundation of America, 2183

South Carolina Department of Health &Environmental Control - SIDS Information, 7054

South Carolina State Library, 8536

South Central Kansas Library System, 8487

South Central Los Angeles Regional Centerfor Devlopmentally Disabled Persons, 8130

South Central Region-Helen Keller NationalCenter, 8409

South Dakota Center For Bleeding Disorders, 4034

South Dakota Department of Health, 5983, 7055

South Dakota Parent Connection, 8398

South Dakota State Library, 8537

South Florida Brain Tumor AssociationLynn Regional Cancer Center, 1161

South Texas Comprehensive Hemophilia andThrombophilia Treatment Center, 4035

Southeast Pennsylvania Support Group, 547

Southeast Regional Genetics Group, 521

Southeastern Brain Tumor Foundation BrainTumor Support Group, 1166

Southeastern Region-Helen Keller NationalCenter, 6125

Southern California Pediatric Brain TumorNetwork, 1142

Southern IL Child and Family Connections, 8204

Southern Illinois University School ofMedicine, 289, 594, 1740, 5517, 6092, 6110, 7236, 7491, 7669, 8661

Southern Nevada 'Grey Matters' ValleyHospital Medical Center, 1212

Southwest Chapter of Crohn's & ColitisFoundation of America, 2168

Southwest Human Development, 8098

Southwest Ohio Brain Tumor Support Group, 1233

Southwest Ohio Chapter of Crohn's &Colitis Foundation of America, 2179

Southwest SIDS Research Institute, 7078

Southwestern Comprehensive Sickle Cell Center, 6656

Southwestern Ohio Chapter of the NationalHemophilia Foundation, 3972

Sparrow Foundation, 8066

Spaulding for Children, 8067

Speak Easy International Foundation, 6958

Speak to Me (Second Edition), 3830

Special Care Dentistry Association, 2427

Special Connections Family Resource Center, 8131

Special Education ActionCommittee Huntsville Outreach Office, 8084

Special Education Administration Kansas State Department of Education, 8234

Special Education Center of Hawaii, 3379

Special Education Division, 8357

Special Education Division StateDepartment of Education, 8132

Special Education Office, 8371

Special Education Office State Departmentof Education, 8309

Special Education Programs - U.S. Dept. ofEducation Office of Special Ed Programs, 8410

Special Education Section State Departmentof Education, 8106

Special Education Services, 8085

Special Education Services Unit, 8414

Special Education Unit, 8333, 8421, 8444

Special Interest Group on Phobias andRelated Anxiety Disorders (SIGPRAD), 5584, 6735

Special Kids Make Special Friends, 2748

A Special Love, 2711

Special Needs Advocate for Parents (SNAP), 8068

Special Needs Branch Department ofEducation, 8184

Special Needs Center/Phoenix PublicLibrary, 8446

Special Needs Library of NE GeorgiaAthens-Clarke County Regional Library, 8468

Special Needs Parent Info Network, 8249

Special Olympics, 8069

Special Parent Involvement Network, 8239

Special Services Division - Indiana StateLibrary, 8482

Specialized Training of Military Parents(STOMP), 8070

Specific Classroom Strategies and Techniques for Students with TS-2nd Edition, 7460

Specific Forms of Psoriasis, 6059
Spectrum Brain Tumor Support Group, 1199
Spectrum Health Research, 4036
Speech and Deafness Newsletter, 3872
Speech and Hearing Clinic, 6777
Speech and the Hearing Impaired Child(Second Edition), 3831
Speech Impairment, 6750
Speech, Language, & Hearing CenterUniversity of Colorado, 6960
Speech, Language, and Hearing Center, 6785
Speechreading: A Way to ImproveUnderstanding, 3832
Speechreading: Methods and Materials, 3894
Spina Bifida, 6806
Spina Bifida Association, 4258, 6816
Spina Bifida Association of Alabama, 6817
Spina Bifida Association of Albany/CapitalDistrict, 6844
Spina Bifida Association of America, 6876
Spina Bifida Association of Arkansas, 6819
Spina Bifida Association of Canton, 6849
Spina Bifida Association of Central Florida, 6824
Spina Bifida Association of Central Indiana, 6830
Spina Bifida Association of Central Ohio, 6850
Spina Bifida Association of Chesapeake-Potomac, 6835
Spina Bifida Association of Cincinnati, 6851
Spina Bifida Association of Colorado, 6822
Spina Bifida Association of Connecticut, 6823
Spina Bifida Association of DelawareValley, 6856
Spina Bifida Association of Georgia, 6828
Spina Bifida Association of Greater Bay Area, 6820
Spina Bifida Association of Greater Dayton, 6852
Spina Bifida Association of Greater FoxValley, 6865
Spina Bifida Association of Greater NewOrleans, 6834
Spina Bifida Association of Greater Pennsylvania, 6857
Spina Bifida Association of Greater Rochester, 6845
Spina Bifida Association of Greater SaintLouis, 6841
Spina Bifida Association of Greater San Diego, 6821
Spina Bifida Association of Houston-GulfCoast, 6859
Spina Bifida Association of Illinois, 6829
Spina Bifida Association of Iowa, 6832
Spina Bifida Association of Jacksonville Nemours Childrens Clinic, 6825
Spina Bifida Association of Kentucky, 6833
Spina Bifida Association of Massachusetts, 6836
Spina Bifida Association of Minnesota, 6839
Spina Bifida Association of Mississippi, 6840
Spina Bifida Association of Nassau County, 6846
Spina Bifida Association of Nebraska, 6842
Spina Bifida Association of North Carolina, 6848
Spina Bifida Association of North Texas, 6860
Spina Bifida Association of North WestOhio, 6853
Spina Bifida Association of NorthernWisconsin, 6831, 6866
Spina Bifida Association of SoutheastFlorida, 6826
Spina Bifida Association of Tampa Bay, 6827
Spina Bifida Association of Tennessee, 6858
Spina Bifida Association of Texas, 6861
Spina Bifida Association of the RoanokeValley, 6863
Spina Bifida Association of the Tri-StateRegion, 6843
Spina Bifida Association of Tri-CountyOhio, 6854
Spina Bifida Association of UpperPeninsula Michigan, 6837
Spina Bifida Association of Utah, 6862
Spina Bifida Association of West Michigan, 6838
Spina Bifida Association of Western NewYork, 6847
Spina Bifida Association of Wisconsin, 6867
Spina Bifida Association Pittsburgh, 6855
SPINAbilities: A Young Person's Guide toSpina Bifida, 6894
Spinal Connection, 6510
Spinal Muscular Atrophies, 6911
Spinal Muscular Atrophy Clinic, 6927
Spinal Muscular Atrophy Coalition (SMA Coalition), 6918
Spinal Muscular Atrophy Foundation, 6919
Spinal Muscular Atrophy Information Page, 6932
Spinal Muscular Atrophy Project, 6928, 6933
Spondylitis Association of America, 254
Springfield Area Support Group, 536
Squirrel Hollow, 996, 4550
Standing on My Own Two Feet, 1924, 2077, 5296, 6225
Stanford CF Center, 2258
Stanford University Center for Narcolepsy, 4891
The Stanley Medical Research Institute, 2475
Star Center for Family Health, 8510
Star-G: Screening, Technology and Research in Genetics, 5555
Starbright, 8071
Starlight Children's Foundation, 8133

Starting Point: To Connect with Resources Related to Pediatric Neuro-oncology, 1264
Starving to Death in a Sea of Objects, 2961
State Board of Education Department ofSpecial Education, 8205
State Department of Education, 8159
State University College at PlattsburghAuditory Research Laboratory, 3573
State University Hospital/Upstate MedicalUniversity, 2314
State University of New York HealthSciences Center, 855, 865
Statewide Parent Advocacy Network, 8329
Statewide Services for Deaf and Hard ofHearing People, 3895
Statewide SIDS Program - IllinoisDepartment of Public Health, 7014
Statewide Technology Access & ResponseSystem for Alabamians with Disabilities, 8086
Steele Children's Research Center, 4037
STEP (Support & Training for ExceptionalParents), 8402
Steps to Independence: Teaching EverydaySkills to Children with Special Needs, 6896
Stereotactic Radiosurgery, 1290
Stop Child Abuse Now, 5706
Stop It Now! (DBA Child Sex Abuse Prevention & Protection, 5668
StopBullying.gov, 7734
Stopping Scoliosis, 6505
Stories About Growing Up, 3668
Strabismus, 4483, 6939
Straight Talk about Psychological Testingfor Kids, 2798
Straight Talk on Stuttering: Information,Encouragement, and Counsel, 6965
Stress and Coping in Autism, 954
Stress Reduction Tapes, Stress ReductionClinic, 8605
Stroke Rehabilitation & Traumatic BrainInjury Research, 3434
Student Study Guide to A Basic Course in American Sign Language, 3833
Student with Prader-Willi Syndrome - Information for Educators, 5886
Students Supporting Brain Tumor Research, 1119
Sturge-Weber Syndrome: A Resource Guidefor a Reason, a Season and a Lifetime, 3927
Stutter No More, 6966
Stuttering, 6950
Stuttering Foundation of America, 6959
Stuttering Foundation of America Newsletter, 6967
Subacute Sclerosing Panencephalitis (SSPE), 6970
Subregional Library for the Blind andPhysically Handicapped, 8469
Substance Abuse and Mental Health ServicesAdministration, 2833
Suburban Audio Visual Service, 8477
A Success Story, 1367
The Successful Parent, 7735
Successful Treatment of MyocardialSarcoidosis with Steriods, 6428
Sudden Arrhythmia Death Syndromes Foundation, 317
Sudden Death in Infancy, Childhood &Adolescence, 7099
Sudden Death of Young Athletes Can BePrevented (Hypertrophic Cardiomyopathy), 4302
Sudden Infant Death Syndrome, 6980
Sudden Infant Death Syndrome (SIDS)Network, 7070
Sudden Infant Death Syndrome Institute ofThe University of Maryland, 7079
Sudden Infant Death Syndrome Risk Factors, 7100
Suicide Awareness Voices of Education, 2473
Suicide Prevention Resource Center, 2474
Suicide, Why?, 2524
Summer Experience, 397, 997, 4551
Summer Wheelchair Sports Camp, 8741
Summit Camp, 398
Sun and Water Therapy, 6060
Suncoast Residential TrainingCenter/Developmental Services Program, 1622, 5371
Sunshine for HIV Kids, 3333
Sunshine Foundation, 8837
SUNY Upstate Medical University ResearchDevelopment, 4033
Superstuff, 492
Support and Educational Exchange forKlinefelter Syndrome, 4443
Support for Asthmatic Youth (SAY) SupportGroups, 427
Support for Asthmatic Youth Pals-Pen Pals, 428
Support for Children with AIDS, 3314
Support for Families of Children withDisabilities, 8134
Support for Parents of Children with BrainTumors, Siblings and Young Adults, 1224
Support Group for Caregivers of BrainTumor Patients, 1143
Support Group for Parents of Children withBrain Tumors, 1144
Support Group for Parents of Childrenwith a Brain Tumor, 1234
Support Group Listing, 6429
Support Organization for Trisomy 18, 13,and Related Disorders (SOFT), 7377, 7501, 7511
Surgery for Epilepsy, 6614

Surprising Truth About Depression: MedicalBreakthroughs That Can Work, 2525
Survival Skills for the Family Unit, 4288
Surviving an Eating Disorder, 2962
Surviving Childhood Cancer: A Guide forFamilies, 111, 164, 4197, 5078, 5179, 6293, 7808
Surviving Coma: the Journey Back, 3443
Surviving Schizophrenia: A Manual forFamilies, Consumers and Providers, 1656
Surviving the Death of a Baby, 7114
SW Michican Spina Bifida & HydrocephalusAssociation, 4231
Sweeney, 2618
Sydenham Chorea Information Page, 1679
Syncope, 7115
Syncope Information Page, 7121
Syndactyly, 7122, 7132
Syndromes Associated with Multiple Congenital Anomalies, 559
Syracuse University, Institute for SensoryResearch, 3574
Systemic Lupus Erythematosus, 7133

T

T-FFED (Trans Folx Fighting Eating Disorders), 2880
Tactic, 1911, 2063, 5285, 6213
TAG Conference, 7272
TAG Newsletter, 7288
Take Charge, 2203
Taking Autism to School, 955
Taking Charge of ADHD: The Complete,Authoritative Guide for Parents, 681
Taking the Mystery Out of SpinalDeformities, 6485
Talisman Programs, 8803
Talisman Summer Camps, 1803, 7771
Talk About Curing Autism, 768
Talk About Sleep, 4952
Talk to Me, 1925, 2078, 5297, 6226
Talk to Me II, 1926, 2079, 5298, 6227
Talking Back to OCD: The Program That HelpKids & Teens Say No Way, 5397
Talking Book Center of NorthwestIllinois, 1852, 1998, 5231, 6159
Talking Book Library at Worcester PublicLibrary, 8506
Talking Book Library, Jacksonville PublicLibrary, 1842, 1988, 5221, 6149
Talking Book Service - Manatee CountyCentral Library, 1843, 1989, 5222, 6150
Talking Book Topics, 1915, 2066, 5287, 6216
Talking Books - National Library Service, 4470
Talking Finger Series - At Grandma's House, 3834
Talking Finger Series - Little Green Monster, 3835
Talking to Your Doctor About SeizureDisorders, 6615
Tampa Bay Area Brain Tumor Support Group, 1162
Tampa Support Group, 517
Tap the Best Resource, 4780
Tay-Sachs & Sandhoff Disease, 7192
Tay-Sachs Disease, 7157, 7185
Tay-Sachs Disease-A Bibliography, MedicalDictionary, & Annotated Research Guide, 7186
TB Skin Test, 7535
TB: What You Should Know, 7536
TBI Challenge, 3466
TBI Support Group for Families & Survivors, 3371
Teach Your Tot to Sign, 3836
Teacher's Guide to Crohn's Disease &Ulcerative Colitis, 2213, 7654
Teacher's Guide to Neuromuscular Disease, 4875
Teacher's Handbook for the Student with PWS (Educator's Resource), 5877
Teaching Children with Autism to Mind-ReadA Pratical Guide for Teachers & Parents, 956
Teaching Coversations to Children WithAutism: Scripts and Script Fading, 957
Teaching Motor Skills to Children with Cerebral Palsy & Similar Movement Disorders, 1530
Teaching Students with Spina Bifida, 6897
Teaching the Tiger, 682, 5398, 7345, 7443
Team Advocates for Special Kids, Anaheim, 8135
Team Advocates for Special Kids, San Diego, 8136
Team of Advocates for Special Kids, 8573
TECH 2000 Project-Michigan DisabilityRights Coalition, 8273
Tech Connection, 8072
Tech-Able, 8470

TechACCESS of Rhode Island, 8534
Technical Assistance Partnership for Childand Family Mental Health, 1777, 7707
Technology Access Center, 8511
Technology Access Center of MiddleTennessee, 8403
Technology Access Center of Tucson, 8447
Technology Access for Life Needs Project, 8376
Technology and Youth - Protecting YourChild, 7760
Technology Assistance for SpecialConsumers, 8073
Technology Assistance Program, 8257, 8334
Technology Partnership Project Instituteon Disability/UAP, 8323
Technology Resource Center, 8528
Techspress Resource Center forIndependent Living, 8523
Ted R. Montoya Hemophilia Program, 4038
Teddi Project, 8838
Teens and Tourette Syndrome, 7462
Teens Talk to Teens About Asthma, 493
TEF/VATER International Support Network, 3101
Telangiectasia, 7195
Telecommunications for the Deaf, 3543
Telecommunications for the Deaf and Hard of Hearing, 3544
Temple University, Section of AuditoryResearch, 3576
Ten Things Every Child With Autism WishesYou Know, 958
Ten Years to Live, 569
Tennesse Hemophilia & Bleeding DisordersFoundation, 3979
Tennessee Chapter of Crohn's &Colitis Foundation of America, 2184
Tennessee Department of HealthImmunization, 5984
Tennessee Saving Little Hearts, 4329
Tennessee SIDS Program, 7056
Teratogen and Birth Defects InformationProject, 8574
Territorial Apprehensiveness (TERRAP)Programs, 5585
Tetanus and Diptheria Vaccine, 6009
Tetralogy of Fallot, 7222
Texas Assistive Technology Partnership, 8411
Texas Association of Retinitis Pigmentosa, 6263
Texas Association on Mental Retardation, 2676
Texas Central Chapter of the NationalHemophilia Foundation, 3981
Texas Children's Cancer Center, 4183
Texas Children's Hospital, 3079
Texas Department of Health - SIDSInformation and Counseling Program, 7060
Texas Department oF HealthImmunization Division, 5985
Texas Heart Institute Journal, 324
Texas Heart to Heart, 4331
Texas Lions Camp, 1935, 2086, 3911, 8817
Texas Perinatal Association, 5907
Texas Prader-Willi Syndrome Association, 5855
Texas State Library, 8541
Textbook of Psoriasis, 6037
Thalassemia Action Group (TAG) Patient Support Group Brochure, 7293
Thalassemias, 7238
Thalassemias Action Group (TAG), 7260, 7279
Therapeutic Strategies for OI: A Guide for Physical and Occupational Therapists, 5470
There are Solutions for the Student with Asthma, 494
There's an S on My Back: S is for Scoliosis, 6506
They're Just Kids, 8606
Things To Avoid During Pregnancy, 3165
Things to Consider, 6061
This Is Mr. TB Germ, 7537
Thomas Jefferson University Brain InjuryRehabilitation Program, 3437
Thomas Jefferson University SleepDisorders Center, 4933
Thorpe Camp, 4728
3D Vision, 4472
Thrombocytopenias, 7295
Thumbsucking, 7310
Thumpers, 4328
Thursday's Child, 8839
Thyroid Federation International, 4355
Thyroid Foundation of America, 4350
Thyroid Society for Education andResearch, 4351
Tick-Borne Disease Alliance, 4614
Tics, 7324
Tics and Tourette's Syndrome Fact Sheet, 7350
Tidewater Center for Technology Access, 8426
TIES, The Children's Hospital, 8572
Tik-A-Witha, 8781
Timbertop Nature Adventure Camp, 8828
TIPS: Talipes Information and ParentalSupport, 1724
Tlane Cancer Center, 1184

TMA Annual Patient Conference, 1585

To Be Me: Understanding What It's Like toHave Asperger's Syndrome, 389

To Give An Edge: A Guide for New Parentsof Children with Down's Syndrome, 2749

Toddlers and Preschoolers, 1712

Together...There Is Hope, 560

Toilet Training for Individuals withAutism and Related Disorders, 960

Tool Box of Hope - For When Your Body Doesn't Feel Good, 5878

Tools for Life Division of RehabilitationServices, 8180

Toothpick, 2367

TOPS Club, 2881

Touch of Nature Environmental Center, 8742

Touched with Fire-Manic DepressiveIllness & the Artistic Temperament, 1070

Touching Tree, 5377

Tourette Syndrome, 7351

Tourette Syndrome and Human Behavior, 7444

Tourette Syndrome and the School Nurse, 7464

Tourette Syndrome and the SchoolPsychologist, 7463

Tourette Syndrome and Tic Disorder Clinic, 7413

Tourette Syndrome Association, 7434

Tourette Syndrome Association - ArizonaChapter, 7383

Tourette Syndrome Association - GreaterNew York State Chapter, 7396, 7402

Tourette Syndrome Association - HudsonValley Chapter, 7403

Tourette Syndrome Association - LongIsland Chapter, 7404

Tourette Syndrome Association - Maine/NewHampshire Chapter, 7392

Tourette Syndrome Association - MinnesotaChapter, 7395

Tourette Syndrome Association - New MexicoChapter, 7400

Tourette Syndrome Association - New YorkCity Chapter, 7405

Tourette Syndrome Association - NorthernCalifornia/Hawaii Chapter, 7384, 7389

Tourette Syndrome Association - RockyMountain Region, 7386, 7397, 7398, 7412

Tourette Syndrome Association - Southern California Chapter, 7385

Tourette Syndrome Association - UtahChapter, 7410

Tourette Syndrome Association - Washingtonand Oregon Chapter, 7407, 7411

Tourette Syndrome Association -Greater Rochester and Finger Lakes Area, 7387, 7401

Tourette Syndrome Association of Florida, 7388

Tourette Syndrome Association of GreaterWashington, 7393

Tourette Syndrome Association of Illinois, 7390

Tourette Syndrome Association of Indiana, 7391

Tourette Syndrome Association of New Jersey, 7399

Tourette Syndrome Association of Ohio, 7406

Tourette Syndrome Association of RhodeIsland, 7409

Tourette Syndrome Association ofMassachusetts, 7394

Tourette Syndrome Camp Organization, 711, 5404, 7466

Tourette Syndrome Online, 7341

Tourette Syndrome: The Facts, 7445

Tourette's Syndrome, 7446

Tourette's Syndrome - Tics, Obsession, Compulsions: Developmental Psychopathology, 7346

Tourettes Syndrome Online, 7435

Toxoplasmosis, 7467

Toxoplasmosis Fact Sheet, 7476, 7477

Train 4 Autism, 773

Train-Ohio Super Computer Center, 8368

Transposition of the Great Arteries, 7478

TransWeb, 8663

Traumatic Brain Injury Model Systems National Data and Statistical Center, 3451

Traumatic Incident Reduction Association, 5788

Travis:I Got Lots of Neat StuffChildren Living with Muscular Dystrophy, 4846

The Treasure Chest, 3677

Treasure Chest of Behavioral Strategiesfor Individuals with Autism, 961

Treasure Valley Brain Injury Support Group, 1168

Treating Abused and Traumatized Children, 5714

Treating Bulimia: A PsychoeducationalApproach, 2963

Treating Depressed Children, 2526

Treating Depression, 2527

Treating IBD, 2201

Treating IBD: A Patient's Guide to theMedical and Surgical Management, 7645

Treating Psychological Trauma and PTSD, 5807

Treating the Headache Patient, 4763

Treating Trauma & Traumatic Grief in Children and Adolescents, 5808

Treatment of Children with Mental Disorder, 1800, 7765

Tri-Services Military CF Center, 2339

Tri-State Bleeding Disorders Chapter ofthe National Hemophilia Foundation, 3973

Tri-State Sleep Disorders CenterCenter for Research in Sleep Disorders, 4943

Tri-State Support Group, 540

TRIAD Project-Advocates for Persons withDisabilities, 8347

Triangle D Camp for Children, 8825

A Tribute to PWS Children from Around theWorld, 5861

TRIP Database, 8662

Trisomy 13 Syndrome, 7505

Trisomy 18 Foundation, 7378, 7414, 7502, 7503

Trisomy 18 Syndrome, 7494

Troll In A Bowl: Games and Card Print Factory, 3716

Trouble with Secrets, 5715

TS International, 7547

TS: A Look at the Interface BetweenTourette Syndrome and the Law, 7461

Tuberculosis, 7514

Tuberous Sclerosis, 7538

Tuberous Sclerosis Alliance, 7379, 7544

Tuberous Sclerosis: 3rd Edition, 7550

Tuberous Sclerosis: Fact Sheet, 7553

Tufts New England Medical CenterFloating Hospital for Children, 2288

Tug McGraw Foundation, 1120

Tulane University Clinical ImmunologySection, 450

Tulane University, US-Japan BiomedicalResearch Laboratories, 3427

Tulsa City-County Library System, 8530

Turner Syndrome, 7554

Turner's Syndrome, 7612

Turner's Syndrome News, 7607

Turner's Syndrome Society - Tampa SupportGroup, 7568

Turner's Syndrome Society of Alaska, 7562

Turner's Syndrome Society of Arizona, 7563

Turner's Syndrome Society of CentralNew York, 7583

Turner's Syndrome Society of Connecticut, 7567

Turner's Syndrome Society of Gulf Coast, 7573

Turner's Syndrome Society of Houston, 7593

Turner's Syndrome Society of InlandNorthwest, 7598

Turner's Syndrome Society of Iowa/NewFound Friends, 7571

Turner's Syndrome Society of Kentucky, 7572

Turner's Syndrome Society of Maryland, 7574

Turner's Syndrome Society of Mid-South, 7591

Turner's Syndrome Society of Minnesota, 7578

Turner's Syndrome Society of NationalCapitol Area, 7597

Turner's Syndrome Society of Nevada, 7580

Turner's Syndrome Society of New England, 7575

Turner's Syndrome Society of New Jersey, 7582

Turner's Syndrome Society of North Texas, 7594

Turner's Syndrome Society of NorthCarolina, 7585

Turner's Syndrome Society of Northern NewEngland, 7581

Turner's Syndrome Society of NorthernFlorida, 7569

Turner's Syndrome Society of Oklahoma, 7587

Turner's Syndrome Society of Philadelphia, 7588

Turner's Syndrome Society of Rhode Island, 7589

Turner's Syndrome Society of RockyMountain, 7566

Turner's Syndrome Society of Salt LakeCity, 7596

Turner's Syndrome Society of San Antonio, 7595

Turner's Syndrome Society of South Florida, 7570

Turner's Syndrome Society of SouthCarolina, 7590

Turner's Syndrome Society of SoutheasternWisconsin, 7576, 7599

Turner's Syndrome Society of SouthernCalifornia, 7565

Turner's Syndrome Society of SouthwesternOhio, 7586

Turner's Syndrome Society of St. Louis/West Illinois, 7579

Turner's Syndrome Society of Tennessee, 7592

Turner's Syndrome Society of the UnitedStates, 7606

Turner's Syndrome Society of the US, 7561

Turner's Syndrome Society of Upstate NewYork, 7584

Turner's Syndrome Society of West Michigan, 7577

Turner's Syndrome Society Resource Center, 7600

Turner's Syndrome Society ResourceBibliographies, 7613

Turner's Syndrome SocietyCentral And Northern, 7564

Turner's Syndrome: A Personal Perspective, 7614

Turner's Syndrome: Guide for Families, 7615

Turner's Syndrome: The Hows and Whys ofthe Missing X Chromosome, 7616

The Turners, 7335, 7426

Twelve Steps and Twelve Traditions of Overeaters Anonymous, 5345

Twelve Steps of Overeaters Anonymous, 2964

Twenty Years At Hull House, 6507

Two Worlds - One Planet, 890

22Q and You Center, 2620

25 Ways to Promote Spoken Language inYour Child with a Hearing Loss, 3874

U

UC Berkeley School of Social Welfare, 5136, 5587, 8575
UCD Hemophilia Treatment Center, 4039
UCP Newsletter, 1535
UCP of Greater Suffolk, 1463
UCP Washington Wire, 1536
UCSD Hemophilia Treatment Center, 4040
UIC Eye Center, 6257
Ulcerative Colitis, 59, 7617, 7655
Ulster County Social Services, 8348
The Ultimate ASL Dictionary, 3715
Un Curso Basico de Lenguaje Americano de Senas, 3846
UNC CF Center, 2317
Under the Microscope, 2204
Understanding and Treating Children withAutism, 962
Understanding and Treating Depression, 2500
Understanding and Treating the HereditaryPsychiatric Spectrum Disorders, 1782, 7712
Understanding Asthma, 483
Understanding Attention Deficit Disorder, 628
Understanding Autism, 891
Understanding Bullying - Fact Sheet, 7766
Understanding Childhood Obesity, 5346
Understanding Crohn Disease andUlcerative Colitis, 2202
Understanding Cystic Fibrosis, 2368
Understanding Dental Health, 2434
Understanding Depression, 2528
Understanding Down Syndrome, 2750
Understanding Glioblastoma Multiforme, 1291
Understanding Herpes, 4154, 4972
Understanding Hyperactivity, 629
Understanding Juvenile RheumatoidArthritis, 4399
Understanding Panic Disorder, 2546
Understanding SBS/Shaken Impact Syndrome Brochure, 5718
Understanding Schizophrenia, 1665
Understanding School Violence Fact Sheet, 7767
Understanding Scoliosis, 6486
Understanding Seizures & Epilepsy, 6562
Understanding Sickle Cell Disease, 6667
Understanding SMA, 6938
Understanding the Defiant Child, 1783, 7713
Understanding Your Child's Education Needs/Individualized Education Program Packet, 4289
Understanding Your Teenager's Depression, 2529
Understanding Youth Violence: Fact Sheet, 7768
UnderstandingPsoriasis.org by Healthology, 6034
United Brachial Plexus Network, 3077
United Cerebral Palsy Associations, 1391, 1510
United Cerebral Palsy Central PA, 1473
United Cerebral Palsy Land of Lincoln, 1432
United Cerebral Palsy Michigan, 1449
United Cerebral Palsy of Alabama, 1393
United Cerebral Palsy of Alaska/PARENTS, 1399
United Cerebral Palsy of Baton RougeMcMains Children's Developmental Center, 1441
United Cerebral Palsy of Berkshire County, 1447
United Cerebral Palsy of Central Arizona, 1400
United Cerebral Palsy of Central Arkansas, 1402
United Cerebral Palsy of Central California, 1403
United Cerebral Palsy of Central Florida, 1421
United Cerebral Palsy of Central Maryland, 1444
United Cerebral Palsy of Central Minnesota, 1451
United Cerebral Palsy of Central Ohio, 1467
United Cerebral Palsy of Cincinnati, 1468
United Cerebral Palsy of Delaware, 1418
United Cerebral Palsy of East CentralFlorida, 1422
United Cerebral Palsy of EasternConnecticut, 1415
United Cerebral Palsy of Florida, 1423
United Cerebral Palsy of Georgia, 1429
United Cerebral Palsy of Greater Chicago, 1433
United Cerebral Palsy of Greater Cleveland, 1469
United Cerebral Palsy of Greater DaneCounty, 1492
United Cerebral Palsy of Greater Hartford, 1416
United Cerebral Palsy of Greater Houston, 1486
United Cerebral Palsy of Greater Indiana, 1437

United Cerebral Palsy of Greater KansasCity, 1439, 1453
United Cerebral Palsy of Greater NewOrleans, 1442
United Cerebral Palsy of Greater St. Louis, 1454
United Cerebral Palsy of GreaterSacramento, 1394, 1404
United Cerebral Palsy of Hawaii, 1430
United Cerebral Palsy of Hudson County, 1457
United Cerebral Palsy of Huntsville &Tennessee Valley, 1395
United Cerebral Palsy of Idaho, 1431
United Cerebral Palsy of Illinois, 1434
United Cerebral Palsy of Kansas, 1440
United Cerebral Palsy of Los Angeles,Ventura and Santa Barbara Counties, 1405
United Cerebral Palsy of MetroBoston, 1448
United Cerebral Palsy of MetropolitanDallas, 1450, 1487
United Cerebral Palsy of Middle Tennessee, 1484
United Cerebral Palsy of Minnesota, 1452
United Cerebral Palsy of Mobile, 1396
United Cerebral Palsy of Nassau County, 1464
United Cerebral Palsy of Nebraska, 1456
United Cerebral Palsy of New York City, 1465
United Cerebral Palsy of North Carolina, 1466
United Cerebral Palsy of North Florida/Tender Loving Care, 1424
United Cerebral Palsy of NortheasternPennsylvania, 1443, 1474
United Cerebral Palsy of Northern, Central& Southern New Jersey, 1458
United Cerebral Palsy of Northwest Alabama, 1397
United Cerebral Palsy of Northwest Florida, 1425
United Cerebral Palsy of NorthwesternPennsylvania, 1475
United Cerebral Palsy of NorthwestMissouri, 1455
United Cerebral Palsy of Oklahoma, 1470
United Cerebral Palsy of Orange County, 1406
United Cerebral Palsy of Oregon & SWWashington, 1471
United Cerebral Palsy of Pennsylvania, 1476
United Cerebral Palsy of Philadelphia & Vicinity, 1477
United Cerebral Palsy of Pittsburgh, 1478
United Cerebral Palsy of Prince Georges &Montgomery Counties, 1445
United Cerebral Palsy of Rhode Island, 1482
United Cerebral Palsy of San Diego County, 1407
United Cerebral Palsy of San Joaquin,Calaveras & Amador Counties, 1408
United Cerebral Palsy of San Luis Obispo, 1409
United Cerebral Palsy of Santa Clara & SanMateo Counties, 1410
United Cerebral Palsy of Sarasota-Manatee, 1426
United Cerebral Palsy of South Carolina, 1483
United Cerebral Palsy of South CentralPennsylvania, 1479
United Cerebral Palsy of South Florida, 1427
United Cerebral Palsy of South Puget Sound, 1491
United Cerebral Palsy of SoutheasternWisconsin, 1493
United Cerebral Palsy of Southern Arizona, 1401
United Cerebral Palsy of Southern Illinois, 1435
United Cerebral Palsy of Southern Maryland, 1446
United Cerebral Palsy of SouthernConnecticut, 1417
United Cerebral Palsy of SouthwesternPennsylvania, 1480
United Cerebral Palsy of Stanislaus CountyStanislaus, 1411
United Cerebral Palsy of Tampa Bay, 1428
United Cerebral Palsy of Texas, 1488
United Cerebral Palsy of the Golden State, 1412
United Cerebral Palsy of the Inland Empire, 1413
United Cerebral Palsy of the Mid-South, 1485
United Cerebral Palsy of the North Bay, 1414
United Cerebral Palsy of the Wabash Valley, 1438
United Cerebral Palsy of Utah, 1489
United Cerebral Palsy of Washington DC &Northern Virginia, 1419
United Cerebral Palsy of Washington DC& Northern Virginia, 1490
United Cerebral Palsy of West Alabama, 1398
United Cerebral Palsy of West CentralWisconsin, 1494
United Cerebral Palsy of WesternPennsylvania, 1481
United Cerebral Palsy of Will County, 1436
United Cerebral Palsy Research andEducational Foundation, 1497
United Health Services Blood DisorderCenter, 4042
United Leukodystrophy Foundation, 4570
United Liver Foundation, 4429, 7819
United Network for Organ Sharing, 7380, 7486, 7492
United Ostomy Association, 4162, 4169
United Ostomy Association Hotline, 7626
United Services, 8296
United Virginia Chapter of the NationalHemophilia Foundation, 3984
Unity Sleep Disorders ClinicUnity Health System, 4915
Univ. of Texas-Southwestern Med. Ctr. at Dallas - Clinical Ctr. for Liver Disease, 1019
University Affiliated Program, School ofMedicine, 8399
University Alabama Birmingham, 4663

University Center for the Development of Language & Literacy, 6786

University of Alabama - Birmingham Arthritis Clinical Intervention Program, 6447

University of Alabama Speech and HearingCenter, 3552

University of Alaska, Fairbanks, 8576

University of California, San FranciscoDermatology Drug Research, 1576, 1582, 3000, 3006, 5629, 5635, 6027

University of Chicago Children's Hospital,Department of Pediatrics, 2272

The University of Chicago Comer Children'sHospital, 6329

University of Chicago-Department of Psychiatry, 5335

University of Cincinnati Adult HemophiliaProgram, 4043

University of Cincinnati College ofMedicine/Division of Pediatrics, 2323

University of Connecticut Health Center, 2260

University of Illinois at Chicago,Craniofacial Center, 2127, 2428, 3423

University of Illinois at ChicagoInstitute for Tuberculosis Research, 7415, 7523

University of Iowa - Wendell Johnson Speech and Hearing Clinic, 3912, 6805, 6969

University of Iowa Birth Defects andGenetic Disorders Unit, 1809, 1855, 1946, 1957, 2001, 8577

University of Iowa Hospitals & Clinics, 2276

The University of Iowa Libraries, 6323

University of Kansas Center for Researchon Learning, 4519

University of Kentucky: Pediatric Pulmonary Medicine, 2279

University of Maine, Conley Speech andHearing Center, 3560

University of Maryland Medical Center, 4942

University of Memphis Neuropsychology Lab, 3438

University of Miami, Mailman Center forChild Development, 8460

University of Miami, Mailman Centerfor Child Development, 8578

University of Michigan Adult Hemophiliaand Cougulation Disorders Program, 4044

University of Michigan Health System, 5896

University of Michigan, Cystic FibrosisCenter, 2293

University of Michigan, Kresge HearingResearch Institute, 3569

University of Mississippi Medical Center, 2295, 2429

University of Missouri-Columbia CysticFibrosis Center, 2298

University of Nebraska at Omaha PediatricPulmonary/Cystic Fibrosis Center, 2300

University of Nebraska, Lincoln BarkleyMemorial Center, 3562

University of Nevada - Department of Speech-Language Pathology, 6788

University of New Mexico School ofMedicine, 2305

University of North Carolina at ChapelHill, Brain Research Center, 866

University of North Carolina SarcoidosisSupport Group, 6368

University of Oklahoma Cystic FibrosisCenter, 2324

University of Pennsylvania Weight andEducation Program, 2902

University of Pennsylvania, DepressionResearch Unit, 2478

University of Pittsburgh Cystic FibrosisCenter/Children's Hospital, 2329

University of Rochester Medical Center, 2315

University of South Florida, 6324

University of Southern CaliforniaComprehensive Sickle Cell Center, 6649

University of Tennessee Hemophilia Clinic, 4045

University of Texas Department ofHematology Research, 4046

University of Texas Medical Branch, 5481

University of Texas Medical Branch atGalveston, Clinical Research Center, 4945

University of Texas Sleep/Wake DisordersCenter, 4938

University of Texas Southwestern MedicalCenter/Asthma & Allergic Diseases, 451

University of Texas, Mental HealthClinical Research Center, 2479

University of Utah, 4834

University of Utah Intermountain CysticFibrosis Center, 2340

University of Virginia General ClinicalResearch Center, 452

University of Washington CF Center, 2345

University of Washington Department of Speech & Hearing Sciences, 6783

University of Washington Speech and Hearing Clinic, 6791

University of Washington: ExperimentalEducation Unit, 2704

University of Wisconsin Asthma andAllergic Disease Center, 453

University of Wisconsin-Madison CysticFibrosis/Pulmonary Center, 2349

University Professor, 3679

University Students with Autism and Asperger's Syndrome Web Site, 379, 905

Unlocking Potential: College and OtherChoices for People with LD and AD/HD, 6898

Unmarking Celiac Disease, 1357

UOAA National Conference, 4165

Upbeat, 2753

Update, 4264

Upper Peninsula Library for the BlindPhysically Handicapped, 1868, 2015, 5247, 6175

Upstate/Northeast New York Chapter of Crohn's & Colitis Foundation of America, 2174

Urinary System, 8858

Urologic Care of the Child with SpinaBifida, 6907

Urticaria, 7656

US Aspergers Association, 368

US Autism & Asperger Association, 369, 774

US Blind Golfers Association, 8174

US Disabled Ski Team, 8415

US Paralympics, 8074

US Rowing Assocation, 8220

US Wheelchair Weightlifting Association, 8385

USC - Neonatology Research Units, 7080

Useful Information on Phobias and Panic, 2547

UT Southwestern Medical Center at Dallas:Hematology-Oncology Research, 4041

Utah Center for Assistive Technology, 8416

Utah Chapter of the National HemophiliaFoundation, 3982

Utah Department of Health, 5986, 7061

Utah Parent Center, 8417

Utah State Library Commission, 8542

Utah Support GroupNational Ataxia Foundation, 551

V

VACC Camp, 299, 498, 1310

Vanderbilt Hemostasis-Thrombosis Clinic, 4047

Variety Audio, 1839, 1985, 5218, 6146

Variety Club Camp & Development Center, 8812

Vascular Anomalies Center, 3926

Vascular Birthmarks Foundation, 3923

VBF Conference, 3925

Ventricular Septal Defects, 7665

Vermont Department of Health - SIDSInformation and Counseling Program, 7062

Vermont Department oF HealthState Immunication Program, 5987

Vermont Department of LibrariesSpecial Service Unit, 8543

Vermont Parent Information Center, 8422

Vermont Regional Hemophilia Center, 4048

Via Christi Specialty Clinics: Cystic Fibrosis, Adult and Pediatrics, 2278

Views from Our Shoes: Growing Up with aBrother or Sister with Special Needs, 6899

Vinland Center, 8281

Violence by Children & Teenagers, 7671

Violence in the Media: A ReferenceHandbook, 7761

Violence Prevention Works, 7736

Violentkids.com, 7737

Viral Hepatitis: Everybody's Problem?, 4122

Virginia Assistive Technology System, 8427

Virginia Beach Public Library, 8549

Virginia Commonwealth UniversityDepartment of Neurosurgery Research, 3440

Virginia Department of HealthBureau of Immunization, 5988

Virginia SIDS Program - VirginiaDepartment of Health, 7063

Virginia State Library for the Visuallyand Physically Handicapped, 1886, 2033, 5265, 6193

Virtual Children's Hospital, 2099

Virtual Children's Hospital: Treatment ofCongenital Clubfoot, 1725

Virtual Childrens Hosptial, 8664

Virtual Pediatric Hospital, 4153, 4575, 4971, 6001

Vision of Children Foundation, 185, 8075

Vision Therapy, 4484

Vision Therapy Success Stories, 4485

Vision USA-American Optometric Association, 4469

VISIONS/Vacation Camp for the Blind, 1936, 2087, 5302, 6231

Visual Strategies for Improving Communication, 963

Visual Systems Research Group, 4471

Vital Options, 1145

Vitamin C Foundation, 6016

Voice Foundation (The), 6772

Voice Health Institute, 6773

Voice of the Diabetic, 2579

Voice of the Retarded, 4709

Volta Bureau Library, 3558

Volta Review, 3873

Volta Voices, 3859

VOR, 4708

Voyageur Outward Bound School, 8282

W

W.M. Krogman Center for Research In ChildGrowth and Development, 3250

Wagon Road, 8801

Waisman Center - Auditory Physiology Research Laboratory, 6792

Walk with Me, 1531

Wallace Memorial Library, 3563

Warmline Family Resource Center, 8137

Washington DC Metropolitan Area SupportGroup, 1154

Washington Library for the Blind andPhysically Handicapped, 1887, 2034, 5266, 6194

Washington PAVE, 8431

Washington State Chapter of Crohn's &Colitis Foundation of America, 2187

Washington State Department of HealthImmunization Program, 5989

Washington University Cystic FibrosisCenter, 2299

Washtenaw County Library, 1869, 2016, 5248, 6176

Washtenaw County Library for the Blind andPhysically Disabled, 1870, 2017, 5249, 6177

Water Balance in Schizophrenia, 1661

Waterville Public Library, 8503

Wayne County Regional Library for theBlind, 1871, 2018, 5250, 6178

Wayne State University, 3334

We Can Hear and Speak, 3847

We Can: Guide for Parents of Childrenwith Arthritis, 4400

We Insist on Natural Shapes (WINS), 2883

WE MOVE (Worldwide Education and Advocacyfor Movement Disorders), 1392, 1511, 1673, 2811, 2823, 7331, 7342, 7381, 8076

We've Climbed Mountains: Increasing Our Understanding of Autism Spectrum Disorders, 892

WebMD Community Services, 8665

Wellness Community, 5171

Wellness Community San Francisco/East Bay, 1146

Wellspring Camps, 5355

Wesley Medical Research Institutes, 8488, 8579

Wesley Woods, 399, 998, 4552

West Central Ohio Hemophilia Center, 4049

West Florida Regional Library, 8461

West Los Angeles Brain Tumor Support Group, 1147

West Michigan Cancer Center Support Group, 1200

West Virginia Assistive Technology System, 8434

West Virginia Department of Health andHuman Services, 7066

West Virginia Library Commission, 8552

West Virginia Parent Training andInformation, 8435

West Virginia School for the Blind, 1888, 2035, 5267, 6195

West Virginia University Cystic FibrosisCenter, 2346

West Virginia University Mountain StateCystic Fibrosis Center, 2347

Westchester Center for Eating Disorders, 2896

Western Kentucky Assistive TechnologyConsortium, 8494

Western New York Chapter ofCrohn's & Colitis Foundation of America, 2175

Western New York SIDS Center, 7044

Western North Carolina Brain Tumor SupportGroup, 1229

Western Pennsylvania Chapter of Crohn's &Colitis Foundation of America, 2182

Western Pennsylvania Chapter of TheNational Hemophilia Foundation, 3977

Western Psychiatric Institute & Clinic,Sleep Evaluation Center, 4934

What Can I Give You?, 6508

What Every Family Should Know, 7193

What Everyone Should Know About Epilepsy, 6617

What Health Care Workers Should Know AboutHepatitis B, 4123

What I Need to Know About Constipation, 3057

What Is AIDS?, 3342

What Is Hemophilia?, 4090

What Is Post Traumatic Stress Disorder?, 5812

What is Tay-Sachs?, 7194

What is Thalassemia Trait?, 7294

What Makes Ryan Tic?, 7347, 7447

What School Bus Drivers Need to Know AboutStudents with Tourette Syndrome, 7465

What School Personnel Should Know About Asthma, 466

What To Do About Your Brain Injured Child, 3460

What to Do When a Friend Is Depressed:Guide for Students, 2548

What You Can Do About AIDS, 3343

What You Need to Know About Brain Tumors, 1292

What You Need To Know About LactoseIntolerance, 4794

What You Should Know About BleedingDisorders, 4091

What's the Best Medicine for My Headaches?, 4781

What's This Thing Called Scoliosis, 6487

Wheeless' Textbook of Orthopaedics, 336, 1726, 3028, 4457, 4563, 4651, 5459, 6497, 6877

When Are Opioid (Narcotic) DrugsAppropriate for Headache?, 4782

When Food is Love, 2965, 5347

When Mom Gets Sick, 7155

When Nothing Matters Anymore: A SurvivalGuide for Depressed Teens, 2530

When Parents Can't Fix It, 8607

When Seizures Don't Look Like Seizures, 6618

When Someone You Know Has AIDS, 3344

When the Spine Curves, 6523

When Your Child Has a Life-ThreateningIllness, 8704

When Your Child is Ready to Return to School, 1293

When Your Student Has Arthritis: Guidefor Teachers, 4407

Where Did AIDS Come From?, 3345

Where's Chimpy?, 2751

Whitney Library for the Blind, 8512

Who Says It Has to Be Fair, 5050

Whoo's Report, 1365

Why Can't Michael Pay Attention?, 630

Why Isn't My Child Happy? A Video GuideAbout Childhood Depression, 2491

Why We Can Hear And Speak, 3680

Why Won't My Child Pay Attention?, 631

Wichita Public Library, 8489

Wide Smiles, 1689, 1699

Wilderness Inquiry, 8283

Wilderness on Wheels Foundation, 8153

Willamette Valley Ataxia Support Group, 544

Williams Syndrome, 7772

Williams Syndrome Association, 7777

Williams Syndrome Foundation, 7778

Williams Syndrome Foundation Home Page, 7785

Williams Syndrome Monthly Medline Alert, 7786

Wilms Tumor, 7789

Wilson Disease, 7813

Wilson's Disease, 7828

Wilson's Disease Association, 7820

Wilson's Disease Association International, 7825

Wilson's Disease Patient InformationExchange, 7826

Windsor Mountain Camp, 3913

Wing of Madness: A Depression Guide, 2501

Winnie-the-Pooh's ABCs, 3848

Winthrop-University Hospital SleepDisorders Center, 4916

Wisconsin Association for Perinatal Care, 5908

Wisconsin Chapter of Crohn's & ColitisFoundation of America, 2188

Wisconsin Lions Camp, 1937, 2088, 3914

Wish Fulfillment Organizations, 8705

Wish Upon a Star, 8840

Wish with Wings, 8841

Wishing Star Foundation, 8842

Wishing Well Foundation, 8843

WisTech, 8441

Withering Child, 2966

WNY Brain Tumor Support Group, 1225

Wolff's Headaches & Other Head Pain, 4764

Wolfner Memorial Library for the Blind, 1875, 2022, 5254, 6182

Women and Headache, 4783

Worcester Public Library, 8507

Word Signs: A First Book of Sign Language, 3849

Working Together, 2973

Working with Children and Adolescents inGroups, 2531

Workshop on Therapeutic Approaches forDuchenne Muscular Dystrophy, 4876

The World According to Pat: Reflections of Residential School Days, 3678

World Allergy Organization, 6319

World Allergy Organization Journal, 6345

World Arnold-Chiari MalformationAssociation, 305

World Association Sarcoidosis OtherGranulatomous, 6430

World Craniofacial Foundation, 4592

World Health Organization, 30, 2094, 3085, 3315, 4103, 4145, 4673, 5477, 5734, 5750, 5953, 6247, 6975, 7382, 7474, 7521

World Institute on Disability, 8077

World of Sound, 3896

World of the Autistic Child, 964

World Research Foundation, 8078

Worthmore Academy, 999, 4553

www.aap.org, 6333

www.acaai.org, 6334
www.Nasal-Allergies.com, 6332
www.pediatriccareonline.org, 6335
www.wrongdiagnosis.com, 6336
Wyoming Department of Health, 7068
Wyoming's New Options in Technology(WYNOT), 8445

Y

Yale Pediatric Hematology/OncologyResearch Center, 4050
Yale University Cystic Fibrosis ResearchCenter, 2261
Yale University School of Medicine, 290, 322, 595, 1741, 4340, 4383, 5518, 7493, 7670
Yale University, Behavioral MedicineClinic, 2480
Yale University, Ribicoff ResearchFacilities, 2481
Yard Sale Coloring Book, 4401
Yesterday's Tomorrow, 2532
York County Parent Awareness, 8250
You and Your ADD Child, 686
You and Your Deaf Child, 3850
You and Your Deaf Child: A Self-Help Guidefor Parents of Deaf and Hard of Hearing, 3851

You Can Control Asthma - Books for theFamily & Kids, 484
You're Bigger than It, 7646
Young Adult Institute, 8079
The Young Deaf Child, 3845
Young Deaf Child, 3852
Young Hearts, 4322
Young People and Chronic Illness: TrueStories, Help and Hope, 4342
Young People with Cancer: A Handbookfor Parents, 8706
Your Adolescent, 7762
Your Child and Asthma, 495
Your Child and Epilepsy, 6591
Your Diet & Psoriasis, 6062
Your Digestive System & How it Works, 60
Your Kidneys and How They Work, 8707
yourtotalhealth.ivillage.com, 6337
Youth Crisis Hotline, 5670

Z

Zero to Three, 8080
Zero-To-3 Hawaii Project, 8185

Alabama

ARC of Morgan County, 8081
Alabama Department of Rehabilitation Services, 3988
Alabama Head Injury Foundation, 3364
Alabama Institute for the Deaf & Blind, 1824, 1969, 3551, 5202, 6121
Alabama/Northwest Florida Chapter of Crohn s Colitis Foundation of
     America, 2144
Autism Society of Alabama, 777
Autism Society of North Alabama, 778
Birmingham Support Group, 503
Camp ASCCA/Easter Seals, 8711
Camp Merrimack, 982, 1538, 2765, 8712
Camp Rap A Hope, 8713
Camp Shocco for the Deaf, 3901
Camp Smile-A-Mile, 8714
Down Syndrome Clinic, Children's Hospital of Alabama, 2677
Early Intervention Program, 8082
Gregory Fleming James Cystic Fibrosis Cent er, 2245
Mobile Association for the Blind, 1891, 1975, 2041, 5208, 5269, 6136
National Child Advocacy Center, 8363
Pediatric Brain Tumor Support Group, 1121
Sickle Cell Foundation of Greater Montgomery, 6632
Special Education Action Committee Huntsville Outreach Office, 8084
Special Education Services, 8085
Spina Bifida Association of Alabama, 6817
Statewide Technology Access & Response System for Alabamians with
     Disabilities, 8086
United Cerebral Palsy of Alabama, 1393
United Cerebral Palsy of Greater Birmingham, 1394
United Cerebral Palsy of Huntsville & Tennessee Valley, 1395
United Cerebral Palsy of Mobile, 1396
United Cerebral Palsy of Northwest Alabama, 1397
United Cerebral Palsy of West Alabama, 1398
University of Alabama - Birmingham Arthrit is Clinical Intervention
     Program, 6447
University of Alabama Speech and Hearing Center, 3552

Alaska

Alaska Chapter of Asthma and Allergy Found ation of America, 429
Alaska Department of Education, 8087
Assistive Technologies of Alaska, 8088
Camp Kushtaka, 2607
Maternal, Child & Family Health, Early Intervention/Infant Learning
     Program, 8090
PARENTS, 8091
Rid Alaska of Child Abuse, 5671
SIDS Information & Counseling Program Alaska Department of Health,
     6997
Turner's Syndrome Society of Alaska, 7562
United Cerebral Palsy of Alaska/PARENTS, 1399
University of Alaska, Fairbanks, 8576

Arizona

Arizona Ataxia Support Group, 504
Arizona Camp Sunrise & Sidekicks, 114, 166, 1294, 3121, 5180, 7809
Arizona Chapter of Crohn's & Colitis Foundation of America, 2145
Arizona Early Intervention Program/ Department of Economic Security,
     8092
Arizona Sleep Disorders Center, 4889
Arizona Spina Bifida Association, 6818
Arizona Technology Access Program Institute for Human Development,
     8093
Autism Society of America Greater Phoenix Chapter, 779
Autism Society of America Southern Arizona Chapter, 780
Blake Foundation Children's Achievement Center, 8094
Brain Injury Association of Arizona, 3365
Brain Tumor Support Group at NovaCare Rehabilitation Institute of
     Tucson, 1122
Brain Tumor Support Group at Phoenix, 1123
Camp Abilities Tucson, 8715
Camp Civitan, 1929, 2081, 3897, 8716
Camp Shane Arizona, 5350
Children's Center for Neurodevelopmental Studies, 862
Crisis Nursery, 5672
Cystic Fibrosis Center: Phoenix Children's Hospital, 2246

Division of Special Education State Department of Education, 8095
Families of SMA - Arizona Chapter, 6920
Injury Prevention Center, 4227
Maricopa Co Childhood Immunization Program, 5954
Mayo Clinic Scleroderma Service, 6448
Mayo Comprehensive Hemophilia Center, 4019
National Center for Neurogenic Communicati on Disorders, 6784
Neurofibromatosis, Inc - Arizona Chapter, 5013
Office of Women's & Children's Health, 6998
Phoenix Center for Cancer and Blood Disorders, 4028
Pilot Parents of Southern Arizona, 8096
Prader-Willi Syndrome Arizona Association, 5821
Raising Special Kids, 8097
Southwest Chapter of Crohn's & Colitis Foundation of America, 2168
Special Needs Center/Phoenix Public Library, 8446
Steele Children's Research Center, 4037
Technology Access Center of Tucson, 8447
The Arizona Partnership for Immunization, 5955
Tourette Syndrome Association - Arizona Chapter, 7383
Turner's Syndrome Society of Arizona, 7563
United Cerebral Palsy of Central Arizona, 1400
United Cerebral Palsy of Southern Arizona, 1401

Arkansas

Arkansas Department of Health - SIDS Information & Counseling Program,
     6999
Arkansas Department of Health Div. of Comm Diseases/Immunizations,
     5956
Arkansas Disability Coalition, 8099
Arkansas Disability Coalition Parent Train ing and Information Center,
     8100
Arkansas Easter Seals Technology Resource Center, 8448
Arkansas Regional Library for the Blind and Physically Handicapped, 1831,
     1977, 5210, 6138
Arkansas Rehabilitation Research and Training Center for Deaf Persons,
     3567
Brain Injury Association of Arkansas, 3366
Camp Aldersgate, 8717
Camp Funshine, 2377
Children's Tumor Foundation-Arkansas Chapt er, 5014
Children's Tumor Foundation-Arkansas Infor www.php.com, 5015
Crowley Ridge Regional Library, 8449
DD Services, Department of Human Services, 8101
Educational Services for the Visually Impaired, 1830, 1976, 5209, 6137,
     8450
Epilepsy Education Association of Arkansas, 6535
FOCUS, 8102
Family-2-Family Health Information Center of Arkansas, 8103
Hemophilia Center of Arkansas, 3943, 4006
Increasing Capabilities Access Network, 8104
Library for the Blind and Handicapped, Southwest, 8451
Parent to Parent Arc of Arkansas, 8105
Special Education Section State Department of Education, 8106
United Cerebral Palsy of Central Arkansas, 1402

California

ARC Family Resource Project, 8107
Ability First, 8718
Ability First, Camp Paivika, 8719
All Kids By Two Health Services Agency, 5957
Allergy and Asthma Medical Group and Resea rch Center, 6325
American Action Fund for Blind Children and Adults, 1978, 3553, 5211,
     6139
American Association for Pediatric Ophthalmology and Strabismus, 1889
Assistive Technology Center Simi Valley Hospital, 8453
Ataxia Telangiectasia Medical Research Foundation, 554
Autism Research Institute, 860
Autism Society of America Coachella Valley, 781
Autism Society of America Greater Long Beach/San Gabriel Valley, 782
Autism Society of America Inland Empire Chapter, 783
Autism Society of America Los Angeles Chapter, 784
Autism Society of America North San Diego County Chapter, 785
Autism Society of America Orange County Chapter, 786
Autism Society of America San Diego Chapter, 787
Autism Society of America San Francisco Bay Chapter, 788
Autism Society of America San Gabriel Valley Chapter, 789

Autism Society of America Santa Barbara Chapter, 790
Autism Society of America Tulare County Chapter, 791
Autism Society of California, 792
Blind Children's Center, 1833, 1979, 5212, 6140
Blind Childrens Center, 6123
Bloomfield, 1927, 2080, 5299, 6228
Braille Institute Desert Center, 1834, 1980, 5213, 6141
Braille Institute Sight Center, 1835, 1981, 5214, 6142
Braille Institute Youth Center, 1836, 1982, 5215, 6143
Brain Imaging Center at the University of California, Irvine, 3424
Brain Research Institute, 3425
Brain Tumor Patient & Family Support Group, 1124
Brain Tumor Support Group at Newport Beach, 1125
Brain Tumor Support Group at San Diego, 1126
Brain Tumor Support Group at San Luis Obispo, 1127
Brain Tumor Support Group at Santa Monica, 1128
Brain Tumor Support Program Cedars-Sinai Neurosurgical Inst. &
    Wellness Communit, 1129
Brain and Spinal Injury Center (BASIC) Research at University of
    California, 3426
Brian Wesley Ray Cystic Fibrosis Center, 2247
CARE Family Resource Center, 8108
California Brain Injury Association, 3367
California Department of Health Services Immunization Branch, 5958
California SIDS Program, 7000
Camp Alex A. Krem, 8721
Camp Crescent Moon, 6669
Camp Grizzly, 3899
Camp Joan Mier, 8722
Camp Kindle- Project Kindle, 3349
Camp Krem, 980
Camp Ronald McDonald at Eagle Lake, 8723
Camp Rubber Soul, 8724
Camp Shane California, 5351
Camp Sunshine Dreams, 118, 169, 1298, 3123, 5182, 7811
Camp Wonder, 6468
Camp de los Ninos - Diabetes Society, 2608
Camp-A-Lot, 8725
Carolyn Kordich Family Resource Center, 8109
Center for Accessible Technology, 8454
Center for the Partially Sighted, 1890, 2036, 2558, 5268, 6197
Center for the Research and Treatment of Anorexia Nervosa, 2907
Central California Chapter of the National Hemophilia Foundation, 3944
Challenged Family Resource Center, 8110
Child Sexual Abuse Treatment Program (Giar retto), 5673
Children Living with Illness, 8111
Children's Hospital & Research Center of Oakland, 2678
Children's Hospital of Los Angeles, 2678
Children's Hospital of Orange County: Depa rtment of Pulmonology -
    Cystic Fibrosis, 2249
Children's Hospital: Pediatric Pulmonary Center, 2250
Christian Berets, 8726
Clearinghouse for Specialized Media and Technology (CSMT), 8455
Comfort Connection Family Resource Center, 8112
Community Health Improvement Partners - Immunize San Diego
    (CHIP-ISD), 5959
Cooley's Anemia Foundation-California, 7261
CorStone-Children & Loss Group, 7001
Cystic Fibrosis Center: Cedars-Sinai Medical Center, 2251
Cystic Fibrosis Center: University of California at San Francisco, 2252
Cystic Fibrosis Research, Inc., 2253
Cystic Fibrosis and Pediatric Respiratory Diseases Center, 2254
Department of Developmental Services of Early Start Program, 8113
Down Syndrome Association of Los Angeles, 2660
Dream Street Foundation, 8727
Early Start Family Resource Network, 8114
Easter Seal Summer Camp Programs, 8728
Eating Disorders Research and Treatment Program, 2909
Enchanted Hills Camp, 1931, 2082, 3906
EpiCenter, 6547
Epilepsy Foundation of Northern California, 6536
Exceptional Family Resource Center, 8115
Exceptional Family Support, Education and Advocacy Center, 8116
Exceptional Parents, 8117
Families Caring for Families, 8118
Families of SMA - Northern California Chap ter, 6921
Family First Program Alpha Resource Center, 8119
Family Focus Resource Center, 8120
Family Resource Center at Lucile Packard Children's Hospital, 1752
Federal Hemophilia Treatment Center Program of Los Angeles, 4003

Firefighters Kids Camp Camp Concord, 1332
Foundation for Glaucoma Research, 2038
Foundation for Prader-Willi Research, 5859
Fragile X Association of Southern California, 3183
Fragile X Center of San Diego, 3184
Francis J. Curry National Tuberculosis Center, 7522
Fresno Brain Tumor Support Group, 1130
Glaucoma Research Foundation, 2040
Gloriana Opera Company, 8729
Greater Los Angeles/Orange County Chapter of Chron's & Colitis
    Foundation, 2146
Greater North Valley California Support Group, 505
Greater San Diego/Desert Chapter of Crohn' s & Colitis Foundation of
    America, 2147
H.E.A.R.T.S. Connection Family Resource Center, 8122
Harbor Regional Center Family and Professional Resource Center, 8123
Hear Center, 3554
Hearing Education & Awareness for Rockers, 3550
Hemophilia Association of San Diego County, 3945
Hemophilia Foundation of Northern California, 3946
Hemophilia Foundation of Southern California, 3947
Hydrocephalus Support Group of Southern California, 4228
Immunization Partnership of Alameda County, 5960
Inland Empire Brain Tumor Support Group, 1131
International Pemphigus Foundation, 5534
Jodi House, 3368
Kaiser Permanente Medical Center, 2255
Kern Autism Network, 793
Little People of America - District 2, 3242, 3243, 3245, 5445, 5446, 5448
Little People of America - District 7, 3237, 3240, 3241, 3244, 5440, 5443
Little People of America - San Francisco Bay Area Chapter, 3238, 5441
Little People of America - Utah Seagulls, 3246, 5449
Loma Linda University Sleep Disorders Cent er, 4890
Los Angeles Ataxia Support Group, 506
MATRIX: Parent Network and Family Resource Center, 8124
Matrix Parents Network and Resource Center, 8125
Memorial Miller Children's Hospital Cystic Fibrosis Center, 2256
National Organization of Parents of Blind Children, 6129
Neurofibromatosis, Inc - California Chapte r, 5016
Neuroscience Institute Brain Tumor Support Group, 1132
New Beginnings - Blind Children's Center, 1837, 1983, 5216, 6144
New Beginnings - The Blind Children's Center, 1892, 2044, 5270, 6199
Northern California Chapter of Asthma and Allergy Foundation of
    America, 430
Northern California Chapter of Crohn's and Colitis Foundation, 2148
Northern California Comprehensive Sickle C ell Center, 6648
Northern California Support Group, 507
Northridge Hospital: Leavey Cancer Center, 1133
Okizu Foundation Camps, 120, 171, 1300, 3124, 5183, 7812
Orange County Support Group, 508
Orthopaedic Biomechanics Laboratory, 1496
Orthopaedic Hospital's Hemophilia Treatment Center, 4026
Pacific Southwest Regional Genetics Group, 509
Palo Alto Brain Tumor Support Group, 1134
Parents Helping Parents of San Francisco, 8126
Parents Helping Parents of Santa Clara, 8127
Pathology Department SIDS/SUDC Research Project, 7076
Peaks and Valleys Family Resource Center, 8128
Pediatric Disabilities Clinic, Down Syndrome Clinic, 2679
Peninsula Support & Education Group for Parents of Children with Brain
    Tumors, 1135
Prader-Willi California Foundation, 5822
Pulmonary Care and Cystic Fibrosis Center, 2257
REACH - Sarcoidosis Support, 6357
Region IX Office Program Consultants for Maternal and Child Health, 7002
SMA Research Group, 6926
Sacramento Area Brain Tumor Support Group Lawrence J Ellison
    Ambulatory Care Ctr, 1136
Sacramento Center for Assistive Technology, 8456
San Diego Support Group, 510
San Fernando Valley Support Group, 511
San Francisco Brain Tumor Support Group, 1137
San Francisco Public Library for the Blind and Print Disabled, 1838, 1984,
    5217, 6145
San Gabriel/Pomona Parents' Place, 8129
Santa Barbara Brain Tumor Support Group, 1138
Santa Cruz County Brain Tumor Support Group, 1139
Santa Rosa Brain Tumor Support Group, 1140
Scleroderma Research Foundation, 6449
Sickle Cell Disease Foundation of California, 6633

South Bay Brain Tumor Support Group, 1141
South Central Los Angeles Regional Center for Devlopmentally Disabled Persons, 8130
Southern California Pediatric Brain Tumor Network, 1142
Special Connections Family Resource Center, 8131
Special Education Division State Department of Education, 8132
Stanford CF Center, 2258
Stanford University Center for Narcolepsy, 4891
Starlight Children's Foundation, 8133
Support Group for Caregivers of Brain Tumor Patients, 1143
Support Group for Parents of Children with Brain Tumors, 1144
Support for Families of Children with Disabilities, 8134
Team Advocates for Special Kids, Anaheim, 8135
Team Advocates for Special Kids, San Diego, 8136
Team of Advocates for Special Kids, 8573
Tourette Syndrome Association - Southern California Chapter, 7385
Turner's Syndrome Society Central And Northern, 7564
Turner's Syndrome Society of Southern California, 7565
UC Berkeley School of Social Welfare, 5136, 5587, 8575
UCD Hemophilia Treatment Center, 4039
UCSD Hemophilia Treatment Center, 4040
USC - Neonatology Research Units, 7080
United Cerebral Palsy of Central California, 1403
United Cerebral Palsy of Greater Sacramento, 1404
United Cerebral Palsy of Los Angeles, Ventura and Santa Barbara Counties, 1405
United Cerebral Palsy of Orange County, 1406
United Cerebral Palsy of San Diego County, 1407
United Cerebral Palsy of San Joaquin, Calaveras & Amador Counties, 1408
United Cerebral Palsy of San Luis Obispo, 1409
United Cerebral Palsy of Santa Clara & San Mateo Counties, 1410
United Cerebral Palsy of Stanislaus County Stanislaus, 1411
United Cerebral Palsy of the Golden State, 1412
United Cerebral Palsy of the Inland Empire, 1413
United Cerebral Palsy of the North Bay, 1414
University of California, San Francisco Dermatology Drug Research, 1576, 1582, 3000, 3006, 5629, 5635
University of Southern California Comprehensive Sickle Cell Center, 6649
Variety Audio, 1839, 1985, 5218, 6146
Vital Options, 1145
Warmline Family Resource Center, 8137
Wellness Community San Francisco/East Bay, 1146
Wellspring Camps, 5355
West Los Angeles Brain Tumor Support Group, 1147

Colorado

Assistive Technology Partners, 8138
Autism Society of America Larimer County Chapter, 794
Autism Society of America Pikes Peak Chapter, 795
Autism Society of America: Colorado Chapter, 796
Autism Society of American Boulder County Chapter, 797
Brain Injury Association of Colorado, 3369
Brain Tumor Patient & Family Support Group, 1148
Brain Tumor Patient/Family Group, 1149
Breckenridge Outdoor Education Center, 1928
Cardiac Kids/Association of Volunteers, 4310
Children's Hospital: Academic Pediatric Surgery Department, 1737
Children's Tumor Foundation - Colorado Cha pter, 5017
Colorado Consortium of Intensive Care Nurseries United Parents (UP), 8139
Colorado Dept. of Public Heand & Environme nt: Immunization Program, DCEED-IMM-A3, 5961
Colorado SIDS Program, 7003
Colorado Support Group, 512
Delta/Montrose Parent to Parent, 8140
Denver Children's Hospital, 2259
Denver Early Childhood Connections, 8141
Denver Sarcoidosis Awareness Support Group, 6358
Disabilities Advocacy & Support Network, 8291
Disability Connection and RAFT, Larimer County's Early Childhood Connection, 8142
Effective Parent Project, 8143
El Groupo Vida, 8144
Help Parent Support Group Hope & Education for Loving Parents, 8145
Hemophilia Society of Colorado, 3948
Little People of America - Front Range Chapter, 3239, 5442
Magic of Music and Dance, 8731
Mile High Down Syndrome Association, 2661

Mountain States Regional Genetics Services Network, 513
National Jewish Center for Immunology and Respiratory Medicine, 447
National Jewish Health, 441
National Jewish Medical & Research Center, 448, 5751, 6376
Oasis, 8146
PEAK Parent Center, 8147
Parent Support Group of Littleton & Auora, 8148
Parents Supporting Parents of Eagle County, 8149
Parents Supporting Parents of Garfield and Pitkin County, 8150
Parents of Asthmatic/Allergic Children, In c., 431, 6320
Prader-Willi Colorado Association, 5823
Prevention Initiatives State Department of Education, 8151
Region VIII Office Program Consultants for Maternal and Child Health, 7004
Resources for Young Children and Families, 8152
Rocky Mountain Chapter of Crohn's & Colitis Foundation of America, 2149
Rocky Mountain Village, 8732
Speech, Language, & Hearing Center University of Colorado, 6960
Speech, Language, and Hearing Center, 6785
Spina Bifida Association of Colorado, 6822
TIES, The Children's Hospital, 8572
Tourette Syndrome Association - Rocky Mountain Region, 7386, 7397, 7398, 7412
Turner's Syndrome Society of Rocky Mountain, 7566
Wilderness on Wheels Foundation, 8153

Connecticut

A.J. Pappanikou Center for Developmental D isabilities, 8154
Assistive Technology Project, 8155
Autism Society of America Connecticut Chapter, 798
Brain Injury Association of Connecticut, 3370
Brain Tumor Support Group, 1150, 1151
CPAC, 8156
Central Connecticut Chapter of Crohn's & Colitis Foundation of America, 2150
Connecticut Brain Tumor Support Group (Adult), 1152
Connecticut Down Syndrome Congress, 2662
Connecticut Lead Poisoning Prevention Program, 4498
Department of Mental Retardation, 8157
Families of SMA - Connecticut Chapter, 6922
Gaylord Hospital Sleep Medicine, 4892
Hemlocks Easter Seals Recreation, 1729, 6524
Hole in the Wall Gang Camp, 3350, 4092
Leukemia & Lymphoma Society - Westchester/ Connecticut/Hudson Valley Chapter, 139
Mansfield's Holiday Hill, 8733
Marvelwood Summer, 2801
Northern Connecticut Affiliate Chapter of Crohn's & Colitis Foundation of America, 2152
Parent to Parent Network of Connecticut the Family Center, 8158
Parents Association of Connecticut Childre n with Visual Impairments (PACVI), 6279
Prader-Willi Connecticut Association, 5824
Region 1 of the National Association for Parents of the Visually Impaired, 6124
Spina Bifida Association of Connecticut, 6823
State Department of Education, 8159
Sudden Infant Death Syndrome (SIDS) Network, 7070
TBI Support Group for Families & Survivors, 3371
Tourette Syndrome Association - Connecticut Chapter, 7387
Turner's Syndrome Society of Connecticut, 7567
United Cerebral Palsy of Eastern Connecticut, 1415
United Cerebral Palsy of Greater Hartford, 1416
United Cerebral Palsy of Southern Connecticut, 1417
University of Connecticut Health Center, 2260
Yale Pediatric Hematology/Oncology Research Center, 4050
Yale University Cystic Fibrosis Research Center, 2261
Yale University, Behavioral Medicine Clinic, 2480
Yale University, Ribicoff Research Facilities, 2481

Delaware

Autism Society of Delaware, 799
Brain Injury Association of Delaware, 3372
Children's Beach House, 3903
Delaware Assisstive Technology Initiative (DATI), 8160

Delaware Division of Libraries for the Blind and Physically Handicapped, 1577, 3001, 5630
Department of Public Instruction, 8161
Parent Information Center of Delaware, 8162
Pediatric Brain Tumor Support Group, 1153
Prader-Willi Delaware Association, 5825
SIDS Information & Counseling - Division of Public Health, 7005
Turner's Syndrome Society of Philadelphia, 7588
United Cerebral Palsy of Delaware, 1418

District of Columbia

Advocates for Justice and Education, 8163
Autism Society of America District of Columbia Chapter, 800
Brain Injury Association of Washington DC, 3373
Brain Research Center, 1257
Center for Auditory and Speech Sciences-Gallaudet University, 3555
Child Welfare Information Gateway, 5682
Children's National Health System, 95, 154, 6326
Commission of Public Health Immunization Program, 5962
Council of Families with Visual Impairment, 1840, 1986, 5219, 6147
Counseling and Research Center for SIDS, 7067
DC Arc, 8164
DC-EIP Services, 8165
Department of Health Division of Immunization, 5963
District of Columbia Public Library/ Librarian for the Deaf Community, 3556
Division of Community Health Nursing, 7006
Georgetown University, 6450
Georgetown University Child Development Center, 8166, 8457, 8561
Georgetown University Sleep Disorders Center, 4893
HEATH Resource Center, 8458
Hemophilia Program at Children's National Medical Center, 4010
Howard University Center for Sickle Cell Disease, 6650
Lab School of Washington Summer Program, 708, 993, 4544
Laurent Clerc National Deaf Education Center-Gallaudet Universty, 3557
National Center for Education in Maternal and Child Health, 5909
National Technical Assistance Center for Children's Mental Health, 1774, 7704
Partnership for Assistive Technology, 8168
Scottish Rite Centers for Childhood Langua ge Disorders, 6782
Spina Bifida Association Pittsburgh, 6855
Spina Bifida Association of Arkansas, 6819
Spina Bifida Association of Greater Bay Ar ea, 6820
Spina Bifida Association of Greater Fox Valley, 6865
Spina Bifida Association of Greater San Di ego, 6821
Spina Bifida Association of Northern Indiana, 6831
Spina Bifida Association of Southeast Florida, 6826
Spina Bifida Association of Tennessee, 6858
Talking Books - National Library Service, 4470
Technical Assistance Partnership for Child and Family Mental Health, 1777, 7707
United Cerebral Palsy of Washington DC & Northern Virginia, 1419
United Cerebral Palsy of Washington DC & Northern Virginia, 1490
Volta Bureau Library, 3558
Washington DC Metropolitan Area Support Group, 1154

Florida

Alliance for Assistive Service and Technology (FAAST), 8169
Alliance for Eating Disorders Awareness, 2903
American SIDS Institute, 7071
Angels in the Sun Brain Tumor Support Group, 1155
Ataxia Telangiectasia Children's Project, 553
Autism Society of America Broward Chapter, 801
Autism Society of America Emerald Coast Chapter, 802
Autism Society of America Florida Chapter, 803
Autism Society of America Jacksonville Chapter, 804
Autism Society of America Panhandle Chapter, 806
Autism Society of Greater Orlando, 807
Brain Injury Association of Florida, 3374
Brain Tumor Support Group, 1156
Brain Tumor Support Group at Miami, 1157
Brain Tumor Support Group at St. Petersburg, 1158
Brain Tumor Support Group at Tampa, 1159
Broward County Support Group, 514
CF & Pediatric Pulmonary Disease Center, 2262
Camp Boggy Creek, 6908

Camp Thunderbird, 8734
Cancer Support Group for Children, 1160
Center for Independence Technology and Education, (CITE), 8459
Child and Family Connections, 8194
Children's Medical Services Program Florida SIDS Program, 7007
Children's Tumor Foundation - Florida Chap ter, 5018
Clearwater, FL Support Group, 515
Coconut Creek Eating Disorders Support Group, 2885
Comprehensive Pediatric Hemophilia Treatment Center, 4000
Cystic Fibrosis Center - All Children's Hospital, 2263
Developmental Center, 704, 988, 4540
Dyslexia Research Institute, 2781
Early Intervention Unit, Division of Children's Medical Services, 8170
Easter Seals Camp Challenge, 8735
Epilepsy Association of the Big Bend, 6537
Epilepsy Foundation of Florida, 6538
Family Network on Disabilities, 8171
Family/Community Support Group of the Brain Injury Association of Florida, 3375
Florida Bureau of Braille and Talking Book Library Services, 1841, 1987, 5220, 6148
Florida Camp for Children and Youth, 2613
Florida Chapter of Crohn's & Colitis Found ation of America, 2153
Florida Department of Education, 8172
Florida Department of Health Immunization Program, 5964
Florida Epilepsy Services Providers Associ ation, 6539
Florida Families of Children with Visual I mpairments, 6280
Florida Hemophilia Association, 3949
Florida Ophthalmic Institute, 2037
Florida School-Deaf and Blind Summer Camp, 1932, 2083, 3907, 5300, 6229
Florida's Collaboration for Young Children and their Families Head State, 8173
Frontier Travel Camp, 396
Gold Coast Down Syndrome Organization, 2663
Goodwill Industries-Suncoast, 2664
Goodwill Industries-Suncoast: Choices for Work Program, 3376
Hemophilia Foundation of Greater Florida, 3950
Hydrocephalus Family Support Group of Central Florida, 4229
Kris' Camp, 992
Miami Children's Hospital, Division of Pulmonology, 2264
Miami Comprehensive Hemophilia Center, 4020
NE Florida Support Group, 516
National Ophthalmic Research Institute, 2043
Neurofibromatosis Center at North Broward Medical Center, 5043
New Heights (formerly Cerebral Palsy of No rtheast Florida), 1420
PWSA Florida Chapter, 5826
Pediatric Heart Foundation, 4311
Prader-Willi Alliance of New York, 5846
Pulmonary Wellness Program, 2265
Renfrew Center of Miami, 2886
Research & Training Center for Children's Mental Health at University of South FL, 1775, 7705
Research and Training Center for Children' Mental Health, 8569
Scleroderma Foundation Southeast Florida Chapter, 6438
Shriners Hospital for Children, 6477
South Florida Brain Tumor Association Lynn Regional Cancer Center, 1161
Spina Bifida Association of Central Florid a, 6824
Spina Bifida Association of Jacksonville N emours Childrens Clinic, 6825
Spina Bifida Association of Tampa Bay, 6827
Suncoast Residential Training Center/Developmental Services Program, 1622
Talking Book Library, Jacksonville Public Library, 1842, 1988, 5221, 6149
Talking Book Service - Manatee County Central Library, 1843, 1989, 5222, 6150
Tampa Bay Area Brain Tumor Support Group, 1162
Tampa Support Group, 517
Tourette Syndrome Association of Florida, 7388
Turner's Syndrome Society - Tampa Support Group, 7568
Turner's Syndrome Society of Northern Florida, 7569
Turner's Syndrome Society of South Florida, 7570
US Blind Golfers Association, 8174
United Cerebral Palsy of Central Florida, 1421
United Cerebral Palsy of East Central Florida, 1422
United Cerebral Palsy of Florida, 1423
United Cerebral Palsy of North Florida/ Tender Loving Care, 1424
United Cerebral Palsy of Northwest Florida, 1425
United Cerebral Palsy of Sarasota-Manatee, 1426
United Cerebral Palsy of South Florida, 1427

United Cerebral Palsy of Tampa Bay, 1428
University of Miami, Mailman Center for Child Development, 8460
University of Miami, Mailman Center for Child Development, 8578
University of South Florida, 6324
VACC Camp, 299, 498, 1310
West Florida Regional Library, 8461

Georgia

Albany Library for the Blind and Physical Handicapped, 1844, 1990, 5223, 6151
All Ages Support Group, 1163
Augusta-Richmond County Public Library, 8462
Autism Society of America Greater Georgia Chapter, 808
Bainbridge Subregional Library for the Blind and Physically Handicapped, 1845, 1991, 5224, 6152
Brain Injury Resource Foundation, 3377
Brain Tumor Foundation for Children, 1164
Brain Tumor Support Group, 1165
CEL Subregional Library for the Blind and Physically Handicapped, 1846, 1992, 5225, 6153
Camp Hawkins, 2763
Camp Juliena, 3900
Camp Kudzu, 2606
Children's Tumor Foundation - Georgia, 5019
Comprehensive Sickle Cell Center, 6651
Cooley's Anemia Foundation-Buffalo Chapter, 7262
DHR/Division of Public Health - Babies Can t Wait Program, 8175
Department for Exceptional Students Georgia Department of Education, 8176
Department of Counseling and Educational Leadership-Columbus State University, 8177
Department of Pediatrics, Medical College of Georgia, 2266
Division of Birth Defects and Genetic Diseases, 8559
Down Syndrome Association of Atlanta, 2665
Egleston Cystic Fibrosis Center: Departmen t of Pediatrics, 2267
Emory Autism Resource Center, 849
Emory Eye Center - Strabismus Research, 6944
Gainesville Subregional LBPH Hall County Public Library, 8463
Georgia Ataxia Support Group, 518
Georgia Chapter of Crohn's & Colitis Foundation of America, 2154
Georgia Department of Human Resources - Center for Family Resource Planning, 7009
Georgia Department of Human Resources Children's Health Services, 7008
Georgia Perinatal Association, 5906
Greater Atlanta Area Support Group, 519
Hemophilia Foundation of Georgia, 3951
La Fayette Subregional Library for the Blind and Physically Disabled, 8464
Macon Subregional Library for the Blind and Handicapped, Washington Memorial, 8465
Macon Support Group, 520
Oconee Regional Library, Library for the Blind and Physically Handicapped, 8466
PWSA of Georgia, 5827
Parent to Parent of Georgia, 8178
Parents Educating Parents and Professional for All Children (PEPPAC), 8179
Pediatric Neurodevelopmental Center at Marcus Institute, 2680
Prevent Child Abuse Georgia, 5674
Region IV Office Program Consultants For Maternal and Child Health, 7010
Rome Subregional Library for the Blind and Physically Handicapped, 8467
Sarcoidosis Support Group, 6359
Sickle Cell Foundation of Georgia, 6635
Southeast Regional Genetics Group, 521
Southeastern Brain Tumor Foundation Brain Tumor Support Group, 1166
Southeastern Region-Helen Keller National Center, 6125
Special Needs Library of NE Georgia Athens-Clarke County Regional Library, 8468
Spina Bifida Association of Georgia, 6828
Squirrel Hollow, 996, 4550
Subregional Library for the Blind and Physically Handicapped, 8469
Tech-Able, 8470
Tools for Life Division of Rehabilitation Services, 8180
United Cerebral Palsy of Georgia, 1429

Hawaii

AWARE, 8181
Aloha Special Technology Access Center, 8471
Assistive Technology Resource Centers of H awaii (ATRC), 8182
Autism Society of Hawaii, 809
Brain Injury Association of Hawaii, 3378
Brain Tumor Support Group, 1167
Camp Erdman YMCA, 8736
Federal Hemophilia Treatment Center of Hawaii, 4004
Hawaii Department of Health Immunization Program, 5965
Hawaii Down Syndrome Congress, 2666
Hawaii SIDS Information & Counseling Project, 7011
Hemophilia Foundation of Hawaii, 3952
Kardiac Kids, 4313
Library for the Blind and Physically Handicapped, Hawaii State Library, 8472
Parents and Children Together (PACT), 8183
Special Education Center of Hawaii, 3379
Special Needs Branch Department of Education, 8184
United Cerebral Palsy of Hawaii, 1430
Zero-To-3 Hawaii Project, 8185

Idaho

Assistive Technology Project, 8186
Autism Society of America Treasure Valley Chapter, 810
Brain Injury Association of Idaho, 3380
Camp Hodia, 2604
Child Health Improvement Program Idaho Department of Health, 7012
Department of Education, 8187
Hemophilia Foundation of Idaho, 3953
Idaho Dept. of Health & Welfare Immunizati on Program, 5966
Idaho Parents Unlimited, 8188
Idaho State Talking Book Library, 1847, 1993, 5226, 6154
Infant/Toddler Program, 8189
Palouse Area Parent To Parent, 8190
Parent Reaching Out to Parents, 8191
Prader-Willi Northwest Association-Idaho, 5829
Treasure Valley Brain Injury Support Group, 1168
United Cerebral Palsy of Idaho, 1431

Illinois

Academy for Eating Disorders (AED), 2887
Adult Down Syndrome Center of Lutheran General Hospital, 2681
Advocate Lutheran General Children's Hospital, Pediatric Research, 2682
Archway, 8192
Assistive Technology Project, 8193
Autism Society of Illinois, 811
Brain Injury Association of Illinois, 3381
Brain Research Foundation, 1258
Brain Tumor Resource & Support Group, 1169
Brain Tumor Support Group, 1170
Brain Tumor Support Group at Northwestern Memorial Hospital, 1171
Brain Tumor Support Group at Park Ridge, 1172
Camp Discovery, 196, 1605, 3019, 5644, 6063, 6467
Camp Horizon, 8709
Camp New Friends, 5060
Camp Roehr, 6622
Center for Narcolepsy Research at the University of Illinois at Chicago, 4939
Central DuPage Hospital Center for Digestive Disorders, 1755
Chicago Library Service for the Blind, 1848, 1994, 5227, 6155
Chicago, IL Area Ataxia Support Group, 522
Children's Tumor Foundation - Illinois, 5020
Children's Tumor Foundation - Illinois Cha pter, 5021
Chilren's Heart Services, 4314
Citizens United for Research in Epilepsy (CURE), 6548
Comprehensive Bleeding Disorder Center, 3999
Craniofacial Center at University of Illin ois, Chicago, 2128
Crohn's & Colitis Foundation of America Carol Fisher Chapter, 2155
Cystic Fibrosis Center: Children's Memoria l Hospital, 2268
Dermatology Information Network (DERMINFONET), 1578, 3002, 5631
Developmental Services Center, 8195
Dystonia Medical Research Foundation, 2813
Easter Seals - Timber Pointe Outdoor Center, 8738
Easter Seals Camp Sunnyside, 8752

Family Resource Center, 8121
Family Resource Center on Disabilities, 8196
Family T.I.E.S. Network, 8197
Greater Interagency Council Parent to Parent Support Network, 8198
Hemophilia Foundation of Illinois, 3954
Illinois State Library, Talkng Book and Braille Service, 1849, 1995, 5228, 6156
International Society for Traumatic Stress Studies, 5789
Jewish Council for Youth Services, 8739
LaRabida Children's Hospital, Down Syndrome Clinic, 2683
Leukemia Research Foundation, 8199
Loyola University Medical Center/ Department of Pediatrics, 2269
Loyola University of Children, Parmly Hearing Institute, 3559
MDA Summer Camp, 4877
Mid Illinois Talking Book System, 1850, 1996, 5229, 6157
Mid-Illinois Talking Book Center, 1851, 1997, 5230, 6158
Mothers of Children with Allergies (MOCHA), 6321
National Center for Latinos with Disabilities, 8200
National Center on Child Abuse Prevention Research, 5683
National Eye Research Foundation, 2042
National Library of Dermatologic Teaching Slides, 1579, 3003, 5632
Neurofibromatosis, Inc - Illinois, 5022
Neurofibromatosis, Inc - Illinois/Midwest, 5023
Neurofibromatosis, Inc - New England/North east, 5029
Next Steps - Parents Reaching Parents, 8201
Northern Illinois Center for Adaptive Technology, 8473
Northwestern University Asthma and Allergy Disease Center, 449
Obsessive Compulsive Foundation of Metropo litan Chicago, 5373
Office of Community Health and Prevention Bureau of Early Intervention, DHR, 8202
Olympia, 8740
PKU Organization of Illinois, 5548
PWSA of Illinois, 5830
Parent to Parent Network, 8203
Parents Alliance Employment Project, 8474
Parents of Children with Brain Tumors (PCBT), 1173
Park Ridge, Cystic Fibrosis Center, 2270
Prevent Child Abuse Illinois, 5675
Professional Assistance Center for Education (PACE), 8475
Region 3 of the National Association for Parents of the Visually Impaired, 6127
Region V Office Program Consultants for Maternal and Child Health, 7013
Saint Francis Medical Center Specialty Clinics, CF Center, 2271
Scleroderma Foundation Chicago Chapter, 6439
Shawnee Library System, 8476
Southern IL Child and Family Connections, 8204
Spina Bifida Association of Illinois, 6829
State Board of Education Department of Special Education, 8205
Statewide SIDS Program - Illinois Department of Public Health, 7014
Suburban Audio Visual Service, 8477
Summer Wheelchair Sports Camp, 8741
Talking Book Center of Northwest Illinois, 1852, 1998, 5231, 6159
The University of Chicago Comer Children's Hospital, 6329
Touch of Nature Environmental Center, 8742
Tourette Syndrome Association of Illinois, 7390
Tourette Syndrome Camp Organization, 711, 5404, 7466
UIC Eye Center, 6257
United Cerebral Palsy Land of Lincoln, 1432
United Cerebral Palsy of Greater Chicago, 1433
United Cerebral Palsy of Illinois, 1434
United Cerebral Palsy of Southern Illinois, 1435
United Cerebral Palsy of Will County, 1436
University of Chicago Children's Hospital, Department of Pediatrics, 2272
University of Chicago-Department of Psychi atry, 5335
University of Illinois at Chicago Institute for Tuberculosis Research, 7415, 7523
University of Illinois at Chicago, Craniofacial Center, 2127, 2428, 3423

Indiana

ATTAIN: Assistive Technology Through Action in Indiana, 8206
About Special Kids (ASK), 8207
Allen County Public Library, 8478
Ann Whitehill Down Syndrome Program, 2684
Assistive Technology Training and Information Center, 8208, 8479
Autism Society of Indiana, 812
Bartholomew County Public Library, 8480
Benign Brain Tumor Support Group, 1174
Brain Injury Association of Indiana, 3382

Brain Tumor Support Group, 1175
Brain Tumor Support Group at Indianapolis, 1176
Camp About Face, 2134
Camp Brave Eagle, 8708
Camp Isanogel, 8743
Camp Millhouse, 8744
Central Indiana Sarcoidosis Support Group, 6360
Central Indiana Support Group, 523
Children's Tumor Foundation - Indiana Affi liate, 5024
Cystic Fibrosis and Chronic Pulmonary Disease Clinic, 2273
Division of Exceptional Learners Indiana Department of Education, 8209
Down Syndrome Association of Central Indiana, 8210
Down Syndrome Association of NWI, 2667
Down Syndrome Support Association of Southern Indiana (DSSASI), 2668
Easter Seal Society, 8745
Elkhart Public Library, 8481
Family Resource Center of Southeast Indiana, 8211
First Direction, 8212
First Steps, 8213
First Steps for Families, 8214
First Steps, Early Interventions, New Horizons Rehabilitation, 8215
Future Choices, 8216
Happiness Bag Incorporated, 8746
Happy Hollow Children's Camp, 8747
Hemophilia Foundation of Indiana, 3955
Indiana Chapter of Crohn's & Colitis Found ation of America, 2156
Indiana Deaf Camp, 3908
Indiana Hemophilia and Thrombosis Center, 4015
Indiana Resource Center for Autism, 850
Indiana State Board of Health - SIDS Project, 7015
Indiana State Dept. of Health Immunization, 5967
John Warvel, 2616
Kiwanis Twin Lakes Camp, 8748
Knox County Advocates, 8217
Methodist Hospital Sleep Disorders Center, 4894
MidWest Medical Center - Sleep Disorders Center, 4895
NE Indiana Support Group, 524
NEO Fight, 8218
Northwest Indiana Subregional Library for Blind and Physically Handicapped, 1853, 1999, 5232, 6160
Our Hearts, 4316
PWSA of Indiana, 5831
Pediatric Ophathalmology and Adult Strabis mus Service Research, 1893
Prevent Child Abuse Indiana, 5676
Primary Brain Cancer Support Group, 1177
Project Special Care, 8219
Riley Cystic Fibrosis Center, 2274
Riley Hemophilia and Thrombophilia Center, 3989
SMA Support Inc, 6923
Sleep Disorder Center, St Elizabeth Medica l Center, 4896
Sleep Disorders Center-Good Samaritan Hospital, 4897
Sleep/Wake Disorders Center-Community Heal th Network, 4898
Special Services Division - Indiana State Library, 8482
Spina Bifida Association of Central Indian a, 6830
Tourette Syndrome Association of Indiana, 7391
United Cerebral Palsy of Greater Indiana, 1437
United Cerebral Palsy of the Wabash Valley, 1438
Worthmore Academy, 999, 4553

Iowa

ARC of East Central Iowa Pilot Parents, 8221
Blank Children's Hospital: Department of P ulmonology, 2275
Brain Injury Association of Iowa, 3383
Brain Tumor Support Group, 1178
Bureau of Children, Family, and Community Services, 8222
Camp Courageous, 8749
Camp Courageous of Iowa, 8750
Camp Tanager, 8751
Children's Tumor Foundation - Iowa Chapter, 5025
Des Moines YMCA Camp, 119, 170, 497, 1299, 2378, 2610
Family & Educator Connection - Cedar Falls /Waterloo Region, 8223
Family & Educator Connection - Clear Lake/ Mason City Region, 8224
Family & Educator Connection - Marshalltow n Region, 8225
Hemophilia Treatment Center at the University of Iowa, 4011
Iowa Department of Public Health Bureau of Immunization, 5968
Iowa Library for the Blind and Physically Handicapped, 1854, 2000, 5233, 6161
Iowa Program for Assistive Technology, 8226

Iowa SIDS Program, 7016
Iowa's System of EI Services, 8227
Mercy Sleep Laboratory, 4940
PWSA of Iowa, 5832
Parent Educator Connection, 8228
Parent Educator Connection Program, 8229
Prevent Child Abuse Iowa, 5677
Quad Cities Brain Tumor Support Group, 1179
Spina Bifida Association of Iowa, 6832
The Link, 814
The University of Iowa Libraries, 6323
Turner's Syndrome Society of Iowa/New Found Friends, 7571
University of Iowa - Wendell Johnson Speech and Hearing Clinic, 3912, 6805, 6969
University of Iowa Birth Defects and Genetic Disorders Unit, 1809, 1855, 1946, 1957, 2001, 8577
University of Iowa Hospitals & Clinics, 2276

Kansas

Assistive Technology for Kansas Project, 8230
Autism Society of the Heartland, 815
Brain Injury Association of Kansas & Greater Kansas City, 3384
CKLS Headquarters, 2002
Camp Discovery American Diabetes Association, 2603
Department of Health & Environment, 8231
Families Together, 8232
Families Together/Parent to Parent of KS, 8233
Great Plains Region-Helen Keller National Center, 6128
Headstrong Brain Tumor Support Group, 1180
Heart to Heart, 4312, 4330, 4332, 4334
Kansas Department of Health & Environment Bureau of Family Health, 7017
Kansas Department of Health & Environment Immunization Program, 5969
Kansas State Library, 8483
Kansas University Medical Center: Departme nt of Pulmonology, 2277
Manhattan Public Library, 8484
Neurofibromatosis, Inc - Kansas & Central Plains, 5026
Prenatal Diagnostic and Genetic Center, 8485, 8567
Services for the Visually Disabled, 1857, 2003, 5235, 6163
Solution Outreach Center at OCCK, Inc., 8486
South Central Kansas Library System, 8487
Special Education Administration Kansas St ate Department of Education, 8234
United Cerebral Palsy of Kansas, 1440
University of Kansas Center for Research on Learning, 4519
Via Christi Specialty Clinics: Cystic Fibr osis, Adult and Pediatrics, 2278
Wesley Medical Research Institutes, 8488, 8579
Wichita Public Library, 8489

Kentucky

AbleData, 3545
Assistive Technology Services Network, 8235
Autism Society of America Bluegrass Chapter, 816
Bethel Mennonite Camp, 8753
Bluegrass Technology Center, 8490
Brain Injury Association of Kentucky, 3385
Brain Injury Support Group, 1181
College of Education - Western Kentucky University, 8236
Division of Preschool Services, 8237
Easter Seal Kysoc, 2612, 3905, 4725, 8754
EnTech: Enabling Technologies of Kentuckiana, 8491
Infant-Toddler Program, Division of Mental Retardation, 8238
Kentucky Chapter of Crohn's & Colitis Foundation of America, 2159
Kentucky Department of Human Resources Bureau of Health Services, 7018
Kentucky Hemophilia Foundation, 3956
Kentucky Library for the Blind and Physically Handicapped, 1858, 2004, 5236, 6164
Life Adventure Center, 1802, 7770
Louisville Talking Book Library, 8492
Northern Kentucky Talking Book Library, 8493
PWSA of Kentucky, 5834
Special Parent Involvement Network, 8239
Spina Bifida Association of Kentucky, 6833
Turner's Syndrome Society of Kentucky, 7572
University of Kentucky: Pediatric Pulmonar y Medicine, 2279

Western Kentucky Assistive Technology Consortium, 8494

Louisiana

Autism Society of Louisiana, 817
Brain Injury Association of Louisiana, 3386
Brain Injury Support And Education Group, 1182
Brain Injury Support Group, 1183
Camp Bon Coeur, 8755
Division of Special Populations, 8240
Families Helping Families of Greater New Orleans, 8241
LA Lions Camp Pelican, 2379
Louisiana Assistive Technology Access Network, 8242
Louisiana Chapter, 525
Louisiana Comprehensive Hemophilia Care Center, 4017
Louisiana Hemophilia Foundation, 3957
Louisiana Lions Camp for Crippled Children, 8756
Louisiana State Library, 8495
Louisiana State University Genetics Section of Pediatrics, 8496, 8564
Louisiana State University Health Sciences Center, 2280
Louisiana Support Group, 526
Louisiana/Mississippi Chapter of Crohn's & Colitis Foundation of America, 2160
Louisiana/Mississippi Chapter of Crohn's & Colitis Foundation of America, 2165
Med-Camps of Louisiana, 8757
NE Louisiana Sickle Cell Anemia Foundation, 6636
Preschool Programs - Division of Special Populations, 8243
Project PROMPT, 8244
Public Health Services of Louisiana, 7019
Spina Bifida Association of Greater New Orleans, 6834
Tlane Cancer Center, 1184
Tulane University Clinical Immunology Section, 450
Tulane University, US-Japan Biomedical Research Laboratories, 3427
Turner's Syndrome Society of Gulf Coast, 7573
United Cerebral Palsy of Baton Rouge McMains Children's Developmental Center, 1441
United Cerebral Palsy of Greater New Orleans, 1442

Maine

Autism Society of Maine, 818
Bangor Public Library, 8497
Brain Tumor Support Group of Maine, 1185
CDC Lincoln County, 8245
Camp Waban, 8758
Cary Library, 8498
Central Maine Medical Center, 2281
Child Department Services, 8246
Child Department Services, Department of Education, 8247
Consumer Information and Technology Training Exchange (Maine CITE), 8248
Department of Human Services, 7020
Eastern Maine Medical Center: Cystic Fibrosis Center, 2282
Jackson Laboratory, 3248
Lewiston Public Library, 8499
Maine Dept. of Human Services: Bureau of Health Immunization Program, 5970
Maine Hemophilia and Thrombosis Center, 4018
Maine State Library, 8500
Maine Support, 527
Open Support Group-All Kinds of Cancer Care of Maine, 1186
Pediatric Cystic Fibrosis Center, 2283
Pine Tree Camp Children - Adults, 8759
Portland Public Library, 8502
Sleep Laboratory, Maine Medical Center, 4941
Special Needs Parent Info Network, 8249
United Cerebral Palsy of Northeastern Maine, 1443
University of Maine, Conley Speech and Hearing Center, 3560
Waterville Public Library, 8503
York County Parent Awareness, 8250

Maryland

ARC Family Connection Parent to Parent Program, 8251
American Action Fund for Blind Children and Adults, 1832
Autism Society of America Baltimore Chesapeake Chapter, 819

Behavioral and Developmental Pediatrics Division, University of Maryland, 2685
Bell's Palsy Research Foundation, 1006
Brain Injury Association of Maryland, 3388
Center for Eating Disorders, 2888
Center for Infant & Child Loss, 7021
Center for Research for Mothers & Children, 7073
Chesapeake Chapter, 529
Cooley's Anemia Foundation-Capital Area (DC, VA, MD), 7263
Dept. of Health & Mental Hygiene-Immunizat ion, 5971
Developmental Pediatrics School of Medicine, University of Maryland, 8252
East Central Region-Helen Keller National Center, 1827, 6133
Easter Seals Camp Fairlee Manor, 8760
Epilepsy Research Laboratory, Department o f Neurology, 6549
Hemophilia Foundation of Maryland, 3958
International Center for Skeletal Dysplasia Registry, 2986
John Hopkins Arthritis Center, 445
John Hopkins Children's Hospital, 2284
Johns Hopkins Arthritis Center, 446
Johns Hopkins Brain Tumor Education Group, 1188
Johns Hopkins Department of Orthopaedics Surgery, 6475
Johns Hopkins Division of Allergy and Clin ical Immunology, 6328
Johns Hopkins University Sleep Disorders Center, 4899
Kamp-A-Kom-Plish, 8761
Kennedy Krieger Institute, 4753
Kennedy Krieger Institute, Down Syndrome Clinic, 2686
Learning Independence Through Computers, 8504
MD Infant/Toddler/Preschool Services Division, 8253
Maryland Infant and Toddlers Program Family Support Network, 8254
Maryland SIDS Information & Counseling Program, 7022
Maryland State Library for the Blind and Physically Handicapped, 1859, 2005, 5237, 6165
Maryland-Greater Washington, DC Chapter As thma and Allergy Foundation of America, 432
Maryland/South Delaware Chapter of Crohn's & Colitis Foundation of America, 2161
NAD Youth Leadership Camp, 3910
NIH/ Eunice Kennedy Shriver National Insti tute of Child Health & Human Development, 5910
NIH/National Institute of Mental Health Eating Disorders Program, 5911
NIH/National Library of Medicine (NLM), 10
NIH/Osteoporosis and Related Bone Diseases National Resource Center, 5450
National Diabetes Information Clearinghouse, 2557
National Digestive Diseases Information Clearinghouse, 31, 269, 1753, 1945, 2189, 2244
National Rehabilitation Information Center, 1495, 3078
Neurofibromatosis, Inc - MidAtlantic, 5027
PWSA of Maryland, Virginia & DC, 5836
Parents Place of Maryland, 8255
Parents of Children with Down Syndrome Arc of Montgomery County, 2669
Partners in Intensive Care, 8256
Patient Recruitment & Public Liaison Office Clinical Center, 7779
Prince George's County Memorial Library Talking Book Center, 1860, 2006, 5238, 6166
Raven Rock Lutheran Camp, 4727
Sarcoidosis Awareness Network, 6361
Sickle Cell Disease Association of America - Connecticut Chapter, 6634
Sickle Cell Disease Association of the Piedmont, 6640
Spina Bifida Association of Chesapeake-Pot omac, 6835
Spinal Muscular Atrophy Project, 6928
Sudden Infant Death Syndrome Institute of The University of Maryland, 7079
Technology Assistance Program Maryland Rehabilitation Center, 8257
The League at Camp Greentop and The Therapeutic Recreation, 8762
Tourette Syndrome Association of Greater Washington, 7393
Turner's Syndrome Society of Maryland, 7574
Turner's Syndrome Society of National Capitol Area, 7597
United Cerebral Palsy of Central Maryland, 1444
United Cerebral Palsy of Prince Georges & Montgomery Counties, 1445
United Cerebral Palsy of Southern Maryland, 1446
University of Maryland Medical Center, 4942

Massachusetts

Association of Gastrointestinal Motility Disorders, 2904
Asthma & Allergy Foundation of America New England Chapter, 433

Autism Research Foundation, 859
Autism Society of America Massachusetts Chapter, 820
Baystate Medical Center, 2285
Berkshire Center, 4517
Boston Children's Hospital Dept. of Otolaryngology & Communication, 3566
Boston Hemophilia Center, 3993
Braille and Talking Book Library Perkins School for the Blind, 1861, 2007, 5239, 6167
Brain Center Brain Tumor Support Group, 1189
Brain Injury Association of Massachusetts, 3389
Brain Tumor Support Group, 1190
Brain Tumor Support Group at Burlington, 1191
Brain Tumor Support Group at Worcester, 1192
Brain Tumor Survivor Support Group, 1193
Brigham and Women's Hospital, Asthma and Allergic Disease Research Center, 443
Bureau of Early Childhood Programs, 8258
Bureau of Family Health Services-Alabama Child Death Review, 6996
CKLS Headquarters, 1856, 5234, 6162
Camp Joslin, 2605
Camp Ramah in New England (Summer), 8764
Camp Ramah in New England (Winter), 8765
Camp Ramah in New England Tikvah Program, 985, 1540, 6621, 8763
Carroll Center for the Blind, 2008, 4518, 5240, 6168
Carroll School Summer Programs, 8766
Center for Digestive Disorders, 7628
Center for Interdisciplinary Research on Immunologic Diseases, 444
Children's Happiness Foundation, 8259
Children's Hospital Boston, 2286
Children's Tumor Foundation - Northern New England, 5028
Clara Barton Camp, 2609
Community Sickle Cell Support Group, 6637
Cooley's Anemia Foundation-Massachusetts Chapter, 7264
Developmental Medicine Center, 3319
Down Syndrome Program, Children's Hospital Boston, 2687
Eagle Hill School - Summer Program, 705, 989, 4541
Early Intervention Services, 8260
Eaton-Peabody Laboratory of Auditory Physiology, 3561
Education Development Center - EDC, 8261
Family Ties at Massachusetts Department of Public Health, 8262
Federation for Children with Special Needs, 8263
Greater Boston Arc Parent Support, 8264
Handi-Kids/King Solomon Foundation, 8767
Hard of Hearing Advocates, 3549
Harold Goodglass Aphasia Research Center, 3428
Heart to Heart Fund, 4317
Hemophilia Center of the New England Medical Center, 4009
Joslin Diabetes Center, 2559
Kingsmont, 5353
Landmark School, 2800
Massachusetts Assistive Technology Partnership, 8265
Massachusetts Association for Parents of t he Visually Impaired (MAPVI), 6281
Massachusetts Chapter of SIDS Alliance, 7023
Massachusetts Down Syndrome Congress (MDSC), 2670
Massachusetts Easter Seals Camping Program, 8768
Massachusetts Eating Disorder Association (MEDA), 2889
Massachusetts General Hospital, 2287
Massachusetts Sudden Infant Death Syndrome, 7074
Massachusetts, New England Hemophilia Association, 3959
National Association for Parents of the Visually Impaired, 1825, 1970, 5203, 6122, 6126
National Birth Defects Center, 8266
National Temporal Bone, Hearing and Balanc e Pathology Resource Registry, 3568
New England Chapter of Crohn's & Colitis Foundation of America, 2162
New England Region-Helen Keller National Center, 6130
New England Regional Genetics Group, 528, 8501, 8565
New England Support Group, 530
Option Institute: Son Rise Program, 821
Parent Education/Support Group, 1194
Pediatric Clinical Trials International, 2697
Pediatric Pulmonary Unit, 7077
Prader-Willi Association of New England (Maine, Mass, RI, NH, VT), 5835, 5837
Region I Office Program Consultants For Maternal and Child Health, 7024
Resources for Rehabilitation, 8505
Sleep Disorders Center, 6679
Sleep Disorders Unit, Beth Israel Hospital, 4900

Spina Bifida Association of Massachusetts, 6836
Talking Book Library at Worcester Public Library, 8506
Tourette Syndrome Association of Massachusetts, 7394
Tufts New England Medical Center Floating Hospital for Children, 2288
Turner's Syndrome Society of New England, 7575
United Cerebral Palsy of Berkshire County, 1447
United Cerebral Palsy of MetroBoston, 1448
Worcester Public Library, 8507

Michigan

Adventure Learning Center Camp Programs, 1801, 7769
Anchor Point Camp, 392, 975, 4533
Apnea Identification Program, 7025
Autism Society of Michigan, 822
Big Crystal Camp, 977
Bioengineering Center of Wayne State University, 3429
Brain Injury Association of Michigan, 3390, 3422
Brain Tumor Networking Club, 1195
Brain Tumor Support Group at Ann Arbor, 1197
Brain Tumor Support Group for Patients & F amilies: University of
    Michigan Med Ctr, 1198
Burger School for the Autistic, 851
Butterworth Hospital, Cystic Fibrosis Center, 2289
CAUSE, 8267
Camp Barakel, 8769
Camp Barefoot, 3470
Camp Catch-A-Rainbow, 116, 167, 1295, 3122, 7810
Camp Fish Tales, 8770
Camp O' Fair Winds, 4538
Camp Tushmehata, 1930
Center for Sleep Science at University of Michigan, 4901
Central Michigan University Summer Clinics, 3902, 6803
Children's Hospital of Michigan Cystic Fibrosis Care, Teaching &
    Resource, 2290
Children's Tumor Foundation - Michigan Cha pter, 5030
Cystic Fibrosis Center/Pediatric Pulmonary and Sleep Medicine, 2291
Detroit Michigian Ataxia Support Group, 531
Downtown Detroit Subregional Library for the Blind and Handicapped,
    1862, 2009, 5241, 6169
Early on Michigan, 8268
Eastern Michigan Hemophilia Center, 4002
Eric RicStar Winter Music Therapy Summer Camp, 1545, 8771
Families at Heart, 4318
Family Support Network of Michigan Parent Participation
    Program-MDCH, 8269
Frederick Douglas Branch for Specialized Services and Physically
    Handicapped, 8508
Genesee County Health Department, 7026
Glaucoma Laser Trabeculoplasty Study, 2039
Hemophilia Foundation of Michigan, 3960
Indian Trails Camp, 8772
Kalamazoo Center for Medical Studies, 2292
Kalamazoo Comprehensive Hemophilia Treatment Center, 4016
Kent County Health Department, 7027
Kent County Library for the Blind, 1863, 2010, 5242, 6170
Library of Michigan Service for the Blind, 1864, 2011, 5243, 6171
Livingston County CMH Services, 8270
Macomb Library for the Blind and Physically Handicapped, 1865, 2012,
    5244, 6172
Michigan Chapter of Allergy and Asthma Foundation of America, 434
Michigan Chapter of Crohn's & Colitis Foundation of America, 2163
Michigan State University Comprehensive Center for Bleeding Disorders,
    4021
Mideastern Michigan Library Co-op, 1866, 2013, 5245, 6173
Muskegon County Library for the Blind, 1867, 2014, 5246, 6174
Northern Regional Bleeding Disorder Center, 4024
Oakland County Health Division - SIDS Project, 7028
PWSA of Michigan, 5838
Parents are Experts, 8272
Regional Hemophilia Program, 4030
Rehabilitation Institute of Michigan, 3391, 3430
SIDS LEAD - Children's Special Health Care Services, 7029
SIDS Nursing Intervention Program, 7030
SW Michican Spina Bifida & Hydrocephalus Association, 4231
Sarcoidosis Awareness Foundation, 6362
Sarcoidosis Resource Support Group, 6363
Sarcoidosis Support - Beaumont, 6364
Seeking Techniques Advancing Research in Shunts (STARS), 4242

Spectrum Brain Tumor Support Group, 1199
Spectrum Health Research, 4036
Spina Bifida Association of Upper Peninsula Michigan, 6837
Spina Bifida Association of West Michigan, 6838
TECH 2000 Project-Michigan Disability Rights Coalition, 8273
Turner's Syndrome Society of Southeastern Michigan, 7576
Turner's Syndrome Society of West Michigan, 7577
United Cerebral Palsy Michigan, 1449
United Cerebral Palsy of Metropolitan Detroit, 1450
University Center for the Development of L anguage & Literacy, 6786
University of Michigan Adult Hemophilia and Cougulation Disorders
    Program, 4044
University of Michigan, Cystic Fibrosis Center, 2293
University of Michigan, Kresge Hearing Research Institute, 3569
Upper Peninsula Library for the Blind Physically Handicapped, 1868, 2015,
    5247, 6175
Washtenaw County Library, 1869, 2016, 5248, 6176
Washtenaw County Library for the Blind and Physically Disabled, 1870,
    2017, 5249, 6177
Wayne County Regional Library for the Blind, 1871, 2018, 5250, 6178
West Michigan Cancer Center Support Group, 1200

Minnesota

ARC Suburban, 8274
Abbott Northwestern Brain Tumor Support Group at Abbott Northwestern
    Hospital, 1201
Autism Society of America Manasota Chapter, 805
Autism Society of Minnesota, 823
Brain Injury Association of Minnesota, 3392
Brain Injury Support Group at Abbott Northwestern Hospital, 1202
Brain Tumor Support Group at Duluth, 1203
Brain Tumor Support Group at Robbinside, 1204
Brain Tumor Support Group at United Hospital, 1205
Camp Buckskin, 701, 978, 4535
Camp Friendship, 979, 2762, 8773
Camp New Hope, 983, 2766, 8774
Camp Winnebago, 8775
Center for Sleep Diagnostics, 4902
Courage Camps, 8776
Courage North, 8777
Department of Children, Family, & Learning, 8275
Down Syndrome Association of Minnesota, 2671
Down Syndrome Clinic of Minneapolis Children's Medical Center, 2688
Eden Wood Center, 2768, 7788, 8778
Family to Family Network ARC of Hennepin County, 8276
Groves Academy, 706, 990, 4542
Hemophilia Foundation of Minnesota and the Dakotas, 3961
Hemophilia and Thrombosis Center at the University of Minnesota Medical
    Center, 4013
Interagency Early Intervention Project, 8277
Knutson, 8779
Mayo Clinic and Foundation, 4828
Minneapolis, MN Support Group, 532
Minnesota Cystic Fibrosis Center, 2294
Minnesota Library for the Blind & Physically Handicapped, 1872, 2019,
    5251, 6179
Minnesota Sudden Infant Death Center, 7031
Minnesota/Dakotas Chapter of Crohn's & Colitis Foundation of America,
    2164
Non-Malignant Brain Tumor Support Group, 1206
PACER Center, 8509
PWSA Chapter - Minnesota, 5839
Parents For Heart of Minnesota, 4319
Parents for Parents, 8278
Pilot Parents in Anoka and Ramsey Counties, 8279
Pilot Parents of Northeast Minnesota, 8280
Search Beyond Adventures, 8780
Spina Bifida Association of Minnesota, 6839
Star Center for Family Health, 8510
Tourette Syndrome Association - Minnesota Chapter, 7395
Turner's Syndrome Society of Minnesota, 7578
United Cerebral Palsy of Central Minnesota, 1451
United Cerebral Palsy of Minnesota, 1452
Vinland Center, 8281
Voyageur Outward Bound School, 8282
Wilderness Inquiry, 8283

Mississippi

Autism Society of Mississippi, 824
Brain Injury Association of Mississippi, 3393
First Steps Program, 8284
Mississippi Chapter, 533
Mississippi Dept. of Health Bureau of Preventative Health Immunization, 5972
Mississippi Hemophilia Foundation, 3962
Mississippi State Department of Health and Child Health Services, 7032
Office of Special Education, 8271, 8285
Parent Partners, 8286
Project Start, 8287
Spina Bifida Association of Mississippi, 6840
Tik-A-Witha, 8781
University of Mississippi Medical Center, 2295, 2429

Missouri

AMOR - A Cancer Support Group for Patients & Their Families, 1207
Adriene Resource Center for Blind Children, 1873, 2020, 5252, 6180
Allergy and Pulmonary Medicine, 435
Assemblies of God National Center for the Blind, 1874, 2021, 5253, 6181
Assistance Technology Project, 8288
Asthma and Allergy Foundation of America - Saint Louis Chapter, 437
Asthma and Allergy Foundation of America Greater Kansas City Chapter, 436
Autism Society of America Gateway Chapter, 825
Brain Cancer Support Group at Mid-America Cancer Center, 1208
Brain Injury Association of Missouri, 3394
Brain Tumor Support Group, 1196, 1209
Brain Tumor Support Group of Greater St Louis, 1210
Central Institute for the Deaf, 3570
Central Missouri Area Support Group, 534
Children's Mercy Hospital, Down Syndrome Clinic, 2689
Children's Mercy Hospital, University of Missouri, 2296
Children's Therapy Center, 8289
Children's Tumor Foundation - Missouri Cha pter, 5031
Council for Extended Care of Mentally Retarded Citizens, 4723
Cystic Fibrosis, Pediatric Pulmonary and Pediatric Gastrointestinal Center, 2297
Department of Elementary and Secondary Education, 8290
Down's Syndrome Medical Clinic, 2690
EDI, 2611
Family Resource Network, 8292
Gateway Hemophilia Association of Missouri, 3963
Heart to Heart - St. Louis, 4320
Hickory Hill, 2615
Hydrocephalus Support Group, 4230, 4232
Judevine Center for Autism, 852
Kansas City, Missouri Support Group, 535
Mid-America Chapter of Crohn's & Colitis F oundation of America, 2158
Missouri Parents Act, 8293
PWSA Missouri Chapter, 5840
Parent Act, 8294
Pediatric Epilepsy Center, 6550
Positive Solutions for Life Challenges, 8295
Prader-Willi Syndrome Advocates, 5833
Region VII Office Program Consultants for Maternal and Child Health, 7033
SIDS Resources, 7034
Saint Louis Chapter of Crohn's & Colitis Foundation of America, 2166
Sidney R. Baer Day Camp, 8782
Spina Bifida Association of Greater Saint Louis, 6841
Springfield Area Support Group, 536
Tourette Syndrome Association - Greater Missouri Chapter, 7396
Turner's Syndrome Society of St. Louis/ West Illinois, 7579
United Cerebral Palsy of Greater Kansas City, 1439, 1453
United Cerebral Palsy of Greater St. Louis, 1454
United Cerebral Palsy of Northwest Missouri, 1455
United Services, 8296
University of Missouri-Columbia Cystic Fibrosis Center, 2298
Washington University Cystic Fibrosis Center, 2299
Whitney Library for the Blind, 8512
Wolfner Memorial Library for the Blind, 1875, 2022, 5254, 6182

Montana

Big Sky Kids Cancer Camp, 115
Brain Injury Association of Montana, 3395
CO-TEACH/Division of Educational Research and Service, 8297
Charles Campbell Children's Camp, 1542
Developmental Disabilities Program, 8298
Division of Special Education, 8299
MonTECH, 8300
Montana Department of Health & Environmental Sciences, 7035
Montana State Library, 8513
Parents Let's Unite for Kids, 8301
Quality Life Concepts, 8302

Nebraska

Assistive Technology Partnership, 8303
Autism Society of Nebraska, 826
Boys Town National Research Hospital, 6787
Brain Tumor Support Group at the Nebraska Medical Center, 1211
Camp Easter Seals, 8783
Camp Kindle, 3348
Floyd Rogers, 2614
Individual and Family Support Arc of Lincoln & Lancaster County, 8304
Iowa Chapter of Crohn's Colitis Foundation of America, 2157
Junior Wheelchair Sports Camp, 8730
Lied Learning and Technology Center for Ch ildhood Deafness and Vision Disorders, 3571
National Camps for Blind Children, 1934, 2085, 5301, 6230
Nebraska Chapter of the National Hemophilia Foundation, 3964
Nebraska Dept. of Health Immunization Prog ram, 5973
Nebraska Library Commission Talking Book & Braille Services, 1876, 2023, 5255, 6183
Nebraska Parents Center, 8305
Nebraska Regional Hemophilia Center, 4022
Nebraska SIDS Foundation, 7036
North Platte Public Library, 8514
PWSA of Nebraska, 5842
Parent Assistance Network, 8306
Parent Support Group, 8307
Special Education Office State Department of Education, 8309
Spina Bifida Association of Nebraska, 6842
United Cerebral Palsy of Nebraska, 1456
University of Nebraska at Omaha Pediatric Pulmonary/Cystic Fibrosis Center, 2300
University of Nebraska, Lincoln Barkley Memorial Center, 3562

Nevada

American Academy of Somnology, 5112, 5135, 6678, 6706
Assistive Technology Collaborative, 8310
Autism Society of Northern Nevada Chapter, 827
Camp Lotsafun, 981
Children's Lung Specialists, 2301
Children's Tumor Foundation - Nevada, 5032
Early Intervention Services Division of Child & Family Services, 8311
Educational Equity, Special Education Branch, 8312
Hemophilia and Thrombosis Center of Nevada, 4014
Las Vegas-Clark County Library District, 8515
Nevada Parent Network, 8313
Nevada Parents Encouraging Parents (PEP), 8314
Nevada State Division of Health, Maternal & Child Health, 7037
Nevada State Health Division Bureau of Com munity Health - Immunization Program, 5974
Nevada State Library and Archives, 8516
Parents Encouraging Parents, 8308, 8315
Scleroderma Foundation Nevada Chapter, 6440
Southern Nevada 'Grey Matters' Valley Hospital Medical Center, 1212
University of Nevada - Department of Speec h-Language Pathology, 6788

New Hampshire

Angels of Hope, 1213
Autism Society of New Hampshire, 828
Brain Injury Association of Maine, 3387
Brain Injury Association of New Hampshire, 3396
Bureau of Early Learning, 8316
Camp Allen, 8784

Camp Dartmouth-Hitchcock, 8785
Crotched Mountain School & Rehabilitation Center, 986, 1543, 3472, 4724, 6623, 8710
Dartmouth-Hitchcock Sleep Disorders Center Dartmouth Medical Center, 4903, 8317
Division of Special Education, 8318
Families with Heart, 4321
Family Center Early Supports & Services, 8319
Hemophilia and Coagulation Programs, 4012
High Hopes Foundation of New Hampshire, 8320
Medical Genetics Clinic, 2691
NH Dept. of Health & Human Services Immunization Program, 5975
New England Retinoblastoma Support Group (NERSG), 6282
New Hampshire Cystic Fibrosis Care and Teaching Center, 2302
New Hampshire SIDS Program, 7038
New Hampshire State Library, 8517
Parent Information Center, 8321
Parent to Parent of New Hampshire, 8322
Sleep/Wake Disorders Center, Hampstead Hospital, 4904
Technology Partnership Project Institute on Disability/UAP, 8323
Turner's Syndrome Society of Northern New England, 7581
Windsor Mountain Camp, 3913

New Jersey

Bancroft Camp, 8787
Blood Research Institute of Saint Michael's Medical Center, 3992
Brain Injury Association of New Jersey, 3397
Brain Tumor Support Group at Plainfield Muhlenberg Medical Center, Neuroscience, 1215
CJ Foundation for SIDS, 7072
CRI Worldwide Pediatric Center for Excellence, 1754
Camp Chatterbox, 8788
Camp Merry Heart/Easter Seals Easter Seal Society, 1297, 1539
Camp Oakhurst, 6909, 8789
Camp Sun 'N Fun, 8793
Camp Vacamas, 496, 6671
Center for Enabling Technology, 8518
Cerebral Palsy Center Summer Program, 1541
Cross Roads Outdoor Ministries, 8790
Division of Student Services, 8324
Early Intervention System, 8325
Eating Disorders Association of New Jersey, 2890
Epilepsy Foundation New Jersey, 6540
Family Support Center of New Jersey, 8326
Hydrocephalus Group - Children's Hospital of New Jersey, 4233
Monmouth Medical Center, Cystic Fibrosis & Pediatric Pulmonary Center, 2303
National Sarcoidosis Resource Center, 6374
New Image Camps, 5354
New Jersey Camp Jaycee, 4726
New Jersey Center for Outreach & Services for the Autism Community (COSAC), 829
New Jersey Center for Outreach and Service s for the Autism Community (COSAC), 853
New Jersey Chapter of Crohn's & Colitis Foundation of America, 2167
New Jersey Department of Health - Child Health Program, 7039
New Jersey Department of Health Immunizations Program, 5976
New Jersey Institute of Technology Center for Biomedical Engineering, 3249
New Jersey Medical School, 2304
New Jersey SIDS Resource Center, 7040
New Jersey Self-Help Clearinghouse, 8327
New Jersey State Library Talking Book and Braille Center, 1877, 2024, 5256, 6184
New Jersey Statewide Parent to Parent, 8328
Newark Sleep Disorders Center, 4905
PWSA - New Jersey Chapter, 5844
Parent Project for Muscular Dystrophy Research, 4831
Renfrew Center of Northern New Jersey, 2891
Round Lake Camp, 710, 995
Sarcoidosis Support Resource Central New J ersey, 6365
Scleroderma Foundation New Jersey Chapter, 6441
Spina Bifida Association of the Tri-State Region, 6843
Statewide Parent Advocacy Network, 8329
Tourette Syndrome Association of New Jersey, 7399
Turner's Syndrome Society of New Jersey, 7582
US Rowing Assocation, 8220
United Cerebral Palsy Research and Educational Foundation, 1497

United Cerebral Palsy of Hudson County, 1457
United Cerebral Palsy of Northern, Central & Southern New Jersey, 1458
Young Hearts, 4322

New Mexico

Brain Injury Association of New Mexico, 3398
Computer Access Center, 8557
EPICS Project-SW Communication Resources, 8330
Long Term Services Division, 8331
NM Alliance for the Neurologically Impaired, 1216
New Mexico Autism Society, 830
New Mexico Department of Health Immunization Program, 5977
New Mexico State Library for the Blind and Physically Handicapped, 1878, 2025, 5257, 6185
Parents Reaching Out, 8332
People Living Through Cancer, 1217
Region 5 of the National Association for Parents of the Visually Impaired, 6131
Santa Fe Mountain Center, 8791
Sickle Cell Council of New Mexico, Inc., 6638
Special Education Unit, 8333
Technology Assistance Program, 8334
Ted R. Montoya Hemophilia Program, 4038
University of New Mexico School of Medicine, 2305

New York

Advocacy Center, 8335
Advocates for Children of New York, 8336, 8792
Albany Medical College Pediatric Pulmonary & Cystic Fibrosis Center, 2306
Albany New York Regional Comprehensive Hemophilia Treatment Center, 3991
American Foundation for AIDS Research, 3317
Arlene R Gordon Research Institute, 6196
Armond V. Mascia CF Center, 2307
Aspire of WNY, 1459
Association for Research of Childhood Cancer, 8554
Aurora of Central New York, 8337
Autism Speaks, 861
Big Hearts for Little Hearts, 4323
Bleeding Disorders Association of Northeas tern New York, 3965
Brady Institute for Traumatic Brain Injury, 3431
Brain Injury Association of New York State, 3399
Brain Tumor Support Group, 1214, 1218
Brain Tumor Support Group at South Nassau Community Hospital, 1219
Bronx Comprehensive Sickle Cell Center, 6652
Brooklyn College Speech and Hearing Center, 6774
CF & Pediatric Pulmonary Care Center, 2308
CF, Pediatric Pulmonary & GI Center, 2309
CMTA Chapter - New York (Greater), 1548
Camp Dunnabeck at Kildonan, 2799
Camp Good Days & Special Times, 6670
Camp Huntington, 2764, 4536, 4722
Camp Northwood, 394
Camp Shane, 5349
Capital Regional Sleep-Wake Disorders Center, 4906
Cardiac Kids, 4324
Cardiovascular Research Foundation, 318
Center for Family Support, 831, 1055, 1619, 2672, 4710, 5111
Center for Hearing and Communication, 3546
Center for Neural Recovery & Rehabilitatio n Research, 6551
Center for Sleep Medicine of the Mount Sinai Medical Center, 4907
Center for the Disabled, 1460
Center for the Study of Anorexia and Bulimia, 2908
Central New York Chapter of Crohn's & Colitis Foundation of America, 2169
Cerebral Palsy Associations of New York State, 1461
Child Abuse Prevention Project: Be'ad HaYeled (For the Sake of the Child), 5678
Child Development Clinical Services, 2692
Children's Clinical Research Center, 3318
Children's Lung and Cystic Fibrosis Center, 2310
Chrissy & Friends, 6541
Columbia Presbyterian Medical Center, 4829
Columbia Presbyterian Medical Center Sleep Disorders Center, 4908
Cooley's Anemia Foundation - Staten Island, 7265

Cooley's Anemia Foundation-Buffalo, 7266
Cooley's Anemia Foundation-Long Island/Bro oklyn Chapter, 7267
Cooley's Anemia Foundation-Queens, 7268
Cooley's Anemia Foundation-Suffolk Chapter, 7269
Cooley's Anemia Foundation-Westchester/Roc kland Chapter, 7270
Crohn's & Colitis Foundation of America, 2190
Dana Alliance for Brain Initiatives, 3432
Depressive and Manic-Depressive Assocation of Mount Sinai, 1056, 2476
Early Intervention Program, 8338
East Central Region-Helen Keller National Center, 1972, 5205
Epilepsy Foundation of Long Island, 6542
Facilitated Communication Institute at Syracuse University, 863
Fairfield/Westchester Chapter of Crohn's & Colitis Foundation of America, 2151, 2170
Families of SMA - Long Island NY Chapter, 6924
Freedom Camp, 8794
Friends for Life Auburn United Methodist Church, 8083
Friends of Karen, 8339
Genetic Network of the Empire State, 537
Gow School Summer Programs, 8795
Greater New York Chapter of Crohn's & Colitis Foundation of America, 2171
Helping Hearts, 4325
Hemophilia Center of Western New York, 3966, 4007
Henry Youngerman Center for Communication Disorders, 6789
Hy Feinstein Clubhouse, 3400
Hypertrophic Cardiomyopathy Program at St. Luke's-Roosevelt Hospital Center, 4295
Inspire - Cerebral Palsy Center, 1462
Institute for Basic Research in Developmental Disabilities, 854, 2693, 8519, 8562
Institute on Communication and Inclusion, 864
International NF Summer Camp, 5061
International Pemphigus Foundation: New Yo rk Support Group, 5532
JGB Cassette Library International, 8520
Keren-Or Jerusalem Center for Multi- Handicapped Blind Children, 8521, 8563
Laboratory of Dermatology Research, 1580, 3004, 5633
Leukemia & Lymphoma Society - Western & Central New York Chapter, 140
Long Island Adult Brain Tumor Support Group, 1220
Long Island Chapter of Crohn's & Colitis Foundation of America, 2172
Long Island College Hospital, 2311
Long Island Sarcoidosis Support, 6366
Lupus Research Institute, 7140
Making Headway Foundation-Family Support Program, 1221
Maplebrook School, 709, 994, 4545
Marist Brothers Mid-Hudson Valley Camp Marist Brothers, 8796
Marty Lyons Foundation, 8340
Mary M Gooley Hemophilia Center of the National Hemophilia Foundation, 3967
Metro Intergroup of Overeaters Anonymous, 2892
Montifiore Medical Center, 3572
Mount Sinai Traumatic Brain Injury, 3401
NHF Camp Directory, 4093
NYS Center for SIDS Office, 7041
NYU Rusk Institute, 4830
Nassau Library System, 8522
National Alliance for Research on Schizophrenia and Depression, 1057, 1620, 1621, 2477, 5374
National Eating Disorder Association of Lo ng Island (NEDA-LI), 2906
National Eating Disorders Association-Long Island (NEDA-LI), 2893
New York Autism Network, 832
New York Brain Tumor Support Group, 1222
New York City Area Support Group, 538
New York City Information & Counseling Program for SIDS, 7042
New York Department of Education, 8341
New York Obesity Research Center, 2910, 5334
New York State Department of Health Immunization Program, 5978
New York State Talking Book & Braille Library, 1879, 2026, 5258, 6186
New York Support Group, 539
New York University Medical Center Auxillary of Tisch Hospital, 4234, 4241
Northwestern Region-Helen Keller National Center, 1974
Oakhurst, 8797
Overeaters Anonymous Support Group, 2894
Parent Network Center, 8342
Parent to Parent of New York State, 8343
Pediatric Pulmonary Center, 2312
People Treated for Brain Tumors and Their Caregivers, 1223

Prevent Child Abuse New York, 5679
Programs for Children with Special Health Care Needs, 8798
Programs for Infants and Toddlers with Disabilities: Ages Birth Through 2, 8799
Ramapo Anchorage Camp, 4548
Region II Office Program Consultants for Maternal and Child Health, 7043
Rehabilitation Research and Training Center on Traumatic Brain Injury, 3433
Renfrew Center of New York City, 2895
Research to Prevent Blindness, 1894, 2045, 5271, 6200
Resources for Children with Special Needs, 8344
Rochester Chapter of Crohn's & Colitis Foundation of America, 2173
Rockefeller University Laboratory for Investigative Dermatology, 1581, 3005, 5634
Rusk Institute of Rehabilitation Medicine, 4827, 8571
SLE Lupus Foundation, 7141
SUNY Upstate Medical University Research Development, 4033
Saint Joseph's Hospital Health Center Sleep Laboratory, 4909
Saint Mary's Healthcare System for Children, 8345
Schneider Children's Hospital of Long Island, 2313
Scleroderma Foundation Tri-State, Inc (NY, NJ, CT), 6442
Sinergia/Metropolitan Parent Center, 8346
Sleep Center, Community General Hospital, 4910
Sleep Disorders Center of Western New York Millard Fillmore Hospital, 4911
Sleep Disorders Center, University Hospital, 4912
Sleep-Wake Disorders Center, Montefiore Sleep Disorders Center, 4913
Sleep-Wake Disorders Center, New York Presbyterian Hospital, 4914
Spina Bifida Association of Albany/Capital District, 6844
Spina Bifida Association of Greater Roches ter, 6845
Spina Bifida Association of Nassau County, 6846
Spina Bifida Association of Western New York, 6847
Spinal Muscular Atrophy Clinic, 6927
State University College at Plattsburgh Auditory Research Laboratory, 3573
State University Hospital/Upstate Medical University, 2314
State University of New York Health Sciences Center, 855, 865
Stroke Rehabilitation & Traumatic Brain Injury Research, 3434
Support for Parents of Children with Brain Tumors, Siblings and Young Adults, 1224
Syracuse University, Institute for Sensory Research, 3574
TRIAD Project-Advocates for Persons with Disabilities, 8347
Techspress Resource Center for Independent Living, 8523
Tourette Syndrome Association - Greater New York State Chapter, 7402
Tourette Syndrome Association - Greater Rochester and Finger Lakes Area, 7401
Tourette Syndrome Association - Hudson Valley Chapter, 7403
Tourette Syndrome Association - Long Island Chapter, 7404
Tourette Syndrome Association - New Mexico Chapter, 7400
Tri-State Support Group, 540
Turner's Syndrome Society of Central New York, 7583
Turner's Syndrome Society of Upstate New York, 7584
UCP of Greater Suffolk, 1463
Ulster County Social Services, 8348
United Cerebral Palsy of Nassau County, 1464
United Cerebral Palsy of New York City, 1465
United Health Services Blood Disorder Center, 4042
Unity Sleep Disorders Clinic Unity Health System, 4915
University of Rochester Medical Center, 2315
Upstate/Northeast New York Chapter of Croh n's & Colitis Foundation of America, 2174
VISIONS/Vacation Camp for the Blind, 1936, 2087, 5302, 6231
WNY Brain Tumor Support Group, 1225
Wagon Road, 8801
Wallace Memorial Library, 3563
Westchester Center for Eating Disorders, 2896
Western New York Chapter of Crohn's & Colitis Foundation of America, 2175
Western New York SIDS Center, 7044
Winthrop-University Hospital Sleep Disorders Center, 4916

North Carolina

Assistive Technology Project, Human Resources, Voc. and Rehab. Services, 8349
Autism Society of North Carolina, 833, 856
Brain Injury Association of North Carolina, 3402
Brain Tumor Support Group of the Carolinas and Virginia Cancer Services, 1226
Camp Shining Stars, 5352

Camp Winding Gap, 8802
Carolina Computer Access Center, 8524
Carolinas Chapter of Crohn's & Colitis Foundation of America, 2176
Communications Disorders Clinic, 6790
Duke Brain Tumor Support Group, 1227
Duke Pediatric Brain Tumor Family Support Program, 1228
Duke University Comprehensive Epilepsy Cen ter, 6552
Duke University Comprehensive Sickle Cell Center, 6653
Duke University Medical Center/ CF Center, 2316
Duke University School of Medicine Pediatr ic and Allergy Immunology, 6327
ECAC, 8350
Eastern North Carolina Chapter (SCDAA), 6639
Exceptional Children Division, 8351
Family Support Network of North Carolina, 8352
Giddings School Special Education Division, 8167
Hemophila Foundation of North Carolina, 3968
Herpes Resource Center, 4146, 4964
Leukemia & Lymphoma Society - North Carolina Chapter, 81, 141
Lipomyelomeningocele Family Support, 4235
North Carolina Library for the Blind, 1880, 2027, 5259, 6187
North Carolina SIDS Information and Counseling Program, 7045
North Carolina Speech, Hearing and Languag e Association, 6775
PWSA of North Carolina, 5847
Partnerships for Inclusion, 8353
Pediatric Rheumatoid Clinic, 4392
Prevent Child Abuse North Carolina, 5680
Rockingham County Schools, 8354
Sarcoidosis Support Group, 6367
Sickle Cell Regional Network, 6641
South Carolina Chapter of Crohn's & Colitis Foundation of America, 2183
Spina Bifida Association of North Carolina, 6848
Talisman Programs, 8803
Talisman Summer Camps, 1803, 7771
Turner's Syndrome Society of North Carolina, 7585
UNC CF Center, 2317
United Cerebral Palsy of North Carolina, 1466
University of North Carolina Sarcoidosis Support Group, 6368
University of North Carolina at Chapel Hill, Brain Research Center, 866
Western North Carolina Brain Tumor Support Group, 1229

North Dakota

Brain Injury Association of North Dakota, 3403
Children's Hospital Merit Care Down Syndrome Service, 2694
Developmental Disabilities Unit, 8355
Interagency Program Assistive Technology, 8356
North Dakota Comprehensive Hemophilia and Thrombosis Treatment Center, 4023
North Dakota SIDS Management Program, 7046
Saint Alexius Medical Center/CF Center, 2318
Special Education Division, 8357

Ohio

American Council of Blind Parents, 1881, 2028, 5260, 6188
Autism Society of Greater Cincinatti, 834
Autism Society of Ohio Tri-County Chapter, 835
Beech Brook, 976, 4534
Bethesda Oak Hospital, Sleep Disorders Center, 4917
Blick Clinic for Developmental Disabilities, 8525
Brain Injury Association of Ohio, 3404
Brain Tumor Support Group, 1230
Bureau of EI Services, 8358
CMTA Chapter - Ohio, 1549
Camp Allyn, 8804
Camp Catch-A-Rainbow, 5181
Camp Emanuel, 3898
Camp Nuhop, 702, 984, 4537
Cancer & Blood Diseases Institute, 3994
Case Western Reserve University, Bolton Brush Growth Study Center, 3247
Case Western Reserve University Cystic Fibrosis Center, 2319
Celebrating Families of Children & Adults with Special Needs, 8359
Center for Sleep & Wake Disorders, Miami Valley Hospital, 4918
Central Ohio Brain Tumor Support Group, 1231
Central Ohio Chapter of Crohn's & Colitis Foundation of America, 2177
Central Ohio Chapter of the National Hemophilia Foundation, 3969

Children's Tumor Foundation - Ohio, 5033
Cincinnati Digestive Health Center, 1756
Cleveland Brain Tumor Patient Network - Adult and Pediatric, 1232
Cleveland Clinic, 4236
Cleveland Clinic Foundation, Sleep Disorders Center, 4919
Cleveland Hearing and Speech Center, 6776
Cleveland Public Library, 8526
Clinical Research Center, Pediatrics, 1018
Columbus Children's Hospital, Cystic Fibrosis Center, 2320
Comprehensive Sickle Cell Center, 6654
Division of Early Childhood Education, 8360
Down Syndrome Clinic, Rainbow Babies and Children's Hospital, 2695
East Central Regional Office, 8361
Family Information Network, 8362
Fragile X Alliance of Ohio, 3185
Highbrook Lodge Camp, 1933, 2084, 8805
Jane and Richard Thomas Center for Down Syndrome, 2696
Kettering Medical Center, Sleep Disorders Center, 4920
Leukemia & Lymphoma Society - Central Ohio Chapter, 82, 142
Leukemia & Lymphoma Society - Northern Ohio Chapter, 83, 143
Leukemia & Lymphoma Society - Tri-State Southern Ohio Chapter, 84, 144
Lewis H. Walker, MD, Cystic Fibrosis Center, 2321
Miami Valley Downs Syndrome Association, 2673
NW Ohio Sleep Disorders Center, 4921
Northeast Ohio Chapter of Crohn's & Colitis Foundation of America, 2178
Northern Ohio Chapter of the National Hemophilia Foundation, 3970
Northwest Ohio Hemophilia Foundation, 3971
Northwest Ohio Hemophilia Treatment Center, 4025
OCECD, 8364
Ohio Department of Health Immunization Program, 5979
Ohio Protection and Advocacy Organization, 8365
Ohio Regional Library for the Blind and Physically Handicapped, 8527
Ohio Sleep Medicine Institute, 4922
Ohio State University Hospitals, Sleep Disorders Center, 4923
Ohio State University Laboratory of Psychobiology, 3435
Ohio Support Group, 541
Operation Liftoff of Ohio, 8366
PWSA of Ohio, 5848
Pediatric Pulmonary Center, 2322
Perinatal and Infant Health Unit - SIDS Information and Counseling Program, 7047
Prader-Willi Families of Ohio, 5849
Region 2 of the National Association for Parents of the Visually Impaired, 1826, 1971, 5204, 6132
Saint Vincent Medical Center, Sleep Disorders Center, 4924
Society for Rehabilitation, 8367
Southwest Ohio Brain Tumor Support Group, 1233
Southwest Ohio Chapter of Crohn's & Colitis Foundation of America, 2179
Southwestern Ohio Chapter of the National Hemophilia Foundation, 3972
Speech and Hearing Clinic, 6777
Spina Bifida Association of Canton, 6849
Spina Bifida Association of Central Ohio, 6850
Spina Bifida Association of Cincinnati, 6851
Spina Bifida Association of Greater Dayton, 6852
Spina Bifida Association of North West Ohio, 6853
Spina Bifida Association of Tri-County Ohio, 6854
Support Group for Parents of Children with a Brain Tumor, 1234
Technology Resource Center, 8528
Tourette Syndrome Association of Ohio, 7406
Tourette Syndrome and Tic Disorder Clinic, 7413
Train-Ohio Super Computer Center, 8368
Tri-State Bleeding Disorders Chapter of the National Hemophilia Foundation, 3973
Tri-State Sleep Disorders Center Center for Research in Sleep Disorders, 4943
Turner's Syndrome Society of Southwestern Ohio, 7586
United Cerebral Palsy of Central Ohio, 1467
United Cerebral Palsy of Cincinnati, 1468
United Cerebral Palsy of Greater Cleveland, 1469
University of Cincinnati Adult Hemophilia Program, 4043
University of Cincinnati College of Medicine/Division of Pediatrics, 2323
Visual Systems Research Group, 4471
West Central Ohio Hemophilia Center, 4049

Oklahoma

Autism Society of Oklahoma, 836
Brain Injury Association of Oklahoma, 3405
Leukemia & Lymphoma Society - Oklahoma Chapter, 85, 145

Neuroscience Institute at Mercy Hospital, 5044
North Central Oklahoma Support Group, 542
Oklahoma ABLE Tech-Wellness Center, 8369
Oklahoma Brain Injury Camp, 3473
Oklahoma Chapter of Crohn's & Colitis Foundation of America, 2180
Oklahoma Chapter of the National Hemophilia Foundation, 3974
Oklahoma Library for the Blind & Physically Handicapped, 8529
Oklahoma State Department of Health - Maternal and Child Health
    Services, 7048
Oklahoma State Department of Health Immunization Division, 5980
PWSA of Oklahoma, 5850
Parents Reaching Out in Oklahoma, 8370
Special Education Office, 8371
Tulsa City-County Library System, 8530
Turner's Syndrome Society of Oklahoma, 7587
United Cerebral Palsy of Oklahoma, 1470
University of Oklahoma Cystic Fibrosis Center, 2324

Oregon

Autism Society of Oregon, 837
Bend Support Group, 1235
Brain Injury Association of Oregon, 3406
Brain Tumor Education & Support Group, 1236
Children's Tumor Foundation - Oregon Suppo rt Group, 5034
Dangerous Decibels Oregon Health & Science University, 3548
Early Childhood CARES Program, 8372
Early Intervention Programs, 8373
Easter Seals Oregon Camping Program, 8806
Hemophilia Foundation of Oregon, 3975
Klamath Falls Support Group, 1237
Legacy Good Samaritan Hospital & Medical C enter, 5035
Leukemia & Lymphoma Society - Oregon Chapter, 86, 146
Meadowood Springs Speech and Hearing Camp, 3909, 6804, 6968
Mt Hood Kiwanis Camp, 8807
Oregon Brain Injury Resource Network, 3407
Oregon Department of Education, 8374
Oregon Health Sciences Unit, 2325
Oregon Health Sciences University Research Center, 3575
Oregon Parent Training and Information Center, 8375
Oregon State Health Division - SIDS Information and Counseling Program,
    7049
Oregon State Library, 8531
Oregon State Library, Talking Book and Braille Services, 1882, 2029,
    5261, 6189
PWSA of Oregon, 5851
Pacific Northwest Regional Genetics Group, 543
Rainrock Treatment Center, 2897
Reading and Speech Clinic, 6779
Regional Resource Center on Deafness, 3564
Research and Training Center on Family Support and Children's Mental
    Health, 1776, 7706, 8570
SIDS Resource of Oregon, 7050
Technology Access for Life Needs Project, 8376
United Cerebral Palsy of Oregon & SW Washington, 1471
Willamette Valley Ataxia Support Group, 544

Pennsylvania

Alleghenies United Cerebral Palsy, 1472
Asthma and Allergy Foundation of America - Southeast Pennsylvania
    Chapter, 438
Autism Society of America Greater Harrisburg Area Chapter, 838
Brain Tumor Support Group at Philadelphia, 1238
Brain Tumor Support Group at Pittsburgh, 1239
Brain Tumor Support Group of the Lehigh Valley, 1240
Briarwood Day Camp, 8808
Bureau of Special Education, 8377
CF Center at The Children's Hospital of Philadelphia, 2326
CMTA Chapter - Pennsylvania, 1550
Camelot For Children, 1241
Camp Achieve, 6619
Camp Frog, 6620
Camp Lee Mar, 8809
Camp PALS, 2767
Camp Yomeca Upper Perkiomen Valley YMCA, 8810
Cardeza Foundation Hemophilia Center, 3995
Central Pennsylvania Area Support Group, 545

Children's Hospital of Philadelphia Hemophilia Program, 3998
Children's Hospital of Pittsburgh General Clinical Research Center, 2698
Children's Seashore House, 2699
Community Medical Center, Sleep Disorders Clinic, 4925
Crozer-Chester Medical Center, 4926
Cystic Fibrosis Center at Polyclinic Medical Center, 2327
Delaware Valley Chapter of the National Hemophilia Foundation, 3976
Division of Early Intervention Services, 8378
Dr. Gertrude A. Barber National Institute, 2700
EFWCP Resource Library, 6546
Epilepsy Foundation Eastern Pennsylvania, 6543
Epilepsy Foundation Western/Central Pennsy lvania, 6544
Fontan Friends, 4327
Free Library of Philadelphia, 8532
Geisinger Wyoming Valley Medical Center, Sleep Disorders Center, 4927
Hemophilia Center of Western Pennsylvania, 4008
Institutes for Achievement of Human Potential, 3436
International Foundation for Genetic Research/Michael Fund, 2701
KenCrest Services, 4711
Keystone Community Resources, 8811
Krancer Center for Inflammatory Bowel Disease Research, 2191
Lankenau Hospital, Sleep Disorders Center, 4928
Lehigh Valley Sickle Cell Support Group, 6642
Leukemia & Lymphoma Society - Western Pennsylvania/West Virginia
    Chapter, 87, 147
Library for the Blind & Physically Handicapped, Leonard C Staisey
    Building, 8533
Medical College of Pennsylvania, Sleep Disorders Center, 4929
Mercy Hospital of Johnstown, Sleep Disorders Center, 4930
Mid-Atlantic Regional Human Genetics Network, 546
Montgomery County Intermediate Unit #23, 8379
NF Clinic - University of Pittsburgh Children's Hospital, 5042
National Registry for Childhood Onset Scleroderma (NRCOS), 6451
PA Tourette Syndrome Alliance, 7408
PWSA of Pennsylvania, 5852
Parent Education Network, 8380
Parent to Parent ARC Allegheny, 8381
Parent to Parent of Pennsylvania, 8382
Parents Union for Public Schools, 8383
Pediatric Hemophilia Program of Pennsylvania, 4027
Pediatric Pulmonary and Cystic Fibrosis Center, 2328
Penn Center for Sleep Disorders, Hospital of the University of
    Pennsylvania, 4931
Penn Neurological Institute, 4832
Pennsylvania Chapter of the American Anorexia Bulimia Association, 2898
Pennsylvania Educational Network for Eating Disorders (PENED), 2899
Pennsylvania SIDS Center, 7051
Pennsylvania's Initiative on Assistive Technology, Institute on Disabilities,
    8384
Pennsylvania/Delaware Valley Chapter of Crohn's & Colitis Foundation of
    America, 2181
Phelps School, 4547
Pittsburgh Area Brain Injury Alliance, 3408
Presbyterian-University Hospital, Pulmonary Sleep Evaluation Center, 4932
Region III Office Program Consultants for Maternal and Child Health, 7052
Renfrew Center of Bryn Mawr, 2900
Renfrew Center of Connecticut, 2884
Renfrew Center of Philadelphia, 2901
Round Lake Camp, 4549
SE Pennsylvania Chapter of Asthma and Allergy Foundation of America,
    439
Sarcoidosis Self-Help, 6369
Sickle Cell Disease Association of America , Philadelphia/Delaware Valley
    Chapter, 6643
Southeast Pennsylvania Support Group, 547
Spina Bifida Association of Delaware Valley, 6856
Spina Bifida Association of Greater Pennsy lvania, 6857
Summer Experience, 397, 997, 4551
Summit Camp, 398
Temple University, Section of Auditory Research, 3576
Thomas Jefferson University Brain Injury Rehabilitation Program, 3437
Thomas Jefferson University Sleep Disorders Center, 4933
Turner's Syndrome Society of Nevada, 7580
US Wheelchair Weightlifting Association, 8385
United Cerebral Palsy Central PA, 1473
United Cerebral Palsy of Northeastern Pennsylvania, 1474
United Cerebral Palsy of Northwestern Pennsylvania, 1475
United Cerebral Palsy of Pennsylvania, 1476
United Cerebral Palsy of Philadelphia & Vicinity, 1477
United Cerebral Palsy of Pittsburgh, 1478

United Cerebral Palsy of South Central Pennsylvania, 1479
United Cerebral Palsy of Southwestern Pennsylvania, 1480
United Cerebral Palsy of Western Pennsylvania, 1481
University of Pennsylvania Weight and Education Program, 2902
University of Pennsylvania, Depression Research Unit, 2478
University of Pittsburgh Cystic Fibrosis Center/Children's Hospital, 2329
W.M. Krogman Center for Research In Child Growth and Development, 3250
Wesley Woods, 399, 998, 4552
Western Pennsylvania Chapter of Crohn's & Colitis Foundation of America, 2182
Western Pennsylvania Chapter of The National Hemophilia Foundation, 3977
Western Psychiatric Institute & Clinic, Sleep Evaluation Center, 4934

Rhode Island

Assistive Technology Access Partnership, 8386
Autism Society of Rhode Island, 839
Brain Injury Association of Rhode Island, 3409
Brain Tumor Support Group at Providence, 1242
Central Region Early Intervention Program, 8387
Children's Neurodevelopment Center at Hasbro Children's Hospital, 2702
Hydrocephalus Association of Rhode Island, 4237
Infant Behavior, Cry and Sleep Clinic, 1757
Office Integrated Social Services, 8388
Rhode Island Arc, 8389
Rhode Island Department of Health, 8390
Rhode Island Department of Health Immunization Program, 5981
Rhode Island Department of Health National SIDS Foundation, 7053
Rhode Island Hemostasis and Thrombosis Center, 4032
Rhode Island Hospital, Cystic Fibrosis Center, 2330
Rhode Island Parent Information Network, 8391
Rhode Island Scleroderma Support Group, 6443
Sleep Disorders Center of Lifespan Hospitals, 4935
TechACCESS of Rhode Island, 8534
Tourette Syndrome Association of Rhode Island, 7409
Turner's Syndrome Society of Rhode Island, 7589
United Cerebral Palsy of Rhode Island, 1482

South Carolina

Assistive Technology Project, 8392
Autism Society of South Carolina, 840
BabyNet, 8393
Brain Injury Alliance of South Carolina, 3410
Brain Injury Association of South Carolina, 3411
Burnt Gin Camp, 8813
CF Center/Medical University of South Carolina, 2331
Carolinas Support Group, 548
Children's Center for Cancer and Blood Disorders, 3924, 3997, 6647
Children's Tumor Foundation - South Carolina Chapter, 5036
Described and Captioned Media Program, 3565
Family Connection of South Carolina, 8535
Hemophilia Association of South Carolina, 3978
International Pemphigus Foundation: South Carolina Support Group, 5533
James R Clark Memorial Sickle Cell Foundation, 6644
Newberry County Memorial Hospital Brain Tumor Support Group, 1243
Office of Exceptional Children South Carolina Department of Education, 8394
PRO-Parents, 8395
PWSA - South Carolina, 5853
Region 4 of the National Association for Parents of the Visually Impaired, 1828, 1973, 5206, 6134
SC Dept. of Health & Environmental Control Immunization Division, 5982
Sarcoidosis Support, 6370
South Carolina Department of Health & Environmental Control - SIDS Information, 7054
South Carolina State Library, 8536
Turner's Syndrome Society of South Carolina, 7590
United Cerebral Palsy of South Carolina, 1483

South Dakota

Autism Society of South Dakota Black Hills Chapter, 841
Communication Service for the Deaf, Inc., 3547
DakotaLink, 8396
Office of Special Education, 8397
Oklahoma Speech Language Hearing Association, 6778
Sioux Valley Hospital, South Dakota Cystic Fibrosis Center, 2332
South Dakota Center For Bleeding Disorders, 4034
South Dakota Department of Health, 7055
South Dakota Department of Health Office of Disease Prevention, 5983
South Dakota Parent Connection, 8398
South Dakota State Library, 8537
Teratogen and Birth Defects Information Project, 8574
Thumpers, 4328
University Affiliated Program, School of Medicine, 8399

Tennessee

ACM Lifting Lives Music Camp, 7787
All Nations Camp, 8720
Alliance for Technology Access (ATA), 8452
Autism Society of America East Tennessee Chapter, 842
Bill Wilkerson Center, 3577
Brain Injury Association of Tennessee, 3412
Camp Easter Seal, 8814
Camp Hickory Wood, 3471
Center for Early Childhood, 8400
Children's Tumor Foundation - Tennessee Affiliate, 5037
Down Syndrome Association of Middle Tennessee, 2674
East Tennessee Comprehensive Hemophilia Center, 4001
East Tennessee Technology Access Center, 8538
Families of SMA - Tennessee Chapter, 6925
First Regional Hemophilia Center, 4005
Leukemia & Lymphoma Society, Tennessee Chapter, 88, 148
Memphis Cystic Fibrosis Center, 2333
Memphis Regional Brain Tumor Survivors Group, 1244
Memphis State University, Center for the Communicatively Impaired, 6780
Middle Tennessee Sarcoidosis Support Group, 6371
Neuroscience Institute, University of Tennessee Health Science Center, 6553
Office of Special Education, State Department of Education, 8401
PWSA - Tennessee, 5854
Pediatric Pulmonary Medicine, 2334
STEP (Support & Training for Exceptional Parents), 8402
Saint Jude Children's Research Hospital, 8539
Sarcoidosis Center, 6375
Sarcoidosis Patient Forum, 6372
Sarcoidosis Research Institute, 6377
Technology Access Center, 8511
Technology Access Center of Middle Tennessee, 8403
Tennesse Hemophilia & Bleeding Disorders Foundation, 3979
Tennessee Chapter of Crohn's & Colitis Foundation of America, 2184
Tennessee Department of Health Immunization, 5984
Tennessee SIDS Program, 7056
Tennessee Saving Little Hearts, 4329
Turner's Syndrome Society of Mid-South, 7591
Turner's Syndrome Society of Tennessee, 7592
United Cerebral Palsy of Middle Tennessee, 1484
United Cerebral Palsy of the Mid-South, 1485
University of Memphis Neuropsychology Lab, 3438
University of Tennessee Hemophilia Clinic, 4045
Vanderbilt Hemostasis-Thrombosis Clinic, 4047

Texas

Arizona HeartLight, 4309
Asthma and Allergy Foundation of America - North Texas Chapter, 440
Ataxia Telangiectasia Project, 555
Autism Society of America Greater Austin Chapter, 843
Baylor College of Medicine, 4833
Baylor College of Medicine Birth Defects Center, 8540, 8555
Baylor Comprehensive Epilepsy Center, 6554
Baylor Sleep Wellness Center, 4944
Benign Essential Blepharospasm Research Foundation, 2812
Brain Injury Association of Texas, 3413
Brain Injury Research Center of the Institute for Rehabilitation & Research, 3439
Brain Tumor Support Group at Dallas, 1245
Brain Tumor Support Group at Plano, 1246
CF Center, Pulmonary Section, 2335
Callier Center for Communication Disorders, 6781
Center for Cancer and Blood Disorders, 6655

Center for Cancer and Blood Disorders at Children's Medical Center in Dallas, 3996

Central Texas Brain Tumor Support Group, 1247

Charis Hills, 395

Children's Association for Maxiumum Potential CAMP, 8815

Children's Cancer Research Institute, 5070, 8556

Cook-Ft. Worth Medical Center, CF Center, 2336

Cooley's Anemia Foundation - Texas, 7271

Cystic Fibrosis Care, Teaching and Research Center, 2337

Cystic Fibrosis-Lung Disease Center Santa Rosa Children's Hospital, 2338

Dallas Academy, 703, 987, 4539

Department of Assistive and Rehabilitation Services, 8404

Down Syndrome Guild of Dallas, 2675

Down Syndrome Specialty Clinic, 2703

HOPE (Helping Oncology Parents Endure) Brain Tumor Foundation of the Southwest, 1248

Harris County Health Department, 7057

Hill School of Fort Worth, 707, 991, 4543

Houston Area Brain Tumor Network, 1249

Houston Ear Research Foundation, 3578

Houston Support Group, 549

Houston-Gulf Coast/South Texas Chapter of Crohn's & Colitis Foundation of America, 2185

Hughen Center, 8816

Hydrocephalus Association of N Texas, 4238

International Pemphigus Foundation: Housto n Support Group, 5536

Leukemia & Lymphoma Society - North Texas Chapter, 89

Leukemia & Lymphoma Society - North Texas Chapter, 149

Leukemia & Lymphoma Society - South Central Texas - San Antonio Chapter, 90, 150

Leukemia & Lymphoma Society - Texas Gulf Coast Chapter, 91, 151

Lone Star Chapter of the National Hemophilia Foundation, 3980

Menninger Child & Family Program, 1773, 7703

North Texas Chapter of Crohn's & Colitis Foundation of America, 2186

North Texas SIDS Information And Counseling Program, 7058

North Texas Support Group, 550

Office of the Dean, University of Texas at Austin, 8405

Parent Case Management, 8406

Partners Resource Network, 8407

Project PODER, 8408

Region VI Office Program Consultants For Maternal and Child Health, 7059

Scleroderma Foundation Texas Bluebonnet Ch apter, 6444

Sickle Cell Association of Austin - Marc Thomas Chapter, 6645

Sickle Cell Association of the Texas Gulf Coast, 6646

Sleep Disorders Center for Children, 4936

Sleep Medicine Associates of Texas, 4937

South Central Region-Helen Keller National Center, 8409

South Texas Comprehensive Hemophilia and Thrombophilia Treatment Center, 4035

Southwest Human Development, 8098

Southwest SIDS Research Institute, 7078

Southwestern Comprehensive Sickle Cell Cen ter, 6656

Spina Bifida Association of Houston-Gulf Coast, 6859

Spina Bifida Association of North Texas, 6860

Spina Bifida Association of Texas, 6861

Sweeney, 2618

Texas Assistive Technology Partnership, 8411

Texas Association on Mental Retardation, 2676

Texas Central Chapter of the National Hemophilia Foundation, 3981

Texas Department oF Health Immunization Division, 5985

Texas Department of Health - SIDS Information and Counseling Program, 7060

Texas Heart to Heart, 4331

Texas Lions Camp, 1935, 2086, 3911, 8817

Texas Perinatal Association, 5907

Texas Prader-Willi Syndrome Association, 5855

Texas State Library, 8541

Tri-Services Military CF Center, 2339

Turner's Syndrome Society Resource Center, 7600

Turner's Syndrome Society of Houston, 7593

Turner's Syndrome Society of North Texas, 7594

Turner's Syndrome Society of San Antonio, 7595

UT Southwestern Medical Center at Dallas: Hematology-Oncology Research, 4041

United Cerebral Palsy of Greater Houston, 1486

United Cerebral Palsy of Metropolitan Dallas, 1487

United Cerebral Palsy of Texas, 1488

Univ. of Texas-Southwestern Med. Ctr. at D allas - Clinical Ctr. for Liver Disease, 1019

University of Texas Department of Hematology Research, 4046

University of Texas Medical Branch at Galveston, Clinical Research Center, 4945

University of Texas Sleep/Wake Disorders Center, 4938

University of Texas Southwestern Medical Center/Asthma & Allergic Diseases, 451

University of Texas, Mental Health Clinical Research Center, 2479

Vitamin C Foundation, 6016

Utah

Baby Watch Early Intervention Program, 8412

Brain Injury Association of Utah, 3414

Camp Kostopulos, 8818

Children's Tumor Foundation - Utah Chapter, 5038

Computer Center for Citizens with Disabilities, 8413

Early Intervention Research Institute, Developmental Center, 8560

Heart of the Matter, 4315

Prader-Willi Utah Association, 5856

Primary Children's Medical Center, 8568

Special Education Services Unit, 8414

Spina Bifida Association of Utah, 6862

Tourette Syndrome Association - Utah Chapter, 7410

Turner's Syndrome Society of Salt Lake City, 7596

US Disabled Ski Team, 8415

United Cerebral Palsy of Utah, 1489

University of Utah, 4834

University of Utah Intermountain Cystic Fibrosis Center, 2340

Utah Center for Assistive Technology, 8416

Utah Chapter of the National Hemophilia Foundation, 3982

Utah Department of Health, 5986, 7061

Utah Parent Center, 8417

Utah State Library Commission, 8542

Utah Support Group National Ataxia Foundation, 551

Vermont

Assistive Technology Project, 8418

Autism Society of Vermont, 844

Brain Injury Association of Vermont, 3415

Camp Akeela, 393

Center on Disabilities and Community Inclusion, 8419

Family, Infant, and Toddler Project, 8420

Farm and Wilderness Camps, 8819

Medical Center Hospital of Vermont, 2341

Special Education Unit, 8421

Thorpe Camp, 4728

Vermont Department oF Health State Immunication Program, 5987

Vermont Department of Health - SIDS Information and Counseling Program, 7062

Vermont Department of Libraries Special Service Unit, 8543

Vermont Parent Information Center, 8422

Vermont Regional Hemophilia Center, 4048

Virginia

Alexandria Library Talking Book Service, 1883, 2030, 5262, 6190

American Diabetes Association, 2602

Arlington County Department of Libraries, 8544

Autism Society of America Northern Virginia Chapter, 845

Brain Injury Association of Virginia, 3416

Brain Tumor Support Group, 1250

Camp Baker Services, 8820

Camp Easter Seal East, Camp Easter Seal We st, 8821

Camp Fantastic, 117, 168, 1296

Camp Holiday Trails, 8822

Childhelp Children's Center of Virginia, 5681

Children's Tumor Foundation - MidAtlantic Region Chapter, 5039

Cystic Fibrosis Center/University of Virginia Health System, 2342

Cystic Fibrosis Program of the Medical College of Virginia, 2343

Division for Research (CEC-DR), 8558

Division for the Visually Handicapped, 1884, 2031, 5263, 6191

Division on Visual Impairments, 1885, 2032, 5264, 6192

ERIC Clearinghouse on Disabilities and Gifted Education, 8545

Eastern Virginia Medical Center, 2344

Fairfax County Public Library, 8546

Families Empowered and Supporting Treatmen t of Eating Disorders, 2905

Hemophilia Association of the Capital Area, 3983

Infant & Toddler Program, 8423
Leukemia & Lymphoma Society - National Capital Area Chapter, 92, 152
Makemie Woods Camp Conference Center, 2617, 8823
National Sudden Infant Death Syndrome Research Center, 7075
National Sudden Infant Death Syndrome Resource Center, 7069
Newport News Public Library System, 8547
Oakland School & Camp, 4546
Office of Special Education, Virginia, 8424
Overlook, 8824
PWSA of Maryland, Virginia & DC, 5857
Parent Educational Advocacy Training Cente r, 8425
Precious Hearts, 4333
Roanoke City Public Library System, 8548
Sarcoidosis Support Group, 6373
Scleroderma Foundation Greater Washington DC Chapter, 6445
Spina Bifida Association of the Roanoke Valley, 6863
Tidewater Center for Technology Access, 8426
Triangle D Camp for Children, 8825
Trisomy 18 Foundation, 7414, 7503
United Virginia Chapter of the National Hemophilia Foundation, 3984
University of Virginia General Clinical Research Center, 452
Virginia Assistive Technology System, 8427
Virginia Beach Public Library, 8549
Virginia Commonwealth University Department of Neurosurgery Research, 3440
Virginia Department of Health Bureau of Immunization, 5988
Virginia SIDS Program - Virginia Department of Health, 7063
Virginia State Library for the Visually and Physically Handicapped, 1886, 2033, 5265, 6193

Washington

Adult Brain Tumor Support Group, 1251
Autism Society of Washington, 846
Bleeding Disorders Foundation of Washington, 3985
Brain Injury Association of Washington, 3417
Brain Tumor Support Group University of Washington Medical Center, 1252
Children's Tumor Foundation - Washington C hapter, 5040
Epilepsy Foundation Northwest, 6545
Evergreen Spina Bifida Association, 6864
Head Injury Hotline, 3418
Healing Hearts, 4326
Hemophilia Foundation of Washington, 3986
Hydrocephalus Support Group of Seattle, 4239
Infant Toddler Early Intervention Program, 8428
Leukemia & Lymphoma Society - Washington/ Alaska Chapter, 80, 93, 8089, 8429
National Foundation for Ectodermal Dysplasias- Regional Office, 2985
National Wilms Tumor Study, 7801
Northwestern Region-Helen Keller National Center, 1829, 5207, 6135
Office of the Superintendent of Public Instruction, 8430
Prader-Willi Northwest Association, 5820, 5828, 5841
Puget Sound Blood Center, 4029
Region X Office Program Consultants for Maternal and Child Health, 7064
SIDS Northwest Regional Center, 7065
Scleroderma Foundation Evergreen Chapter, 6446
Seattle Area Support Group, 552
Tourette Syndrome Association - Washington and Oregon Chapter, 7407, 7411
Turner's Syndrome Society of Inland Northwest, 7598
United Cerebral Palsy of South Puget Sound, 1491
University of Washington CF Center, 2345
University of Washington Department of Spe ech & Hearing Sciences, 6783
University of Washington Speech and Hearin g Clinic, 6791
University of Washington: Experimental Education Unit, 2704
Washington Library for the Blind and Physically Handicapped, 1887, 2034, 5266, 6194
Washington PAVE, 8431
Washington State Chapter of Crohn's & Colitis Foundation of America, 2187
Washington State Department of Health Immunization Program, 5989

West Virginia

Autism Services Center, 857

Autism Society of West Virginia, 847
Autism Training Center, 858
Brain Injury Association of West Virginia, 3419
Cabell County Public Library, 8550
Early Intervention Program, 8432
Kanawha County Public Library, 8551
Mountain Milestones Stepping Stones, 8826
Mountaineer Spina Bifida Camp, 6910
Office of Special Education Administration, 8433
West Virginia Assistive Technology System, 8434
West Virginia Department of Health and Human Services, 7066
West Virginia Library Commission, 8552
West Virginia Parent Training and Information, 8435
West Virginia School for the Blind, 1888, 2035, 5267, 6195
West Virginia University Cystic Fibrosis Center, 2346
West Virginia University Mountain State Cystic Fibrosis Center, 2347

Wisconsin

Autism Society of Wisconsin, 848
Birth to 3 Program, 8436
Brain Injury Association of Wisconsin, 3420
Brain Tumor Support Group, 1253
Brain Tumor Support Group at Milwaukee, 1254
Brain Tumor Support Group at Wauwatosa Froederdt Memorial Lutheran Hospital, 1255
Brown County Library, 8553
Camp Heartland, 3347
Camp Joy, 8827
Center for the Study of Bioethics, 2705
Children's Tumor Foundation - Wisconsin Ch apter, 5041
Development and Training Center, 8437
Division of Community Services, 8438
Early Childhood Handicapped Prgrams, 8439
Easter Seals Wisconsin Camp Respite, 1544
Fox Valley Hydrocephalus Support Group, 4240
Great Lakes Hemophilia Foundation, 3987
Hemophilia Outreach Center, 3990
International Bone Marrow Transplant Registry, 96
John Sierzant Brain Tumor Support Group, 1256
Kids With Heart, 4335
Left Hearts, 4336
Leukemia & Lymphoma Society - Wisconsin Chapter, 94, 153
Medical College of Wisconsin Cystic Fibrosis Center, 2348
National Center for the Study of Wilson's Disease, 7822
PWSA of Wisconsin, 5858
Parent Education Project of Wisconsin, 8440
Physician Referral and Information Line, 442
Regional Epilepsy Center, 6555
Research at BloodCenter of Wisconsin, 4031
Scoliosis Research Society, 6476
Spina Bifida Association of Northern Wisconsin, 6866
Spina Bifida Association of Wisconsin, 6867
Timbertop Nature Adventure Camp, 8828
Turner's Syndrome Society of Southeastern Wisconsin, 7599
United Cerebral Palsy of Greater Dane County, 1492
United Cerebral Palsy of Southeastern Wisconsin, 1493
United Cerebral Palsy of West Central Wisconsin, 1494
University of Wisconsin Asthma and Allergic Disease Center, 453
University of Wisconsin-Madison Cystic Fibrosis/Pulmonary Center, 2349
Waisman Center - Auditory Physiology Resea rch Laboratory, 6792
WisTech, 8441
Wisconsin Association for Perinatal Care, 5908
Wisconsin Chapter of Crohn's & Colitis Foundation of America, 2188
Wisconsin Lions Camp, 1937, 2088, 3914

Wyoming

Brain Injury Association of Wyoming, 3421
Division of Developmental Disabilities, 8442
Parent Information Center, 8443
Parent and Information Center, 8566
Special Education Unit, 8444
Wyoming Department of Health, 7068
Wyoming's New Options in Technology (WYNOT), 8445

A

Accommodation strabismus, 6939
ACM, 300
Acquired hypothyroidism, 4344
Acquired Immune Deficiency Syndrome, 3279
Acquired ptosis, 6064
Acrocephaly, 2112
Acute ascending polyneuritis, 3271
Acute febrile polyneuritis, 3271
Acute gastrointestinal infection, 21
Acute granulocytic leukemia, 121
Acute hepatitis, 4094
Acute idiopathic polyneuritis, 3271
Acute infectious diarrhea, 21
Acute lymphoblastic leukemia, 61
Acute lymphocytic leukemia, 61
Acute myeloblastic leukemia, 121
Acute myelocytic leukemia, 121
Acute myelogenous leukemia, 121
Acute myeloid leukemia, 121
Acute myelomonocytic leukemia, 121
Acute otitis media, 5471
Acute postinfectious polyneuropathy, 3271
ADHD, 597
Adrenoleukodystrophy (ALD), 4564
Adrenomyeloneuropathy, 4564
Adult Gaucher's disease, 3212
Agranulocytosis, genetic infantile, 5080
Agyria, 4577
AHF, 3937
AIDS, 3279
Albinism, 172
Albino, 172
Albright syndrome, 4654
ALL, 61
Allergic reaction, 6314
Allergic rhinitis, 6314
Alopecia areata, 197
Alopecia circumscripta, 197
Alopecia totalis, 197
Alopecia universalis, 197
Alpha-1-antitrypsin deficiency, 210
Alpha-thalassemia, 7238
Amaurosis congenita, 6251
Amaurosis fugax, 4746
Amblyopia, 4458, 6113
AMC, 326
AML, 121
Amyoplasia, 326
Anaclitic depression of infancy, 2435
Anal atresia, 258
Anal fistula, 258
Anal stenosis, 258
Androgenetic alopecia, 197
Anencephaly, 222
Angioedema, 7656
Angioneurotic edema, 7656
Anhidrotic ectodermal dysplasia, 2976
Aniridia, 233
Aniridia-cerebellar ataxia, 233
Anisometropia, 6113
Ankylosing spondylitis, 247
Anorectal malformations, 258
Anorexia nervosa, 2830, 5356
Antihemophilic factor deficiency, 3937
Anus, ectopic, 258
Anus, imperforate, 258
Aortic arch obstruction, 1730
Aortic coarctation, 1730
Aortic stenosis, 281
Aortic valve stenosis, 281
Aphasia, 6750
Apnea of prematurity, 292
Apnea of prematurity, idiopathic, 292
Apnea, central, 292
Apnea, obstructive, 292
Arnold-Chiari deformity, 300
Arnold-Chiari malformation, 300, 4215
Arnold-Chiari malformation type I, 300

Arnold-Chiari malformation type II, 300
Arnold-Chiari syndrome, 300
Arrhythmias, 311
Arthrogryposis multiplex congenita, 326
Articulation, 6750
AS, 247
ASD, 586
Asperger syndrome, 338
Aspiration pneumonia, 5746
Asthma, 400
Asthma, bronchial, 400
Astigmatism, 6113
AT, 499
Ataxia, 499
Ataxia-telangiectasia, 499, 7195
Ataxias, hereditary, 499
Ataxias, spinocerebellar, 499
Ataxic cerebral palsy, 1375
Athetosis, 1666
Atrial septal defects, 586
Atrioseptal defects, 586
Attention deficit disorder, 597
Attention deficit hyperactivity disorder, 597
Atypical pneumonia, 5746
Autism, 338
Autism, infantile, 712
Autistic disorder, 712

B

Baby bottle tooth decay, 2388
Bacterial gastroenteritis, 21
Bacterial pneumonia, 5746
Baldness, 197
Basilar migraine, 4746
BDLS, 2100
Becker muscular dystrophy, 4820
Beckwith-Wiedemann syndrome, 5405
Bed-wetting, 5148
Behavioral abnormalities, 3050
Bell's palsy, 1000, 4600
Benign familial pemphigus, 5520
Beta-thalassemia, 7238
Beta-thalassemia major, 7238
Beta-thalassemia minor, 7238
Bicuspid aortic valve, 281
Biliary Atresia, 1012
Bilirubin, 4973
Bilirubin encephalopathy, 4423
Binge eating, 2830
Bipolar disorder, 1028
Blepharoptosis, 6064
Blepharospasm, 2802
Blood cancer, 61, 121
Bone tumor, 3102
BPD, 1301
Brain infection, 4665
Brain injuries, 3351
Brain trauma, 3351
Brain tumors, 1075
Branched chain ketoaciduria, 4633
Bretonneau's disease, 5924
Brittle bone disease, 5431
Bronchiolitis, 6242
Bronchopulmonary dysplasia, 1301
Bruxism, 2388
Bulimia nervosa, 2830
Burn injuries, 1311

C

CAH, 1804
Cataplexy, 4878
Cataracts, 1816
Cavernous hemangiomas, 3915
CD, 1333
CDH, 1938, 1950
CdLS, 2100
Celiac disease, 1333

Celiac sprue, 1333
Central precocious puberty, 5887
Cerebellar astrocytoma, 1075
Cerebral diseases, 4564
Cerebral infections, 4665
Cerebral palsy, 1375
Cerebral trauma, 3351
CF, 2237
Chelation, 4495
Cheloids, 4415
Chiari malformation, 300
Chickenpox, 5924
Child abuse, 5645
Child care virus, 2380
Childhood dermatomyositis, 1568
Cholestasis, Neonatal, 210
Chorea, 1666
Chorea, benign familial, 1666
Chorea, drug-induced, 1666
Choreoathetoid cerebral palsy, 1375
Christ-Siemens-Touraine syndrome, 2976
Christmas disease, 3937
Chromosome 13, monosomy 13q syndrome,
    6266
Chromosome 13, trisomy 13, 7505
Chromosome 18, trisomy 18, 7494
Chromosome 21, trisomy 21, 2632
Chromosome 45,X syndrome, 7554
Chromosome XXY, 4435
Chronic Gaucher's disease, 3212
Chronic hepatitis, 4094
Chronic otitis media, 5471
Chronic relapsing polyradiculoneuropathy, 3271
Chronic unremit'g polyradiculoneuropathy,
    3271
Class I histiocytoses, 4174
Class I malocclusion, 2388
Class II malocclusion, 2388
Class III malocclusion, 2388
Classic galactosemia, 3197
Classic Gaucher's disease, 3212
Classic hemophilia, 3937
Classic homocystinuria, 4199
Classic migraine, 4746
Classic MSUD, 4633
Classic phenylketonuria, 5544
Cleft lip, 1680
Cleft lip with cleft palate, 1680
Cleft palate, 1680
Closed-head injury, 3351
Clouston's syndrome, 2976
Clubfoot, 1713
CMV, 2380
Coarctation of the aorta, 1730
Cold Sore, 4140
Colic, 1743
Collodion baby, 4359
Common migraine, 4746
Communicating hydrocephalus, 4215
Compensatory scoliosis, 6469
Concussion, 3351
Conduct disorder, 1761
Conductive deafness, 3474
Conductive hearing loss, 3474
Congenital adrenal hyperplasia, 1804
Congenital amaurosis, 6251
Congenital biliary obstruction, 1012
Congenital cataracts, 1816
Congenital diaphragmatic hernia, 1938
Congenital dislocation of the hip, 1950
Congenital dysplasia of the hip, 1950
Congenital generalized phlebectasia, 7195
Congenital glaucoma, 1961
Congenital heart disease, 281
Congenital herpes, 4140, 4959
Congenital hip dysplasia, 1950
Congenital hypothyroidism, 4344
Congenital kyphosis, 6469
Congenital liver disease, 1012
Congenital malformation of palate/lip, 1680
Congenital oculocutaneous albinism, 172

Congenital ptosis, 6064
Congenital scoliosis, 6469
Congenital synostosis, 4448
Congenital talipes equinovarus, 1713
Congenital toxoplasmosis, 7467
Conjunctivitis, 2089
Constipation, 3050
Convulsions, 6525
Cornelia de Lange syndrome, 2100
Cot death, 6980
CP, 1375
Cradle cap, 2994
Craniopharyngioma, 1075
Craniostenosis, 2112
Craniostosis, 2112
Craniosynostosis, 2112
Crib death, 6980
Crohn's disease, 2135
Cryptorchidism, 2214
Cryptorchidy, 2214
Cryptorchism, 2214
Cushing's basophilism, 2224
Cushing's syndrome, 2224
Cutaneous diphtheria, 5924
Cutis marmorata telangiectatica, 7195
Cystathionine synthase deficiency, 4199
Cystic fibrosis, 2237
Cystic hygromas, 3915
Cytomegalic inclusion disease, 2380
Cytomegalovirus, 2380

D

D1 trisomy syndrome, 7505
Dawson's encephalitis, 6970
DDH, 1950
De Lange syndrome, 2100
Deafness, 3474
Deer tick disease, 4600
Deficiency of fructose-1,6-bisphosphate, 4124
Deficiency of phosphofructaldolase, 4124
Deficiency of uridyl diphosphogalactose, 3197
Dental caries, 2388
Dental mottling, 2388
Denys-Drash syndrome, 7789
Depression, 2435
Depth perception, 4458
Dermatitis, allergic contact, 2994
Dermatitis, atopic, 2994
Dermatitis, contact, 2994
Dermatitis, eczematous, 2994
Dermatitis, irritant contact, 2994
Dermatitis, seborrheic, 2994
Dermatomyositis, childhood, 1568
Dermatomyositis, juvenile, 1568
Developmental dysplasia of the hip, 1950
Diabetes, 2549
Diabetes mellitus, 2549
Diaphragmatic hernia, congenital, 1938
Diarrhea, 21
DiGeorge sequence, 2619
DiGeorge syndrome, 2619
Diphtheria, 5924
Distomolar, 2388
DMD, 2802
Dopa-responsive dystonia, 2802
Down syndrome, 2632
DRD, 2802
Drooping eyelid, 6064
Duchenne muscular dystrophy, 4820
Dysarthria, 6750
Dyscalculia, 4502
Dysgraphia, 4502
Dyshidrosis, 2994
Dyslexia, 2769, 4502
Dysphasia, 6750
Dystonia, 2802
Dystonia musculorum deformans, 2802
Dystonia, buccomandibular, 2802
Dystonia, cervical, 2802

Dystonia, dopa-responsive, 2802
Dystonia, drug-induced, 2802
Dystonia, focal, 2802
Dystonia, torsion, 2802

E

Eating disorders, 2830
Ectodermal dysplasias, 2388, 2976
Ectrodactyly-ectodermal dysplasia, 2976
Eczema, 2994
Eczema herpeticum, 4140
Eczema, infantile, 2994
Edwards syndrome, 7494
EEC syndrome, 2976
Ehlers-Danlos syndrome, 3020
EI, 3081
Embryopathy, etretinate, 3166
Embryopathy, isotretinoin, 3166
Embryopathy, retinol, 3166
Encephalocele, 3030, 6806
Encopresis, 3050
Enteritis, regional, 2135
Enterobiasis, 5730
Enterobius vermicularis, 5730
Enuresis, 5148
Enuresis, nocturnal, 6698
Eosinophelia syndrome (NARES), 6314
Eosinophilic granuloma, 4174
Epidemic parotitis, 5924
Epidermolysis bullosa, 3061
Epidermolysis bullosa dystrophica, 3061
Epidermolysis bullosa simplex, 3061
Epidermolytic hyperkeratosis, 4359
Epidural hematoma, 3351
Epilepsy, 5356, 6525
Epilepsy, idiopathic, 6525
EPP, 5768
Erb's palsy, 3072
Erb-Duchenne paralysis, 3072
Erythema infectiosum, 3081
Erythema migrans, 4600
Erythroblastosis fetalis, 3929
Erythroblastosis neonatorum, 3929
Erythrohepatic protoporphyria, 5768
Erythropoietic protoporphyria, 5768
Esophageal atresia, 3089
Ewing's sarcoma, 3102
Ewing's tumor, 3102
Exomphalos-macroglossia-gigantism, 5405
Extrapulmonary tuberculosis, 7514

F

Facial nerve paralysis, 1000
Facioscapulohumeral muscular dystrophy, 4820
Factor IX deficiency, 3937
Factor VIII deficiency, 3937
Factor VIIIR deficiency, 3937
FAE, 3135
Fainting, 7115
Fallot's syndrome, 7222
Familial dysautonomia, 3125
Farsightedness, 6113
FAS, 3135
Fazio-Londe disease, 6911
FD, 3125
Fecal incontinence, 3050
Female Pseudo-Turner syndrome, 5184
Ferrochelatase deficiency, 5768
Fetal acquired immune deficiency, 3279
Fetal AIDS, 3279
Fetal alcohol effect, 3135
Fetal alcohol syndrome, 3135
Fetal retinoid syndrome, 3166
Fifth disease, 3081
First degree burns, 1311
Food poisoning, 21
45,X/46,XY/47,XXY mosaicism, 4435

46,XX/47,XXY mosaicism, 4435
46,XY/47,XXY mosaicism, 4435
46,XY/48,XXYY mosaicism, 4435
48,XXXY, 4435
49,XXXYY, 4435
Fragile X syndrome, 3176
Friedereich's ataxia, 499
Fungal pneumonia, 5746

G

Galactokinase deficiency, 3197
Galactose epimerase deficiency, 3197
Galactosemia, 3197
Gastroenteritis, 21
Gaucher disease, 3212
GBS, 3271
Gelineau's syndrome, 4878
Generalized essential telangiectasia, 7195
Generalized tetanus, 5924
Genital herpes, 4140
Geophagia, 5719
German measles, 5924
Germinal matrix hemorrhage, 4374
GH deficiency, 3227
Gilles de la Tourette syndrome, 7351
Globoid cell leukodystrophy, 4564
Glucosyl cerebroside lipidosis, 3212
Glucosylceramide lipidosis, 3212
Gluten-sensitive enteropathy, 1333
GM2 gangliosidosis, type I, 7157
GM2 gangliosidosis, type III, 7157
GMH, 4374
Group conduct disorder, 1761
Growth hormone deficiency, 3227
Growth hormone deficiency, isolated, 3227
GSE, 1333
GTS, 7351
Guillain-Barre syndrome, 3271

H

Hailey-Hailey disease, 5520
Hallervorden-Spatz disease, 2802
Hand-Schüller-Christian disease, 4174
Harlequin fetus, 4359
Hashimoto's disease, 4344
Hay fever, 6314
Head injuries, 3351
Head trauma, 3351
Hearing impairment, 3474
Hearing loss, 3474
Hemangiomas, 3915
Hemangiomas, capillary, 3915
Hemangiomas, mixed, 3915
Hemangiomatosis, disseminated, 3915
Hemiplegic migraine, 4746
Hemolytic anemia, 6624
Hemolytic disease of the newborn, 3929
Hemophilia, 3937
Hemophilia A, 3937
Hemophilia B, 3937
Hepatitis, 4094
Hepatitis A, 4094
Hepatitis B, 4094
Hepatitis C, 4094
Hepatitis D, 4094
Hepatitis E, 4094
Hepatolenticular degeneration, 7813
Hepatotropic virus, 4094
Hereditary benign telangiectasia, 7195
Hereditary fructose intolerance, 4124
Hereditary hemorrhagic telangiectasia, 7195
Hereditary sensory and autonomic neuropa, 3125
Herpes labialis, 4140
Herpes simplex, 4140, 4959
Herpes simplex virus, 4140, 4959
Herpetic gingivostomatitis, 4140

Herpetic whitlow, 4140
Heterotropia, 6939
Hexa deficiency, 7157
Hexosaminidase A deficiency, 7157
Hidrotic ectodermal dysplasia, 2976
Hip dislocation, 1950
Hip dysplasia, 1950
Hirschsprung disease, 4155
Histiocytosis, 4174
Histiocytosis X, 4174
HIV, 3279
Hives, 7656
HLHS, 4305
HMD, 6232
Hodgkin's disease, 4185
Hodgkin's disease, lymphocyte depletion, 4185
Hodgkin's disease, lymphocyte predominan, 4185
Homocystinuria Type I, 4199
Homocystinuria Type II, 4199
Homocystinuria Type III, 4199
Homozygous Hb S, 6624
HSAN-III, 3125
HSV-1, 4140, 4959
HSV-2, 4140, 4959
Human immunodeficiency virus infection, 3279
Hunter syndrome, 4808
Hurler syndrome, 4808
Hyaline membrane disease, 1301, 6232
Hydrocephalus, 4215
Hydrocephalus, acute, 4215
Hydrocephalus, occult tension, 4215
Hydrocephalus, overt tension, 4215
Hydrocephaly, 4215
Hyperactive child syndrome, 597
Hyperadrenocorticism, 2224
Hyperbilirubinemia, 4423, 4973
Hyperkinetic syndrome, 597
Hyperopia, 6113
Hyperphenylalaninemia, 5544
Hypertrophic cardiomyopathy, 4290
Hypertrophy, 4290
Hypnagogic hallucinations, 4878
Hypnolepsy, 4878
Hypohidrotic ectodermal dysplasia, 2976
Hypopituitarism, 3227
Hypoplasia of thymus and parathyroids, 2619
Hypoplastic Left Heart Syndrome, 4305
Hypothyroidism, 4344

I

IBD, 2135, 7617
Ichthyosiform erythroderma, bullous, 4359
Ichthyosiform erythroderma, congenital, 4359
Ichthyosiform erythroderma, nonbullous, 4359
Ichthyosis, 4359
Ichthyosis simplex, 4359
Ichthyosis vulgaris, 4359
Ichthyosis, lamellar, 4359
Ichthyosis, X-linked, 4359
Icterus neonatorum, 4973
Idiopathic kyphosis, 6469
Idiopathic scoliosis, 6469
Idiopathic thrombocytopenia purpura, 7295
IGHD, 3227
Immunodeficiency, thymic agenesis, 2619
Imperforate anus, 258
Infant respiratory distress syndrome, 6232
Infantile colic, 1743
Infantile glaucoma, 1961
Infantile hypertrophic pyloric stenosis, 6094
Infantile pyloric stenosis, 6094
Infantile spasms, 6525
Infectious conjunctivitis, 2089
Infectious gastroenteritis, 21
Infectious parotitis, 5924
Inflammatory bowel disease, 2135, 7617
Inherited absence of skin pigment, 172
Insulin-dependent diabetes, 2549

Intermediate MSUD, 4633
Intermittent MSUD, 4633
Intraventricular hemorrhage, 4374
Iris, hypoplasia of, 233
Isolated lissencephaly sequence, 4577
ITP, 7295
IVH, 4374

J

Jaundice, 4973
JDMS, 1568
JRA, 4384
Junctional epidermolysis bullosa, 3061
Juvenile rheumatoid arthritis, 4384

K

Kanner's syndrome, 712
Kawasaki disease, 4408
Keloids, 4415
Kernicterus, 4423
KFS, 4448
Kidney tumor, 7789
Kleeblattschadel deformity, 2112
Klinefelter syndrome, 4435
Klippel-Feil syndrome, 4448
Klippel-Feil syndrome Type I, 4448
Klippel-Feil syndrome Type II, 4448
Klippel-Feil syndrome Type III, 4448
Kostmann's disease, 5080
Krabbe disease, 4564
Kugelberg-Welander disease, 6911
Kyphosis, 6469

L

Lactose intolerance, 4784
Landouzy-Dejerine disease, 4820
Landry's paralysis, 3271
Langerhans cell histiocytosis, 4174
Language, 6750
Laron syndrome, 3227
Lazy eye, 4458
LCH, 4174
LCPD, 4554
LDD, 4502
Lead exposure, 4495
Lead poisoning, 4495
Lead toxicity, 4495
Learning disability, 2769, 4502
Learning disorder, 4502
Leber congenital retinal amaurosis, 6251
Left heart obstruction, 281
Legg-Calve-Perthes disease, 4554
Lens opacities, 1816
Letterer-Siwe disease, 4174
Leukemia, 61
Leukodystrophies, 4564
Limb-girdle muscular dystrophy, 4820
Lissencephaly, 4577
Liver, inflammation of, 4094
Localized tetanus, 5924
Loss of hair, 197
Lupus, 7133
Lyme disease, 4600
Lymphangiomas, 3915
Lymphatic malformations, 3915
Lymphoma, Hodgkin's, 4185
Lysosomal storage disorders, 4798

M

Macrocephalia, 4625
Macrocephaly, 4215, 4625
Macrocephaly, benign familial, 4625
Major depressive disorder, 2435

Male Turner syndrome, 5184
Manic-depressive disorder, 1028
Manic-depressive illness, 1028
Manic-depressive psychosis, 1028
Manifest deviation, 6939
Maple syrup urine disease, 4633
Marfan syndrome, 4644
Marfan syndrome, infantile, 4644
Marfan syndrome, neonatal, 4644
Marie-Strumpell spondylitis, 247
Marker X syndrome, 3176
Martin-Bell syndrome, 3176
MAS, 4654
Maternal phenylketonuria, 5544
McCune-Albright syndrome, 4654
MCNS, 4990
Measles, 5924, 6970
Meckel-Gruber syndrome, 3030
Meconium aspiration syndrome, 6232
Medulloblastoma, 1075
Megacolon, aganglionic, 4155
Megacolon, congenital aganglionic, 4155
Megalocephaly, 4625
Meningitis, 4665
Meningitis, bacterial, 4665
Meningitis, chronic, 4665
Meningitis, neonatal, 4665
Meningitis, viral, 4665
Meningocele, 6806
Meningomyelocele, 6806
Mental deficiency, 4675
Mental retardation, 4675
Mesiodens, 2388
Metachromatic leukodystrophy, 4564
Methionine, 4199
Methylcobalamin defect, 4199
Methylenetetrahydrofolate reductase, 4199
MFS, 4644
Microcephalia, 4729
Microcephalism, 4729
Microcephaly, 4729
Microdontia, 4738
Microdontism, 4738
Middle ear, inflammation of, 5471
Migraine headaches, 4746
Migraine with aura, 4746
Migraine without aura, 4746
Mild MSUD, 4633
Milk protein allergy, 4784
Miller-Dieker lissencephaly syndrome, 4577
Miller-Fisher syndrome, 3271
Minimal change nephrotic syndrome, 4990
Mixed cerebral palsy, 1375
Mixed hearing loss, 3474
ML, 4798
MLNS, 4408
Mood disturbance, 2435
Morbilli, 5924
Morphea, 6431
Movement disorders, 1666, 2802
MPS, 4808
MSUD, 4633
Mucocutaneous lymph node syndrome, 4408
Mucolipidoses, 4798
Mucopolysaccharidoses, 4808
Mucoviscidosis, 2237
Mumps, 5924
Muscular dystrophy, 4820
Mycobacterium africanum, 7514
Mycobacterium bovis, 7514
Mycobacterium tuberculosis, 7514
Myelocele, 6806
Myelomeningocele, 300, 6806
Myopia, 6113

N

Narcolepsy, 4878
Natal teeth, 2388
NB, 5062

Nearsightedness, 6113
Neonatal conjunctivitis, 2089
Neonatal herpes simplex, 4959
Neonatal jaundice, 4973
Neonatal opthalmia, 2089
Neonatal pemphigus vulgaris, 5520
Neonatal tetanus, 5924
Nephroblastoma, 7789
Nephrotic syndrome, 4990
Neural tube defect, 222, 3030
Neuroblastoma, 5062
Neurocardiogenic syncope, 7115
Neurofibromatosis, 5005
Neurofibromatosis type I, 5005
Neurofibromatosis type II, 5005
Neuromuscular scoliosis, 6469
Neutropenia, 5080
Neutropenia, chronic, 5080
Neutropenia, cyclic, 5080
Neutropenia, transient, 5080
Nevi, strawberry, 3915
Newborn respiratory distress, 6232
NF1, 5005
NF2, 5005
NHL, 5163
Night terrors, 5122, 6698
Nightmares, 5092
Nine-day measles, 5924
Nocturnal enuresis, 5148
Non-allergic rhinitis, 6314
Non-communicating hydrocephalus, 4215
Non-Hodgkin's lymphoma, 5163
Non-Hodgkin's lymphoma, Burkitt's type, 5163
Non-Hodgkin's lymphoma, large cell type, 5163
Non-Hodgkin's lymphoma, small noncleaved, 5163
Non-Hodgkin's lymphoma, SNCC type, 5163
Noninfectious conjunctivitis, 2089
Nonparalytic strabismus, 6939
Nontropical sprue, 1333
Noonan syndrome, 5184
Norman-Roberts lissencephaly syndrome, 4577
NS, 5184
Nystagmus, 5195
Nystagmus, acquired, 5195
Nystagmus, congenital, 5195
Nystagmus, convergent, 5195
Nystagmus, jerky, 5195
Nystagmus, pendular, 5195

O

Obesity, 5303
Obsessive-compulsive disorder, 5356
Obsessive-compulsive neurosis, 5356
Obstructive sleep apnea, 6672
OCD, 5356
Ocular albinism, 172
Ocular herpes, 4140
Oculocutaneous albinism, 172
Oculocutaneous albinism, type I, 172
Oculocutaneous albinism, type II, 172
ODD, 5418
OI, 5431
Olivopontocerebellar atrophy, 499
Omphalocele, 5405
OPCA, 499
OPCA of neonatal onset, 499
Open-head injury, 3351
Ophiasis, 197
Ophthalmia neonatorum, 2089
Ophthalmoplegic migraine, 4746
Oppositional Defiant Disorder, 5418
Oral herpes, 4140
OSA, 6672
Osteochondroses, 4554
Osteogenesis imperfecta, 5431
Otitis, 6314
Otitis media, 5471
Otitis media with effusion, 5471

Oxycephaly, 2112
Oxyuriasis, 5730

P

Paralytic strabismus, 6939
Paramolar, 2388
Parasitic gastroenteritis, 21
Paroxysmal sleep, 4878
Paroxysmal SVT, 311
Partial albinism, 172
Parvovirus B19, 3081
Passive-aggressive behavior, 5485
Patau syndrome, 7505
Patent ductus arteriosus, 5509
Pauciarticular JRA, 4384
Pavor nocturnus, 5122
PC deficiency, 6010
PDA, 5509
Pediatric AIDS, 3279
Pelade, 197
Pelizaeus-Merzbacher disease, 4564
Pemphigus, 5520
Pemphigus foliaceus, 5520
Pemphigus vegetans, 5520
Pemphigus vulgaris, 5520
Peridens, 2388
Peripheral precocious puberty, 5887
Periventricular hemorrhage, 4374
Permanent discoloration of the teeth, 2388
Persistent fetal circulation, 6073
Perthes disease, 4554
Pertussis, 5924
Pervasive developmental disorder, 338
PFC, 6073
PFD, 4654
Pharynx and larynx hypoplasia, 5405
Phenylalanine hydroxylase deficiency, 5544
Phenylketonuria, 5544
Phobias, 5559
Phobic disorder, 5559
Photoallergic reaction, 5621
Photosensitivity, 5621
Phototoxic reaction, 5621
Physical abuse, 5645
PICA, 5719
Piebaldism, 172
Pinkeye, 2089
Pinworm, 5730
Pituitary basophilism, 2224
Pituitary dwarfism, 3227
Pityriasis rosea, 5738
PKU, 5544
Plagiocephaly, frontal, 2112
Pneumocystis pneumonia, 5746
Pneumonia, 5746
POFD, 4654
Polio, 5924
Polyarticular JRA, 4384
Polydactylia, 5758
Polydactylism, 5758
Polydactyly, 5758
Polydontia, 2388
Polymorphous light eruption, 5621
Polyostotic fibrous dysplasia, 4654
Polysyndactyly, 7122
Pompholyx, 2994
Porphyrias, 5768
Port-wine stains, 3915
Post traumatic stress disorder, 5778
Postural kyphosis, 6469
Prader-Willi syndrome, 5813
Precocious pseudopuberty, 5887
Precocious puberty, 5887
Prematurity, 5898
Primary glaucoma, 1961
PROC deficiency, 6010
Prognathism, 2388
Progressive bulbar palsy of childhood, 6911
Progressive obliterative cholangiopathy, 1012

Protein C deficiency, 6010
Protoporphyria, 5768
Psoriasis, 6024
Ptosis, 6064
PTSD, 5778
Pubertas praecox, 5887
Pulmonary hypertension, primary, 6073
Pulmonary tuberculosis, 7514
Pulmonary valve stenosis, 6083
Pulmonic stenosis, critical, 6083
PVH, 4374
PWS, 5813
Pyloric stenosis, 6094

R

Rachioscoliosis, 6469
RDS, 6232
Reactive airway disease, 400
Reading problems, 4502
Refraction abnormalities, 6113
Refraction errors, 6113
Renal tumor, 7789
Rendu-Osler-Weber disease, 7195
Respiratory distress syndrome, 1301, 6232
Respiratory syncytial virus infection, 6242
Respiratory tract diphtheria, 5924
Retinitis pigmentosa, 6251
Retinoblastoma, 6266
Retinopathy of prematurity, 6299
Retrognathis, 2388
Retromolar, 2388
Rheumatic fever, 1666
Rhinitis, 6314
Rhinorrhea, 6314
Riley-Day syndrome, 3125
ROP, 6299
Roussy-Levy syndrome, 499
RP, 6251
RSV infection, 6242
Rubella, 5924
Rubeola, 5924

S

Salmon stains, 3915
Sanfilippo syndrome, 4808
Sarcoid of Boeck, 6349
Sarcoidosis, 6349
Scaphocephaly, 2112
Schaumann's disease, 6349
Scheuermann's disease, 6469
Schizophrenia, childhood, 1606
Scleroderma, 6431
Scleroderma, linear, 6431
Scoliosis, 6469
Second degree burns, 1311
Secondary glaucoma, 1961
Secretory otitis media, 5471
Segawa syndrome, 2802
Seizures, 6525
Seizures, absence, 6525
Seizures, complex partial, 6525
Seizures, febrile, 6525
Seizures, generalized, 6525
Seizures, generalized tonic-clonic, 6525
Seizures, grand mal, 6525
Seizures, partial, 6525
Seizures, petit mal, 6525
Seizures, simple partial, 6525
Sensorineural deafness, 3474
Sensorineural hearing loss, 3474
Sexual abuse, 5645
Sheie syndrome, 4808
Shprintzen omphalocele syndrome, 5405
Sickle cell anemia, 6624
Sickle cell disease, 6624
Sickle cell trait, 6624
SIDS, 6980

Simple phobias, 5559
Skull fracture, 3351
Slapped cheek, 3081
SLE, 7133
Sleep apnea, 6672
Sleep disturbances, 5092, 5122
Sleep paralysis, 4878
Sleep-terror disorder, 5122
Sleepwalking, 6698
SMA, 6911
SMA type I, 6911
SMA type II, 6911
SMA type III, 6911
Social phobias, 5559
Soiling, 3050
Solitary aggressive conduct disorder, 1761
Somnambulism, 6698
Spasmodic torticollis, 2802
Spasmus nutans, 5195
Spastic cerebral palsy, 1375
Speech, 6750
Speech dysfunction, 6750
Speech impairment, 6750
Spider angioma, 7195
Spider nevus, 7195
Spider telangiectasia, 7195
Spina bifida, 3030, 6806
Spina bifida occulta, 6806
Spinal muscular atrophies, 6911
Squint, 6939
SSPE, 6970
Stammering, 6950
Status epilepticus, 6525
Sticker's disease, 3081
Still's Disease, 4384
Strabismus, 6939
Strawberry hemangioma, 3915
Stuttering, 6950
Subacute sclerosing leukoencephalopathy, 6970
Subacute sclerosing panencephalitis, 6970
Subdural hematoma, 3351
Sudden infant death syndrome, 6980
Supplementary teeth, 2388
Supraventricular tachycardia, 311
Surfactant deficiency, 1301
SVT, 311
Swallowing abnormality in the newborn, 3089
Sydenham's chorea, 1666
Syncope, 7115
Syndactylia, 7122
Syndactylism, 7122
Syndactyly, 7122
Syndrome-associated scoliosis, 6469
Synostosis, 4448
Systemic lupus erythematosus, 7133
Systemic sclerosis, 6431
Systemic-onset JRA, 4384

T

Talipes, 1713

Tay-Sachs disease, 7157
Tay-Sachs disease, infantile type, 7157
Tay-Sachs disease, juvenile type, 7157
TB, 7514
TED, 6010
Teeth, 4738
Teeth, Absence of, 2388
Temporary discoloration of the teeth, 2388
Teratologic congenital dysplasia of the, 1950
Testes, ectopic, 2214
Testes, maldescended, 2214
Testes, true undescended, 2214
Tetanus, 5924
Tetralogy of Fallot, 7222
Thalassemia, 7238
Thiamine-responsive MSUD, 4633
Third and fourth pharyngeal pouch, 2619
Third degree burns, 1311
Threadworm, 5730
Three-day measles, 5924
Three-month colic, 1743
Thrombocytopenia, 7295
Thromboembolic disease, 6010
Thrombotic disorder, 6010
Thumbsucking, 7310
Tic disorder, chronic motor, 7324
Tics, 7324, 7351
Tics of childhood, transient, 7324
Tooth decay, 2388
Tourette syndrome, 5356, 7324, 7351
Toxoplasmosis, 7467
Tracheoesophageal fistula, 3089
Transposition of the great arteries, 7478
Transposition of the great vessels, 7478
Traumatic brain injury, 3351
Trigonocephaly, 2112
Trisomy 13 syndrome, 7505
Trisomy 18 mosaicism, 7494
Trisomy 18 syndrome, 7494
Trisomy 21 mosaicism, 2632
Trisomy 21 syndrome, 2632
Trisomy 21 translocation, 2632
True precocious puberty, 5887
TS, 7538
TSD, 7157
Tuberculosis, 7514
Tuberous sclerosis, 7538
Tumor, benign, 1075
Tumor, malignant, 1075
Turner phenotype with normal chromosomes, 5184
Turner syndrome, 7554
Turricephaly, 2112
Tympanitis, 5471
Tyrosinase neg.oculocutaneous albinism, 172
Tyrosinase pos.oculocutaneous albinism, 172

U

Ulcerative colitis, 7617
Uncoordinated movements, 499

Undescended testes, 2214
Undifferentiated conduct disorder, 1761
Unilateral neviod telangiectasia, 7195
Unstable gait, 499
Urticaria pigmentosa, 7656

V

VACTERL association, 258
Van Bogaert's encephalitis, 6970
Vasodepressor syncope, 7115
Ventricular septal defects, 7665
Vertebrae, fused, 4448
Viral gastroenteritis, 21
Viral infections of childhood, 3081
Viral pneumonia, 5746
Vision, 4458
Visual disturbances, 6113
Visual impairment, 4458
Von Recklinghausen disease, 5005
Von Willebrand's disease, 3937
VSDs, 7665

W

Waardenburg syndrome, 172
WAGR syndrome, 233, 7789
Walker-Warburg syndrome, 4577
WBC, 7772
WD, 7813
Weber-Cockayne syndrome, 3061
Werdnig-Hoffmann disease, 6911
White matter diseases, 4564
Whooping cough, 5924
Williams syndrome, 7772
Williams-Beuren syndrome, 7772
Wilms tumor, 7789
Wilson disease, 2802, 7813
WMS, 7772
WND, 7813
Wohlfart-Kugelberg-Welander disease, 6911
Wolff-parkinson-white syndrome, 311
WPW, 311
Writer's cramp, 2802
WS, 7772

X

X-linked lissencephaly, 4577
XO syndrome, 7554
XXY syndrome, 4435

Z

Zygosyndactyly, 7122

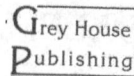

2017 Title List

Visit www.GreyHouse.com for Product Information, Table of Contents, and Sample Pages.

General Reference
An African Biographical Dictionary
America's College Museums
American Environmental Leaders: From Colonial Times to the Present
Encyclopedia of African-American Writing
Encyclopedia of Constitutional Amendments
An Encyclopedia of Human Rights in the United States
Encyclopedia of Invasions & Conquests
Encyclopedia of Prisoners of War & Internment
Encyclopedia of Religion & Law in America
Encyclopedia of Rural America
Encyclopedia of the Continental Congress
Encyclopedia of the United States Cabinet, 1789-2010
Encyclopedia of War Journalism
Encyclopedia of Warrior Peoples & Fighting Groups
The Environmental Debate: A Documentary History
The Evolution Wars: A Guide to the Debates
From Suffrage to the Senate: America's Political Women
Gun Debate: An Encyclopedia of Gun Control & Gun Rights
Political Corruption in America
Privacy Rights in the Digital Era
The Religious Right: A Reference Handbook
Speakers of the House of Representatives, 1789-2009
This is Who We Were: 1880-1900
This is Who We Were: A Companion to the 1940 Census
This is Who We Were: In the 1900s
This is Who We Were: In the 1910s
This is Who We Were: In the 1920s
This is Who We Were: In the 1940s
This is Who We Were: In the 1950s
This is Who We Were: In the 1960s
This is Who We Were: In the 1970s
This is Who We Were: In the 1980s
This is Who We Were: In the 1990s
U.S. Land & Natural Resource Policy
The Value of a Dollar 1600-1865: Colonial Era to the Civil War
The Value of a Dollar: 1860-2014
Working Americans 1770-1869 Vol. IX: Revolutionary War to the Civil War
Working Americans 1880-1999 Vol. I: The Working Class
Working Americans 1880-1999 Vol. II: The Middle Class
Working Americans 1880-1999 Vol. III: The Upper Class
Working Americans 1880-1999 Vol. IV: Their Children
Working Americans 1880-2015 Vol. V: Americans At War
Working Americans 1880-2005 Vol. VI: Women at Work
Working Americans 1880-2006 Vol. VII: Social Movements
Working Americans 1880-2007 Vol. VIII: Immigrants
Working Americans 1880-2009 Vol. X: Sports & Recreation
Working Americans 1880-2010 Vol. XI: Inventors & Entrepreneurs
Working Americans 1880-2011 Vol. XII: Our History through Music
Working Americans 1880-2012 Vol. XIII: Education & Educators
Working Americans 1880-2016 Vol. XIV: Industry Through the Ages
World Cultural Leaders of the 20th & 21st Centuries

Education Information
Charter School Movement
Comparative Guide to American Elementary & Secondary Schools
Complete Learning Disabilities Directory
Educators Resource Directory
Special Education: Policy and Curriculum Development

Health Information
Comparative Guide to American Hospitals
Complete Directory for Pediatric Disorders
Complete Directory for People with Chronic Illness
Complete Directory for People with Disabilities
Complete Mental Health Directory
Diabetes in America: Analysis of an Epidemic
Directory of Health Care Group Purchasing Organizations
HMO/PPO Directory
Medical Device Market Place
Older Americans Information Directory

Business Information
Complete Television, Radio & Cable Industry Directory
Directory of Business Information Resources
Directory of Mail Order Catalogs

Directory of Venture Capital & Private Equity Firms
Environmental Resource Handbook
Food & Beverage Market Place
Grey House Homeland Security Directory
Grey House Performing Arts Directory
Grey House Safety & Security Directory
Hudson's Washington News Media Contacts Directory
New York State Directory
Sports Market Place Directory

Statistics & Demographics
American Tally
America's Top-Rated Cities
America's Top-Rated Smaller Cities
Ancestry & Ethnicity in America
The Asian Databook
Comparative Guide to American Suburbs
The Hispanic Databook
Profiles of America
"Profiles of" Series – State Handbooks
Weather America

Financial Ratings Series
TheStreet Ratings' Guide to Bond & Money Market Mutual Funds
TheStreet Ratings' Guide to Common Stocks
TheStreet Ratings' Guide to Exchange-Traded Funds
TheStreet Ratings' Guide to Stock Mutual Funds
TheStreet Ratings' Ultimate Guided Tour of Stock Investing
Weiss Ratings' Consumer Guides
Weiss Ratings' Financial Literary Basic Guides
Weiss Ratings' Guide to Banks
Weiss Ratings' Guide to Credit Unions
Weiss Ratings' Guide to Health Insurers
Weiss Ratings' Guide to Life & Annuity Insurers
Weiss Ratings' Guide to Property & Casualty Insurers

Bowker's Books In Print® Titles
American Book Publishing Record® Annual
American Book Publishing Record® Monthly
Books In Print®
Books In Print® Supplement
Books Out Loud™
Bowker's Complete Video Directory™
Children's Books In Print®
El-Hi Textbooks & Serials In Print®
Forthcoming Books®
Law Books & Serials In Print™
Medical & Health Care Books In Print™
Publishers, Distributors & Wholesalers of the US™
Subject Guide to Books In Print®
Subject Guide to Children's Books In Print®

Canadian General Reference
Associations Canada
Canadian Almanac & Directory
Canadian Environmental Resource Guide
Canadian Parliamentary Guide
Canadian Venture Capital & Private Equity Firms
Financial Post Directory of Directors
Financial Services Canada
Governments Canada
Health Guide Canada
The History of Canada
Libraries Canada
Major Canadian Cities

Grey House Publishing | **Salem Press** | **H.W. Wilson** | 4919 Route, 22 PO Box 56, Amenia NY 12501-0056

2017 Title List

Visit **www.SalemPress.com** for Product Information, Table of Contents, and Sample Pages.

Science, Careers & Mathematics

Ancient Creatures
Applied Science
Applied Science: Engineering & Mathematics
Applied Science: Science & Medicine
Applied Science: Technology
Biomes and Ecosystems
Careers in The Arts: Fine, Performing & Visual
Careers in Building Construction
Careers in Business
Careers in Chemistry
Careers in Communications & Media
Careers in Environment & Conservation
Careers in Financial Services
Careers in Healthcare
Careers in Hospitality & Tourism
Careers in Human Services
Careers in Law, Criminal Justice & Emergency Services
Careers in Manufacturing
Careers in Overseas Jobs
Careers in Physics
Careers in Sales, Insurance & Real Estate
Careers in Science & Engineering
Careers in Sports & Fitness
Careers in Technology Services & Repair
Computer Technology Innovators
Contemporary Biographies in Business
Contemporary Biographies in Chemistry
Contemporary Biographies in Communications & Media
Contemporary Biographies in Environment & Conservation
Contemporary Biographies in Healthcare
Contemporary Biographies in Hospitality & Tourism
Contemporary Biographies in Law & Criminal Justice
Contemporary Biographies in Physics
Earth Science
Earth Science: Earth Materials & Resources
Earth Science: Earth's Surface and History
Earth Science: Physics & Chemistry of the Earth
Earth Science: Weather, Water & Atmosphere
Encyclopedia of Energy
Encyclopedia of Environmental Issues
Encyclopedia of Environmental Issues: Atmosphere and Air Pollution
Encyclopedia of Environmental Issues: Ecology and Ecosystems
Encyclopedia of Environmental Issues: Energy and Energy Use
Encyclopedia of Environmental Issues: Policy and Activism
Encyclopedia of Environmental Issues: Preservation/Wilderness Issues
Encyclopedia of Environmental Issues: Water and Water Pollution
Encyclopedia of Global Resources
Encyclopedia of Global Warming
Encyclopedia of Mathematics & Society
Encyclopedia of Mathematics & Society: Engineering, Tech, Medicine
Encyclopedia of Mathematics & Society: Great Mathematicians
Encyclopedia of Mathematics & Society: Math & Social Sciences
Encyclopedia of Mathematics & Society: Math Development/Concepts
Encyclopedia of Mathematics & Society: Math in Culture & Society
Encyclopedia of Mathematics & Society: Space, Science, Environment
Encyclopedia of the Ancient World
Forensic Science
Geography Basics
Internet Innovators
Inventions and Inventors
Magill's Encyclopedia of Science: Animal Life
Magill's Encyclopedia of Science: Plant life
Notable Natural Disasters
Principles of Astronomy
Principles of Biology
Principles of Chemistry
Principles of Physical Science
Principles of Physics
Principles of Research Methods
Principles of Sustainability
Science and Scientists
Solar System
Solar System: Great Astronomers
Solar System: Study of the Universe
Solar System: The Inner Planets
Solar System: The Moon and Other Small Bodies
Solar System: The Outer Planets
Solar System: The Sun and Other Stars
World Geography

Literature

American Ethnic Writers
Classics of Science Fiction & Fantasy Literature
Critical Approaches: Feminist
Critical Approaches: Multicultural
Critical Approaches: Moral
Critical Approaches: Psychological
Critical Insights: Authors
Critical Insights: Film
Critical Insights: Literary Collection Bundles
Critical Insights: Themes
Critical Insights: Works
Critical Survey of Drama
Critical Survey of Graphic Novels: Heroes & Super Heroes
Critical Survey of Graphic Novels: History, Theme & Technique
Critical Survey of Graphic Novels: Independents/Underground Classics
Critical Survey of Graphic Novels: Manga
Critical Survey of Long Fiction
Critical Survey of Mystery & Detective Fiction
Critical Survey of Mythology and Folklore: Heroes and Heroines
Critical Survey of Mythology and Folklore: Love, Sexuality & Desire
Critical Survey of Mythology and Folklore: World Mythology
Critical Survey of Poetry
Critical Survey of Poetry: American Poets
Critical Survey of Poetry: British, Irish & Commonwealth Poets
Critical Survey of Poetry: Cumulative Index
Critical Survey of Poetry: European Poets
Critical Survey of Poetry: Topical Essays
Critical Survey of Poetry: World Poets
Critical Survey of Science Fiction & Fantasy
Critical Survey of Shakespeare's Plays
Critical Survey of Shakespeare's Sonnets
Critical Survey of Short Fiction
Critical Survey of Short Fiction: American Writers
Critical Survey of Short Fiction: British, Irish, Commonwealth Writers
Critical Survey of Short Fiction: Cumulative Index
Critical Survey of Short Fiction: European Writers
Critical Survey of Short Fiction: Topical Essays
Critical Survey of Short Fiction: World Writers
Critical Survey of World Literature
Critical Survey of Young Adult Literature
Cyclopedia of Literary Characters
Cyclopedia of Literary Places
Holocaust Literature
Introduction to Literary Context: American Poetry of the 20th Century
Introduction to Literary Context: American Post-Modernist Novels
Introduction to Literary Context: American Short Fiction
Introduction to Literary Context: English Literature
Introduction to Literary Context: Plays
Introduction to Literary Context: World Literature
Magill's Literary Annual 2015
Magill's Survey of American Literature
Magill's Survey of World Literature
Masterplots
Masterplots II: African American Literature
Masterplots II: American Fiction Series
Masterplots II: British & Commonwealth Fiction Series
Masterplots II: Christian Literature
Masterplots II: Drama Series
Masterplots II: Juvenile & Young Adult Literature, Supplement
Masterplots II: Nonfiction Series
Masterplots II: Poetry Series
Masterplots II: Short Story Series
Masterplots II: Women's Literature Series
Notable African American Writers
Notable American Novelists
Notable Playwrights
Notable Poets
Recommended Reading: 600 Classics Reviewed
Short Story Writers

Grey House Publishing | Salem Press | H.W. Wilson | 4919 Route, 22 PO Box 56, Amenia NY 12501-0056